Atherosclerosis
and
Coronary Artery Disease

ATHEROSCLEROSIS AND CORONARY ARTERY DISEASE

Volume One

Editors

VALENTIN FUSTER, M.D., PH.D.
Arthur M. and Hilda A. Master
Professor of Medicine
Director
Cardiovascular Institute
Mount Sinai Medical Center
New York, New York

RUSSELL ROSS, PH.D.
Professor and Director
Center for Vascular Biology
Department of Pathology
University of Washington School of Medicine
Seattle, Washington

ERIC J. TOPOL, M.D.
Chairman
Department of Cardiology
Director
Joseph J. Jacobs Center for Thrombosis and Vascular Biology
The Cleveland Clinic
Cleveland, Ohio

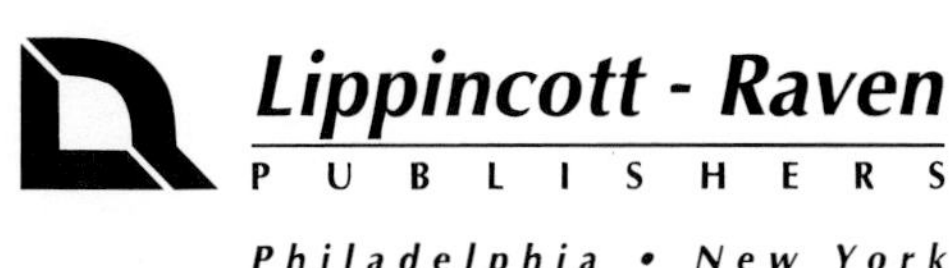

Philadelphia • New York

Lippincott-Raven Publishers, 227 East Washington Square, Philadelphia, Pennsylvania 19106

Made in the United States of America

Library of Congress Cataloging-in-Publication Data

Atherosclerosis and coronary artery diseases / editors, Valentin
Fuster, Russell Ross, Eric J. Topol.
p. cm.
Includes bibliographical references and index.
ISBN 0-7817-0266-6
1. Atherosclerosis. 2. Coronary heart disease. I. Fuster,
Valentin. II. Ross, Russell. III. Topol, Eric J., 1954– .
[DNLM: 1. Atherosclerosis—complications. 2. Coronary Disease—
complications. WG 550 A86749 1996]
RC692.A7297 1996
616.1'36—dc20
DNLM/DLC
for Library of Congress 95-21178
CIP

9 8 7 6 5 4 3 2 1

Contents

Hypertension

II. Pathogenesis of Atherosclerosis

General Principles

The Normal Artery

The Lesions of Atherosclerosis

Special Pathogenetic Factors: Inflammation and Immunity

III. Acute Myocardial Infarction

Pathophysiology

Contributing Authors

John A. Ambrose, M.D.
Professor of Medicine
Director, Cardiac Catheterization Laboratory
Mount Sinai Hospital
One Gustave L. Levy Place
New York, New York 10029

Doron Aronson, M.D.
Fellow in Endocrinology and Metabolism
Department of Medicine
Mount Sinai School of Medicine
New York, New York 10029

Alvaro Avezum, M.D.
Research Fellow
Division of Cardiology
McMaster University
HGH-McMaster Clinic
Hamilton General Hospital
237 Barton Street, East
Hamilton, Ontario
L8L 2X2 CANADA

Lina Badimon, Ph.D.
Professor and Director
Cardiovascular Research Center
Consejo Superior de Investigaciones Científicas
Hospital Santa Creu i San Pau
Autonomous University of Barcelona
Jordi Girona 18–26
08034 Barcelona, SPAIN

Juan Jose Badimon, Ph.D.
Associate Professor of Medicine
Director, Experimental Research
Cardiovascular Institute
The Mount Sinai Medical Center
One Gustave L. Levy Place
New York, New York 10029

Donald S. Baim, M.D.
Professor of Medicine
Harvard Medical School;
Chief, Interventional Cardiology Section
Beth Israel Hospital
330 Brookline Avenue
Boston, Massachusetts 02215

S. Serge Barold, M.B.
Professor of Medicine
University of Rochester School of Medicine and Dentistry;
Chief of Cardiology
The Genesee Hospital
224 Alexander Street
Rochester, New York 14607

Carl G. Becker, M.D.
Department of Pathology, 5152
Medical College of Wisconsin
Milwaukee, Wisconsin 53226

George A. Beller, M.D.
Ruth C. Heede Professor of Cardiology
Chief, Cardiovascular Division
Department of Medicine
University of Virginia Health Sciences Center
Charlottesville, Virginia 22908

Thomas P. Bersot, M.D., Ph.D.
Associate Professor of Medicine
Department of Medicine
University of California, San Francisco; and
Scientist II
Gladstone Institute of Cardiovascular Disease
San Francisco General Hospital
1001 Potrero Avenue
San Francisco, California 94110

Anil K. Bhandari, M.D.
Clinical Associate Professor of Medicine
Section of Cardiology
University of Southern California
1245 Wilshire Boulevard
Los Angeles, California 90017

Henri Bounameaux, M.D.
Priv.-Docent
Division of Angiology and Hemostasis
University Hospital of Geneva
24, Rue Micheli-du-Crest
CH-1211 Geneva 14
SWITZERLAND

Eugene Braunwald, M.D., M.A.(Hon.), M.D.(Hon.), ScD.(Hon.)
Hersey Professor of the Theory and Practice of Medicine
Chairman, Department of Medicine
Harvard Medical School;
Brigham and Women's Hospital
75 Francis Street
Boston, Massachusetts 02115

Sorin Brenner
Department of Cardiology
The Cleveland Clinic Foundation
9500 Euclid Avenue
Cleveland, Ohio 44195

Jan L. Breslow, M.D.
Professor
Laboratory of Biochemical Genetics and Metabolism
The Rockefeller University
1230 York Avenue
New York, New York 10021

Brian Brewer, M.D.
NIH/NHBLI
Molecular Disease Branch
9000 Rockville Pike
Building 10, Room 7N115
Bethesda, Maryland 20892

B. Greg Brown, M.D., Ph.D.
Professor of Medicine and Cardiology
Department of Medicine
Cardiology Division
University of Washington School of Medicine
1959 N.E. Pacific Street
Seattle, Washington 98195

Robert Califf, M.D.
Professor of Medicine
Duke University Medical Center
Box 31223
Durham, North Carolina 27710

Richard O. Cannon III, M.D.
Head, Clinical Service and Cardiovascular Diagnosis Section
Cardiology Branch
National Heart, Lung, and Blood Institute
National Institutes of Health
10 Center Drive, MSC-1650
Bethesda, Maryland 20892-1650

James H. Chesebro, M.D.
Professor of Medicine
Cardiovascular Institute
The Mount Sinai Medical Center
One Gustave L. Levy Place, Box 1030
New York, New York 10029-6574

Guy M. Chisolm III, Ph.D.
Staff, Department of Vascular Cell Biology
The Cleveland Clinic Foundation Foundation, NC10
9500 Euclid Avenue
Cleveland, Ohio 44195

Aram V. Chobanian, M.D.
Dean and Professor of Medicine
Boston University School of Medicine
80 East Concord Street
Boston, Massachusetts 02118

Mina K. Chung, M.D.
Department of Cardiology
Cardiac Pacing and Electrophysiology
The Cleveland Clinic Foundation
9500 Euclid Avenue
Cleveland, Ohio 44195

Alexander W. Clowes, M.D.
Professor of Surgery
Department of Surgery, RF25
Division of Vascular Surgery
The University of Washington Medical Center
Seattle, Washington 98195

Marc Cohen, M.D.
Division of Cardiology
Department of Medicine
Hahnemann University Hospital
Broad and Vine Streets
Philadelphia, Pennsylvania 19102-1192

Peter F. Cohn, M.D.
Professor of Medicine
Department of Medicine
Division of Cardiology
University Medical Center at Stony Brook
Health Sciences Center
Stony Brook, New York 11794-8171

Myron I. Cybulsky, M.D.
Assistant Professor of Pathology
Department of Pathology
Harvard Medical School;
Brigham and Women's Hospital
221 Longwood Avenue, LMRC-4
Boston, Massachusetts 02115-5817

Marilyn M. Dammerman, Ph.D.
Assistant Professor
Laboratory of Biochemical Genetics and Metabolism
The Rockefeller University
1230 York Avenue
New York, NY 10021

Pim J. de Feyter, M.D., Ph.D.
ThoraxCenter
Department of Cardiology
University Hospital Dijkzigt
Erasmus University Rotterdam
Dr. Molewaterplein 40
3015 GD Rotterdam
NETHERLANDS

Anthony C. DeFranco, M.D.
Assistant Professor of Medicine
Staff, Interventional Cardiology
The Cleveland Clinic Foundation
Cleveland, Ohio 44195

Louis J. Dell'Italia, M.D.
Associate Professor of Medicine
Division of Cardiology
University of Alabama at Birmingham
701 S. 19th Street, LMRB Rm. 310
Birmingham, Alabama 35294-0007

Joseph A. Diamond, M.D.
Instructor of Medicine
Hypertension Section
Department of Medicine
Cardiovascular Institute
The Mount Sinai Medical Center
One Gustave L. Levy Place, Box 1030
New York, New York 10029-6574

Paul E. DiCorleto, Ph.D.
Chairman, Department of Cell Biology
The Cleveland Clinic Research Institute
9500 Euclid Avenue
Cleveland, Ohio 44195

Victor J. Dzau, M.D.
Falk Cardiovascular Research Center
Standford University School of Medicine
300 Pasteur Drive, Room 269
Stanford, California 94305-5246

Stephen G. Ellis, M.D.
Director, Sones Cardiac Catheterization Laboratory
Department of Cardiology
The Cleveland Clinic Foundation, Foundation F-25
9500 Euclid Avenue
Cleveland, Ohio 44195

Erling Falk, M.D., Ph.D.
Professor of Cardiovascular Pathology
DHF Cardiovascular Pathology Unit
Skejby University Hospital
8200 Aarhus N
DENMARK

Jay Fallon, M.D.
Professor of Pathology
Cardiovascular Institute
The Mount Sinai Medical Center
One Gustave L. Levy Place
New York, New York 10029

John A. Farmer, M.D.
Associate Professor,
Department of Medicine
Baylor College of Medicine
The Methodist Hospital
6565 Fannin 601
Houston, Texas 77030

Mark C. Fishman, M.D.
Associate Professor of Medicine
Harvard Medical School;
Cardiovascular Research Center
Massachusetts General Hospital
149 13th Street
Charlestown, Massachusetts 02129

Marcus D. Flather, M.B.B.S., M.R.C.P.
Senior Research Fellow
Division of Cardiology
McMaster University
HGH-McMaster Clinic
Hamilton General Hospital
237 Barton Street E.
Hamilton, Ontario
L8L 2X2 CANADA

James S. Forrester, M.D.
Director of Cardiology
Cedars-Sinai Medical Center
8700 Beverly Boulevard
Los Angeles, California 90048

Michael R. Freeman, M.D.
St. Michael's Hospital
Office 701A
30 Bond Street
Toronto, Ontario
M5B 1W8 CANADA

William H. Frishman, M.D.
Professor and Associate Chairman
Department of Medicine
Albert Einstein College of Medicine
Montefiore Medical Center
1825 Eastchester Road
Bronx, New York 10461

Edward D. Frohlich, M.D.
Professor
Departments of Medicine and Physiology
Louisiana State University; and
Clinical Professor of Medicine and Adjunct Professor of Pharmacology
Tulane University; and
Vice President for Academic Affairs
Alton Ochsner Medical Foundation
1516 Jefferson Highway
New Orleans, Louisiana 70121

Valentin Fuster, M.D., Ph.D.
Arthur M. and Hilda A. Master Professor of Medicine
Director, Cardiovascular Institute
The Mount Sinai Medical Center
One Gustave L. Levy Place
New York, New York 10029-6574

W. Bruce Fye, M.D.
Adjunct Professor of the History of Medicine
University of Wisconsin;
Chairman, Cardiology Department
Marshfield Clinic
1000 N. Oak Avenue
Marshfield, Wisconsin 54449

William Ganz, M.D., C.Sc.
Professor of Medicine
Department of Medicine
University of California, Los Angeles;
Cedars-Sinai Medical Center
8700 Beverly Boulevard
Los Angeles, California 90048

Bernard J. Gersh, MB, ChB, DPhil, FRCP
Division of Cardiology
Georgetown University Medical Center
5 Pasquerilla Healthcare Center
3800 Resevoir Road N.W.
Washington, D.C. 20007-2197

Henry Gewirtz, M.D.
Associate Professor
Harvard Medical School;
Department of Nuclear Cardiology
Massachusetts General Hospital
32 Fruit Street, VB301
Boston, Massachusetts 02114

Robert S. Gibson, M.D.
Lockhart B. McGuire Professor of Medicine and Vice Chair
Department of Medicine
University of Virginia Health Sciences Center
Charlottesville, Virginia 22908

Michael A. Gimbrone, Jr., M.D.
Elsie T. Friedman Professor of Pathology
Harvard Medical School;
Director, Vascular Research Division
Brigham and Women's Hospital
221 Longwood Avenue
Boston, Massachusetts 02115

J. Anthony Gomes, M.D.
Professor of Medicine
Cardiovascular Institute
Mount Sinai School of Medicine
The Mount Sinai Medical Center
One Gustave L. Levy Place
New York, New York 10029

David Gordon, M.D.
Associate Professor of Pathology
Department of Pathology
University of Michigan Medical School
1301 Catherine Road
Ann Arbor, Michigan 48108

Avrum I. Gotlieb, M.D., C.M.
Professor of Pathology
Vascular Research Laboratory
Department of Pathology
Banting and Best Diabetes Centre;
The Toronto Hospital Research Institute,
Centre for Cardiovascular Research
University of Toronto;
200 Elizabeth Street, CCRW 1-857
Toronto, Ontario M5G 2C4
CANADA

Antonio M. Gotto, Jr., M.D., D.Phil.
Distinguished Service Professor of Medicine
The Bob and Vivian Smith Professor and Chairman
Department of Medicine
Baylor College of Medicine;
Chief, Internal Medicine Service
The Methodist Hospital
6550 Fannin, MS1423
Houston, Texas 77030

Scott M. Grundy, M.D., Ph.D.
Professor of Internal Medicine and Biochemistry
Center for Human Nutrition
University of Texas Southwestern Medical School at Dallas
5353 Harry Hines Boulevard
Dallas, Texas 75235-9052

David P. Hajjar, Ph.D.
Professor of Biochemistry and Pathology
Department of Pathology
Cornell University Medical College
1300 York Avenue
New York, New York 10021

Jonathan L. Halperin, M.D.
Mount Sinai Medical Center
One Gustave Levy Place
New York, New York 10029

Goran K. Hansson, M.D., Ph.D.
Director of Graduate Program Department of Clinical Chemistry
Gothenburg University
Sahlgren's Hospital S-413
45 Gothenburg, SWEDEN

Donald C. Harrison, M.D.
Professor of Medicine and Cardiology
University of Cincinnati Medical Center
250 Health Professionals Building
P.O. Box 670663
Cincinnati, Ohio 45267-0663

J. Warren Harthorne, M.D.
Associate Professor of Medicine
Departments of Cardiology and Medicine
Massachusetts General Hospital
15 Parkman Street
Boston, Massachusetts 02114

Jeffrey M. Hoeg, M.D.
Chief, Cell Biology Section
Molecular Disease Branch
National Heart, Lung and Blood Institutes
National Institutes of Health
10 Center Drive MSC, Bldg. 10/7N115
Bethesda, Maryland 20892-1666

David R. Holmes, Jr., M.D.
Professor of Medicine
Department of Cardiovascular Diseases and Internal Medicine
Mayo Clinic
200 First Street S.W.
Rochester, Minnesota 55905

Paul N. Hopkins, M.D., M.S.P.H.
Associate Professor of Medicine
Department of Cardiovascular Genetics
University of Utah
410 Chipeta Way
Salt Lake City, Utah 84108

Gordon S. Huggins, M.D.
Clinical and Research Fellow
Department of Cardiology
Harvard University;
Massachusetts General Hospital
55 Fruit Street
Boston, Massachusetts 02114

Laura Hiltscher, A.A., A.S.C.P. Certified
Research Assistant
Department of Pathology
University of Chicago
5841 South Maryland
Chicago, Illinois 60637

Steven C. Hunt, Ph.D.
Professor of Internal Medicine
Department of Internal Medicine
Cardiology Division
University of Utah
410 Chipeta Way
Salt Lake City, Utah 84108

John P. Kane, M.D., Ph.D.
Professor of Medicine and of Biochemistry and Biophysics
Departments of Medicine, Biochemistry, and Biophysics
University of California, San Francisco
San Francisco, California 94143-0130

Robert J. Kaner, M.D.
Assistant Professor of Medicine
Pulmonary Service
Department of Medicine
Memorial Sloan-Kettering Cancer Center
1275 York Avenue
New York, New York 10021

William B. Kannel, M.D.
Department of Medicine
Evans Memorial Research Foundation
Boston University Medical Center
88 East Newton Street
Boston, Massachusetts 02118-2334

Howard L. Kantor, M.D., Ph.D.
Massachusetts General Hospital
Department of Cardiology
32 Fruit Street
Jackson 14
Boston, Massachusetts 02114

Norman M. Kaplan, M.D.
Professor of Medicine
Department of Internal Medicine
University of Texas Southwestern Medical Center
5323 Harry Hines Boulevard
Dallas, Texas 75235-8899

Joel S. Karliner, M.D.
Professor of Medicine
University of California, San Francisco;
Chief, Cardiology Section
San Francisco VA Medical Center
4150 Clement Street
San Francisco, California 94121

Juan Carlos Kaski, M.D.
Senior Lecturer
Department of Cardiological Science
St. George's Hospital Medical School
Cranmer Terrace
London SW17 ORE
UNITED KINGDOM

Gregory A. Kidwell, M.D.
Department of Cardiology
The Cleveland Clinic Foundation
9500 Euclid Avenue
Cleveland, Ohio 44195

Spencer B. King III, M.D.
Professor of Medicine
Departments of Medicine and Interventional Cardiology
Emory University Hospital
1364 Clifton Road
Atlanta, Georgia 30322

James K. Kirklin, M.D.
Professor of Surgery
Director of Cardiothoracic Transplantation
Department of Surgery
University of Alabama at Birmingham
739 Zeigler Building
Birmingham, Alabama 35294

J. Philip Kistler, M.D.
Associate Professor
Department of Neurology
Harvard Medical School
Massachusetts General Hospital
32 Fruit Street, VBK 802
Boston, Massachusetts 02114

Neal S. Kleiman, M.D.
Methodist Hospital
Cardiology Division
6535 Fannin, Ms F-905
Houston, Texas 77030

Larry W. Kraiss, M.D.
Senior Fellow
Department of Surgery
University of Washington School of Medicine
Seattle, Washington 98195-6410

Frederick E. Kuhn, M.D.
St. Agnes Hospital
Baltimore, Maryland
Division of Cardiology
Georgetown University Medical Center
Washington DC 20007

Anatoly Langer, M.D.
St. Michael's Hospital
Office 701A
30 Bond Street
Toronto, Ontario
CANADA M5B 1W8

B. Lowell Langille, Ph.D.
Professor of Pathology
Vascular Research Laboratory
Department of Pathology
Banting and Best Diabetes Centre
The Toronto Hospital Research Institute
Centre for Cardiovascular Research
200 Elizabeth Street, CCRW 1-856
Toronto, Ontario M5G 2C4
CANADA

Richard M. Lawn, Ph.D.
Professor of Medicine
Division of Cardiovascular Medicine
Stanford University School of Medicine
300 Pasteur Drive
Stanford, California 94305

Martin B. Leon, M.D.
Director, Cardiovascular Research
Washington Hospital Center
110 Irving Street N.W.
Washington, DC 20010

Peter Libby, M.D.
Director of Vascular Medicine and Atherosclerosis Unit
Brigham & Women's Hospital
221 Longwood Avenue LMRC307
Boston, Massachusetts 02115

A. Michael Lincoff, M.D.
Assistant Professor of Medicine
Department of Cardiology
The Cleveland Clinic Foundation
9500 Euclid Avenue
Cleveland, Ohio 44195

David T. Linker, M.D.
Associate Professor of Medicine
Department of Cardiology
University of Washington
1959 N.E. Pacific Street
Seattle, Washington 98195

Thomas F. Luscher, M.D.
Division of Cardiology
University Hospital
CH-3010 Bern
SWITZERLAND

Robert W. Mahley, M.D., Ph.D.
Professor of Pathology and Medicine
Director, Gladstone Institute of Cardiovascular Disease
University of California, San Francisco
Department of Pathology
P.O. Box 419100
San Francisco, California 94141-9100

Aaron J. Marcus, M.D.
Professor of Medicine and Pathology
Cornell University Medical College; and
Chief, Hematology and Oncology
Department of Veterans Affairs Medical Center
423 East 23rd Street
New York, New York 10010

Daniel B. Mark, M.D.
Box 3485
Duke University Medical Center
Durham, North Carolina 27710

David C. McGiffin, M.D.
Associate Professor of Surgery
Department of Surgery
Univ. of Alabama at Birmingham
701 S. 19th Street
Birmingham, Alabama 35294

Henry C. McGill, Jr., M.D.
Senior Scientist and Chairman
Department of Physiology and Medicine
Southwest Foundation for Biomedical Research
7620 N.W. Loop 410, P.O. Box 28147
San Antonio, Texas 78228-0147

Murray A. Mittleman, M.D.C.M., Ph.D.
Instructor in Medicine
Harvard Medical School; and
Cardiovascular Division
Institute for Prevention of Cardiovascular Disease
New England Deaconess Hospital
One Autumn Street
Boston, Massachusetts 02215

David J. Moliterno, M.D.
Assistant Professor of Medicine
Department of Cardiology
Ohio State University;
Cleveland Clinic Health Sciences Center
9500 Euclid Avenue, F-25
Cleveland, Ohio 44195

Arthur J. Moss, M.D.
Professor of Medicine
University of Rochester Medical Center
601 Elmwood Avenue
Rochester, New York 14642

James E. Muller, M.D.
Associate Professor of Medicine
Harvard Medical School; and
Institute for Prevention of Cardiovascular Disease
New England Deaconess Hospital
One Autumn Street
Boston, Massachusetts 02215

Robert J. Myerburg, M.D.
Professor of Medicine and Physiology
Director, Division of Cardiology
University of Miami School of Medicine; and
Jackson Memorial Hospital
1611 N.W. 12th Avenue
Miami, Florida 33136

Elizabeth G. Nabel, M.D.
Professor of Medicine
Department of Internal Medicine
Director, Cardiovascular Research Center
University of Michigan Medical Center
1150 West Medical Center Drive
Ann Arbor, Michigan 48109-0644

Gary J. Nabel, M.D., Ph.D.
Professor of Internal Medicine and Biological Chemistry
Department of Internal Medicine
University of Michigan Medical Center
1150 W. Medical Center Drive
Ann Arbor, Michigan 48109-0644

Yoshifumi Naka, M.D., Ph.D.
Department of Physiology
College of Physicians & Surgeons of Columbia University
630 West 168th Street
New York, New York 10032

G. Noll
Cardiology and Cardiovascular Research
University Hospital
CH-3010 Bern, SWITZERLAND

Rick A. Nishimura, M.D.
Professor of Medicine
Division of Cardiovascular Diseases and Internal Medicine
Mayo Clinic
200 First Street S.W.
Rochester, Minnesota 55905

Steven E. Nissen, M.D.
The Cleveland Clinic Foundation
Department of Cardiology
9500 Euclid Avenue F15
Cleveland, Ohio 44195

Masakiyo Nobuyoshi, M.D., Ph.D.
Chairman of Heart Center
Director of Cardiology
Kokura Memorial Hospital
1-1 Kifune-machi, Kokurakita-ku
Kitakyushu 802
JAPAN

Patrick T. O'Gara, M.D.
Assistant Professor of Medicine
Harvard Medical School;
Director, Clinical Cardiology
Brigham and Women's Hospital
75 Francis Street
Boston, Massachusetts 02115

Toshinori Oinuma, M.D.
Post-doctoral Research Fellow
Department of Pathology
University of Chicago
5841 South Maryland
Chicago, Illinois 60637

Robert A. O'Rourke, M.D.
Charles Conrad Brown Distinguished Professor in Cardiovascular Disease
Department of Medicine and Cardiology
University of Texas Health Science Center at San Antonio
7703 Floyd Curl Drive
San Antonio, Texas 78284-7872

Gary K. Owens, Ph.D., MS.
Professor
Department of Molecular Physiology and Biological Physics
University of Virginia
Box 449
Charlottesville, Virginia 22908

Fredric J. Pashkow, M.D.
Medical Director of Cardiac Health Improvement and Rehabilitation Program
Department of Cardiology
The Cleveland Clinic Foundation
9500 Euclid Avenue
Cleveland, Ohio 44195

Richard C. Pasternak, M.D.
Assistant Professor of Medicine
Harvard Medical School; and
Director of Preventive Cardiology and Cardiac Rehabilitation
Massachusetts General Hospital
32 Fruit Street
Boston, Massachusetts 02114

Marc S. Penn
Department of Cell Biology
Cleveland Clinic Foundation, NC10
9500 Euclid Avenue
Cleveland, Ohio 44195

Carl J. Pepine, M.D.
Professor of Medicine
University of Florida
Box J-277
Gainesville, Florida 32610

Marc A. Pfeffer, M.D., Ph.D.
Cardiovascular Division
Brigham & Women's Hospital
75 Francis Street
Boston, Massachusetts 02115

Robert A. Phillips, M.D., Ph.D.
Associate Professor of Medicine
Cardiovascular Institute
Mount Sinai School of Medicine
One Gustave L. Levy Place, Box 1085
New York, New York 10029-6574

David M. Pinsky, M.D.
Department of Physiology
College of Physicians & Surgeons of Columbia University
630 West 168th Street
New York, New York 10032

Andrew S. Plump, Ph.D.
Laboratory of Biochemical Genetics and Metabolism
The Rockefeller University
1230 York Avenue
New York, New York, 10021-6399

Eric N. Prystowsky, M.D.
Northside Cardiology
8402 Harcourt
Suite 300
Indianapolis, IN 46260

Shahbudin H. Rahimtoola, M.D.
Distinguished Professor
George C. Griffith Professor of Cardiology
Department of Medicine
University of Southern California
2025 Zonal Avenue
Los Angeles, California 90033

Elaine W. Raines, M.S.
Research Professor of Pathology
Department of Pathology
University of Washington School of Medicine
1959 N.E. Pacific Street
Seattle, Washington 98195

Elliot J. Rayfield, M.D.
Clinical Professor
Mount Sinai Medical School
Adjunct Physician
Rockefeller University
New York, New York 10128

Michael Reidy, M.D.
Department of Pathology
Mail Stop SJ-60
University of Washington School of Medicine
Seattle, Washington 98195

William J. Rogers, M.D.
Professor of Medicine
Department of Medicine
University of Alabama Medical Center
334 LHR Building
Birmingham, Alabama 35223

Michael E. Rosenfeld, Ph.D.
Associate Professor Department of Pathobiology and Interdisciplinary Program in Nutritional Sciences
University of Washington School of Medicine
Box 353410
Seattle, Washington 98195-3410

Russell Ross, Ph.D.
Professor and Director
Center for Vascular Biology
Department of Pathology
University of Washington School of Medicine
Seattle, Washington 98195-7470

John D. Rutherford, M.D.
University of Texas Southwestern
Division of Cardiology
5323 Harry Hines Boulevard
Dallas, Texas 75235-9047

Siliva M. Santamarina-Fojo, M.D., Ph.D.
Chief, Molecular Biology Section
Molecular Disease Branch
National Heart, Lung and Blood Institute
National Institutes of Health
10 Center Drive MSC, Bldg. 10/7N 115
Bethesda, Maryland 20892-1666

Angelo M. Scanu, M.D.
Professor
Department of Medicine, Biochemistry and Molecular Biology
The University of Chicago
5841 S. Maryland Avenue MC5041
Chicago, Illinois 60637

Hartzell V. Schaff, M.D.
Stiart W. Harrington Professor of Surgery
Division of Cardiovascular and Thoracic Surgery
Mayo Medical School
200 First Street, S.W.
Rochester, Minnesota 55905

Heinrich R. Schelbert, M.D., Ph.D.
Professor of Pharmacology and Radiological Sciences
Department of Molecular and Medical Pharmacology
UCLA School of Medicine
10833 LeConte Avenue
Los Angeles, California 90024-1735

Gregory G. Schwartz, M.D., Ph.D.
Associate Professor of Medicine
Division of Cardiology
University of California, San Francisco; and
San Francisco VA Medical Center
4150 Clement Street
San Francisco, California 94121

Stephen M. Schwartz, M.D., Ph.D.
Professor of Pathology
Department of Pathology
University of Washington
1959 N.E. Pacific Street
Seattle, Washington 98195

Rafael F. Sequeira, M.D.
Associate Professor of Medicine
Department of Medicine
Division of Cardiology
University of Miami/Jackson Memorial Hospital
1611 N.W. 12th Avenue, D-62
Miami, Florida 33136

Patrick W. Serruys, M.D., Ph.D.
Professor of Interventional Cardiology
Thorax Center
University Hospital Dijkzigt
Erasmus University Rotterdam
Dr. Molewaterplein 40
3015 Rd Rotterdam
THE NETHERLANDS

Prediman K. Shah, M.D.
Professor of Medicine
UCLA School of Medicine; and
Shapell and Webb Family Chair in Cardiology and
Director, In-Patient Cadiology
Cedars-Sinai Medical Center
8700 Beverly Boulevard
Los Angeles, California 90048

Timothy A. Springer, Ph.D.
Latham Family Professor of Pathology
Department of Pathology
Harvard Medical School;
Center for Blood Research
200 Longwood Avenue
Boston, Massachusetts 02115

Randall S. Stafford, M.D., Ph.D.
General Internal Medicine Unit
Department of Medicine
Massachusetts General Hospital
Fruit Street
Boston, Massachusetts 02114

Herbert C. Stary, M.D.
Professor
Department of Pathology
Louisiana State University Medical Center
1901 Perdido Street
New Orleans, Louisiana 70112

David M. Stern, M.D.
Associate Professor Department of Physiology
Columbia University
630 West 168th Street
New York, New York 10032

Alan R. Tall, M.D.
Professor of Medicine
Department of Medicine
Columbia University
630 West 168 Street, PH 8 East 101
PNS Bldg 9-501
New York, New York 10032

Geoffrey H. Tofler, M.B.B.S.
Assistant Professor of Medicine
Harvard Medical School; and
Institute for Prevention of Cardiovascular Disease
New England Deaconess Hospital
One Autumn Street
Boston, Massachusetts 02215

Eric J. Topol, M.D.
Chairman, Department of Cardiology
Director, Joseph J. Jacobs Center for Thrombosis and Vascular Biology
The Cleveland Clinic Foundation
9500 Euclid Avenue
Cleveland, Ohio 44195

J. F. Toussaint
Cochin Hospital
Paris, FRANCE

E. Murst Tuczu, M.D.
Department of Cardiology
The Cleveland Clinic Foundation
9500 Euclid Avenue
Cleveland, Ohio 44195

Douglas E. Vaughan, M.D.
Cardiology Division
Vanderbilt University Med. Center
CC-2218 Medical Center North
Nashville, Tennessee 37232-2170

Raymond H. Verhaeghe, M.D.
Associate Professor of Medicine
Department of Molecular and Vascular Biology
University Hospital Gasthuisberg
Herestraat 49
3000 Leuven, BELGIUM

Marc Verstraete, M.D., Ph.D.
Professor of Medicine
Center for Molecular and Vascular Biology
University of Leuven
K.U.L. Campus Gasthuisberg-Herestraat 49
B-3000 Leuven, BELGIUM

Thomas N. Wight, Ph.D.
Department of Pathology, SM30
University of Washington
School of Medicine
Seattle, Washington 98195

James T. Willerson, M.D.
Director, Cardiology Division
University of Texas
Health Sciences Center at Houston
P.O. Box 20708
Houston, Texas 77225

Roger Williams, M.D.
Professor of Cardiovascular Genetics
University of Utah School of Medicine
410 Chipeta Way, Room 161
Salt Lake City, Utah 84108

Robert W. Wissler, M.D., Ph.D.
Distinguished Service Professor of Pathology
Department of Pathology
University of Chicago Medical Center
5841 South Maryland Avenue
Chicago, Illinois 60637

Salim Yusuf, M.B.B.S., D.Phil.
Professor of Medicine
Director, Division of Cardiology
Department of Medicine
McMaster University
HGH-McMaster Clinic
Hamilton General Hospital
237 Barton Street E.
Hamilton, Ontario L8L 2X2
CANADA

Preface

Fully cognizant of the multiple sources of biomedical information in the mid-1990s, particularly in the field of cardiovascular medicine, we were naturally reluctant to think about another new textbook. Yet coronary atherosclerosis is quite a unique topic, owing to its pervasiveness and significance, and the rapidity in which new data and understanding become available—especially in recent years. In considering ischemic heart disease and the broad discipline of coronary atherosclerosis, we were aware that there was no monograph fully devoted to this entity. Accordingly, we set out to provide a comprehensive assessment of this topic from bench to bedside, providing as much depth on the underlying pathophysiology as the clinical management. We were fortunate with the different and complementary expertise of the three of us, and this facilitated considerable crosstalk and learning about the whole range of topics from molecular biology to randomized clinical trials.

The book starts with a historical perspective and overview of the epidemiology of coronary atherosclerotic disease. Following this introduction, each of the known risk factors is addressed, with particular concentration on lipoprotein abnormalities and hypertension—areas which have made substantive progress in refining the pathophysiology and treatment. The second section covers the pathogenesis of the atherosclerotic lesion, with review of the normal artery, embryogenesis, experimental models, and the entire gamut of lesions from fatty streaks to frank plaque rupture. Each of the specific cellular components and related disorders are reviewed separately.

Section Three deals with acute myocardial infarction, with its pathophysiology, representing transition from the previous section, to clinical presentation and acute management. Recognizing that the acute phase is often just the beginning of awareness that a patient suffers from this disease, we have also provided in-depth consideration of secondary prevention measures and subsequent management.

This same clinical template follows in the fourth section for unstable angina and in the next for chronic stable angina. A paramount therapeutic goal for these latter subsets of presentation is to avoid myocardial infarction and establish stability of the atherosclerotic process. Because such patients often have non-coronary atherosclerotic disease as well, we have included the last Section to discuss cerebrovascular and peripheral arterial disease, along with the epidemiologic relationship between coronary and non-coronary atherosclerotic involvement.

With these over 100 chapters and contributions from over 200 authors, we hope that you will find that we have been able to achieve the unique and inaugural objective of a monograph that fully covers atherosclerosis and coronary artery disease. To achieve uniformity in presentation, we have incorporated chapter outlines and a closing part of future directions.

Should this treatise prove to be as useful as we intend, we hope to keep abreast of the explosion of knowledge at the cellular and molecular levels as they impact technological and clinical advances in diagnosis and therapy with updated versions at appropriate intervals.

We are indebted to all of our co-authors who have provided state-of-the-art reviews of their respective fields of expertise. We gratefully acknowledge the staff at Lippincott-Raven Publishers, including Lisa Berger and Kathleen Lyons, who made production of this endeavor a reality. We truly hope that you will find the book a valuable reference source and that it accesses the whole spectrum of this critical topic in your work as a scientist, clinician, or both.

Valentin Fuster, M.D., Ph.D.
Russell Ross, Ph.D.
Eric J. Topol, M.D.

Atherosclerosis and Coronary Artery Disease

Atherosclerosis and Coronary Artery Disease,
edited by V. Fuster, R. Ross, and E. J. Topol.
Lippincott-Raven Publishers, Philadelphia © 1996.

CHAPTER 1

A Historical Perspective on Atherosclerosis and Coronary Artery Disease

W. Bruce Fye

Key Words: Aneurysm; angina pectoris; anticoagulants; arrhythmia; arteriography; atherosclerosis; electrocardiogram; embolism; myocardial infarction; occlusion; reperfusion; thrombosis.

INTRODUCTION

This historical summary focuses on angina pectoris and acute myocardial infarction, the main cardiac manifestations of atherosclerosis. The pathological features of atherosclerosis were recognized long before the clinical syndromes of angina pectoris and acute myocardial infarction were described in the literature. Even after these clinical conditions were recognized, there was prolonged debate about their pathophysiology. This review provides some insights into the origins of the present understanding of atherosclerosis, angina pectoris, and acute myocardial infarction. It was a challenge to decide which advances to include in this chapter because over the centuries thousands of scientists and clinicians from around the world have contributed to our present understanding of the pathophysiology, diagnosis, and treatment of coronary artery disease. Inevitably, some well-known names are missing, and some minor individuals are included. Space constraints also made it necessary to exclude several topics and to focus on the period from the mid-18th to the mid-20th century.

W. B. Fye: Department of Cardiology, Marshfield Clinic, Marshfield, Wisconsin 54449.

ANEURYSMS, VASCULAR DISEASE, AND ATHEROSCLEROSIS

Atherosclerosis is a pathological condition that underlies several important disorders including coronary artery disease, cerebrovascular disease, and diseases of the aorta and peripheral arterial circulation. It is not a new problem. Using sophisticated histological techniques, paleopathologist A. T. Sandison recently confirmed that some Egyptian mummies had evidence of atherosclerosis (1). Paleopathologist Roy Moodie concluded that atherosclerosis in ancient Egyptians followed exactly the same course as it does today (2). Galen, the most influential physician of ancient Greece, described vascular aneurysms, but there is no evidence that he recognized other forms of atherosclerotic cardiovascular disease (3). Galen's teachings dominated medical theory and practice, such as they were, until the Renaissance.

Several 16th century anatomists, including Andreas Vesalius and Gabriele Falloppio, described aneurysms of the aorta and peripheral arteries (4,5). By the beginning of the 17th century, it was recognized that the aorta and other major arteries degenerated with advancing age, but the pathophysiology of this process was unknown. This is not surprising when it is recalled that William Harvey first proposed that the heart propelled blood through a closed vascular circuit in 1628 (6).

Because aneurysms of the peripheral arteries were visible and could be treated surgically, even before the advent of anesthesia or antisepsis, several articles and books appeared on this subject during the 18th century. An 1844 work by British surgeon John Erichsen provides valuable insight into early observations on arterial disease. This book includes nearly two dozen papers on aneurysms from antiquity to the late 18th century (7). The authors (and the original publication dates of their works) include Daniel Sennert (1628), Giovanni Maria Lancisi (1728), Alexander Monro (1733), Albrecht von Haller (1749), Pierre Foubert (1753), William Hunter (1757), Donald Monro (1760), Carlo Guattani (1772), John Hunter (1786), and Jacques Louis Dechamps (1799). In his 1628 publication, German chemist and physician Daniel Sennert described two layers in arteries. Sennert's work contained some practical information: he warned practitioners that an aneurysm might result if an artery instead of a vein was accidentally punctured during bloodletting, a popular therapy at the time.

Swiss physiologist Albrecht von Haller made several important observations on the cardiovascular system. In his 1755 monograph, *Opuscula Pathologica,* Haller described progressive atherosclerotic changes in arteries of the elderly. Six years later, Italian physician and pathologist Giovanni Battista Morgagni published *The Seats and Causes of Disease,* a book that inaugurated the modern era of pathological anatomy. Morgagni emphasized the value of the microscope as a tool for studying disease processes and stressed the importance of clinicopathological correlation (Fig. 1). Pathologist and historian Esmond Long thought Morgagni's studies of the vascular system were his most significant contribution to special pathology and characterized his observations on aneurysms as "magnificent" (8).

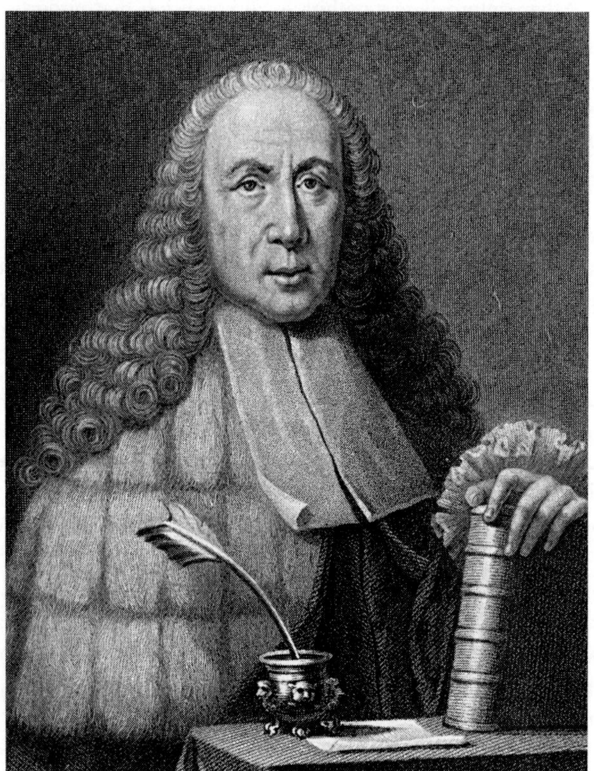

FIG. 1. Giovanni Battista Morgagni (1682–1771). The founder of modern pathology, Morgagni emphasized the importance of clinicopathological correlation. His most significant scientific contributions related to pathology of the vascular system. (From the collection of W. Bruce Fye.)

Atherosclerosis was more than an incidental finding at the dissecting table; it sometimes caused diseases that 18th century physicians and surgeons tried to treat. Their approaches reflected contemporary medical theories rather than a sophisticated understanding of the pathophysiology of diseases of the heart and vascular system. Although these practitioners did not understand the relationship between cerebral atherosclerosis and apoplexy or coronary artery disease and angina pectoris, they surely saw some patients who suffered from these conditions.

Morgagni's pupil Antonio Scarpa, an Italian anatomist and surgeon, extended his mentor's observations on vascular disease. In his 1804 monograph on aneurysms, Scarpa sought to prove that earlier concepts regarding the etiology of aneurysms were incorrect. After carefully studying the various layers of arteries, he concluded that the most common and important antecedent to aneurysm formation was an ulcerated atheromatous lesion. Scarpa emphasized that an aneurysm was not simply a dilated portion of normal artery; it was the result of localized disease of the arterial wall (9).

Although interest in vascular disease remained focused on aneurysms throughout much of the 19th century, some individuals turned their attention to the pathophysiology of atherosclerosis. London surgeon Joseph Hodgson published an important monograph on vascular disease in 1815. Reflecting contemporary medical theory, Hodgson claimed that inflammation was the underlying cause of atheromatous arteries. By this time, it was known that arteries consisted of three distinct layers. Hodgson identified atheromatous material between the intima and media and proposed that these changes could be traced an abnormality of the intima. Reflecting a growing appreciation of the value of chemistry in medicine, he also first reported the results of chemical analysis of atherosclerotic lesions.

In an 1829 monograph on pathological anatomy, French pathologist Jean Lobstein introduced the term "arteriosclerosis" and, like Hodgson, published the results of a chemical analysis of calcified arterial plaques. Several atlases of pathological anatomy were published in Europe during the 19th century, and some of them included illustrations of atherosclerotic arteries. Striking engravings of vascular lesions and the cerebral and cardiac complications of atherosclerosis appeared in the spectacular atlas published by French pathologist Jean Cruveilhier between 1829 and 1842. One hand-colored plate depicted a ventricular aneurysm containing thrombus.

Viennese pathologist Carl Rokitansky's comprehensive monograph on pathological anatomy (1842–1846) included an extensive section on atherosclerosis. Although much of his theory regarding the cause of atherosclerotic lesions was later proved false, Rokitansky's descriptions of the lesions are striking and accurate. He also recognized that there was

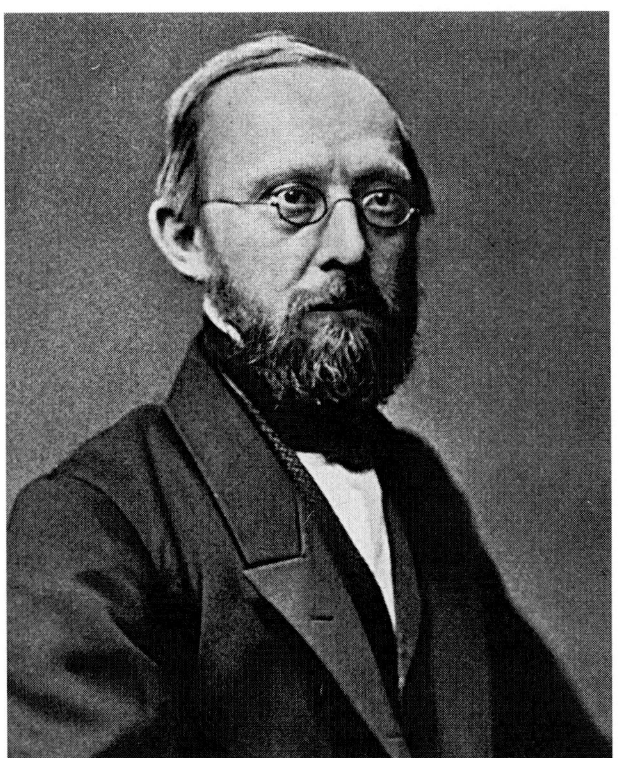

FIG. 2. Rudolf Virchow (1821–1902). Virchow's 1858 book on cellular pathology signaled the end of humoralism. He made classic observations on thrombosis (a term he coined) and embolism. (From the collection of W. Bruce Fye.)

a thrombogenic component to the progression of atherosclerosis. In 1852, he published a monograph on arterial diseases that included 61 spectacular illustrations. The book also contained clear descriptions of atheroma and intimal calcification.

It is hard to overestimate German pathologist Rudolf Virchow's significance in the history of medicine (Fig. 2). Esmond Long called him "the greatest figure in the history of pathology." Virchow's 1858 book *Cellular Pathology* signaled the end of humoralism and inaugurated a new era in the conceptualization of disease. Reflecting his enthusiasm for microscopy, Virchow used the instrument to study blood vessels. He concluded from these researches that atherosclerotic lesions were located within the intimal layer. He believed that these intimal deposits stimulated the proliferation of connective tissue, which triggered further degenerative changes of the vessel wall.

Virchow made pioneering observations on thrombosis and embolism. The first volume of his *Handbuch der Speciellen Pathologie und Therapie,* published in 1854, contained important sections on thrombosis (a term he coined), embolism, and vascular obstruction (10). Virchow described the process of thrombosis in this work. He explained,

> The coagulation of blood within vessels takes place in accord with the same laws as outside the vessels, in that the dissolved fibrin, which does not require the access of atmospheric air, alters its state of aggregation and becomes solid. . . . This coagulum we call a blood-clot, a thrombus, and accordingly we suggest for the process the designation clot-formation, thrombosis (11).

During the final decades of the 19th century, several theories were advanced to attempt to explain the pathophysiology of the various forms of arterial disease that pathologists had identified. Although attention was initially focused on visible lesions of the aorta, the expanding use of the microscope led to the recognition of vascular disease involving the small blood vessels of the kidneys and other organs. This led to the introduction of the concept of arteriosclerosis. Gradually, pathologists abandoned the view that atherosclerosis was the result of inflammation and adopted the view that it was a degenerative process.

The modern era of atherosclerosis research began in 1908, when Russian scientist Alexander Ignatovski showed that he could experimentally induce atherosclerosis in rabbits by feeding them a diet of milk and egg yolk. Extending these experiments, Nikolai Anitschkov showed that a diet rich in cholesterol caused atherosclerosis in experimental animals. German chemist and Nobel Prize winner Adolf Windaus showed that cholesterol was present in atherosclerotic lesions in humans in 1910. Anitschkov published a valuable summary in English of the early experimental studies of atherosclerosis in 1933 (12).

There was growing interest in the clinical and scientific aspects of atherosclerosis during the early 20th century (13). In part, this is explained by the gradually declining morbidity and mortality from infectious diseases that resulted from better nutrition, improved sanitation, and various public health measures. As people lived longer, "degenerative" diseases such as cancer and disorders of the cardiovascular system became more important to patients and physicians alike. Some authorities viewed atherosclerosis as inevitable. But German pathologist Ludwig Aschoff did not. In 1933, he claimed, "The widespread belief that arteriosclerosis is merely a manifestation of old age does not tally with the actual facts." Aschoff thought such a fatalistic attitute was inappropriate: "If arteriosclerosis were merely a phenomenon of aging, neither remedies nor prophylactics would be of any avail, for no one can escape age and death" (14). Researchers were motivated to search for clues to the pathophysiology of this disease process because they did not view it as a simple manifestation of aging that could not be modified in some fashion.

Philadelphia pharmacologist Thomas H. F. Smith, claimed in 1960 that "atherosclerosis had emerged by the end of the 1930s from the position of a medical curiosity. It was no longer considered a casual observation at autopsies but was now regarded as a major cause of death" (15). Scientists sought to understand the pathophysiology of atherosclerosis, and patients and their doctors were eager for effective remedies for the many clinical problems that resulted from this process. This growing interest in atherosclerosis was reflected in the publication of a 617-page book on the subject in 1933 (16). Like the present volume, that work included contributions by leaders in the field who discussed both the scientific and clinical aspects of atherosclerosis and its complications. Still, effective therapy lagged behind the understanding of the pathology of atherosclerosis and coronary artery disease. This is apparent if one reviews Paul Dudley White's classic book on heart disease, first published in 1931, and other texts from the first half of the 20th century (17).

Breakthroughs were being made, however, and at an ever-increasing rate. In 1933, the year Cowdry's book appeared, New York bacteriologist William Tillett reported his discovery of the fibrinolytic activity of β-hemolytic streptococci (18). It would be nearly half a century before this observation was translated into the routine use of thrombolytic therapy for acute myocardial infarction, however. During this time many important discoveries would be made. Initially, these resulted largely from the explosive growth of the biomedical research community in the United States, expansion fueled by generous government funding of academic medical centers following World War II. In recent decades workers in many other nations contributed increasingly to new knowledge (13,19).

ANGINA PECTORIS AND CORONARY ARTERY DISEASE

Renaissance artist Leonardo Da Vinci was the first to describe and illustrate the coronary arteries accurately (20). They were also accurately depicted by Italian anatomist Andreas Vesalius in his monumental work *De Humani Corporis Fabrica* published in 1543. Best known for his discovery of the circulation, reported in 1628 in his monumental book *De Motu Cordis,* English physician and anatomist William Harvey also first described the coronary circulation (Fig. 3). In a 1649 book he described the anatomy of the coronary arteries and veins and proposed that the coronary circulation nourished the heart (21). Using injection techniques, British physician and anatomist Richard Lower described coronary anastomoses two decades later (22). Although other physicians and scientists extended these observations on the anatomy of the coronary circulation, little was known about the functional significance of the coronary arteries until the 19th century.

English physician William Heberden first described angina pectoris in a talk presented to members of the College of Physicians of London in July 1768 (Fig. 4). His paper, published 4 years later, is still recognized as one of the most classic clinical descriptions in medicine (23,24). Speaking of the condition he called angina pectoris, Heberden claimed:

> There is a disorder of the breast, marked with strong and peculiar symptoms, considerable for the kind of danger belonging to it, and not extremely rare, of which I do not recollect any mention among medical authors. The seat of it, and sense of strangling and anxiety with which it is attended, may make it not improperly be called Angina pectoris.
>
> Those, who are afflicted with it, are seized, while they are walking, and more particularly when they walk soon after eating, with a painful and most disagreeable sensation in the breast, which seems as if it would take their life away, if it were to increase or to continue: the moment they stand still, all this uneasiness vanishes. In all other respects the patients are at the beginning of this disorder perfectly well, and in particular have no shortness of breath, from which it is totally different.
>
> After it has continued some months, it will not cease so instantaneously upon standing still; and it will come on, not only when the persons are walking, but when they are lying down and oblige them to rise up out of their beds every night for many months together. . . . When a fit of this sort comes on by walking, its duration is very short, as it goes off almost immediately upon stopping. If it come on in the night, it will last an hour or two. . . . The os sterni is usually pointed to as the seat of this malady, but it seems sometimes as if it was under the lower part of it, and at other times under the middle or upper part, but always inclining more to the left side, and sometimes there is joined with it a pain about the middle of the left arm.

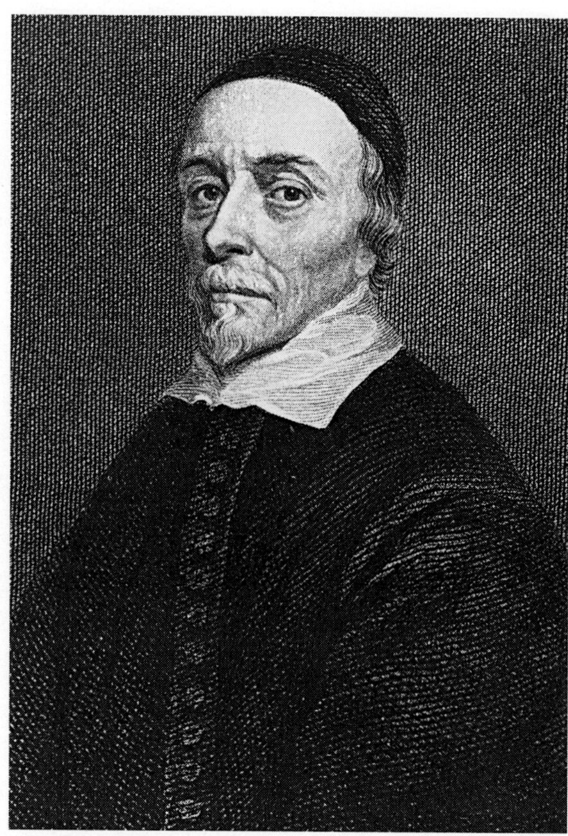

FIG. 3. William Harvey (1578–1657). Best known for his discovery of the circulation, reported in 1628 in *De Motu Cordis,* Harvey also first described the coronary circulation. Those observations were published in 1649. (From the collection of W. Bruce Fye.)

By the time Heberden described the syndrome of angina pectoris to his fellow London physicians, he had seen more than 20 patients with the condition. He thought that most

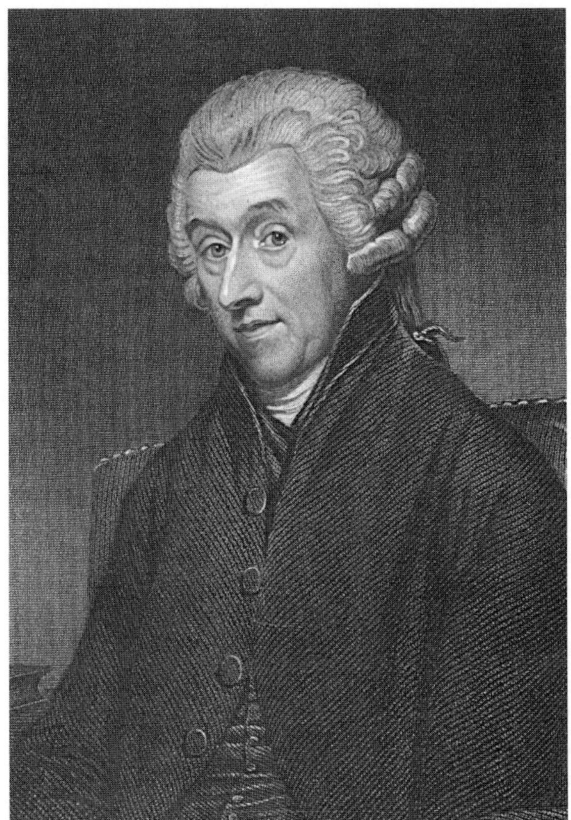

FIG. 4. William Heberden (1710–1801). British physician who is remembered eponymically for first describing angina pectoris (1772). (From the collection of W. Bruce Fye.)

people with angina had a poor prognosis and noted that they were prone to sudden death. Still, Heberden recognized that some individuals would survive for many years despite the presence of typical anginal symptoms. Heberden had never seen an autopsy performed on anyone suffering from angina and was unsure of the cause of the dramatic clinical picture. His management of angina reflected contemporary thought about the mechanism of disease. Although Heberden found that bleeding and purging did not help his patients, he discovered that opiates seemed to prevent nocturnal episodes of angina. Specific remedies for angina would not be introduced for more than a century.

Heberden remained interested in angina. His posthumous book *Commentaries on the History and Cure of Diseases,* published in 1802, included additional observations on the malady (25). By the time he finished the manuscript in 1782, Heberden had seen about 100 patients suffering from the disorder. Although Heberden's clinical description of angina pectoris was masterful, he did not speculate on its pathophysiology. Shortly after Heberden published his original observations on angina, he received an anonymous letter from a 52-year-old physician who suffered from the condition. The doctor urged Heberden to perform an autopsy on him in the event of his death, hoping that this might help clarify the cause of the malady. When "Dr. Anonymous" died 3 weeks later, Heberden asked surgeon and anatomist John Hunter to perform the autopsy. Edward Jenner, best remembered for his introduction of vaccination a few years later, assisted Hunter in the postmortem examination and later recalled that this was the first case of angina he had seen (Fig. 5). Hunter and Jenner found no abnormalities in the heart or other organs to explain the doctor's death, however. Because of Heberden's (as well as Hunter and Jenner's) lack of recognition that coronary artery disease was the cause of angina, the anonymous doctor's coronary arteries were not examined (26).

After serving as Hunter's assistant for 2 years, Jenner returned to his hometown of Gloucestershire to begin his career as a country doctor. Once in practice, Jenner saw more patients with angina. His interest in the condition was further stimulated when he realized that his friend John Hunter suffered from the disorder. By 1786, Jenner had witnessed three autopsies of patients who had suffered from anginal attacks. The postmortem on the last of these patients led Jenner to conclude that the symptoms were related to coronary artery disease. He explained that the autopsy revealed "a kind of firm fleshy tube, formed within the [coronary] vessel, with a considerable quantity of ossific matter dispersed irregularly through it." Jenner proposed that this pathological finding had been overlooked in other patients who had suffered from angina because the coronary arteries were often covered by epicardial fat.

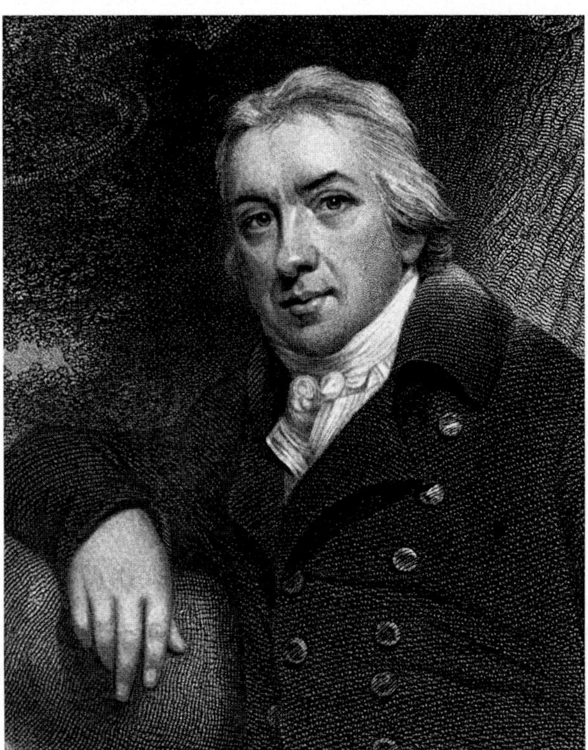

FIG. 5. Edward Jenner (1749–1823). Best known for introducing vaccination, this British physician was the first to attribute angina pectoris to coronary artery disease. (From the collection of W. Bruce Fye.)

In a letter to Heberden, Jenner explicitly linked coronary artery disease to angina; he was the first to do so. Jenner explained, "the importance of the coronary arteries, and how much the heart must suffer from their not being able to perform their functions, (we cannot be surprised at the painful spasms) is a subject I need not enlarge upon, therefore shall only just remark that it is possible that all the symptoms may arise from this one circumstance." Jenner also told Heberden of his reluctance to share his beliefs with Hunter because "it may deprive him of the hopes of a recovery," as there was no remedy for coronary artery disease (27).

Jenner's friend, Bath physician Caleb Hillier Parry, published the first book on angina pectoris in 1799. Parry credited Jenner with first attributing angina to coronary artery disease. Jenner had told Parry that while carefully dissecting the heart of a patient he had seen with angina, his "knife struck something so hard and gritty, as to notch it." At first Jenner thought a piece of ceiling plaster had fallen into his dissecting field, but on closer inspection he discovered that the "coronaries were become bony canals." It was this case that led Jenner to conclude that angina was caused by "malorganization of these [coronary] vessels" (28).

Parry accepted Jenner's hypothesis that angina was caused by coronary artery disease. He was surprised, however, that angina was not described earlier. "Although there can be no reason to doubt," Parry explained, "that mankind must have been subject to this disorder from the remotest antiquity, it is somewhat extraordinary that so many ages should have elapsed without any notice of its existence either as a distinct disease, or as a variety of one commonly known." After a thorough review of the literature, Parry concluded that only ten assays on angina had been published by 1799, and only nine patients with anginal attacks had undergone autopsy.

Parry's case reports were remarkably detailed and, reflecting growing interest in clinicopathological correlation, included the relevant pathological findings. He concluded "that there is an important connection between the rigid and obstructed state of these vessels, and the disease in question [angina pectoris]." Parry attributed angina to "induration" and "ossification" of the coronary arteries and proposed that they might be "so obstructed as to intercept the blood, which should be the proper support of the muscular fibres of the heart that [the] organ must become thin and flaccid, and unequal to the task of circulation" (28).

Scottish anatomist and physician Allan Burns published the first book on heart disease in the English language in 1809. Burns agreed with Parry that angina was caused by "some organic lesions of the nutrient vessels of the heart." He emphasized that because the heart was primarily a muscle, it was "regulated by the same laws which govern other muscles." Burns drew an analogy between coronary artery disease and the ligation of a peripheral artery in order to support his view of the pathophysiology of angina pectoris (29).

Although the contributions of Jenner, Parry, and Burns seemed to document a relationship between coronary artery disease and angina pectoris, other observations made during the 19th century undermined the coronary theory of angina. For example, in his 1813 book on dropsy, a condition we now know is usually caused by congestive heart failure, British physician John Blackall described one patient with typical angina who had only trivial coronary artery disease but whose ascending aorta was severely atherosclerotic. The apparent inconsistent relationship between coronary artery disease found at autopsy and symptoms thought to represent angina was an important factor in the long delay between Heberden's description of angina in 1772 and the widespread acceptance of the coronary theory of its etiology a century later.

The introduction of mediate auscultation by French physician René Laennec gave physicians a powerful diagnostic tool to help them evaluate diseases of the heart and lungs. But the stethoscope, first described in Laennec's two-volume book on auscultation in 1819, contributed to a shift in emphasis in heart disease. Using a stethoscope, doctors could identify abnormal heart sounds and murmurs. It also helped them correlate their patient's complaints and physical findings with autopsy results. For several decades the literature of heart disease reflected this new orientation toward valvular heart lesions.

Although relatively little progress was made during the 19th century with regard to understanding the pathophysiology of angina, an empirical observation led to the use of vasodilators for its treatment. Scottish medical student Thomas Lauder Brunton introduced amyl nitrite for the treatment of angina pectoris in 1867 (30) (Fig. 6). Brunton's mentors at the University of Edinburgh had been experimenting with the substance and were impressed by the immediate and profound effects that followed its inhalation. Using a new instrument, the sphygmograph, they found that amyl nitrate predictably lowered the arterial tension in animals and humans.

Brunton found that the blood pressure rose and the pulse quickened during anginal attacks. He thought angina was caused by a "derangement of the vaso-motor system" that resulted in increased vascular tone and high arterial tension. This theory eventually proved false, but it was a critical factor in Brunton's decision to try amyl nitrite in patients with angina. Although the popularity of therapeutic bleeding had declined by the late 1860s, some doctors still used the procedure in angina because it was thought to reduce arterial tension. When Brunton bled patients with angina, some of them seemed to improve. Recognizing that amyl nitrite was a vasodilator, he thought it might be useful in the treatment of the disorder. When Brunton gave amyl nitrite to patients with angina, their chest discomfort often disappeared within a minute.

Twelve years later, British physician and pharmacologist William Murrell reported that nitroglycerin was an effective treatment for angina. Murrell became interested in nitroglycerin, a homeopathic remedy first used by Constantine Hering

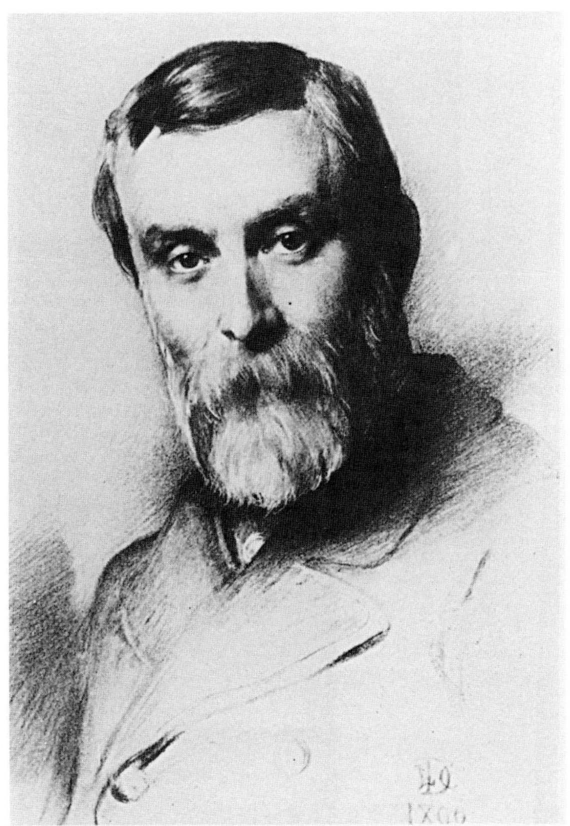

FIG. 6. Thomas Lauder Brunton (1844–1916). Scottish physician and pharmacologist who first advocated vasodilator therapy (amyl nitrite) for angina pectoris in 1867. (From the collection of W. Bruce Fye.)

in the 1840s, because he found that its effect on heart rate and arterial tension was similar to amyl nitrite's (31). Murrell found that nitroglycerin relieved angina promptly, although its effects came on more slowly and lasted longer than those of amyl nitrite. Following Murrell's 1879 report in the *Lancet,* nitroglycerin's value in angina was rapidly and widely acknowledged. This was true, in large part, because its beneficial effects were immediate, dramatic, and reproducible.

By the 20th century, most physicians and medical scientists interested in heart disease accepted the coronary theory of angina. A few did not, however. Clifford T. Allbutt, Regius Professor of Medicine at Cambridge and a prolific author, published several papers on angina and held steadfastly to the belief that it was caused by disease of the aortic root until his death in 1925. By this time, however, there was growing understanding about the pathophysiology of coronary artery disease and its complications. Much of this new insight about angina pectoris came from pathological and physiological research on coronary occlusion and myocardial infarction.

ACUTE MYOCARDIAL INFARCTION

The clinical syndrome we term acute myocardial infarction was first clearly described in the 20th century. Several factors contributed to the delay between Heberden's 1772 paper on angina pectoris and James Herrick's classic description of acute myocardial infarction in 1912. Probably the most important factor in this delay was the belief that sudden coronary occlusion was invariably fatal. That view predominated until the early 20th century. Other reasons included the inconsistent relationship of symptoms to pathological findings in ischemic heart disease, the reliance of 19th century physicians on auscultation as an indicator of heart disease, the failure to examine the coronary arteries and myocardium routinely at autopsy, the lag between pathological and physiological discoveries and their incorporation into medical practice, the preoccupation of late 19th century physicans with the new field of bacteriology, and the lack of any diagnostic tool to help physicians identify coronary artery obstruction or its consequences during life (32).

European and American medical scientists and clinicians made several observations during the second half of the 19th century that ultimately led to a recognition of the clinical and pathological sequelae of coronary occlusion (33). British surgeon John Erichsen investigated the relationship of cardiac arrest and experimental coronary occlusion in the early 1840s. In 1850, British physician Richard Quain described "fatty degeneration" of the myocardium, a process he associated with coronary artery disease. In 1866, French physician Edme Vulpain reported the case of a 75-year-old woman found at autopsy to have cardiac rupture at the site of a dramatically thin left ventricular segment supplied by an occluded coronary artery. Vulpian concluded that a thrombus had formed at the site of an atherosclerotic plaque and occluded the coronary artery, causing the myocardium to become thin and friable. Although Vulpian's interpretation of the pathophysiology of coronary occlusion and its consequences was advanced for the time, he did not address the clinical aspects of the condition or suggest how physicians might recognize coronary occlusion during life (24).

By the end of the 19th century, many pathologists had concluded that there was a causal relationship between thrombotic coronary occlusion and the degenerative changes of the myocardium that were seen using a microscope and were visible to the naked eye. Despite this, clinicians were either unaware of these conclusions or were unimpressed by them. In 1880, Carl Weigert, who worked with German pathologist Julius Cohnheim, published a paper that included a clear description of the pathophysiology of thrombotic occlusion of atherosclerotic coronary arteries leading to myocardial necrosis. Weigert differentiated gradual, progressive obstruction of a coronary artery from abrupt occlusion of the vessel. His paper is a milestone in the description of the pathological aspects of coronary thrombosis and myocardial infarction.

Weigert's clinical colleague Karl Huber extended these observations and claimed, in 1882, that angina pectoris and myocardial infarction were both manifestations of coronary artery disease. These important observations on the pathophysiology of occlusive coronary artery disease had essentially no impact on contemporary medical practice, however. In retrospect, some authors described symptoms that we now recognize as consistent with acute myocardial infarction, but they did not distinguish those episodes from prolonged attacks of angina pectoris.

William Osler, the leading internist of his generation, had studied with Cohnheim and Weigert and appreciated the significance of their observations on coronary artery disease. As early as 1889, Osler observed in an editorial, "The local disturbances of nutrition caused by the blocking of a terminal branch of the coronary artery produces the condition known as infarct of the heart" (34). But Osler was referring to the *pathological* findings of myocardial infarction; he did not comprehend that there was a distinct *clinical* syndrome that accompanied acute coronary occlusion.

American physiologist William Porter performed a series of experiments in the late 19th century that were critical for Herrick's formulation of the clinical syndrome of acute myocardial infarction. For more than a decade, Porter studied the effects of experimental occlusion of the coronary arteries. He documented the results of sudden occlusion (produced by ligation or embolization) of them on the heart rhythm, hemodynamics, and the histology and gross pathology of the organ (35). Porter's assistant Walter Baumgarten studied the effect of myocardial ischemia on contractility and raised issues that are today of great interest in terms of myocardial viability following acute coronary thrombosis and reperfusion therapy. In 1900, Baumgarten found that following acute coronary occlusion, "portions of the mammalian ventricle will resume their contractions if fed with defibrinated blood." Based on experiments he and Porter performed, he concluded that the loss of contractility that resulted from experimentally induced ischemia was reversible for up to 11 hr. Baumgarten also claimed that contractility was most impaired in the central zone of the ischemic area and least affected at the periphery (36).

Gradually, clinicians acknowledged that acute coronary thrombosis was not invariably fatal, but there was no recognition of the clinical syndrome of acute myocardial infarction until Russian physicians W. P. Obrastzow and N. D. Straschesko published the first description of this dramatic event in 1910. They believed that two specific findings were characteristic of acute coronary thrombosis: prolonged chest discomfort, "status anginosus," and persistent dyspnea, "status dyspnoeticus." After presenting cases with autopsy correlations, Obrastzow and Straschesko concluded, "the differential diagnosis of coronary thrombosis from angina pectoris is made by the presence of status anginosus with coronary thrombosis and its absence with isolated attacks of angina pectoris" (37,38).

Although this paper, published in German, attracted little attention, it was known to Chicago internist James Herrick, who eventually convinced the medical community that acute coronary thrombosis could be recognized during life (Fig. 7). Herrick's 1912 paper "Certain Clinical Features of Sudden Obstruction of the Coronary Arteries" (39) is a milestone in our understanding of the pathophysiology of coronary artery disease, angina pectoris, and myocardial infarction. It contained the first description in English of the clinical syndrome of acute myocardial infarction.

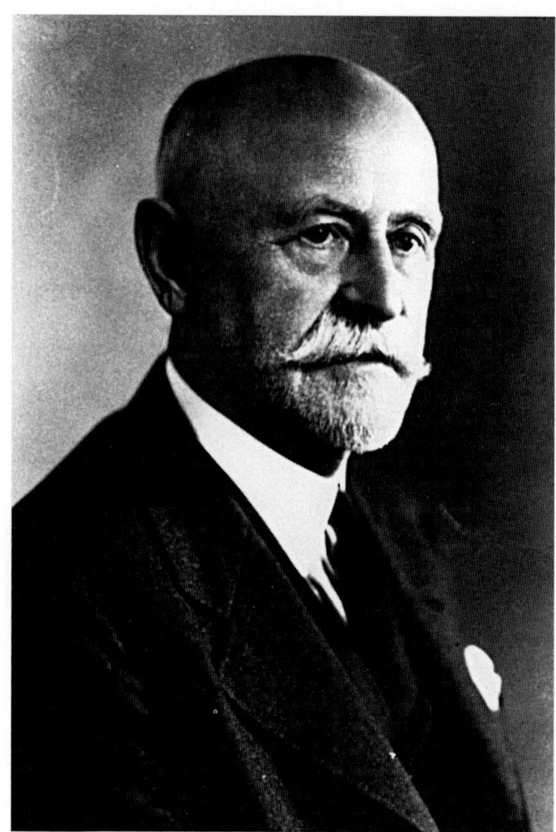

FIG. 7. James B. Herrick (1861–1954). Chicago internist who published, in 1912, the first description of the clinical syndrome of acute myocardial infarction in English. He was among the first to advocate using the electrocardiograph to help confirm the diagnosis. (From the National Library of Medicine.)

Herrick had reviewed experimental, clinical, and pathological reports from Europe and America and concluded that acute thrombosis of a major coronary artery did not invariably cause sudden death. He also provided an explanation of the spectrum of symptoms that could accompany coronary thrombosis. "The clinical manifestations of coronary obstruction will evidently vary greatly," Herrick claimed, "depending on the size, location and number of vessels occluded. The symptoms and end-result must also be influenced by blood-pressure, by the condition of the myocardium not immediately affected by the obstruction, and by the ability of the remaining vessels properly to carry on their work, as determined by their health or disease" (39).

Despite his vivid description, Herrick's report on the clinical features of acute coronary thrombosis attracted little attention until doctors had an objective tool to demonstrate that their patients' chest discomfort and associated symptoms were unequivocally cardiac in origin. Electrocardiogra-

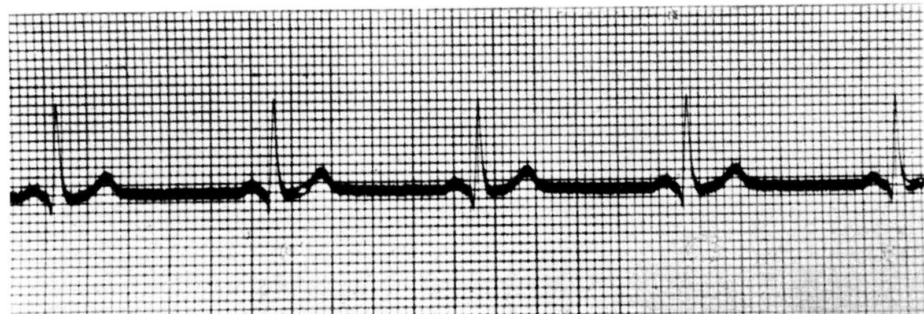

FIG. 8. Einthoven's first published electrocardiographic tracing using a string galvanometer. (From W. Einthoven, "Galvanometrische Registratie van Het Manschelijk Electrocardiogram" in Herrineringsbundel. Professor S. S. Rosenstein. Leiden: Eduard Ijdo; 1902:107.)

phy, introduced by Dutch physiologist Willem Einthoven in 1902, eventually provided clinicians with a powerful tool to help them recognize acute myocardial infarction and differentiate it from angina pectoris and noncardiac conditions causing chest pain (Fig. 8). Initially, the electrocardiogram was used to evaluate cardiac arrhythmias.

Herrick and his assistant Fred Smith were among the first to study the electrocardiographic (ECG) manifestations of experimental coronary occlusion (40). Their findings led Herrick to claim that characteristic ECG changes accompanied acute coronary occlusion, and these typical findings should help physicians recognize acute coronary thrombosis. So Herrick provided clinicians with both an intellectual framework for conceptualizing survival following coronary thrombosis and a new diagnostic approach to help them recognize the event. Other investigators extended Herrick's observations during the 1920s and 1930s. The introduction of the precordial leads by Charles Wolferth and Francis Wood in 1932 was a major advance in the ECG diagnosis of myocardial infarction.

Boston cardiologist Samuel Levine published the first book in English devoted to coronary thrombosis in 1929. He addressed the concept of what we now term cardiac risk factors and claimed that heredity, male sex, obesity, diabetes, and hypertension predisposed patients to coronary thrombosis. Levine identified a broad spectrum of complications that might result from coronary thrombosis and myocardial infarction. He explained that cardiac arrhythmias, cardiac rupture, and thromboembolic events could follow coronary thrombosis in addition to the well-known complication of sudden death (41).

The routine treatment of myocardial infarction in the 1930s and 1940s consisted mainly of prolonged bed rest, oxygen, and narcotics. Quinidine was used to treat ventricular tachycardia, but arrhythmia was rarely detected because continuous electrocardiographic monitoring had not yet been introduced. Prolonged bed rest (up to 6 weeks) was routinely advocated following acute myocardial infarction. Growing awareness of pulmonary emboli and other complications resulting from prolonged immobilization led to a gradual reduction in the time of hospitalization and strict bed rest following myocardial infarction.

During the 1960s the treatment of acute myocardial infarction changed dramatically. American cardiologist Mason Sones first performed selective coronary arteriography in 1958 and reported the technique 4 years later (42) (Fig. 9). This procedure, an extension of angiographic techniques that had evolved over three decades, revolutionized the evaluation and management of patients with known or suspected coronary artery disease (22). It provided researchers with a powerful tool to study ischemic heart disease and was critical for the development of coronary bypass surgery, percutaneous transluminal coronary angioplasty, and thrombolytic therapy.

In 1960, William Kouwenhoven and his colleagues published their method of external cardiac massage that inaugurated the modern era of cardiopulmonary resuscitation (43). Around this time pacemakers and defibrillators were introduced into clinical practice, approaches that enabled physicians to effectively treat bradyarrhythmias and tachyarrhythmias. Advances in the pharmacological treatment of arrhythmias were reported as well: lidocaine and procainamide were shown to be effective for ventricular arrhythmias (44).

In 1962, Kansas cardiologist Hughes Day introduced the concepts of the cardiac arrest team and the coronary care unit (CCU) into the United States. These innovations dramatically changed the management of patients with acute myocardial infarction (45). Continuous ECG monitoring, a critical part of the CCU concept, alerted a specially trained staff to the onset of potentially life-threatening arrhythmias or cardiac arrest. They responded quickly using new mechanical and pharmacological approaches to treat these problems. Early detection and aggressive management of arrhythmias significantly reduced mortality from acute myocardial infarction, and the CCU concept spread rapidly throughout the nation.

Although early deaths from arrhythmias resulting from acute myocardial infarction were reduced, many patients still died as a result of cardiogenic shock and other less dramatic consequences of extensive myocardial necrosis. The introduction of the flow-directed balloon-tipped catheter in 1970 facilitated the assessment of the hemodynamic consequences of acute myocardial infarction. This new approach made it possible to evaluate left ventricular filling pressure and cardiac output at the bedside so the physician could adjust therapy to treat specific hemodynamic abnormalities.

Beginning in the 1950s, various techniques were introduced to estimate infarct size. These approaches included serum enzyme assays, electrocardiographic mapping, and

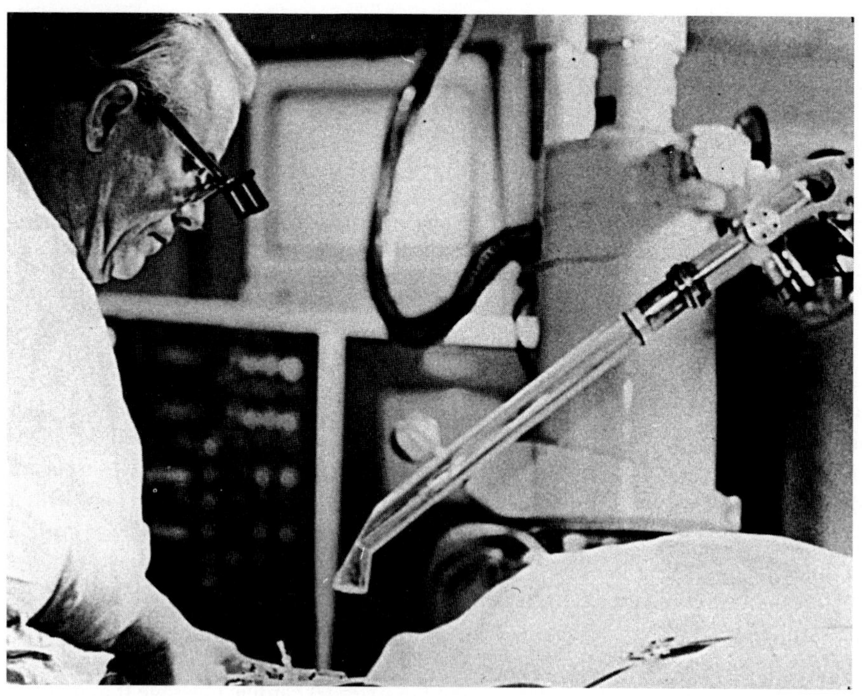

FIG 9. F. Mason Sones, Jr. (1918–1985). American cardiologist who developed the technique of selective coronary arteriography. Reported in 1962, this technique was critical for the future development of coronary bypass surgery, percutaneous transluminal coronary angioplasty, and thrombolytic therapy. (From *Modern Medicine,* with permission.)

evaluation of myocardial performance using radioisotopes, ultrasound, and angiocardiography. They improved the physician's ability to establish a prognosis and helped clinical scientists evaluate new approaches to myocardial preservation. Although several pharmacological and mechanical approaches introduced during the 1970s to limit myocardial necrosis failed to show any significant effect on survival, one strategy—thrombolytic therapy—seemed promising.

As noted earlier, some 19th century pathologists thought that thrombus played a critical role in causing coronary occlusion, which they believed resulted in the myocardial necrosis identified at autopsy. By 1920, as a result of the observations of Herrick and others, the view that sudden thrombotic occlusion of the diseased coronary artery triggered acute myocardial infarction was widely accepted. Soon after the anticoagulants heparin and bishydroxycoumarin (Dicumarol) were developed in the 1930s, some clinicians and medical scientists thought they might be useful in the treatment of acute myocardial infarction. Based on a study of 800 patients reported in 1948, Irving Wright advocated the routine use of anticoagulants following acute myocardial infarction to prevent the extension of coronary thrombosis and the development of mural thrombi (46). Hemorrhagic complications limited the acceptance of this approach, however. Another factor that contributed to the decline in the routine use of oral anticoagulants was the recognition that venous thrombosis and pulmonary emboli occurred less frequently following myocardial infarction once early ambulation became standard.

Modern thrombolytic therapy can be traced to 1933, when New York bacteriologist William Tillett discovered that β-hemolytic streptococci produced a fibrinolytic substance that he termed fibrinolysin (later renamed streptokinase) (47). Extending Tillett's work, Sol Sherry, Anthony Fletcher, and their associates reported on the administration of intravenous streptokinase in 24 patients with acute myocardial infarction in 1958. In this, the first on thrombolytic therapy for myocardial infarction, they proposed that "the rapid dissolution of a coronary thrombus by enzymatic means could result in reduction of the final area of muscle infarction, reduction of the degree of electrical instability present during the early critical phase of infarction and prevent the appearance of or lyse mural thrombi." (48)

The pyrogenicity of the streptokinase then available retarded further clinical studies using this agent. In 1960, Miami cardiologist Robert Boucek and his associates reported administering fibrinolysin, a mixture of human plasmin and streptokinase, to eight patients following acute myocardial infarction (49). They used a novel approach to deliver the thrombolytic agent: it was administered through a catheter placed in one of the sinuses of Valsalva. Boucek's enthusiasm for the procedure was limited by his recognition that he could not prove that a coronary thrombus was present in any of the patients or whether it was lysed as a result of the administration of fibrinolysin. To understand these concerns, it is important to recognize that Boucek and his associates did not perform coronary arteriograms as part of their study. That procedure was rarely performed in 1960, and when it was used everyone but Mason Sones used a nonselective technique that generally provided inadequate visualization of the coronary circulation.

During the middle of the 20th century, some influential clinicians and pathologists began to question the role of coronary thrombosis in acute myocardial infarction. In 1939,

New York cardiologist Charles Friedberg reported that one-third of a series of 37 patients thought to have died of acute myocardial infarction did not have evidence of a fresh coronary thrombus at autopsy (50). A quarter of a century later, San Francisco cardiologist Meyer Friedman, reporting a study of the pathogenesis of coronary thrombus, acknowledged that there was "considerable argument" regarding the relationship of thrombus formation and underlying atherosclerosis and "even between thrombosis and infarction." Friedman's findings supported the view held by some, but by no means all, pathologists that "the thrombus lay in direct communication with a preexisting intramural atheromatous process." He concluded that "fracture" of the atheromatous plaque preceded and was "responsible for the formation of thrombus" (51).

Some pathologists questioned the causal role of coronary thrombosis in acute myocardial infarction during the 1960s and 1970s, however. One of them, William Roberts of the National Institutes of Health, wrote several papers on the subject. In 1972, he explained that a variety of postmortem findings "suggest that coronary thrombi are consequences rather than causes of acute myocardial infarction" (52). Spokane cardiologist Marcus DeWood was aware of this controversy when he published a report on the prevalence of total coronary occlusion during the early hours of myocardial infarction. DeWood performed coronary arteriograms in these patients and found that 87% of those studied within 4 hr of the onset of symptoms had occlusion of the infarct-related artery (53).

The first report of the intracoronary administration of a thrombolytic agent into a coronary artery was published in 1976 by E. I. Chazov and colleagues from Russia. They reported on two patients in whom coronary angiograms were performed before and after the administration of thrombolytic therapy. Reperfusion was demonstrated in one patient when the lytic therapy was administered 4 hr after the onset of symptoms. Lytic therapy was unsuccessful in a second case when it was administered 10 hr following the onset of symptoms. This paper, published in Russian with a brief English summary, was apparently unknown to American workers. This situation is reminiscent of James B. Herrick's original description of acute myocardial infarction, which was preceded by the observations of two Russians a few months earlier (54).

The English-speaking world first learned of the technique of intracoronary thrombolytic therapy in 1979, when German cardiologist Peter Rentrop reported the intracoronary administration of streptokinase in five patients with acute myocardial infarction. He concluded that the infarct was precipitated by thrombus in four of his patients and found that symptoms improved in each of them when the infarct-related artery was reperfused (55). This report, together with DeWood's paper, inaugurated the modern era of treatment of acute myocardial infarction, which places emphasis on prompt reperfusion. Many multicenter clinical trials of thrombolytic therapy have been undertaken since 1971, when the European Working Party reported on a trial they conducted in nine hospitals. They concluded that streptokinase was superior to heparin in reducing mortality and reinfarction following acute myocardial infarction (56).

CONCLUSIONS

The subsequent developments in the dynamic field of thrombolytic therapy are beyond the scope of this historical review. This is also true of immediate or direct percutaneous transluminal coronary angioplasty, an increasingly popular alternative to thrombolytic therapy for achieving reperfusion following acute myocardial infarction. Of necessity, many significant topics have been excluded from this brief review of atherosclerosis and coronary artery disease. The remainder of this book provides a state-of-the-art review of basic and clinical research, diagnostic techniques, and therapeutic approaches in the areas of atherosclerosis and coronary artery disease. As you read it, I urge you to reflect on the provocative question "Where does the review of the literature end and history begin?" The distinction is really quite artificial. History is actually everything that happened before the moment you read this. This historical review emphasizes events that occurred several years to several centuries ago, but my approach has been similar to that used when one prepares a review of the literature. This concept emphasizes the continuity of current knowledge with concepts and practices of earlier generations of physicians and scientists.

REFERENCES

1. Sandison AT. Degenerative vascular disease. In: Brothwell D, Sandison AT, eds. *Diseases in Antiquity: A Survey of the Diseases, Injuries and Surgery of Early Populations.* Springfield, IL: Charles C Thomas; 1967:474–488.
2. Moodie RL. *Paleopathology: An Introduction to the Study of Ancient Evidences of Disease.* Urbana: University of Ilinois Press; 1923.
3. Harris CRS. *The Heart and Vascular System in Ancient Greek Medicine from Alcmaeon to Galen.* Oxford: Clarendon Press; 1973.
4. Bing RJ. Atherosclerosis. In: Bing RJ, ed. *Cardiology: The Evolution of the Science and the Art.* Philadelphia: Harwood Academic Publishers; 1992:127–143.
5. Long ER. Development of our knowledge of arteriosclerosis. In: Blumenthal HT, ed. *Cowdry's Atherosclerosis.* Springfield, IL: Charles C Thomas; 1967:5–20.
6. Harvey W. *Exercitatio Anatomica. De Motu Cordis et Sanguinis in Animalibus.* Springfield, IL: Charles C Thomas; 1928. Leake C, translator.
7. Erichsen JE. *Observations on Aneurism Selected from the Works of the Principal Writers on that Disease from the Earliest Periods to the Close of the Last Century.* London: Sydenham Society; 1844.
8. Long ER. *A History of Pathology.* New York: Dover Publications; 1965.
9. Scarpa A. *A Treatise on the Anatomy, Pathology, and Surgical Treatment of Aneurism, with Engravings.* Edinburgh: Mundell, Doig, & Stevenson; 1808. Wishart JH, translator.
10. Virchow R. Örtliche Störungen des Kreislaufes. In: Virchow R, Vogel J, Stiebel SFS, eds. *Handbuch der Speciellen Pathologie und Therapie,* Vol. 1. Erlangen: Ferdinand Enke; 1854:95–270.
11. Rather LJ. *A Commentary on the Medical Writings of Rudolf Virchow.* San Francisco: Norman Publishing; 1990.
12. Anitschokow N. Experimental arteriosclerosis in animals. In: Cowdry

EV, ed. *Arteriosclerosis: A Survey of the Problem.* New York: Macmillan; 1933:271–322.
13. Dock W. Research in arteriosclerosis—the first fifty years. *Ann Intern Med* 1958;49:699–705.
14. Aschoff L. Introduction. In: Cowdry EV, ed. *Arteriosclerosis: A Survey of the Problem.* New York: Macmillan; 1933:1–18.
15. Smith THF. A chronology of atherosclerosis. *Am J Pharmacy* 1960; 132:390–405.
16. Cowdry EV, ed. *Arteriosclerosis: A Survey of the Problem.* New York: Macmillan; 1933.
17. White PD. *Heart Disease.* New York: Macmillan; 1931.
18. Tillett WS, Garner RL. The fibrinolytic activity of hemolytic streptococci. *J Exp Med* 1933;58:485–502.
19. Ahrens EH Jr. The Crisis in Clinical Research: Overcoming Institutional Obstacles. New York: Oxford University Press; 1992.
20. Keele KD. *Leonardo da Vinci on the Movement of the Heart and Blood.* London: Harvey and Blythe Ltd.; 1952.
21. Bedford DE. Harvey's third circulation. De circulo sanguinis in corde. *Br Med J* 1968;4:273–277.
22. Fye WB. Coronary arteriography: It took a long time. *Circulation* 1984; 70:781–787.
23. Heberden W. Some account of a disorder of the breast. *Med Trans Coll Physicians Lond* 1772;2:59–67.
24. Leibowitz JO. *The History of Coronary Heart Disease.* London: Wellcome Institute of the History of Medicine; 1970.
25. Heberden W. *Commentaries on the History and Cure of Diseases.* London: T. Payne; 1802.
26. Kligfield P. The early pathophysiologic understanding of angina pectoris. *Am J Cardiol* 1982;50:1433–1435.
27. Baron J. *The Life of Edward Jenner, M.D.* London: Henry Colburn; 1827.
28. Parry CH. *An Inquiry into the Symptoms and Causes of the Syncope Anginosa Commonly Called Angina Pectoris.* Bath, England: R. Cruttwell; 1799.
29. Burns A. *Observations on Some of the Most Frequent and Important Diseases of the Heart.* Edinburgh: Bryce & Co.; 1809.
30. Fye WB. T. Lauder Brunton and amyl nitrite: A Victorian vasodilator. *Circulation* 1986;74:222–229.
31. Fye WB. Nitroglycerin: A homeopathic remedy. *Circulation* 1986;73: 21–29.
32. Fye WB. The delayed diagnosis of acute myocardial infarction: It took half a century. *Circulation* 1985;72:262–271.
33. Fye WB, ed. Classic Papers on Coronary Thrombosis and Myocardial Infarction. Birmingham, AL: Classics of Cardiology Library; 1991.
34. [Osler W]. Rupture of the heart. *Med News* 1889;54:129–130.
35. Fye WB. Acute coronary occlusion always results in death, or does it? *Circulation* 1985;71:4–10.
36. Baumgarten W. Infarction in the heart. *Am J Physiol* 1899;2:243–265.
37. Obrastzow WP, Straschesko ND. Zue Kenntnis der Thrombose der Koronararterien des Herzens. *Z Klin Med* 1910;71:116–132.
38. Muller JE. Diagnosis of myocardial infarction: Historical notes from the Soviet Union and the United States. *Am J Cardiol* 1977;40: 269–271.
39. Herrick JB. Certain clinical features of sudden obstruction of the coronary arteries. *JAMA* 1912;59:2015–2020.
40. Howell JD. Early perceptions of the electrocardiogram: From arrhythmia to infarction. *Bull Hist Med* 1984;58:83–98.
41. Levine SA. *Coronary Thrombosis: Its Various Clinical Features.* Baltimore: Williams & Wilkins; 1929.
42. Sones FM Jr, Shirey EK. Cine coronary arteriography. *Mod Concepts Cardiovasc Dis* 1962;31:735–738.
43. Fye WB. Ventricular fibrillation and defibrillation: Historical perspectives. *Circulation* 1985;71:858–865.
44. Fye WB. Disorders of the heartbeat: A historical overview from antiquity to the mid-20th century. *Am J Cardiol* 1993;72:1055–1070.
45. Day HW. A cardiac resuscitation program. *Lancet* 1962;82:153–156.
46. Wright IS, Marple CD, Beck DF. Report of the committee for the evaluation of anti-coagulants in the treatment of coronary thrombosis with myocardial infarction. *Am Heart J* 1948;36:801–815.
47. Mueller RL, Scheidt S. History of drugs for thrombotic disease: Discovery, development, and directions for the future. *Circulation* 1994;89: 432–449.
48. Fletcher AP, Alkjaersig N, Smyrniotis F, et al. The treatment of patients suffering from early myocardial infarction with massive and prolonged streptokinase therapy. *Trans Assoc Am Physicians* 1958;71:287–296.
49. Boucek RJ, Murphy WP, Sommer LS, et al. Segmental perfusion of the coronary arteries with fibrinolysin in man following a myocardial infarction. *Am J Cardiol* 1960;6:525–533.
50. Friedberg CK, Horn H. Acute myocardial infarction not due to coronary artery occlusion. *JAMA* 1939;112:1675–1679.
51. Friedman M, Van den Bovenkamp GJ. The pathogenesis of a coronary thrombus. *Am J Pathol* 1966;48:19–44.
52. Roberts WC, Buja LM. The frequency and significance of coronary arterial thrombi and other observations in fatal acute myocardial infarction: A study of 107 necropsy patients. *Am J Med* 1972;52:425–443.
53. DeWood MA, Spores J, Notske R, et al. Prevalence of total coronary occlusion during the early hours of transmural myocardial infarction. *N Engl J Med* 1980;303:897–902.
54. Chazov EI, Matveeva LS, Mazaev AV, Sargin KE, Sadovskaya GV, Ruda MY. Intracoronary administration of fibrinolysin in acute myocardial infarction. *Terap Arkh* 1976;48:8–19.
55. Rentrop KP, Blanke H, Karsch KR, et al. Acute myocardial infarction: Intracoronary application of nitroglycerin and streptokinase. *Clin Cardiol* 1979;2:354–363.
56. Streptokinase in recent myocardial infarction: A controlled multicentre trial. European working party. *Br Med J* 1971;3:325–331.

Atherosclerosis and Coronary Artery Disease,
edited by V. Fuster, R. Ross, and E. J. Topol.
Lippincott-Raven Publishers, Philadelphia © 1996.

CHAPTER 2

Prevalence, Incidence, and Mortality of Coronary Heart Disease

William B. Kannel

Key Words: Coronary disease; Incidence; Risk factors; Mortality; Secular trends.

INTRODUCTION

Life expectancy in the United States is now at its highest, chiefly as a consequence of the improved living conditions. Most of the improvement over the past 25 years has resulted from the 49% decline in the age-adjusted death rate for the cardiovascular diseases. This indicates the extent to which these leading causes of death are subject to preventive and therapeutic measures. The residual magnitude of the problem is, however, substantial, requiring vigorous preventive measures.

GENERAL CARDIOVASCULAR MORBIDITY AND MORTALITY

Despite major reductions in death rates for the various forms of cardiovascular disease over the past 25 years in the United States, cardiovascular disease remains the most serious threat to life and health (1,2). A third of men in the United States currently develop a major cardiovascular disease before reaching age 60; the odds for women are 1 in 10 (3). Coronary heart disease in particular is a major cause of death after age 40 years in men and 64 years in women (4).

Cardiovascular disease is an expanding problem in the elderly, causing 70% of all deaths beyond age 75 (4). Coronary heart disease is the most common and most lethal cardiovascular event in each sex, causing much disability in old age. Unrecognized myocardial infarctions are especially common in the elderly (5). Beyond age 65, women become as vulnerable to cardiovascular mortality as men (4–7). The predisposing modifiable risk factors for coronary disease are similar in young and old and in men and women. The relevant risk factors include hypertension, dyslipidemia, impaired glucose tolerance, physical indolence, and cigarette smoking. A lower risk ratio for some risk factors in the elderly is offset by a greater absolute risk of cardiovascular disease in advanced age. As a result, the attributable risk and the potential benefit of treatment rise with age (8). In the elderly, average atherogenic cholesterol and low-density lipoproteins are often unacceptable and higher in women than men. About 10 million of the elderly and two women for every man require further investigation and treatment for dyslipidemia by National Heart, Lung and Blood Institute guidelines.

Multivariate risk profiles composed of the major risk factors predict coronary heart disease as efficiently in the elderly as in the young. This, and the fact that the decline in cardiovascular mortality has included the elderly, suggests

W. B. Kannel: Department of Medicine, Section of Preventive Medicine and Epidemiology, Evans Memorial Research Foundation, Boston University School of Medicine, Boston, Massachusetts 02118.

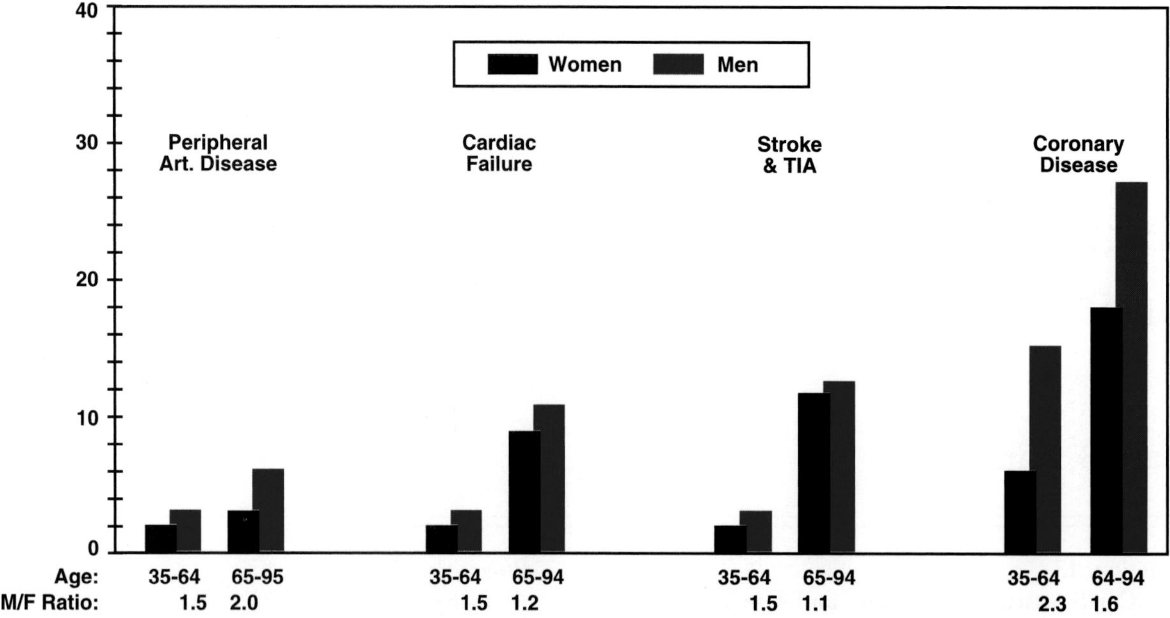

FIG. 1. Incidence of cardiovascular events by age and sex (Framingham Study 36-year follow-up). (From Kannel, ref. 25, with permission.)

efficacy for intervention even in the elderly. Because of the preponderance of women in the elderly population, trials testing the efficacy of correcting risk factors have not included, but should include, women.

Cardiovascular disease accounts for 44% of the nation's mortality and much of the nation's morbidity. Its cost to the nation's economy is by far the largest for any diagnostic group, amounting to an estimated $144 billion in 1988 (9). The 5-year medical cost of a myocardial infarction (for diagnostic and therapeutic services) is $51,211 in 1986 dollars (10).

Data from the Framingham Study provide reliable estimates of cardiovascular morbidity and mortality based on 36 years of follow-up of a defined population sample of 5,209 men and women aged 35 to 94 years. These data indicate that average annual rates of first major cardiovascular events increase from five per 1,000 men at ages 35 to 44 years to 59 per 1,000 at ages 85 to 94 years (Fig. 1). For

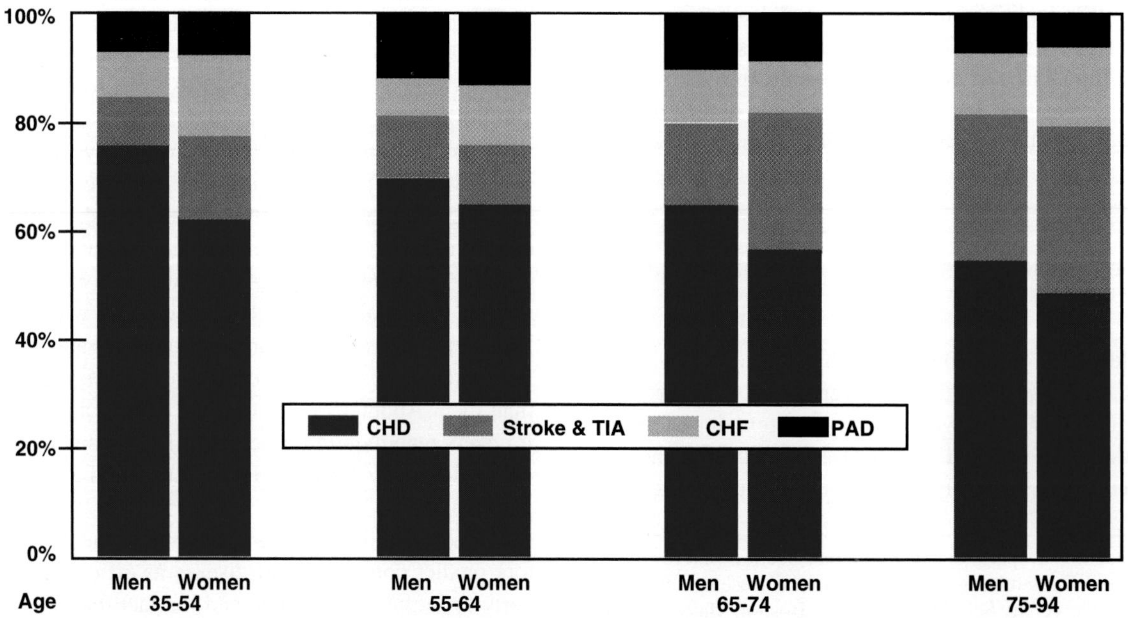

FIG. 2. Percentage of first cardiovascular events by type (Framingham Study 36-year follow-up).

women, comparable rates are achieved 10 years later in life, with the gap in incidence closing with advancing age. Coronary heart disease is the event comprising almost two-thirds of all cardiovascular disease both in men and women under age 75 years (Fig. 2). The fraction of cardiovascular events resulting from coronary heart disease declines with age, whereas the proportions from stroke and cardiac failure increase with age. Under age 75 a higher proportion of cardiovascular events result from coronary heart disease in men than women.

SECULAR TRENDS

A downward trend in mortality from the cardiovascular diseases has occurred since about 1940 (Fig. 3). Long-term declines have been noted for rheumatic, cerebrovascular, and hypertensive diseases, and a decline for coronary heart disease since the mid-1960s (Fig. 3). The coronary heart disease (CHD) decline antedates widespread thrombolytic and antihypertensive treatment. Prior to 1940, cardiovascular mortality rose steeply to become the dominant cause of death as the infectious and parasitic diseases came under control and were replaced by an epidemic increase in fatal coronary attacks. Cardiovascular mortality thereafter declined about 1% per year in the 1950s and 1960s (2) and accelerated in the 1970s to 3% per year since then. For CHD there has been over a 50% decline in the age-adjusted death rate since the peak in 1963. The current rate of decline is about 3–4% per year.

A noteworthy feature of the recent decline in cardiovascular mortality is that it has declined in all races, both sexes, all age groups, and all geographic areas in the United States. Greatest declines have been noted in young adults and the higher socioeconomic segments of the population. There are also geographic differences in the rate of decline (2,11). In recent years the largest absolute decline in cardiovascular mortality has been in coronary heart disease. Because cardiovascular diseases cause one-half of all deaths, declines in these diseases are chiefly responsible for the improvement of average life expectancy, which by 1989 was 75.2 years (12).

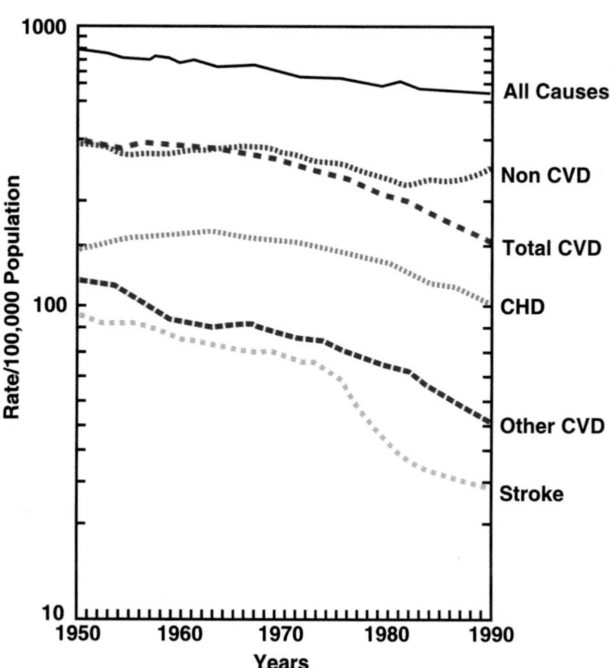

FIG. 3. Age-adjusted death rates for selected causes of death, United States, 1950–1990.

The decline in coronary heart disease mortality reverses the epidemic rise of the 1940s into the 1960s and coincides with reductions in the major cardiovascular risk factors, more effective treatment or coronary events, and greater efforts at secondary prevention (11,13). The reduction in coronary heart disease mortality in the United States exceeds that observed in most countries (14). Many Western countries have only recently experienced a downward trend in coronary heart disease mortality, and the trend is still upward in countries of Eastern Europe.

There are very few uniform statistics on trends in morbidity. This is unfortunate because reduction in mortality without a decline in the attack rate would indicate that better medical care was responsible, whereas a reduction in both morbidity and mortality suggests that environmental influences and/or preventive measures have improved.

CORONARY HEART DISEASE

Coronary heart disease in particular kills and disables Americans in their most productive years and, by National Heart, Lung and Blood Institute estimates, cost $21 billion for medical care and $31 billion in indirect economic costs in 1988. Coronary disease is the third most frequent cause of short-stay hospitalizations and costs among the highest per hospital admission (15). It is also the leading cause of premature permanent disability in the American labor force, accounting for 19% of disability allowances by the Social Security Administration (24).

Prevalence

The National Health Interview Survey estimates that the prevalence of coronary heart disease in 1989 was 6.9 million or 3% of the population (6,7). For men, the prevalence was 86 per 1,000 at ages 45–64 years and 169 at 65 years and over. For women the corresponding estimates by age are 26 at 45–64 years and 113.0 at 65 and over, a prevalence substantially lower than in men.

Incidence of Clinical Manifestations

Coronary artery disease causes about 800,000 new heart attacks each year and 450,000 recurrent attacks (2). The inci-

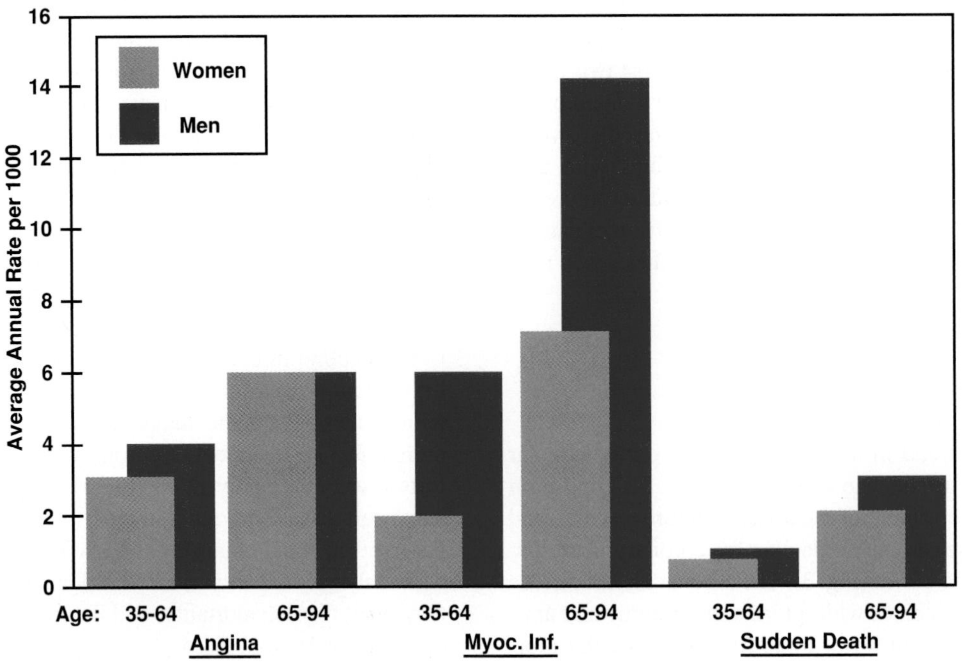

FIG. 4. Incidence of clinical manifestation of coronary heart disease by age and sex.

dence in women lags behind that in men by 10 years for total coronary heart disease and by 20 years for myocardial infarction and sudden death (Figs. 1 and 4). The male predominance is least evident for uncomplicated angina pectoris (Fig. 4).

The first coronary manifestation in women is more likely to be angina, whereas in men it more often presents as a myocardial infarction (Table 1). More angina in men occurs after a myocardial infarction than before. Only one in five coronary attacks are preceded by long-standing angina, and even fewer if the infarction is silent or unrecognized. Serious manifestations of coronary disease such as myocardial infarction or sudden death are rare in premenopausal women. The incidence and severity of coronary heart disease increase with age in both sexes. The coronary heart disease incidence rate in postmenopausal women is two to three times that of women the same age who remain premenopausal (16), and this applies whether the menopause is natural or surgical. The male-predominant sex ratio in incidence narrows progressively with advancing age.

Unrecognized myocardial infarctions are common, numbering about one in every three infarctions (Fig. 5). Half of the unrecognized infarctions are silent, and the rest so atypical that neither the patient nor the physician considers the possibility. More than half of these subjects subsequently develop overt clinical manifestations of coronary heart disease and hence eventually come under medical care. Angina is a less frequent accompaniment of unrecognized infarction than recognized symptomatic myocardial infarction. Despite the apparent innocuousness of unrecognized infarction, the subsequent long-term mortality experienced is nearly the same as that with recognized infarction (Table 2). Diabetic men and hypertensive persons of both sexes are particularly susceptible to silent or unrecognized infarctions.

TABLE 1. *Percentage of first CHD events by type of event*[a]

	Percent	
	Men	Women
Total no. of CHD events	905	692
Myocardial infarction	49.5%	34.9%
Angina pectoris	31.0%	47.7%
Coronary insufficiency syndrome	4.8%	5.9%
Sudden death	10.9%	8.7%
Nonsudden CHD death	3.8%	2.8%

[a] Framingham Study 36-year follow-up; subject ages 35–94 years.

TABLE 2. *Prognosis following recognized versus unrecognized myocardial infarction in men and women*[a]

	Standardized risk ratio			
	Recognized myocardial inf.		Unrecognized myocardial inf.	
Outcome	Men	Women	Men	Women
Death	2.6	3.9	2.7	2.5
Sudden death	4.0	4.4	4.8	6.2
Myocardial inf.	2.8	8.5	2.0	4.8
Angina pectoris	6.2	5.7	2.7	4.9
Cardiac failure	4.2	7.7	5.8	5.3
Stroke	2.7	5.1	4.3	2.6

[a] Framingham Study 30-year follow-up.

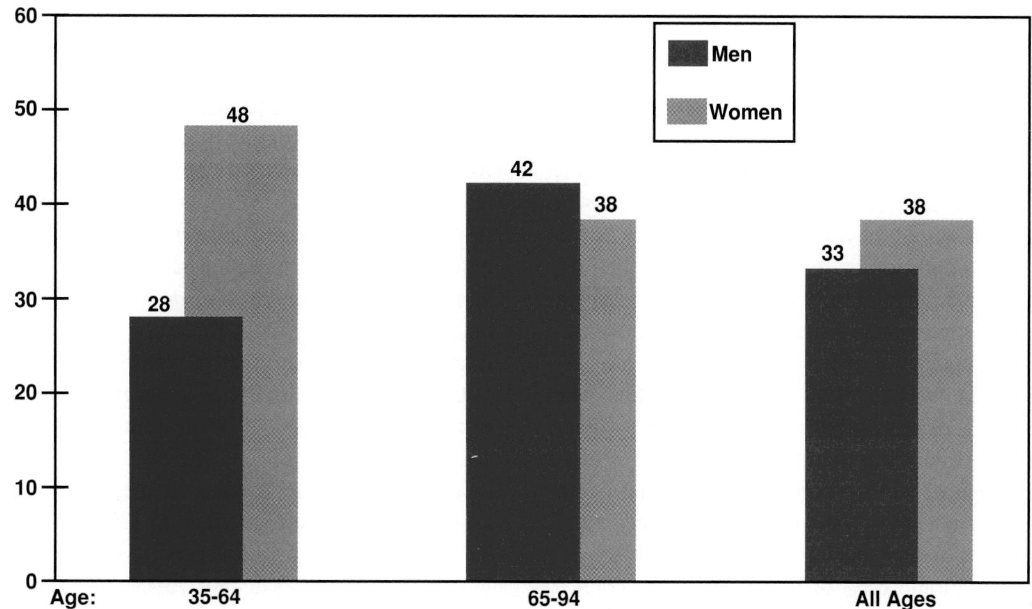

FIG. 5. Percentage of myocardial infarctions that are unrecognized (Framingham Study 36-year follow-up).

Prognosis

Even after surviving the acute stage of a myocardial infarction morbidity and mortality are two to nine times those of the general population (Fig. 6) (17). The incidence of reinfarction, sudden death, angina pectoris, cardiac failure, and stroke are all substantial, and the relative and absolute risks of these occurrences are as great in women as in men. Following a recognized myocardial infarction, 23% of men and 31% of women will have a recurrent infarction within 6 years, and 41% of men and 34% of women will develop angina. About 20% will be disabled with cardiac failure, and 9% of men and 18% of women will sustain a stroke. Sudden death will occur in 13% of men and 6% of women. The outlook is no better following an unrecognized infarction (Table 2). Although about two-thirds of myocardial infarction patients do not make a complete recovery, 88% under age 65 are able to return to their usual occupations (18).

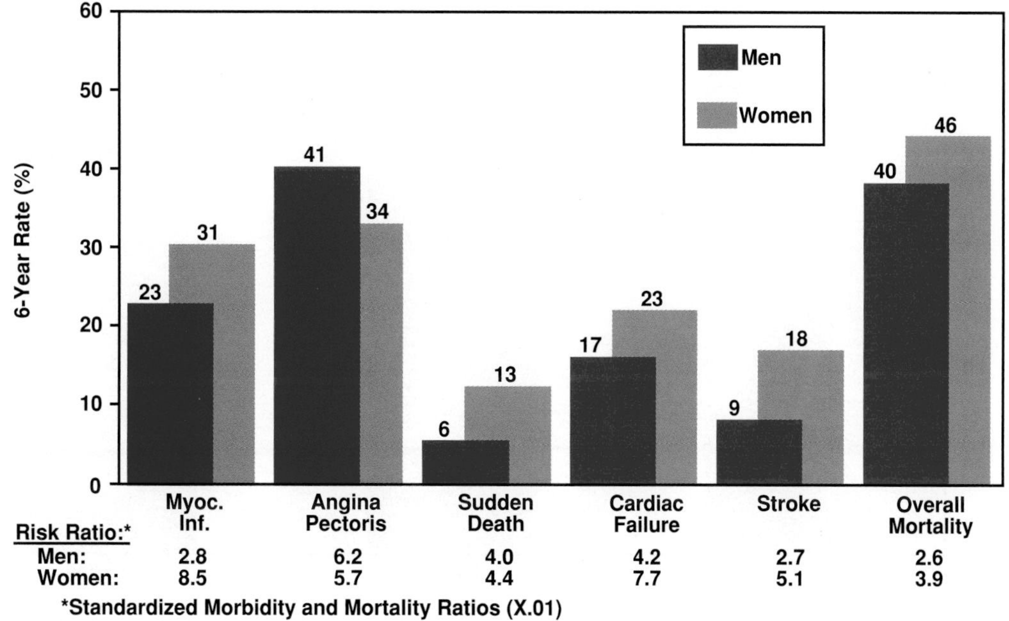

FIG. 6. Prognosis following overt myocardial infarction (Framingham Study 36-year follow-up).

Mortality

Coronary heart disease is the leading cause of death in American adults, accounting for more than 25% of the deaths in persons over age 35 (4). In 1989, there were 498,000 coronary deaths (12). Mortality from this disease increases steeply with age and also causes many deaths in adults at the peak of their productive lives.

In a substantial proportion of coronary fatalities, the progression from inapparent disease to death is abrupt. Much of the premature coronary mortality surfaces with little warning. Sudden, unexpected, out-of-hospital coronary deaths account for more than one-half of all coronary fatalities. The fraction of coronary deaths that are sudden deaths is lower in women than men and lower in elderly men (Fig. 7). However, the percentage of sudden coronary deaths that occur without prior overt coronary heart disease is much greater in women than men and greater in younger than older persons. In 48% of men and 63% of women who experience sudden deaths, these happen without prior indication of overt coronary disease. About 80% of coronary fatalities in persons under age 65 occur at the time of the initial coronary attack (3). Thus, despite a higher death rate following a prior coronary attack, most coronary deaths arise from the segment of the population who are free of symptomatic coronary heart disease.

After myocardial infarction, sudden deaths occur at four to six times the rate in the general population. Including all deaths in and out of hospital, the first year following a recognized myocardial infarction is especially dangerous, with 27% of men and 44% of women succumbing (Fig. 8). Most of these deaths occur within the first 30 days. In contrast to initial myocardial infarction incidence, where women have an advantage, survival following recognized myocardial infarction in women is not as good as in men at all ages (Fig. 9). This may be because women tend to have a higher burden of risk factors at time of infarction as well as the fact that they have smaller coronary arteries (10). Long-term survival following unrecognized myocardial infarction is little better than for recognized infarctions, and survival is better for women than men (5). Following uncomplicated angina pectoris, the survival rates for men under age 65 is nearly the same as it is for recognized infarctions and is much worse than survival in women with angina (Fig. 9).

Coronary heart disease is either the leading cause or one of the leading causes of death in men and women of every racial or ethnic group (2). The death rate for coronary heart disease is 4.5 times higher in men than women at ages 25–34, but that ratio declines to 1.5 by ages 75–84 years. The coronary death rate is reported to be twice as high in blacks than in whites at ages 25–34, but that difference disappears by age 75. Heart disease mortality is not quite as high among the Hispanic population as it is among blacks and whites (20).

Cardiac Failure

Heart failure is the end stage of coronary disease after the myocardium has used all its reserve and compensatory mechanisms. Once overt indications appear, half of the patients will be dead within 5 years despite modern medical management (21). Risk of cardiac failure is increased two- to sixfold with coronary disease, with angina conferring half

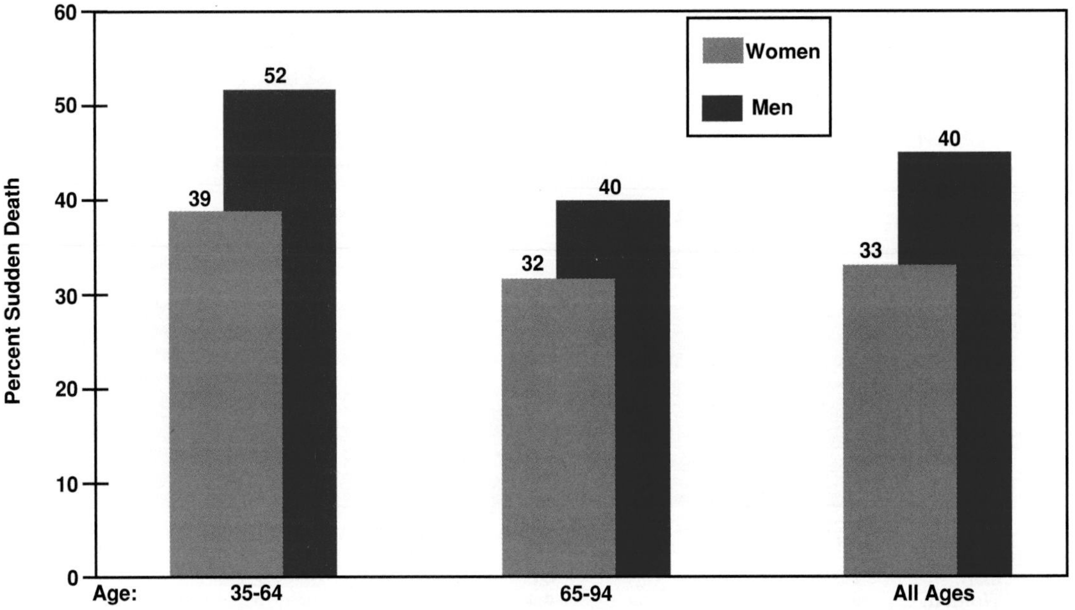

FIG. 7. Percentage of coronary heart disease deaths as sudden death (Framingham Study 36-year follow-up).

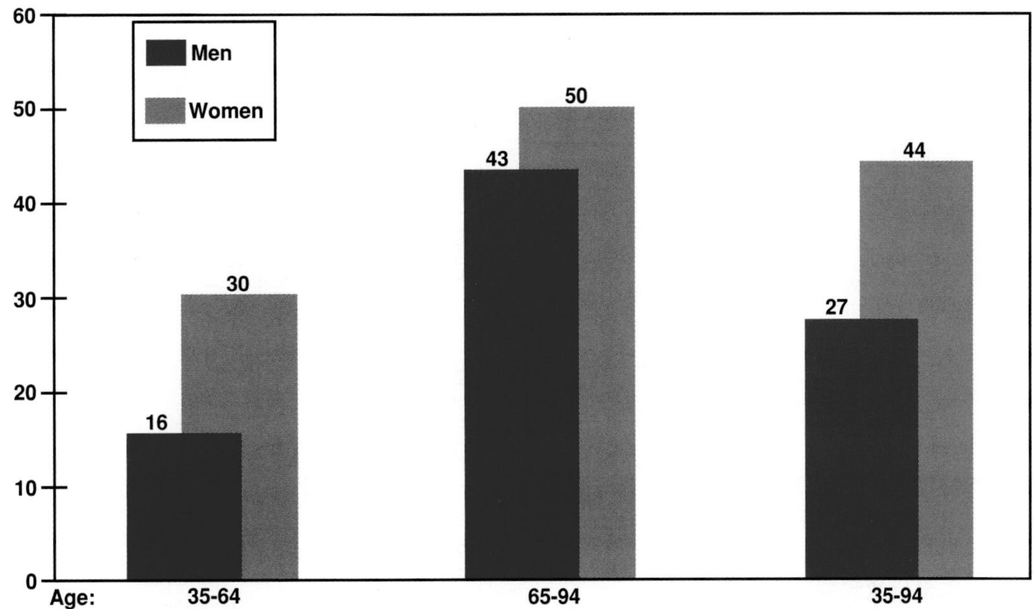

FIG. 8. Percentage dead within 1 year following initial myocardial infarction by age and sex (Framingham Study 36-year follow-up).

the risk of a myocardial infarct. Coronary heart disease, generally accompanied by hypertension, is responsible in 39% of cardiac failure (22). Sudden death is a common feature of cardiac failure, occurring at six to nine times the general population rate.

Mortality and hospital discharge rates for cardiac failure have failed to decline substantially since 1970 despite a marked decline in coronary heart disease mortality and marked improvement in hypertension control (22). This cannot be readily explained. Some postulate that improved survival of cases of angina, myocardial infarction, and hypertensive heart disease may result in an increased prevalence of chronic heart disease and ultimately cardiac failure (38). There is also uncertainty about the prevalence of underlying

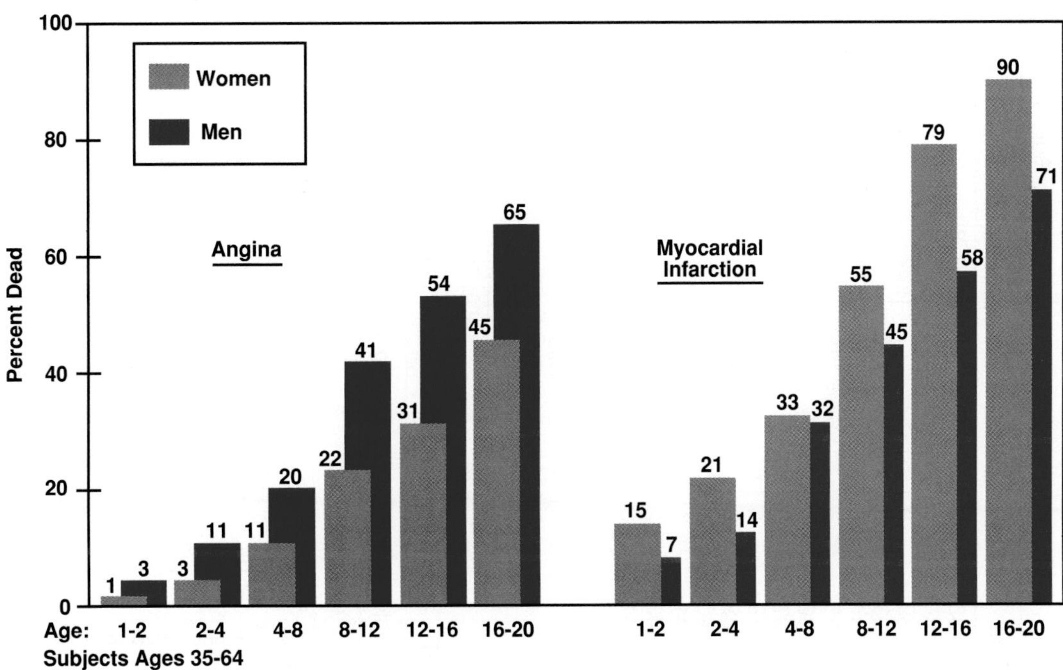

FIG. 9. Mortality following angina pectoris and myocardial infarction by sex (Framingham Study 36-year follow-up).

TABLE 3. *Coronary heart disease risk factor prediction chart*[a]

1. Find Points For Each Risk Factor

Age (If Female)				Age (If Male)				HDL-Cholesterol		Total-Cholesterol		Systolic Blood Pressure		
Age	Pts.	Age	Pts.	Age	Pts.	Age	Pts.	HDL-C	Pts.	Total-C	Pts.	SBP	Pts.	Other
30	−12	47–48	5	30	−2	57–59	13	25–26	7	139–151	−3	98–104	−2	Cigarettes
31	−11	49–50	6	31	−1	60–61	14	27–29	6	152–166	−2	105–112	−1	Diabetic-male
32	−9	51–52	7	32–33	0	62–64	15	30–32	5	167–182	−1	113–120	0	Diabetic-female
33	−8	53–55	8	34	1	65–67	16	33–35	4	183–199	0	121–129	1	ECG-LVH
34	−6	56–60	9	35–36	2	68–70	17	36–38	3	200–219	1	130–139	2	
35	−5	61–67	10	37–38	3	71–73	18	39–42	2	220–239	2	140–149	3	0 pts for each
36	−4	68–74	11	39	4	74	19	43–46	1	240–262	3	150–160	4	
37	−3			40–41	5			47–50	0	263–288	4	161–172	5	
38	−2			42–43	6			51–55	−1	289–315	5	173–185	6	
39	−1			44–45	7			56–60	−2	316–330	6			
40	0			46–47	8			61–66	−3					
41	1			48–49	9			67–73	−4					
42–43	2			50–51	10			74–80	−5					
44	3			52–54	11			81–87	−6					
45–46	4			55–56	12			88–96	−7					

2. Sum Points For All Risk Factors

_____ Age + _____ HDL-C + _____ Total-C + _____ SBP + _____ Smoker + _____ Diabetes + _____ ECG-LVH = _____ Point Total

NOTE: *Minus Points Subtract From Total.*

3. Look Up Risk Corresponding To Point Total

Probability			Probability			Probability			Probability		
Pts.	5 Yr.	10 Yr.	Pts.	5 Yr.	10 Yr.	Pts.	5 Yr.	10 Yr.	Pts.	5 Yr.	10 Yr.
≤1	<1%	<2%	10	2%	6%	19	8%	16%	28	19%	33%
2	1%	2%	11	3%	6%	20	8%	18%	29	20%	36%
3	1%	2%	12	3%	7%	21	9%	19%	30	22%	38%
4	1%	2%	13	3%	8%	22	11%	21%	31	24%	40%
5	1%	3%	14	4%	9%	23	12%	23%	32	25%	42%
6	1%	3%	15	5%	10%	24	13%	25%			
7	1%	4%	16	5%	12%	25	14%	27%			
8	2%	4%	17	6%	13%	26	16%	29%			
9	2%	5%	18	7%	14%	27	17%	31%			

4. Compare To Average 10 Year Risk

Probability		
Age	Women	Men
30–34	<1%	3%
35–39	<1%	5%
40–44	2%	6%
45–49	5%	10%
50–54	8%	14%
55–59	12%	16%
60–64	13%	21%
65–69	9%	30%
70–74	12%	24%

[a] These charts were prepared with the help of William B. Kannel, M.D., Professor of Medicine and Public Health, and Ralph D'Agostino, Ph.D., Head, Department of Mathematics, both at Boston University; Keaven Anderson, Ph.D., Statistician, NHLBI, Framingham Study; Daniel McGee, Ph.D., Associate Professor, University of Arizona, based on data from the Framingham Heart Study. © 1990, American Heart Association. Reprinted with permission.

etiologies for congestive heart failure. Etiologies may have shifted in recent years from predominantly hypertension to coronary heart disease (24).

PREVENTIVE IMPLICATIONS

Examination of the incidence, prevalence, mortality, and natural history of coronary disease suggests the need for a preventive approach. Further innovations in diagnosis and treatment for coronary disease will undoubtedly improve the outlook of patients surviving the initial attack, but this can have only a limited impact because of the high unheralded initial mortality. When the heart is infarcted, no therapy can be expected to restore full function. If the initial presentation is sudden death, therapy after onset is frequently futile. A preventive approach involving detection and correction of predisposing conditions before the advent of overt clinical disease is required for a substantial impact.

Coronary heart disease often emerges without warning. One in five coronary attacks presents as a sudden death, and two-thirds of the fatalities occur too precipitously to be brought under medical attention.

Awaiting overt signs and symptoms of coronary disease before treatment is no longer justified. In some respects, the occurrence of symptoms may be regarded more properly as a medical failure than as the initial indication for treatment. High-risk candidates for preventive management can be detected from a coronary risk profile made up of ingredients easily obtained by office procedures (Table 3).

ACKNOWLEDGMENTS

The work reported here was supported by the Framingham Visiting Scientist Program, Pfizer, Merck, Sharpe and Dohme, ICI, and NIH Grant Nos. NO1-HV-92922, NO1-HV-52971, and 5T32-HL-07374-13.

REFERENCES

1. National Center for Health Statistics. *United States, 1990. DHHS Pub. No. (HS) 91-1232.* Washington: U.S. Government Printing Office; 1991.
2. National Heart, Lung and Blood Institute. *Morbidity and Mortality Chartbook on Cardiovascular, Lung, and Blood Diseases, 1990.* Washington: U.S. Department of Health and Human Services; 1990.
3. Gordon T, Kannel WB. Premature mortality from coronary heart disease: The Framingham Study. *JAMA* 1971;215:1617–1625.
4. National Center for Health Statistics. *Vital Statistics of the United States, 1988, Vol. II, Mortality, Part A.* Washington: USDHHS; 1991.
5. Kannel WB, Cupples LA, Gagnon DR. Incidence, precursors and prognosis of unrecognized myocardial infarction. *Adv Cardiol* 1990;37: 202–214.
6. National Center for Health Statistics, Adams PF, Benson V. *Current Estimates from the National Heart Interview Survey, United States, 1989. Vital and Health Statistics. DHHS Pub. No. (PHS) 90-1504.* Washington: U.S. Government Printing Office; 1990.
7. National Center for Health Statistics, Collins JG. *Prevalence of Selected Chronic Conditions, United States, 1986–88. Vital and Health Statistics.* Washington: USDHHS; 1989.
8. National Heart, Lung and Blood Institute. Proceedings of the workshop on cholesterol and heart disease in older persons and women. *Ann Epidemiol* 1992;2:5–14.
9. National Heart, Lung and Blood Institute. *NHLBI Fact Book, Fiscal Year 1990.* Washington: USDHHS, NIH; 1991.
10. Wittels EH, Hay JW, Gotto AM. Medical costs of coronary artery disease in the United States. *Am J Cardiol* 1990;65:432–440.
11. Thom TJ, Kannel WB. Factors in the decline of coronary disease mortality. In: Connor WE, Bristow JD, eds. *Coronary Heart Disease: Prevention, Complications and Treatment.* Philadelphia: JB Lippincott; 1985:5–20.
12. National Center for Health Statistics. *Annual Summary of Births, Marriages, Divorces and Deaths: United States, 1989. Monthly Vital Statistics Report, Vol. 38, No. 13.* Washington: USDHHS; 1990.
13. Burke GL, Sprafka JM, Folsom AR, Luepker RV, Norsted SW, Blackburn H. Trends in CHD mortality, morbidity and risk factor levels from 1960 to 1986: The Minnesota Heart Survey. *Int J Epidemiol* 1989; 81(Suppl 3):573–581.
14. Uemura K, Pisa Z. Trends in cardiovascular disease mortality in industrialized countries since 1950. *World Health Stat Q* 1988;41:155–177.
15. National Center for Health Statistics, Graves EJ. *Detailed Diagnosis and Procedures. National Hospital Discharge Survey 1989. Vital and Health Statistics. 1991. Series 13, No. 107. DHHS Publication No. (PHS) 91 1768.* Washington: USDHHS; 1991.
16. Gordon T, Kannel WB, Hjortland MC, et al. Menopause and coronary heart disease. *Ann Intern Med* 1978;89:157–161.
17. Cupples LA, D'Agostino RB. Survival following initial cardiovascular events: 30-year follow-up. Framington Heart Study, Section 35. In: Kannel WB, Wolf PA, Garrison RJ, eds. *The Framingham Study: An Epidemiological Investigation of Cardiovascular Disease, NIH publication no. 88-2969.* Bethesda; National Heart, Lung, and Blood Institute; 1988.
18. Kannel WB. *The Natural History of Myocardial Infarction: The Framingham Study.* Leiden: Leiden University Press; 1973.
19. Wong ND, Cupples LA, Ostfeld AM, Levy D, Kannel WB. Risk factors for long-term coronary prognosis after initial myocardial infarction. The Framingham Study. *Am J Epidermiol* 1989;130:469–480.
20. National Center for Health Statistics. *Deaths of Hispanic Origin, 15 Reporting States, 1979–81. Vital and Health Statistics, Series 20, No. 18, DHHS Publication No. (PHS) 91-1855,* Washington: USDHHS; 1990.
21. Kannel WB, Belanger AJ. Epidemiology of heart failure. *Am Heart J* 1991;121(3):951–957.
22. Kannel WB, Castelli WP, McNamara PM, et al. Role of blood pressure in the development of congestive heart failure: The Framingham Study. *N Engl J Med* 1972;287:781–787.
23. Gillum RF. Heart failure in the United States, 1970–1985. *Am Heart J* 1987;113:1043–1045.
24. Turlink JR, Goldhaber SJ, Pfiffer MA. An overview of contemporary etiologies of congestive heart failure. *Am Heart J* 1991;121: 1852–1853.
25. Kannel WB. The natural history of cardiovascualr risk. In: Braunwald E, Hollenberg NK, eds. *Atlas of Heart Diseases, Vol. 1, Hypertension: Mechanisms and Therapy.* Philadelphia: Current Medicine 1995.

PART I

Major Risk Factors and Primary Prevention

Atherosclerosis and Coronary Artery Disease,
edited by V. Fuster, R. Ross, and E. J. Topol.
Lippincott-Raven Publishers, Philadelphia © 1996.

CHAPTER 3

Overview

Henry C. McGill, Jr.

Key Words: Coronary heart disease; atherosclerosis; risk factor; primary prevention.

DETERMINING PROBABILITY OF DISEASE

The concept of risk determination by measuring variables associated with the occurrence of disease was formed early in the development of epidemiology. The variables are commonly classified under the major categories of person, place, and time. A variable that predicts *relative risk,* the ratio of disease incidence among exposed persons to that among unexposed persons, is useful in generating hypotheses about etiology. For example, among 1.2 million persons observed between 1982 and 1988, the ratio of rate of death from coronary heart disease in 35- to 64-year-old male smokers (exposed) to that in nonsmokers (unexposed) was 2.81 (relative risk). For former smokers, the relative risk was 1.75 (1).

H. C. McGill, Jr.: Department of Physiology and Medicine, Southwest Foundation for Biomedical Research, San Antonio, Texas 78228-0147.

In contrast, the degree to which a variable determines *attributable risk,* the total incidence of disease associated with that variable, is useful in selecting targets for preventive programs. Attributable risk takes into account the proportion of persons exposed as well as the relative risk. For example, in 1985, 35% of adult men under 65 were current smokers and 26% were former smokers. Combining prevalence rates with relative risks yields the astonishing estimate that, in 1985, 45% of coronary heart disease deaths in United States men under 65 years of age occurred in smokers (1).

Epidemiology initially focused on outbreaks of acute infectious disease. As these diminished in importance, the scope of epidemiology was extended to chronic diseases, particularly cardiovascular disease and cancer. The insights and information gained from epidemiologic methods provided knowledge essential to the primary prevention of atherosclerosis and coronary heart disease. The concept of relative risk was incorporated into the term ''risk factor,'' which infiltrated the language of clinical medicine and became part of the public's vocabulary.

ATHEROSCLEROSIS AS A PREVENTABLE DISEASE

Until the middle of the 20th century, age was considered the major determinant of atherosclerosis, and prevention was not discussed. The abundance of cholesterol in human atherosclerotic lesions was well known shortly after the turn of the century (2), and Anitschow produced an experimental animal model of atherosclerosis in 1913 by feeding cholesterol to rabbits (3). However, it remained difficult to believe that this common and essential component of animal tissues could cause a lethal disease in humans.

A Dutch physician who practiced in Java, De Langen, published in 1916 the observation that Javanese had lower blood cholesterol levels and also had a lower frequency of atherosclerotic disease and gallstones than persons in the Netherlands (4). This report lay unnoted in an obscure journal until cited in 1941 by Snapper in support of his observation that the low frequency of atherosclerotic disease among the Chinese was associated with their low intake of fat (5).

The rising incidence of coronary heart disease, which reached epidemic proportions among the industrialized countries by midcentury, commanded the attention of physicians and scientists after World War II. Several observers attributed the decline in frequency of coronary heart disease in the Scandinavian countries during the war to reduced availability of butter, eggs, and meat (6–9). There were many problems with the quality of both the dietary and mortality data, but, regardless of their validity, the reports stimulated the idea that atherosclerosis and its sequelae might be prevented by modifying dietary fat. Wide variations in coronary heart disease morbidity and mortality among countries provided further evidence that atherosclerosis was not inevitable with aging.

In 1953, Ancel Keys, one of the pioneers in the investigation of coronary heart disease, wrote, ''[C]linical coronary disease usually represents the cumulative effect of a factor, or factors, operating over a period of years.'' The major problem in prevention was ''. . . the question of predicting the threat of coronary disease'' (10).

DEVELOPMENT OF THE RISK FACTOR CONCEPT FOR CORONARY HEART DISEASE

Early Observations

Between 1930 and 1950, a number of reports indicated that persons with coronary heart disease had higher levels of serum cholesterol than other patients (11). A systematic case-control study (comparison of characteristics in persons having a disease with those in age- and sex-matched healthy persons) found higher serum cholesterol concentrations among survivors of myocardial infarction than among control subjects (12). Others observed that coronary heart disease subjects were predominantly male and that they frequently had hypertension (13). The associations indicated that serum cholesterol levels, elevated blood pressure, and maleness predicted a higher risk of coronary heart disease, and the strength and consistency of these associations suggested a causal relationship. However, conclusions were limited by the case-control study design because serum cholesterol and blood pressure were measured after myocardial infarction had occurred, and the disease may have caused their elevations.

The Framingham Study

To demonstrate conclusively that serum cholesterol concentration or blood pressure predicted coronary heart disease, it was necessary to measure these variables in healthy persons, measure the subsequent incidence of coronary heart disease, and relate the incidence of disease to the previously measured variables (a longitudinal study). Such a study was initiated by the Division of Chronic Disease of the United States Public Health Service among the residents of Framingham, Massachusetts, in 1948. The project was transferred to the newly established National Heart Institute in 1949 (14). The Framingham Study, as it came to be known, enrolled about 5,000 adults 30 to 59 years of age and free of cardiovascular disease and examined them for the first time in 1950.

Framingham Results

In 1957, when 90% of the subjects had been followed for 4 years, the number of coronary heart disease events was sufficient to conduct a preliminary analysis of results from the 45- to 62-year age group (15). One-third of the new events were sudden cardiac death, and another one-fifth of the new events were asymptomatic. The rate of new events in men was about twice that in women. Men with hypertension, obesity, or elevated serum cholesterol concentration at the initial examination had from two- to sixfold higher rates of new coronary heart disease events. The effect of obesity was largely accounted for by its association with hypertension. Coronary heart disease was more frequent in heavy smokers, but the association was not statistically significant. This first Framingham report discussed the traits associated with higher rates of coronary heart disease as "factors" and referred to their power to predict risk but did not use the term "risk factor." Two years later, a report based on 6 years of follow-up added smoking as a predictor of coronary heart disease (16).

Other Longitudinal Studies

During the 1950s and early 1960s, other similar longitudinal epidemiologic studies were started in Albany, New York (17); Tecumseh, Michigan (18); Chicago, Illinois (19,20); and San Francisco, California (21). Later, a similar longitudinal study of Japanese men living in Japan, Hawaii, and California began (22). Reports from these studies soon confirmed the Framingham results regarding serum cholesterol, hypertension, and smoking.

In 1978, the data from five major longitudinal studies were pooled for a combined analysis of observations on 8,422 men over 72,011 person-years (23). This report firmly established blood pressure, serum cholesterol concentration, and smoking (in addition to age and male sex) as predictors of the incidence of coronary heart disease and added diabetes mellitus.

The "Risk Factor" Concept

The term "risk factor" first appeared in the title of a journal article in 1963 (24). Subsequently, the risk factor concept was widely accepted and the term was extended to the other sequelae of atherosclerosis, stroke and peripheral arterial disease. It was also extended to other diseases, such as the various forms of cancer. Research was directed toward the mechanisms of action of the risk factors, while the search for new risk factors continued. It was proposed that risk factor modification would prevent coronary heart disease, but evidence was not sufficient to warrant action.

DO THE RISK FACTORS CAUSE CORONARY HEART DISEASE?

Definition of Risk Factor

A risk factor is defined by common usage as any measurable trait or characteristic of an individual that predicts that individual's probability of developing clinically manifest disease. The definition is broad and does not necessarily imply a causal relationship. The characteristic may be exposure to an environmental agent (tobacco smoke), an intervening variable (serum cholesterol concentration) resulting from an environmental agent (dietary lipids) or a genetic variant (low-density lipoprotein receptor defect), another disease (hypertension or diabetes), or an early or preclinical manifestation of coronary heart disease (electrocardiographic abnormality).

This broad definition of a risk factor is useful in the early stages of investigating a disease, when etiology and pathogenesis are uncertain. However, the ultimate objective is to prevent the disease, and prevention requires identification of causes. Therefore, much effort has been devoted to ascertaining whether the risk factors, particularly those that can be modified, are truly causes of coronary heart disease. Although a risk factor such as male sex cannot be modified, knowledge of why it predicts the occurrence of coronary heart disease may suggest other preventive strategies.

Criteria for Causal Relationship

The group that evaluated evidence relating smoking to health in 1964 developed criteria to judge the causal significance of an association (25). These criteria were amplified by Hill (26) and have been widely used to determine whether associations, such as those of the risk factors with coronary heart disease, represent causal relationships. The criteria are usually stated as follows:

1. Strength. The relative risk associated with the trait is high. Smoking, for example, predicts a twofold or greater risk of coronary heart disease, depending on age. Continuous variables, such as serum cholesterol concentration and blood pressure, predict twofold or greater risk at high levels. Many traits are associated with slight or moderate increases in risk of coronary heart disease and may be causal but have not been included in preventive programs because of their small attributable risk.
2. Dose response. The more severe the trait, the greater is the relative risk. Serum cholesterol, blood pressure, and smoking meet this criterion. If most persons in a population are exposed to a degree that produces a maximal effect, a dose–response relationship may be difficult to demonstrate. When populations or groups consume saturated fatty acids or cholesterol in amounts that elicit a maximal elevation of serum cholesterol, individual dietary intakes may not predict risk of coronary heart disease because variability among individuals results largely from genetic variability.
3. Temporal sequence. The trait precedes the disease. Case-control studies, which initially showed that persons with coronary heart disease had elevated serum cholesterol levels, could not provide this information. Longitudinal epidemiologic studies measured the trait in healthy persons before clinically manifest disease appeared.

4. Consistency. The association appears in studies involving different populations, different racial groups, and groups living under different conditions. Hundreds of studies have found that the major risk factors predict the risk of coronary heart disease in many different geographic, ethnic, and racial groups. However, the predictive power of some risk factors varies among populations, for example, among blacks as compared to whites; among Japanese as compared to Western populations; or among Mexican Americans as compared to whites. Smoking is not associated with increased risk of coronary heart disease in populations with low serum cholesterol levels and low overall frequency of coronary heart disease.

5. Independence. The trait is associated with increased risk when the effects of other known or suspected causes or risk factors are removed. When variables are tested for their association with disease occurrence one at a time (univariate analysis), analyses may yield misleading results if two or more variables are associated with another. Correction is accomplished by statistical methods that consider the effects of several independent variables in the same analysis (multivariate analysis). For example, the effect of obesity on risk of coronary heart disease frequently is eliminated when hypertension and diabetes are included in multivariate analyses. However, because obesity is a risk factor for hypertension and diabetes, it should still be considered a risk factor for coronary heart disease.

6. Coherence. The association is consistent with the results of other sources of evidence: clinical investigation, animal experimentation, or in vitro research. Abundant clinical and animal experimentation support the relationship of serum cholesterol concentration and hypertension to atherosclerosis and coronary heart disease. The effects of smoking and diabetes on atherosclerosis and coronary heart disease have not been reproduced in experimental animals, but there are potential plausible mechanisms. There is a rapidly growing body of knowledge from cellular and molecular biology that helps to explain how the risk factors affect atherosclerosis.

7. Specificity. The trait predicts the occurrence of only one disease. The effects of elevated serum cholesterol concentration are limited to the atherosclerotic diseases, of which coronary heart disease is the major variety. Hypertension is associated with cardiac hypertrophy, renal failure, and stroke as well as coronary heart disease. Smoking, on the other hand, predisposes to a variety of diseases, ranging from oral, lung, and bladder cancer to emphysema and chronic bronchitis. Smoking probably affects many different organ systems because tobacco smoke contains thousands of different chemical compounds, each of which may affect a different organ. Diabetes also affects multiple organ systems, but the major effect of treated diabetes is to accelerate atherosclerosis.

8. Reversibility. Reduced incidence of disease when the trait is removed or ameliorated provides the most convincing evidence of a causal relationship. Application of this criterion requires an experiment, either naturally occurring or planned. The decrease in coronary heart disease risk among persons who quit smoking fulfills this criterion and compensates for the lack of experimental animal evidence and specificity. Experiments in humans (controlled clinical trials) to lower serum cholesterol or reduce blood pressure are laborious, expensive, and require long follow-up periods but provide the strongest evidence for a causal relationship.

REFINING RISK FACTOR MEASUREMENTS

Serum Cholesterol

Accurate measurement of serum (or plasma) cholesterol became a major concern when its usefulness in predicting coronary heart disease risk was established (27). The intraindividual coefficient of variation from day to day is 6% (28). Plasma yields slightly lower values than does serum, and the difference varies with the anticoagulant used. Improvements in analytical methods, including automated analyzers and enzymatic assays (29), have greatly improved the precision and accuracy of the measurement of serum cholesterol.

Lipoproteins

The initial observations that serum cholesterol predicted risk of coronary heart disease were made on the basis of total cholesterol because methods were not available for measuring subclasses of plasma lipoproteins in large numbers of persons. Results from the analytical ultracentrifuge (30,31) and, later, paper electrophoresis (32) indicated that the distribution of cholesterol among the lipoproteins also predicted risk (33). The heparin–manganese precipitation method of measuring high-density lipoprotein (HDL) cholesterol and of estimating low-density lipoprotein (LDL) cholesterol (34) facilitated measurement of lipoprotein cholesterol in large numbers. In longitudinal studies, LDL cholesterol was directly and HDL cholesterol was inversely associated with coronary heart disease (35–38).

An immunologically distinctive form of LDL, lipoprotein (a) [Lp(a)], discovered over 30 years ago (39), was associated with increased incidence of coronary heart disease in Finnish subjects independently of plasma LDL cholesterol levels (40,41). Despite a few confirmatory reports, Lp(a) received little attention until the gene for its distinctive protein, apolipoprotein(a), was sequenced and its structure found to be similar to that for plasminogen (42). This similarity provided a plausible mechanism of action: attenuation of clot lysis by competing with plasminogen for its binding to fibrin (43). Further confirmation of its predictive power, combined with a plausible mechanism, has now made Lp(a) a candidate for risk factor status (44). However, until a way to modify it is available, we cannot conduct a controlled clinical trial as a definitive test of its causal relationship to coronary heart disease.

The search for a definition of the lipoprotein profile that more accurately predicts risk of coronary heart disease continues. For example, a heritable class of small, dense LDL (45,46) is associated with higher risk of coronary heart disease (47).

The discovery of a chemically modified lipoprotein, oxidized LDL (48), led to extensive investigation of its properties and its putative role in atherogenesis (49). As yet, it is not measurable in the plasma of healthy persons and cannot be identified as a risk factor for coronary heart disease but is a candidate for risk factor status. The various subclasses of HDL are also believed to be associated with different levels of risk (50).

These refinements are not yet sufficiently established to be practical for widespread application in preventive programs based on risk factor modification, but they are useful in examining mechanisms of action. In the future, we may anticipate a sharper definition of plasma lipoprotein levels as risk predictors.

Blood Pressure

Physicians formerly believed that diastolic blood pressure was a more reliable indicator of hypertensive disease than systolic pressure and, consequently, a better predictor of risk of coronary heart disease. However, the Framingham study found that systolic blood pressure was as good a predictor of coronary heart disease risk as diastolic blood pressure, and in some respects better (14). At one time, limited evidence indicated that plasma renin activity, a mediator of blood pressure control, directly augmented atherosclerosis and therefore might predict risk of coronary heart disease better than blood pressure alone (51). However, this relationship was not supported in subsequent studies (52), and no other trait has approached the practical utility of blood pressure as a predictor of risk.

Smoking

Many of the earlier reports of cigarette smoking effects did not find increased risk of coronary heart disease with pipe and cigar smoking as with cigarette smoking (53). Later studies found risk associated with pipe and cigar smoking to be intermediate between that for cigarette smokers and nonsmokers (54). The risk probably was lower because pipe and cigar smokers inhale less tobacco smoke than cigarette smokers. Blood levels of cotinine, a metabolite of nicotine, or of thiocyanate, a metabolite of cyanide, are more objective and reliable indicators of exposure to tobacco smoke than self-reported smoking behavior (55) but should not be necessary for preventive programs or for clinical practice.

Male Sex

Male sex is one of the best-documented and strongest risk factors for coronary heart disease, but the least understood (56). Intuitively, the relative immunity of premenopausal women is attributed to the female sex steroid hormones, but paradoxically, men treated with estrogen after a myocardial infarct had more frequent recurrent coronary heart disease, not less (57). On the other hand, there is compelling evidence from uncontrolled observational studies that estrogen replacement therapy reduces the incidence of coronary heart disease in postmenopausal women (58).

The sex differential in incidence of coronary heart disease is not universal. The difference is greatest among whites and is attenuated in blacks and other nonwhite groups. The rate at which incidence increases declines after middle age in men but continues to increase in women during and after the menopause, so that the rates become nearly equal in men and women in the older ages.

The predictive power of the other risk factors is about the same in men and women. The male–female difference is accounted for in part by differences in the other risk factors; for example, women have higher HDL cholesterol levels than men. However, known risk factors do not account for the entire sex difference. A more complete explanation of the sex differential would be valuable in designing preventive regimens, and a controlled clinical trial of postmenopausal estrogen replacement therapy in women is necessary to establish conclusively its protective power.

Family History

Coronary heart disease, particularly that occurring in younger persons, has long been recognized as clustering in families. The first step in explaining the physiological basis of familial aggregation was the identification of individuals with very high serum cholesterol levels (59), a syndrome transmitted as an autosomal dominant trait that became known as familial hypercholesterolemia. This condition was ultimately traced to a defect in the LDL receptor gene (60).

Subsequently, investigators have found many genetic variants that are associated with lipid and lipoprotein abnormalities and with probability of coronary heart disease. These variations include polymorphisms in apolipoproteins, B, E, A-I, A-II, C-II (61); apolipoprotein(a) (62); and cholesterol ester transfer protein, lipoprotein lipase, hepatic lipase, and lecithin:cholesterol acyltransferase (63).

The application of molecular genetic methods combined with progress in mapping the human genome assure that many more genetic variants contributing to atherosclerosis and to coronary heart disease will be discovered. We will probably find genes that modulate or interact with risk factors other than serum lipids, such as hypertension, smoking, and diabetes (64). The emerging knowledge of the molecular and cellular metabolism of the atherosclerotic lesion will lead to new candidate genes that influence atherosclerosis at the vessel wall level.

Meanwhile, family history of coronary heart disease, particularly of precocious events, remains a powerful predictor of risk of coronary heart disease independently of the other known risk factors (65). We may expect this residual unexplained risk to diminish as genetic control of physiological processes is further defined.

CONTROVERSIAL RISK FACTORS

Dietary Fat and Cholesterol

It may seem strange to include diet in the category of "controversial" risk factors in view of the overwhelming evidence implicating dietary intake of saturated fatty acids and cholesterol as the major environmental causes of elevated serum cholesterol, atherosclerosis, and coronary heart disease. Diet has long been cited as a risk factor under the broadest definition of the term as a characteristic or trait associated with the disease. The strong and consistent association was based on correlations among average intakes of fat and cholesterol, average serum cholesterol levels, average severity of atherosclerosis, and morbidity and mortality rates for *groups,* as demonstrated in the Seven Countries Study (66).

In contrast, dietary intakes of *individuals* were weakly or not at all associated with either individual serum cholesterol levels or probability that the individual will develop coronary heart disease. Thus, the strict definition of a risk factor, ability of the trait (dietary lipid consumption) to predict risk of disease in individuals, was not fulfilled.

The first definitive evidence that began to fill this gap came in 1981 from the Western Electric Study. Risk of death from coronary heart disease was positively correlated with the diet score, based on cholesterol and fat intake, determined 19 years previously (67). Similar analyses from four other longitudinal studies showed positive, but weak, associations of fat and cholesterol intake with subsequent incidence of coronary heart disease (68–71). The associations were further weakened in multivariate analyses.

Dietary fat and cholesterol intake measured in individuals of one population does not predict risk of coronary heart disease well because there is high individual variability in responses to diet, probably because of genetic variability, and there is large measurement error in assessing dietary intakes. These sources of error degrade correlations (72,73). Ecological correlations, those based on group averages or rates, conceal most of this interindividual and intraindividual variability and yield higher correlations.

Taken together, all types of evidence accumulated over nearly 50 years lead to the conclusion that dietary type of fat and cholesterol intake are major determinants of atherosclerosis and the risk of coronary heart disease. Whether individual dietary lipid intake should be classified as a risk factor according to the strictest definition remains the only controversy.

Triglycerides

Since the late 1950s, many reports have described an association of plasma triglyceride concentrations with coronary heart disease in either case-control or longitudinal studies, but many others have found no association (74–77). Most studies find an association in univariate analyses, but multivariate analyses that include LDL and HDL cholesterol and diabetes result in greatly attenuated or insignificant associations.

Many theoretical considerations and in vitro observations provide plausible mechanisms by which plasma triglycerides may contribute to atherogenesis. A major reason for the difficulty in detecting an association for triglycerides is the large hourly and daily variability in serum triglyceride concentrations. Furthermore, no intervention trials have attempted to lower plasma triglyceride levels in either primary or secondary prevention trials, and, therefore, there has been no experimental test of the hypothesis.

Obesity

Obesity is one of the most plausible, yet inconsistent, of all the suspected risk factors for coronary heart disease (78). Results from both longitudinal and case-control studies have included a positive and independent relationship of weight to coronary heart disease; a univariate relationship that disappears when hypertension, diabetes, and serum cholesterol levels are included in a multivariate analysis; and no relationship under any conditions. Analysis of the effect of obesity is subject to confounding because it is associated with hypertension and diabetes and is a risk factor for those diseases. Furthermore, smoking, a powerful risk factor itself, is associated with leanness. The issue may be clarified in the future by classifying obesity according to the distribution of adipose tissue: upper-body, or central, fat is associated with risk of coronary heart disease, whereas lower-body fat is not (79). The weight of present evidence indicates that obesity contributes to risk of coronary heart disease through its effect on hypertension and diabetes; whether there is another mechanism is not clear.

Lack of Physical Activity

An early study comparing the incidence of coronary heart disease between bus drivers (sedentary) and conductors (active) suggested that physical activity protected men from coronary heart disease (80). Many reports showing no association with physical activity appeared, for example, the Seven Countries Study (66); but other longitudinal studies found physical activity to be associated with decreased risk of coronary heart disease (81). Moderate physical activity favorably affects HDL cholesterol, blood pressure, body weight, and insulin resistance, mechanisms by which it may reduce risk of coronary heart disease (82). Physical activity may also protect from myocardial infarction by improving the efficiency of cardiac function. Physical activity, a readily modifiable trait, has emerged with persuasive evidence that it is protective against coronary heart disease.

THE SEARCH FOR OTHER RISK FACTORS

In 1981, Hopkins and Williams (83) accumulated a list of 246 risk factors for coronary heart disease. This review used a broad definition of "risk factor" that included traits associated with the established risk factors, characteristics associated with atherosclerosis in animal studies, and factors predicted from theoretical considerations. A similar review 10 years later would probably include another hundred or so factors fitting this definition. Representative examples of a few recently identified potential risk factors follow.

Fibrinogen

The plasma fibrinogen level predicts coronary heart disease independently of other risk factors (84,85). Interpretation is complicated by the strong association of smoking with plasma fibrinogen levels, and an effect on fibrinogen may be one of the mechanisms by which smoking increases the probability of coronary heart disease. Increased plasma fibrinogen could accelerate the progression of atherosclerotic lesions, particularly the formation of advanced fibrous plaques, or it could increase the probability of a terminal occlusive thrombosis over an established plaque.

Leukocyte Count

The leukocyte count independently predicts myocardial infarction (86–88). The relationship is partially explained by an association with smoking. Leukocytosis may produce such an effect by a number of potential mechanisms, such as vascular injury or adherence to endothelium (89). It may also be a marker for a more serious but undetected abnormality. Its present usefulness is primarily as an indicator of smoking exposure.

Baldness

A case-control study showed an excess of vertex baldness among men surviving myocardial infarction (90). A review of eight previous similar studies concluded that baldness was associated with slightly greater risk of coronary heart disease (91). Speculation regarding mechanisms centers around the relationship of baldness to the metabolism of male sex steroid hormones. Baldness may be a phenotypic marker for another abnormality directly linked to coronary heart disease. Because it is easy and inexpensive to recognize, its present usefulness is limited to identifying persons who are at very high risk and who should take above-average precautions to control the mutable risk factors.

Homocysteinemia

The demethylation of methionine produces the amino acid homocysteine, which is oxidized to a mixture of disulfides commonly designated "homocyst(e)ine." A rare genetic disorder results in high levels of plasma homocyst(e)ine, a condition associated with mental retardation and precocious arteriosclerosis. Smaller but more frequent elevations of plasma homocyst(e)ine are associated with heterozygosity of the gene for cystathionine β-synthase, an enzyme involved in metabolism of sulfur-containing amino acids (92). A number of case-control studies have shown an association of elevated plasma homocyst(e)ine levels with atherosclerotic disease, including coronary artery disease (93). The association was independent of other established risk factors. The risk factor status of hyperhomocyst(e)inemia was strengthened by observing a similar association in a longitudinal study (94). Several biologically plausible mechanisms involving endothelial injury and thrombosis have been suggested, but none is clearly established. Hyperhomocyst(e)inemia is readily treated with folate (95). A plausible mechanism and experimental results from a randomized clinical trial would complete the story.

These examples of emerging risk factors are selected from among many to illustrate the process by which new risk factors are identified and how they are evaluated for usefulness in prevention. They also illustrate the complexity of processes involved in the etiology of coronary heart disease.

DO RISK FACTORS AFFECT ATHEROSCLEROSIS OR CLINICAL DISEASE?

Natural History

Atherosclerosis begins as intimal lipid deposits (fatty streaks) in childhood and adolescence (Fig. 1) (96). Fatty streaks in some arterial sites are converted into fibrous plaques by continued accumulation of lipid, smooth muscle, and connective tissue. In middle age, fibrous plaques undergo a variety of changes (hemorrhage, ulceration, thrombosis, or calcification), some of which produce occlusion, ischemia, and clinical disease. Typically, clinical disease occurs 30 or more years after the process begins as fatty streaks, but it may be greatly accelerated in persons with severe hypercholesterolemia.

The major risk factors were identified on the basis of their ability to estimate the probability of coronary heart disease, the syndrome resulting from occlusion of a coronary artery. The use of clinical disease as an endpoint did not permit direct inferences about the association of risk factors with the preclinical stages of atherosclerotic lesions. The presence of severe coronary atherosclerosis in many persons dying

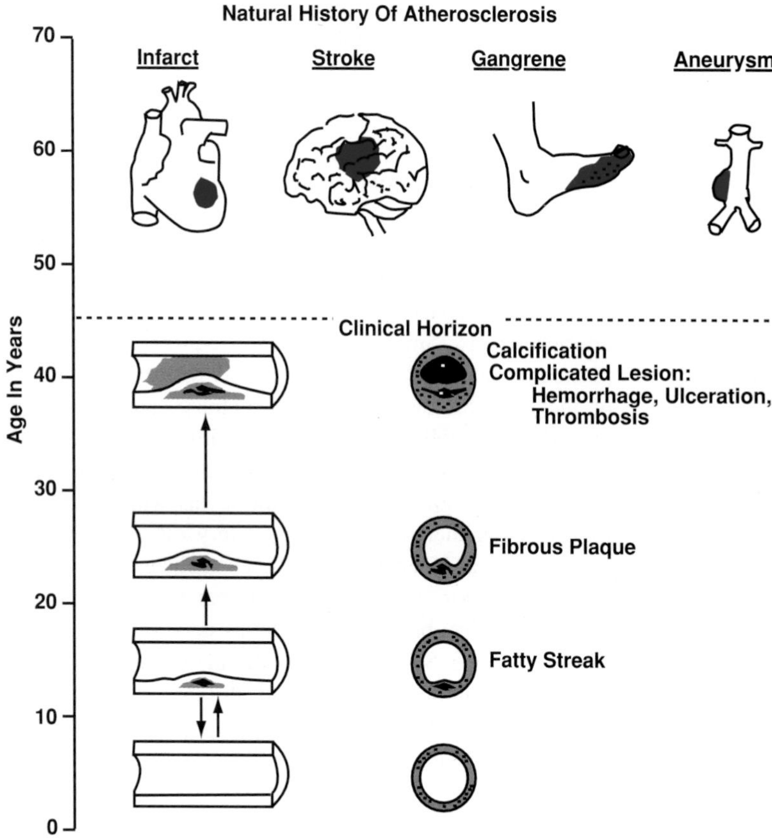

FIG. 1. Natural history of human atherosclerosis. The earliest detectable lesion is a deposit of lipid, principally cholesterol and its esters, in the intima and inner media of large muscular and elastic arteries. These appear in the aorta during the first decade of life; in the coronary arteries during the second decade; and in the cerebral arteries during the third decade. The process is similar in molecular and cellular characteristics in all three arterial systems. Continued accumulation of lipid and proliferation of smooth muscle and connective tissue form fibrous plaques, which undergo a variety of changes. The terminal occlusive episode usually results from rupture of a plaque and thrombosis on its intimal surface. Clinical manifestations vary with the artery involved. Risk factors may affect one, several, or all stages of the process. (Redrawn from McGill et al., ref. 96, and published with permission.)

of other causes and having no symptoms of coronary heart disease raised questions about the relationship of atherosclerosis to coronary heart disease and whether the risk factors for clinical disease influenced the initiation and progression of atherosclerosis. For example, did serum cholesterol concentration affect only fatty streaks, did it affect progression to fibrous plaques, or did it precipitate occlusive thrombosis? Did the other risk factors, such as hypertension and smoking, affect fatty streaks or the conversion of fatty streaks to fibrous plaques or both? Did any risk factors affect only the final terminal episode—plaque rupture and occlusive thrombosis? Answers to these questions were important in determining which should be modified to prevent coronary heart disease, and when the modification should begin.

These answers have been difficult to obtain. Early efforts before 1970 focused on the association of serum cholesterol levels, measured either before or after death, with the extent and severity of atherosclerotic lesions in autopsied persons. The subjects were predominantly older persons dying of natural causes, including atherosclerotic diseases. The results were mixed, with a preponderance of studies finding no association.

Geographic Distribution of Atherosclerosis

An international survey of atherosclerosis in autopsied persons showed a threefold variation in extent of coronary artery raised lesions (fibrous plaques, complicated lesions, and calcified lesions combined) in persons dying of accidents and of noncardiovascular disease from 19 geographic and ethnic groups (97) (Fig. 2). Lesions were positively correlated with coronary heart disease mortality rates, average serum cholesterol levels, and dietary fat intakes of the corresponding populations (98). These results were consistent with the hypothesis that diet, serum cholesterol, and atherosclerosis were causally related to coronary heart disease, but they were subject to the limitations of other ecological correlations and did not show that the relationship was true for individuals within a population.

Individual Correlations

Five reports appearing between 1979 and 1987 related risk factors, measured during life in longitudinal epidemiologic studies, with atherosclerotic lesions measured after death and autopsy (99–103). There was general agreement that serum cholesterol concentration and elevated blood pressure were positively correlated with atherosclerosis in the coronary arteries, particularly with raised lesions. The HDL cholesterol was inversely correlated with lesions in the one study in which it was measured. Smoking was associated with aortic lesions in all groups but with coronary artery lesions in only one (104). Relative body weight was associated with coronary artery lesions in only one group.

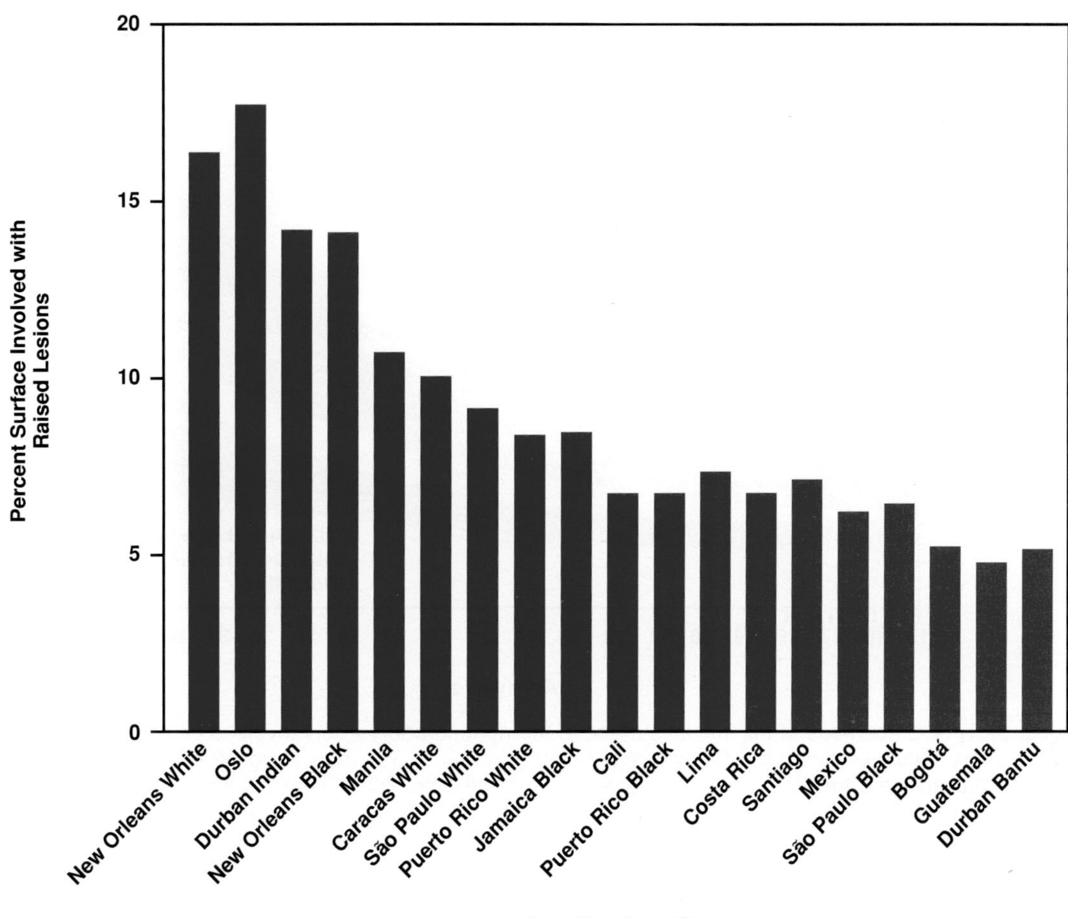

FIG. 2. Percentage of the intimal surface of coronary arteries involved by raised lesions (fibrous plaques and complicated lesions) in persons 25 through 64 years of age, dying of noncardiovascular causes, from 19 geographic and ethnic groups. The threefold difference parallels incidence of coronary heart disease in the corresponding populations. Drawn from results reported by the International Atherosclerosis Project (97).

Smoking was assessed by interviewing surviving relatives of over 1,300 autopsied men. Raised lesions were consistently more extensive in the coronary arteries of smokers, and smokers had much more extensive lesions in the aorta (105). Cholesterol concentrations in postmortem serum samples were associated with coronary artery raised lesions in white men but not in black men (106).

Coronary artery angiography and quantitative evaluation techniques confirmed the association of coronary artery lesions with serum cholesterol, blood pressure, diabetes, smoking, and male sex (107). However, the results were not always consistent. For example, one large study found no association with smoking, although the usual associations with other risk factors were present (108). These scattered negative results did not negate the positive findings, however, because of the nature of the sample. Angiograms cannot be performed in randomly selected healthy individuals but only in persons suspected of having one or more manifestations of coronary heart disease.

Risk Factors and Atherosclerosis in Childhood

A longitudinal study of risk factors in children and young adults provided the opportunity to relate serum cholesterol and blood pressure measured during life to arterial lesions in subjects who later died and were autopsied (109). In 57 individuals averaging 20 years of age, antemortem LDL cholesterol levels were positively associated, and HDL cholesterol/LDL cholesterol ratios were inversely associated with coronary artery fatty streaks. Systolic blood pressure was also associated with atherosclerotic lesions.

A recent project collected arteries and blood from about 400 young men dying of accidents, homicide, and suicide between the ages of 15 and 34 and measured serum lipoprotein cholesterol and thiocyanate (a marker for smoking) levels in postmortem blood (110). Their VLDL + LDL cholesterol levels were positively correlated, and HDL cholesterol levels were negatively correlated, with the extent of all types of atherosclerotic lesions (principally fatty streaks) in the

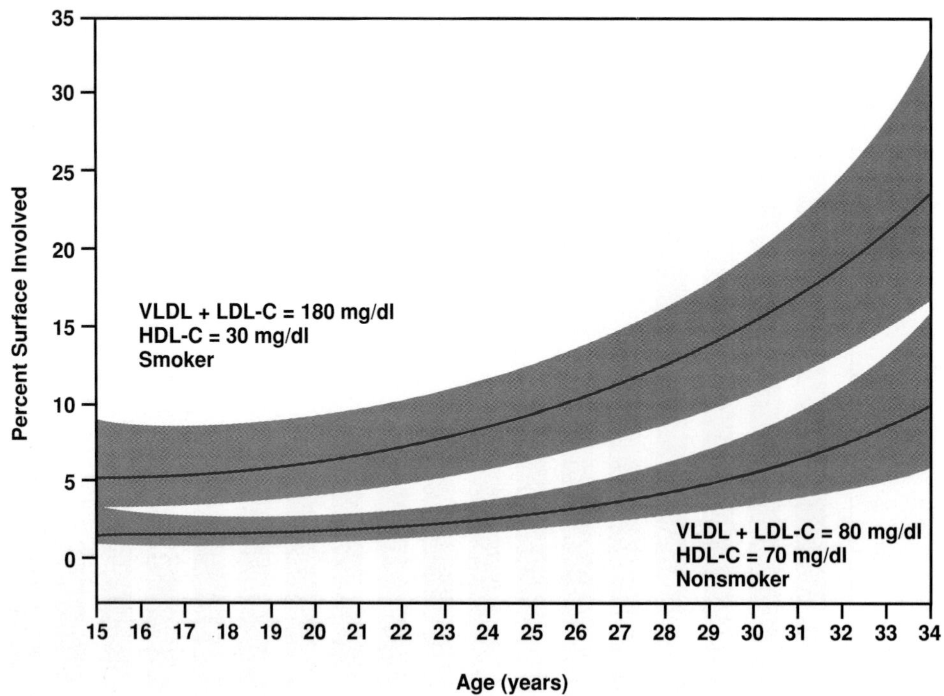

FIG. 3. Total percentage of the intimal surface of the right coronary artery involved by atherosclerosis at two risk levels, predicted by multiple regression analysis of 351 men 15 to 34 years of age. The values are adjusted for race. The *upper line* represents the predicted extent of lesions at a high risk level with VLDL + LDL cholesterol 1 SD above the mean, HDL cholesterol 1 SD below the mean, and smoking status indicated by the serum thiocyanate concentration. The *lower line* represents the predicted extent of lesions at a contrasting low risk level with VLDL + LDL cholesterol 1 SD below the mean, HDL cholesterol 1 SD above the mean, and no smoking. The shaded bands represent 95% confidence intervals. Drawn from results reported by the Pathobiological Determinants of Atherosclerosis in Youth Research Group (110).

right coronary artery. Smoking, as indicated by the thiocyanate level, was positively associated with the extent of all lesions and with the prevalence of fibrous plaques in the right coronary artery. High VLDL + LDL cholesterol, low HDL cholesterol, and smoking, compared to low VLDL + LDL cholesterol, high HDL cholesterol, and nonsmoking, predicted a substantial difference in extent of coronary atherosclerosis throughout the 15- to 34-year age group (Fig. 3).

Thus, evidence is accumulating that serum lipoproteins, smoking, and blood pressure influence the early stages of atherosclerosis 30 or more years before clinical coronary heart disease appears. This association with the early stages of atherogenesis strengthens the conclusion that the relationship is causal and encourages the belief that risk factor modification early in life will contribute to primary prevention of coronary heart disease.

Gene Polymorphisms and Lesions

Gene polymorphisms that affect lipid metabolism, blood pressure, or other risk factors have also become known as risk factors, and evidence has begun to accumulate regarding their association with atherosclerotic lesions. Three common alleles of apolipoprotein E (apo E) that determine six phenotypes have a substantial effect on serum cholesterol levels and lipoprotein profiles (111). Early reports of the association of apo E genotypes with coronary artery lesions assessed by angiography yielded mixed results. Methods to determine apo E genotype from liver DNA of autopsied persons made it possible to relate genotypes to arterial lesions (112). Apo E genotypes were associated with up to threefold differences in extent of atherosclerotic lesions in the abdominal aorta, and an effect remained after adjustment for serum cholesterol levels. A similar trend in the right coronary artery was not statistically significant.

More genetic polymorphisms that account for unexplained familial aggregation of coronary heart disease are certain to emerge as research identifies genes influencing not only lipid metabolism and blood pressure but also the cellular and molecular processes in the atherosclerotic lesion—growth factors, cytokines, adhesion molecules, and enzymes. Genetic variation also may affect blood coagulability. As this knowledge accumulates, it will become possible to describe a constellation of risk factors by analysis of DNA at birth. The technical problems will be simple compared to the ethical, legal, and economic problems associated with genetic testing that predicts probability of disease (113).

RISK FACTORS IN CHILDREN AND ADOLESCENTS

The realization that atherosclerosis begins early in life and that young American adults have a remarkably high prevalence of advanced coronary atherosclerotic lesions (114–116) stimulated interest in whether the risk factors for adult clinically manifest coronary heart disease might exist in some form in children. Serum cholesterol levels in children of underdeveloped countries, where coronary heart disease was rare, were much lower than those of children in the developed countries (117). However, the fatty streaks of childhood did not vary among populations to the same degree as adult coronary heart disease (118), and the significance of the higher serum cholesterol levels was not clear.

In the early 1970s, several centers in the United States, Europe, and Australia surveyed children and adolescents for levels of serum lipids and lipoproteins, blood pressure, obesity, smoking, and other characteristics related to adult risk factors (119–122). Although the average values and ranges of most variables were lower than in adults, there was considerable variability. Smoking began by age 12 and increased to a prevalence approaching 40% by the end of the second decade (123). High levels of risk factor variables tended to cluster in individual children (124).

Furthermore, the risk factors tracked: children with high values tended to stay high, and the low, low, within childhood (125–127) and from childhood into young adulthood (128). Serum lipid and lipoprotein levels were higher in children of parents who had experienced precocious coronary heart disease (129,130), an observation consistent with the identification of family history as a risk factor. During puberty, serum cholesterol and HDL cholesterol levels fell, and the LDL cholesterol-to-HDL cholesterol ratio rose in boys, but both variables remained stable in girls (131).

Community intervention programs directed at children and adolescents showed favorable changes in serum lipids and smoking (132). Symposia and workshops were organized, and monographs and books were written about the potential for long-range primary prevention of atherosclerosis and atherosclerotic disease through control of risk factors in children (133–136). The American Heart Association published recommendations for dietary modification in children with hyperlipidemia (137) and, later, in healthy children (138). The National Cholesterol Education Program published similar recommendations in 1991 (139).

Eventually, the variables in children derived from risk factors for adult coronary heart disease were shown to be correlated with fatty streaks in children and with progression of fatty streaks to fibrous plaques in young adulthood (see previous section, "Do Risk Factors Affect Atherosclerosis or Clinical Disease?"). These associations, occurring 30 years before the appearance of clinical disease, provide further evidence of their causal relationship to atherosclerosis and coronary heart disease and expand the meaning of the term "risk factor."

RISK FACTORS AND THE GREAT DECLINE

In the mid-1960s, a remarkable decline in mortality from coronary heart disease began in most of the industrialized countries (140). The decline in the United States has continued until 1988, the most recent year for which data are available (141), and now approaches a nearly 50% decrease from peak rates. All socioeconomic, racial, and geographic groups have participated in the decline, although the magnitude and time of onset have varied (142).

The magnitude and consistency of the declining rates indicate that they were real. Was the decline a result of better care (emergency medical services, intensive care, improved medical management, drugs, percutaneous transluminal angioplasty, bypass surgery, and others), of reduction in risk factors (serum lipids, blood pressure, smoking, and others), both improved care and risk factor reduction, or from other unknown causes? In the first decade of the decline, observed changes in serum cholesterol and smoking alone predicted about half the actual observed decline (143). Subsequent continued reductions in serum cholesterol levels (144,145) and smoking (146) have accompanied the continued decline in mortality.

The decline gave a powerful stimulus to the belief that primary prevention of coronary heart disease was feasible, and the association of decreased mortality with favorable trends in risk factor levels supported the concept that risk factor modification would be beneficial.

THE CONCEPT OF PRIMARY PREVENTION

Treatment and Secondary Prevention

As the frequency of coronary heart disease increased in the technically developed countries during the first half of the 20th century, most efforts were directed toward diagnosing, treating, and preventing recurrence. Electrocardiographic and imaging techniques for identifying ischemic myocardium were refined. Intensive care units focused on the care of patients with myocardial infarction were designed. Emergency medical services provided immediate supportive care to myocardial infarct victims and transported them rapidly to specialized care centers. Coronary angiography visualized obstructive atherosclerotic lesions in patients with angina and myocardial infarction and also in asymptomatic patients. Percutaneous transluminal angioplasty and coronary bypass procedures relieved obstructions. Thrombolytic agents dissolved thrombi. Drug treatments to prevent recurrent infarction were tested. However, nearly one-third of all new events were sudden cardiac death, as in the original Framingham Study report (15), and atherosclerotic cardiovascular disease continued to be the leading cause of death, particularly before age 65.

Primary Prevention

Primary prevention of coronary heart disease, as contrasted with preventing recurrence of disease (secondary prevention), was proposed as a goal shortly after World War II (10). The feasibility of primary prevention depended on whether the risk factors were causal and whether they could be modified. Elevated serum cholesterol concentration was the most prevalent risk factor and fulfilled most of the criteria for a causal relationship, but the most persuasive evidence, results from a controlled clinical trial showing that reduction of serum cholesterol reduced coronary heart disease, was lacking.

Dietary Recommendations

Despite the lack of experimental proof, the American Heart Association in 1957 recommended that individuals should reduce the total dietary fat intake from the average 40% to 25% or 30% of calories (147). No recommendation was made regarding type of fat or amount of cholesterol. The American Heart Association revised and republished similar recommendations periodically thereafter. Subsequent statements included more specific recommendations about limiting saturated fatty acid and cholesterol intake (148).

A number of small clinical investigations in free-living and metabolic ward subjects indicated that reducing saturated fatty acid and cholesterol intakes lowered serum cholesterol concentrations. Two controlled diet trials with institutionalized men showed reductions in coronary heart disease (149,150).

A trial of fat-modified diets in over 2,000 free-living men in five cities confirmed the feasibility of lowering serum cholesterol in free-living persons by limiting fat and cholesterol intake (151). However, an expert group concluded that a definitive trial of diet as a means of preventing coronary heart disease in noninstitutionalized subjects was not feasible because of the large sample size required and recommended instead that trials be conducted in persons with high levels of risk factors (152).

Lipid-Lowering Clinical Trials

The Lipid Research Clinics Coronary Primary Prevention Trial tested a bile acid sequestrant in about 4,000 men with high LDL cholesterol levels (153). In 7 years, an 11% reduction in LDL cholesterol was accompanied by a 19% reduction in coronary heart disease. The reduction in incidence of coronary heart disease was proportional to the reduction in LDL cholesterol (154). A trial of intervention in men with the three major risk factors—hypercholesterolemia, hypertension, and smoking—showed no reduction in coronary heart disease after 7 years (155) but did show reduction after 10 years (156). Other clinical trials in Europe with clofibrate (157) and gemfibrozil (158) yielded similar favorable effects of serum cholesterol-lowering regimens on cardiovascular endpoints but raised the specter of increased overall mortality, especially with clofibrate.

Hypertension Treatment

Remarkably effective drugs alleviated hypertension and prevented cardiac failure, renal failure, and stroke. However, their ability to prevent coronary heart disease was disappointing (159,160). The reasons for this failure to reverse the effects of hypertension on coronary heart disease risk remain unclear.

Other Developments

Between 1975 and 1985, other developments gave impetus to the concept of primary prevention by risk factor control. The discovery of the LDL cell surface receptor and its role in regulating cholesterol and lipoprotein metabolism (60) provided a plausible mechanism linking diet, plasma lipoproteins, and atherosclerosis. A new class of cholesterol-lowering drugs that lowered serum cholesterol by inhibiting 3-hydroxy-3-methylglutaryl coenzyme A reductase was introduced (161). Numerous studies showed that cessation of smoking led to reduction in frequency of coronary heart disease (53).

National Campaigns for Primary Prevention

In the United States, Canada, and Europe, many national voluntary health agencies and professional organizations endorsed the recommendations for reducing dietary fat and cholesterol intake to lower serum cholesterol; controlling elevated blood pressure through weight control, physical activity, and drugs; and cessation of smoking in order to reduce the risk of coronary heart disease (162). The recommendations differed in details and points of emphasis, but all agreed that high-risk persons—defined by having high serum cholesterol concentration, high blood pressure, and smoking—would benefit from risk factor reduction.

Public Health versus Clinical Medicine Strategies

The major difference among the recommended preventive programs was whether risk factor control should be directed toward the entire population, the strategy of public health engineering, or only toward persons at high risk, the strategy of clinical medicine (163). Attributable risk is useful in deciding between these two divergent approaches. Because the high-risk individuals are less numerous, they contribute a smaller proportion of the overall disease in the population than the much more numerous persons at moderate and low risk. Therefore, although treatment through risk factor modification might be of great benefit to those persons at high risk, it would have a disappointingly small effect in reducing the overall frequency of disease. In contrast, smaller reductions in risk among the more numerous persons at moderate risk would have a greater effect in reducing disease frequency in the population.

The two strategies are not incompatible with one another, but they compete for scarce resources in conducting preventive campaigns. The debate continues.

The National Institutes of Health Consensus Conference

In 1985, the National Institutes of Health convened a group of scientists and physicians in order to reach a consensus on the question of whether serum cholesterol levels should be reduced to prevent coronary heart disease (164). The panel concluded that serum cholesterols above the 90th percentile should be treated intensively by diet and drugs; that those between the 75th and 90th percentiles should treated by diet; and that all persons should be advised to reduce total fat, saturated fatty acid, and cholesterol intakes. Dietary recommendations applied to children over the age of 2 years. These recommendations adopted both the clinical medicine and the public health strategies.

National Cholesterol Education Program

A smaller panel focused on the high-risk, clinical medicine strategy and prepared detailed specifications for the "detection, evaluation, and treatment of high blood cholesterol in adults" (165). The manual included algorithms for decision making in the management of hyperlipidemia. The manual was revised and updated in 1993, 5 years later (166).

ADVERSE EFFECTS OF RISK FACTOR MODIFICATION: THE LOW BLOOD CHOLESTEROL SCARE

When any change in the habits of a large number of people is advocated, or when changes in medical practice are advised, a major concern is the possibility, however, remote, of violating the command, "*Primum non nocere.*" In 1971, two reports from opposite sides of the Pacific aroused alarm by reporting associations of low serum cholesterol levels with stroke (167) and of fat-modified diets with cancer (168). Subsequent reports indicated associations of low serum cholesterol with colon cancer and noncardiovascular deaths in both observational studies and cholesterol-lowering clinical trials. A combined analysis of results of 19 longitudinal studies from around the world in 1990 showed an inverse relationship of serum cholesterol with lung cancer (but not colon cancer), respiratory disease, digestive disease, trauma, and residual deaths (169). Excluding early deaths, among whom the low cholesterol may have been the result of preexisting disease, did not change the results.

A conference reviewing these results (169) concluded that the inverse association was probably caused by some form of confounding but recommended a continued search for the reason for the observed association. The magnitude of the observed effect of low serum cholesterol was not sufficient to indicate a change in public health policy with regard to cholesterol lowering. No adverse effects have been reported to result from cessation of smoking or control of hypertension.

THE FUTURE OF RISK FACTORS AND PRIMARY PREVENTION

The risk factor concept is firmly established in public health, in clinical medicine, and in public perception. The role of the major risk factors as causal is also firmly established. Persuasive evidence indicates that modification of the major risk factors reduces risk of coronary heart disease. Primary care and specialist physicians have accepted responsibility for managing patients at high risk with techniques known to be effective in modifying risk factors—diet for hyperlipidemia; weight control, physical activity, and drugs for hypertension and hyperlipidemia; diet and drugs for diabetes; and various techniques for smoking cessation. These functions of the medical care system are likely to intensify in all of the industrialized countries with the increasing emphasis on primary care, health maintenance, and cost control.

Many voluntary, professional, and government groups have recommended nationwide changes in diet to prevent coronary heart disease, and many changes have taken place. However, this movement will progress more slowly. Its progress will depend on the public's perceptions and its motivation to act on those perceptions. If evidence continues to indicate that high fat intake is also a risk factor for cancer, and if the low serum cholesterol–cancer association turns out to be spurious, the convergence of reasons to reduce fat intake will strengthen those motivations. As market demands change, industry will be willing and able to provide foods to meet those demands.

New risk factors will be identified, and proposed risk factors will be evaluated by ongoing research. The criteria for a causal relationship, which determine their usefulness in primary prevention, remain the same. The most likely new risk factors will be genetic polymorphisms that affect established risk factors or affect atherogenesis directly. Genetic markers of risk will be useful in identifying the high-risk individual for medical care but will be of little value in the population-based strategy. A simple genetic marker for the individual who is highly sensitive to the lipemic effects of dietary saturated fatty acids or cholesterol would be useful.

Modifying dietary intakes of children over age 2 years of age to maintain lower serum lipid levels and preventing smoking among teenagers offer the greatest long-range potential benefit at least cost and also offer health benefits other than retarding the onset of coronary heart disease. However, experimental proof of effectiveness is lacking, and rigorous proof, such as that gained from a controlled clinical trial, is not likely ever to be available. As with most medical decisions, action must be taken in the absence of ultimate proof.

Cost-effectiveness remains a major issue for drug treatment of the medically managed hyperlipidemic patient and for mass dietary modification for the entire population. Estimates for both strategies vary widely, depending on the assumptions used (170,171).

The long-term results of all preventive efforts depend on the assumptions that lifetime exposure to serum cholesterol concentration, hypertension, and smoking determine the extent of advanced atherosclerotic lesions, particularly fibrous plaques in the coronary arteries; that the probability of clinical coronary heart disease rises rapidly when about 60% of the coronary artery intimal surface is involved by lipid-rich fibrous plaques; and that reducing the duration or intensity of exposure to these three agents will substantially delay the age at which coronary atherosclerosis reaches that level of severity (172). Abundant evidence from over 50 years of research supports the validity of these assumptions.

REFERENCES

1. U.S. Department of Health and Human Services, Public Health Service, Office of the Surgeon General. *Reducing the Health Consequences of Smoking: 25 Years of Progress: A Report of the Surgeon General,* Chapter 3: *Changes in Smoking-Attributable Mortality,* DHHS publ. no. (CDC) 89-8411, 1989 executive summary. Rockville, MD: U.S. Department of Health and Human Services, Public Health Service, Centers for Disease Control, Center for Chronic Disease Prevention and Health Promotion, Office on Smoking and Health; 1989: 117–169.
2. Windaus A. Ueber den Gehalt normaler und atheromatoser Aorten an Cholesterin und Cholesterinestern. *Z Physiol Chem* 1910;67:174–176.
3. Anitschkow N, Chalatow S. Ueber experimentelle Cholesterinsteatose und ihre Bedeutung fur die Entstehung einiger pathologischer Prozesse. *Zentralbl Allg Pathol Pathol Anat* 1913;24:1–9. [Anitschkow N, Chalatow S. On experimental cholesterin steatosis and its significance in the origin of some pathological processes. *Arteriosclerosis* 1983;3:178–182.]
4. Langen CD de. Cholesterine-stofwisseling en rassenpathologie. *Geneeskd Tydsch V Nederl Indie.* 1916;56:1–34.
5. Snapper I. *Chinese Lessons to Western Medicine.* New York: Interscience Publishers; 1941:30–31, 160–161.
6. Vartiainen I. War-time and the mortality in certain diseases in Finland. *Ann Med Intern Fenn* 1946;35:234–240.
7. Vartiainen I, Kanerva K. Arteriosclerosis and war-time. *Ann Med Intern Fenn* 1947;36:748–758.
8. Malmros H. The relation of nutrition to health: A statistical study of the effect of the wartime on arteriosclerosis, cardiosclerosis, tuberculosis and diabetes. *Acta Med Scand* 1950;246(Suppl):137.
9. Strom A, Jensen RA. Mortality from circulatory diseases in Norway 1940–1945. *Lancet* 1951;1:126–129.
10. Keys A. Prediction and possible prevention of coronary disease. *Am J Public Health* 1953;43:1399–1407.
11. Steiner A, Domanski B. Serum cholesterol level in coronary arteriosclerosis. *Arch Intern Med* 1943;71:397–402.
12. Gertler MM, Garn SM, Lerman J. The interrelationships of serum cholesterol, cholesterol esters and phospholipids in health and in coronary artery disease. *Circulation* 1950;2:205–214.
13. Master AM, Dack S, Jaffe HL. Age, sex and hypertension in myocardial infarction due to coronary occlusion. *Arch Intern Med* 1939;64: 767–786.
14. Dawber TR. *The Framingham Study; The Epidemiology of Atherosclerotic Disease.* Cambridge: Harvard University Press; 1980.
15. Dawber TR, Moore FE, Mann GV. Coronary heart disease in the Framingham Study. *Am J Public Health* 1957;47(Suppl):4–23.
16. Dawber TR, Kannel WB, Revotskie N, Stokes J III, Kagan A, Gordon T. Some factors associated with the development of coronary heart disease. Six years' follow-up experience in the Framingham Study. *Am J Public Health* 1959;49:1349–1356.
17. Hilleboe HE, James G, Doyle JT. Cardiovascular health center. I. Project design for public health research. *Am J Public Health* 1954; 44:851–863.
18. Epstein FH, Ostrander LD Jr, Johnson BC, Payne MW, Hayner NS, Keller JB, Francis T Jr. Epidemiological studies of cardiovascular disease in a total community—Tecumseh, Michigan. *Ann Intern Med* 1965;62:1170–1187.
19. Paul O, Lepper MH, Phelan WH, Dupertuis GW, MacMillan A, McKean H, Park H. A longitudinal study of coronary heart disease. *Circulation* 1963;28:20–31.
20. Stamler J, Lindberg HA, Berkson DM, Shaffer A, Miller W, Poindexter A. Prevalence and incidence of coronary heart disease in strata of the labor force of a Chicago industrial corporation. *J Chron Dis* 1960;11:405–420.
21. Rosenman RH, Friedman M, Straus R, Wurm M, Kositchek R, Hahn W, Worthessen NT. A predictive study of coronary heart disease. The Western Collaborative Group Study. *JAMA* 1964;189:15–26.
22. Syme SL, Marmot MG, Kagan A, Kato H, Rhoads G. Epidemiologic studies of coronary heart disease and stroke in Japanese men living in Japan, Hawaii, and California; Introduction. *Am J Epidemiol* 1975; 102:477–480.
23. Pooling Project Research Group. Relationship of blood pressure, serum cholesterol, smoking habit, relative weight and ECG abnormalities to incidence of major coronary events: Final report of the Pooling Project. *J Chron Dis* 1978;31:201–306.
24. Doyle JT. Risk factors in coronary heart disease. *NY State J Med* 1963;63:1317–1320.
25. Surgeon General's Advisory Committee on Smoking and Health. *Smoking and Health; Report of the Advisory Committee to the Surgeon General of the Public Health Service.* Chapter 3: *Criteria for Judgment,* PHS publ. no. 1103. Washington: U.S. Government Printing Office; 1964;19–21.
26. Hill AB. The environment and disease: Association or causation? *Proc R Soc Med* 1965;58:295–300.
27. Cooper GR, Myers GL, Smith J, Schlant RC. Blood lipid measurements; variations and practical utility. *JAMA* 1992;267:1652–1660.
28. Smith JS, Cooper GR, Myers GL, Sampson EJ. Biological variability in concentrations of serum lipids: Sources of variation among results from published studies and composite predicted values. *Clin Chem* 1993;39:1012–1022.
29. Richmond W. Preparation and properties of a bacterial cholesterol oxidase from *Nocardia* sp. and its application to the enzymatic assay of total cholesterol in serum. *Clin Chem* 1973;19:1350.
30. Lindgren FT, Elliott HA, Gofman JW. The ultracentrifugal characterization and isolation of human blood lipids and lipoproteins, with applications to the study of atherosclerosis. *J Phys Colloid Chem* 1951; 55:80–93.
31. Gofman JW, Glazier F, Tamplin A, Strisower B, De Lalla O. Lipoproteins, coronary heart disease, and atherosclerosis. *Physiol Rev* 1954; 34:589–607.
32. Less RS, Hatch FT. Sharper separation of lipoprotein species by paper electrophoresis in albumin-containing buffer. *J Lab Clin Med* 1963; 61:518–528.
33. Rosenfeld L. Lipoprotein analysis. Early methods in the diagnosis of atherosclerosis. *Arch Pathol Lab Med* 1989;113:1101–1110.
34. Burstein M, Scholnick HR, Morfin R. Rapid method for the isolation of lipoproteins from human serum by precipitation with polyanions. *J Lipid Res* 1970;11:583–595.
35. Miller GJ, Miller NE. Plasma-high-density-lipoprotein concentration and development of ischaemic heart-disease. *Lancet* 1975;1:16–19.
36. Rhoads GG, Gulbrandsen CL, Kagan A. Serum lipoproteins and coronary heart disease in a population study of Hawaii Japanese men. *N Engl J Med* 1976;294:293–298.
37. Gordon T, Kagan A, Garcia-Palmieri M, Kannel WB, Zukel WJ, Til-

lotson J, Sorlie P, Hjortland M. Diet and its relation to coronary heart disease and death in three populations. *Circulation* 1981;63:500–515.
38. Castelli WP, Doyle JT, Gordon T, Hames CG, Hjortland MC, Hulley SB, Kagan A, Zukel WJ. HDL cholesterol and other lipids in coronary heart disease. The Cooperative Lipoprotein Phenotyping Study. *Circulation* 1977;55:767–772.
39. Berg K. A new serum type system in man—the Lp system. *Acta Pathol Microbiol Scand* 1963;59:369–382.
40. Berg K, Dahlen G, Frick MH. Lp(a) lipoprotein and pre-β_1-lipoprotein in patients with coronary heart disease. *Clin Genet* 1974;6:230–235.
41. Dahlen G, Berg K, Frick MH. Lp(a) lipoprotein/pre-β_1-lipoprotein, serum lipids and atherosclerotic disease. *Clin Genet* 1976;9:558–566.
42. McLean JW, Tomlinson JE, Kuang W-J, Eaton DL, Chen EY, Fless GM, Scanu AM, Lawn RM. cDNA sequence of human apolipoprotein(a) is homologous to plasminogen. *Nature* 1987;330:132–137.
43. Loscalzo J, Weinfeld M, Fless GM, Scanu AM. Lipoprotein(a), fibrin binding, and plasminogen activation. *Arteriosclerosis* 1990;10: 240–245.
44. Howard GC, Pizzo SV. Biology of disease; lipoprotein(a) and its role in atherothrombotic disease. *Lab Invest* 1993;69:373–386.
45. Krauss RM, Burke DJ. Identification of multiple subclasses of plasma low density lipoproteins in normal humans. *J Lipid Res* 1982;23: 97–104.
46. Austin MA, King M-C, Vranizan KM, Krauss RM. Atherogenic lipoprotein phenotype. A proposed genetic marker for coronary heart disease risk. *Circulation* 1990;82:495–506.
47. Austin MA, Breslow JL, Hennekens CH, Curing JE, Willett WC, Krauss RM. Low-density lipoprotein subclass patterns and risk of myocardial infarction. *JAMA* 1988;260:1917–1921.
48. Henriksen T, Mahoney EM, Steinberg D. Enhanced macrophage degradation of low density lipoprotein previously incubated with cultured endothelial cells: Recognition by receptors for acetylated low density lipoproteins. *Proc Natl Acad Sci USA* 1981;78:6499–6503.
49. Steinberg D, Witztum JL. Lipoproteins and atherogenesis. Current concepts. *JAMA* 1990;264:3047–3052.
50. Miller NE, Hammett F, Saltiss S, Rao S, Van Zeller H, Coltart J, Lewis B. Relation of angiographically defined coronary artery disease to plasma lipoprotein subfractions and apolipoproteins. *Br Med J* 1981;282:1741–1744.
51. Brunner HR, Laragh JH, Baer L, Newton MA, Goodwin FT, Krakoff LR, Bard RH, Buhler FR. Essential hypertension: Renin and aldosterone, heart attack and stroke. *N Engl J Med* 1972;286:441–449.
52. Kirkendall WM, Hammond JJ, Overturf ML. Renin as a predictor of hypertensive complications. *Ann NY Acad Sci* 1978;304:147–160.
53. United States Office on Smoking and Health. *The Health Consequences of Smoking; Cardiovascular Disease; A Report of the Surgeon General*. Rockville, MD: U.S. Department of Health and Human Services, Public Health Service, Office on Smoking and Health; 1983.
54. Carstensen JM, Pershagen G, Eklund G. Mortality in relation to cigarette and pipe smoking: 16 years' observation of 25,000 Swedish men. *J Epidemiol Community Health* 1987;41:166–172.
55. Haley NJ, Axelrod CM, Tilton KA. Validation of self-reported smoking behavior: Biochemical analyses of cotinine and thiocyanate. *Am J Public Health* 1983;73:1204–1207.
56. McGill HC Jr, Stern MP. Sex and atherosclerosis. *Atheroscler Rev* 1979;4:157–242.
57. Coronary Drug Project Research Group. The Coronary Drug Project. Initial findings leading to modifications of its research protocol. *JAMA* 1970;214:1303–1313.
58. Barrett-Connor E, Bush TL. Estrogen and coronary heart disease in women. *JAMA* 1991;265:1861–1867.
59. Müller C. Xanthomata, hypercholesterolemia, angina pectoris. *Acta Med Scand* 1938;Suppl 89:75–84.
60. Brown MS, Goldstein ML. Familial hypercholesterolemia. Genetic, biochemical, and pathophysiologic considerations. *Adv Intern Med* 1975;20:273–296.
61. Breslow JL. Apolipoprotein genetic variation and human disease. *Physiol Rev* 1988;68:85–132.
62. Scanu AM. Lipoprotein(a). A genetic risk factor for premature coronary heart disease. *JAMA* 1992;267:3326–3329.
63. Lusis AJ. Genetic factors affecting blood lipoproteins: The candidate gene approach. *J Lipid Res* 1988;29:397–429.
64. Perkins KA. Family history of coronary heart disease: Is it an independent risk factor? *Am J Epidemiol* 1986;124:182–194.
65. Jorde LB, Williams RR. Relation between family history of coronary artery disease and coronary risk variables. *Am J Cardiol* 1988;62: 708–713.
66. Keys A. *Seven Countries. A Multivariate Analysis of Death and Coronary Heart Disease*. Cambridge: Harvard University Press; 1980.
67. Shekelle RB, Shryock AM, Paul O, Lepper M, Stamler J, Shuguey Liu, Raynor WJ Jr. Diet, serum cholesterol, and death from coronary heart disease. The Western Electric Study. *N Engl J Med* 1981;304: 65–70.
68. Gordon T, Castelli WP, Hjortland MC, Kannel WB, Dawber TR. High density lipoprotein as a protective factor against coronary heart disease. The Framingham Study. *Am J Med* 1977;62:707–714.
69. McGee DL, Reed DM, Yano K, Kagan A, Tillotson J. Ten-year incidence of coronary heart disease in the Honolulu Heart Program. Relationship to nutrient intake. *Am J Epidemiol* 1984;119:667–676.
70. Kromhout D, de Lezenn Coulander C. Diet, prevalence and 10-year mortality from coronary heart disease in 871 middle-aged men. *Am J Epidemiol* 1984;119:733–741.
71. Kushi LH, Lew RA, Stare FJ, Ellison CR, Lozy ME, Bourke G, Daly L, Graham I, Hickey N, Mulcahy R, Kevaney J. Diet and 20-year mortality from coronary heart disease. The Ireland–Boston Diet–Heart Study. *N Engl J Med* 1985;312:811–818.
72. McGill HC Jr, MacMahan CA, Wene JD. Unresolved problems in the diet–heart issue. *Arteriosclerosis* 1981;1:164–176.
73. Jacobs DR, Anderson JT, Blackburn H. Diet and serum cholesterol. Do zero correlations negate the relationship? *Am J Epidemiol* 1979; 110:77–87.
74. Hulley SB, Rosenman RH, Bawol RD, Brand RJ. Epidemiology as a guide to clinical decisions; the association between triglyceride and coronary heart disease. *N Engl J Med* 1980;302:1383–1389.
75. Lippel K, Tyroler H, Eder H, Gotto A Jr, Vahouny G. Relationship of hypertriglyceridemia to atherosclerosis. *Arteriosclerosis* 1981;1: 406–417.
76. Austin MA. Plasma triglyceride and coronary heart disease. *Arterioscler Thromb* 1991;11:2–14.
77. NIH Consensus Development Panel on Triglyceride, High-Density Lipoprotein, and Coronary Heart Disease. Triglyceride, high-density lipoprotein, and coronary heart disease. *JAMA* 1993;269:505–510.
78. Barrett-Connor EL. Obesity, atherosclerosis, and coronary artery disease. *Ann Intern Med* 1985;103:1010–1019.
79. Pi-Sunyer FX. Medical hazards of obesity. *Ann Intern Med* 1993;119: 655–660.
80. Morris JN, Heady JA, Raffle PAB, Roberts CG, Parks JW. Coronary heart disease and physical activity of work. *Lancet* 1953;2: 1053–1057.
81. Paffenbarger RS Jr, Hale WE. Work activity and coronary heart mortality. *N Engl J Med* 1975;292:545–550.
82. Berlin JA, Colditz GA. A meta-analysis of physical activity in the prevention of coronary heart disease. *Am J Epidemiol* 1990;132: 612–628.
83. Hopkins PN, Williams RR. A survey of 246 suggested coronary risk factors. *Atherosclerosis* 1981;40:1–52.
84. Wilhelmsen L, Svardsudd K, Korsan-Bengtsen K, Larsson B, Welin L, Tibblin G. Fibrinogen as a risk factor for stroke and myocardial infarction. *N Engl J Med* 1984;311:501–505.
85. Kannel WB, Wolf PA, Castelli WP, D'Agostino RB. Fibrinogen and risk of cardiovascular disease. The Framingham Study. *JAMA* 1987; 258:1183–1186.
86. Friedman GD, Klatsky AL, Siegelaub AB. The leukocyte count as a predictor of myocardial infarction. *N Engl J Med* 1974;290: 1275–1278.
87. Zalokar JB, Richard JL, Claude JR. Leukocyte count, smoking, and myocardial infarction. *N Engl J Med* 1981;304:465–468.
88. Grimm RH, Neaton JD, Ludwig W. Prognostic importance of the white blood cell count for coronary, cancer, and all-cause mortality. *JAMA* 1985;254:1932–1937.
89. Ernst E, Hammerschmidt DE, Bagge U, Matria A, Dormandy JA. Leukocytes and the risk of ischemic diseases. *JAMA* 1987;257: 2318–2324.
90. Lesko SM, Rosenberg L, Shapiro S. A case-control study of baldness in relation to myocardial infarction in men. *JAMA* 1993;269: 998–1003.
91. Herrera CR, Lynch C. Is baldness a risk factor for coronary artery

disease? A review of the literature. *J Clin Epidemiol* 1990;43: 1255–1260.
92. Wilcken DEL, Reddy SG, Gupta VJ. Homocysteinemia, ischemic heart disease, and the carrier state for homocystinuria. *Metabolism* 1983;32:363–370.
93. Malinow MR. Hyperhomocyst(e)inemia. A common and easily reversible risk factor for occlusive atherosclerosis. *Circulation* 1990; 81:2004–2006.
94. Stampfer MJ, Malinow MR, Willett WC, Newcomer LM, Upson B, Ullmann D, Tishler PV, Hennekens CH. A prospective study of plasma homocyst(e)ine and risk of myocardial infarction in US physicians. *JAMA* 1992;268:877–881.
95. Brattstrom LE, Israelsson B, Jeppsson J-O, Hultberg BL. Folic acid—an innocuous means to reduce plasma homocysteine. *Scand J Clin Lab Invest* 1988;48:215–221.
96. McGill HC, Geer JC, Strong JP. Natural history of human atherosclerotic lesions. In: Sandler M, Bourne GH, eds. *Atherosclerosis and Its Origin.* New York: Acadmic Press; 1963:43–52.
97. Tejada C, Strong JP, Montenegro MR, Restrepo C, Solberg LA. Distribution of coronary and aortic atherosclerosis by geographic location, race, and sex. *Lab Invest* 1968;18:509–526.
98. Scrimshaw NS, Guzman MA. Diet and atherosclerosis. *Lab Invest* 1968;18:623–628.
99. Feinleib M, Kannel WB, Tedeschi CG, Landau TK, Garrison RJ. The relation of antemortem characteristics to cardiovascular findings at necropsy. The Framingham Study. *Atherosclerosis* 1979;34:145–157.
100. Holme I, Solberg LA, Weissfeld L, Helgeland A, Hjermann I, Leren P, Strong JP, Williams OD. Coronary risk factors and their pathway of action through coronary raised lesions, coronary stenoses and coronary death. Multivariate statistical analysis of an autopsy series; The Oslo Study. *Am J Cardiol* 1985;55:40–47.
101. Sternby NH. Atherosclerosis, smoking and other risk factors. In: Gotto AM Jr, Smith LC, Allen B, eds. *Atherosclerosis V.* New York: Springer-Verlag; 1980:67–70.
102. Sorlie PD, Garcia-Palmieri MR, Castillo-Staab MI, Costas R Jr, Oalmann MC, Havlik R. The relation of antemortem factors to atherosclerosis at autopsy. The Puerto Rico Heart Health Program. *Am J Pathol* 1981;103:345–352.
103. Reed DM, MacLean CJ, Hayashi T. Predictors of atherosclerosis in the Honolulu Heart Program. I. Biologic, dietary, and lifestyle characteristics. *Am J Epidemiol* 1987;126:214–225.
104. Solberg LA, Strong JP. Risk factors and atherosclerotic lesions: A review of autopsy studies. *Arteriosclerosis* 1983;3:187–198.
105. Strong JP, Richards ML. Cigarette smoking and atherosclerosis in autopsied men. *Atherosclerosis* 1976;23:451–476.
106. Oalmann MC, Malcolm GT, Toca VT, Guzman MA, Strong JP. Community pathology of atherosclerosis and coronary heart disease: Post mortem serum cholesterol and extent of coronary atherosclerosis. *Am J Epidemiol* 1981;113:396–403.
107. Bonnet J, Couffinal T, Tourtoulou V, Benchimol D. A cardiologist looks at the importance of being able to quantify the patient's plaque size. In: Wissler RW, ed. *NATO Advanced Research Workshop on Progress, Problems, and Promises for an Effective Quantitative Evaluation of Atherosclerosis in Living and Autopsied Experimental Animals and Man, Siena, Italy, 1990: Atherosclerotic Plaques: Advances in Imaging for Sequential Quantitative Evaluation.* New York: Plenum Press; 1991:9–16.
108. Vlietstra RE, Kronmal RA, Frye RL, Seth AK, Tristani FE, Killip T III. Factors affecting the extent and severity of coronary artery disease in patients enrolled in the Coronary Artery Surgery Study. *Arteriosclerosis* 1982;2:208–215.
109. Berenson GS, Wattigney WA, Tracy RE, Newman WP III, Srinivasan SR, Webber LS, Dalferes ER Jr, Strong JP. Atherosclerosis of the aorta and coronary arteries and cardiovascular risk factors in persons aged 6 to 30 years and studied at necropsy (The Bogalusa Heart Study). *Am J Cardiol* 1992;70:851–858.
110. Pathobiological Determinants of Atherosclerosis in Youth (PDAY) Research Group. Relationship of atherosclerosis in young men to serum lipoprotein cholesterol concentrations and smoking. A preliminary report from the Pathobiological Determinants of Atherosclerosis in Youth (PDAY) Research Group. *JAMA* 1990;264:3018–3024.
111. Davignon J, Gregg RE, Sing CF. Apolipoprotein E polymorphism and atherosclerosis. *Arteriosclerosis* 1988;8:1–21.
112. Hixson JE, Pathobiological Determinants of Atherosclerosis in Youth (PDAY) Research Group. Apolipoprotein E polymorphisms affect atherosclerosis in young males. *Arterioscler Thromb* 1991;11: 1237–1244.
113. NoWak R. Genetic testing set for takeoff. *Science* 1994;265:464–467.
114. Enos WF, Holmes RH, Beyer J. Coronary disease among United States soldiers killed in action in Korea. Preliminary report. *JAMA* 1953;152:1090–1093.
115. Holman RL, McGill HC Jr, Strong JP, Geer JC. The natural history of atherosclerosis. The early aortic lesions as seen in New Orleans in the middle of the 20th century. *Am J Pathol* 1958;34:209–235.
116. Strong JP, McGill HC Jr. The natural history of coronary atherosclerosis. *Am J Pathol* 1962;40:37–49.
117. Scrimshaw NS, Balsam A, Arroyave G. Serum cholesterol levels in school children from three socio-economic groups. *Am J Clin Nutr* 1957;5:629–633.
118. McGill HC Jr. Fatty streaks in the coronary arteries and aorta. *Lab Invest* 1968;18:560–564.
119. Frerichs RR, Srinivasan SR, Webber LS, Berenson GS. Serum cholesterol and triglyceride levels in 3,446 children from a biracial community. The Bogalusa Heart Study. *Circulation* 1976;54:302–309.
120. Srinivasan SR, Frerichs RR, Webber LS, Berenson GS. Serum lipoprotein profile in children from a biracial community. The Bogalusa Heart Study. *Circulation* 1976;54:309–318.
121. Lauer RM, Connor WE, Leaverton PE, Reiter MA, Clarke WR. Coronary heart disease risk factors in school children: The Muscatine Study. *J Pediatr* 1975;86:697–706.
122. Vartiainen E, Puska P, Salonen JT. Serum total cholesterol, HDL cholesterol and blood pressure levels in 13-year-old children in eastern Finland. *Acta Med Scand* 1982;211:95–103.
123. Webber LS, Hunter SM, Johnson CC, Srinivasan SR, Berenson GS. Smoking, alcohol, and oral contraceptives. Effects on lipids during adolescence and young adulthood—Bogalusa Heart Study. *Ann NY Acad Sci* 1991;623:135–154.
124. Webber LS, Voors AW, Srinivasan SR, Frerichs RR, Berenson GS. Occurrence in children of multiple risk factors for coronary artery disease: The Bogalusa Heart Study. *Prev Med* 1979;8:407–418.
125. Clarke WR, Schrott HG, Leaverton PE, Connor WE, Lauer RM. Tracking of blood lipids and blood pressures in school age children: The Muscatine Study. *Circulation* 1978;58:626–634.
126. Frerichs RR, Weber LS, Voors AW, Srinivasan SR, Berenson GS. Cardiovascular disease risk factor variables in children at two successive years—The Bogalusa Heart Study. *J Chron Dis* 1979;32: 251–262.
127. Webber LS, Cresanta JL, Voors AW, Berenson GS. Tracking of cardiovascular disease risk factor variables in school-age children. *J Chron Dis* 1983;36:647–660.
128. Orchard TJ, Donahue RP, Kuller LH, Hodge PN, Drash AL. Cholesterol screening in childhood: Does it predict adult hypercholesterolemia? The Beaver County experience. *J Pediatr* 1983;103:687–691.
129. Tamir I, Bojanower Y, Levtow O, Heldenberg D, Dickerman Z, Werbin B. Serum lipids and lipoproteins in children from families with early coronary heart disease. *Arch Dis Child* 1972;47:808–810.
130. Boulton TJC. Serum cholesterol in early childhood: Familial and nutritional influences and the emergence of tracking. *Acta Pediatr Scand* 1980;69:441–445.
131. Berenson GS, Srinivasan SR, Cresanta JL, Foster TA, Webber LS. Dynamic changes of serum lipoproteins in children during adolescence and sexual maturation. *Am J Epidemiol* 1981;113:157–170.
132. Puska P, Vartiainen E, Pallonen U, Salonen JT, Poyhia P, Koskela K, McAlister A. The North Karelia Youth Project: Evaluation of two years of intervention on health behavior and CVD risk factors among 13- to 15-year old children. *Prev Med* 1982;11:550–570.
133. Lauer RM, Shekelle RB. *Childhood Prevention of Atherosclerosis and Hypertension.* New York: Raven Press; 1980.
134. Berenson GS, McMahan CA, Voors AW, Webber LS, Srinivasan SR, Frank GC, Foster TA, Blonde CV. *Cardiovascular Risk Factors in Children: The Early Natural History of Atherosclerosis and Essential Hypertension.* New York: Oxford University Press; 1980.
135. Berenson GS, ed. *Causation of Cardiovascular Risk Factors in Children: Perspectives on Cardiovascular Risk in Early Life.* New York: Raven Press; 1986.
136. Williams CL, Wynder EL, eds. Hyperlipidemia in childhood and the development of atherosclerosis. *Ann NY Acad Sci* 1991;623:1–482.
137. Steering Committee for Medical and Community Program of the

American Heart Association. The value and safety of diet modification to control hyperlipidemia in childhood and adolescence. A statement for physicians. *Circulation* 1978;58:381A.
138. American Heart Association, Nutrition Committee and the Cardiovascular Disease in the Young Council. Diet in the healthy child. *Circulation* 1983;67:1411A–1414A.
139. U.S. National Cholesterol Education Program. *Report of the Expert Panel on Blood Cholesterol Levels in Children and Adolescents. Blood Cholesterol Levels in Children and Adolescents. NIH publ. no. 91-2732.* Bethesda, MD: U.S. Department of Health and Human Services, Public Health Service, National Institute of Health, National Heart, Lung and Blood Institute; 1991.
140. Havlik RJ, Feinleib M, eds. *Proceedings of the Conference on the Decline in Coronary Heart Disease Mortality. NIH publ. no. 79-1610.* Bethesda, MD: National Institutes of Health; 1979.
141. National Center for Chronic Disease Prevention and Health Promotion, CDC. Trends in ischemic heart disease mortality—United States, 1980–1988. *JAMA* 1992;268:1837.
142. Wing S, Barnett E, Casper M, Tyroler HA. Geographic and socioeconomic variation in the onset of decline of coronary heart disease mortality in white women. *Am J Public Health* 1992;82:204–209.
143. Stern MP. The recent decline in ischemic heart disease mortality. *Ann Intern Med* 1979;91:630–640.
144. Johnson CL, Rifkind BM, Sempos CT, Carroll MD, Bachorik PS, Briefel RR, Gordon DJ, Burt VL, Brown CD, Lippel K, Cleeman JI. Declining serum total cholesterol levels among US adults. The National Health and Nutrition Examination Surveys. *JAMA* 1993;269:3002–3008.
145. National Center for Health Statistics–National Heart, Lung, and Blood Institute Collaborative Lipid Group. Trends in serum cholesterol levels among US adults aged 20 to 74 years. Data from the National Health and Nutrition Examination Surveys, 1960 to 1980. *JAMA* 1987;257:937–942.
146. National Center for Health Statistics, CDC. Cigarette smoking among adults—United States, 1991. *JAMA* 1993;269:1931.
147. Page IH, Stare FJ, Corcoran AC, Pollack H, Wilkinson CF Jr. Atherosclerosis and the fat content of the diet. *Circulation* 1957;16:163–178.
148. American Heart Association, Committee on Nutrition. *Diet and Heart Disease.* New York: American Heart Association; 1965.
149. Dayton S, Pearce ML, Hashimoto S, Dixon WJ, Tomiyasu U. A controlled clinical trial of a diet high in unsaturated fat in preventing complications of atherosclerosis. *Circulation* 1969;40(Suppl II):II-1–II-63.
150. Turpeinen O, Karvonen MJ, Pekkarinen M, Miettinen M, Elosuo R, Paavilainen E. Dietary prevention of coronary heart disease: The Finnish Mental Hospital Study. *Int J Epidemiol* 1979;8:99–118.
151. National Diet–Heart Study Research Group. The National Diet–Heart Study final report. *Circulation* 1968;37(Suppl 1):1–428.
152. National Heart and Lung Institute, Task Force on Arteriosclerosis. *Arteriosclerosis; a report, Vol. 1 DHEW publ. no. (NIH) 72-137.* Bethesda, MD: National Institutes of Health; 1971.
153. Lipid Research Clinics Program. The Lipid Research Clinics Coronary Primary Prevention Trial results. I. Reduction in incidence of coronary heart disease. *JAMA* 1984;251:351–364.
154. Lipid Research Clinics Program. The Lipid Research Clinics Coronary Primary Prevention Trial results. II. The relationship of reduction in incidence of coronary heart disease to cholesterol lowering. *JAMA* 1984;251:365–374.
155. Multiple Risk Factor Intervention Trial Research Group. Multiple risk factor intervention trial. Risk factor changes and mortality results. *JAMA* 1982;248:1465–1477.
156. Multiple Risk Factor Intervention Trial Research Group. Mortality rates after 10.5 years for participants in the Multiple Risk Factor Intervention Trial. *JAMA* 1990;263:1795–1801.
157. Oliver MF, Heady JA, Morris JN, Cooper J. A co-operative trial in the primary prevention of ischaemic heart disease using clofibrate: Report from the Committee of Principal Investigators. *Br Heart J* 1978;40:1069–1118.
158. Frick MH, Elo O, Haapa K, Heinonen OP, Heinsalmi P, Helo P, Huttunen JK, Kaitaniemi P, Koskinen P, Manninen V, Maenpaa H, Malkonen M, Manttari M, Norola S, Pasternack A, Pikkarainen J, Romo M, Sjoblom T, Nikkila EA. Helsinki Heart Study: Primary-prevention trial with gemfibrozil in middle-aged men with dyslipidemia. Safety of treatment, changes in risk factors, and incidence of coronary heart disease. *N Engl J Med* 1987;317:1237–1245.
159. Samuelsson O, Wilhelmsen L, Andersson OK, Pennert K, Berglund G. Cardiovascular morbidity in relation to change in blood pressure and serum cholesterol levels in treated hypertension. *JAMA* 1987;258:1768–1776.
160. Miall WE. The effects on coronary artery disease of treatment for mild hypertension. *Atheroscler Rev* 1990.
161. Grundy SM. HMG-CoA reductase inhibitors for treatment of hypercholesterolemia. *N Engl J Med* 1988;319:24–33.
162. Brooks JG, Rifkind BM. Cholesterol and coronary heart disease prevention—a transatlantic consensus. *Eur Heart J* 1989;10:702–711.
163. Rose G. Strategy of prevention: Lessons from cardiovascular disease. *Br Med J* 1981;282:1847–1851.
164. National Institutes of Health, Office of Medical Applications of Research. Lowering blood cholesterol to prevent heart disease. *JAMA* 1985;253:2080–2086.
165. National Cholesterol Education Program. *Report of the Expert Panel on Detection, Evaluation, and Treatment of High Blood Cholesterol in Adults. NIH publ. no. 88-2925.* Bethesda, MD: National Heart, Lung and Blood Institute; 1988.
166. National Cholesterol Education Program. *Second Report of the Expert Panel on Detection, Evaluation, and Treatment of High Blood Cholesterol in Adults (Adult Treatment Panel II). NIH publ. no. 93-3095.* Bethesda, MD: National Heart, Lung and Blood Institute; 1993.
167. Komachi Y, Iida M, Shimamoto T, et al. Geographic and occupational comparisons of risk factors in cardiovascular diseases in Japan. *Jpn Circ J* 1971;35:189–207.
168. Pearce ML, Dayton S. Incidence of cancer in men on a diet high in polyunsaturated fat. *Lancet* 1971;1:464–467.
169. Jacobs D, Blackburn H, Higgins M, Reed D, Iso H, McMillan G, Neaton J, Nelson J, Potter J, Rifkind B, Rossouw J, Shekelle R, Yusuf S. Report of the conference on low blood cholesterol: Mortality associations. *Circulation* 1992;86:1046–1060.
170. Goldman L, Sia STB, Cook EF, Rutherford JD, Weinstein MC. Costs and effectiveness of routine therapy with long-term beta-adrenergic antagonists after acute myocardial infarction. *N Engl J Med* 1988;319:152–157.
171. Kristiansen IS, Eggen AE, Thelle DS. Cost effectiveness of incremental programmes for lowering serum cholesterol concentration: Is individual intervention worth while? *Br Med J* 1991;302:1119–1122.
172. Grundy SM. Cholesterol and coronary heart disease. A new era. *JAMA* 1986;256:2849–2858.

PART I

Major Risk Factors and Primary Prevention

Atherosclerosis and Coronary Artery Disease,
edited by V. Fuster, R. Ross, and E. J. Topol.
Lippincott-Raven Publishers, Philadelphia © 1996.

CHAPTER 4

Lipids, Nutrition, and Coronary Heart Disease

Scott M. Grundy

Key Words: Dyslipidemia; Fat, saturated; Fat, monounsaturated; Fat, polyunsaturated; Hypercholesterolemia; Lipoproteins, high-density; Lipoproteins, intermediate-density; Lipoproteins, low-density; Lipoproteins, very low density; Metabolism; Regression dilution bias; Serum cholesterol level; Triglycerides.

INTRODUCTION

Nutrition is the cornerstone of the prevention of coronary heart disease (CHD). This claim is based primarily on a large body of epidemiological data indicating that the incidence of CHD in various countries correlates closely with the type of diet consumed in these countries (1–3). Although confounding factors other than nutrition may affect rates of CHD, a mass of epidemiological evidence leaves little doubt that nutrition contributes importantly to coronary atherosclerosis and CHD. Moreover, there is growing evidence that several different dietary factors play a role in atherogenesis, and the mechanisms whereby various factors impart their effects are becoming better understood. Although diet may influence atherogenesis and risk for CHD in ways that have not been uncovered, the diet also affects the known risk factors. The present chapter will focus mainly on the link between nutrition and these major risk factors. The influence of the diet on each of these will be considered below.

Scott M. Grundy: Center for Human Nutrition, University of Texas Southwestern Medical Center at Dallas, Dallas, Texas 75235-9052.

HIGH SERUM CHOLESTEROL AND LOW-DENSITY LIPOPROTEINS

A positive relationship exists between serum total cholesterol levels and risk of CHD (4–7). That a high serum cholesterol can induce atherosclerosis was demonstrated first when rabbits were fed cholesterol in the diet (8). Many studies in experimental animals, including primates, subsequently showed that diet-induced hypercholesterolemia will produce arterial lesions resembling human atherosclerosis (9–11). Moreover, a human condition first called familial xanthomatosis was early noted to be characterized by very high levels of serum cholesterol and premature coronary atherosclerosis. A number of epidemiological surveys, including those carried out between populations (12,13), within countries (4,7), and in migrating populations (14), subsequently revealed a positive association between serum total cholesterol and rates of atherosclerotic CHD. In more recent years, several controlled clinical trials found that lowering cholesterol levels reduces risk for CHD and can retard the progression of atherosclerosis (15–17). These clinical trials largely confirm the etiological connections among high serum cholesterol, coronary atherosclerosis, and CHD. The sum of accumulated data thus proves beyond a reasonable doubt that elevated serum total cholesterol is a major risk factor for CHD.

Although *total* cholesterol levels correlate with risk, it must be recognized that serum cholesterol is not homogeneous. Since cholesterol is completely insoluble in aqueous solutions, special mechanisms are needed to keep it in solution. This is accomplished by complexing it with other lipids and proteins. These complexes are called lipoproteins. There are several major categories of lipoproteins that typically are distinguished by their densities. These are low-density lipoproteins (LDL), high-density lipoproteins (HDL), very low density lipoproteins (VLDL), and intermediate-density lipoproteins (IDL). In normal persons, about two-thirds of the total cholesterol is carried in LDL. This lipoprotein contains mostly cholesterol ester in its lipid core, and it has unesterified cholesterol, phospholipids, and protein in its surface coat (Fig. 1). The only protein present in LDL is apolipoprotein B-100 (apo B-100). Data indicate that LDL cholesterol contributes predominantly to the relationship between total cholesterol and CHD. For example, among genetic forms of hyperlipidemia, the greatest risk for premature CHD occurs in those in whom elevated LDL cholesterol is the only significant abnormality (18–22). Moreover, in epidemiological studies in which lipoprotein fractions were measured, LDL cholesterol usually emerged as the major correlate with CHD. In recent years, many investigations in experimental animals and in vitro systems have provided insights into the mechanisms whereby an elevated LDL promotes atherogenesis. Finally, clinical trials in which LDL levels were lowered document that both risk for CHD is reduced (15,16) and progression of coronary atherosclerosis is retarded (23–25). Thus, LDL cholesterol is the major serum cholesterol fraction linked to coronary atherosclerosis. Consequently, the National Cholesterol Education Program (NCEP) (26) has identified LDL cholesterol as the primary target of cholesterol-lowering therapy.

To understand the influence of nutrition on LDL-cholesterol levels, a review of the key steps in LDL metabolism may be helpful. These steps are outlined in Fig. 2. The LDL derives from catabolism of precursor lipoproteins (VLDL and VLDL remnants). The liver secretes VLDL as a triglyc-

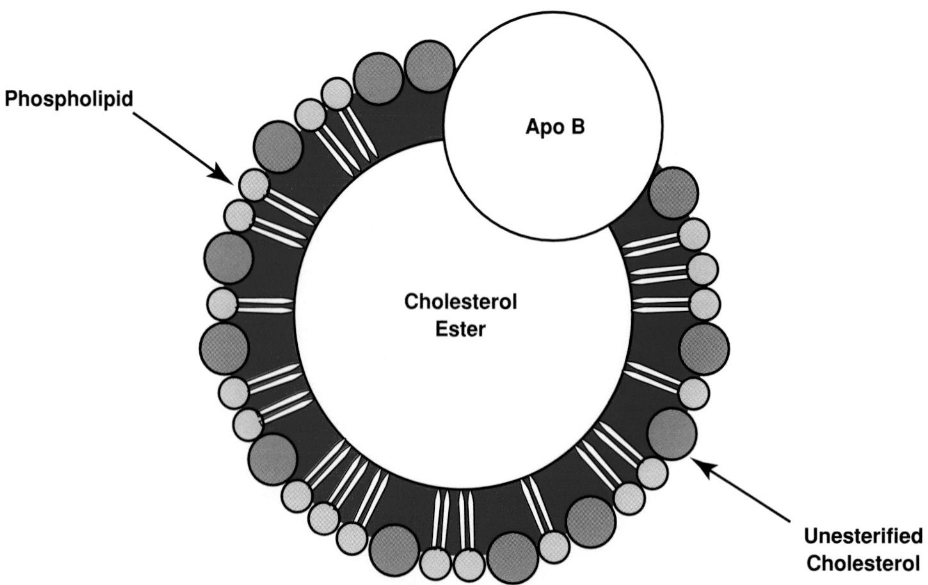

FIG. 1. Schematic picture of the structure of LDL. The LDL particle consists of a cholesterol-ester-rich core and a more polar coat containing unesterified cholesterol and phospholipids. There is one molecule of apolipoprotein B (apo B) embedded into the surface coat.

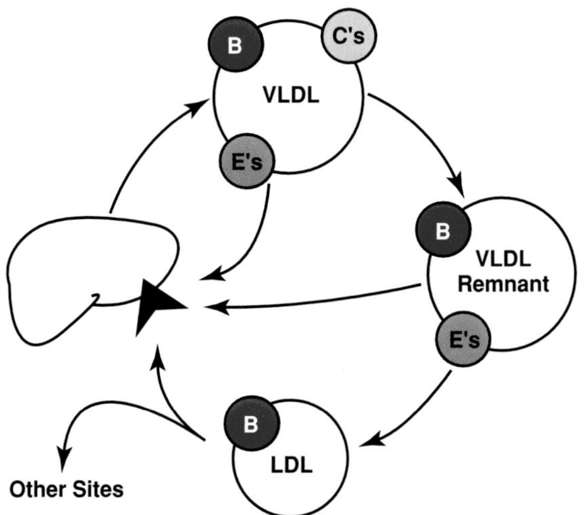

FIG. 2. Pathways for lipid transport in apolipoprotein B-containing lipoproteins. The liver secretes very low-density lipoproteins (LDL), which contain apo B *(B)*, apo C's *(C's)*, and apo E's *(E's)*. VLDL are triglyceride-rich lipoproteins. Triglycerides are hydrolyzed by lipoprotein lipase converting VLDL to VLDL remnants. Most apo C's are lost. VLDL remnants can have two fates, either direct removal by the liver or conversion to LDL. LDL has only one apolipoprotein, apo B. Most LDL particles are removed by the liver through LDL receptors.

eride-rich lipoprotein. VLDL contains apo B-100 (apo B) as the major apolipoprotein, but other apolipoproteins (apo C's and apo E) also are present. As VLDL circulates in plasma they interact with an enzyme, lipoprotein lipase, located on the surface of capillary endothelial cells and their triglycerides are progressively removed. Lipoprotein lipase is activated by one of the apo C's—apo C-II. Partial removal of triglycerides results in formation of VLDL remnants. These immediate precursors of LDL (VLDL remnants) can either be taken up by the liver or converted to LDL. The mechanism for hepatic uptake of VLDL remnants is not fully understood; the process appears to be mediated by receptors that recognize apo E. VLDL remnants also can be converted to LDL. Most of LDL is removed by the liver, but small amounts enter other tissues. Hepatic uptake of LDL is mediated largely by LDL receptors.

Serum levels of LDL depend in large part on metabolism of apo B. Three parameters of apo B metabolism affect LDL levels. These are (a) hepatic secretion rates of apo B-containing lipoproteins, (b) the fraction of these lipoproteins converted to LDL, and (c) LDL-receptor activity. Another factor affecting LDL-cholesterol levels is the amount of cholesterol carried in each LDL particle (27,28). Only one molecule of apo B is present per LDL particle, but the quantity of cholesterol per particle can vary considerably. Normal people have about 1.5 times the mass of cholesterol per LDL particle as apo B. However, as shown by a recent study from our laboratory (28), even in people who have normal LDL-cholesterol levels, LDL-cholesterol/apo B ratios can vary from 1.3 to 1.7. Our studies suggest that about 85% of the variation in LDL-cholesterol levels is explained by variation of LDL-apo B metabolism, whereas the remaining 15% depends on LDL-cholesterol/apo B ratios.

The latter ratios correlate with the size of LDL particles. In general low LDL-cholesterol/apo B ratios reflect relatively *small* LDL particles. Smaller LDL usually have higher density. Some investigators contend that small, dense LDL particles are more atherogenic than normal-sized LDL (29–31). Besides epidemiological support for this relationship (29–31), at least two mechanisms can be visualized to explain the link. First, small, dense LDL particles may filter unusually rapidly into the arterial wall and thereby promote atherogenesis. Second, smaller LDL particles appear to be particularly susceptible to oxidation (32), which may be another atherogenic property (33). The role of oxidation of LDL in development of arterial lesions will be briefly discussed later in this chapter as well as elsewhere in this volume.

In contrast, cholesterol-enriched LDL also may be more atherogenic than normal-sized LDL. When primates are fed excess cholesterol, their LDL particles become enriched with cholesterol ester, and these cholesterol-enriched LDL seemingly produce more severe atherosclerosis than do normal-sized LDL (34). Thus, any factor, such as diet, that either increases or decreases the amount of cholesterol carried in LDL particles may enhance the atherogenic potential of LDL.

Definitions of Serum Cholesterol Levels

Three categories of serum total cholesterol are defined by the NCEP (26): desirable (<200 mg/dl), borderline-high (200–239 mg/dl), and high (≥240 mg/dl). Corresponding definitions for LDL-cholesterol levels are as follows: desirable (<130 mg/dl), borderline-high-risk (130–159 mg/dl), and high-risk (≥160 mg/dl). For the population as a whole, the total cholesterol level correlates highly with LDL cholesterol within each category. For individuals, however, the correlation may not be as tight. In this chapter, the term "hypercholesterolemia" generally is used to indicate a high-risk LDL-cholesterol level of ≥160 mg/dl. "Moderate hypercholesterolemia" signifies an LDL-cholesterol level of 160–220 mg/dl, whereas "severe hypercholesterolemia" applies when LDL-cholesterol levels exceed 220 mg/dl.

Relation of Serum Cholesterol Levels to Coronary Heart Disease

Epidemiological studies (1,35) suggest that for every 1% increase in total cholesterol the risk for CHD rises by 2%. Clinical trial data (15,16) support this relationship; they show that for every 1% reduction in cholesterol levels, risk decreases by 2%. This relationship can be called the 1%/2% rule. Furthermore, a 1% change in serum cholesterol level generally corresponds to an approximately 2 mg/dl change. Thus, the 1%/2% rule can be expressed alternatively as a

(1 mg/dl)/1% rule, i.e., for every 1 mg/dl change in serum cholesterol the risk for CHD changes by 1% in the same direction. According to recent analysis (35), the 1%/2% rule may actually underestimate the relationship between cholesterol levels and risk. This is because of a phenomenon called "regression dilution bias," which means that single measurements generally underestimate the strength of biological links; if a correction is made for this bias, a 1% change in serum cholesterol level appears to account for a 3% change in risk. Although this correction possibly provides a more accurate assessment of the cholesterol–CHD link, the more conventional 1%/2% [(1 mg/dl)/1%] rule will be applied in this chapter. Employing these rules, we can say that compared to desirable cholesterol levels, people with a borderline-high cholesterol have an approximately 1.5-fold increase in risk; those with moderate hypercholesterolemia have a two- to fourfold higher risk, whereas those with severe hypercholesterolemia have a greater than fourfold increment in risk. These increments represent relative increases in risk, and they apply mainly to CHD risk below age 65 years. In elderly people, differences in relative risk at different cholesterol levels are reduced; however, since absolute risk is so much higher in elderly people, the *absolute* increase in risk imparted by higher cholesterol levels actually is greater in older people than in middle-age individuals (36).

Causes of Borderline-High Cholesterol Levels

Approximately 40% of American adults have borderline-high cholesterol levels (26). Even these higher levels contribute significantly to the relatively high rates of CHD in the United States. One factor responsible for higher total and LDL cholesterol is the relatively high background level for LDL cholesterol in humans compared to other species (37). For example, a 20-year-old man who is not obese and who consumes a diet low in saturated fatty acids and cholesterol will have a total cholesterol level of about 140 mg/dl (38,39). This corresponds to an LDL-cholesterol in the range of 75–90 mg/dl. A total cholesterol of 140 mg/dl is still considerably below the borderline-high range (200–230 mg/dl); and those populations who maintain cholesterol levels of 140–160 mg/dl into middle age develop little clinical CHD. Only when levels rise well above 160 mg/dl does the risk begin to increase significantly (5).

But what about the risk associated with total cholesterol levels in the range of 160–200 mg/dl? Epidemiological surveys indicate that people with levels in the range of 160–200 mg/dl have somewhat higher CHD rates than do those with lower levels (5). Incidence of atherogenesis seemingly is proportional to cholesterol levels over a broad range, from high to low (40). Even so, the relative and absolute risks for CHD accompanying concentrations in this slightly elevated zone are not great. In fact, after the pooling of a large body of epidemiological data, Jacobs et al. (41) reported that the lowest total mortality in adult men was found in those with total cholesterol levels of 160–200 mg/dl. For practical purposes, therefore, it seems warranted to designate total cholesterol levels in this range as "desirable," as done by the NCEP (26).

The first level of definite elevation thus corresponds to a borderline-high total cholesterol (200–239 mg/dl). Although genetic factors may help to raise concentrations into this range, other factors common in the general population appear to be mainly responsible. These include the diet, obesity, aging, and, in postmenopausal women, loss of estrogens. For example, excess cholesterol in the American diet, which is about 200 mg/day higher than optimal, raises the total cholesterol by about 6 mg/dl (42). Moreover, the excess cholesterol-raising fatty acids (mostly saturated fatty acids), which exceed optimal intakes by approximately 7% of total calories (26), increase total cholesterol levels by another 19 mg/dl (43). The precise contribution of the rise of body weight with age is not known, but increasing body weights probably account for another 25 mg/dl increment in middle-age Americans compared to 20-year olds (44,45). A further rise associated with aging appears to be due to metabolic aging per se (44,45). This adds another 30 mg/dl. Finally, loss of estrogens after the menopause in women frequently yields another increment of about 20 mg/dl (26). Because of these several factors, middle-aged Americans typically have total cholesterol levels that are 80–100 mg/dl higher than baseline levels.

The probable mechanisms whereby these factors increase cholesterol concentrations are becoming better understood. Most of them apparently decrease the expression of LDL receptors. Compared to other species, humans may inherently have a low activity of LDL receptors, accounting for relatively high levels of LDL compared to other species. In addition, dietary cholesterol (46–48), saturated fatty acids (49–51), aging per se (52–54), and loss of estrogens (after the menopause in women) (55,56) all seemingly decrease the activity of LDL receptors. Obesity, in contrast, enhances the secretion of VLDL-apo B (57,58), leading to increased formation of LDL (59). Whether the greater synthesis of cholesterol occurring in obese people also suppresses expression of LDL receptors is uncertain.

Approximately 25% of middle-aged and older Americans have a high serum cholesterol (≥240 mg/dl) (26). These high levels represent an increment above borderline-high levels, which are due to previously discussed factors. Presumably these still higher concentrations result from genetic factors. Two genetic factors have been mainly implicated. These are (a) a further reduction in LDL-receptor activity (18,27) and (b) a greater hepatic secretion of apo B-containing lipoproteins beyond that induced by obesity. Two other mechanisms also deserve consideration: (c) a decreased clearance of LDL due to the presence of LDL particles that are poor ligands for LDL receptors (19,20) and (d) an enhanced conversion of VLDL to LDL, leading to an overproduction of LDL particles (27,37). Mechanisms related to decreased clearance of LDL (i.e., reduced activity of LDL receptors and LDL particles having low affinity for receptors) have been identified with certainty, whereas those responsible for an overproduction of LDL (i.e., increased hepatic secretion of lipoproteins and increased conversion of VLDL to LDL) are more problematic. Identified genetic causes of reduced LDL clearance involve defects in the gene encoding for LDL receptors (familial hypercholesterolemia) (18) and abnormalities in the apo B molecule imparting poor binding of LDL to receptors (familial defective apo B) (19,20). Specific genetic defects leading to overproduction of LDL have not been identified, but indirect evidence for their existence comes from isotope kinetic studies (60–62).

An important question is whether some people are genetically hyperresponsive to the LDL-raising effects of diet and obesity. Limited data indicate that genetic hyperresponsiveness to diet does exist. For example, some people respond to dietary cholesterol and saturated fatty acids with a greater rise in LDL levels than do others (63). Recently we reported that hypercholesterolemic patients with a relatively low clearance capacity for LDL tend to be hyperresponsive to saturated fatty acids (64). Nonetheless, the molecular basis for hyperresponsiveness to diet has not been elucidated.

Role of Diet Composition and Specific Nutrients

Although saturated fatty acids as a group undoubtedly raise LDL-cholesterol levels (65), the issue of what is their best replacement in the diet is a subject of ongoing interest and controversy. Since the protein content of the diet must be kept relatively constant, possible replacements include both carbohydrates and/or other types of fats. In fact, the issue is broader than just replacement of saturated fatty acids because of the possibility that other nutrients have health benefits or detrimental effects themselves. For this reason, it is necessary to consider the overall composition of the diet as well as specific nutrients.

Dietary Fat

The fat in the diet consists mainly of triglycerides made up of three fatty acid molecules esterified to glycerol. Different types of dietary fat contain different patterns of fatty acids. There are three basic kinds of fatty acids—saturated, monounsaturated, and polyunsaturated. Each kind contains two or more different subtypes (Table 1). Each fatty acid seemingly has unique effects on lipid and lipoprotein metabolism, and perhaps other unique metabolic actions as well; therefore each fatty acid deserves to be considered separately.

TABLE 1. *Dietary fatty acids*

Dietary fatty acids
Saturated fatty acids
Stearic acid (18:0)
Palmitic acid (16:0)
Myristic acid (14:0)
Lauric acid (12:0)
Medium-chain fatty acids (8:0 and 10:0)
Monounsaturated fatty acids
Oleic acid (16:cis 1)
Trans fatty acids (16:trans 1)
Polyunsaturated fatty acids
Omega-6 fatty acids
Linoleic acid (18:2)
Omega-3 fatty acids
Linolenic acid (18:3)
Eicosapentanoic acid (EPA) (20:5)
Docosahexanoic acid (DHA) (22:6)

The first number indicates the number of carbon atoms; the second denotes the number of double bonds per molecule.

Saturated Fatty Acids

Palmitic Acid. The major saturated fatty acid in the American diet is palmitic acid (16:0; see footnote to Table 1); it makes up about 60% of total saturates. Palmitic acid is high in most meats and dairy fats, but some also occurs in plant products. A large quantity of data indicates that palmitic acid raises the serum total cholesterol level; this has been demonstrated by specifically comparing palmitic acid with unsaturated fatty acids and carbohydrates. The hypercholesterolemic effect of palmitic acid has been documented best in metabolic ward studies (66–69). Increments in total cholesterol occur almost entirely in LDL, with little change in HDL or VLDL. This fatty acid seemingly suppresses the expression of LDL receptors (49–51).

Some researchers question whether palmitic acid truly raises the serum LDL cholesterol. This issue has been raised because of the observation that in some animal species, including some primates, high intakes of palmitic acid have only a small cholesterol-raising action, seemingly smaller than reported for humans. Moreover, when the experimental design in human studies has not been rigorous, the cholesterol-raising effect of palmitic acid may appear to be small. On the other hand, more definitive human studies (63,68,69) show clearly that this fatty acid raises LDL-cholesterol levels compared to unsaturated fatty acids (or carbohydrate). Indeed, palmitic acid is the predominant dietary saturated fatty acid, and thus it is the major cholesterol-raising fatty acid in the American diet.

Myristic Acid. A second saturated fatty acid is myristic acid (14:0). It occurs in appreciable amounts in butter fat and in certain tropical oils (coconut oil and palm kernel oil). Limited evidence indicates that myristic acid raises cholesterol levels at least as much as palmitic acid (66), or perhaps even more (67). Still, myristic acid is less important as a cholesterol-raising fatty-acid than palmitic acid because it is ingested in much smaller amounts.

Lauric Acid. Saturated fatty acids can be divided into two groups: long-chain [stearic acid (18:0), palmitic acid (16:0), and myristic acid (14:0)] and medium-chain fatty acids of eight to ten carbon atoms. An intermediate-length fatty acid falling between these two groups is lauric acid (12:0). The long-chain groups are absorbed with triglycerides in chylomicrons, whereas medium-chain fatty acids enter directly into the portal circulation as free fatty acids. Lauric acid, however, is absorbed partly with chylomicron triglycerides and partly as a free fatty acid. It has been suggested that medium-chain saturates do not raise cholesterol levels (70,71). If lauric acid belongs in the medium-chain category, it might not be hypercholesterolemic. Earlier, limited data (66,67) failed to provide a solid answer on the effects of lauric acid. If lauric acid does not raise cholesterol levels, it could be useful as a substitute for the cholesterol-raising saturated fatty acids.

To resolve this uncertainty, we recently carried out a study in which lauric acid was incorporated into a synthetic fat and tested for its effects on cholesterol levels (72). Essentially the only fatty acids present in this test fat were lauric acid and oleic acid. They were provided in equal proportions. This high-lauric fat was compared to palm oil; the latter differed only by having palmitic acid in the place of lauric acid. These two fats also were compared to high-oleic safflower oil, which consists almost entirely of oleic acid. As expected, palm oil strikingly raised LDL-cholesterol levels compared to the safflower oil. The lauric acid-enriched oil also raised LDL-cholesterol levels compared to safflower oil, but only about two-thirds as much as did palm oil. Even so, lauric acid *did* raise LDL-cholesterol level relative to oleic acid; consequently, lauric acid definitely must be considered a cholesterol-raising fatty acid; and it would not be an acceptable substitute for palmitic acid in the diet.

Medium-Chain Fatty Acids. The actions of medium-chain fatty acids (8:0 and 10:0) on serum cholesterol levels remain to be determined with certainty. Early workers (73) argued that these fatty acids are hypercholesterolemic. This was thought to be so because butter fat, which is rich in medium-chain fatty acids, is especially hypercholesterolemic compared to other hard fats. Nonetheless, as already mentioned, at least two studies (70,71) failed to document a cholesterol-raising effect of these medium-chain acids. Thus the current general view holds that medium-chain fatty acids do not increase cholesterol levels, but this issue is not fully resolved; further investigations are needed.

Stearic Acid. Early research in humans by Ahrens et al. (73), Keys et al. (66), and Hegsted et al. (67) along with animal research (74) suggested that stearic acid, contrary to other saturated fatty acids, does not increase serum cholesterol levels. This suggestion was confirmed more recently by our laboratory (69,75). Neither does stearic acid raise LDL-cholesterol levels (69,37). Although one recent study (76) reported a mild LDL-raising action compared to linoleic acid, most data indicate that stearic acid is "neutral" on LDL-cholesterol levels (66,67,69,73–75). In this regard, stearic acid is similar to oleic acid, the effects of which will be discussed below.

The reason stearic acid does not increase LDL levels whereas other long-chain saturates do, is not completely understood. Contrary to early evidence in laboratory animals, over 90% of stearic acid in the human diet is absorbed (69). Investigations in both laboratory animals (77,78) and in humans (69) have noted that much of stearic acid is rapidly transformed into oleic acid. Seemingly, stearic acid does not remain long in the body as a saturated fatty acid, and this could account for its failure to raise LDL levels.

Monounsaturated Fatty Acids

Two types of monounsaturated fatty acids occur in the diet. The major kind is omega-9, *cis* 18:1 (oleic acid). It is present in both animal and vegetable products. In fact, oleic acid is the predominant fatty acid in the American diet. A lesser group of monounsaturates consists of the *trans* 18:1 fatty acids. They are produced by hydrogenation of polyunsaturated oils. The most common is elaidic acid (omega-9, *trans* 18:1), but other *trans* isomers are formed during hydrogenation. The actions of these two types of monounsaturates on serum cholesterol levels can be reviewed separately.

Dietary *oleic acid* is considered to be "neutral," neither raising nor lowering serum cholesterol levels. As indicated before, most saturated fatty acids raise the serum cholesterol relative to oleic acid (66–69). This neutrality appears to extend to all lipoproteins—VLDL, LDL, and HDL—although the primary focus in this section is on LDL. Just why oleic acid does not increase serum LDL-cholesterol levels is not fully understood. One reason may be that oleic acid is the favored substrate for acyl cholesterol acyl transferase (ACAT) in the liver (79). A large amount of oleic acid in the liver may promote the esterification of cholesterol by ACAT; this should decrease unesterified cholesterol in the liver cell, and if so, the suppressive action of unesterified cholesterol on LDL-receptor transcription could be withdrawn (37,79). Alternative LDL-lowering mechanisms for oleic acid have been envisioned. For example, enrichment of cell membranes with oleic acid might promote receptor-mediated uptake of LDL (80). Moreover, the secretion of lipoproteins by the liver could be reduced, although there is not strong evidence to support this mechanism. A complete understanding of how oleic acid effects LDL metabolism awaits further investigation.

Trans monounsaturated fatty acids have recently received considerable attention. There has long been uncertainty about their effects on cholesterol levels in humans. Until recently it was generally assumed that *trans* monounsaturates are "neutral," similar to the *cis* variety, oleic acid. Recent evidence, however, indicates that this is not true (81); *trans* fatty acids raise LDL levels relative to oleic acid. The LDL rise induced by *trans* fatty acids may be somewhat less than that caused by palmitic acid (81), but even so, all monounsaturates cannot be lumped together as "neutral" fatty acids. The *cis* and *trans* forms of monounsaturated fatty acids must be considered separately for their effects on LDL levels.

The reasons *trans* fatty acids raise LDL levels compared to oleic acid are not clear. Clearly *cis* and *trans* fatty acids differ in their steric configurations. Oleic acid molecules do not pack tightly, which explains why high-oleic oils, like olive oil, are liquids at room temperature. *Trans* monounsaturated fatty acid molecules, in contrast, fit together compactly and impart solidity to their oils. In terms of physical properties, *trans* monounsaturates behave similarly to saturated fatty acids; this similarity might explain why *trans* fatty acids have an LDL-raising property like that of saturated acids, i.e., they might have a similar effect on cholesterol distribution in the liver cell.

Polyunsaturated Fatty Acids

These are of two types: omega-6 and omega-3 acids. The major omega-6 fatty acid is linoleic acid (ω-6, 18:2). The predominant omega-3 fatty acid found in plants is linolenic acid (ω-3, 18:3); but longer-chain, omega-3 fatty acids, notably eicosapentanoic acid (EPA) (ω-3, 20:5) and docosahexanoic acid (DHA) (ω-3, 22:6), occur in fish oils. EPA and DHA comprise about 26% of the total fatty acids of fish oils.

For many years *linoleic acid* was the preferred dietary fatty acid because it was thought to be the best cholesterol-lowering fatty acid. Several early studies (66,67) reported that linoleic acid lowers total cholesterol levels compared to oleic acid. This observation contributed to recommendations for increased use of polyunsaturated vegetable oils in the diets of Americans and Europeans. Indeed, during the past 40 years, linoleic acid intakes have increased from about 4% to about 7% of total calories in the American diet. Paradoxically, at the same time, there has been a growing reservation about the safety of increased linoleate consumption. First, there has been concern on epidemiological grounds: no large population has ever consumed high amounts of linoleic acid with proven long-term safety. Moreover, in laboratory animals, diets high in linoleic acid promote chemical carcinogenesis (82,83) and suppress the immune system (84). In humans, large amounts of linoleic acid in the diet can lower HDL-cholesterol levels (68,85–87) and possibly predispose to cholesterol gallstones (88,89). Finally, enrichment of LDL lipids with linoleic acid makes them more likely to be oxidized (90,91); this action might promote atherogenesis. These possible side effects of high intakes of linoleic acid have led to modified recommendations that linoleic acid intake probably should be limited to no more than 7% of total calories.

Moreover, recent reports (68,92–94) note that linoleic acid provides little additional cholesterol lowering compared to oleic acid. In particular, LDL cholesterol appears to be reduced similarly (68,92–94). The total cholesterol lowering of linoleic acid occurs mostly in VLDL and HDL fractions (85–87). Thus, because of the possible long-term adverse effects of high intakes of linoleic acid, there is little reason to advocate higher intakes than currently exist.

The other category of polyunsaturated fatty acids—omega-3—has generated considerable interest as well. The major focus of this interest has been on EPA and DHA. These fatty acids, found in fish oils, have been claimed to improve the lipoprotein profile, reduce the danger of thrombosis, and slow down the development of atherosclerosis. The major action of omega-3 fatty acids on plasma lipids is to decrease serum triglyceride levels (95,96). Otherwise, however, EPA and DHA appear to have little beneficial effect on lipoprotein metabolism. In fact, in patients with high triglycerides, when triglycerides are reduced by omega-3 fatty acids, LDL-cholesterol concentrations often rise (97). Also, in the absence of high triglycerides, these fatty acids do not uniquely reduce LDL cholesterol. When they are exchanged for saturated fatty acids, LDL-cholesterol levels decline, but this effect is no different from that found with other types of unsaturated fatty acids.

Carbohydrates

Although much attention has been paid to dietary cholesterol and fats, the role of carbohydrates must not be overlooked. Carbohydrates are the major source of dietary calories, even in populations consuming high-fat diets. Carbohydrates provide 45–60% of the total calories in the diet. Moreover, they occur in several forms. These include simple sugars (monoglycerides and diglycerides), complex digestible carbohydrates (starches), and nondigestible carbohydrate (fiber). Fiber is present in soluble and insoluble forms; being undigestible, fiber does not contribute to total caloric intake. Generally, the complex digestible carbohydrates have been lumped together as a single group. However, it may be useful for practical purposes to divide the sources of complex carbohydrates into (a) starchy foods and (b) fruits and vegetables. The starchy foods consist of refined starches (breads and pasta) or foods of concentrated carbohydrate content (rice, potatoes, and legumes). Starchy foods contrast to fruits and vegetables in that the latter contain a significant amount of other nutrients besides their complex-carbohydrate content. Although carbohydrates from the various sources differ little in their effects on serum cholesterol levels, the *overall* nutritional benefits of different carbohydrate-rich foods probably do differ from one another, as will be discussed later.

Digestible carbohydrates as a class appear to affect total cholesterol and LDL-cholesterol levels similarly to oleic acid (66,67,98–101). They neither raise nor lower the levels, hence they, too, are called "neutral." Further, no strong evidence indicates that different types of digestible carbohydrates (simple sugars or complex carbohydrates) affect LDL-cholesterol levels differently from one another. This is not to say that carbohydrates and oleic acid have identical effects on LDL metabolism. Carbohydrates tend to raise serum triglyceride concentrations (98,102), an effect that may reduce LDL particle size and lower LDL-cholesterol/apo B ratios. For example, Kuusi et al. (103) reported that high-carbohydrate (low-fat) diets reduce LDL-cholesterol levels more than they lower LDL-apo B levels when compared to a diet high in saturated fats. In contrast, a previous study (68) showed that replacement of saturated fatty acids with oleic acid lowers levels of LDL cholesterol without reducing LDL-cholesterol/apo B ratios, i.e., LDL-apo B and LDL-cholesterol levels are lowered equally. An important question is whether high-carbohydrate diets produce any lowering of apo B levels relative to saturated fatty acids. Abbott et al. (104) reported that carbohydrates, compared to saturated fatty acids, modestly reduce LDL-apo B concentrations, but two recent reports (105,106) indicate that replacement of saturated fatty acids with carbohydrate produces no reduction in apo B levels in spite of lowering LDL-cholesterol concentrations. These latter findings raise questions about the utility of carbohydrates as a substitute for saturated fatty acids in the diet, although they do not preclude benefit.

Another unresolved issue has to do with the influence of undigestible fiber on cholesterol levels. Several reports have suggested that dietary fiber actively lowers serum cholesterol levels (107–111). This action appears to be greater for soluble fiber than for the insoluble form. A recent review (111) of all available data indicates that raising intakes of soluble fiber has the potential to lower total cholesterol levels by about 3–5% or perhaps somewhat less.

Table 2 summarizes the influence of the specific nutrients discussed above on serum levels of lipids and lipoproteins. It can be seen that each nutrient has a different action, and the net effect of the diet depends on the total amount of each nutrient consumed. The evidence indicates that each nutrient is relatively independent of the others in this effect.

TABLE 2. *Summary of influence of specific nutrients on serum lipid and lipoprotein levels*

Specific nutrient	Serum lipids and lipoproteins: Total cholesterol	Triglycerides	LDL	HDL
Dietary cholesterol	↑↑	—	↑↑	↑
Saturated fatty acids				
Palmitic acid	↑↑↑	—	↑↑↑	↑
Myristic acid	↑↑↑↑	—	↑↑↑↑	—
Lauric acid	↑↑	—	↑↑	—
Medium-chain fatty acids	↑	↑	↑	—
Stearic acid	—	—	—	—
Monounsaturated fatty acids				
Oleic acid	—	—	—	—
Trans fatty acids	↑↑	—	↑↑	↓
Polyunsaturated fatty acids				
Omega-6 (linolenic acid)	↓	↓	↓	↓
Omega-3 (EPA, DHA)	↓	↓↓↓	—	—
Carbohydrates	—	↑↑	—	↓↓

Symbols: ↑, Increase (number of arrows indicates relative increase); ↓, decrease; —, no change.

Overnutrition and Obesity

More attention generally has been given to the composition of the diet than to intake of total calories for their effects on serum cholesterol. A few early reports claimed that obesity per se has little or no effect on cholesterol levels. Most epidemiological studies, however, have found a positive correlation between body weight and cholesterol levels (12,112–116). Recently, Denke et al. (44,45) examined the link between body weight, expressed as body mass index, and serum cholesterol in both men and women. These results were derived from the large database of the Second National Health and Nutrition Examination Survey (NHANES II). Serum cholesterol levels correlated positively with body mass index for both sexes. The link, however, was more pronounced in younger adults than in older ones. A greater increment in cholesterol levels, moreover, occurred as body weight rose from lean weight to mild obesity than from the latter to marked obesity.

Only a few investigations have addressed whether weight gain per se will increase cholesterol levels. However, Anderson, et al. (117) reported that for young adult men the total cholesterol increases approximately 4 mg/dl for every kilogram of weight gain. This change is consistent with the population data reported by Denke et al. (44); both studies suggest that cholesterol concentrations in young adult men are particularly sensitive to weight gain. Although no metabolic ward studies are available in older adults, population evidence suggests a less pronounced effect of weight gain in older age groups (44).

The primary mechanism whereby obesity increases cholesterol levels seemingly is an enhancement of hepatic secretion of lipoproteins. Isotope kinetic studies indicate that the obese state promotes secretion of VLDL (57,58), and this in turn provides more VLDL for conversion to LDL (59). In many obese people, this effect raises total cholesterol and LDL-cholesterol levels (44,45). The extent to which the LDL-cholesterol level rises in response to obesity depends on one's ability to clear LDL from the circulation. If the LDL-receptor activity is high, LDL particles should be removed efficiently, and LDL-cholesterol levels therefore should not rise to abnormally high levels. On the other hand, if LDL-receptor activity is relatively suppressed, onset of obesity seemingly can produce a substantial rise in LDL levels.

Clinical experience suggests that individuals vary in their LDL-cholesterol response to changes in body weight. Some people are highly sensitive to slight increases in weight, and small weight gains induce a substantial increase in LDL levels. Others appear to be more resistant and manifest little if any increase in cholesterol concentrations with weight gain. This difference in responsiveness could have a genetic basis. Two mechanisms can be visualized. First, development of obesity could stimulate the secretion of apo B-containing lipoproteins more in some people than in others. Alternatively, there almost certainly is variability in different people's inherent LDL-receptor activity; those having a relatively low activity should demonstrate a greater hypercholesterolemic response to the development of obesity than would those with a higher baseline activity. The response in LDL levels to weight reduction may vary in a reverse way.

Although LDL responsiveness to weight reduction may be influenced by genetic factors, it also depends on diet composition. For example, in both the Multiple Risk Factor Intervention Trials (118) and in the National Diet–Heart Study (119), serum-cholesterol lowering induced by removing saturated fatty acids from the diet was doubled when patients simultaneously lost weight. In a metabolic ward study, Wolf and Grundy (120) found that weight reduction in obese, normolipidemic patients often did not lower LDL-cholesterol levels when there was no change in diet composition, i.e., no reduction in intake of saturated fatty acids. Thus, to achieve the maximal benefit for LDL lowering from weight reduction, a simultaneous decrease in intake of saturated fatty acids and cholesterol appears to be necessary.

Dietary Antioxidants

A strong body of evidence indicates that lowering LDL-cholesterol levels will reduce risk for CHD by curtailing atherogenesis. Seemingly LDL filters into the arterial wall where it participates in the development of atherosclerotic lesions. The precise mechanism whereby LDL plays this role, however, is not understood. Most investigators believe that LDL must be modified in some way to become atherogenic. Recently an intriguing hypothesis has been put forward, namely, that the oxidation of LDL is a key and crucial intermediate modification promoting atherogenesis (33). Oxidized LDL may be more susceptible than normal LDL to uptake by macrophages, and hence to foam cell formation. But oxidized LDL also may be a pathologic agent itself and may set into motion several elements of the atherogenic process. Oxidized LDL has been shown to be chemotactic and may recruit monocytes into the arterial wall where they can be transformed into foam cells. It also may be cytotoxic and damage endothelial cells and/or promote cellular secretion of several potentially atherogenic molecules. At the present time, the LDL-oxidation theory of atherogenesis is just that—a theory. But growing evidence supports this theory, and if correct, it could open a door to new therapeutic approaches to the prevention of atherosclerosis.

One of these approaches might be the use of antioxidants to prevent the formation of oxidized LDL. Support for this concept was the observation that an antioxidant drug, probucol, will prevent atherosclerosis in hypercholesterolemic rabbits (121,122). The diet itself, however, contains several antioxidants that potentially could inhibit the oxidation of LDL. Three of these are vitamins: vitamin C, vitamin E, and beta-carotene. All three will prevent the oxidation of LDL in vitro (123–125). Furthermore, high doses of vitamin E fed to humans have been shown to retard the oxidation of LDL (126,127). However, both animal studies and clinical trials will be required to prove that these antioxidants actually prevent the development of atherosclerosis. If the studies reveal benefit in retarding atherogenesis, the antioxidant vitamins could become an adjunct to cholesterol-lowering therapy for prevention of atherosclerosis. Their use would be another important step in the dietary prevention of CHD.

ATHEROGENIC DYSLIPIDEMIA

Besides an elevation of LDL-cholesterol levels, several other types of lipoprotein disorders appear to predispose to premature CHD. One pattern appears to be particularly implicated. This is the coexistence of increased VLDL remnants (usually manifest as mild hypertriglyceridemia), increased small, dense LDL particles, and low HDL levels. This lipoprotein pattern can be called *atherogenic dyslipidemia,* because of its frequent association with premature CHD. It can be classified along with hypercholesterolemia (increased LDL-cholesterol levels) as the two major patterns of atherogenic lipoprotein disorders. Some investigators believe that the atherogenic dyslipidemia pattern rivals hypercholesterolemia as a risk factor for CHD. One possibility is that a common metabolic defect underlies this dyslipidemia. If so, this single defect would have to affect the metabolism of all the lipoproteins. There is no doubt that the metabolisms of all the different lipoprotein classes are interrelated. However, it is perhaps more likely that in populations the pattern of dyslipidemia represents a constellation of disorders that produce a similar lipoprotein phenotype. In this section, two major features of the atherogenic dyslipidemic pattern—hypertriglyceridemia and low HDL cholesterol—will be addressed separately. This will allow for a more complete examination of the effects of nutrition on two major lipoprotein systems, VLDL and HDL, which may be separately involved in atherogenesis.

TRIGLYCERIDES AND VERY LOW DENSITY LIPOPROTEINS

The potential link between serum triglycerides and CHD has been a subject of great interest and considerable investigation. A large number of prospective and case–control studies reveal that serum triglyceride levels are positively correlated with CHD rates. This positive correlation is highly consistent by univariate analysis (128). The relation, however, is not so clear-cut when multivariate analysis is carried out (129,130); in such analysis total cholesterol and HDL-cholesterol levels are given priority over triglycerides because of their tighter links with CHD rates. In several studies subjected to multivariate analysis, triglyceride levels retain an "independent" relation to CHD risk, but in others they do not (see ref. 128 for review). Some investigators, however, believe that multivariate analysis may underestimate the true strength of the association between triglyceride levels and CHD risk. In so doing they mask a causative connection. It must be remembered that most serum triglycerides are carried in VLDL particles, and some forms of VLDL may be more atherogenic than others. For example, larger VLDL particles, which are rich in triglycerides but poor in cholesterol, probably are less atherogenic than are smaller VLDL particles, which tend to be enriched in cholesterol (131).

Various clinical conditions support these generalizations about the variable atherogenicity of different VLDL particles. For example, in *familial lipoprotein lipase (LDL) deficiency,* triglyceride levels are extremely elevated, but significant atherosclerosis does not develop; in this condition, the triglycerides are carried predominantly in large chylomicron particles that are poor in cholesterol; furthermore, chylomicrons probably are too large to penetrate through the intima of the arterial wall. Similarly, in *familial hypertriglyceridemia,* VLDL particles are large and triglyceride-rich (132), and risk for CHD appears to be only modestly increased (133). In contrast, with *familial combined hyperlipidemia,* the VLDL particles are smaller and contain more cholesterol (132); this disorder more strongly predisposes to premature CHD (133). Smaller VLDL particles also are found in many patients with *non-insulin-dependent diabetes mellitus* (NIDDM); elevated triglyceride concentrations have been reported to be a strong "independent" risk factor for CHD in NIDDM patients (134). Finally, in the genetic disorder called *familial dysbetalipoproteinemia,* VLDL particles are relatively small and are greatly enriched with cholesterol. These particles, called beta-VLDL, appear to be particularly atherogenic; familial dysbetalipoproteinemia is definitely accompanied by increased risk for CHD (135). Thus, enrichment of VLDL with cholesterol apparently enhances the atherogenic potential of this class of lipoproteins.

Besides the potential atherogenicity of VLDL particles, the presence of elevated triglycerides may induce other abnormalities in serum lipoproteins that promote atherosclerosis (131). For example, elevated VLDL triglycerides often delay the lipolysis of chylomicron triglycerides, and the accumulation of partially catabolized chylomicron particles (chylomicron remnants) could promote atherogenesis. High serum triglycerides also induce the formation of small, dense LDL particles that have been reported to be unusually atherogenic (29–31). Further, elevated triglycerides usually are accompanied by low HDL-cholesterol concentrations, another risk factor for CHD. Finally there is growing evidence that elevated triglycerides induce a mildly hypercoaguable state that could predispose to coronary thrombosis (136–140). Although the relative contributions of these various abnormalities to the increment in CHD risk induced by high triglycerides are difficult to define, taken together they probably raise the risk beyond that caused by elevated VLDL cholesterol alone.

To better understand the effects of nutrition on raised triglyceride and VLDL levels, the mechanisms underlying these abnormalities should be considered. Three factors determine steady-state concentrations of VLDL triglycerides: (a) rates of hepatic secretion of VLDL triglycerides, (b) rates of triglyceride lipolysis, and (c) rates of processing of VLDL remnants that are the products of this lipolysis. Processing of VLDL remnants involves either their direct removal by the liver or their conversion to LDL. Rates of hepatic secretion of VLDL triglycerides theoretically can be increased in two different ways. First, the liver might secrete an increased number of VLDL particles; as a result, input rates for both VLDL triglycerides and VLDL apo B are raised. This mechanism has been proposed as the underlying defect in familial combined hyperlipidemia. Unfortunately, available methods for studying lipoprotein kinetics cannot define precisely rates of hepatic secretion of VLDL apo B. Nonetheless, indirect evidence suggests that oversecretion of apo B-containing lipoproteins may be one cause of familial combined hyperlipidemia (60–62,141). A second mechanism for increased hepatic secretion of VLDL triglycerides is enrichment of VLDL particles with triglycerides. In this case, the number of particles secreted by the liver is not necessarily increased; instead, each particle contains increased amounts of triglyceride. This abnormality may be one cause of familial hypertriglyceridemia (132,141).

Defective lipolysis of serum triglycerides is another cause of hypertriglyceridemia. Its most severe form is found with familial LPL deficiency (142,143). This condition is accompanied by a marked elevation of chylomicrons, but VLDL triglycerides also may be elevated. A similar pattern occurs with familial deficiency of apo C-II, the apolipoprotein required for activation of LPL (142,143). Less marked deficiencies of LPL may manifest by only moderately severe hypertriglyceridemia.

Defective processing of VLDL remnants occurs in familial dysbetalipoproteinemia. Affected patients possess a defective form of apolipoprotein E (called apo E2) (144). This apolipoprotein binds poorly to hepatic receptors; consequently, removal of VLDL particles by the liver is delayed, and VLDL accumulate in the circulation. Their prolonged circulation leads to cholesterol accumulation and conversion of VLDL remnants to beta-VLDL. Less severe increases in VLDL remnants occur in hepatic triglyceride lipase deficiency, presumably because of the absence of the enzyme involved in converting VLDL to LDL.

Effects of Diet on Triglyceride Metabolism

Dietary factors are known to affect triglyceridemic metabolism. In some cases they raise triglycerides, and in others they lower triglyceride levels. Four factors affecting triglyceride levels can be considered: (a) dietary fat, (b) carbohydrates, (c) ethanol, and (d) obesity.

Dietary Fat

When patients have defective lipolysis of plasma triglycerides (e.g., LPL or apo CII deficiency), removal of chylomicrons derived from dietary fat is greatly delayed. Severe hypertriglyceridemia is the result. On the other hand, in patients with milder defects in triglyceride metabolism, dietary fat *does not* raise fasting triglyceride levels. In fact, for reasons not fully understood, high-fat diets actually produce lower triglyceride levels than do low-fat, high-carbohydrate diets (145).

The different categories of long-chain fatty acids have not been studied for their effects on triglyceride levels as systematically as they have for cholesterol levels. Data indicate that saturated fatty acids do not uniquely raise triglyceride levels compared to monounsaturated fatty acids. On the other hand, polyunsaturated fatty acids may lower serum triglycerides, at least in some individuals (146). The triglyceride-lowering action of omega-6 polyunsaturates (linoleic acid) is relatively mild (146,147), whereas omega-3 polyunsaturates (EPA and DHA) have a much more pronounced effect (147–149). The omega-3 fatty acids in particular interfere with synthesis of VLDL triglycerides in the liver. Even though omega-3 polyunsaturates lower triglyceride concentrations, they do not reduce serum total apo B levels (150). Thus, these fatty acids seemingly reduce the triglyceride content of each VLDL particle secreted into plasma, but they do not necessarily decrease the total number of VLDL particles being secreted. Thus, their utility for prevention of CHD by this mechanism can be questioned.

Carbohydrates

Compared to dietary fat, carbohydrates in the diet tend to raise triglyceride levels (151–153). Two possible mechanisms may account for this effect. First, high-carbohydrate diets may stimulate the synthesis of VLDL triglycerides by the liver (154,155); in addition, they may reduce the synthesis of LPL by adipose tissue (156). High-carbohydrate diets seemingly do not increase the number of VLDL particles being secreted by the liver, as suggested by the finding that they do not raise serum total apo B levels even when triglyceride concentrations rise (157).

Alcohol

The intake of alcohol stimulates the synthesis of triglycerides by the liver, and one manifestation of this effect is an overproduction of VLDL triglycerides (158). High intakes of alcohol usually cause a moderate rise in triglyceride levels, but in patients with an underlying hypertriglyceridemia, the response can be marked, i.e., severe hypertriglyceridemia may develop. Alcohol apparently does not raise the number of VLDL particles secreted by the liver, because it does not raise LDL concentrations (158). Although some investigators have speculated that alcohol may interfere with LPL function, its primary action for raising triglycerides almost certainly is an increased hepatic secretion of VLDL triglycerides.

Overnutrition and Obesity

It is well known that obese people frequently have high triglyceride levels. These high levels are related in part to overnutrition, because levels begin to fall immediately with the institution of caloric restriction. The obese state almost certainly increases the number of VLDL particles secreted by the liver (57–59). Previous investigations (57–59) provide three types of evidence to support this mechanism. In VLDL particles of obese people, the triglyceride content is not disproportionately increased compared to apo B, as occurs with high-carbohydrate diets or high alcohol intakes. In addition, isotope kinetic studies (57–59) suggest that hepatic secretion rates of VLDL-apo B are increased. Finally, total apo B levels often are abnormally high in obese individuals (59). Thus, elevated triglyceride concentrations found in obese individuals seemingly arise by a fundamentally different mechanism than do high triglycerides accompanying an increased intake of carbohydrate or alcohol. By the same token, obesity-induced hypertriglyceridemia probably is a more atherogenic condition.

HIGH-DENSITY LIPOPROTEINS

Levels of HDL cholesterol are inversely correlated with risk for CHD (159–161). This inverse relationship has been noted in many epidemiological studies, and it is particularly strong in high-risk populations, such as in the United States and northern Europe. In these populations, low HDL-cholesterol levels rival high LDL-cholesterol concentrations as predictors of CHD. Prospective studies (162) in the United States reveal that for every 1 mg/dl fall in HDL-cholesterol concentrations the risk for CHD increased by 2–3%. Because of the growing evidence for a link between low HDL levels and CHD, the NCEP has designated a low HDL cholesterol as a major risk factor, and recently the NCEP (26) has put increased emphasis on HDL levels for identifying and treating high-risk patients.

Nature of High-Density Lipoprotein–Coronary Heart Disease

The mechanisms whereby low HDL levels enhance risk are not as well understood as they are for elevated LDL.

Four different mechanisms have been proposed. First, a low concentration of HDL may directly promote the development of atherosclerosis; this is because HDL or its components may stimulate reverse cholesterol transport, i.e., promote the removal of cholesterol from the arterial wall (163–165). In the presence of a low HDL, this removal action may be impaired. Second, HDL may prevent the oxidation or self-aggregation of LDL within the arterial wall and thereby reduce the atherogenicity of LDL (33). Another connection may be in the link between HDL and other atherogenic lipoproteins. In particular, HDL-cholesterol concentrations frequently are inversely related to those of VLDL remnants (166–168) and small, dense LDL (29–31). In this case, the low HDL level may simply be a marker for other atherogenic factors. Third, other CHD risk factors—cigarette smoking, obesity, and lack of exercise—often are accompanied by reduced levels of HDL. Again, a low HDL cholesterol would be more of a marker than a direct cause. Thus, the possibility must be considered that several different factors account for the HDL–CHD connection, and all of them may not be due to the action of HDL to prevent directly the development of atherosclerosis.

Certain evidence nonetheless supports a direct connection between HDL levels and atherogenesis. These include animal studies in which HDL concentrations are correlated inversely with the severity of atherosclerosis (169,170). In addition, in patients in whom HDL is deficient on a genetic basis, premature CHD often is present (171–173). Third, in several clinical trials of cholesterol lowering (15–17), reduction in CHD events by therapy has been correlated with an increase in HDL levels concomitantly with a reduction in LDL concentrations. In spite of this supporting evidence, questions still remain about the precise nature of the connection between HDL and atherogenesis. For example, in some animal models, low HDL levels are not accompanied by increased atherogenesis; and some genetic forms of low HDL levels in humans seemingly do not raise CHD risk. HDL particles consist of several subspecies and contain different apolipoproteins. Only certain HDL species may actively protect against atherogensis, although the critical species have not been specifically identified.

Causes of Low High-Density Lipoprotein-Cholesterol Levels

The metabolism of HDL is complex, and it would not be surprising if low HDL levels have different causes. On the clinical level, several causes of a low HDL cholesterol have been identified. Genetic factors undoubtedly are important; in fact, about half of the variation in low HDL-cholesterol concentrations is explained by genetic variability (174). The three major nongenetic influences leading to a low HDL level are cigarette smoking, lack of exercise, and obesity (26). Further, an inverse relationship between HDL-cholesterol and triglyceride levels is well-documented; patients with high triglycerides typically have a low HDL level. Finally, certain drugs—beta-adrenergic blocking agents (beta-blockers), anabolic steroids, and progestational agents—decrease HDL concentrations. In line with the HDL-lowering action of anabolic steroids and progestational agents, it should be noted that men have lower HDL levels than do women. This difference possibly can be explained by an HDL-lowering action of androgens. In accord, HDL-cholesterol levels fall by about 10 mg/dl as boys enter puberty. These nongenetic factors acting on one's genetic constitution appear to account for most of the low HDL levels in the general population.

Precisely how these different factors lower HDL concentrations remains to be determined. However, understanding of the regulation of HDL metabolism is growing, and it may soon be possible to explain the known clinical causes of low HDL levels in mechanistic terms. A brief review of HDL metabolism may allow for speculation about molecular mechanisms and for the effects of diet on HDL metabolism. One classification divides HDL particles into more-dense (HDL_3) and less-dense (HDL_2) lipoproteins. Recently each class has been shown to consist of two subspecies, i.e., particles containing apolipoprotein (apo) AI only (LpAI) and those having both apo AI and apo AII (LpAI:AII). HDL_3 is enriched in the LpA:AII species, whereas HDL_2 contains relatively more LpAI. An early investigation (175) suggested that LpAI levels are better correlated with CHD risk than are LpAI:AII levels. More recent studies (176–180) have not fully supported this concept, but it nonetheless remains an interesting hypothesis, and deserves further investigation. A recent report from our laboratory (181) indicated that patients with low HDL levels have a greater reduction in LpAI levels than LpAI:AII levels. This observation correlates well with the well-known finding that HDL_2 levels are preferentially reduced in many patients with low HDL concentrations.

Figure 3 shows a schematic representation of the metabolism of LpAI particles. A similar pathway probably exists for LpAI:AII particles. The concepts presented are derived from a large body of evidence. The figure suggests that HDL particles containing only apo AI move in a circular pathway (the HDL cycle). Apo AI enters the circulation from the liver and gut and becomes incorporated into existing HDL_3 particles. These smaller particles acquire core cholesterol esters through the action of lecithin-cholesterol acyl transferase (LCAT); in the process, HDL_3 is expanded into HDL_{2a}. This species of HDL_2 contains mainly cholesterol ester in its core. As HDL_{2a} circulate, some of the cholesterol esters are replaced by triglycerides; this substitution occurs through interaction with triglyceride-rich particles, such as VLDL. The exchange is promoted by cholesterol ester transfer protein (CETP). In the process, HDL_{2a} is transformed into HDL_{2b}. Finally, HDL_{2b} is degraded back into HDL_3. Hepatic triglyceride lipase (HTGL) seemingly plays a major role in this conversion; this enzyme has the capability to hydrolyze both the core triglycerides and surface-coat phos-

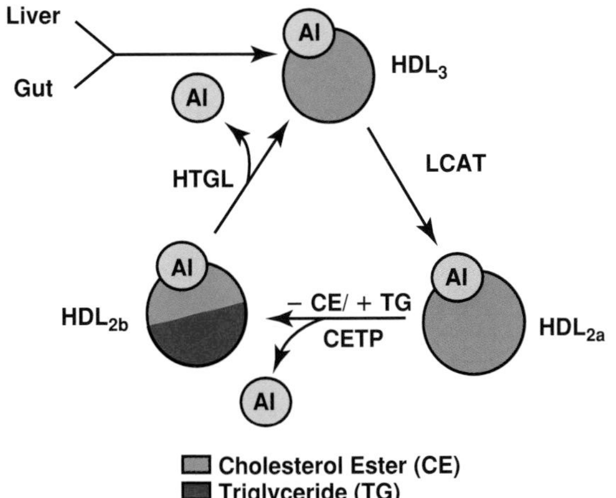

FIG. 3. The high-density lipoprotein (HDL) cycle. The pathways for metabolism of apo AI *(AI)*. The liver and gut secrete apo AI, which is first incorporated in small HDL particles *(HDL_3)*. HDL_3 is expanded by cholesterol ester through the action of lecithin-cholesterol acyl transferase *(LCAT)*. The result is a larger HDL particle *(HDL_{2a})*. This particle undergoes cholesterol ester-triglyceride exchange with triglyceride-rich lipoproteins through the action of cholesterol ester transfer protein *(CETP)*. The result is a triglyceride-enriched HDL *(HDL_{2b})*. The latter is then degraded, with loss of triglycerides, by hepatic triglyceride lipase *(HTGL)*. This results in the formation of HDL_3 again to complete the HDL cycle. At each turn of the cycle, some apo AI is lost from HDL particles.

pholipids of HDL_{2b}. We postulate that at each turn of the HDL cycle, some apo AI is freed from the particles and is lost from the circulation. Presumably, the more rapidly this cycle turns, the greater will be the amount of apo AI lost. Thus, a rapid rotation of the cycle should cause a shrinkage of the HDL pool, resulting in a fall in HDL-cholesterol levels.

In Fig. 4, the various abnormalities that may lead to a reduction in HDL-cholesterol levels are shown. First, there could be a reduction in synthesis of apo AI. Although this mechanism is attractive, most metabolic studies (182–184) have shown that patients with low HDL levels are more likely to have enhanced catabolism of apo AI than decreased input as the cause of their low HDL. Nonetheless, our investigations have revealed that individual variations in input rates for apo AI do occur, and these can affect steady-state concentrations of HDL (183). Even so, it appears that enhanced catabolism of apo AI is a more consistent cause of low HDL levels. One mechanism for an enhanced catabolism of apo AI could be an increased rate of conversion of HDL_{2a} to HDL_{2b}. This might be brought about in several ways. First, in the presence of hypertriglyceridemia, the exchange of cholesterol ester for triglycerides appears to be increased. An elevated triglyceride level is known to be associated with low HDL levels in many people. In some cases this may be the result of a deficiency of LPL, because an inverse correlation between HDL-cholesterol levels and activity of LPL has been reported (185–187). Another mechanism could be the direct transfer of apo AI from HDL particles to the surface coat of triglyceride-rich lipoproteins. Finally, an increased concentration of CETP could promote cholesterol ester–triglyceride exchange at this step. At the next step in the HDL cycle, an increased activity of HTGL may enhance the conversion of HDL_{2b} to HDL_3 with loss of apo AI. Several studies (188–190), including a recent report from our laboratory (187), have noted that increased HTGL activity is accompanied by a reduction in HDL levels. Indeed, our studies (187) suggested that an increased HTGL activity is the prime cause of reduced HDL concentrations. Of interest, men usually have higher HTGL activities than do women, a difference that could explain why men typically have lower HDL levels than do women.

The same nutritional factors that affect other lipoprotein fractions also influence HDL levels. These will be reviewed briefly. But first, an important and unresolved question is whether diet-induced alterations in HDL-cholesterol levels affect the antiatherogenic potential of HDL. For example, if a dietary change lowers HDL-cholesterol levels, does this change increase the risk for CHD? If so, recommendations about dietary modifications for the general public might have to be altered because low-fat diets, which reduce LDL cholesterol, also lower HDL levels (38,39,98,100,101). An argument against the possibility that diet-induced alterations in HDL have public health significance comes from worldwide population studies. Those populations consuming low-fat diets usually have lower rates of CHD than do populations eating high-fat diets; this is so even though average HDL levels usually are lower in the former populations (38,39). This of course does not necessarily mean that HDL lowering by diet is harmless in high-risk populations. Further, HDL lowering could be more harmful by certain dietary changes than by others. These issues will be considered in the following.

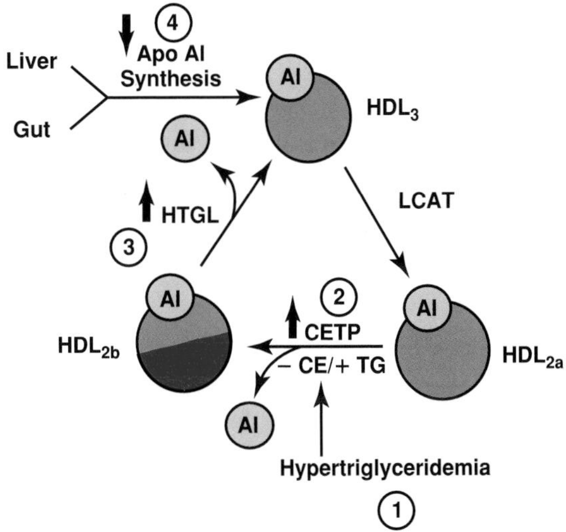

FIG. 4. Causes of low HDL cholesterol. These include (a) hypertriglyceridemia, (b) increased CETP, (c) increased HTGL, and (d) decreased apo AI synthesis.

Dietary Fat

Different dietary fats do not have identical effects on HDL-cholesterol levels. The highest HDL levels are found in populations that consume diets high in saturated fatty acids (39). This may be due in part to higher intakes of cholesterol that go along with saturated fats and also tend to raise HDL concentrations. Even so, in the metabolic ward setting, diets high in saturated fatty acids often produce the highest HDL levels (94). At the same time, these diets produce the highest LDL levels as well. The *cis* monounsaturated fatty acids (i.e., oleic acid) may yield slightly lower levels of HDL cholesterol than do saturates, but in metabolic ward investigations (98), the differences usually are not statistically significant. In contrast, *trans* monounsaturated fatty acids have been reported to cause a significant reduction in HDL levels (81). The omega-6 polyunsaturates (specifically linoleic acid) also lower HDL cholesterol when compared to oleic acid. The literature suggests that for every 2% of total calories consumed as linoleic acid, HDL-cholesterol levels decrease by about 1% (85–87,191,192). Thus, small changes in linoleic acid intake generally do not give detectable changes in HDL levels, but higher intakes do. Isotope kinetic studies indicate that high intakes of linoleic acid reduce the input of apo AI (193).

Dietary Carbohydrate

As noted before, when carbohydrates are substituted for fat in the diet, the HDL-cholesterol level declines (98–100). Apo AI and apo AII levels fall as well (101). These changes are not dependent on the type of carbohydrate (98–100) nor on duration of feeding (39). They are observed in short-term, metabolic ward studies; in addition, populations that consume low-fat, high-carbohydrate diets have relatively low HDL levels compared to those eating high-fat diets (38,39). One mechanism for reduced HDL concentrations on low-fat diets appears to be a reduced production of apo AI (193), whereas another may be the HDL-lowering effect of higher triglyceride levels induced by high-carbohydrate diets (Fig. 3).

Alcohol

Consumption of alcohol raises HDL-cholesterol levels. This effect is readily apparent in populations consuming varying amounts of alcohol. It further has been observed during feeding of alcohol to subjects on a metabolic ward (158). The precise mechanism whereby alcohol raises HDL-cholesterol levels is not known, but alcohol excess has been reported to reduce circulating levels of CETP (194). Whether alcohol also decreases the synthesis of HTGL or increases apo AI synthesis is uncertain.

Obesity

Obesity is accompanied by a reduction in HDL-cholesterol levels (44,45). A significant portion of the low HDL levels occurring in the American population is undoubtedly the result of obesity. The reasons whereby obesity reduces HDL levels could be multiple. Obesity stimulates the synthesis of VLDL triglycerides and thereby raises triglyceride levels; this effect could lower HDL concentrations (Fig. 3). Furthermore, isotope kinetic studies (132,183) indicate that even in the absence of hypertriglyceridemia, the obese state induces an increased catabolism of apo AI. This action could be related to increased synthesis of CETP and HTGL, although these possibilities have not been documented. Weight reduction causes a slow but progressive rise in HDL-cholesterol levels, and in most obese patients having low HDL levels, weight reduction restores the levels to normal (120).

NONLIPID CORONARY HEART DISEASE RISK FACTORS

The effects of nutrition on CHD risk are not confined to the lipid risk factors. The nonlipid risk factors also are affected by diet. In fact, modification of the diet can reduce the risk for CHD acting through these factors almost as much as by modifying lipid and lipoprotein levels. Two other diet-related, nonlipid risk factors are hypertension and non-insulin-dependent diabetes mellitus (NIDDM). As for total impact on CHD risk in the general population, hypertension ranks well above diabetes mellitus because it occurs more frequently. The role of nutrition in the genesis of NIDDM will be considered in another chapter in this volume. The importance of hypertension as a risk factor can be considered here briefly. A positive correlation between hypertension and CHD rates has been identified in many population studies. In a recent meta-analysis of nine major prospective studies, MacMahon et al. (195) found no evidence for a threshold relation between diastolic blood pressure and CHD rates. Using an improved statistical analysis that corrected for regression dilution bias, these workers found that prolonged differences in diastolic blood pressure of 5.0, 7.5, and 10.0 mm Hg are accompanied by at least 21%, 29%, and 37% differences in CHD rates. These estimates are higher than in older calculations that failed to correct for regression dilution bias. Thus, relatively modest reductions in blood pressure brought about by dietary change—weight loss and sodium restriction—could have a significant impact on total CHD rates in the population.

POTENTIAL FOR DIETARY PREVENTION OF CORONARY HEART DISEASE

To estimate the extent to which dietary modification theoretically could reduce CHD in our society, it is necessary first to project the contribution of diet to current CHD rates. To make this estimate, a division of coronary heart disease into premature CHD and CHD in the elderly may be helpful. The first goal of prevention is to reduce the burden of premature CHD (i.e., CHD before age 65 years). Secondary emphasis can be given to delaying the onset of CHD in older people. In all populations, even in those at lowest risk, there is progressive development of coronary atherosclerosis throughout life. However, in many low-risk populations, the severity of atherosclerosis usually does not reach a critical point at which coronary events occur in large numbers (40). Three factors besides aging seemingly account for differences in CHD rates between low-risk and high-risk populations. These are cigarette smoking, genetic susceptibility, and dietary excesses.

There is widespread agreement that cigarette smoking contributes importantly to premature CHD. Thus the first goal for prevention of CHD is to reduce smoking habits. A beneficial effect is certain. The quantitative contribution of genetic susceptibility to development of CHD in high-risk populations is less well known. Some investigators believe that high-risk populations have increased genetic susceptibility for risk factors (e.g., hypertension and hypercholesterolemia) compared to low-risk populations. Others believe that genetic makeup of different populations is basically similar and environmental factors therefore account for most of the difference in risk. Regardless, there is a general agreement that much of the difference in risk among populations is mediated through the known CHD risk factors (elevated blood pressures and cholesterol). According to the data of the Framingham Heart Study (196), the three major risk factors—cigarette smoking, hypertension, and dyslipidemia (high cholesterol and low HDL)—each contributes about one-third to excess deaths resulting from premature CHD. Thus, the essential question to address is how much do the current American and northern European diets contribute to these risk factors.

In the past there has been an uncertainty about how much the known major risk factors—cigarette smoking, hypertension, and cholesterol disorders—contribute overall to CHD rates. Estimates as low as 50% have been suggested. However, if we introduce the concept of excess deaths, i.e., deaths from CHD that can be attributed to smoking plus elevations of blood pressure and cholesterol above desirable levels of the latter two, estimates of 85–90% contribution to excess deaths have been obtained (5). These high values assume that a desirable blood pressure is below 120/80 mm Hg and a desirable total cholesterol is below 160 mg/dl. The contribution of risk factors to excess deaths would be somewhat less if the desirable blood pressure is set somewhat higher (<140/90 mm Hg) and desirable total cholesterol at <200 mg/dl; the contribution would be perhaps 70–80%.

Since diet affects both blood pressure and cholesterol levels, we can review the effects of several dietary factors (e.g., dietary cholesterol, cholesterol-raising fatty acids, obesity, and sodium chloride) on these two risk factors. Estimates of the contribution of each dietary factor are primarily for premature CHD (before age 65 years) because most available epidemiological data relate to this age group.

Dietary Cholesterol

Data accumulated over the past two decades has clarified the impact of dietary cholesterol on serum total cholesterol levels. If the results of best studies are combined (42), we can surmise that for every 100 mg of cholesterol per 1,000 calories per day, the serum total cholesterol will rise by about 6–10 mg/dl. This means that if cholesterol intakes were to be reduced by an average of 200 mg/day from current levels, the total cholesterol would fall by at least 6 mg/dl. If we employ the previously mentioned (1 mg/dl)/1% rule, then a 6 mg/dl fall in cholesterol levels would equate with a 6% reduction in CHD risk.

Cholesterol-Raising Fatty Acids

Two types of fatty acids belong in this category: three long-chain saturates [lauric acid (12:0), myristic acid (14:0), and palmitic acid (16:0)] and *trans* monounsaturated fatty acid. The current American diet contains about 14% of total calories from these fatty acids. A realistic reduction in their intake would be to decrease them by approximately 7% of total calories. According to current data on effects of cholesterol-raising fatty acids on total cholesterol levels, a 7% reduction in intake of these fatty acids should lower total cholesterol levels by about 19 mg/dl. Again the (1 mg/dl)/1% rule suggests that a 19 mg/dl reduction in cholesterol levels will decrease risk for CHD by about 19%.

Obesity and Serum Cholesterol

Obesity can adversely affect serum cholesterol levels in several ways, i.e., it can increase VLDL- and LDL-cholesterol levels and decrease HDL-cholesterol levels. To define the impact of obesity on cholesterol-related risk, we can attempt to estimate the effects of being 20 lb overweight, because this is the average degree of overweight of American men. From epidemiological data (44,45), being 20 lb overweight will raise VLDL + LDL-cholesterol levels on the average by at least 10 mg/dl and will reduce HDL cholesterol by at least 3 mg/dl. A 10 mg/dl increase in cholesterol levels will increase CHD risk by about 10%, whereas a 3 mg/dl reduction in HDL cholesterol will raise risk by at least 6%. Thus, on the average, 20 lb of overweight should increase CHD risk by about 16% via its actions on cholesterol concentrations in all lipoprotein fractions.

Obesity and Blood Pressure

A recent meta-analysis of weight reduction trials by MacMahon et al. (197) revealed a variable response in blood

TABLE 3. *Impact of dietary modification on risk for premature coronary heart disease*

Dietary change	Effect	Change in coronary heart disease risk (%)
Dietary cholesterol: 200 mg/d decrease	Serum cholesterol: 6 mg/dl decrease	−6
Cholesterol-raising fatty acids: 7% of total calorie decrease	Serum cholesterol: 19 mg/dl decrease	−19
Weight reduction: 20 lb loss	Serum cholesterol: 10 mg/dl decrease	−10
	HDL cholesterol: 3 mg/dl rise	−6
	Blood pressure: 3 mm Hg fall in diastolic pressure	−13
Dietary salt: 3 g/day decrease	Blood pressure: 5 mm Hg fall in mean blood pressure	−13
Total risk reduction		−67

pressure to weight loss. However, they estimated that on the average a 20-lb weight loss would reduce diastolic blood pressure by at least 3 mm Hg. It was further estimated that a permanent reduction in diastolic blood pressure of 3 mm Hg should decrease CHD risk by about 13%.

Dietary Salt and Blood Pressure

Although the quantitative relationship between dietary salt and blood pressure has been a disputed issue, a recent analysis and review of 33 clinical trials by Law et al. (198–200) revealed that a 50 mmol/day reduction in dietary sodium (about 3 g of salt/day) would decrease mean blood pressure by about 5 mm Hg, or, in hypertensive patients, about 7 mm Hg. Law et al. (200) estimated that this decline in blood pressure should reduce CHD risk by an amount similar to the estimated 13% decrease using the meta-analysis data of MacMahon et al. (197).

Combined Dietary Reduction of Premature CHD

Table 3 sums the reductions in risk for premature CHD that should accompany the dietary changes discussed above. For example, a 200 mg/day decrease in intake of cholesterol should reduce risk for premature CHD by approximately 6%. Decreasing cholesterol-raising fatty acids by 7% of total calories will provide another 19% decrease in risk. A 20-lb weight loss will lower risk in three ways: approximately 10% by lowering VLDL + LDL cholesterol, about 6% by raising HDL cholesterol, and another 13% by decreasing blood pressure. Finally, a 3 gm/day decrease in salt intake should add still another 13% to the reduction in CHD risk. Together these changes should produce an approximately 67% decrease in risk for premature CHD. Of interest, this estimate approximates the two-thirds of excess risk for premature CHD attributed to hypertension and cholesterol disorders in the Framingham Heart Study (196). It also is consistent with the lower rates of CHD found in populations in which the habitual diet is one that minimizes the modifiable risk factors. Certainly genetic factors affect cholesterol and blood pressure levels, but on a population basis, the excess risk attributable to the standard risk factors appears to be explained largely by dietary habits.

When considering the impact of diet on the development of premature CHD, the question naturally will arise as to the relative contributions of nutrition and genetics. Some individuals are genetically predisposed to either dyslipidemia or hypertension, and they will be unusually susceptible to the development of premature CHD. Notable examples are people who have monogenic causes of severe hypercholesterolemia (18,20). In addition, some people with elevated cholesterol (or blood pressure) are resistant to dietary change and will remain at high risk in spite of adopting a risk-reducing diet. On the other hand, for a large number of people with a genetic predisposition to CHD, it may be possible to prevent the development of premature disease by adopting healthy life habits. This point is illustrated by whole populations which have a low incidence of CHD because of their cultural eating and exercising habits. Genetic disposition to premature CHD appears to be masked by these habits.

Diet and Prevention of Coronary Heart Disease in the Elderly

Since rates of CHD rise progressively throughout life, the aging factor assumes increasing importance as a risk factor for CHD in the elderly, and the diet will decline in relative importance. Moreover, there is a natural tendency for blood pressure and cholesterol to rise with age, and these late increments appear to be less susceptible to modification by dietary intervention. The rise in cholesterol with aging occurs earlier in men, but it becomes more pronounced after the menopause in women (26). Serum total cholesterol levels in elderly women actually exceed those of men and probably contribute importantly to increasing rates of CHD in women. Furthermore, as other life-threatening illnesses in older people are controlled, atherosclerotic diseases will assume increased importance as a cause of morbidity and mortality in the elderly. This will be true even in those who have minimized their risk factors and are able to prevent premature CHD.

The above leads to the question of whether CHD rates in the elderly can be reduced significantly. Almost certainly the best way to prevent CHD in the elderly is to prevent premature CHD. Through changes in life habits initiated early in life, the rate of atherogenesis should be slowed, and this retardation should pay off in the elderly as well as in middle age. But with the rise of blood pressure and cholesterol with age, changes in life habits may not be sufficient to prevent CHD in later years. An additional approach, pharmacological control of risk factors, may be required to have a major effect on the incidence of CHD in elderly people. A good example of the pharmacological approach was the Systolic Hypertension in the Elderly Program (SHEP) (201). This trial employed low doses of diuretics and/or beta-blockers and these agents significantly reduced *both* stroke and CHD. A similar reduction in CHD events might be obtained by reducing elevated serum cholesterol with drugs in older people. The clinical benefit achieved with cholesterol lowering in secondary prevention trials suggests that efficacy would be extended to older, high-risk people. Thus, to reduce significantly the burden of CHD in the elderly, the judicious use of cholesterol-lowering drugs and antihypertensive agents may be required in a large segment of the older population.

PRACTICAL APPROACHES TO DIETARY PREVENTION OF CORONARY HEART DISEASE

Dietary Treatment of High Blood Cholesterol

The previous considerations indicate that prevention of CHD through cholesterol lowering requires several specific dietary modifications. These employ changes in diet composition, weight reduction in the obese, and reduction in salt intake. In addition, increased exercise adds further benefit. Under the category of diet composition, we can review the role of dietary cholesterol, fat, and carbohydrate.

Dietary Cholesterol

Four major sources of dietary cholesterol include (a) egg yolk, (b) animal fat, (c) animal flesh (muscle), and (d) internal organs (liver, pancreas, kidney, and brain). A practical reduction in cholesterol intake should focus on decreasing consumption of egg yolk, animal fat, and internal organs. If these sources of cholesterol are largely eliminated, the cholesterol present in animal muscle (lean meat) should not provide more than 200 mg/day of cholesterol. With this approach a sufficient decrease in cholesterol should be acceptable for most people.

Dietary Fat

The primary goal for fat modification is to reduce intake of cholesterol-raising fatty acids. These include saturated fatty acids of C12 to C16 and *trans* monounsaturates. A reasonable aim is to cut in half intakes of cholesterol-raising fatty acids. The primary focus of change will be to reduce intakes of animal fats. These include the fat associated with meats as well as milk fat. The former requires use of lean meat and avoidance of processed high-fat meats. The use of low-fat or, preferably, nonfat milk products is especially important. This calls for a marked reduction in intakes of whole milk, butter, ice cream, cream, and cheese, a challenge to the dairy industry to develop acceptable low-fat, milk-based products that can be substituted for high-fat products. Finally, the major sources of *trans* fatty acids—hard margarines, shortenings, and bakery goods rich in *trans* fatty acids—will have to be decreased. Alternative products that are low in cholesterol-raising fatty acids ought to be developed to use in their place. Consideration can be given to substituting stearic acid for cholesterol-raising fatty acids in some food products because it has similar physical properties but not a cholesterol-raising potential. It might be noted that beef fat is high in stearic acid, which enhances the acceptability of lean-meat products. The small amount of meat fat that remains in lean meat will have less effect on cholesterol levels than was previously thought.

Recently there has been a controversy about the utility of hydrogenated vegetable oils in the American diet. Without question, currently available products—margarines and shortenings—have the ability to raise LDL-cholesterol levels. This is due to their content of *trans* fatty acids. The stearic acid produced in hydrogenation does not increase LDL levels. It is important to compare hydrogenated vegetable oils with the animal fats they replace in their cholesterol-raising potential. Butter and tropical oils are the most potent cholesterol-raising fats, more so than even the most hydrogenated shortenings. The latter have about the same cholesterol-raising potential as beef and pork fat. The soft margarines have only a modest cholesterol-raising property. Thus, there is a marked difference between the effects of butter and soft margarines on cholesterol levels, and the latter is preferable in cholesterol-lowering diets.

Although it was previously believed that linoleic acid is the best fatty acid replacement for cholesterol-raising fatty acids, the growing concern about possible adverse effects of its long-term ingestion has led to a more cautious recommendation. Intakes of oils high in linoleic acid (e.g., corn oil and high-linoleic acid forms of safflower oil, sunflower seed oil, and soybean oil) therefore should be limited. They can be replaced with oils higher in oleic acid (e.g., olive oil, canola oil, and high-oleic forms of safflower oil and sunflower seed oil). In the future industry should be able to provide both processed food and animal products that are enriched in oleic acid. The introduction of these products will make possible more variety in cholesterol-lowering diets.

Carbohydrates

Another potential replacement for fatty acids that increase cholesterol is carbohydrate. Its use will reduce LDL-cholesterol levels as much as oleic acid. However, its effects on total apo B levels appear to be less pronounced. One question that generates great interest is what should be the relative proportions of total fat and total carbohydrate in the diet. Some investigators believe that simple exchange of unsaturated fatty acids for cholesterol-raising fatty acids will *not* produce the greatest benefit from diet change, even though it should produce a maximal reduction in LDL cholesterol that can be achieved with diet. Instead, they believe that carbohydrate should primarily replace the offending fatty acids. The latter view has largely prevailed as reflected by current diet recommendations. These are based on three arguments. First, replacement of cholesterol-raising fatty acids with carbohydrate will lower LDL-cholesterol levels. Second, it may be difficult to completely replace fat calories with carbohydrate calories, hence total caloric intake may fall; this should promote weight reduction. Third, low-fat diets may reduce the risk for cancer. Each of these arguments is worthy of more careful examination.

There is no question that substitution of carbohydrate for the cholesterol-raising fatty acids will lower LDL-cholesterol levels. The reduction will be similar to that produced by unsaturated fatty acids. However, carbohydrates have several effects on lipoprotein levels that are potentially adverse. They tend to raise VLDL levels, lower HDL levels, and may induce small, dense LDL particles. In addition, they may not lower the level of total apo B. All of these changes have been reported to increase CHD risk. Whether risk is raised when this ''atherogenic'' profile is induced by carbohydrate is unknown, but at least their presence does introduce a note of caution.

The proposition that reducing fat intake will lead to weight loss in overweight persons deserves consideration. The basic notion is that carbohydrates are calorically less dense than fats, and people have a natural tendency to overingest fat calories. Consequently, when carbohydrate replaces fat in the diet, total caloric intake will unconsciously be reduced, and weight reduction will occur. Although this concept is widely accepted, very few data actually support it. Of particular interest, over the past decade there has been a progessive decline in percentage of total calories as fat in the general population, but surprisingly, the average body weight of Americans has been increasing. This raises the possibility that Americans have overcompensated to a lower fat intake and have actually increased total calories through a greater consumption of carbohydrate. Thus, reducing fat intake may not ''automatically'' cause weight reduction as some have proposed.

Finally, do low-fat diets reduce the risk for cancer compared to high-fat diets? This question has not been answered adequately; it is a complex issue having several components. For example, certain types of fatty acids, such as saturates and polyunsaturates, may promote the development of cancer. On the other hand, there is no evidence that dietary oleic acid predisposes to cancer. Also to be considered is the possibility that factors in certain high-carbohydrate foods may protect against cancer. Epidemiological studies strongly suggest that high intakes of fruits and vegetables provide a barrier against certain forms of cancer. The critical factor might be antioxidant vitamins, but perhaps there are other protective agents.

If fruits and vegetables do contain anticancer factors, these must be differentiated from carbohydrates per se. Fruits and vegetables tend to be high in other compounds relative to their carbohydrate content. There is little likelihood that overconsumption of fruits and vegetables per se will promote obesity. On the other hand, increased intakes of calorically dense carbohydrates (e.g., sugars and starchy foods) could lead to increasing body weight without providing any extra benefit. Thus, any recommendation to increase carbohydrate intake in a cholesterol-lowering diet probably should be restricted to fruits and vegetables.

Weight Reduction

There is a widespread pessimism about the possibility of successful weight loss in obese patients. This pessimism, however, may not be justified for many overweight persons. For example, whereas severely overweight people often have great difficulty in losing weight, less obese persons are much more likely to be successful. Overweight men, who tend to suffer the cardiovascular complications of obesity earlier than women, often are particularly successful in losing weight. It must be remembered that only mild degrees of obesity, 10–20 lb overweight, can unfavorably affect both lipid levels and blood pressure, and removal of this excess weight can significantly lower risk. A few points need to be made about weight-loss therapy. Greater success is usually achieved when a patient works with a trained nutritionist on a long-term basis. Attempts at rapid weight loss with very low calorie diets almost always are unsuccessful; these efforts do not modify long-term eating habits. Programs using a slower weight loss and behavioral modification techniques under professional guidance are more likely to be successful. Patients should set long-term goals for weight loss and should strive to reach these goals over a period of many months, or years if necessary.

Three Patterns of Cholesterol-Lowering Diets

Epidemiological studies point to two different eating patterns in large populations that are associated with low rates of CHD. One of these is the ''Asian diet'' that is typical of the diet consumed in China and Japan. This diet is a low-fat diet: fat intakes of 10–20% of total calories are typical. Intakes of dietary cholesterol and cholesterol-raising fatty acids also are low. The other pattern is the ''Mediterranean diet,'' which is the traditional diet of Greece, Crete, and southern Italy. It is relatively high in fat (30–40% of total calories), but most of the fat calories come from olive oil. Intakes of dietary cholesterol and fatty acids that raise cholesterol also are low, as are rates of CHD. Either of these

TABLE 4. *Recommended dietary modifications to lower serum cholesterol*

	Choose	Decrease
Fish, chicken, turkey, and lean meats	Fish, poultry without skin, lean cuts of beef, lamb, pork or veal, shellfish	Fatty cuts of beef, lamb, pork; spare ribs, organ meats, regular cold cuts, sausage, hot dogs, bacon, sardines, roe
Skim and low-fat milk, cheese, yogurt, and dairy substitutes	Skim or 1% fat milk (liquid, powdered, evaporated)	Whole milk (4% fat): regular, evaporated, condensed; cream, half and half, 2% milk, imitation milk products, most nondairy creamers, whipped toppings
	Buttermilk	
	Nonfat (0% fat) or low-fat yogurt	Whole-milk yogurt
	Low-fat cottage cheese (1% or 2% fat)	Whole-milk cottage cheese (4% fat)
	Low-fat cheeses, farmer, or pot cheeses (all of these should be labeled no more than 2–6 g fat/oz)	All natural cheeses (e.g. blue, roquefort, camembert, cheddar, swiss)
	Low-fat or "Light" cream cheese, low-fat or "Light" sour cream	Cream cheeses, sour cream
	Sherbet	Ice cream
	Sorbet	
Eggs	Egg whites (2 whites = 1 whole egg in recipes), cholesterol-free egg substitutes	Egg yolks
Fruits and vegetables	Fresh, frozen, canned, or dried fruits and vegetables	Vegetables prepared in butter, cream, or other sauces
Breads and cereals	Homemade baked goods using unsaturated oils sparingly, angel food cake, low-fat crackers, low-fat cookies	Commercial baked goods: pies, cakes, doughnuts, croissants, pastries, muffins, biscuits, high-fat crackers, high-fat cookies
	Rice, pasta	Egg noodles
	Whole-grain breads and cereals (oatmeal, whole wheat, rye, bran, multigrain, etc.)	Breads in which eggs are major ingredient
Fats and oils	Baking cocoa	Chocolate
	Unsaturated vegetable oils: corn, olive, rapeseed (canola oil), safflower, sesame, soybean, sunflower	Butter, coconut oil, palm oil, palm kernel oil, lard, bacon fat
	Margarine or shortening made from one of the unsaturated oils listed above	
	Diet margarine	
	Mayonnaise, salad dressings made with unsaturated oils listed above	Dressings made with egg yolk
	Low-fat dressing	
	Seeds and nuts	Coconut

Adapted from ref. 201.

two eating patterns appears to be acceptable for dietary prevention of CHD. Both may be attractive to many Americans as alternatives to the typical America diet.

Nonetheless, it is not necessary for Americans to completely reject their traditional eating habits in favor of diets typical of populations living elsewhere in the world. Many Americans may want to incorporate components of the Asian or Mediterranean diets into their eating habits. but it is not necessary to do away with traditional foods. What is needed is to modify these foods in such a way as to make them less atherogenic. This essentially means to reduce their contents of cholesterol and cholesterol-raising fatty acids. Practical suggestions for modifying the diet are listed in Table 4. In particular, animal products need to be modified to decrease their fat content. Egg yolks should be reduced and replaced with cholesterol-free substitutes. Animal products (meat and milk products) should be modified by removal of fat. This fat can either not be replaced or be replaced with unsaturated fat. Margarines and shortenings can be produced with natural oils that do not employ *trans* fatty acids. To some extent stearic acid may be used in the place of *trans* fatty acids. These changes will allow Americans to continue to consume traditional foods without their current drawbacks. Even so, there is a need for the introduction of more fruits and vegetables into the American diet at the expense of concentrated carbohydrate sources (starchy food and simple sugars).

Finally, a greater effort must be made to reverse the trend toward increasing obesity and decreasing exercise. Overweight has emerged as the foremost nutritional problem in the United States, and new strategies to reversing obesity through public health and clinical approaches are a challenge to future research. CHD risk can be further reduced by combining regular exercise with improved nutrition.

Dietary Treatment of Atherogenic Dyslipidemia

Although the pattern of atherogenic dyslipidemia (increased VLDL remnants, increased small, dense LDL, and low HDL levels) is being recognized increasingly as a risk factor, less attention has been given to its dietary control than for hypercholesterolemia. In the past few years, however as more attention has been drawn to the risk accompanying atherogenic dyslipidemia, the issue of its dietary management has come under focus. Ideally, the nutritional control of hypercholesterolemia and atherogenic dyslipidemia would be the same. To some extent, a common approach may be possible. However, some modifications to current recommendations may be necessary for those individuals who have this lipoprotein pattern. First, common approaches can be addressed, and second, differences can be considered.

In patients who have atherogenic dyslipidemia, weight reduction deserves first consideration. Weight loss will lower VLDL triglycerides, raise HDL cholesterol, and perhaps convert small, dense LDL into normal-sized LDL particles. These beneficial effects of weight reduction may be amplified by regular physical activity. Exercise likewise will help to lower triglycerides and raise HDL levels. Thus, the combination of weight reduction and exercise is the principal approach to the dietary management of atherogenic dyslipidemia.

A reduction in intake of saturated fatty acids and cholesterol also can be recommended for patients with this lipoprotein pattern. This dietary change will help to lower LDL-cholesterol levels. However, replacement of saturated fatty acids with carbohydrate may not be appropriate. Low-fat, high-carbohydrate diets tend to further raise triglycerides and to lower HDL levels. A better replacement for saturated fatty acids will be unsaturated fatty acids. Among the latter, linoleic acid may more effectively reduce triglycerides than will oleic acid, but the former may carry more side effects as discussed before. Therefore, oleic acid probably is preferable as a substitute for cholesterol-raising fatty acids. Omega-3 fatty acids will produce the best lowering of triglycerides, but they have certain drawbacks for long-term use: they are inconvenient to take, they may be accompanied by unpleasant side effects, and they do not reduce total apo B levels. Therefore, they generally are not employed in dietary treatment of hypertriglyceridemia.

Finally, there is the question of whether moderate amounts of alcohol should be recommended for patients with low HDL-cholesterol levels. Alcohol is known to raise HDL levels and several epidemiological studies indicate that a relatively high consumption of alcohol, especially wine, is associated with a reduced risk for CHD. The latter observation in particular has led some investigators to advocate a daily consumption of moderate amounts of alcohol. However, before such a recommendation can be made, several caveats must be mentioned. Excess alcohol consumption has many potential side effects, and any prescription to increase its use carries the risk of misuse. Certainly its putative value in preventing CHD has never been documented in a controlled clinical trial. Also, alcohol has triglyceride-raising effects, and particularly in patients with atherogenic dyslipidemia, who have relatively high triglyceride levels, consumption of alcohol often will further raise the levels. For these reasons, the use of alcohol for the purpose of CHD prevention must be individualized and made with the understanding that it remains to be proven that its benefits overweigh its side effects.

REFERENCES

1. National Cholesterol Education Program. Report of the Expert Panel on Population Strategies for Blood Cholesterol Reduction. *Circulation* 1991;83:2154.
2. Grundy SM, Bilheimer D, Blackburn H, et al. Rationale of the diet–heart statement of the American Heart Association: Report of Nutrition Committee. *Circulation* 1982;65:839A–854A.
3. National Research Council, Committee on Diet and Health, Food and Nutrition Board, and Commission on Life Sciences. *Diet and health: Implications for reducing chronic disease risk.* Washington, D.C.: National Academy Press; 1989:749.
4. Gordon T, Kannel WB, Castelli WP, Dawber TR. Lipoproteins, cardiovascular disease, and death: The Framingham Study. *Arch Intern Med* 1981;141:1128–1131.
5. Stamler J, Wentworth D, Neaton J. Is the relationship between serum cholesterol and risk of death from CHD continuous and graded? *JAMA* 1986;256:2823–2328.
6. Pooling Project Research Group. Relationship of blood pressure, serum cholesterol, smoking habit, relative weight and ECG abnormalities to incidence of major coronary events: Final report of the Pooling Project. *Am Heart Assoc Monograph* 1978;60.
7. Anderson KM, Castelli WP, Levy DL. Cholesterol and mortality: 30 years of follow-up from the Framingham Study. *JAMA* 1987;257: 2176–2180.
8. Anitschkow N, Chalatow S. Ueber experimentelle cholesterinseatose und ihre bedeutung fur die entstehung einiger pathologisher prozesse. *Zentralbl Allg Pathol Pathol Anat* 1913;24:1–9.
9. Strong JP, McGill HC. Diet and experimental atherosclerosis in baboons. *Am J Pathol* 1967;50:669–690.
10. Strong JP. Atherosclerosis in primates. Introduction and overview. *Primates Med* 1976;9:1–15.
11. McGill HC Jr, McMahan CA, Kruski AW, Mott GE. Relationship of lipoprotein cholesterol concentrations to experimental atherosclerosis in baboons. *Arteriosclerosis* 1981;1:3–12.
12. Keys A. *Seven countries: a multivariate analysis on death and coronary heart disease.* Cambridge, Massachusetts: Harvard University Press; 1980:132.
13. Keys A, Menotti A, Aravanis C, et al. The Seven Countries Study: 2,289 deaths in 15 years. *Prev Med* 1984;13:141–154.
14. Kagan A, Harris BR, Winkelstein W Jr, et al. Epidemiologic studies of coronary heart disease and stroke in Japanese men living in Japan, Hawaii and California: Demographic physical, dietary and biochemical characteristics. *J Chron Dis* 1974;27:345–364.
15. Lipid Research Clinics Program. The Lipid Research Clinics coronary primary prevention trial results: I. Reduction in the incidence of coronary heart disease. *JAMA* 1984;251:351–364.
16. Lipid Research Clinics Program. The Lipid Research Clinics coronary primary prevention trial results: II. The relationship of reduction in incidence of coronary heart disease to cholesterol lowering. *JAMA* 1984;251:365–374.
17. Frick MH, Elo MO, Haapa K, et al. Helsinki Heart Study: primary prevention trial with gemfibrozil in middle-aged men with dyslipidemia. *N Engl J Med* 1987;317:1237–1245.
18. Goldstein JL, Brown MS. Familial hypercholesterolemia. In: Scriver CR, Beaudet AL, Sly WS, Valle D, eds. *The Metabolic Basis of Inherited Disease.* New York: McGraw-Hill; 1989:1215–1250.
19. Vega GL, Grundy SM. *In vivo* evidence for reduced binding of low density lipoproteins to receptors as a cause of primary moderate hypercholesterolemia. *J Clin Invest* 1986;78:1410–1414.
20. Innerarity TL, Mahley RW, Weisgraber KH, et al. Familial defective apolipoprotein B-100: a mutation of apolipoprotein B that causes hypercholesterolemia. *J Lipid Res* 1990;31:1337–1349.
21. Rauh G. Familial defective apolipoprotein B100: clinical characteristics of 54 cases. *Atherosclerosis* 1992;92(2–3):233–241.

22. Tybjaerg-Hansen A, Humphries SE. Familial defective apolipoprotein B-100: a single mutation that causes hypercholesterolemia and premature coronary artery disease. *Atherosclerosis* 1992;96:91–107.
23. Blankenhorn DM, Nessim SA, Johnson RL, Sanmarco ME, Azen SP, Cashin-Hemphill L. Beneficial effects of combined colestipol–niacin therapy on coronary atherosclerosis and coronary venous bypass grafts. *JAMA* 1987;257:3233–3240.
24. Brown G, Albers JJ, Fisher LD, et al. Regression of coronary artery disease as a result of intensive lipid-lowering therapy in men with high levels of apolipoprotein B. *N Engl J Med* 1990;323:1289–1298.
25. Buchwald H, Varco RL, Matts JP, et al. Effect of partial ileal bypass surgery on mortality and morbidity from coronary heart disease in patients with hypercholesterolemia. Report of the Program on the Surgical Control of Hyperlipidemias (POSCH). *N Engl J Med* 1990; 323:946–955.
26. Expert Panel on Detection, Evaluation, and Treatment of High Blood Cholesterol in Adults. National Cholesterol Education Program: second report of the Expert Panel on Detection, Evaluation, and Treatment of High Blood Cholesterol in Adults (Adult Treatment Panel II). *Circulation* 1994;89:1329–1445.
27. Vega GL, Denke MA, Grundy SM. Metabolic basis of primary hypercholesterolemia. *Circulation* 1991;84:118–128.
28. Abate N, Vega GL, Grundy SM. Variability in cholesterol content and physical properties of lipoproteins containing apolipoprotein B-100. *Atherosclerosis* 1993;104:159–171.
29. Austin MA, Breslow JL, Hennekens CH, Buring JE, Willett KC, Krauss RM. Low-density lipoprotein subclass patterns and risk of myocardial infarction. *JAMA* 1988;260:1917–1921.
30. Austin MA, King MC, Vranizan KM, Newman B, Krauss RM. Inheritance of low density lipoprotein subclass patterns: Results of complex segregation analysis. *Am J Hum Genet* 1988;43:838–846.
31. Austin MA, King MC, Vranizan KM, Krauss RM. Atherogenic lipoprotein phenotype: A proposed genetic marker for coronary heart disease risk. *Circulation* 1990;82:495–506.
32. De Graaf J, Hak-Lemmers HLM, Hectors MPC, Demacker PNM, Henricks JCM, Stalenhoef AFH. Enhanced susceptibility to *in vitro* oxidation of the dense low density lipoprotein subfraction in healthy subjects. *Arterioscler Thromb* 1991;11:298–306.
33. Steinberg D, Parthasarathy S, Carew TE, Khoo JC, Witztum JL. Beyond cholesterol: modifications of low-density lipoprotein that increase its atherogenicity. *N Engl J Med* 1989;320:915–923.
34. Rudel LL, Pitts LL II, Nelson CA. Characterization of plasma low density lipoproteins of nonhuman primates fed dietary cholesterol. *J Lipid Res* 1977;18:211–222.
35. Davis C, Rifkind B, Brenner H, Gordon D. A single cholesterol measurement underestimates the risk of CHD. An empirical example from the Lipid Research Clinics mortality follow-up study. *JAMA* 1990; 264:3044–3046.
36. Malenka DJ, Baron JA. Cholesterol and coronary heart disease. The importance of patient-specific attributable risk. *Arch Intern Med* 1988; 148:2247–2252.
37. Grundy SM. Multifactorial etiology of hypercholesterolemia: implications for prevention of coronary heart disease. *Arterioscler Thromb* 1991;11:1619–1635.
38. Kesteloot H, Huang DX, Yang XS, et al. Serum lipids in the People's Republic of China: Comparison of western and eastern populations. *Arteriosclerosis* 1985;5:427–433.
39. Knuiman JT, West CE, Katan MB, Hautvast JGA. Total cholesterol and high density lipoprotein cholesterol levels in populations differing in fat and carbohydrate intake. *Arteriosclerosis* 1987;7:612–619.
40. Grundy SM. Cholesterol and coronary heart disease: a new era. *JAMA* 1986;256:2849–2858.
41. Jacobs D, Blackburn H, Higgins M. Report of the Conference on Low Blood Cholesterol: Mortality association. *Circulation* 1992;86: 1046–1060.
42. Grundy SM, Barrett-Connor E, Rudel LL, Miettinen T, Spector AA. Workshop on the impact of dietary cholesterol on plasma lipoproteins and atherogenesis. *Arteriosclerosis* 1988;8:95–101.
43. Mensink RP, Katan MB. Effects of dietary fatty acids on serum lipids and lipoproteins: A meta-analysis of 27 trials. *Arterioscler Thromb* 1992;12:911–919.
44. Denke MA, Sempos CT, Grundy SM. Excess body weight: An underrecognized contributor to high blood cholesterol in Caucasian American men. *Arch Intern Med* 1993;153:1093–1103.
45. Denke MA, Sempos CT, Grundy SM. Excess body weight: an underrecognized contributor to dyslipidemia in white American women. *Arch Intern Med* 1994;401–410.
46. Goldstein JL, Brown MS. The low density lipoprotein receptor and its relation to atherosclerosis. *Annu Rev Biochem* 1977;46:879–930.
47. Kovanen PT, Brown MS, Basu SK, Bilheimer DW, Goldstein JL. Saturation and suppression of hepatic lipoprotein receptors: A mechanism for the hypercholesterolemia of cholesterol-fed rabbits. *Proc Natl Acad Sci USA* 1981;78:1396–1400.
48. Sorci-Thomas M, Wilson MD, Johnson FL, Williams DL, Rudel LL. Studies on the expression of genes encoding apolipoproteins B100 and B48 and the low density lipoprotein receptor in nonhuman primates. *J Biol Chem* 1989;264(15):9039–9045.
49. Spady DK, Dietschy JM. Dietary saturated triglycerides suppress hepatic low density lipoprotein receptors in the hamster. *Proc Natl Acad Sci USA* 1985;82:4526–4530.
50. Fox JC, McGill HC Jr, Carey KD, Getz GS. *In vivo* regulation of hepatic LDL receptor mRNA in the baboon: Differential effects of saturated and unsaturated fat. *J Biol Chem* 1987;262:7014–7020.
51. Nicolosi RJ, Stucchi AF, Kowala MC, Hennessy LK, Hegsted DM, Schaefer EJ. Effect of dietary fat saturation and cholesterol on LDL composition and metabolism. *Arteriosclerosis* 1990;10:119–128.
52. Miller NE. Why does plasma low density lipoprotein concentration in adults increase with age? *Lancet* 1984;1:263–266.
53. Grundy SM, Vega GL, Bilheimer DW. Kinetic mechanisms determining variability in low density lipoprotein levels and their rise with age. *Arteriosclerosis* 1985;5:623–630.
54. Ericsson S, Eriksson M, Vitols S, Einarsson K, Berglund L, Angelin B. Influence of age on the metabolism of plasma low density lipoproteins in healthy males. *J Clin Invest* 1991;87:591–596.
55. Ma PT, Yamamoto T, Goldstein JL, Brown MS. Increased mRNA for low density lipoprotein receptor in livers of rabbits treated with 17 alpha-ethinyl estradiol. *Proc Natl Acad Sci USA* 1986;83:792–796.
56. Eriksson M, Berglund L, Rudling M, Henriksson P, Angelin B. Effects of estrogen on low density lipoprotein metabolism in males: Short-term and long-term studies during hormonal treatment of prostatic carcinoma. *J Clin Invest* 1989;84:802–810.
57. Kesaniemi YA, Beltz WF, Grundy SM. Comparisons of metabolism of apolipoprotein B in normal subjects, obese patients, and patients with coronary heart disease. *J Clin Invest* 1985;76:586–595.
58. Egusa G, Beltz WF, Grundy SM, Howard BV. Influence of obesity on the metabolism of apolipoprotein B in man. *J Clin Invest* 1985; 76:596–603.
59. Kesaniemi YA, Grundy SM. Increased low density lipoprotein production associated with obesity. *Arteriosclerosis* 1983;3:170–177.
60. Janus ED, Nicoll AM, Turner PR, Magill P, Lewis B. Kinetic basis of the primary hyperlipidaemias: Studies of apolipoprotein B turnover in genetically-defined subjects. *Eur J Clin Invest* 1980;10:161–171.
61. Teng B, Sniderman AD, Soutar AK, Thompson GR. Metabolic basis of hyperapobetalipoproteinemia: turnover of apolipoprotein B in low density lipoproteins and its precursors and subfractions compared with normal and familial hypercholesterolemia. *J Clin Invest* 1986;77: 663–672.
62. Kissebah AH, Alfarsi S, Evans DJ. Low density lipoprotein metabolism in familial combined hyperlipidemia: mechanism of the multiple lipoprotein phenotypic expression. *Arteriosclerosis* 1984;4:614–624.
63. Grundy SM, Vega GL. Plasma cholesterol responsiveness to saturated fatty acids. *Am J Clin Nutr* 1988;47:822–824.
64. Denke MA, Grundy SM. Individual responses to a cholesterol-lowering diet in fifty men with moderate hypercholesterolemia. *Arch Intern Med* 1994;154:317–325.
65. Grundy SM, Denke MA. Dietary influence on serum lipids and lipoproteins. *J Lipid Res* 1990;31:1149–1192.
66. Keys A, Anderson JT, Grande F. Serum cholesterol response to changes in the diet. IV. Particular saturated fatty acids in the diet. *Metabolism* 1965;14:776–787.
67. Hegsted DM, McGandy RB, Myers ML, Stare FJ. Quantitative effects of dietary fat on serum cholesterol in man. *Am J Clin Nutr* 1965;17: 281–295.
68. Mattson FH, Grundy SM. Comparison of effects of dietary saturated, monounsaturated, and polyunsaturated fatty acids on plasma lipids and lipoproteins in man. *J Lipid Res* 1985;26:194–202.
69. Bonanome A, Grundy SM. Effect of dietary stearic acid on plasma

cholesterol and lipoprotein levels. *N Engl J Med* 1988;318: 1244–1248.
70. Grande F. Dog serum lipid responses to dietary fats differing in the chain length of the saturated fatty acids. *J Nutr* 1962;76:255–264.
71. Hashim SA, Arteaga A, van Itallie TB. Effect of a saturated medium-chain triglyceride on serum-lipids in man. *Lancet* 1960;1:1105–1108.
72. Denke MA, Grundy SM. Comparison of effects of lauric acid and palmitic acid on plasma lipids and lipoproteins. *Am J Clin Nutr* 1992; 56:895–898.
73. Ahrens EH, Hirsch J, Insull W, Tsaltas TT, Blomstrand R, Peterson ML. The influence of dietary fats on serum-lipid levels in man. *Lancet* 1957;1:943–953.
74. Kritchevsky D, Tepper SA, Bises G, Kleinfeld DM. Experimental atherosclerosis in rabbits fed cholesterol-free diets. Part 10. Cocoa butter and palm oil. *Atherosclerosis* 1982;41:279–284.
75. Denke MA, Grundy SM. Effects of fats high in stearic acid on lipid and lipoprotein concentrations in men. *Am J Clin Nutr* 1991;54: 1036–1040.
76. Zock PL, Katan MB. Hydrogenation alternatives: effects of *trans* fatty acids and stearic acid versus linoleic acid on serum lipids and lipoproteins in humans. *J Lipid Res* 1992;33:399–410.
77. Elovson J. Immediate fate of albumin bound [I-14C] stearic acid following its intraportal injection into carbohydrate refed rats. Early course of desaturation and esterification. *Biochim Biophys Acta* 1965; 106:480–494.
78. Bonanome A, Bennett M, Grundy SM. Metabolic effects of dietary stearic acid in mice: changes in the fatty acid composition of triglycerides and phospholipids in various tissues. *Atherosclerosis* 1992;94: 119–127.
79. Daumeri CM, Woollett LA, Dietary JM. Fatty acids regulate hepatic low density lipoprotein receptor activity through redistribution of intracellular cholesterol pools. *Proc Natl Acid Sci USA* 1992;89: 10797–10801.
80. Loscalzo J, Fredman J, Rudd RM, Barsky-Vasserman I, Vaughan DE. Unsaturated fatty acids enhance low density lipoprotein uptake and degradation by peripheral blood mononuclear cells. *Arteriosclerosis* 1987;7:450–455.
81. Mensink RP, Katan MB. Effect of dietary *trans* fatty acids on high-density and low-density lipoprotein cholesterol levels in healthy subjects. *N Engl J Med* 1990;323:439–445.
82. Carroll KK, Khor HT. Effects of level and type of dietary fat on incidence of mammary tumors induced in female Sprague-Dawley rats by 7, 12-dimethylbenz (alpha) anthracene. *Lipids* 1971;6:415–420.
83. Reddy BS. Amount and type of dietary fat and colon cancer: Animal model studies. *Prog Clin Biol Res* 1986;222:295–309.
84. Weyman C, Berlin J, Smith AD, Thompson RSH. Linoleic acid as an immunosuppressive agent. *Lancet* 1975;2:33–34.
85. Vega GL, Groszek E, Wolf R, Grundy SM. Influence of polyunsaturated fats on composition of plasma lipoproteins and apolipoproteins. *J Lipid Res* 1982;23:811–822.
86. Shepherd J, Packard CJ, Patsch JR, Gotto AM Jr, Taunton OD. Effects of dietary polyunsaturated and saturated fat on the properties of high density lipoprotein and the metabolism of apolipoprotein. *J Clin Invest* 1978;60:1582–1592.
87. Jackson RL, Kashyap ML, Barnhart RL, Allen C, Hogg E, Glueck CJ. Influence of polyunsaturated and saturated fats on plasma lipids and lipoproteins in man. *Am J Clin Nutr* 1984;39:589–597.
88. Grundy SM. Effects of polyunsaturated fats on lipid metabolism in patients with hypertriglyceridemia. *J Clin Invest* 1975;55:269–282.
89. Sturdevant RAL, Pearce ML, Dayton S. Increased prevalence of cholelithiasis in men ingesting a serum cholesterol-lowering diet. *N Engl J Med* 1973;288:24–27.
90. Parthasarathy S, Khoo JC, Miller E, Barnett J, Witztum JL. Low density lipoprotein rich in linoleic acid is protected against oxidative modification: Implications for dietary prevention of atherosclerosis. *Proc Natl Acad Sci USA* 1990;87:3894–3898.
91. Berry E, Kaufman N, Friedlander Y, Eisenberg S, Stein Y. The effect of dietary substitution of monounsaturated with polyunsaturated fatty acids on lipoprotein levels, structure, and function in free-living population. *Circulation* 1989;80:11–85.
92. Mensink RP, Katan MB. Effect of a diet enriched with monounsaturated or polyunsaturated fatty acids on levels of low-density and high-density lipoprotein cholesterol in healthy women and men. *N Engl J Med* 1989;321:436–441.
93. Valsta LM, Jauhiainen M, Mutanen M, Aro A, Katan MB. Effects of a monounsaturated rapeseed oil and a polyunsaturated sunflower oil diet on lipoprotein levels in humans. *Artherioscler Thromb* 1992;12: 50–57.
94. Mensink RP, Katan MB Effects of dietary fatty acids on serum lipids and lipoproteins: a meta-analysis of 27 trials. *Arteriosclerosis* 1992; 12:911–919.
95. Connor WE. Effects of omega-3 fatty acids in hypertriglyceridemic states. *Semin Throm Hemostasis* 1988;14:271–284.
96. Sanders TAB, Sullivan DR, Reeve J, Thompson GR. Triglyceride-lowering effect of marine polyunsaturates in patients with hypertriglyceridemia. *Arteriosclerosis* 1985;5:459–465.
97. Sullivan DR, Sanders TAB, Trayner IM, Thompson GR. Paradoxical elevation of LDL apoprotein B levels in hypertriglyceridemic patients and normal subjects ingesting fish oil. *Atherosclerosis* 1986;61: 129–134.
98. Grundy SM. Comparison of monounsaturated fatty acids and carbohydrates for lowering plasma cholesterol. *N Engl J Med* 1986;314: 745–748.
99. Grundy SM, Florentin L, Nix D, Whelan MF. Comparison of monounsaturated fatty acids and carbohydrates for reducing raised levels of plasma cholesterol in man. *Am J Clin Nutr* 1988;47:965–969.
100. Mensink RP, Katan MB. Effect of monounsaturated fatty acids versus complex carbohydrates on high-density lipoproteins in healthy men and women. *Lancet* 1987;1:122–125.
101. Mensink RP, de Groot MJM, van den Broeke LT, Severijnen-Nobels JP, Demacker PNM, Katan MB. Effects of monounsaturated fatty acids and complex carbohydrates on serum lipoproteins and apoproteins in healthy men and women. *Metabolism* 1989;38:172–178.
102. Knittle JL, Ahrens EH Jr. Carbohydrate metabolism in two forms of hyperglyceridemia. *J Clin Invest* 1964;43:485–495.
103. Kuusi T, Ehnholm C, Huttunen JK, et al. Concentration and composition of serum lipoproteins during a low-fat diet at two levels of polyunsaturated fat. *J Lipid Res* 1985;26:360–367.
104. Abbott WGH, Swinburn B, Ruotolo G, Hara H, Patti L, Harper I, Grundy SM, and Howard BV. Effect of a high-carbohydrate, low saturated-fat diet on apolipoprotein and triglyceride metabolism in Pima Indians. *J Clin Invest* 1990;150:1313–1319.
105. Dreon DM, Fernstrom HA, Miller B, Krauss RM. Low density lipoprotein subclass patterns and lipoprotein response to a reduced-fat diet in men. *FASEB J* 1994;8:121–126.
106. Ginsberg HN, Karmally W, Barr SL, Johnson C, Holleran S, Ramakrishnan R. Effects of increasing dietary unsaturated fatty acids within guidelines of the AHA Step I diet on plasma lipid and lipoprotein levels in normal males. *Arterioscler Thomb* 1994;14:892–901.
107. Bell LP, Hectorn KJ, Reynold H, Hunninghake DB. Cholesterol-lowering effects of soluble-fiber cereals as part of a prudent diet for patients with mild to moderate hypercholesterolemia. *Am J Clin Nutr* 1990;52:1020–1026.
108. Anderson JW, Garrity TF, Wood CL, White SE, Smith BM, Oeltgen PR. Prospective, randomized, controlled comparison of the effects of low-fat and low-fat plus high-fiber diets on serum lipid concentrations. *Am J Clin Nutr* 1992;56:887–894.
109. Lepre F, Crane S. Effect of oatbran on mild hyperlipidaemia. *Med J Aust* 1992;157:305–308.
110. Whyte JL, McArthur R, Topping D, Nestel P. Oat bran lowers plasma cholesterol levels in mildly hypercholesterolemic men. *J Am Diet Assoc* 1992;92:446–449.
111. Ripsin CM, Keenan JM, Jacobs DR Jr. Oat products and lipid lowering: a meta-analysis. *JAMA* 1992;267(24):3317–3325.
112. Ashley FW Jr, Kannel WB. Relation of weight change to changes in atherogenic traits: the Framingham Study. *J Chron Dis* 1974;27: 103–114.
113. Kannel WB, Gordon T, Castelli WP. Obesity, lipids, and glucose intolerance: the Framingham Study. *Am J Clin Nutr* 1979;32: 1238–1245.
114. Garrison RJ, Wilson PW, Castelli WP, Feinleib M, Kannel WB, McNamara PM. Obesity and lipoprotein cholesterol in the Framingham Offspring Study. *Metabolism* 1980;29:1053–1060.
115. Shekelle RB, Shryock AM, Paul O, et al. Diet, serum cholesterol, and death from coronary heart disease: the Western Electric Study. *N Engl J Med* 1981;304:65–70.
116. Stamler J. Overweight, hypertension, hypercholesterolemia and coronary heart disease. In: Mananni M, Lewis B, Contaldo F, eds. *Medical*

Complications of Obesity. New York: Academic Press; 1979: 191–216.

117. Anderson JT, Lawler A, Keys A. Weight gain from simple overeating. II. Serum lipids and blood volume. *J Clin Invest* 1957;36:81–88.
118. Caggiula AW, Christakis G, Farrand M, et al. The Multiple Risk Factor Intervention Trial (MRFIT) IV. Intervention blood lipids. *Preventive Med* 1981;10:443–475.
119. National Diet–Heart Study Research Group: the National Diet–Heart Study final report. *Circulation* 1968;Monograph 18:I–201.
120. Wolf R, Grundy SM. Influence of weight reduction on plasma lipoproteins in obese patients. *Arteriosclerosis* 1983;3:160–169.
121. Carew TE, Schwenke DC, Steinberg D. Antiatherogenic effect of probucol unrelated to its hypocholesterolemic effect: Evidence that antioxidants *in vivo* can selectively inhibit low density lipoprotein degradation in macrophage-rich fatty streaks and slow the progression of atherosclerosis in the Watanabe heritable hyperlipidemic rabbit. *Proc Natl Acad Sci USA* 1987;84:7725–7729.
122. Kata T, Nagano Y, Yokode M, Isshii K, Kume N, Ooshima A, Yoshida H, Kawai C. Probucol prevents the progression of atherosclerosis in Watanabe heritable hyperlipidemic rabbit, and animal model for familial hypercholesterolemia. *Proc Natl Acad Sci USA* 1987;84: 5928–5931.
123. Jialal I, Vega GL, Grundy SM. Physiologic levels of ascorbate inhibit the oxidative modification of low density lipoprotein. *Atherosclerosis* 1990;82:185–191.
124. Jialal I, Grundy SM. Preservation of the endogenous antioxidants in low density lipoprotein by ascorbate but not probucol during oxidative modification. *J Clin Invest* 1991;87:597–601.
125. Jialal I, Norkus EP, Coristol L, Grundy SM. B-Carotene inhibits the oxidative modification of low-density lipoprotein. *Biochim Biophys Acta* 1991;1086:134–138.
126. Jialal I, Grundy SM. Effect of dietary supplementation with alpha-tocopherol an oxidative modification of low density lipoproteins. *J Lipid Res* 1992;33:899–906.
127. Jialal I, Grundy SM. Effect of combined supplementation with alpha-tocopherol, ascorbate, and beta-carotene on low-density lipoprotein oxidation. *Circulation* 1993;88:2780–2786.
128. Austin MA. Plasma triglyceride and coronary heart disease. *Arterioscler Thromb* 1991;11:2–14.
129. Hulley SB, Rosenman RH, Bawol RD, Brand RJ. Epidemiology as a guide to clinical decisions: The association between triglyceride and coronary heart disease. *N Engl J Med* 1980;302:1383–1389.
130. Hulley SB, Avins AL. Asymptomatic hypertriglyceridemia: Insufficient evidence to treat. *Br Med J* 1992;304:394–396.
131. Grundy SM, Vega GL. Two different views of the relationship of hypertriglyceridemia to coronary heart disease: implications for treatment. *Arch Intern Med* 1992;94:119–127.
132. Brunzell JD, Albers JJ, Chait A, Grundy SM, Groszek E, McDonald GB. Plasma lipoproteins in familial combined hyperlipidemia and monogenic familial hypertriglyceridemia. *J Lipid Res* 1983;24: 147–155.
133. Brunzell JD, Schrott HG, Motulsky AG, Bierman EL. Myocardial infarction in familial forms of hypertriglyceridemia. *Metabolism* 1976;25:313–320.
134. Garg A, Grundy SM. Management of dyslipidemia in NIDDM. *Diabetes Care* 1990;13:153–169.
135. Brown MD, Goldstein JL, Fredrickson DS. Familial type 3 hyperlipoproteinemia (dysbeta lipoproteinemia). In: Stanburg JB, Wyngaarden JB, Fredrickson DS, Goldstein JL, Brown MS, eds. *The Metabolic Basis of Inherited Disease,* 5th ed. New York: McGraw-Hill; 1983: 665–671.
136. Barrowcliffe TW, Gray E, Kerry PJ, Gutteridge JMC. Triglyceride-rich lipoproteins are responsible for thrombin generation induced by lipid peroxides. *Thromb Haemostasis* 1984;52:7–10.
137. Miller GJ, Walter SJ, Stirling Y, Thompson SG, Esnouf MP, Meade TW. Assay of factor VII activity by two techniques: Evidence for increased conversion of VII to XII in hyperlipidemia with possible implications for ischaemic heart disease. *Br J Haematol* 1985;59: 249–258.
138. Miller GJ, Martin JC, Webster J, et al. Association between dietary fat intake and plasma factor VII coagulant activity—a predictor of cardiovascular mortality. *Atherosclerosis* 1986;60:269–277.
139. De Sousa JC, Soria C, Ayrault-Jarrier M, et al. Association between coagulation factors VII and X with triglyceride rich lipoproteins. *J Clin Pathol* 1988;41:940–944.
140. Simpson BCR, Meade TW, Stirling Y, Mann JL, Chakrabarit R, Woolf L. Hypertriglyceridaemia and hypercoagulability. *Lancet* 1983; 1:786–789.
141. Chait A, Albers JJ, Brunzell JD. Very low density lipoprotein overproduction in genetic forms of hypertriglyceridemia. *Eur J Clin Invest* 1980;10:17–22.
142. Nikkila EA. Familial lipoprotein lipase deficiency and related disorders in chylomicron metabolism. In: Stanbury JB, Wyngaarden JB, Fredrickson DS, Goldstein JL, Brown MS, eds. *The Metabolic Basis of Inherited Disease*. New York: McGraw-Hill; 1983:622–642.
143. Brunzell JD. Familial lipoprotein lipase deficiency and other causes of the chylomicronemia syndrome. In: Scriver CR, Beaudet AL, Sly WS, Valle D, eds. *The Metabolic Basis of Inherited Disease*. New York: McGraw-Hill; 1989:1165–1180.
144. Mahley RW, Rall SC Jr. Type III hypolipoproteinemia (dysbetalipoproteinemia): the role of apolipoprotein E in normal and abnormal lipoprotein metabolism. In: Scriver CR, Beaudet AL, Sly WS, Valle D, eds. *The Metabolic Basis of Inherited Disease*. New York: McGraw-Hill; 1989:1195–1213.
145. Garg A, Bantel JP, Henry RR, Coulston AM, Brinkley L, Chen I, Grundy SM, Huet BA, Reaven GM. Effects of varying carbohydrate content of diet in patients with noninsulin dependent diabetes mellitus. *JAMA* 1994;271:1421–1428.
146. Grundy SM. Effects of polyunsaturated fats on lipid metabolism in patients with hypertriglyceridemia. *J Clin Invest* 1975;55:269–282.
147. Phillipson BE, Rothrock DW, Connor WE, Harris WS, Illingworth DR. Reduction of plasma lipids, lipoproteins, and apoproteins by dietary fish oils in patients with hypertriglyceridemia. *N Engl J Med* 1985;312:1210–1216.
148. Harris WS. Fish oils and plasma lipid and lipoprotein metabolism in humans: a critical review. *J Lipid Res* 1989;30:785–807.
149. Nozaki S, Vega GL, Grundy SM. Postheparin lipolytic activity and plasma lipoprotein response to omega-3 polyunsaturated fatty acids in patients. *Am J Clin Nutr* 1991;53:638–643.
150. Failor RA, Childs MT, Bierman EL. The effects of omega-3 and omega-6 fatty acid-enriched diets on plasma lipoproteins and apoproteins in familial combined hyperlipidemia. *Metabolism* 1988;37: 1021–1028.
151. Knittle JL, Ahrens EH Jr. Carbohydrate metabolism in two forms of hyperglyceridemia. *J Clin Invest* 1964;43:485–495.
152. Ahrens EH Jr, Hirsch J, Oette K, Farquhar JW, Stein Y. Carbohydrate-induced and fat-induced lipemia. *Trans Assoc Am Physicians* 1961; 74:134–146.
153. Garg A, Bonanome A, Grundy SM, Zhang ZJ, Unger RH. Comparison of a high-carbohydrate diet with a high-monounsaturated-fat diet in patients with non-insulin-dependent diabetes mellitus. *N Engl J Med* 1988;391:829–834.
154. Nestel PJ, Hirsch EZ. Triglyceride turnover after diets rich in carbohydrate or animal fat. *Australasian Ann Med* 1965;14:265–269.
155. Nestel PJ, Carroll KF, Havenstein N. Plasma triglyceride response to carbohydrates, fats, and caloric intake. *Metabolism* 1970;19:1–18.
156. Jackson RL, Yates MT, McNerney CA, Kashyap ML. Diet and HDL metabolism: high carbohydrate vs. high fat diets. *Adv Exp Med Biol* 1987;210:165–172.
157. Mellish J, Le N-A, Ginsberg H, Steinberg D, Brown MV. Dissociation of apoprotein B and triglyceride production in very-low density lipoproteins. *Am J Physiol* 1980;239:E354–E362.
158. Crouse JR, Grundy SM. Effects of alcohol on plasma lipoproteins and cholesterol and triglyceride metabolism in man. *J Lipid Res* 1984; 25:486–496.
159. Miller GJ, Miller NE. Plasma high density lipoprotein concentration and development of ischaemic heart disease. *Lancet* 1975;1:16–19.
160. Gordon T, Castelli WP, Hjortland MC, Kannel WB, Dawber TR. High density lipoprotein as a protective factor against coronary heart disease: the Framingham Study. *Am J Med* 1977;62:707–714.
161. Goldbourt V, Holtzman E, Neufeld HN. Total and high density lipoprotein cholesterol in the serum and risk of mortality: Evidence of a threshold effect. *Br Med J* 1985;290:1239–1243.
162. Gordon DJ, Probstfeld JL, Garrison RJ, et al. High-density lipoprotein cholesterol and cardiovascular disease. Four prospective American series. *Circulation* 1989;79:8–15.

163. Glomset JA. The plasma lecithin: Cholesterol acyltransferase reaction. *J Lipid Res* 1968;9:155–167.
164. Rothblat GH, Bamberger M, Phillips MC. Reverse cholesterol transport. In: Alber JJ, Segrest JP, eds. *Methods in enzymology,* Vol 129. London: Academic Press; 1986:628–644.
165. Van Tol A. Reverse cholesterol transport. In: Steinmetz A, Kaffarnik H, Schneider J, eds. *Cholesterol Transport Systems and Their Relation to Atherosclerosis.* Berlin: Springer-Verlag; 1989:85–91.
166. Gofman J, Lindgren F, Elliott H, et al. The role of lipids and lipoproteins in atherosclerosis. *Science* 1950:111:166–171, 186.
167. Tatami R, Mabuchi H, Ueda K, et al. Intermediate-density lipoprotein and cholesterol-rich very low density lipoprotein in angiographically determined coronary artery disease. *Circulation* 1981;64:1174–1184.
168. Reardon MF, Nestel PJ, Craig H, Harper RW. Lipoprotein predictors of the severity of coronary artery disease in men and women. *Circulation* 1985;71:881–888.
169. Badimon JJ, Badimon L, Fuster V. Regression of atherosclerotic lesions by high density lipoprotein plasma fraction in the cholesterol-fed rabbit. *J Clin Invest* 1990;85:1234–1241.
170. Rubin EM, Krauss RM, Spangler EA, Verstuyft JG, Clift SM. Inhibition of early atherogenesis in transgenic mice by human apolipoprotein A-I. *Nature* 1991;353:265–267.
171. Karathanasis SK, Ferris E, Haddad IA. DNA inversion within the apolipoproteins AI/CIII/AIV encoding gene cluster of certain patients with premature atherosclerosis. *Proc Natl Acad Sci USA* 1987;84: 7198–7202.
172. Ordovas JM, Cassidy DK, Civeira F, Bisgaier CL, Schaefer EJ. Familial apolipoprotein A-I, C-III, and I-IV deficiency and premature atherosclerosis due to deletion of a gene complex on chromosome 11. *J Biol Chem* 1989;264:16339–16342.
173. Matsunaga T, Hiasa Y, Yanagi H. Apolipoprotein A-I deficiency due to a codon 84 nonsense mutation of the apolipoprotein A-I gene. *Proc Natl Acad Sci USA* 1991;88:2793–2797.
174. Heller DA, de Faire U, Petersen NL, Dahlen G, McClern GE. Genetic and environmental influences on serum levels in twins. *N Engl J Med* 1993;328:1150–1166.
175. Puchois P, Kandoussi A, Fievet P, et al. Apolipoprotein A-I containing lipoproteins in coronary artery disease. *Atherosclerosis* 1987;68: 35–40.
176. Coste-Burel V, Mainard F, Chivot L, Auget JL, Madec Y. Study of lipoprotein particles LpAI and LpAI:AII in patients before coronary bypass surgery. *Clin Chem* 1990;36:1889–1891.
177. Genest JJ, Bard JM, Fruchart JC, Ordovas JM, Wilson PFW, Schaefer E. Plasma apolipoprotein AI, AII, B, E and CIII containing particles in men with premature coronary artery disease. *Atherosclerosis* 1991; 90:149–157.
178. Parra HJ, Arveiler D, Evans AE, et al. A case–control study of lipoprotein particles in two populations at contrasting risk for coronary heart disease: the ECTIM study. *Arterioscler Thromb* 1992;12:701–707.
179. Cheung MC, Brown BG, Wolf A, Albers JJ. Altered particle size distribution of apolipoprotein A-I containing lipoproteins in subjects with coronary artery disease. *J Lipid Res* 1991;32:383–394.
180. Marques-Vidal P, Ruidavets JB, Jaureguy MN, Perret B, Cambou JP, Chap H. Lipids and lipoproteins as risk factors for myocardial infarction in a population of Haute-Garonne. In: *Proceedings 9th International Symposium on Atherosclerosis.* 1991; p. 153 (abstr).
181. Montali A, Vega GL, Grundy SM. Concentrations of apolipoprotein AI-containing particles in patients with hypoalphalipoproteinemia. *Arterioscler Thromb* 1994;14:511–517.
182. Brinton EA, Eisenberg S, Breslow JL. Increased apo AI and AII fractional catabolic rate in patients with low high density lipoprotein cholesterol levels with and without hypertriglyceridemia. *J Clin Invest* 1991;87:536–544.
183. Gylling H, Vega GL, Grundy SM. Physiologic mechanisms for reduced apolipoprotein AI concentrations associated with low levels of high density lipoprotein cholesterol in patients with normal plasma lipids. *J Lipid Res* 1992;33:1527–1539.
184. Vega GL, Grundy SM. Two patterns of LDL metabolism in normotriglyceridemic patients with hypoalphalipoproteinemia. *Arterioscler Thromb* 1993;13:579–589.
185. Nikkila EA, Taskinen M-R, Rehunen S, Harkonen M. Lipoprotein lipase activity in adipose tissue and skeletal muscle of runners: Relation to serum lipoproteins. *Metabolism* 1978;27:1661–1671.
186. Nikkila EA, Taskinen MR, Kekki M. Relation of plasma high-density lipoprotein cholesterol to lipoprotein lipase activity in adipose tissue and skeletal muscle of man. *Atherosclerosis* 1978;29:497–501.
187. Blades B, Vega GL, Grundy SM. Activities of lipoprotein lipase and hepatic triglyceride lipase in postheparin plasma of patients with low concentrations of HDL cholesterol. *Arterioscler Thomb* 1993;13: 1227–1235.
188. Tikkanen MJ, Nikkila EA, Kuusi T, Sipinen S. High density lipoprotein 2 and hepatic lipase: reciprocal changes produced by estrogen and norgestrel. *J Clin Endocrinol Metab* 1982;54:1113–1117.
189. Kuusi T, Kesaniemi YA, Vueristo M, Miettinen TA, Koskenvuo M. Inheritance of high density lipoprotein and lipoprotein lipase and hepatic lipase activity. *Arteriosclerosis* 1987;7:421–425.
190. Laakso M, Sarlund H, Ehnholm C, Voutilainen E, Aro A, Pyorala K. Relationship between postheparin plasma lipases and high density lipoprotein cholesterol in different types of diabetes. *Diabetologia* 1987;30:703–706.
191. Hjermann I, Enger SC, Helgeland A, Holme I, Leren P, Trygg K. The effect of dietary changes on high density lipoprotein cholesterol. *Am J Med* 1979;66:105–109.
192. Shepherd J, Packard CJ, Grundy SM, Yeshurun D, Gotto AM Jr, Taunton OD. Effects of saturated and polyunsaturated fat diets on the chemical composition and metabolism of low density lipoproteins in man. *J Lipid Res* 1980;21:91–99.
193. Brinton EA, Eisenberg S, Breslow JL. Elevated high density lipoprotein cholesterol levels correlate with decreased apolipoprotein AI and AII fractional catabolic rate in women. *J Clin Invest* 1989;84: 262–269.
194. Hannuksela M, Marcel YL, Kesaniemi YA, Savolainen M. Reduction in the concentration and activity of plasma cholesterol esterol transfer protein by alcohol. *J Lipid Res* 1992;33:737–744.
195. MacMahon S, Peto R, Cutler J, et al. Blood pressure, stroke, and coronary heart disease. *Lancet* 1990;335:765–774.
196. Stokes J, Kannel WB, Wolf PA. The relative importance of selected risk factors for various manifestations of cardiovascular disease among men and women from 35 to 64 years old: 30 years of follow-up in the Framingham Study. *Circulation* 1987;75:V-65–V-73.
197. MacMahon S, Cutler J, Brittain E, Higgins M. Obesity and hypertension: epidemiological and clinical issues. *Eur Heart J* 1987;8(Suppl B):57–70.
198. Law MR, Frost CD, Wald NJ. By how much does dietary salt reduction lower blood pressure? I—Analysis of observational data among populations. *Br Med J* 1991;302:811–815.
199. Frost CD, Law MR, Wald NJ. II—Analysis of observational data within populations. *Br Med J* 1991;302:815–818.
200. Law MR, Frost CD, Wald NJ. III—Analysis of data from trials of salt reduction. *Br Med J* 1991;302:819–824.
201. SHEP Cooperative Research Group. Prevention of stroke by antihypertensive drug treatment in older persons with isolated systolic hypertension. *JAMA* 1991;265:3255–3264.
202. The report of the Expert Panel on Detection, Evaluation and Treatment of High Blood Cholesterol in Adults; 1988. NIH publication no. 88-2925.

Atherosclerosis and Coronary Artery Disease,
edited by V. Fuster, R. Ross, and E. J. Topol.
Lippincott-Raven Publishers, Philadelphia © 1996.

CHAPTER 5

Genetic Dyslipoproteinemias

H. B. Brewer, Jr., Siliva M. Santamarina-Fojo, Jeffrey M. Hoeg

Key words: Apolipoproteins; Dyslipoproteinemia; Lipoprotein lipase; Hepatic lipase; Familial hypercholesterolemia; Dysbetalipoproteinemia; Tangier disease; Hypoalphalipoproteinemia.

INTRODUCTION

Plasma lipids are transported by lipoproteins composed of several classes of lipids and proteins designated apolipoproteins. There are six major classes of human plasma lipoproteins, including chylomicrons, very low density lipoproteins (VLDL), intermediate-density lipoproteins (IDL), low-density lipoproteins (LDL), high-density lipoproteins (HDL), and lipoprotein(a) [Lp(a)] (1,2). HDL can be further separated by hydrated density into HDL_2 and HDL_3. Over the last two decades the roles of apolipoproteins, enzymes, lipoprotein receptors, and transfer proteins in lipoprotein metabolism have been elucidated, and this new information provides a conceptual framework for understanding lipid transport in normal individuals and in patients with the genetic dyslipoproteinemias.

H. B. Brewer, Jr.: Molecular Disease Branch, NIH/National Heart, Lung, and Blood Institute, Bethesda, Maryland 20892.
S. M. Santamarina-Fojo: Molecular Biology Section, NIH/National Heart, Lung, and Blood Institute, Bethesda, Maryland 20892.
J. M. Hoeg: Cell Biology Section, NIH/National Heart, Lung, and Blood Institute, Bethesda, Maryland, 20892.

LIPOPROTEIN METABOLISM

Based on current information the metabolism of the human plasma lipoproteins can be conceptually separated into two separate pathways. One pathway is composed of the apolipoprotein B (apoB)-containing lipoproteins (chylomicrons, VLDL, IDL, and LDL) and the second pathway involves HDL. Schematic overviews of the two metabolic pathways for lipoprotein biosynthesis, transport, and catabolism in normal subjects are illustrated in Figs. 1 and 2.

Apolipoprotein B-Lipoprotein Metabolic Pathways

The metabolism of the plasma lipoproteins containing the B apolipoproteins, apoB-48 and apoB-100, consists of two separate pathways (for general reviews see refs. 3–6). The first apoB pathway involves the stepwise delipidation of triglyceride-rich chylomicron particles containing apoB-48, which transport dietary cholesterol and triglycerides from the intestine to peripheral tissues and finally to the liver. Following secretion, chylomicrons acquire two apolipoproteins, apoE and apoC-II, present on HDL. ApoC-II activates

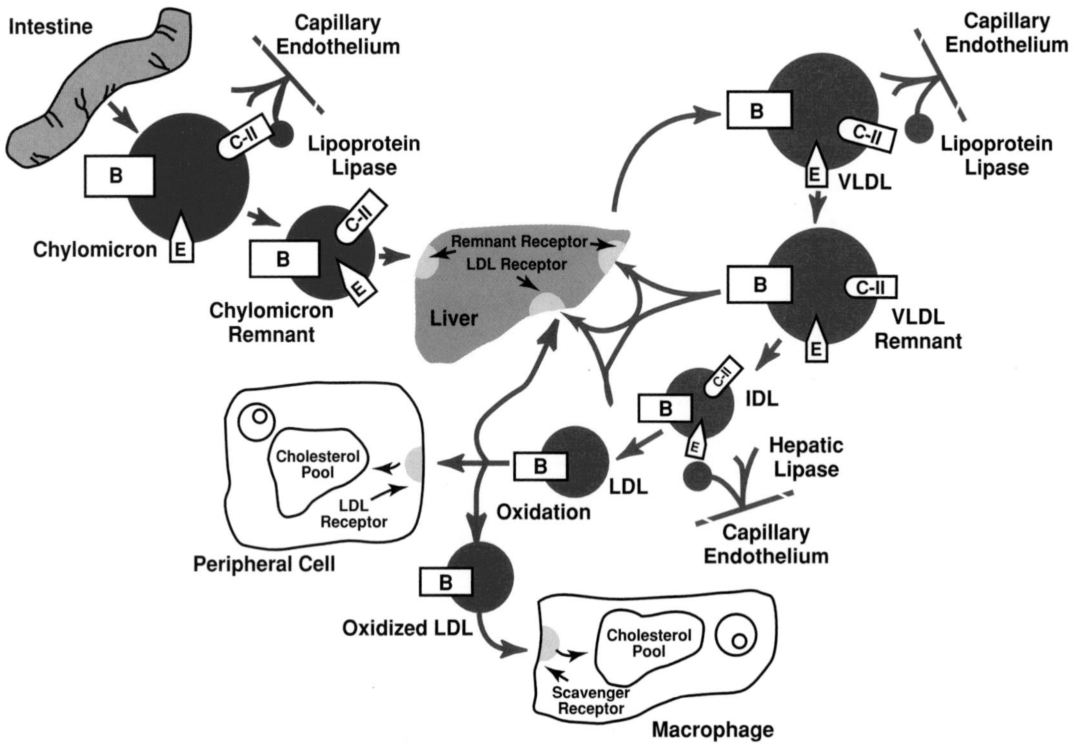

FIG. 1. Overview of the metabolic pathways of the major apoB-containing lipoprotein particles, including chylomicrons, very low density lipoproteins *(VLDL),* intermediate-density lipoproteins *(IDL),* and low-density lipoproteins *(LDL).* The intestinal apoB pathway involves the stepwise delipidation of intestinal-derived triglyceride-rich chylomicrons by lipoprotein lipase and its cofactor apoC-II with the formation of chylomicron remnants. Chylomicron remnants are taken up by the liver primarily by the remnant receptor. ApoE is the major ligand on chylomicron remnants which interacts with the remnant receptor. In the hepatic apoB pathway, triglyceride-rich VLDL are secreted from the liver and undergo delipidation by lipoprotein lipase with conversion of VLDL to VLDL remnants, IDL, and finally LDL. A second lipolytic enzyme, hepatic lipase, plays a key role in the conversion of IDL to LDL. During the conversion of VLDL to LDL approximately half of the lipoproteins are removed by the liver either by the LDL or remnant receptors. LDL interact with LDL receptors, which initiates receptor-mediated cellular uptake and degradation. LDL may also undergo oxidation with the formation of oxidized LDL, which is cleared up by the macrophage via the scavenger receptor.

the lipolytic enzyme lipoprotein lipase (LPL), which is attached to the capillary endothelium. Activation of lipoprotein lipase results in triglyceride hydrolysis and remodeling of the triglyceride-rich lipoprotein particles. Concomitant with the hydrolysis of triglycerides, apolipoproteins as well as lipid constituents are transferred from chylomicrons to HDL. With lipolysis the chylomicrons are converted to small chylomicron remnants with a hydrated density of initially VLDL and then IDL.

The second apoB pathway involves triglyceride-rich VLDL containing apoB-100 secreted by the liver. ApoC-II and apoE dissociate from HDL and reassociate with the hepatogenous triglyceride-rich VLDL secreted from the liver. ApoC-II activates LPL as outlined above and VLDL are serially converted to VLDL remnants, IDL, and finally LDL. Hepatic lipase, a second lipolytic enzyme, and apoE have been proposed to be required for the efficient conversion of IDL to LDL. Hepatic lipase plays an important role in lipoprotein metabolism as both a phospholipase and triacylglycerol hydrolase. During the metabolic conversion of VLDL to LDL approximately 50% of VLDL remnants and IDL are removed from the plasma by the liver.

Remnants of both the chylomicron and VLDL pathways have been proposed to be removed from the plasma primarily by the interaction of either apoE or apoB-100 with the hepatic remnant or LDL receptors. The LDL receptor has been extensively characterized and two apolipoproteins on the triglyceride remnants, apoB-100 and apoE, serve as ligands for the LDL receptor (7–10).

The identification and definitive characterization of the remnant receptor has been a challenge. The current best candidate for the putative remnant receptor is a glycosylated 600-kDa protein designated the LDL receptor-related protein (LRP) (11,12). The major apolipoprotein ligand for the putative remnant receptor is apoE, and a major pathway for clearance of triglyceride-rich remnants involves apoE-mediated cellular uptake.

LDL, the final lipoprotein in the VLDL cascade, contains

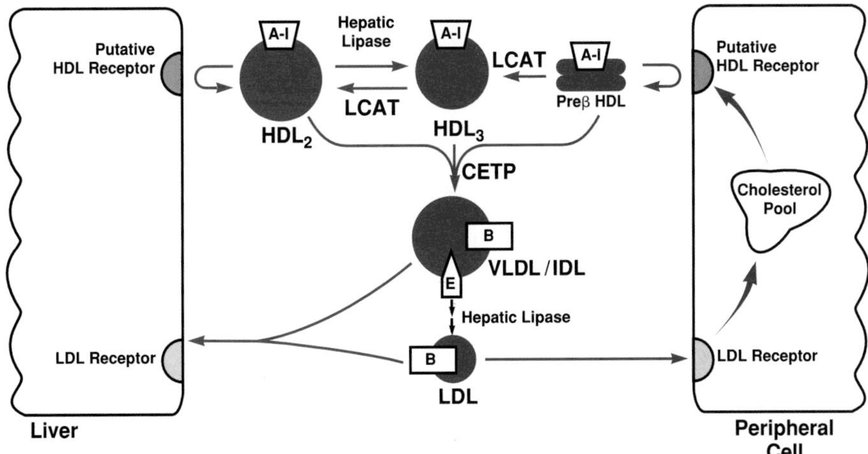

FIG. 2. General overview of high-density lipoprotein *(HDL)* and reverse cholesterol transport. Excess cellular cholesterol is removed from peripheral cells (e.g., fibroblasts, smooth muscle cells, and macrophages) by nascent preβ-HDL following interaction with a putative HDL receptor. Cholesterol is converted to cholesteryl esters by lecithin cholesterol acyltransferase *(LCAT)* and the nascent HDL is converted to particles with a hydrated density of HDL_3 and then HDL_2. Cholesteryl esters are transported directly from HDL to the liver or are transferred to the apoB-containing lipoproteins, VLDL–IDL–LDL, by cholesterol ester transfer protein *(CETP)*. LDL plays an important role in reverse cholesterol transport by delivering the cholesterol esters derived from HDL back to the liver via the LDL receptor pathway.

virtually only apoB-100 and interacts primarily with the LDL receptor present on the plasma membrane of the liver (Fig. 1). In addition, LDL interacts with the LDL receptor on peripheral cells, including adrenal, fibroblasts, and smooth muscle cells (8,9). The interaction of LDL with the LDL receptor initiates receptor-mediated endocytosis and transport of LDL to intracellular lysosomes, where the protein moiety is degraded and cholesteryl esters are hydrolyzed to free cholesterol, which are then transferred to the intracellular cholesterol pool. An additional pathway for LDL metabolism is the uptake by macrophages with the formation of foam cells in the arterial wall. Native LDL is not readily taken up by macrophages. However, oxidative modification of LDL results in markedly enhanced LDL uptake by the scavenger receptor on macrophages with foam cell formation (13–16). Oxidative modifications of LDL were observed following *in vitro* incubation with endothelial cells, smooth muscle cells, and macrophages, or following modification with malondialdehyde. Recent studies have indicated that oxidized lipids within LDL may play an important role in the pathophysiology of the atherosclerotic lesion by stimulating the secretion of cytokines and other factors which modulate endothelial cell function as well as facilitate the recruitment of plasma monocytes into the vessel wall (17). Based on current data it has been proposed that oxidative modification of LDL may be a prerequisite for the macrophage uptake of LDL, foam cell formation, and the development of the atherosclerotic lesion.

High-Density-Lipoprotein Metabolism

The major role of HDL in lipoprotein metabolism is to transport cholesterol from peripheral tissues back to the liver, where it is removed from the body following conversion to bile acids or as biliary cholesterol. This hypothetical process, termed reverse cholesterol transport (18,19), is summarized schematically in Fig. 2. Nascent HDL, composed primarily of apo-A-I phospholipid discs, are secreted from both the human intestine and liver. Nascent HDL acquire excess cholesterol from tissues, and the enzyme lecithin cholesterol acyltransferase (LCAT) catalyzes the esterification of plasma lipoprotein cholesterol to cholesteryl esters. With the formation of cholesteryl esters the nascent HDL are converted to spherical lipoproteins with a hydrated density of HDL_3. HDL_3 are converted to the larger HDL_2 by the acquisition of apolipoproteins and lipids released during the stepwise delipidation and remodeling of the triglyceride-rich chylomicrons and VLDL as well as by the esterification of the cholesterol removed from peripheral tissues. HDL is proposed to transfer the cholesterol removed from the peripheral tissues to the liver. HDL_2 are converted back to HDL_3 by hepatic lipase through the removal of phospholipids and triglycerides and the generation of nascent apoA-I HDL (3,18–23). The cycle of uptake of cholesterol from the peripheral tissues and then transport of cholesteryl to the liver is repeated. An additional pathway for transport of cholesterol to the liver is the transfer of cholesterol esters in HDL to VLDL–IDL–LDL by the cholesterol ester transfer protein (CETP) with ultimate transfer of cholesterol to the liver by the apoB-containing lipoproteins (24). In this proposed model of reverse cholesterol transport HDL interacts with a putative HDL receptor on peripheral cells and the liver. The precise nature of the specific HDL receptor involved in the transport of cholesterol from peripheral cells back to the liver where it can be excreted from the body remains to be definitively established.

Lipoprotein(a)

Lipoprotein(a) a cholesterol-rich atherogenic lipoprotein that closely resembles LDL in lipid composition, has a hydrated density intermediate between LDL and HDL. The protein moiety of Lp(a) consists of apoB-100 and a unique apolipoprotein, designated apo(a) (25,26). Apo(a) is linked by a single disulfide bridge to apoB-100 on LDL to form Lp(a). Apo(a) is a large glycoprotein ranging in size from 400 to 700 kDa. The amino acid sequence of apo(a) is similar to the sequence of plasminogen and contains cysteine-rich domains of 80–114 amino acids in length termed kringles (27,28). Apo(a) contains a variable number of copies of kringle 4, and a single copy of kringle 5 followed by the protease domain of plasminogen. In contrast to plasminogen, apo(a) has no serine protease enzymic activity, and it cannot be converted to an active plasminlike enzyme by tissue plasminogen activator, streptokinase, or urokinase. Current data suggest that apo(a) is synthesized and directly secreted into plasma independent of the biosynthetic pathways of the apoB-containing lipoproteins. An elevated plasma level of Lp(a) is an independent risk factor for the development of premature cardiovascular disease (29–33). The precise physiologic function(s) of Lp(a) in lipoprotein metabolism remains to be established.

The rapid expansion of our knowledge of the pathways for lipoprotein metabolism has permitted the classification of the molecular defects in patients with the genetic dyslipoproteinemias into defects in either lipoprotein receptors, apolipoproteins, enzymes, or transfer proteins. The major genetic dyslipoproteinemias associated with an increased risk of premature cardiovascular disease are summarized in Table 1. Each of these genetic dyslipoproteinemias has characteristic clinical features as well as lipoprotein profiles and will be summarized in this chapter.

HYPERLIPOPROTEINEMIAS

Familial Hypercholesterolemia

The elucidation of the molecular defect in familial hypercholesterolemia (FH) has provided an understanding of the role of receptor-mediated endocytosis in lipoprotein metabolism, the importance of phenotypic heterogeneity in the expression of genetic diseases, and the development of therapies that can halt the progression of atherosclerosis.

Young adults with homozygous FH have total and LDL cholesterol concentrations four- to sevenfold greater than normal and a constellation of physical findings that bring them to medical attention (Fig. 3; see Colorplate 1). The raised, yellowish-beige, rugous xanthomas on the knuckles and in the interdigital web of the fingers (Fig. 3A) are often the initial manifestation of the disease. By the ages of 5–12 years the other stigmata, including arcus cornea (Fig. 3B), tuberous xanthomas (Fig. 3C), and planar xanthomas (Fig. 3D), appear. Histologic analysis reveals that these xanthomas are from cells derived from the deposition of LDL-derived lipid in monocyte-macrophages (34). Lipid deposition is a key component of the atherosclerotic lesion in the arterial wall. The lesions in the coronary arteries are readily detectable by coronary angiography. The premature atherosclerosis in FH is illustrated in Fig. 4A (white arrows) in an angiogram of the left coronary artery in the left anterior oblique position, which contains a 50–70% stenosis in a homozygous FH patient who developed angina at the age of 20 years. These lesions, as well as lesions not detectable by angiography, can now be detected noninvasively by electron beam tomography. (Electron beam tomography [EBT] was previously termed ultrafast computed tomography [CT].) In contrast to conventional CT, the x-rays are generated by a beam of electrons which are focused by a magnet,

TABLE 1. *Genetic dyslipoproteinemias*

Disorder	Inheritance	Genetic defect	Frequency in population
Hyperlipoproteinemias			
Familial hypercholesterolemia	AD	Receptor: LDL receptor	1/500
Familial defective apoB-100	AD	Apolipoprotein: ApoB	1/500
Familial combined hyperlipidemia	AD	Unknown	3–5/1,000
Familial dysbetalipoproteinemia	D or AR	Apolipoprotein: ApoE	1/5,000
Familial hyperchylomicronemia			
Apolipoprotein C-II deficiency	AR	Apolipoprotein: ApoC-II	Rare
Lipoprotein lipase deficiency	AR	Enzyme: lipoprotein lipase	Rare
Hepatic lipase deficiency	AR	Enzyme: hepatic lipase	Rare
Elevated lipoprotein (a)	AD	—	20%[a]
β-Sitosterolemia	AR	Unknown	Rare
Hypolipoproteinemias			
Tangier disease	AD	Unknown	Rare
Apolipoprotein A-I deficiency	AR	Apolipoprotein: ApoA-I	Rare
Familial hypoalphalipoproteinemia	AR	Unknown	Rare

AD, Autosomal dominant; AR, autosomal recessive.

[a] Twenty percent of the population has lipoprotein (a) greater then 30 mg/dl, which is associated with an increased risk of premature cardiovascular disease.

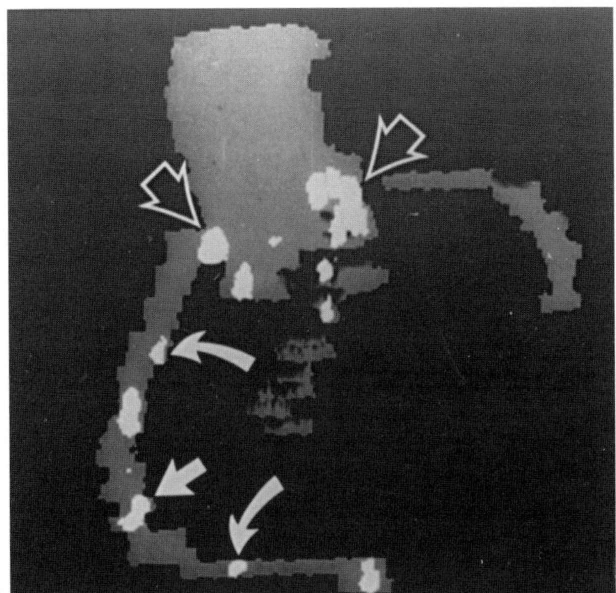

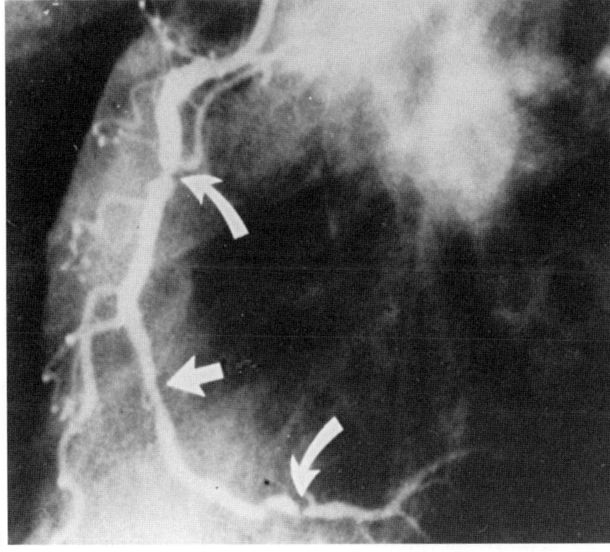

FIG. 4. Cardiovascular disease in homozygous familial hypercholesterolemia demonstrated **(A)** coronary angiography and **(B)** electron beam tomography. The stenotic lesions in the left coronary artery by angiography are indicated by the solid white arrows (panel A). These same lesions are calcific, as indicated by the solid arrows for the same location in the electron beam tomography observed in this same patient (panel B). In addition, additional calcific lesions which were not detected by angiography are observed in both the coronary artery as well as in the coronary ostia and ascending aortic root as highlighted by the large open arrows (panel B).

analogous to that used in standard television cathode-ray tubes. This permits the acquisition of images within 50–100 msec. This fast focusing is then gated to the electrocardiogram and the heart can be imaged in a freeze-frame, stroboscopic manner. This permits fine resolution of all of the structures of the mediastinum, including the coronary arteries. In addition to the coronary artery lesions observed by angiography, this new method can both detect and quantitate the calcific atherosclerosis in the coronary ostia and the ascending aortic root (Fig. 4B, large open arrows). The severity of calcific atherosclerosis is highly correlated with both the severity of the hypercholesterolemia as well as the duration of exposure of the endothelium to the high concentrations of LDL particles (35). This formulation has led to the concept of the cholesterol-year score (35,36), which parallels the cigarette pack-year score for assessing the risk for pulmonary disease.

The human LDL receptor gene is located on chromosome 1 (37) and is 45.5 kb in length. The gene contains 18 exons ranging in size from 78 to 2,535 nucleotides, which are separated by 17 introns (38). The single-chain nascent protein has a molecular weight of 93 kDa and the glycosylated receptor has an apparent molecular weight of 164 kDa by sodium dodecyl sulfate–polyacrylamide gel electrophoresis (39,40). The deduced protein structure of both the bovine (41) and human LDL receptors (42) suggests several functional domains (Fig. 5). The LDL receptor is an acidic protein (Pi = 4.6) which contain 839 amino acids, and cysteine residues comprise 15% of the 322 amino-terminal residues. In the amino-terminal domain there are seven 40-amino acid, cysteine-rich repeated cassettes (9,41). Monoclonal antibodies against the amino-terminal domain are variable in their ability to impair LDL binding (43). Deletion of one or more of the seven 40-amino acid, cysteine-rich repeats abolishes binding of LDL to the LDL receptor (44).

In addition to the ligand-binding domain, the LDL receptor contains four other domains. The second 350-amino acid domain, like the cysteine-rich ligand-binding domain, resides on the extracellular side of the plasma membrane and contains a high degree of homology with the epidermal growth factor precursor (40). The third domain is rich in serine and threonine residues, which are glycosylation sites (39,45). Using site-directed mutagenesis, Davis and coworkers established that this 48-amino acid region was the site of the majority of the glycosylation (46). The fourth domain consists of 22 hydrophobic amino acid residues which span the plasma membrane. Finally, the fifth domain, a 50-amino acid carboxyl-terminus domain, is important for the cellular metabolism of the LDL receptor. This latter domain permits the generation of dimers and multimers of LDL receptors at the cell surface that is important for receptor internalization (47). In addition, the LDL receptor is phosphorylated at serine residue 833, which resides in the cytoplasmic domain (48). Up to two-thirds of isolated bovine adrenal cortex LDL receptors are phosphorylated (48). A specific LDL receptor kinase has been purified and LDL receptor phosphorylation by this kinase requires a heat-stable activator protein (49). In addition, this domain has been shown to target the receptor to the sinusoidal surface of polarized hepatocytes in transgenic mice (50).

The study of skin fibroblasts from FH patients provided the first insight into the abnormalities in cellular cholesterol

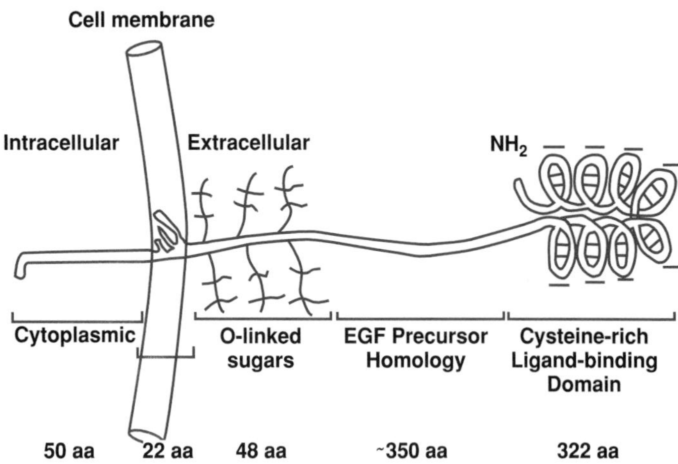

FIG. 5. Schematic representation of the structural features of the LDL receptor. The proposed protein structural domains were determined by analysis of the amino acid *(aa)* sequence derived from the determination of the LDL-receptor cDNA structure. *EGF,* Epidermal growth factor.

metabolism. In contrast to fibroblasts from normolipidemic controls, cells from FH patients did not downregulate endogenous cholesterol biosynthesis in the presence of LDL (51). This cellular defect was shown to be due to mutations in the gene encoding for cell surface LDL receptors which resulted in the inability of the LDL-derived cholesterol to enter the cell and undergo lysosomal degradation (52).

Since the initial studies, more than 150 different mutations in the LDL receptor have been characterized which result in FH (53,54). Point mutations as well as insertional and deletional mutations have been reported (53,54). These mutations can be classified based upon the aberrant function of the cellular metabolism of the LDL receptor (Table 2). Class 1 mutations lead to the failure to synthesize the LDL receptor protein, while class 2 mutations lead to the synthesis of an LDL receptor that cannot be effectively transported from the endoplasmic reticulum to the cell surface. Class 2a mutations lead to a complete block in transport, while class 2b mutations lead to a partial block in transport. In the case of class 3 mutations, the LDL receptor reaches the cell surface, but cannot bind normally to LDL. The inability of LDL receptors to cluster into coated pits derives from mutations designated as class 4. Finally, the normal life cycle of LDL receptors involves the uptake of the membrane-bound receptor by endocytosis and the recycling of the internalized LDL receptors back to the plasma membrane. Mutations which lead to receptors that cannot be normally recycled are termed class 5 mutations.

Heterozygotes for FH have elevated LDL cholesterol concentrations and a four- to sixfold increased risk for premature cardiovascular disease; further, by age 39 years, 90% of heterozygous FH patients have detectable tendon xanthomas. The heterozygotes have one normal allele, and therapy can be effective in reducing the concentration of LDL by upregulating the activity of the normal LDL receptors. The hepatocyte is the principal cell type expressing LDL receptors (55). Use of bile acid sequestrants and inhibitors of 3-hydroxy-3-methylglutaryl coenzyme A (HMG-CoA) reductase can effectively increase the expression of hepatic LDL receptors. Combined, these drugs are additive in both expressing LDL receptors and in reducing the concentration of plasma LDL cholesterol. Diet plus a combination of niacin, an inhibitor of HMG-CoA reductase, and a bile acid sequestrant can reduce the total and LDL-cholesterol concentrations in heterozygous FH by 35–50% (56,57). Although the majority of patients have a substantial improvement in their plasma lipoprotein concentrations, a large fraction of these patients do not achieve the goal LDL-cholesterol concentrations outlined by the Adult Treatment Panel of the National Cholesterol Education Program (58). These therapies can retard the progression of atherogenesis and even reduce cardiovascular and all-cause mortality (59); however, even more aggressive

TABLE 2. *Classification of low-density-lipoprotein receptor mutations leading to familial hypercholesterolemia*

Mutation class	Cellular LDL-receptor metabolism	Cellular receptor location: Intracellular	Coated pits	Noncoated regions	Extracellular	Frequency in FH (%)
Class 1	No protein synthesis					34
Class 2a	Complete block in transport	+				7
Class 2b	Partial block in transport	+	±			39
Class 3	Defective LDL binding		+			9
Class 4	Defective clustering into coated pits			+	+	6
Class 5	Failure to recycle receptor		+	+		12

LDL, Low-density lipoprotein; FH, familial hypercholesterolemia.

measures may be required to halt as well as reverse the atherosclerotic process. A variety of techniques have been used to remove atherogenic lipoproteins from patients heterozygous for FH. Plasma exchange, heparin extracorporeal lipoprotein precipitation, and dextran-sulfate LDL adsorption are all effective in both reducing LDL-cholesterol concentrations and affecting the angiographic progression of coronary artery disease. The use of LDL apheresis is being advocated as a useful adjunct to diet and pharmacologic therapy in treating heterozygous FH patients who have established coronary artery disease (60).

Individuals inheriting mutant LDL receptor genes in both alleles are either homozygous for the same mutation or are termed compound heterozygotes. A founder effect has been observed in unique populations such as in Quebec and South Africa, where virtually all of the FH patients have the same mutation. In these regions of the world there is a high likelihood that patients presenting with total cholesterol concentrations >600 mg/dl and classical xanthomas are true homozygotes. In contrast, in more outbred populations and in the absence of consanguinity, there is a greater likelihood that FH patients are compound heterozygotes. Rather than the specific mutation, the residual activity of the LDL receptors in both true homozygotes and compound heterozygotes is the major determinant of the severity of the atherosclerotic process. Fibroblast LDL-receptor activity correlates with plasma LDL-cholesterol concentration and with the response to dietary and drug therapy (61). A variety of dietary and pharmacologic interventions have been tested in patients with homozygous FH (62). In addition, more aggressive and experimental therapies such as partial ileal bypass, portacaval shunt, plasma exchange (63–65) or apheresis utilizing dextran-sulfate adsorption (66,67), heparin precipitation (68), or immunosorption (69,70), and liver transplantation have all been used to prevent the cardiovascular sequelae of this disease. At present the removal of LDL particles by either plasma exchange or LDL apheresis is the treatment of choice for homozygous FH. LDL apheresis is preferable since it removes only the atherogenic lipoprotein particles. With these apheresis techniques there is not only a profound reduction in LDL-cholesterol concentrations, there is also regression of the skin xanthomas, stabilization of the coronary atherosclerosis, and even regression of substantial, flow-limiting coronary artery lesions (65,66,71).

Recently, experimental gene therapy involving the replacement of defective LDL receptors within the hepatocytes has been undertaken. With the initial identification of human hepatic LDL receptors and their deficiency in patients with FH (55,72–74), initial attempts at hepatic LDL-receptor replacement involved liver transplantation (75–77). The effect of liver transplant has been to normalize the plasma lipoprotein concentrations as well as to induce regression of the tissue deposition of cholesterol in xanthomas as well as in the coronary arteries (78).

Another way of repleting hepatic LDL receptors has been to use *ex vivo* gene therapy (79). Hepatocytes isolated from homozygous FH patients have been cultured, transformed by retroviral infection, selected for transformation, and reinfused into the portal circulation. This therapy appears to have been successful in reducing the total and LDL-cholesterol concentrations in the plasma of an animal model for FH, the Watanabe heritable hyperlipidemic rabbit (80,81). The initial case report indicated a 15–20% reduction in total and LDL-cholesterol concentrations after gene therapy (82). A great deal remains to be done to evaluate both the safety and efficacy of gene therapy in this disease.

In addition to the overexpression of the LDL-receptor gene as a form of replacement therapy, it may be possible to express other candidate genes that could modulate atherogenesis (36,83). At the level of atherosclerosis, only about half of the variability is due to the LDL-cholesterol concentrations (84). Recent studies indicated, for example, that both lipoprotein lipase and hepatic lipase can account for a substantial degree of variability of calcific atherosclerosis in homozygous FH (84). These findings suggest that the overexpression of genes other than that for the LDL receptor could be useful therapeutically in these patients with markedly accelerated atherogenesis.

Familial Defective ApoB-100

In addition to genetic defects in the LDL receptor, structural mutations in the ligand-binding domain of apoB-100 can also lead to hypercholesterolemia and xanthomatosis. The metabolic defect in familial defective apoB-100 (FDB) is reduced clearance of autologous LDL compared to LDL from normolipidemic study subjects (85). LDL from one of these probands and from the proband's first-degree relatives had substantially reduced binding to LDL receptors expressed in normal skin fibroblasts (86). Sequence analysis of the two alleles of the apoB gene of a subject heterozygous for this disorder revealed a glutamine-for-arginine substitution in the codon for amino acid 3,500 (87). This same mutant allele was found in six unrelated subjects and in eight affected relatives in two of these kindreds. Based on these results this disease has been designated familial defective apolipoprotein B-100. A monoclonal antibody (88) whose epitope was within residues 3,350 and 3,506 of apolipoprotein B has been isolated and characterized. This antibody, MB47, bound with a higher affinity to abnormal LDL compared to normal LDL, permitting the development of a useful assay for clinical and epidemiologic studies.

One additional mutation has recently been described (89) in which the change of a C to a T at nucleotide 10,800 leads to a substitution of a cysteine for an arginine at amino acid residue 3,531. This has been observed in 2 of 1,400 patients screened in a lipid clinic population. Like the mutation at amino acid 3,500, this amino acid substitution leads to hypercholesterolemia and a significant reduction in LDL-receptor binding affinity. As in patients heterozygous for FH, heterozygotes for familial defective apoB-100 also have been observed to have tendon xanthomas and premature cardiovascular disease. These combined results now indicate that patients with type II hyperlipoproteinemia may have either a defect in the LDL receptor resulting in familial hypercholesterolemia, or the ligand, apoB-100, for the LDL receptor leading to FDB.

Like patients heterozygous for FH, patients with FDB respond to drug therapy. However, their response to specific therapy differs. FDB patients appear to be more resistant to lovastatin compared to heterozygous FH patients. At 40 mg/day of lovastatin heterozygous FH patients had LDL-cholesterol concentrations decline by 32% compared to only a 22% decrease in FDB patients (90). In contrast, FDB patients appeared to respond more favorably to both niacin (FDB vs FH, 24% vs 14% LDL reduction) (91) and bile acid sequestrant therapy (FDB vs FH, 32% vs 22% LDL reduction) (92) than did heterozygous FH patients. These data suggest that the specific molecular defect in the LDL-receptor-ligand pathway may have important therapeutic implications.

Familial Combined Hyperlipidemia

Familial combined hyperlipidemia (FCH) is one of the most common monogenetic disorders in humans, with a gene frequency assuming a single defect as high as 3–5/1,000 (93–98). The clinical features of FCH usually are expressed in the fourth and fifth decades. A characteristic feature of FCH is the presence of multiple lipoprotein profiles in the proband and affected relatives. The lipoproteins which are most frequently elevated are VLDL, LDL, or LDL + VLDL (lipoprotein phenotypes IV, IIa, or IIb, respectively). Patients with FCH have two changes in their plasma lipoproteins that can be utilized to establish the diagnosis of FCH. The first is a cholesterol-rich plasma LDL containing an abnormal cholesterol-to-apoB ratio (normal, <1.3; FCH, >1.3), which is designated ''dense LDL.'' The second is an LDL-apoB level greater than 130 mg/dl. In addition, HDL levels are frequently reduced, particularly in patients with hypertriglyceridemia. The most important clinical sequela of FCH is the development of premature coronary heart disease, which is similar in severity and clinical course to the cardiovascular disease present in FH heterozygotes.

A subset of patients with FCH has been identified having normal LDL cholesterol levels but elevated levels of LDL apoB >130 mg/dl. This syndrome, termed hyperapobetalipoproteinemia, is characterized by increased plasma levels of LDL-apoB and the presence of dense LDL in the absence of hyperlipidemia (97,98). Kinetic studies of radiolabeled VLDL and LDL revealed an increase in VLDL-apoB synthesis and a relatively normal rate of LDL catabolism (99,100). Of particular clinical importance is the development of premature cardiovascular disease in patients with hyperapobetalipoproteinemia. These patients can mistakenly be considered not to have a dyslipoproteinemia which requires a treatment, since they may have ''normal LDL-cholesterol levels.''

The clinical features of patients with FCH include arcus cornea and xanthelasma; however, tendon xanthomas are unusual. The lack of tendon xanthomas in a patient with hypercholesterolemia is a useful clinical feature to differentiate FCH from FH.

The molecular defect(s) in patients with FCH has not been definitively established. The presumptive diagnosis of FCH can be established only by the identification of a characteristic pattern of dyslipoproteinemia in the propositus and family members. No homozygotes for FCH have been identified. Affected individuals in a number of kindreds with FCH may be genetic compounds, containing two defective genes, one for FCH and second one for another underlying genetic dyslipoproteinemia.

Familial Hyperchylomicronemia

Familial chylomicronemia, a rare genetic syndrome inherited as an autosomal recessive trait, is characterized by severe fasting hypertriglyceridemia and massive accumulations of chylomicrons in plasma (101,102). Affected individuals often present early in childhood with recurrent episodes of abdominal pain and/or pancreatitis frequently precipitated by the ingestion of a fatty meal. In these patients, both serum and urine amylase levels may appear normal due to interference by the plasma lipids and/or by circulating inhibitors with the amylase assays (102–105). Thus, classic pancreatitis may be difficult to diagnose. The major clinical findings seen in patients with chylomicronemia are illustrated in Fig. 6 (Colorplate 2). Lipid accumulation in the liver and spleen of some patients leads to hepatosplenomegaly as well as mild but reversible elevation of liver transaminase. Eruptive xanthomas, small yellow papular skin lesions localized primarily over the buttocks and extensor surfaces, appear when plasma triglyceride levels exceed 1,000–2,000 mg/dl, and usually regress within a few weeks after triglyceride levels are lowered (106). Similarly, lipemia retinales may be detected by funduscopic examination when triglyceride values are greater than 2,000–3,000 mg/dl. The retinal vessels in these patients appear lipemic, and the fundus has a pale pink appearance due to light scattering by circulating chylomicrons. All of these clinical features are reversible and do not lead to either progressive liver dysfunction or visual impairment. Patients with familial chylomicronemia do not appear to be at risk for developing premature cardiovascular disease. The major morbidity associated with this disorder is recurrent episodes of pancreatitis, which in some affected individuals have resulted in pancreatic insufficiency.

Abnormalities in the lipid profile of patients presenting with familial chylomicronemia include severe fasting hypertriglyceridemia, with levels between 500 and 5,000 mg/dl, and plasma cholesterol concentrations that range from normal to as high as 1,000 mg/dl. Chylomicrons, which are normally rapidly cleared from the circulation, are present in the patient's plasma after a 12-hr fast, and VLDL concentrations are also frequently increased. In addition, LDL- and HDL-cholesterol values are reduced as a result of both decreased synthesis and increased catabolism (101). The two major molecular defects that lead to the familial chylomicronemia are a deficiency of lipoprotein lipase (LPL) or of its cofactor, apoC-II. These two genetic disorders are summarized in the following sections.

ApoC-II Deficiency

ApoC-II is a small, 8,800-molecular weight protein that is present in plasma associated with chylomicrons, VLDL, and HDL. It is synthesized primarily by the liver (107) and serves as a cofactor for the lipolytic enzyme. In the presence of apoC-II, LPL hydrolyses triglycerides present in chylomicrons and VLDL to monoglycerides and diglycerides as well as free fatty acids which can be utilized as sources of energy or reesterified for storage in adipose tissue (101,102). Thus, a deficiency of apoC-II results in marked derangements of both triglyceride and lipoprotein metabolism.

Deficiency of apoC-II is a very rare cause of familial chylomicronemia, with fewer than ten kindreds reported (108). With rare exceptions (109,110), this genetic disorder is inherited as an autosomal recessive trait and affected homozygous individuals present with many of the classical features of familial chylomicronemia as described previously (101,102). The diagnosis of apoC-II deficiency is made when the plasma of a patient presenting with the chylomicronemia syndrome is unable to activate LPL *in vitro,* suggesting a functional deficiency of apoC-II. In addition, a deficiency of apoC-II or an apoC-II variant can be identified by analysis of the patient's plasma by isoelectric focusing or two-dimensional gel electrophoresis. Postheparin plasma LPL activity in the presence of exogenous apoC-II is normal to increased in these individuals.

The underlying molecular defects that lead to a functional deficiency of apoC-II have been identified in several kindreds by sequence analysis of the apoC-II gene of affected family members (102,111). The location of these mutations in the apoC-II gene are summarized in Fig. 7. Most of the identified gene defects are single point mutations that result in decreased expression of the apolipoprotein and thus lead to markedly reduced concentrations or total absence of plasma apoC-II. These include mutations in the apoC-II gene that either introduce a premature termination codon (apoC-$II_{Nijmegen}$, apoC-II_{Padova}, apoC-II_{Bari}, and apoC-II_{Paris2}), substitute the initiation codon (apoC-II_{Paris1}), or disrupt a donor splice site (apoC-$II_{Hamburg}$) (102,111). The defects in the Japanese and Venezuelan kindreds are unique in that four to five different mutations were identified in the apoC-II gene of the homozygous probands, resulting in a deficiency of apoC-II (102,111). In the case of apoC-$II_{Toronto}$ and apoC-$II_{St.Michael}$ (102,111), frameshift mutations in the proposed LPL binding domain (residues 65–79) of apoC-II result in the synthesis of an altered protein that cannot activate bovine LPL *in vitro.* Unlike the situation in most apoC-II-deficient patients, significant amounts of a nonfunctional apoC-II are detected in the plasma of affected individuals. Characterization of the various kindreds indicates that the underlying molecular defects that lead to apoC-II deficiency are heterogeneous with no evidence of a founder gene effect that would permit rapid screening of affected individuals or identification of carriers for the trait.

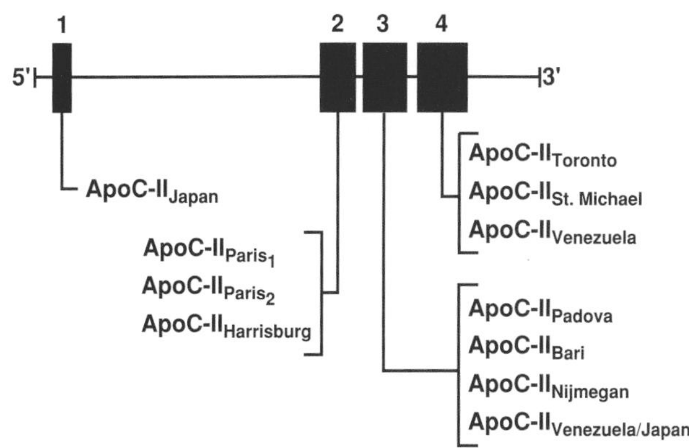

FIG. 7. Schematic representation of the apoC-II gene. *Solid boxes:* exons 1–4. The locations of the different mutations in the apoC-II gene are illustrated.

Lipoprotein Lipase Deficiency

Human LPL is a glycoprotein of approximately 55,000 daltons (112) that is synthesized primarily by adipocytes, heart and skeletal muscle, macrophages, and mammary gland (113). The active enzyme is a noncovalent homodimer which is anchored to the endothelial cell surface by a membrane-bound heparin sulfate proteoglycan. In the presence of its cofactor, apoC-II, LPL hydrolyses the 1- and 3-ester bonds in triglycerides present in chylomicrons and VLDL to monoglycerides, diglycerides, and free fatty acids. In the process, LPL in combination with apoC-II facilitates the intravascular remodeling of lipoprotein particles and the ultimate clearance of remnant lipoproteins from the circulation.

The majority of patients presenting with the familial chylomicronemia syndrome have a deficiency of LPL. Unlike apoC-II deficiency, LPL deficiency is a relatively common disorder, with a frequency of 1:5,000 to 1:10,000 in some populations (114). The carrier state for LPL deficiency is as prevalent as, and in some areas more prevalent (114–116) than, the heterozygous state for familial hypercholesterolemia. The diagnosis of LPL deficiency is suspected from the clinical presentation and established by finding markedly reduced or absent LPL activity in the patient's postheparin plasma. A bolus of 60 U/kg of heparin sulfate will release LPL bound to the endothelial vessel wall into the circulation,

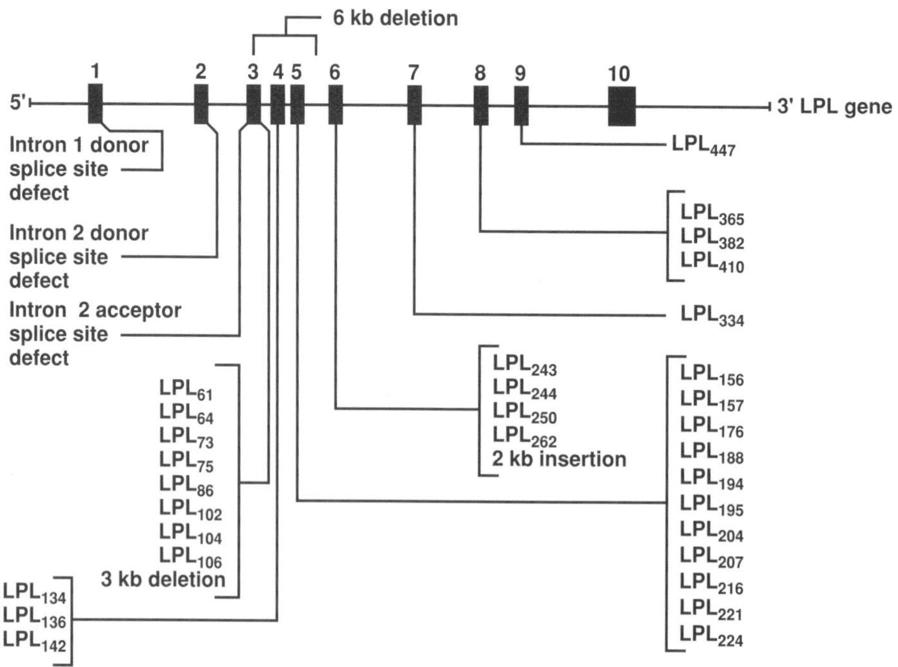

FIG. 8. Schematic representation of the LPL gene. *Solid boxes:* exons 1–10. The locations of the different mutations in the LPL gene are illustrated.

where it can be easily quantitated (101,102). Determination of adipocyte LPL activity obtained from a fat biopsy can also be used to make the diagnosis (101,102).

A large number of mutations in the LPL gene that lead to the expression of familial chylomicronemia have been identified (108,117,118) and are summarized in Fig. 8. Several major gene rearrangements involving a 2-kb, 3 kb-deletion and a 6-kb insertion have been described in several kindreds (119,120). The 2-kb insertion involves a partial duplication of exon 6, while the 6-kb deletion involves exons 3–6 of the LPL gene (121). In addition, a large deletion of exon 9 in LPL has been described (122). These defects result in markedly reduced levels of LPL in the postheparin plasma of affected individuals. Point mutations that lead to the substitution of a single amino acid in LPL and to the synthesis of a nonfunctional enzyme have also been reported. These include substitutions of LPL residues 69, 75, 86, 136, 142, 156, 157, 162, 176, 188, 194, 195, 204, 207, 216, 224, 243, 244, 250, 334, 365, and 410 (122–126). Interestingly, these mutations are all clustered around the highly conserved fourth, fifth, and sixth exons of the LPL gene, which encode for amino acids involved in the catalytic function (127). Defects that result in the introduction of a premature stop codon at positions 61, 64, 73, 106, 146, 221, 224, 262, and 447 (117,118), as well as splicing defects, have also been reported. Unlike apoC-II, evidence for a founder gene effect as a cause for LPL deficiency has been identified in the French Canadian and other populations which have mutations at positions 188 and 207 of LPL (115,116,125,126).

Although many carriers for the LPL deficiency trait appear to have normal plasma lipids, analysis of several extended kindreds with different mutations in the LPL gene indicate that the heterozygous state for LPL deficiency may underlie some of the more common hyperlipidemic disorders found in the general population (117,121,128). Thus, a significant association is present between the carrier state for LPL deficiency and familial hypertriglyceridemia (129), familial combined hyperlipidemia (130), and postprandial lipemia (126). Given the high frequency of the carrier state for LPL deficiency in the general population, mutations in LPL alone or through interactions with either environmental or genetic factors may account for a significant proportion of hyperlipidemias within a given population.

Homozygous individuals with LPL deficiency do not appear to be at an increased risk for developing premature cardiovascular disease (117). It is unclear, however, if the partial LPL deficiency observed in carriers for the trait may result, at least in a subset of patients, in an increased risk of atherosclerosis. Recent studies have provided some insights into this question. The synthesis of LPL by either macrophages or smooth muscle cells present in atherosclerotic lesions has been demonstrated (117). Enhanced lipolysis mediated by LPL may, in turn, increase the accumulation of cholesteryl esters in these cells and ultimately result in enhanced foam cell formation in the arterial wall. In addition, the presence of LPL in the subendothelial space may promote the binding and retention of LDL (131) and VLDL (132) to the subendothelial matrix, potentially enhancing the conversion of these lipoproteins to more atherogenic forms. LPL also appears to enhance the binding of atherogenic lipoproteins to smooth muscle cells (133) as well as increase monocyte adhesion to aortic endothelial cells (134). More recent studies indicate a significant association between high levels of LPL synthesis as well as secretion in macrophages and susceptibility to atherosclerosis in inbred murine strains (135), providing further evidence for a potential role of LPL in atherosclerosis.

Characterization of transgenic mice overexpressing LPL primarily in adipose tissue, heart, and skeletal muscle (134,136) suggests that expression of LPL in tissues other than those found in the arterial wall may, in fact, be beneficial. Thus, these animals have a markedly improved lipid profile, including elevations in total HDL (137) and HDL_2-cholesterol (136) as well as reduction in plasma triglyceride and cholesterol-rich LDL and appear to be protected against diet-induced hypertriglyceridemia and hypercholesterolemia. Although studies analyzing the effect of LPL overexpression on atherosclerosis are not available, it appears that in this setting, increased LPL activity may be beneficial. In other studies (138), the treatment of rats with the novel compound NO-1886, which increases LPL activity, leads to higher levels of HDL as well as protection against the development of coronary artery lesions.

Thus, LPL may play a dual role in the development of atherosclerosis. The synthesis of LPL by cells present in the arterial wall may promote the atherosclerotic process, whereas LPL-mediated lipoprotein uptake by the liver may result in enhanced catabolism of atherogenic particles, thereby reducing lesion formation. Ultimately, the role of LPL in the development of or protection against atherosclerosis may be dictated by its site of synthesis as well as interaction with other genetic and environmental factors.

Hepatic Lipase Deficiency

Hepatic lipase (HL) deficiency, a rare genetic disorder first described in 1982 by Breckenridge et al. (139), has been identified to date in only four different kindreds (139–144). The frequency of this disorder in the general population, however, may be underestimated due to the difficulty in identifying affected individuals. HL is an important enzyme which mediates the hydrolysis of triglycerides and phospholipids present in plasma lipoproteins (145–147). Its action as both an acylglycerol hydrolase and phospholipase results in the conversion of IDL to LDL and HDL_2 to HDL_3 (148–150). Thus, HL plays an important role in the metabolism of remnant lipoproteins and HDL.

The diagnosis of HL deficiency is established by finding markedly reduced or absent HL activity but normal LPL activity in the patient's postheparin plasma. Individuals with a deficiency of HL may present with features characteristic of type III hyperlipoproteinemia, including hypercholesterolemia, hypertriglyceridemia, accumulation of triglyceride-rich lipoproteins as well as β-VLDL, palmar xanthomas, and premature cardiovascular disease (139–144). Triglyceride levels have ranged from normal to 4,000 mg/dl in affected individuals. In addition, pancreatitis has been described in a patient presenting with severe hypertriglyceridemia due to combined HL deficiency and partial deficiency of LPL (141,142). However, unlike patients with type III hyperlipoproteinemia, patients with a deficiency of HL have triglyceride-enriched lipoproteins and a normal VLDL-cholesterol/total triglyceride ratio of <0.3, a finding which is useful in distinguishing the two genetic syndromes (140,141,144). In addition, many patients with HL deficiency have increased plasma apoB concentrations (139,141,151), which appears to be the result of a reduced fractional clearance rate of apoB from VLDL and IDL (151).

The underlying molecular defects which lead to HL deficiency have been investigated in several independent kindreds (152–156). Two mutations resulting in the replacement of Ser^{267} by Phe and Thr^{383} by Met have been described in the affected proband from the Ontario kindred (155). In the kindred from Quebec, a mutation which leads to the substitution of Thr^{383} by Met was identified in only one of two alleles (155). The authors thus speculated that the deficiency imparted by this mutation might be modulated by other factors such as age, gender, or the effect of variation at other genes (152–154). The proband from a third kindred was shown to be homozygous for a single A → G substitution in intron 1 of the HL gene which resulted in alternative splicing, premature termination of translation, and the synthesis of a truncated, nonfunctional enzyme (156). Additional sequence variants of the HL gene which have been identified in normolipidemic subjects with normal HL activity involve mutations in exon 3 (Val^{73}→Met) and in exon 5 (Asn^{193}→Ser) (153,154).

Although several patients with HL deficiency have developed premature cardiovascular disease (139,141), the role that a deficiency of this enzyme plays in the development of atherosclerosis remains to be established. Of interest, however, is the recent generation of transgenic mice overexpressing the human HL gene (157). Although the mouse strain utilized in these studies is not susceptible to the development of diet-induced lesions, the authors described decreased cholesterol accumulation in the vessels of transgenic mice compared to control animals, suggesting that elevated HL levels reduced cholesterol deposition in the arterial wall (157). Further studies will be required to evaluate definitively the role of HL in atherosclerosis.

Familial Dysbetalipoproteinemia

Individuals with familial dysbetalipoproteinemia have a delayed clearance of remnants of triglyceride-rich lipoproteins, resulting in the accumulation of remnants from both the hepatic VLDL as well as chylomicron pathways. Several different nomenclatures have been used for the codification of familial dysbetalipoproteinemia (158–160). Patients with this disorder have been classified as having dysbetalipoproteinemia when low or normal plasma lipid values are present and as having type III hyperlipoproteinemia when hyperlipidemia has developed. The remnant lipoproteins have the hydrated density of VLDL and IDL, but have the electrophoretic mobility of β rather than the usual pre-β lipoproteins. These cholesterol-rich, β electrophoretically migrating lipoproteins are present with the density <1.006 g/ml. As a result of the change in VLDL electrophoretic mobility, patients with this disease have also been classified as having β-VLDL, floating β lipoproteins (density <1.006 g/ml), or broad-beta disease. Additional important diagnostic features of familial dysbetalipoproteinemia include an elevation of cholesterol and triglycerides with a ratio of approximately 1:1 and a VLDL-cholesterol to plasma-triglyceride ratio >0.3 (control subjects <0.3). Patients with dysbetalipoproteinemia often develop hyperlipidemia as well as other clinical symptomatology in the fourth and fifth decades. The major clinical feature of this disorder is an increased risk of both premature coronary heart disease and peripheral vascular disease.

One of the fascinating clinical features of dysbetalipoproteinemia is the presence of palmar xanthomas (xanthoma striata palmaris), which are virtually pathognomonic of this dyslipoproteinemia (Fig. 9; see Colorplate 3). Palmar xanthomas are frequently accompanied by tuberous lesions over the elbows, knees, and buttocks. Occasionally, the patients may develop achilles tendon xanthomas, characteristic of patients with FH.

The underlying metabolic defect in familial dysbetalipoproteinemia is the presence of a defective apoE, which plays a key role in the metabolism and cellular uptake of remnants of triglyceride-rich lipoproteins (161). Population studies have indicated that apoE is controlled at a single genetic locus with an unusual degree of polymorphism (162–165). There are three common alleles in the general population, which have been designated $\Sigma 2$, $\Sigma 3$, and $\Sigma 4$. The three E apolipoproteins encoded by these three alleles are separable by isoelectrofocusing and are designated apoE2, apoE3, and apoE4, respectively. Six major apoE phenotypes are present in the population, including homozygotes for apolipoproteins E2, E3, and E4 as well as heterozygotes for apolipoproteins E2,3, E2,4, and E3,4. The structural differences in the apoE isoproteins have been shown to be due to one or two amino acid substitutions involving cysteine and arginine exchanges at amino acid residues 112 and 158.

The predominant E isoprotein in the normolipidemic population is apoE3 and it is considered the normal or parent isoprotein. Two different modes of inheritance have been identified in hyperlipidemic patients with familial dysbetalipoproteinemia (Table 3). The majority of individuals who have hyperlipidemia have the autosomal recessive form of the disease. An increased frequency of the E2 allele (apoE2,2 phenotype) (7,163–165) or E^0 allele (apoE absence) (166–169) has been observed in hyperlipidemic patients with familial dysbetalipoproteinemia. However, the majority of individuals with the apoE2,2 phenotype are normocholesterolemic or hypocholesterolemic (4,7,165). Subjects with the apoE2,2 phenotype and no hyperlipidemia have been

TABLE 3. *Inheritance in hyperlipidemic patients with familial dysbetalipoproteinemia*

Mutation	ApoE phenotype	Receptor binding activity (%)
Recessive inheritance		
ApoE ($Arg^{158} \rightarrow Cys$)	E2	<2
Dominant inheritance		
$ApoE_{Harrisburg}$ ($Lys^{146} \rightarrow Glu$)	E1	—
ApoE ($Lys^{146} \rightarrow Gln$)	E2	40
ApoE ($Arg^{142} \rightarrow Cys$)	E3	—
$ApoE_{Leiden}$ (7 aa insertion at aa 121)	E3	40
$ApoE_{Philadelphia}$ ($Glu^{13} \rightarrow Lys$, $Arg^{145} \rightarrow Cys$)	E4	—
ApoE ($Cys^{112} \rightarrow Arg$, $Arg^{142} \rightarrow Cys$)	E3	4

aa, Amino acid.

categorized as normolipidemic E2 dysbetalipoproteinemic homozygotes. The development of hyperlipidemia in the recessive form of familial dysbetalipoproteinemia has been proposed to require the presence of an additional environmental or genetic abnormality such as obesity, hypothyroidism, or a second dyslipoproteinemia, particularly familial combined hyperlipidemia. Thus, a second genetic defect may be required for the apoE2,2 subject to become hyperlipidemic.

Patients with the dominant form of inheritance of familial dysbetalipoproteinemia develop hyperlipidemia as heterozygotes. The apoE mutations associated with the dominant form of this dyslipoproteinemia include mutations at residue 142, residue 146, or a seven-amino acid insertion at residue 121 of apoE (Table 3) (7,170–173). The hyperlipidemia observed in some cases of the dominant form of the disease often appears at an earlier age and is associated with significant cardiovascular disease.

Individuals with the apoE4 variant have elevated plasma levels of total as well as LDL cholesterol when compared to subjects with the apoE3,3 phenotype. Kinetic studies utilizing radiolabeled apoE isoproteins have established that apoE4 is catabolized more rapidly than apoE3 (10,174). Based on these results, it has been proposed that patients with the apoE4 phenotype have a more rapid clearance of plasma chylomicrons and VLDL remnants by the liver than do apoE3 subjects. The increased rate of hepatic clearance of the remnant particles leads to downregulation of the LDL receptor, resulting in higher plasma concentrations of cholesterol, LDL, and remnant particles. An increased level of plasma LDL would be expected to increase the risk of premature cardiovascular disease in patients with the apoE4 phenotype. It is also of interest that patients with Alzheimer's disease have an increased frequency of the apoE4 allele (175,176). The role of apoE4 in Alzheimer's disease is not completely understood.

Hypertriglyceridemia–Low-HDL Syndrome

A common lipoprotein profile present in patients with established coronary heart disease is elevated triglycerides and decreased HDL-cholesterol levels (177). There are no characteristic clinical features and the patients have a significantly increased risk of premature heart disease. The lipid and lipoprotein profiles in these patients may vary depending on the diet and lifestyle, as well as the presence of a second genetic dyslipoproteinemia. The mode of inheritance of this syndrome has not been established and there may be several different molecular defects resulting in this lipoprotein phenotype. The increased risk in the development of premature cardiovascular disease may be due to the elevation of atherogenic remnants of triglyceride-rich particles or low HDL, or a combination of both.

Elevated Lipoprotein(a)

Elevated plasma levels of Lp(a) have been proposed to be an important independent risk factor for the development of premature cardiovascular disease. Plasma Lp(a) levels range from <1 to >100 mg/dl. Of clinical importance is the correlation of the size of the apo(a) isoprotein and the plasma Lp(a) levels (178). The different molecular weights of Lp(a) in human plasma are due to a variable number of copies of kringle 4 in the amino acid sequence of apo(a) (179,180). Lp(a) isoproteins of higher and lower molecular weights are associated with lower and higher plasma concentrations, respectively. The molecular size and plasma levels of Lp(a) are inheritable. Approximately 20% of the population have levels above 30 mg/dl, which is associated with a twofold increase in the relative risk of premature cardiovascular disease. The mechanism(s) by which elevated plasma levels of Lp(a) increase the risk of premature heart disease has not been definitively ascertained. Lp(a) may be taken up by macrophages resulting in cholesterol deposition and foam cell formation. Alternatively, its atherogenic properties may be related to its role in increasing thrombosis. Lp(a) has been reported to interact with fibrin peptides, inhibit thrombolysis, and be a competitive inhibitor of plasminogen for the plasminogen receptor present on endothelial cells (181,182). Individuals with elevated plasma Lp(a) levels have no diagnostic clinical features and subjects with relatively normal total cholesterol levels may have elevated plasma levels of Lp(a) which increase the risk of premature heart disease.

β-Sitosterolemia

β-Sitosterolemia is a rare autosomal recessive disease characterized by plasma and tissue accumulation of plant sterols, including sitosterol, campesterol, and stigmasterol, as well as other sterols, including shellfish sterols (183,184). The defect in this disease can more appropriately be considered a pansterol defect in which all of the dietary sterols are absorbed by the intestine. The increased plasma concentrations of sterols are frequently accompanied by an increase in cholesterol levels. The clinical manifestations of β-sitosterolemia begin in childhood or the first and second decades of life. Tendon xanthomas may develop even if the plasma cholesterol concentrations are relatively normal. The presence of tendon xanthoma in a child without hypercholesterolemia may also be a clue to the diagnosis of β-sitosterolemia. In addition, the disease should also be considered in young patients with tendon xanthomas and hypercholesterolemia. In these individuals LDL-receptor function is normal and some of these patients have been classified as "pseudo-familial hypercholesterolemia."

The diagnosis of β-sitosterolemia can be definitively ascertained by the determination of the plasma levels of plant sterols (upper limit of normal is 0.5% of total plasma sterols), which are transported primarily within LDL. The fecal bile acid pattern is unusual, with increased levels of deoxycholic and lithocholic acids and fecal bile alcohols.

The characteristic clinical features of β-sitosterolemia in addition to the tendon xanthomas are tuberous xanthomas, arcus cornea, xanthelasma, and premature cardiovascular disease (Fig. 10; see Colorplate 4). Hemolytic anemia may also occur in β-sitosterolemia.

The molecular defect in β-sitosterolemia has not been determined. A very low rate of hepatic and intestinal cholesterol synthesis has been reported due to low HMB-CoA reductase activity, which is accompanied by increased intestinal absorption of all sterols, including cholesterol and plant and shellfish sterols (185,186). In addition, a defect in the hepatic excretion of plant and shellfish sterols has been observed which results in delayed hepatic clearance of all absorbed sterols (187,188). Treatment of homozygous β-sitosterolemia patients with bile acid sequestrants results in substantial lowering of plasma sterols and regression of xanthomas, suggesting that treatment may be effective in reducing the risk of premature heart disease.

HYPOALPHALIPOPROTEINEMIAS

The genetic dyslipoproteinemias which are characterized by abnormally low concentrations of plasma lipoproteins and an increased risk of early heart disease involve primarily genetic defects in HDL.

Tangier Disease

Tangier disease is a genetic dyslipoproteinemia characterized clinically by orange tonsils, cloudy corneas, hepatosplenomegaly, lymphadenopathy, intermittent peripheral neuropathy, and a mild increase in risk of premature cardiovascular disease (189,190). Tangier disease should be suspected when the plasma cholesterol is below 120 mg/dl and the triglycerides are normal or slightly elevated. Marked decreases in the plasma levels of HDL cholesterol, apoA-I, and apoA-II (<2–5% of normal) are the lipoprotein profile hallmark of patients with Tangier disease.

The onset of the clinical features of Tangier disease is insidious, presumably reflecting the slow tissue accumulation of cholesteryl esters. The most characteristic site of deposition is the pharyngeal tonsils and the presence of orange tonsils is virtually pathognomonic and can provide the diagnosis of Tangier disease at a glance. Frequently, however, the tonsils have been removed prior to the physician examining the patient. Hepatosplenomegaly, due to lipid accumulation in the reticuloendothelial system, is often present. Hypersplenism is rare; however, removal of the spleen for splenomegaly may lead to hyperplasia of the reticuloendothelial cells in the omentum or other areas of the body. Tangier patients may present with transient recurrent peripheral neuropathy which is also due to an accumulation of lipid within the nerve sheaths. Neurologic symptoms including motor weakness, paresthesia, and dysesthesia may occur, but often wax and wane. The clinical course of patients with Tangier disease is extremely variable, and the diagnosis may not be made until the third or fourth decade. Despite the low plasma HDL levels, the risk of premature cardiovascular disease is only minimal. Heterozygotes have plasma HDL, apoA-I, and apoA-II that are approximately 50% of normal levels and triglyceride levels that are mildly elevated. Heterozygotes have no significant clinical sequelae.

On physical examination the unique clinical feature of homozygotes with Tangier disease is the presence of lobulated, bright orange-yellow tonsils (Fig. 11; see Colorplate 5). If the tonsils have been removed, pharyngeal tags of orange-yellow tissue may still be evident upon examination. The rectal mucosa may have a similar orange appearance, and the identification of cholesteryl esters in foam cells in the rectal mucosa may be used to establish the diagnosis. Asymptomatic corneal opacities often require slit-lamp examination for identification. Mild hepatosplenomegaly and lymphadenopathy may also be present. The neuropathy in Tangier disease may be detected by decreased deep tendon reflexes and sensory motor abnormalities.

The molecular defect in Tangier disease have not been elucidated. Kinetic studies using radiolabeled HDL have established that the low plasma HDL levels in Tangier disease are due to markedly increased HDL catabolism (191,192). Recent *in vitro* studies analyzing HDL-facilitated cholesterol efflux from cholesterol-loaded fibroblasts from Tangier patients and control subjects revealed decreased cholesterol efflux from cells from Tangier disease patients when compared to control cells, suggesting that the molecular defect in Tangier disease is an intracellular defect in cholesterol metabolism (193).

Apolipoprotein A-I Deficiency

ApoA-I, a major apolipoprotein of HDL, is of clinical importance due to the inverse association of plasma apoA-I levels and the development of premature coronary heart disease. The majority of structural mutations which have been identified in apoA-I do not affect HDL levels and have apparently little clinical significance. However, identification of structural mutations in apoA-I which lead to decreased plasma HDL levels and premature cardiovascular disease have important clinical implications for the diagnosis and treatment of patients with early heart disease. Two point mutations in the amino acid sequence of apoA-I, the deletion of apoA-I lysine 107 and the substitution of proline 165 for arginine, are associated with reduced levels of HDL cholesterol (194).

Mutations in the apoA-I + apoC-III + apoA-IV gene complex on chromosome 11 which lead to the virtual absence of plasma apoA-I and HDL cholesterol are associated with severe premature heart disease. Four illustrative kindreds will be reviewed with premature coronary heart disease, markedly decreased plasma HDL levels, and a deficiency of apoA-I alone or in combination with apoC-III or apoC-III + apoA-IV.

ApoA-I Deficiency

Two representative kindreds with apoA-I deficiency will be summarized. In the first kindred the proband with apoA-I deficiency was a 5-year-old Turkish girl with planar xanthomas and a markedly reduced level of plasma HDL (195). Family history was positive for early heart disease. Clinical features included mild hepatomegaly, but no splenomegaly, neuropathy, or orange tonsils. Plasma apoA-I was absent, apoA-II was reduced to 10% of controls, and apoC-III as well as apoA-IV levels were within the control range. The molecular defect in the proband was identified as a deletion of a base resulting in a frameshift introducing a premature stop codon at residue 27 in apoA-I.

The proband in a second kindred with apoA-I deficiency was a 25-year-old man of Philippine origin with planar xanthomas (196) and established coronary heart disease based on ultrafast computed tomography (Fig. 12; see Colorplate 6). The lipoprotein profile included normal plasma triglycerides, reduced total cholesterol, and markedly decreased HDL cholesterol (<3 mg/dl) and apoA-II (7–13 mg/dl) and absence of plasma apoA-I. The proband's 62-year-old aunt also had no plasma apoA-I and had coronary artery bypass surgery at age 61 years. The structural defect in the apoA-I gene in this kindred has not been reported.

ApoA-I + ApoC-III Deficiency

The affected individuals in this kindred are two sisters identified at ages 31 and 32 years with mild corneal opacities and planar xanthomas on the trunk, neck, and eyelids and severe coronary artery disease (197,198). Plasma levels of VLDL were reduced, LDL was normal, and HDL was severely decreased (6 mg/dl). ApoA-I and apoC-III were absent and apoA-II was reduced to <5% of normal. The molecular defect in this kindred was a rearrangement in the apoA-I and apoC-III genes resulting in the failure of synthesis of both apoA-I and apoC-III.

ApoA-I + ApoC-III + ApoA-IV Deficiency

The proband was a 45-year-old woman with mild corneal opacities and severe premature heart disease (199,200). There were no xanthomas, orange tonsils, or organomegaly. Plasma triglycerides and VLDL were reduced, LDL and plasma apoB were normal, and HDL was markedly decreased. Plasma apolipoproteins A-I, C-III, and A-IV were absent from plasma, and apoA-II was decreased to <10% of normal. The genetic defect in this kindred is a 7.5-kb deletion that results in the failure of synthesis of all three apolipoproteins, A-I, C-III, and apoA-IV.

These kindreds with apoA-I deficiency illustrate two clinically important points. First, the close proximity and tandem array of the genes for apolipoproteins A-I, C-III, and A-IV on chromosome 11 permits the loss of the expression of up to three apolipoproteins by a single mutation. Second, the absence of synthesis of plasma apoA-I and markedly decreased HDL-cholesterol levels due to a genetic defect in the apoA-I gene alone or in combination with a deficiency of apoC-III or apoC-III + apoA-IV results in the development of severe premature heart disease. Thus, apoA-I is necessary for normal plasma levels of HDL, and a defect in the apoA-I gene that results in decreased apoA-I synthesis dramatically increases the risk of premature cardiovascular disease.

Familial Hypoalphalipoproteinemia

Kindreds with familial hypoalphalipoproteinemia have been identified with normal plasma triglycerides and decreased plasma HDL-cholesterol levels (201,202). A subset of these kindreds has cosegregation of low plasma HDL levels and an increased risk of premature cardiovascular disease. There are no characteristic clinical features and the plasma lipids and lipoproteins are often normal except for the reduced plasma levels of HDL cholesterol. The genetic defect(s) leading to familial hypoalphalipoproteinemia has not been identified. Patients with coronary artery disease with "normal lipids" may be members of kindreds with familial hypoalphalipoproteinemia.

SUMMARY

During the last two decades there has been a progressive increase in our knowledge of the pathways of cholesterol and triglyceride metabolism. The detailed information now available on the role of the plasma lipoproteins in lipid transport and the specific functions in metabolism of lipoprotein receptors, enzymes, transfer proteins, and apolipoproteins has provided the framework for a detailed understanding of lipid transport. In addition, the role of the plasma lipoproteins, enzymes, and receptors in the development of the atherosclerotic process has been more clearly defined. This new knowledge has markedly facilitated the elucidation of the molecular defects in patients with genetic dyslipoproteinemias. Identification of the specific gene defects and the resulting clinical phenotypes now provides the opportunity to develop improved methods for identification of the individual at risk for developing a dyslipoproteinemia and the potential for more selective and specific treatment programs. The ultimate goal of these studies is to identify and treat effectively the patient with a potential risk of premature cardiovascular disease. The current availability of more effective drugs for the treatment of the dyslipoproteinemias and the ultimate ability to correct gene defects by gene therapy provide an encouraging future for the eventual reduction in atherosclerosis and the prevention of premature cardiovascular disease.

REFERENCES

1. Gofman JW, deLalla O, Glazier F, et al. The serum lipid transport system in health, metabolic disorders, atherosclerosis, and coronary artery disease. *Plasma* 1954;2:413–484.
2. Berg K, Dahlen G, Frick MH. Lp(a) lipoprotein and pre-beta 1-lipoprotein in patients with coronary heart disease. *Clin Genet* 1974;6: 230–235.
3. Brewer HB, Jr, Gregg RE, Hoeg JM, Fojo SS. Apolipoproteins and lipoproteins in human plasma: an overview. *Clin Chem* 1988;34:4–8.
4. Brewer HB, Jr, Gregg RE, Hoeg JM. Apolipoproteins, lipoproteins, and atherosclerosis. In: Braunwald E, ed. *Heart disease: a textbook of cardiovascular medicine*. Philadelphia: Saunders; 1989:121–144.
5. Vega GL, Denke MA, Grundy SM. Metabolic basis of primary hypercholesterolemia. *Circulation* 1991;84:118–128.
6. Schaefer EJ. Diagnosis and management of lipoprotein disorders. In: Rifkind BM, ed. *Drug treatment of hyperlipidemia*. New York: Dekker; 1991:17–52.
7. Davignon J, Gregg RE, Sing CF. Apolipoprotein E polymorphism and atherosclerosis. *Arteriosclerosis* 1988;8:1–21.
8. Goldstein JL, Brown MS. The LDL receptor locus and the genetics of familial hypercholesterolemia. *Annu Rev Genet* 1979;13:259–289.
9. Goldstein JL, Brown MS, Anderson RG, Russell DW, Schneider WJ. Receptor-mediated endocytosis: concepts emerging from the LDL receptor system. *Annu Rev Cell Biol* 1985;1:1–39.
10. Gregg RE, Brewer HB, Jr. The role of apolipoprotein E and lipoprotein receptors in modulating the *in vivo* metabolism of apolipoprotein B-containing lipoproteins in humans. *Clin Chem* 1988;34:28–32.
11. Herz J, Hamann U, Rogne S, Myklebos O, Gausepohl H, Stanley KK. Surface location and high affinity for a calcium of a 500 kDa liver membrane protein closely related to the LDL receptor suggest a physiological role as a lipoprotein receptor. *EMBO J* 1988;7:4119–4127.
12. Strickland DK, Ashcom JD, Williams S, Burgess WH, Migliorini M, Argraves WS. Sequence identity between alpha2-macroglobulin receptor and low density lipoprotein receptor-related protein suggests that this molecule is a multifunctional receptor. *J Biol Chem* 1990; 265:17401–17404.
13. Steinberg D. Lipoproteins and atherosclerosis. A look back and a look ahead. *Arteriosclerosis* 1983;3:283–301.
14. Steinberg D. Antioxidants and atherosclerosis: a current assessment. *Circulation* 1991;84:1420–1425.
15. Van Lenten BJ, Fogelman AM. Processing of lipoproteins in human monocyte-macrophages. *J Lipid Res* 1990;31:1455–1466.
16. Haberland ME, Fogelman AM. The role of altered lipoproteins in the pathogenesis of atherosclerosis. *Am Heart J* 1987;113:573–557.

17. Navab M, Hama SY, Nguyen TB, Fogelman AM. Monocyte adhesion and transmigration in atherosclerosis. *Coron Artery Dis* 1994;5: 198–204.
18. Glomset JA, Janssen ET, Kennedy R, Dobbins J. Role of plasma lecithin:cholesterol acyltransferase in the metabolism of high density lipoproteins. *J Lipid Res* 1966;7:638–648.
19. Glomset JA. The plasma lecithins:cholesterol acyltransferase reaction. *J Lipid Res* 1968;9:155–167.
20. Eisenberg S. High density lipoprotein metabolism. *J Lipid Res* 1984; 25:1017–1058.
21. Rader DJ, Castro G, Zech LA, Fruchart JC, Brewer HB, Jr. *In vivo* metabolism of apolipoprotein A-I on high density lipoprotein particles LpA-I and LpA-I, A-II. *J Lipid Res* 1991;32:1849–1859.
22. Brinton EA, Eisenberg S, Breslow JL. Human HDL cholesterol levels are determined by apoA-I fractional catabolic rate, which correlates inversely with estimates of HDL particle size: effects of gender, hepatic and lipoprotein lipases, triglyceride and insulin levels, and body fat distribution. *Arterioscler Thromb* 1994;14:707–720.
23. Grundy SM. Multifactorial etiology of hypercholesterolemia: implications for prevention of coronary heart disease. *Arterioscler Thromb* 1991;11:1619–1635.
24. Tall AR. Plasma cholesteryl ester transfer protein. *J Lipid Res* 1993; 34:1255–1274.
25. Utermann G, Weber W. Protein composition of Lp(a) lipoprotein from human plasma. *FEBS Lett* 1983;154:357–361.
26. Fless GM, Rolih CA, Scanu AM. Heterogeneity of human plasma lipoprotein (a). Isolation and charcterization of the lipoprotein subspecies and their apoproteins. *J Biol Chem* 1984;259:11470–11478.
27. Eaton DL, Fless GM, Kohr WJ, McLean JW, Xu QT, Miller CG. Partial amino acid sequence of apolipoprotein(a) shows that it is homologous to plasminogen. *Proc Natl Acad Sci USA* 1987;84: 3224–3228.
28. McLean JW, Tomlinson JE, Kuang WJ, Eaton DL, Chen EY, Fless GM. cDNA sequence of human apolipoprotein(a) is homologous to plasminogen. *Nature* 1987;330:132–137.
29. Kostner GM, Avagaro P, Zazzolato G, Marth E, Bittolo-Bon G, Quinci GB. Lipoprotein Lp(a) and the risk for myocardial infarction. *Arteriosclerosis* 1981;38:51–61.
30. Armstrong VW, Cremer P, Eberle E, Manke A, Schulze F, Wieland H. The association between serum Lp(a) concentrations and angiographically assessed coronary atherosclerosis. Dependence on serum LDL levels. *Atherosclerosis* 1986;62:249–257.
31. Utermann G. The mysteries of lipoprotein(a). *Science* 1989;246: 904–910.
32. Scanu AM. Genetic basis and pathophysiological implications of high plasma Lp(a) levels. *J Intern Med* 1992;231:679–683.
33. Schaefer EJ, Lamon-Fava S, Jenner JL, McNamara JR, Ordovas JM, Davis CE. Lipoprotein(a) levels and risk of coronary heart disease in men: the Lipid Research Clinics Coronary Primary Prevention Trial. *JAMA* 1994;271:999–1003.
34. Bulkley BH, Buja LM, Ferrans VJ, Bulkley GB, Roberts WC. Tuberous xanthoma in homozygous type II hyperlipoproteinemia. A histologic, histochemical, and electron microscopical study. *Arch Pathol* 1975;99:293–300.
35. Hoeg JM, Feuerstein IM, Tucker EE. Detection and quantitation of calcific atherosclerosis by ultrafast CT in children and young adults with homozygous familial hypercholesterolemia. *Arterioscler Thromb* 1994;14:1066–1074.
36. Hoeg JM. Familial hypercholesterolemia: what the zebra can teach us about the horse. *JAMA* 1994;271:543–546.
37. Lindgren V, Luskey KL, Russell DW, Franke U. Human genes involved in cholesterol metabolism: chromosomal mapping of the loci for the low density lipoprotein receptor and 3-hydroxy-3-methylglutaryl coenzyme A reductase with cDNA probes. *Proc Natl Acad Sci USA* 1985;82:8567–8571.
38. Sudhof TC, Goldstein JL, Brown MS, Russell DW. The LDL receptor gene: a mosiac of exons shared with different proteins. *Science* 1985; 228:815–822.
39. Schneider WJ, Beisiegel U, Goldstein JL, Brown MS. Purification of the low density lipoprotein receptor, an acidic glycoprotein of 164,000 molecular weight. *J Biol Chem* 1982;257:2664–2673.
40. Cummings RD, Kornfield S, Schneider WJ, Hobgood KK. Tolleshaug H, Brown MS. Biosynthesis of N- and O-linked oligosaccharides of the low density lipoprotein receptor. *J Biol Chem* 1983;258: 15261–15273.
41. Russell DW, Schneider WJ, Yamamoto T, Luskey KL, Brown MS, Goldstein JL. Domain map of the LDL receptor: sequence homology with the epidermal growth factor precursor. *Cell* 1984;37:577–585.
42. Yamamoto T, Davis CG, Brown MS, Schneider WJ, Casey ML, Goldstein JL. The human LDL receptor: a cysteine-rich protein with multiple *Alu* sequences in its mRNA. *Cell* 1984;39:27–38.
43. Van Driel IR, Goldstein JL, Sudhof TC, Brown MS. First cysteine-rich repeat in ligand-binding domain of low density lipoprotein receptor binds Ca2+ and monoclonal antibodies, but not lipoproteins. *J Biol Chem* 1987;262:17443–17449.
44. Hobbs HH, Brown MS, Goldstein JL, Russell DW. Deletion of exon encoding cysteine-rich repeat of low density lipoprotein receptor alters its binding specificity in a subject with familial hypercholesterolemia. *J Biol Chem* 1986;261:13114–13120.
45. Tolleshaug H, Goldstein JL, Schneider WJ, Brown MS. Posttranslational processing of the LDL receptor and its genetic disruption in familial hypercholesterolemia. *Cell* 1982;30:715–724.
46. Davis CG, Elhammer A, Russell DW, Schneider WJ, Kornfield S, Brown WS. Deletion of the clustered O-linked carbohydrates does not impair function of the low density lipoprotein receptor in transfected fibroblasts. *J Biol Chem* 1986;261:2828–2838.
47. Davis CG, van Driel IR, Russell DW, Brown MS, Goldstein JL. The low density lipoprotein receptor. Identification of amino acids in cytoplasmic domain required for rapid endocytosis. *J Biol Chem* 1987; 262:4075–4082.
48. Kishimoto A, Brown MS, Slaughter CA, Goldstein JL. Phosphorylation of serine 833 in cytoplasmic domain of low density lipoprotein receptor by a high molecular weight enzyme resembling casein kinase II. *J Biol Chem* 1987;262:1344–1351.
49. Kishimoto A, Goldstein JL, Brown MS. Purification of catalytic subunit of low density lipoprotein receptor kinase and identification of heat-stable activator protein. *J Biol Chem* 1987;262:9367–9373.
50. Yokode M, Pathak RK, Hammer RE, Brown MS, Goldstein JL, Anderson RGW. Cytoplasmic sequence required for basolateral targeting of LDL receptor in livers of transgenic mice. *J Cell Biol* 1992;117: 39–46.
51. Brown MS, Goldstein JL. Familial hypercholesterolemia: defective binding of lipoproteins to cultured fibroblasts associated with impaired regulation of 3-hydroxy-3-methylglutaryl coenzyme A reductase activity. *Proc Natl Acad Sci USA* 1974;71:788–792.
52. Brown MS, Goldstein JL. Analysis of a mutant strain of human fibroblasts with a defect in the internalization of receptor-bound low density lipoprotein. *Cell* 1976;9:663–674.
53. Hobbs HH, Brown MS, Goldstein JL. Molecular genetics of the LDL receptor gene in familial hypercholesterolemia. *Hum Mutat* 1992;1: 445–446.
54. Goldstein JL, Hobbs HH, Brown MS. Familial hypercholesterolemia. In: Scriver CR, Beaudet AL, Sly WS, Valle D, Stanbury JB, Wyngaarden JB, eds. *The metabolic and molecular bases of inherited disease.* New York: McGraw-Hill; 1995:1981–2030.
55. Edge SB, Hoeg JM, Triche T, Schneider PD, Brewer HB Jr. Cultured human hepatocytes. Evidence for metabolism of low density lipoproteins by a pathway independent of the classical low density lipoprotein receptor. *J Biol Chem* 1986;261:3800–3806.
56. Witztum JL, Simmons D, Steinberg D, Beltz WF, Weinreb R, Young SG. Intensive combination drug therapy of familial hypercholesterolemia with lovastatin, probucol, and colestipol hydrochloride. *Circulation* 1989;79:16–28.
57. Illingworth DR. Management of hyperlipidemia: goals for the prevention of atherosclerosis. *Clin Invest Med* 1990;13:211–218.
58. Summary of the second report of the National Cholesterol Education Program (NCEP) Expert Panel on detection, evaluation, and treatment of high blood cholesterol in adults (Adult Treatment Panel II). *JAMA* 1993;269:3015–3023.
59. Scandinavian Simvastatin Survival Study Group. Randomized trial of cholesterol lowering in 4444 patients with coronary heart disease: the Scandinavian Simvastatin Survival Study (4S). *Lancet* 1994;344: 1383–1389.
60. Gordon BR, Stein E, Jones P, Illingworth DR. Indications for low-density lipoprotein apheresis. *Am J Cardiol* 1994;74:1109–1112.
61. Sprecher DL, Hoeg JM, Schaefer EJ, Zech LA, Gregg RE, Lakatos E. The association of LDL receptor activity, LDL cholesterol level,

and clinical course in homozygous familial hypercholesterolemia. *Metabolism* 1985;34:294–299.
62. Hoeg JM. Pharmacologic and surgical treatment of dyslipidemic children and adolescents. *Ann N Y Acad Sci* 1991;623:275–284.
63. Postiglione A, Thompson GR. Experience with plasma-exchange in homozygous familial hypercholesterolemia. *Prog Clin Biol Res* 1985; 188:213–220.
64. Stein EA, Glueck CJ, Wesselman A, Owens ER, Nichols S, Vink P. Repetitive intermittent flow plasma exchange in patients with severe hypercholesterolemia. *Atherosclerosis* 1981;38:149–164.
65. Stein EA, Adolph R, Rice V, Glueck CJ, Spitz HB. Nonprogression of coronary aretery atherosclerosis in homozygous familial hypercholesterolemia after 31 months of repetitive plasma exchange. *Clin Cardiol* 1986;9:115–119.
66. Tatami R, Inoue N, Itoh H, Kishino B, Koga N, Nakashima Y. Regression of coronary atherosclerosis by combined LDL-apheresis and lipid-lowering drug therapy in patients with familial hypercholesterolemia: a multicenter study. *Atherosclerosis* 1992;95:1–13.
67. Gordon BR, Kelsey SF, Bilheimer DW, Brown DC, Dau PC, Gotto AM, Jr. Treatment of refractory familial hypercholesterolemia by low-density lipoprotein apheresis using an automated dextran sulfate cellulose adsorption system. *Am J Cardiol* 1992;70:1010–1016.
68. Eisenhauer T, Schuff-Werner P, Armstrong VW, Talartschik J, Scheler F, Seidel D. Long-term experience with the HELP system for treatment of severe familial hypercholesterolemia. *Am Soc Artificial Organs Trans* 1987;33:395–397.
69. Stoffel W, Borberg H, Greve V. Application of specific extracorporeal removal of low density lipoprotein in familial hypercholesterolemia. *Lancet* 1981;2:1005–1007.
70. Borberg H, Gaczkowski A, Oette K, Stoffel W. Immunosorptive apheresis of LDL. *Prog Clin Biol Res* 1990;337:163–167.
71. Borberg H, Gaczkowski A, Hombach V, Oette K, Stoffel W. Regression of atherosclerosis in patients with familial hypercholesterolemia under LDL-apheresis. *Prog Clin Biol Res* 1988;255:317–326.
72. Harders-Spengel K, Wood CB, Thompson GR, Myant NB, Soutar AK. Difference in saturable binding of low density lipoprotein to liver membranes from normocholesterolemic subjects and patients with heterozygous familial hypercholesterolemia. *Proc Natl Acad Sci USA* 1982;79:6355–6369.
73. Hoeg JM, Demosky SJ Jr, Schaefer EJ, Starzl TE, Brewer HB Jr. Characterization of hepatic low density lipoprotein binding and cholesterol metabolism in normal and homozygous familial hypercholesterolemic subjects. *J Clin Invest* 1984;73:429–436.
74. Hoeg JM, Demosky SJ Jr, Gregg RE, Schaefer EJ, Brewer HB Jr. Distinct hepatic receptors for low density lipoprotein and apolipoprotein E in humans. *Science* 1985;227:759–761.
75. Starzl TE, Bilheimer DW, Bahnson HT, Shaw BW Jr, Hardesty RL, Griffith BP. Heart–liver transplantation in a patient with familial hypercholesterolemia. *Lancet* 1984;1:1382–1383.
76. Bilheimer DW, Goldstein JL, Grundy SM, Starzl TE, Brown MS. Liver transplantation to provide low-density-lipoprotein receptors and lower plasma cholesterol in a child with homozygous familial hypercholesterolemia. *N Engl J Med* 1984;311:1658–1664.
77. Hoeg JM, Starzl TE, Brewer HB Jr. Liver transplantation for treatment of cardiovascular disease: comparison with medication and plasma exchange in homozygous familial hypercholesterolemia. *Am J Cardiol* 1987;59:705–707.
78. Sorci-Thomas M, Prack MM, Dashti N, Johnson F, Rudel LL, Williams DL. Apolipoprotein (apo) A-I production and mRNA abundance explain plasma apoA-I and high density lipoprotein differences between two nonhuman primate species with high and low susceptibilities to diet-induced hypercholesterolemia. *J Biol Chem* 1988;263: 5183–5189.
79. Wilson JM, Chowdhury JR. Prospects for gene therapy of familial hypercholesterolemia. *Mol Biol Med* 1990;7:223–232.
80. Chowdhury JR, Grossman M, Gupta S, Chowdhury NR, Baker JR Jr, Wilson JM. Long-term improvement of hypercholesterolemia after *ex vivo* gene therapy in LDLR-deficient rabbits. *Science* 1991;254: 1802–1805.
81. Wilson JM, Grossman M, Wu CH, Chowdhury NR, Wu GY, Chowdhury JR. Hepatocyte-directed gene transfer *in vivo* leads to transient improvement of hypercholesterolemia in low density lipoprotein receptor-deficient rabbits. *J Biol Chem* 1992;267:963–967.
82. Grossman M, Raper SE, Kozarsky K, Stein EA, Engelhardt JF, Muller D. Successful *ex vivo* gene therapy directed to liver in a patient with familial hypercholesterolemia. *Nature Genet* 1994;6:335–341.
83. Hoeg JM. Homozygous familial hypercholesterolemia: a paradigm for phenotypic variation. *Am J Cardiol* 1993;72:11D–14D.
84. Dugi KA, Feuerstein IM, Santamarina-Fojo S, Brewer HB Jr, Hoeg JM. Lipoprotein lipase may contribute to the variant degree of atherosclerosis in homozygous familial hypercholesterolemia. *Circulation* 1994;90:I-405.
85. Vega GL, Grundy SM. *In vivo* evidence for reduced binding of low density lipoproteins to receptors as a cause of primary moderate hypercholesterolemia. *J Clin Invest* 1986;78:1410–1414.
86. Innerarity TL, Weisgraber KH, Arnold KS, Mahley RW, Krauss RM, Vega GL. Familial defective apolipoprotein B-100: low density lipoproteins with abnormal receptor binding. *Proc Natl Acad Sci USA* 1987;84:6919–6923.
87. Soria LF, Ludwig EH, Clarke HR, Vega GL, Grundy SM, McCarthy BJ. Association between a specific apolipoprotein B mutation and familial defective apolipoprotein B-100. *Proc Natl Acad Sci USA* 1989;86:587–591.
88. Weisgraber KH, Innerarity TL, Newhouse YM, Young SG, Arnold KS, Krauss RM. Familial defective apolipoprotein B-100: enhanced binding of monoclonal antibody MB47 to abnormal low density lipoproteins. *Proc Natl Acad Sci USA* 1988;85:9758–9762.
89. Kane JP, Havel RJ. Disorders of the biogenesis and secretion of lipoproteins containing the B apolipoproteins. In: Scriver CR, Beaudet AL, Sly WS, Valle D, Stanbury JB, Wyngaarden JB, eds. *The metabolic and molecular bases of inherited disease*. New York: McGraw-Hill; 1995:1853–1885.
90. Illingworth DR, Vakar F, Mahley RW, Weisgraber KH. Hypocholesterolemia effects of lovastatin in familial defective apolipoproteinemia B-100. *Lancet* 1992;339:598–600.
91. Schmidt EB, Illingworth DR, Bacon S, Russell SJ, et al. Hypolipidemic effects of nicotinic acid in patients with familial defective apolipoprotein B-100. *Metabolism* 1993;42:137–139.
92. Schmidt EB, Illingworth DR, Bacon S, Mahley RW, Weisgraber KH. Hypocholesterolemia effects of cholestyramine and colestipol in patients with familial defective apolipoprotein B-100. *Atherosclerosis* 1993;98:213–217.
93. Goldstein JL, Schrott HG, Hazzard WR, Bierman EL, Motulsky AG. Hyperlipidemia in coronary heart disease. II. Genetic analysis of lipid levels in 176 families and delineation of a new inherited disorder, combined hyperlipidemia. *J Clin Invest* 1973;52:1544–1568.
94. Rose HG, Kranz P, Weinstock M, Juliano J, Haft JI. Inheritance of combined hyperlipoproteinemia: evidence for a new lipoprotein phenotype. *Am J Med* 1973;54:148–160.
95. Nikkila EA, Aro A. Family study of serum lipids and lipoproteins in coronary heart-disease. *Lancet* 1973;1:954–959.
96. Brunzell JD, Albers JJ, Chait A, Grundy SM, Groszek E, McDonald GB. Plasma lipoproteins in familial combined hyperlipidemia and monogenic familial hypertriglyceridemia. *J Lipid Res* 1983;24: 147–155.
97. Sniderman A, Shapiro S, Marpole D, Skinner B, Teng B, Kwiterovich PJ Jr. Association of coronary atherosclerosis with hyperapobetalipoproteinemia [increased protein but normal cholesterol levels in human plasma low density (beta) lipoproteins]. *Proc Natl Acad Sci USA* 1980; 77:604–608.
98. Sniderman AD, Wolfson C, Teng B, Franklin FA, Bachorik PS, Kwiterovich PJ Jr. Association of hyperapolipoproteinemia with endogenous hypertriglyceridemia and atherosclerosis. *Ann Intern Med* 1982; 97:833–839.
99. Janus ED, Nicoll AM, Turner PR, Magill P, Lewis B. Kinetic bases of the primary hyperlipidaemias: studies of apolipoprotein B turnover in genetically defined subjects. *Eur J Clin Invest* 1980;10:161–172.
100. Thompson GR, Teng B, Sniderman AD. Kinetics of LDL subfractions. *Am Heart J* 1987;113:514–557.
101. Brunzell JD. Familial lipoprotein lipase deficiency and other causes of the chylomicronemia syndrome. In: Scriver CR, Beaudet AL, Sly WS, Valle D, eds. *The metabolic basis of inherited disease*. New York: McGraw-Hill; 1989:1165–1180.
102. Fojo SS, Brewer HB Jr. The familial hyperchylomicronemia syndrome. *JAMA* 1991;265:904–908.
103. Fallat RW, Vester JW, Glueck CJ. Suppression of amylase activity by hypertriglyceridemia. *JAMA* 1973;225:1331–1334.

104. Lesser PB, Warshaw AL. Diagnosis of pancreatitis masked by hyperlipemia. *Ann Intern Med* 1975;82:795–798.
105. Warshaw AL, Bellini CA, Lesser PB. Inhibition of serum and urine amylase activity in pancreatitis with hyperlipemia. *Ann Surg* 1975; 182:72–75.
106. Parker F, Bagdade JD, Odland GF, Bierman EL. Evidence for the chylomicron origin of lipids accumulating in diabetic eruptive xanthomas: a correlative lipid biochemical, histochemical, and electron microscopic study. *J Clin Invest* 1970;49:2172–2187.
107. Wu AL, Windmueller HG. Relative contributions by liver and intestine to individual plasma apolipoproteins in the rat. *J Biol Chem* 1979; 254:7316–7322.
108. Santamarina-Fojo S. Genetic dyslipoproteinemias: role of lipoprotein lipase and apoC-II. *Curr Opin Lipidol* 1992;3:186–195.
109. Brunzell JD, Miller NE, Alaupovic P, St. Hilaire RJ, Wang CS, Sarson DL. Familial chylomicronemia due to a circulating inhibitor of lipoprotein lipase activity. *J Lipid Res* 1983;24:12–19.
110. Kihara S, Matsuzawa Y, Kubo M, Nozaki S, Funahashi T, Yamashita S. Autoimmune hyperchylomicronemia. *N Engl J Med* 1989;320: 1255–1259.
111. Fojo SS, Brewer HB Jr. Hypertriglyceridaemia due to genetic defects in lipoprotein lipase and apolipoprotein C-II. *J Intern Med* 1992;231: 669–677.
112. Cheng C, Bensadoun A, Bersot T, Hsu JST, Melford KH. Purification and characterization of human lipoprotein lipase and hepatic triglyceride lipase. *J Biol Chem* 1985;260:10720–10727.
113. Wion KL, Kirchgessner TG, Lusis AJ, Schotz MC, Lawn RM. Human lipoprotein lipase complementary DNA sequence. *Science* 1987;235: 1638–1641.
114. Gagne C, Brum LDF, Julien P, Moorjani S, Lupien PJ. Primary lipoprotein lipase activity deficiency: clinical investigation of a French Canadian population. *Can Med Assoc J* 1989;140:405–411.
115. Julien P. High frequency of lipoprotein lipase deficiency in the Quebec population. *Can J Cardiol* 1992;8:675–676.
116. Dionne C, Gagne C, Julien P, Murthy MR, et al. Geneaology and regional distribution of lipoprotein lipase deficiency in French-Canadians of Quebec. *Hum Biol* 1993;65:29–39.
117. Santamarina-Fojo S, Dugi K. Structure, function and role of lipoprotein lipase in lipoprotein metabolism. *Curr Opin Lipidol* 1994;5: 117–125.
118. Santamarina-Fojo S, Brewer HB Jr. Lipoprotein lipase: structure, function and mechanism of action. *Int J Clin Lab Res* 1994;24: 143–147.
119. Langlois S, Deeb S, Brunzell JD, Kastelein JJ, Hayden MR. A major insertion accounts for a significant proportion of mutations underlying human lipoprotein lipase deficiency. *Proc Natl Acad Sci USA* 1989; 86:948–952.
120. Benlian P, Loux N, De Gennes JL. A homozygous deletion of exon 9 in the lipoprotein lipase gene causes type I hyperlipoproteinemia. *Arterioscler Thromb* 1991;11:1465a (abst).
121. Devlin RH, Deeb S, Brunzell J, Hayden MR. Partial gene duplication involving exon–*Alu* interchange results in lipoprotein lipase deficiency. *Am J Hum Genet* 1990;46:112–119.
122. Foubert L, Benlian P, deGennes JL. Molecular genetics and lipoprotein lipase deficiency. *Bull Acad Natl Med* (Paris) 1994;178:405–413.
123. Bruin T, Tuzgöl S, Mulder WJ, Van den Ende AE, Jansen H, Hayden MR. A compound heterozygote for lipoprotein lipase deficiency, Val^{69}→Leu and Gly^{188}→Glu: correlation between *in vitro* LPL activity and clinical expression. *J Lipid Res* 1994;35:438–445.
124. Pepe G, Chimienti G, Resta F, Di Perna V, Tarricone C, Lovecchio M. A new Italian case of lipoprotein lipase deficiency: A Leu^{365}→Val change resulting in loss of enzyme activity. *Biochem Biophys Res Commun* 1994;199:570–576.
125. Normand T, Bergeron J, Fernandez-Margallo T, Bharucha A, Ven Murthy MR, Julien P. Geographic distribution and genealogy of mutation 207 of the lipoprotein lipase gene in the French Canadian population of Québec. *Hum Genet* 1992;89:671–675.
126. Dionne C, Gagne C, Julien P, Murthy MR, et al. Genetic epidemiology of lipoprotein lipase deficiency in Saguenay-Lac-St-Jean. *Ann Genet* 1992;35:89–92.
127. Emmerich J, Beg OU, Peterson J, Previato L, Brunzell JD, Brewer HB Jr, Human lipoprotein lipase. Analysis of the catalytic triad by site-directed mutagenesis of Ser-132, Asp-156, and His-241. *J Biol Chem* 1992;267:4161–4165.
128. Miesenboeck G, Hoelzl B, Foeger B, Brandstaetter E, Paulweber B, Sandhofer F. Heterozygous lipoprotein lipase deficiency due to a missense mutation as the cause of impaired triglyceride tolerance with multiple lipoprotein abnormalities. *J Clin Invest* 1993;91:448–455.
129. Gagne C, Brun D. Primary lipoprotein lipase deficiency. *Presse Med* 1993;22:212–217.
130. Wilson DE, Emi M, Iverius P-H, Hata A, Wu LL, Hillas E. Phenotypic expression of heterozygous lipoprotein lipase deficiency in the extended pedigree of a proband homozygous for a missense mutation. *J Clin Invest* 1990;86:735–750.
131. Saxena U, Klein MG, Vanni TM, Goldberg IJ. Lipoprotein lipase increases low density lipoprotein retention by subendothelial cell matrix. *J Clin Invest* 1992;89:373–380.
132. Saxena U, Ferguson E, Auerbach BJ, Bisgaier CL. Lipoprotein lipase facilitates very low density lipoprotein binding to the subendothelial cell matrix. *Biochem Biophys Res Commun* 1993;194:769–774.
133. Tabas I, Li Y, Brocia RW, Xu SW, Swenson TL, Williams KJ. Lipoprotein lipase and sphingomyelinase synergistically enhance the association of atherogenic lipoproteins with smooth muscle cells and extracellular matrix. *J Biol Chem* 1993;268:20419–20432.
134. Saxena U, Kulkarni NM, Ferguson E, Newton RS. Lipoprotein lipase-mediated lipolysis of very low density lipoproteins increase monocyte adhesion to aortic endothelial cells. *Biophys Res Commun* 1992;189: 1653–1658.
135. Renier G, Skamene E, DeSanctis JB, Radzioch D. High macrophage lipoprotein lipase expression and secretion are associated in inbred murine strains with susceptibility to atherosclerosis. *Arterioscler Thromb* 1993;13:190–196.
136. Shimada M, Shimano H, Gotoda T, Yamamoto K, Kawamura M, Inaba T. Overexpression of human lipoprotein lipase in transgenic mice. *J Biol Chem* 1993;268:17924–17929.
137. Hayden MR, Liu MS, Jirik F, Ma Y, LeBouef R, Brunzell JD. Expression of human lipoprotein lipase in transgenic mice. *J Cell Biochem* 1993;17E:242.
138. Tsutsumi K, Inoue Y, Shima A, Iwasaki K, Kawamura M, Murase T. The novel compound NO-1886 increases lipoprotein lipase activity with resulting elevation of high density lipoprotein cholesterol, and long-term administration inhibits atherogenesis in the coronary arteries of rats with experimental atherosclerosis. *J Clin Invest* 1993;92: 411–417.
139. Breckenridge WC, Little JA, Alaupovic P, Wang CS, Kuksis A, Kakis G. Lipoprotein abnormalities associated with a familial deficiency of hepatic lipase. *Atherosclerosis* 1982;45:161–179.
140. Carlson LA, Holmquist L, Nilsson-Ehle P. Deficiency of hepatic lipase activity in post-heparin plasma in familial hyper-α-triglyceridemia. *Acta Med Scand* 1986;219:435–447.
141. Auwerx JH, Marzetta CA, Hokanson JE, Brunzell JD. Large buoyant LDL-like particles in hepatic lipase deficiency. *Arteriosclerosis* 1989; 9:319–325.
142. Auwerx JH, Babirak SP, Hokanson JE, Stahnke G, Will H, Deeb SS. Coexistence of abnormalities of hepatic lipase and lipoprotein lipase in a large family. *Am J Hum Genet* 1990;46:470–477.
143. Ikeda Y, Takagi A. Hypertriglyceridemia in a deficiency of lipoprotein lipase and hepatic lipase. *Tanpakushitsu Kakusan Koso* 1988;33: 783–790 [in Japanese].
144. Connelly PW, Maguire GF, Lee M, Little JA. Plasma lipoproteins in familial hepatic lipase deficiency. *Arteriosclerosis* 1990;10:40–48.
145. Kuusi T, Nikkila EA, Taskinen MR, Somerharju P, Ehnholm C. Human postheparin plasma hepatic lipase activity against triacylglycerol and phospholipid substrates. *Clin Chim Acta* 1982;16:39–45.
146. Jensen GL, Daggy B, Bensadoun A. Triacylgycerol lipase, monoacylglycerol lipase and phospholipase activities of highly purified rat hepatic lipase. *Biochim Biophys Acta* 1982;710:464–470.
147. Laboda HM, Glick JM, Phillips MC. Hydrolysis of lipid monolayers and the substrate specificity of hepatic lipase. *Biochim Biophys Acta* 1986;876:233–242.
148. Kuusi T, Saarinen P, Nikkila EA. Evidence for the role of hepatic endothelial lipase in the metabolism of plasma high density $lipoprotein_2$ in man. *Atherosclerosis* 1980;36:589–593.
149. Rao SN, Cortese C, Miller NE, Levy Y, Lewis B. Effects of heparin infusion on plasma lipoproteins in subjects with lipoprotein lipase deficiency. Evidence for a role of hepatic endothelial lipase in the metabolism of high-density lipoprotein subfractions in man. *FEBS Lett* 1982;150:255–259.

150. Kinnunen PKJ. Hepatic endothelial lipase: isolation, some characteristics, and physiological role. In: Borgstrom B, Brockman HL, eds. *Lipases*. New York: Elsevier; 1984:307–328.
151. Demant T, Carlson LA, Holmquist L, Karpe F, Nilsson-Ehle P, Packard CJ. Lipoprotein metabolism in hepatic lipase deficiency: studies on the turnover of apolipoprotein B and on the effect of hepatic lipase on high density lipoprotein UK. *J Lipid Res* 1988;29:1603–1611.
152. Hegele RA, Little JA, Vezina C, Maguire GF, Tu L, Wolever TS. Hepatic lipase deficiency: clinical, biochemical, and molecular genetic characteristics. *Arterioscler Thromb* 1993;13:720–728.
153. Hegele RA, Little JA, Connelly PW. Compound heterozygosity for mutant hepatic lipase in familial hepatic lipase deficiency. *Biochem Biophys Res Commun* 1991;179:78–84.
154. Hegele RA, Vezina C, Moorjani S, Lupien PJ, Gagne C, Brun LD. A hepatic lipase gene mutation associated with heritable lipolytic deficiency. *J Clin Endocrinol* 1991;72:730–732.
155. Durstenfeld A, Ben-Zeev O, Reue K, Stahnke G, Doolittle MH. Molecular characterization of human hepatic lipase deficiency. *In vitro* expression of two naturally occurring mutations. *Arterioscler Thromb* 1994;14:381–385.
156. Brand K, Dugi KA, Brunzell JD, Nevin DN, Brewer HB Jr, Santamarina-Fojo S. Alternative splicing: a novel mechanism leading to deficiency of hepatic lipase. *Circulation* 1993;88:I-178.
157. Busch SJ, Barnhart RL, Martin GA, Fitzgerald MC, Yates MT, Mao SJT. Human hepatic triglyceride lipase expression reduces high density lipoprotein and aortic cholesterol in cholesterol-fed transgenic mice. *J Biol Chem* 1994;269:16376–16382.
158. Mahley RW. Dietary, fat, cholesterol, and accelerated atherosclerosis. *Atheroscler Rev* 1979;5:1–34.
159. Brewer HB Jr, Zech LA, Gregg RE, Schwartz D, Schaefer EJ. Type III hyperlipoproteinemia: diagnosis, molecular defects, pathology, and treatment. *Ann Intern Med* 1983;98:623–640.
160. Havel RJ. Familial dysbetalipoproteinemia. New aspects of pathogenesis and diagnosis. *Med Clin N Am* 1982;66:441–454.
161. Gregg RE, Zech LA, Schaefer EJ, Brewer HB Jr. Type III hyperlipoproteinemia: defective metabolism of an abnormal apolipoprotein E. *Science* 1981;211:584–586.
162. Rall SC Jr, Weisgraber KH, Innerarity TL, Mahley RW. Structural basis for receptor binding heterogeneity of apolipoprotein E from type III hyperlipoproteinemic subjects. *Proc Natl Acad Sci USA* 1982;79: 4696–4700.
163. Utermann G, Vogelberg KH, Steinmetz A, Schoenborn W, Pruin N, Jaeschke M. Polymorphism of apolipoprotein E. II. Genetics of hyperlipoproteinemia type III. *Clin Genet* 1979;15:37–62.
164. Zannis VI, Just PW, Breslow JL. Human apolipoprotein E isoprotein subclasses are genetically determined. *Am J Hum Genet* 1981;33: 11–24.
165. Mahley RW, Innerarity TL, Rall SC Jr, Weisgraber KH. Plasma lipoproteins: apolipoprotein structure and function. *J Lipid Res* 1984;25: 1277–1294.
166. Schaefer EJ, Gregg RE, Ghiselli G, Forte TM, Ordovas JM, Zech LA. Familial apolipoprotein E deficiency. *J Clin Invest* 1986;78: 1206–1219.
167. Lohse P, Brewer HB III, Meng MS, Skarlatos SI, LaRosa JC, Brewer HB Jr. Familial apolipoprotein E deficiency and type III hyperlipoproteinemia due to a premature stop codon in the apolipoprotein E gene. *J Lipid Res* 1992;33:1583–1590.
168. Mabuchi H, Itoh H, Takeda M, Kajinami K, Wakasugi T, Koizumi J. A young type III hyperlipoproteinemic patient associated with apolipoprotein E deficiency Medicine, Kanazawa, Japan. *Metabolism* 1989;38:115–119.
169. Kurosaka D, Teramoto T, Matsushima T, Yokoyama T, et al. Apolipoprotein E deficiency with a depressed mRNA of normal size. *Atherosclerosis* 1991;88:15–20.
170. Mann WA, Gregg RE, Sprecher DL, Brewer HB Jr. Apolipoprotein $E\text{-}1_{Harrisburg}$: a new variant of apolipoprotein E dominantly associated with type III hyperlipoproteinemia. *Biochim Biophys Acta* 1989;1005: 239–244.
171. Rall SC Jr, Newhouse YM, Clarke HR, Weisgraber KH, McCarthy BJ, Mahley RW. Type III hyperlipoproteinemia associated with apolipoprotein E phenotype E3/3. Structure and genetics of an apolipoprotein E3 variant. *J Clin Invest* 1989;83:1095–1101.
172. Wardell MR, Weisgraber KH, Havekes LM, Rall SC Jr. Apolipoprotein E3-Leiden contains a seven-amino acid insertion that is a tandem repeat of residues 121–127. *J Biol Chem* 1989;264:21205–21210.
173. Brewer HB Jr, Santamarina-Fojo S, Hoeg JM. Genetic defects in the human plasma apolipoproteins. *Atheroscler Rev* 1991;23:51–61.
174. Gregg RE, Zech LA, Schaefer EJ, Stark D, Wilson D, Brewer HB Jr. Abnormal *in vivo* metabolism of apolipoprotein E4 in humans. *J Clin Invest* 1986;78:815–821.
175. Lohse P, Mann WA, Stein EA, Brewer HB Jr. Apolipoprotein $E\text{-}4_{Philadelphia}$ ($Glu^{13} \rightarrow Lys, Arg^{145} \rightarrow Cys$). Homozygosity for two rare point mutations in the apolipoprotein E gene combined with severe type III hyperlipoproteinemia. *J Biol Chem* 1991;266:10479–10484.
176. Roses AD. Apolipoprotein E affects the rate of Alzheimer disease expression: beta-amyloid burden is a secondary consequence dependent on APOE genotype and duration of disease. *J Neuropathol Exp Neurol* 1994;53:429–437.
177. Schaefer EJ, Genest JJ Jr, Ordovas JM, Salem DN, Wilson PWF. Familial lipoprotein disorders and premature coronary artery disease. *Atherosclerosis* 1994;108(Suppl):S41–S54.
178. Utermann G, Menzel HJ, Kraft HG, Duba HC, Kemmler HG, Seitz C. Lp(a) glycoprotein phenotypes. Inheritance and relation to Lp(a)-lipoprotein concentrations in plasma. *J Clin Invest* 1987;80:458–465.
179. Koschinsky ML, Beisiegel U, Henne-Bruns D, Eaton DL, Lawn RM. Apolipoprotein(a) size heterogeneity is related to variable number of repeat sequences in its mRNA. *Biochemistry* 1990;29:640–644.
180. Azrolan N, Gavish D, Breslow JL. Lp(a) levels correlate inversely with apo(a) size and KIV copy number but not with apo(a) mRNA levels in a cynomolgus monkey model. *Circulation* 1990;82:III-90.
181. Loscalzo J. Lipoprotein(a). A unique risk factor for atherothrombotic disesase. *Arteriosclerosis* 1990;10:672–679.
182. Miles LA, Plow EF. Lp(a): an interloper in the fibrinolytic system. *Thromb Haemostasis* 1990;63:331–335.
183. Salens G, Shefer S, Nguyen L, Ness GC, et al. Sitosterolemia. *J Lipid Res* 1992;33:945–955.
184. Bjorkhem I, Boberg KM. Inborn errors in bile acid biosynthesis and storage of sterols other than cholesterol. In: Scriver CR, Beaudet AL, Sly WS, Valle D, Stanbury JB, Wyngaarden JB, eds. *The metabolic and molecular bases of inherited disease*. New York: McGraw-Hill; 1995:2073–2099.
185. Nguyen LB, Salen G, Shefer S, Bullock J, Chen T, Tint GS. Deficient ileal 3-hydroxy-3-methylglutaryl coenzyme A reductase activity in sitosterolemia: sitosterol is not a feedback inhibitor of intestinal cholesterol biosynthesis. *Metabolism* 1994;43:855–859.
186. Shefer S, Salen G, Bullock J, Nguyen LB, Ness GC, Vhao Z. The effect of increased hepatic sitosterol on the regulation of 3-hydroxy-3-methylglutaryl-coenzyme A reductase and cholesterol 7 alpha-hydroxylase in the rat and sitosterolemic homozygotes. *Hepatology* 1994;20:213–219.
187. Bhattacharyya AK, Connor WE, Lin DS, McMurry MM, Shulman RS. Sluggish sitosterol turnover and hepatic failure to excrete sitosterol into bile cause expansion of body pool of sitosterol in patients with sitosterolemia and xanthomatosis. *Arterioscler Thromb* 1991;11: 1287–1294.
188. Salens G, Tint GS, Shefer S, et al. Increased sitosterol absorption is offset by rapid elimination to prevent accumulation in heterozygotes with sitosterolemia. *Arterioscler Thromb* 1992;12:563–568.
189. Assmann G, Schmitz G, Brewer HB Jr. Familial high density lipoprotein deficiency: Tangier disease. In: Scriver CR, Beaudet AL, Sly WS, Valle D, eds. *The metabolic basis of inherited disease*. New York: McGraw-Hill; 1989:1267–1282.
190. Schaefer EJ, Zech LA, Schwartz DE, Brewer HB Jr. Coronary heart disease prevalence and other clinical features in familial high-density lipoprotein deficiency (Tangier disease). *Ann Intern Med* 1980;93: 261–266.
191. Serfaty-Lacrosniere C, Civeira F, Lanzberg A, Isaia P, Berg J, Janus ED. Homozygous Tangier disease and cardiovascular disease. *Atherosclerosis* 1994;107:85–98.
192. Bojanovski D, Gregg RE, Zech LA, Meng MS, Bishop C, Ronan R. *In vivo* metabolism of proapolipoprotein A-I in Tangier disease. *J Clin Invest* 1987;80:1742–1747.
193. Francis GA, Oram JF. Defective excretion of cholesterol from Tangier patients' fibroblasts to apolipoprotein A-I: a potential cause of hypoalphalipoproteinemia. *Circulation* 1994;90:I-241.
194. von Eckardstein A, Funke H, Henke A, Altland K, Benninghoven A, Assmann G. Apolipoprotein A-I variants. Naturally occurring substi-

tutions of proline residues affect plasma concentration of apolipoprotein A-I. *J Clin Invest* 1989;84:1722–1730.

195. Schmitz G, Lackner K. High density lipoprotein deficiency with xanthomas: a defect in apoA-I synthesis. In: Crepaldi G, Baggio G, eds. *Atherosclerosis VIII*. Rome: Tekno Press; 1989:399–403.
196. Bekaert ED, Alaupovic P, Knight-Gibson CS, Laux MJ, Pelachyk JM, Norum RA. Characterization of apoA- and apoB-containing lipoprotein particles in a variant of familial apoA-I deficiency with planar xanthoma: the metabolic significance of LP-A-II particles. *J Lipid Res* 1991;32:1587–1599.
197. Norum RA, Lakier JB, Goldstein S, Angel A, Goldberg RB, Block WD. Familial deficiency of apolipoproteins A-I and C-III and precocious coronary-artery disease. *N Engl J Med* 1982;306:1513–1519.
198. Karathanasis SK, Zannis VI, Breslow JL. A DNA insertion in the apolipoprotein A-I gene of patients with premature atherosclerosis. *Nature* 1983;305:823–825.
199. Schaefer EJ, Ordovas JM, Law SW, Ghiselli G, Kashyap ML, Srivastava LS. Familial apolipoprotein A-I and C-III deficiency, variant II. *J Lipid Res* 1985;26:1089–1101.
200. Ordovas JM, Cassidy DK, Civeira F, Bisgaier CL, Schaefer EJ. Familial apolipoprotein A-I, C-III, and A-IV deficiency and premature atherosclerosis due to deletion of a gene complex on chromosome 11. *J Biol Chem* 1989;264:16339–16342.
201. Third JL, Montag J, Flynn M, Freidel J, Laskarzewski P, Glueck CJ. Primary and familial hypoalphalipoproteinemia. *Metabolism* 1984;33: 136–146.
202. Genest J Jr, Bard JM, Fruchart JC, Ordovas JM, Schaefer EJ. Familial hypoalphalipoproteinemia in premature coronary artery disease. *Arterioscler Thromb* 1993;13:1728–1737.

Atherosclerosis and Coronary Artery Disease,
edited by V. Fuster, R. Ross, and E. J. Topol.
Lippincott-Raven Publishers, Philadelphia © 1996.

CHAPTER 6

Structure and Function of the Plasma Lipoproteins and Their Receptors

John P. Kane

Key Words: Apoliprotein; Chylomicrons; Lipids; Lipoprotein—high-density, intermediate-density, low-density, very low-density; Phospholipids; Triglycerides.

OVERVIEW

It is estimated that as much as 80% of the carbon and hydrogen in energy substrates used by the human body passes through lipid intermediaries at some point before being oxidized to terminal products. Most of that lipid transits the blood in the form of free fatty acids or triglycerides. Furthermore, there is a constant bidirectional movement of the lipid constituents of membranes between cells and the blood. The lipids of plasma are virtually all solubilized and dispersed by association with a highly evolved group of proteins. The simplest association among these is that between unesterified fatty acids and albumin, which has three high-affinity sites that are characterized by hydrophobic clefts with cationic amino acid side chains so disposed as to permit association with the carboxylate function (1). Another example is the transport of retinol by retinol binding protein in association with prealbumin.

J. P. Kane: Cardiovascular Research Institute, University of California, San Francisco, San Francisco, California 94143.

The transport of more complex lipids, however, is chiefly accomplished by lipoproteins (Table 1, Table 2). These generally take the form of spherical microemulsion particles, comprised of a core region containing the hydrophobic cholesteryl esters and triglycerides in variable proportions, surrounded by a mixed monolayer of phospholipids and unesterified cholesterol (2). The charged head groups of the various phospholipid species and the free hydroxyl group of cholesterol associate with water dipoles in the surrounding aqueous medium while the hydrophobic fatty acid chains of phospholipids and the sterol ring structure are in contact with each other and with the hydrophobic core lipids. Certain lipoproteins have the lipid moiety organized as a bilayer disk composed of phospholipid and unesterified cholesterol with apolipoproteins disposed on the surface. Examples of this type of structure are found in several quantitatively minor species of high-density lipoproteins (HDL).

In accordance with its distribution isotherms, some unesterified cholesterol enters the hydrophobic core of lipoproteins of the microemulsion type. This component becomes more significant in lipoproteins with large diameters. Conversely, a small amount of triglyceride and cholesteryl ester are present in the surface monolayers. A number of specific proteins (apolipoproteins) (Table 2) that have evolved to interact with the lipid microemulsions associate primarily

TABLE 1. *Properties of human plasma lipoproteins*

Class	Density (g/ml)	Electrophoretic mobility	Range of diameters (nm)	Molecular weight
Chylomicrons	0.93	Remain at origin	75–1,200	50–1,000 × 10^6
VLDL	0.93–1.006	Pre-β	30–80	10–80 × 10^6
IDL	1.006–1.019	Slow pre-β	25–35	5–10 × 10^6
LDL	1.019–1.063	β	18–25	2–3 × 10^6
HDL	1.063–1.21	α	5–12	65–386 × 10^3

with the surface monolayers. Proteins of one group contain several sequences that form amphipathic helices, are between 6 and 50 kDA, and are capable of moving among lipoprotein species in blood. In contrast, the B apolipoproteins have much greater molecular weights, few amphipathic helices, and a large content of β structure. They penetrate at certain points to substitute for the monolayer, interacting directly with core lipids (3). The B apolipoproteins remain with the lipoprotein particles on which they were secreted throughout their lifetimes in plasma. The plasma lipoproteins vary greatly in diameter. The principal core constituent of the largest species is triglyceride, whereas smaller lipoproteins contain a progressively higher mole fraction of cholesteryl esters in the cores such that these lipids are nearly the exclusive core constituents of the classes with diameters below 230 Å (low-density lipoproteins, LDL). The densities of lipoproteins increase progressively as particle diameters decrease, chiefly because the proportion of protein and monolayer lipid to core lipid increases. Preparative ultracentrifugation, a technique employed for four decades to separate classes of lipoproteins, has provided a widely used operational approach to lipoprotein classification (4). The lipoprotein classes separated from human plasma by this technique are described in Tables 1 and 2.

The apolipoproteins associated with human lipoproteins represent several evolutionary classes. A group of seven with relatively small molecular weights (apolipoproteins A-I, A-II, A-IV, C-1, C-II, C-III, and E) are members of a gene family characterized by tandem repeats of 11 codons (5). Each contains a number of amphipathic helices that can associate with zwitterionic head groups of phospholipids of the surface monolayer (6,7). Each of these proteins binds with relatively high affinity to the lipoprotein particle but has a measurable solubility in the molecularly dispersed state and is readily exchangeable among lipoprotein particles. The B apolipoprotein group is comprised of two very large proteins, apo B-100 and apo B-48, products of a single gene. They contain a large amount of β structure and relatively few amphipathic helices. Unlike the other apolipoproteins, they have extremely high affinity for the lipoprotein particle and are unexchangeable among lipoprotein particles (3,8). A group of relatively hydrophobic proteins that are associated with the lipoprotein system, including apolipoprotein D, cholesteryl ester transfer protein, and phospholipid transfer protein (9,10), appear to function primarily in lipid exchange. Last, a number of proteins that are largely present in molecular dispersion in plasma and that have known functions outside of lipid transport associate with lipoproteins to a limited extent and may play special roles in the lipoprotein context. These include transferrin, ceruloplasmin, haptoglobin, factor VII, complement 4 component binding protein, lipopolysaccharide binding protein (LBP), and others (11,12). The apolipoproteins of human plasma are described in Table 3.

There are four general thematic roles for plasma lipoproteins in lipid transport. The first two involve the transport of exogenous and endogenous triglycerides, respectively, to body tissue. The third is the delivery of cholesterol to tissues via LDL, and the forth is the retrieval of lipids from peripheral tissue via HDL. Chylomicrons are the large triglyceride-rich lipoproteins of enteric origin that carry exogenous triglycerides into plasma (8,13), whereas very low-density lipoproteins (VLDL) originate in liver and carry endogenous triglycerides to similar fates (Table 1). Free fatty acids (FFA) for triglyceride synthesis by liver come in large part from peripheral adipocytes, where they are released by hydrolysis of stored triglycerides. A variable portion of plasma free fatty acids comes from the intravascular hydrolysis of the triglycerides of VLDL and chylomicrons. Hydrolysis of the triglycerides of adipose tissue is mediated by an intracellular, hormonally regulated lipase. Intracellular lipolysis is stimulated by catecholamines, growth hormone, glucagon, and

TABLE 2. *Composition of normal plasma lipoproteins (percent of mass)*

	Unesterified cholesterol	Cholesteryl esters	Phospholipids	Triglycerides	Protein
Chylomicrons	2	3	7	86	2
VLDL	7	12	18	55	8
IDL	9	29	19	23	19
LDL	8	42	22	6	22
HDL	4	14	34	4	45

TABLE 3. *Apolipoproteins of human blood plasma*

	Average concentration in plasma (mg/dl)	Aminoacyl molecular weight
Apo A-I[a]	130	29,016
Apo A-II[a]	40	8,700
Apo A-IV[a]	40	44,465
Apo C-I[a]	6	6,630
Apo C-II[a]	3	8,900
Apo C-III[a]	12	8,800
Apo D	10	19,000
Apo E[a]	5	34,145
Apo B-100	85	512,723
Apo B-48	Variable	240,800

[a] Denotes members of multigene family.

other hormones and by afferent autonomic stimulation. It is suppressed by insulin. On release from adipose tissue, the fatty acids are transported in plasma in complex with albumin. About one-third of the fatty acid burden of blood that perfuses the liver is removed in each circulatory pass, relatively independent of plasma level. Thus, a high rate of peripheral lipolysis tends to increase FFA uptake by liver, providing fatty acids for oxidation, export of triglycerides, or ketogenesis, depending on the status of the hepatic substrate economy. Chylomicrons and VLDL both marginate in capillaries, where they are subject to lipolysis by lipoprotein lipase, liberating fatty acids that are chiefly taken up locally (Fig. 1). As a result of lipolysis, the particles decrease in size, and the cores become relatively enriched in cholesteryl esters. The resultant particles are termed remnants.

Chylomicron remnants are removed quantitatively by endocytosis into hepatocytes, where the remaining triglycerides and the cholesteryl esters and surface lipids enter hepatic pools. A major portion of VLDL remnants, perhaps half, are similarly endocytosed, whereas the remainder undergo further depletion of triglycerides and emerge as still smaller, cholesteryl ester-rich low-density lipoprotein particles (LDL) (8). The LDL are removed from plasma and the extracellular space in large part by endocytosis via the LDL receptor, present in all nucleated cells. They are degraded within lysosomes, yielding cholesterol, which is largely utilized in cell membranes. About half of the uptake of LDL is accounted for by the liver.

Nascent VLDL and chylomicrons contain apolipoproteins that are destined to emerge in the protein moieties of high-density lipoproteins (HDL). These proteins, with surface phospholipids and free cholesterol, migrate away from the triglyceride-rich lipoproteins during lipolysis to become part of the HDL mass (Fig. 1). Cholesterol and phospholipids are also added to HDL from peripheral tissues. Free cholesterol is esterified by lecithin cholesterol acyl transferase (LCAT) (14) to form cholesteryl esters that are the chief core constituent of some spherical HDL species. Cholesteryl esters are then transferred to VLDL, intermediate-density lipoproteins (IDL), and LDL under the influence of cholesteryl ester transfer protein (CETP). Finally, the endocytosis of these acceptor proteins by hepatocytes provides what is probably the principal route for retrieval of cholesterol from peripheral tissues to liver. Direct hepatic uptake of certain HDL species probably contributes to this centripetal pathway as well. These pathways are described in detail below.

Modern models of atherogenesis place the lipoproteins that contain apolipoprotein B in an etiological role. There is also convincing evidence that some role or roles played by HDL act to countervail to varying degrees the atherogen-

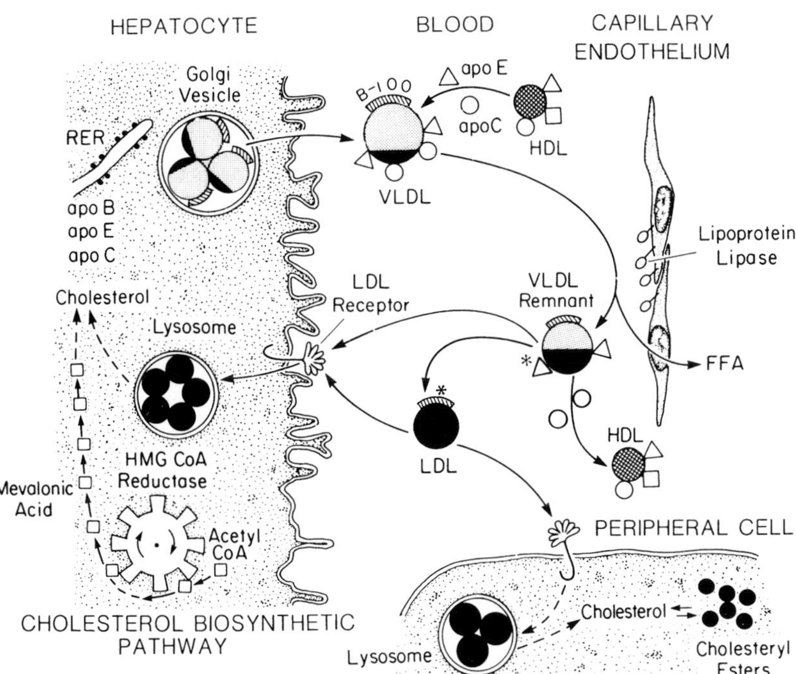

FIG. 1. Metabolism of lipoproteins of hepatic origin. Nascent VLDL are secreted via the Golgi apparatus. They acquire additional C apolipoproteins and apo E from HDL. Lipolysis by lipoprotein lipase produces remnant particles, which yield C apolipoproteins and a portion of their apo E to HDL. A portion of VLDL remnants is endocytosed in liver following binding of their apo E moieties to receptors. The remaining VLDL remnants are converted to LDL by further loss of triglycerides and loss of apo E. A major pathway for LDL degradation involves the endocytosis of LDL by LDL receptors, for which B100 is the ligand. *Black areas* denote cholesteryl esters; *stippled areas,* triglycerides; *cross-hatched areas,* high-density lipoprotein particles; asterisk denotes a functional ligand for LDL receptor; *triangles* indicate apolipoprotein E; *open circles and squares* represent C apolipoproteins.

icity of the apo-B-containing particles. This may be effected by improving the retrieval of cholesterol from peripheral sites or by inhibition of the oxidation of LDL, or both. Thus, defects in a number of these processes could influence the course of atherogenesis.

Emerging functions of lipoproteins outside of lipid transport suggest that they have broader biological involvement than was previously appreciated. For example, human HDL have been found to be profoundly cytocidal versus *Trypanosoma brucei,* a property that may have evolved during a period of residence by early humans in a predominantly tropical environment (15). Furthermore, it is now recognized that chylomicrons and VLDL, and other lipoproteins to a lesser extent, can bind lipopolysaccharide endotoxins and, in the case of triglyceride-rich lipoproteins, remove them from plasma via endocytosis of remnant particles by hepatocytes (16). Thus, increases in plasma triglycerides that occur during acute inflammation, which reflect both increased VLDL synthesis and decreased intravascular lipolysis, may have evolved adaptively to protect against endotoxemia (17). Thus, it is probable that some of the determinants of lipoprotein secretion and metabolism may emanate from other systems in which lipoproteins play a role. Other emerging functions of lipoproteins outside of lipid transport include involvement in blood clotting (18–20) and thrombolysis and in the inhibition of the infectivity of endogenous C viruses (21).

TRANSPORT OF EXOGENOUS LIPIDS

Secretion of Chylomicrons

Ingested triglycerides are hydrolyzed by pancreatic lipase to form a mixture of β-monoglycerides and unesterified fatty acids, which are both absorbed by the enterocyte. Unesterified cholesterol is present as such in foods of animal origin and is liberated from ingested cholesteryl esters by a cholesteryl esterase. Enterocytes selectively absorb unesterified cholesterol while virtually excluding phytosterols. This process appears to involve one or more transmembrane proteins (22). The intracellular transport of free fatty acids derived originally from ingested triglycerides is probably facilitated by one or more fatty acid binding proteins (23,24). After esterification with CoA, the fatty acyl groups directly transacylate the β-monoglyceride to triglycerides. Some free cholesterol is esterified, chiefly with oleic and linoleic acids, by acyl CoA: cholesterol acyl transferase (ACAT) to yield esters that will appear in the chylomicron.

The form of apolipoprotein B, apo B48, that is found in chylomicrons is a transcription product of the same gene that produces apo B100, a protein of 4,536 amino acids. Apo B48, so named because it is completely homologous with the N-terminal 48% of B100, results from a tissue-specific editing process that introduces a stop codon in the transcript, thus producing a truncated version of the protein (25,26). This posttranscriptional process involves a sequence-specific cytidine deaminase that transverts cytidine to uracil at residue 6,666, converting a gln codon to a stop (27,28). Introduction of the stop codon activates cryptic polyadenylation sites that produce a message of about 7 kb in the intestine of humans and rabbits. Synthesis of apo B100 by human intestine occurs but is probably less than 5% of total B protein.

The B48 protein is synthesized in ribosomes attached to the endoplasmic reticulum. Some of the process of the lipidation of apo B in intestine must be inferred from more detailed knowledge of the process of formation and secretion of VLDL by the hepatocyte. However, available observations on intestine suggest that the processes are similar. Caution is indicated in equating the hepatic and intestinal processes completely, though, because there is a disorder, chylomicron retention disease (also termed Anderson's syndrome), in which there is selective inability to secrete chylomicrons, though VLDL synthesis and secretion proceed in an apparently normal fashion (29,30). This suggests that at least one element in the process must be different between the two tissues. As described in more detail below, scission of a 27-amino-acid signal peptide probably occurs cotranslationally, and partial lipidation of the nascent apo B48 chain proceeds as the protein is translocated across the membrane of the endoplasmic reticulum, probably by a pause transfer mechanism, forming a small spherical precursor of the chylomicron. In a second step, a lipid particle fuses with the partially lipidated apo B (31). The fusion appears to require the microsomal triglyceride transport protein MTP, a heterodimeric protein that includes a protein disulfide isomerase subunit (32,33). It is probable that the MTP–PDI complex may be involved in both steps of lipidation. The nascent particles are then transported to the Golgi apparatus where a further complement of phospholipid may be added, and where other apolipoproteins are found in association with the particle.

Secretion of chylomicrons into the extracellular space occurs when membranes of the *trans*-cisternae of the Golgi fuse with the basolateral membrane. The chylomicrons then pass into the intestinal lacteals and transit the thoracic duct to spill ultimately into blood in the subclavian vein. In addition to the apo B48, nascent chylomicrons contain newly synthesized apo A-I, apo A-II, and apo A-IV. Because the rates of synthesis of apolipoproteins C and apo E are very low in intestine (34,35), it is likely that limited amounts of these proteins are present on the nascent chylomicrons. The capillaries of intestine are fenestrated such that macromolecules in the size range of HDL can pass into the lymph spaces (34). This allows an extensive exchange of phospholipid from chylomicrons to HDL and acquisition of C apolipoproteins and apo E by chylomicrons. Apolipoproteins A-I, A-II, and A-IV dissociate very rapidly on exposure of nascent chylomicrons to lymph and plasma and enter the HDL pool. Access of HDL to the intestinal lymph space may also facilitate interaction of HDL that contain lipopolysaccharide binding protein with bacterial endotoxins that have transited the enterocyte (12).

The principal mechanism by which intestine accommodates large fluxes of triglyceride transport is by increasing the particle volumes of the chylomicrons secreted. Synthesis of apo B48 appears to be increased only minimally or not at all with fat feeding in the rat (34), whereas triglyceride transport can increase as much as 20-fold.

Intravascular Lipolysis of Chylomicrons

Lipolysis of lipoprotein-borne triglycerides proceeds at the vascular endothelium. By electron microscopy, chylomicrons and VLDL can be seen to marginate on capillary walls in adipose tissue and in skeletal and cardiac muscle. Evidence is gathering to indicate that a complex interaction of lipoproteins, lipoprotein lipase, and endothelial proteoglycans is involved (36), with the lipase binding both to heparan sulfate and to lipoproteins (37–39). Lipoprotein lipase (LPL) is a member of a family of lipases that includes hepatic lipase (HL) and pancreatic lipase. They appear to have evolved from a primordial serine protease. The active sites of all are highly homologous and are each in the N-terminal domain. The C-terminal domains appear to be required for appropriate interaction with lipid substrates. The active form of LPL is a homodimer. Appropriate glycosylation of the enzyme is also required for activity (40). Apolipoprotein C-II is an obligate activator of the enzyme, binding by its C-terminal region to the lipase. The LPL is synthesized and secreted most significantly in adipose tissue, striated muscle, and mammary gland. It moves across endothelium to the luminal surface in each of these tissues. The LPL activity is regulated by as yet poorly defined metabolic and endocrine signals. There appear to be gender-based differences (41) in the ratio of activity in central and peripheral adipocytes. Fasting decreases LPL activity in adipose tissue, whereas it increases activity on cardiac and skeletal muscle (42,43). This effect would spare FFA for use in skeletal and cardiac muscle when energy substrates are not abundant. Insulin deficiency results in vanishingly low levels of LPL activity in adipose tissue (44). The regulation of LPL activity under different conditions appears to involve transcriptional control, posttranslational processes, or both.

A number of mutations that result in impaired function of LPL are now recognized. In the homozygous state, they cause severe chylomicronemia. They might also contribute to significant lipemia in the heterozygous state if aggravating factors such as pregnancy, poorly controlled diabetes, or alcohol abuse are present. Individuals homozygous for mutations causing deficiency of apolipoprotein C-II also have severe impairment of removal of chylomicrons and VLDL.

Intravascular hydrolysis of triglycerides ultimately liberates free fatty acids and glycerol. The major fraction of liberated fatty acids is taken up in the tissue where hydrolysis occurred, and glycerol is removed by tissues that possess glycerokinase activity, principally liver and intestine. Albumin appears to be a transient ligand for at least a portion of the fatty acids, whence they proceed to cell membranes where a lipid binding protein may facilitate their uptake (24). The marked albumin deficiency that occurs in severe nephrosis causes significant impairment of lipolysis as a result of product inhibition of LPL by fatty acids.

Depletion of core triglycerides leads to the production of progressively smaller, spherical particles until about 70% of the core triglyceride has been removed. The surface monolayer of phospholipid and free cholesterol sheds amphipathic lipids to HDL apace with the decrease in particle diameters. This process, until recently regarded as passive, is obligatorily dependent on phospholipid transfer protein, an 81-kDa protein of 476 amino acids (10,45). This protein has no significant homology with smaller intracellular phospholipid transfer proteins but appears to have an evolutionary relationship to lipopolysaccharide binding protein (LBP) (46), bacterial permeability-increasing protein (BPI) (47), and cholesteryl ester transfer protein. Phospholipid transfer protein (PLTP) appears to be synthesized in a number of tissues including placenta, pancreas, lung, kidney, liver, and brain. Deficiency of PLTP leads to retention of phospholipids in chylomicron and VLDL remnant particles (48). The importance of PLTP in maintaining HDL levels is underscored by the virtual absence of HDL in homozygous PLTP deficiency.

As triglyceride hydrolysis proceeds, the C apolipoproteins and a portion of the complement of apo E dissociate from the particles to associate with HDL. The small (circa 500 to 800 Å diameter) triglyceride-depleted lipoprotein products of lipolysis that contain apo B48 and apo E are termed chylomicron remnants. The process of lipolysis from secretion to the remnant stage requires about 15 min in normal individuals (49).

Metabolism of Chylomicron Remnants

Chylomicron remnants are removed from blood categorically and with great efficiency via endocytosis into the hepatocytes (50). The process is still poorly understood but is clearly mediated by a receptor or receptors for which apo E is the ligand. Though chylomicron remnants bind to the LDL receptor with high affinity, the absence of significant retention of chylomicron remnants in homozygous LDL-receptor-defective animals and humans points to the existence of an additional receptor. The LDL-receptor-like protein (LRP) may be the responsible receptor (51,52). This protein contains 4,525 amino acids and has a number of structurally distinct regions (51,53). Four of these contain cysteine-rich repeats homologous to those on the LDL receptor and other sequences homologous to EGF, a membrane-spanning region, and a cytoplasmic domain that includes sequence targeting to coated pits. The protein recycles through endosomal compartments in a fashion analogous to the LDL receptor (54). The protein is synthesized as a 600-kDa precursor that undergoes selective proteolysis to yield subunits of 515 and 85 kDa that remain noncovalently associated. It binds apo E and is found in hepatic endosomes (54). Though it binds chylomicron remnants of plasma poorly, they may improve their ligand property by acquiring apo E from a pool located on the hepatic microvilli. This alteration of the remnants may occur during interaction of the remnants with hepatic lipase (55,56) and may be facilitated by interaction of the remnant particles with heparan sulfate (50,57,58). The presence of hepatic lipase in endosomal compartments is compatible with this model (59). The observation that the 39-kDa inhibitor of LRP reduces endocytosis of chylomicron remnants (60) indicates that the LRP or a related receptor is involved. It is possible that LPL bound to lipoproteins may also be a ligand for LRP (52,61).

Kinetic studies of endocytosis of chylomicron remnants by liver reveals a delay after binding, suggesting that modification of the particles is required before endocytosis proceeds. Unlike the metabolism of VLDL remnants, no circulating daughter particles such as LDL are formed from chylomicron remnants. Both the triglycerides and the cholesterol of chylomicron remnants are used in the secretion of VLDL by the liver. Tocopherols also enter the hepatocyte in endocytosed chylomicron remnants, to be sorted on the basis of stereoisomerism and resecreted in VLDL (62).

A common variant allele of apo E, apo E_2, has very low affinity for the LDL receptor and also, apparently, for the functional chylomicron remnant receptor. In individuals homozygous for apo E_2, remnant particles of chylomicrons and VLDL can accumulate in plasma if additional factors that potentiate lipemia are present. This disorder is termed familial dysbetalipoproteinemia.

TRANSPORT OF ENDOGENOUS TRIGLYCERIDES

The Hepatic Triglyceride Economy

The secretion of triglyceride-rich VLDL provides a pathway by which the liver can export calories in the form of triglyceride fatty acids and also export cholesterol, certain exchangeable apolipoproteins, and tocopherol (Fig. 1). The production rate of VLDL varies greatly, reflecting the supply of disposable energy substrate. It is significantly increased by estrogens and alcohol. The fatty acids employed in triglyceride synthesis come from several sources. Free fatty acids released by the activity of intracellular (hormone-sensitive) lipase in adipose tissue are transported in plasma, bound to albumin. The fraction extracted from blood by liver is about one-third, independent of level. Hence, situations in which lipolysis in adipocytes is increased will present the hepatocyte with an increased influx of FFA. The most potent down-regulator of the intracellular lipase is insulin. Biosynthesis of fatty acids also proceeds using carbon sources derived from the catabolism of glucose, amino acids, and ethanol. Fatty acid synthesis is enhanced in the fed state and is suppressed during prolonged fasting, when ketogenesis is active.

Assembly and Secretion of VLDL

Though the livers of several mammalian species secrete both apo B48 and B100, apo B100 is the sole B protein produced in human liver. B48 is undetectable in the plasma of patients with abetalipoproteinemia who have undergone liver transplant despite normal production of B100. Each nascent VLDL particle contains a single copy of apo B100 (8). The gene for apo B extends over 43 kbp of DNA on the short arm of chromosome 2. It is comprised of 29 exons, one of which contains over 7,500 base pairs (63). Both positive and negative transcriptional regulatory sites have been described in the 5′ flanking region of the gene. The mRNA from human liver is 14 kbp in length. No editing of the message is apparent in human liver.

The B100 protein is approximately 549 kDa including carbohydrate linked at up to 16 sites. The protein contains about 40 lipophilic sequences distributed rather evenly through the molecule that allow it to associate with the microemulsion moieties of VLDL, IDL, and LDL with such high affinity that it remains with a single lipoprotein particle from secretion to ultimate endocytosis. These sequences include several amphipathic helices and a large number of sequences yielding amphipathic β structure. Apo B100 is synthesized on ribosomes attached to the endoplasmic reticulum (64). It may be partially lipidated cotranslationally during transmembrane transfer into the endoplasmic reticulum by a ''pause transfer'' mechanism (65,66). The lipids in this stage of lipidation probably come from the inner leaflet of the endoplasmic membrane (67). A substantial fraction of newly synthesized apo B is degraded without being secreted, suggesting that lipidation may induce conformational changes that allow it to proceed to a second stage of lipidation (68,69).

The lipidation of apo B100 has been postulated to be a two-step process (70). The first phase of lipidation by HepG2 cells appears to produce spherical particles of about 220 Å diameter. These cells appear to lack the ability to carry out the second stage of lipidation and consequently secrete LDL-like nascent particles (71,72). The second phase appears to involve the coalescence of the small spherical particles with triglyceride-rich spherical particles produced in the smooth endoplasmic reticulum. The microsomal triglyceride transfer protein (MTP), which is a heterodimer with disulfide isomerase (PDI) (32), appears to be involved in the first step and perhaps is involved with formation of the triglyceride-rich particle as well. Perhaps the disulfide isomerase subunit of the heterodimer of MTP is required to establish intramolecular disulfide bonds in apo B100. The strongest evidence supporting the involvement of MTP in lipidation of apo B is the finding that functional MTP was absent in several cases of recessive abetalipoproteinemia, a condition in which no apo-B-containing lipoproteins can be secreted from the liver or intestine (32,33). Fully lipidated VLDL normally are transported to the Golgi vesicles, where glycosylation of apolipoproteins proceeds, before the VLDL are transported to the plasma membrane and released into the space of Disse.

Nascent VLDL

Nascent VLDL isolated from the Golgi apparatus contain newly synthesized apolipoprotein E and the C apolipoproteins. Their surface monolayers contain about twofold more phospholipid and much less unesterified cholesterol than plasma VLDL (73,74). Thus, as soon as they emerge from the hepatocyte, exchanges with HDL probably commence in which phospholipid migrates to the HDL, possibly nucleating new HDL particles; unesterified cholesterol may move from HDL to VLDL, and VLDL may gain apolipoproteins C and E from HDL (73). It appears that the transfer of phospholipid to HDL is highly dependent on phospholipid transfer protein (45,48). In contrast to other species that have high levels of ACAT activity in liver, human VLDL contain relatively little cholesteryl ester (75).

Regulation of VLDL Synthesis

Increases of triglyceride secretion in VLDL are largely accommodated by increases in particle volume, though a modest increase in secretion of apo B100 can take place when triglyceride secretion is maximal. Apo B100 message appears to be constitutively expressed in HepG2 cells (76). Because so much apo B100 is degraded intracellularly, it is possible that increases in secretion of apo B100 may reflect changes in the rate of degradation. The fact that apo B100 message increases in abetaliopoproteinemia suggests that there is significant regulation of expression or degradation (77). Also, insulin is known to inhibit synthesis and secretion of apo B from rat hepatocytes (78,79). Estrogens increase synthesis of apo B in HepG2 cells (80), perhaps related to the estrogen response observed in ancestral vertebrates in support of ovigenesis. The most commonly encountered form of hyperlipidemia in humans, familial combined hyperlipoproteinemia, appears to involve an increased secretion rate for VLDL.

Metabolism of VLDL

The VLDL are subject to lipolysis by lipoprotein lipase (LPL), which is bound to capillary endothelium of skeletal and cardiac muscle and adipose tissue, as described above for chylomicrons. The circulating half-life of VLDL particles is about 30 to 60 min in normal humans (49). The rate of hydrolysis of triglycerides is regulated partly by the inhibitory effects of apo C-III. This protein is synthesized largely in liver. Its gene is situated on chromosome 11 near those of apo A-I and A-IV (81,82). This protein, rich in amphipathic helical structure, inhibits the premature binding of VLDL to the LDL receptor. Progressive hydrolysis of core triglycerides leads to a cascade of successively smaller spherical particles. As this proceeds, lipids of the surface monolayers are transferred to HDL, a process that appears to be dependent on PLTP. During the course of lipolysis, the C apolipoproteins are lost from the particle, including apo C-II, the activator of the enzyme. Thus, lipolysis by LPL becomes less efficient as the triglyceride is depleted. At this point, the particles have become intermediate-density lipoproteins (IDL), enriched in cholesteryl esters, and retaining a portion of the original complement of apo E in addition to one copy of apo B100. The fate of these remnant particles is dichotomous at this point. Approximately half, perhaps those with a larger complement of apo E, are endocytosed in liver; the remainder are converted to cholesteryl-ester-rich daughter particles, LDL. Because it is recognized that a subpopulation of VLDL that contains no apolipoprotein E exists in human plasma, it is possible that this subclass may be converted quantitatively to LDL. Endocytosis of VLDL remnants is mediated by the LDL receptor, with apo E as the ligand (67,83). The receptors cluster in coated pits, which subsequently are endocytosed as coated vesicles. The receptors are dissociated with the CURL (compartment for uncoupling of receptor and ligand) and return to the cell surface (67), whereas the remnants are degraded, returning triglycerides and cholesterol to hepatic pools.

Apolipoprotein E, a protein of 34.2 kDa, contains 299 amino acids. Its gene is located on chromosome 19 close to genes for apo C-II and the LDL receptor (82,84). Apo E contains two independently folded domains (85). The carboxy-terminal domain associates with lipids, whereas the larger amino-terminal domain contains a linear sequence rich in basic residues that functions as ligand for the LDL receptor and for the LRP protein. In this domain, helices are arranged in a 2×2 bundle presenting a dense cluster of positive charge that appears to be the receptor interactive site (86). Apo E is synthesized in a number of tissues including liver, intestine, and the central nervous system. Expression is greatest in liver, where a tissue-specific regulatory domain located 18 kb downstream directs expression of both the apo E and apo C-I genes (87,88).

Formation of LDL

The VLDL remnant particles that are not endocytosed as such lose further triglycerides via hepatic lipase (HL). The loss of C apoproteins relieves inhibition of the lipase, allowing hydrolysis of most of the remaining triglycerides. Though HL is in the family of lipases to which LPL and pancreatic lipase belong, it has several distinct properties that comport with its role in lipolysis in remnants. Its gene is located on chromosome 15 (89,90). This protein of 499 amino acids does not require apo C-II as cofactor and, in contrast, is activated by apo E (91). It also has significantly more activity as a phospholipase than does LPL (92). Evidence adduced from several experimental approaches indicates that it plays a major role in the formation of LDL. This appears to involve interaction of remnants with heparan sulfate on the surface of the hepatocyte, a process mediated by apo E. Apo E binds poorly to the terminal lipoprotein products of lipolysis, probably accounting for their release from liver membranes. These mature LDL particles, of approximately 215 Å diameter with a cholesteryl-ester-rich core containing only 3–6% triglycerides, have apo B100 as essentially the sole apolipoprotein. Both HDL and IDL accumulate in the plasma of individuals who lack active HL, indicating a double role for the enzyme in the metabolism of remnant particles and HDL. Overexpression of HL in transgenic rabbits leads to a marked reduction in both HDL and intermediate-density lipoproteins (93).

CENTRIFUGAL TRANSPORT OF CHOLESTEROL

Structure of LDL

Each LDL particle contain one copy of apo B100 (8). Therefore, two populations of LDL exist in plasma containing apo B100 molecules that are products of different alleles. The apo B100 appears to be disposed in a circumferential distribution around the spherical microemulsion particle representing the lipid core of LDL (3,94,95), whereas a more extended disposition would be required in VLDL. Endoprotease probes reveal two superdomains in VLDL and three in LDL, suggesting that major conformational rearrangement takes place as VLDL particles are converted to LDL (96). Three-dimensional mapping with monoclonal antibodies supports a model of protein domains connected by peptide sequences present in the surface monolayer and interacting with core lipids (94,97), a finding consistent with the induced circular dichroic behavior of a carotenoid probe (98). In the presence of hypertriglyceridemia, the LDL content of triglycerides is increased, and the particles assume smaller diameters within an array of five quantized states (99). Conformational differences in apo B100 characterize these states, and two with the smallest diameters have diminished affinity for the LDL receptor (99).

Metabolism of LDL

The circulating half-life of LDL is approximately 2.5 days in normal humans. The principal mechanism by which these lipoproteins are removed from blood is endocytosis into nucleated cells via the LDL receptor, for which apo B100 is the ligand. Endocytosis by hepatocytes accounts for approximately half of the uptake. The ligand domain remains latent in VLDL and IDL of larger particle diameters but then conforms or is exposed in LDL. It is clearly a complex domain containing, at minimum, sequence elements located around the interdomain loop in the carboxyl-terminal region of the protein (8).

Receptor-mediated endocytosis of LDL provides a major source of cholesterol to cells for the maintenance of cell membranes. Because LDL contain tocopherols, this mechanism serves to deliver them to cells as well (62). It has been estimated that individual human fibroblasts contain from 10^4 to 10^5 receptor molecules (100,101). Receptor number is increased during cell division and under other circumstances when an increased supply of cholesterol is required. The highest levels of receptor expression occur in malignant cells. The LDL-receptor-mediated endocytosis also plays an important role in delivery of cholesterol to steroidogenic tissues. Expression of LDL receptors is regulated transcriptionally by an as yet unidentified sterol interacting with sterol response elements (102). One regulatory element in the 5′ flanking sequence interacts with the transcription factor Sp1 (103). The protein SREBP-1, attached to the nuclear envelope, undergoes proteolysis when sterols are depleted, releasing a 68 kda fragment that migrates into the nucleus and activates transcription of the LDL receptor-, and HMGCOA reductase genes (178). The de novo synthesis of cholesterol is controlled by transcriptional regulation of HMGCoA reductase and HMGCoA synthase (102). HMGCoA reductase activity is also regulated by degradation of the enzyme. This mechanism is activated by both sterol and isoprenoid compounds (104–107).

The LDL receptor gene contains 18 exons and is located on chromosome 19. Five exons encode the ligand interactive domain (108). The gene product contains a signal sequence of 21 amino acids that is rapidly hydrolyzed (109). Glycosylation raises the apparent molecular mass of the receptor protein from 120 kDa to 160 kDa. Interaction with the ligands, apo B100 and apo E, occurs via an amino-terminal domain consisting of seven repeating units, rich in exposed negative charges, and rigidly constrained by disulfide bridges (110). This domain is connected to a region of 400 amino acids that shares some homology with a protein considered to be a precursor of epidermal growth factor. This is followed, respectively, by a short domain that bears O-linked carbohydrate and a membrane-spanning domain. A carboxyl-terminal domain projects within the cell and is believed to be critical to clustering of receptors in coated pits (Fig. 2).

The fate of endocytosed LDL in most cells is similar to that described above for VLDL remnants. Decreasing pH in endosomes causes dissociation of ligand and receptor. The receptors are returned to the cell surface via the CURL compartment, whereas the lipoprotein particles undergo proteolytic degradation, a process that is probably initiated by cathepsin D (111) and finally results in complete hydrolysis to amino acids. Cholesteryl esters are hydrolyzed to free cholesterol by acid esterase activity, and the cholesterol enters cellular pools. Cholesterol can then be esterified, largely with oleic acid, by ACAT, providing for storage of cholesterol in the ester form.

A large number of mutations of the LDL receptor gene

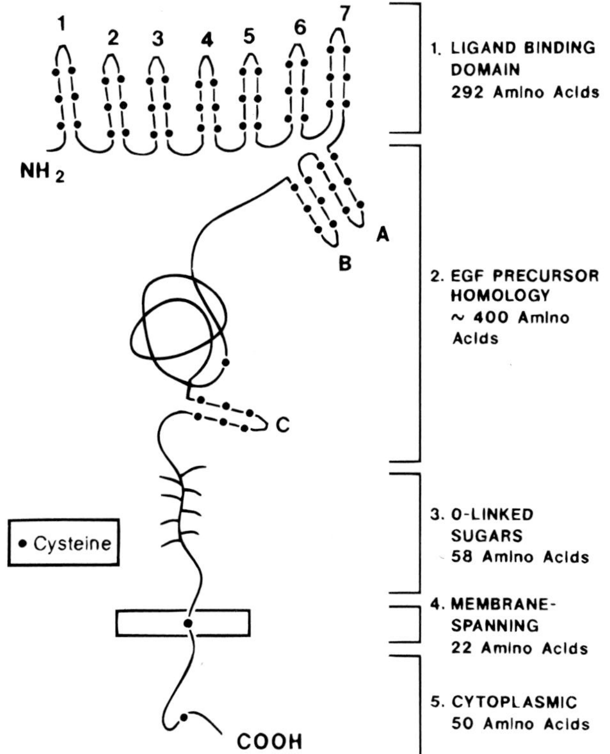

FIG. 2. The LDL receptor, showing five structural domains of the protein.

have been described that result, variously, in failure to produce the protein, failure of glycosylation or transport of the receptor to the cell surface, failure of the receptor to localize in coated pits or to endocytose, and, most common, failure to bind ligand lipoproteins with normal affinity. Phenotypically, any of these mutations can lead to accumulation of LDL in plasma, even in the heterozygous state, a condition termed familial hypercholesterolemia (82,112). Elevated levels of LDL in plasma are also the consequence of mutations that impair the ligand properties of apo B100 for the LDL receptor (113–115). In addition to endocytosis via the LDL receptor, LDL can be taken up in all nucleated cells by non-receptor-mediated processes that are of low efficiency but that become significant as the LDL concentration in extracellular fluid increases greatly, as in familial hypercholesterolemia. Furthermore, macrophages and transformed smooth muscle cells can endocytose chemically or physically modified LDL via a pair of structurally interrelated scavenger receptors (116,117) These receptors are coiled coils or superhelices of three monomeric units. Each has a cytoplasmic amino-terminal domain, a single transmembrane sequence, a spacer followed by an α-helical coiled coil, and a collagenous supercoil. The two receptor types differ in that one has an additional carboxyl-terminal cysteine-rich domain. They appear to be products of a single gene. Two mRNA species have been observed. Still other receptors on macrophages are capable of endocytosis of oxidized LDL (118,119).

HDL METABOLISM

Origins of HDL

Proteins and lipid constituents that will form HDL originate in both hepatocytes and absorptive enterocytes in the intestine. Bilayer discoidal particles composed of phospholipid and free cholesterol with apolipoproteins A-I and E, thought to be nascent particles, have been isolated and found to be excellent substrates for LCAT (120–122). Esterification of cholesterol generates a hydrophobic phase that accumulates in the interlamellar space, forming spherical microemulsion particles typical of plasma HDL. However, the apparent absence of discoidal particles in the Golgi apparatus suggests that these particles are formed after exocytosis of apolipoproteins E and A-I. In fact, there is also evidence to support the hypothesis that apo A-I can be secreted in a poorly lipidated form that subsequently recruits lipids to form small particles including discoidal forms that are substrates for LCAT (123). The association of some apo A-I and E with nascent VLDL (73) suggests that some of the origins of HDL are to be found in VLDL and presumably, by analogy, in chylomicrons. Thus, under normal conditions the most likely model is the secretion of triglyceride-rich lipoproteins, rich in surface phospholipid, with associated apolipoproteins A-I, A-II, E, and C (73).

As VLDL reach the space of Disse and chylomicrons enter the intestinal lymphatics, phospholipid begins to dissociate from the surface with apolipoproteins A-I, A-II, and possibly E, to nucleate new HDL particles or to join existing HDL. Nascent VLDL are enriched in phosphatidylethanolamine (124), which is selectively depleted during the loss of phospholipids from VLDL. It is likely that PLTP is an obligatory participant, catalyzing phospholipid transfer (48). Lecithin–cholesterol acyl transferase (LCAT) then esterifies free cholesterol acquired during dissociation of phospholipids from the nascent triglyceride-rich lipoprotein and probably also acquired by transfer from other lipoproteins. Other sources also contribute lipid to the HDL of plasma. In the centripetal transport pathway described below, both unesterified cholesterol and phospholipid move from peripheral cells to HDL. Also, macrophages have the ability to secrete discoidal particles that contain phospholipid and cholesterol accompanied by apo E (125), which is synthesized and secreted by the macrophages. These particles probably contribute lipid substrates for LCAT and merge into the circulating mass of HDL, though some particles may be endocytosed directly in liver via the LDL receptor. The process of secretion of precursors of HDL from liver is not dependent on secretion of apo-B-containing lipoproteins, however, as the accumulation of apo-A-I, phospholipid, and cholesterol is normal in perfusates of liver in which apo B secretion is completely blocked by orotic acid (126).

HDL Structure

Apolipoprotein A-I appears to be present in nearly all HDL molecular species as a primary structural element. This

28-kDa protein contains 243 amino acids and is rich in amphipathic helical structure (127,128), presenting as eight repeats of 22 amino acids and two of 11 amino acids. Apo A-I is synthesized in liver and intestine (82) and is secreted with a six amino acid prosequence that is cleaved by proteolysis in plasma to form the mature protein (129). Apo A-I can apparently assume several conformations in accommodating to different lipid-to-protein ratios. The apo A-I gene is clustered on the long arm of chromosome 11 with the genes for apo C-III and apo A-IV (130). Transcription appears to be regulated by nutritional and endocrine factors. Overexpression of apo A-I in transgenic mice appears to retard atherogenesis (131,132).

Apolipoprotein A-II is also a major protein constituent of HDL but is not present in all of the molecular species. It is a disulfide-bridged homodimer of a monomeric chain of only 77 amino acids (133). This monomeric unit also forms heterodimers with the E_2 and E_3 isoforms of apo E. Its gene is located on chromosome 1. Apo A-II is secreted as a proprotein that undergoes proteolytic cleavage of a five-amino-acid sequence at the amino terminus to form the mature protein (134). Apolipoprotein A-IV is a 46-kDa protein found in both HDL and chylomicrons (135–137). Like apo A-I, with which it has extensive homology, it is rich in amphipathic helix (138,139). In humans, it is synthesized largely in the intestine and occurs in a number of isoforms. It is capable of activating LCAT with some substrates.

All of the C apoproteins are found in HDL, which serves as a reservoir of C proteins and apo E for recycling to nascent VLDL and chylomicrons. Unlike apolipoproteins C-II and C-III, apo C-I is predominantly associated with HDL. This protein, containing only 57 amino acids, is synthesized in the liver (140,141). It has three amphipathic helices. Overexpression of apo C-I in transgenic mice causes hypertriglyceridemia. Its gene is closely linked to apo C-II and the LDL receptor on chromosome 19.

Most HDL particles appear to contain cores of cholesteryl esters and monolayers of phospholipid and unesterified cholesterol with which the helical apolipoproteins associate. The core domains can contain significant amounts of triglycerides, especially in the presence of hypertriglyceridemia. When plasma triglyceride levels are abnormally increased, triglycerides exchange for a portion of the cholesteryl esters of HDL, providing the basis for a log-inverse relationship between HDL cholesterol levels and total plasma triglycerides (142).

The Centripetal Transport Pathway

Centripetal transport of cholesterol begins with its association with one or more molecular species of HDL (120). Substantial quantities of several phospholipid species are also transferred to HDL from cells (143). It remains uncertain whether this involves direct contact of the acquiring species with cell membranes. Calculations of the rate of spontaneous desorption of free cholesterol from cell membranes suggests that the process would not have to depend on contact. The potential role of HDL receptors on cells is supported by observations that cell membranes contain high-affinity binding sites that appear to increase numerically in cholesterol-laden cells. A 100-kDa membrane protein that binds HDL with high affinity has been identified. It has been inferred that the function of the protein is to facilitate the movement of cholesterol to the cell surface via a protein kinase C-mediated signaling mechanism (144–146). However, data from several laboratories do not support a link between binding of HDL to cell membranes and efflux of cholesterol (147,148).

Whether free cholesterol desorbs spontaneously or its movement is facilitated by an HDL binding event, much of its appears to bind to a newly discovered molecular species of HDL, the 65-kDa pre-β HDL (149–151) (Fig. 3). This molecular species of HDL probably remained uncharacter-

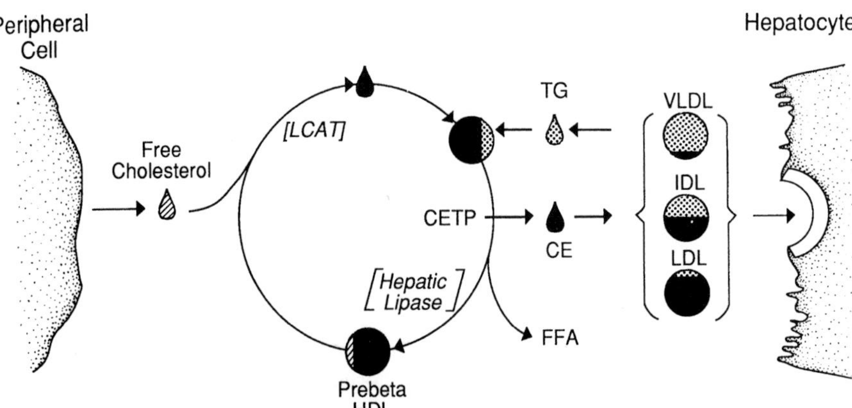

FIG. 3. The role of pre-β high-density lipoprotein (HDL) in reverse cholesterol transport. *Black areas* denote cholesteryl esters; *stippled areas,* triglycerides; *hatched areas,* free cholesterol. LCAT, lecithin–cholesterol acyl transferase; CETP, cholesteryl ester transfer protein; TG, triglycerides; CE, cholesteryl esters; FFA, free fatty acid; VLDL, very low-density lipoproteins; IDL, intermediate-density lipoproteins; LDL, low-density lipoproteins.

ized for many years because it is not retrieved in the classical HDL density interval on ultracentrifugation. The particle contains only apo A-I, phospholipid, cholesterol, and a very small amount of cholesteryl ester. It binds free cholesterol with high affinity and is an excellent substrate for LCAT (151–153). Esterification of cholesterol in 65-kDa HDL leads to its ultimate appearance in HDL species of α mobility (153,154). The cholesteryl esters are then transferred to acceptor lipoproteins, which include VLDL, chylomicrons, and their remnants as well as LDL. The endocytosis in liver of remnants of chylomicrons and VLDL and of LDL provides the means by which much of the cholesterol acquired from peripheral tissues is ultimately delivered to the liver. The transport system is entropically driven: esterification of cholesterol by LCAT reduces its local chemical potential, maintaining a diffusion gradient from the cell membranes. The increase in entropy associated with the transfer of cholesteryl esters into the cores of acceptor lipoproteins provides the energy for the transfer process. As cholesteryl esters are transferred to acceptor lipoproteins, triglycerides are transferred from VLDL and chylomicrons to the cores of α species of HDL (153). It appears that hepatic lipase is chiefly responsible for the removal of these triglycerides from HDL. As cholesteryl esters and triglycerides are removed from HDL, 65-kDa pre-β HDL is regenerated, contributing the final portion of a newly recognized metabolic cycle (Fig. 3) (153). Classes of HDL particles with and without apo A-II are both capable of forming 65-kDa pre-β HDL as cholesteryl esters are transferred to lipoprotein acceptors (155).

Lecithin–cholesterol acyl transferase is a hydrophobic protein comprised of 416 amino acids that is secreted by the liver. The LCAT gene is on chromosome 16 (156,157). Apolipoprotein A-I is a required cofactor (152), though apolipoproteins C-I, A-IV, and E also stimulate its activity under some conditions. LCAT catalyzes the transacylation of a fatty acid from the *sn*-2 position of lecithin to cholesterol. Integrated transesterification and centripetal movement of cholesterol in plasma appear to involve two additional elements, apolipoprotein D and cholesteryl ester transfer protein. Apo D is a highly glycosylated protein of 33 kDa that is the product of a gene on chromosome 3 (158). It is synthesized by many tissues including placenta, liver, and intestine. Cholesteryl ester transfer protein has a molecular mass of 53 kDa and contains 476 amino acids (9). The protein is more hydrophobic than other apolipoproteins, consistent with its function as a lipid transfer protein. It is apparently synthesized in liver, intestine, adrenals, and probably in macrophages. The gene is located on chromosome 16 (159). This protein catalyzes the transfer of triglycerides and, to a lesser extent, phospholipids as well as cholesteryl esters. It appears that alternative splicing mechanisms may yield intracellular lipid transfer proteins from the same structural gene that yields the plasma protein. Deficiencies of LCAT and CETP activities have both been identified in human subjects. In LCAT deficiency, abnormal lamellar lipoproteins containing unesterified cholesterol and phospholipid accumulate in plasma in place of spherical cholesteryl-ester-rich HDL (14). In CETP deficiency, there is a marked accumulation of cholesteryl ester-rich HDL in plasma (160,161).

In addition to the centripetal transport process described above, it appears that HDL may interact with liver in at least two ways to deliver cholesterol. HDL species that contain apo E can be endocytosed directly by the HDL receptor. HDL can also transfer sterol to liver without being endocytosed. It is likely that this transfer involves some binding event (162–164). The observation that CETP can facilitate transfer of cholesteryl esters directly to hepatocytes in culture suggests that it may be involved in transfers to the liver (165). Still other putative mechanisms have been partially characterized (166–168). However, the technique of radiation inactivation has yielded data that suggest that the principal HDL binding site in liver has a molecular weight too small to be a receptor protein (169). It is possible that a specific cluster of lipid molecules could serve as a binding site for HDL.

Speciation of HDL

The realization that ultracentrifugation causes the denaturation and loss of some elements of HDL (170) led to the development of the technique of selected affinity immunosorption for isolation of the native particle species of HDL (171). Nondenaturing gel electrophoresis of HDL isolated by this technique reveals up to eight discrete lipoprotein species, and two-dimensional isoelectric focusing and electrophoresis separate many more proteins than are found on ultracentrifugally prepared HDL. A number of these proteins are known to exist in a state of molecular dispersion in plasma in addition to a fraction that is bound to HDL (11). These include haptoglobin, both subunits of the SP 40/40 sulfated glycoprotein (also termed apo J) (172), fibrinogen, the binding protein for complement component 4 (C4BP), and lipopolysaccharide binding protein (LBP) (12). In addition, two HDL species that contain tightly bound transferrin and ceruloplasmin chelate transition metals and inhibit the oxidation of LDL (173). Additional, yet uncharacterized, proteins are also associated with immunosorbed HDL.

The best characterized of the newly recognized species of HDL is the 65-kDa pre-β HDL (149). This particle contains about 85% protein. Because apo A-I is the only detectable protein, this is assumed to represent two copies of that protein. Two-dimensional separation reveals two additional particles of slightly greater mobility (174). Analysis by FPLC indicates that these other elements comprise no more than 10% of pre-β HDL. The conformation of apo A-I in the 65-kDa species is markedly different from that in other HDL species (175), and its binding affinity for hepatic membranes is much lower than that of other HDL species (176). Discrete HDL species that contain apo E and apo A-IV are also being characterized (177).

The finding that a number of discrete HDL particle species exist in plasma reflects interactions among the lipid and protein components of HDL such that complexes of unique stoichiometries are formed with low structural free energies within the array of sterically permissable stoichiometries. The activities of transfer proteins such as PLTP and CETP overcome energy barriers to transfer, allowing the most stable complexes to form. The quantitative distribution of HDL species probably reflects in part the relative rates of processes such as esterification and lipid transfer as well as the absolute pool sizes of apolipoproteins. The observation that species distribution changes spontaneously over time after blood is drawn indicates the dynamic nature of these processes and demonstrates that the species distribution in plasma is not at its lowest free energy state. The study of HDL species distribution is likely to provide important insights into the major processes in which HDL are involved.

REFERENCES

1. He X-M, Carter DC. Atomic structure and chemistry of human serum albumin. *Nature* 1992;358:209–215.
2. Miller KW, Small DM. Structure of triglyceride-rich lipoproteins: An analysis of core and surface phases. In: Gotto AM, ed. *Plasma Lipoproteins: New Comprehensive Biochemistry*. Amsterdam: Elsevier; 1987.
3. Schumaker VN, Phillips ML, Chatterton JE. Apolipoprotein B and low density lipoprotein structure: Implications for biosynthesis of triglyceride-rich lipoproteins. *Adv Protein Chem* 1994;45:205–248.
4. Havel RJ, Eder HA, Bragdon JH. The distribution and chemical composition of ultracentrifugally separated lipoproteins in human serum. *J Clin Invest* 1955;34:1345–1353.
5. Luo C-C, Li W-H, Moore MN, et al. Structure and evolution of the apolipoprotein multigene family. *J Mol Biol* 1986;187:325–340.
6. Segrest JP, Garber DW, Brouilette CG, et al. The amphipathic alpha-helix: A multifunctional structural motif in plasma apolipoproteins. *Adv Protein Chem* 1994;45:303–369.
7. Segrest JP, Jones MK, Loof HD, et al. The amphipathic helix in the exchangeable apolipoproteins: A review of secondary structure and function. *J Lipid Res* 1992;33:141–166.
8. Kane JP, Havel RJ. Disorders of the biogenesis and secretion of lipoproteins containing the B-apolipoproteins. In: Scriver CR, Beaudet AL, Sly WS, et al, eds. *The Metabolic Basis of Inherited Disease*. New York: McGraw-Hill; 1994.
9. Drayna D, Jarnagin AS, McLean J, et al. Cloning and sequencing of human cholesteryl ester transfer protein cDNA. *Nature* 1987;327:632–634.
10. Day JR, Albers JJ, Lofton-Day CE, et al. Complete cDNA encoding human phospholipid transfer protein from human endothelial cells. *J Biol Chem* 1994;269:9388–9391.
11. Kunitake ST, Carilli CT, Lau K, et al. Identification of proteins associated with apolipoprotein A-I-containing lipoproteins purified by selected affinity immunosorption. *Biochemistry* 1994;33:1988–1993.
12. Wurfel MM, Kunitake ST, Lichenstein H, et al. Lipopolysaccharide (LPS) binding protein is carried on lipoproteins and acts as a cofactor in the neutralization of LPS. *J Exp Med* 1994;180:1025–1035.
13. Havel RJ, Kane JP. Introduction: Structure and metabolism of plasma lipoproteins. In: Scriver CR, Beaudet AL, Sly WS, et al, eds. *The Metabolic Basis of Inherited Disease*. New York: McGraw-Hill; 1994.
14. Glomset JA, Assman G, Gjone E, and Norum KR. Lecithin-cholesterol acyltransferase deficiency and fisheye disease. In: Scriver CR, Beaudet AL, Sly WS, et al., eds. *The Metabolic and Molecular Basis of Inherited Disease*. New York: McGraw-Hill, 1995.
15. Hager KM, Pierce MA, Moore DR, et al. Endocytosis of a cytotoxic human high density lipoprotein results in disruption of acidic intracellular vesicles and subsequent killing of African trypanosomes. *J Cell Biol* 1994;126:155–167.
16. Read TE, Harris HW, Grunfeld C, et al. Chylomicrons enhance endotoxin excretion in bile. *Infect Immun* 1993;61:3496–3502.
17. Feingold KR, Staprans I, Memon RA, et al. Endotoxin rapidly induces changes in lipid metabolism that produce hypertriglyceridemia: Low doses stimulate hepatic triglyceride production while high doses inhibit clearance. *J Lipid Res* 1992;33:1765–1776.
18. Bowie EJ. Lipid-related clotting reactions of clinical significance. *Arch Pathol Lab Med* 1992;116:1345–1349.
19. Sakai T, Kisiel W. Formation of tissue factor activity following incubation of recombinant human tissue factor apoprotein with plasma lipoproteins. *Thromb Res* 1990;60:213–222.
20. Wun TC, Huang MD, Kretzmer KK, et al. Immunoaffinity purification and characterization of lipoprotein associated coagulation factors from HepG2 hepatoma, Chang liver, and SK hepatoma cells, a comparative study. *J Biol Chem* 1990;265:16096–16101.
21. Levy JA, Dimpfl J, Hardman DA, et al. Transfer of mouse antixenotropic virus neutralizing factor to human lipoproteins. *J Virol* 1982; 42:365–371.
22. Thurnhofer H, Schabel J, Botz M, et al. Cholesterol transfer protein located in the intestinal brush border membrane. Partial purification and characterization. *Biochim Biophys Acta* 1991;1064:275–286.
23. Xu Z, Bernlohr DA, Banaszak IJ. Crystal structure of recombinant murine adipocyte lipid-binding protein. *Biochemistry* 1992;31: 3484–3492.
24. Schaffer TE and Lodish HF. Expression cloning and characteristic of a novel adipocyte lung chain fatty acid transport protein. *Cell* 1994; 79:427–436.
25. Powell LM, Wallis SC, Pease RJ, et al. A novel form of tissue-specific RNA processing produces apolipoprotein B-48 in intestine. *Cell* 1987; 50:831–840.
26. Driscoll DM, Cassanova E. Characterization of the apolipoprotein B mRNA editing activity in enterocyte extracts. *J Biol Chem* 1990;265: 21401–21403.
27. Bostrom K, Garcia Z, Poksay KS, et al. Apolipoprotein B mRNA editing. *J Biol Chem* 1990;265:22446–22452.
28. Hardman DA, Protter AA, Schilling JW, et al. Carboxyl terminal analysis of human B-48 protein confirms the novel mechanism proposed for chain termination. *Biochem Biophys Res Commun* 1987; 149:1214–1219.
29. Lacaille F, Bratos M, Bouma M-E, et al. La maladie d'Anderson. *Arch Fr Pediatr* 1989;46:491–498.
30. Roy CC, Levy E, Green PHR, et al. Malabsorption, hypocholesterolemia, fat-filled enterocytes with increased intestinal apoprotein B: Chylomicron retention disease. *Gastroenterology* 1987;92:390–399.
31. Christensen NJ, Rubin CE, Cheung MC, et al. Ultrastructural immunolocalization of apolipoprotein B within human jejunal absorptive cells. *J Lipid Res* 1983;24:1229–1242.
32. Wetterau JR, Aggerbeck LP, Bouma ME, et al. Absence of microsomal triglyceride transfer protein in individuals with abetalipoproteinemia. *Science* 1992;258:999–1001.
33. Hamilton RL, Havel RJ. Is microsomal triglyceride transfer protein the missing link in abetalipoproteinemia? *Hepatology* 1993;18:460.
34. Imaizumi K, Havel RJ, Fainaru M, et al. Origin and transport of the A-I and arginine-rich apolipoproteins in mesenteric lymph of rats. *J Lipid Res* 1978;19:1038–1046.
35. Imaizumi K, Fainaru M, Havel RJ. Composition of proteins of mesenteric lymph chylomicrons in the rat and alterations produced upon exposure of chylomicrons to blood serum and serum proteins. *J Lipid Res* 1978;19:712–722.
36. Olivecrona T, Bengtsson-Olivecrona G. Lipoprotein lipase and hepatic lipase. *Curr Opin Lipidol* 1993;4:187–196.
37. Eisenberg S, Sehayek E, Olivecrona T, et al. Lipoprotein lipase enhances binding of lipoproteins to heparan sulphate on cell surfaces and extracellular matrix. *J Clin Invest* 1992;90:2013–2021.
38. Mulder M, Lombardi P, Jansen H, et al. Heparan sulphate proteoglycans are involved in the lipoprotein lipase-mediated enhancement of the cellular binding of very low density and low density lipoproteins. *Biochem Biophys Res Commun* 1992;185:582–587.
39. Williams KJ, Fless GM, Petrie KA, et al. Mechanisms by which lipoprotein lipase alters cellular metabolism of lipoprotein(s). Low density lipoprotein, and nascent lipoproteins. Roles for low density lipoprotein receptors and heparan sulphate proteoglycans. *J Biol Chem* 1992;267: 13284–13292.
40. Braun JEA, Severson DL. Regulation of the synthesis, processing and translocation of lipoprotein lipase. *Biochem J* 1992;287:337–347.
41. Arner P, Lithell H, Wahrenberg H, et al. Expression of lipoprotein

lipase in different human subcutaneous adipose tissue regions. *J Lipid Res* 1991;32:423–429.
42. Enerback S, Semb H, Tavernier J, et al. Tissue-specific regulation of guinea pig lipoprotein lipase: Effects of nutritional state and of tumor necrosis factor on mRNA levels in adipose tissue, heart and liver. *Gene* 1988;64:97–106.
43. Doolittle MH, Ben-Zeev O, Elovson J, et al. The response of lipoprotein lipase to feeding and fasting. Evidence for posttranslational regulation. *J Biol Chem* 1990;265:4570–4577.
44. Frayn KN. Insulin resistance and lipid metabolism. *Curr Opin Lipidol* 1993;4:197–204.
45. Tollefson JH, Ravnik S, Albers JJ. Isolation and characterization of a phospholipid transfer protein (LTP-II) from human plasma. *J Lipid Res* 1988;15:1593–1602.
46. Schumann RR, Leong SR, Flaggs GW, et al. Structure and function of lipopolysaccharide binding protein. *Science* 1990;249:1429–1431.
47. Gray PW, Flaggs G, Leong SR, et al. Cloning of the cDNA of a human neutrophil bactericidal protein: Structural and functional correlations. *J Biol Chem* 1989;264:9505–9509.
48. Malloy MJ, Zoppo A, Tu AY, et al. A new metabolic disorder: Phospholipid transfer protein deficiency. *Clin Res* 1994;42:85A.
49. Stalenhoef AFH, Malloy MJ, Kane JP, et al. Metabolism of apolipoprotein B-48 and B-100 of triglyceride-rich lipoproteins in normal and lipoprotein lipase-deficient humans. *Proc Natl Acad Sci USA* 1984;81:1839–1843.
50. Shafi S, Brady SE, Bensadoun A, et al. Role of hepatic lipase in the uptake and processing of chylomicron remnants in rat liver. *J Lipid Res* 1994;35:709–720.
51. Herz J, Hamann U, Rogne S. Surface location and high affinity for calcium of a 500-kD liver membrane protein closely related to the LDL-receptor suggest a physiological role as lipoprotein receptor. *EMBO J* 1988;7:4119–4127.
52. Brown MS, Herz J, Kowal RC, et al. The low density lipoprotein receptor-related protein: Double agent or decoy? *Curr Opin Lipidol* 1991;2:65–72.
53. Herz J, Kowal RC, Goldstein JL, et al. Proteolytic processing of the 600 kD low density lipoprotein receptor-related protein (LRP) occurs in a *trans*-Golgi compartment. *EMBO J* 1990;9:1769–1776.
54. Lund H, Takahashi K, Hamilton RL, et al. Lipoprotein binding and endosomal itinerary of the low density lipoprotein receptor-related protein in rat liver. *Proc Natl Acad Sci USA* 1989;86:9318–9322.
55. Sultan F, Lagrange D, Jansen H, et al. Inhibition of hepatic lipase activity impairs chylomicron remnant-removal in rats. *Biochim Biophys Acta* 1990;1042:150–152.
56. Borensztajn J, Kotlar TJ, Chang S. Apoprotein-independent binding of chylomicron remnants to rat liver membranes. *Biochem J* 1991;279:769–773.
57. Oswald B, Shelburne F, Landis B. The relevance of glycosaminoglycan sulfates to apo E induced lipid uptake by hepatocyte monolayers. *Biochem Biophys Res Commun* 1986;141:158–164.
58. Stow JL, Kjellen L, Unger E. Heparan sulfate proteoglycans are concentrated on the sinusoidal plasmalemmal domain and in intracellular organelles of hepatocytes. *J Cell Biol* 1985;100:975–980.
59. Belcher JD, Hamilton RL, Brady SE, et al. Hepatic endosomes have hepatic lipase. *Circulation* 1988;28:II, 145.
60. Mokuno H, Brady S, Kotite L, et al. Effect of the 39 kDa receptor-associated protein on the hepatic uptake and endocytosis of chylomicron remnants and low density lipoproteins in the rat. *J Biol Chem* 1994;269:13238–13243.
61. Beisiegel U, Weber W, Bengtsson-Olivecrona G. Lipoprotein lipase enhanced the binding of chylomicrons to low density receptor-related protein. *Proc Natl Acad Sci USA* 1991;88:8342–8346.
62. Kayden HJ, Traber MG. Absorption, lipoprotein transport and regulation of plasma concentrations of vitamin E in humans. *J Lipid Res* 1993;34:343–358.
63. Blackhart BD, Ludwig EH, Pierotti VR, et al. Structure of the human apolipoprotein B gene. *J Biol Chem* 1986;261:15364–15367.
64. Alexander CA, Hamilton RL, Havel RJ. Subcellular localization of "B" apoprotein of plasma lipoproteins in rat liver. *J Cell Biol* 1976;69:241–263.
65. Chuck SL, Yao Z, Blackhart BD, et al. New variation on the translocation of proteins during early biogenesis of apolipoprotein B. *Nature* 1990;346:382–385.
66. Dorsey CA, Lingappa VR. Co-translational and post-translational control of early steps in protein biogenesis: Implications for the liver. In: Blair JL, Ockner RK, eds. *Progress in Liver Diseases*. Philadelphia: WB Saunders; 1992.
67. Havel RJ. Role of the liver in hyperlipidemia. *Semin Liver Dis* 1992;12:356–363.
68. Thrift RN, Drisko J, Dueland S, et al. Translocation of apolipoprotein B across the endoplasmic reticulum is blocked in a nonhepatic cell line. *Proc Natl Acad Sci USA* 1992;89:9161–9165.
69. Dixon JL, Ginsberg HN. Regulation of hepatic secretion of apolipoprotein B-containing lipoproteins: Information obtained from cultured liver cells. *J Lipid Res* 1993;34:167–179.
70. Hamilton RL. Apolipoprotein-B-containing plasma lipoproteins in health and in disease. *Trends Cardiovasc Med* 1994;4:131–139.
71. Yao Z, Blackhart BD, Linton MF, et al. Expression of carboxyl-terminally truncated forms of human apolipoprotein B in rat hepatoma cells. *J Biol Chem* 1991;266:3300–3308.
72. Spring DJ, Chen-Liu LW, Chatterton JE, et al. Lipoprotein assembly. Apolipoprotein B size determines lipoprotein core circumference. *J Biol Chem* 1992;267:14839–14845.
73. Hamilton RL, Moorehouse A, Havel RJ. Isolation and properties of nascent lipoproteins from highly purified rat hepatocytic Golgi fractions. *J Lipid Res* 1991;32:529–543.
74. Marsh JB, Diffenderfer MR. Isolation of nascent high-density lipoprotein from rat liver perfusates by immunoaffinity chromatography: Effects of oleic acid infusions. *Metabolism* 1991;40:26–30.
75. Erickson SK, Cooper AD. Acyl-coenzyme A:cholesterol acyltransferase in human liver. In vivo detection and some characteristics of the enzyme. *Metabolism* 1980;29:991–996.
76. Pullinger C, North J, Teng B, et al. The apolipoprotein B gene is constitutively expressed in HepG2 cells: Regulation of secretion by oleic acid, albumin and insulin, and measurement of the mRNA half-life. *J Lipid Res* 1989;30:1065–1077.
77. Lackner KJ, Monge JC, Gregg RE, et al. Analysis of the apolipoprotein B gene and messenger ribonucleic acid in abetalipoproteinemia. *J Clin Invest* 1986;78:1707–1712.
78. Patsch W, Franz S, Schonfeld G. Role of insulin in lipoprotein secretion by cultured hepatocytes. *J Clin Invest* 1983;71:1161–1174.
79. Sparks CE, Sparks JD, Bolognino M, et al. Insulin effects on apolipoprotein B lipoprotein synthesis and secretion by primary cultures of rat hepatocytes. *Metabolism* 1986;35:1128–1136.
80. Tam S-P, Archer TK, Deeley RG. Biphasic effects of estrogen on apolipoprotein synthesis in human hepatoma cells: Mechanisms of antagonism by testosterone. *Proc Natl Acad Sci USA* 1986;83:3111–3115.
81. Karathanasis SK, McPherson J, Zannis VI, et al. Linkage of human apolipoproteins A-I and C-III genes. *Nature* 1983;304:371–373.
82. Zannis VI, Kardassis D, Zanni EE. Genetic mutations affecting human lipoproteins, their receptors, and their enzymes. In: Harris H, Hirschhorn K, eds. *Advances in Human Genetics*. New York: Plenum Press; 1993.
83. Havel RJ, Hamilton RL. Hepatocytic lipoprotein receptors and intracellular lipoprotein catabolism. *Hepatology* 1988;8:1689–1704.
84. Das HK, McPherson J, Bruns GAP, et al. Isolation, characterization, and mapping to chromosome 19 of the human apolipoprotein E gene. *J Biol Chem* 1985;260:6240–6246.
85. Weisgraber KH. Apolipoprotein E: Structure–function relationships. *Adv Protein Chem* 1994;45:249–302.
86. Wilson C, Wardell MR, Weisgraber KH, et al. Three dimensional structure of the LDL receptor binding domain of human apolipoprotein E. *Science* 1991;252:1817–1822.
87. Simonet WS, Bucay N, Pitas RE, et al. Multiple tissue-specific elements control the apolipoprotein E/C-I gene locus in transgenic mice. *J Biol Chem* 1991;266:8651–8654.
88. Simonet WS, Bucay N, Lauer SJ, et al. A far-downstream hepatocyte-specific control region directs expression of the linked human apolipoprotein E and C-I genes in transgenic mice. *J Biol Chem* 1993;268:8221–8229.
89. Sparkes RS, Zollman S, Klisak I, et al. Human genes involved in lipolysis of plasma lipoproteins. Mapping of loci for lipoprotein lipase to 8p22 and hepatic lipase to 15q21. *Genomics* 1987;1:138–144.
90. Datta S, Luo CC, Li WH, et al. Human hepatic lipase. Cloned cDNA sequence, restriction fragment length polymorphisms, chromosomal localization, and evolutionary relationships with lipoprotein lipase and pancreatic lipase. *J Biol Chem* 1988;263:1107–1110.

91. Thuren T, Weisgraber KH, Sisson P, et al. Role of apolipoprotein E in hepatic lipase catalyzed hydrolysis of phospholipid in high density lipoproteins. *Biochemistry* 1992;31:2332–2338.
92. Deckelbaum RJ, Ramakrishnan R, Eisenberg S, et al. Triacylglycerol and phospholipid hydrolysis in human plasma lipoproteins. Role of lipoprotein and hepatic lipase. *Biochemistry* 1992;31:8544–8551.
93. Fan J, Wang J, Bensadoun A, et al. Overexpression of hepatic lipase in transgenic rabbits leads to a marked reduction of plasma high density lipoproteins and intermediate density lipoproteins. *Proc Natl Acad Sci USA* 1994;91:8724–8728.
94. Chatterton JE, Phillips ML, Curtiss LK, et al. Mapping apolipoprotein B on the low density lipoprotein surface by immunoelectron microscopy. *J Biol Chem* 1991;266:5955–5962.
95. Phillips ML, Schumaker VN. Conformation of apolipoprotein B after lipid extraction of low density lipoproteins attached to an electron microscope grid. *J Lipid Res* 1989;30:415–422.
96. Chen GC, Zhu S, Hardman DA, et al. Structural domains of human apolipoprotein B-100. Differential accessibility to limited proteolysis of B-100 in low density and very low density lipoproteins. *J Biol Chem* 1989;264:14369–14375.
97. Bastiaens P, de Beus A, Lacker M, et al. Resonance energy transfer from a cylindrical distribution of donors to a plane of acceptors. Location of apo-B-100 protein on the human low-density lipoprotein particle. *Biophys J* 1990;58:665–675.
98. Chen GC, Chapman MJ, Kane JP. Secondary structure and thermal behavior of trypsin-treated low-density lipoproteins from human serum, studied by circular dichroism. *Biochim Biophys Acta* 1983; 754:451–456.
99. Chen GC, Liu W, Duchateau P, et al. Conformational differences in human apolipoprotein B-100 among subspecies of low density lipoproteins (LDL). *J Biol Chem* 1994;269:29121–29128.
100. Brown MS, Goldstein JL. Regulation of the activity of the low density lipoprotein receptor in human fibroblasts. *Cell* 1975;6:307–316.
101. Goldstein JL, Basu SK, Brunschede GY, et al. Release of low density lipoprotein from its cell surface receptor by sulfated glycosaminoglycans. *Cell* 1976;7:85–95.
102. Goldstein JL, Brown MS. Regulation of the mevalonate pathway. *Nature* 1990;343:425–430.
103. Dawson PA, Hofmann SL, Vander-Westhuyzen DR, et al. Sterol-dependent repression of low density lipoprotein receptor promoter mediated by 16-base pair sequence adjacent to binding site for transcription factor Sp1. *J Biol Chem* 1988;263:3372–3379.
104. Inoue S, Simoni RD. 3-Hydroxy-3-methylglutaryl-coenzyme-A reductase and T cell receptor alpha subunit are differentially degraded in the endoplasmic reticulum. *J Biol Chem* 1992;267:9080–9086.
105. Roitelman J, Olender EH, Bar-Nun S, et al. Immunological evidence for eight spans in the membrane domain of 3-hydroxy-3-methylglutaryl coenzyme-A reductase: Implications for enzyme degradation in the endoplasmic reticulum. *J Cell Biol* 1992;117:959–973.
106. Roitelman J, Simoni RD. Distinct sterol and non-sterol signals for the regulated degradation of 3-hydroxy-3-methylglutaryl coenzyme-A reductase. *J Biol Chem* 1992;267:25264–25273.
107. Rudney H, Panini SR. Cholesterol biosynthesis. *Curr Opin Lipidol* 1993;4:230–237.
108. Sudhof TC, Goldstein JL, Brown MS, et al. The LDL receptor gene: A mosaic of exons shared with different proteins. *Science* 1985;228: 815–822.
109. Brown MS, Goldstein JL. A receptor-mediated pathway for cholesterol homeostasis. *Science* 1986;232:34–47.
110. Yamamoto T, Davies CG, Brown MS, et al. The human LDL receptor: A cysteine-rich protein with multiple Alu sequences in its mRNA. *Cell* 1984;39:27–38.
111. Runquist EA, Havel RJ. Acid hydrolases in early and late endosome fractions from rat liver. *J Biol Chem* 1992;266:22557–22563.
112. Hobbs HH, Brown MS, Goldstein JL. Molecular genetics of the LDL receptor gene in familial hypercholesterolemia. *Hum Mutation* 1992; 1:445–466.
113. Innerarity TL, Weisgraber KH, Arnold KS, et al. Familial defective apolipoprotein B-100: Low density lipoproteins with abnormal receptor binding. *Proc Natl Acad Sci USA* 1987;84:6919–6923.
114. Soria LF, Ludwig EH, Clarke HRG, et al. Association between a specific apolipoprotein B mutation and familial defective B-100. *Proc Natl Acad Sci USA* 1989;86:587–591.
115. Pullinger CR, Hennessy LK, Chatterton JE, et al. Familial ligand-defective apolipoprotein B: Identification of a new mutation that decreses LDL receptor binding affinity. *J Clin Invest* 1995;95: 1225–1234.
116. Kodama T, Freeman M, Rohrer L, et al. Type I macrophage scavenger receptor contains alpha helical and collagen-like coiled coils. *Nature* 1990;343:531–535.
117. Rohrer L, Freeman M, Kodama T, et al. Coiled-coil fibrous domains mediate ligand binding by macrophage scavenger receptor type II. *Nature* 1990;343:570–572.
118. Endemann G, Stanton LW, Madden KS, et al. CD36 is a receptor for oxidized low density lipoprotein. *J Biol Chem* 1993;268:11811.
119. Stanton LW, White RT, Bryant CM, et al. A macrophage Fc receptor for IgG is also a receptor for oxidized low density lipoprotein. *J Biol Chem* 1992;267:22446–22451.
120. Kane JP. High-density lipoproteins. In: Kreisberg RA, Segrest J, eds. *Plasma Lipoproteins and Coronary Artery Disease.* Boston: Blackwell Scientific Publications; 1992.
121. Glickman RM, Magun AM. High density lipoprotein formation by the intestine. *Methods Enzymol* 1986;129:519–536.
122. Hamilton RL, Williams MC, Fielding CJ, et al. Discoidal bilayer structure of nascent high density lipoproteins from perfused rat liver. *J Clin Invest* 1976;58:667–680.
123. Forte TM, Goth-Goldstein R, Nordhausen RW, et al. Apolipoprotein A-I-cell membrane interaction: Extracellular assembly of heterogeneous nascent HDL particles. *J Lipid Res* 1993;34:317–324.
124. Hamilton RL, Fielding PE. Nascent very low density lipoproteins from rat hepatocytic Golgi fractions are enriched in phosphatidylethanolamine. *Biochem Biophys Res Commun* 1989;160:162–167.
125. Basu SK, Goldstein JL, Brown MS. Independent pathways for secretion of cholesterol and apolipoprotein E by macrophages. *Science* 1983;219:871–873.
126. Hamilton RL, Guo LSS, Felker TE, et al. Nascent high density lipoproteins from liver perfusates of orotic acid-fed rats. *J Lipid Res* 1986; 27:967–978.
127. Baker HN, Gotto J, Jackson RL. The primary structure of human plasma high density apolipoprotein glutamine I (apo A-I). II. The amino acid sequence and alignment of cyanogen bromide fragments IV, III, and I. *J Biol Chem* 1975;250:2725–2738.
128. Barker WC, Dayhoff MO. Evolution of lipoproteins deduced from protein sequence data. *Comp Biochem Physiol* 1977;57:309–315.
129. Edelstein C, Gordon JI, Toscas K, et al. In vitro conversion of proapoprotein A-I. Partial characterization of an extracellular enzyme activity. *J Biol Chem* 1983;258:1430–1433.
130. Cheung P, Kao FT, Law ML, et al. Localization of the structural gene for human apolipoprotein A-I on the long arm of human chromosome 11. *Proc Natl Acad Sci USA* 1984;81:508–511.
131. Walsh A, Ito Y, Breslow JL. High levels of human apolipoprotein A-I in transgenic mice result in increased plasma levels of small high density lipoprotein (HDL) particles comparable to human HDL3. *J Biol Chem* 1989;264:6488–6494.
132. Rubin EM, Ishida BY, Clift SM, et al. Expression of human apolipoprotein A-1 in transgenic mice results in reduced plasma levels of murine apolipoprotein A-I and the appearance of two new high density lipoprotein size subclasses. *Proc Natl Acad Sci USA* 1991;88: 434–438.
133. Brewer HB Jr, Lux SE, Roman R, et al. Amino acid sequence of human apoLp-Gln-II (apo A-II), an apolipoprotein isolated from the high density lipoprotein complex. *Proc Natl Acad Sci USA* 1972;69: 1304–1308.
134. Gordon JI, Sims HF, Edelstein C, et al. Extracellular processing of proapolipoprotein A-II in HepG2 cell cultures is mediated by a 54 kDa protease immunologically related to cathepsin B. *J Biol Chem* 1985;260:14824–14831.
135. Swaney JB, Reese H, Eder HA. Polypeptide composition of rat high density lipoprotein: Characterization by SDS-gel electrophoresis. *Biochem Biophys Res Commun* 1974;59:513–519.
136. Green PHR, Glickman RM, Sauder CD, et al. Human intestinal lipoproteins. Studies in chyluric subjects. *J Clin Invest* 1979;64:233–242.
137. Gordon JI, Budelier CL, Sims HF, et al. Biosynthesis of human preproapolipoprotein A-IV. *J Biol Chem* 1984;259:468–474.
138. Li WH, Tanimura M, Luo CC, et al. The apolipoprotein multigene family: Biosynthesis, structure, structure–function relationships, and evolution. *J Lipid Res* 1988;29:245–271.
139. Elshourbagy NA, Walker DW, Boguski MS, et al. The nucleotide and

derived amino acid sequence of human apolipoprotein A-IV mRNA and the close linkage of its gene to the genes of apolipoprotein A-I and C-III. *J Biol Chem* 1986;261:1998–2002.

140. Jackson RL, Sparrow JT, Baker HN, et al. The primary structure of apolipoprotein-serine. *J Biol Chem* 1974;249:5308–5313.
141. Wu AI, Windmueller HG. Relative contribution of liver and intestine to individual plasma apolipoproteins in the rat. *J Biol Chem* 1979; 254:6316–7322.
142. Myers LH, Phillips NR, Havel RJ. Mathematical evaluation of methods for estimation of the concentration of the major lipid components of human serum lipoproteins. *J Lab Clin Med* 1976;88:491–505.
143. Bielicki JK, Johnson WJ, Glick JM, et al. Efflux of phospholipids from fibroblasts with normal and elevated levels of cholesterol. *Biochem Biophys Acta* 1991;1084:7–14.
144. Slotte JP, Oram JF, Bierman EL. Binding of high density lipoproteins to cell receptors promotes translocation of cholesterol from intracellular membranes to the cell surface. *J Biol Chem* 1987;262: 12904–12907.
145. Oram JF, Mendez AJ, Slotte JP, et al. High density lipoprotein apolipoprotein mediate removal of sterol from intracellular pools but not from plasma membranes of cholesterol-loaded fibroblasts. *Arterioscler Thromb* 1991;11:403–414.
146. Mendez AJ, Oram JF, Bierman EL. Protein kinase C as a mediator of high density lipoprotein receptor-dependent efflux of intracellular cholesterol. *J Biol Chem* 1991;266:10104–10111.
147. Mendel CM, Kunitake ST. Cell-surface binding sites for high density lipoproteins do not mediate efflux of cholesterol from human fibroblasts in tissue culture. *J Lipid Res* 1988;29:1171–1178.
148. Karlin JB, Johnson WJ, Benedict CR, et al. Cholesterol flux between cells and high density lipoprotein: Lack of relationship to specific binding of the lipoprotein to the cell surface. *J Biol Chem* 1987;262: 12557–12564.
149. Kunitake ST, La Sala KJ, Kane JP. Apoprotein A-I-containing lipoproteins with pre-beta electrophoretic mobility. *J Lipid Res* 1985;26: 549–553.
150. Ishida BY, Frohlich J, Fielding CJ. Prebeta-migrating high density lipoprotein: Quantitation in normal and hyperlipemic plasma by solid phase radioimmunoassay following electrophoretic transfer. *J Lipid Res* 1987;28:778–786.
151. Ishida BY, Albee D, Paigen B. Interconversion of prebeta-migrating lipoproteins containing apolipoprotein A-I and HDL. *J Lipid Res* 1990;31:227–236.
152. Fielding CJ, Shore VG, Fielding PD. A protein cofactor of lecithin: cholesterol acyltransferase. *Biochem Biophys Res Commun* 1972;46: 1943–1949.
153. Kunitake ST, Mendel CM, Hennessy LK. Interconversion between apolipoprotein A-I-containing lipoproteins of pre-beta and alpha electrophoretic mobilities. *J Lipid Res* 1992;33:1807–1816.
154. Kunitake ST, La-Sala KJ, Mendel CM, et al. Some unique properties of apo A-I-containing lipoproteins with prebeta electrophoretic mobility. In: *NIH Workshop on Lipoprotein Heterogeneity*. 1987:419–427.
155. Hennessy LK, Kunitake ST, Kane JP. Apolipoprotein A-I-containing lipoproteins, with or without apolipoprotein A-II, as progenitors of pre-beta HDL particles. *Biochemistry* 1993;32:5759–5765.
156. Warden CH, Langner CA, Gordon JI, et al. Tissue-specific expression, developmental regulation, and chromosomal mapping of the lecithin: cholesterol acyltransferase gene. Evidence for expression in brain and testes as well as liver. *J Biol Chem* 1989;264:21573–21581.
157. McLean J, Wion K, Drayna D, et al. Human lecithin–cholesterol acyltransferase gene: Complete gene sequence and sites of expression. *Nucl Acids Res* 1986;14:9397–9406.
158. Drayna D, Fielding C, McLean J, et al. Cloning and expression of human apolipoprotein D cDNA. *J Biol Chem* 1986;261:16535–16538.
159. Lusis AJ, Zollman S, Sparkes RS, et al. Assignment of the human gene for cholestryl ester transfer protein to chromosome 16. *Genomics* 1987;1:232–235.
160. Koizumi J, Mabuchi H, Yoshimura A, et al. Deficiency of serum cholesteryl-ester transfer activity in patients with familial hyperalphalipoproteinemia. *Atherosclerosis* 1985;58:175–186.
161. Kurasawa T, Yokoyama S, Miyake Y, et al. Rate of cholesteryl ester transfer between high and low density lipoproteins in human serum and a case with decreased transfer rate in association with hyperalphalipoproteinemia. *J Biochem* 1985;98:1499–1508.
162. Pittman RC, Knecht TP, Rosenbaum MS, et al. A nonendocytotic mechanism for the selective uptake of high density lipoprotein-associated cholesterol esters. *J Biol Chem* 1987;262:2443–2450.
163. Glass C, Pittman RC, Weinstein DB, et al. Dissociation of tissue uptake of cholesterol ester from that of apoprotein A-I of rat plasma high density lipoprotein: Selective delivery of cholesterol ester to liver, adrenal, and gonad. *Proc Natl Acad Sci USA* 1983;80: 5435–5439.
164. Stein Y, Dabash Y, Hollander G, et al. Metabolism of HDL-cholesteryl ester in the rat, studied with a nonhydrolyzable analog, cholesteryl linoleyl ether. *Biochim Biophys Acta* 1983;752:98–105.
165. Granot E, Tabas I, Tall AR. Human plasma cholesteryl ester transfer protein enhances the transfer of cholesteryl ester from high density lipoproteins into cultured HepG2 cells. *J Biol Chem* 1987;262: 3182–3187.
166. Tozuka M, Fidge N. Purification and characterization of two high-density-lipoprotein-binding proteins from rat and human liver. *Biochem J* 1989;261:239–244.
167. Kambouris AM, Roach PD, Calvert GD, et al. Retroendocytosis of high density lipoproteins by the human hepatoma cell line, HepG2. *Arteriosclerosis* 1990;10:582–590.
168. Schouten D, Kleinherenbrink-Stins MF, Brouwer A, et al. Characterization in vitro of interaction of human apolipoprotein E-free high density lipoprotein with human hepatocytes. *Arteriosclerosis* 1990; 10:1127–1135.
169. Mendel CM, Kunitake ST, Kane JP, et al. Radiation inactivation of binding sites for high density lipoproteins in human fibroblast membranes. *J Biol Chem* 1988;263:1314–1319.
170. Kunitake ST, Kane JP. Factors affecting the integrity of high density lipoproteins in the ultracentrifuge. *J Lipid Res* 1982;23:936–940.
171. McVicar JP, Kunitake ST, Hamilton RL, et al. Characteristics of human lipoproproteins isolated by selected-affinity immunosorption of apolipoprotein A-I (high density lipoproteins). *Proc Natl Acad Sci USA* 1984;81:1356–1360.
172. de Silva HV, Stuart WD, Duvic CR, et al. A 70-kDa apolipoprotein designated apoJ is a marker for subclasses of human plasma high density lipoproteins. *J Biol Chem* 1990;265:13240–13247.
173. Kunitake ST, Jarvis M, Hamilton RL, et al. Binding of transition metals by apolipoprotein A-I-containing plasma lipoproteins: Inhibition of oxidation of low density lipoproteins. *Proc Natl Acad Sci USA* 1992;89:6993–6997.
174. Francone OL, Gurakar A, Fielding C. Distribution and function of lecithin: cholesterol acyltransferase and cholesteryl ester transfer protein in plasma lipoproteins. *J Biol Chem* 1989;264:7066–7072.
175. Kunitake ST, Young SG, Chen GC, et al. Conformation of apolipoprotein B-100 in the low density lipoproteins of Tangier disease. *J Biol Chem* 1990;265:20739–20746.
176. Mendel CM, Kunitake ST, Kane JP. Discrimination between subclasses of human high density lipoproteins by the HDL binding sites of bovine liver. *Biochim Biophys Acta* 1986;875:59–68.
177. Duverger N, Ghalim N, Ailhaud G, et al. Characterization of apo A-IV containing lipoprotein particles isolated from human plasma and intestinal fluid. *Arterioscler Thromb* 1993;13:126–132.
178. Wang X, Sato R, Brown MS, Hua X, and Goldstein JL. SREBP-1 a membrane-bound transcription factor released by sterol-regulated proteolysis. *Cell* 1994;77:53–62.

Atherosclerosis and Coronary Artery Disease,
edited by V. Fuster, R. Ross, and E. J. Topol.
Lippincott-Raven Publishers, Philadelphia © 1996.

CHAPTER 7

Plasma High-Density Lipoproteins and Atherogenesis

Alan R. Tall and Jan L. Breslow

Key Words: High density lipoproteins (HDL); Cholesteryl ester transfer protein (CETP); Atherosclerosis; Transgenic mouse; Lipoprotein lipase (LPL); Lecithin: cholesterol acyl transferase (LCAT).

A.R. Tall: Department of Medicine, Columbia University, New York, New York 10032.

J.L. Breslow: Laboratory of Biochemical Genetics and Metabolism, The Rockefeller University, New York, New York 10021.

INTRODUCTION

The high-density lipoproteins (HDL) were first identified as a discrete class of lipoproteins when plasma was analyzed in the analytical ultracentrifuge (1). With the introduction of the preparative ultracentrifuge, it became possible to isolate HDL and to define its composition. The HDL was found to comprise two major subclasses, called HDL_2 and HDL_3. Early research on HDL led to the hypothesis that HDL were formed as a byproduct of the lipolysis of triglyceride-rich lipoproteins and suggested that increased HDL levels might be associated with a lower rate of coronary heart disease (CHD) (2). In the 1960s, Glomset developed the concept that HDL played a central role in the reverse transport of cholesterol from peripheral tissues back to the liver (reverse cholesterol transport) and suggested that reverse cholesterol transport may have an antiatherogenic role (3). These concepts have remained embedded in HDL research, even though the relationship between reverse cholesterol transport and atherogenesis has still not been completely clarified.

The year 1976 saw the first clear documentation of the inverse relationship between HDL levels and the prevalence of CHD in a population-based study of Japanese men living in Hawaii (4). In this decade the general structure of HDL was clarified, the apoproteins of HDL were purified and sequenced, metabolic studies on HDL confirmed the close relationship between HDL and the triglyceride-rich lipoproteins, and cell culture studies began to define mechanisms involved in the removal of cellular cholesterol by HDL (5).

With the introduction of molecular genetics in the 1980s, the cDNAs and genes of the major HDL proteins and processing enzymes were cloned, leading to the discovery of genetic deficiency states of HDL (6). The development of transgenic mouse models of lipoprotein metabolism in the 1990s has helped to unravel some of the complexities of HDL metabolism and has provided clear evidence of a direct and antiatherogenic role of HDL (7,8). On the clinical front, studies such as the Helsinki Heart Study, designed primarily as LDL-lowering interventions, have provided indirect evidence suggesting that pharmacological intervention that raises HDL may have benefits for CHD (9). The National Cholesterol Education Panel has placed increased emphasis on the use of HDL cholesterol levels in assessing risk of CHD and in guiding the type of lipid-lowering therapy to be employed in subjects with hyperlipidemia (10).

HDL COMPOSITION AND STRUCTURE

Plasma HDL are small, dense, spherical lipid–protein complexes consisting of about 50% protein and 50% lipid (5). The major lipids are phosphatidylcholine, cholesterol, cholesteryl ester, and triglyceride. The two main structural apoproteins of HDL are apo A-I (M_r 28,000) and apo A-II (M_r 17,000). In addition, HDL contains small amounts of apo C proteins (apo C-I, apo C-II, and apo C-III), apo E, and apo A-IV and trace quantities of cholesteryl ester transfer protein (CETP), phospholipid transfer protein (PLTP), and lecithin : cholesterol acyl transferase (LCAT). These minor protein components play an important part in the regulation of HDL and lipoprotein metabolism. HDL also contains several components of unknown function, including apo D and apo J (or clusterin), apo SAA (an acute-phase reactant), and PI-glycan-specific phospholipase D.

High-density lipoprotein newly formed by secretion or as a byproduct of lipolysis has a distinctive discoidal structure (11). Discoidal HDL contains phospholipid, cholesterol, and HDL apolipoproteins but lacks neutral lipids. Nascent discoidal HDL are excellent substrates for LCAT, leading to the generation of cholesteryl esters and the conversion of discoidal particles into spherical structures. Thus, nascent discoidal HDL are rapidly converted into mature spherical HDL. Studies of the structure of discoidal particles by negative-stain electron microscopy, X-ray scattering, and scanning calorimetry showed that they consist of phospholipid bilayer disks circumscribed by a peripheral ring of apolipoprotein (12). The main structural protein of HDL, apo A-I, is thought to form an extended series of interconnected amphipathic helical segments arrayed around the edge of the disks like a picket fence (13). The hydrophobic faces of the amphipathic segments are in contact with the hydrocarbon chains of the phospholipid molecules. Neutral lipids generated by LCAT action have limited solubility in the phospholipid bilayer and hence give rise to an oil droplet that splits the bilayer and generates the mature spherical HDL containing a core of neutral lipid and a surface monolayer of phospholipid with the apolipoprotein helices intercalated between the splayed head groups of the phospholipids.

HDL SUBCLASSES

The major subclassification of HDL has been based on the separation of HDL_2 and HDL_3 in the preparative ultracentrifuge, between densities 1.063 to 1.125 and 1.125 to 1.210 g/ml, respectively (5). Whereas HDL_2 contains about 60% lipid and 40% protein, HDL_3 consists of about 45% lipid and 55% protein. The mean diameter of HDL_2 particles is about 10–12 nm, and that of HDL_3 is about 8–9 nm. Much finer subclassification of HDL particles can be achieved by native polyacrylamide gel electrophoresis, which separates particles of different hydrodynamic radius (14). By this technique, the HDL is found to encompass distinct particles from about 10 to 14 nm (called HDL_{2b}-gge) as well as several partially separated peaks between about 10 and 7.6 nm called HDL_{2a}, HDL_{3a}, HDL_{3b}, and HDL_{3c}, in decreasing order of size.

An important and distinctive subclassification of HDL is based on immunochemical differences between HDL particles. The primary classification is based on differences in content of apo A-I and apo A-II (15–18). HDL consists of particles containing apo A-I (LpA-I) or apo A-I and apo A-II (LpA-I/A-II). There may also be a small number of particles containing apo A-II only (LpA-II), but these probably constitute less than 10% of the total mass of HDL. Although centrifugally isolated HDL-2 is somewhat enriched in LpA-I compared to LpA-I/A-II, there is no exact correspondence between the subclassification based on size and density and that based on apoprotein composition. When analyzed by native polyacrylamide gradient gel electrophoresis, LpA-I is found to contain particles of both large and small size, as does LpA-I/A-II. There is increasing evidence that LpA-I and LpA-I/A-II have somewhat distinctive metabolic properties as well as possible differences in their relationship to atherogenesis (see below).

Another mode of classifying lipoproteins and HDL is according to their electrophoretic mobility in agarose gels. Although HDL was originally defined as an α migrating particle, a significant subfraction of apo A-I is found in particles with pre-β (or α_2) mobility (19,20). The pre-β migrating HDL fraction appears to be labile and may be formed during incubation of plasma. The pre-β HDL can represent anywhere from a few percent up to 10% or more of the total HDL. LCAT activity converts pre-β into α HDL, whereas CETP activity converts α into pre-β HDL (21). Pre-β HDL appears to have distinctive structural and metabolic properties and may have particular importance in mediating cellular cholesterol efflux (19,20). Both free apo A-I and discoidal particles have pre-β mobility (19), but it is uncertain to what extent the pre-β fraction of plasma HDL represents discoidal particles or free apo A-I.

HDL APOPROTEINS AND PROCESSING ENZYMES: GENES, STRUCTURES, AND FUNCTIONS

Structure and Function of Apo A-I

The apo A-I gene is located on the long arm of chromosome 11 in region q23 in a cluster with the apo C-III and apo A-IV genes (22–25). The gene order is apo A-I, apo C-III, apo A-IV, with the apo C-III gene in the opposite orientation to the other two genes. The apo A-I gene is 1,863 bp in length and comprises four exons and three introns. Mature apo A-I is 243 amino acids in length and consists largely of eight 22-amino-acid-long amphipathic α helices separated by helix-breaking proline residues (26–30). The hydrophobic face of the helix is thought to bind to neutral lipids and hydrocarbon regions of phospholipids. The polar face may interact with the zwitterionic polar head groups of the phospholipids and with water. The apo A-I molecule has a low free energy of stabilization in water but becomes more stable and develops increased helical content on interaction with lipids (12,31).

The human apo A-I gene is transcribed largely in the human liver and intestine (32). The *cis*-acting DNA elements required for liver expression reside 5′ to the gene within the proximal 256 bp (33). The apo A-I promoter binds a complex array of transcription factors, including positive regulators such as HNF4 and retinoic acid receptors RXR-α and RAR-α, and negative regulators including Arp-I, Ear-2, and Ear-3, which belong to the steroid hormone receptor superfamily (34–38). These findings may explain apo A-I gene regulation during development or in response to retinoids. There are one or more distinct *cis*-acting DNA elements required for intestinal expression that are distinct from the liver elements (39). The region encompassing these elements lies 3′ to the apo A-I gene in the intergenic region between the apo C-III and apo A-IV genes. This region may control the intestinal expression of the entire apo A-I, apo C-III, apo A-IV gene locus (40). A detailed understanding of the transcriptional control of the apo A-I gene may lead to therapies that increase apo A-I production and HDL cholesterol levels. However, many of the factors that regulate apo A-I production rates, such as a high-fat diet or probucol therapy, do not influence the level of apo A-I mRNA, indicating important regulation of apo A-I production on a posttranscriptional level (see below).

In addition to its role as the major structural protein of HDL, apo A-I can activate LCAT. However, this property is shared by apo A-IV, other apolipoproteins, and synthetic peptides containing amphipathic helices, indicating that the activation is unlikely to reflect highly specific protein–protein interactions. Different apo A-I monoclonal antibodies (mAbs) have been identified that either inhibit or stimulate the activation of LCAT by apo A-I. Overall, the data suggest that apo A-I may help to organize the lipid substrates for optimal presentation to LCAT. Some regions of apo A-I, possibly because of secondary structural features, appear to be more important than other regions.

Structure and Function of Apo A-II

Apolipoprotein A-II is the second most abundant HDL structural protein. The apo A-II gene is found on the long arm of chromosome 1 (q21–q23) (41). The mature apo A-II polypeptide chain contains 77 amino acids (42–44). However, human apo A-II contains a single cysteine at residue 6 and exists in plasma primarily as a homodimer. Like apo A-I, apo A-II contains regions of amphipathic α helices, but many fewer of them (45). Apo A-II can displace apo A-I from HDL particles (46). Some species such as the dog do not have apo A-II in their HDL (46). Although the metabolic functions of apo A-II are poorly understood, recent studies in transgenic mice suggest that apo A-II may inhibit the remodeling of HDL particles by hepatic lipase (see below). This property could help to preserve a minimum amount of LpA-I/A-II in plasma.

HDL Processing Enzymes: LCAT

The human LCAT gene is found on chromosome 16q22 (47) and encompasses six exons (48). The major site of LCAT mRNA expression is the liver (48); in the rat there is also some expression of LCAT mRNA in brain and testis (49). The mature LCAT enzyme contains 416 amino acids and has a M_r approximately 63,000 (50). The LCAT enzyme is responsible for almost all of the cholesteryl ester found in human plasma (3).

Lipid Transfer Proteins: CETP and PLTP

The CETP gene encompasses 16 exons and is found on chromosome 16q12–16q21 near the LCAT locus (52). The CETP gene belongs to an ancient gene family that includes lipopolysaccharide binding proteins (such as the plasma lipopolysaccharide binding protein) and the plasma phospholipid transfer protein (PLTP) (53–56). The CETP cDNA encodes a 476-amino-acid polypeptide that is N-glycosylated at four sites, giving rise to the mature form of plasma CETP of M_r approximately 70,000 (57,58). The CETP mRNA is expressed in the liver and small intestine and a variety of peripheral organs, with prominent expression in spleen (51) and adipose tissue (59). Hepatic and peripheral CETP mRNA are increased in response to a high-cholesterol diet, leading to increased plasma CETP levels (59,60). Hepatic CETP mRNA is down-regulated in response to corticosteroids or bacterial lipopolysaccharides (61).

The PLTP cDNA encodes a mature protein of 476 amino acids and M_r approximately 78,000 (56). The PLTP cDNA was cloned from an endothelial cell library, and the major sites of expression of the PLTP mRNA are the placenta, lung, liver, and pancreas. The PLTP gene is found on chromosome 20, where the LBP and BPI genes are also found. The exon/intron structures of the CETP and PLTP genes appear to be similar (unpublished data).

The plasma CETP mediates all neutral lipid transfer events in human plasma, including the transfer of cholesteryl esters from HDL and LDL to VLDL and the reciprocal transfer of triglycerides in the opposite direction (62,63). The CETP also mediates phospholipid exchange between lipoproteins. By contrast, the PLTP mediates net transfer of phospholipids between lipoproteins (64) as well as HDL size changes (''conversion'' events) (65). By contrast, CETP has no ability to mediate net phospholipid transfer into HDL (64). These distinctive biochemical properties suggest that although CETP may be able to alter the molecular species of phospholipid in HDL, PLTP mediates net phospholipid movements between HDL and other lipoproteins or even between HDL and certain cells.

HDL–CELL INTERACTIONS

Cholesterol Efflux Studies

High-density lipoprotein plays a central role in the removal of cholesterol from cells. In early studies Werb and Cohn (66) loaded mouse peritoneal macrophages with cholesterol and studied its efflux. Macrophages promptly excreted cholesterol as long as serum was present in the culture medium. Ho et al. (67) loaded macrophages with cholesteryl esters by incubation with acetyl-LDL and showed that hydrolysis and excretion of stored cholesteryl esters were stimulated by the presence of cholesterol acceptors in the culture medium. Several agents were found to be effective as cholesterol acceptors, including HDL, whole serum, the $d > 1.21$ g/ml fraction, intact erythrocytes, casein, and thyroglobulin. In contrast, LDL and some other factors were found to be ineffective. HDL was thought to stimulate the net hydrolysis of cholesteryl esters by removing unesterified cholesterol from cells and thus interrupting the cholesteryl ester cycle within macrophages, i.e., the continuous cycle of cholesterol esterification by cellular ACAT followed by hydrolysis of cholesteryl esters by cholesteryl ester hydrolase. These studies provided a potential mechanism by which HDL may reverse atheroma foam cell formation, thereby limiting formation or promoting regression of atheromata.

Many studies have demonstrated a central role of plasma cholesterol esterification in the stimulation of net cellular cholesterol efflux. Using cultured rat hepatoma cells, Rothblat's group (68) showed that the reduction in cellular cholesterol content mediated by fresh serum was correlated with the extent of serum lipoprotein modification by LCAT. Unmodified serum in which LCAT had been inactivated depressed cellular cholesterol synthesis and increased cellular cholesterol content. LCAT was shown to decrease the influx of cholesterol into cells, thereby decreasing net cellular cholesterol efflux. Some studies have also suggested that the LCAT reaction on nascent HDL particles may be stimulated by CETP-mediated cholesteryl ester transfer from HDL to other lipoproteins (69). However, direct inhibition of CETP by mAbs in human plasma does not modify the rate of the LCAT reaction, and plasma from subjects with a genetic deficiency of CETP shows a normal rate of plasma cholesterol esterification (63,70,71). Thus, in whole plasma there does not appear to be tight biochemical linkage between LCAT and CETP activities. Nonetheless, it remains plausible that CETP stimulates LCAT action on nascent HDL in vivo, thereby promoting reverse cholesterol transport.

Several studies have attempted to define subclasses of HDL that act as preferred acceptors of cellular cholesterol in plasma (20,72). Serum pre-β HDL has been identified as an important early acceptor of cellular cholesterol (20). Purified apo A-I can also mediate cellular cholesterol efflux from macrophages but not smooth muscle cells, most likely by forming pre-β HDL-like particles (73). Other studies have attempted to determine if there is HDL apoprotein specificity by studying cellular cholesterol efflux using immunochemically defined HDL subclasses. Although some authors have reported that LpA-I is more effective at stimulating cellular cholesterol efflux than LpA-I/A-II, others have obtained different results using different conditions (74). Some of the important variables that may influence the outcome of such experiments include the use of different cell types and also the activity of LCAT in the lipoprotein preparations employed. Because LpA-I normally contains the bulk of plasma LCAT activity, LpA-I may be more active in stimulating net cholesterol efflux if LCAT is active in the preparation. Also, the mechanisms of cholesterol efflux may be different in various cell types, dependent on the different domains of lipid in the cells (see below). Studies with reconstituted discoidal HDL particles have indicated that particles reconstituted with apo A-I are the most effective stimulators of cellular cholesterol efflux (75). It is worth noting that there is a major conceptual hiatus between the detailed studies of cholesterol efflux by HDL subfractions in cell culture and epidemiologic investigations of HDL, where the vast majority of studies have relied on total HDL cholesterol measurements, and the evidence that a specific subfraction of HDL is antiatherogenic is weak (see below).

The molecular mechanisms by which HDL mediates cholesterol efflux have been the subject of intensive investigation, as recently reviewed by Rothblat et al. (74). Three general models for cholesterol efflux have been proposed: (a) HDL receptor-mediated cholesterol translocation and efflux (75,76), (b) acceptor retroendocytosis (77), and (c) passive diffusion of free cholesterol through the aqueous phase between the plasma membrane and acceptor particles (78,79), called aqueous diffusion. Although HDL binding proteins have been described (80), there is substantial evidence that efflux of plasma membrane cholesterol does not require binding of HDL to specific receptors (81), and the results from studies of the intracellular movement and efflux of the lysosomal pool of cholesterol are thought not to be consistent with a triggering of intracellular cholesterol transport by binding of HDL to a receptor (82). Retroendocytosis of HDL has been demonstrated in macrophages by electron microscopy, and a defect in this process has been proposed in Tangier disease (77). However, the quantitative importance of retroendocytosis and its role in Tangier disease remain uncertain.

The aqueous diffusion model of cholesterol efflux has obtained substantial experimental support. As predicted by this model, the efficiency of a particle in stimulating cholesterol efflux depends in large part on physical parameters such a size and surface area (74). However, a number of experimental results indicate a difference in acceptor efficiency that cannot be attributed solely to the physical properties of the acceptors (74). For example, the apolipoprotein content of acceptor particles influences the rate of efflux from macrophages: particles reconstituted with apo A-I show more rapid efflux than those reconstituted with apo A-II or apo Cs. However, this difference was not observed with some other cell types, suggesting that additional factors such as apolipoprotein structure and plasma membrane organization might be involved in cellular cholesterol efflux.

These considerations have led Rothblat, Phillips, and coworkers (74) to propose a model in which heterogeneous domains of cholesterol within the plasma membrane interact differently with HDL (Fig. 1). These workers propose that cholesterol efflux from cholesterol-rich membrane regions involves the aqueous diffusion mechanism. By contrast, cholesterol efflux from cholesterol-poor membrane regions is mediated by the insertion of segments of apolipoprotein into the phospholipid membrane, stimulating cholesterol movement into HDL. This model is appealing and has the ability to describe many experimental observations. Kinetic studies of cholesterol efflux from cellular membranes indicate the existence of several different exponential components, consistent with the existence of specific domains of cholesterol. HDL particles are dynamic structures on which the apolipoproteins can undergo conformational changes (83,84). One of the most dramatic examples of this apoprotein plasticity is the postulated ''hinged domain'' of apo A-I. It has been proposed that this domain is comprised of at least one pair of helical segments located in the region of residue 100 of

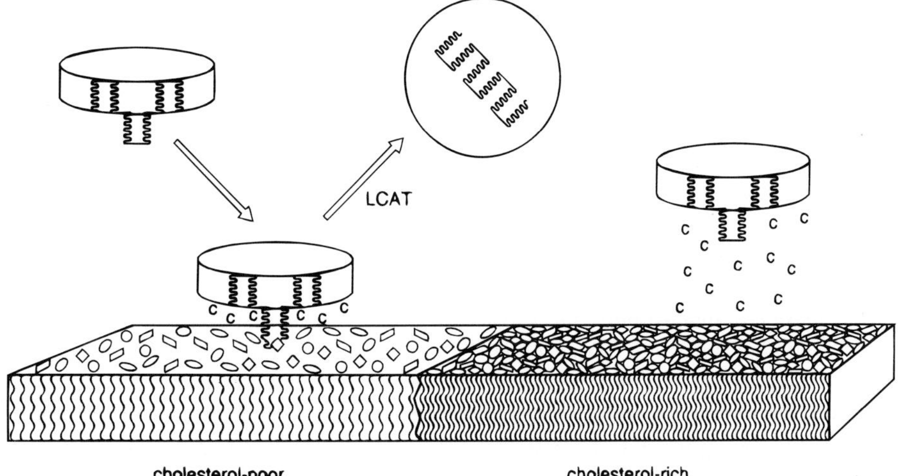

FIG. 1. Model for the efflux of cholesterol from cholesterol-poor and cholesterol-rich plasma membrane domains and the interaction with acceptors containing apo A-I. Hinged region of apo A-I on HDL disk interacts with cholesterol-poor domain of the plasma membrane. Cholesterol molecules (C) move from membrane to the acceptor. Through the action of LCAT, the disk is converted to a spherical HDL. The apoA-I does not interact with the cholesterol-rich domain because of the increased lateral packing density, and thus flux from this domain occurs through a large unstirred water layer. From ref. 74, with permission.

apo A-I (83,84). Depending on the packing of the apolipoprotein on the surface of the particle, this segment would be either associated with the lipid in HDL or released from the surface and extending into the aqueous phase surrounding the particle (83,84).

As noted above, in nascent discoidal HDL, the apoprotein forms an annulus around the edge of the disk (12). In large disks with a high phospholipid/protein ratio, all of the apoprotein amphipathic helices are thought to be in contact with the disk edge. In smaller discoidal particles, the hinged region of apo A-I may be in an open configuration, i.e., removed from contact with disk lipids. It could be this extended hinge region that would interact with specific lipid domains in the plasma membrane (74). It would be easier for such an apoprotein segment to insert itself into a cholesterol-poor region of membrane, because the lateral packing pressure in such regions is reduced, and it is known that cholesterol-rich membranes resist penetration by apo A-I. This type of lipoprotein–membrane interaction would be considerably less stringent than classical ligand–receptor interaction and would be consistent with the nonspecific nature of HDL binding to cells, as suggested by Tabas and Tall (85). This model may also be consistent with the observation that small pre-β HDL particles are the initial cholesterol acceptors in plasma (20).

Recent experiments using apo A-I monoclonal antibodies have provided strong support for the concept of a flexible domain of apo A-I involved in cellular cholesterol efflux (86). Two specific apo A-I mAbs inhibited cholesterol efflux from macrophages to HDL by about 50%, but six other apo A-I mAbs had no effect. These inhibitory antibodies recognize epitopes localized to residues 74 to 105 and 96 to 111, i.e., the region previously proposed to contain the flexible hinge region of apo A-I (83,84).

Subsequent to cholesterol uptake by discoidal HDL particles, these particles are acted on by LCAT, which converts discoidal to spherical particles. The CETP may be accommodated into discoidal HDL particles without displacement of apo A-I (C. Bruce, A. Tall, and M. Phillips, unpublished data). By analogy, LCAT may also bind to HDL by a similar accommodation. The accommodation process may also involve flexible segments in the apo A-I structure that make room for the CETP or LCAT molecules at the edge of discoidal particles or between the splayed phospholipid head groups of spherical HDL particles. Interestingly, the same apo A-I mAbs that inhibit cellular cholesterol efflux either stimulate or inhibit LCAT activity on discoidal particles, suggesting that the antibodies may be fixing the apo A-I in conformations either favorable or unfavorable for the accommodation of LCAT (86).

We propose the hypothesis that the different functions of a common flexible region of apo A-I (i.e., binding to cells or accommodation of CETP/LCAT) could be mutually exclusive. For example, small discoidal particles with a displaced flexible segment of apo A-I may be optimized for interaction with cells but may not be able to bind LCAT or CETP. Subsequent to cellular interaction, these particles may become enlarged as a result of the addition of extra phospholipids and cholesterol, leading to the apposition of flexible apo A-I segments to lipid. These flexible segments would then be available for accommodation of moderately surface-active molecules such as LCAT or CETP. In this way, small discoidal HDL may be optimized for cellular cholesterol efflux while larger particles are more readily available for cholesteryl ester formation and transfer.

Prostanoid Release and Signal Transduction

High-density lipoproteins can induce the secretion of cellular prostanoids (87,88). Thus, HDL stimulated the release of prostacyclin from endothelial cells and prostaglandin E_2 from smooth muscle cells. Part of the mechanism involves the transfer of arachidonate moieties contained in HDL phospholipids or cholesteryl esters into the cell. LDL can also provide a source of arachidonate for cellular prostanoid synthesis (89). This process is more active in PDGF-treated cells with up-regulated LDL receptors that are actively metabolizing LDL (89). Because most cells have down-regulated LDL receptors in vivo, the delivery of phospholipids and cholesteryl esters to cells by HDL may be more important. HDL can deliver lipids to cells by multiple mechanisms including exchange of phospholipids, selective uptake of cholesteryl esters, or uptake by the LDL receptor of HDL-containing multiple copies of apo E (90). In addition to stimulating the release of cellular prostanoids, HDL may also bind and stabilize prostacyclin (91). Prostacyclin has vasodilatory and platelet antiaggregatory properties. The release of prostanoids by HDL may contribute to the hydrolysis of stored cholesteryl esters in smooth muscle cells (91), because prostacyclin increases cholesteryl ester hydrolase activity (92). Although speculative, these studies suggest a novel mechanism involving prostacyclin release, by which HDL may protect against myocardial infarction, a process usually involving formation of a thrombus on a preexisting atherosclerotic plaque.

There is some limited evidence that HDL can mediate cellular signal transduction (93–96). In addition to delivering lipids to cells, this mechanism could be involved in the stimulation of cellular prostanoid release. It presently seems unlikely that HDL mediates cellular signal transduction events by interaction with specific receptors. However, changes in membrane lipid domains, resulting from the interaction of amphipathic helices of apoproteins with the plasma membrane, could influence the activity of cell membrane-associated phospholipases, leading to the generation of lipid second messengers and signal transduction events (74). Such events could be responsible for a variety of cellular responses that have been reported to be triggered by HDL (93–96). An interesting recent example of such responses involves the interaction of HDL with alveolar type II cells (97). These cells store phospholipid (primarily dipalmitoyl phosphatidylcholine) as intracellular membranous whorls called lamellar bodies, which is a source of lipid components of lung surfactant. Inositol phospholipid catabolism, calcium mobilization, and protein kinase C activity are linked to surfactant secretion in cultured type II pneumocytes (97). Phosphatidylcholine/apo A-I or phosphatidylcholine/apo E complexes stimulated signal transduction by these pathways as well as phospholipid secretion when incubated with type II pneumocytes. Whether these HDL-mediated events are interdependent is presently unknown. The in vivo relevance of HDL stimulation of prostanoid secretion or HDL signal transduction events is also unknown.

HDL LEVELS IN HUMAN POPULATIONS

The distribution of HDL cholesterol levels in the population was determined in the Lipid Research Clinic Prevalence Study (98). For men aged 45 to 49 years, the average HDL cholesterol level is 45 mg/dl, with the bottom decile below 33 mg/dl and the top decile above 60 mg/dl. For women the average is 56 mg/dl, the bottom decile is below 39 mg/dl, and the top decile above 78 mg/dl. Among white Americans, mean HDL cholesterol levels are similar in boys and girls before puberty (about 58 mg/dl) but diverge at puberty, when HDL levels fall by about 10 to 15 mg/dl in boys and remain at these lower levels throughout adult life (99,100). These differences are probably related to the rise in testosterone levels in boys. The absence of similar changes associated with a rise or fall in estrogen levels at menarche or menopause in women suggests that physiological estrogen levels may not be a major contributor to the differences in HDL cholesterol between the sexes. By contrast, postmenopausal estrogen replacement, which exposes the liver to supraphysiological levels, can result in increases of 10 to 20 mg/dl in HDL cholesterol. Black Americans, especially black men, have higher levels of HDL cholesterol than whites, and the difference in levels between black men and black women is less than for whites (101).

Analysis of HDL subclasses indicates that HDL_3 levels are fairly constant in different individuals (13). In subjects with higher HDL levels much of the increment in HDL occurs in larger subspecies of HDL (HDL_2). There is a general inverse relationship between plasma triglyceride and HDL cholesterol levels (102). Thus, hypertriglyceridemic subjects typically have lower levels of HDL cholesterol. There is also an inverse relationship between plasma triglyceride and apo A-I levels, but this relationship is not as strong as that between triglycerides and HDL cholesterol (102), possibly because the proximate cause of low HDL cholesterol in many hypertriglyceridemic subjects is accelerated transfer of cholesteryl esters from HDL to triglyceride-rich lipoproteins (103).

Plasma levels of LpA-I/A-II are generally higher and more stable than levels of LpA-I (104). Much of the difference in HDL levels between men and women appears to result from lower levels of LpA-I in men (105). In subjects with low HDL, both LpA-I and LpA-I/AII may be decreased, but changes in LpA-I appear to be larger (106). Although it appears that hypertriglyceridemic subjects have increased amounts of pre-β HDL particles (21), there is a paucity of information on pre-β HDL in population studies.

HDL METABOLISM

Secretion and Remodeling

The major apoprotein of HDL, apo A-I, is synthesized in approximately equal proportions by the liver and small intestine (5,90). By contrast, the second most abundant apoprotein of HDL, apo A-II, is made exclusively in the liver. A major portion of the apolipoprotein and phospholipid destined to become HDL is initially secreted on large, triglyceride-transporting VLDL (derived from the liver) or chylomicrons (derived from the small intestine). During lipolysis of chylomicrons and VLDL, surface lipids (phospholipid and cholesterol) and proteins (apo A-I, apo A-II, and apo Cs) are transferred into the HDL fraction. These components may form nascent discoidal HDL particles, which are rapidly acted on by LCAT to generate mature spherical HDL, or they may be incorporated into preexisting HDL particles. The latter process results in an increase in size and decrease in density of HDL particles, leading to conversion of preexisting HDL_3 into HDL_2. High-density lipoprotein can also probably be formed as a direct result of cellular secretion. Secretory nascent HDL appear as spherical particles containing neutral lipid or as apolipoprotein/phospholipid bilayer disks and can be visualized in liver perfusates or in mesenteric lymph derived from the small intestine. Spherical HDL may be seen in the secretory organelles of hepatocytes or enterocytes, suggesting intracellular assembly. However, discoidal HDL have not been identified within cells and thus are probably formed extracellularly, either by lipolysis of newly secreted triglyceride-rich lipoproteins or as a result of the interaction of newly secreted apoproteins with cellular plasma membranes.

The lipolysis of chylomicrons and VLDL by lipoprotein lipase (primarily in adipose tissue, heart, and skeletal muscle) results in a net transfer of phospholipid into HDL (Fig. 2). Free cholesterol diffuses into HDL from other lipoproteins, erythrocytes, and endothelial cells. The HDL-associated enzyme LCAT uses phospholipid and cholesterol, generating cholesteryl esters (CE) and lysophospholipid and driving the influx of additional phospholipid and cholesterol into HDL. Plasma lipid transfer proteins play an important part in the transfer of phospholipids and neutral lipids between HDL and other plasma lipoproteins. The net movement of phospholipids between HDL and other lipoproteins is thought to be facilitated by the PLTP. Phospholipid exchange, mediated by both CETP and PLTP, might be important in replenishing HDL with unsaturated phospholipids optimal for the LCAT reaction. In humans, a major part of the

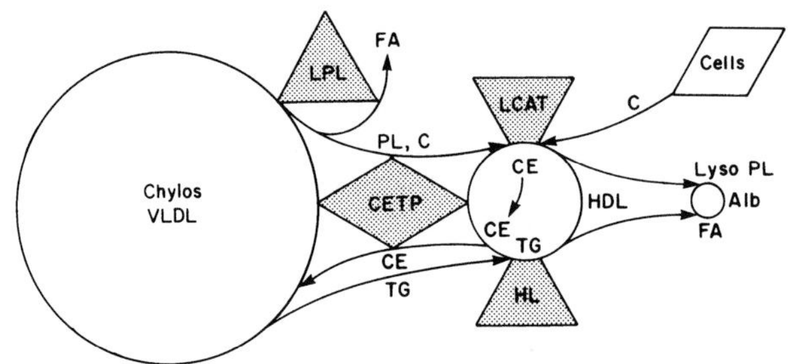

FIG. 2. Enzymatic modification of HDL. The lipolysis of chylomicrons and VLDL by LPL in tissues (adipose, muscle) results in uptake of fatty acids (FA) by the tissues and transfer of PL and C into HDL. Plasma LCAT uses PL and C as substrates, forming CE. The plasma CETP facilitates the transfer of PL, CE, and TG as shown. HL hydrolyzes HDL, PL, and TG in the liver. Lysophospholipids ($_{\text{Lyso}}$Pl) and FA formed by LCAT, and HL may be bound to albumin (alb). From ref. 11, with permission.

CE formed within HDL is transferred into larger triglyceride-rich lipoproteins as a result of CETP activity. The CETP mediates the heteroexchange of HDL CE with triglycerides (TG) of VLDL or chylomicrons, resulting in cholesteryl ester depletion and triglyceride enrichment of HDL.

The combined effects of lipolysis and lipid transfer result in the formation of HDL particles that are enlarged and enriched with additional apoproteins and lipids (5,90). These HDL_2 particles then undergo remodeling by hepatic lipase, an enzyme found primarily on the endothelial cells of the liver sinusoids. Hepatic lipase has both triglyceride hydrolase and phospholipase activity, resulting in a depletion of HDL triglycerides and phospholipids and a decrease in HDL size. Hepatic lipase activity is probably also accompanied by a loss of apoproteins from HDL, resulting in catabolism of apo A-I in the liver and kidney. Overall, there is a cycle of enlargement of HDL from influx of lipids, apoproteins, and LCAT activity, followed by CE–TG exchange and then shrinkage of HDL and loss of lipid and protein components subsequent to hepatic lipase activity. Normally the enlargement and shrinkage processes are balanced so that HDL composition and size remain fairly stable in an individual. The balance of the cycle may be shifted so that larger HDL may be formed during alimentary lipemia, and smaller HDL during fasting. Differences in the activity of lipases and of lipid transfer processes appear to underlie many of the differences in HDL levels between different individuals, and these processes appear to be influenced by environmental and genetic factors influencing HDL levels.

Metabolism of HDL Cholesterol and Cholesteryl Ester

In mammalian species the major portion of body cholesterol synthesis occurs in peripheral tissues (107). The movement of cholesterol from the periphery to the liver via the plasma compartment is called reverse cholesterol transport. The initial step in reverse cholesterol transport involves the transfer of cholesterol from cellular plasma membranes into HDL; this process is described in detail above. The HDL-associated LCAT converts cholesterol to cholesteryl ester and thereby provides a driving force for the net movement of cholesterol into HDL.

The metabolism of HDL lipids is a dynamic process, and normally the CE of HDL is turned over 10–40 times more rapidly than apo A-I or apo A-II (5,90). The CE formed in HDL as a result of LCAT activity can undergo three fates. First, it can be transferred to VLDL or chylomicrons by cholesteryl ester transfer protein (CETP); second, it can be transferred into cells in a variety of tissues in a process of selective CE uptake; and third, it can be catabolized with HDL particles. The relative importance of these three different pathways varies in different species, depending on whether CETP activity is present in plasma. In humans, the CETP pathway is of major importance in HDL CE catabolism, as illustrated by the marked increase in HDL CE in genetic CETP deficiency (108). The selective uptake process has been demonstrated in rats and rabbits, using radiolabeled cholesteryl ethers to trace the tissue uptake of HDL CE (109,110), but the mechanisms and significance of selective uptake are not well understood. Catabolism of HDL particles may be mediated by uptake of large, apo-E-enriched HDL by LDL receptors in the liver or elsewhere. This pathway is particularly important in species with low plasma CETP activity but probably does not normally play a major role in HDL catabolism in humans, except in individuals with low CETP activity from genetic or other causes. Although cellular HDL binding proteins have been described (111), their importance in the metabolism or overall regulation of HDL levels is poorly understood.

In addition to reverse cholesterol transport involving HDL CE, there appears to be a net flux of unesterified cholesterol from HDL into the liver. Attempts to model the metabolism of plasma cholesterol suggest that there is a net transfer of cholesterol from tissues to liver via HDL, of similar magnitude to the net transfer of CE through VLDL + LDL to liver (112). Following injection of HDL-containing radiolabeled cholesterol in humans, there is a rapid appearance of cholesterol radioactivity in bile, suggesting mechanisms for its rapid uptake and transfer into bile (112). Although not well understood, one plausible mechanism whereby HDL cholesterol may be taken up by liver cells involves hepatic lipase. Hydrolysis of HDL phospholipids by hepatic lipase may drive the uptake of HDL cholesterol in the liver (113). Also, there are HDL binding proteins in the liver (111), but a functional role for these proteins has not been proven.

Catabolism of HDL Proteins

The catabolic half-lives of apo A-I and apo A-II in normal humans is about 4–5 days (5,114). Careful studies of HDL catabolism in humans have revealed that the residence time of apo A-I is slightly less than that of apo A-II (115). This may reflect the more rapid catabolism of LpA-I compared to LpA-I/A-II. Thus, mean residence time of apo A-I injected with LpA-I is shorter than that of apo A-I injected with LpA-I/A-II (115). Studies in animals suggest that the major catabolic sites of apo A-I are the liver and the kidney (5).

METABOLIC REGULATION OF HDL

Much of the information describing the normal regulation of HDL levels in humans has been obtained from metabolic turnover studies (114–116). Alterations of HDL cholesterol and protein concentrations may be associated with changes in synthesis or catabolism of HDL proteins. The less common mode of regulation appears to be variation in the synthesis of apo A-I or apo A-II. Examples of this mode of regulation include diets highly enriched in polyunsaturated fatty acids, which cause decreases in HDL cholesterol and apo A-I as a result of decreased transport rate of apo A-I without any changes in fractional catabolism. A low-fat diet decreases HDL cholesterol levels by decreasing HDL apolipoprotein transport rate (116). The increase in HDL caused by estrogen therapy may be caused by increased synthesis of apo A-I (118,119). Species differences in HDL levels in monkeys may be related to differences in apo A-I synthesis and secretion rates (90). A family with hyperalphalipoproteinemia from increased apo A-I production has been described (120).

Variations in HDL cholesterol, apo A-I, and apo A-II between individuals are more generally correlated with differences in the fractional catabolic rate (FCR) of these apolipoproteins and not with variations in synthetic rate (116). Thus, factors that affect the catabolism of apo A-I (or HDL cholesterol) may be important regulators of HDL levels. Breslow and colleagues (116) have carried out metabolic turnover studies on a large number of subjects with a wide range of HDL cholesterol values (20 to 120 mg/dl). These studies confirmed a strong correlation of HDL cholesterol and apo A-I levels and a lack of correlation of HDL cholesterol and apo A-II levels. There was a strong inverse correlation between HDL cholesterol levels and the FCRs of apo A-I and apo A-II ($r = -0.81$ and -0.76, respectively). In contrast, there was little or no association between HDL cholesterol levels and the transport rates of apo A-I and apo A-II ($r = 0.06$ and -0.35, respectively). Women showed lower FCR for apo A-I than men. Subjects with hypoalphalipoproteinemia (low HDL cholesterol) also have increased FCR for apo A-I and apo A-II compared to subjects with normal HDL cholesterol values. This is true in both normo- and hypertriglyceridemic subjects with reduced HDL levels.

Thus, a variety of observations indicate that factors influencing the catabolism of apo A-I and apo A-II are important in the modulation of HDL levels in humans. Because HDL cholesterol and apo A-I levels are highly correlated, it is impossible to discern from turnover data whether changes in apo A-I catabolism cause changes in HDL cholesterol or vice versa. However, a number of considerations suggest that catabolism of apo A-I may be regulated indirectly, at least in part by factors than affect the turnover of HDL cholesterol. Reduced HDL cholesterol and apo A-I levels are commonly associated with hypertriglyceridemia in humans. Hypertriglyceridemia from a variety of causes results in accelerated transfer of CE from HDL to triglyceride-rich lipoproteins, as demonstrated in the majority of in vitro studies of incubated plasma (121). The accelerated CE transfer is associated with a reciprocal transfer of triglyceride, resulting in enrichment of HDL with triglyceride. The more triglyceride-enriched the HDL particles, the more susceptible they are to reductions in size and apoprotein content as a result of lipoprotein or hepatic lipase action (5,90,116,121). Thus, Goldberg et al. (122) have shown that acute hypertriglyceridemia, resulting from antibody inhibition of LPL, produces a marked decrease in HDL CE with a secondary acceleration of apo A-I catabolism. It is likely that hypertriglyceridemia causes increased CETP-mediated exchange of HDL CE with triglyceride, followed by lipolysis (by hepatic lipase) of the triglyceride-enriched HDL. Factors that decrease the size of HDL, or the ratio of HDL CE/apo A-I plus apo A-II in HDL, appear to promote the removal of apoproteins from HDL, leading to their catabolism (116). The data from the turnover studies are consistent with these proposed mechanisms. Thus, two estimates of HDL size or density, the HDL cholesterol/apo A-I + apo A-II ratio and the percentage of the apo

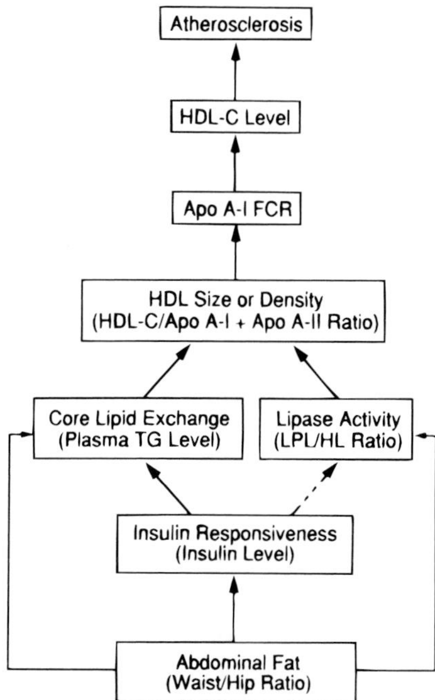

FIG. 3. Hypothetical schema of the factors influencing the metabolism and levels of high-density lipoprotein (HDL), expanded from Heikki Frick et al. (9) to show the proposed interaction of the additional parameters reported in this study. HDL-C, HDL cholesterol; Apo, apolipoprotein; FCR, fractional catabolic rate; TG, triglyceride; LPL, lipoprotein lipase; HL, hepatic lipase. From ref. 116, with permission.

A-I tracer found in the $d > 1.21$ g/ml fraction were correlated strongly with apo A-I FCR ($r = -0.81$ and 0.62, respectively). Investigations of HDL metabolism in human genetic CETP deficiency provide direct evidence that the catabolism of apo A-I and apo A-II can be delayed by a defect in CE transfer (123).

Thus, it appears that processes regulating the rate of transfer of CE from HDL to other lipoproteins may play a critical role in determining the size of the HDL CE pool, the size of HDL particles, and the catabolic rates of apo A-I and apo A-II (Fig. 3). The CE transfer process is mediated by CETP, but the transfer rate is ordinarily influenced primarily by the concentrations of acceptor lipoproteins (VLDL and chylomicrons). Another important factor determining the size of the HDL core lipid pool may be the activity of hepatic lipase. Thus, major correlates of HDL cholesterol/apo A-I + apo A-II were fasting triglyceride levels and the ratio of LPL/HL activities, which together predicted 70% of the variability (116). Waist-to-hip ratio and fasting insulin in turn predicted 46% of the variability in the ratio of LPL/HL. Based on these correlations, it was hypothesized that abdominal fat, insulin sensitivity, lipase activity, and triglyceride levels regulate HDL size, which in turn regulates HDL cholesterol and apo A-I levels (Fig. 3). Thus, genetic or environmental factors that influence obesity, insulin sensitivity, and lipase activities regulate HDL cholesterol levels.

GENETIC REGULATION OF HDL CHOLESTEROL LEVELS

Although environmental and hormonal influences account for a significant fraction of the variance of HDL cholesterol levels in the population, there is evidence from family studies that genetic factors are also important. For example, twin studies have indicated a high degree of heritability of HDL cholesterol levels. These studies have shown a much higher correlation between HDL cholesterol levels of monozygotic than dizygotic twin pairs. In three different studies the correlation of HDL cholesterol levels in monozygotic twins ranged from 0.68 to 0.74, whereas in dizygotic twins the correlation was only 0.34–0.46 (124–126). These studies are highly suggestive of genetic influences on HDL cholesterol levels, although it is also possible that monozygotic twins share a more similar environment than dizygotic twins. Other studies of familial aggregation of HDL cholesterol values, using path analysis, have estimated the heritability of HDL cholesterol values at 0.55, divided between genetic, 0.36, and cultural, 0.19, components (124). Taken together, these studies suggest a large genetic component in the determination of HDL cholesterol levels.

An assessment of major genetic locus effects on HDL cholesterol levels can be derived by complex segregation analysis (127–134). This approach has revealed no major gene for high HDL cholesterol levels and relatively uncommon recessive genes for low HDL cholesterol levels varying in allele frequencies from 0.028 to 0.116. Thus, homozygosity for the minor allele required to influence phenotype would exist in 1% or less of individuals. This would not explain a significant fraction of the phenotypic variation in HDL cholesterol levels in the population. However, complex segregation analysis consistently indicates significant polygenic inheritance of HDL cholesterol levels, accounting for 40% to 60% of the phenotypic variance. Thus, HDL cholesterol levels are highly heritable. The polygenic component in complex segregation analysis is defined as being linked to an infinitely large number of genetic factors. However, this analysis only distinguishes a single major locus from polygenes but does not actually provide information on the number of loci involved. It remains to be determined whether we are dealing with severe loci with appreciable effects in humans or many loci, each with an unmeasurable effect in clinical situations.

Common Genes That Might Regulate HDL Cholesterol Levels in the General Population

Apolipoprotein A-I

Commonly observed genetic variations in the promoter sequence of the human apo A-I gene lead to differences of apo A-I transport rate (195,196). However, it is controversial whether these differences result in differences in HDL levels.

Cholesteryl Ester Transfer Protein

An important exception to the generalization that the heritability of HDL cholesterol values is largely a result of polygenic influences is the recent finding of highly prevalent mutations of the cholesteryl ester transfer protein (CETP) gene in the Japanese (137). Two different mutations of the CETP gene are sufficiently common to influence the distribution of HDL cholesterol values in the general Japanese population (137). These mutations are present in about 6% of the Japanese population and account for about 10% of the variance of HDL cholesterol values. In an earlier study of 500 families of Japanese ancestry living in Hawaii, using complex segregation analysis, no major locus effect on HDL cholesterol levels was found, and polygenic inheritance was estimated to be 0.385 (127). The failure of this methodology to detect the influence of CETP gene mutations in this population raises a question about the sensitivity of the method. A recent set of studies by Assman and colleagues (personal communication) has identified several distinct CETP gene mutations in the German population and has suggested that CETP gene mutations may not be uncommon in this population as well.

Genes Causing Hypertriglyceridemia

There is an inverse relationship between plasma triglyceride levels and HDL cholesterol values in the general population. Thus, common genetic factors influencing triglyceride levels may also be determinants of HDL cholesterol. Hypertriglyceridemia is common, affecting 10% of men between ages 35 and 39 [triglycerides >250 mg/dl (98)], but the known genetic causes, homozygosity for LPL or apo C-II mutations, are rare (<1 per million). Recent evidence has implicated the apo C-III gene in the regulation of triglyceride levels in the general population. In Caucasians, hypertriglyceridemia has been strongly associated with a DNA polymorphism in the apo A-I, apo C-III, apo A-IV gene complex (138,139). This is an SstI RFLP in the 3′ untranslated region of the apo C-III gene. Polymorphisms in the promoter of the apo C-III gene have been used in conjunction with the SstI polymorphism to create apo C-III gene haplotypes and identify three classes of alleles that confer susceptibility, resistance, or neutrality with regard to hypertriglyceridemia (140). Moreover, transgenic mice expressing apo C-III are hypertriglyceridemic, and triglyceride levels are proportional to the amount of apo C-III in plasma and are very sensitive to small increments in apo C-III levels (141). These human and animal studies suggest that genetic variation in the apo C-III gene or in other genes affecting apo C-III expression could influence triglyceride and thus HDL cholesterol levels in the population. However, causative mutations at the apo C-III gene locus have not yet been identified.

There are several other reports of genes that might influence triglyceride and/or HDL cholesterol levels. These include carriers of the apo E_4 allele, who were found to be at increased risk for hypertriglyceridemia (142,143), other polymorphisms of the apo A-I, apo C-III, apo A-IV gene locus (6), and alleles of highly polymorphic markers surrounding the LPL gene, associated with altered levels of HDL_2 chol (144). Recently, sib-pair analysis has been used to implicate the apo A-II gene locus in the regulation of apo A-II and FFA levels but not HDL cholesterol levels (145). However, the causative mutations and mechanisms are not known.

GENETIC DEFICIENCY STATES AFFECTING HDL

Mutations of the Apo A-I Gene

Apolipoprotein A-I Gene Cluster Mutations

A DNA inversion involving the apo A-I and C-III genes resulted in a complete deficiency of apo A-I and apo C-III and HDL cholesterol levels between 0 and 7 mg/dl (146–151). Two sisters with this defect had xanthomas and premature coronary artery disease. Their LDL cholesterol and apo B levels were normal. Lipoprotein turnover studies indicated a three- to nine-fold increase in their VLDL FCR with rapid conversion to LDL but normal LDL FCR. These studies as well as recent transgenic mouse data indicate that apo C-III may delay VLDL clearance. A deletion of the entire apo A-I, apo C-III, apo A-IV gene locus resulted in HDL-C of 1 mg/dl, LDL cholesterol and triglycerides at the 25th percentile, premature coronary artery disease, and diffuse generalized atherosclerosis (152). These mutations suggest that complete apo A-I deficiency predisposes to premature atherosclerosis, but the rapid catabolism of VLDL because of apo C-III deficiency is probably also an atherogenic factor in these patients.

Isolated Apo A-I Gene Mutations Resulting in Complete Deficiency of Apo A-I

A Japanese female homozygous for a codon 84 nonsense mutation (Gln:stop) had absent plasma apo A-I and HDL cholesterol, premature coronary heart disease (CHD), and planar xanthomas. The LDL cholesterol was 198 mg/dl, and triglycerides 107 mg/dl (153). A Turkish girl with apo A-I deficiency caused by frameshift mutation resulting in a premature termination codon had planar xanthomas and corneal clouding but no evidence of CHD, presumably because of her young age (154). Recently a large Canadian family with an apo A-I gene mutation resulting in complete deficiency of apo A-I was described (155). Two homozygous sisters had xanthomas and premature CHD, while other homozygous family members appeared to be healthy. The sisters with low HDL cholesterol and premature CHD also had elevated LDL cholesterol. Thus, complete deficiency of apo A-I is a strong predisposing factor to xanthomatosis and premature atherosclerosis. However, the rate of disease development is variable and may be modified by other factors such as elevated LDL cholesterol levels.

Apolipoprotein A-I Gene Mutations Resulting in Partial Deficiency of Apo A-I

A missense mutation of the apo A-I gene (173 arg:cys) called apo A-I Milano resulted in an average 40% decrease in apo A-I and apo A-II levels, a 67% decrease in HDL cholesterol, increased VLDL triglyceride, and normal LDL levels (6,156–160). However, both LDL and HDL were triglyceride-enriched. The defects in apo A-I Milano reflect both the change in one of the amphipathic α-helical regions of apo A-I as well as the introduction of a cysteine residue into the apo A-I amino acid sequence, allowing disulfide bonding to other apolipoproteins. Despite the low HDL cholesterol levels, subjects with apo A-I Milano do not have increased coronary artery disease; in fact, the opposite is suspected, with longevity noted in some family members. A case of apo A-I deficiency resembling fish eye disease has been described as a result of a frameshift mutation with introduction of cysteines and premature termination at codon 230. This 42-year-old man had massive corneal opacifications, complete absence of HDL, and half-normal LCAT activity but no overt coronary artery disease. His LDL cholesterol was 203 mg/dl, and triglycerides were 196 mg/dl.

The LCAT gene was normal, indicating that LCAT deficiency was secondary to the defect of apo A-I. Other interesting apo A-I gene mutations include an in-frame deletion with apparent dominant expression arising from the fact that each HDL contains more than one apo A-I molecule (161) and two missense mutations that result in familial amyloidosis associated with deposition of amino-terminal fragments of apo A-I in amyloid fibrils in various tissues (162,163).

Mutations of the Apo A-II Gene

Two Japanese sisters homozygous for an apo A-II gene-splicing defect were found to have no detectable apo A-II, 33% reductions in apo A-I, but normal HDL cholesterol values (164). These sisters were clinically normal and had normal coronary angiograms.

Lipoprotein Processing Gene Mutations

Tangier Disease

In this disorder there is an unknown genetic defect leading to rapid catabolism of apo A-I and markedly reduced plasma apo A-I, and HDL cholesterol levels. The apo A-I gene is normal. The LDL levels are low, and LDL is triglyceride-enriched. Although there is no general evidence of premature atherosclerosis, cholesteryl-ester-enriched foam cells accumulate in the tonsils, liver, and spleen, resulting in enlargement of these organs. Defective metabolism of HDL in macrophages has been reported in Tangier disease (77).

LPL Deficiency

Subjects with homozygous structural mutations of the LPL gene, or of the gene of the LPL activator apo C-II, have marked hypertriglyceridemia and markedly depressed LDL and HDL cholesterol (6). The decrease in HDL may reflect defective formation secondary to the lipolytic defect. These conditions do not predispose to premature atherosclerosis.

Hepatic Lipase Deficiency

Hepatic lipase (HL) deficiency caused by structural mutations in the HL gene is a very rare recessive condition resulting in increased VLDL and IDL, β-migrating VLOL, and increased triglyceride-rich HDL_2 (6). The phenotype indicates a role of HL in the clearance of chylomicron remnants and IDL and in the hydrolysis of HDL triglycerides and phospholipids, resulting in interconversion of HDL_2 into HDL_3. Despite the increased HDL levels in these subjects, some of these individuals have premature coronary artery disease.

LCAT Deficiency

LCAT deficiency is a recessive condition resulting from structural mutations of the LCAT gene (6). The phenotypic manifestations of LCAT deficiency are variable in severity, depending on whether the defect in LCAT activity is complete (classical LCAT deficiency) or partial (fish eye disease). Patients with total LCAT deficiency develop corneal opacities, anemia, and renal failure. Foam cells are present in the bone marrow and glomeruli. The HDL cholesterol levels are markedly reduced (1–10 mg/dl), and apo A-I levels are 25–30% of normal. The HDL consists of disk-shaped particles resembling nascent HDL and small spherical HDL; VLDL and LDL are also abnormal. The typical spherical LDL is highly triglyceride-enriched. Premature atherosclerosis may develop in classical LCAT deficiency. Several large Dutch kindreds with LCAT deficiency and clearly increased premature CHD have recently been discovered by J. Kastelein et al. (personal communication). Coronary artery disease has also been reported in fish eye disease.

CETP Deficiency

Four different CETP gene mutations have been described in Japanese subjects. Two of the mutations result in gene-splicing defects at the intron 14 splice donor (137,165), one produces a missense change in the coding sequence (aspartate 442 : glycine), and the other produces a nonsense mutation at codon 309. The initially described intron 14 mutation (int 14 G : A) as well as the codon 442 missense mutation are common in Japan, with heterozygotes constituting about 1% and 6% of the general population of Japan, respectively (137). Although these mutations have not been found in Caucasian subjects (168), several distinctive CETP gene mutations have been discovered in a small screening of the German population, suggesting that genetic CETP deficiency may be not uncommon in non-Asian populations (G. Assman, personal communication).

All forms of genetic CETP deficiency causes increases in plasma HDL cholesterol and apo A-I levels. The degree of elevation of HDL cholesterol is inversely related to the residual CETP activity in plasma. Homozygosity for null alleles such as the two intron 14 splicing defects results in HDL cholesterol of 100–200 mg/dl, and heterozygous deficiency typically results in HDL cholesterol of 50–90 mg/dl, with increased prominence of the HDL_2 fraction. Genetic CETP deficiency also results in decreased levels of CE in VLDL and IDL (171). When homozygotes, heterozygotes, and unaffected family members are compared, the CE/TG ratio of VLDL and IDL shows a strong gene dosage effect (71). Homozygous deficiency of CETP typically results in decreased LDL cholesterol and apo B levels, but this is probably seen only with complete absence of plasma CETP.

Although the D442G missense mutation also causes increases in HDL cholesterol, there are distinctive aspects of the phenotype (137,166). Heterozygotes with the missense mutation have reduced plasma CETP concentration and specific activity and have substantially increased HDL cholesterol levels (typically 50–90 mg/dl). By contrast, homozygotes have residual plasma CETP activity and have HDL cholesterol levels similar or only slightly higher than heterozygotes. Cellular expression of the missense mutant cDNA results in decreased secretion and specific activity compared to wild type (166). When coexpressed with the wild type, the mutant cDNA appears to cause decreased secretion and activity of the wild-type protein, suggesting a dominant inhibitory effect. Thus, the phenotype is consistent with the results of cell transfection experiments and suggests that the mutant allele is partially defective and has dominant expression. The biochemical basis of genetic dominance is poorly understood but could indicate that multimeric forms of CETP are present in the cellular secretory pathway.

GENETIC DEFICIENCY STATES AFFECTING HDL AND ATHEROGENESIS

The description above indicates that the absence of apo A-I as a result of A-I gene mutations predisposes to accelerated atherogenesis. The individuals reported with apo A-I deficiency and accelerated atherosclerosis also have moderate elevations of LDL cholesterol. In contrast, genetic deficiency states that result in very low apo A-I and HDL cholesterol levels, such as Tangier disease, apo A-I Milano, and fish eye disease do not appear to predispose to accelerated atherosclerosis. However, in these states LDL is abnormal and highly triglyceride-enriched. This suggests that HDL particles containing apo A-I have a direct protective effect against the development of atherosclerosis. This protective effect becomes apparent only in the face of a stimulus to atherogenesis such as increased LDL cholesterol levels. These observations are also consistent with human studies showing that groups consuming very low-fat diets have both low HDL cholesterol and LDL cholesterol but are not predisposed to atherogenesis (11,120). Also, consistent with this hypothesis, overexpression of apo A-I in transgenic mice directly protects against atherogenesis in hypercholesterolemic apo E knockout mice (167a), but apo A-I knockout mice with low VLDL and LDL cholesterol do not develop atherosclerosis (168). How apo A-I and HDL modify the atherogenic stimulus is uncertain. Several possibilities exist, such as the removal of cholesterol from cells in atherosclerotic lesions or the limitation of oxidative modifications of LDL (see below).

STUDIES OF HDL METABOLISM IN TRANSGENIC MICE

Transgenic and gene knockout technology provides the tools to study the functions of single genes or the interaction of a few genes in complex physiological settings. This approach has provided invaluable insights into lipoprotein metabolism and atherogenesis, where many of the important genes have been identified but their functions in vivo and modes of interaction have not been well understood. The use of transgenic technology has been especially fruitful in studies of HDL metabolism and the role of HDL in atherogenesis. Transgenic mouse lines have been established that express several of the lipoprotein transport genes involved in HDL metabolism, including apo A-I, apo A-II, apo C-II, apo C-III, LPL, and CETP (7). The major findings in these mice are described in another chapter (20).

ENVIRONMENTAL FACTORS INFLUENCING HDL LEVELS

Table 1 lists some of the factors influencing HDL cholesterol levels. Exercise and the consumption of ethanol raise HDL cholesterol levels. These changes may be related to increases in activity of LPL and decreases in plasma CETP concentrations (11,90). Obesity and smoking are associated with lower levels of HDL cholesterol. Vegetarians and others who habitually consume high-carbohydrate, low-fat diets with high P/S ratios tend to have low levels of both HDL cholesterol and LDL cholesterol, but their overall coronary risk is also low (189–193). Low levels of HDL cholesterol are commonly found in diabetics (194).

Alcohol intake is an important factor contributing to increased HDL cholesterol. The mechanisms by which alcohol increases HDL levels may involve alterations in triglyceride metabolism as well as changes in lipase and CETP activity (195–197). Moderate doses of alcohol administered to normal medical students initially resulted in increased plasma triglyceride levels (195), probably reflecting increased hepatic VLDL triglyceride output. As alcohol intake was continued, however, plasma triglyceride levels fell, in association with an increase in lipoprotein lipase activity in adipose tissue. At the same time HDL cholesterol levels were increased. Thus, it is likely that increased VLDL turnover associated with more effective lipolysis leads to increased formation of HDL as a byproduct of lipolysis. Another factor likely to be involved in the increase in HDL levels is a decrease

TABLE 1. *Some factors that alter HDL levels*

Increased HDL
Female sex
Exercise conditioning
Alcohol intake
Nicotinic acid, fibrates, phenytoin
Estrogens
Decreased HDL
Low-fat diet
High-polyunsaturated-fat diet
Obesity, especially truncal
Probucol, β-blockers, progestins, and androgens
Smoking
Diabetes

in plasma CETP levels (196,197). Alcohol intake has been associated with decreased plasma CETP levels, and plasma CETP levels are inversely correlated with HDL cholesterol levels.

Several currently used hypolipidemic drugs also affect HDL cholesterol levels (198). Niacin and gemfibrozil raise HDL cholesterol levels by 10% to 15%. Bile acid sequestrants and inhibitors of HMGCoA reductase also tend to increase HDL cholesterol, but the effects are smaller and more variable. Probucol typically causes a 10–30% lowering of HDL cholesterol. Oral estrogens and diphenylhydantoin raise HDL cholesterol levels, and androgens, some progestins, and β-blockers lower HDL cholesterol.

HDL AS A RISK FACTOR FOR CORONARY HEART DISEASE IN HUMANS

Epidemiologic Studies

Although several earlier studies suggested a protective effect of HDL in coronary artery disease, the first major population-based case-control study to document this effect was the Honolulu Heart Program study, based on a cohort of about 1,500 men of Japanese ancestry living in Hawaii (199). Relative risk of coronary heart disease, based on 264 prevalence cases, was found to be about 0.46 between the upper and lower quartiles of HDL cholesterol. Subsequently, numerous prospective epidemiologic investigations in North America and elsewhere have shown a significant and independent inverse relationship between HDL cholesterol levels and the incidence of coronary artery disease (200). For example, in a 12-year follow-up of the Framingham study, this relationship held after multivariate adjustment for total cholesterol, systolic blood pressure, cigarette smoking, and body mass index. The HDL cholesterol levels showed a strong inverse relationship with coronary artery disease at low (<200 mg/dl), medium, and high (>260 mg/dl) total cholesterol levels.

The change in risk associated with increasing levels of HDL cholesterol can be estimated (198). A standardized analysis of the incidence of fatal and nonfatal myocardial infarction in four large American studies showed a decrement of about 2.5% in coronary risk for each 1 mg/dl increase in HDL cholesterol levels. According to limited data, the relationship of HDL cholesterol to coronary disease appeared to be even stronger in women than men, and, unlike LDL cholesterol, it did not decline with increasing age. In the four studies, similar trends relating lower HDL-cholesterol to mortality from cardiovascular diseases and from all causes was statistically significant only in the LRC Follow-up Study (200).

Because low levels of HDL (as well as total) cholesterol are common in nonindustrialized countries where both the consumption of fat (198) and the rates of coronary heart disease are low, cross-cultural comparisons often do not confirm the prevailing evidence on the inverse relationship of HDL cholesterol and coronary heart disease in the industrialized world. However, cross-cultural comparison of coronary mortality rates in 19 industrialized countries showed a significant inverse correlation with HDL ($r = -0.57$) and total cholesterol ($r = 0.67$). The differing results in industrialized and nonindustrialized countries suggest that low levels of HDL cholesterol may be a risk factor mainly in populations that consume a high fat diet. These observations may be consistent with studies on genetic deficiency states affecting HDL as well as experiments in genetically manipulated animal models, which indicate that low HDL cholesterol (see above) is a risk factor for atherosclerosis only in the context of atherogenic levels of LDL cholesterol. Atherogenic levels of LDL cholesterol would include values often considered normal in industrialized societies.

An Apparent Protective Effect of HDL in Lipid-Lowering Studies

Although no clinical trials have set out specifically to test the benefit of raising low HDL levels, post-hoc analyses of various cholesterol-lowering trials do suggest a beneficial effect of raising HDL cholesterol levels. Several trials that achieved a beneficial effect on coronary artery disease from lowering LDL cholesterol also reported increases in HDL cholesterol (201–204). Analysis of data by proportional hazards regression analysis suggested that in the two cholestyramine trials the changes in HDL cholesterol made a significant contribution. In the Helsinki Heart Study (9), gemfibrozil administration to asymptomatic middle-aged men with increased non-HDL cholesterol resulted in a decrease in LDL cholesterol of 8% and an increase in HDL cholesterol of 10%. The 5-year incidence of myocardial infarction was 34% lower in the group receiving gemfibrozil compared to placebo. In this study the changes in LDL cholesterol, when considered alone, seemed insufficient to account for the decrease in coronary artery disease. Proportional-hazards regression analyses of the men who received gemfibrozil indicated that HDL increases were the single most significant predictor of a favorable treatment outcome (205). Although this is suggestive, changing HDL was not part of the original study design in these investigations, and the post-hoc analysis could be subject to various kinds of bias. There is a need to carry out an intervention trial specifically aimed at raising HDL, preferably in subjects selected for low HDL cholesterol.

Alcohol, HDL, and Coronary Heart Disease

Moderate alcohol intake is associated with a protective effect against coronary artery disease, apparently mediated in large part by alcohol-induced increases in HDL cholesterol levels (206). The evidence from both observational studies and experimental trials suggests that alcohol raises the level of total HDL and that approximately 50% of the reduction in risk attributable to alcohol consumption is explained by the changes in total HDL. In a case-control study conducted in six suburban Boston hospitals, 340 patients with myocardial infarctions were compared to an equal number of age- and sex-matched controls (206). There was a significant inverse association between alcohol consumption and the risk of myocardial infarction, which remained highly significant after control for known coronary risk factors. In multivariate analysis the relative risk for the highest intake category (subjects who consumed three or more drinks per day) as compared with the lowest (those who had less than one drink per month) was 0.45. The levels of total HDL cholesterol and its HDL_2 and HDL_3 subfractions were strongly associated with alcohol consumption. The addition of HDL or either of its subfractions to the multivariate model substantially reduced the inverse association between alcohol intake and myocardial infarction, whereas the addition of other plasma lipid measurements did not materially alter the relationship.

Although the effects of moderate alcohol may be beneficial, heavy alcohol intake increases overall morbidity and mortality from cardiovascular diseases (206). The harmful effects of heavy alcohol intake on the heart occur primarily with heavy drinking. These include dilated cardiomyopathy, dysrhythmias, and hypertensive heart disease. Alcohol can have opposite effects on the occurrence of stroke; it may promote cerebral hemorrhage, for instance, but protect against cerebrovascular occlusion.

Low HDL Cholesterol Associated with Other Lipoprotein Abnormalities

It should be pointed out that decreased levels of HDL cholesterol are usually associated with other lipoprotein abnormalities such as elevated levels of triglycerides, increased VLDL cholesterol, IDL cholesterol, and increased amounts of small, dense LDL (207,208). Low HDL cholesterol may also be associated with increased levels of postprandial lipoproteins (209). In one case-control study, the pattern of low HDL cholesterol, high triglycerides, increased VLDL and IDL cholesterol, and dense LDL was present in 50% of patients with first myocardial infarction and 26% of sex- and age-matched neighborhood controls (208). In this study it was not possible to separate statistically the coronary heart disease (CHD) risk of each of these lipoprotein abnormalities, and it is possible that the heart disease risk of low HDL cholesterol might be related in part to increased levels of other lipoproteins that are themselves atherogenic. Finally, in epidemiologic studies, HDL cholesterol levels are not correlated with LDL cholesterol levels, which are directly related to coronary heart disease risk (210). Consequently, the ratio of level of LDL to HDL cholesterol is a better predictor of risk than either measurement alone.

Austin (211) reviewed the relationship among triglycerides, HDL cholesterol, and CHD risk. Most studies have found a significant univariate relationship between triglyceride and CHD risk. However, in some studies, after controlling for HDL cholesterol, this association remained significant, whereas in other studies it did not. Austin has shown that the large variability of triglyceride measurements and the correlation of triglyceride values with other lipid measures appear to result in underestimation of the association between triglyceride and disease in multivariate analysis. Genetic factors, such as those determining the high-triglyceride, small-LDL, low-HDL-cholesterol phenotype may play an important role in determining CHD susceptibility in some individuals with elevated triglyceride levels.

Some authors have attempted to consider both triglycerides and HDL cholesterol in the assessment of CHD risk (212). For example, in the Helsinki Heart Study, subjects initially identified as having high VLDL + LDL cholesterol (more than 5.2 mmol/liter) had a relative risk of CHD of 3.8 if they had LDL/HDL cholesterol >5 and triglycerides >2.3 mmol/liter (200 mg/dl) compared with subjects with LDL/HDL cholesterol <5 and triglyceride <200 mg/dl). The high-risk group benefited most from lipid lowering with gemfibrozil, with a 71% lower incidence of CHD than a corresponding placebo group. Thus, serum triglyceride concentration was found to have prognostic value, especially when used in conjunction with HDL and LDL cholesterol.

HDL Subfractions and Risk of Coronary Heart Disease

Attempts to relate coronary heart disease risk to levels of subfractions of HDL have yielded somewhat conflicting results. Some prospective and case-control epidemiologic studies show that HDL_2 cholesterol levels are a better discriminator of risk than low HDL_3 cholesterol levels. Compatible with this notion, women who are at lower risk of CHD than men have higher HDL_2 cholesterol levels. However, other studies show that both HDL_2 and HDL_3 cholesterol levels are diminished in subjects with CHD, and neither subfraction is better than total HDL cholesterol levels in predicting risk (213). With regard to the HDL apoproteins, apo A-I levels are highly correlated with HDL cholesterol levels and predict risk equally well. On the other hand, apo A-II levels are not correlated with HDL cholesterol levels and do not predict CHD risk. Some case-control studies have suggested that LpA-I levels are predictive of CHD risk but that LpA-I/A-II levels are not. However, these findings were not confirmed in another investigation. Because LpA-I and LpA-I/A-II are metabolically distinct, there is a need to carry out more extensive measurements of these subfractions in epidemiologic studies.

WHY IS THERE AN INVERSE RELATIONSHIP BETWEEN HDL CHOLESTEROL AND CORONARY ARTERY DISEASE?

There are several different theories that have attempted to explain the relationship between HDL levels and atherogenesis observed in human and animal studies. These may be divided into theories that postulate a direct antiatherogenic action of HDL versus those that say that HDL is merely a metabolic marker for some other event, such as a defect in the metabolism of triglyceride-rich lipoprotein metabolism. Because of the close links between HDL and the metabolism of triglyceride-rich lipoproteins, this has been difficult to sort out using epidemiologic approaches. As indicated above, however, recent genetic evidence in humans with isolated apo A-I deficiency as well as in transgenic mice overexpressing apo A-I clearly indicate direct atherogenic effects of complete apo A-I deficiency as well as antiatherogenic effects of apo A-I overexpression. However, these examples may represent extreme situations, because the common situation of low HDL cholesterol in humans involves accelerated HDL catabolism secondary to defects in triglyceride metabolism and/or lipid transfer processes. In this instance, low HDL cholesterol may be a marker of atherogenic particles such as chylomicron or VLDL remnants, IDL, or small, dense LDL (11).

Reverse Cholesterol Transport Hypothesis

This hypothesis states that reverse cholesterol transport mediates removal of cholesterol from atheromata and that the level of plasma HDL determines the efficiency of this process. Despite the appeal of this theory, the evidence supporting it is fairly limited. As outlined above, HDL can remove cholesterol from cells, including cholesteryl-ester-loaded macrophage foam cells resembling those found in atheromata. These cells also secrete apo E and phospholipids, giving rise to locally formed apo-E-containing HDL particles. These particles may become enriched with CE as a result of LCAT action, driving net cholesterol efflux. Large cholesteryl-ester-rich HDL particles containing multiple copies of apo E can be removed by hepatic LDL receptors. In animal models of atherogenesis, the infusion of HDL-like particles (liposomes) or HDL itself has been reported to result in accelerated regression of atherosclerosis. Less directly, in animal models and in humans, regression of atherosclerosis occurs in settings where LDL is lowered and HDL is increased. It is likely that regression involves removal of cholesterol from lesions by HDL. Thus, it appears likely that HDL is directly involved in a process of reverse cholesterol transport from atheromata into plasma and back to the liver.

What is less clear is the extent to which the "protective" effect of HDL noted in human epidemiologic studies is mediated by changes in the efficiency of the reverse cholesterol transport system. For example, it has never been shown that variations in HDL cholesterol concentrations similar to those in plasma modulate cholesterol removal from cells of the arterial wall. Furthermore, the original finding of an inverse relationship between HDL cholesterol levels and human tissue cholesterol stores (as measured in isotopic cholesterol turnover studies) was not confirmed in more definitive studies of a larger number of subjects using more appropriate modeling of cholesterol pools (11). However, these measurements are macroscopic in nature, and no kinetic parameter accurately measures the pool of cholesterol in atheromata. Thus, some authors have hypothesized that the common inverse relationship between HDL and CHD is observed because HDL is acting as a marker for abnormal metabolism resulting in accumulation of atherogenic lipoproteins.

Atherogenic Remnant Hypothesis

Zilversmit originally proposed that some chylomicrons bearing dietary cholesterol would be hydrolyzed on large blood vessels and subsequently enter the arterial wall and promote atheroma formation (11). The atherogenic remnant hypothesis was subsequently modified to say that low HDL levels might be a marker for the accumulation of chylomicron or VLDL remnants in plasma. In addition to bearing dietary cholesterol, the remnants would become enriched in CE derived from HDL and LDL as a result of CETP activity. The concentration of chylomicron or VLDL remnants might be increased through overproduction of VLDL, inefficient lipolytic processing, or defective receptor-mediated clearance. The cholesterol- and cholesteryl-ester-enriched remnants would enter the artery wall and contribute to atheroma foam cell formation. The low levels of HDL could result from both inefficient lipolytic transfer of lipids into HDL and accelerated CE–TG interchange with the accumulation of TG-rich lipoproteins.

A clear example of accumulation of atherogenic remnants in association with low HDL cholesterol levels is seen in type III hyperlipoproteinemia. In this disorder there is overproduction of VLDL and decreased hepatic removal of remnants because of a genetic defect in apo E leading to accumulation of chylomicron and VLDL remnants. There is accelerated transfer of CE from HDL into remnants contributing to reduced levels of HDL CE (11). This was originally demonstrated by incubation of plasma from type III patients and has been confirmed in transgenic mouse models of type III, where expression of CETP with mutant apo E leads to reduced HDL and enrichment of remnants with cholesteryl esters.

Direct evidence of a more general link between accumulation of postprandial triglyceride-rich lipoproteins and low HDL levels has been obtained by Patsch and co-workers (209). These workers showed that the degree of elevation of postprandial triglyceride levels is strongly inversely correlated with fasting HDL_2, HDL cholesterol, and apo A-I levels. The postprandial triglyceridemia was correlated relatively weakly with fasting TG levels, suggesting that the measurement of postprandial triglyceridemia might be more readily able to identify atherogenic risk arising from accumulation of remnants. In a small case-control study, postprandial triglyceride and retinyl ester levels were found to be higher in cases than controls and inversely correlated with HDL_2 concentrations. In a larger case-control study, Ginsberg H., et al. (unpublished) recently found that men with coronary artery disease had higher postprandial triglyceride levels than controls and that postprandial TG measurements were strong independent predictors of CHD.

These studies appear to confirm an atherogenic role of postprandial triglyceride-transporting lipoproteins. However, the inverse relationship between postprandial triglyceride levels and HDL cholesterol has not been observed consistently in subsequent studies. For example, Cohen and Grundy (214) and others (215) studied plasma TG and retinyl palmitate responses to 50-g fat meals and found similar postprandial triglyceride and retinyl palmitate clearance in men with normal triglycerides and either normal HDL or low HDL. In contrast the postprandial lipemia was markedly higher in hypertriglyceridemic men. These authors concluded that defects in chylomicron triglyceride clearance that give rise to excess postprandial lipemia are not a common occurrence in normolipidemic men with low HDL cholesterol concentration.

HDL and Oxidative Modifications of LDL

A large body of evidence suggests that oxidation of LDL is involved in atherogenesis (see the chapter by Chisolm, *this volume*). Extensively oxidized LDL may be recognized by receptors on macrophages promoting atheroma foam cell formation, or it may be cytotoxic to endothelial and other cells. Minimally oxidized LDL also has important biological properties that may be involved in atherogenesis, such as the stimulation of MCP-1 synthesized in cocultures of endothelial and smooth muscle cells, promoting macrophage chemotaxis (see the chapter by Rosenfeld et al., *this volume*). Similar events in the arterial wall may promote the localization of foam-cell-forming macrophages in the arterial intima. In vitro experiments indicate that HDL can inhibit many of the effects of LDL oxidation. Parthasarathy et al. (216) showed that inclusion of HDL in incubations containing Cu and LDL had a profound inhibitory effect on the subsequent degradation of LDL by macrophages while having no effect on the generation of TBARS or conjugated dienes (measures of lipid oxidation). The HDL itself was relatively resistant to oxidative modification. These workers suggested that HDL may play a protective role in atherogenesis by preventing the generation of oxidatively modified LDL. Navab et al. (217) showed that HDL inhibits the stimulation of macrophage chemotaxis induced by minimally modified LDL in macrophage–endothelial cell cocultures, and Chisholm and colleagues demonstrated that HDL inhibits the LDL-mediated cytotoxicity of vascular smooth muscle and endothelial cells (218).

There are several potential mechanisms by which HDL may modify the formation or properties of oxidized LDL. These include (a) an exchange of lipid peroxidation products between HDL and LDL, sequestering oxidized lipids away from apo B and limiting apo B modification (216); (b) binding of oxidation-promoting transition metals by apo A-I (219); and (c) HDL contains paraoxonase activity, which may be able to inhibit the generation of oxidized lipids (220). The paraoxonase resides in a fraction of HDL containing apo A-I and apo J (221). Although paraoxonase is known to be genetically regulated, the true function of this enzyme is unknown. In fresh plasma, HDL carries most (85%) of the oxidized core lipoprotein lipids, and HDL lipid is preferentially oxidized under mild conditions (222), reflecting the lack of natural antioxidants in HDL CE. Oxidized lipids could be taken up from HDL by hepatocytes, raising the possibility that rapid hepatic clearance of CE peroxides in HDL could ameliorate the buildup of oxidized lipids in LDL. Another possibility is that myeloperoxidase secreted by activated macrophages oxidizes HDL tyrosine residues, which enhances the ability of HDL to remove sterol from cells (223). Although supported by considerable experimental evidence, the hypothesis that HDL protects against oxidative modifications of LDL or its consequences is currently lacking proof of in vivo relevance.

HDL CHOLESTEROL LEVELS IN THE EVALUATION OF DYSLIPIDEMIA

The second report of the National Cholesterol Education Panel (Adult Treatment Panel II) places increased emphasis on HDL cholesterol in the evaluation and treatment of dyslipidemia in the American population (224). Consistent with earlier recommendations, this report continues to identify LDL as the primary target of cholesterol-lowering therapy. However, more attention is paid to HDL cholesterol as a CHD risk factor, including the following: (a) addition of HDL cholesterol to initial cholesterol screening; (b) designation of high HDL-cholesterol as a negative risk factor (in the earlier set of recommendations HDL cholesterol <35 mg/dl was considered a positive risk factor); and (c) consideration of HDL cholesterol in the choice of drug therapy. The panel recommends measurements of both total serum cholesterol and HDL cholesterol in all adults of age 20 at least once every 5 years, assuming accurate HDL cholesterol measurements are available. The way this information is to be used in screening and subsequent evaluation is summarized in Fig. 4.

Patients with low HDL cholesterol are advised to lose weight if overweight and to increase physical activity. These hygienic measures will have the beneficial effects of promoting reduction of cholesterol levels and increasing HDL cholesterol levels. For individuals who have low HDL cholesterol and who need drugs to lower LDL cholesterol to acceptable levels, hypolipidemic agents that have the most beneficial effects on HDL cholesterol are recommended, i.e., nicotinic acid or a fibric acid derivative such as gemfibrozil (however, gemfibrozil has only modest LDL-C lowering capacity). Drugs that lower HDL cholesterol such as probucol

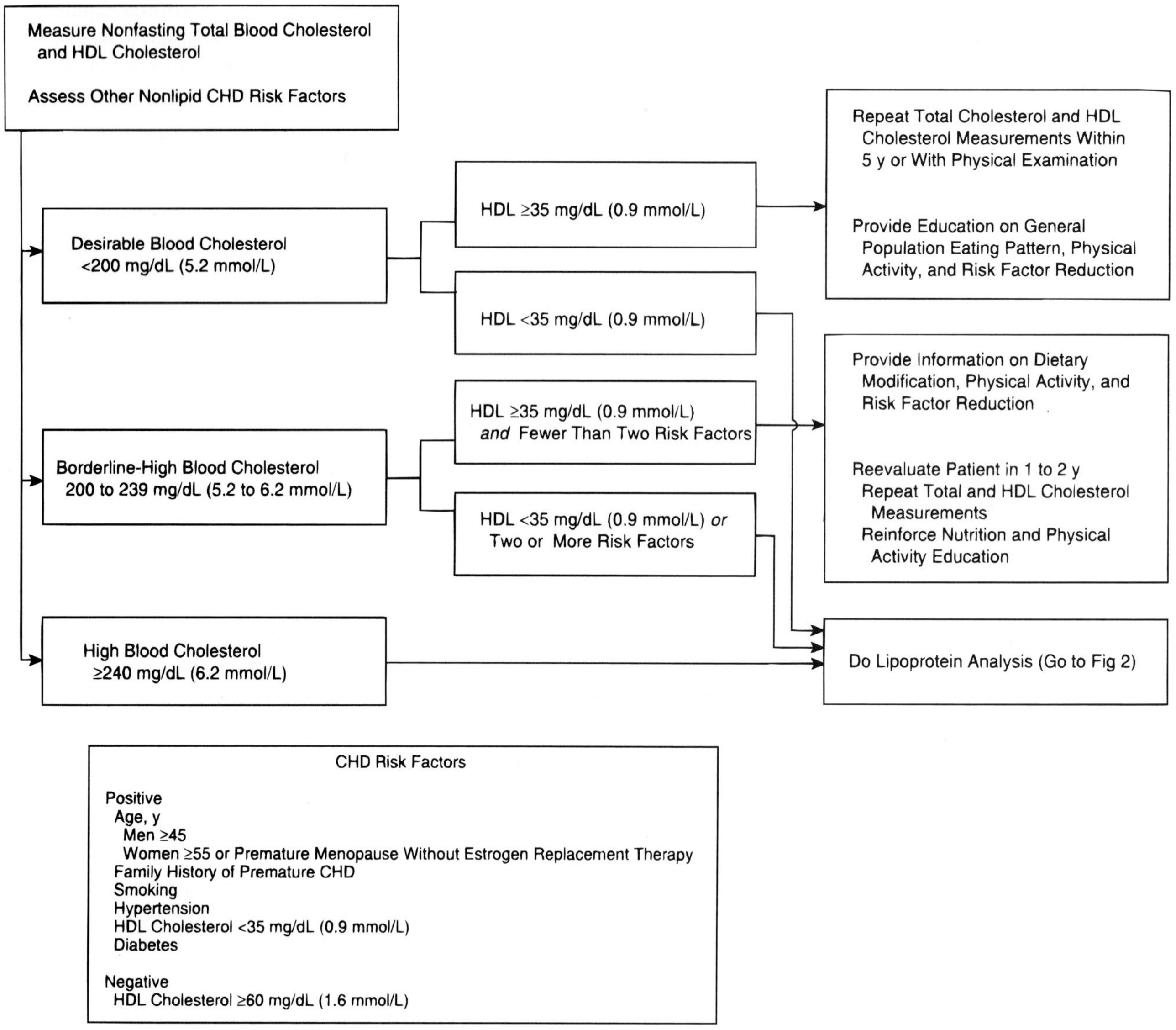

FIG. 4. Primary prevention in adults without evidence of coronary heart disease (CHD). Initial classification is based on total cholesterol and high-density lipoprotein (HDL) cholesterol levels. From ref. 10, with permission.

should be avoided. Although improved, the recommendations on ATP-II are likely to be further revised as more information becomes available, particularly from intervention trials that identify low HDL as the primary abnormality for treatment. The recommendations do not provide advice on how to treat individuals with isolated low HDL cholesterol or the more common example of high-triglyceride–low-HDL cholesterol with normal LDL cholesterol levels. Many clinicians currently feel that such individuals should be treated for low HDL cholesterol, especially if the individual is known to have or is at increased risk for CHD.

FUTURE DIRECTIONS

Further insights into the metabolic regulation of plasma HDL levels will require a better understanding of the factors regulating lipoprotein triglyceride levels, lipid transfer processes, and synthesis of apolipoprotein genes. This will require a molecular understanding of the transcriptional and posttranscriptional regulation of genes such as apo A-I, lipoprotein lipase, hepatic lipase, apo C-III, and CETP.

The mechanism by which HDL protects against atherosclerosis is still poorly understood. Studies in transgenic and knockout mice may help to elucidate these mechanisms. In addition to stimulating reverse cholesterol transport and preventing oxidative modifications of LDL, other novel mechanisms may be involved.

Clinical intervention trials in which subjects identified with low HDL are subjected to changes in life style or given drugs in order to raise HDL levels are badly needed. Once this information is available, therapeutic recommendations concerning HDL can be made on a more rational basis.

Drugs that increase HDL levels by a variety of different mechanisms are likely to be developed. These may include agents that increase apo A-I synthesis, increase lipoprotein lipase activity, or decrease plasma CETP levels. Some of these may prove to have antiatherogenic actions, filling a major gap in the current therapy of coronary heart disease.

SUMMARY

The plasma HDL are small, spherical lipoproteins consisting of about 50% protein and 50% lipid. The major lipids are phospholipids, cholesterol, and cholesteryl esters. The major apoproteins are apo A-I and apo A-II. The HDL also contains proteins of central importance in lipoprotein metabolism, namely, the enzyme lecithin : cholesterol acyl transferase (LCAT) and the plasma lipid transfer proteins, cholesteryl ester transfer protein (CETP) and phospholipid transfer protein (PLTP).

The lipolysis of triglyceride-rich lipoproteins represents an important source of HDL. Thus, during triglyceride hydrolysis, phospholipids and soluble apoproteins are shed from chylomicrons and VLDL and incorporated in the HDL fraction. The LCAT enzyme acts on phospholipid and cholesterol, generating cholesteryl esters, which are redistributed to triglyceride-rich lipoproteins as a result of the activity of CETP. The CETP exchanges HDL CE for triglyceride. The triglyceride-rich HDL is subsequently acted on by lipases leading to the release and catabolism of apo A-I.

The overall metabolic function of HDL may be related to a process of reverse cholesterol transport, i.e., the centripetal movement of cholesterol from the periphery back to the liver. The HDL can remove cholesterol from cells, either by a process of simple diffusion or by nonspecific contact between HDL and cell surface. The flexibility of HDL apolipoproteins, particularly apo A-I, may be important in mediating these HDL–cell interactions. The cholesterol in HDL may become esterified and transferred to other lipoproteins for subsequent clearance by the liver, or the HDL cholesterol and cholesteryl ester may be more directly removed in the liver.

The HDL cholesterol levels show considerable variability in human populations and are influenced by factors such as gender, obesity, alcohol intake, cigarette smoking, and diabetes. Genetic factors also play an important role in the determination of HDL levels, but the genetic determinants of HDL levels are generally poorly understood. However, in some populations genetic deficiency of cholesteryl ester transfer protein, causing elevated HDL levels, is sufficiently common to have a major influence on HDL levels. Metabolic turnover studies in humans indicate that differences in HDL levels between different individuals are generally related to differences in catabolic rates of apo A-I and apo A-II. These differences may be related to variation in the activities of lipoprotein and hepatic lipase, which may influence HDL levels indirectly by an effect on plasma triglyceride levels or, more directly, may catabolize HDL lipids. Differences in lipid transfer rate from HDL to triglyceride-rich lipoprotein represent an important mechanism mediating the high-triglyceride–low-HDL relationship commonly observed in human populations. Lipid transfer rates may depend on plasma triglyceride levels or on CETP levels when the latter are decreased from genetic or other causes.

A strong independent inverse relationship between HDL levels and coronary heart disease has been noted in numerous cross-sectional and prospective epidemiologic studies. In general, a rise in HDL cholesterol of 1 mg/dl results in a 2.5% decrease in coronary heart disease risk. Indirect evidence from drug intervention trials such as the Helsinki Heart Study suggests that raising HDL levels will be beneficial for coronary artery disease. Available ways to raise HDL include hygienic measures and use of some triglyceride- or LDL-lowering drugs that cause relatively small increases in HDL cholesterol.

The mechanism of the apparent protective effect of HDL on coronary artery disease is incompletely understood. Evidence from human genetic deficiency states of apo A-I, as well as recent data obtained in transgenic mice, indicates a direct effect of HDL to reverse or prevent atherosclerosis. This could be related to increased reverse cholesterol transport or to the ability of HDL to prevent oxidative modifications of LDL that promote atherogenesis or to some other factor. In addition to these direct effects of HDL, it remains likely that low HDL levels in human populations commonly indicate accelerated lipid transfer from HDL to triglyceride-rich lipoproteins, which are themselves atherogenic. Thus, low HDL may be a marker for a tendency to accumulate atherogenic chylomicron or VLDL remnants or a tendency to accumulate atherogenic small, dense LDL particles, both processes reflecting accelerated lipid transfer processes.

REFERENCES

1. Gofman JW, Lindgren F, Elliott H, et al. The role of lipids and lipoproteins in atherosclerosis. *Science* 1950;111:166–171.
2. Gofman JW, de Lalla O, Glazier F, Freeman NK, Lindgren FT, Nichols AV, Strisower EH, Tamplin AR. The serum lipoprotein transport system in health, metabolic disorders, atherosclerosis and coronary artery disease. *Plasma* 1954;2:413–484.
3. Glomset JA. The plasma lecithin : cholesterol acyltransferase reaction. *J Lipid Res* 1968;9:155–167.
4. Rhoads GG, Gulbrandsen CL, Kagan A. Serum lipoproteins and coronary heart disease in a population study of Hawaii Japanese men. *N Engl J Med* 1976;294:293–298.
5. Eisenberg S. High density lipoprotein metabolism. *J Lipid Res* 1984; 25:1017–1058.
6. Breslow JL. Familial disorders of high density lipoprotein metabolism. In: Scrivner CR, Beaudet AL, Sly WS, Valle D, eds. *The Metabolic Basis of Inherited Disease.* New York: McGraw-Hill; 1989: 1251.
7. Breslow JL. Transgenic mouse models of lipoprotein metabolism and atherosclerosis. *Proc Natl Acad Sci USA* 1993;90:8314–8318.
8. Rubin EM, Krauss RM, Spangler EA, Verstuyft JG, Clift SM. Inhibition of early atherogenesis in transgenic mice by human apolipoprotein AI. *Nature* 1991;353:265.
9. Heikki Frick M, Elo O, Haapa K, et al. Helsinki Heart Study: Preliminary prevention trial with gemfibrozil in middle-aged men with dyslipidemia. *N Engl J Med* 1987;317:1237–1245.
10. Expert Panel on Detection, Evaluation, and Treatment of High Blood Cholesterol in Adults. Summary of the Second Report of the National Cholesterol Education Program (NCEP) Expert Panel on Detection,

Evaluation, and Treatment of High Blood Cholesterol in Adults (Adult Treatment Panel II). *JAMA* 1993;269:3015–3023.
11. Tall AR. Plasma high density lipoprotein metabolism and relationship to atherogenesis. *J Clin Invest* 1990;86:379–384.
12. Tall AR, Deckelbaum RJ, Small DM, Shipley GG. Structure and thermodynamic properties of high density lipoprotein recombinants. *J Biol Chem* 1977;252:4701–4711.
13. Jonas A, Steinmetz A, Churgay L. The number of amphipathic α-helical segments of apolipoproteins A-I, E, and A-IV determines the size and functional properties of their reconstituted lipoprotein particles. *J Biol Chem* 1993;268:1596–1602.
14. Blanche PJ, Gong EL, Forte TM, Nichols AV. Characterization of human high-density lipoproteins by gradient gel electrophoresis. *Biochim Biophys Acta* 1981;665:408–419.
15. Cheung MC, Albers JJ. Distribution of high density lipoprotein particles with different apoprotein composition: Particles with A-I and A-II and particles with A-I but no A-II. *J Lipid Res* 1982;23:747–753.
16. Cheung MC, Albers JJ. Characterization of lipoprotein particles isolated by immunoaffinity chromatography. *J Biol Chem* 1984;259: 12201–12209.
17. Cheung MC, Brown BG, Wolf AC, Albers JJ. Altered particle size distribution of apolipoprotein A-I-containing lipoproteins in subjects with coronary artery disease. *J Lipid Res* 1991;32:383–394.
18. Duverger N, Rader D, Duchateau P, Fruchart J-C, Castro G, Brewer HB Jr. Biochemical characterization of the three major subclasses of lipoprotein A-I preparatively isolated from human plasma. *Biochemistry* 1993;32:12372–12379.
19. Davidson WS, Sparks DL, Lund-Katz S, Phillips MC. The molecular basis for the difference in charge between pre-β and α-migrating high density lipoproteins. *J Biol Chem* 1994;269:8959–8965.
20. Castro GR, Fielding CJ. Early incorporation of cell-derived cholesterol into pre-β-migrating high-density lipoprotein. *Biochemistry* 1988;27:25–29.
21. Kunitake ST, Mendel CM, Hennessy LK. Interconversion between apolipoprotein A-I-containing lipoproteins of pre-beta and alpha electrophoretic mobilities. *J Lipid Res* 1992;33:1807–1816.
22. Karathanasis SK, McPherson J, Zannis VI, Breslow JL. Linkage of human apolipoproteins A-I and C-III genes. *Nature* 1983; 2093;304: 371.
23. Bruns GAP, Karathanasis SK, Breslow JL. Human apolipoprotein AI–CIII gene complex is located on chromosome 11. *Arteriosclerosis* 1984;4:97–102.
24. Karathanasis SK. Apolipoprotein multigene family: Tandem organization of human apolipoprotein AI, CIII, and AIV genes. *Proc Natl Acad Sci USA* 1985;82:6374–6378.
25. Karathanasis SK, Zannis VI, Breslow JL. Isolation and characterization of the human apolipoprotein A-I gene. *Proc Natl Acad Sci USA* 1983;80:6147–6151.
26. Breslow JL, Ross D, McPherson J, Williams H, Kurnit D, Nussbaum AL, Karathanasis SK, Zannis VI. Isolation and characterization of cDNA clones for human apolipoprotein A-I. *Proc Natl Acad Sci USA* 1982;79:6861–6865.
27. Zannis VI, Karathanasis SK, Keutmann HY, Goldberger G, Breslow JL. Intracellular and extracellular processing of human apo A-I. Secreted apo A-I isoprotein 2 is a propeptide. *Proc Natl Acad Sci USA* 1983;80:2574–2578.
28. Fitch WM. Phylogenies constrained by the crossover process as illustrated by human hemoglobins and a thirteen-cycle, eleven-amino-acid repeat in human apolipoprotein A-I. *Genetics* 1977;86:623–644.
29. McLachlan AD. Repeated helical pattern in apolipoprotein A-I. *Nature* 1977;267:465–466.
30. Segrest JP, Jackson RL, Morrisett JD, Gotto AM Jr. A molecular theory of lipid–protein interactions in the plasma lipoproteins. *FEBS Lett* 1974;38:247–258.
31. Tall AR, Shipley GG, Small DM. Conformational and thermodynamic properties of apoprotein A-I of human high density lipoproteins. *J Biol Chem* 1976;251:3749–3755.
32. Zannis VI, Cole FS, Jackson CL, Kurnit CL, Karathanasis SK. Distribution of apo A-I, apoC-II, apoC-III, and apoE mRNA in human tissues, time dependent induction of apoE mRNA by cultures of human monocyte–macrophages. *Biochemistry* 1985;24:4450–4455.
33. Walsh A, Ito Y, Breslow JL. High levels of human apolipoprotein A-I in transgenic mice result in increased plasma levels of small high density lipoprotein (HDL) particles comparable to human HDL3. *J Biol Chem* 1989;264:(11)6488–6494.
34. Ogami K, Kardassi D, Cladara C, Zannis VI. Purification and characterization of a heat stable nuclear factor CIIIB1 involved in the regulation of the human ApoC-III gene. *J Biol Chem* 1991;266:9640–9646.
35. Widon RL, Ladias JA, Kouidou S, Karathanasis SK. Synergistic interactions between transcription factors control expression of the apolipoprotein AI gene in liver cells. *Mol Cell Biol* 1991;11:677–687.
36. Papazasfiri P, Ogami K, Ramji DP, Nicosia A, Monaci P, Cladaras C, Zannis VI. Promoter elements and factors involved in hepatic transcript of the human apoA-I gene positive and negative regulators bind to overlapping sites. *J Biol Chem* 1991;266:5790–5797.
37. Rottman JN, Widom RL, Nadal-Ginard B, Mahdavi V, Karathanasis SK. A retinoic acid-responsive element in the apolipoprotein AI gene distinguishes between two different retinoic acid response pathways. *Mol Cell Biol* 1991;11:3814–3820.
38. Ladias JA, Karathanasis SK. Regulation of the apolipoprotein AI gene by ARP-1, a novel member of the steroid receptor superfamily. *Science* 1991;251:561–565.
39. Walsh A, Azrolan N, Wang K, Marcigliano A, O'Connell A, Breslow JL. Intestinal expression of the human apoA-I gene in transgenic mice is controlled by a DNA region 3′ to the gene in the promoter of the adjacent convergently transcribed apoC-III gene. *J Lipid Res* 1993; 34:617–623.
40. Lauer SJ, Simonet WS, Bucay N, De Silva HV, Taylor JM. Tissue-specific expression of the human apolipoprotein A-IV gene in transgenic mice. *Circulation* 1991;84(Suppl II):17.
41. Moore MN, Kao FT, Tsao YK, Chan L. Human apolipoprotein A-II: Nucleotide sequence of a cloned cDNA, and localization of its structural gene on human chromosome 1. *Biochem Biophys Res Commun* 1984;(11)123:1–7.
42. Knott TJ, Priestley LM, Urdea M, Scott J. Isolation and characterisation of a cDNA encoding the precursor for human apolipoprotein AII. *Biochem Biophys Res Commun* 1984(3):734–740.
43. Lackner KJ, Law SW, Brewer HB Jr. Human apolipoprotein A-II: Complete nucleic acid sequence of preproapo A-II. *FEBS Lett* 1984; 175(1):159–164.
44. Brewer HB Jr, Lux SE, Ronan R, John KM. Amino acid sequence of human apoLp-Gln-II (apo AII) an apolipoprotein isolated from the high-density lipoprotein complex. *Proc Natl Acad Sci USA* 1972;69: 1304–1308.
45. Sharpe CR, Sidoli A, Shelley CS, Lucero MA, Shoulders CC, Baralle FE. Human apolipoproteins AI, AII, CII, CIII. cDNA sequences and mRNA abundance. *Nucleic Acids Res* 1984;12(9):3917–3932.
46. Lagocki PA, Scanu AM. *In vitro* modulation of the apolipoprotein composition of high density lipoprotein. *J Biol Chem* 1980;255: 3701–3706.
47. Azoulay M, Henry I, Tata F, Weil D, Grzeschik KH, Chaves ME, McIntyre N, Williamson R, Humphries SE, Junien C. The structural gene for lecithin : cholesterol acyl transferase (LCAT) maps to 16q22. *Ann Hum Genet* 1987;51(pt. 2):129–136.
48. McLean J, Wion K, Drayna D, Fielding C, Lawn R. Human lecithin–cholesterol acyltransferase gene: Complete gene sequence and sites of expression. *Nucl Acids Res* 1986;14(23):9397–9408.
49. Warden CH, Langner CA, Gordon JI, Taylor BA, McLean JW, Lusis AJ. Tissue-specific expression, developmental regulation, and chromosomal mapping of the lecithin : cholesterol acyltransferase gene. *J Biol Chem* 1989;264(36):21573–21581.
50. McLean J, Fielding C, Drayna D, Dieplinger H, Baer B, Kohr W, Henzel W, Lawn R. Cloning and expression of human lecithin–cholesterol acyltransferase cDNA. *Proc Natl Acad Sci USA* 1986;83: 2335–2339.
51. Agellon L, Quinet E, Gillette T, Drayna D, Brown M, Tall AR. Organization of the human cholesteryl ester transfer protein gene. *Biochemistry* 1990;29:1372–1376.
52. Lusis AJ, Zollman S, Sparkes RS, Klisak I, Mohandas T, Drayna D, Lawn RM. Assignment of the human gene for cholesteryl ester transfer protein to chromosome 16q12–16q21. *Genomics* 1987;1:232–235.
53. Gray PW, Flaggs G, Leong SR, Weiss J, Ooi E, Elsbach P. Cloning of the cDNA of a human neutrophil bactericidal protein. *J Biol Chem* 1989;264:9505–9509.
54. Schumann RR, Leong RSR, Flaggs GW, Gray PW, Wright SD, Mathison JC, Tobias PS, Ulevitch RJ. Structure and function of lipopolysaccharide binding protein. *Science* 1990;249:1429–1431.
55. Tobias PS, Mathison JC, Ulevich RJ. A family of lipopolysaccharide binding proteins involved in responses to gram-negative sepsis. *J Biol Chem* 1988;263(27):13479–13481.

56. Day JR, Albers JJ, Lofton-Day CE, Gilbert TE, Ching AFT, Grant FJ, O'Hara PJ, Marcovina SM, Adolphson JL. Complete cDNA encoding human phospholipid transfer protein from human endothelial cells. *J Biol Chem* 1994;269:9388–9391.
57. Drayna D, Jarnagin AS, McLean J, Henzel W, Kohr W, Fielding C, Lawn R. Cloning and sequencing of human cholesteryl exter transfer protein cDNA. *Nature* 1987;327:632–634.
58. Hesler C, Swenson T, Tall AR. Purification and characterization of human plasma cholesteryl ester transfer protein. *J Biol Chem* 1987; 262:2275–2282.
59. Jiang X, Moulin P, Quinet E, Goldberg IJ, Yacoub LK, Agellon LB, Compton D, Polokoff R, Tall AR. Mammalian adipose tissue and muscle are major sources of lipid transfer protein mRNA. *J Biol Chem* 1991;266:4631–4639.
60. Quinet E, Agellon L, Marcel Y, Milne R, Kroon, Tall AR. Atherogenic diet increases cholesteryl ester transfer protein mRNA in rabbit liver. *J Clin Invest* 1990;85:357–363.
61. Masucci-Magoulas L, Moulin P, Jiang XC, Richardson H, Walsh AM, Breslow J, Tall A. Decreased cholesteryl ester transfer (CETP) mRNA, and protein and increased HDL following lipopolysaccharide or corticosteroid administration: Studies in human CETP transgenic mice. *J Clin Invest [in press]*.
62. Hesler CB, Milne RW, Swenson TL, Weech PK, Marcel YL, Tall AR. Monoclonal antibodies to the M_r 74,000 cholesteryl ester transfer protein neutralize all of the cholesteryl ester and triglyceride transfer activities in human plasma. *J Biol Chem* 1988;263:5020–5023.
63. Yen FY, Deckelbaum RJ, Mann CJ, Marcel YL, Milne RW, Tall AR. Inhibition of cholesteryl ester transfer protein activity by monoclonal antibody: Effects on cholesteryl ester formation and neutral lipid mass transfer in human plasma. *J Clin Invest* 1989;83:2018–2024.
64. Tall AR, Abreu E, Shuman JS. Separation of plasma phospholipid transfer protein from cholesterol ester/phospholipid exchange protein. *J Biol Chem* 1983;258:2174–2186.
65. Jauhiainen M, Metso J, Pahlman R, Blomqvist S, van Tol A, Ehnholm C. Human plasma phospholipid transfer protein causes high density lipoprotein conversion. *J Biol Chem* 1993;268:4032–4036.
66. Werb Z, Cohn ZA. Cholesterol metabolism in the macrophage. II. Ingestion and intracellular fate of cholesterol and cholesterol esters. *J Exp Med* 1972;135:21–44.
67. Ho YK, Brown MS, Goldstein JL. Hydrolysis and excretion of cytoplasmic cholesteryl esters by macrophages: Stimulation by high density lipoprotein and other agents. *J Lipid Res* 1980;21:391–398.
68. Ray E, Bellini F, Stoudt G, Hemperly S, Rothblat G. Influence of lecithin : cholesterol acyltransferase on cholesterol metabolism in hepatoma cells and hepatocytes. *Biochim Biophys Acta* 1980;617: 318–334.
69. Chajek T, Aron L, Fielding CJ. Interaction of lecithin : cholesterol acyltransferase and cholesteryl ester transfer protein in the transport of cholesteryl ester into sphingomyelin liposomes. *Biochemistry* 1980; 19:3673–3877.
70. Koizumi J, Mabuchi H, Yoshimura A, Michishita I, Takeda M, Itoh H, Sakai Y, Ueda K, Takeda R. Deficiency of serum cholesteryl ester transfer activity in patients with familial hyperalphalipoproteinemia. *Atherosclerosis* 1985;58:175–186.
71. Koizumi J, Inazu A, Kunimas Y, Ichiro K, Uno Y, Jakinami K, Miyamoto S, Moulin P, Tall AR, Mabuchi H, Takeda R. Serum lipoprotein lipids concentrations and composition in homozygous and heterozygous patients with cholesteryl ester transfer protein deficiency. *Atherosclerosis* 1991;90:189–196.
72. Huang Y, von Eckardstein A, Wu S, Maeda N, Assmann G. A plasma lipoprotein containing only apolipoprotein E and with γ mobility on electrophoresis releases cholesterol from cells. *Proc Natl Acad Sci USA* 1994;91:1834–1838.
73. Komaba A, Li Q, Hara H, Yokoyama S. Resistance of smooth muscle cells to assembly of high density lipoproteins with extracellular free apolipoproteins and to reduction of intracellularly accumulated cholesterol. *J Biol Chem* 1992;267:17560–17566.
74. Rothblat GH, Mahlberg FH, Johnson WJ, Phillips MC. Apolipoproteins, membrane cholesterol domains, and the regulation of cholesterol efflux. *J Lipid Res* 1992;33:1091–1097.
75. Mahlberg FH, Rothblat GH. Cellular cholesterol efflux; role of cell membrane kinetic pools and interaction with apolipoproteins AI, AII, and Cs. *J Biol Chem* 1992;267:4541–4550.
76. Oram JF. Cholesterol trafficking in cells. *Curr Opin Lipidol* 1990;1: 416–421.
77. Schmitz G, Assmann G, Robenek H, Brennhausen B. Tangier disease: A disorder of intracellular membrane traffic. *Proc Natl Acad Sci USA* 1985;82:6305–6309.
78. Phillips MC, McLean LR, Soudt GW, Rothblat GH. Mechanism of cholesterol efflux from cells. *Atherosclerosis* 1980;36:409–422.
79. Rothblat GH, Phillips MC. Mechanism of cholesterol efflux from cells. Effects of acceptor structure and concentration. *J Biol Chem* 1982;257:4775–4782.
80. Slotte JP, Oram JF, Bierman EL. Binding of high density lipoproteins to cell receptors promotes translocation of cholesterol from intracellular membranes to the cell surface. *J Biol Chem* 1987;262: 12904–12907.
81. Johnson WJ, Mahlberg FH, Chacko GK, Phillips MC, Rothblat GH. The influence of cellular and lipoprotein cholesterol contents on the flux of cholesterol between fibroblasts and high density lipoprotein. *J Biol Chem* 1988;263:14099–14106.
82. Johnson WJ, Chacko GK, Phillips MC, Rothblat GH. The efflux of lysosomal cholesterol from cells. *J Biol Chem* 1990;265:5546–5553.
83. Segrest JP, Jones MK, DeLoof H, Brouillette CG, Venkatachalapathi YV, Anantharamaiah GM. The amphipathic helix in the exchangeable apolipoproteins: A review of secondary structure and function. *J Lipid Res* 1992;33:141–166.
84. Jonas A, Kezdy KE, Wald JH. Defined apolipoprotein A-I conformations in reconstituted high density lipoprotein discs. *J Biol Chem* 1989; 264:4818–4824.
85. Tabas I, Tall AR. Mechanism of the association of HDl_3 with endothelial cells, smooth muscle cells, and fibroblasts. *J Biol Chem* 1984; 259:13897–13905.
86. Banka CL, Black AS, Curtiss LK. Localization of an apolipoprotein A-I epitope critical for lipoprotein-mediated cholesterol efflux from monocyte cells. *J Biol Chem* 1994;269:10288–10297.
87. Fleisher LN, Tall AR, Witte LD, Miller RW, Cannon PJ. Stimulation of arterial endothelial cell prostacyclin synthesis by high density lipoproteins. *J Biol Chem* 1982;257:6653–6655.
88. Pomerantz K, Tall AR, Feinmark SJ, Cannon P. Stimulation of vascular smooth muscle prostacyclin and prostaglandin E_2 synthesis by plasma high and low density lipoproteins. *J Biol Chem* 1984;259: 9587–9594.
89. Habenicht AJR, Salbach P, Goerig M, Zeh W, Janssen-Timmen U, Blattner C, King WC, Glomset JA. The LDL receptor pathway delivers arachidonic acid for eicosanoid formation in cells stimulated by platelet-derived growth factor. *Nature* 1990;345:634–636.
90. Tall AR. Plasma high density lipoproteins—metabolism and relationship to atherogenesis. *J Clin Invest* 1990;86:379–384.
91. Morishita H, Yui Y, Hattori R, Aoyama T, Kawai C. Increased hydrolysis of cholesteryl ester with prostacyclin is potentiated by high density lipoprotein through the prostacyclin stabilization. *J Clin Invest* 1990;86:1885–1891.
92. Hajjar DP, Weksler BB, Falcone DJ, Hefton JM, Tack-Goldman K, Minick CR. Prostacyclin modulates cholesteryl ester hydrolytic activity by its effect on cyclic AMP in rabbit aortic smooth muscle cells. *J Clin Invest* 1982;70:479–488.
93. Jorgensen EV, Anantharamaiah GM, Segrest JP, Gwynne JT, Handwerger S. Synthetic amphipathic peptides resembling apolipoproteins stimulate the release of human placental lactogen. *J Biol Chem* 1989; 264:9215–9219.
94. Jurgens G, Xu-Q-B, Huber LA, Bock G, Howanietz H, Wick G, Traill KN. Promotion of lymphocyte growth by high density lipoproteins (HDL). *J Biol Chem* 1989;264:8549–8556.
95. Blackburn WD, Dohlman JG, Venkatachalapathi YV, Pillion DJ, Koopman WJ, Segrest JP, Anantharamaiah GM. Apolipoprotein A-I decreases neutrophil degranulation and superoxide production. *J Lipid Res* 1991;32:1911–1928.
96. Porn MI, Akerman KEO, Slotte JP. High-density lipoproteins induce a rapid and transient release of CA^{2+} in cultured fibroblasts. *Biochem J* 1991;279:29–33.
97. Voyno-Yasenetskaya TA, Dobbs LG, Erickson SK, Hamilton RL. Low density lipoprotein- and high density lipoprotein-mediated signal transduction and exocytosis in alveolar type II cells. *Proc Natl Acad Sci USA* 1993;90:4256–4260.
98. Lipid Research Clinics Program. *The Prevalence Study, Population Studies Data Book I*. Bethesda: US Department of Health and Human Services, National Institues of Health; 1980:1527.
99. Heiss G, Johnson NJ, Reiland S, Davis CE, Tyroler HA. The epidemiology of plasma high-density lipoprotein cholesterol levels: The

Lipid Research Clinics Program Prevalence Study: Summary. *Circulation* 1980;62(Suppl IV):IV-116–IV-136.
100. Godsland IF, Wynn V, Crook D, Miller NE. Sex, plasma lipoproteins, and atherosclerosis: Prevailing assumptions and outstanding questions. *Am Heart J* 1987;114:1467–1503.
101. Tyroler HA, Glueck CJ, Christensen B, Kwiterovich PO Jr. Plasma high-density lipoprotein cholesterol comparisons in black and white populations: The Lipid Research Clinics Program Prevalence Study. *Circulation* 1980;62(Suppl IV):IV-99–IV-107.
102. Phillips NR, Havel RJ, Kane JP. Serum apolipoprotein A-I levels: Relationship to lipoprotein lipid levels and selected demographic variables. *Am J Epidemiol* 1982;116:302–313.
103. Tall AR. Plasma cholesteryl ester transfer portion. *J Lipid Res* 1993; 34:1255–1274.
104. Cheung MC, Brown BG, Wolf AC, Albers JJ. Altered particle size distribution of apolipoprotein A-I containing lipoproteins in subjects with coronary artery disease. *J Lipid Res* 1991;32:383–394.
105. Moulin PM, Cheung MC, Bruce C, Zhong S, Cocke T, Richardson H, Tall AR. Gender effects on the distribution of the cholesteryl ester transfer protein in apolipoprotein A-I defined lipoprotein subpopulations. *J Lipid Res* 1994;35:793–802.
106. Montali A, Vega GL, Grundy SM. Concentrations of apolipoprotein A-I-containing particles in patients with hypoalphalipoproteinemia. *Arterioscler Thromb* 1994;14:511–517.
107. Dietschy JM, Turley SD, Spady DK. Role of liver in the maintenance of cholesterol and low density lipoprotein homeostasis in different animal species, including humans. *J Lipid Res* 1993;34:1637–1659.
108. Brown ML, Inazu A, Hesler CB, Agellon LB, Mann C, Whitlock ME, Marcel YL, Milne RW, Koizumi J, Mabuchi H, Takeda R, Tall AR. Molecular basis of lipid transfer protein deficiency in a family with increased high density lipoproteins. *Nature* 1989;342:448–451.
109. Glass C, Pittman RC, Weinstein DB, Steinberg D. *Proc Natl Acad Sci USA* 1983;80:5435–5439.
110. Pittman RC, Knecht TP, Rosenbaum MS, Taylor CA Jr. A nonendocytotic mechanism for the selective uptake of high-density lipoprotein-associated cholesterol esters. *J Biol Chem* 1987;262:2443–2450.
111. McKnight GL, Reasoner J, Gilbert T, Sundquist KO, Hokland B, McKernan PA, Champagne J, Johnson CJ, Bailey MC, Holly R, O'Hara PJ, Oram J. Cloning and expression of a cellular high density lipoprotein-binding protein that is up-regulated by cholesterol loading of cells. *J Biol Chem* 1992;267:12131–12141.
112. Schwartz LC, Zech LA, Vandenbroek JM, Cooper PS. In: Milner N, ed. *High Density Lipoprotein and Atherosclerosis*. New York: Elsevier Science Publishing Co.; 1989:321–329.
113. Bamberger M, Lund-Katz S, Phillips MC, Rothblat GH. Mechanism of the hepatic lipase induced accumulation of high-density lipoprotein cholesterol by cells in culture. *Biochemistry* 1985;24:3693–3701.
114. Blum CB, Levy RI, Eisenberg S, Hall M III, Goebel RH, Berman M. High density lipoprotein metabolism in man. *J Clin Invest* 1977;60: 795–807.
115. Rader DJ, Castro G, Zech LA, Fruchart J-C, Brewer HB Jr. In vivo metabolism of apolipoprotein A-I on high density lipoprotein particles LpA-I and LpA-I, A-II. *J Lipid Res* 1991;32:1849–1859.
116. Brinton EA, Eisenberg S, Breslow JL. Human HDL cholesterol levels are determined by apoA-I fractional catabolic rate, which correlated inversely with estimates of HDL particle size. *Arterioscler Thromb* 1994;14:707–720.
117. Brinton EA, Eisenberg S, Breslow JL. A low-fat diet decreases high density lipoprotein (HDL) cholesterol levels by decreasing HDL apolipoprotein transport rates. *J Clin Invest* 1980;85:144.
118. Schaefer EJ, Foster DM, Zech LA, Lindgren FT, Brewer HB Jr, Levy RI. The effects of estrogen administration on plasma lipoprotein metabolism in premenopausal females. *J Clin Endocrinol Metab* 1983; 57:262–267.
119. Walsh BW, Sacks FM. Estrogen treatment raises plasma HDL concentrations by increasing HDL production. *Arterioscler Thromb* 1991; 11:140a.
120. Gordon DJ, Rifkind BM. High density lipoprotein—the clinical implications of recent studies. *N Engl J Med* 1989;321:1311–1316.
121. Tall AR. Plasma cholesteryl ester transfer protein. *J Lipid Res* 1993; 34:1255–1274.
122. Goldberg IJ, Blaner WS, Vanni TM, Moukides M, Ramakrishnan R. Role of lipoprotein lipase in the regulation of high density lipoprotein apolipoprotein metabolism. *J Clin Invest* 1990;86:463–473.
123. Ikewaki K, Rader DJ, Sakamot T, Nishiwaki M, Wakimot N, Schaefer JR, et al. Delayed catabolism of high density lipoprotein apolipoproteins A-I and A-II in human cholesteryl ester transfer protein deficiency. *J Clin Invest* 1993;93:1650–1658.
124. McGue M, Rao DC, Iselius L, Russell JM. Resolution of genetics and cultural inheritance in twin families by path analysis: Application to HDL-cholesterol. *Am J Hum Genet* 1985;37:998–1014.
125. Feinleib M, Garrison RJ, Fabsitz R, Christian JC, Hrubec Z, Bohrani NO, Kannel WB, Rosenman R, Schwartz JT, Wagner JO. The NHLBI twin study of cardiovascular disease risk factors: Methodology and summary of results. *Am J Epidemiol* 1977;106:284–285.
126. Austin MA, King M-C, Bawol RD, Hulley SB, Friedman GD. Risk factors for coronary heart disease in adult female twins: Genetic heritability and shared environmental influences. *Am J Epidemiol* 1987; 125:308–318.
127. Morton NE, Gulbrandsen CL, Rhoads GG, Kagan A, Lew R. Major loci for lipoprotein concentrations. *Am J Hum Genet* 1978;30: 583–589.
128. Lalouel JM, Morton NE. Complex segregation analysis with pointers. *Hum Hered* 1981;31:312–321.
129. Iselius L, Lalouel JM. Complex segregation analysis of hyperalphalipoproteinemia. *Metabolism* 1982;31:521–523.
130. Byard PJ, Borecki IB, Glueck CJ, Laskarzewski PM, Third JLHC, Roa DC. A genetic study of hypoalphalipoproteinemia. *Genet Epidemiol* 1984;1:43–51.
131. Friedlander Y, Kark JD, Stein Y. Complex segregation analysis of low levels of plasma high-density lipoprotein cholesterol in a sample of nuclear families in Jerusalem. *Genet Epidemiol* 1986;3:285–297.
132. Hasstedt SJ, Ash KO, Williams RR. A re-examination of major locus hypothesis for high density lipoprotein cholesterol level using 2,170 persons screened in 55 Utah pedigrees. *Am J Med Genet* 1986;24: 57–67.
133. Friedlander Y, Kark JD. Complex segregation analysis of plasma lipid and lipoprotein variables in a Jerusalem sample of nuclear families. *Hum Hered* 1987;37:7–19.
134. Bucher KD, Kaplan EB, Naboodiri KK, Glueck CJ, Laskarzewski P, Rifkind BM. Segregation analysis of low levels of high-density lipoprotein cholesterol in the collaborative Lipid Research Clinics Program family study. *Am J Hum Genet* 1987;40:489–502.
135. Smith JD, Brinton EA, Breslow JL. Polymorphisms in the human apolipoprotein A-I gene promoter region. *J Clin Invest* 1992;89: 1796–1800.
136. Angotti E, Mele E, Costanzo F, Avvedimento EV. A polymorphism (G→A transition) in the −78 position of apolipoprotein A-I promoter increases transcription efficiency. *J Biol Chem* 1994;269: 17371–17374.
137. Inazu A, Jiang X-C, Haraki T, Kamon N, Koizumi J, Mabuchi H, Takeda R, Takata K, Moriyama Y, Doi M, Tall AR. Genetic cholesteryl ester transfer protein deficiency caused by two prevalent mutations as a major determinant of increased levels of high density lipoprotein cholesterol. *J Clin Invest JCI* 1994;94:1872–1882.
138. Rees A, Shoulders CC, Stocks J, Galton DJ, Baralle FE. DNA polymorphism adjacent to the human apoprotein AI gene: Relation to hypertriglyceridemia. *Lancet* 1983;1:444–446.
139. Ordovas JM, Civeira F, Genest J Jr, et al. Restriction fragment length polymorphisms of the apolipoprotein AI, CIII, AIV gene locus. Relationships with lipids, apolipoproteins and premature coronary artery disease. *Atherosclerosis* 1991;87:75–86.
140. Dammerman N, Sandkuijl LA, Halaas J, Chung W, Breslow JL. An apolipoprotein CIII haplotype protective against hypertriglyceridemia is specified by promoter and 3′ untranslated region polymorphisms. *Proc Natl Acad Sci USA* 1993;90:4562–4566.
141. Ito Y, Azrolan N, O'Connell A, Walsh A, Breslow JL. Hypertriglyceridemia as a result of human apolipoprotein CIII gene expression in transgenic mice. *Science* 1990;249:790–793.
142. Ghiselli G, Schaefer EJ, Zech LA, Gregg RE, Brewer HB Jr. Increased prevalence of apolipoprotein E_4 in type V hyperlipoproteinemia. *J Clin Invest* 1982;70:474–477.
143. Kuusi T, Taskinen M-R, Solakivi T, Kauppinen-Maeklin R. Role of apolipoproteins E and C in type V hyperlipoproteinemia. *J Lipid Res* 1988;29:293–298.
144. Coresh J, Svenson KL, Beaty TH, Kwiterovich PO, Lusis AJ. Sib-pair linkage analysis of the lipoprotein lipase gene and lipoprotein levels: The Johns Hopkins Coronary Artery Disease Family Study. *Am J Hum Genet* 1993;53(Suppl):788.
145. Warden CH, Daluiski A, Bu X, et al. Evidence for linkage of apolipo-

protein A-II locus to plasma apolipoprotein A-II and free fatty acid levels in mice and humans. *Proc Natl Acad Sci USA* 1993;90: 10886–10899.

146. Norum RA, Lakier JB, Goldstein S, Angela A, Goldberg RB, Block WD, Noffze DK, Dolphin PJ, Edelglass J, Bogorad DD, Alaupovic P. Familial deficiency of apolipoproteins A-I and C-III precocious coronary-artery disease. *N Engl J Med* 1982;306:1513–1519.
147. Forte TM, Nichols AV, Krauss RM, Norum RA. Familial apolipoprotein AI and apolipoprotein CIII deficiency. *J Clin Invest* 1984;74: 1601–1603.
148. Ginsberg HN, Le N-A, Goldberg IJ, Gibson JC, Rubinstein A, Wang-Iverson O, Norum R, Brown WV. Apolipoprotein B metabolism in subjects with deficiency of apolipoproteins CII and AI. *J Clin Invest* 1986;78:1287–1295.
149. Karathanasis SK, Norum RA, Zannis VI, Breslow JL. An inherited polymorphism in the human apolipoprotein A-I gene locus related to the development of atherosclerosis. *Nature* 1983;301:718–720.
150. Karathanasis SK, Zannis VI, Breslow JL. A DNA insertion in the apolipoprotein A-I gene of patients with premature atherosclerosis. *Nature* 1983;305:823–825.
151. Karathanasis SK, Ferris E, Haddad IA. DNA inversion within the apolipoproteins AI/CIII/AIV-encoding gene cluster of certain patients with premature atherosclerosis. *Proc Natl Acad Sci USA* 1987;84: 7198–7202.
152. Ordovas JM, Cassidy DK, Civeira F, Bisgaier CL, Schaefer EJ. Familial apolipoprotein A-I, C-III, and A-IV deficiency and premature atherosclerosis due to deletion of a gene complex on chromosone 11. *J Biol Chem* 1989;264:16339–16342.
153. Matsunaga T, Hiasa Y, Yanagi Y, Maeda T, Hattori N, Yamakawa K, Yamanouchi Y, Tanaka I, Obara T, Hamaguchi H. Apolipoprotein A-I deficiency due to a codon 84 nonsense mutation of the apolipoprotein A-I gene. *Proc Natl Acad Sci USA* 1991;88:2793–2797.
154. Lackner KJ, Dieplinger H, Nowicka G, Schmitz G. High density lipoprotein deficiency with xanthomas. *J Clin Invest* 1993;92:2262–2273.
155. Ng DS, Leiter LA, Vezina C, Connelly PW, Hegele RA. Apolipoprotein A-I Q[−2]X causing isolated apolipoprotein A-I deficiency in a family with analphalipoproteinemia. *J Clin Invest* 1994;93:223–229.
156. Franceschini G, Sirtori CR, Capurso A, Weisgraber KH, Mahley RW. AI_{Milano} apoprotein. Decreased high density lipoprotein cholesterol levels with significant lipoprotein modifications and without clinical atherosclerosis in an Italian family. *J Clin Invest* 1980;66:892–900.
157. Orsini GB, Cerrone A, Menottia A. AI_{Milano} apoprotein identification of the complete kindred and evidence of a dominant genetic transmission. *Am J Hum Genet* 1985;37:1083–1097.
158. Franceschini G, Sirtori M, Gianfranceschi G, Sirtori CR. Relation between the HDL apoproteins and AI isoproteins in subjects with the AI_{Milano} abnormality. *Metabolism* 1981;30:502–509.
159. Gualandri V, Orsini GB, Cerrone A, Franceschini G, Sirtori CR. Familial associations of lipids and lipoproteins in a highly consanguineous population: The Limone sul Garda study. *Metabolism* 1984;34: 212–221.
160. Franceschini G, Sirtori CR, Bosisio E, Gualandri V, Orsini GB, Mogavero AM, Capurso A. Relationship of the phenotypic expression of the AI_{Milano} apoprotein with plasma lipid and lipoprotein patterns. *Atherosclerosis* 1985;58:159–174.
161. Deeb SS, Cheung MC, Peng R, Wolf AC, Stern R, Albers JJ, Knopp RH. A mutation in the human apolipoprotein A-I gene. *J Biol Chem* 1991;266:13654–13660.
161. Nichols WC, Dwulet FE, Liepnieks J, Benson MD. Variant apolipoprotein AI as a major constituent of a human hereditary amyloid. *Biochem Biophys Res Commun* 1988;156:762–768.
163. Nichols WC, Gregg RE, Brewer HB Jr, Benson MD. A mutation on apolipoprotein A-I in the Iowa type of familial amyloidotic polyneuropathy. *Genomics* 1990;8:318–323.
164. Soutar AK, Hawkins PN, Vigushin DM, Tennent GA, Booth SE, Hutton T, Nguyen O, Totty NF, Feest TG, Hsuan JJ, Pepys MB. Apolipoprotein AI mutation Arg-60 causes autosomal dominant amyloidosis. *Proc Natl Acad Sci USA* 1992;89:7389–7393.
164a. Deeb SS, Takata K, Peng RL, Kajiyama G, Albers JJ. A splice-junction mutation responsible for familial apolipoprotein A-II deficiency. *Am J Hum Genet* 1990;46:822–827.
165. Brown ML, Inazu A, Hesler CB, Agellon LB, Mann C, Whitlock ME, et al. Molecular basis of lipid transfer protein deficiency in a family with increased high density lipoproteins. *Nature* 1989;342:448–451.
166. Takahashi K, Jiang X-C, Sakai N, Yamashita S, Hirao K, Bujo H, et al. A missense mutation in the cholesteryl ester transfer protein gene with possible dominant effects on plasma high density lipoprotein. *J Clin Invest* 1993;92:2060–2064.
167. Gotoda T, Knoshita M, Shimano H. Cholesteryl ester transfer protein deficiency caused by a nonsense mutation detected in the patient's macrophage mRNA. *Biochem Biophys Res Commun* 1993;194: 519–524.
167a. Paszty C, Maeda N, Verstuyft J, Rubin EM. Apolipoprotein AI transgene corrects apolipoprotein E deficiency-induced atherosclerosis in mice. *J Clin Invest* 1994;94:899–903.
167b. Plump AS, Scott CJ, Breslow JL. Human apolipoprotein A-I gene-expression increases high density lipoprotein and suppresses atherosclerosis in the apolipoprotein E-deficient mouse. *Proc Nat'l Acad Sci USA* 1994;91:9607–9611.
168. Li H, Reddick RL, Maeda N. Lack of apoA-I is not associated with increased susceptibility to atherosclerosis in mice. *Arterioscler Thromb* 1993;13:1814–1821.
168a. Inazu A, Brown ML, Hesler CB, Agellon LB, Koizumi J, Takata K, et al. Increased high density lipoprotein caused by a common cholesteryl ester transfer protein gene mutation. *N Engl J Med* 1990;323: 1234–1238.
169. Plump AS, Smith JD, Hayek T, Aalto-Setala K, Walsh A, Verstuyft JG, Rubin EM, Breslow JL. Severe hypercholesterolemia and atherosclerosis in apolipoprotein E-deficient mice created by homologous recombination in ES cells. *Cell* 1992;71:343–353.
170. Zhang SH, Reddick RL, Piedrahita JA, Maeda N. Spontaneous hypercholesterolemia and arterial lesions in mice lacking apolipoprotein E. *Science* 1992;258:468–471.
171. Rubin EM, Ishida BY, Clift SM, Krauss RM. Expression of human apolipoprotein A-I in transgenic mice results in reduced plasma levels of murine apolipoprotein A-I and the appearance of two new high density lipoprotein size subclasses. *Proc Natl Acad Sci USA* 1991; 88:434–438.
172. Hayek T, Ito Y, Azrolan N, Verdery RB, Aalto-Setala K, Walsh A, Breslow JL. Dietary fat increases high density lipoprotein (HDL) levels both by increasing the transport rates and decreasing the fractional catabolic rates of HDL cholesterol ester and apolipoprotein (apo) A-I. *J Clin Invest* 1993;93:1665–1699.
172a. Swanson ME, Hughes TE, St Denny I, France DS, Paternity JR Jr, Tapparelli C, Gfeller Berki K. High level expression of human apolipoprotein A-I in transgenic rats raises total serum high density lipoprotein cholesterol and lowers rat apolipoprotein A-I. *Transgen Res* 1992; 1:142–147.
173. Chajek-Shaul T, Hayek T, Walsh A, Breslow JL. Expression of the human apolipoprotein A-I gene in transgenic mice alters high density lipoprotein (HDL) particle size distribution and diminishes selective uptake of HDL cholesteryl esters. *Proc Natl Acad Sci USA* 1991;88: 6731–6735.
173a. Williamson R, Lee D, Hagaman J, Maeda N. Marked reduction of high density lipoprotein cholesterol in mice genetically modified to lack apolipoprotein A-I. *Proc Natl Acad Sci USA* 1992;89:7134–7138.
174. Plump AS, Hayek T, Walsh A, Breslow JL. Diminished HDL cholesterol ester flux in apo A-I deficient mice. *Circulation* 1993;88:2266a.
174a. Schultz JR, Gong EL, McCall MR, Nichols AV, Clift SM, Rubin EM. Expression of human apolipoprotein A-II and its effect on high density lipoproteins in transgenic mice. *J Biol Chem* 1992;267:21630–21660.
175. Hedrick CC, Castellani LW, Warden CH, Puppione DL, Lusis AJ. Influence of mouse apolipoprotein A-II on plasma lipoproteins in transgenic mice. *J Biol Chem* 1993;268:20676–20682.
176. Shimada M, Shimano H, Gotoda T, Yamamoto K, Kawamura M, Inaba T, Yazaki Y, Yamada N. Overexpression of human lipoprotein lipase in transgenic mice. *J Biol Chem* 1993;268:17924–17929.
177. Agellon LB, Walsh A, Hayek T, Moulin P, Jiang X, Shelanski SA, Breslow JL, Tall AR. Reduced high density lipoprotein cholesterol in human cholesteryl ester transfer protein transgenic mice. *J Biol Chem* 1991;266:10796–10801.
178. Hayek T, Chajek-Shaul T, Walsh A, Agelon LB, Moulin P, Tall AR, Breslow JL. An interaction between the human cholesteryl ester transfer protein (CETP) and apolipoprotein A-I genes in transgenic mice results in a profound CETP-mediated depression of HDL cholesterol levels. *J Clin Invest* 1992;90:505–510.
179. Hayek T, Azrolan N, Verdery RB, Walsh A, Chajek-Shaul T, Agellon LB, Tall AR, Breslow JL. Hypertriglyceridemia and cholesteryl ester

transfer protein interact to dramatically alter high density lipoprotein levels, particle sizes and metabolism. *J Clin Invest* 1993;13: 1359–1367.
180. Zhong S, Goldberg IJ, Bruce C, Rubin E, Breslow J, Tall A. Human apoA-II inhibits the hydrolysis of HDL triglyceride and the decrease of HDL size induced by hypertriglyceridemia and cholesteryl ester transfer protein in transgenic mice. *J Clin Invest [in press].*
181. Thuren T, Wilcox RW, Sisson P, Waite P. Hepatic lipase hydrolysis of lipid. Regulation by apolipoproteins. *J Biol Chem* 1991;266: 4853–4861.
182. Warden CH, Hedrick CC, Qiao J-H, Castellani LW, Lusis AJ. Atherosclerosis in transgenic mice overexpressing apolipoprotein A-II. *Science* 1993;261:469–472.
183. Marotti KR, Castle CK, Murray RW, Rehberg EF, Polites HG, Melchior GW. The role of cholesteryl ester transfer protein in primate apolipoprotein A-I metabolism—insights from studies with transgenic mice. *Arterioscler Thromb* 1992;12:736–744.
184. Jiang X-C, Masucci-Magoulas L, Mar J, Lin M, Walsh A, Breslow JL, Tall A. Down-regulation of LDL receptor mRNA in human cholesteryl ester transfer protein transgenic mice: Mechanism to explain accumulation of lipoprotein B particles. *J Biol Chem* 1993;268: 27406–27412.
185. Paigen B, Mitchell D, Reue K, Morrow A, Lusis A, Leboeuf RC. Ath-1, a gene determining atherosclerosis susceptibility and high density lipoprotein levels in mice. *Proc Natl Acad Sci USA* 1987;84: 3763–3767.
186. Schultz JR, Versuyft JG, Gong EL, Nichols AV, Rubin EM. Protein composition determines the anti-atherogenic properties of HDL in transgenic mice. *Nature* 1993;365:762–764.
187. Marotti KR, Castle CK, Boyle TP, Lin AH, Murray RW, Melchior GW. Severe atherosclerosis in transgenic mice expressing simian cholesteryl ester transfer protein. *Nature* 1993;364:73–75.
188. Ishibashi S, Goldstein JL, Brown MS, Herz J, Burns DK. Massive xanthomatosis and atherosclerosis in cholesterol-fed low density lipoprotein receptor-negative mice. *J Clin Invest* 1994;93:1885–1893.
189. Ernst N, Fisher M, Smith W, et al. The association of plasma high-density lipoprotein cholesterol with dietary intake and alcohol consumption: the Lipid Research Clinics Program Prevalence Study. *Circulation* 1980;62(Suppl IV):IV-41–IV-52.
190. Dwyer T, Calvert GD, Baghurst KI, Leitch DR. Diet, other lifestyle factors and HDL-cholesterol in a population of Australian male service recruits. *Am J Epidemiol* 1981;114:683–696.
191. Sacks FM, Ornish D, Rosner B, McLanahan S, Castelli WP, Kass EH. Plasma lipoprotein levels in vegetarians: The effects of ingestion of fats from dairy products. *JAMA* 1985;254:1337–1341.
192. Thorogood M, Carter R, Benfield R, McPherson K, Mann JI. Plasma lipids and lipoprotein cholesterol concentrations in people with different diets in Britain. *Br Med J* 1987;295:351–353.
193. Arntzenius AC, Kromhout D, Barth JD, et al. Diet, lipoproteins, and the progression of coronary atherosclerosis: The Leiden Intervention Trial. *N Engl J Med* 1985;312:805–811.
194. Howard BV. Lipoprotein metabolism in diabetes mellitus. *J Lipid Res* 1987;28:613–628.
195. Belfrage P, Berg B, Hagerstrand I, Nilsson-Ehle P, Tornqvist H, Wiebe T. Alterations of lipid metabolism in healthy volunteers during long-term ethanol intake. *Eur J Clin Invest* 1977;7:127–131.
196. Savolainen MJ, Hannuksela M, Seppaenen S, Kervinen K, Kesaeniemi YA. Increased high-density lipoprotein cholesterol concentration in alcoholics is related to low cholesteryl ester transfer protein activity. *Eur J Clin Invest* 1990;20:593–599.
197. Hannuksela M, Marcel YL, Kesaeniemi YA, Savolainen MJ. Reduction in the concentration and activity of plasma cholesteryl ester transfer protein by alcohol. *J Lipid Res* 1992;33:737–744.
198. Gordon DJ, Rifkind BM. High density lipoprotein—the clinical implications of recent studies. *N Engl J Med* 1989;321:1311–1316.
199. Rhoads GG, Gulbrandsen CL, Kagan A. Serum lipoproteins and coronary heart disease in a population study of Hawaii Japanese men. *N Engl J Med* 1976;294:293–298.
200. Gordon DJ, Probstfield JL, Garrison RJ, Neaton JD, Castelli WP, Knoke JD, Jacobs DR Jr, Bangdiwala S, Tyrole HA. High-density lipoprotein cholesterol and cardiovascular disease. *Circulation* 1989; 79:8–15.
201. Gordon DJ, Knoke J, Probstfield JL, Superko R, Tyroler HA. High density lipoprotein cholesterol and coronary heart disease in hypercholesterolemic men: The Lipid Research Clinics Coronary Primary Prevention trial. *Circulation* 1986;74:1217–1225.
202. Canner PL, Berge KG, Wenger NK, et al. Fifteen year mortality in Coronary Drug Project patients: Long-term benefit with niacin. *J Am Coll Cardiol* 1986;8:1245–1255.
203. Levy RI, Brenske JF, Epstein SE, et al. The influence of changes in lipid values induced by cholestyramine and diet on progression of coronary artery disease: Results of the NHLBI Type II Coronary Intervention study. *Circulation* 1984;69:325–327.
204. Blakenhorn DH, Nessim SA, Johnson RL, Sammarco ME, Azen SP, Cashin-Hemphill L. Beneficial effects of combined colestipol–niacin therapy on coronary atherosclerosis and coronary venous bypass grafts. *JAMA* 1987;257:3233–3240.
205. Manninen V, Elo MO, Frick MH, et al. Lipid alterations and decline in the incidence of coronary heart disease in the Helsinki Heart Study. *JAMA* 1988;260:641–651.
206. Gaziano JM, Buring JE, Breslow JL, Goldhaber SZ, Rosner B, VanDenburgh M, Willett W, Hennekens H. Moderate alcohol intake, increases levels of high-density lipoprotein and its subfractions, and decreased risk of myocardial infarction. *N Engl J Med* 1993;329: 1829–1834.
207. Genest JJ Jr, Martin-Munley SS, McNamara JR, et al. Familial lipoprotein disorders in patients with premature coronary artery disease. *Circulation* 1992;85:2025–2033.
208. Austin MA, Breslow JL, Hennekens CH, Buring JE, Willet WC, Krauss RM. Low-density lipoprotein subclass patterns and risk of myocardial infarction. *JAMA* 1988;260:1917–1921.
209. Patsch JR, Karlin JB, Scott LW, Smith LC, Gotto AM Jr. Inverse relationship between blood levels of high density lipoprotein subfraction 2 and magnitude of postprandial lipemia. *Proc Natl Acad Sci USA* 1983;80:1449–1453.
210. Castelli WP, Abbott RF, McNamara PM. Summary estimates of cholesterol used to predict coronary heart disease. *Circulation* 1983;67: 730–734.
211. Austin MA. Plasma triglyceride and coronary heart disease. *Arterioscler Thromb* 1991;11:2–14.
212. Manninen V, Tenkanen L, Koskinen P, Huttunen JK, Maenttaeri M, Heinone OP, Frick MH. Joint effects of serum triglyceride and LDL cholesterol and HDL cholesterol concentrations on coronary heart disease risk in the Helsinki Heart Study. *Circulation* 1992;85:37–45.
213. Stampfer MJ, Sacks FM, Ssalvini S, Willett WC, Hennekens CH. A prospective study of cholesterol, apolipoproteins, and the risk of myocardial infarction. *N Engl J Med* 1991;325:373–381.
214. Cohen JC, Grundy SM. Normal postprandial lipemia in men with low plasma HDL concentrations. *Arterioscler Thromb* 1992;12:972–975.
215. Miller M, Kwiterovich O Jr, Bachorik PS, Georgopoulos A. Decreased postprandial response to a fat meal in normotriglyceridemic men with hypoalphalipoproteinemia. *Arterioscler Thromb* 1993;13:385–392.
216. Parthasarathy S, Barnett J, Fong LG. High-density lipoprotein inhibits the oxidative modification of low-density lipoprotein. *Biochim Biophys Acta* 1990;1044:275–283.
217. Navab M, Imes SS, Hama SY, et al. Monocyte transmigration induced by modification of low density lipoprotein in cocultures of human aortic wall cells is due to induction of monocyte chemotactic protein 1 synthesis and is abolished by high density lipoprotein. *J Clin Invest* 1991;88:2039–2046.
218. Hessler JR, Robertson AL, Chisholm GM. LDL-induced cytotoxicity and its inhibition by HDL in human vascular smooth muscle and endothelial cell in culture. *Atherosclerosis* 1979;32:213–229.
219. Kunitake ST, Jarvis MR, Hamilton RL, Kane JP. Binding of transition metals by apolipoprotein A-I containing plasma lipoproteins: Inhibition of oxidation of low density lipoproteins. *Proc Natl Acad Sci USA* 1992;89:6993–6997.
220. Mackness MI, Arrol S, Abbott C, Durrington PN. Protection of low-density lipoprotein against oxidative modification by high-density lipoprotein associated paraoxonase. *Atherosclerosis* 1993;104: 129–135.
221. Kelso GJ, Stuart WD, Richter RJ, Furlong CE, Jordan-Starck TC, Harmony JAK. Apolipoprotein J is associated with paraoxonase in human plasma. *Biochemistry* 1994;33:832–839.
222. Bowry W, Stanley KK, Stocker R. High density lipoprotein is the major carrier of lipid hydroperoxides in human blood plasma from fasting donors. *Proc Natl Acad Sci USA* 1992;89:10316–10320.
223. Francis GA, Mendez AJ, Bierman EL, Heinecke JW. Oxidative tyrosylation of high density lipoprotein by peroxidase enhances cholesterol removal from cultured fibroblasts and macrophage foam cells. *Proc Natl Acad Sci USA* 1993;90:6631–6635.

Atherosclerosis and Coronary Artery Disease, edited by V. Fuster, R. Ross, and E. J. Topol. Lippincott-Raven Publishers, Philadelphia © 1996.

CHAPTER 8

Oxidized Lipoproteins and Atherosclerosis

Guy M. Chisolm III and Marc S. Penn

Key Words: Antioxidant; Cholesterol; Lipoproteins; Low-density lipoproteins; Oxidation.

INTRODUCTION

The concept that oxidized lipoproteins are involved in atherosclerosis lesion development was formulated from demonstrations (a) that low-density lipoprotein (LDL) can injure cells under certain conditions (1,2), which were later shown to be conditions that facilitated oxidation of the lipoprotein (3,4); (b) that LDL modified by malondialdehyde, a product of the oxidation of unsaturated fatty acids, was taken up by monocyte/macrophages via scavenger receptors (5); and (c) that macrophages will also take up via scavenger receptors LDL that was modified by cultured endothelial cells (6). Endothelial modification of LDL was later shown to be via oxidation, mediated by reactive oxygen species produced by the cells (7,8). Cultured smooth muscle cells (7,9), stimulated monocytes (10), neutrophils (10), and macrophages (11) were also shown to oxidize LDL. Since these discoveries, research on lipoprotein oxidation has undergone a virtual explosion. Mechanisms for LDL oxidation have been explored, the dozens of products of this oxidation have been partially identified, and numerous effects of oxidized LDL on cultured cells have been described. Among the latter are a number of cell-altering phenomena that appear to be atherogenic in nature and that do not appear duplicable by exposing cells to native LDL. Thus, even based only on work in vitro, one could speculate that LDL oxidation might play a causal role in atherogenesis and even in later lesion development.

For years it has been demonstrated that LDL-like material extracted from vascular lesions of humans and animals had properties distinct from those of plasma LDL (12,13). Changes in charge, density, and lipid composition had been reported. This literature has been more recently reinterpreted to be indicative of the oxidation of this lesion component. Indeed, recent data examining such arterial lipoprotein fractions for direct signs of oxidation show that the resident arterial lipoprotein pool is at least in part oxidized. These examinations include studies showing that antibodies recognizing oxidized but not native LDL bind epitopes in human and animal atherosclerotic lesions (14–18). Whether the lipoprotein pool is oxidized locally at a lesion or prelesion

G. M. Chisolm III and M. S. Penn: Department of Cell Biology, Cleveland Clinic Foundation, Cleveland, Ohio 44195.

site, or whether an oxidized subfraction of circulating plasma LDL is selectively retained in the vessel wall, has not been determined, although, as mentioned above, the cell types populating an early lesion site have been shown in culture to be capable of LDL oxidation.

The congruence of the actions of oxidized LDL on cells with the known features of atherosclerotic lesions and the evidence that LDL in lesions is oxidized suggest strongly an atherosclerotic role for the altered lipoprotein. Perhaps the most compelling data are a growing number of studies showing that antioxidant administration retards the progression of atherosclerosis. Although many antioxidants are known to have other actions that could perhaps explain their antiatherosclerotic activities, the fact that decreased atherosclerosis has been observed with a wide variety of antioxidants, including probucol (19–21), α-tocopherol (22–24), diphenylphenylenediamine (DPPD) (25), butylated hydroxytoluene (BHT) (26), and β-carotene (27), and the fact that this has been demonstrated in rats (28), rabbits (19–21,25,26), primates (22,29), and humans (23,24,27) does not disprove but lessens the likelihood that alternate mechanisms can explain each of these results. Nevertheless, we must remain critical of the data and unconvinced that oxidized LDL is the perpetrator of atherosclerosis until definitive proof has been obtained. To date we can say that oxidized lipoproteins reside in atherosclerotic lesions and that antioxidant data in vivo and cell function data in culture indirectly support the hypothesis that oxidized LDL is a mediator of the disease.

The focus of the literature on oxidized lipoproteins has centered on LDL because it serves as the principal carrier of cholesterol in normal human plasma and because of the strong correlations between elevated plasma LDL or cholesterol levels and increased atherosclerosis risk. But there are interesting data accumulating on the effects of oxidized forms of VLDL and HDL, and it is appropriate to speculate that they may become oxidized by similar mechanisms and that their altered biochemical characteristics may also adversely affect physiological processes.

WHAT ARE OXIDIZED LIPOPROTEINS?

As with many complex biochemical systems, the beginning approaches to the topic of oxidized lipoproteins introduced ambiguities that have been difficult to resolve. The terms oxidized HDL, oxidized LDL, and oxidized VLDL are useful terms only to the extent that they signify the type of modification to the native lipoprotein; they are imprecise in many aspects that are important to our understanding of lipoprotein oxidation. For example, the term oxidized LDL does not indicate the degree to which the lipoprotein is oxidatively modified. It is clear that LDL oxidation can be regarded as a continuum. One can oxidize LDL in vitro to a desired level and then block the progression. It is possible, therefore, to introduce into an experiment LDL that is oxidized to an infinite number of different levels. These differentially oxidized preparations can evoke different responses in cells and in vivo. This is illustrated by several diverse studies. In one of these, for example, LDL that was oxidized to a relatively low degree, so that it was still recognized by the LDL (B/E) receptor, has been referred to as "minimally modified" LDL. This preparation induced monocyte adhesion in endothelial cells, whereas native LDL or LDL that was oxidized to a greater extent did not (30).

In addition, the term oxidized LDL is used to describe the oxidized lipoprotein irrespective of the means by which the oxidation was mediated. There are indications that LDL oxidized by metal ions or by ultraviolet light may have quite different properties. For example, B/E receptor recognition is destroyed in the first process but not the second at comparable levels of lipid peroxidation (31). Furthermore, the same term has been applied to describe LDL-like extracts from vascular lesions identified by antibodies that recognize oxidized LDL but not native LDL. Although this would suggest that the epitope to which the antibody would bind, e.g., a lipid peroxidation product linked to a particular amino acid residue (32), was in common with LDL oxidized in vitro, it does not validate further similarities between LDL oxidized in vitro and oxidized LDL residing in a lesion.

Finally, the term oxidized LDL does not distinguish between LDL subjected to free-radical-initiated lipid peroxidation and LDL that has taken up, or gained by exchange, various lipid oxidation products from cells, tissue sites, or other lipoproteins.

These considerations make generalizations about oxidized LDL difficult with respect to its categorization, its biochemical properties, its effects on cell functions, and its disposition in vivo. Until more is determined about the nature of oxidized LDL in vivo in terms of measurable parameters, one should maintain a healthy skepticism about extrapolating findings in vitro to an in vivo setting.

Some studies refer to oxidized LDL as modified LDL; however, this term is also used to describe more specific forms of chemically modified LDL, such as acetylated LDL, malondialdehyde (MDA)-modified LDL, or methylated LDL. As with increasing oxidation, increasing modification with acetic anhydride or MDA decreases recognition by B/E receptors and increases recognition by scavenger receptors on macrophages. Oxidized LDL appears to be modified, in part, by MDA (15), but similarities between oxidized LDL and MDA-modified LDL beyond this are few. The amino acid residues of oxidized LDL appear modified by multiple lipid oxidation products in addition to MDA (33). Although acetylated LDL was a ligand used to define scavenger receptors, acetylation of LDL does not appear to occur in vivo (34). Thus, chemically modified forms of LDL cannot be expected to share many biological properties with oxidized LDL but may be useful to link specific biological properties to specific types of chemical change.

Oxidation of LDL leads to dramatic changes in both the apolipoprotein apo B100 and virtually all of the lipid moieties of the lipoprotein. There appear to be two distinct classes of changes that take place in the apoprotein. Oxidative fragmentation takes place nonenzymatically, rendering the single polypeptide chain in pieces but still associated with the surface of the particle (35). Second, reactive residues of the apoprotein, lysine and histidine, for example, bind to lipid peroxidation products, including MDA and 4-hydroxynonenal (4-HNE) (33), both of which are aldehyde breakdown products of polyunsaturated fatty acyl moieties. These changes increase the net negative charge of the lipoprotein from its native state, alter receptor recognition, and thereby increase the rate at which oxidized LDL is removed from plasma (36,37).

It is perhaps not surprising that numerous new lipid products are formed when LDL is oxidized, because the native lipoprotein contains dozens of distinct lipids including cholesterol, various cholesterol esters, several classes of phospholipids, each potentially with a variety of fatty acid moieties, and various triglycerides. Furthermore, numerous other lipophilic substances are formed, including vitamins and carotenoids, some of which are antioxidants. Each of these substances can potentially form multiple products on oxidation. It has been shown, for example, that both cupric ion and cell-mediated oxidation of LDL transform its free cholesterol component into numerous oxysterols, including 7-ketocholesterol, 7α- and 7β-hydroxycholesterol, epoxysterols, and 7α- and 7β-hydroperoxycholesterols (38–40).

A variety of carbonyls are formed from the oxidation of unsaturated fatty acids, including 4-HNE, MDA, hexanal, and 2,4-heptadienal, among many others (33). α-Tocopherol is consumed as LDL oxidation proceeds (41), as is the antioxidant ubiquinol (42). It is of potential importance to recognize that α-tocopherol has been shown to have both oxidant and antioxidant capabilities under different circumstances (43). As the antioxidant capacity of the lipoprotein diminishes, the lipid oxidation products formed include hydroperoxides of cholesteryl esters, phospholipids, and triglycerides (44) as well as various oxysterols and carbonyls.

In addition to the formation of numerous potentially bioactive lipid oxidation products, another lipid, lysophosphatidylcholine (lysoPC), is formed indirectly, secondary to the oxidation of LDL. A phospholipase A_2 activity was discovered in association with LDL during oxidation (8) and has subsequently been characterized (45–49). This platelet-activating factor hydrolase-like activity (45) has been described as an enzymatic activity inherent to apo B (48) that appears to prefer phosphatidylcholine as substrate only after oxidation of the unsaturated fatty acid in the 2-position. The lysoPC thus formed has the potential to alter a number of cell functions, many of which are described below.

THE OCCURRENCE OF OXIDIZED LDL IN VIVO

Although the unknown nature of oxidized LDL in vivo complicates its definition, and although the relationship of LDL oxidized in vivo to that oxidized in vitro is poorly understood, there is, nevertheless, general agreement that a form of oxidized LDL does in fact exist in vivo. Evidence most strongly supports that it resides in atherosclerotic lesions, but there are also instances in which it has been reported in plasma and other tissue sites. Antibodies that recognize specific lipid peroxidation products bound to lysyl residues of polypeptides, e.g., MDA, 4-HNE (15), recognize oxidized but not native LDL and have been shown to bind sites in human (18) and animal (15,18,50) atherosclerotic lesions. Antibodies have also been made against oxidized LDL that do not recognize native LDL and that bind unknown epitopes of oxidized LDL and also bind to sites in lesions (14,16). That the binding sites for the antibodies in lesions are at least in part on LDL and do not simply reflect lipid oxidation products bound to nonlipoprotein proteins is suggested by studies showing partial colocalization with antibodies recognizing apo B (15) and those showing that LDL-like fractions extracted from lesions also bind to these antibodies (51).

Other properties of such LDL-like preparations from lesions corroborate the notion that oxidized lipoproteins reside in lesions. For example, LDL from arterial lesions has been shown to have reduced α-tocopherol, increased TBA reactivity, increased negative net charge, and increased uptake by macrophages compared to plasma LDL (51–53), all of which are traits in common with oxidized LDL.

There are studies that suggest that oxidized forms of lipoproteins also exist in plasma. One general group of these shows that a variety of parameters used to quantify lipoprotein oxidation indicate elevated plasma levels of oxidized lipoproteins accompanying diabetes in subjects in poor glycemic control (for reviews, see refs. 54,55) and in diabetic experimental animals (56–58).

There is speculation that oxidized forms of LDL also circulate in normal human plasma. This speculation is based on the separation from human and primate LDL of a small subfraction, referred to as LDL$^-$, that has characteristics in common with LDL oxidized in vitro (59,60). In primates, these characteristics included increased negative charge, increased amounts of cholesterol oxides, and enhanced toxicity to cultured endothelial cells in comparison to native LDL. In both hypercholesterolemic and normocholesterolemic primates, the LDL$^-$ subfraction constituted about 5% of total LDL; however, over 50% of the cholesterol of LDL$^-$ was oxidized, whereas only about 10% of the native LDL cholesterol was oxidized (60).

In addition to these instances, there have been reports of increased lipid oxidation products in the plasma of patients with higher risk of myocardial infarction (61,62). Interestingly, antibodies that recognize oxidized LDL (and MDA-modified protein in general) but not native LDL have been measured in the plasma of normal humans (63). The antibody levels have been shown to be elevated in the plasma of patients with advancing carotid atherosclerosis (63). The role of these antibodies in disease is uncertain but is the subject of further research.

The above reports suggesting the existence of plasma-borne oxidized lipoproteins invite speculation that the oxidized forms of LDL accumulating in lesions could have resulted from the selective intimal sequestration of plasma-borne oxidized LDL. To date it is difficult to differentiate this possibility from the hypothesis that the arterial pool of oxidized LDL is derived from LDL that entered the intima from plasma as native LDL but was then oxidized locally by the cells in the lesion site. Reports showing that oxidized forms of lipoproteins circulate in the plasma of diabetic or hypercholesterolemic subjects are difficult to interpret. Some of the assays used to track lipid oxidation products in plasma are believed inaccurate because of interfering substances from the plasma. Furthermore, those studies that find oxidation products in isolated plasma lipoprotein preparations must contend with the caveat that the oxidation products they measure may have formed during isolation as a result of an enhanced susceptibility to oxidation rather than have circulated in vivo as an oxidized entity. These two alternatives may be difficult to distinguish, although either could certainly have important implications. The concept that a subfraction of human LDL is more susceptible to oxidation than the remainder has been demonstrated in humans and shown attributable to a small, dense subpopulation of LDL, the concentration of which correlates with vascular disease (64,65).

In summary, we can say with confidence that a form of oxidized LDL exists in atherosclerotic lesions, and there are indications that oxidized LDL or a subfraction of LDL highly susceptible to oxidation circulates in plasma under certain conditions. Whether the oxidized LDL causes atherosclerosis or causes certain aspects of lesion development is currently only a hypothesis, but one for which supporting indirect data are accumulating. These indirect data include the atherogenic nature of the changes in cell function that can be induced in vitro by oxidized but not native LDL and the effectiveness of antioxidants to retard lesion progression, both of which are reviewed in subsequent sections.

OXIDATION OF LDL BY CELLS

That vascular cells can mediate the oxidation of LDL was shown by two groups simultaneously in 1984 (7,8). Both of these studies showed that the previously reported modification of LDL by endothelial cells (6) resulted from LDL oxidation; endothelial-cell-modified LDL and LDL oxidized in cell-free systems were revealed to be identical with respect to transforming LDL into both a ligand for scavenger receptors (8) and a potent cytotoxin (7). In the latter study vascular smooth muscle cells were shown to oxidize LDL as well as endothelial cells, and both endothelial and smooth muscle cells were shown to be more potent than fibroblasts at mediating the oxidative changes. Subsequent studies showed that activated monocytes (10), neutrophils (10), and macrophages (11), all known to produce reactive oxygen species, were capable of LDL oxidation. It has been recognized through more recent studies that the mechanisms by which these different cells oxidize LDL may be distinct from one another.

In addition, the metal ion content of the medium may influence which among multiple possible mechanisms of oxidation prevails in LDL oxidation by cells. Metal-ion-containing media were used in the studies first reporting LDL oxidation by vascular cells (7,8). The presence of metal ions is believed to play an essential role in the oxidation of LDL by both endothelial and smooth muscle cells (9,66). A variety of mechanisms have been proposed to explain LDL oxidation by these cells, but these remain the subject of speculation. Complications include the fact that free metal ions can facilitate the oxidation of LDL in the absence of cells, albeit more slowly. Even if metal-ion-dependent mechanisms could be elucidated unequivocally in culture, their relevance would require identifying the in vivo source and form of the metal.

Superoxide anion has been proposed to be essential in endothelial cell oxidation of LDL by some researchers (67) but deemed unnecessary by others (68). 15-Lipoxygenase has been suggested as an essential component of endothelial cell oxidation of LDL (68), but lipoxygenase involvement has been refuted in metal-ion-dependent mechanisms of cell-mediated LDL oxidation (69). Nitric oxide, combined with superoxide to form peroxynitrite, has been studied as an oxidant capable of oxidizing LDL, but there are also data to support a role for NO as an antioxidant (70,71). Thiols have been proposed to play an essential role in metal-ion-dependent smooth muscle cell oxidation of LDL (72–74). The role of the cells was linked to conversion of cystine to cysteine, which generated radicals capable of initiating peroxidation (73,74). There are, however, apparent shortcomings in this scheme as well (70).

Efforts to determine the mechanisms of macrophage oxidation of LDL show similarities to endothelial-cell-mediated oxidation in that most have been delineated in metal-ion-containing media. Additional mechanisms have been proposed involving hydrogen peroxide and peroxidases (70). Recently it has been demonstrated that myeloperoxidase, a secreted heme protein product of activated macrophages, is present in human atherosclerotic lesions and that myeloperoxidase can generate reactive agents that can oxidize LDL (75).

One of the unsettled issues surrounding the likelihood of vascular cells mediating lipoprotein oxidation in a lesion site in vivo is whether or not there is a physiological source of metal ions. Unlike many of the culture media used to study LDL oxidation, circulating plasma and interstitial fluid are not believed to carry free cupric ion. Of particular interest, then, is the mechanism by which cells in culture can oxidize LDL in metal-ion-free medium. One cell type shown capable of this is the adherent human monocyte (10). The mechanism by which monocytes oxidize LDL has been shown to require stimulation of the monocytes, for example, with phagocytic stimuli (10) and release by the monocytes of superoxide anion (76,77). There are also data suggesting that stimulation of monocyte 15-lipoxygenase may be involved (78). Although metal ion putatively is not present in the culture medium used in these studies, it is nevertheless required for monocyte oxidation of LDL, suggesting that the monocytes themselves supply metal ion to the reaction. It was recently demonstrated that the copper-carrying acute-phase protein ceruloplasmin, formerly characterized predominantly as an antioxidant, is actually capable of oxidizing LDL, even in a cell-free system (79), suggesting ceruloplasmin to be a physiological supplier of metal ion to lipoprotein oxidation reactions. Studies have recently been performed that demonstrate that U937 cells, a monocytoid cell line that behaves similar to monocytes with respect to LDL oxidation (80), can oxidize LDL only after secretion of ceruloplasmin following stimulation (81). Thus, one hypothetical mechanism for oxidation of LDL by monocyte-derived macrophages includes enhanced lipoxygenase activity, superoxide anion production, and ceruloplasmin secretion, all secondary to stimulation.

Although the evidence that a small fraction of circulating LDL may be oxidized allows speculation that arterial oxidized LDL is selectively sequestered in the artery wall, there is other evidence suggesting that arterial tissue components could facilitate local oxidation of plasma LDL that entered the tissue unaltered. It was demonstrated long ago that plasma LDL enters the interstitial space of the normal intima and media, and it was shown by acute elevation of plasma LDL that the rate of entry is proportional to the plasma concentration (82). The concept that the interstitial space of even normal intima contains LDL is accepted. It was also demonstrated long ago that connective tissue elements present in the interstitium had the capacity to bind LDL. Proteoglycans, collagen, and elastin have all been shown to bind lipids and lipoproteins. The role played by these phenomena in lipoprotein oxidation is uncertain, but a number of possibilities have been demonstrated. The susceptibility of LDL to oxidation increases markedly after binding to proteoglycans (83,84). This increase pertains even after the lipoprotein is dissociated from the proteoglycan (84). This invites speculation that native LDL bound to proteoglycan not only would increase the residence time of the lipoprotein in the tissue pool and thereby enhance the probability that it could be oxidized but also would alter the lipoprotein to a more susceptible state. It has been shown that once oxidized, LDL binds more readily to collagen (85).

METABOLISM OF OXIDIZED LDL BY CELLS

Cellular Recognition and Uptake of Oxidized LDL

The extent of LDL oxidation correlates with decreasing recognition by the B/E (LDL) receptor. The B/E receptor thus recognizes only lightly oxidized (''minimally modified'') forms of oxidized LDL. Other potential pathways for oxidized lipoprotein delivery to cellular compartments include receptor-mediated internalization by other receptors, direct delivery of the more polar oxidized lipids via the aqueous phase, direct delivery of the more lipophilic surface-oriented lipids by collision with the cell membrane, and nonspecific phagocytosis of aggregated oxidized lipoproteins. These are represented pictorially in Fig. 1.

The discoveries that receptors other than the B/E and scavenger receptors exist that recognize oxidized LDL emanated from data showing that oxidized LDL could not be completely displaced from the scavenger receptors by acetylated LDL. This suggested the existence of additional scavenger receptors that recognize oxidized, but not acetylated, LDL (86,87). Later, however, such nonreciprocal competition between these two ligands was also shown to be exhibited by each of two forms of scavenger receptors when exclusively overexpressed after transfection into Chinese hamster ovary cells (88). As LDL oxidation progresses (by means other than ultraviolet irradiation), the lipoprotein loses its ability to be recognized by the B/E receptor, and its affinity increases for other receptors, including the class A scavenger receptors types I and II (SR-AI and SR-AII), which also recognize acetylated LDL (6,89), a subclass of Fc receptors, FcγRII–B2 (90), CD36, which recognizes lightly oxidized LDL (91), and SR-BI, a CD36-related (class B) scavenger receptor that recognizes acetylated LDL, oxidized LDL, and native LDL (92). These receptors are depicted in Fig. 1. As a consequence of enhanced uptake, receptor recognition of oxidized LDL can increase its biological impact in certain contexts. For example, the level of suppression of PDGF activity produced by endothelial cells is related to the extent of LDL oxidation; however, the same level of suppression achieved with highly oxidized LDL was obtained using only lightly oxidized acetyl-LDL (93), presumably because the enhanced uptake of acetylated LDL via the scavenger receptor increased the delivery of the suppressive moiety.

Mechanisms for oxidized LDL uptake by macrophages have been identified that are distinct from receptor recognition of the modified lipoprotein. One of these derives from the observation that oxidized LDL more readily aggregates than does native LDL. Thus, oxidized LDL uptake may proceed in part via nonspecific phagocytosis of these aggregated forms (94). Aggregates may also be formed or enlarged by binding to large proteoglycans, which would increase the susceptibility of LDL to oxidation (84). Human plasma contains antibodies that recognize oxidized LDL but not native LDL (63), inviting speculation that oxidized LDL uptake by macrophages could take place via Fc receptor recognition of oxidized LDL–antibody complexes. Which, if any, of these mechanisms for the macrophage uptake of oxidized LDL dominates in vivo in foam cell formation is not currently known.

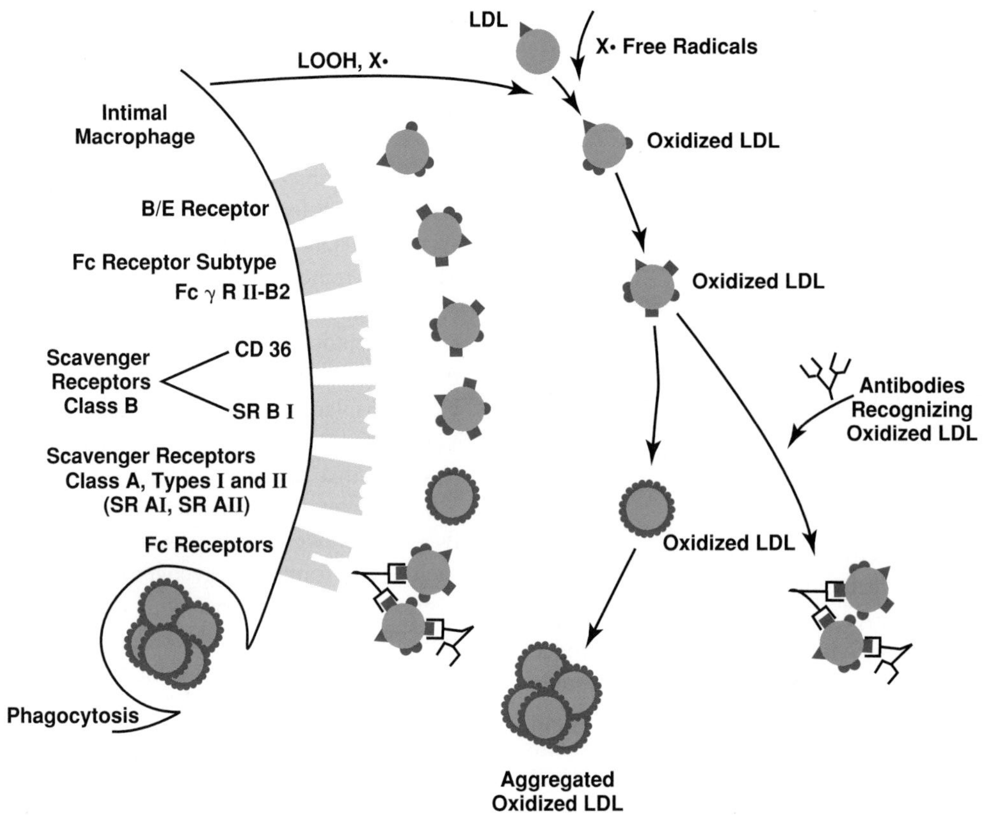

FIG. 1. Diagram of some of the potential means of oxidized LDL uptake by macrophages. These include uptake after B/E receptor recognition of mildly oxidized forms, uptake by several receptors that bind oxidized LDL, uptake by Fc receptors that bind oxidized LDL–antibody complexes, and uptake by phagocytosis of aggregates containing oxidized LDL.

Catabolism of Oxidized LDL

Once ingested by cells, oxidized LDL is metabolized distinctly from either native LDL or acetylated LDL (95–101). Oxidized LDL is catabolized more slowly, a phenomenon that may enhance its accumulation in macrophages. This decreased catabolism is not secondary to a relative decrease in uptake compared with an unoxidized counterpart ligand such as acetylated LDL because the delay has been noted when normalized for internalization. A possible mechanism to explain this decrease is based on the observation that components of oxidized LDL can inhibit lysosomal proteases required for optimal lipoprotein degradation, in particular, cathepsin B (97). The rate and mechanism of catabolism of the components of oxidized LDL may also be altered from those that pertain in native LDL lipid metabolism because, for example, certain oxysterols are known to interfere with cellular cholesterol metabolism.

It is also possible that enzymes distinct from those catabolizing native LDL lipids could participate in the catabolism of oxidized LDL components. Glutathione peroxidase could be expected to degrade fatty acid hydroperoxides following the action of esterases on the hydroperoxides of cholesteryl esters, triglycerides and phospholipids. In addition, phospholipid hydroperoxide glutathione peroxidase, a selenoperoxidase distinct from glutathione peroxidase that is capable of reducing cholesterol hydroperoxidase and hydroperoxides of phospholipids, triglycerides, or cholesteryl esters without prior esterase activity (102,103), also may play a role in oxidized LDL lipid metabolism and oxidized LDL detoxification (104).

EFFECTS OF OXIDIZED LDL ON VASCULAR CELL AND MACROPHAGE FUNCTION

Even prior to reports that cells could oxidize LDL (7,8), LDL oxidized in cell-free systems had been shown to injure cells (2–4). Since these studies, however, it has been shown that sublethal levels of oxidized LDL markedly alter numerous functions in a variety of cells and tissues in ways that are distinct from the effects of native LDL and unrelated to cell injury. These functions include the induction or suppression of the expression of several genes, changes in cell motility, changes in cell–cell adhesion, changes in growth factor and cytokine production, influences on cellular lipid metabolism, and alterations in enzyme activities. Many but not all of these findings can be fit into a hypothetical sequence in which oxidized LDL exacerbates atherosclerosis. Much of the focus of research related to the role of oxidized LDL in atherosclerosis has been on characterizing these cell function changes, identifying the oxidized LDL moieties responsible for the effects, and determining the mechanisms by which these components act. The following are summaries of some of these attempts. Although these effects are of pathophysiological interest, it should be pointed out that their occurrence in vivo is for most only a matter of speculation.

Cell Injury by Oxidized LDL

Cells can be killed by concentrations of oxidized LDL below the estimated concentrations of total LDL (native plus oxidized) in interstitial space (1–4). This has invited speculation that if LDL in the intimal interstitium were to become oxidized, it could participate in the dysfunction of endothelium believed to occur in early atherosclerosis (105,106) or in the accumulation of dead cell debris known to occur in later stages of lesion development. Injury to endothelium could lead, for example, to increased entry of lipoproteins into the intima from the lumen, or it could impair the other important functions of this cell layer.

The capacity of oxidized LDL to injure or kill cells appears to be a general result of oxidation that develops regardless of the mode of oxidation. In cell-free systems it has been shown that LDL becomes toxic after oxidation in oxygenated solution (3,4), by metal-ion-supplemented solutions (107), by ultraviolet irradiation (108), or by the action of lipoxygenase (109). In cell-mediated oxidation, LDL becomes toxic after oxidation by endothelial cells (7), smooth muscle cells (7), activated monocytes (10), or neutrophils (10). Supplementation of these systems with a variety of (antioxidants or HDL blocks these reactions (2–4,110). In general, the potency of oxidized LDL to kill cells is related to the degree of oxidation, but even moderately oxidized LDL can kill cells (3,4).

In early studies, the toxicity of oxidized LDL was demonstrated with cultured vascular smooth muscle cells, endothelium, and fibroblasts as target cells (1–4), but it appears to be a general phenomenon. Proliferating cells are more susceptible (2,107), and it was shown for human fibroblasts that the DNA synthesis phase of the cell cycle correlated with highest vulnerability (107). B/E receptors are not required for toxicity since receptor negative cells can be killed by oxidized LDL (1,111), and cells are vulnerable to the organic solvent extracts of oxidized LDL (3). Furthermore, cells without scavenger receptors (e.g., foreskin fibroblasts) are susceptible (4). On the other hand, if LDL is oxidized in such a way as to preserve B/E receptor recognition, as has been reported for ultraviolet-irradiated LDL, the killing of cells expressing the B/E receptor is enhanced (108). These results suggest that internalization of the entire lipoprotein may not be required for cell injury but that receptor-mediated uptake can increase the delivery of the cytotoxins.

Attempts have been made to identify the cytotoxic lipids that are formed during LDL oxidation. Many of the lipid oxidation products known to be produced during LDL oxidation have previously been demonstrated to kill cells. Several oxysterols, including 7α- and 7β-hydroxycholesterol, 7-ketocholesterol, epoxycholesterols (38,39), as well as non-sterol-derived oxidation products such as lysoPC, oxidized fatty acids, and 4-HNE (33) are among substances formed in oxidized LDL that are known toxins (33,112). Attempts to identify the major cytotoxins of LDL oxidized in vitro have variably suggested that 7β-hydroperoxycholesterol (40) and 7β-hydroxycholesterol (113) play major roles. It is possible that different toxic lipids dominate under different circumstances, or the vulnerability of various cell types to different oxidized lipids may vary. In addition, the relative amounts of the toxic lipids formed can vary with the degree or the mode of LDL oxidation. Many of the toxic lipids formed on oxidized LDL are known to exist in vivo. 7β-Hydroperoxycholesterol, for example, has been shown to reside in human atherosclerotic lesions (40).

The mechanism by which oxidized LDL kills cells is unknown, and this too may be different for different cells. It appears that selected antioxidants can inhibit cell killing (104,114,115). The use of a variety of inhibitors has led to a proposed mechanism whereby the lipid hydroperoxides of LDL initiate a free-radical-mediated chain reaction of metal-ion-dependent peroxidation of cellular lipids and ultimate cell death (104). It has been reported that injury of lymphoid target cells by UV-irradiated LDL may be via apoptosis or programmed cell death (116). Whether an apoptotic mechanism of cell death can be more generally attributed to oxidized LDL toxicity in other cell types is unknown.

The Effects of Oxidized Lipoproteins on Cell Motility

Oxidized LDL has been shown to have varied effects on the motility of the cell types known to exist in normal and atherosclerotic vessel walls including endothelial cells (117), smooth muscle cells (118), and monocyte/macrophages (119,120). As discussed above, these cell types are capable of oxidizing LDL. Therefore, by acting as a chemotactic or chemostatic factor, oxidized LDL may initiate a positive feedback loop whereby the presence of more oxidized LDL leads to the attraction and immobilization of cells capable of forming additional oxidized LDL.

Oxidized LDL has been shown to have chemotactic and chemostatic effects on monocytes and macrophages, respectively (119,120). These processes may explain in part how atherosclerotic lesions become enriched in monocyte-derived macrophages. The chemotactic effects of oxidized LDL are mediated by a direct effect of oxidized LDL on monocytes and by an indirect effect on endothelial cells. The direct chemotactic and chemostatic effects of oxidized LDL have been shown to be contained in the lipid fraction of oxidized LDL and are thought to be related to lysoPC. LysoPC was shown to be a specific chemoattractant for monocytes (121), and oxidized LDL was shown to immobilize macrophages in the presence of known chemoattractants (119). Thus, oxidized LDL itself could theoretically attract monocytes to a lesion and then inhibit the movement of the macrophages. This effect was not mediated solely by interactions of oxidized LDL with scavenger receptors, because acetylated LDL and other ligands for the receptor did not influence movement of these cells.

Oxidized LDL has also been shown to alter monocyte motility indirectly by inducing the increased production and release of monocyte chemotactic protein 1 (MCP-1) by endothelial cells and smooth muscle cells (30,122). That this observation may have relevance in vivo is suggested by Northern blot analysis of atherosclerotic lesions that revealed significant levels of MCP-1 messenger RNA; MCP-1 mRNA could not be detected in normal intima (123). Furthermore, in situ hybridization of atherosclerotic lesions demonstrated colocalization of MCP-1 mRNA with epitopes recognized by antibodies to oxidized LDL (124).

In contrast, oxidized LDL, but not native LDL, is a potent inhibitor of endothelial cell migration. This was demonstrated in an in vitro wound-healing model in which portions of endothelial monolayers were scraped away and migration was quantified across the wound edge (117). The inhibitory activity resides in the lipid portion of the oxidized LDL and was shown by several criteria to be independent of cell injury (117). LysoPC appears to be responsible for at least a portion of the inhibitory activity (125). Interestingly, an opposing effect of oxidized LDL has been reported on vascular smooth muscle cells. Oxidized LDL was observed to be chemotactic for arterial smooth muscle cells (126), an effect that may be related to the oxidized LDL enhancement of PDGF receptor expression and PDGF AA production in smooth muscle cells (127).

The Effects of Oxidized Lipoproteins on Growth Factors and Cytokines

That oxidized LDL can change growth factor production was first demonstrated in a study in which oxidized LDL potently suppressed PDGF produced by endothelial cells grown in culture (93). The suppression depended on the degree of oxidation of the LDL. Oxidized acetylated LDL also exhibited the suppressive property and was more potently suppressive than oxidized LDL at low levels of oxidation, presumably because of enhanced uptake of acetylated LDL by scavenger receptors. Since this study, suppression of PDGF production by oxidized LDL in macrophages has been reported (128), and, more generally, both positive and negative effects on the production, release, or activity of different growth factors and cytokines in various cell types have been observed. Oxidized LDL alteration in growth factor production could play a major role in the pathogenesis of atherosclerosis, because many of the growth factors influenced by oxidized LDL stimulate smooth muscle cell proliferation or migration.

Contrary to the suppressive effect of oxidized LDL on endothelial cell PDGF, it has been shown that lysoPC increases mRNA levels of PDGF A and B chains in cultured human endothelial cells (129). The apparent inconsistency may be explained by the fact that there are lipids residing on oxidized LDL that are stimulatory, such as lysoPC, and those that are inhibitory, such as cholesteryl linoleic acid hydroperoxides (130), and that the relative amounts of these lipids may vary in different oxidized LDL preparations. Further experimentation evaluating the effects of various oxidized LDL lipid fractions on growth factor production will be necessary before the effects of oxidized LDL on PDGF production are fully understood.

Although oxidized LDL decreases PDGF production in endothelial cells and macrophages in vitro, it appears to have an opposite effect on vascular smooth muscle cells. It has been reported that relatively low concentrations of native or oxidized LDL increased PDGF AA production and PDGF receptor expression in human smooth muscle cells (127). Induction by oxidized LDL was found to be more potent than that by native LDL. This observation suggests the possibility of an oxidized-LDL-induced autocrine action of PDGF. Oxidized LDL has been shown to have a proliferative effect on vascular smooth muscle cells at subtoxic concentrations (131,132).

Oxidized LDL may indirectly stimulate smooth muscle proliferation by increasing heparin-binding epidermal growth factor (HB-EGF) production from adjacent vascular cell types. LysoPC has recently been shown to increase mRNA levels for HB-EGF as well as its release from human monocytes (133) and endothelial cells (129). The effects of lysoPC on HB-EGF production are thought to result from altered processing or degradation of the transcripts, because nuclear run-on assays did not reveal an effect of lysoPC on HB-EGF transcription (133). In endothelial cells, lysoPC increased the level of transcription (129).

Endothelin production by both macrophages and endothelial cells has been shown to be altered by oxidized LDL, although the reports are somewhat contradictory in the case of endothelial cells, in that both suppression (134) and stimulation (135) have been observed. Oxidized LDL has been shown to enhance macrophage production of endothelin (136).

Relatively low concentrations of oxidized LDL increase the production of granulocyte–monocyte colony-stimulating factor (GM-CSF), macrophage CSF (M-CSF), and granulocyte CSF (G-CSF) by aortic endothelial cells from humans and rabbits (137). However, in another study showing that a variety of cytokines induced M-CSF in both endothelial and smooth muscle cells, oxidized LDL was found not to increase M-CSF consistently (138). M-CSF enhances the proliferation and differentiation of monocytes and plays a role in their survival and activation; M-CSF administered to Watanabe heritable hyperlipemia (WHHL) rabbits inhibited the progression of atherosclerotic lesions (139).

Oxidized LDL has recently been shown to increase the production of IL-8, a potent chemoattractant for T lymphocytes, by human monocytes (140). The level of production of IL-8 correlated with the level of LDL oxidation, and this activity of oxidized LDL was found to be partly related to lysoPC.

Pretreatment of mouse peritoneal macrophages with oxidized LDL leads to potent inhibition of the gene expression of certain cytokines after macrophage stimulation (141,142). The gene expression of tumor necrosis factor-α, interleukin-1α (142), IL-1β, and IL-6 (141) were suppressed. The suppression was independent of cell injury and not the result of a more general inhibition of protein synthesis (142). The inhibitory moiety resided in the lipid portion of the lipoprotein (142).

More recently, it has become clear that this cytokine suppression by oxidized LDL is not a general suppression of macrophage stimulation; it appears instead to be selective for particular stimulation pathways and particular cytokines (143). For example, increases in TNF-α, and IL-110 nRNA induced by IFN-γ plus IL-2 were more sensitive to oxidized LDL suppression than the induction of these genes by LPS. Stimulation of iNOS gene expression by IFN-γ plus LPS was suppressed by oxidized LDL, but the antagonistic effect of IFN-γ on LPS-induced gene expression of the TNF receptor, TNFRII, was unaffected by oxidized LDL (143). These data suggest that oxidized LDL lipid components can interfere with specific intracellular pathways and exert selective control over cytokine gene expression.

Potential Effects of Oxidized LDL on Thrombotic Events

It has previously been suggested that the fibrinolytic capacity is decreased in patients with hypertriglyceridemia or hypercholesterolemia (144). Furthermore, epidemiologic studies have suggested that patients with coronary artery disease may be hypercoagulable. The decrease in the fibrinolytic capacity of these patients is thought to stem from an increase in plasminogen activator inhibitor-1 (PAI-1) levels (145), whereas the hypercoagulable state in patients with coronary artery disease is thought to be mediated by an increase in tissue factor activity. Because oxidized LDL is known to exist in arterial lesions, the possibility that oxidized LDL may mediate blood coagulation or the fibrinolytic pathway has been investigated.

It has been demonstrated that human umbilical vein endothelial cells (HUVEC) exposed to oxidized LDL increased PAI-1 synthesis, but native LDL had no effect (146). The oxidized LDL used in these studies was obtained by peroxidation with ultraviolet light, which should not have interfered with B/E receptor recognition. However, coincubation of cells with ultraviolet-oxidized LDL and antibodies directed against the native LDL receptor did not diminish the increased synthesis of PAI-1, suggesting that cellular recognition by the B/E receptor was not necessary. In another study, oxidized LDL prepared by dialysis against cupric ions, when added to cultures of HUVEC, not only stimulated the production of PAI-1 but also decreased the synthesis and release of tissue-type plasminogen activator (t-PA) (147). Native LDL again had no effect on either PAI-1 or t-PA synthesis. This study demonstrated that lipids from oxidized LDL prepared by chloroform–methanol extraction contained the activity that the intact lipoprotein complex had on the fibrinolytic system. As discussed above, oxidized LDL is rich in lysoPC and numerous oxysterols. When oxidized LDL was depleted of lysoPC by pretreatment with phospholipase B, its ability to stimulate PAI-1 synthesis was blunted with no change in the inhibitory effect on t-PA synthesis. 25-Hydroxycholesterol and 7-ketocholesterol were found to be inhibitory to t-PA synthesis without altering PAI-1 synthesis from control (147). 7-Ketocholesterol is a known constituent of oxidized LDL.

In contrast another study demonstrated that native and acetylated LDL exposure to HUVEC increased PAI-1 synthesis but that the incubation of highly oxidized LDL with HUVEC decreased PAI-1 expression (148). The exposure times used in these studies were on the order of 16–18 h, potentially allowing the native and acetylated LDL to become oxidized; HUVEC are known to oxidize LDL in culture (7). The increases in PAI-1 synthesis observed in these studies were possibly caused by oxidized LDL formed during the incubation period. The fact that incubation with highly oxidized LDL resulted in decreased PAI-1 synthesis brings into question whether the oxidized LDL was toxic to the cells; however, this was deemed unlikely, because cell viability was tested by multiple means, including lactate dehydrogenase release. The above phenomena were observed whether pooled LDL or LDL obtained from patients with known defects in apo B100 was used. The finding that native LDL and acetylated LDL had similar effects indicated that these phenomena were independent of B/E receptor recognition. The apparent discrepancies with other studies are unresolved.

The above studies focus on the effects of oxidized LDL on the fibrinolytic system; however, other studies have focused on the effects of oxidized LDL on tissue factor expression. The incubation of subtoxic concentrations of oxidized LDL with HUVEC resulted in a concentration-dependent increase in the cell surface (149) and total cell (150) expression of tissue factor. This effect was found to peak between 4 and 8 h (149,150) with an increase in tissue factor mRNA levels at 2 h. These results demonstrate that oxidized LDL is capable of inducing tissue factor expression in vitro. If oxidized LDL were to induce tissue factor expression in vivo, it could possibly explain the hypercoagulable nature of atherosclerotic arteries; however, in situ hybridization and immunohistochemical studies have failed to demonstrate tissue factor expression by endothelial cells in normal or atherosclerotic vessels (151). These studies instead revealed elevated tissue factor expression in the arterial media and in proximity to cholesterol clefts in lesions. It has been demonstrated that arterial smooth muscle cells rapidly express tissue factor in response to balloon injury in vivo (152,153) as well as in response to several mitogens (e.g., angiotensin II, thrombin, and fetal bovine serum) in vitro (154). It has recently been shown that copper-oxidized LDL, but not native LDL, stimulates the surface expression of tissue factor activity in rabbit smooth muscle cells in a concentration-dependent fashion with a peak at 4–6 h (155). Chloroform–methanol extracts of oxidized LDL elicited tissue factor activity in these arterial smooth muscle cells (155). These findings, combined with others (151,154), invite speculation that fissure formation in atherosclerotic plaques or balloon angioplasty may expose plasma to increased levels of oxidized-LDL-induced tissue factor, which could result in thrombosis.

An oxidized-LDL-mediated increase in tissue factor expression may have implications for lesion development independent of its effects on blood coagulation. A product of the blood coagulation cascade initiated by tissue factor is the cleavage of prothrombin to thrombin, and thrombin is reported to be a mitogen for arterial smooth muscle cells (156). Therefore, an increase in tissue factor expression by oxidized LDL or arterial injury may result in a local increase in smooth muscle cell proliferation via this mechanism.

The Effects of Oxidized Lipoproteins on Vascular Reactivity

The tone of the smooth muscle cell-rich arterial media in the normal artery is directly influenced by the endothelium lining the vessel via endothelial cell production and release of endothelium-derived relaxing factors (EDRF) such as nitric oxide (NO). However, atherosclerotic vessels have impaired endothelium-dependent vasodilation as well as an increased sensitivity to drugs which cause vasoconstriction (157). It has been demonstrated that oxidized LDL has many effects on the vascular tone of arteries, including effects on the nitric oxide pathway, calcium ion exchange, and prostaglandin and endothelin production.

Oxidized LDL has been demonstrated to have an overall negative effect on the EDRF-mediated relaxation of arterial smooth muscle cells. Studies have suggested that oxidized LDL may interfere with multiple steps, including the synthesis of nitric oxide synthase, the transport of nitric oxide from the endothelial cell, and the responsiveness of the smooth muscle cell. Pig coronary arteries incubated with native LDL in the absence of antioxidants showed a slow but sustained increase in arterial muscle tone in organ culture; however, in the presence of antioxidants such as BHT or EDTA, the phenomenon was diminished, suggesting a role for oxidized LDL in determining vascular tone (158). This concept was further supported by the observation that lipid peroxide levels were elevated in those cultures without antioxidant supplement. Other studies have shown that oxidized LDL, but not native LDL, is a potent inhibitor of EDRF-mediated vasodilation (159,160). The mediators of the effects of oxidized LDL were shown to be contained in the lipid moiety and absent in the protein portion of the lipoprotein (160).

These findings are consistent with studies that indicate that lysoPC may be a mediator of this biological function of oxidized LDL (159–163). Oxidized LDL that was depleted of lysoPC by incubation with phospholipase B failed to inhibit the vasorelaxation of EDRF. It has been suggested that lysoPC blocks the EDRF response by stimulating the protein kinase C (PKC) signaling pathway, because the addition of inhibitors of PKC attenuated the effect of oxidized LDL (161). Stimulation of the PKC pathway with phorbol 12-myristate 13-acetate caused an inhibition of EDRF similar to that seen with oxidized LDL.

Also, consistent with the demonstration that lysoPC is the biological mediator of EDRF inhibition by oxidized LDL is the finding that HDL inhibited the effects of oxidized LDL on the smooth muscle cell response to EDRF (163,164). HDL may block the effect of oxidized LDL by sequestering lysoPC in the lipid core of HDL. LysoPC was shown to partition into the lipid core of HDL from the oxidized LDL molecule as well as from cell membranes after incubation with oxidized LDL. As would be expected, HDL incubation reversed the inhibition imparted by either lysoPC or oxidized LDL (163).

Studies have been performed to evaluate the mechanism by which oxidized LDL inhibits the action of EDRF, for example, whether it inhibits EDRF production or promotes degradation, or whether it alters the responsiveness of arterial smooth muscle cells to vasodilators. It has been demonstrated that preincubation of arterial tissue with either native LDL or oxidized LDL did not inhibit the formation of EDRF (165). Preincubation of arterial segments with either native LDL or oxidized LDL did not alter nitroglycerin-induced relaxation, demonstrating that oxidized LDL did not cause decreased sensitivity of the arterial smooth muscle cells to endothelium-independent vasodilators (160). There is evidence that oxidized LDL can influence guanylate cyclase, resulting in decreased substrate turnover (166). This suggests that oxidized LDL may increase vascular tone by altering smooth muscle cell metabolism of NO-containing compounds. Oxidized LDL, and possibly native LDL, may interfere with the relaxation of arterial smooth muscle cells by inactivating EDRF directly after release from endothelial cells. It has been suggested that nitric oxide may partition into the hydrophobic core of these macromolecules (165,167).

The presence of oxidized LDL has been shown to increase the sensitivity of vascular smooth muscle to vasoconstrictor agents in both intact and endothelium-denuded arteries (165). The oxidized-LDL-mediated hypersensitivity of arterial segments to various vasoconstrictor substances is independent of the ability of oxidized LDL to sequester EDRF.

Rather, the observed hypersensitivity can be suppressed by the addition of calcium channel blockers to the media, suggesting that oxidized LDL incubation results in increased transmembrane calcium influx or release from intracellular stores (168). Oxidized LDL has been shown to increase cytoplasmic calcium (169), and, under the influence of this increase, smooth muscle cells may increase their responsiveness to vasoconstrictor agents. This biological function of oxidized LDL has been shown to be localized to the lipid fraction, and in particular, lysoPC has been shown to increase intracellular calcium levels in smooth muscle cells (170). The intracellular signaling mechanism involves the cGMP pathway, and the lysoPC-induced increase in intracellular calcium can be blocked by verapamil.

Paradoxically, in response to oxidized LDL exposure, human saphenous vein endothelial cells increased their production and release of the potent dilator PGI_2 with a biphasic temporal response (171). The degree to which PGI_2 synthesis was increased correlated with the degree of lipoprotein oxidation. Incubation with native LDL resulted in a small, monophasic rise in PGI_2. The mechanism responsible for oxidized LDL stimulation of PGI_2 production is unclear, but the response was inhibited by indomethacin, an antagonist of cyclooxygenase. It was suggested that the second PGI_2 peak may result from oxidized-LDL-induced cytotoxicity.

Studies have been undertaken to evaluate the role of oxidized LDL in regulating the gene expression and secretion of endothelin, a potent vasoconstrictor with mitogenic properties (172). Endothelin may be of particular interest in restenosis after angioplasty because increased levels have been detected in the coronary sinus in patients after PTCA (173). Oxidized LDL, but not native LDL, induced endothelin secretion in human macrophages at levels equal to those obtained with phorbol myristate acetate (136). Similar results were obtained with acetylated LDL, suggesting that the scavenger receptor is involved in the pathway of lipoprotein-induced endothelin secretion. Analogous effects of oxidized LDL on endothelin gene expression and secretion in porcine and human endothelial cells were reported (135). This group further confirmed the likely role of the scavenger receptor in this pathway by showing that the addition of dextran sulfate, a scavenger receptor antagonist, blocked the effects of oxidized LDL on endothelin secretion. The effects of oxidized LDL on endothelin secretion by endothelial cells is not a settled issue because it has also been reported that the lyso PC in oxidized LDL suppressed endothelin-1 secretion by endothelial cells (134). The authors mentioned the possibility of a role for lipoprotein-associated endotoxin in the former studies because endotoxin readily associates with LDL and HDL.

Effect of Oxidized LDL on Leukocyte Adhesion

Early atherosclerotic lesions are characterized by increased monocyte adhesion to the overlying endothelium (105). Areas near arterial branch points such as the intercostal ostia of the aorta are known to be predisposed to atherosclerosis (174). These areas have been shown to have increased lipoprotein accumulation in the intima as well as an increased number of monocytes attached to the endothelium. A possible explanation for the increased monocyte adhesion is the presence of oxidized LDL in the prelesion intima. Moderately oxidized LDL has been shown to stimulate monocyte adhesion to endothelial cells in culture (30,175) by the induction of a monocyte-specific binding protein on the endothelial cell surface (30,176), and HDL has been shown to block the effects of oxidized LDL on the expression of adhesion molecules (177).

Injections of oxidized LDL have been shown to induce binding of leukocytes to the endothelial cell surface in vivo (178). Furthermore, it has been demonstrated that the injection of antibodies to platelet-activating factor (179) and CD11b/CD18 (180) blocked this leukocyte adhesion, suggesting a role for the latter receptor complexes in the binding of leukocytes to the endothelial cell surface. The addition of sugars to the above receptors blocked early (4-h) oxidized-LDL-induced monocyte adhesion (181). Whether the effect of the sugars was on glycoprotein carbohydrate chains on monocytes or endothelial cells is unknown, but in this system, monocyte adhesion was blocked by treatment with low levels of trypsin. Similarly, another study demonstrated an ECAM-1-, ICAM-1-, and VCAM-1-independent increase in monocyte adhesion early in response to oxidized LDL that was completely suppressed by the presence of HDL (177). The specific surface receptor responsible for early monocyte adhesion in response to oxidized LDL is unknown; however, it appears that oxidized LDL increases monocyte adhesion by multiple mechanisms (182).

The ability of oxidized LDL to induce monocyte adhesion is, at least in part, associated with lysoPC (183). Both VCAM-1 and ICAM-1 expression have been shown to be increased on endothelial cells when exposed to lysoPC. This effect is generalizable to phospholipase A_2 activity, because stimulators of phospholipase A_2, such as interleukin-1-β and tumor necrosis factor, have also been shown to increase surface adhesion molecule expression. Furthermore, inhibitors of phospholipase A_2 block the effects of phospholipase A_2 stimulators but not of lysoPC.

Finally, there are recent data suggesting that monocytes exposed to oxidized LDL may contribute to the expression of adhesion molecules on the endothelial cell surface (184). The subsequent exposure of endothelial cells to conditioned media from cultures of monocytes incubated with copper-oxidized LDL resulted in the increased expression of VCAM-1, ICAM-1, and ELAM-1 on their surface (184). Monocytes grown in the presence of native LDL had no effect. Furthermore, the exposure of endothelial cells to non-conditioned media containing oxidized LDL resulted in no increase in monocyte adhesion. These results may lead to the identification of oxidized-LDL-induced monocyte-derived cytokines that regulate the surface expression of adhesion molecules on endothelial cells.

OXIDIZED LDL AND ATHEROSCLEROSIS

A Theory of Atherosclerosis Suggesting a Role for LDL Oxidation

Certainly part of the attraction of the theory that oxidized LDL is responsible for some of the pathological features of atherosclerotic lesions derives from the findings in cultured cell systems that oxidized LDL causes the aforementioned cellular changes that correlate with known aspects of arterial lesions but are not induced by native LDL. Endothelial injury, LDL retention in intimal interstitium, monocyte recruitment into intima, engorgement of macrophages with lipoprotein-derived lipid, smooth muscle cell migration and proliferation, accumulation of necrotic cell debris, and tendencies toward vasoconstriction and procoagulant activity are characteristics of atherosclerosis that can be predicted by oxidized LDL interactions with cultured cells or isolated vascular tissue. From these findings of altered cell function, a theory of atherosclerosis based on LDL oxidation can be constructed. The theory is similar in many aspects to updated versions of the "response to injury" theory of atherogenesis, with oxidized LDL playing a central role as an agent that causes injury to, or dysfunction of, the endothelium as an early event (105,106). One version of many possible variants of the oxidative theory is presented below and is illustrated in Figs. 2A–C.

It is known that LDL enters the normal arterial wall interstitium and accumulates in amounts that are regulated by the endothelium and likely the internal elastic lamina (185). Elevations in the level of plasma LDL proportionately increase the rate of LDL entry (82). Thus, high interstitial LDL secondary to high plasma LDL, and the tendency for LDL to bind proteoglycans, would increase the residence time for an LDL molecule entering the tissue (186) and increase the probability of opportunistic LDL oxidation, perhaps by free radical production from adjacent endothelium or smooth muscle cells or an isolated macrophage (7,8,10,11). This effect could also be exacerbated by the enhanced susceptibility of LDL to oxidation after binding to proteoglycans (84) and the tendency of oxidized LDL to bind more readily to collagen (85). In addition, small, dense LDL, which has been shown to signal increased risk of atherosclerosis and to be more readily oxidized than other LDL subfractions (64,65), may be able to pass the endothelium more readily. Once LDL is oxidized, injury to endothelium may lead to local increases in endothelial cell turnover and enhanced entry of lipoproteins.

Oxidized LDL may participate in a number of actions that encourage monocyte invasion of intima. Oxidized LDL causes monocyte chemotactic protein-1 to be produced by endothelium (122); it causes expression by endothelium of monocyte binding proteins (30,175,176) and it acts as a monocyte chemoattractant (119). Once recruited to the in-

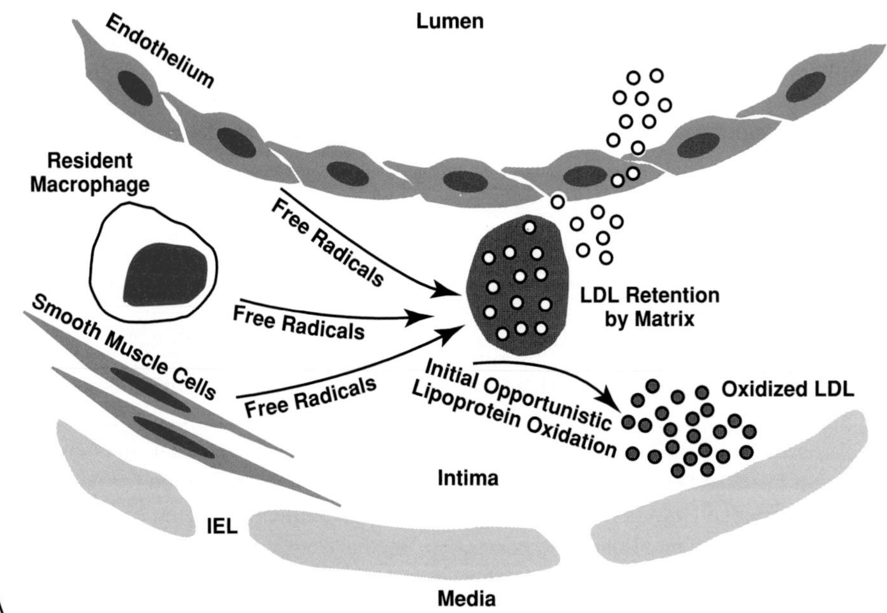

FIG. 2. (A) Schematic of a hypothetical sequence in which lipoprotein oxidation causes atherosclerosis. VLDL and LDL enter into and accumulate in the arterial intima, processes that are governed by endothelial vesicular transport rates, local endothelial cell turnover, the plasma concentration of the lipoproteins, and the size of intima, which may be increased near branches of the arterial vasculature. Increases in the intimal pool size of these lipoproteins from increases in the four factors above and binding to connective tissue elements increase the residence time of the lipoprotein in the intima, which, in turn, increases the probability of opportunistic oxidation. The oxidation may be by reactive oxygen from isolated macrophages or intimal smooth muscle cells or from the endothelium.

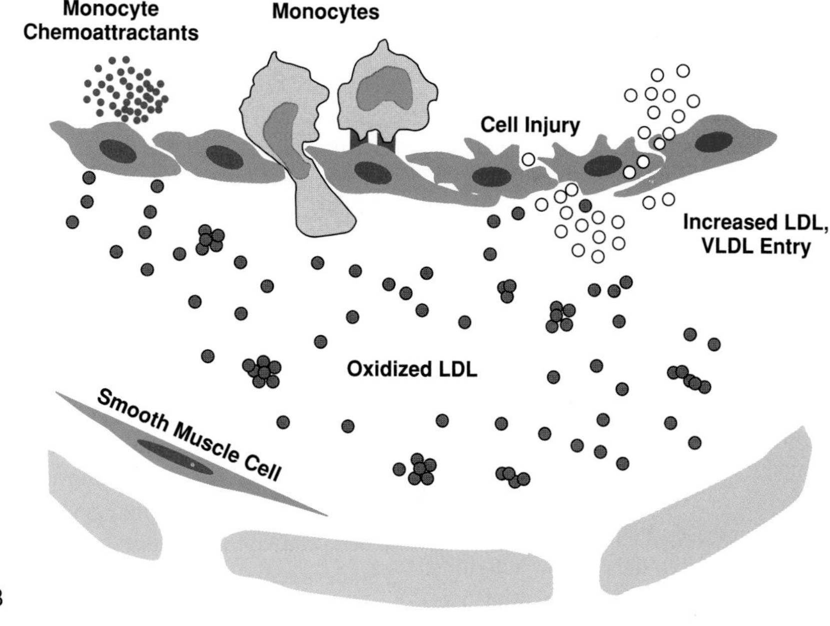

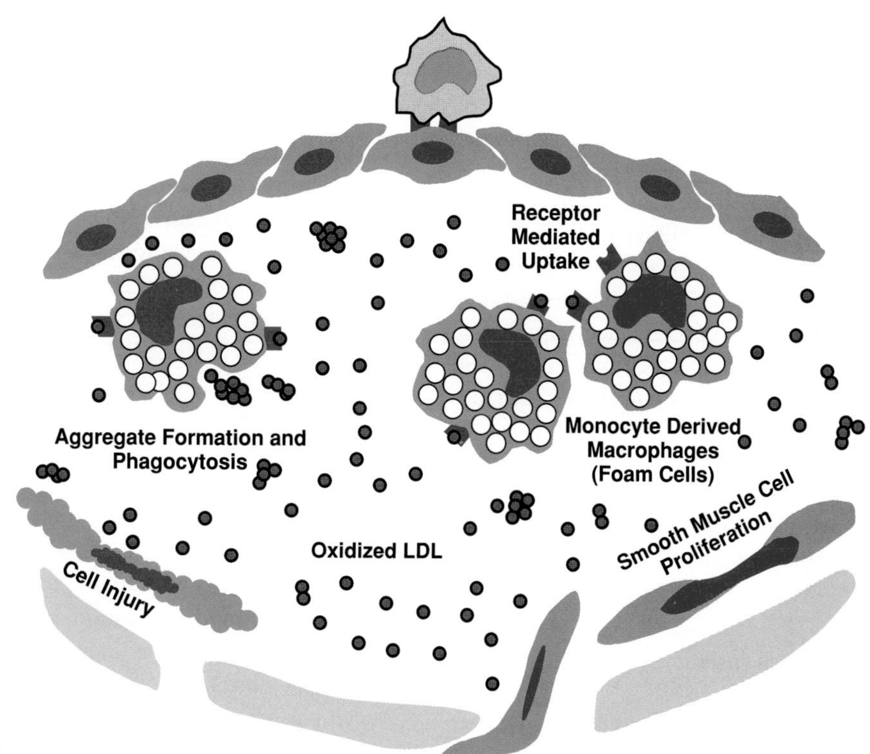

FIG. 2. *Continued.* **(B)** Once oxidized, the modified lipoproteins may injure or activate endothelium, increasing the turnover of these cells and allowing the entry of more plasma macromolecules. Oxidized LDL can also facilitate monocyte invasion of the intima by eliciting secretion of monocyte chemoattractants (MCP-1) and surface expression of monocyte binding proteins. Oxidized LDL and the lysophosphatidylcholine emanating from it may act as chemoattractants for monocytes. **(C)** Further potential atherogenic actions of oxidized LDL include serving as ligand for foam cell formation via the pathways pictured in Fig. 1, by promoting migration and proliferation of smooth muscle cells, and by killing cells and thereby contributing to the accumulation of dead-cell debris.

tima, the monocyte-derived phagocytes can internalize oxidized LDL by a number of receptor-mediated pathways, including class A scavenger receptors SR-AI and SR-AII (88), CD36 (91), FcRII-B2 (90), and SR-BI (92), all of which recognize oxidized LDL and Fc receptors that bind oxidized LDL complexed with antibodies that have been demonstrated in plasma and shown to bind oxidized but not native LDL (63). The tendency of LDL to aggregate on oxidation suggests the additional possibility for uptake via phagocytosis (94). As a result of encountering phagocytic stimuli, these resident macrophages may participate in further LDL oxidation, mediated by the reactive oxygen species these cells are known to produce (10,11).

The presence of smooth muscle cells in the intima may be facilitated by a chemoattractant effect (126) as well as by the proliferative influence of oxidized LDL (131,132). In addition, oxidized LDL increases PDGF expression by smooth muscle cells (187). In general, the cellular activities may be influenced indirectly by the various effects of oxidized LDL on growth factor and cytokine induction and suppression shown to occur in vascular cells and macrophages. Once recruited into the intima, smooth muscle cells may develop into foam cells by an oxidized-LDL-facilitated process. Smooth muscle cells have been shown to express receptors in vitro that recognize modified lipoprotein (188,189), and scavenger receptors are induced on smooth muscle cells in vivo by atherogenic diets (189).

Other atherosclerotic actions of oxidized LDL that may speed lesion development include killing of proliferating smooth muscle cells (2), contributing to a necrotic core; inhibition of endothelial migration (117), slowing the healing after endothelial injury; induction of tissue factor production (149,150,155), leading to a procoagulant environment; and suppression of endothelium-dependent relaxation (162), potentially leading to a narrowed lumen.

Obviously which of these effects pertains in vivo is the subject of extensive research, and due caution should be taken in extrapolating to the living system results derived from cultured cells or isolated tissues.

Antioxidants and Atherosclerosis

The proposal that antioxidants may retard the progression of atherosclerosis is not a new one. There is a literature of studies examining the effects on experimental atherosclerosis of vitamins A, C, and E as well as BHT and other antioxidants that extends from the 1940s through the 1970s (for review, see ref. 190), prior to the recent emphasis on this topic. The results emanating from these studies are inconsistent.

The equivocal nature of the outcomes of these prior studies was later countered with nearly simultaneous independent reports from two groups that probucol, an antioxidant drug that lowers lipids by an unknown mechanism, markedly reduced fatty streak formation in the WHHL rabbit (19,21), an experimental model in which receptor-mediated lipoprotein metabolism is impaired and that serves in some respects as a model for human familial hypercholesterolemia. The two studies suggested that the retardation of fatty streak development was independent of the lipid-lowering effect of probucol. In one of the studies (19) a control group of animals was given lovastatin, an HMG-CoA reductase inhibitor, to lower total cholesterol to levels comparable to those in the probucol group, and fatty streak formation was significantly reduced by probucol even in comparison to lovastatin. Before these studies probucol had been shown capable of protecting lipids and lipoproteins from oxidation, including a study in humans showing that oxidation in vitro of LDL isolated from patients taking probucol was inhibited compared to that of untreated controls (191). Probucol has since been shown to be a successful antiatherogenic agent in other experimental models, including the cholesterol-fed rabbit (20) and primates fed an atherogenic diet (29); however, probucol has not been shown to be an antiatherosclerotic agent in all studies (see below).

The antioxidant effects of probucol have been attributed to its capacity to scavenge peroxyl radicals and lipid radicals; however, it also has numerous other effects on cell function. The attribution of its antiatherogenic effects to its antioxidant properties has gained strength in part from the finding that other antioxidants with peroxyl-radical-scavenging capacities, such as BHT and DPPD, neither of which lowers lipids, have also been shown to reduce lesion formation in atherogenic rabbit models (25,26). The effectiveness of probucol also rekindled interest in vitamin E, a scavenger of peroxyl and, to a lesser extent, alkoxyl radicals. Vitamin E has been reported to retard atherosclerosis progression in certain arteries of primates fed an atherogenic diet (22) as well as a modified WHHL rabbit model of atherosclerosis (192).

Different approaches have been taken to examine the effects of antioxidants on atherosclerosis in humans. Among multiple national populations, indices of cardiovascular mortality and vitamin consumption revealed a significant correlation between reduced cardiovascular disease and vitamin E consumption that was independent of other risk factors (193). The correlation appeared stronger than that with reduced plasma cholesterol. More recently, large populations of men and women were studied in order to test heart disease risk and various nutritional parameters. Both women and men exhibited reduced vascular disease parameters with high ingestion rates of vitamin E (23,24). Particularly strong were the reduced cardiovascular risks with vitamin E supplementation to the diet. β-Carotene was also reported to correlate with reduction in cardiovascular events in humans (27).

Not all studies report the effectiveness of antioxidants against atherosclerosis. Several studies with vitamin E have been negative (190). In a study of probucol in cholesterol-fed rabbits, in which untreated animals were fed cholesterol intermittently to maintain total plasma cholesterol levels comparable to those of animals continuously fed cholesterol with probucol, probucol did not decrease fatty streak development (194). Whether intermittent feeding reduced atherosclerosis independent of cholesterol level, or whether the aspects of the experimental design are responsible for the apparent disparity between this study and others (e.g., ref. 20), has not been determined. Probucol effectively lowers HDL cholesterol as well as other lipoproteins, complicating the interpretation of its effectiveness as an antiatherogenic antioxidant. Probucol given to primates fed an atherogenic diet reduced lesions in thoracic aorta but not abdominal aorta or iliac arteries (29). The intimal lesion size correlated inversely with resistance of LDL to oxidation in vitro, but other effects of probucol could not be ruled out as having played a role in the results. No antiatherosclerotic effect was attributable to probucol in a study testing whether probucol would affect femoral atherosclerosis when given to hypercholesterolemic patients with cholestyramine, a bile acid sequestrant (195).

It is perhaps too early to generalize on the findings of antioxidant-mediated antiatherosclerotic effects. Balancing the numerous studies with positive outcomes is a group with negative outcomes. None of the antioxidants used is free of multiple functional effects independent of antioxidant properties, and some are known to be harmful (25,26). The various studies have been performed and analyzed using diverse criteria for atherosclerosis progression, which complicates comparisons among studies and generalizations. The data, however, invite speculation that lipophilic scavengers of lipid radicals that can associate with lipoproteins and that interfere with the propagation of lipid peroxidation in the lipoprotein particles appear to retard fatty streak development.

Oxidants and Antioxidants in Restenosis After Angioplasty

Restenosis of coronary and peripheral arteries after balloon dilation is a major clinical problem. It would be misleading to imply that the processes involved in atherosclerosis lesion development are equivalent to those that govern the restenotic lesion that forms after angioplasty. The time frames for lesion formation are disparate, as are some of the features of the lesions. On the other hand, some similarities do exist. Lipid and lipoprotein oxidation products are present in both. Considering the damage done to endothelium, intima, and media by the balloon, both at the lesion site and to the adjacent uninvolved regions, it is not surprising that phagocytic leukocytes and higher levels of plasma lipoproteins readily enter the "wound." Thus, at the inception of the restenotic lesion, lipid substrate and cells known to produce reactive oxygen species are in ample supply. One could readily speculate that the opportunity exists for the resulting lipid oxidation products to alter cellular behavior locally (132). The debate continues as to whether restenosis is determined by smooth muscle cell proliferation, vascular remodeling, vasoconstriction, or a combination (196–199), but there are sequences of events that can be proposed based on known in vitro effects of oxidized lipoproteins that are consistent with a role of oxidized lipoproteins. Although speculative, these ideas are stimulating research in this direction.

Hypothetical mechanisms of restenosis can be constructed from the multiple effects of oxidized LDL described above. Because oxidized LDL has been shown in cultures to be a chemoattractant for smooth muscle cells (126), a deterrent to endothelial cell migration (117), and a stimulant of smooth muscle cell proliferation (131,132), perhaps through the release of autocrine or paracrine (187) growth factors, it has both the capacities to retard healing of the balloon-induced endothelial cell injury and to stimulate indirectly smooth muscle cell proliferation. In addition, by interfering with endothelium-dependent relaxation (162), oxidized LDL may facilitate luminal narrowing by deterring vasorelaxation.

There are a limited number of studies demonstrating that antioxidants may retard restenosis. Interestingly, some of the same lipophilic antioxidants shown to inhibit atherosclerosis progression also appear to limit vascular regrowth after balloon injury. Probucol (200), BHT (201), and vitamin E (132) have each been shown to reduce significantly the intimal thickening following balloon injury of the arteries of cholesterol-fed rabbits. Probucol was also reported to be of benefit after angioplasty in a limited human study (202). Vitamins E and C together, but neither alone, were able to limit luminal narrowing in porcine coronary arteries after balloon injury, independent of any inhibition of intimal thickening (203). In addition, desferal, a chelator of iron, has been shown to inhibit stenosis in a vascular injury model and to inhibit smooth muscle cell proliferation in vitro (204). Because desferal can block metal ion participation in lipid peroxidation reactions, the effect of desferal could be related to its antioxidant activity as well as to the sequestration of cellular iron needed for cell cycle progression. Ebselen, a compound that reduces lipid hydroperoxides, has been reported to limit restenosis after angioplasty in a small group of humans (205). One study in humans showed limited benefit of vitamin E treatment, but in this group of patients, the vitamin E treatment was not offered in advance of angioplasty (206). Lipophilic substances such as vitamin E and probucol would be expected to require significant time to reach elevated antioxidant levels in tissue.

Thus, although unproven, it is consistent with in vitro data that lipid oxidation products could induce an exaggerated stenosis after balloon injury. The success of certain antioxidants in animal models suggests further research; however, there are numerous studies of therapies that effectively inhibit stenosis after injury in animals but are ineffective in humans.

SUMMARY

The data regarding antiatherosclerotic effects of antioxidants are strong enough to warrant continued research of a lipoprotein oxidation theory of atherosclerosis; however, caution needs to be applied to avoid embracing the concept without proof. Decades of research have demonstrated that atherogenesis, the progression of lesions, their calcification, and thrombotic complications are likely mediated by multiple factors. To believe all are mediated by or derived from uncontrolled oxidative events is perhaps naive.

REFERENCES

1. Henriksen T, Evensen SA, Carlander B. Injury to human endothelial cells in culture induced by low density lipoproteins. *Scand J Clin Lab Invest* 1979;39:361–368.
2. Hessler JR, Robertson AL Jr, Chisolm GM. LDL-induced cytotoxicity and its inhibition by HDL in human vascular smooth muscle and endothelial cells in culture. *Atherosclerosis* 1979;32:213–229.
3. Hessler JR, Morel DW, Lewis LJ, Chisolm GM. Lipoprotein oxidation and lipoprotein-induced cytotoxicity. *Arteriosclerosis* 1983;3: 215–222.
4. Morel DW, Hessler JR, Chisolm GM. Low density lipoprotein cytotoxicity induced by free radical peroxidation of lipid. *J Lipid Res* 1983;24:1070–1076.
5. Schechter I, Fogelman AM, Haberland ME, Seager J, Hokom M, Edwards PA. The metabolism of native and malondialdehyde altered low density lipoproteins by human monocyte–macrophages. *J Lipid Res* 1981;22:63–71.
6. Henriksen T, Mahoney EM, Steinberg D. Enhanced macrophage degradation of low density lipoprotein previously incubated with cultured endothelial cells: Recognition by receptors for acetylated low density lipoproteins. *Proc Natl Acad Sci USA* 1981;78:6499–6503.
7. Morel DW, DiCorleto PE, Chisolm GM. Endothelial and smooth muscle cells alter low density lipoprotein in vitro by free radical oxidation. *Arteriosclerosis* 1984;4:357–364.
8. Steinbrecher UP, Parthasarathy S, Leake DS, Witzum LJ, Steinberg D. Modification of low density lipoprotein by endothelial cells involves lipid peroxidation and degradation of low density lipoprotein phospholipids. *Proc Natl Acad Sci USA* 1984;81:3883–3887.
9. Heinecke JW, Rosen H, Chait A. Iron and copper promote modification of low density lipoprotein by human arterial smooth muscle cells in culture. *J Clin Invest* 1984;74:1890–1894.
10. Cathcart MK, Morel DW, Chisolm GM. Monocytes and neutrophils oxidize low density lipoprotein making it cytotoxic. *J Leukocyte Biol* 1985;38:341–350.
11. Parthasarathy S, Printz DJ, Boyd D, Joy L, Steinberg D. Macrophage oxidation of low density lipoprotein generates a form recognized by the scavenger receptor. *Arteriosclerosis* 1986;6:505–510.
12. Smith EB, Slater RS. Relationship between low density lipoprotein in aortic intima and serum lipid levels. *Lancet* 1972;1:463–468.
13. Hoff HF, Gaubatz JW. Isolation of a low density lipoprotein from atherosclerotic vascular tissue of WHHL rabbits. *Atherosclerosis* 1982;42:272–297.
14. Boyd HC, Gown AM, Wolfbauer G, Chait A. Direct evidence for a protein recognized by a monoclonal antibody against oxidatively modified LDL in atherosclerotic lesions from a Watanabe heritable hyperlipidemic rabbit. *Am J Pathol* 1989;135:815–825.
15. Haberland ME, Fong D, Cheng L. Malondialdehyde-altered protein occurs in atheroma of Watanabe heritable hyperlipidemic rabbits. *Science* 1988;241:215–218.
16. Mowri H, Ohkuma S, Takano T. Monoclonal DLR1a/104G antibody recognizing peroxidized lipoproteins in atherosclerotic lesions. *Biochim Biophys Acta* 1988;963:239–245.
17. Palinski W, Rosenfeld ME, Yla-Herttuala S, Gurtner GC, Socher SS, Butler SW, Parthasarathy S, Carew TE, Steinberg D, Witztum JL. Low density lipoprotein undergoes oxidative modification in vivo. *Proc Natl Acad Sci USA* 1989;86:1372–1376.
18. Ylä-Herttuala S, Palinski W, Rosenfeld ME, Parthasarathy S, Carew TE, Butler S, Witztum JL, Steinberg D. Evidence for the presence of oxidatively modified low density lipoprotein in atherosclerotic lesions of rabbit and man. *J Clin Invest* 1989;84:1086–1095.
19. Carew TE, Schwenke DC, Steinberg D. Antiatherogenic effect of probucol unrelated to its hypocholesterolemic effect: Evidence that antioxidants in vivo can selectively inhibit low density lipoprotein degradation in macrophage-rich fatty streaks and slow the progression of atherosclerosis in the Watanabe heritable hyperlipidemic rabbit. *Proc Natl Acad Sci USA* 1987;84:7725–7729.
20. Daugherty A, Zweifel BS, Schonfeld G. Probucol attenuates the development of aortic atherosclerosis in cholesterol-fed rabbits. *Br J Pharmacol* 1989;98:612–618.
21. Kita T, Nagano Y, Yokode M, Ishii K, Kume N, Ooshima A, Yoshida H, Kawai C. Probucol prevents the progression of atherosclerosis in Watanabe heritable hyperlipidemic rabbit, an animal model for familial hypercholesterolemia. *Proc Natl Acad Sci USA* 1987;84: 5928–5931.
22. Verlangieri AJ, Bush MJ. Effects of *d*-α-tocopherol supplementation on experimentally induced primate atherosclerosis. *J Am Coll Nutr* 1992;11:131–138.
23. Stampfer MJ, Hennekens CH, Manson JE, Colditz GA, Rosner B, Willett WC. Vitamin E consumption and the risk of coronary disease in women. *N Engl J Med* 1993;328:1444–1449.
24. Rimm EB, Stampfer MJ, Ascherio A, Giovannucci E, Colditz GA, Willett WC. Vitamin E consumption and the risk of coronary disease in men. *N Engl J Med* 1993;328:1450–1456.
25. Sparrow CP, Doebber TW, Olszewski J, Wu MS, Ventre J, Stevens KA, Chao Y. Low density lipoprotein is protected from oxidation and the progression of atherosclerosis is slowed in cholesterol-fed rabbits by the antioxidant N,N′-diphenylphenylenediamine. *J Clin Invest* 1992;89:1885–1891.
26. Bjorkhem I, Henriksson-Freyschuss A, Breuer O, Diczfalusy U, Berglund L, Henriksson P. The antioxidant butylated hydroxytoluene protects against atherosclerosis. *Arterioscler Thromb* 1991;11:15–22.
27. Gaziano JM, Manson JE, Kidker PM, Buring JE, Hennekens CH. Beta carotene therapy for chronic stable angina. *Circulation* 1990;82: III-201 (abstr).
28. Shankar R, Sallis JD, Stanton H, Thomson R. Influence of probucol on early experimental atherogenesis in hypercholesterolemic rats. *Atherosclerosis* 1989;78:91–97.
29. Sasahara M, Raines EW, Chait A, Carew TE, Steinberg D, Wahl PW, Ross R. Inhibition of hypercholesterolemia-induced atherosclerosis in the nonhuman primate by probucol. I. Is the extent of atherosclerosis related to resistance of LDL to oxidation? *J Clin Invest* 1994;94: 155–164.
30. Berliner JA, Territo MC, Sevanian A, Ramin S, Kim JA, Bamshad B, Esterson M, Fogelman AM. Minimally modified low density lipoprotein stimulates monocyte endothelial interactions. *J Clin Invest* 1990;85:1260–1266.
31. Dousset N, Negre-Salvayre A, Lopez M, Salvayre R, Douste-Blazy L. Ultraviolet-treated lipoproteins as a model system for the study of the biological effects of lipid peroxides on cultured cell. I. Chemical modifications of ultraviolet-treated low-density lipoproteins. *Biochim Biophys Acta* 1990;1045:219–223.
32. Palinski W, Ylä-Herttuala S, Rosenfeld ME, Butler SW, Socher SA, Parthasarathy S, Curtiss LK, Witztum JL. Antisera and monoclonal antibodies specific for epitopes generated during oxidative modification of low density lipoprotein. *Arteriosclerosis* 1990;10:325–335.
33. Jürgens G, Hoff HF, Chisolm GM, Esterbauer H. Modification of human serum low density lipoprotein by oxidation—characterization and pathophysiologic implications. *Chem Phys Lipids* 1987;45: 315–336.
34. Brown MS, Goldstein JL. Lipoprotein metabolism in the macrophage: Implications for cholesterol deposition in atherosclerosis. *Annu Rev Biochem* 1983;52:223.
35. Fong LG, Parthasarathy S, Witzutum JL, Steinberg D. Nonenzymatic oxidative cleavage of peptide bonds in apoprotein B-100. *J Lipid Res* 1987;28:1466–1477.
36. Steinbrecher UP, Witztum JL, Parthasarathy S, Steinberg D. Decrease in reactive amino groups during oxidation or endothelial cell modifica-

tion of LDL. Correlation with changes in receptor-mediated catabolism. *Arteriosclerosis* 1987;7:135–143.
37. Nagelkerke JF, Havekes L, van Hinsbergh VWM, van Berkel TJC. In vivo catabolism of biologically modified LDL. *Arteriosclerosis* 1984;4:256–264.
38. Bhadra S, Arshad MAQ, Rymaszewski Z, Norman E, Wherley R, Subbiah MTR. Oxidation of cholesterol moiety of low density lipoprotein in the presence of human endothelial cells or Cu^{+2} ions: Identification of major products and their effects. *Biochem Biophys Res Commun* 1991;176:431–440.
39. Zhang H, Basra HJK, Steinbrecher UP. Effects of oxidatively modified LDL on cholesterol esterification in cultured macrophages. *J Lipid Res* 1990;31:1361–1369.
40. Chisolm GM, Ma G, Irwin KC, Martin LL, Gunderson KG, Linberg LF, Morel DW, DiCorleto PE. 7β-Hydroperoxycholest-5-en-3β-ol, a component of human atherosclerotic lesions, is the primary cytotoxin of oxidized human low density lipoprotein. *Proc Natl Acad Sci USA* 1994;91:11452–11456.
41. Esterbauer H, Jürgens G, Quehenberger O, Koller E. Autoxidation of human low density lipoprotein: Loss of polyunsaturated fatty acids and vitamin E and generation of aldehydes. *J Lipid Res* 1987;28: 495–509.
42. Stocker R, Bowry VW, Frei B. Ubiquinol-10 protects human low density lipoprotein more efficiently against lipid peroxidation than does alpha-tocopherol. *Proc Natl Acad Sci USA* 1991;88:1646–1650.
43. Ingold KU, Bowry VW, Stocker R, Walling C. Autoxidation of lipids and antioxidation by alpha-tocopherol and ubiquinol in homogeneous solution and in aqueous dispersions of lipids. Unrecognized consequences of lipid particle size as exemplified by oxidation of human low density lipoprotein. *Proc Natl Acad Sci USA* 1993;90:45–49.
44. Wagner JR, Motchnik PA, Stocker R, Sies H, Ames BN. The oxidation of blood plasma and low density lipoprotein components by chemically generated singlet oxygen. *J Biol Chem* 1993;268:18502–18506.
45. Steinbrecher UP, Pritchard PH. Hydrolysis of phosphatidylcholine during LDL oxidation is mediated by platelet-activating factor acetylhydrolase. *J Lipid Res* 1989;30:305–315.
46. Parthasarathy S, Steinbrecher UP, Barnett J, Witztum JL, Steinberg D. Essential role of phospholipase A_2 activity in endothelial cell-induced modification of low density lipoprotein. *Proc Natl Acad Sci USA* 1985;82:3000–3004.
47. Stafforini DM, Carter ME, Zimmerman GA, McIntyre TM, Prescott SM. Lipoproteins alter the catalytic behavior of the platelet-activating factor acetylhydrolase in human plasma. *Proceedings of the National Academy of Sciences of the United States of America.* 1989;86: 2393–2397.
48. Parthasarathy S, Barnett J. Phospholipase A_2 activity of low density lipoprotein: Evidence for an intrinsic phospholipase A_2 activity of apoprotein B-100. *Proc Natl Acad Sci USA* 1990;87:9741–9745.
49. Stafforini DM, Prescott SM, McIntyre TM. Human platelet activating factor acetylhydrolase: Association with lipoprotein particles and role in the degradation of platelet-activating factor. *J Biol Chem* 1987; 262:4223–4230.
50. Rosenfeld ME, Palinski W, Ylä-Herttuala S, Butler S, Witztum JL. Distribution of oxidized proteins and apolipoprotein B in atherosclerotic lesions of varying severity from WHHL rabbits: Immunocytochemical analysis using antibodies generated against modified and native LDL. *Arteriosclerosis* 1990;10:336–349.
51. YlaP-Herttuala S, Palinski W, Rosenfeld ME, Steinberg D, Witztum JL. Isolation and characterization of lipoproteins from normal and atherosclerotic arteries. *Eur Heart J* 1990;11:88–99.
52. Daugherty A, Zwiefel BS, Sobel BE, Schonfeld G. Isolation of low density lipoprotein from atherosclerotic vascular tissue of Watanabe heritable hyperlipidemic rabbits. *Arteriosclerosis* 1990;10:336–349.
53. Hoff HF, O'Neil J. Lesion-derived low density lipoprotein and oxidized low density lipoprotein share a lability for aggregation, leading to enhanced macrophage degradation. *Arterioslcer Thromb* 1991;11: 1209–1222.
54. Lyons TJ. Glycation and oxidation: A role in the pathogenesis of atherosclerosis. *Am J Cardiol* 1993;71:26B–31B.
55. Chisolm GM, Irwin KC, Penn MS. Lipoprotein oxidation and lipoprotein-induced cell injury in diabetes. *Diabetes* 1992;41(Suppl 2): 61–66.
56. Morel DW, Chisolm GM. Antioxidant treatment of diabetic rats inhibits lipoprotein oxidation and cytotoxicity. *J Lipid Res* 1989;30: 1827–1834.
57. Higuchi Y. Lipid peroxides and α-tocopherol in rat streptozotocin-induced diabetes mellitus. *Acta Med Okayama* 1982;3:165–175.
58. Karpen CW, Pritchard KA Jr, Arnold JH, Cornwell DG, Panganamala RV. Restoration of protacyclin/thromboxane A_2 balance in the diabetic rat. Influence of dietary vitamin E. *Diabetes* 1982;31:947–951.
59. Avogaro P, Bon GB, Cazzolato G. Presence of a modified low density lipoprotein in humans. *Arteriosclerosis* 1988;8:79–87.
60. Hodis HN, Kramsch DM, Avogaro P, Bittolo-Bon G, Cazzolato G, Hwang J, Sevanian A. Biochemical and cytotoxic characteristics of an in vivo circulating oxidized low density lipoprotein (LDL^-). *J Lipid Res* 1994;35:669–677.
61. Stringer MD, Gorog PG, Freeman A, Kakkar VV. Lipid peroxides and atherosclerosis. *Br Med J* 1989;298:281–284.
62. Liu K, Cuddy TE, Pierce GN. Oxidative status of lipoproteins in coronary disease patients. *Am Heart J* 1992;123:285–290.
63. Salonen JT, Yla-Herttuala S, Yamamoto R, Butler S, Korpela H, Salonen R, Nyyssonen K, Palinski W, Witztum JL. Autoantibody against oxidised LDL and progression of carotid atherosclerosis. *Lancet* 1992; 339:883–887.
64. Tribble DL, Holl LG, Wood PD, Krauss RM. Variations in oxidative susceptibility among six low density lipoprotein subfractions of differing density and particle size. *Atherosclerosis* 1992;93:189–199.
65. Chait A, Brazg RL, Tribble DL, Krauss RM. Susceptibility of small, dense, low-density lipoproteins to oxidative modification in subjects with the atherogenic lipoprotein phenotype, pattern B. *Am J Med* 1993;94:350–356.
66. Parthasarathy S, Fong LG, Quinn MT, Steinberg D. Oxidative modification of LDL: Comparison between cell-mediated and copper-mediated modification. *Eur Heart J* 1990;11:83–87.
67. Steinbrecher UP. Role of superoxide in endothelial-cell modification of low-density lipoproteins. *Biochim Biophys Acta* 1988;959:20–30.
68. Parthasarathy S, Wieland E, Steinberg D. A role for endothelial cell lipoxygenase in the oxidative modification of low density lipoprotein. *Proc Natl Acad Sci USA* 1989;86:1046–1050.
69. Sparrow CP, Olszewski J. Cellular oxidative modification of low density lipoprotein does not require lipoxygenases. *Proc Natl Acad Sci USA* 1992;89:128–131.
70. Parthasarathy S. Mechanism(s) of cell-mediated oxidation of low density lipoprotein. In: Nohl H, Esterbauer H, Rice-Evans C, eds. *Free Radicals in the Environment, Medicine and Toxicology.* London: Richelieu Press; 1994:163–179.
71. Jessup W, Mohr D, Gieseg SP, Dean RT, Stocker R. The participation of nitric oxide in cell-free and its restriction of macrophage-mediated oxidation of low-density lipoprotein. *Biochim Biophys Acta* 1992; 1180:73–82.
72. Parthasarathy S. Oxidation of low-density lipoprotein by thiol compounds leads to its recognition by the acetyl LDL receptor. *Biochim Biophys Acta* 1987;917:337–340.
73. Heinecke JW, Rosen H, Suzuki LA, Chait A. The role of sulfur-containing amino acids in superoxide production and modification of low density lipoprotein by arterial smooth muscle cells. *J Biol Chem* 1987;262:10098–10103.
74. Sparrow CP, Olszewski J. Cellular oxidation of low density lipoprotein is caused by thiol production in media containing transition metal ions. *J Lipid Res* 1993;34:1219–1228.
75. Daugherty A, Dunn JL, Rateri DL, Heinecke JW. Myeloperoxidase, a catalyst for lipoprotein oxidation, is expressed in human atherosclerotic lesions. *J Clin Invest* 1994;94:437–444.
76. Cathcart MK, McNally AK, Morel DW, Chisolm GM. Superoxide anion participation in human monocyte-mediated oxidation of low-density lipoprotein and conversion of low-density lipoprotein to a cytotoxin. *J Immunol* 1989;142:1963–1969.
77. Hiramatsu K, Rosen H, Heinecke JW, Wolfbauer G, Chait A. Superoxide initiates oxidation of low density lipoprotein by human monocytes. *Arteriosclerosis* 1987;7:55–60.
78. McNally AK, Chisolm GM, Morel DW, Cathcart MK. Activated human monocytes oxidize low-density lipoprotein by a lipoxygenase-dependent pathway. *J Immunol* 1990;145:254–259.
79. Ehrenwald E, Chisolm GM, Fox PL. Intact human ceruloplasmin oxidatively modifies low density lipoproteins. *J Clin Invest* 1994;93: 1493–1501.
80. Cathcart MK, Chisolm GM, McNally AK, Morel DW. Oxidative modification of low density lipoprotein (LDL) by activated human

monocytes and the cell lines U937 and HL60. *In Vitro Cell Dev Biol* 1988;24:1001–1008.

81. Ehrenwald E, Fox P. Endogenous ceruloplasmin is required for monocyte cell oxidation of low densitiy lipoprotein (LDL). *FASEB J* 1994; 8:A803.
82. Bratzler RL, Chisolm GM, Colton CK, Smith KA, Lees RS. The distribution of labeled low-density lipoprotein across the rabbit thoracic aorta in vivo. *Atherosclerosis* 1977;28:289–307.
83. Camejo G, Hurt-Camejo E, Rosengren B, Wiklund O, López F, Bondjers G. Modification of copper-catalyzed oxidation of low density lipoprotein by proteoglycans and glycosaminoglycans. *J Lipid Res* 1991; 32:1983–1991.
84. Hurt-Camejo E, Camejo G, Rosengren B, López F, Ahlström C, Fager G, Bondjers G. Effect of arterial proteoglycans and glycosaminoglycans on low density lipoprotein oxidation and its uptake by human macrophages and arterial smooth muscle cells. *Arterioscler Thromb* 1992;12:569–583.
85. Kalant N, McCormick S, Parniak MA. Effects of copper and histidine on oxidative modification of low density lipoprotein and its subsequent binding to collagen. *Arterioscler Thromb* 1991;11:1322–1329.
86. Arai H, Kita T, Yokode M, Narumiya S, Kawai C. Multiple receptors for modified low density lipoproteins in mouse peritoneal macrophages: Different uptake mechanisms for acetylated and oxidized low density lipoproteins. *Biochem Biophys Res Commun* 1989;159: 1375–1382.
87. Sparrow CP, Parthasarathy S, Steinberg D. A macrophage receptor that recognizes oxidized low density lipoprotein but not acetylated low density lipoprotein. *J Biol Chem* 1989;264:2599–2604.
88. Freeman M, Ekkel Y, Rohrer L, Penman M, Freedman NJ, Chisolm GM, Krieger M. Expression of type I and type II bovine scavenger receptors in Chinese hamster ovary cells: Lipid droplet accumulation and nonreciprocal cross competition by acetylated and oxidized low density lipoprotein. *Proc Natl Acad Sci USA* 1991;88:4931–4935.
89. Esbach S, Pieters MN, van der Boom J, Schouten D, van der Heyde MN, Roholl PJ, Brouwer A, Van Berkel TJ, Knook DL. Visualization of the uptake and processing of oxidized low-density lipoproteins in human and rat liver. *Hepatology* 1993;18:537–545.
90. Stanton LW, White RT, Bryant CM, Protter AA, Endemann G. A macrophage Fc receptor for IgG is also a receptor for oxidized low density lipoprotein. *J Biol Chem* 1992;267:22446–22451.
91. Endemann G, Stanton LW, Madden KS, Bryant CM, White RT, Protter AA. CD36 is a receptor for oxidized low density lipoprotein. *J Biol Chem* 1993;268:11811–11816.
92. Acton SL, Scherer PE, Lodish HF, Krieger M. Expression cloning of SR-BI, a CD36-related Class B scavenger receptor. *J Biol Chem* 1994; 269:21003–12009.
93. Fox PL, Chisolm GM, DiCorleto PE. Lipoprotein mediated inhibition of endothelial cell production of platelet-derived growth factor-like proteins depends on free radical lipid peroxidation. *J Biol Chem* 1987; 262:6046–6054.
94. Hoff HF, Whitaker TE, O'Neil J. Oxidation of low density lipoprotein leads to particle aggregation and altered macrophage recognition. *J Biol Chem* 1992;267:602–609.
95. Lougheed M, Zhang H, Steinbrecher UP. Oxidized low density lipoprotein is resistant to cathepsins and accumulates within macrophages. *J Biol Chem* 1991;266:14519–14525.
96. Jialal I, Chait A. Differences in the metabolism of oxidatively modified low density lipoprotein and acetylated low density lipoprotein by human endothelial cells. Inhibition of cholesterol esterification by oxidatively modified low density lipoprotein. *J Lipid Res* 1989;30: 1561–1568.
97. Hoppe G, O'Neil J, Hoff HF. Inactivation of lysosomal proteases by oxidized low density lipoprotein is partially responsible for its poor degradation by mouse peritoneal macrophages. *J Clin Invest* 1994; 94:1506–1512.
98. Jessup W, Mander EL, Dean RT. The intracellular storage and turnover of apolipoprotein B of oxidized LDL in macrophages. *Biochim Biophys Acta* 1992;1126:167–177.
99. Roma P, Bernini F, Fogliatto R, Bertullli SM, Negri S, Fumagalli R, Catapano AL. Defective catabolism of oxidized LDL by J774 murine macrophages. J Lipid Res 1992;33:819–829.
100. Mander LE, Dean RT, Stanley KK, Jessup W. Apolipoprotein B of oxidized LDL accumulates in the lysosomes of macrophages. *Biochim Biophys Acta* 1994;1212:80–92.
101. Roma P, Catapano AL, Bertulli SM, Varesi L, Fumagalli R, Bernini F. Oxidized LDL increase free cholesterol and fail to stimulate cholesterol esterification in murine macrophages. *Biochem Biophys Res Commun* 1990;171:123–131.
102. Thomas JP, Geoger PG, Maiorino M, Ursini F, Girotti AW. Enzymatic reduction of phospholipid and cholesterol hydroperoxides in artificial bilayers and lipoproteins. *Biochim Biophys Acta* 1990;1045:252–260.
103. Thomas JP, Maiorino M, Ursini F, Girotti AW. Protective action of phospholipid hydroperoxide glutathione peroxidase against membrane-damaging lipid peroxidation. In situ reduction of phospholipid and cholesterol hydroperoxides. *J Biol Chem* 1990;265:454–461.
104. Thomas JP, Geiger PG, Girotti AW. Lethal damage to endothelial cells by oxidized low density lipoprotein: Role of selenoperoxidases in cytoprotection against lipid hydroperoxide- and iron-mediated reactions. *J Lipid Res* 1993;34:479–490.
105. Ross R. The pathogenesis of atherosclerosis: An update. *N Engl J Med* 1986;314:488–500.
106. Ross R. The pathogenesis of atherosclerosis: A perspective for the 1990s. *Nature* 1993;362:801–809.
107. Kosugi K, Morel DW, DiCorleto PE, Chisolm GM. Toxicity of oxidized low-density lipoprotein to cultured fibroblasts is selective for S phase of the cell cycle. *J Cell Physiol* 1987;130:311–320.
108. Negre-Salvayre A, Lopez M, Levade T, Pieraggi M-T, Dousset N, Douste-Blazy L, Salvayre R. Ultraviolet-treated lipoproteins as a model system for the study of the biological effects of lipid peroxides on cultured cell. II. Uptake and cytotoxicity of ultraviolet-treated LDL on lymphoid cell lines. *Biochim Biophys Acta* 1990;1045:224–232.
109. Cathcart MK, McNally AK, Chisolm GM. Lipoxygenase-mediated transformation of human low density lipoprotein to an oxidized and cytotoxic complex. *J Lipdi Res* 1991;32:63–70.
110. Henriksen T, Evensen SA, Carlander B. Injury to cultured endothelial cells induced by low density lipoproteins: Protection by high density lipoproteins. *Scand J Clin Lab Invest* 1979;39:369–375.
111. Borsum T, Henriksen B, Carlander B, Reisvaag A. Injury to human cells in culture induced by low density lipoprotein: An effect independent of receptor binding and endocytotic uptake of low density lipoprotein. *Scand J Clin Lab Invest* 1982;42:75–81.
112. Chisolm GM. Cytotoxicity of oxidized lipoproteins. *Curr Opin Lipidol* 1991;2:311–316.
113. Hughes H, Mathews B, Lenz ML, Guyton JR. Cytotoxicity of oxidized LDL to porcine aortic smooth muscle cells is associated with the oxysterols 7-ketocholesterol and 7-hydroxycholesterol. *Arterioscler Thromb* 1994;14:1177–1185.
114. Kuzuya M, Naito M, Funaki C, Hayashi T, Asai K, Kuzuya F. Probucol prevents oxidative injury to endothelial cells. *J Lipid Res* 1991; 32:197–204.
115. Negre-Salvayre A, Alomar Y, Troly M, Salvayre R. Ultraviolet-treated lipoproteins as a model system for the study of the biological effects of lipid peroxides on cultured cells. III. The protective effect of antioxidants (probucol, catechin, vitamin E) against the cytotoxicity of oxidized LDL occurs in two different ways. *Biochim Biophys Acta* 1991;1096:291–300.
116. Escargueil I, Nègre-Salvayre A, Pieraggi M-T, Salvayre R. Oxidized low density lipoproteins elicit DNA fragmentation of cultured lymphoblastoid cells. *FEBS Lett* 1992;305:155–159.
117. Murugesan G, Chisolm GM, Fox PL. Oxidized low density lipoprotein inhibits the migration of aortic endothelial cells in vitro. *J Cell Biol* 1993;120:1011–1019.
118. Autio I, Jaakkola O, Solakivi T, Nikkari T. Oxidized low-density lipoprotein is chemotactic for arterial smooth muscle cells in culture. *FEBS Lett* 1990;277:247–249.
119. Quinn MT, Parthasarathy S, Fong LG, Steinberg D. Oxidatively modified low density lipoproteins: A potential role in recruitment and retention of monocyte/macrophages during atherogenesis. *Proc Natl Acad Sci USA* 1987;84:2995–2998.
120. Quinn MT, Parthasarathy S, Steinberg D. Endothelial cell-derived chemotactic activity for mouse peritoneal macrophages and the effects of modified forms of low density lipoprotein. *Proc Natl Acad Sci USA* 1985;82:5949–5953.
121. Quinn MT, Parthasarathy S, Steinberg D. Lysophosphatidylcholine: A chemotactic factor for human monocytes and its potential role in atherogenesis. *Proc Natl Acad Sci USA* 1988;85:2805–2809.
122. Cushing SD, Berliner JA, Valente AJ, Territo MC, Navab M, Parhami F, Gerrity R, Schwartz CJ, Fogelman AM. Minimally modified low

denstiy lipoprotein induces monocyte chemotactic protein 1 in human endothelial cells and smooth muscle cells. *Proc Natl Acad Sci USA* 1990;87:5134–5138.
123. Ylä-Herttuala S, Lipton BA, Rosenfeld ME, Sarkioja T, Yoshimura T, Leonard EJ, Witztum JL, Steinberg D. Expression of monocyte chemoattractant protein 1 in macrophage-rich areas of human and rabbit atherosclerotic lesions. *Proc Natl Acad Sci USA* 1991;88: 5252–5256.
124. Bruckdorfer KR, Jacobs M, Rice-Evans C. Endothelium-derived relaxing factor (nitric oxide), lipoprotein oxidation and atherosclerosis. *Biochem Soc Trans* 1990;18:1061–1063.
125. Murugesan G, Chisolm GM, Fox PL. Oxidized low density lipoprotein inhibits the migration of aortic endothelial cells in vitro. *J Cell Biol* 1993;120:1011–1019.
126. Autio I, Jaakkola O, Solakivi T, Nikkari T. Oxidized low-density lipoprotein is chemotactic for arterial smooth muscle cells in culture. *FEBS Lett* 1990;277:247–249.
127. Stiko-Rahm A, Hultgardh-Nilsson A, Regnstrom J, Hamsten A, Nilsson J. Native and oxidized LDL enhances production of PDGF AA and the surface expression of PDGF receptors in cultured human smooth muscle cells. *Arterioscler Thromb* 1992;12:1099–1109.
128. Malden LT, Chait A, Raines EW, Ross R. The influence of oxidatively modified low density lipoproteins on expression of platelet-derived growth factor by human monocyte-derived macrophages. *J Biol Chem* 1991;266:13901–13907.
129. Kume N, Gimbrone MA Jr. Lysophosphatidylcholine transcriptionally induces growth factor gene expression in cultured human endothelial cells. *J Clin Invest* 1994;93:907–911.
130. Van Heek M, Schmitt D, DiCorleto PE. Oxidized cholesteryl linoleate mediates the inhibition by oxidized LDL of platelet-derived growth factor (PDGF) production by bovine aortic endothelial cells (BAEC). *J Cell Biol* 1991;115:367a (abstr).
131. Chatterjee S. Role of oxidized human plasma low density lipoproteins in atherosclerosis: Effects on smooth muscle cell proliferation. *Mol Cell Biochem* 1992;111:143–147.
132. Lafont A, Chai YC, Cornhill JF, Whitlow PL, Howe PH, Chisolm GM. Effect of alpha-tocopherol on restenosis after angioplasty in a model of experimental atherosclerosis. *J Clin Invest* 1995;95: 1018–1025.
133. Nakano T, Raines EW, Abraham JA, Klagsbrun M, Ross R. Lysophosphatidylcholine upregulates the level of heparin-binding epidermal growth factor-like growth factor mRNA in human monocytes. *Proc Natl Acad Sci USA* 1994;91:1069–1073.
134. Jougasaki M, Kugiyama K, Saito Y, Nakao K, Imura H, Yasue H. Suppression of endothelin-1 secretion by lysophosphatidylcholine in oxidized low density lipoprotein in cultured vascular endothelial cells. *Circ Res* 1992;71:614–619.
135. Boulanger CM, Tanner FC, Béa M-L, Hahn AWA, Werner A, Lüscher TF. Oxidized low density lipoproteins induce mRNA expression and release of endothelin from human and porcine endothelium. *Circ Res* 1992;70:1191–1197.
136. Martin-Nizard F, Houssaini HS, Lestavel-Delattre S, Duriez P, Fruchart JC. Modified low density lipoproteins activate human macrophages to secrete immunoreactive endothelin. *FEBS Lett* 1991;293: 127–130.
137. Rajavashisth TB, Andalibi A, Territo MC, Berliner JA, Navab M, Fogelman AM, Lusis AJ. Induction of endothelial cell expression of granulocyte and macrophage colony-stimulating factors by modified low-density lipoproteins. *Nature* 1990;344:254–257.
138. Clinton SK, Underwood R, Hayes L, Sherman ML, Kufe DW, Libby P. Macrophage colony-stimulating factor gene expression in vascular cells and in experimental and human atherosclerosis. *Am J Pathol* 1992;140:301–316.
139. Inoue I, Inaba T, Motoyoshi K, Harada K, Shimano H, Kawamura M, Gotoda T, Cka T, Shiomi M, Watanabe Y, et al. Macrophage colony stimulating factor prevents the progression of atherosclerosis in Watanabe heritable hyperlipidemic rabbits. *Atherosclerosis* 1992; 93:245–254.
140. Terkeltaub R, Banka CL, Solan J, Santoro D, Brand K, Curtiss LK. Oxidized LDL induces monocytic cell expression of interleukin-8, a chemokine with T-lymphocyte chemotactic activity. *Arterioscler Thromb* 1994;14:47–53.
141. Fong LG, Fong TA, Cooper AD. Inhibition of lipopolysaccharide-induced interleukin-1 beta mRNA expression in mouse macrophages by oxidized low density lipoprotein. *J Lipid Res* 1991;32:1899–1910.
142. Hamilton TA, Ma GP, Chisolm GM. Oxidized low density lipoprotein suppresses the expression of tumor necrosis factor-alpha mRNA in stimulated murine peritoneal macrophages. *J Immunol* 1990;144: 2343–2350.
143. Hamilton TA, Major JA, Chisolm GM. The effects of oxidized LDL on inducible mouse macrophage gene expression are gene and stimulus dependent. *J Clin Invest* 1995;95:2004–2011.
144. Crutchley DJ, McPhee GV, Terris MF, Canossa-Terris MA. Levels of three hemostatic factors in relation to serum lipids. Monocyte procoagulant activity, tissue plasminogen activator, and type-1 plasminogen activator inhibitor. *Arteriosclerosis* 1989;9:934–939.
145. Olofsson BO, Dahlen G, Nilsson TK. Evidence for increased levels of plasminogen activator inhibitor and tissue plasminogen activator in plasma of patients with angiographically verified coronary artery disease. *Eur Heart J* 1989;10:77–82.
146. Latron Y, Chautan M, Anfosso F, Alessi MC, Nalbone G, Lafont H, Juhan-Vague I. Stimulating effect of oxidized low density lipoproteins on plasminogen activator inhibitor-1 synthesis by endothelial cells. *Arterioscler Thromb* 1991;11:1821–1829.
147. Kugiyama K, Sakamoto T, Misumi I, Sugiyama S, Ohgushi M, Ogawa H, Horiguchi M, Yasue H. Transferable lipids in oxidized low-density lipoprotein stimulate plasminogen activator inhibitor-1 and inhibit tissue-type plasminogen activator release from endothelial cells. *Circ Res* 1993;73:335–343.
148. Tremoli E, Camera M, Maderna P, Sironi L, Prati L, Colli S, Piovella F, Bernini F, Corsini A, Mussoni L. Increased synthesis of plasminogen activator inhibitor-1 by cultured human endothelial cells exposed to native and modified LDLs: An LDL receptor-independent phenomenon. *Arterioscler Thromb* 1993;13:338–346.
149. Weis JR, Pitas RE, Wilson BD, Rodgers GM. Oxidized low-density lipoprotein increases cultured human endothelial cell tissue factor activity and reduces protein C activation. *FASEB J* 1991;5:2459–2465.
150. Drake TA, Hannani K, Fei HH, Lavi S, Berliner JA. Minimally oxidized low-density lipoprotein induces tissue factor expression in cultured human endothelial cells. *Am J Pathol* 1991;138:601–607.
151. Wilcox JN, Smith KM, Schwartz SM, Gordon D. Localization of tissue factor in the normal vessel wall and in the atherosclerotic plaque. *Proc Natl Acad Sci USA* 1989;86:2839–2843.
152. Taubman MB. Tissue factor regulation in vascular smooth muscle: A summary of studies performed using in vivo and in vitro models. *Am J Cardiol* 1993;72:55C–60C.
153. Marmur MB, Rossikhina M, Guha A, Fyfe B, Friedich V, Mendlowitz M, Nemerson Y, Taubman MB. The induction of tissue factor in arterial media following balloon injury. *J Clin Invest* 1993;91: 2253–2259.
154. Taubman MB, Marmur JD, Rosenfield CL, Guha A, Nihctberger S, Nemerson Y. Agonist-mediated tissue factor expression in cultured vascular smooth muscle cells: Role of Ca^{2+} mobilization and protein kinase C activation. *J Clin Invest* 1993;91:547–552.
155. Penn MS, DiCorleto PE, Chisolm GM. Oxidized low density lipoprotein induces tissue factor expression by rabbit aortic smooth muscle cells. *Circulation* 1994;90:I-353 (abstr).
156. McNamara CA, Sarembock IJ, Gimple LW, Fenton JW, Coughlin SR, Owens GK. Thrombin stimulates proliferation of cultured rat aortic smooth muscle cells by a proteolytically activated receptor. *J Clin Invest* 1993;91:94–98.
157. Tomoike H, Egashira K, Yamamoto Y, Nakamura M. Enhanced responsiveness of smooth muscle, impaired endothelium-dependent relaxation and the genesis of coronary spasm. *Am J Cardiol* 1989;63: 33E–39E.
158. Simon BC, Cunningham LD, Cohen RA. Oxidized low density lipoproteins cause contraction and inhibit endothelium-dependent relaxation in the pig coronary artery. *J Clin Invest* 1990;86:75–79.
159. Chin JH, Azhar S, Hoffman BB. Inactivation of endothelial derived relaxing factor by oxidized lipoproteins. *J Clin Invest* 1992;89:10–18.
160. Yokoyama M, Hirata K, Miyake R, Akita H, Ishikawa Y, Fukuzaki H. Lysophosphatidylcholine: Essential role in the inhibition of endothelium-dependent vasorelaxation by oxidized low density lipoprotein. *Biochem Biophys Res Commun* 1990;168:301–308.
161. Ohgushi M, Kugiyama K, Fukunaga K, Murohara T, Sugiyama S, Miyamoto E, Yasue H. Protein kinase C inhibitors prevent impairment

of endothelium-dependent relaxation by oxidatively modified LDL. *Arterioscler Thromb* 1993;13:1525–1532.
162. Kugiyama K, Kerns SA, Morrisett JD, Roberts R, Henry PD. Impairment of endothelium-dependent arterial relaxation by lysolecithin in modified low-density lipoproteins. *Nature* 1990;344:160–162.
163. Matsuda Y, Hirata K, Inoue N, Suematsu M, Kawashima S, Akita H, Yokoyama M. High density lipoprotein reverses inhibitory effect of oxidized low density lipoprotein on endothelium-dependent arterial relaxation. *Circ Res* 1993;72:1103–1109.
164. Matsuda Y. High density lipoprotein and low density lipoprotein attenuate the inhibitory effects of oxidized low density lipoprotein on endothelium-dependent arterial relaxation. *Kobe J Med Sci* 1993;39: 1–14.
165. Galle J, Mülsch A, Busse R, Bassenge E. Effects of native and oxidized low density lipoproteins on formation and inactivation of endothelium-derived relaxing factor. *Arteriosclerosis* 1991;11:198–203.
166. Schmidt K, Graier WF, Kostner GM, Mayer B, Kukovetz WR. Activation of soluble guanylate cyclase by nitrovasodilators is inhibited by oxidized low-density lipoprotein. *Biochem Biophys Res Commun* 1990;172:614–619.
167. Jacobs M, Plane F, Bruckdorfer KR. Native and oxidized low-density lipoproteins have different inhibitory effects on endothelium-derived relaxing factor in the rabbit aorta. *Br J Pharmacol* 1990;100:21–26.
168. Galle J, Bassenge E, Busse R. Oxidized low density lipoproteins potentiate vasoconstrictions to various agonists by direct interacion with vascular smooth muscle. *Circ Res* 1990;66:1287–1293.
169. Negre-Salvayre A, Salvayre R. Protection by Ca^{2+} channel blockers (nifedipine, diltiazem and verapamil) against the toxicity of oxidized low density lipoprotein to cultured lymphoid cells. *Br J Pharmacol* 1992;107:738–744.
170. Stoll LL, Spector AA. Lysophosphatidylcholine causes cGMP-dependent verapamil-sensitive Ca^{2+} influx in vascular smooth muscle cells. *Am J Physiol* 1993;264:C885–C893.
171. Triau JE, Meydani SN, Schaefer EJ. Oxidized low density lipoprotein stimulates prostacyclin production by adult human vascular endothelial cells. *Arteriosclerosis* 1988;8:810–818.
172. Douglas SA, Louden C, Vickery-Clark LM, Sotrer BL, Hart T, Feuerstein GZ, Elliott JD, Ohlstein EH. A role for endogenous endothelin-1 in neointimal formation after rat carotid artery balloon angioplasty. *Circ Res* 1994;75:190–197.
173. Tahara A, Kohno M, Yanagi S, Itagane H, Toda I, Akioka K, Teragaki M, Yasuda M, Takeuchi K, Takeda T. Circulating immunoreactive endothelin in patients undergoing percutaneous transluminal coronary angioplasty. *Metabolism* 1991;40:1235–1237.
174. Schwenke DC, Carew TE. Quantification in vivo of increased LDL content and rate of LDL degradation in normal rabbit aorta occurring at sites susceptible to early atherosclerotic lesions. *Circ Res* 1988;62: 699–710.
175. Frostegård J, Nilsson J, Haegerstrand A, Hamsten A, Wigzell H, Gidlund M. Oxidized low density lipoprotein induces differentiation and adhesion of human monocytes and the moncytic cell line U937. *Proc Natl Acad Sci USA* 1990;87:904–908.
176. Kume N, Cybulsky MI, Gimbrone MA Jr. Lysophosphatidylcholine, a component of atherogenic lipoproteins, induces mononuclear leukocyte adhesion molecules in cultured human and rabbit arterial endothelial cells. *J Clin Invest* 1992;90:1138–1144.
177. Maier JA, Barenghi L, Pagani F, Bradamante S, Comi P, Ragnotti G. The protective role of high-density lipoprotein on oxidized-low-density-lipoprotein-induced U937/endothelial cell interactions. *Eur J Biochem* 1994;221:35–41.
178. Lehr HA, Hubner C, Nolte D, Finckh B, Beisiegel U, Kohlschutter A, Messmer K. Oxidatively modified human low-density lipoprotein stimulates leukocyte adherence to the microvascular endothelium in vivo. *Res Exp Med* 1991;191:85–90.
179. Lehr HA, Seemuller J, Hubner C, Menger MD, Messmer K. Oxidized LDL-induced leukocyte/endothelium interaction in vivo involves the receptor for platelet-activating factor. *Arterioscler Thromb* 1993;13: 1013–1018.
180. Lehr H-A, Kröber M, Hübner C, Vajkoczy P, Menger MD, Nolte D, Kohlschütter A, Messmer K. Stimulation of leukocyte/endothelium interaction by oxidized low-density lipoprotein in hairless mice: Involvement of CD11b/CD18 adhesion receptor complex. *Lab Invest* 1993;68:388–395.
181. Kim JA, Territo MC, Wayner E, Carlos TM, Parhami F, Smith CW, Haberland ME, Fogelman AM, Berliner JA. Partial characterization of leukocyte binding molecules on endothelial cells induced by minimally oxidized LDL. *Arterioscler Thromb* 1994;14:427–433.
182. Chisolm GM. Oxidized lipoproteins and leukocyte-endothelial interactions: Growing evidence for multiple mechanisms [editorial]. *Lab Invest* 1993;68:369–371.
183. Yokote K, Morisaki N, Zenibayashi M, Ueda S, Kanzaki T, Saito Y, Yoshida S. The phospholipase-A_2 reaction leads to increased monocyte adhesion of endothelial cells via the expression of adhesion molecules. *Eur J Biochem* 1993;217:723–729.
184. Frostegard J, Wu R, Haegerstrand A, Patarroyo M, Lefvert AK, Nilsson J. Mononuclear leukocytes exposed to oxidized low density lipoprotein secrete a factor that stimulates endothelial cells to express adhesion molecules. *Atherosclerosis* 1993;103:213–219.
185. Penn MS, Saidel GM, Chisolm GM. Relative significance of endothelium and internal elastic lamina in regulating the entry of macromolecules into arteries in vivo. *Circ Res* 1993;74:74–82.
186. Schwenke DC, Carew TE. Initiation of atherosclerotic lesions in cholesterol-fed rabbits. II. Selective retention of LDL vs. selective increases in LDL permeability in susceptible sites of arteries. *Arteriosclerosis* 1989;9:908–918.
187. Stiko-Rahm A, Hultgardh-Nilsson A, Regnstrom J, Hamsten A, Nilsson J. Native and oxidized LDL enhances production of PDGF AA and the surface expression of PDGF receptors in cultured human smooth muscle cells. *Arterioscler Thromb* 1992;12:1099–1109.
188. Pitas RE, Innnerarity TL, Mahley RW. Foam cells in explants of atheroslerotic rabbit aortas have receptors for β-very low density lipoproteins and modified low density lipoproteins. *Arteroisclerosis* 1983; 3:2–12.
189. Li H, Freeman MW, Libby P. Regulation of smooth muscle cell scavenger receptor expression in vivo by atherogenic diets and in vitro by cytokines. *J Clin Invest* 1995;95:122–133.
190. Chisolm GM. Antioxidants and atherosclerosis: A current assessment. *Clin Cardiol* 1991;14:I-25–I-30.
191. Parthasarathy S, Young SG, Witztum JL, Pittman RC. Probucol inhibits oxidative modification of low density lipoprotein. *J Clin Invest* 1986;77:641–644.
192. Williams RJ, Motteram JM, Sharp CH, Gallagher PJ. Dietary vitamin E and the attenuation of early lesion development in modified Watanabe rabbits. *Atherosclerosis* 1992;94:153–159.
193. Gey KF. The antioxidant hypothesis of cardiovascular disease: Epidemiology and mechanisms. *Biochem Soc Trans* 1990;18:1041–1045.
194. Stein Y, Stein O, Delplanque B, Fesmire JD, Lee DM, Alaupovic P. Lack of effect of probucol on atheroma formation in cholesterol-fed rabbits kept at comparable plasma cholesterol levels. *Atherosclerosis* 1989;75:145–155.
195. Walldius G, Erikson U, Olsson AG, Bergstrand L, Hadell K, Johansson J, Kaijser L, Lassvik C, Molgaard J, Nilsson S, et al. The effect of probucol on femoral atherosclerosis: The Probucol Quantitative Regression Swedish Trial (PQRST). *Am J Cardiol* 1994;74:875–883.
196. Kakuta T, Currier JW, Haudenschild CC, Ryan TJ, Faxon DP. Differences in compensatory enlargement, not intimal formation, accounts for restenosis after angioplasty in the atherosclerotic rabbit model. *Circulation* 1994;89:2809–2815.
197. Gertz SD, Gimple LWS, Banai S, Ragosta M, Powers ER, Roberts WC, Perez LS, Sarembock IJ. Geometric remodeling is not the principal atherogenic process in restenosis after balloon angioplasty. Evidence from correlative angiographic–histomorphometric studies of atherosclerotic arteries in rabbits. *Circulation* 1994;90:3001–3008.
198. Glagov S. Intimal hyperplasia, vascular remodeling, and the restenosis model. *Circulation* 1994;89:2888–2891.
199. Lafont A, Guzman L, Whitlow PL, Goormastic M, Cornhilll JF, Chisolm GM. Restenosis after experimental angioplasty: Intimal medial and adventitial changes associated with constrictive remodeling. *Circ Res* 1995;76:996–1002.
200. Ferns GAA, Forster L, Stewart-Lee A, Konneh M, Nourooz-Zadeh J, Änggård EE. Probucol inhibits neointimal thickening and macrophage accumulation after balloon injury in the cholesterol-fed rabbit. *Proc Natl Acad Sci USA* 1992;89:11312–11316.
201. Freyschuss A, Stiko-Rahm A, Swedenborg J, Henriksson P, Björkhem I, Berglund L, Nilsson J. Antioxidant treatment inhibits the development of intimal thickening after balloon injury of the aorta in hypercholesterolemic rabbits. *J Clin Invest* 1993;91:1282–1288.
202. Lee YJ, Yamaguchi H, Daida H, Yokol H, Miyano H, Takaya J, Sakurai H, Noma A. PTCA: Pharmacological interventions to modify restenosis. *Circulation* 1991;84:II-298 (abstr).

203. Nunes GL, Sgoutas DS, Sigman SR, Britt B, Gravanis MB, King III SB, Berk BC. Vitamins C and E improve the response to coronary balloon injury in the pig: Effect of vascular remodeling. *Circulation* 1993;88:I-372 (abstr).
204. Porreco E, Ucchino S, Di Febbo C, Di Bartolomeo N, Angelucci D, Napolitano AM, Mezzetti A, Cuccutullo F. Antiproliferative effect of desferrioxamine on vascular smooth muscle cells in vitro and in vivo. *Arterioscler Thromb* 1994;14:299–304.
205. Hirayama A, Nanto S, Ohara T, Nishida K, Okuyama Y, Kodama K. Preventive effect on restenosis after PTCA by Ebselen: A newly synthesized anti-inflammatory agent. *J Am Coll Cardoil* 1992;19: 259A (Abstr).
206. DeMaio SJ, King SB, Lembo NJ, Roubin GS, Hearn JA, Bhagavan HN, Sgoutas DS. Vitamin E supplementation, plasma lipids and incidence of restenosis after percutaneous transluminal coronary angioplasty (PTCA). *J Am Coll Nutr* 1992;11:68–73.

Atherosclerosis and Coronary Artery Disease,
edited by V. Fuster, R. Ross, and E. J. Topol.
Lippincott-Raven Publishers, Philadelphia © 1996.

CHAPTER 9

Lipoprotein (a)

Richard M. Lawn and Angelo M. Scanu

Key Words: Lipoprotein (a); Lipoprotein; Apolipoprotein (a); Apolipoprotein; Atherosclerosis.

INTRODUCTION

The role of plasma lipoproteins in the development of atherosclerosis has become increasingly well understood in recent decades. Previous chapters have discussed the transport and delivery of cholesterol to peripheral tissues by apo-B-containing lipoproteins [postprandial triglyceride-rich particles and their remnants, endogenous low-density lipoproteins (LDL) produced from the very low- to intermediate density lipoprotein (VLDL–IDL) pathway] as well as the "protective" functions of high-density lipoproteins (HDL) in reverse cholesterol transport and lipoprotein oxidation. In the past 30 years, a distinct lipoprotein, lipoprotein (a) [Lp(a)], has moved from its initial discovery phase to the recognition by most investigators as one of the major independent risk factors for atherosclerotic cardiovascular disease (ASCVD). The Lp(a) lipoprotein was discovered in 1963 by Kåre Berg and his colleagues at the University of Oslo as part of a search for variant forms of β-lipoproteins in the human population (1). Those investigators injected the β-lipoprotein fraction isolated from the plasma of different human subjects into rabbits and then tested the reactivity of the rabbit antisera to human plasma samples. About one-third of the subjects exhibited a novel antigen that was given the name Lp(a). Quantitative techniques subsequently showed that nearly all human subjects possess Lp(a) in their circulation, in widely varying amounts. In the following years, Berg's groups and others demonstrated that Lp(a) was a quantitative genetic trait transmitted in an autosomal codominant fashion. The biomedical interest in Lp(a) increased in 1974 when Berg, Dahlen, and Frick (2) reported an association between high plasma Lp(a) levels and coronary heart disease, an observation subsequently confirmed by a number of retrospective (3–10) and prospective (11–17) studies. However, two prospective studies failed to see a significant association (18,19). The reasons underlying the discrepancy in results among investigators are several, but they are likely to be related to genotypic and phenotypic variations among the patients selected, differences in ethnic background, effect of age and sex, lack of standardized methodology, and lack of an established cutoff point for "normal" plasma Lp(a) levels. An additional confounding factor is our current limited knowledge on the mechanism(s) underlying the cardiovascular pathogenicity of Lp(a), an issue that is addressed later in this chapter.

R. M. Lawn: Falk Cardiovascular Research Center, Stanford, California 94305.
A. M. Scanu: University of Chicago, Chicago, Illinois 60637.

LIPOPROTEIN (a) STRUCTURE

Lipoprotein (a) has a basic lipoprotein structure that resembles that of native LDL in cholesterol and phospholipid distribution and in the presence of apolipoprotein B100 (apo B100) (Fig. 1). In addition, Lp(a) contains a specific glycoprotein called apolipoprotein (a) or apo (a), which, in spite

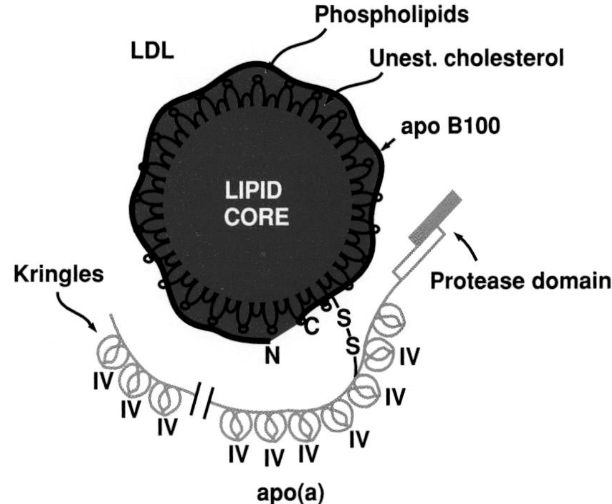

FIG. 1. Schematic model of the structure of human Lp(a). Lipoprotein(a) is made up of an LDL-like particle containing cholesterol, phospholipids, and apo B100, to which is covalently linked apo (a), the glycoprotein that is the specific marker of Lp(a). The dominant structural motif of apo(a) is a large domain made up of a number of kringles that resemble the kringle 4 of plasminogen. Individual alleles of apo (a) contain a range of from 13 to 40 kringle 4-like units and a single kringle 5 homolog. Kringles are looped structures stabilized by three disulfide bridges. Kringles are also found in a proteins of the coagulation/fibrinolytic system. The homologous protease-like domain of apo (a) appears to be enzymatically inactive, suggesting that apo (a) may share substrates of plasminogen and compete for its binding and activation. (Adapted from Scanu and Fless, ref. 105.)

of its name, is neither lipophilic nor bears resemblance to any other known plasma apolipoprotein. What makes Lp(a) unique is the attachment by a disulfide bridge and nonpolar interactions of a single copy of apo B100, approximately 500 kDa, to apo (a), varying in mass between 300 and 800 kDa. As a consequence of the marked size polymorphism of apo (a), the Lp(a) particle exhibits an important variability in density and molecular weight (20) and, from the functional viewpoint, impaired binding to the LDL receptor and an enhanced affinity to a number of cell and extracellular surfaces (21–24). Whereas apo B100 wraps about the lipid sphere, making multiple contacts within and below the particle surface, apo (a) is a highly elongated protein that greatly increases the intrinsic viscosity of Lp(a) (25). The bulk of circulating apo (a) exists in association with LDL-like particles; however, in hypertriglyceridemic states, a small portion of the apo B–apo (a) complex is also present in triglyceride-rich particles with a hydrated density lower than that of LDL (26). Usually, there is little or no unassociated apo (a) in the circulation, probably because of the high affinity of this glycoprotein for the surface of apo-B100-containing lipoproteins and rapid clearance from the plasma.

The uncommon structural features of apo (a) emerged from the studies of the cloning and sequencing of its cDNA. Limited protein sequence analysis of apo (a) allowed the design of oligonucleotide probes that were used to screen cDNA libraries from human tissues (27,28). Ultimately, overlapping clones from the RNA of a single human liver sample revealed the complete cDNA and inferred protein sequence of human apo (a). The complete sequence analysis of the apo (a) mRNA had several surprises (28) (Fig. 2). The first was the occurrence of numerous exact or nearly exact repeats of a 342-base sequence. Indeed, most of the 14,000 base pairs of cDNA consisted of 22 tandem exact repeats and 15 modified repeats. Although a number of proteins contain internally repeated subunits, the extent and fidelity of the repeated sequences in apo (a) were unprecedented. The second unexpected result was that the sequence of apo (a) closely resembles that of plasminogen, which is a protease zymogen whose active form, plasmin, cleaves fibrin to dissolve blood clots. Plasminogen is activated by tissue and urokinase plasminogen activators, by cleavage at a specific arginine residue. Plasminogen consists of an amino-terminal domain followed by five ''kringle'' units and a catalytic region that is related to the serine protease trypsin.

Apoprotein (a) is a much larger protein than plasminogen. Some of the structural properties of the two proteins are similar, but distinctive features are also present. Both proteins have identical secretion signal peptides. Plasminogen contains an amino-terminal preactivation region and three kringles that have no close counterpart in apo (a). The fourth

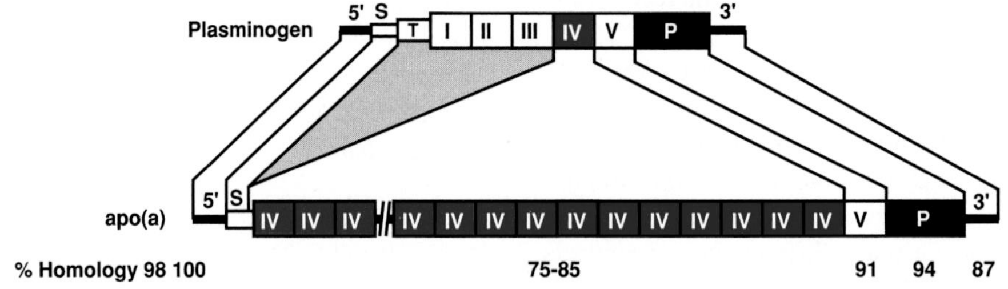

FIG. 2. Comparison of the sequence of apo (a) and plasminogen cDNA. Connecting lines indicate regions of homology with the percentage of DNA sequence identity for each domain shown below. Domain symbols refer to the 5′ untranslated, signal sequence, tail (or preactivation peptide), kringles 1–5, protease and 3′ untranslated regions. The apo (a) probably evolved from a duplicated plasminogen gene that has subsequently undergone deletion of several exons, multiplication of kringle-encoding domains, and base substitutions. (Reprinted from McLean et al., ref. 28, with permission.)

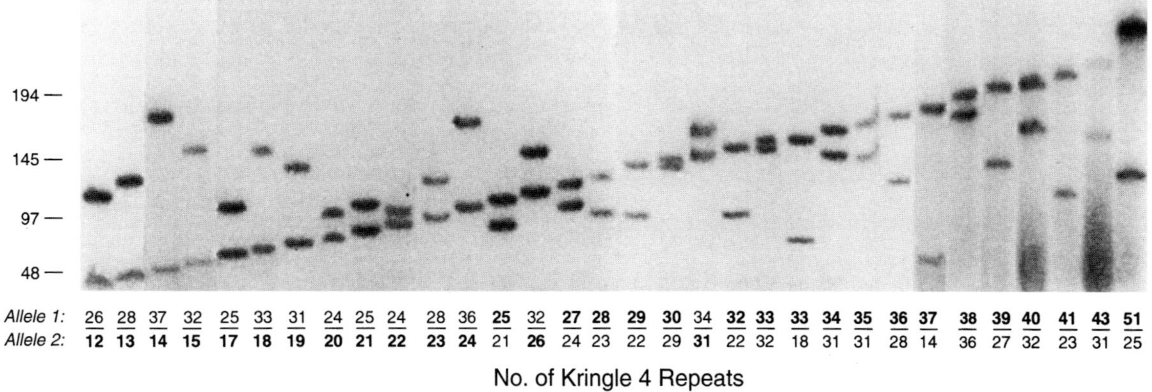

FIG. 3. Variation in the number of kringle repeats in the apo (a) gene leads to variation in the size of the protein. Genomic blots of the apo (a) gene after pulse-field electrophoresis from different human subjects shows that copies of the apo (a) gene may contain from about 15 to 40 kringles, encoding proteins with molecular mass ranging from about 300,000 to 800,000. (Reprinted from Lackner et al., ref. 33, with permission.)

and fifth kringle and protease domains have been conserved in apo (a). The originally described apo (a) cDNA contains 37 copies of a sequence that ranges from 75–85% nucleotide and 61–75% amino acid identity to plasminogen kringle 4 and single domains even more closely related to kringle 5 and the protease regions of plasminogen. There are 22 exact tandem copies of a kringle-4-like sequence, and 15 more varied repeats. Some sequence differences among the kringles of apo (a) and plasminogen presumably lead to distinctive properties. For instance, the kringle-4-like domains of apo (a) contain glycosylation sites, whereas kringle 4 of plasminogen does not. Apo (a) is a highly glycosylated (about 30% by weight) protein whose binding characteristics may be influenced by its high content of sialic acid and resulting negative charge. Only the final kringle-4-like repeat of apo (a), kringle 4_{37}, contains the key amino acid residues that in the homologous kringle of plasminogen form the binding site for lysine and fibrin. Moreover, kringle 4_{36}, the apo (a) kringle preceding kringle 4_{37}, contains an "extra" cysteine residue, a candidate for the covalent linkage of apo (a) to apo B100 (28). The predictions concerning kringles 4_{36} and 4_{37} have been supported by subsequent studies (see below). McLean et al. (28) also proposed that variable numbers of repeated domains exist in the apo (a) genes to account for the large variation of the protein's size among individuals. It has now been confirmed that alleles of the apo (a) gene in the human population contain from about 15 to 40 kringle domains, encoding proteins that range in molecular mass from about 300 to 800 kDa (29–33) (Fig. 3).

SYNTHESIS AND METABOLISM OF LIPOPROTEIN (a)

All components of the Lp(a) particle are synthesized in the liver. The hepatic site of synthesis of apo (a) was first demonstrated by the cloning of apo (a) cDNA from liver-derived RNA (28) and dramatically confirmed by liver transplantation results showing a switch of plasma apo (a) isoform from that of the recipient to that of the liver donor (34). Currently, it is not established whether the assembly and maturation of Lp(a) occur within or outside the hepatocyte itself, or both. Cell culture studies employing either the human cell line HepG2 (35) or primary baboon hepatocytes (36) detected disulfide-linked apo B100 and apo (a) in the cell supernatants but not within the lysed cells, although subsequent studies with the baboon cells supported the assembly at the cell surface (37). In contrast, Edelstein et al. (38) were able to detect some of the disulfide-linked complex in the lysates of long-term primary human hepatocytes. These studies suggest that although some apo (a) may be disulfide-linked to apo B within the cell, much of the maturation of the Lp(a) particle can occur in the circulation after the secretion of its components, as can occur in transgenic mice (39).

In terms of catabolism, the major routes of plasma clearance of Lp(a) remain unknown. Contrary to LDL, which is catabolized chiefly by the LDL receptor, the metabolic fate of Lp(a) appears to be to a large extent independent of this receptor, because of both its reduced binding affinity and the lower plasma concentration of Lp(a) than LDL (22,40). This conclusion is supported by genetic studies showing no linkage between variation in plasma Lp(a) levels and the LDL receptor gene locus (21) and also by the analysis of families carrying genes for either defective LDL receptor or defective apo B100. In these families the marked elevation of plasma LDL does not appear to influence the plasma Lp(a) concentrations (41). Finally, drugs that increase LDL receptor activity, such as bile acid resins or HMG-CoA reductase inhibitors, have no significant effect on Lp(a). An intriguing possibility raised by a study of lipoprotein turnover in humans is that apo (a) can detach from the Lp(a) particle in the circulation, resulting in a conversion of some Lp(a) to an LDL-like particle (42). Experimental support for this hypothesis is awaited with interest.

Control of Apo (a) Synthesis

The unexpected similarity of apo (a) to plasminogen has suggested clues for the understanding of the activity of Lp(a). The availability of the cloned apo (a) cDNA provided the beginning of a molecular approach to study the control of synthesis of this gene and the resulting lipoprotein particle. Plasma Lp(a) concentrations vary widely in the human population, ranging from less than 0.1 to more than 200 mg/dl. Because blood levels of Lp(a) appear to be major contributors to morbidity, it is important to understand the factors regulating these levels. Metabolic and genetic studies have provided evidence that synthesis of apo (a), rather than catabolism, is the key determinant for plasma Lp(a) concentrations (42–44), and the apo (a) component of the lipoprotein particle is the most important determinant of the final Lp(a) plasma concentration (45,46). Studies in human populations have shown that a general inverse relationship exists between apo (a) size and plasma Lp(a) concentrations (29,47,48). Analyses of cultured baboon hepatocytes demonstrated that this inverse relationship may be accounted for by the size-dependent maturation of apo (a) in the endoplasmic reticulum (49). However, it has also been shown that even within a given apo (a) isoform size class, a great deal of variation in plasma Lp(a) concentration exists, emphasizing the contribution of distinct regulatory elements in the apo (a) gene. This is supported by observations in both humans and cynomolgus monkeys that show that hepatic apo (a) mRNA levels are related to Lp(a) concentration (31,50,51), and by genetic studies that conclude that nearly 100% of the interindividual variation in plasma Lp(a) concentration is attributable to the apo (a) gene locus (46,52,53). Thus, the disparate levels of Lp(a) in the population may largely result from a combination of inherited differences in transcriptional control elements of the apo (a) gene and the number of kringle domains encoded by the gene. To test this hypothesis, and to aid in the search for means to reduce plasma apo (a) concentration, the 5′ region of the human apo (a) gene was cloned and subjected to molecular analysis.

A segment of 1,400 bp of genomic DNA was linked to a reporter gene and transfected into cultured hepatocytes, where it was shown to promote transcription of RNA. In vitro mutagenesis and nuclear protein binding experiments demonstrated that the transcriptional activity in this region is predominantly dependent on the binding of the liver-enriched transcription factor HNF-1 to a region near the transcription start site (54). Studies of individual apo (a) genes have identified a limited number of variants in this region that affect expression. However, the complete delineation of the control elements of the apo (a) gene awaits further studies, which should also prove valuable in identifying means for therapeutically modulating its expression.

Environmental and Hormonal Influences on Lipoprotein (a) Concentration

Although it is generally true that Lp(a) levels remain constant throughout life, several exceptions have been observed. Maeda et al. (55) reported that plasma Lp(a) levels doubled transiently after myocardial infarction or surgery. Subsequently, Slunga et al. (56) and Mbewu et al. (57) observed only a weak or no significant acute-phase response of Lp(a) after myocardial infarction, respectively, and von Rijn et al. (58) reported a mean increase of 59% in Lp(a) concentration in a group of young women 8 days after cesarean section. Thus, it appears that some individuals undergo a weak acute-phase response of plasma Lp(a), although it is quite modest compared to other acute-phase reactants.

More consistently, it has been noted that treatment with estrogen, progesterone, and other sex hormones depresses plasma Lp(a) levels by roughly 50% (59–61). This is consistent with the reports that plasma Lp(a) levels increase after menopause (62). Estrogen also causes a decrease in plasma LDL. In contrast, growth hormone has opposite effects on the two lipoproteins, causing an increase in plasma Lp(a) and a decrease in LDL (63). This results from the dual capacity of the growth hormone to increase the hepatic lipoprotein production and increase the LDL receptor number, which markedly enhances the clearance of LDL but not Lp(a) from plasma, pointing again to the different metabolic pathways of these two lipoprotein species.

A disease state that has consistently been shown to affect circulating Lp(a) levels is kidney failure. Wanner and colleagues (64) reported an elevation in plasma Lp(a) levels in patients with nephrotic syndrome and decreased levels in sustained remission. A number of other studies have also reported that Lp(a) plasma concentrations are elevated in patients with end-stage renal disease or microalbuminuria (65,66). Whether there is a regulatory feedback between renal protein loss and enhanced Lp(a) synthesis remains to be established.

LIPOPROTEIN (a) AS A CARDIOVASCULAR PATHOGEN

An understanding of the normal physiological role of Lp(a) would help to elucidate the pathophysiology associated with the elevated plasma levels of Lp(a). However, the normal function of Lp(a) is yet unknown. Individuals with complete or near absence of Lp(a) suffer no apparent ill effects. The unexpected homology of apo (a) with plasminogen has inspired several hypotheses about the function(s) of Lp(a) and the speculation that apo (a) might serve as a link between the processes of thrombosis and atherosclerosis. As a molecular relative of plasminogen, apo (a) might modulate fibrinolysis or enhance the delivery of cholesterol-rich particles to sites of fibrin deposition. This latter possibility has led to speculation that apo (a) may have evolved to play a role in wound healing by delivering cholesterol to sites where new membrane biosynthesis is required (67).

Although the amino acid sequence of apo (a) is approximately 80% similar to that of plasminogen, there are significant differences between the two. Among these differences is the loss of the activation site where the zymogen form of plasminogen is cleaved by plasminogen activators. As a result of this and other sequence differences, apo (a) is unable to function as an active plasmin-like protease. However, numerous studies have shown that Lp(a) can interfere with the binding of plasminogen to substrates such as fibrin, cell surfaces, and extracellular matrix. The Lp(a) may act as a competitive inhibitor of the process of plasmin generation, clot lysis, and the binding of plasminogen to endothelial and monocytoid cells and platelets, thus promoting a prothrombotic state (see for review ref. 68). However, such effects have not been seen in all studies (69), and in humans there has been no clear detection of a correlation between high plasma Lp(a) levels and fibrinolytic parameters such as euglobin clot lysis time, fibrin split products, or α_2-antiplasmin (70–75). Furthermore, studies by Smith and Crosbie (76) found that in samples of atherosclerotic vessels from individuals with a wide range of plasma Lp(a) concentrations, there was no inverse correlation between the amount of extractable plasminogen and Lp(a), inconsistent, according to the authors, with the hypothesis that Lp(a) blocks plasminogen binding to fibrin in vivo. However, the reported studies have not taken into account the recently reported variable effect on the fibrinolytic process of the size and sequence polymorphs of apo (a), thus calling for caution until more critical studies in this direction are conducted (77,78).

In addition, the atherothrombogenic action of Lp(a) may be more topical than generalized. For instance, at a given arterial site, Lp(a) may favor the formation of thrombi that, in turn, could be a key driving force in the process of plaque formation. Thrombi are often present on the surface of coronary vessels and within existing plaque (Fig. 4). These thrombi might play a role in triggering repair processes such as the proliferation and migration of smooth muscle cells and the production of extracellular matrix via chemical messengers derived from platelets or fibrin breakdown products. Elevated Lp(a) concentrations at the tissue level could inhibit the lysis of these thrombi, prolong the process of vessel repair, and lead to an accelerated atherosclerotic process, especially in the presence of other cardiovascular risk factors such as hyperlipidemia, diabetes, and cigarette smoking.

More compelling evidence for a relationship between plasma Lp(a) levels and thrombosis derives from studies on nonhuman primates that showed a direct correlation between elevated plasma levels of Lp(a) and enhancement of thrombosis in a segment of carotid artery with a clamp-induced injury (79). Thus, under defined settings, Lp(a) can have an atherothrombogenic action. It is possible that some of the

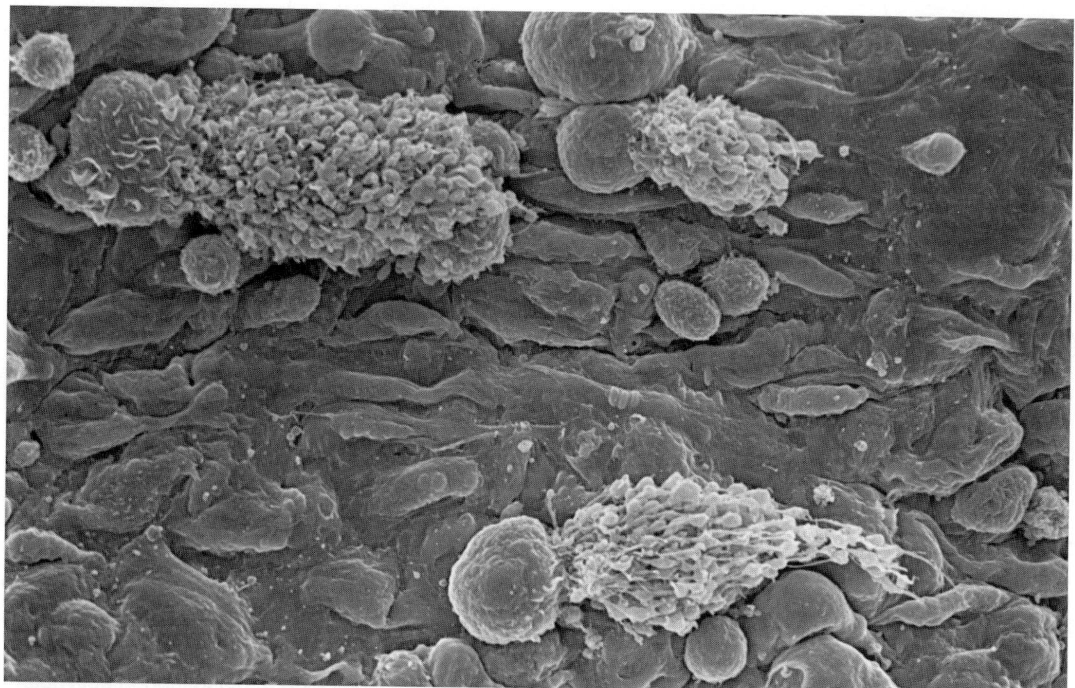

FIG. 4. Mural thrombi on the surface of vessel lesions, such as these seen here by scanning electron microscopy, may be a driving force in the growth of atherosclerotic plaque. Such thrombi might persist longer in individuals with elevated levels of Lp(a) because of inhibition of plasminogen activation. (Reprinted from Ross, ref. 106, with permission.)

inconsistencies in the literature may depend on the heterogeneity of the subjects studied in terms of differences in Lp(a) species and apo (a) phenotype, with a varying effect on function (see below) as well as on differences in experimental models and procedures. However, what is apparent is that measurements based on whole human blood samples may not detect possible antifibrinolytic effects of Lp(a), which may be localized to sites on vessel walls. A direct effect of Lp(a) on clot lysis in vivo has recently been demonstrated using transgenic mice. Lysis of radiolabeled clots in apolipoprotein (a) transgenic mice was shown to be significantly retarded in comparison to control animals (80).

OTHER ACTIVITIES OF LIPOPROTEIN (a)

The inhibition of plasminogen activation by Lp(a) may have repercussions beyond clot lysis. Transforming growth factor-β (TGF-β) is a multipotential cytokine that inhibits cell proliferation in a number of cell types. The TGF-β is synthesized as a latent molecule that requires cleavage of its propeptide region by proteases such as plasmin. Grainger and colleagues (81) reported that Lp(a) and recombinant apo (a) stimulate proliferation of cultured human vascular smooth cells in a dose-dependent manner, whereas LDL does not. This effect results from inhibition of plasminogen activation and, consequently, the activation of plasmin, a latent TGF-β. In a similar fashion, apo (a) in addition to TGF-β activation, increases the motility of smooth muscle cells co-cultured with endothelial cells in a wound response model (82). Since smooth muscle proliferation and migration are hallmarks of atherosclerosis and restenosis, these results point to other possible mechanisms for the atherothrombogenic action of Lp(a). This scenario has now been extended to transgenic mouse models (83) and may be responsible for part of the association between low levels of active TGF-β and triple vessel coronary disease in a human study (84).

The presence of apo (a) in Lp(a) enhances the binding of this cholesterol-rich lipoprotein particle to extracellular matrix components typically found in atherosclerotic plaques such as fibrin, glycosaminoglycans, and fibronectin, accounting for the increased accumulation of Lp(a) as compared to LDL in the atherosclerotic lesions (85–87) (Fig. 5;

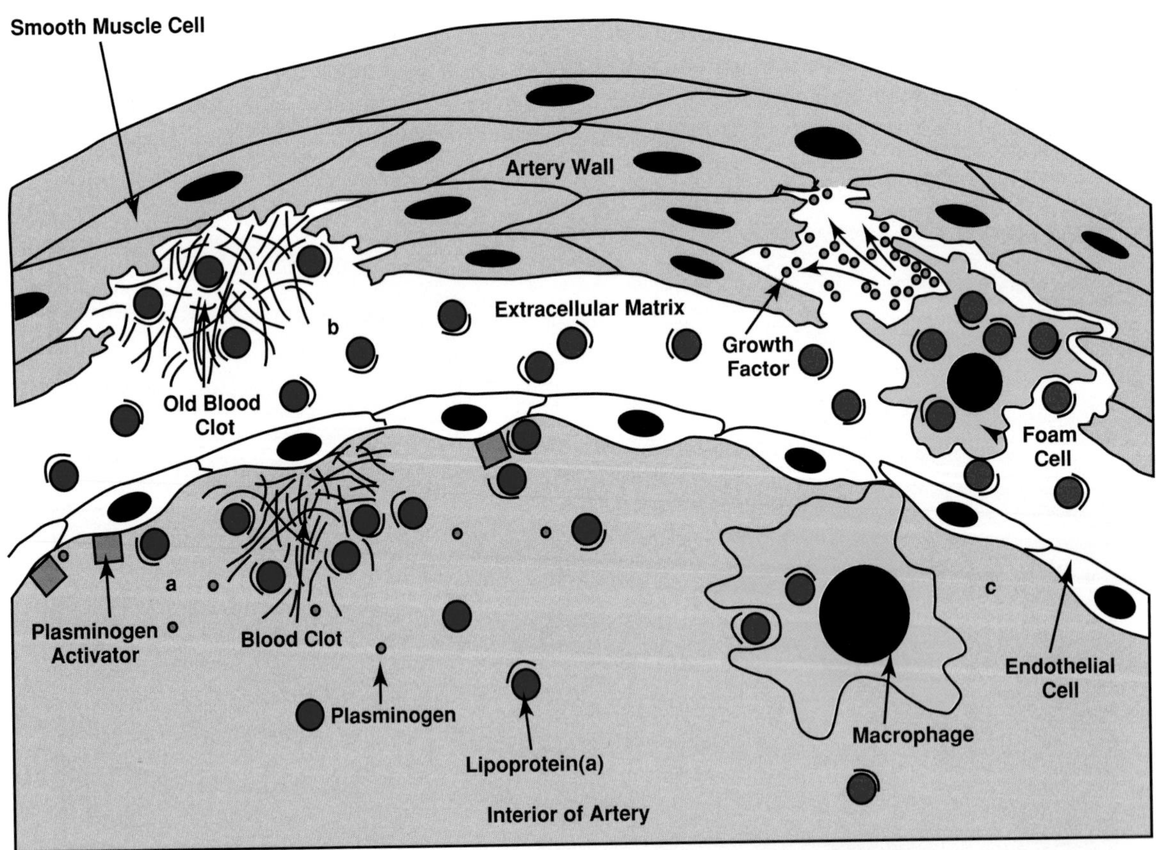

FIG. 6. Lipoprotein(a) promotes heart disease by a number of possible mechanisms. Lipoprotein(a) binds to plasminogen-binding sites on blood clots and cell surfaces. Inhibition of plasminogen activation can impair clot lysis and contribute to smooth muscle cell proliferation and migration in the developing atherosclerotic plaque. Lipoprotein(a) can also contribute to the uptake of lipids by macrophages. The resulting foam cells might accelerate atherosclerosis by cytotoxic effects and the release of growth factors and cytokines. (Reprinted from Lawn, ref. 107, with permission.)

see Colorplate 7). In addition, Lp(a) has been shown to be readily bound and internalized by macrophages, leading to foam cell formation, after oxidation or prior stimulation of the cells (Fig. 6) (88,89). These cholesterol-laden macrophages may play a major role in triggering the process of plaque development through release of growth and chemotactic factors as well cytokines (90). To evaluate the many possible functions of Lp(a) in vivo, there has been a recent emphasis on the development of suitable animal models.

ANIMAL MODELS

The apo (a) gene appears to be a relative newcomer during the evolution of primates. Consistent with its high degree of sequence similarity to plasminogen, the apo (a) gene may have developed from a duplicated plasminogen gene during the course of evolution of primates. With only one well-supported exception to date, Lp(a) has been detected only in monkeys, apes, and humans. The exception is the insectivore, the hedgehog (91). If this animal proves to possess apo (a) that resembles the primate protein, the information would suggest that either the apo (a) gene is indeed of ancient lineage, although not expressed in most current species, or that such a gene arose twice in the course of evolution from a plasminogen-like precursor.

Nonhuman primate studies have made several contributions to the understanding of Lp(a). Tomlinson et al. (92) utilized the rhesus monkey to demonstrate that liver, brain, and testes are the sources of apo (a) mRNA. Baboons were used to show the relationship of mRNA to protein isoform size and, more recently, to study the hepatic assembly of the Lp(a) particle (37,49,93). Cynomolgus monkey studies have emphasized the role of transcription regulation in the determination of circulating Lp(a) levels (51), and rhesus monkey families were utilized to help elucidate the inheritance patterns of Lp(a) concentration (94). Recently, by combining the lysine/fibrin-binding property of Lp(a) with sequence analysis of rhesus monkey apo (a), Scanu et al. (78) demonstrated that the rhesus monkeys under their study were lysine/fibrin-binding defective and exhibited a mutation (trp^{72}–arg) in the lysine binding pocket of kringle 4_{37} of apo (a). Subsequently the same authors found examples of such a mutation in 100% lysine-binding-defective human subjects (94,95) along with subjects with only a partial defect in lysine binding unrelated to the trp^{72}–arg mutation. The mechanism(s) underlying these defects have not been clarified but may be dependent on mutations in other amino acids of the lysine-binding pocket or exogenous factors capable of destabilizing the kringle 4 structure (see following section).

The transgenic mouse has become a valuable tool in the study of apo (a) and its interactions with other gene products involved in lipid transport and metabolism. The human apo (a) gene has been successfully introduced into the mouse, an animal species that normally lacks this protein. In contrast to the human model, the apo (a) circulating in the mouse was almost entirely free of lipid association because of the lack of affinity of the human recombinant for mouse LDL (39). Interestingly, these transgenic mice developed extensive fatty-streak-type vascular lesions when maintained on a high-fat diet for 3 months (96) (Fig. 7; see Colorplate 8). However, no lesion development was noted when the transgenic animals were fed a low-fat diet. The results of these studies suggest that apo (a), unincorporated into a Lp(a) particle, can be atherogenic provided that a hyperlipidemic state is created by fat feeding.

As mentioned above, these transgenic mice have subsequently been used to study the effects of apo (a) on clot lysis (80) and TGF-β activation (83) in vivo. They also have the potential for evaluating the positive or negative effect of the interaction of apo (a) with other proteins. For instance, when mated to transgenic mice overexpressing human apo -AI–containing HDL, the atherogenic activity of apo (a) is counteracted (97). In addition, a double transgenic mouse expressing both human apo (a) and human apo B100 has been shown to be capable of forming a complete Lp(a) particle with disulfide linkage between the two apolipoproteins (99,100). The possible effects of this linkage on atherosclerosis can now be investigated.

HUMAN VARIANTS

Apolipoprotein (a) is an extremely polymorphic protein, in terms of its size, primary structure, and plasma concentration (Fig. 8; see Colorplate 9). Even before its sequence was determined, apo (a) was noted to occur in widely varying molecular weights contributing to the density heterogeneity of the Lp(a) particle (20). The cloning and sequencing of the apo (a) cDNA provided a ready explanation for this size polymorphism (28). The occurrence of numerous, tandemly repeated exact copies of kringle-encoding domains suggested that homologous DNA recombination would lead to alleles of the apo (a) gene in existing populations with a range of kringle copies unless a strong selective pressure for a precise size of the product was present. This predicted size polymorphism of apo (a) has been borne out by several studies (29–33). Moreover, the exploration of the effect of this polymorphism on lysine/fibrin binding and other functional properties of apo (a) has just begun. In the future we should be able to determine which isoform is ''more atherogenic'' and provide relatively more accurate estimates of the cardiovascular pathogenicity of Lp(a), now only based on plasma concentrations.

It is now apparent that single nucleotide substitutions in the apo (a) gene can occur. However, because of the large size of the apo (a) gene, the search of these substitutions has to be limited to regions of suspected functional importance. In this respect, the region of the apo (a) gene coding for the lysine-binding pocket of kringle 4_{37} can now be readily amplified (101), and the technique has been used successfully to identify a mutation in the lymphocyte DNA of human subjects exhibiting an Lp(a) with a functional defect in lysine binding (95). Scanu et al. (95) have found an important variation in lysine binding among subjects, and the heterogeneity motif is likely also to apply for other functions of apo (a). As we continue to develop suitable techniques to correlate given apo (a) functions to specific domains in the apo (a) gene, we should be in a position to assess the actual frequency of the sequence-dependent functional polymorphism of apo (a) and of its role in atherothrombogenesis. However, it is important to realize that changes in apo (a) function may not all be secondary to mutations at the gene level and depend, for instance, on reductive and/or oxidative events occurring in the circulation leading to changes in the structural organization and stability of the kringles of apo (a). These events are more likely to occur in disease states and/or during the administration of pharmacological agents capable of interacting with kringle structures (i.e., N-acetylcysteine).

THERAPEUTIC APPROACHES

If one concurs with the notion that the cardiovascular pathogenicity of Lp(a) is related to its high plasma levels, then lowering them should represent a desirable therapeutic goal. However, to try to achieve such a goal requires deciding on the plasma Lp(a) levels to be treated, the desirable values to achieve, and the means for achieving satisfactory results. Dietary and/or physical fitness programs commonly used in the treatment of dyslipoproteinemic states have little effect on plasma Lp(a) levels. In general, this also is true for pharmacological agents such as HMG-CoA reductase inhibitors and fibrates, although some isolated, unconfirmed reports to the contrary have appeared (102). An exception is niacin, which, in dosages of 3 to 4 g daily, has been shown to decrease the plasma levels of Lp(a) by about 30% (103,104). However, this experience is not universal and may depend on pretreatment plasma Lp(a) levels, apo (a) phenotype, dosage, and length of treatment. Because of the potential side effects of high dosages of niacin, the risk/benefit relationships must be carefully evaluated with particular reference to impaired liver function, glucose intolerance, hyperuricemia, and dermatological changes. Because of these potential adverse effects, the use of niacin may be confined to those cases with high plasma levels of Lp(a) and a personal and/or family history of ASCVD. In such cases dyslipidemic states may be also present, and they may be helped at least in part by the administration of niacin. In general, in the presence of high plasma levels of Lp(a), correctable risk factors must be treated more aggressively.

Several reports have shown that hormones, and in particular estrogens, may lower significantly plasma Lp(a) (59–61); however, their safety in a sustained treatment program remains to be established. Also untested is the use of antioxidants in the form of supplements of vitamin C, E, and β-carotene, or probucol on the premise that the cardiovascular pathogenicity of Lp(a) depends on its oxidized form.

In view of the present uncertainties, any successful medical treatment of high Lp(a) must rely on the acquisition of further knowledge on the factors controlling the production and secretion of apo (a) and the formation of the Lp(a) complex. While waiting for these developments, in severe cases an efficient way to markedly decrease the plasma levels of Lp(a) inclusive of LDL is by the technique of LDL-apheresis. However, this technique is only available in specialized centers, is invasive, costly and demanding of patient time and commitment.

FUTURE DIRECTIONS

Since the discovery of the previously unsuspected homology between apo (a) and plasminogen about 6 years ago, much progress has been made in the understanding of the structural properties of this unique glycoprotein, particularly in terms of its marked kringle-4-dependent size polymorphism affecting the hydrated density of whole Lp(a) and its plasma levels. Information is emerging on the factors controlling the expression of the apo (a) gene, on the biosynthesis and maturation of apo (a) in the hepatocyte, and on the incorporation of apo (a) into an Lp(a) particle either intracellularly, extracellularly, or both. It is also becoming apparent that the structural polymorphism of apo (a) can be associated with a functional polymorphism, lysine/fibrin binding being the most extensively studied parameter thus far. Questions are now being asked whether the atherothrombogenic potential of Lp(a) is a simple function of the whole lipoprotein class or also varies with its subspecies, differing with density and apo (a) size. The contribution of this type of Lp(a) polymorphism to cardiovascular pathogenicity is now amenable to exploration both in man and in the experimental animal. The investigation of the structural and functional heterogeneity of Lp(a) may provide an important insight into the mechanisms by which Lp(a) acts as a cardiovascular pathogen and to help explain the current uncertainties on the subject. An increased understanding of the basic biology of Lp(a) should also help in designing pharmacological agents able to modulate effectively the levels of Lp(a) in the plasma or reduce its pathological effects.

REFERENCES

1. Berg K. A new serum type system in man—the Lp system. *Acta Pathol Microbiol Scand* 1963;59:369–382.
2. Berg K, Dahlen G, Frick MH. Lp(a) lipoprotein and pre-β-lipoprotein in patients with coronary heart disease. *Clin Genet* 1974;230–235.
3. Rhoads GG, Dahlen G, Berg K, Morton NE, Dannenberg AL. Lp(a) lipoprotein as a risk factor of myocardial infarction. *JAMA* 1986;256: 2540–2544.
4. Armstrong VW, Cremer P, Eberle E, Manke A, Schulze F, Wieland H, Kreuzer H, Seidel D. The association between serum Lp(a) concentrations and angiographically assessed coronary atherosclerosis: Dependence on serum LDL levels. *Atherosclerosis* 1986;62:249–257.

5. Dahlen GH, Guyton JR, Attra M, Farmer JA, Kautz JA, Gotto AM Jr. Association of levels of lipoprotein Lp(a), plasma lipids, and other lipoproteins with coronary artery disease documented by angiography. *Circulation* 1986;74:758–765.
6. Durrington PN, Ishola M, Hunt L, Arrol S, Bhatnagar D. Apolipoproteins(a), AI, and B and parental history in men with early onset ischaemic heart disease. *Lancet* 1988;1070–1073.
7. Genest J Jr, Jenner JL, McNamara JR, Ordovas JM, Silberman SR, Wilson PWF, Schaefer EJ. Prevalence of lipoprotein(a) [Lp(a)] excess in coronary artery disease. *Am J Cardiol* 1991;67:1039–1045.
8. Genest J Jr, Martin-Munley SS, McNamara JR, Ordovas JM, Jenner JL, Meyers RH, Silberman SR, Wilson PW, Salem DN, Schaefer EJ. Familial lipoprotein disorders in patients with premature coronary artery heart disease. *Circulation* 1992;85:2025–2033.
9. Schreiner PJ, Morrisett JD, Sharrett AR, Patsch W, Tyroler HA, Wu K, Heiss G. Lipoprotein(a) as a risk factor for preclinical atherosclerosis. *Arterioscler Thromb* 1993;13:826–833.
10. Solymoss BC, Marcil M, Wesolowska E, Gilfix BM, Lesperance J, Campeau L. Relation of coronary artery disease in women <60 years of age to the combined elevation of serum lipoprotein(a) and total cholesterol to high-density cholesterol ratio. *Am J Cardiol* 1993;72: 1215–1219.
11. Rosengren A, Wilhelmsen L, Eriksson E, Risberg B, Widel H. Lipoprotein(a) and coronary heart disease: A prospective case-control study in a population sample of middle aged men. *Br Med J* 1990; 301:1248–1251.
12. Bostom AG, Gagnon DR, Cupples LA, Wilson PW, Jenner JL, Ordovas JM, Schaefer EJ, Castelli WP. A prospective investigation of elevated lipoprotein(a) detected by electrophoresis and cardiovascular disease in women. *Circulation* 1994;90:1688–1695.
13. Sigurdsson G, Baldursdottir A, Sigvaldsonason H, Agnarsson U, Thorgeirsson G, Sigfusson N. Predictive value of apolipoproteins in a prospective study of coronary artery disease in men. *Am J Cardiol* 1992;69:1251–1254.
14. Wald NJ, Law M, Ledue TB, Haddow JE. Apolipoproteins and ischemic heart disease: Implications for screening. *Lancet* 1994;343: 75–79.
15. Schaefer EJ, Lamon-Fava S, Jenner JL, McNamara JR, Ordovas JM, Davis CE, Abolafia JM, Lippel K, Levy RI. Lipoprotein(a) levels and risk for coronary heart disease in men: The Lipid Research Clinics Primary Prevention Trial. *JAMA* 1994;271:999–1003.
16. Cantin B, Moorjani S, Despres J-P, Dagenias GR, Lupien P-L. Lp(a) in ischemic heart disease: The Quebec Cardiovascular Study. *J Am Coll Cardiol* 1994;23:482A.
17. Cremer P, Nagel D, Labrot B, Mann H, Muche R, Elster H, Seidel D. Lipoprotein Lp(a) as predictor of myocardial infarction: Results from the prospective Gottingen Risk Incidence and Prevention Study. *Eur J Clin Invest* 1994;24:444–453.
18. Jauhiainen M, Koskinen P, Ehnholm C, Frick MH, Manttari M, Manninen V, Huttunen JK. Lipoprotein(a) and coronary heart disease risk: A nested case-control study of the Helsinki Heart Study participants. *Atherosclerosis* 1991;89:59–67.
19. Ridker PM, Hennekens CH, Stampfer MJ. A prospective study of lipoprotein(a) and the risk of myocardial infarction. *JAMA* 1993;270: 2195–2199.
20. Fless GM, Rolih CA, Scanu AM. Heterogeneity of human plasma lipoprotein(a). Isolation and characterization of the lipoprotein subspecies and their apoproteins. *J Biol Chem* 1984;259:11470–11478.
21. Maartmann-Moe K, Berg K. Lp(a) lipoprotein enters cultured fibroblasts independently of the plasma membrane low density lipoprotein receptor. *Clin Genet* 1981;20:352–362.
22. Armstrong VW, Walli AK, Seidal D. Isolation characterization and uptake into human fibroblasts of an apo(a)-free lipoprotein obtained on reduction of lipoprotein(a). *J Lipid Res* 1985;26:1314–1323.
23. Harpel PC, Gordon BR, Parker TS. Plasmin catalyzes binding of lipoprotein(a) to immobilized fibrinogen and fibrin. *Proc Natl Acad Sci USA* 1989;86:3847–3851.
24. Salonen EM, Jauhianen L, Zardi L, Vaheri A, Enholm C. Lipoprotein(a) binds to fibronectin and serine proteinase capable of cleaving it. *EMBO J* 1989;8:4035–4040.
25. Phillips ML, Lembertas A, Schumaker V, Lawn RM, Shire S, Zioncheck TF. Physical properties of recombinant apolipoprotein(a) and its association with LDL to form an Lp(a)-like complex. *Biochemistry* 1993;32:3722–3728.
26. Scanu A, Pfaffinger D, Edelstein C. Postprandial Lp(a): Identification of a triglyceride-rich particle containing apo E. *Chem Phys Lipids* 1994;67/68:193–198.
27. Eaton DL, Fless GM, Kohr WJ, McLean JW, Xu QT, Miller CG, Lawn RM, Scanu AM. Partial amino acid sequence of apolipoprotein(a) shows that it is homologous to plasminogen. *Proc Natl Acad Sci USA* 1987;84:3224–3228.
28. McLean JW, Tomlinson JE, Kuang WJ, Eaton DL, Chen EY, Fless GM, Scanu AM, Lawn RM. Human apolipoprotein(a): cDNA sequence of an apolipoprotein homologous to plasminogen. *Nature* 1987;330:132–137.
29. Gavish D, Azrolan N, Breslow JL. Plasma Lp(a) concentration is inversely correlated with the ratio of kringle IV/kringle V encoding domains in the apo(a) gene. *J Clin Invest* 1989;84:2021–2027.
30. Koschinsky ML, Beisiegel U, Henne-Bruns D, Eaton DL, Lawn RM. Apolipoprotein(a) size heterogeneity is related to variable number of repeat sequences in its mRNA. *Biochemistry* 1990;29:640–644.
31. Lindahl G, Gersdorf E, Menzel HJ, Seed M, Humphries S, Utermann G. Variation in the size of human apolipoprotein(a) is due to a hypervariable region in the gene. *Hum Genet* 1990;84:563–567.
32. Lackner C, Boerwinkle E, Leffert CC, Rahmig T, Hobbs HH. Molecular basis of apolipoprotein(a) isoform size heterogeneity as revealed by pulsed-field gel electrophoresis. *J Clin Invest* 1991;87:2153–2161.
33. Lackner C, Cohen JC, Hobbs HH. Molecualr definition of the extreme size polymorphism in apolipoprotein(a). *Hum Mol Genet* 1993;2: 933–940.
34. Kraft HG, Menzel HJ, Hoppichler F, Vogel W, Utermann G. Changes of genetic apolipoprotein phenotypes caused by liver transplantation. Implications for apolipoprotein synthesis. *J Clin Invest* 1989;83: 137–142.
35. Koschinsky M, Côté G, Gabel V, van der Hoek YY. Identification of the cysteine residue in apolipoprotein(a) that mediates extracellular coupling with apolipoprotein B-100. *J Biol Chem* 1993;268: 19819–19825.
36. White AL, Rainwater DL, Lanford RE. Intracellular maturation of apolipoprotein(a) and assembly of lipoprotein(a) in primary baboon hepatocytes. *J Lipid Res* 1993;34:509–517.
37. White AL, Lanford RE. Cell surface assembly of lipoprotein(a) in primary cultures of baboon hepatocytes. *J Biol Chem* 1994;269: 28716–28723.
38. Edelstein C, Davidson NO, Scanu AM. Oleates stimulates the formation of triglyceride-rich particles containing apoB-100 -apo(a) in long-term primary cultures of human hepatocytes. *Chem Phys Lipids* 1994; 67/68:135–143.
39. Chiesa G, Hobbs HH, Koschinsky ML, Lawn RM, Maika SD, Hammer RE. Reconstitution of lipoprotein(a) by infusion of human LDL into transgenic mice expressing human apolipoprotein(a). *J Biol Chem* 1992;267:24369–24374.
40. Snyder ML, Polacek D, Scanu AM, Fless GM. Comparative binding and degradation of lipoprotein(a) and low density lipoprotein by human monocyte-derived macrophages. *J Biol Chem* 1992;267: 339–346.
41. Soutar AK, McCarthy SN, Seed M, Knight BL. Relationship between apolipoprotein(a) phenotype, lipoprotein(a) concentration in plasma, and low density lipoprotein receptor function in a large kindred with familial hypercholesterolemia due to the pro^{664}–leu mutation in the LDL receptor gene. *J Clin Invest* 1991;88:483–492.
42. Knight BL, Perombelon YF, Soutar AK, Wade DP, Seed M. Catabolism of lipoprotein (a) in familial hypercholesterolaemic subjects. *Atherosclerosis* 1991;87:227–237.
43. Krempler F, Kostner GM, Bolzano K, Sandhofer F. Turnover of Lp(a) in man. *J Clin Invest* 1980;65:1483–1490.
44. Rader DJ, Cain W, Zech LA, Usher D, Brewer HB Jr. Variation in lipoprotein(a) concentrations among individuals with the same apolipoprotein(a) isoform is determined by the rate of lipoprotein(a) production. *J Clin Invest* 1993;91:443–447.
45. Utermann G, Kraft HG, Menzel JH, Hopferwieser T, Seitz C. Genetics of the quantitative Lp(a) lipoprotein trait. I. Relation of Lp(a) glycoprotein phenotypes to Lp(a) lipoprotein concentrations in plasma. *Hum Genet* 1988;78:41–46.
46. Boerwinkle E, Leffert CC, Lin J, Lackner C, Chiesa G, Hobbs HH. Apolipoprotein(a) gene accounts for greater than 90% of the variation in plasma lipoprotein(a) concentratinos. *J Clin Invest* 1992;90:52–60.
47. Utermann G, Duba C, Menzel HJ. Genetics of the quantitative Lp(a)

lipoprotein trait. II. Inheritance of Lp(a) glycoprotein phenotypes. *Hum Genet* 1988;78:47–50.
48. Gaubatz JW, Ghanem KI, Guevara J Jr, Nava ML, Patsch W, Morrisett JD. Polymorphic forms of human apolipoprotein(a) inheritance and relationship of their molecular weight to plasma levels of lipoprotein(a). *J Lipid Res* 1990;31:603–613.
49. White A, Hixson J, Rainwater D, Lanford R. Molecular basis for "null" lipoprotein(a) phenotypes and the influence of apolipoprotein(a): Size on plasma lipoprotein (a) level in baboon. *J Biol Chem* 1994;269:9060–9066.
50. Wade DP, Knight BL, Harders-Spengel K, Soutar AK. Detection and quantitation of apolipoprotein(a) mRNA in human liver and its relationship with plasma lipoprotein(a) concentratin. *Atherosclerosis* 1991;91:63–72.
51. Azrolan N, Gavish D, Breslow JL. Plasma lipoprotein(a) concentration is controlled by apolipoprotein (a) [apo(a)] protein size and abundance of hepatic apo(a) mRNA levels in cynomolgus monkey model. *J Biol Chem* 1991;266:13866–13872.
52. Kraft HG, Kochl S, Menzel JH, Sandholzer C, Utermann G. The apolipoprotein(a) gene: A transcribed hypervariable locus controlling plasma lipoprotein(a) concentration. *Hum Genet* 1992;90:220–230.
53. DeMeester CA, Bu X, Puppione D, Gray RM, Lusis AJ, Rotter JI. Genetic variation in lipoprotein(a) levels in families enriched for coronary artery disease is determined almost entirely by the apolipoprotein(a) gene locus. *Hum Genet* 1995;56:675–679.
54. Wade DP, Lindahl GE, Lawn RM. Apolipoprotein(a) gene transcription is regulated by liver-enriched trans-acting factor HNF-1α. *J Biol Chem* 1994;269:19757–19765.
55. Maeda S, Abe A, Seishima M, Makino K, Noma A, Kawade M. Transient changes of serum lipoprotein(a) as an acute phase protein. *Atherosclerosis* 1989;78:145–150.
56. Slunga L, Johnson O, Dahlen GH, Eriksson S. Lipoprotein(a) and acute-phase proteins in acute myocardial infarction. *Scand J Clin Lab Invest* 1992;52:95–101.
57. Mbewu AD, Durrington PN, Bulleid S, Mackness MI. The immediate effect of streptokinase on serum lipoprotein(a) concentration and the effect of myocardial infarction on serum lipoprotein(a), apolipoproteins AI and B, lipids and C-reactive protein. *Atherosclerosis* 1993; 103:65–71.
58. von Rijn H, Kimmel C, Gimpel JA, Kortlandt W, Bruinse HW. Does Lp(a) act as an acute phase reactant in healthy young women who underwent cesarian section? *Clin Chem Enzyme Commun* 1993;5: 157–162.
59. Henriksson P, Angelin B, Berglund L. Hormonal regulation of serum Lp(a) levels: Opposite effects after estrogen treatment and orchidectomy in males with prostatic carcinoma. *J Clin Invest* 1992;89: 1166–1171.
60. Soma MR, Osnago-Gadda I, Paoletti R, Fumagalli R, Morrisett JD, Meschia M, Crosignani P. The lowering of lipoprotein(a) induced by estrogen plus progesterone replacement therapy in postmenopausal women. *Arch Intern Med* 1993;153:1462–1468.
61. Crook D, Sidhu M, Seed M, O'Donnell M, Stevenson JC. Lipoprotein Lp(a) levels are reduced by danazol, an anabolic steroid. *Atherosclerosis* 1992;92:41–47.
62. Jenner JL, Ordovas JM, Lamon-Fava S, Schaefer MM, Wilson PW, Castelli WP, Schaefer EJ. Effects of age, sex, and menopausal status on plasma lipoprotein(a) levels: The Framingham Offspring Study. *Circulation* 1993;87:1135–1141.
63. Eden S, Wiklund O, Oscarsson J, Rosen T, Bengtsson BA. Growth hormone treatment of growth hormone-deficient adults results in a marked increase in Lp(a) and HDL cholesterol concentrations. *Arterioscler Thromb* 1993;13:296–301.
64. Wanner C, Rader D, Bartens W, Kramer J, Brewer HB, Schollmeyer P, Wieland H. Elevated plasma lipoprotein(a) in patients with the nephrotic syndrome. *Ann Intern Med* 1993;119:263–269.
65. Dieplinger H, Lackner C, Kronenberg F, Sandholzer C, Lhotta K, Hoppichler F, Graf H, Konig P. Elevated plasma concentrations of lipoprotein(a) in patients with end-stage renal disease are not related to the size polymorphism of apolipoprotein(a). *J Clin Invest* 1993;91: 397–401.
66. Black IW, Wilcken DE. Decreases in apolipoprotein(a) after renal transplantation: Implications for lipoprotein(a) metabolism. *Clin Chem* 19923;38:353–357.
67. Brown MS, Goldstein JL. Plasma lipoproteins: Teaching old dogmas new tricks. *Nature* 1987;330:113–114.
68. Howard GC, Pizzo SV. Lipoprotein(a) and its role in atherothrombotic disease. *Lab Invest* 1993;69:373–386.
69. Liu JN, Harpel PC, Pannell R, Gurewich V. Lipoprotein(a): A kinetic study of its influence on fibrin-dependent plasminogen activation by prourokinase or tissue plasminogen activator. *Biochemistry* 1993;32: 9694–9700.
70. Garcia Frade LJ, Alvarez JJ, Rayo I, Torrado MC, Lasuncion MA, Garcia Avello A, Hernandez A, Marin E. Fibrinolytic parameters and lipoprotein(a) levels in plasma of patientes with coronary artery disease. *Thromb Res* 1991;63:407–418.
71. Alessi MC, Parra HJ, Joly P, Vu-Dac N, Bard JM, Fruchart JC, Juhan-Vague I. The increased plasma Lp(a):B lipoprotein particle concentration in angina pectoris is not associated with hypofibrinolysis. *Clin Chim Acta* 1990;188:119–127.
72. Sundell IB, Nilsson TK, Hallmans G, Hellsten G, Dahlen GH. Interrelationships between plasma levels of plasminogen activator inhibitor, tissue plasminogen activator, lipoprotein(a), and established cardiovascular risk factors in a North Swedish population. *Atherosclerosis* 1989;80:9–16.
73. Glueck CJ, Glueck HI, Tracy T, Speirs J, McCray C, Stroop D. Relationships between lipoprotein(a), lipids, apolipoproteins, basal and stimulated fibrinolytic regulators, and D-dimer. *Metabolism* 1993;42: 236–246.
74. von Eckardstein A, Heinrich J, Funke H, Schulte H, Schonfeld R, Kohler E, Steinmetz A, Assmann G. Glutamine/histidine polymorphism in apo A-IV affects plasma concentrations of lipoprotein(a) and fibrin split products in coronary heart disease patients. *Arterioscler Thromb* 1993;13:240–246.
75. Oshima S, Uchida K, Yasu T, Uno K, Nonogi H, Haze K. Transient increase of plasma lipoprotein(a) in patients with unstable angina pectoris. Does lipoprotein(a) alter fibrinolysis? *Arterioscler Thromb* 1991;11:1772–1777.
76. Smith EB, Crosbie L. Does lipoprotein(a) [Lp(a)] compete with plasminogen in human atherosclerotic lesions and thrombi? *Atherosclerosis* 1991;89:127–136.
77. Leerink C, Duif P, Gimpel J, Kortlandt W, Bouma BN, von Rijn H. Lysine-binding heterogeneity of Lp(a): Consequences for fibrin binding and inhibition of plasminogen activation. *Thromb Haemost* 1992;68:185–188.
78. Scanu AM, Miles L, Fless GM, Pfaffinger D, Eisenbart J, Jackson E, Hoover-Plow JL, Brunck T, Plow EF. Rhesus monkey lipoprotein(a) binds to lysine sepharose and U937 monocytoid cells less efficiently than human lipoprotein(a). *J Clin Invest* 1993;91:283–291.
79. Williams JK, Bellinger DA, Nichols TC, Griggs TR, Bumol TF, Fouts RL, Clarkson TB. Occlusive arterial thrombosis in cynomolgus monkeys with varying plasma concentrations of lipoprotein(a). *Arterioscler Thromb* 1993;13:548–554.
80. Palabrica TM, Liu AC, Aronovitz MJ, Furie B, Lawn RM, Furie BC. Antifibrinolytic activity of apolipoprotein(a) in vivo: Human apolipoprotein(a) transgenic mice are resistant to tissue plasminogen activator-mediated thrombolysis. *Nature Med* 1995;1.
81. Grainger DJ, Kirschenlohr HL, Metcalfe JC, Weissberg PL, Wade DP, Lawn RM. The proliferation of human smooth muscle cells is promoted by lipoprotein(a). *Science* 1993;260:1655–1658.
82. Kojima S, Harpel PC, Rifkin DB. Lipoprotein(a) inhibits the generation of transforming growth factor beta: An endogenous inhibitor of smooth muscle cell migration. *J Cell Biol* 1991;113:1439–1445.
83. Grainger DJ, Kemp PR, Liu AC, Lawn RM, Metcalfe JC. Activation of transforming growth factor-β is inhibited in apoliprotein(a) transgenic mice. *Nature* 1994;370:460–462.
84. Grainger DJ, Kemp PR, Metcalfe JC, Liu AC, Lawn RM, Williams NR, Grace AA, Schofield PM, Cauhan A. The serum concentration of active transforming growth factor-β is severely depressed in advanced atherosclerosis. *Nature Med* 1995;1:74–79.
85. Rath M, Niendorf A, Reblin T, Dietel M, Krebber HJ, Beisiegel U. Detection and quantification of lipoprotein(a) in the arterial wall of 107 coronary bypass patients. *Arteriosclerosis* 1989;9:579–592.
85a. Neindorf A, Rath M, Wolf K, Peters S, Harmut A, Beisiegel U, Dietel M. Morphological detection and quantification of lipoprotein(a) deposition in atheromatous lesions of human aorta and coronary arteries.
86. Cushing GL, Gaubatz JW, Nava ML, Burdick BJ, Bocan TMA, Guyton JR, Weilbaecher D, DeBakey ME, Lawrie GM, Morrisett JD.

Quantitation and localization of apolipoprotein(a) and B in coronary artery bypass vein grafts resected at re-operation. *Arteriosclerosis* 1989;9:593–603.

87. Pepin JM, O'Neil JA, Hoff HF. Quantification of apo(a) and apoB in human atherosclerotic lesions. *J Lipid Res* 1991;32:317–326.
88. Haberland ME, Fless GM, Scanu AM, Fogelman AM. Malondialdehyde modification of lipoprotein(a) produces avid uptake by human monocyte-macrophages. *J Biol Chem* 1992;267:4143–4151.
89. Bottalico LA, Keesler GA, Fless GM, Tabas I. Cholesterol loading of macrophages leads to marked enhancement of native lipoprotein(a) and, apoprotein(a) internalization and degradation. *J Biol Chem* 1993; 268:8569–8573.
90. Witztum J, Steinberg D. Role of oxidized low density lipoprotein in atherogenesis. *J Clin Invest* 1991;88:1785–1792.
91. Laplaud PM, Beaubatie L, Rall SJ, Luc G, Sbaboureau M. Lipoprotein(a) is the major apoB-containing lipoprotein in the plasma of a hibernator, the hedgehog (*Erinaceus europaeus*). *J Lipid Res* 1988; 29:1157–1170.
92. Tomlinson JE, McLean JW, Lawn RM. Rhesus apolipoprotein(a): Sequence, evolution and sites of synthesis. *J Biol Chem* 1989;264: 5957–5965.
93. Hixson JE, Britten ML, Manis GS, Rainwater DL. Apolipoprotein(a) (Apo(a)) glycoprotein isoforms result from size differences in Apo(a) mRNA in baboons. *J Biol Chem* 1989;264:6013–6016.
94. Scanu AM, Khalil A, Neven L, Tidore M, Dawson G, Pfaffinger D, Jackson E, Carey KD, McGill HC, Fless GM. Genetically determined hypercholesterolemia in a rhesus monkey family due to a deficiency of the LDL receptor. *J Lipid Res* 1988;29:1671–1681.
95. Scanu AM, Pfaffinger D, Lee JC, Hinman J. A point mutation (Trp72-Arg) in human apolipoprotein(a) kringle 4-37 associated with a lysine binding defect in Lp(a). *Biochim Biophys Acta* 1994;1227:41–45.
96. Lawn RM, Wade DP, Hammer RE, Chiesa G, Verstuyft JG, Rubin EM. Atherogenesis in transgenic mice expressing human apolipoprotein(a). *Nature* 1992;360:670–672.
97. Liu AC, Lawn RM, Verstuyft JG, Rubin EM. Human apolipoprotein A-I prevents atherosclerosis associated with apolipoprotein(a) in transgenic mice. *J Lipid Res* 1994;35:2263–2267.
98. Linton MF, Farese RV, Chiesa G, Grass DS, Chin P, Hammer RE, Hobbs HH, Young SG. Transgenic mice expressing high plasma concentrations of human apolipoprotein B100 and lipoprotein(a). *J Clin Invest* 1993;92:3029–3037.
99. Callow M, Stoltzfus L, Lawn RM, Rubin EM. Expression of human apolipoprotein B and assembly of lipoprotein (a) in transgenic mice. *Proc Natl Acad Sci USA* 1994;91:2130–2134.
100. Linton MF, Farese RV, Chiesa G, Grass DS, Chin P, Hammer RE, Hobbs HH, Young SG. Transgenic mice expressing high plasma concentrations of human apolipoprotein B100 and lipoprotein(a). *J Clin Invest* 1993;92:3029–3037.
101. Pfaffinger D, McLean J, Scanu AM. Amplification of human apo(a) kringle 4-37 from blood lymphocyte DNA. *Biochim Biophys Acta* 1993;1225:107–109.
102. Scanu AM. Lipoprotein(a): A genetic risk for premature coronary heart disease. *JAMA* 1992;267:3326–3329.
103. Gurakar A, Hoeg JM, Kostner G, Papadopoulos NM, Brewer HB. Levels of lipoprotein Lp(a) decline with neomycin and niacin treatment. *Atherosclerosis* 1985;57:293–301.
104. Carlson LA, Hamsten A, Asplund A. Pronounced lowering of serum levels of lipoprotein Lp(a) in hyperlipidaemic subjects treated with nicotinic acid. *J Int Med Res* 1989;226:271–276.
105. Scanu AM, Fless GM. Lipoprotein(a): Heterogeneity and biological relevance. *J Clin Invest* 1990;85:1709–1715.
106. Ross R. The pathogenesis of atherosclerosis: A perspective for the 1990s. *Nature* 1993;362:801–809.
107. Lawn RM. Lipoprotein(a) in heart disease. *Sci Am* 1992;266:54–60.

Atherosclerosis and Coronary Artery Disease,
edited by V. Fuster, R. Ross, and E. J. Topol.
Lippincott-Raven Publishers, Philadelphia © 1996.

CHAPTER 10

Clinical Classifications of Lipid Abnormalities

Thomas P. Bersot and Robert W. Mahley

Key Words: Dyslipidemia; Lipoprotein phenotyping; Atherogenic dyslipidemia; Remnant lipoproteins; Xanthoma.

INTRODUCTION

About 170 years ago, physicians began to make observations associating xanthomas with certain disease processes, some of which were recognized to be familial. Although physicians of that era had no knowledge of dyslipidemia or its pathophysiological role in these disorders, these reports constitute the earliest descriptions of dyslipidemic syndromes. Most of the progress from these early beginnings to today's understanding of the pathophysiology of lipid disorders and their classification has occurred in the past 50 years with the advent of modern scientific methods and their application to problems in clinical medicine (1).

XANTHOMAS ASSOCIATED WITH HYPERLIPIDEMIA

The classification of clinical syndromes associated with hyperlipidemia began with descriptions of xanthomas, which are still useful in categorizing dyslipidemia (Table 1 and Fig. 1; see Colorplates 10A–K). In the 19th century, planar xanthomas (xanthomas within the plane of the skin, panels A and B of Fig. 1) were described in association with biliary tract disease, and eruptive xanthomas (Fig. 1, panels J and K) in association with diabetes mellitus (2). Subsequently tuberous xanthomas (Fig. 1, panels E–G) were recognized in siblings who died sudden deaths in childhood, establishing that this type of xanthoma occurred on a familial basis and heralded serious medical consequences. It is likely that these children had homozygous familial hypercholesterolemia (2). Analysis of the lipid content of tuberous xanthomas revealed high cholesterol contents, which ultimately led to the correlation between this xanthoma type and severe hypercholesterolemia (2). Rare patients with severe hyperlipemia and eruptive xanthomas in the absence of diabetes mellitus were also discovered, prompting the suggestion that hypertriglyceridemia might also play a role in the formation of certain types of xanthomas. However, real progress in the classification of lipid disorders began with application of techniques for measuring concentrations of blood lipids and the recognition that the metabolism of blood lipids is governed by the metabolism of the plasma lipoproteins.

LIPOPROTEIN IDENTIFICATION AND HYPERLIPOPROTEINEMIA PHENOTYPING

Lipoproteins were first isolated by salting out and separated by electrophoresis into crude, impure α and β compo-

T. P. Bersot and R. W. Mahley: Gladstone Institute of Cardiovascular Disease, Gladstone Foundation Labs, San Francisco, California 94140.

TABLE 1. *Classification of xanthomas associated with primary and secondary dyslipidemia*

Xanthoma	Location	Associated with
Planar	Palmar and intertriginous creases of the extremities	Primary dyslipidemia: type III hyperlipoproteinemia Secondary dyslipidemia: obstructive liver disease, multiple myeloma, hypothyroidism
Tuberous or tuberoeruptive	Elbow, dorsum of hand, knee, buttocks	Type III hyperlipoproteinemia, homozygous familial hypercholesterolemia
Tendon	Extensor tendons of hands, Achilles tendon	Familial hypercholesterolemia, familial defective apolipoprotein B100, type III hyperlipoproteinemia (rare), β-sitosterolemia
Eruptive	Arm and thigh (posterolateral surface), back, buttocks	Primary dyslipidemia: lipoprotein lipase deficiency, apolipoprotein C-II deficiency Secondary dyslipidemia: diabetes mellitus, pancreatitis, dysproteinemia (myeloma, lupus)

nents. However, it was not until the application of analytical ultracentrifugation to the separation of plasma lipoproteins that the major classes of lipoproteins were recognized and their concentrations quantitated (3). After the analytical ultracentrifuge was used to define the lipoproteins' respective densities of flotation, the technique of sequential flotation was developed for the more widely available preparative ultracentrifuge (4). The four lipoprotein classes described were chylomicrons, very-low-density lipoproteins (VLDL), low-density lipoproteins (LDL), and high-density lipoproteins (HDL) (Table 2). As the HDL were studied further, two major subfractions were defined, HDL_2 and HDL_3. Almost immediately, the LDL (for review, see ref. 5) were found to have a direct relationship with atherosclerosis, and the HDL an inverse relationship (3,6,7).

These findings set the stage for studies that determined plasma concentrations of the various lipoproteins in familial dyslipidemic states and allowed the characterization of abnormal lipoproteins. In 1967, a diagnostic and treatment classification system was proposed based on identification of the specific lipoprotein abnormalities causing hyperlipidemia in patients (8). The plasma lipoprotein abnormalities were identified by fat staining of electrophoretically separated plasma and estimation of the cholesterol concentrations of VLDL, LDL, and HDL (9). This approach was extremely useful because it focused attention on the importance of lipoprotein pathophysiology in abnormalities of plasma cholesterol and triglyceride metabolism. The rationale for focusing treatment on the lipoproteins was that the metabolism of the lipoproteins dictates blood lipid levels, and specific lipoproteins modulate atherogenesis. Six common phenotypes were described (Table 3), and these phenotypes became quite useful as a shorthand method of describing the lipoprotein abnormalities of hyperlipidemic patients. For each specific phenotype, disorders causing secondary phenocopies were identified, and it was suggested that one or more genetic disorders may produce the same lipoprotein phenotype.

TABLE 2. *Ultracentrifugal and electrophoretic terminology describing plasma lipoproteins*

Lipoprotein	Density of flotation	Electrophoretic mobility
Chylomicrons	$d < 0.94$[a] $S_f > 400$[b]	Origin
Very low density	$0.94 < d < 1.006$ S_f 20–400	pre-β or α_2
Low density	$1.006 < d < 1.063$ S_f 0–20	β
High density	$1.063 < d < 1.21$ $F^{\circ}_{1.20}$ 0–9	α_1
HDL_2	$1.063 < d < 1.125$ $F^{\circ}_{1.20}$ 5–9	α_1
HDL_3	$1.125 < d < 1.21$ $F^{\circ}_{1.20}$ 0–4	α_1

[a] Density in g/ml.
[b] S_f = Svedberg units of flotation; $F^{\circ}_{1.20}$ = corrected flotation rate at d = 1.20 g/ml.

GENETIC DIVERSITY OF LIPOPROTEIN PHENOTYPES

Studies of the lipid and lipoprotein abnormalities in myocardial infarction survivors and their family members provided evidence that multiple lipoprotein phenotypes could exist in the same kindred (10,11). Later it was found that mutations of separate genes, the genes encoding lipoprotein

TABLE 3. *Lipoprotein phenotyping system*

Phenotype	Lipoprotein concentration increased	Electrophoretic mobility
I	Chylomicrons	Origin[a]
IIa	LDL	β
IIb	VLDL and LDL	VLDL—α_2 LDL—β
III	Remnant lipoproteins	"Broad beta"[b]
IV	VLDL	α_2
V	Chylomicrons and VLDL	Chylomicrons—origin VLDL—α_2

[a] Chylomicrons remain at the site of application if paper or agarose is the electrophoresis medium.
[b] Migration from the β position to the α_2 position, representing chylomicron remnants and VLDL remnants.

lipase and apolipoprotein C-II, produced the same type I lipoprotein phenotype (12). These observations proved the lack of utility of lipoprotein phenotyping as a means of identifying specific genetic disorders that cause hyperlipidemia. However, the phenotyping system proved to be a highly efficacious method of teaching health professionals about the clinical relevance of the lipoproteins. The system remains in use today as a shorthand method for conveying information about lipoprotein abnormalities.

SINGLE-GENE MUTATIONS FOR LIPID DISORDERS

During the decade in which the phenotyping system enjoyed widespread use, investigators studied the structure, composition, and metabolism of the lipoproteins associated with hyperlipidemia among the six phenotypes. Many important proteins were purified and characterized, including the apolipoproteins (13–15), lipoprotein receptors (16), the lipoprotein and hepatic lipases (17), lecithin:cholesterol acyltransferase (18), and cholesteryl ester transfer protein (19). Among the first and best-characterized single-gene mutations are those responsible for the disorders familial hypercholesterolemia (FH) and type III hyperlipoproteinemia (20,21).

Discovery of the LDL receptor and that mutations of the LDL receptor gene are responsible for raised LDL concentrations in FH provided powerful insights into the regulation of plasma LDL levels and intracellular cholesterol metabolism. These insights included recognition that plasma LDL levels are inversely related to the number of LDL receptors expressed on the cell surfaces within the body, the finding that depletion of intracellular cholesterol and inhibition of cholesterol biosynthesis results in enhanced LDL receptor expression by cells, discovery of cholesterol biosynthesis inhibitors (the statins) that are the most potent and clinically useful cholesterol-lowering drugs, recognition of the liver as the organ with most (more than 50%) of the body's complement of LDL receptors, and the determination that dietary saturated fatty acids of 12-, 14-, and 16-carbon chain lengths and dietary cholesterol influence plasma cholesterol levels by reducing hepatic expression of LDL receptor (5,22,23).

Type III hyperlipoproteinemia was found to be associated with mutations of the apolipoprotein E (apo E) gene (21). The accumulation of remnant lipoproteins in type III patients with apo E gene mutations suggested that apo E plays a role in the clearance of these lipoproteins. It was also observed that apo E binds to the LDL receptor, but the lack of substantial remnant accumulation in homozygous FH patients with few, if any, functional LDL receptors suggested that apo-E-enriched remnant lipoproteins are not removed from the blood exclusively by apo-E–LDL receptor interactions. Ultimately, a remnant receptor, the LDL-receptor-related protein (LRP), was identified, and apo E was found to be the ligand that binds remnant lipoproteins to the LRP (24,25).

ATHEROGENIC DYSLIPIDEMIA

Accumulated remnant lipoproteins and LDL, associated with type III hyperlipoproteinemia and FH, respectively, represent two of four currently recognized dyslipidemic states associated with accelerated atherogenesis. A third is low HDL concentrations, which occur on a familial basis or in conjunction with other disorders such as diabetes mellitus. The fourth is elevation of the concentration of lipoprotein (a) [Lp(a)].

The mechanism by which remnant lipoproteins initiate atheroma formation involves the uptake of remnant lipoproteins by macrophages in the arterial wall (26,27). This uptake results in the delivery of remnant cholesterol and the accumulation of excessive intracellular cholesterol. This excessive macrophage cholesterol content transforms the macrophage into the conductor of the symphony of events that leads to atheroma formation (28).

Unlike remnants, plasma LDL were noted to be incapable of binding to macrophages, precluding cholesterol accumulation and initiation of atherogenesis. Subsequently, investigators found that modifications of LDL in vitro produced LDL that are bound by specific receptors on macrophages and internalized (29). The mechanism by which in vivo LDL modification occurs is still under active investigation (30).

The pathophysiology remains relatively obscure for the causes of reduced HDL concentrations and the role of low HDL levels in atherogenesis. It is clear, based on studies of families with low HDL levels and upon population studies (31–35), that low HDL concentrations, especially of the HDL_2 subfraction, are associated with accelerated coronary atherosclerosis. Recent investigations of the HDL from patients with familial low-HDL kindreds suggest that the reduction in HDL_2 levels is specifically caused by low concentrations of HDL particles containing only apo A-I (36).

Although much has been learned about the structure of Lp(a) in recent years, its precise role in atherogenesis is unclear (37,38). Most studies examining Lp(a) concentrations have found that myocardial infarction survivors have higher Lp(a) levels than the general population. However, recently developed knowledge that Lp(a) is an acute-phase reactant and a prospective study that found no correlation between Lp(a) levels at baseline and the risk of developing a subsequent myocardial infarction challenge the concept of Lp(a) as a universal risk factor for atherosclerosis (39). It may be that high Lp(a) levels confer additional risk only in those patients with elevated total cholesterol levels or other atherosclerosis risk factors (40). Because of the uncertainty regarding the role of Lp(a) in the atherogenesis, routine clinical assessment of Lp(a) levels does not appear to be warranted at the present time.

TREATMENT-ORIENTED CLASSIFICATION OF DYSLIPIDEMIA: A CONTEMPORARY APPROACH

At the current time, clinical classification of dyslipidemia for management purposes does not require establishing the

TABLE 4. *Classification of dyslipidemia according to triglyceride, total cholesterol, and HDL cholesterol concentrations*

Cholesterol disorders[a]	Cholesterol level elevated and exceeds triglyceride concentration
Triglyceride disorders[b]	Triglyceride level elevated and exceeds cholesterol concentration
HDL cholesterol concentration reduced	<35 mg/dl

[a] Total cholesterol: ideal <200 mg/dl; borderline high, 200–239 mg/dl; high risk ≥240 mg/dl. LDL cholesterol: ideal <130 mg/dl; borderline high, 130–159 mg/dl; high risk ≥160 mg/dl.

[b] Triglyceride: ideal <200 mg/dl; high risk >400 mg/dl.

precise genetic diagnosis. However, knowledge of the particular genetic diagnosis may be helpful for genetic counseling, and it will assume great importance when gene-transfer therapy becomes possible. Currently, the classification depends on measurement of the concentrations of plasma triglycerides, total cholesterol, and HDL cholesterol (Table 4). If the cholesterol concentration is elevated to a greater extent than the triglyceride concentration, the patient's hypercholesterolemia is caused by an increased LDL level, usually as a result of one of the disorders listed in Table 5. On the other hand, the fasting triglyceride concentration exceeds the cholesterol level in patients with any of the genetic disorders causing predominant hypertriglyceridemia (Table 6).

Effective treatment can be prescribed based on assignment of each patient to the cholesterol disorders group, the triglyceride disorders group, or the low-HDL group and subsequent use of the National Cholesterol Education Program treatment guidelines for initiating therapy and establishing treatment goals (41). All patients should be managed with reductions in total dietary fat, saturated fat, and cholesterol. In addition, the patients with elevated triglyceride concentrations should lose weight if indicated and restrict their alcohol intake. Lipid-lowering drugs for patients with cholesterol disorders include three first-choice drugs: niacin, resins, and statins. Probucol may be used in selected patients. For triglyceride problems, niacin and the fibrates are the drugs of choice.

Patients with reduced HDL cholesterol concentrations deserve further consideration. Often these patients have normal total cholesterol concentrations and normal or only slightly elevated LDL cholesterol levels. As a consequence, their LDL levels may not be elevated enough to meet the National Cholesterol Education Program guidelines for drug therapy despite the well-accepted fact that these patients are at increased risk of developing coronary heart disease. To guide effective treatment of these patients, it is useful to compute the ratio of the total cholesterol level to the HDL-cholesterol concentration. Data from the Framingham study revealed that ratios greater than 4.5 are associated with increased coronary heart disease risk and that an optimal ratio is less than 3.5 (42).

TABLE 5. *Genetic causes of cholesterol disorders*

Familial hypercholesterolemia (16,20)
Familial defective apolipoprotein B100 (53)
Familial combined hyperlipidemia (10)
Polygenic hypercholesterolemia (10)

TABLE 6. *Genetic causes of triglyceride disorders*

Familial hypertriglyceridemia (10)
Familial combined hyperlipidemia (10)
Familial type III hyperlipoproteinemia (21)
Chylomicronemia syndrome (54)
  Apo C-II mutations
  Lipoprotein lipase mutations

However, some caveats apply in using the total cholesterol : HDL cholesterol ratio. First is the difficulty of obtaining accurate, reproducible HDL cholesterol determinations. Careful attention is required in the laboratory for the reliable measurement of HDL cholesterol levels. Errors can drastically affect the ratio. Another important concern is that no clinical trials have been designed solely to determine the benefit of reducing the total cholesterol : HDL cholesterol ratio of patients with low HDL concentrations as their only dyslipidemic problem. Other trials suggest that drug-induced increases in HDL are beneficial, but concomitant reductions of LDL levels or LDL levels plus triglyceride levels in these trials preclude assigning benefit solely to increases in HDL levels (43). Nevertheless it seems prudent to extend the potential benefit of lipid management to these high-risk patients until definitive therapeutic trials have been conducted.

Special treatment provisions have been recommended for patients with established atherosclerotic vascular disease or multiple risk factors (41). These provisions include reducing the LDL cholesterol concentration below 100 mg/dl for patients with vascular disease and below 130 mg/dl for patients with two or more risk factors. Clinical trial data support vigorous cholesterol lowering for the purpose of secondary prevention, and reanalyses of the data from primary and secondary prevention trials suggest a much greater benefit from cholesterol reduction than was appreciated previously (44).

SECONDARY CAUSES OF HYPERLIPIDEMIA

Secondary causes of hyperlipidemia should be sought and excluded immediately when dyslipidemia is identified initially. Causes of secondary hyperlipidemia are listed in Table 7.

LOW BLOOD LIPID LEVEL—A HEALTH HAZARD?

Hypolipidemia, unusually low concentrations of cholesterol or cholesterol and triglycerides, occurs as a result of

TABLE 7. *Secondary causes of dyslipidemia*

Associated with hypercholesterolemia
Nephrotic syndrome
Hypothyroidism
Dysglobulinemia
Acute intermittent porphyria
Hepatoma
Obstructive jaundice
Multiple myeloma
Associated with hypertriglyceridemia
Diabetes mellitus
Uremia
Renal transplantation
Chronic dialysis
Nephrotic syndrome
Contraceptive steroids
Alcohol
Dysglobulinemia
Cushing's syndrome

genetic disorders affecting certain apolipoproteins (apo B100, apo A-I) and the microsomal triglyceride transfer protein (Table 8). These disorders are relatively rare. Hypocholesterolemia is much more common in the general population in persons consuming low-fat diets. It has been speculated that low total cholesterol levels may be associated with excess mortality from a variety of causes (45). However, a recent comprehensive meta-analysis of pertinent studies suggests that only hemorrhagic stroke appears to be increased in persons with low total cholesterol levels if they also are hypertensive (46). Although of concern, the enhanced risk of stroke is more than compensated for by a tenfold reduction in coronary heart disease events relative to the increase in the incidence of stroke.

UNCERTAINTIES OF TREATMENT

The classification of dyslipidemia is most important for the purpose of making rational treatment choices for dyslipidemic patients. Brewer *(this volume)* provides the details needed to evaluate patients for specific genetic disorders, and Farmer and Gotto *(this volume)* describe the detailed use of appropriate therapeutic strategies. It is important to keep in mind that clinical trials provide evidence that coronary disease events can be prevented by lowering LDL levels and VLDL levels (43,47–52). On the other hand, clinical trials have not been conducted to prove the value of cholesterol-lowering therapy in patients with low concentrations of HDL, in patients above age 65 with lipid abnormalities, or in patients with diabetes mellitus who have elevated VLDL and reduced HDL concentrations. Because atherosclerosis in elderly patients is probably very similar to that seen in younger patients, it seems rational to extend the benefits of lipid lowering to elderly persons. In the case of patients with low HDL concentrations, treatment guidelines that focus solely on reducing LDL cholesterol concentrations may not be adequate. Many of these patients have LDL cholesterol concentrations within the National Cholesterol Education Program's treatment guidelines yet are at substantial risk because of reduced HDL concentrations. Treatment of these patients should focus on reducing LDL concentrations to correct the ratio of total cholesterol:HDL cholesterol rather than raising the HDL cholesterol concentration.

TABLE 8. *Causes of hypolipidemia*

Genetic
Hypobetalipoproteinemia: Truncations of apo B100 (55)
Abetalipoproteinemia: Mutations of microsomal triglyceride transfer protein gene (56)
Hypoalphalipoproteinemia: Tangier disease (57)
Mutations of the apo A-I gene (58)
Nutritional
Low-fat diets

FUTURE DEVELOPMENT OF CLINICAL CLASSIFICATIONS OF LIPID DISORDERS

The clinical classification of lipid disorders is proceeding on two fronts. First, scientists are attempting to identify the mutations that underlie familial lipid disorders. The value of this approach is that therapeutic efforts can be targeted with a greater chance of efficacy when the metabolic bases of the disorders are understood. The advantage of this approach is obvious when one considers the possibilities of gene-transfer therapy. The second approach to clinical classification that is evolving is the identification of additional atherogenic dyslipidemic states. A better understanding of the role of HDL in atherogenesis will lead to the identification of abnormalities of HDL metabolism that accelerate coronary heart disease. Discoveries likely to be made regarding postprandial lipoprotein metabolism will enhance our understanding and treatment of blood lipids and their role in coronary heart disease. The ability to identify concentrations of modified LDL or to evaluate the processes that lead to LDL modification may also shape future diagnostic and treatment paradigms.

REFERENCES

1. Selzer A. Fifty years of progress in cardiology: A personal perspective. *Circulation* 1988;77:955–963.
2. Fredrickson DS, Goldstein JL, Brown MS. The familial hyperlipoproteinemias. In: Stanbury JB, Wyngaarden JB, Fredrickson DS, eds. *The Metabolic Basis of Inherited Disease,* 4th ed. New York: McGraw-Hill; 1978:604–655.
3. Gofman JW, deLalla O, Glazier F, Freeman NK, Lindgren FT, Nichols AV, Strisower B, Tamplin AR. The serum lipoprotein transport system in health, metabolic disorders, atherosclerosis and coronary heart disease. *Plasma* 1954;2:413–484.
4. Havel RJ, Eder HA, Bragdon JH. The distribution and chemical composition of ultracentrifugally separated lipoproteins in human serum. *J Clin Invest* 1955;34:1345–1353.
5. Brown MS, Goldstein JL. A receptor-mediated pathway for cholesterol homeostasis. *Science* 1986;232:34–47.

6. Gofman JW, Young W, Tandy R. Ischemic heart disease, atherosclerosis, and longevity. *Circulation* 1966;34:679–697.
7. Barr DP, Russ EM, Eder HA. Protein–lipid relationships in human plasma. II. In atherosclerosis and related conditions. *Am J Med* 1951; 11:480–493.
8. Fredrickson DS, Levy RI, Lees RS. Fat transport in lipoproteins—an integrated approach to mechanisms and disorders. *N Engl J Med* 1967; 276:34–44,94–103,148–156,215–225,273–281.
9. Friedewald WT, Levy RI, Fredrickson DS. Estimation of the concentration of low-density lipoprotein cholesterol in plasma, without use of the preparative ultracentrifuge. *Clin Chem* 1972;18:499–502.
10. Goldstein JL, Hazzard WR, Schrott HG, Bierman EL, Motulsky AG. Hyperlipidemia in coronary heart disease. I. Lipid levels in 500 survivors of myocardial infarction. *J Clin Invest* 1973;52:1533–1543.
11. Goldstein JL, Schrott HG, Hazzard WR, Bierman EL, Motulsky AG. Hyperlipidemia in coronary heart disease. II. Genetic analysis of lipid levels in 176 families and delineation of a new inherited disorder, combined hyperlipidemia. *J Clin Invest* 1973;52:1544–1568.
12. Breckenridge WC, Little JA, Steiner G, Chow A, Poapst M. Hypertriglyceridemia associated with deficiency of apolipoprotein C-II. *N Engl J Med* 1978;298:1265–1273.
13. Mahley RW, Innerarity TL, Rall SC Jr, Weisgraber KH. Plasma lipoproteins: Apolipoprotein structure and function. *J Lipid Res* 1984;25: 1277–1294.
14. Breslow JL. Lipoprotein transport gene abnormalities underlying coronary heart disease susceptibility. *Annu Rev Med* 1991;42:357–371.
15. Zannis VI, Kardassis D, Cardot P, Hadzopoulou-Cladaras M, Zanni EE, Cladaras C. Molecular biology of the human apolipoprotein genes: Gene regulation and structure/function relationship. *Curr Opin Lipidol* 1992;3:96–113.
16. Hobbs HH, Russell DW, Brown MS, Goldstein JL. The LDL receptor locus in familial hypercholesterolemia: Mutational analysis of a membrane protein. *Annu Rev Genet* 1990;24:133–170.
17. Olivecrona T, Bengtsson-Olivecrona G. Lipoprotein lipase and hepatic lipase. *Curr Opin Lipidol* 1993;4:187–196.
18. Glomset JA. The plasma lecithin:cholesterol acyltransferase reaction. *J Lipid Res* 1968;9:155–167.
19. Fielding CJ. Lipid transfer proteins: Catalysts, transmembrane carriers and signaling intermediates for intracellular and extracellular lipid reactions. *Curr Opin Lipidol* 1993;4:218–222.
20. Goldstein JL, Brown MS. Familial hypercholesterolemia. In: Scriver CR, Beaudet AL, Sly WS, Valle D, eds. *The Metabolic Basis of Inherited Disease,* 6th ed. New York: McGraw-Hill; 1989:1215–1250.
21. Mahley RW, Rall SC Jr. Type III hyperlipoproteinemia (dysbetalipoproteinemia): The role of apolipoprotein E in normal and abnormal lipoprotein metabolism. In: Scriver CR, Beaudet AL, Sly WS, Valle D, eds. *The Metabolic Basis of Inherited Disease,* 6th ed. New York: McGraw-Hill; 1989:1195–1213.
22. Grundy SM, Vega GL. Influence of mevinolin on metabolism of low density lipoproteins in primary moderate hypercholesterolemia. *J Lipid Res* 1985;26:1464–1475.
23. Dietschy JM, Turley SD, Spady DK. Role of liver in the maintenance of cholesterol and low density lipoprotein homeostasis in different animal species, including humans. *J Lipid Res* 1993;34:1637–1659.
24. Brown MS, Herz J, Kowal RC, Goldstein JL. The low-density lipoprotein receptor-related protein: Double agent or decoy? *Curr Opin Lipidol* 1991;2:65–72.
25. Mahley RW, Hussain MM. Chylomicron and chylomicron remnant catabolism. *Curr Opin Lipidol* 1991;2:170–176.
26. Innerarity TL, Arnold KS, Weisgraber KH, Mahley RW. Apolipoprotein E is the determinant that mediates the receptor uptake of β-very low density lipoproteins by mouse macrophages. *Arteriosclerosis* 1986; 67:114–122.
27. Koo C, Wernette-Hammond ME, Garcia Z, Malloy MJ, Uauy R, East C, Bilheimer DW, Mahley RW, Innerarity TL. The uptake of cholesterol-rich remnant lipoproteins by human monocyte-derived macrophages is mediated by low density lipoprotein receptors. *J Clin Invest* 1988;81:1332–1340.
28. Mahley RW, Weisgraber KH, Innerarity TL, Rall SC Jr. Genetic defects in lipoprotein metabolism: Elevation of atherogenic lipoproteins caused by impaired catabolism. *JAMA* 1991;265:78–83.
29. Steinberg D, Parthasarathy S, Carew TE, Khoo JC, Witztum JL. Beyond cholesterol. Modifications of low-density lipoprotein that increase its atherogenicity. *N Engl J Med* 1989;320:915–924.
30. Steinberg D, Witztum JL. Lipoproteins and atherogenesis. Current concepts. *JAMA* 1990;264:3047–3052.
31. Miller GJ, Miller NE. Plasma-high-density-lipoprotein concentration and development of ischaemic heart-disease. *Lancet* 1975;1:16–19.
32. Montag J, Flynn M, Freidel J, Laskarzewski P, Glueck CJ. Primary and familial hypoalphalipoproteinemia. *Metabolism* 1984;33:136–146.
33. Gordon DJ, Probstfield JL, Garrison RJ, Neaton JD, Castelli WP, Knoke JD, Jacobs DR Jr, Bangdiwala S, Tyroler HA. High-density lipoprotein cholesterol and cardiovascular disease. Four prospective American studies. *Circulation* 1989;79:8–15.
34. Assmann G, Funke H. HDL metabolism and atherosclerosis. *J Cardiovasc Pharmacol* 1990;16(Suppl 9):S15–S20.
35. Miller NE. Associations of high-density lipoprotein subclasses and apolipoproteins with ischemic heart disease and coronary atherosclerosis. *Am Heart J* 1987;113:589–597.
36. Fruchart J-C, Ailhaud G, Bard J-M. Heterogeneity of high density lipoprotein particles. *Circulation* 1993;87:III-22–III-27.
37. Utermann G. The mysteries of lipoprotein(a). *Science* 1989;246: 904–910.
38. Scanu AM. Genetic basis and pathophysiological implications of high plasma Lp(a) levels. *J Intern Med* 1992;231:679–683.
39. Ridker PM, Hennekens CH, Stampfer MJ. A prospective study of lipoprotein(a) and the risk of myocardial infarction. *JAMA* 1993;270: 2195–2199.
40. Seed M, Hoppichler F, Reaveley D, McCarthy S, Thompson GR, Boerwinkle E, Utermann G. Relation of serum lipoprotein(a) concentration and apolipoprotein(a) phenotype to coronary heart disease in patients with familial hypercholesterolemia. *N Engl J Med* 1990;322: 1494–1499.
41. National Cholesterol Education Program. Second report of the Expert Panel on Detection, Evaluation, and Treatment of High Blood Cholesterol in Adults (Adult Treatment Panel II). *Circulation* 1994;89: 1329–1445.
42. Castelli WP. The folly of questioning the benefits of cholesterol reduction. *Am Fam Physician* 1994;49:567–574.
43. Manninen V, Tenkanen L, Koskinen P, Huttunen JK, Mänttäri M, Heinonen OP, Frick MH. Joint effects of serum triglyceride and LDL cholesterol and HDL cholesterol concentrations on coronary heart disease risk in the Helsinki Heart Study. Implications for treatment. *Circulation* 1992;85:37–45.
44. Law MR, Wald NJ, Wu T, Hackshaw A, Bailey A. Systematic underestimation of association between serum cholesterol concentration and ischaemic heart disease in observational studies: Data from the BUPA study. *Br Med J* 1994;308:363–366.
45. Jacobs D, Blackburn H, Higgins M, Reed D, Iso H, McMillan G, Neaton J, Nelson J, Potter J, Rifkind B, Rossouw J, Shekelle R, Yusuf S. Report of the Conference on Low Blood Cholesterol: Mortality Associations. *Circulation* 1992;86:1046–1060.
46. Law MR, Thompson SG, Wald NJ. Assessing possible hazards of reducing serum cholesterol. *Br Med J* 1994;308:373–379.
47. Lipid Research Clinics Program. The Lipid Research Clinics Coronary Primary Prevention Trial results. II. The relationship of reduction in incidence of coronary heart disease to cholesterol lowering. *JAMA* 1984;251:365–374.
48. Lipid Research Clinics Program. The Lipid Research Clinics Coronary Primary Prevention Trial results. I. Reduction in incidence of coronary heart disease. *JAMA* 1984;251:351–364.
49. Frick MH, Elo O, Haapa K, Heinonen OP, Heinsalmi P, Helo P, Huttunen JK, Kaitaniemi P, Koskinen P, Manninen V, Mäenpää H, Mälkönen M, Mänttäri M, Norola S, Pasternack A, Pikkarainen J, Romo M, Sjöblom T, Nikkilä EA. Helsinki Heart Study: Primary-prevention trial with gemfibrozil in middle-aged men with dyslipidemia. Safety of treatment, changes in risk factors, and incidence of coronary heart disease. *N Engl J Med* 1987;317:1237–1245.
50. Brown G, Albers JJ, Fisher LD, Schaefer SM, Lin J-T, Kaplan C, Zhao X-Q, Bisson BD, Fitzpatrick VF, Dodge HT. Regression of coronary artery disease as a result of intensive lipid-lowering therapy in men with high levels of apolipoprotein B. *N Engl J Med* 1990;323:1289–1298.
51. Buchwald H, Varco RL, Matts JP, Long JM, Fitch LL, Campbell GS, Pearce MB, Yellin AE, Edmiston WA, Smink RD Jr, Sawin HS Jr, Campos CT, Hansen BJ, Tuna N, Karnegis JN, Sanmarco ME, Amplatz K, Castaneda-Zuniga WR, Hunter DW, Bissett JK, Weber FJ, Stevenson JW, Leon AS, Chalmers TC, the POSCH Group. Effect of partial

ileal bypass surgery on mortality and morbidity from coronary heart disease in patients with hypercholesterolemia. Report of the Program on the Surgical Control of the Hyperlipidemias (POSCH). *N Engl J Med* 1990;323:946–955.

52. Kane JP, Malloy MJ, Ports TA, Phillips NR, Diehl JC, Havel RJ. Regression of coronary atherosclerosis during treatment of familial hypercholesterolemia with combined drug regimens. *JAMA* 1990;264: 3007–3012.
53. Innerarity TL, Mahley RW, Weisgraber KH, Bersot TP, Krauss RM, Vega GL, Grundy SM, Friedl W, Davignon J, McCarthy BJ. Familial defective apolipoprotein B100: A mutation of apolipoprotein B that causes hypercholesterolemia. *J Lipid Res* 1990;31:1337–1349.
54. Chait A, Brunzell JD. Chylomicronemia syndrome. *Adv Intern Med* 1991;37:249–273.
55. Young SG. Recent progress in understanding apolipoprotein B. *Circulation* 1990;82:1574–1594.
56. Wetterau JR, Aggerbeck LP, Bouma M-E, Eisenberg C, Munck A, Hermier M, Schmitz J, Gay G, Rader DJ, Gregg RE. Absence of microsomal triglyceride transfer protein in individuals with abetalipoproteinemia. *Science* 1992;258:999–1001.
57. Assmann G, Schmitz G, Brewer HB Jr. Familial high density lipoprotein deficiency: Tangier disease. In: Scriver CR, Beaudet AL, Sly WS, Valle D, eds. *The Metabolic Basis of Inherited Disease,* 6th ed. New York: McGraw-Hill; 1989:1267–1282.
58. Breslow JL. Familial disorders of high density lipoprotein metabolism. In: Scriver CR, Beaudet AL, Sly WS, Valle D, eds. *The Metabolic Basis of Inherited Disease,* 6th ed. New York: McGraw-Hill; 1989: 1251–1266.

Atherosclerosis and Coronary Artery Disease,
edited by V. Fuster, R. Ross, and E. J. Topol.
Lippincott-Raven Publishers, Philadelphia © 1996.

CHAPTER 11

Management

John A. Farmer and Antonio M. Gotto, Jr.

Key Words: Coronary artery disease; Atherosclerosis; Risk factors; Dyslipidemia; Dietary therapy; Drug therapy.

INTRODUCTION

Despite the progress that has been made in elucidating the underlying mechanisms of atherogenesis, no single, cogent hypothesis has been described that accounts for all clinical, epidemiologic, and laboratory observations. However, it is clear that certain clinically discernible factors participate intimately in the development of coronary artery disease (CAD). Management of these risk factors has gained acceptance as a means of reducing the likelihood of coronary events. Major modifiable and nonmodifiable CAD risk factors are presented in Table 1 [criteria for assessing the causal significance of these statistical associations have been reviewed by Stamler (1)]. Although therapeutic options are limited to the control of modifiable risk factors, nonmodifiable risk factors must also be identified to best determine the intensity of therapy. Clinical trial data establish the benefit of interventions targeting hypercholesterolemia, hypertension, and tobacco use.

Because of the prevalence of dyslipidemia in the United States and other developed nations, ongoing public health efforts continue to emphasize the education of physicians and the general population on the importance of managing lipid risk factors. A number of lipid abnormalities are associated with increased risk. These lipid abnormalities can be consequences of genetic or environmental factors or secondary to other disease states. The strongest evidence of atherogenicity exists for elevated levels of low-density lipoprotein (LDL) cholesterol, although low levels of high-density lipoprotein (HDL) cholesterol and elevated triglyceride levels are also targets of intervention. Clinical trials have demonstrated that CAD morbidity and mortality may be reduced by antilipidemic therapy in both primary and secondary prevention, and have shown that the progression of established CAD may be slowed or even reversed by aggressive interventions. As research advances, treatment guidelines may incorporate other factors associated with atherogenesis that are currently under scrutiny, such as apolipoprotein levels or lipoprotein[a] levels.

In 1988, the National Cholesterol Education Program (NCEP), an organization of the National Institutes of Health, released recommendations for the treatment of adults with dyslipidemia (2). The Adult Treatment Panel (ATP I) recommended that routine screening of adults be conducted to

John A. Farmer: Section of Cardiology, Ben Taub General Hospital, and Department of Medicine, Baylor College of Medicine, Houston, Texas 77030.

Antonio M. Gotto, Jr: Internal Medicine Service, Methodist Hospital, Houston, Texas, and Department of Medicine, Baylor College of Medicine, Houston, Texas 77030.

TABLE 1. *Major risk factors for coronary artery disease*

Age[a]
Family history of premature CAD
Elevated LDL cholesterol
Low HDL cholesterol
Cigarette smoking
Hypertension
Diabetes mellitus

CAD, Coronary artery disease; LDL, low-density lipoprotein; HDL, high-density lipoprotein.

[a] Adult Treatment Panel (ATP) II-defined cutpoints for increased risk are ≥45 years in men and ≥55 years in women, or premature menopause without estrogen-replacement therapy.

identify subjects at high risk for CAD, and presented LDL-cholesterol values at which hygienic and pharmacologic therapy should be considered.

In 1993, these guidelines were updated to reflect the most recent consensus of experts on the treatment of dyslipidemia (3). The Adult Treatment Panel II (ATP II) guidelines differ from the ATP I report in several aspects. The ATP II provides separate treatment algorithms for primary and secondary prevention and places increased emphasis on overall risk status in determining follow-up. An increased emphasis on HDL cholesterol is also evident: HDL cholesterol is incorporated in the initial screening process (in part due to the improved accuracy and lower cost of the measurement), and enhanced recognition is given to HDL cholesterol as a risk factor.

This chapter reviews current approaches to the clinical management of dyslipidemia in primary and secondary prevention of CAD, including the screening and treatment recommendations of the ATP II.

RISK STATUS AS A GUIDE TO THERAPY

Because both lipid and nonlipid risk factors can increase risk synergistically, individual risk factors should not be considered in isolation, but as part of a complete risk factor profile. Patients can then be stratified according to total risk for CAD to guide the type and intensity of therapy. The most aggressive therapy is reserved for those at highest risk, i.e., those patients at increased short-term risk for future events due to the presence of established CAD. Risk of infarction is five to seven times greater in persons with symptomatic coronary disease than in asymptomatic persons (4). The risk status of patients with dyslipidemia but without CAD lies within a range from relatively low to greatly increased, depending on the number and severity of concomitant risk factors. Young men and premenopausal women without severe elevations of LDL cholesterol or multiple risk factors are at low short-term risk, and a conservative approach is warranted in these patients. However, patients with multiple risk factors, diabetes mellitus, a family history of premature CAD, or certain genetic disorders are likely to have significant atherosclerosis, and more aggressive therapy is often necessary. The distinction between primary and secondary prevention of CAD is therefore somewhat artificial, in that a stark contrast in the extent of atherosclerosis between asymptomatic and symptomatic patients with similar risk profiles is not observed. In fact, angiographically monitored clinical trials have suggested that coronary events are more closely related to the presence of lesions with certain morphologic characteristics than to the extent of stenosis (5). Nevertheless, the known presence of atherosclerotic disease remains the strongest indicator of overall risk for future coronary events.

In addition to LDL cholesterol, the risk factors defined for use in the ATP II algorithm are age (≥45 years in men and ≥55 years in women, or premature menopause without estrogen-replacement therapy), cigarette smoking, hypertension or the use of antihypertensive agents, a family history of premature coronary heart disease, diabetes mellitus, and HDL cholesterol <35 mg/dl. High HDL cholesterol (>60 mg/dl) is considered a negative risk factor, i.e., the number of risk factors considered to be present is reduced by one when determining follow-up. Obesity and sedentary lifestyle should also be considered because they are frequently associated with other risk factors such as low HDL cholesterol, hypertension, and diabetes mellitus. This tabulation of risk is not meant to be rigid or comprehensive, but rather serves to identify the presence of major risk factors known to contribute to CAD morbidity and mortality. The simplicity of the ATP II algorithm favors its clinical utility, but it also requires clinical judgment for its successful implementation.

The significance of triglyceride as a risk factor for CAD remains controversial. On univariate analysis, elevated fasting triglyceride level is strongly associated with the presence and extent of coronary atherosclerosis. However, patients whose lipid profile is predominantly characterized by elevated triglyceride frequently are obese, are sedentary, or have low HDL cholesterol. On multivariate analysis that corrects for these variables, the predictive power of fasting triglyceride level diminishes or disappears. However, as reviewed by Austin (6,7), these analyses may be inadequate means of assessing the relation between triglyceride and CAD risk because of the close metabolic relation between HDL cholesterol and triglyceride, and because the atherogenic potential of the postprandial state is not considered.

SCREENING

The ATP II guidelines represent a two-tiered strategy for reducing the toll of coronary disease. First, they give population-wide recommendations that promote vascular health, i.e., adoption of a low-fat, low-cholesterol diet, regular exercise, weight control, and cessation of tobacco use. Patients should be routinely educated on the importance of these lifestyle habits in preventing coronary disease. It has been estimated that the number of coronary events in the United

States would be reduced 50% if the entire population adhered to these recommendations (8,8a). Second, the ATP II presents criteria for identifying specific individuals at high risk for CAD and for instituting therapy.

Primary Prevention

In primary prevention, the ATP II advocates that all adults over age 20 have their serum total cholesterol level checked every 5 years. If accurate methods are available, HDL-cholesterol level should also be determined at this time. Nonlipid risk factors should be identified as well. Follow-up based on these measurements is shown in Table 2. Total cholesterol is classified as desirable (<200 mg/dl), borderline-high (200–239 mg/dl), or high (≥240 mg/dl), and follow-up is determined by this classification and by HDL-cholesterol level. Individuals with desirable levels of total cholesterol and HDL cholesterol (≥35 mg/dl) should be reevaluated within 5 years. However, if HDL cholesterol is low, a fasting lipoprotein analysis should be performed to estimate LDL-cholesterol level.

Individuals with borderline-high total cholesterol, HDL cholesterol ≥35 mg/dl, and fewer than two other risk factors should repeat screening in 1–2 years. However, patients with borderline-high total cholesterol who have either low HDL cholesterol or two or more other risk factors should have a fasting lipoprotein analysis performed.

Fasting lipoprotein analysis is necessary for all patients with high total cholesterol, regardless of HDL-cholesterol level.

Because a complete lipoprotein analysis requires a fasting measurement of triglyceride levels, the sample must be drawn after a fast of at least 9–12 hr. The LDL cholesterol is estimated by the Friedewald formula, based on measured levels of total and HDL cholesterol and triglyceride (in mg/dl):

$$\text{LDL cholesterol} \approx \text{total cholesterol} - \text{HDL cholesterol} - (\text{triglycerides}/5)$$

This formula is not accurate for patients with triglyceride levels exceeding 400 mg/dl or with type III hyperlipidemia (dysbetalipoproteinemia), in which case ultracentrifugation is required to determine LDL-cholesterol level.

Follow-up based on LDL cholesterol is illustrated in Table 3. The LDL-cholesterol level is classified as desirable (<130 mg/dl), borderline-high (130–159 mg/dl), or high (≥160 mg/dl); this classification of risk supplants that initially made based on total cholesterol. Patients with desirable levels of LDL cholesterol should be counseled on risk reduction and should repeat testing within 5 years. Borderline-high LDL cholesterol is followed up according to the presence of other risk factors. If fewer than two are present (including low HDL cholesterol), the patient should receive information on the Step I Diet (see Table 8) and risk reduction, but specific therapy is unnecessary; lipoprotein analysis should be repeated in 1 year. If two or more risk factors are present, or if the subject has high LDL cholesterol, dietary therapy is indicated; a second estimate of LDL cholesterol by lipoprotein analysis should be made in 1–8 weeks, so that treatment can be correctly initiated. A variance greater than 30 mg/dl requires that a third estimate be obtained, and the average of the three used. If the patient remains categorized at high risk due to high LDL cholesterol or borderline-high LDL cholesterol and the presence of two other risk factors, a clinical evaluation should be performed and dietary therapy initiated.

TABLE 2. *ATP II recommendations for primary prevention based on total and HDL cholesterol*

Result of nonfasting analysis		Recommendation
Total cholesterol <200	HDL-C ≥35	Repeat testing in 5 years
	HDL-C <35	Perform fasting lipoprotein analysis
Total cholesterol 200–239	HDL-C ≥35, and <2 other risk factors present	Repeat testing in 12 years
	HDL-C <35, or 2 other risk factors present	Perform fasting lipoprotein analysis
Total cholesterol ≥240		Perform fasting lipoprotein analysis regardless of other risk factors

All lipid values in mg/dl.

TABLE 3. *ATP II recommendations for primary prevention based on LDL-cholesterol level*

Result of lipoprotein analysis (mg/dL)		Recommendation
LDL-C <130		Repeat nonfasting screen in 5 years
LDL-C 130–159	<2 other risk factors	Repeat lipoprotein analysis in 1 year
	≥2 other risk factors	Initiate dietary therapy
LDL-C ≥160		Initiate dietary therapy

Secondary Prevention

A fasting lipoprotein analysis should be obtained annually for all patients with established CAD or clinical atherosclerotic disease of the aorta, arteries of the limbs, or carotid arteries. Patients with optimal LDL cholesterol (<100 mg/dl) should receive personalized instruction on lifestyle

TABLE 4. *ATP II recommendations for secondary prevention*

Result of fasting lipoprotein analysis (mg/dl)	Recommendation
LDL-C ≤100	Individualized instruction on diet and physical activity; repeat lipoprotein analysis annually
LDL-C >100	Initiate dietary therapy

Fasting lipoprotein analysis is the initial screening analysis in secondary prevention.

changes, including diet modification, weight control, and exercise, but specific LDL-cholesterol-lowering therapy is not required. Patients with higher than optimal LDL cholesterol are to receive a complete clinical evaluation so that an appropriate therapeutic regimen may be selected (Table 4). Lipid values are usually depressed for several weeks after myocardial infarction and should be interpreted cautiously (9). It nonetheless may be appropriate to initiate antilipidemic therapy during this period if LDL cholesterol is likely to be elevated, given the motivation frequently demonstrated by these patients in adhering to therapy.

CLINICAL EVALUATION

The clinical evaluation includes a history, physical examination, and basic laboratory tests. In addition to characterizing more accurately the patient's risk status, the evaluation should determine whether the dyslipidemia is primary or secondary, and if the former, whether it is familial. If secondary dyslipidemia is present, therapy should first be directed at the underlying condition. If the dyslipidemia persists, it then should be treated as a primary condition. Common causes of secondary dyslipidemia are listed in Table 5. Numerous medications may adversely affect the lipid profile; these effects are of particular concern in diabetes and hypertension, because of the frequency of dyslipidemia in patients with these disorders.

It is useful to classify lipid abnormalities by Fredrickson phenotype (10), which indicates the lipoprotein or lipoproteins elevated (Table 6). However, the Fredrickson system classifies hyperlipidemias only, i.e., low HDL cholesterol is not incorporated. Types IIa and IIb are the most frequently observed hyperlipidemic phenotypes. In addition to environmental factors and causes of secondary hypercholesterolemia, the type IIa phenotype can be caused by polygenic hypercholesterolemia or specific genetic disorders such as familial hypercholesterolemia, familial combined hyperlipidemia, or dysbetalipoproteinemia. Familial hypercholesterolemia and familial combined hyperlipidemia can also present as type IIb.

In both primary and secondary prevention, the average of two or three LDL-cholesterol estimates must be obtained

TABLE 5. *Selected causes of secondary hyperlipidemia*

Related to serum cholesterol level	Related to serum triglyceride level
Diet rich in saturated fatty acids	Chronic renal failure
Hypothyroidism	Excessive alcohol consumption
Nephrotic syndrome	Estrogen use (contraceptive or replacement)
Chronic liver disease (mainly primary biliary cirrhosis)	Beta-blocker, diuretic use
Cholestasis	Obesity
Dysglobulinemia	Pregnancy
Cushing's syndrome	Cushing's syndrome
Porphyria (acute intermittent)	Glucocorticoid use
Anorexia nervosa	Isotretinoin use
Diabetes mellitus	Hypopituitarism
	Hypothyroidism
	Pancreatitis
	Dysglobulinemia
	Glycogen storage disease
	Lipodystrophy
	Porphyria (acute intermittent)
	Uremia
	Systemic lupus erythematosus
	Bulimia

before any decision to initiate or change therapy can be made. However, for general monitoring, total cholesterol is usually an adequate and economical surrogate for LDL cholesterol (see Table 7).

DIETARY THERAPY

A variety of dietary factors influence circulating lipid levels, including the amount of fat and cholesterol in the diet, the relative intake of saturated, monounsaturated, and polyunsaturated fatty acids, carbohydrate intake, and body weight. Dietary therapy, including exercise and weight control, is the initial step in the management of dyslipidemia and is sufficient in most cases. In primary prevention, the goal of dietary therapy is to lower LDL cholesterol below 160 mg/dl, or below 130 mg/dl if two or more risk factors are present. The goal of dietary therapy in secondary prevention is an LDL-cholesterol level below 100 mg/dl (Table 7).

In primary prevention, the initial level of dietary therapy recommended by the ATP II is the Step I Diet. The more intensive Step II Diet should be initiated if the Step I Diet does not achieve the LDL-cholesterol goal after an adequate trial, usually 6 months. In cases of severe dyslipidemia, dietary therapy may begin with the Step II Diet if the Step I Diet is likely to be insufficient. The Step II Diet also serves as dietary therapy in secondary prevention. The dietary goals of the Step I and Step II Diets are given in Table 8.

The Step I Diet requires that ≤30% of calories be obtained from fat and 8–10% of calories be derived from saturated fat (the typical American diet derives 35–40% of calories from fat and approximately 13–14% of calories from saturated fat). Complex carbohydrates should be substituted

TABLE 6. *Fredrickson classification of the hyperlipidemias*

Phenotype	Lipoprotein(s) elevated	Blood cholesterol level	Blood triglyceride level	Atherogenicity
I	Chylomicrons	Normal to ↑	↑↑↑↑	None seen
IIa	LDL	↑↑	Normal	+ + +
IIb	LDL and VLDL	↑↑	↑↑	+ + +
III	IDL	↑↑	↑↑↑	+ + +
IV	VLDL	Normal to ↑	↑↑	+
V	VLDL and chylomicrons	Normal to ↑	↑↑↑↑	+

Adapted from Fredrickson et al., ref. 10, and Gotto and Pownall, ref. 80.
VLDL, Very low density lipoprotein; IDL, intermediate-density lipoprotein.

where possible to reduce the calories derived from fat. Both monounsaturated fat and polyunsaturated fat lower LDL cholesterol when substituted for saturated fat in the diet. However, increased intake of polyunsaturated fat is potentially detrimental because HDL cholesterol is also lowered. The ATP II recommends that 7% of total calories be derived from polyunsaturated fat in both the Step I and Step II Diets. Compared with polyunsaturated fat, monounsaturated fat is a preferable substitute for saturated fat and can account for up to 15% of total calories. In populations with relatively high intakes of monounsaturated fat, hypercholesterolemia and CAD appear to be less common than in populations consuming more saturated fat (11). Oleic acid is the major monounsaturated fatty acid found naturally in foods and is present at high levels in oils such as canola oil and olive oil.

Although dietary cholesterol has a major effect on serum cholesterol concentration in several animal models, some investigators question whether restricting dietary cholesterol intake significantly lowers circulating levels in humans. Response varies widely, but a 10 mg/dl increase in serum total cholesterol may generally be expected per 100 mg/kcal decrease in dietary cholesterol (12). The Step I Diet limits dietary cholesterol to less than 300 mg/day.

Additionally, the Step I Diet recommends that carbohydrates make up 55% of calories and protein makes up 15% of calories. To achieve dietary goals, grains, legumes, and fruits should be emphasized, supplemented by low-fat dairy products, fish, poultry, and lean cuts of other meats.

Soluble fiber, such as psyllium and guar gums, has been shown to produce a mild but statistically significant decrease in LDL cholesterol (13). The ATP II recommends a total fiber intake of 20–30 g/day, of which 25% should be soluble fiber. Although the cholesterol-lowering effect of soluble fiber is small, inclusion of fiber-rich foods should facilitate adherence to a low-fat, low-cholesterol diet. A high-fiber diet can cause nonspecific gastrointestinal symptoms, however.

After initiation of dietary therapy, efficacy should be assessed at approximately 4–6 weeks and again at 3 months. This frequent evaluation permits an accurate assessment of efficacy and adherence, and provides opportunity for encouraging and motivating the patient. Because dietary cholesterol is difficult to quantitate, an accurate assessment of dietary habits is required. Monitoring the exact amount and type of food ingested over several days is a useful means of estimating fat and cholesterol intake.

The efficacy of dietary therapy varies considerably among individuals. Some patients show complete normalization of lipid levels with diet, whereas others show no response. This variation is a function of compliance, initial lipid levels, and genetically mediated differences in metabolism. On average, a reduction in total cholesterol of approximately 5–7% may be expected.

If there is insufficient improvement in the lipid profile after an adequate trial of the Step I Diet, progression to the Step II Diet is indicated. To ensure adequate nutrition, the

TABLE 7. *ATP II initiation and target levels for therapy*

	Initiation (LDL cholesterol)	Target (LDL cholesterol)	Monitoring goal (total cholesterol)
No CHD, <2 risk factors			
Diet	≥160	<160	<240
Drug	≥190	<160	<240
No CHD, ≥2 risk factors			
Diet	≥130	<130	<200
Drug	≥160	<130	<200
CHD present			
Diet	≥100	<100	<160
Drug	≥130	<100	<160

All lipid values in mg/dl.

TABLE 8. *NCEP Step I and Step II Diets*

Nutrient	Recommended intake: Step I	Step II
Total fat	30% of total calories	
Saturated fat	8–10% of total calories	≤7% of total calories
Polyunsaturated fat	≤10% of total calories	
Monounsaturated fat	≤15% of total calories	
Carbohydrate	≥55% of total calories	
Protein	Approximately 15% of total calories	
Cholesterol	<300 mg/day	<200 mg/day
Total calories	To achieve and maintain desirable body weight	

Step II Diet does not further restrict the percent of total calories derived from fat; the percent of calories derived from protein and carbohydrates is also the same in both diets. However, the Step II Diet lowers saturated fat intake to <7% of total calories and limits dietary cholesterol to <200 mg/day. An additional 3–7% reduction in serum total cholesterol may be anticipated with the Step II Diet.

A similar pattern of diet modification is effective in treating elevated triglyceride, although a high intake of carbohydrates can aggravate hypertriglyceridemia and reduce HDL cholesterol. Dietary therapy for hypertriglyceridemia should therefore place increased emphasize on raising the ratio of monounsaturated fat to saturated fat and on increasing the portion of calories derived from complex carbohydrates without increasing the portion of calories derived from all carbohydrates. Alcohol consumption may need to be restricted in some patients.

Frequently, physicians do not have adequate training in dietary therapy or are unable to devote the considerable time and effort required to formulate and monitor a dietary plan. In such cases it is often desirable to enlist the services of a registered dietician to maximize adherence, particularly if the Step II Diet has been prescribed.

Ornish and Brown (14) have argued that dietary therapy can achieve LDL-cholesterol reductions and vascular improvement comparable with drug therapy if more intensive lifestyle changes are undertaken than those represented by the Step I and Step II Diets, e.g., a very low-fat, vegetarian diet and measures designed to promote psychological health, such as stress reduction. Although this approach requires unusually close monitoring and a high degree of determination on the part of the patient, Ornish and Brown emphasize that therapy is not a decision based on preference but on medical indication. Nevertheless, such a dramatic diet modification may pose the risk of nutritional inadequacy if professional guidance is not provided.

In contrast, some researchers have suggested that pharmacologic measures should be implemented sooner in patients at high risk. In a recent study conducted in outpatient lipid clinics, Step II dietary therapy produced only a 5% decrease in LDL cholesterol in a free-living patient population with moderate hypercholesterolemia compared with matched patients receiving a high-fat diet representative of the average American diet (15). A significant 6% decrease in HDL cholesterol was also noted, and triglyceride levels were not significantly altered. These findings suggest that metabolic-ward estimates of efficacy may have limited applicability to the typical clinical environment, and that a low-fat, low-cholesterol diet is only mildly effective in lowering LDL cholesterol in the general population. Nevertheless, the efficacy of diet varies widely in individuals: some patients exhibit dramatic benefit, while others show little or no response. A full trial of dietary therapy is warranted in all patients because the potential benefit is quite great.

Weight Loss and Physical Activity

An integral part of dietary therapy is weight reduction in obese persons. It has been estimated that 25% of the U.S. population is definitely obese and another 25% may be considered mildly overweight (16). In addition to other health problems, obesity is associated with several other contributors to premature CAD, including hypertriglyceridemia, low HDL cholesterol, hypertension, and poor glucose control or frank diabetes.

Obesity-associated hypertriglyceridemia is common and is caused primarily by an overproduction of very low density lipoprotein (VLDL). Lipoprotein lipase activity is also frequently decreased in obese subjects, resulting in decreased VLDL catabolism. Low HDL cholesterol often occurs concomitantly with hypertriglyceridemia, although obesity per se may be associated with decreased production of HDL and its associated apolipoproteins. Abnormal glucose tolerance or overt diabetes mellitus, characterized by peripheral insulin resistance and perhaps decreased secretion of insulin by the pancreas, is common in obese persons, and hypertension is also common. In fact, the clustering of these risk factors is often associated with a distinct syndrome (17) that is intimately related to insulin resistance and may be associated with increased risk for CAD.

Increased exercise and weight reduction usually normalize obesity-related dyslipidemia, although overzealous restriction of caloric intake in overweight subjects should not be encouraged. A gradual weight loss of approximately ½–1 lb/week is desirable unless the patient is morbidly obese.

Recent studies have demonstrated that the anatomic distribution of adipose tissue may have clinical importance (16). Truncal adipose tissue appears to be more active metabolically than gluteal–femoral adipose tissue. Truncal obesity is associated with an increased concentration of free fatty acids in the circulation, which potentiates triglyceride synthesis, and with secondary hyperinsulinemia due to decreased hepatic extraction of insulin. Hence, the distribution of adipose tissue should also be considered when setting goals for weight loss. The waist–hip ratio is a useful parameter for monitoring the success of weight-reduction efforts.

Regular exercise is also an integral part of dietary therapy. In the Multiple Risk Factor Intervention Trial (MRFIT), patients who performed regular, moderate physical activity had 30% fewer fatal cardiac events and a significant decrease in total mortality compared with less active patients (18). It has been suggested that subjects able to perform strenuous exercise may be less prone to coronary disease because of a number of potentially confounding factors, and that these epidemiologic data may be biased by selection criteria. However, in a study of almost 17,000 healthy subjects of diverse ages, adoption of moderate sporting activity during a 4-year interval correlated with lower mortality over a subsequent 9-year follow-up, and demonstrated that regular exercise is associated with longevity independently of the age at which it is begun (19).

The mechanism by which exercise protects against cardiovascular disease is probably multifactorial and may be due to beneficial effects on blood pressure, glucose tolerance, and serum lipids. As with most other factors that raise HDL cholesterol, exercise predominantly increases HDL_2 cholesterol, which is more strongly associated with reduced CAD risk compared with other HDL subfractions.

DRUG THERAPY

Because patients who receive pharmacologic therapy will generally require it for life, the initiation of such therapy should be considered carefully. Drug therapy is usually lifelong because dyslipidemia that is resistant to hygienic measures often has a strong genetic component, compounded by the fact that LDL-cholesterol levels tend to increase with age. Drug therapy also entails significant cost and the possibility of side effects. It is therefore important that concerted efforts be made to maximize the benefit of hygienic measures before considering drugs. If pharmacologic therapy is initiated, hygienic measures should continue to be followed, as the effects of diet and drug are additive.

Available Drugs

From a pharmacologic standpoint, it is of benefit to consider agents as predominantly cholesterol-lowering or predominantly triglyceride-lowering therapies. The bile acid sequestrants, the 3-hydroxy-3-methylglutaryl coenzyme A (HMG-CoA) reductase inhibitors (also called statins), and probucol predominantly lower LDL cholesterol, whereas nicotinic acid and the fibric acid derivatives (also called fibrates) are the major triglyceride-lowering drugs (Table 9).

Because of its emphasis on LDL-cholesterol lowering, the ATP II has classified pharmacologic agents into major and minor drugs (Table 10). Major drugs are the bile acid sequestrants (cholestyramine, colestipol), nicotinic acid, and the HMG-CoA reductase inhibitors (fluvastatin, lovastatin, pravastatin, simvastatin). Other drugs are the fibric acid derivatives (clofibrate, fenofibrate, gemfibrozil) and probucol. This classification reflects the lower priority assigned to triglyceride lowering by the ATP II. Estrogen-replacement therapy is also an option in postmenopausal women.

Bile Acid Sequestrants

Clinical experience with the bile-acid-sequestering resins is extensive, and the efficacy and safety of this class of antilipidemic drugs are well documented. Although they differ in structure, cholestyramine and colestipol are similar in mechanism and effects on lipid levels (20).

The bile acid sequestrants stimulate the conversion of cholesterol to bile acids, compounds secreted into the duodenum that assist the solubilization of dietary fat and cholesterol (21). Normally, bile acids are efficiently reabsorbed (only 3% are lost in the feces) and the bulk of the reabsorbed bile acid pool is recycled. The bile-acid-sequestering resins bind the negatively charged bile acids, blocking reabsorption and reducing the bile acid pool available for reuse. The hepatic level of bile acids modulates the subsequent synthesis of bile acids by negative feedback on the rate-limiting enzyme in the conversion of cholesterol to bile acids, cholesterol 7α-hydroxylase. The LDL receptor expression in hepatocytes is consequently increased, resulting in increased uptake of apolipoprotein (apo) B- and apo E-containing lipoproteins from the circulation.

Because of the diffuse nature of the absorption process and the relative inefficiency of the drugs, large doses are required to bind effectively the intestinal bile acid pool. Overall efficacy of the drug is further blunted by a compensatory increase in hepatic cholesterol synthesis stimulated by HMG-CoA reductase, the rate-limiting enzyme in cholesterol synthesis. Bile acid sequentrants lower total and LDL cholesterol by 15–25% at maximum dosage. Triglyceride levels are generally unaffected, although occasionally a significant increase occurs. The HDL cholesterol may increase mildly, generally <5%. As with several of the lipid-lowering drugs, the dose–response relation of the resins is not linear: much of the effect on LDL cholesterol is achieved at lower dosages, with a declining relative benefit at higher doses.

The safety of this class of drug is its primary advantage. Since the agents do not enter the systemic circulation, nonspecific gastrointestinal symptoms are the predominant adverse effects observed. However, these side effects may seriously hinder compliance, as may the difficulty of administration and low palatability. Gastrointestinal side effects may be eased by administering the drug with food, administering stool softeners, and increasing the amount of fiber in the diet. Efforts to improve the tolerability of the drugs have

TABLE 9. *Effects of lipid-lowering drugs on plasma lipid values*

Drug	Effect on: Total cholesterol	LDL-C	HDL-C	Triglyceride	Patient tolerability
Bile-acid resins	↓20%	↓20–25%	↑35%	Neutral or ↑	Poor
Nicotinic acid	↓25%	↓25%	↑15–30%	↓20–50%	Poor to reasonable
Fibric acid derivatives	↓10–20%	↓5–25%	↑10–30%	↓20–60%	Good
Probucol	↓25%	↓10–15%	↓20–30%	Neutral	Reasonable
Reductase inhibitors	↓15–30%	↓20–35%	↑2–12%	↓10–25%	Good

TABLE 10. *Lipid-lowering drugs: dosage and side effects*

Drug class	Usual daily dosage	Tolerability/side effects
Nicotinic acid (niacin), crystalline	200 mg (100 mg b.i.d.) initially, increasing gradually to 2–4 g (divided doses) Avoid time-release preparations (increased risk of hepatotoxicity)	Tolerability poor to reasonable Flushing, hepatotoxicity, hyperglycemia, hyperuricemia or gout, upper GI complaints, rare acanthosis nigricans, rare retinal edema To minimize flushing: initial dose titration, take with meals, as necessary aspirin, ibuprofen, or indomethacin 30 min before administration
Bile-acid sequestrants (resins)	Cholestyramine 8–16 g (max 32 g) Colestipol 10–20 g (max 30 g) Divided doses if not low dose	Tolerability poor Upper and lower GI complaints, chiefly constipation and indigestion (no systemic toxicity); decrease absorption of other drugs (digitalis preparations, warfarin, thyroxine, thiazide diuretics, beta-blockers); may decrease absorption of folic acid Take other drugs 1–3 hr before resin; bulking laxatives for constipation; folic acid supplementation in pediatric patients
HMG-CoA reductase inhibitors (statins)	Fluvastatin 20–40 mg Lovastatin 10–40 mg (max 80 mg) Pravastatin 10–40 mg Simvastatin 5–20 mg	Tolerability good A few patients have reversible creatine kinase elevations; rare myopathy (possible when combined with cyclosporine, fibrate, or perhaps nicotinic acid or erythromycin); minor elevations of serum transaminases, usually transient, can occur; prolongation of prothrombin time may occur when lovastatic given with coumarin; do not use in women of childbearing age unless contraception fully satisfactory
Fibric acid derivatives (fibrates)	Gemfibrozil 1,200 mg (600 mg b.i.d.) Clofibrate 2 g (1 g b.i.d.) Benzafibrate[a] 600 mg (200 mg t.i.d.) Fenofibrate[b] 300 mg (100 mg t.i.d.) Ciprofibrate[a] 100–200 mg	Tolerability good Transient transaminase increases not infrequent; can potentiate effects of oral anticoagulants; use with caution with statins; all rare—nausea, diarrhea, gallstones, alopecia, muscle weakness with increased CK
Probucol	1,000 mg (500 mg b.i.d.)	Tolerability reasonable Side effects usually infrequent and of short duration; chiefly GI (diarrhea, abdominal pain, flatulence, nausea, and vomiting); prolongation of QT interval has occurred; serious ventricular arrhythmias have been reported

HMG-CoA, 3-Hydroxy-3-methylglutaryl coenzyme A; b.i.d., twice a day; max, maximum; t.i.d., three times a day; GI, gastrointestinal.

For all drugs, consult product labeling.

[a] Not presently approved by the U.S. Food and Drug Administration.

[b] Approved by the U.S. Food and Drug Administration, but not presently available in the United States.

included the development of confectionary gum preparations and low-calorie formulations, but have only modestly improved patient acceptance.

Other possible side effects include nonspecific binding of fat-soluble vitamins and orally administered drugs such as coumadin, diuretics, digitalis preparations, β-adrenergic blocking agents, and thyroid hormones. The resins should be administered at least 1 hr after or 4 hr before other orally administered medications to avoid binding.

Bile acid sequestrants have been used as monotherapy or in combination with other agents in a number of primary- and secondary-prevention trials. The double-blind, placebo-controlled Lipid Research Clinics Coronary Primary Prevention Trial (LRC-CPPT) (22) evaluated the clinical benefit of cholestyramine therapy in 3,806 men with primary hypercholesterolemia (type IIa hyperlipidemia) over a mean follow-up period of 7.4 years. Many patients randomized to cholestyramine therapy were unable to tolerate the 24 g/day dose, resulting in a wide variation in mean dose per patient over the trial period. Mean levels of serum total cholesterol and LDL cholesterol fell 13% and 20%, respectively, in the cholestyramine group. A significant 19% reduction in combined risk for CHD death and nonfatal myocardial infarction was observed in the treatment group. Additionally, need for coronary artery bypass surgery was decreased by 17%, and other physiologic parameters such as progression to a positive treadmill and the incidence of new-onset angina also showed improvement. Although there was no beneficial effect of cholestyramine therapy on total mortality, the LRC-CPPT conclusively established the benefit of cholesterol lowering on cardiac event rates in primary prevention.

The efficacy of the bile acid sequestrants in combination with other antilipidemic drugs has been demonstrated in several secondary-prevention trials. The 3-year St Thomas' Atherosclerosis Regression Study (STARS) (23) evaluated the effect on atherosclerosis progression of dietary therapy alone or with cholestyramine (16 g/day) compared with normal care in 90 men with coronary disease and hypercholesterolemia. In both active-therapy groups, vascular benefit and a reduction in clinical events were observed. In the group receiving diet and cholestyramine therapy, the mean absolute width of the coronary segments studied increased 0.103 mm, compared with an increase of 0.003 mm in the group receiving dietary therapy only and a decrease of 0.201 mm in the normal-care group ($p < 0.05$). One cardiac event was recorded in the diet-plus-cholestyramine group and three in the diet-only group, compared with ten in the normal care group. This significant benefit ($p < 0.05$) was greater than expected given the modest absolute changes in width of coronary segments.

HMG-CoA Reductase Inhibitors

The advent of pharmacologic inhibitors of HMG-CoA reductase has been a major advance in the treatment of dyslipidemia; these agents have proven to be extremely effective in lowering LDL cholesterol and their efficacy does not appear to attenuate over time. The first HMG-CoA reductase inhibitor to be discovered was mevastatin, a fungal metabolite isolated from extracts of *Penicillium citrinum* in 1976. Currently, fluvastatin, lovastatin, pravastatin, and simvastatin are approved for use by the U.S. Food and Drug Administration for treatment of dyslipidemia. Structurally, fluvastatin and pravastatin are open acids, whereas lovastatin and simvastatin are lactone derivatives. Of these agents, fluvastatin is the only synthetic compound and consists of a racemic mixture of an active and an inactive isomer.

The LDL cholesterol is lowered 25–40% with statin use. The HDL cholesterol is raised 5–10% and triglyceride is lowered 10–20% (24). Lovastatin, pravastatin, and simvastatin are roughly equipotent at recommended doses; fluvastatin appears to be somewhat less potent at equivalent doses.

It is generally accepted that these drugs lower circulating cholesterol levels by inhibiting HMG-CoA reductase, the rate-limiting enzyme of cholesterol synthesis, thereby reducing the cellular production of cholesterol. Consequently, the number or competence of LDL receptors is increased, enhancing the clearance of lipoproteins containing apo B or apo E. However, the mechanism of these agents may be more complex than originally thought. The hepatic production of apo B-100 may be decreased and the subsequent production of apo B-100-containing lipoproteins may be altered (25). Some data suggest that the drugs inhibit absorption of dietary cholesterol, although this is not considered a major mechanism (26). The mechanism for the increase in HDL cholesterol is unclear; reductase-inhibitor therapy may alter the production of HDL by the liver or gastrointestinal tract, or the increase may be associated with the decrease in VLDL and LDL levels.

The safety profile of the statins is favorable, although a few serious side effects have been reported and long-term safety data are limited. Initially, there was concern that pharmacologic inhibition of cholesterol synthesis might alter steroid production or affect lens integrity, but this has not been observed. Rather, hepatotoxicity and myopathy are the two major adverse effects reported to date. In the Extended Clinical Evaluation of Lovastatin (EXCEL) Study (27), which investigated the safety and efficacy of various doses of lovastatin in 8,245 patients over 48 weeks, hepatotoxicity was the most common serious side effect. Overall, transaminase elevations >3 times the upper limit of normal occur in approximately 1% of patients, and are slightly more frequent at maximum dosages. The transaminase elevations usually occur within the first 12 months. It has not been determined whether the transaminitis is a direct result of drug toxicity or secondary to a loss of hepatocyte integrity and enzyme leakage. Liver enzyme levels appear to normalize on discontinuation of the drugs. Since these alterations of liver function are usually asymptomatic, periodic monitoring of liver enzymes is necessary. Statins should be used with caution in patients with preexisting liver disease.

Creatine kinase elevations in patients taking a statin are difficult to evaluate. Although a marker of overt muscle damage due to drug toxicity, creatine kinase levels may also be increased by exercise, trauma, and other conditions not related to drug therapy. Overall clinical experience indicates that the frequency of significant myopathy, defined as creatine kinase levels >10 times the upper limit of normal, is approximately 0.1% with statin use. Rhabdomyolysis and other severe reactions have occurred, but generally in patients with multiple health problems or receiving other medications. Concomitant use of gemfibrozil, erythromycin, nicotinic acid, or cyclosporine increases the possibility of myopathy. Because many patients not receiving medications also have intermittent elevations of creatine kinase, intermittent creatine kinase measurements are not sufficiently discriminating for monitoring drug safety, and moderate elevations do not themselves require discontinuation of the drug.

Preliminary reports indicate these agents may rarely be involved in hypersensitivity reactions such as arthralgias, although this risk has not been clearly delineated (28). Sleep disturbances have occasionally been reported with statin use, and it has been suggested that these disorders may occur more frequently with the hydrophobic agents lovastatin and simvastatin than with the hydrophilic agents fluvastatin and pravastatin, which presumably are excluded from the central nervous system. However, studies have not shown a definite advantage of the hydrophilic statins.

Although the clinical benefit of these agents in primary prevention has not been evaluated in a large, double-blind, placebo-controlled trial, a number of angiographically monitored secondary-prevention trials have been conducted using statins as monotherapy or in combination with other drugs. These trials show that aggressive antilipidemic therapy slows the progression of atherosclerosis and increases the frequency of regression, as determined by the change in angiographically measured stenosis of lesions. Furthermore, the clinical benefit observed in several of these trials exceeded expectation given the modest degree of anatomic benefit and short duration of the trials. For example, in two recent regression studies utilizing pravastatin, the Pravastatin Limitation of Atherosclerosis in the Coronary Arteries (PLAC I) (29) and Pravastatin, Lipoproteins, and Atherosclerosis in the Carotids (PLAC III) (30) studies, a significant clinical benefit was observed within 6 months of active therapy. PLAC I was a 3-year randomized, placebo-controlled trial in 408 patients with documented CAD and LDL cholesterol of 130–189 mg/dl after dietary therapy alone. After 90 days, 5 myocardial infarctions were recorded in the treatment group, compared with 17 in the control group ($p = 0.005$). It has been suggested that aggressive cholesterol lowering stabilizes a subgroup of lesions frequently associated with clinical events, via a number of possible mechanisms (5). Thus, these trials have further clarified the role of pharmacotherapy in reducing CAD risk, and have demonstrated the importance of aggressive management of patients with established atherosclerotic disease.

Probucol

Although probucol has been utilized in clinical medicine for several decades, its therapeutic role remains controversial and its mechanism of action unclear. The drug lowers LDL cholesterol 10–20%, although compared with other agents, patient response to probucol is much less predictable. It has been hypothesized that this variation in response is related to genetic differences in apo E structure, because patients with the apo E_4/E_4 isomorph appear more responsive to probucol therapy (31). Despite its LDL-cholesterol-lowering activity, probucol is not considered a first-line agent, because it also lowers HDL cholesterol 20–30%. Triglyceride levels are generally unaffected. However, unlike the other lipid-lowering agents, probucol apparently does not require functioning LDL receptors to lower LDL cholesterol. The drug may therefore be useful in familial hypercholesterolemia, in which there is a deficiency of functioning LDL receptors. The drug has been reported to retard atherosclerosis in animal models of familial hypercholesterolemia such as the Watanabe heritable hyperlipidemic rabbit (32). In humans, regression of tendinous xanthomas in patients with familial hypercholesterolemia has been documented (33).

Probucol increases the fractional catabolic rate of LDL (34), possibly by modifying the LDL particle itself (35) and thereby enhancing its removal from the circulation. At least part of the drug's LDL-lowering effect may be secondary to a decrease in cholesterol synthesis by the liver or an effect on bile-salt production, although the data remain controversial (36). *In vitro* studies suggest that hepatic production of triglyceride-rich lipoproteins is decreased by probucol.

The decrease in HDL cholesterol does not appear to eliminate the possibility of atherosclerosis reversal with probucol use. For example, the transfer of cholesteryl ester from HDL to apo B-containing lipoproteins, especially LDL, is reportedly enhanced by probucol. This may reflect an increase in reverse cholesterol transport via an increase in the flux of cellular cholesterol into the circulation (37). It has also been reported that probucol stimulates cholesteryl ester transfer protein, an effect which may promote reverse cholesterol transport. However, much investigation is still required to clarify the effects of probucol on lipoprotein metabolism.

In addition to its effect on lipid levels, probucol is a potent antioxidant and may inhibit the oxidative modification of LDL believed to be necessary for its internalization by macrophages (38) (as also discussed elsewhere in this volume). Several other mechanisms by which oxidized LDL may contribute to atherogenesis have been proposed as well, and would also presumably be inhibited by probucol.

Probucol appears to cause few side effects at the recommended dose of 500 mg b.i.d. The most frequently noted side effects are nonspecific gastrointestinal discomforts such as nausea, constipation, or heartburn. Probucol can cause prolongation of the QT interval, although serious ventricular arrhythmias are rare. When not administered with a fatty meal, absorption of probucol is decreased (39) and the increase in QT levels does not appear to be significant. Nevertheless, an electrocardiogram should be obtained prior to initiating probucol therapy, and use of the drug should be restricted if prolongation of the QT interval is observed.

There are few clinical trial data on the benefit of probucol in reducing CAD. The Probucol Quantitative Regression Swedish Trial (PQRST) (40) was a 3-year, double-blind, placebo-controlled trial that evaluated the effect of probucol therapy on the progression of atherosclerosis in patients with hypercholesterolemia and femoral atherosclerosis. Although the trial confirmed that probucol inhibits lipoprotein oxidation *in vivo,* no clinical benefit was observed.

Nicotinic Acid

Nicotinic acid (niacin), an essential B vitamin, favorably affects all major lipid subfractions at pharmacologic doses. Frequently a dose in excess of 4.5 g/day is required for maximum efficacy, although adequate responses are occasionally seen at lower doses. Triglyceride is lowered 40–60%, LDL cholesterol is lowered up to 25%, and an increase in HDL cholesterol of 25–30% can be achieved (41). Moreover, the ratio of HDL_2 to HDL_3 is increased severalfold (42).

The mechanism of action of nicotinic acid is complex and not well understood (43). Most studies indicate that decreased VLDL production is the predominant mechanism, thereby lowering the concentrations of the products of VLDL catabolism, intermediate-density lipoprotein (IDL), and LDL. Contributing effects include a reduction in the release of free fatty acids by adipocytes, which decreases the availability of these particles in lipoprotein synthesis and lipid metabolism. Some of the increase in HDL cholesterol may be secondary to the reduction in VLDL, although the fractional catabolic rate of apo A-I is reportedly decreased by the drug.

Unfortunately, the side effects of nicotinic acid are numerous and may seriously impair long-term efficacy due to reduced compliance. Although some of these side effects are minor irritants and do not seriously affect long-term tolerability, nicotinic acid has been associated with severe, occasionally life-threatening complications. Thus, close monitoring and careful patient education are essential. Crystalline nicotinic acid is rapidly absorbed following oral administration, reaching a peak plasma level in 45 min. This rapid absorption contributes to some of the untoward side effects of nicotinic acid, and may be slowed by administering the drug at mealtimes. Extended-release preparations are available, but appear to be highly hepatotoxic and should be avoided (44). It is recommended that nicotinic acid therapy be initiated at a low, divided dose and gradually increased at weekly intervals until maximum benefit is obtained.

The most common side effects of nicotinic acid are cutaneous and gastrointestinal manifestations. Cutaneous vasodilation and flushing is virtually universal but frequently attenuates over time. This prostaglandin-mediated flushing can be extremely troublesome, but can be blunted by premedication with aspirin or other prostaglandin inhibitors. Rarely, dermatologic manifestations may include acanthosis nigricans.

Nicotinic acid exacerbates ulcer diathesis and should be used with extreme caution in patients with a history of peptic ulcer disease.

Hepatotoxicity can occur and although it is usually mild, it can result in fulminant hepatic failure. Because nicotinic acid-induced hepatoxicity is often asymptomatic or associated with mild nonspecific symptoms, periodic monitoring of liver enzymes is necessary. Mild transaminase elevations do not obligate discontinuation of therapy, but closer observation and dose reduction may be required.

Nicotinic acid therapy is associated with a variety of metabolic effects, including hyperuricemia and worsened glucose tolerance. This impairment of glucose metabolism is especially problematic in insulin-resistant individuals, and use of the drug is relatively contraindicated in patients with diabetes mellitus. If used in diabetes, frequent monitoring of blood sugar is required and dosages of insulin or oral hypoglycemics may need to be adjusted; inability to maintain glycemic control mandates discontinuation of the drug.

Creatine kinase elevations may occur with nicotinic acid use, although myopathy is rare. The possibility of myopathy is increased with concomitant use of a statin or certain other compounds, and most reported cases of nicotinic acid-induced myopathy may in fact be attributable to drug–drug interactions. In the Coronary Drug Project (45), the largest clinical trial completed to date utilizing nicotinic acid as pharmacologic monotherapy, there was no documented case of rhabdomyolysis in patients receiving 3 g/day nicotinic acid for an average of 6 years.

A large body of data exists regarding the use of nicotinic acid in primary and secondary prevention. The Coronary Drug Project randomized over 5,000 male survivors of myocardial infarction to one of five active treatment groups, one of which received 3 g/day nicotinic acid. A sixth group, containing 2,789 patients, received a placebo. Because a considerable number of patients receiving nicotinic acid dropped out or were unable to tolerate the maximum dose, the therapeutic response was less than anticipated. Total cholesterol fell approximately 10% in the nicotinic acid group, and triglyceride fell approximately 25%. Total and cardiovascular mortality were not significantly affected by nicotinic acid therapy during the trial, although significantly fewer myocardial infarctions were noted in this treatment group compared with the placebo group. Interestingly, a follow-up study (46) completed 9 years after the treatment regimens were discontinued reported that total mortality in the nicotinic acid group was a significant 11% less than in the placebo group.

In the Familial Atherosclerosis Treatment Study (FATS) (47), which investigated the effects of aggressive antilipidemic therapy on the progression of atherosclerotic lesions in men with CAD and elevated apo B, patients were randomized to placebo or one of two treatment groups: 4 g/day nicotinic acid and 40 mg/day lovastatin or 4 g/day nicotinic acid and 30 g/day colestipol. Both treatment groups showed angiographically measured regression, whereas progression was observed in the placebo group. Additionally, 10 of 52 patients in the placebo group had cardiovascular events during the trial, but only 3 of 46 in the lovastatin–nicotinic acid group and 2 of 48 in the colestipol–nicotinic acid group experienced events. This clinical benefit was significant despite the short duration of the trial (2 years).

Fibric Acid Derivatives

The fibric acid derivatives currently approved for use in the United States are fenofibrate (not yet marketed), gemfibrozil, and clofibrate. Other fibrates in use elsewhere include bezafibrate and ciprofibrate.

Although this class of antilipidemic drug has been in use for several decades and their clinical effects are well documented, their precise mechanism remains unclear and is believed to be multifactorial (48,49). The major effect of the drugs is to decrease circulating levels of triglyceride-rich lipoproteins by activating lipoprotein lipase, the key enzyme in VLDL catabolism. Other potential mechanisms include decreased hepatic activity of acetyl-coenzyme A carboxylase, a major enzyme involved in fatty acid synthesis, thereby reducing the availability of this substrate for triglyceride production. Fibrates may also reduce the production and release of free fatty acids by adipocytes. It had previously been thought that these drugs reduce HMG-CoA reductase activity, but more recent studies have shown no change in the urinary excretion of mevalonic acid (a marker of HMG-CoA reductase activity) following fibrate administration (50).

The efficacy of fibrate therapy varies somewhat by lipid phenotype. In type IIa hyperlipidemia, fibrates lower LDL cholesterol 10–20% and increase HDL cholesterol approximately 10%. A decrease in circulating apo B-100 levels generally accompanies this reduction in LDL cholesterol. The drugs are also effective if both VLDL and LDL are elevated (type IIb hyperlipidemia), although response varies widely. In type IV hyperlipidemia (moderate hypertriglyceridemia), triglyceride is lowered 40–60%, with a concomitant rise in HDL cholesterol of 20–30%. However, in both type IV and type IIB hyperlipidemia, LDL cholesterol can occasionally be increased. Interestingly, bezafibrate (51) and gemfibrozil (52) have been shown to shift the composition of LDL toward larger, less-dense species. Small, dense LDL is associated with elevated triglyceride and low HDL cholesterol, and is believed to be more atherogenic than normal LDL. For example, the susceptibility of LDL to oxidation has been shown to increase with density.

The most common adverse effects of the fibrates are gastrointestinal. Increased lithogenicity of the bile has also been associated with these agents. Rarely, reversible myopathy with creatine kinase elevation may occur, particularly if renal function is impaired, hypoalbuminemia is present, or a statin is also administered. The drugs can potentiate the action of warfarin-type oral anticoagulants, and should be used cautiously in patients receiving a sulfonylurea, because of the possibility of hypoglycemia.

The safety of the fibrates has been questioned because of an observed increase in all-cause mortality in analyses of pooled clinical trial data. Much of this concern derives from the World Health Organization (WHO) Cooperative Trial (53), which investigated the effects of clofibrate in primary prevention. The double-blind WHO trial randomized over 5,000 middle-aged men with hypercholesterolemia to either 1,600 mg/day clofibrate or placebo. Despite a modest 9% decrease in serum cholesterol achieved over the 5-year trial, ischemic heart disease incidence was 20% lower in the intervention group, largely due to a 25% reduction in nonfatal myocardial infarction. An increased risk of noncardiovascular death was also noted in this group, particularly due to cancer and to complications of cholelithiasis. Several potential design flaws in the WHO trial mitigate this finding, however, including a failure to analyze the data on an intent-to-treat basis (54). Furthermore, other trials of clofibrate therapy in primary prevention also achieved reductions in cardiovascular events, but did not observe excess noncardiovascular mortality (55,56). Nonetheless, because of the possibility of drug-related mortality, clofibrate is little used in the United States today.

The Helsinki Heart Study evaluated gemfibrozil therapy in primary prevention, randomizing over 4,000 men to either 600 mg b.i.d. gemfibrozil or placebo (57). Roughly two-thirds of participants had primary hypercholesterolemia, and the rest had either hypertriglyceridemia or combined hyperlipidemia. The LDL cholesterol fell 10%, triglyceride fell 43%, and HDL cholesterol increased roughly 10% over the 5-year trial. A 34% reduction in CHD incidence was observed in the gemfibrozil group. A later analysis indicated that gemfibrozil therapy was particularly effective in patients at increased risk due to the presence of mixed dyslipidemia (58). Most of the clinical benefit observed was confined to the 10% of treated subjects with triglyceride >200 mg/dl and an LDL : HDL cholesterol ratio >5; in this group, a 71% reduction in CHD incidence was noted.

Other Agents

Estrogen-Replacement Therapy

Postmenopausal women with elevated LDL may benefit from estrogen-replacement therapy (ERT); some experts believe that ERT is the therapy of choice if hygienic measures are insufficient. ERT reduces LDL-cholesterol levels by approximately 15% by stimulating a promoter region on the LDL-receptor gene, resulting in increased LDL clearance. The HDL cholesterol is raised 15%, but oral estrogens may also increase triglyceride. In the Lipid Research Clinics Program Follow-up Study, the risk ratio for cardiovascular death was 0.34 in estrogen users compared with those who did not take estrogen (59). The benefit was attributed to the increase in HDL cholesterol associated with estrogen. Additionally, ERT is associated with protection from osteoporosis. However, the risk–benefit ratio of ERT has been questioned because risk for endometrial carcinoma and risk for breast cancer are increased. Nonetheless, it is estimated that only a 10% reduction in CAD risk is needed to offset the increased risk for cancer, because of the high prevalence of CAD in older women, and reductions of that magnitude seem readily attainable with ERT. The risk of estrogen-induced carcinoma is reduced by the addition of progestin, but the benefit on lipid levels is also lessened, and there are few data on the effect of the combined use of estrogen and progestin on CAD risk. Several clinical trials of ERT are currently under way.

Omega-3 Fatty Acids

Several investigators have recommended increased intake of omega-3 polyunsaturated fatty acids because of epidemiologic associations between a high intake of these compounds and a low occurrence of ischemic heart disease. For example, MRFIT showed an inverse relation between dietary intake of omega-3 fatty acids and ischemic heart disease over a 10-year follow-up (60). The benefit of these compounds may be attributable to their strong hypotriglyceridemic effect, which is due to a decrease in VLDL production. Additionally, omega-3 fatty acids exert effects on hemostasis that may be beneficial in both acute and chronic coronary syndromes. Platelet function may be altered, resulting in decreased platelet aggregation. However, whether this hypoaggregability is clinically significant, especially when compared with other agents such as aspirin, is not clear.

Omega-3 fatty acids are abundant in marine fish. Omega-3 fatty acid supplements are available as well, and can lower serum triglyceride 50% at a dose of 5 g/day, although efficacy varies interindividually and by phenotype. There is evidence that HDL cholesterol may be increased as well (61). However, because of its high energy content, omega-3 fatty acid supplementation may interfere with efforts to control caloric intake. Furthermore, no controlled clinical trials have been performed to evaluate the effect of omega-3 fatty acids in the primary prevention of CHD. It has been suggested that increased intake of omega-3 fatty acids may promote LDL oxidation.

Selection of Drugs

Elevated LDL Cholesterol

In primary prevention, at least 6 months of intensive dietary therapy should precede consideration of drugs in most cases. However, individuals with severe genetic abnormalities such as familial hypercholesterolemia or who are otherwise at very high risk and unlikely to achieve acceptable lipid levels with dietary therapy alone may be considered candidates for drug therapy after a shorter trial of hygienic measures alone. Drugs should be considered in patients without atherosclerotic disease and with fewer than two other risk factors if LDL cholesterol remains ≥190 mg/dl after lifestyle changes are fully implemented. The goal of therapy is to lower LDL cholesterol below 160 mg/dl. If the patient has two or more risk factors, a more aggressive approach is recommended: drugs should be considered if LDL cholesterol remains ≥160 mg/dl, with a goal of <130 mg/dl.

In secondary prevention, drug therapy should be considered if LDL cholesterol remains ≥130 mg/dl, with a goal of <100 mg/dl.

In both primary and secondary prevention, if LDL cholesterol is below the initiation level for drug therapy but above the goal of dietary therapy, the clinician may also opt to initiate drug therapy if, in his or her judgment, sufficient benefit would be obtained.

Although LDL cholesterol remains the primary target of therapy, the ATP II places increased emphasis on total risk status to further identify the therapeutic needs of the patient and to guide the selection and intensity of treatment. Thus, patients with moderately elevated LDL cholesterol that is resistant to dietary therapy, but who are otherwise at low short-term risk, i.e., young men (<35 years of age) and premenopausal women with LDL cholesterol ≤190 mg/dl and fewer than two other risk factors, would generally not proceed to pharmacologic therapy given the low benefit-to-risk ratio of such therapy. However, it is often prudent to consider pharmacologic therapy in these patients in the presence of a genetic dyslipidemia associated with CAD, a family history of CAD, or diabetes mellitus.

Initially, the statins were not considered first-line agents because of the lack of long-term safety data. However, clinical experience has continued to be favorable and many experts now prefer these agents as initial therapy because of their established efficacy and the low incidence of side effects. Bile acid sequestrants are also effective and are free of systemic side effects, but their use has declined because of poor tolerability and the absence of any cost advantage. The ATP II recommends that the bile acid sequestrants be favored in primary prevention, especially in young men and premenopausal women. Statins are preferred in secondary prevention and in primary prevention if multiple risk factors are present.

The aggressive LDL-cholesterol goal of <100 mg/dl recommended by the ATP II for patients with established CAD frequently may require combination therapy. Even if tolerable, the maximum dose of a bile acid sequestrant or nicotinic acid will generally lower LDL cholesterol no more than 25%. A statin may also be insufficient if LDL cholesterol is severely elevated. A combination of two or possibly three drugs may then be considered if the clinician believes sufficient benefit would be obtained. A combination of nicotinic acid and a bile acid sequestrant is useful because the drugs' LDL-cholesterol-lowering effects are additive, and because triglyceride and HDL cholesterol are also favorably affected. This combination may be more tolerable than if only one of the drugs were taken, because a lower dose of each drug is required to achieve a given reduction in LDL cholesterol. This combination was effective in several secondary-prevention trials, including FATS (47) and the Cholesterol Lowering Atherosclerosis Study (CLAS) (62).

A more potent LDL-cholesterol-lowering combination is a bile acid sequestrant and a statin. The effects of these drugs also appear to be additive, and LDL cholesterol may be lowered up to 60% at maximum doses. This combination has been utilized in FATS and other trials. In the University of California, San Francisco, Arteriosclerosis Specialized Center of Research Intervention Trial (63), a combined regimen of a bile acid sequestrant, nicotinic acid, and a statin was used to treat severe LDL-cholesterol elevations in some patients with heterozygous familial hypercholesterolemia. The role of probucol in combination therapy has not been well delineated.

A variety of nonconventional agents have been used as antilipidemic therapy in isolated instances, including ketoconazole, neomycin, and sitosterol. The clinical role and safety of these agents in the management of dyslipidemia have not been fully assessed.

Extracorporeal LDL apheresis is an option for very severe hypercholesterolemia, predominantly homozygous familial hypercholesterolemia. An immunoabsorption process is employed utilizing apo B antibodies to selectively remove LDL from the plasma. This process has largely supplanted plasma filtration, which uses a nonspecific partitioning mechanism modulated to the molecular size of LDL.

The use of heparin-induced extracoporeal LDL precipitation in patients with severe, recalcitrant hypercholesterolemia has been investigated. In one study (64) in 51 patients with coronary disease and very high LDL cholesterol after conventional therapy, mean LDL cholesterol was lowered by the procedure from 283 mg/dl at baseline to 203 mg/dl at 12 months. Additionally, the mean LDL : HDL cholesterol ratio decreased from 7 to 3.5 after 1 year of treatment.

Combined Hyperlipidemia and Hypertriglyceridemia

The ATP II classifies triglyceride level as desirable (<200 mg/dl), borderline-high (200–400 mg/dl), high (400–1,000 mg/dl), and very high (>1,000 mg/dl) (Table 11).

Borderline-high triglyceride is frequently associated with secondary dyslipidemia, and is often accompanied by low HDL cholesterol. A thorough clinical evaluation is necessary to identify any underlying disorders such as hypertension, truncal obesity, excessive alcohol intake, glucose intolerance, or other conditions that may alter VLDL production or catabolism. Borderline-high triglyceride may require drug therapy if it is due to a genetic disorder associated with increased CAD risk. In primary prevention, the presence of a positive family history for premature CAD is extremely valuable in identifying such atherosclerosis-prone individuals. Borderline-high triglyceride in patients with established CAD is likely a contributing factor and should be treated. Drug therapy may also be an option if multiple risk factors are present, particularly high total or LDL cholesterol and concomitant low HDL cholesterol. In the Helsinki Heart Study (58) subjects in the placebo group with an LDL : HDL cholesterol ratio >5 and triglyceride >200 mg/dl had a relative risk for CHD of 3.8 compared with those with an LDL : HDL cholesterol ratio ≤5 and triglyceride ≤200 mg/dl; in the intervention group, this increased risk was almost completely alleviated by gemfibrozil therapy. In the Prospective Cardiovascular Münster (PROCAM) Study (65), subjects with moderately (160–189 mg/dl) or severely (≥190 mg/dl) elevated LDL cholesterol and triglyceride ≥200 mg/dl were at a 2.5-fold greater risk for CHD than those with triglyceride <200 mg/dl. If pharmacologic therapy is indicated for elevated triglyceride levels, a fibric acid derivative is the first-choice drug. Nicotinic acid may also be selected. In addition to their hypotriglyceridemic action, both drugs raise HDL cholesterol in patients with elevated triglyceride.

TABLE 11. *ATP II classification of triglyceride levels*

Level (mg/dl)		Comments
Desirable	<200	
Borderline-high	200–400	Treat with hygienic measures; if elevation persists, drugs may be appropriate if patient has CAD or multiple severe risk factors; HDL cholesterol often low when triglyceride is elevated
High	400–1,000	Generally indicates concomitant primary hypertriglyceridemia and secondary hypertriglyceridemia; treat with hygienic measures after correcting underlying disorders; drugs may be needed to reduce risk for pancreatitis if levels persist
Very high	>1,000	Immediate attention required; drugs often needed concurrently with hygienic measures to reduce risk for pancreatitis

High triglyceride most typically is due to a mixture of primary and secondary factors; of the latter, obesity is particularly common. Treatment should be similar to that for borderline-high triglyceride, with an emphasis on controlling causes of secondary hypertriglyceridemia. Patients with high triglyceride levels may quickly develop very high triglyceride levels, which increase risk for chylomicron-induced pancreatitis. It therefore may be advisable to initiate drug therapy in these patients with high triglyceride if hygienic measures are insufficient, particularly if a history of acute pancreatitis is present.

Similarly, triglyceride-lowering measures should be instituted immediately in patients who already have very high triglyceride. Triglyceride levels >1,000 mg/dl are frequent in the type I and type V phenotypes. Type I hyperlipidemia is rare and is characterized by the accumulation of chylomicrons in the circulation due to deficient activity of lipoprotein lipase. It can result from the genetic absence of lipoprotein lipase, an autosomal recessive defect, or it may be secondary to a deficiency of apo C-II or other activators of lipoprotein lipase, or to other rare genetic abnormalities. Inhibition of lipoprotein lipase activity occasionally occurs in systemic lupus erythematous or multiple myeloma. In addition to the possibility of pancreatitis, lipemia retinalis and diffuse eruptive xanthoma are symptoms of type I hyperlipidemia. These clinical manifestations are reversible if the underlying lipid abnormality can be successfully managed. Because drug therapy is ineffective in patients lacking lipoprotein lipase, dietary fat and cholesterol must be severely restricted. Short- to moderate-chain fatty acids should be emphasized because they are not reformed into chylomicrons by the intestinal lacteals, but are instead absorbed directly into the portal circulation. If an activator of lipoprotein lipase is absent and symptoms of pancreatitis occur, plasma infusion of apo C-II may suffice to clear the chylomicrons from the circulation.

Type V hyperlipidemia in adults is most often associated with untreated or poorly controlled diabetes. Glucose control and hygienic measures, particularly weight loss in obese persons, often normalize lipid levels. Alcohol intake should be restricted. A fibrate is usually effective if these measures are insufficient. Nicotinic acid and omega-3 fatty acid supplements have been used, but both drugs worsen control of diabetes.

Concomitant elevation of LDL cholesterol and triglyceride (combined hyperlipidemia) is common and is associated with numerous clinical conditions. Underlying causes of the dyslipidemia should be identified and treated (Table 5). Familial combined hyperlipidemia is a genetic disorder that causes an overproduction of apo B-containing lipoproteins by the liver, and appears to be one of the most common genetic disorders found in patients with premature CAD. Although elevated LDL cholesterol and triglyceride is the disorder most frequently observed, the phenotype of afflicted individuals may vary over time and may differ from that of other family members.

The pharmacologic treatment of primary combined hyperlipidemia is controversial because monotherapy does not usually lower both lipid fractions adequately. If one lipid abnormality predominates, the drug should be selected accordingly, i.e., a statin if LDL cholesterol is predominantly elevated and a fibrate or nicotinic acid if triglyceride is the major target of therapy. The bile acid sequestrants are not recommended as monotherapy, because they tend to raise triglyceride. Combination therapy may be considered if monotherapy inadequately lowers both lipids. The combination of a bile acid sequestrant and nicotinic acid is very effective, but patient compliance is often poor. The combination of a bile acid sequestrant and a fibrate has also been used in combined hyperlipidemia. Although the combination of a statin and a fibrate is theoretically attractive, the use of this regimen is controversial because of the possibility of myopathy or rhabdomyolysis. However, several recent studies have demonstrated that the combination of these two agents may be a suitable therapeutic alternative with proper patient selection and careful monitoring. For example, in a double-blind, placebo-controlled trial in 290 patients with type IIa or type IIb hyperlipidemia, combination therapy with pravastatin and gemfibrozil was very effective: LDL cholesterol, VLDL cholesterol, and apo B were lowered 37%, 49%, and 31%, respectively. The HDL cholesterol increased 17% and the LDL:HDL cholesterol ratio improved (66). No case of severe myopathy was reported in this short-term study. Nevertheless, use of this combination requires very careful monitoring and patient education.

Type III hyperlipidemia is caused by dysbetalipoproteinemia, an uncommon genetic abnormality characterized by elevated cholesterol and triglyceride. The underlying genetic defect is homozygosity for the apo E_2 isomorph, which results in reduced binding affinity and hence reduced clearance of VLDL and chylomicron remnants. Dietary therapy alone is frequently effective, but drugs should be considered if lifestyle changes are insufficient. Drug therapy is similar to that for other forms of combined hyperlipidemia.

Low HDL Cholesterol

The ATP II considers low HDL cholesterol (<35 mg/dl) to be a significant risk factor for CAD. The HDL-cholesterol level is roughly equally dependent on genetic and environmental factors; it is associated with hypertriglyceridemia, overweight, a sedentary lifestyle, tobacco use, the use of certain drugs such as androgens and noncardioselective beta-blockers, and a variety of specific genetic disorders. The ratio of LDL cholesterol to HDL cholesterol is sometimes used as an indicator of risk as well; epidemiologic evidence and clinical-trial data indicate that, in general, a ratio >5 is undesirable.

It has been estimated that subjects with familial hypoalphalipoproteinemia, an autosomal dominant disorder associated with isolated low HDL cholesterol, constitute 5% of the patient population with premature atherosclerosis (67). Subjects with apo A-I/C-III/A-IV deficiency have low HDL cholesterol and are prone to severe atherosclerosis. However, some genetic disorders associated with low HDL cholesterol, such as Tangier disease, fish-eye disease, and the mutation apo A-I_{Milano} are not associated with premature atherosclerosis. Isolated low HDL cholesterol associated with genetic disorders is often resistant to pharmacologic therapy. A comparison of the effects of gemfibrozil and lovastatin on primary hypoalphalipoproteinemia revealed little difference in the limited efficacy of these agents in this disorder (68).

If HDL cholesterol is low due to environmental factors, hygienic measures are usually very effective and should emphasize diet modification, exercise, weight control, and cessation of tobacco use. However, no clinical trials have been conducted that specifically investigate the clinical benefit of interventions that raise HDL cholesterol. The ATP II therefore does not recommend pharmacologic therapy for isolated low HDL cholesterol in primary prevention. However, if other lipid abnormalities are present, particularly elevated LDL cholesterol, drug therapy may be indicated if hygienic measures are insufficient. LDL cholesterol remains the target of therapy, but agents that also increase HDL cholesterol should be selected. Hygienic measures are also emphasized in secondary prevention if low HDL cholesterol is present, but because drugs are frequently necessary to achieve the LDL-cholesterol goal for patients with CAD, agents that also raise HDL cholesterol should be considered. Nicotinic acid and gemfibrozil are particularly effective in this regard if triglyceride is elevated. The statins have only a modest benefit on HDL cholesterol, but significantly improve the LDL:HDL cholesterol ratio. If LDL cholesterol is sufficiently high, combination therapy may be required. A combination of a bile acid sequestrant and nicotinic acid is possible, but a combination of a statin and a fibrate should be avoided in most cases because of the possibility of myopathy.

SPECIAL ISSUES IN THE MANAGEMENT OF DYSLIPIDEMIA

Management of Dyslipidemia in the Elderly

Cardiovascular disease is a major cause of morbidity and mortality in the elderly, a rapidly growing segment of the population of developed countries. The U.S. Census Bureau estimates that by the year 2030, 20% of this country's population will be 65 years of age or older. Because cholesterol levels tend to increase with age, dyslipidemia is particularly prevalent in this group. The management of CAD risk factors in this group is therefore a major challenge for public health.

Despite the high percentage of elderly Americans with dyslipidemia, the value of preventive interventions in this group has been questioned. Some have argued that because the relative risk for CAD associated with cholesterol level declines with age, and because many elderly have frail constitutions or competing illnesses, antilipidemic interventions do not provide sufficient benefit in the elderly to justify the potential rigors. However, the ATP II has reaffirmed that age is not itself a basis for excluding patients from therapy. Although relative risk declines with age, the attributable risk—the absolute increase in the number of patients with CAD per increment of serum cholesterol—increases with age (69). Hence, potentially there are more elderly individuals who may benefit from preventive therapy than there are younger individuals. Furthermore, the life expectancy of a 65-year-old man in good health is approximately 15 years, suggesting that most elderly candidates for therapy will be able to realize the benefit of such therapy. The ATP II emphasizes the concept of biological age, i.e., relative physiologic strength, rather than chronologic age in determining whether and what type of therapy are warranted in an elderly patient.

Total cholesterol increases with age in both men and women. In men, the rate of increase begins to subside somewhat after age 50 years. However, in women, mean serum cholesterol continues to increase into the seventh decade and eventually exceeds that of men. The increase in mean serum cholesterol in women predominantly reflects an increase in LDL cholesterol following menopause. The HDL cholesterol remains relatively constant in males and females after puberty; the lower levels found in men are believed to be caused by androgens. Thus, the LDL:HDL cholesterol ratio increases with the aging process in both men and women.

Data from the Framingham Heart Study and MRFIT suggest that lowering serum cholesterol from 285 to 200 mg/dl would reduce risk for coronary heart disease by 33% in the 65- to 74-year-old age group and 23% in the 75- to 84-year-old age group (69). According to these data, the estimated number of preventable coronary heart disease deaths per thousand patient-years in men and women is 9.5 and 3.8, respectively, in the 65- to 74-year-old age group and 12.7 and 6.5, respectively, in the 75- to 84-year-old age group. Analyses of elderly cohorts in clinical trials have shown that the benefit of antilipidemic therapy experienced by these patients is similar to that experienced by younger patients. In the Stockholm Ischaemic Heart Disease Trial (70), which enrolled survivors of acute myocardial infarction ≤70 years of age, total mortality in the 60- to 70-year-old age group fell 28% compared with matched subjects in the placebo group, reflecting a large reduction in ischemic heart disease mortality. Nonetheless, no double-blind, placebo-controlled trial has been completed that specifically investigates the value of antilipidemic therapy in the elderly, although several ongoing clinical trials are addressing this question. However, there is no evidence that the process of atherosclerosis or the risk factors that promote the disease are different in younger and older subjects. For example, the Systolic Hypertension in the Elderly Program (71) demonstrated that antihypertensive therapy in primary prevention was effective in reducing the incidence of cardiovascular disease in the elderly.

Hygienic measures such as diet, exercise, and smoking cessation should continue to be emphasized. The frequency of gastrointestinal problems in the elderly makes the bile acid sequestrants difficult to administer at maximum dose. Tolerability may be increased by increasing fluid intake or adding stool softeners. As mentioned previously, ERT is often useful in postmenopausal women with elevated LDL cholesterol.

Diabetes Mellitus

Both insulin-dependent diabetes mellitus (IDDM) and non-insulin-dependent diabetes mellitus (NIDDM) are major risk factors for CAD: atherosclerotic disease is the cause of death in 75–80% of adults with diabetes mellitus (72). It occurs not only more often, but also earlier in diabetes. The risk for CAD is 2–3 times greater in diabetic men than in nondiabetic men, and a somewhat greater increase in risk is seen in diabetic women compared with nondiabetic women, effectively negating the delay in CAD onset in women compared with men. The diabetic patient may therefore be a candidate for more aggressive management of hyperglycemia and of CAD risk factors associated with diabetes such as hypertension and dyslipidemia.

Numerous lipid-based mechanisms have been proposed to explain the increased risk associated with diabetes. These include increased coagulability, altered clearance of glucosylated lipoproteins, and increased susceptibility of LDL to oxidation. The lipid profile in the diabetic is frequently characterized by elevated triglyceride, low HDL cholesterol, and a normal LDL-cholesterol level. However, diabetics frequently have small, dense LDL and increased apo B levels. These lipid abnormalities are compounded by the coexistence of other CAD risk factors such as hypertension.

Despite the increased risk for CAD and the frequent presence of dyslipidemia in diabetes, no large, prospective, double-blind clinical trial has been performed evaluating the impact of antilipidemic therapy in NIDDM. Dietary therapy and glucose control are the basic steps of therapy in diabetes. The lipid profile of patients with IDDM is often normal if glucose control is good.

If hygienic measures do not normalize the lipid profile, pharmacologic therapy should be strongly considered. In fact, many investigators recommend an LDL-cholesterol goal of <100 mg/dl due to the high rate of CAD in these patients. In 1992, the American Diabetes Association (ADA) convened a consensus panel on diabetic dyslipidemia (72). The ADA group recommended an LDL-cholesterol goal of <130 mg/dl and a triglyceride goal of <200 mg/dl in primary prevention, and goals of <100 and <150 mg/dl, respectively, in secondary prevention. However, the ATP II does not provide recommendations specific to diabetic dyslipidemia.

Drug selection depends on the phenotype. Because triglyceride is usually the predominant lipid elevated, the fibric acid derivatives are first-line agents. Nicotinic acid is relatively contraindicated because it usually worsens glucose control. If used, the doses of hypoglycemics and insulin may need to be adjusted. Continued poor glucose control mandates discontinuation of nicotinic acid. Hypercholesterolemia is uncommon in diabetes, occurring in less than 10% of patients with the disease. In these instances, the statins are first-line agents. Although the bile acid sequestrants are not ideal as monotherapy because they often raise triglyceride, the combination of a fibrate and a bile acid sequestrant is often effective, particularly if both LDL cholesterol and triglyceride are elevated. This phenotype is typical in nephrotic syndrome.

Because of the frequency of hypertension in diabetics, the effects of antihypertensives on serum lipids and glucose control should be considered. High-dose diuretic therapy may worsen glucose tolerance in patients with diabetes, resulting in a secondary increase in triglyceride. Noncardioselective beta-blockers partially inhibit lipoprotein lipase activity, resulting in a secondary increase in triglyceride and decrease of HDL cholesterol. Calcium-channel blockers do not affect the lipid profile in diabetes. Angiotensin-converting-enzyme (ACE) inhibitors have been shown to increase insulin sensitivity and also have a beneficial impact on diabetic nephropathy, and therefore are preferred in diabetes (73).

The complexity of the metabolic abnormalities in diabetes requires that these patients be monitored closely.

Hyperlipidemia in Children

Numerous pathologic studies have demonstrated that the earliest lesions of atherosclerosis occur during adolescence. The Bogalusa Heart Study (74) investigated the extent of fatty streak development in the aorta in subjects aged 6–30 years who had died at a young age of trauma or unrelated illness. The extent of fatty streak development correlated with antemortum serum lipid levels in male subjects. Although not all fatty streaks progress to advanced atherosclerotic lesions, it is thought that all advanced atherosclerotic lesions originate as fatty streaks. However, despite the importance of lipid-loading of cells in lesion development, it has not been conclusively proven that altering serum lipid levels is of clinical benefit in children or free from untoward effects on growth or steroid production. Additionally, individuals with dyslipidemia in childhood do not always have dyslipidemia in adulthood. A conservative approach to treatment of dyslipidemia in children and adolescents is therefore prudent until clinical evidence of safety and benefit is available.

The NCEP convened a panel to formalize recommendations, which were released in 1991, for the management of dyslipidemia in children and adolescents (75). The panel recommended that in all children over the age of 3 years saturated fat should be limited to ≤10% of total calories and cholesterol to <300 mg/day. Screening was recommended only if a family history of genetic dyslipidemia or premature CAD is present. Total cholesterol <170 mg/dl is considered acceptable, whereas levels of 170–199 mg/dl are borderline-high and levels >200 mg/dl are high. If total cholesterol is high, a fasting lipoprotein analysis should be conducted. If total cholesterol is borderline-high, a second total cholesterol measurement should be obtained; if the average of the two measurements is borderline-high or high, a fasting lipoprotein analysis is necessary. An LDL-cholesterol level is acceptable if <110 mg/dl, borderline-high if between 110 and 129 mg/dl, and high if >130 mg/dl.

The goal of therapy if LDL cholesterol is borderline high is a level <110 mg/dl. For high LDL cholesterol, a level below 130 mg/dl is a minimal goal; ideally, a level below 110 mg/dl is preferred. The Step I Diet is the initial level of dietary therapy. If the LDL-cholesterol goal is not met with this diet after at least 3 months, the Step II Diet should be initiated.

The NCEP limits use of pharmacologic therapy to patients >10 years of age at high risk after intensive dietary therapy alone. For such patients, LDL cholesterol ≥160 mg/dl is considered the value at which drugs should be considered if a genetic abnormality associated with CAD, a positive family history of CAD, or two or more other CAD risk factors are present. Otherwise, drugs should be considered if LDL cholesterol remains ≥190 mg/dl. The panel recommends that the minimum goal of drug therapy be LDL cholesterol <130 mg/dl, although a goal of <110 mg/dl is preferable. However, many experts feel this is an overly aggressive approach, and would not subject children to pharmacologic therapy in the absence of proven clinical benefit. In children and adolescents, the bile acid sequestrants are the drugs of choice because they lack systemic effects. However, because binding of vitamins and other nutrients may occur, careful monitoring and possibly vitamin supplements are required.

It is not clear whether therapy is needed for elevated triglyceride in children and adolescents, except in severe instances.

Blood Cholesterol and Noncoronary Mortality

Several epidemiologic studies have correlated low serum cholesterol (levels below approximately 160 mg/dl) with increased risk for noncoronary mortality. However, a causal relation between low cholesterol and noncoronary mortality is unlikely, and the data are probably confounded by other factors (76,77). In several but not all of the studies with prolonged follow-up, the correlation attenuated over time, suggesting that preexisting conditions associated with hypocholesterolemia, such as cancer, attributed to the association. Furthermore, the association is not consistent regarding the cause of the increased mortality; rather, the increased risk has been variously observed in deaths from trauma, a variety of digestive diseases, lung cancer, liver cancer, and suicide. No plausible biological mechanism has been suggested that could explain the alleged toxicity of the blood cholesterol levels implicated. Additionally, there is no convincing evidence of excess mortality in geographic populations that have low cholesterol levels, such as those of China and Japan.

A separate issue is the failure of cholesterol-lowering therapy to favorably impact total mortality, leading some to question the value of such therapy. Increased noncoronary mortality has been observed in some primary-prevention trials, particularly the WHO Cooperative Trial (54), although methodologic flaws cast doubt on the significance of these findings. In one meta-analysis of controlled trials (78), the odds ratio for mortality from causes other than coronary heart disease in patients at lower risk (defined as fewer than 10 deaths per 1,000 patient-years in matched controls) and receiving drug therapy was 1.21 compared with placebo; no difference in relative risk was seen between low-risk patients receiving dietary therapy and low-risk control patients, suggesting that drug toxicity was the cause of the increased risk in patients receiving drug therapy. However, meta-analyses that exclude the WHO data have not found significant increases in noncardiovascular mortality. In fact, a meta-analysis by Law et al. (79) calculated a nonsignificant 4% decrease in total mortality per 0.6 mmol/L (23 mg/dl) decrease in total cholesterol with active treatment, which is comparable to the 6% decrease that was expected based on a 10% decrease in ischemic heart disease per 0.6 mmol/L decrease in cholesterol. The effect of cholesterol lowering on total mortality remains largely unresolved because of the weakness of the data; no clinical trial has been conducted with sufficient statistical power to determine conclusively the effects of therapy on total mortality. Nevertheless, the possibility of drug toxicity cannot be ignored, and pharmacologic intervention should be limited to those at high risk for coronary events to ensure sufficient benefit.

FUTURE DIRECTIONS

Further refinement of treatment guidelines is an ongoing obligation as our understanding of the factors that promote CAD risk increases. The significance of triglyceride as a risk factor must be more clearly elucidated, and the role of other factors such as serum levels of lipoprotein[a], fibrinogen, and apolipoproteins are under investigation. Future directions in antilipidemic therapy include the development of more potent antilipidemic drugs, such as more effective inhibitors of HMG-CoA reductase or drugs that intervene elsewhere in the biosynthesis of cholesterol. Other potential targets of intervention include raising HDL levels or inhibiting lipoprotein oxidation. Gene therapy has many potential applications, such as altering the production or activity of receptors, apolipoproteins, and enzymes important in lipoprotein production and metabolism.

SUMMARY

It is clear that certain clinically discernible factors participate intimately in the development of coronary artery disease. Management of these risk factors has gained acceptance as a means of reducing the likelihood of coronary events. Clinical trial data establish the benefit of interventions targeting hypercholesterolemia, hypertension, and tobacco use.

A number of lipid abnormalities are associated with increased risk. The strongest evidence of atherogenicity exists for elevated levels of LDL cholesterol, although low levels of HDL cholesterol and elevated triglyceride levels are also targets of intervention. Clinical trials have demonstrated that CAD morbidity and mortality may be reduced by antilipidemic therapy in both primary and secondary prevention, and have shown that the progression of established CAD may be slowed or even reversed by aggressive interventions.

In 1993, these adult treatment guidelines of the National Cholesterol Education Program were updated to reflect the most recent consensus of experts on the treatment of dyslipidemia. The ATP II provides separate treatment algorithms for primary and secondary prevention and places increased emphasis on overall risk status in determining follow-up.

The decline in morbidity and mortality from atherosclerotic disease is one of the major advances in medicine achieved over the past several decades. The ability to decrease the complications of atherosclerosis by modification of risk factors is an accepted strategy to improve both the length and quality of life. Along with the management of hypertension, stable angina, and acute coronary syndromes, management of dyslipidemia has advanced rapidly over the past 10 years. However, unresolved issues remain, including the impact of cholesterol lowering on noncardiovascular mortality and the role of other factors such as apolipoprotein levels and lipoprotein[a] levels in screening and risk stratification.

REFERENCES

1. Stamler J. Epidemiology, established major risk factors, and the primary prevention of coronary heart disease. In: Chatergee K, Cheitlin MD, Karliner J, Parmley WW, Rapaport E, Scheinman M, eds. *Cardiology—an illustrated text.* Philadelphia: Lippincott; 1991;7.2–7.35.
2. National Cholesterol Education Program. Report of the National Cho-

lesterol Education Program Expert Panel on Detection, Evaluation, and Treatment of High Blood Cholesterol in Adults. *Arch Intern Med* 1988; 148:36–69.

3. National Cholesterol Education Program. Second report of the Expert Panel on Detection, Evaluation, and Treatment of High Blood Cholesterol in Adults (Adult Treatment Panel II). *Circulation* 1994;89: 1329–1445.
4. Rossouw JE, Lewis B, Rifkind BM. The value of lowering cholesterol after myocardial infarction. *N Engl J Med* 1990;323:1112–1119.
5. Brown BG, Zhao X-Q, Sacco DE, Alberts JJ. Lipid lowering and plaque regression. New insights into prevention of plaque disruption and clinical events in coronary disease. *Circulation* 1993;87:1781–1791.
6. Austin MA. Plasma triglyceride and coronary heart disease. *Arterioscler Thromb* 1991;11:2–14.
7. Austin MA. Plasma triglyceride as a risk factor for coronary heart disease: the epidemiologic evidence and beyond. *Am J Epidemiol* 1989; 129:249–259.
8. National Research Council. 1989.

8a. U.S. Department of Health and Human Services.

9. Ballantyne FC, Melville DA, McKenna JP, Morrison BA, Ballantyne D. Response of plasma lipoproteins and acute phase proteins to myocardial infarction. *Clin Chim Acta* 1979;99:85–92.
10. Fredrickson DS, Levy RI, Lees RS. Fat transport in lipoproteins—an integrated approach to mechanisms and disorders. *N Engl J Med* 1967; 276:34–42, 94–103, 148–156, 215–225, 273–281.
11. Schmidt EB. n-3 polyunsaturated fatty acids and ischemic heart disease. *Curr Opin Lipidol* 1993;4:27–33.
12. Grundy SM, Barrett-Conner E, Rudel LL, Miettinen T, Spector AA. Workshop on the impact of dietary cholesterol on plasma lipoproteins and atherogenesis. *Arteriosclerosis* 1988;8:95–101.
13. Glore SR, Van Treeck D, Knehans AW, Guild M. Soluble fiber and serum lipids: a literature review. *J Am Diet Assoc* 1994;94:425–436.
14. Ornish D, Brown SE. Treatment of and screening for hyperlipidemia [letter; comment]. *N Engl J Med* 1993;329:1124–1125.
15. Hunninghake DB, Stein EA, Dujovne CA, et al. The efficacy of intensive dietary therapy alone or combined with lovastatin in outpatients with hypercholesterolemia. *N Engl J Med* 1993;328:1213–1219.
16. Grundy SM, Barnett JP. Metabolic and health complications of obesity. *Dis Mon* 1990;36:643–731.
17. Zavaroni I, Bonini L, Fantuzzi M, Dall Aglio E, Passeri M, Reaven GM. Hyperinsulinemia, obesity, and syndrome X. *J Intern Med* 1994; 235:51–56.
18. Leon AS, Connett J, Jacobs DR Jr, Rauramaa R. Leisure-time, physical activity levels and risk of coronary heart disease and death. The Multiple Risk Factor Intervention Trial. *JAMA* 1987;258:238–2395.
19. Paffenbarger RS Jr, Hyde RT, Wing AL, Lee IM, Jung DL, Kampert JB. The association of changes in physical-activity level and other lifestyle characteristics with mortality among men. *N Engl J Med* 1993; 328:538–545.
20. Einarsson K, Ericsson S, Ewerth S, et al. Bile acid sequestrants: mechanisms of action on bile acid and cholesterol metabolism. *Eur J Clin Pharmacol* 1991;40(Suppl 1):S53–S58.
21. Einarsson K, Angelin B. The catabolism of cholesterol. *Curr Opin Lipidol* 1991;2:190–196.
22. Lipid Research Clinics Program. The Lipid Research Clinics Coronary Primary Prevention Trial Results. I. Reduction in incidence of coronary heart disease. II. The relationship of reduction in incidence of coronary heart disease to cholesterol lowering. *JAMA* 1984;251:351–374.
23. Watts GF, Lewis B, Brunt JNH, et al. Effects on coronary artery disease of lipid-lowering diet, or diet plus cholestyramine, in the St Thomas' Atherosclerosis Regression Study (STARS). *Lancet* 1992;339: 563–569.
24. Hunninghake DB. HMG-CoA reductase inhibitors. *Curr Opin Lipidol* 1992;3:22–28.
25. Arad Y, Ramakrishnan R, Ginsberg HN. Lovastatin therapy reduces low density lipoprotein apoB levels in subjects with combined hyperlipidemia by reducing the production of apoB-containing lipoproteins: implications for the pathophysiology of apoB production. *J Lipid Res* 1990;31:567–582.
26. Miettinen TA. Inhibition of cholesterol absorption by HMG-CoA reductase inhibitor. *Eur J Clin Pharmacol* 1991;40(Suppl I):S19–S21.
27. Bradford RH, Shear CL, Chremos AN, et al. Extended Clinical Evaluation of Lovastatin (EXCEL) Study results. I. Efficacy in modifying plasma lipoproteins and adverse event profile in 8245 patients with moderate hypercholesterolemia. *Arch Intern Med* 1991;151:43–49.
28. Mantell G, Burke MT, Staggers K. Extended clinical safety profile of lovastatin. *Am J Cardiol* 1990;66:11B–15B.
29. Pitt B, Mancini GBJ, Ellis SG, Rosman HS, McGovern ME. Pravastatin limitation of atherosclerosis in the coronary arteries (PLAC I). *J Am Coll Cardiol* 1994;23(Suppl):131A(abst).
30. Furberg CD, Crouse JR, Byington RP, Bond G, Espeland MA. PLAC-2: effects of pravastatin on progression of carotid atherosclerosis and clinical events. *J Am Coll Cardiol* 1993;21(Suppl):71A(abst).
31. Nestruck AC, Bouthillier D, Sing CF, Davignon J. Apolipoprotein E polymorphism and plasma cholesterol response to probucol. *Metabolism* 1987;36:743–747.
32. Kita T, Nagano Y, Yokode M, et al. Probucol prevents the progression of atherosclerosis in the Watanabe heritable hyperlipidemic (WHHL) rabbit, an animal model for familial hypercholesterolemia. *Proc Natl Acad Sci USA* 1987;84:5928–5931.
33. Baker SG, Joffe BI, Mendelsohn D, Seftel HC. Treatment of homozygous familial hypercholesterolaemia with probucol. *S Afr Med J* 1988; 62:7–11.
34. Kesaniemi YA, Grundy SM. Effect of probucol on cholesterol and lipoprotein metabolism in man. *J Lipid Res* 1984;25:780–790.
35. Narreszewicz M, Carew TE, Pittman RC, Witzteem JL, Steinberg D. A novel mechanism by which probucol lowers low density lipoprotein levels demonstrated in the LDL receptor deficient rabbit. *J Lipid Res* 1984;25:1206–1213.
36. De la Vega FM, Mendoza-Figueroa T. Effects of probucol on lipid metabolism and secretion in long-term cultures of adult rat hepatocytes. *Biochim Biophys Acta* 1991;1081:293–300.
37. Franceschini G, Sirtori M, Vaccarino V, et al. Mechanisms of HDL reduction after probucol. Changes in HDL subfractions and increased reverse cholesteryl ester transfer. *Arteriosclerosis* 1989;9:462–469.
38. Kuzuya M, Kuzuya F. Probucol as an antioxidant and antiatherogenic drug. *Free Radic Biol Med* 1993;14:67–77.
39. Eder HA. The effect of diet on the transport of probucol in monkeys. *Artery* 1982;10:105–107.
40. Walldius G, Regnstrom J, Nilsson J, et al. The role of lipids and antioxidative factors for development of atherosclerosis. The Probucol Quantitative Regression Swedish Trial (PQRST). *Am J Cardiol* 1993; 71(Suppl):15B–19B.
41. Figge HL, Figge J, Souney PF, Mutnick AH, Sacks F. Nicotinic acid: a review of its clinic use in the treatment of lipid disorders. *Pharmacotherapy* 1988;8:287–294.
42. Shepherd J, Packard CJ, Patsch JR, Gotto AM, Taunton OD. Effects of nicotinic acid therapy on plasma high-density lipoprotein subfraction distribution and composition and on apolipoprotein A metabolism. *J Clin Invest* 1979;63:858–867.
43. Drood JM, Zimetbaum PJ, Frishman WH. Nicotinic acid for the treatment of hyperlipoproteinemia. *J Clin Pharmacol* 1991;31:641–650.
44. McKenney, et al. (1994).
45. Coronary Drug Project Research Group. Clofibrate and niacin in coronary heart disease. *JAMA* 1975;231:360–381.
46. Canner PL, Berge KG, Wenger NK, et al. Fifteen year mortality in coronary drug project patients: long-term benefit with niacin. *J Am Coll Cardiol* 1986;8:1245–1255.
47. Brown BG, Alberts JJ, Fisher LD, et al. Regression of coronary artery disease as a result of intensive lipid lowering therapy in men with high levels of apolipoprotein B. *N Engl J Med* 1990;323:1289–1298.
48. Davignon J. Fibrates: a review of important issues and recent findings. *Can J Cardiol* 1994;10:61B–71B.
49. Illingworth DR. Fibric acid derivatives. In: Rifkind BM, ed. *Drug treatment of hyperlipidemia.* New York: Marcel Dekker; 1991:103–138.
50. Beil FV, Schrameyer-Wernecke A, Beisiegel U, et al. Lovastatin versus bezafibrate: efficacy, tolerability and effect on urinary mevalonate. *Cardiology* 1990;77(Suppl 4):22–32.
51. Homma Y, Ozawa H, Kobayashi T, et al. Effects of bezafibrate therapy on subfractions of plasma low-density lipoprotein and high-density lipoprotein, and on activities of lecithin : cholesterol acyltransferase and cholesteryl ester transfer protein in patients with hyperlipoproteinemia. *Atherosclerosis* 1994;106:191–201.
52. Tsai MY, Yuan J, Hunninghake DB. Effect of gemfibrozil on composition of lipoproteins and distribution of LDL subspecies. *Atherosclerosis* 1992;95:35–42.
53. Committee of Principal Investigators. A co-operative trial in the pri-

mary prevention of ischaemic heart disease using clofibrate. *Br Heart J* 1978;40:1069–1118.
54. Committee of Principal Investigators. WHO cooperative trial on primary prevention of ischaemic heart disease with clofibrate to lower serum cholesterol. Final mortality followup. *Lancet* 1984;2:600–604.
55. Group of Physicians on the Newcastle upon Tyne Region. Trial of clofibrate in the treatment of ischaemic heart disease. *Br Med J* 1971; 4:767–775.
56. Research Committee of the Scottish Society of Physicians. Ischaemic heart disease: a secondary prevention trial using clofibrate. Report by a research committee of the Scottish Society of Physicians. *Br Med J* 1971;4:775–784.
57. Frick MH, Elo O, Haapa K, et al. Helsinki Heart Study: Primary-prevention with gemfibrozil in middle-aged men with dyslipidemia. *N Engl J Med* 1987;317:1237–1245.
58. Manninen V, Tenkanen L, Koskinen P, et al. *Circulation* 1992;85: 37–45.
59. Bush TL, Barrett-Conner E, Cowan LD, et al. Cardiovascular mortality and noncontraceptive use of estrogen in women: results from the Lipid Research Clinic Program Follow-Up Study. *Circulation* 1987;75: 1102–1109.
60. Dolecek TA. Epidemiological evidence of relationships between dietary polyunsaturated fatty acids and mortality in the Multiple Risk Factor Intervention Trial. *Proc Soc Exp Biol Med* 1992;200:177–182.
61. Saynor R, Gillott T. Changes in blood lipids and fibrinogen with a note on safety in a long term study on the effects of n-3 fatty acids in subjects receiving fish oil supplements and followed for seven years. *Lipids* 1992;27:533–538.
62. Cashin-Hemphill L, Mack WJ, Pogoda JM, Sanmarco ME, Azen SP, Blankenhorn DH. Beneficial effects of colestipol–niacin on coronary atherosclerosis: a 4-year follow-up. *JAMA* 1990;264:3013–3017.
63. Kane JP, Malloy MJ, Ports TA, Phillips NR, Diehl JC, Havel RJ. Regression of coronary atherosclerosis during treatment of familial hypercholesterolemia with combined drug regimens. *JAMA* 1990;264: 3007–3012.
64. Seidel D, Armstrong VW, Scheeff-Werner P. The HELP–LDL Apheresis multicenter study, an angiographically assessed trial on the role of LDL-apheresis in the secondary prevention of coronary heart disease. I. Evaluation of safety and cholesterol lowering during the first 12 months. *Eur J Clin Invest* 1991;21:375–383.
65. Assmann G, Schulte H. Relation of high-density lipoprotein cholesterol and triglycerides to incidence of atherosclerotic coronary artery disease (the PROCAM experience). *Am J Cardiol* 1992;10:733–737.
66. Wiklund O, Angelin B, Bergman M, et al. Pravastatin and gemfibrozil alone and in combination for the treatment of hypercholesterolemia. *Am J Med* 1993;94:13–20.
67. Genest JJ, Martin-Murley S, McNamara JR, Salam DH, Schaefer EJ. Frequency of genetic dyslipidemia in patients with premature coronary disease. *Circulation* 1989;9:707A.
68. Vega GL, Grundy SM. Comparison of lovastatin and gemfibrozil in normolipidemic patients with hypoalphalipoproteinemia. *JAMA* 1989; 262:3148–3153.
69. Gordon DJ, Rifkind BM. Treating high blood cholesterol in the older patient. *Am J Cardiol* 1989;63:48H–52H.
70. Carlson LA, Rosenhamer G. Reduction of mortality in the Stockholm Ischaemic Heart Disease Secondary Prevention Study by combined treatment with clofibrate and nicotinic acid. *Acta Med Scand* 1988; 223:405–418.
71. SHEP Cooperative Research Group. Prevention of stroke by antihypertensive drug treatment in older persons with isolated systolic hypertension: final results of the Systolic Hypertension in the Elderly Program (SHEP). *JAMA* 1991;265:3255–3264.
72. American Diabetes Association. Detection and management of lipid disorders in diabetes. *Diabetes Care* 1993;16(Suppl 2):106–112.
73. Carella MJ, Gossain VV, Rovner DR. Early diabetic nephropathy. Emerging treatment options. *Arch Intern Med* 1994;154:625–630.
74. Berenson GS, Wattigney WA, Tracy RE, et al. Atherosclerosis of the aorta and coronary arteries and cardiovascular risk factors in persons aged 6 to 30 years and studied at necropsy. (The Bogalusa Heart Study). *Am J Cardiol* 1992;70:851–858.
75. National Cholesterol Education Program. Report of the Expert Panel on Blood Cholesterol Levels in Children and Adolescents. *Pediatrics* 1992;89:525–584.
76. Rossouw JE, Gotto AM Jr. Does low cholesterol cause death? [Editorial]. *Cardiovasc Drugs Ther* 1993;789–793.
77. Stamler J, Stamler R, Brown WV, et al. Serum cholesterol: doing the right thing [Editorial]. *Circulation* 1993;88:1954–1960.
78. Davey Smith G, Song F, Sheldon TA. Cholesterol lowering and mortality: The importance of considering initial level of risk. *Br Med J* 1993; 306:1367–1373.
79. Law MR, Thompson SG, Wald NJ. Assessing possible hazards of reducing serum cholesterol. *Br Med J* 1994;308:373–379.
80. Gotto AM, Pownell HJ. 1992.
81. Frank JW, Reed DM, Grove JS, Benfante R. Will lowering population levels of serum cholesterol affect total mortality? Expectations from the Honolulu Heart Program. *J Clin Epidemiol* 1992;45:333–346.
82. MacMahon S, Cutler J, Brittain EL, Higgins M. *Eur Heart J* 1987; 8(Suppl B):57–70.
83. Miettinen TA, Huttunen JK, Naukkarinen V, Strandberg T, Vanhanen H. Long-term use of probucol in the multifactorial prevention of vascular disease. *Am J Cardiol* 1986;57:49H–54H.
84. Prihoda JS, Illingsworth DR. Drug therapy of hyperlipidemia. In: O'Rourke RA, ed. *Current problems in cardiology.* St. Louis: Year Book Medical Publishers; 1992;17(9):547–592.
85. Witztum JL, Simmons D, Steinberg D, et al. Intensive combination drug therapy of familial hypercholesterolemia with lovastatin, probucol, and colestipol hydrochloride. *Circulation* 1989;79:16–28.

Atherosclerosis and Coronary Artery Disease,
edited by V. Fuster, R. Ross, and E. J. Topol.
Lippincott-Raven Publishers, Philadelphia © 1996.

CHAPTER 12

Impact of Management in Stabilization of Coronary Disease

B. Greg Brown and Valentin Fuster

Key Words: Regression trials; Quantitative arteriography; Plaque stability; Plaque disruption; Foam cells; Core lipids; Fibrous Cap.

INTRODUCTION

The past two decades have witnessed important advances in the understanding of the vascular biology of atherogenesis and the dynamic interplay among atherosclerotic plaque size, vasomotor tone, blood flow, thrombosis, and, most recently, the pathological processes that lead to plaque disruption and clinical ischemic events. This chapter reviews a series of angiographic ''regression'' trials completed in the past decade. It interprets these studies from the perspective of the underlying pathological processes that promote coronary atherosclerosis regression and retard its progression. In it, we present the evidence supporting the unifying hypothesis that lipid depletion from two important plaque pools results in plaque stability and reduced clinical events.

B. G. Brown: Department of Medicine, Cardiology Division, University of Washington School of Medicine, Seattle, Washington 98195.

V. Fuster: Cardiovascular Institute, Department of Medicine, Mount Sinai School of Medicine, New York, New York, 10029.

MANAGEMENT OBJECTIVES FOR PATIENTS WITH CORONARY ARTERY DISEASE

Comprehensive management of coronary artery disease (CAD) has two fundamental objectives. The first of these is to reduce the severity of ischemic symptoms caused by arterial obstructive disease. The presence of ischemia indicates that the capacity of the vascular bed to fully meet the varying oxygen demands of the myocardium is impaired by one or more of the following mechanisms:

- A fixed flow-limiting coronary stenosis (1,2).
- Abnormal epicardial vessel tone (3,4).
- Intermittent arterial vasospasm (5).
- Microvascular dysfunction (6,7).
- Incomplete collateral development.

A variety of medical approaches are now used to relieve symptoms by favorably altering the O_2 supply–demand imbalance. Alternatively, this objective of symptom relief may be accomplished through more direct structural and/or physiological changes favorably affecting the diminished vascular flow capacity. These include development of collaterals, relaxation of excess vasoconstrictor tone, or improvement in the severity of flow-limiting stenosis (''regression''). Regression has been questioned as a possible mechanism for symptom relief. In this chapter, the evidence for the occurrence of regression is reviewed, together with the role of lipid lowering in achieving it; mechanisms contributing to regression are also discussed.

The second fundamental management objective in CAD is to prevent the anticipated worsening of symptoms, or progression to a *clinical event* such as cardiac death, myocardial infarction, or worsening angina requiring bypass surgery or angioplasty. In this chapter, the mechanisms of gradually progressive arterial obstruction are briefly reviewed, together with the mechanism of plaque disruption resulting in abrupt worsening of arterial obstruction. Evidence is presented that indicates a linkage between lipid lowering and stabilization of the plaque structure. This set of observations supports the idea that lipid-lowering therapy prevents clinical events by selectively lipid-depleting or ''regressing'' a relatively small subgroup of lipid-rich plaques that are at high risk of plaque disruption, ulceration, and hemorrhage, and which account for the great majority of clinical events.

EVIDENCE FOR REGRESSION

Our understanding of atherosclerosis regression derives from animal experiments and from clinical arteriographic studies. There are important biological differences between the various experimental models of atherosclerosis and the human disease. And there are significant differences among the methods for assessing disease. Accordingly, concepts emerging from these two perspectives are not always equivalent. Even the basic term *regression* means something quite different to the experimental pathologist than to the clinician, as can be seen in terms of the histological sections of Fig. 1. To the pathologist, regression means shrinkage of intimal plaque through a reduction in its major components—smooth muscle, macrophages, connective tissues, and lipid. To the physician interpreting human disease from its arteriographic appearance, regression is defined as an enlargement in the caliber of the narrowed arterial lumen. Such improvement occurs infrequently in the natural course of the disease (8). Atherosclerosis regression may occur by the process of plaque shrinkage but also by a variety of other possible mechanisms. For example, lysis of fully occlusive thrombi or of mural thrombi is commonly observed in the course of unstable ischemic syndromes (9–11). Wound healing may favorably remodel an acutely disrupted plaque (11). Remodeling of the underlying arterial architecture (Glagov phenomenon) can improve arteriographic lumen caliber independently of changes in plaque size (11–14). Relaxation of arterial vasomotor tone can similarly improve lumen caliber (3,4). The role of the endothelium and the relationship(s) of therapy to its function have been shown to be important in many of these processes (4,7,13,15–18). Because these arteriographic images do not permit an easy distinction among the various mechanisms of regression, our understanding of the principal process(es) by which it occurs in patients is limited.

Thus, the key question is not ''Does arteriographic regression occur in patients?'' (it does), but, ''Can such regression be promoted with a sufficiently great magnitude and frequency to justify a major therapeutic strategy?'' Important related questions are, ''What are its mechanisms?'' and ''Does regression provide clinical benefits?'' and ''If so, how?'' Although there is not yet a consensus, the emerging evidence is encouraging.

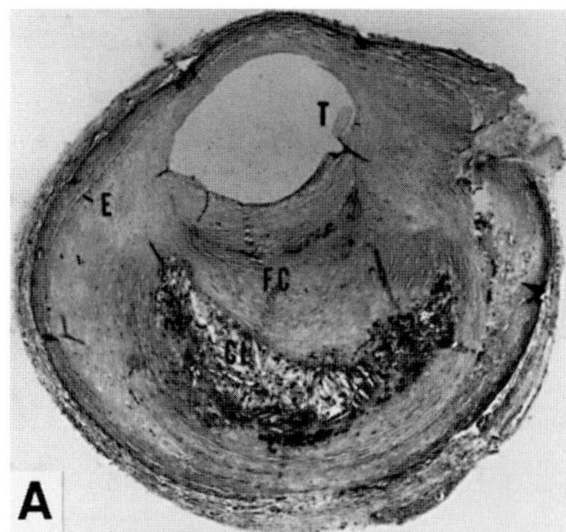

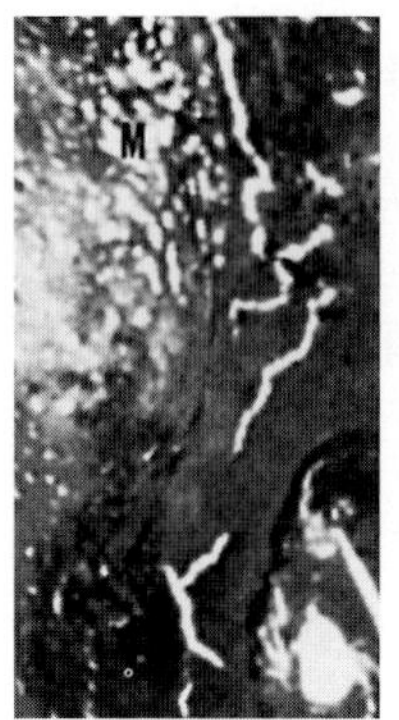

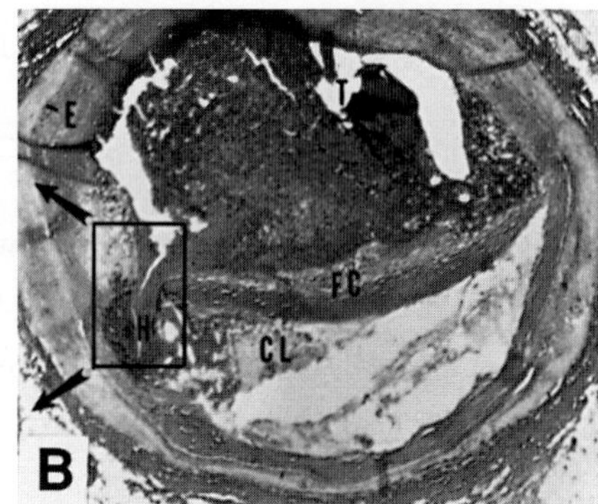

FIG. 1. A: Histological section through a structurally stable coronary plaque in a patient with vasospastic angina. Morphological features include: E, internal elastic lamina; FC, a thick fibrous cap composed largely of collagen and smooth muscle cells (SMC); CL, core lipid, here largely crystalline; T, a small tag of thrombus. **B:** Section through a structurally unstable coronary plaque in a patient dying from myocardial infarction. The lumen, only moderately narrowed by the plaque, is acutely occluded by thrombus (T). There are many features in common with the section in **A.** In the unstable plaque, core lipid (some dislodged by sectioning artifact) comprises a much larger fraction of the plaque. The fibrous cap is much thinner than in **A**, is fissured (or vented) at its left shoulder, permitting a small pocket of hemorrhage (H) in the plaque. This fissure, the associated hemorrhagic pocket, and the plaque shoulder, here rich in lipid-laden macrophages (M) (round, bright spots), are shown at increased magnification in the inset. Also at higher magnification (not shown), the fibrous cap has few SMC but many M. (**B** reproduced from Brown et al., ref. 35, with permission.)

Evidence in Experimental Models

Atherosclerosis has been shown convincingly to regress with lipid lowering in the nonhuman primate studies of Armstrong, Wissler, Clarkson, and Small and their colleagues (19–23). In the typical regression experiment, the amount and composition of intimal growth is assessed among cholesterol-fed animals at specified times, using group-averaged chemical and histological endpoints. During a sustained exposure to an "atherogenic" diet, plasma cholesterol may increase to more than 600 mg/dl, and there are substantial increases in coronary artery content of collagen (threefold), elastin (fourfold), and cholesterol (sevenfold, mostly esterified). On return to a native vegetarian "regression" diet, plasma cholesterol falls quickly to normal (140 mg/dl), and the arterial lipid and connective tissue accumulates partially regress over 20–40 months. Collagen content does not decline much from its peak value (−20%), but elastin (−50%) and cholesterol (−60%) do (21,23); and there is a fibrous transformation that thins the myointimal cellular response (24). Not all forms of cholesterol are readily depleted from these lipid-rich intimal deposits. The more mobile forms, including cholesteryl esters in foam cells, lipoproteins, and cholesteryl ester droplets, are known to diminish in response to lowered plasma cholesterol (22), but the cholesterol monohydrate crystals of the core lipid region are relatively resistant to mobilization (22,24). Histological morphometry shows that plaque mass is reduced during regression therapy (20,22,25).

Evidence in the Human

As late as 1987, there was only anecdotal evidence that the observations of regression in animals could be extended to patients with atherosclerotic disease. Kuo et al. (26), Brensike et al. (27), Duffield et al. (28), Nash et al. (29) and Nikkila et al. (30) had pioneered the use of arteriographic studies. In general, these studies concluded that lipid-lowering therapy reduced the frequency of disease progression, but regression was rarely observed and was not increased by the therapies tested. A more recent series of randomized clinical arteriographic trials has provided a perspective on the magnitude, frequency, and conditions under which regression can occur in patients. The more recent trials have incorporated more powerful therapeutic combinations to modify lipids and more objective methods for analysis of the arteriogram. These trials and their lipid response data are summarized in Table 1. Their results, based on arteriographic and clinical outcomes, are summarized in Table 2. In order of their publication, they are:

- *NHLBI Type II.* The National Heart, Lung and Blood Institute's 5-year comparison of diet versus diet and cholestyramine among patients selected for >90th percentile LDL cholesterol and some evidence for coronary disease (27).

TABLE 1. *Summary descriptions for 15 reported arteriographic lipid-lowering trials: Lipid response to treatments*

Study[a]	*n*	Entry requirements	Control regimen[b]	Treatment regimen	Treatment response LDL	Treatment response HDL	Years
Combination therapy studies							
CLAS	188	CABG[c]	D (−)	D + R + N[c]	−43%	+37%	2
POSCH	838	MI, chol	D	D + PIB ± R	−42%	+5%	9.7
Lifestyle	48	CAD	U	V + M + E	−37%	−3%	1
FATS (N + C)	146	CAD, apo B	D ± R	D + R + N	−32%	+43%	2.5
FATS (L + C)	146	CAD, apo B	D ± R	D + R + L	−46%	+15%	2.5
CLAS II	138	CABG	D	D + R + N	−40%	+37%	4
UC-SCOR	97	FH	U	D + R + N ± L	−39%	+25%	2
STARS (D + R)	90	CAD, chol	U	D + R	−36%	−4%	3
SCRIP	300	CAD	U	D + (R/N/LF) + E, BP	−22%	+12%	4
Heidelberg	113	CAD	U	D + Ex	−8%	+3%	1
HARP	91	CAD "NL" lipids	D ± R	P ± N ± R ± F	−41%	+13%	2.5
Monotherapy studies							
NHLBI	143	CAD, LDL	D	D + R	−31%	+8%	5
STARS (D)	90	CAD, chol	U	D	−16%	0%	3
MARS	270	CAD	D	D + L	−38%	+9%	2
CCAIT	331	CAD, chol	D	D + L	−29%	+7%	2
PLAC I	408	CAD, LDL	D	D + P	−28%	+9%	3
MAAS	381	CAD	D	D + S	−31%	+9%	4
REGRESS	885	CAD	D	D + P	−29%	+10%	2

[a] See text for the details and full names of these studies.
[b] Mean LDL cholesterol response to control regimen, −7%; mean HDL cholesterol response, 0%.
[c] Abbreviations: CAD, coronary artery disease; LDL, low-density lipoprotein >90th percentile; CABG, coronary artery bypass graft surgery; MI, myocardial infarction; apo B, apolipoprotein B ≤125 mg/dl; FH, familial hypercholesterolemia; chol, cholesterol >220 mg/dl; D, diet; U, usual care; R, resin (colestipol or cholestyramine); N, nicotinic acid; PIB, partial ileal bypass; V, vegetarian diet <10% fat; M, relaxation techniques; Ex, exercise program; L, lovastatin; S, simvastatin; C, colestipol; F, fibrate-type drugs; BP, blood pressure therapy.

TABLE 2. *Summary of arteriographic outcomes, treatment lipid response, and frequencies of reported clinical events in 15 lipid-lowering coronary arteriographic trials*

	Control patients				Changes among treated patients				
Study[a]	Progression	Regression	Δ%S[c]	Δ MLD (mm)	Progression	Regression	Δ%S(P)[d]	Δ MLD (mm) (P)	"Event"[b] reduction (%)
Combination therapy studies									
CLAS	61%	2%	—	—	39%	16%	—	—	25%
POSCH (10 yr)	65%	6%	—	—	37%	14%	—	—	35% (62%[y])[f]
Lifestyle	32%	32%	+3.4%	—	14%	41%	−2.2 (0.001)[e]	—	0 vs 1 (↑)
FATS (N + C)	46%	11%	+2.1%	−0.05	25%	39%	−0.9 (0.005)	+0.035 (0.005)	80%§
FATS (L + C)	46%	11%	+2.1%	−0.05	22%	32%	−0.7 (0.02)	+0.012 (0.06)	70%
CLAS II	83%	6%	—	—	30%	18%	—	—	43%
UC-SCOR	41%	13%	+0.8%	—	20%	33%	−1.5 (0.04)	—	1 vs 0
STARS (D + R)	46%	4%	+5.8%	−0.23	12%	33%	−1.9 (0.01)	+0.12 (0.001)	89%[f]
SCRIP	50%	10%	+3.2%	−0.20	50%	20%	+1.2 (0.02)	−0.08 (.003)	50%
Heidelberg	42%	4%	+3.0%	−0.13	20%	30%	−1.0 (0.05)[e]	0.00 (0.05)	−27%(↑)[g]
HARP	38%	15%	+2.4%	−0.17	33%	13%	+2.1 (NS)	−0.12 (NS)	33%
Monotherapy studies									
NHLBI	49%	7%	—	—	32%	7%	—	—	33%
STARS (D)	46%	4%	+5.8%	−0.23	15%	38%	−1.1 (NS)	+0.03 (0.05)	69%[f]
MARS	41%	12%	+2.2%	−0.06	29%	23%	+1.6% (0.2)	−0.03 (0.2)	29%
CCAIT	50%	7%	+2.9%	−0.09	33%	10%	+1.7% (0.04)	−0.05 (0.01)	22%
PLAC I	38%	14%	+3.4%	−0.15	26%	14%	+2.1% (0.13)	−0.09 (0.04)	13% (54%[x])
MAAS	32%	12%	3.6%	−0.13	23%	19%	1.0 (0.006)	−0.04 (0.007)	22%
REGRESS	NA	NA	NA	−0.09	NA	NA	NA	−0.03 (0.001)	39%[f]

[a] See text for the details, abbreviations, and full name of these studies. Progression and regression are variably defined, per patient, in each study.

[b] Events are variably defined in these studies; in general, the frequency of cardiovascular events (death, MI, unstable ischemia requiring revascularization or hospitalization, or both) in control and treated groups are compared using the sometimes sketchy details and definitions provided.

[c] Δ(%S) is usually reported as the average change in percent stenosis over all the lesions measured per patient. A positive (+) value represents "progression"; (−), "regression."

[d] P = Value for comparison of Δ%S or ΔMLD in control versus treated groups.

[e] Statistical comparison in Lifestyle uses a lesion-based method.

[f] Studies for which the reduction in cardiovascular clinical events was statistically significant.

[g] ↑ An increase of −27% reduction means 27% increase (NS).

[x] 54% reduction in CHD death and non-fatal MI.

[y] 62% reduction in coronary bypass surgery.

- *CLAS*. The Cholesterol-Lowering Atherosclerosis Study compared diet with diet, niacin, and colestipol for 2 years among male post-coronary-bypass patients (31).
- *POSCH*. The Program of Surgical Control of the Hyperlipidemias was a 9.7-year mean follow-up of patients with cholesterol >220 who had survived a first myocardial infarction and who were randomly assigned either to partial ileal bypass or to medical management in a "usual care" strategy (32).
- *Lifestyle*. The Lifestyle Heart Trial compared usual care with a variety of hygienic changes including a very low-fat vegetarian diet plus moderate exercise and relaxation techniques among patients with clinically manifest coronary disease (33).
- *FATS*. The Familial Atherosclerosis Treatment Study compared a moderate approach to lipid lowering with two more intensive drug regimens among men with elevated apolipoprotein B (≥125 mg/dl), and coronary disease (34,35).
- *CLAS II*. An extension of the CLAS trial to 4 years among about three-fourths of the original participants (36).
- *UC SCOR*. The University of California San Francisco investigators, as part of their Atherosclerosis SCOR Program Project, compared usual care with combined diet, colestipol, niacin, and possibly lovastatin among men and women followed in a lipid clinic for the genetic disorder familial hypercholesterolemia. Coronary disease was rarely clinically manifest among these severely hyperlipidemic subjects (37).
- *STARS*. The St. Thomas Atherosclerosis Regression Study compared usual care with dietary counseling or with diet plus cholestyramine among male patients with coronary disease and with cholesterol exceeding 220 mg/dl (38).
- *SCRIP*. The Stanford Coronary Risk Intervention Project studied patients with clinically established coronary disease. The usual-care control group was compared to those given a risk reduction regimen targeted at hyperlipidemia, hypertension, obesity, and cigarette use, and including dietary counseling plus a structured exercise program (39).
- *Heidelberg*. In this study, regular programmed physical exercise plus an AHA phase 3 diet are compared with the usual-care approach among 113 men routinely catheterized for stable angina pectoris (40).
- *HARP*. In the Harvard Atherosclerosis Reversal Program, 91 patients were selected for coronary disease and apparently "normal" lipids; a composite medical regimen (diet plus pravastatin, ± niacin, ± cholestyramine, ± a fibric acid derivative) targeted at LDL cholesterol ≤90 mg/dl and LDL cholesterol/HDL cholesterol ratio ≤2.0 was compared with dietary counseling ± cholestyramine (41).

More recently, a series of trials have examined the effect of monotherapy with one of the HMG-CoA reductase inhibitors on atherosclerosis, as assessed quantitatively from the coronary arteriogram or from percutaneous β-mode ultrasound of the carotid bifurcation. Those include:

- *MARS*. In the Monitored Atherosclerosis Regression Study, 280 patients with angiographic and symptomatic CAD were counseled in diet and given lovastatin (80 mg) or its placebo over a 2-year interval. Cholesterol at entry ranged from 190 to 295 mg/dl (42).
- *CCAIT*. In the Canadian Coronary Atherosclerosis Intervention Trial, 331 patients with CAD and cholesterol ranging from 220 to 300 mg/dl took lovastatin with dosage adjusted to a target LDL <130 mg/dl, or took its placebo. An average lovastatin dose of 36 mg was taken over the 2-year angiographic interval (43).
- *PLAC I*. In the Pravastatin Limitation of Atherosclerosis in the Coronary Arteries Study, 408 patients with angiographic and symptomatic CAD and LDL cholesterol ranging between 130 and 190 mg/dl were treated with diet and pravastatin, 40 mg/day, or its placebo, over a 3-year angiographic interval (44).
- *MAAS*. In the Multicentre Anti-Atheroma Study (45), 381 patients with coronary heart disease were assigned to treatment with diet and either simvastatin 20 mg daily or placebo, for 4 years. Entry cholesterol was required to lie in the range 5.5 mmol/liter (210 mg/dl) to 8.0 (310); entry triglycerides must not exceed 4.0 mmol/l (350 mg/dl).
- *REGRESS*. In the Regression Growth Evaluation Statin Study (46), 885 male patients were diet treated and randomly assigned to either pravastatin or its placebo. These patients were evenly divided among post-coronary-bypass, postangioplasty, and medical management. The study has been presented but not published.

In the NHLBI II, CLAS, CLAS II, MARS (secondary), and POSCH trials, change in disease severity was assessed visually, using panels of experts blinded to patient identity, randomization, and temporal sequence of the film pair. In the others, a similarly blinded analysis incorporated techniques of computer-assisted quantitative arteriography (47). Of interest, there was an entry requirement for even modest hyperlipidemia in only five of these nine trials (48). Despite the diversity among these trials in clinical presentation, lipid entry requirements, treatment regimens, and methods for arteriographic analysis, the outcomes, summarized in Table 2, are surprisingly consistent. Each study demonstrated a benefit from treatment, whether by diet or by diet supplemented by other life-style changes or by lipid-lowering drugs. As a generalization of the composite of results (not a meta-analysis), 8% of the control group patients were considered to have improvement in arterial obstruction ("regression"), and over half had worsening ("progression") during the study period. By contrast, about one-fourth of treated patients regressed. This type of comparison is illustrated using FATS data in Fig. 2.

As a generalization from Table 2, averaged estimates of disease severity, per patient, worsened (progressed) by about 3% stenosis among the controls while improving (regressing) by 1% to 2% stenosis among the treated patients. The "monotherapy" studies with somewhat less pro-

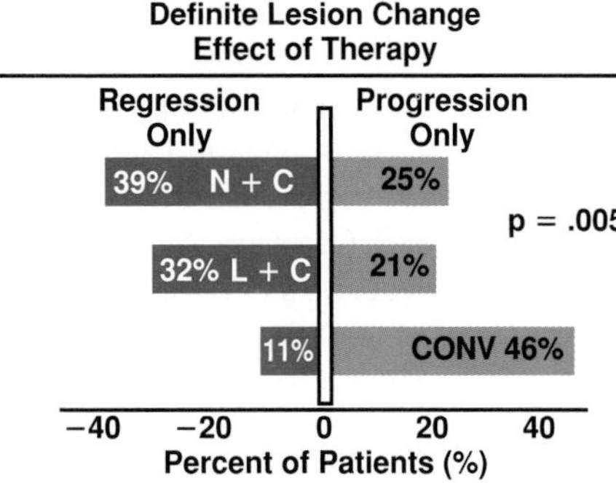

FIG. 2. Effect of therapy in FATS on the per-patient frequency of proximal lesion progression (worsening by ≥10% of at least one of nine lesions without any improving by that much), or of regression (converse of above). In comparison with conventional treatment, the frequency of per-patient progression is halved, and regression is tripled with the two more intensive lipid-altering strategies. See Table 2 for comparable data in other studies.

nounced LDL cholesterol and/or HDL cholesterol changes, did not achieve net regression among treated patients. These treatment benefits were statistically significant because the group variance of this estimate of disease change is also quite small, a testament to the precision of the quantitative coronary angiographic methods. In nearly every study the frequency of clinical cardiovascular events was reduced substantially, although the reductions achieved statistical significant in only 40%. Failure to confirm a significant clinical benefit is not unexpected because the trials using arteriographic endpoints were powered to demonstrate arteriographic benefits and used patient samples with marginal power to detect clinical benefits.

Multivariate statistical analysis has been used to identify those factors correlated with change in disease severity. Such change was usually characterized, per patient, either as the mean difference (final to baseline) in percentage stenosis among all lesions measured or as a visually derived global change estimate. In NHLBI-II, changes in the ratios HDL cholesterol/total cholesterol or HDL cholesterol/LDL cholesterol were the only significant negative correlates of disease change among the study cohort (49). In CLAS, non-HDL cholesterol best correlated with global change among placebo patients, as did the level of apo C-III in HDL among treated patients (50). In Lifestyle, an index of adherence to all aspects of the program best correlated with arteriographic outcome. In FATS, as shown in Fig. 3, the multivariate expression including the treatment-induced change in apo B (or LDL cholesterol), HDL cholesterol, systolic blood pressure, and baseline ischemia on the exercise treadmill test, predicting the change in mean proximal stenosis ($\Delta\%S_{prox}$) correlated well with the observed change ($r = 0.51$; $p < 0.001$). In these men with CAD and elevated LDL cholesterol, Lp(a) levels were dominant correlates of baseline disease severity, its progression, and event rate over 2.5 years. However, among patients with substantial treatment-induced LDL cholesterol reductions and HDL cholesterol increases, persistent elevations of Lp(a) were no longer atherogenic or clinically threatening (51). In UC-SCOR, only in-treatment LDL cholesterol correlated with arteriographic outcome. In STARS, change in LDL cholesterol/HDL cholesterol ratio and mean BP change during therapy were significant independent correlates of disease change. In Heidelberg, in which only three severe lesions per patient were measured, risk factors including lipids and exercise intensity were not associated with disease change. In NHLBI-II, FATS, UC-SCOR, Lifestyle, and STARS, the insertion of these predictive variables in the analysis abolished the association of benefit with treatment group, implying that the effect of therapy on arterial disease was mediated by its effect on the risk variable(s) identified.

We may conclude that reduction of LDL cholesterol or its components (apo B) or reduction of the LDL cholesterol/HDL cholesterol ratio has been a frequently observed correlate of arterial benefit. Blood pressure reduction, apo C-III distribution, Lp(a) levels, and compliance with life-style changes have also emerged in one or more studies. It appears from the more recent "monotherapy" studies that the magnitude of arterial and clinical benefit is somewhat reduced when LDL cholesterol and/or HDL cholesterol is less intensively altered. HARP (41) and CCAIT (43) call into question the merits of treating patients with more normal lipid levels,

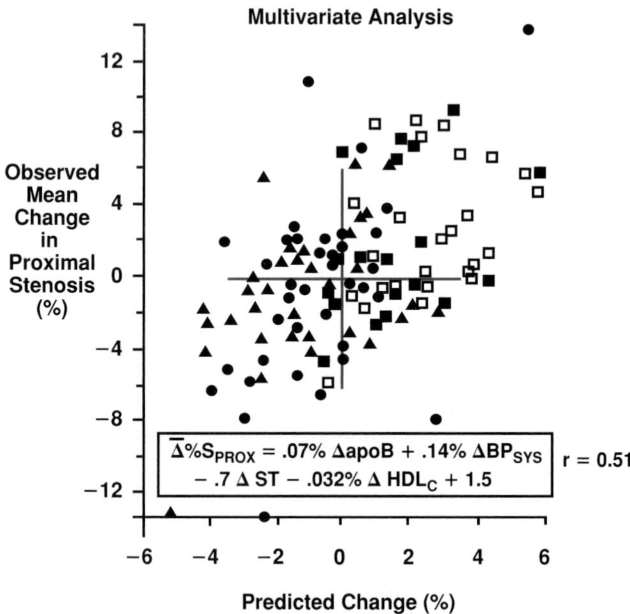

FIG. 3. Multivariate statistical analysis in FATS. The observed mean change, per patient, in proximal stenosis severity ($\Delta\%S_{prox}$) is plotted against a value estimated by the above expression (Δ, change from baseline; apoB, apolipoprotein B; SBP, systolic BP; ST, ECG ST-segment level during treadmill test). Changes during treatment in apo B, SBP, HDL cholesterol, and treadmill ischemia were thus independent and significant correlates of change in obstructive disease. The LDL cholesterol may be substituted for apo B with little change in correlation (34).

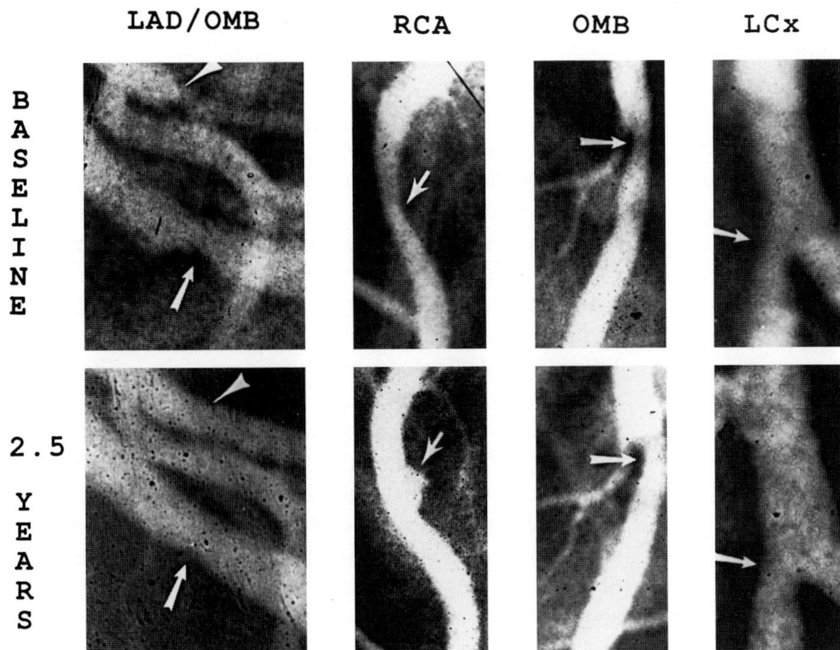

FIG. 4. Examples of definite regression in intensively treated patients in FATS. **Top row:** baseline. **Bottom row:** 2.5 years later. LAD *(top arrow),* left anterior descending artery (100 → 20%S); OMB *(bottom arrow),* obtuse marginal branch (39 → 18%S); RCA, right coronary artery (48 → 30%S) (note plaque ulcer at 2.5 years); OMB (69% → 37%); LCx, left circumflex artery (44 → 30%S). (Modified from Brown et al. ref. 34, with permission.)

although CLAS (31) and FATS (34) support this approach. When women are included in these studies (37,39), the arterial treatment benefits appear comparable to those in men.

Figure 4 illustrates cases of lesion regression seen in intensively treated FATS patients over a 2.5-year period. As Figs. 4 and 5 indicate, regression may occur in mild, moderate, and severe lesions. Although regression was somewhat more frequent among the more severe lesions, the relative benefit

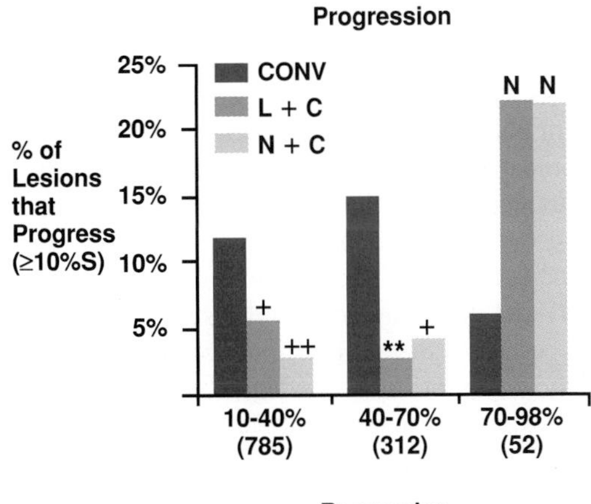

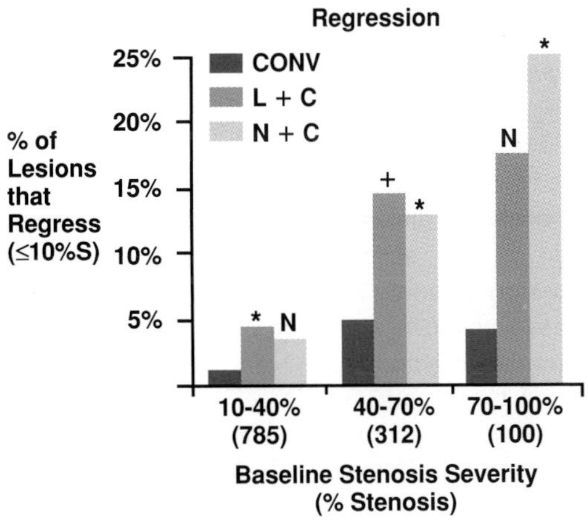

FIG. 5. Frequency of definite lesion change in FATS, expressed as the percentage of lesions that decrease in severity (regress) by a measured 10% stenosis or more. Lesions from 120 patients are subgrouped into 785 mild stenoses (10–40%S), 312 moderate stenoses (40–70%S), and 52 severe stenoses (70–98%S). Also, 48 lesions, initially totally occluded, are added to the severe lesion regression analysis because these may "regress" by recanalization. In general, change is relatively infrequent. The more severe the lesion at baseline, the more likely its change. Intensive lipid-lowering therapy increases regression frequency at all levels of severity. See Table 1 for abbreviations. χ^2 statistical comparisons versus control group (CONV) frequency: $^*p < 0.05$; $^+p < 0.02$; $^{**}p < 0.005$; $^{++}p < 0.001$; N, not significant).

from therapy was roughly uniform over the spectrum of disease severity. Those lesions that did regress improved by an average of 19 ± 12 (SD)% stenosis or by an average of 16 ± 5% stenosis after exclusion of regression from recanalization of 12 initially occluded arteries. Thus (Fig. 5), only a few lesions (about 5%) undergo natural, or spontaneous regression by the criterion amount of ≤10% S. Although this number can be significantly increased (to about 12%) by lipid-lowering therapy, the great majority of stenoses do not improve even with "intensive" regimens that result in marked alterations in the lipid and lipoprotein profile. Yet, these regimens are commonly associated with much more substantial reductions in clinical event rate (Table 2). We will return later to this apparent paradox.

PREVENTING PROGRESSION

Pathological Processes

This section focuses briefly on several clinically important aspects of plaque biology: lipid accumulation in the foam cells and core region, disruption of plaques and their healing, and variation in vasoconstrictor tone.

Arterial Lipid Accumulation

Both LDL and, more recently, Lp(a) have been localized in the intimal extracellular space, the cholesterol content of which has been shown to originate from plasma LDL cholesterol (52–55). Intimal lipid also accumulates in subendothelial monocyte-derived macrophages (56,57). Such "foam cell" formation is thought to occur by unregulated scavenger receptor uptake of oxidized LDL (58,59) and possibly of Lp(a) (60,61) by macrophages. Smooth muscle cells may also become foam cells. Foam cells are abundant in precursor fatty streak lesions (62), in the cap of early fibrous plaques, and in the shoulders, cap, and basilar neovascular complex of advanced plaques (63). Lipid may enter the core region of the fibrous plaque by transmural flux (64) of its more mobile forms (lipoprotein particles, droplets, and vesicles) (65,66), or it may be deposited there as a result of foam cell necrosis (62,67). There, lipids coalesce into lower-energy phases dictated by the local cholesterol, phospholipid, and cholesteryl ester concentrations (22). Cholesteryl ester droplets and vesicles and cholesterol monohydrate crystals are the dominant core lipids (22,63). The flux of small perifibrous lipid droplets through the endothelium has been thought to initiate core lipid accumulation in the earliest human aortic lesions (65,68). The subsequent contribution of foam cell necrosis to its continued accumulation in the larger mature fibrous plaques remains to be determined. This last question is a key one because of the proposed therapeutic role of antioxidants (58), which, by preventing LDL oxidation, may act to prevent foam cell formation and, ultimately, core lipid accumulation.

Arterial Lipid Content

It is unclear why certain patients or certain arterial segments develop lipid-rich plaques while adjacent segments have the more stable fibrous intimal involvement. Roberts and co-workers (69,72) have studied plaque composition as it relates to certain aspects of the spectrum of clinical atherosclerosis. Briefly, by quantitative morphometry of the histological section, they have determined the proportion of intimal area that is contributed by each of the principal plaque components: (a) dense fibrous tissue, (b) cellular fibrous tissue, (c) calcific deposits, (d) inflammatory infiltrates, (e) extracellular core lipid (as "pultaceous debris"), and (f) foam cell lipid (69). They separated serially sampled arterial sections into four ranges of lumen area reduction. They found, on average, that early intimal involvement is almost entirely fibrocellular, but at the stage of severe arterial obstruction, the cellular contribution has declined to about 25% of total intimal area while dense fibrous tissue occupies about 50%. Foam cells appear in some numbers when intimal involvement is moderate; their fraction increases to 10% of the area in the more severe stages and then declines in the most severe. Calcific deposits and extracellular lipid become relatively abundant in the more severe stages; each increases progressively to contribute about 10% of intimal area in the most severe. Younger women (<40 years) with CAD were found to have significantly less dense fibrous tissue and more cellular connective tissue and lipid-rich foam cells than their older male counterparts, suggesting a greater potential for reversibility (70). Conversely, the very elderly showed a tendency toward a more fibrotic disease and had significantly fewer foam cells than younger men and women (71). A single patient with plasma cholesterol exceeding 700 mg/dl as a result of homozygous familial hypercholesterolemia had advanced diffuse and focal intimal disease that, surprisingly, consisted almost entirely of dense fibrous tissue (72). This finding is consistent with the idea that intimal cholesterol is fibrogenic (24) and that more advanced disease is more fibrous but also points out that intimal lipid accumulation may not be strongly determined by the degree of plasma lipid elevation. Indeed, age or antioxidant status or the specific lipid phenotype or tissue genotype may be a more important determinant of lipid content. Further studies are needed.

Plaque Disruption

As described below, the structural disruption, or fissuring, of plaques is now recognized as the critical event triggering abrupt arterial occlusion and ischemia. Also, "silent" fissuring can occur in the absence of ischemic symptoms (11,73,74), possibly defining another mechanism of plaque growth. By this mechanism, mural thrombus, or that formed at sites of intraplaque hemorrhage, can undergo ingrowth and organization by smooth muscle cells, thus expanding the plaque connective tissue mass. Evidence supporting this proposed mechanism of fibrogenesis is described elsewhere (11,74,75).

Vasoconstrictor Tone

Increased vasoconstrictor tone may contribute to progressive luminal narrowing. Atherosclerosis affects vascular tone by interfering with the endothelial production and normal release of the endogenous vasodilator, EDRF, which is nitric oxide (NO) or an analog (15–18,76–78). Endothelial NO dysfunction appears to account for the apparently paradoxical epicardial coronary vasoconstrictor effects of isometric and aerobic exercise in patients with CAD (79,80). Because the impairment of vasodilatory function is experimentally reversed by reducing dietary cholesterol (81) despite persistence of intimal thickening, and because vascular smooth muscle responsiveness to direct dilators is largely unaltered by atherosclerosis, it is felt that vasorelaxant dysfunction is caused by a direct effect of the atherogenic state on the endothelial release of EDRF. The mechanism of impairment is unknown, but LDL cholesterol and, more specifically, oxidized LDL have been implicated (81–83).

Evidence in Humans

Evidence that lipid-lowering therapy can effectively retard progression of atherosclerotic arterial obstruction in patients dates to 1979 (26). The composite of such data from randomized arteriographic trials is summarized in Table 2. Again, despite the diversity of these trials, the evidence for reduced lesion progression in the treated patients is surprisingly consistent. Approximately one-half of the control group patients in Table 2 were judged to have worsening arterial obstruction during the study period; by contrast, about one-fourth of the treated patients worsened (a 50% reduction from control). Again, the data of Fig. 2 from FATS illustrate this comparison (34).

Figure 5 shows that the likelihood of a lesion's progression is, in part, determined by its baseline severity. Intensive lipid-lowering therapy decreases, by about fourfold, the likelihood of definite lesion progression among mild and moderate lesions but does not appear to similarly benefit the severe lesions studied, although the number studied was too small to reach any conclusions.

PREVENTING PLAQUE DISRUPTION AND CLINICAL EVENTS

Prevention of Clinical Events

The landmark Lipid Research Clinics Coronary Primary Prevention Trial (84) demonstrated that clinical coronary events, but not cardiac or total mortality, were significantly reduced (−19%) in association with a 9% reduction, relative to the dietary control, in total cholesterol and a 13% reduction in LDL cholesterol, accomplished with diet and cholestyramine. Importantly, the magnitude of cardiovascular benefit correlated with the degree of total and of LDL cholesterol reduction (85). The Helsinki Heart Trial (86) also achieved a significant reduction in total cardiac events but not mortality. And the 15-year follow-up of the Coronary Drug Project showed highly significant 11% reductions in cardiac and all-cause mortality attributable to niacin therapy (87).

Table 2 provides additional evidence that clinical cardiac events are decreased by lipid-lowering therapy. Each trial reports events somewhat differently. In general, when reported, we have classified as clinical events cardiac death, confirmed myocardial infarction, and progressive or unstable ischemia requiring revascularization. The data from FATS in Table 2 demonstrate a 70–80% reduction in event rate ($p < 0.01$) compared to control among intensively treated patients. Thus, clinical cardiovascular events are clearly reduced by lipid-lowering therapy in the primary prevention trials and in the angiographic trials. The recently published 4S Study (88) adds to the now-irrefutable evidence that secondary prevention with lipid-lowering therapy provides major clinical benefit. In this group of 4,444 men and women with a history of myocardial infarction, a 38% LDL cholesterol reduction with simvastatin in the treated group was associated with a 42% reduction, relative to the control group, in cardiac death and a 30% reduction in all-cause mortality ($p = 0.003$). It is noteworthy that clinical benefits have been statistically significant only in trials with an entry requirement for lipid elevation. Indeed, the amount of risk reduction seems out of proportion, with the average regression in lesion severity being only 1–2% stenosis and with the fact that only about 12% of all intensively treated lesions actually regress (Fig. 5). To understand how regression of a small number of lesions can result in a substantial clinical benefit, we must understand the series of events in the plaque that turn a stable quiescent lesion into an unstable culprit lesion triggering a clinical event.

Determinants of Plaque Disruption

Acute ischemic syndromes are most commonly precipitated when sites of mild or moderate atherosclerotic narrowing become disruptively transformed into severely obstructive culprit lesions. As seen in Fig. 1B, such a transformation usually involves fissuring of the fibrous cap of the atheroma, often with intramural hemorrhage and mural or occlusive thrombus. The plaque at high risk for such fissuring and subsequent hemorrhage or thrombosis usually has a large core lipid pool and a structurally weakened fibrous cap. The cap can be weakened by the migration or death of its smooth muscle cells, by an accumulation of lipid-laden macrophages, or by proteolytic or mechanical damage to its collagen. Evolving insights into three major aspects of atherosclerosis have greatly altered our understanding of the precipitation of plaque events leading to acute clinical events.

First, mild and moderate coronary lesions (<70% stenosis) may progress abruptly to severe obstruction, with resulting unstable angina, myocardial infarction, or death. In fact, a majority of clinical events occur under these circumstances (9,89–91). Among 32 patients undergoing successful thrombolytic therapy for acute MI, the severity of the atherosclerotic stenosis underlying the thrombotic occlusion was measured at less than 50% diameter stenosis in one-third of cases and between 50% and 60% stenosis in another third (9). Similarly, when the lesion precipitating an MI has, by chance, been seen on a recent angiogram, its preinfarct severity averages 50% stenosis, and its morphology will not usually suggest that it is destined soon to become occluded (9,89–91). Although a given severe (≥70%) lesion is more likely to progress or totally occlude than those of the less severe variety, clinical events are more frequently triggered by lesions that are initially mild or moderate, because (a) these are much more numerous in the patient's anatomy (92), and (b) because the majority of occlusions of severe stenoses occur without an event (93).

A second insight was originally brought into focus by Constantinides (94) but has received renewed attention (11,73,74,95–100). It is that, for the great majority of ischemic coronary events, a "culprit" lesion can be identified with variations of the following morphological features at histological examination, as illustrated in Fig. 1B: (a) a fissure, tear, or vent in the fibrous cap overlying the core lipid pool, (b) a thrombus adherent at the site of the fissure, (c) bleeding into the core lipid region, and (d) severe arterial obstruction by the composite mass of expanded plaque and thrombus. Angiographic examples of plaques that have become unstable and caused a clinical event are shown in Fig. 6. One can imagine the pathogenesis of each of these arteriographic examples in terms of the histologic section in Fig. 1B. Figure 6A shows a hemorrhagic pocket in the atheroma connected to the lumen by a narrow-necked fissure or vent. In such cases, it has long been debated whether increased internal pressure in the plaque (from bleeding or an inflammatory abscess) has burst the fibrous cap into the lumen or whether a primary fissure in the plaque permits bleeding into its core region. Figure 6B is almost certainly an example of hemorrhage into the plaque, via an upstream fissure from the lumen, with resultant expansion of the plaque and ob-

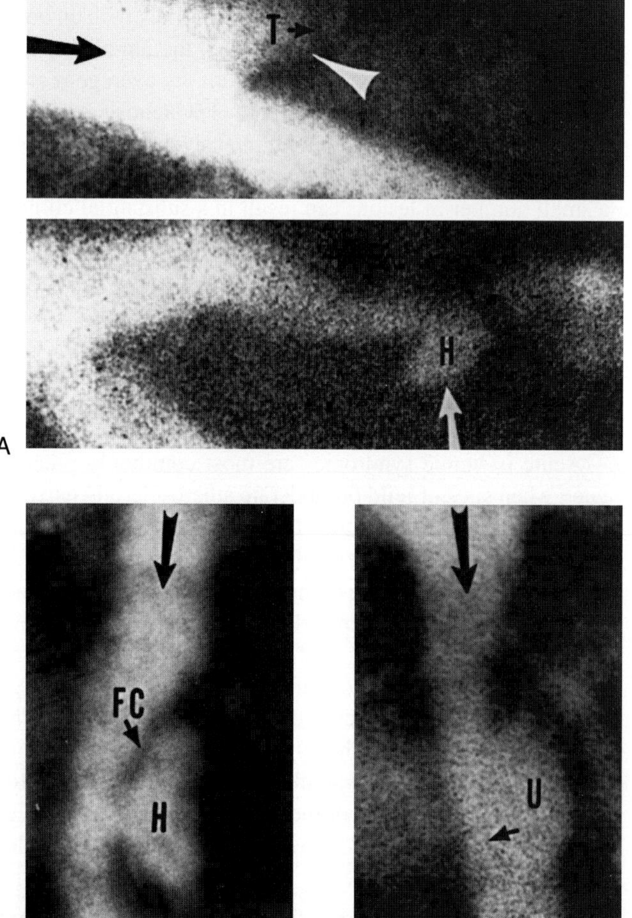

FIG. 6. Highly magnified arteriographic images of structurally unstable plaques causing unstable angina or myocardial infarction. **A:** This LAD is acutely occluded; 24 h after t-PA IV, the thrombotic component (T) of the obstruction is lysed, revealing a pocket of contrast (H) protruding beyond the lumen boundaries into presumed plaque and fed through a narrow-necked fissure. This appears to be the arteriographic counterpart of the hemorrhagic pocket (H) in Fig. 1B. **B:** Angiographically visualized plaque hemorrhage. Bleeding into the lipid-rich core of the plaque appears to have formed a hemorrhagic pocket (H), which has driven the thin fibrous cap (FC) into the lumen, progressively obstructing it. The opposite wall has been remodeled, curving outward in order to preserve lumen size in the face of the expanding plaque. On cine, contrast enters this pocket from the lumen via small breaks or channels at its upstream shoulder and exits via a mid-FC vent. **C:** A large ulcer (U) is seen after t-PA for unstable angina. This image appears to have been created by full-length erosion or eruption of the fibrous cap, of which only a thin arteriographic vestige remains *(arrow).*

struction of flow when the fibrous cap was forced into the lumen. Figure 6C illustrates an angiographic finding described as "ulceration of the plaque." It may have been formed by mechanical or proteolytic erosion of a thin fibrous cap to unroof the core lipid region or by an eruptive venting of a hemorrhagic plaque.

A third insight is that there are features of plaque structure and lipid composition that predict the risk of fissuring. Fissures of the arterial intima rarely occur in the absence of atheroma. Among patients dying of noncardiac causes, new fissures can be found in 9–17%, suggesting that not all fissures progress to severe obstruction (74). The greater the core lipid content, the greater the likelihood of fissuring. In a detailed histological assessment of 86 infarct lesions, an intimal fissure extended from the lumen into an unstructured pool of extracellular lipid in 83% of cases (97,99), as illustrated in Fig. 1B. Yet, in any given patient, only a small subgroup of all plaques (perhaps one in eight) has a substantial core lipid accumulation. Certain aspects of fibrous cap composition also heighten the risk of fissuring. The macrophage density in fissured caps is greater than that in intact caps (95,96). Fissuring occurs most commonly at the shoulder of an eccentric lipid-rich plaque (Fig. 1B), a location of high macrophage density (97) and also of high circumferential stress when there is significant core lipid, according to computer models of cyclic pulsatile distention of the diseased arterial cross section (97,98). Finally, the fibrous cap is thinned and weakened by the disappearance of smooth muscle cells and by lysis of collagen. Cytotoxic agents, including macrophage secretory products and oxidatively modified LDL (105–108), can transform a viable and structurally intact cap (Fig. 1A) into one that is thinned and acellular and thus much more susceptible to fissuring (Fig. 1B).

This perception of plaque disruption as a "passive" process related to the softness and size of the core lipid pool and the strength of the fibrous cap is being refined as our understanding of the "active" macrophage inflammatory mechanisms evolves. Atherectomy specimens from culprit lesions for unstable angina have a significantly higher macrophage content than those from stable angina lesions (101). Macrophages release metalloproteinases such as interstitial collagenase, gelatinase, and stromalysin, all of which have been identified in atherosclerotic plaques (102) and in cultured macrophages (103). The inflammatory aspect of macrophages and T cells is emphasized by Van der Wal et al. (100), who found intimal rupture into a large core lipid pool in only 12 (60%) of 20 infarct lesions but uniformly identified increased macrophage density at focal sites of plaque erosion or disruption and also demonstrated focal expression of HLA-DR inflammatory antigens. This emphasis is supported by the seminal studies of Davies et al. (104) and by Fuster et al. (11). The extent to which these inflammatory changes occur after the rupture remains to be determined.

Prevention of Plaque Disruption

As described above, plaque fissuring is predicted by certain lipid-related plaque features including macrophage foam cell density, core lipid pool size, and possible cytotoxicity from oxidized LDL. Reduction of plasma LDL would be expected to reduce the likelihood of fissuring because of the experimentally documented favorable effects of LDL lowering on these predictors. As a clinical consequence, LDL-lowering therapy ought to decrease the frequency of abrupt progression to clinical events. Indeed, this has been the case. Analysis of 13 coronary events among 146 FATS patients reveals that each event was precipitated by a culprit coronary lesion in the distribution of worsening ischemia that had progressed significantly in severity from the baseline stenosis measurement to that at the time of the event (34). As seen in Fig. 7, the "culprit" lesions causing the great majority (eight of nine) of cardiac events among the conventionally treated patients, arose from a pool of 414 lesions that were mild or moderate at baseline. By comparison, only one of 683 such lesions progressed to an event in the two intensively treated patient groups ($p < 0.004$ per patient or per lesion). However, lesions severe (≥70% stenosis) at baseline did not appear to benefit from lipid lowering; three of 36 such lesions among the intensively treated and one of 16 among conventionally treated patients progressed to cause an event (p = NS).

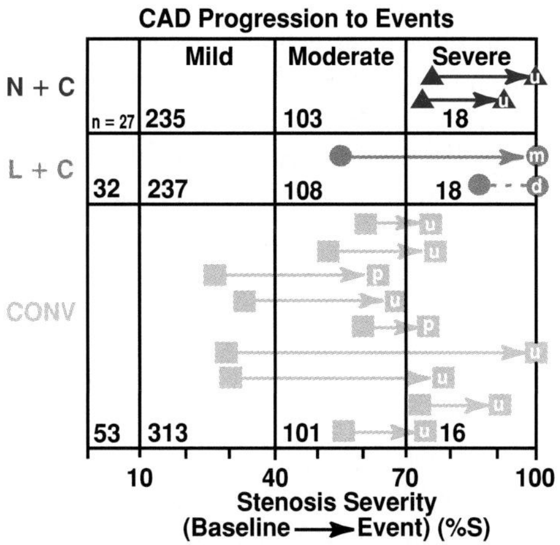

FIG. 7. Lesion changes associated with the 13 coronary events as measured from 1,316 lesions in 120 FATS patients. Among lesions exposed to intensive lipid-lowering therapy, only one of 683 mild or moderate lesions, at baseline, among 74 such patients progressed to a clinical event (see Fig. 5 for definitions), while eight of 414 such lesions among 46 conventionally treated patients did so (per patient or per lesion, $p < 0.004$). By this standard, severe lesions did not appear to benefit from therapy. N, niacin; C, colestipol; L, lovastatin; CONV, conventional therapy; U, unstable angina event; M, myocardial infarction; D, death; P, progressive angina; %S, percentage diameter stenosis. The number in each panel represents the number of lesions at risk, at baseline, in each subgroup.

LIPID DEPLETION FOR PLAQUE AND CLINICAL STABILITY: A HYPOTHESIS THAT FITS THE FACTS

Observations

- Of unstable clinical episodes (e.g., myocardial infarction), 60% to 90% result from disruption and thrombosis of lipid-rich plaques (73,94–96,99–101,104).
- Plaque lipid may be depleted by normalizing elevated plasma cholesterol (19–23):
  - —Lipid-laden macrophages (foam cells) disappear within 6 months (20–22).
  - —Core lipid volume begins to diminish after 6 months (22).
  - —After 2 years, 60% of plaque cholesterol is depleted (20).
  - —Plaque shrinkage is primarily caused by cholesteryl ester depletion (20,22).
- Plaque instability is predicted by its lipid-related features (73):
  - —Area of the core lipid region as a percentage of total plaque area (104).
  - —Foam cell content of fibrous cap and shoulder regions (73,94–97,99–101).
  - —Foam cell stromalysin, one of a family of inflammatory metalloproteinases that can weaken the fibrous cap (102,103).
- Only about 15% of human coronary lesions are lipid-rich plaques (more than 50% lipid by volume) (104).
- Only about 12% of all coronary lesions visibly regress (≥10% stenosis change) with intensive lipid lowering (34).
- Clinical benefits from intensive lipid lowering are associated with a 10-fold reduction in the frequency of abrupt progression of mild or moderate coronary lesions to become severe lesions (34; Fig. 7).

Unifying Hypothesis

Angiographic coronary stenosis regression, seen in 12% of all coronary lesions during intensive lipid-lowering therapy, reflects depletion of cholesteryl esters selectively from the "vulnerable" subgroup of lipid-, and foam-cell-rich lesions, which comprise about 15% of all visible coronary lesions. Such lipid depletion typically reduces stenosis severity by 10–20% but, more importantly, stabilizes the plaque in terms of its mechanical strength and endothelial functional integrity. The plaque fibrous cap is strengthened by favorable geometric changes and by a marked reduction in the number of intimal inflammatory cells (macrophages and T lymphocytes) that secrete proteolytic enzymes. Plaque stabilization by these mechanisms appears to explain the substantial reduction of clinical events associated with intensive lipid lowering.

SUMMARY

The consensus of evidence from angiographic trials demonstrates both coronary artery and clinical benefits from lipid lowering, using any of a variety of treatment regimens. The findings of decreased arterial disease progression and increased regression have been convincing but, at best, modest in their magnitude. For example, among those treated intensively in FATS, the mean improvement in proximal stenosis severity was less than 1% stenosis per patient, and only 12% of all lesions showed convincing regression. In view of these modest arterial benefits, the associated reductions in cardiovascular events have been surprisingly great. For example, coronary events were reduced 75% in FATS; this was entirely explained by a 93% reduction in the likelihood that a mildly or moderately diseased arterial segment would experience substantial progression to become the severe lesion that triggered the clinical event.

We believe the magnitude of the clinical benefit is best explained in terms of this observation, using the following lines of reasoning. Clinical events most commonly spring from lesions that are initially of mild or moderate severity and that abruptly undergo a disruptive transformation to a severe "culprit" lesion. The process of plaque fissuring leading to plaque disruption and thrombosis triggers most clinical coronary events. Fissuring is predicted by a large accumulation of core lipid in the plaque and by a high density of plaque-laden macrophages in its thinned fibrous cap. Lesions with these characteristics comprise only 10–20% of the overall lesion population but account for 80–90% of the acute clinical events. In the experimental setting, normalization of an atherogenic lipid profile substantially decreases the number of lipid-laden intimal macrophages (foam cells) and gradually depletes cholesterol from the core lipid pool. In the clinical setting, intensive lipid lowering virtually halts the progression of mild and moderate lesions to severe obstructions precipitating clinical events.

In conclusion, the reduction in clinical events observed in these trials appears to be best explained by the relationship of the lipid and foam cell content of the plaque to its likelihood of fissuring and by the effects of lipid-lowering therapy on these "high-risk" features of plaque morphology. The composite of data presented here supports the hypothesis that lipid-lowering therapy selectively lipid-depletes (regresses) that relatively small but dangerous subgroup of fatty lesions containing a large lipid core and dense clusters of intimal macrophages. These lesions are thereby effectively stabilized, and clinical event rate is accordingly decreased.

FUTURE DIRECTIONS

The concept that abrupt disruption of the atherosclerotic plaque, with associated thrombosis, precipitates cardiovascular events is now firmly embedded in our understanding of the pathogenesis of clinical coronary disease. Several current lines of investigation relate to mechanisms of plaque instability. These include studies of (a) histocytochemistry and in situ hybridization to identify biochemical or cellular markers of plaque vulnerability; (b) plaque structure and connective tissue strength as determinants of plaque instability; (c) the role of endothelial functional in vasorelaxation and resistance to thrombosis; (d) the role of the various plaque lipid pools in relation to plaque vulnerability; (e) the role of circulating lipid levels (both LDL cholesterol and HDL cholesterol and their subfractions) in the dynamics of plaque lipid accumulation or depletion; (f) the role of antioxidants in the process(es) of plaque lipid accumulation in these pools; and (g) the role of arterial remodeling as a means of adapting to these pathological processes.

In the coming decade, it appears likely that the human intrusive atherosclerotic plaque and its associated diffuse intimal disease, vasomotor dysfunction, and adaptive remodeling will be intensively probed using newly emerging techniques, which include intravascular ultrasound, magnetic resonance imaging, catheter-based segmental therapy including gene transfer techniques, and examination of plaque tissues obtained at directional coronary atherectomy.

Based on our current understanding, we believe that these methods will be applied to test the clinically relevant hypothesis that cholesteryl ester depletion from foam cells and from the core lipid region of plaques will stabilize the plaque against clinically important disruptive changes. Further studies will address means for enhancing such lipid depletion. The role of HDL, especially apo A-I, and Lp(a) in these processes will be better defined.

ACKNOWLEDGMENTS

The efforts of Robert P. Kelly, Betsy Sayler, Lynn Hillger, and Dianne Sacco in preparing this manuscript are greatly appreciated. This chapter has been extensively modified from an article published previously (35).

This work was supported in part by NIH grants R01 HL 19451, P01 HL 30086, and R01 HL 42419 from the National Heart, Lung and Blood Institute, in part by the University of Washington Clinical Research Center (NIH #RR37), by a grant (NIH DK 35816) to the Clinical Nutrition Research Unit, and in part by a grant from the John L. Locke, Jr. Charitable Trust, Seattle, Washington.

REFERENCES

1. Demer LL, Gould KL, Goldstein RA, Kirkeeide RL, Mullani NA, Smalling RW, Nishikawa A, Merhige ME. Assessment of coronary artery disease severity by positron emission tomography. Comparison with quantitative arteriography in 193 patients. *Circulation* 1989;79: 825–835.
2. Klocke FJ. Measurements of coronary flow reserve: Defining pathophysiology versus making decisions about patient care. *Circulation* 1987;76:1183–1189.
3. Ludmer PL, Selwyn AP, Shook TL, et al. Paradoxical vasoconstriction induced by acetylcholine in atherosclerotic coronary arteries. *N Engl J Med* 1986;315:1046–1051.
4. Nabel EG, Selwyn AP, Ganz P. Large coronary arteries in humans are responsive to changing blood flow: An endothelium-dependent mechanism that fails in patients with atherosclerosis. *J Am Coll Cardiol* 1990;16:349–356.
5. Kaski JC, Crea F, Meran DO, Rodriguez LG, Aranjo L, Chierchia S, Davies G, Maseri A. Local coronary supersensitivity to diverse vasoconstrictive stimuli in patients with variant angina. *Circulation* 1986;74:1255–1265.
6. Cannon RO, Camici PG, Epstein SE. Pathophysiological dilemma of syndrome X. *Circulation* 1992;85:883–892.
7. Loscalzo J, Dzau VJ. Flow activates an endothelium potassium channel to release an endogenous nitrovasodilator. *J Clin Invest* 1991;88: 1663–1671.
8. Brown BG, Bolson EL, Pierce CD, Peterson RB, Dodge HT. Regression of atherosclerosis in man: Current data and their methodological limitations. In: Malinkow MR, Blaton VH, eds. *Regression of Atherosclerotic Lesions*. New York: Plenum Press; 1984:289–310.
9. Brown BG, Gallery CA, Badger RS, Kennedy JW, Mathey D, Bolson EL, Dodge HT. Incomplete lysis of thrombus in the moderate underlying atherosclerotic lesion during intracoronary infusion of streptokinase for acute myocardial infarction: Quantitative angiographic observations. *Circulation* 1986;73:653–661.
10. TIMI IIIA Investigators. Early effects of tissue-type plasminogen activator added to conventional therapy on the culprit coronary lesion in patients presenting with ischemic cardiac pain at rest. Results of the Thrombolysis in Myocardial Ischemia (TIMI IIIA) Trial. *Circulation* 1993;87:1–14.
11. Fuster V, Badimon L, Badimon JJ, Chesebro JH. The pathogenesis of coronary artery disease and the acute coronary syndromes. *N Engl J Med* 1992;326:242–250;310–318.
12. Glasgov S, Weisenberg E, Zarins CK, Stankunavicius R, Kolettis GJ. Compensatory enlargement of human atherosclerotic coronary arteries. *N Engl J Med* 1987;316:1371–1375.
13. Langille BL, O'Donnell F. Reductions in arterial diameter produced by chronic decreases in blood flow are endothelium-dependent. *Science* 1986;231:405–407.
14. Jaffe RB, Glancy DC, Epstein SE, Brown BG, Morrow AG. Coronary arterial-right heart fistulae: Long-term observations in seven patients. *Circulation* 1973;47:133–143.
15. McLenachan JM, Williams JK, Fish RD, Ganz P, Selwyn AP. Loss of flow-mediated endothelium-dependent dilation occurs early in the development of atherosclerosis. *Circulation* 1991;84:1273–1278.
16. Furchgott RF, Zawadzki JV. The obligatory role of endothelial cells in the relaxation of arterial smooth muscle by acetylcholine. *Nature* 1980;299:373–376.
17. Furchgott RF, Vanhoutte PM. Endothelium-derived relaxing and contracting factors. *FASEB J* 1989;3:2007–2018.
18. Selke FW, Armstrong ML, Harrison DG. Endothelium-dependent vascular relaxation is abnormal in the coronary microcirculation of atherosclerotic primates. *Circulation* 1990;81:1568–1593.
19. Wissler RW, Vesselinovitch D. Can atheroscleroic plaques regress? Anatomic and biochemical evidence from nonhuman animal models. *Am J Cardiol* 1990;65:33–40.
20. Armstrong ML, Megan MB. Lipid depletion in atheromatous coronary arteries in rhesus monkeys after regression diets. *Circ Res* 1972;30: 675–680.
21. Clarkson TB, Bond MG, Bullock BC, Marzetta CA. A study of atherosclerosis regression in *Macaca mulatta*. IV. Changes in coronary arteries from animals with atherosclerosis induced for 19 months and then regressed for 24 or 48 months at plasma cholestrol concentrations of 300 or 200 mg/dl. *Exp Mol Pathol* 1981;34:345–368.
22. Small DM, Bond MG, Waugh D, Prack M, Sawyer JK. Physiochemical and histological changes in the arterial wall of nonhuman primates during progression and regression of atherosclerosis. *J Clin Invest* 1984;73:1590–1605.
23. Armstrong MC, Megan MB. Arterial fibrous protein in cynomolgus monkeys after atherogenic and regression diets. *Circ Res* 1975;36: 256–261.
24. Brown BG, Fry DL. The fate and fibrogenic potential of subintimal implants of crystalline lipid in the canine aorta. Quantitative histological and autoradiographic studies. *Circ Res* 1978;43:261–273.
25. Carew TE, Schwenke DC, Steinberg D. An antiatherogenic effect of

probucol unrelated to its hypocholesterolemic effect: Evidence that antioxidants *in vivo* can selectively inhibit low density lipoprotein degradation in macrophage-rich streaks slowing the progression of atherosclerosis in the WHHL rabbit. *Proc Natl Acad Sci USA* 1987; 84:7725–7729.

26. Kuo PT, Hayase K, Kostic JB, Moreyra AE. Use of combined diet and colestipol in long-term (7–7.5 years) treatment of patients with Type II hyperlipoproteinemia. *Circulation* 1979;59:199–214.
27. Brensike JF, Levy RI, Kelsey SF, et al. Effects of therapy with cholestyramine on progression of coronary atherosclerosis: Results of the NHLBI Type II coronary intervention study. *Circulation* 1984;69: 313–324.
28. Duffield RGM, Lewis B, Miller NE, Jamieson CW, Brunt JNH, Colchester ACF. Treatment of hyperlipidemia retards progression of symptomatic femoral atherosclerosis. *Lancet* 1983;ii:639–642.
29. Nash DT, Gensini G, Esente P. Effect of lipid lowering therapy on the progression of coronary atherosclerosis assessed by scheduled repetitive coronary arteriography. *Int J Cardiol* 1982;2:43–55.
30. Nikkila EA, Viikinkoski P, Valle M, Frick MH. Prevention of progression of coronary atherosclerosis by treatment of hyperlipidemia: A seven-year prospective angiographic study. *Br Med J* 1984;289: 220–223.
31. Blankenhorn DH, Nessim SA, Johnson RL, Sanmarco ME, Azen SP, Cachin-Hamphill L. Beneficial effects of colestipol niacin therapy on coronary atherosclerosis and coronary venous bypass grafts. *JAMA* 1987;257:3233–3240.
32. Buchwald H, Matts JP, Ritch LL, Compos CT, et al. Effect of partial ileal bypass on mortality and morbidity from coronary heart disease in patients with hypercholesterolemia—Report of the Program on Surgical Control of the Hyperlipidemias (POSCH). *N Engl J Med* 1990;323:946.
33. Ornish D, Brown SE, Scherwitz LW, et al. Can lifestyle changes reverse coronary heart disease? *Lancet* 1990;336:129–133.
34. Brown BG, Albers JJ, Fisher LD, et al. Regression of coronary artery disease as a result of intensive lipid-lowering therapy in men with high levels of apolipoprotein B. *N Engl J Med* 1990;323:1289–1298.
35. Brown BG, Zhao X-Q, Sacco DE, Albers JJ. Lipid lowering and plaque regression. New insights into prevention of plaque disruption and clinical events in coronary disease. *Circulation* 1993;87: 1781–1791.
36. Cashin-Hemphill L, Mack WJ, Pogoda MJ, Sanmarco ME, Azen SP, Blankenhorn DH. Beneficial effects of colestipol–niacin on coronary atherosclerosis. *JAMA* 1990;264:3013–3017.
37. Kane JP, Malloy MJ, Ports TA, et al. Regression of coronary atherosclerosis during treatment of familial hypercholesterolemia with combined drug regimens. *JAMA* 1990;264:3007.
38. Watts GF, Lewis B, Brunt JNH, Lewis ES, et al. Effects on coronary artery disease of lipid-lowering diet, or diet plus cholestyramine, in the St. Thomas' Atherosclerosis Regression Study (STARS). *Lancet* 1992;339:563–569.
39. Alderman E, Haskell WL, Fain JM, Superko HR, Maron DJ, Champagne MA, Mackey SF, Williams PT, Krauss RM, Farquhar JW, et al. Beneficial angiographic and clinical response to multifactor modification in the Stanford Coronary Risk Intervention Project (SCRIP). *Circulation* 1991;84(Suppl II):II-140 (asbtr).
40. Schuler G, Hambrecht R, Schlierf G, Niebauer J, Hauer K, Neumann J, Hoberg E, Drinkmann A, Bacher F, Grunze M, Kubler W. Regular physical exercise and low-fat diet. Effects on progression of coronary artery disease. *Circulation* 1992;86:1–11.
41. Sacks F, Pasternak RC, Gibson CM, Rosner B, Stone PH. Effect on coronary atherosclerosis of decrease in plasma cholesterol concentrations in normocholesterolemic patients. *Lancet* 1994;344:1182–1186.
42. Blankenhorn DH, Azen SP, Kramsch DM, Mack WJ, Cashin-Hemphill L, Hodis HN, DeBoer LWV, Makrer PR, Masteller MJ, Vailas LI, Alaupovic P, Hirsch LJ. Coronary angiographic changes with lovastatin therapy: The Monitored Atherosclerosis Regression Study (MARS). *Ann Intern Med* 1993;119:967–976.
43. Waters D, Higginson L, Gladstone P, Kimball B, LeMay M, Boccuzzi JJ, Lesperance J. Effect of monotherapy with an HMG-CoA reductase inhibitor on the progression of coronary atherosclerosis as assessed by serial quantitative arteriography: The Canadian Coronary Atherosclerosis Intervention Trial. *Circulation* 1994;89:959–968.
44. Pitt B, Mancini GBJ, Ellis SG, Rosman HS, McGovern ME. Pravastatin Limitation of Atherosclerosis in the Coronary Arteries (PLAC I). *J Am Coll Cardiol* 1994;23(Suppl): 131A (abstr).
45. The MAAS Investigators. Effect of simvastatin on coronary atheroma: The Multicenter Anti-Atheroma Study (MAAS). *Lancet* 1994;344: 633–638.
46. Barth JD, Zanjee MMB, The REGRESS Research Group. Regression Growth Evaluation Statin Study (REGRESS). Study design and baseline characteristics in 600 patients. *Can J Cardiol* 1992;8:925–931.
47. Brown BG, Bolson EL, Dodge HT. Quantitative computer techniques for analyzing coronary arteriograms. *Prog Cardiovasc Dis* 1986;28: 403–418.
48. Stewart BF, Brown BG, Zhao X-Q, Hillger LA, Sniderman AD, Dowdy A, Fisher LD, Albers JJ. Benefits of lipid-lowering therapy in men with elevated apolipoprotein B are not confined to those with very high LDL-cholesterol. *J Am Coll Cardiol* 1994;23:899–906.
49. Levy RI, Brensike JF, Epstein SE, Kelsey SF, Passamani ER, Richardson JM, et al. The influence of changes in endothelial values induced by cholestyramine and diet on progression of coronary artery disease: Results of the NHLBI Type II Coronary Intervention Study. *Circulation* 1984;69:325–337.
50. Blankenhorn DH, Alaupovic P, Wickham E, Chin HP, Azen SP. Prediction of angiographic change in native human coronary arteries and aortocoronary bypass grafts. Lipid and non-lipid factors. *Circulation* 1990;81:470–476.
51. Maher VMG, Brown BF, Marcovina SM, Sacco D, Lin JT, Hillger LA, Alberts JJ. The adverse effect of lipoprotein (a) on coronary atherosclerosis and clinical events is eliminated by substantially lowering LDL cholesterol. *J Am Coll Cardiol* 1994;23:131A (abstr).
52. Smith EB. The relationship between plasma and tissue lipids in human atherosclerosis. *Adv Lipid Res* 1974;12:1–49.
53. Walton KW, Williamson N. Histological and immunofluorescent studies on the evolution of the human atheromatous plaque. *J Atheroscler Res* 1968;8:599–624.
54. Rath M, Niendorf A, Reblin T, Dietel M, Krebber H-J, Beisiegel U. Detection and quantification of lipoprotein (a) in the arterial wall of 107 coronary bypass patients. *Arteriosclerosis* 1989;9:579–592.
55. Cushing GL, Gaubatz JW, Nava ML, Burdick BJ, Bocan TMA, Guyton JR, Weilbaecker D, DeBakey ME, Lawrie GM, Morrisett JD. Quantitation and localization of apolipoproteins (a) and B in coronary artery bypass vein grafts resected at operation. *Arteriosclerosis* 1989; 9:593–603.
56. Gerrity RG. The role of monocyte in atherogenesis. I. Transition of blood-borne monocytes into foam cells in fatty lesions. *Am J Pathol* 1981;103:181–190.
57. Ross R. The pathogenesis of atherosclerosis—an update. *N Engl J Med* 1986;314:488–500.
58. Steinberg D, Parthasarathy S, Carew TE, Khoo JC, Witztum JL. Beyond cholesterol: Modifications of low-density lipoprotein that increase its atherogenicity. *N Engl J Med* 1989;320:915–924.
59. Berliner JA, Territo MC, Sevanian A, Ramin S, Kim JA, Barnshad B, Esterson M, Fogelman AM. Minimally modified LDL stimulates monocyte endothelial interactions. *J Clin Invest* 1990;85:1260–1266.
60. Yamaguchi J, Hoff MF. Apolipoprotein B accumulation and development of foam cell lesions in coronary arteries of hypercholesterolemic swine. *Lab Invest* 1984;51:325–332.
61. Krempler F, Kostner GM, Roscher A, Bolzano K, Sandhofer F. The interaction of human apoB containing lipoproteins with mouse peritoneal macrophages: A comparison of Lp(a) with LDL. *J Lipid Res* 1984;25:283–287.
62. Stary HC. Changes in the cells of atherosclerotic lesions as advanced lesions evolve in coronary arteries of children and young adults. In: *Pathobiology of the Human Atherosclerotic Plaque*. Glagou S, Newman WP, Schaffer SA, eds. New York: Springer-Verlag; 1989: 93–106.
63. Guyton JR, Klemp KF. The lipid-rich core region of human atherosclerotic fibrous plaques. *Am J Pathol* 1989;1343:705–717.
64. Fry DL. Mass transport, atherogenesis, and risk. *Arteriosclerosis* 1987;7:88–100.
65. Guyton JR, Bocan TMA. Human aortic fibrolipid lesions. Progenitor lesions for fibrous plaques, exhibiting early formation of the cholesterol-rich core. *Am J Pathol* 1985;120:193–206.
66. Smith EB, Evans PH, Pownham MD. Lipid in the aorta intima: The correlation of morphologcial and chemical characteristics. *J Atheroscler Res* 1967;7:171–186.

67. Haust MD. The morphogenesis and fate of potential and early atherosclerotic lesions in man. *Hum Pathol* 1971;2:1–29.
68. Guyton JR, Bocan TM, Schifani TA. Quantitative ultrastrutcural analysis of perifibrous lipid and its association with elastin in nonatherosclerotic human aorta. *Arteriosclerosis* 1985;5:644–652.
69. Kragel AH, Reddy SG, Wittes JT, Roberts WC. Morphometric analysis of the composition of atherosclerotic plaques in the four major epicardial coronary arteries in acute myocardial infarction and in sudden coronary death. *Circulation* 1989;80:1747–1756.
70. Dollar AL, Kragel AH, Fernicola DJ, Waclaview MA, Roberts WC. Composition of atherosclerotic plaques in coronary arteries in women less than 40 years of age with fatal coronary artery disease and implications for plaque reversibility. *Am J Cardiol* 1991;67:1223–1227.
71. Gertz SD, Malezadah S, Dollar MA, Kragel AH, Roberts WC. Composition of atherosclerotic plaques in the four major epicardial coronary arteries in patients greater than or equal to 90 years of age. *Am J Cardiol* 1991;67:1228–1233.
72. Kragel AH, Roberts WC. Composition of atherosclerotic plaques in the coronary arteries in homozygous familial hypercholesterolemia. *Am Heart J* 1991;121:210–211.
73. Tracey RE, Devaney K, Kissling G. Characteristics of the plaque under a coronary thrombus. *Virchows Arch Pathol Anat* 1985;405: 411–427.
74. Davies MJ, Krikler DM, Katz D. Atherosclerosis: Inhibition or regression as therapeutic possibilities. *Br Heart J* 1991;65:302–310.
75. Duguid JB. Thrombosis as a factor in the pathogenesis of aortic atherosclerosis. *J Pathol Bacteriol* 1948;60:57–69.
76. Moncada S, Palmer RM, Higgs EA. Nitric oxide physiology, pathophysiology, and pharmacology. *Pharmacol Rev* 1991;43:109–142.
77. Stamler JS, Simon DI, Osborne JA, Mullins ME, Jaraki O, Michel T, Singel DJ, Loscalzo J. S-Nitrosylation of proteins with nitric oxide—synthesis and characterization of novel biologically active compounds. *Proc Natl Acad Sci USA* 1992;89:444–448.
78. Chilian WM, Dellsperger KC, Layne SM, Eastham CL, Armstrong MA, Marcus ML, Heistad DD. Effects of atherosclerosis on the coronary micro-circulation. *Am J Physiol* 1990;258:H529–539.
79. Brown BG, Lee AB, Bolson EL, Dodge HT. Reflex constriction of significant coronary stenosis as a mechanism contributing to ischemic ventricular dysfunction during isometric exercise. *Circulation* 1984; 70:18–24.
80. Hess OM, Bortone A, Eid K, Gage JE, Nonogi H, Grimm J, Krayenbuehl HP. Coronary vasomotor tone during static and dynamic exercise. *Eur Heart J* 1989;10(suppl F):105–110.
81. Harrison DG, Armstrong ML, Freeman PC, Heistad DD. Restoration of endothelium-dependent relaxation by dietary treatment of atherosclerosis. *J Clin Invest* 1987;80:808–811.
82. Vita JA, Treasure CB, Nabel EG, McLenachan JM, Fish RD, Yeung AC, Veksktein VI, Selwyn AP, Ganz P. Coronary vasomotor response to acetylcholine relates to risk factors for coronary artery disease. *Circulation* 1990;81:491–491.
83. Muegge A, Edwell JH, Peterson TE, Hofmeyer TG, Heistad DD, Harrison DD. Chronic treatment with polyethylene-glycolated superoxide dismutase partially restores endothelium-dependent vascular relaxations in cholesterol-fed rabbits. *Circ Res* 1991;69:1293–1300.
84. The Lipid Research Clinics Program. The Lipid Research Clinics Coronary Primary Prevention Trial Results: I. Reduction in incidence of coronary heart disease. *JAMA* 1984;251:351–364.
85. The Lipid Research Clinics Program. The Lipid Research Clinics Coronary Primary Prevention Trial Results: II. The relationship of reduction in incidence of coronary heart disease to cholesterol lowering. *JAMA* 1984;251:365–374.
86. Manninen V, Elo MO, Frick MH, et al. Lipid alterations and decline in the incidence of coronary heart disease in the Helsinki Heart Study. *JAMA* 1988;260:641–651.
87. Canner PL, Berge KG, Wenger NK, et al. Fifteen year mortality in Coronary Drug Project Patients: Long-term benefit with niacin. *J Am Coll Cardiol* 1986;8:1245–1255.
88. The 4S Investigators. Randomized trial of cholesterol lowering in 4,444 patients with coronary heart disease: The Scandinavian Simvastatin Survival Study (4S). *Lancet* 1994;344:1383–1389.
89. Ambrose JA, Tannenbaum MA, Alexopoulos D, et al. Angiographic progression of coronary artery disease and the develoment of myocardial infarction. *J Am Coll Cardiol* 1988;12:56–62.
90. Little WC, Constantinescu M, Applegate RM, et al. Can coronary angiography predict the site of a subsequent myocardial infarction in patients with mild-to-moderate coronary artery disease? *Circulation* 1988;78:1157–1166.
91. Little WC. Angiographic assessment of the culprit coronary artery lesion before acute myocardial infarction. *Am J Cardiol* 1990;66: 44G–47G.
92. Brown BG, Lin J-T, Kelsey S, Passamani ER, Levy RI, Dodge HT, Detre KM. Progression of coronary atherosclerosis in patients with probable familial hypercholesterolemia. Quantitative arteriographic assessment of patients in NHLBI Type II Study. *Arteriosclerosis* 1989;9(Suppl I):I-81–I-90.
93. Webster MWI, Chesebro JH, Smith HC, et al. Myocardial infarction and coronary artery occlusion: A prospective 5-year angiographic study. *J Am Coll Cardiol* 1990;15(Suppl A):218A (abstr).
94. Constantinides P. Plaque fissures in human coronary thrombosis. *J Atheroscler Res* 1966;6I:1–17.
95. Constantinides P. Plaque hemorrhages, their genesis and their role in supraplaque thrombosis and atherogenesis. In: Glagov S, Newman W, Schaffer SA, eds. *Pathobiology of the Human Atherosclerotic Plaque*. New York: Springer-Verlag; 1990:393–411.
96. Lendon CL, Davies MJ, Born GVR, Richardson PD. Atherosclerotic plaque caps are locally weakened when macrophage density is increased. *Atherosclerosis* 1991;87:87–90.
97. Richardson PD, Davies MJ, Born GVR. Influence of plaque configuration and stress distribution on fissuring of coronary atherosclerotic plaques. *Lancet* 1989;334:941–944.
98. Loree HM, Kamm RD, Strongfellow RG, Lee RT. Effects of fibrous cap thickness on peak circumferential stress in model atherosclerotic vessels. *Circ Res* 1992;71:850–858.
99. Davies MJ. A macro and micro view of coronary vascular insult in ischemic heart disease. *Circulation* 1990;82(Suppl II):II38–II46.
100. Van der Wal AC, Becker AE, Van der Loos CM, Das PK. Site of intimal rupture or erosion of thrombosed coronary atherosclerotic plaques is characterized by an inflammatory process irrespective of the dominant plaque morphology. *Circulation* 1994;89:36–44.
101. Moreno PR, Falk E, Palacios IF, Newell JB, Fuster V, Fallon JT. Macrophage infiltration in acute coronary syndromes: Implications for plaque rupture. *Circulation* 1994;90:775–778.
102. Shah PK, Falk E, Badimon JJ, Levy G, Fernandez-Oritz A, Fallon J, Fuster V. Human monocyte-derived macrophages express collagenase and induce collagen breakdown in atherosclerotic fibrous caps: Implication for plaque rupture. *Circulation* 1993;88(Suppl I):I-254 (abstr).
103. Henney AM, Wakeley PR, Davies MJ, Foster K, Hembrey R, Murphy G, Humphries S. Location of stromelysin gene in atherosclerotic plaques using in-site hybridization. *Proc Natl Acad Sci USA* 1991; 88:8154–8158.
104. Davies MJ, Richardson PD, Woolf N, Katz DR, Mann J. Risk of thrombosis in human atherosclerotic plaques: Role of extracellular lipid, macrophages, and smooth muscle cell content. *Br Heart J* 1993; 69:377–381.
105. Hessler JR, Morel DW, Lewis LJ, Chisolm GM. Lipoprotein oxidation and lipoprotein-induced cytotoxicity. *Arteriosclerosis* 1983;3: 215–222.
106. Kugiyama K, Kerns SA, Morrisett JD, Roberts R, Henry PD. Impairment of endothelium-dependent arterial relaxation by lysolecithin in modified low-density lipoproteins. *Nature* 1990;344:160–162.
107. Yla-Herttuala S, Palinski W, Rosenfeld ME, Parthasarathy S, Carew TE, Butler S, Witztum JL, Steinberg D. Evidence for the presence of oxidatively modified low density lipoprotein in atherosclerotic lesions of rabbit and man. *J Clin Invest* 1989;84:1086–1095.
108. Haberland M, Fong D, Cheng L. Malondialdehyde-altered protein occurs in atheroma of Watanabe heritable hyperlipidemic rabbits. *Science* 1988;24:215–218.

Hypertension

Atherosclerosis and Coronary Artery Disease,
edited by V. Fuster, R. Ross, and E. J. Topol.
Lippincott-Raven Publishers, Philadelphia © 1996.

CHAPTER 13

Genetics and Mechanisms

Steven C. Hunt, Paul N. Hopkins, and Roger R. Williams

Key Words: Genetic marker; Genetic linkage; Genetic association; Na–Li countertransport, Na–K ATPase transport; Familial dyslipidemic hypertension.

INTRODUCTION

Blood pressure is controlled by multiple physiologic systems, each with many components and all interrelated. Part of the difficulty in studying the causes of hypertension is that unless specific variables can be studied in isolation from other variables, their characteristics will be confounded by those other variables. At the same time, hypertension may result from defective interactions among variables, so that isolating a single variable may make it impossible to identify any defect. By studying the genetic mechanisms related to specific components of blood pressure control, specific abnormalities may be identified which can then be studied in combination with modifying factors.

Steven C. Hunt, Paul N. Hopkins, and Roger R. Williams: Department of Internal Medicine, University of Utah School of Medicine, Salt Lake City, Utah 84108.

Progress has been made in identifying specific variables that seem to be genetically controlled. Some of these variables show evidence of a single gene with large effects on the variation of a related phenotype. Some of these variables are also risk factors for cardiovascular disease. Whether these common factors lead directly to both hypertension and cardiovascular disease or whether they lead to hypertension which increases risk of cardiovascular disease is still being determined. This chapter will review the basic blood pressure control systems which have large genetic determination. The hypotheses relating high blood pressure to atherosclerosis and cardiovascular endpoints will also be discussed.

Knowledge about the basic physiology of blood pressure control is extensive and continues to increase as additional hormones, vessel responses, and receptors are identified. The multitude of control systems involved in regulation of blood pressure makes the study of the genetics of hypertension a challenge. The control system diagrams used by Guyton (1) have quantified many of the physiologic relationships and provide clues as to likely components of the blood pressure system that may be abnormal, resulting in elevated blood pressures. This chapter will review some of the basic mechanisms that have been suggested as candidates for abnormal blood pressure control due to genetic factors. The relationship of hypertension and these proposed genetic abnormalities to the development of cardiovascular disease will also be discussed.

Cardiovascular disease may develop from the direct effects of hypertension. Chronic elevation of blood pressure is known to induce structural alterations in the vasculature and in other organs. Hypertension may also cause associated physiologic systems to respond to the higher pressures, thereby changing other components related to increased risk of coronary disease. There may also be factors that lead to the development of both hypertension and coronary heart disease (CHD) independently, not requiring a direct relationship to exist between elevated pressure and coronary disease.

Hypertension clearly has multiple causes and is heterogeneous even within defined populations. One of the major research questions has been whether there are genes that have large, identifiable effects on the variation in blood pressure among individuals or whether genetic control is a result of small effects from many genes. Two problems with these studies are the heterogeneity of defects in blood pressure control and definition of the phenotype that should be used in the genetic studies. Heterogeneity masks the effects of any particular gene being studied because of the variation in a phenotype which is independent of the genetic mechanism of interest. Unless the genetic effect is strong or unless the population is subdivided to reduce heterogeneity, studies using blood pressure as a phenotype, or even using intermediate phenotypes associated with blood pressure, will be difficult. The epidemiology of blood pressure and its relationship to cardiovascular disease will be addressed to provide the rationale for phenotype definition and selection of candidate genes that are being investigated as contributors to hypertension development. It is not the purpose of this chapter to review the basic physiology of each system; however, major components that could be altered by a genetic abnormality will be described.

BLOOD PRESSURE AS A MAJOR CARDIOVASCULAR RISK FACTOR

Both coronary artery disease (CAD) and stroke are strongly and positively associated with blood pressure in a graded, independent, and consistent fashion, as shown in a meta-analysis of nine major prospective studies (2) (Fig. 1). Moreover, treatment of hypertension markedly decreased risk of stroke and modestly reduced coronary artery disease endpoints in multiple studies (3–6). Considering these trials together, treatment resulted in a significant reduction of coronary artery disease endpoints by 17% (95% confidence interval, CI, 10–23%), while stroke incidence declined 38% (95% CI 30–44%) (7). These results establish hypertension as a major, causal risk factor for cardiovascular disease. Systolic blood pressure is at least as predictive a risk factor as diastolic blood pressure, as shown in numerous prospective studies (8,9) and by the positive benefits realized by treating isolated systolic hypertension (4). In fact, CAD risk increases progressively with systolic pressure independently of diastolic pressure (10). Including systolic blood pressure

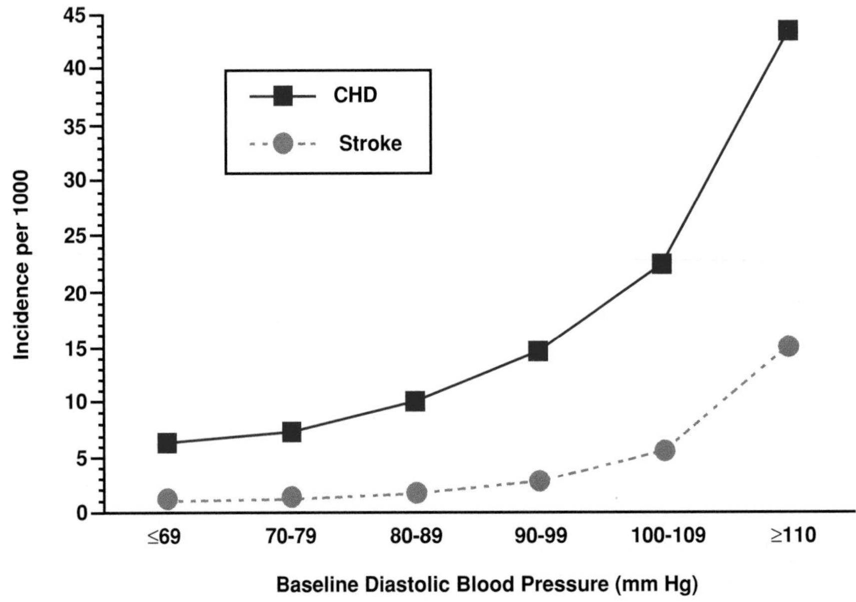

FIG. 1. Stroke and coronary heart disease (CHD) incidence rates (per 1,000 individuals) as a function of baseline diastolic blood pressure from nine prospective studies. Shown are raw, unadjusted incidence rates for men and women ages 25–84 years (though in most studies participants were males age 40–60 years). (Data from MacMahon et al., ref. 2.)

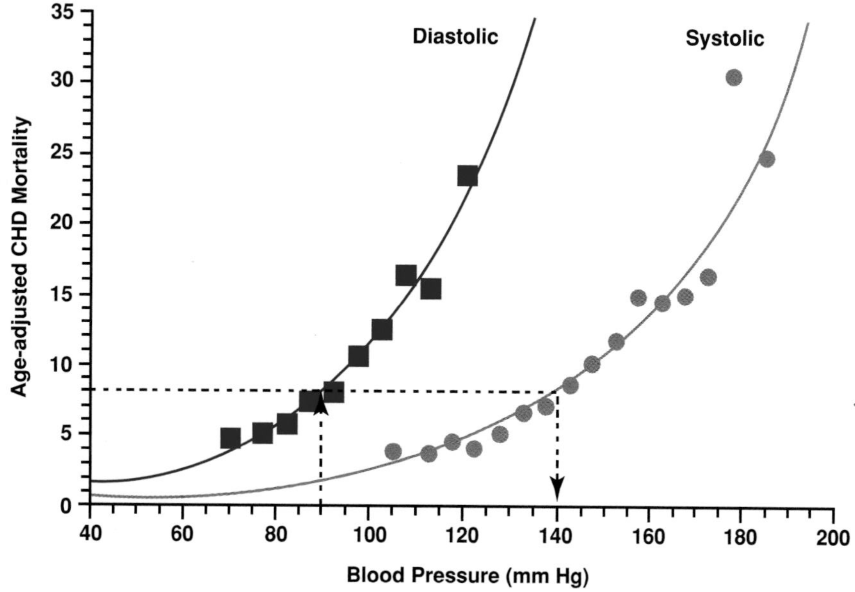

FIG. 2. Age-adjusted coronary heart disease mortality in 6 years (per 1,000 individuals) as a function of systolic and diastolic blood pressure among the 356,222 men age 35–57 years screened and free of myocardial infarction in the MRFIT trial. (Data from Stamler, ref. 9.)

into the staging scheme for severity of hypertension in the most recent report of the Joint National Committee on Detection, Evaluation, and Treatment of High Blood Pressure (11) was long overdue and is amply justified by epidemiological observations (Fig. 2).

In the Multiple Risk Factor Intervention Trial (MRFIT) 6-year follow-up of 356,222 middle-age men, ideal ranges for systolic and diastoic blood pressures were under 120 and 80 mm Hg, respectively. Only 25% of the men had systolic blood pressures in this ideal range (9). Importantly, the blood pressure strata where the attributable risk for CHD was highest (a function of both prevalence and relative risk) was in the high normal range (85–89 mm Hg) of diastolic blood pressure and in the low hypertensive range for systolic blood pressure (140–144 mm Hg). Based on these MRFIT data, 32% of all the CHD deaths could be attributed to diastolic blood pressure greater than 80 mm Hg and 42% to systolic blood pressure above 120 (9).

Relative risks associated with hypertension are typically greater for stroke than for CHD (2). This appears to be true of atherothrombotic stroke as well as other forms of stroke. However, atherosclerosis in hypertensive individuals is not more extensive in carotid or intracerebral vessels than in coronary arteries. Rather, hypertension largely reverses the relative protection against atherosclerosis which the carotid and intracerebral vessels normally enjoy (12,13). This is graphically illustrated in Fig. 3. The increased relative risk is therefore due to a low baseline risk of cerebral atherosclerosis in normotensives rather than markedly elevated absolute risks in hypertensive individuals. In patients with familial hypercholesterolemia, who generally are not hypertensive (14), the cerebral vessels are relatively spared compared to coronary arteries (15).

Some international studies have reported no association between clinically defined coronary heart disease endpoints and high blood pressure where serum cholesterol is consistently low. For example, in the 15-year follow-up of the Seven Countries Study, the multiple logistic coefficient for systolic blood pressure was highest in the United States, followed by northern Europe, and then southern Europe (all still statistically significant), but was not significant for Japan, where too few deaths from CHD occurred for any risk factor to be significant (16). In other studies in Japan and Puerto Rico, where serum cholesterol levels were low, high blood pressure was not a significant CHD risk factor (17–19). Possibly, there were too few CHD events to detect the effect of blood pressure in these studies. In autopsy, hypertension was associated with more raised coronary lesions even in countries with a very low incidence of clinical disease (12). More recently, high-resolution carotid ultrasound revealed an excess of plaques in patients with hypertension (20,21). However, if these raised lesions did not progress sufficiently rapidly because of low plasma cholesterol, they may not lead to a statistically significant excess of clinically detectable disease. Alternatively, blood pressure may only foster atherosclerosis when serum cholesterol levels are sufficiently high. Indeed, in animal experiments among various species, hypertension accelerated the development of atherosclerosis, but usually only when serum cholesterol levels were above some permissive level (22). Hypertension clearly accelerated plaque formation in Watanabe heritable hyperlipidemic rabbits (23) and cynomolgus monkeys fed an atherogenic diet (24).

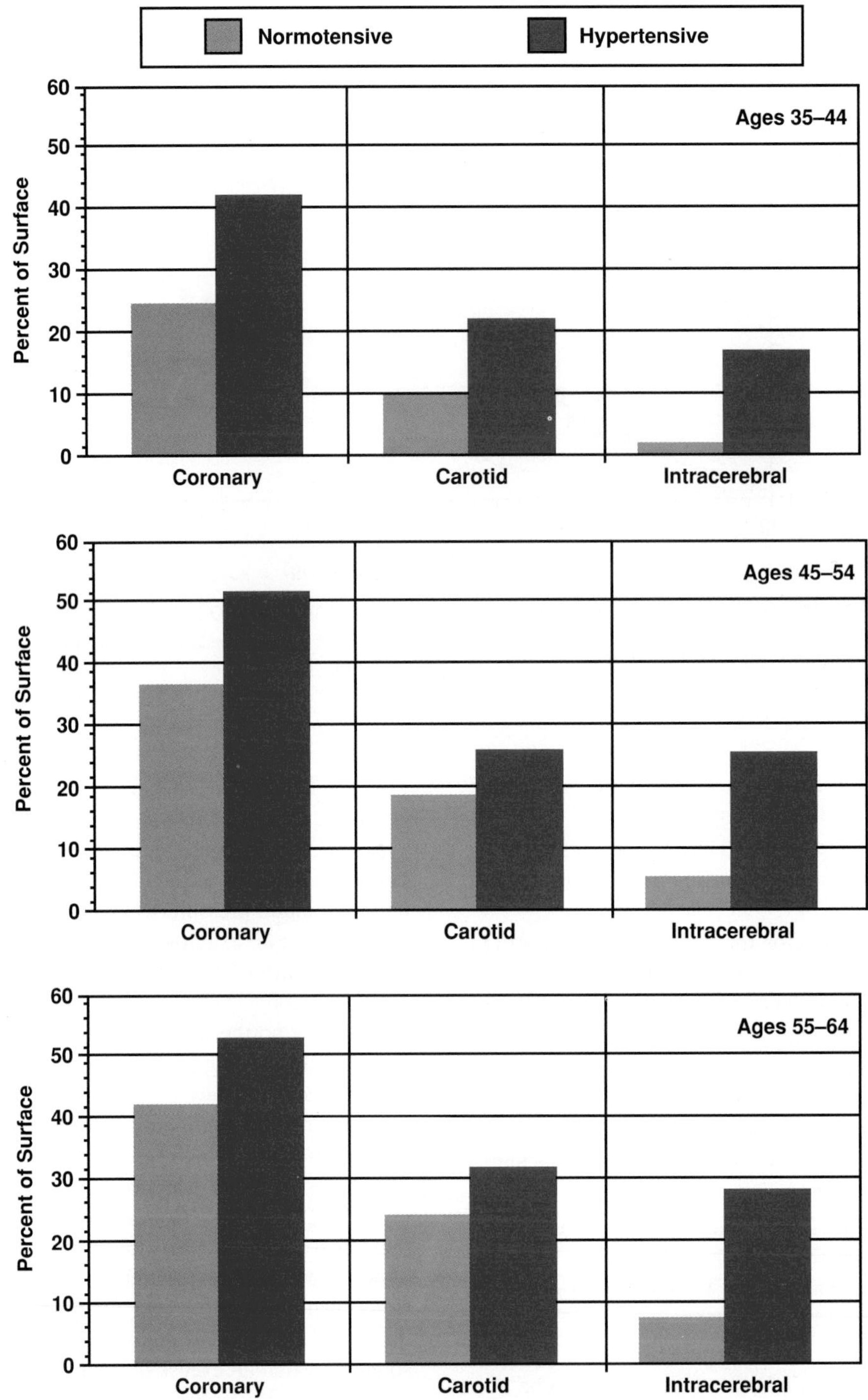

FIG. 3. Percent of surface involved in raised atherosclerotic lesions at autopsy among men from Oslo, Norway, with and without diagnosed hypertension in the International Atherosclerosis Project. (Data from Robertson and Strong, ref. 12, and Solberg and McGarry, ref. 13.)

FAMILIAL AGGREGATION OF CARDIOVASCULAR ENDPOINTS

Coronary heart disease, hypertension, and stroke all aggregate within families, suggesting that genetic factors and/or shared common environmental factors make significant contributions to each of these endpoints. A family history of hypertension is an independent predictor of the development of hypertension (25–27). Family history as a prediction variable also has advantages over biochemical, anthropometric, or other risk factors in the sense that it is not confounded by heterogeneity between families (28). Since the endpoint of hypertension is used, two families may have different causes of their positive family history, but each cause will increase the probability that other family members will become hypertensive at early ages.

Using a sample of 15,250 families from the Utah population, different definitions of a family history of CHD and hypertension were compared to determine which was the most predictive of future incidence of these diseases (29). Table 1 shows the relative risks associated with two of these definitions, for men and women. A positive family history of either hypertension or CHD increases the risk of disease onset in family members unaffected at the time of family history determination after 13 years of follow-up. The increased risk was mostly confined to the younger ages and was higher for the stronger definition of a positive family history. In families with two or more members with CHD before age 55 years, male first-degree relatives had up to 12.7 times the risk of developing CHD after 13 years compared to men in families with no CHD events. A weaker definition of family history (any first-degree relative with CHD at any age) increased the risk up to 2.9 times. Table 1 also shows that persons over age 70 years have little or no greater risk of CHD or hypertension than the general population regardless of the definition of family history. This suggests that relatives who have no disease by age 70 likely do not have the genetic factors causing the positive family history in the family.

Not only does the same disease aggregate within a family, but a positive family history of one disease increases the likelihood of a positive family history of another disease. Correlations of a quantitative family history score (which compares the observed number of events and person-years of experience in the family to age- and gender-specific population rates) between CHD and hypertension, stroke, and diabetes are 0.23, 0.18, and 0.12, respectively. Table 2 shows that the prevalence of a positive family history of CHD (≥2 affected) is increased threefold if the family has a positive family history of hypertension, stroke, or diabetes and suggests that there are probably genetic components that are common to the development of both hypertension and CHD in the same family. As discussed below, there is evidence for such a common genetic component (30).

TABLE 1. *Relative risks of coronary heart disease and hypertension after 13 years of follow-up for persons in families with a positive family history of coronary heart disease or hypertension*

Age (yr)	CHD ≥2 Early events	CHD ≥1 Event	HBP ≥2 Early events	HBP ≥1 Event
Men				
20–39	12.7*	2.9*	4.1*	2.5*
50–59	2.9*	1.3*	2.4*	1.7*
≥70	0.7	1.3*	0.8	0.9
Women				
20–39	8.0*	1.4	5.0*	2.8*
50–59	3.7	1.2	1.5	1.5*
≥70	1.5	1.1	0.8	1.0
Percent of population	1.7	38.1	11.4	53.1

Adapted from Hunt et al., ref. 29.
Relative risks of a positive family history compared to families with no events.
CHD, Coronary heart disease; HBP, high blood pressure.
* $p < 0.05$.

TABLE 2. *Relative risk of a positive family history of coronary heart disease by family history status of hypertension, stroke, and adult-onset diabetes*

Family history status	Percent with a positive CHD family history	Relative risk of positive CHD family history
Positive HBP family history	11.8	3.3
Negative HBP family history	3.6	Referent
Positive stroke family history	11.8	3.3
Negative stroke family history	3.6	Referent
Positive diabetes family history	14.7	3.3
Negative diabetes family history	4.4	Referent

HEMODYNAMIC FACTORS AND ATHEROGENESIS

Blood pressure in the arterial range appears to be an essential requirement for the development of atherosclerosis. Venous atherosclerosis does not develop even in patients with homozygous familial hypercholesterolemia (31). The relatively rapid progression of atherosclerosis in saphenous veins used in coronary artery bypass suggests there is nothing uniquely resistant about veins themselves. The normal pulmonary arterial circulation with its systolic pressures of 12–22 mm Hg is another protected site. Nevertheless, with pulmonary hypertension, atherosclerotic plaques are commonly seen (32).

Recent studies have provided further insights into the roles of blood pressure and hemodynamics in atherogenesis. In one study, rabbit aorta was isolated in vitro and pressurized to either 70 to 160 mm Hg pressure. The penetration of radiolabeled low-density lipoprotein (LDL) into layers of the artery wall was determined at the two pressures. LDL concentration in the intima and inner media was increased 44-fold at the higher pressure. LDL concentration decreased rapidly in more peripheral layers until, in the adventitia, LDL concentrations at the two pressures were nearly equal. In contrast, albumin concentration was increased tenfold at the high pressure, but was distributed evenly throughout the arterial wall layers. The investigators suggested that at higher pressures, the subintimal tissues are compacted and thereby retard the movement of the relatively large LDL particles retard the movement of the relatively large LDL particles through the wall. Thus, trapping of LDL at the internal elastic lamina together with pressure-driven convection of LDL into the artery wall appear to be the major mechanisms underlying the relationship between blood pressure and atherosclerosis (33). These findings are consistent with a mathematical model derived by Fry (34) in which the trapping effects of the internal elastic lamina led to increasing LDL accumulation in the intima as plasma concentration increased and as pressure increased. The presence of endothelial cells paradoxically increased LDL accumulation by preventing backdiffusion from the intima into the bloodstream. Maximal accumulation of LDL was predicted when endothelial cells covered 97% of the surface and were separated by small gaps. Sufficient pressure-driven convection of LDL into the intima may therefore be a key limiting factor in atherogenesis.

Sites of atherosclerosis predilection can largely be explained by hemodynamic models. Plaques are much more frequent in areas *opposite* flow dividers—in areas of slow flow (low shear) or eddy currents (Fig. 4). Turbulence is not a feature of flow in these sites. In fact, essentially no turbulence is seen in most of the normal cardiovascular system (35). These observations are directly opposed to the intuitive expectation that atherosclerosis should appear at sites of high shear stress or turbulent flow. When clear plastic replicas of human carotid arteries are perfused with fluid at typical arterial pressures in a pulsatile pattern, tiny bubbles injected into the stream revealed flow patterns as diagrammed in Fig. 4 (36). At the flow divider, the pattern revealed by the bubbles is laminar and fast. The shearing forces along the vessel wall in such areas are relatively high. While intimal thickening is stimulated early at arterial sites exposed to high shear stress (primarily from smooth muscle cell accumulation), the process does not proceed on to atherosclerosis. Release of growth factors may mediate this early proliferation of smooth muscle cells. Indeed, increased replication and LDL binding capacity has been reported for smooth muscle cells from hypertensive rats (37,38). However, these proliferative effects probably do not explain excess atherosclerosis in hypertensive patients. (Rather, they may more directly relate to myointimal hyperplasia.) Endothelial prostacyclin (39) and nitric oxide (40) production are stimulated by increased shear forces, perhaps mitigating other factors which might otherwise continue to stimulate intimal proliferation. Increased nitric oxide production by endothelial cells exposed to high shear has been shown recently to inhibit monocyte adhesion (41). In addition, high shear might make adhesion or penetration into the arterial wall mechanically more difficult for monocytes, platelets, LDL, or other lipoproteins.

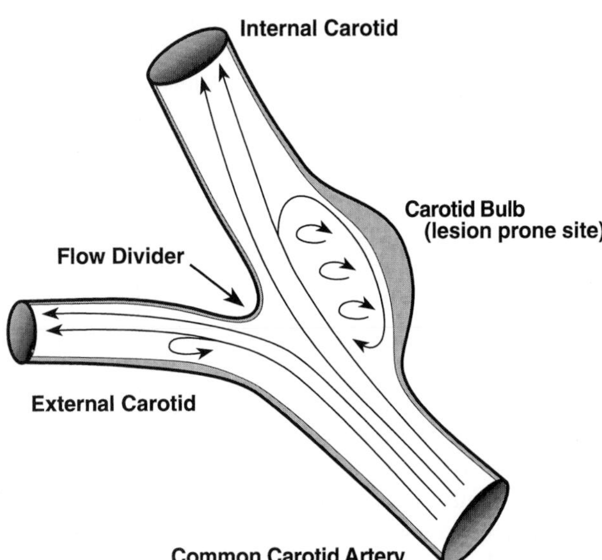

FIG. 4. Hemodynamic factors favoring development of atherosclerosis. Lesion-prone sites are characterized by slow flow, eddy currents, prolonged residence time for formed blood elements, potentially higher side pressures, and increased adhesion of monocytes mediated in part by lower rates of production of NO and prostacyclin. *Arrows:* Streamlines and flow patterns of bubbles injected into glass casts of human arteries.

In slow-flow areas of glass cast models, bubbles swirl languidly around in a stable eddy pattern. Their clearance from the artery was clearly delayed until well into the next pulsation. In a mathematical model with parameters fit to human autopsy findings, intimal thickening was stimulated to the greatest extent in such areas of slow flow as shown in Fig. 4. Intimal thickening increased gradually with age to a point when macrophages became trapped at a critical intimal thickness, at which time intimal thickness increased rapidly as macrophages accumulated (42). Increased residence time near the artery wall might promote penetration by blood components such as LDL, monocytes, and platelets into the intima. Indeed, a variety of marker molecules were found to penetrate the areas of slow flow much more readily than at the flow dividers or along smooth-walled arteries (43). Intimal plaques accumulated exclusively in areas of low shear created experimentally by aortic stenoses placed in hypercholesterolemic beagles (44). Finally, low-shear stress, calculated by anatomic features in 20 arterial segments, was strongly correlated with greater progression of coronary atherosclerosis over 3 years among patients in the Harvard Atherosclerosis Reversibility Project (45). The unique hemodynamics of the coronary circulation, with near cessation of flow during systole, together with the high pressures generated at the aortic root may explain the predilection of coronary arteries to atherosclerosis. As heart rate increases, relatively more time is spent in systole with proportionately more time for penetration of blood elements into the arterial wall. This may help explain the fourfold increase in coronary disease risk as resting heart rate increased from under 60 to over 100 beats per minute (46).

In the 19th century the noted collector and writer of limericks Edward Lear penned:

The principle preached by Bernoulli
Can lead to results most pecoulli,
It may favor stenosis
And lead to thrombosis
If the blood flow is increased undoulli

In older literature, Bernoulli's principle is cited (as the above limerick intimates) as a factor that could promote atherogenesis and cause disruption of plaque by causing discrete areas of low pressure at sites of stenosis (47). While plaque rupture or hemorrhage might possibly be precipitated by uneven pressures if flow were sufficiently fast, plaque growth would certainly not be promoted by hemodynamic factors at points of maximum stenosis. (Plaque growth is promoted just beyond such points.) Nevertheless, Bernoulli's principle may further explain the predilection for atherosclerosis in some regions of slow flow, or more precisely, the lack of atherosclerosis in regions of rapid flow. Blood velocity will be much greater at a flow divider than at the opposite wall. This increased velocity results in lower side pressure (that is, pressure felt perpendicular to flow). If flow is 100 cm/sec (blood velocity in the aorta) at a flow divider and just 0–10 cm/sec at the outer wall, the Bernoulli equation predicts that the side pressure would be 7–8 mm Hg higher at the outer wall. (The same principle allows airplanes to fly.) The reduction of pressure at points of rapid flow may contribute to relative protection of these sites, but only at velocities seen in the largest arteries. At flow velocities found in coronary arteries (about 30 cm/sec), differences in side pressures will amount to something less than 1 mm Hg (comparing flow at 30 versus 0 cm/sec), probably too small to contribute meaningfully to divergent rates of atherogenesis. Since low shear still predicts areas of accelerated plaque growth even in the coronary arteries, endothelial effects and mechanical factors other than Bernoulli's principle must predominate.

DYSLIPIDEMIA AND HYPERTENSION

Epidemiological studies have clearly shown consistent associations between hypertension and dyslipidemia as have been reported from Framingham (48), the Lipid Research Clinic (LRC) population (49), and Stanford subjects (50,51). Abnormalities associated with hypertension have included increased levels of cholesterol, LDL cholesterol, apolipoprotein B, triglycerides, and very low density lipoprotein (VLDL) cholesterol, as well as decreased levels of high-density lipoprotein (HDL) cholesterol and apolipoprotein A-I. Various names have been given to this syndrome, which is the most common syndrome associated with hypertension. Perhaps the most descriptive of these names is the multiple metabolic syndrome.

Multiple Metabolic Syndrome

Twin and family studies suggest that genetic factors play an important role in the coaggregation of lipid abnormalities and hypertension, as shown from the National Heart, Lung, and Blood Institute (NHLBI) twin cohort (52) and Utah families (53–55). Sibling aggregation of both hypertension and lipid abnormalities occurred more often than expected by chance (53). In Utah sibling pairs ascertained only for the diagnosis of hypertension before age 60 years in both siblings, high triglycerides and low HDL-C were found three times more often than expected ($p < 0.0001$). These abnormalities occurred in persons with normal weight as well as in the obese. This syndrome was descriptively labeled "familial dyslipidemic hypertension" (FDH) and occurs in about 12% of persons with essential hypertension and 1–2% of the general population.

Siblings with this syndrome had increased fasting triglycerides, VLDL cholesterol, and apolipoprotein B and decreased HDL-C (55). The syndrome itself appears heterogeneous, as about one-third of siblings with familial dyslipidemic hypertension met LDL-C and triglyceride criteria for having familial combined hyperlipidemia. Hypertensive sibships with high triglyceride and low HDL-C but normal LDL-C had greater obesity, especially central obesity, than hypertensive sibships with familial combined hyperlipidemia. While fasting insulin levels were elevated in both groups, they were related more closely to obesity in the high-triglyceride and low-HDL-C group. Adjustment for obesity in this group decreased the estimated mean insulin levels almost to the normolipidemic group level, while adjustment of insulin levels for obesity in the familial combined group had only minor effects on the elevated mean insulin levels. Therefore, elevated insulin levels appear to have different causes in the two subsets of patients, justifying the separation of hypertensive families into those with and without FCHL.

Results from the NHLBI twin study confirmed the Utah findings (52) (Table 3). In addition, this study showed that

TABLE 3. *Familial dyslipidemic hypertension in the NHLBI twins versus Utah siblings*

Characteristic tabulated	NHLBI	Utah
Study subjects	Twins	Siblings
Number of hypertensives tested	185	131
Frequency of FDH		
In general population (%)	2	1.5
In all hypertensives (%)	10	12
Frequency of lipid abnormalities		
HDL-C below 10th percentile (%)	83	62
Triglyceride above 90th percentile (%)	33	45
LDL-C above 90th percentile (%)	22	22

Adapted from Selby et al., ref. 52, and Williams et al., ref. 129.

NHLBI Twin Concordance for FDH: monozygotes three times dizygotes ($p = 0.06$).

occurrence of CHD after 16 years of follow-up was much greater in persons with both hypertension and dyslipidemia than in persons with only hypertension or dyslipidemia. Two other similar studies have clearly shown that familial combined hyperlipidemia is one of the most common lipid syndromes associated with CHD, and that the majority of families with this syndrome of high LDL-C and triglycerides also have low HDL-C (54,56). A 6-year prospective study has shown that while only 4.3% of the study participants had elevated baseline triglycerides and a baseline LDL-C/HDL-C ratio greater than 5, 25% of all definite myocardial infarctions occurred in this subgroup (57). Elevated triglycerides greatly increased the risk of CHD when other lipids were also abnormal.

In persons receiving common antihypertensive medications, the observed tendency of some diuretics and beta-blockers to elevate cholesterol and triglyceride levels, to depress HDL cholesterol, and to promote insulin resistance may make additional contributions to the dyslipidemia observed in persons with hypertension (58). While antihypertensive medications may contribute to the dyslipidemia in some persons with hypertension, they do not explain the familial coaggregation of dyslipidemia in the hypertensive NHLBI twins, 80% of whom had never been on treatment, or in the hypertensive Utah siblings with highly significant dyslipidemia even after their lipid levels were adjusted for the published effects of specific medications they were taking.

In addition to abnormal levels of lipids and lipoproteins, LDL particles tend to be more dense and smaller in size in individuals with the multiple metabolic syndrome (55,59). This atherogenic lipid profile has been shown to segregate as a major-gene trait in two studies. One study estimated dominant inheritance (60), while another estimated recessive inheritance (61). Dense LDL increased the risk of coronary heart disease threefold in a cross-sectional study (62). There is a high correlation between LDL density and triglyceride levels, explaining why dense LDL is so common in the multiple metabolic syndrome (63). The dense LDL are more prone to oxidation and their smaller size may promote infiltration into endothelial layers, contributing to atherosclerosis. In addition, small intracellular amounts of LDL appear to increase intracellular free calcium levels in vascular smooth muscle and alter the cellular pH by way of the Na–H antiporter (64).

The dense LDL phenotype was linked to the LDL-receptor locus on chromosome 19 in one study (65). However, it is not clear how the LDL-receptor locus, which affects binding of the LDL cholesterol and removal, could affect a syndrome such as familial dyslipidemic hypertension or familial combined hyperlipidemia, which more often have triglyceride and HDL abnormalities than the LDL-cholesterol abnormality (66). In addition, persons with familial hypercholesterolemia tend to have a lighter, more buoyant LDL rather than the more dense LDL as seen in this syndrome.

Other linkage studies have suggested that this syndrome is linked to the apo A1, C3, A4 locus, which is involved in HDL, triglyceride, and insulin metabolism (67,68). It is likely that the heterogeneity of this syndrome results from multiple loci. It is also possible that the appearance of multiple lipid abnormalities defining this syndrome may result from multiple common genetic abnormalities within a family and that individuals within this family who have only one genetic abnormality express only high triglyceride or high LDL or low HDL.

A number of candidate genes have been proposed for familial combined hyperlipidemia, which is phenotypically overlapping with familial dyslipidemic hypertension. Linkage of familial combined hyperlipidemia has been reported to the apolipoprotein A1–C3–A4 complex on chromosome 11 (69), following a previous positive association study (70), but contradictory results exist. Other candidate genes have been considered for familial combined hyperlipidemia (71). While apo B has been suggested as a candidate gene, it appears from subsequent study that it is unlikely that this gene would be a major cause of familial combined hyperlipidemia even though apo B levels are usually elevated (72). The lipoprotein lipase (LPL) gene might be associated with increased blood pressures (73,74) and familial combined hyperlipidemia (75) in heterozygous carriers. Involvement of LPL would also explain the syndrome of higher triglyceride levels and lower HDL levels because of a defect in conversion of VLDL and chylomicrons to LDL and intermediate-density lipoproteins. The lipid abnormalities seen in familial combined hyperlipidemia and familial dyslipidemic hypertension may be related to hypertension through various pathways, such as alteration of ion transport systems, structural changes in the vasculature, or increasing responsiveness of vascular smooth muscle to hormonal or other factors in addition to shared associations with obesity. Some of these are discussed later in this chapter.

Heterozygous Lipoprotein Lipase Deficiency

Lipoprotein lipase is a triglyceride hydrolase responsible for the processing of triglyceride-rich lipoproteins, chylomicrons, and VLDL. Rare homozygotes have nearly complete deficiency of LPL manifest by fat intolerance, episodic abdominal pain, severe hypertriglyceridemia, and fasting hyperchylomicronemia classically presenting in infancy (76). In studies of close relatives, obligate carriers have shown mean adipose-tissue LPL activities reduced about 50% (77), but individual measurements have shown considerable overlap with levels in normal persons (78). Observations (79) indicate that the heterozygous state for a lipoprotein lipase mutation constitutes a latent metabolic defect which can lead to manifest hypertriglyceridemia.

Recent determinations of the cDNA sequence for the normal human enzyme (80) and the structure of the human gene (81) now permit unambiguous genetic characterization of carriers of mutant alleles. Five distinct molecular variants of the LPL gene being studied in Utah pedigrees include the following: a glycine-to-glutamic acid substitution at position

TABLE 4. *Frequency of dyslipidemia and hypertension by LPL 188 mutation status*

Abnormality	Frequency, age ≥40 yr (%) Carriers (N = 12)	Noncarriers (N = 43)	p Value
VLDL-C > 90th percentile	83	37	0.004
Triglyceride > 90th percentile	67	21	0.01
HDL-C < 10th percentile	58	35	0.04
LDL-C > 90th percentile	8	9	N.S.
Confirmed hypertension	68	25	0.02

Adapted from Williams et al., ref. 73.
Levels of significance were estimated by Fisher's Exact Test.

188 of the mature enzyme, leading to synthesis and secretion of an inactive enzyme (82); an internal duplication of a 2-kilobase (kb) fragment leading to partial duplication of exon 6 and associated with no detectable immunoreactive material in postheparin plasma samples (83); an asparagine-to-serine substitution at position 291 of the mature enzyme (84); an exon 3 missense mutation producing mostly inactive LPL enzyme; and an exon 3 truncation mutation that causes a stop codon (84).

A significant association was noted between the heterozygous state for LPL deficiency and essential hypertension and lipid abnormalities (73,79). In vitro expression of the gene with the 188 mutation resulted in the production of immunoreactive but functionally defective LPL (82). A homozygous proband was identified for this mutation and subsequent sequential screening of aunts, uncles, and cousins of the proband in the two branches of the proband's pedigree led to the evaluation of 126 subjects and the finding of 29 heterozygous carriers of this mutation (79). As shown in Table 4, lipid abnormalities and hypertension were approximately twice as frequent among carriers over age 40 years as among noncarriers. Subsequent expansion of this and other pedigrees including 121 carriers have shown that expression of the abnormal phenotype was also observed among participants under age 40 years. Table 5 shows mean levels for blood pressure and other variables. LPL-mutation carriers over age 40 years show nonsignificant trends toward higher blood pressures. Body mass index, fasting glucose, and insulin levels were not different between carriers and noncarriers in this study.

These preliminary findings based on 12 carriers over age 40 years of one LPL point mutation suggest that heterozygous lipoprotein lipase deficiency together with age-related influences may predispose persons to the development of dyslipidemia and hypertension. Pedigrees are being screened for each of the other mutations and preliminary results suggest that each acts similarly to the 188 mutation. It is also noteworthy that six of the seven probands independently identified so far by screening persons for triglycerides greater than the 99th percentile and HDL-C below the 5th percentile had essential hypertension. The possibility that LPL mutations result in familial dyslipidemic hypertension is suggested by the parallel findings of predominant elevations in triglycerides and VLDL cholesterol as well as depression in HDL cholesterol. As another interesting parallel, LDL-cholesterol abnormalities are not prominent in either FDH or LPL mutations tested so far. Studies suggest that insulin directly affects the action of LPL in adipose tissue (85). Others have reported support for heterozygous LPL deficiency as one cause of familial combined hyperlipidemia (86). An abstract reports linkage of a marker at the LPL locus to blood pressure in diabetic families (74).

VASOACTIVE SUBSTANCES AND ATHEROGENESIS

The effects of a number of vasoactive substances in both hypertension and atherogenesis have been the subject of much recent research.

Insulin

Insulin resistance is closely related to several metabolic and clinical conditions, including hyperinsulinemia, hypertension, coronary heart disease, diabetes, and obesity (87).

TABLE 5. *Mean levels (± S.D.) of variables tested in carriers and noncarriers*

Variable	Subjects age ≥40 yr Carriers (N = 12)	Subjects age ≥40 yr Noncarriers (N = 43)	Subjects age <40 yr Carriers (N = 17)	Subjects age <40 yr Noncarriers (N = 54)
Age (yr)	57 ± 9	56 ± 11	27 ± 10	25 ± 10
SBP (mm Hg)	151 ± 31	136 ± 18	118 ± 11	115 ± 12
DBP (mm Hg)	89 ± 15	83 ± 9	71 ± 10	72 ± 9
Glucose (mg/dl)	104 ± 17	102 ± 53	86 ± 10	86 ± 28
Insulin (μU/ml)	18 ± 12	17 ± 12	11 ± 7	11 ± 11
BMI (kg/m^2)	31.5 ± 5.6	30.4 ± 6.5	22.2 ± 4.3	24.0 ± 6.4

Adapted from Williams et al., ref. 73.
SBP, Systolic blood pressure; DBP, diastolic blood pressure; BMI, body mass index.

Insulin resistance has been included as part of the Deadly Quartet (88) and suggested as the basis of syndrome X (51,89). At least three prospective studies have shown plasma insulin associated with coronary heart disease (90–92). Additionally, high insulin levels have been shown to be predictive of the development of diabetes in a number of different populations (93–96).

A few prospective studies have shown insulin related to the development of hypertension (97–100). Niskanen et al. found that the postglucose 1-hr insulin level was higher among both diabetic and nondiabetic subjects who developed hypertension over a 5-year follow-up period (98). In a 10-year prospective study of hypertension in men of ages 48–51 years, Skarfors et al. found that both fasting and challenged insulin levels predicted the development of hypertension independently of other risk factors except baseline blood pressure, with relative risks around 1.1, $p = 0.007$, for a 2.6 μU/L insulin difference (97). Lissner et al. found that women in the top quartile of the fasting insulin distribution developed three times as much hypertension over 12 years as women in the lowest insulin quartile (100). The increased risk from high insulin levels and an association with diastolic blood pressure remained after adjustment for baseline blood pressure.

While it is clearer how the altered lipid levels of the multiple metabolic syndrome could affect the risk for coronary disease, it is less clear how these lipid abnormalities are translated into increased risk for hypertension. Insulin resistance is hypothesized to promote hypertension in various ways, including (a) stimulation of cation transport and Na reabsorption in the distal and proximal tubule causing renal Na retention and hypertension (101,102), (b) stimulation of norepinephrine excretion and increased blood pressure (103), (c) stimulation of vascular endothelium and smooth muscle cells to hypertrophy, increasing peripheral vascular resistance and blood pressure (i.e., growth factor-like effect of insulin) (104,105), (d) stimulation of intracellular calcium and increased smooth muscle contractility (106,107), and (e) obesity-related angiotensinogen production in adipose tissue leading to insulin resistance (108).

Many studies have shown that untreated hypertensive individuals have higher insulin levels than do normotensive control subjects (89,109–111). Furthermore, treatment of hypertension does not necessarily normalize the insulin levels (111). There is evidence that abnormalities in glucose and insulin metabolism precede and may play a role in the causes of hypertension.

Insulin resistance and hypertension have been described in relation to the sympathetic nervous system. Increased dietary intake of calories increases insulin levels and sympathetic response (112). This sympathetic response increases thermogenesis to burn off the excess calories, preventing further weight gain. However, increased norepinephrine also increases vasoconstriction and sodium retention, further increasing blood pressure. Catecholamines also buffer the insulin effects on glucose metabolism (113), increasing insulin resistance (114,115). Body fat distribution as measured by waist-to-hip ratio also plays an important role relating sympathetic response to systolic and diastolic blood pressure (116). The amount of intraabdominal fat correlates with the insulin response to a glucose load (117), indicating that upper or central obesity may aggravate preexisting insulin resistance or be responsible for part of the initiation of that resistance. Euglycemic clamp studies have shown increases in blood pressure and sympathetic stimulation as the insulin levels increased in nonobese subjects (103), indicating that insulin resistance also occurs in the absence of obesity.

Studies suggest that high plasma triglycerides and/or fatty acids promote insulin resistance (118–121). Persons with type V hyperlipoproteinemia have high triglycerides from both increased chylomicrons and high VLDL and also develop insulin resistance. In one study, half of 95 adults with type V had hypertension (122). Insulin resistance itself can aggravate lipid levels, creating a vicious circle. Increased insulin levels increase the synthesis and secretion of VLDL-TG by the liver, possibly explaining some of the observed hypertriglyceridemia commonly seen in hypertension (123,124). After weight loss, which increases the effectiveness of insulin, VLDL-TG secretion and plasma triglyceride concentration decrease (125). In fructose-fed rats, blocking the production of insulin decreased the plasma triglyceride concentration and reduced blood pressure, indicating that the hypertension may be secondary to the insulin and/or lipid abnormalities (126). It has been shown that blood pressure in the obese could be lowered by physical training without a loss of weight, but only in those who were hyperinsulinemic and hypertriglyceridemic at baseline (127). Insulin sensitivity defects appear to occur in skeletal muscle of hypertensive subjects even in those of normal weight (110). Insulin resistance and hypertriglyceridemia also exist in hypertensive individuals who are not obese (51).

Most evidence points to lipid or lipoprotein abnormalities resulting from insulin resistance, rather than causing that resistance. There may be a subset of individuals who have primary lipid abnormalities (perhaps due to polygenes or major genes) which promote insulin resistance and hyperinsulinemia resulting in future hypertension. By varying the amount of free fatty acids in the diet, it was shown that there was a dose-dependent decrease in glucose uptake when dietary free fatty acid was increased (128). The insulin resistance was caused by decreased glycogen synthesis and carbohydrate oxidation. Insulin resistance occurred in both peripheral and hepatic tissues. Therefore, there is evidence that some type of lipid-metabolism defect could be related to increased insulin resistance and hypertension. Further evidence is needed to determine in what proportion of individuals hyperinsulinemia precedes lipid or lipoprotein abnormalities, or vice versa, or whether they are simultaneous occurrences.

Figure 5 shows the close association of obesity, hypertriglyceridemia, and hyperinsulinemia with hypertension (129). Hypertensives have a greater prevalence of 90th per-

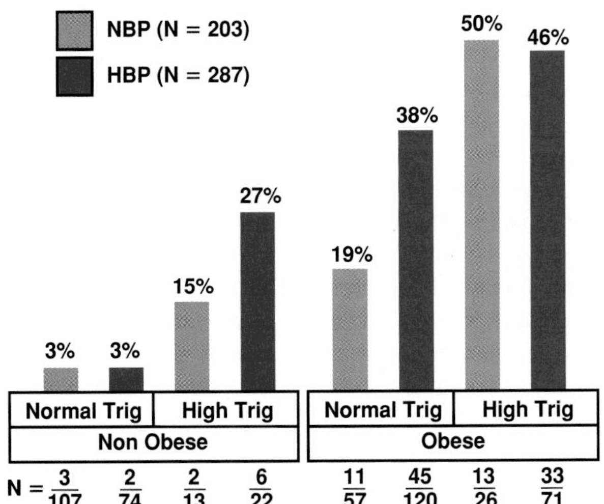

FIG. 5. Prevalence of high fasting insulin levels greater than the 90th percentile. Obesity is defined as body mass index greater than 27.8 kg/m^2 for men and greater than 27.3 kg/m^2 for women. High- and low triglyceride (Trig) levels are greater than or less than the age- and gender-specific 90th percentiles from the Lipid Research Clinic data. NBP, Normal blood pressure; HBP, high blood pressure. (From Williams et al., ref. 129.)

centile fasting insulin levels than do normotensives. Increased insulin is rare in nonobese, normal-triglyceride individuals, but quite common in the high-triglyceride group. Obesity and high triglyceride levels appear to overwhelm the insulin response, removing the difference between normotensive and hypertensive subjects.

Insulin resistance and hyperinsulinemia are not always synonymous. For example, patients with insulinomas have hyperinsulinemia without hypertension or insulin resistance, and patients with pheochromocytoma have insulin resistance and hypertension without hyperinsulinemia (130). Neither rats nor humans with renal vascular hypertension have hyperinsulinemia (131,132). Therefore, hypertension appears to be more related to an underlying cause of insulin resistance than to hyperinsulinemia.

Even though studies in both rats and humans have shown that hypertensive individuals have resistance to insulin-stimulated glucose uptake, not all evidence points to a clear link between insulin levels (representing insulin resistance) and high blood pressure. A relative risk of hypertension of 2.24 ($p = 0.03$) was found for fasting insulin in the nonobese, but no association in the obese ($RR = 1.32$, $p =$ N.S.) (99,133). Hypertensive and normotensive rats with acutely elevated insulin levels do not increase sodium reabsorption (134). Chronic insulin infusion (28 days) in normal dogs does not increase blood pressure or sympathetic stimulation (135,136). This group of researchers has also shown conflicting results in rats and reviewed some of the differences among rats, dogs, and humans (137).

A more recent study in rats showed that after 10 days of elevated insulin levels caused by increased dietary glucose intake, blood pressure increased 6.0/2.2 mm Hg (138). If physiologic amounts of insulin were also infused, there was a greater blood pressure increase (8.6/2.9 mm Hg). An in vivo study on humans showed that insulin infusion with a glucose clamp did decrease sodium excretion even though there was decreased sodium reabsorption in the proximal tubule of the kidney (139). The decreased net sodium excretion occurred because there was increased distal tubule reabsorption of sodium which more than counterbalanced the decreased reabsorption in the proximal tubule. Further studies on hypertension incidence are needed to clarify the role of insulin levels as an independent risk factor in both men and women of all ages. However, whatever the causes of insulin resistance, dyslipidemia, and hyperinsulinemia, these phenotypes are clearly associated with hypertension and coronary heart disease and are highly familial.

From segregation analyses after adjusting for age, gender, and body mass index, evidence was found for a major genetic locus determining both fasting and stimulated insulin levels in normoglycemic members of pedigrees ascertained for diabetes (140). High gene frequencies were found for the hyperinsulinemic allele among family members with normal glucose tolerance ($q = 0.25$). A high frequency might explain the high prevalence of non-insulin-dependent diabetes mellitus (NIDDM) and insulin resistance in the Pima, but a single genetic mutation with such a high frequency seems unlikely in the general Caucasian population. Reaven (87) has suggested that up to one-third of the nondiabetic population may be hyperinsulinemic, in which case the locus segregating in the NIDDM pedigrees represents an additive contribution to perhaps another major gene involved with diabetes. The sources of variance in fasting insulin were estimated as 33.1% due to the major-gene locus, 11.4% due to polygenic inheritance, and 55.5% due to other, unmeasured effects (140). Thus, despite the many factors contributing to insulin levels which were not controlled, such as body fat distribution and physical activity, 44.5% of the variance in fasting insulin levels was explained by genetic inheritance.

A gene for high insulin levels may contribute to the concordance of hypertension and diabetes. Between 30% and 50% of those with NIDDM are hypertensive (141). Approximately 40% of hypertensives have lipid abnormalities and 46% of those with high cholesterol (>240 mg/dl) have hypertension (>140/90 mm Hg) (142), indicating a strong clustering of these disorders. An analysis of the National Academy of Sciences twin registry showed that there was evidence for a common genetic determinant of hypertension, obesity, and diabetes (30). Fifty-nine percent of the variation in a common factor underlying the concordance of these three conditions was estimated to be explained by genetics. The genetic portion of the common factor explained 21% of the variance in hypertension, 11% for diabetes, and 6% for obesity. Each of the three conditions also had significant contributions from genes that were not common to the other conditions. The remaining variance was explained by environmental factors that were not shared by the twins.

Endothelin

Endothelin is a potent vasoconstricting peptide of 21 amino acids which is also mitogenic for smooth muscle cells. It has been found to occur in at least three forms, called endothelin-1, 2, and 3. Endothelial cells produce only endothelin-1 (143). Endothelin-converting-enzyme inhibitors and endothelin antagonists have shown some efficacy in reducing blood pressure in certain genetic animal models of hypertension (144,145). Whether endothelin plays an important role in human essential hypertension remains enigmatic because plasma levels (which are variably elevated or normal in human hypertension) do not necessarily reflect endothelial production rates since most endothelin is probably not secreted luminally. Nevertheless, several interesting observations suggest potential roles in promoting both hypertension and atherosclerosis. Endothelin production by cultured endothelial cells and intact aorta is stimulated by oxidized LDL (146) as well as by hypoxia (147), thrombin, transforming growth factor-β, interleukin-1, epinephrine, angiotensin II, vasopressin, calcium ionophore, and phorbol ester. Whether increased endothelin production may be involved in the hypertension associated with dyslipidemia is not known, but is an attractive hypothesis. Proliferating smooth muscle cells can also produce endothelin (148). Production of endothelin is inhibited by cyclic guanosine monophosphate (cGMP) and cyclic adenosine monophosphate (cAMP). Serum and vascular concentrations of endothelin were increased in patients with atherosclerosis (149). Endothelin may thus promote excess vasoconstriction known to occur at diseased vascular sites, especially if unopposed by nitric oxide (see below).

Interestingly, endothelin synthesis by endothelial cells is induced by cyclosporin (150). Indeed, endothelin may mediate, in large part, the salt-sensitive hypertension caused by cyclosporin. Both endothelin infusion and cyclosporin cause renal afferent vasoconstriction, decreased glomerular filtration rate, salt retention, and hypertension (150,151). This salt-sensitive hypertension, which develops after endothelin infusion in animals, is prevented by captopril, implicating the renin–angiotensin system as a mediator of the hypertensive effects of endothelin (152). These findings illustrate the intricate and sometimes unpredictable interplay among various systems which affect blood pressure.

Linkage analyses have not been done for endothelin, although genes have been cloned for endothelin and for two endothelin receptors, ETA and ETB. An association study of endothelin-1 and blood pressure (153) did not show that the particular polymorphism within the endothelin-1 gene on chromosome 6 was related to blood pressure.

Nitric Oxide in Blood Pressure Control

The potent vasodilator nitric oxide (NO) is yet another vasoactive substance with roles in hypertension and atherosclerosis. Furchgott and Zawadzki (154) first described the necessity of having an intact endothelium for acetylcholine to cause vasodilatation. If the endothelium was removed, acetylcholine caused constriction. The vasodilating substance released by endothelial cells after stimulation of muscarinic receptors was called endothelial-derived relaxing factor. Endothelial-derived relaxing factor was soon shown to be NO and/or adducts of NO. In fact, NO may circulate primarily as a nitrosothiol adduct after combining with sulfhydryl groups on proteins or free amino acids. Recently, plasma albumin was suggested to provide a buffer or pool of NO while free amino acids such as cysteine shuttle the NO to intracellular sites. Both the protein and free amino acid adducts are biologically active and have a significantly longer active half-life than free NO (155). NO is produced by several isozymes, among them two constitutively synthesized, noninducible NO synthases (one cytosolic and another membrane-bound obtained from endothelial cells and producing picomolar quantities of NO) and two inducible enzymes which predominate in smooth muscle cells (156). The inducible enzymes can produce sufficient NO (nanomolar quantities of NO) to cause shock when production is sufficiently stimulated by endotoxin or several cytokines including tumor necrosis factor, interleukin-1, and lipopolysaccharide.

The constitutive endothelial NO synthase is calcium and calmodulin dependent, and is stimulated by a variety of hormones (acetylcholine, bradykinin, serotonin, norepinephrine, histamine, ADP), peptides (endothelin, vasopressin, substance P), and mechanical factors such as flow or shear stress, all of which mediate increased intracellular calcium concentrations. Nitric oxide synthases oxidize the guanidine nitrogen of L-arginine to form citrulline and NO. These enzymes can be inhibited by certain arginine derivatives such as L-N^G-monomethyl arginine (L-NMMA), L-nitro arginine methyl ester (L-NAME), and L-*N*-nitro arginine (LNA). Nitric oxide diffuses across cell membranes and binds to the heme portion of soluble guanylate cyclase resulting in increased production of cGMP. In smooth muscle cells, increased cGMP activates cGMP kinase, which can then act on many proteins. Among the effects are increased permeability of potassium channels, increased calcium ATPase, decreased phospholipase C activity with reduced concentration of inositol phosphatides, and decreased phosphorylation of myosin light chain. In smooth muscle these effects lead directly and indirectly to relaxation. In platelets NO leads to decreased aggregation and adherence. Interestingly, in endothelial and smooth muscle cells, increased cGMP inhibits endothelin production, resulting in a negative feedback loop (since endothelin increases activity of the constitutive NO synthase in endothelial cells). In general, the endothelium provides a buffer to many potentially vasoconstricting agents by producing NO in response to the same intracellular signal (increasing calcium concentration) that causes vasoconstriction in smooth muscle cells. Hence, for example, acetylcholine or serotonin cause vasodilatation in an intact artery, but constriction if the endothelium is removed or impaired.

Nitric oxide may be unique among vasoactive substances in that tonic production appears to be involved in maintenance of normal blood pressure in animals (157–159) and humans (160) since infusion of NO synthase inhibitors raises blood pressure and vascular resistance even in normal individuals. Several studies suggest impaired NO production in hypertensive individuals (161–163). At least part of the impaired NO production appears to be due to the high blood pressure itself, being in part reversible with lowered pressure (164). Yet, sustained hypertension in normal rats was induced by prolonged administration of an NO synthase inhibitor (165,166). In humans, the increased blood pressure caused by NO synthesis inhibition by L-NMMA infusion did not result in increased central sympathetic outflow, though this mechanism may contribute to the hypertension caused by L-NMMA in several animal models (167). Interestingly, the vasodilatation of muscle vascular beds by insulin has been reported to be mediated by NO release (168). Defective NO release could promote insulin resistance by limiting blood flow to muscle cells when insulin levels are high, thereby decreasing delivery of glucose.

In kidneys, several mechanisms may contribute to antihypertensive effects of NO. Renal blood flow appears to be controlled by the balance between angiotensin II and NO. A 3-day infusion of L-NAME in conscious dogs at doses below the threshold to acutely affect blood pressure led to a 35% decrease in glomerular filtration rate, a 32% decrease in urinary sodium excretion, a sustained reduction in urine flow rate, and a 45% increase in plasma renin activity. These effects were reversible with administration of L-arginine (169). In normal rats, similar renal blood flow decrements were induced by NO synthesis inhibition. However, there was no effect on renal plasma flow if the animals were previously treated with a converting-enzyme inhibitor or an angiotensin II receptor antagonist. Interestingly, peripheral resistance and blood pressure were still raised by NO synthesis inhibition in these rats even after blocking angiotensin II production, suggesting different constricting factors may be counterbalanced by NO in the peripheral circulation (170). In two-kidney, one-clip renovascular hypertension, NO appears to be an important counterbalance to elevated circulating angiotensin II in keeping perfusion normal in the nonclipped kidney (171). Part of the reduction in sodium excretion caused by NO inhibitors may be due to alterations in renal interstitial fluid pressure which accompany other renal hemodynamic changes, but direct tubular effects are also possible, since increased cGMP decreases tubular sodium reabsorption (172). In addition, part of the increase in sodium excretion induced by volume loading was shown to be mediated by NO in dogs (173).

Although not clear at this time, it seems likely that the endothelial NO synthase is an important contributor to the effects noted in the above paragraph. However, NO is also produced by an enzyme in macula densa cells that is distinct from the endothelial constitutive NO synthase. This macula densa NO synthase is induced by a high-salt diet and stimulated by perfusion of macula densa cells with a high-sodium solution. Production of NO by the macula densa counteracted the vasoconstriction observed in the afferent arterioles when the macula densa was perfused with a solution of higher salt concentration. Inhibition of NO production had no effect when the macula densa was perfused with a low-salt solution. The vasoconstrictor acting when NO synthesis was inhibited was not identified (174).

Of great interest are the recent findings of a possible defect in NO production as a cause of the hypertension of the Dahl salt-sensitive rat. Hypertension in these animals has been prevented by long-term oral or parenteral administration of L-arginine but not D-arginine (156,175). Other studies demonstrated correction of shifted pressure–natriuresis curves by L-arginine administration in salt-sensitive animals (176). No effect of L-arginine was seen in the salt-resistant rats in these studies. Administration of dexamethasone in a dose sufficient to suppress inducible NO synthases prevented the ameliorating effect of L-arginine in the salt-sensitive animals. That is, an inducible enzyme was implicated as deficient in the salt-sensitive animals rather than the constitutive endothelial NO synthase (156).

Because of nitric oxide's important blood pressure effects, genes regulating nitric oxide have been suggested as candidate genes involved with the development of hypertension. The gene coding for this enzyme has been cloned (177) and an informative polymorphism has been identified within the 22-kb gene on chromosome 7 (178). However, the constitutive gene was not linked to hypertension in two studies (ref. 179, and S. C. Hunt, *unpublished results*), paralleling the salt-sensitive animal study results above.

Nitric Oxide in Atherosclerosis

Several investigators have reported abnormally decreased vasodilatation or frank constriction of coronary arteries in patients with atherosclerotic coronary artery disease after infusion of acetylcholine, bradykinin, substance P, or other endothelium-dependent vasodilators (180–182). Abnormal endothelial-dependent vasodilatation appears to extend to the arteriolar and microvascular level when epicardial atherosclerosis or hypercholesterolemia is present (183–186). Furthermore, abnormal vasodilatation of coronary arteries is significantly correlated to coronary risk factors (especially male gender, age, hypercholesterolemia, and hypertension) even when coronary arteries appear angiographically normal (184,187–189). Low HDL (190) also appears to cause endothelial dysfunction. High lipoprotein (a) levels in children with heterozygous familial hypercholesterolemia were associated with impaired endothelial-dependent vasodilatation (191). By this mechanism both atherosclerosis and its risk factors may predispose to vasoconstriction and arterial spasm.

Multiple animal studies document the adverse effects of hypercholesterolemia on endothelial-dependent relaxation (185). A marked impairment of endothelial-dependent relaxation occurred after just 4 weeks of cholesterol feeding in rabbits, while fish oil was found to be protective (192). Dietary (193,194) or drug (195) treatment of hyperlipidemia in animals restores endothelial-dependent vascular reactivity back toward normal. Importantly, this occurs before visually apparent regression of lesions has occurred, though cholesterol ester content of lesions is reduced (196). Observations in human hypercholesterolemic subjects also demonstrate endothelial dysfunction in hypercholesterolemia (197–201). Treatment of hypercholesterolemic patients with diet and cholestyramine (with an LDL reduction of 36%) resulted in improved coronary endothelial function (202). In another study, positron emission tomography demonstrated improvement in cardiac perfusion in just 90 days of vigorous cholesterol-lowering therapy. Cardiac perfusion reverted back to baseline values within 2 months after discontinuing the lipid-lowering treatment (203). Patients in this study reported a 51% reduction in angina episodes during their treatment. These results may help explain the marked reduction in angina reported by others after only 1 month of vigorous dietary cholesterol-lowering intervention (204) and the marked decrease in silent ischemia detected by ambulatory ECG monitoring after just 4 months of lovastatin therapy (205).

How does hyperlipidemia cause endothelial dysfunction? In cholesterol-fed rabbits, NO production by vessel walls was actually found to be increased despite dramatic impairment in release of endothelial-derived relaxing factor activity as assessed by a bioassay, suggesting increased degradation of the NO that was produced (206). Others have found that oxidized lipoproteins may quench or inactivate available NO (207–209), though increased levels of native LDL also appear to interfere with its activity (207). Experimental evidence suggests lysolecithin as a key toxic component of oxidized LDL (210,211) and that HDL can remove lysolecithin and reverse its inhibition of endothelial-dependent relaxation (212). Additionally, endothelium from hypercholesterolemic, cholesterol-fed rabbits was found to produce excess superoxide anion, probably via increased xanthine oxidase activity (213). NO is known to be rapidly destroyed by superoxide anions and appears to be protected by vascular superoxide dismutase.

Recently, estradiol has been shown to reverse abnormal coronary responses to acetylcholine in postmenopausal women (214,215). Furthermore, estrogen administration resulted in significant enhancement of NO release in other vascular beds (216,217). Endogenous estrogen appears to reverse the adverse endothelial effects of hypercholesterolemia in premenopausal women (218). These studies provide important insights into gender differences in risk of coronary atherosclerosis.

While impaired endothelium-dependent relaxation is characteristic of atherosclerotic arteries and is associated with coronary risk factors, perhaps of greater importance are the arterioprotective effects of NO itself. Recently, marked reduction in atherosclerosis was seen when cholesterol-fed rabbits were supplemented with L-arginine, the precursor of NO (219). Thus, oral L-arginine (2.25% in drinking water resulting in a sixfold increase in oral intake and two- to threefold increases in plasma arginine) in rabbits fed a 1% cholesterol diet resulted in a reduction in plaque area to about 9% in the descending thoracic aorta compared to 38% in cholesterol-fed controls without arginine supplements. More recent studies demonstrate that the same dose of oral L-arginine also reduces neointimal thickening after balloon dilation in normocholesterolemic rabbits (220). Decreased platelet aggregation and adhesion, decreased monocyte adherence, or decreased proliferation of smooth muscle cells, effects of NO that have been demonstrated in vitro (221), may all have contributed to the beneficial outcomes in these animal experiments. Conversely, inhibition of NO synthesis promoted atherosclerosis in cholesterol-fed rabbits (222). Evidence that the direct NO donor molsidomine has a beneficial effect in preventing restenosis after coronary angioplasty has already been presented (223). Whether arginine supplements might inhibit human atherogenesis remains an intriguing and important question.

RENIN–ANGIOTENSIN–KALLIKREIN SYSTEMS

The renin–angiotensin system plays an important role in salt and water homeostasis and the maintenance of vascular tone. Each component of this system represents a potential candidate in the etiology of hypertension. Accordingly, genetic investigations of renin activity, angiotensin-converting-enzyme activity, angiotensinogen, and angiotensin II have been done. Most work on the molecular genetics of human hypertension has concentrated on variables in these control systems. Details of these studies are covered in another chapter in this volume. Briefly, linkage of plasma renin activity and angiotensin-converting enzyme (ACE) to hypertension has been rejected (224,225). Although the renin gene has not been linked to hypertension, renin levels are important in the pathophysiology of hypertension, as they are modulated by genetic and phenotypic variation of other, related variables. Also, high renin activity has been related to the development of coronary heart disease in a prospective study (226). Because angiotensinogen has been reported to be linked and associated with hypertension or blood pressure, and kallikrein levels have been suggested to segregate as a major gene, the mechanisms relating these two variables to hypertension will be reviewed. Relationships to cardiovascular disease will also be proposed.

Plasma Angiotensinogen and Angiotensin II

Linkage of hypertension to angiotensinogen levels has been demonstrated in multiple populations (227–230). Association of the M235T variant within the angiotensinogen gene has been found in some studies (227–229), but not in others (230–234).

Angiotensin II is formed after cleavage of angiotensinogen by renin and cleavage of angiotensin I by ACE. Cleavage by renin is usually the rate-limiting step in plasma angiotensin II formation. Because the plasma concentration of angiotensinogen is close to the Michaelis constant of the enzymatic reaction between renin and angiotensinogen (235), a rise or fall in angiotensinogen can lead to a parallel change in the formation of angiotensin II (236,237). There is also a direct positive feedback mechanism of increasing angiotensin II levels on increased formation of angiotensinogen.

In normal physiology, the renin conversion of angiotensinogen to angiotensin I decreases the amount of angiotensinogen. Increased angiotensin II levels stimulate hepatic angiotensinogen production and release, returning angiotensinogen levels to normal. Angiotensin II-stimulated angiotensinogen production seems to occur by stabilization of the mRNA for angiotensinogen, not by activation of transcription by any known DNA sequence (238). Renin is normally regulated by sodium loads sensed by the macula densa in the juxtaglomerular apparatus in the kidney or by reduced perfusion pressure. In the presence of decreased pressure or sodium loads, plasma renin is increased, producing more angiotensin II (239). Vasoconstriction occurs reducing the renin levels and replenishing the angiotensinogen levels through the angiotensin II positive feedback loop. A genetic abnormality in angiotensinogen production appears to increase angiotensinogen levels resulting in higher amounts converted to angiotensin II. The higher angiotensinogen levels would also be maintained through higher feedback by angiotensin II. Increased angiotensin II stimulates aldosterone release, increasing sodium and water retention, which increases blood pressure.

Long-term administration of angiotensin II at subpressor doses has been shown to elevate blood pressure (240). It is hypothesized that the increased blood pressure resulting from chronic angiotensinogen elevation would tend to reduce the renin released in the kidney. Higher angiotensin II levels also have a negative feedback on renin, decreasing renin levels (241). Since it has been shown that increased amounts of angiotensinogen are associated with higher blood pressure, this implies that if renin activity is reduced, it is still sufficient to maintain the increased conversion of angiotensinogen to angiotensin I. Preliminary results from a rat study suggest that if plasma renin activity remains low, there is no relationship between blood pressure and angiotensinogen, while for rats with high renin there was a strong relationship (242). High renin led to angiotensinogen depletion.

Other evidence supports the relationship between angiotensinogen and hypertension. Plasma angiotensinogen was higher in hypertensive subjects and in the offspring of hypertensive parents than in normotensive controls (243). The 235T allele at the angiotensinogen locus is associated with higher angiotensinogen levels and with increased blood pressure levels in French subjects (244). In the Four Corners Study (245), angiotensinogen concentrations were significantly associated with higher blood pressure in the subset most likely to show genetic predisposition, namely the high-blood-pressure offspring of parents with high blood pressure. The correlation between angiotensinogen levels and blood pressure in another study was $r = 0.39$ (246). An injection of angiotensinogen increases blood pressure (247), while if angiotensinogen antibodies are administered, blood pressure is decreased (248). Vascular injury induces angiotensinogen gene expression (249). Finally, blood pressure is elevated in transgenic animals who are overexpressing angiotensinogen (250). Thus, many different studies have provided evidence that angiotensinogen is associated with blood pressure levels and with risk of hypertension.

Obesity appears to be an important promotor of hypertension. One mechanism through which obesity may increase blood pressure is by way of the angiotensinogen system, especially in those who may have the AGT gene that elevates angiotensinogen levels. Even in those without the defective AGT gene, significant obesity may induce elevated blood pressure through the angiotensinogen pathway. Therefore, obesity may either add to genetic influences or may mimic genetic influences even when they are not present.

In a rat feeding experiment, it was shown that fasted rats decreased the production of mRNA for angiotensinogen in adipose cells, decreased the cellular release of angiotensinogen into the local circulation, and decreased central blood pressure (108). It was hypothesized that decreased local angiotensinogen led to local vasodilatation and increased tissue perfusion allowing (a) free fatty acids to be removed from the tissue into the general circulation for fuel use, (b) increased insulin-stimulated glucose uptake by the adipose tissue, and (c) decreased blood pressure from the decreased vasoconstriction of vessels surrounded by adipose tissue. When the rats were overfed, angiotensinogen mRNA increased 16-fold from fasted levels and over twofold above control levels, with increased cellular release of angiotensinogen. This may represent local vasoconstriction resulting in the observed increase in systemic blood pressure, reduced fatty acid removal from the tissues (even though cellular release was increased), and decreased glucose uptake by adipose tissue due to the local vasoconstriction preventing glucose delivery to the adipose tissue. These changes would result in insulin resistance and hyperinsulinemia. In spite of the increased local release of angiotensinogen and increased blood pressure, there was no increase in systemic circulating levels of angiotensinogen.

Therefore an environmental response to overfeeding had similar responses on adipocyte angiotensinogen control that a gene for high angiotensinogen levels would have—a chronically overstimulated local angiotensinogen system that increased blood pressure and resulted in insulin resistance and decreased central utilization of free fatty acids. The gene for angiotensinogen would have greater effects, since it appears that hepatic release of angiotensinogen is also increased in those with the gene, resulting in elevated circulating levels of angiotensinogen, while circulating levels were not increased by overfeeding. In addition, differentiation of preadipocytes to adipocytes is related to the activation of the angiotensinogen promoter (251), suggesting that the greater the accrual of adipocytes, the greater the activation of the angiotensinogen gene.

Not only was there an acute overfeeding effect on angiotensinogen release, there were chronic differences in mRNA expression between *ob/ob* and lean control mice. One hypothesis, but not shared by all investigators, is that excess calories, available either through excess diet or decreased expenditure, causes insulin resistance resulting in hyperinsulinemia and higher catecholamine release. This would lead to increased metabolic rate to compensate for the excess calories, but also result in increased blood pressure as a result of increased Na and volume retention and catecholamine-induced vasoconstriction (252). Hyperinsulinemia can aggravate free fatty acid levels and vice versa (121) and may directly relate to abnormal adipose tissue angiotensinogen levels. In humans, glucose infusion reduced free fatty acid levels due to increased reesterification to triglycerides (253), a common feature of the dyslipidemic syndrome. Although human data have yet to be reported, it would appear that at least during periods of chronic weight gain in persons with the high-angiotensinogen gene, the effects of the gene and diet would be additive and may represent the increased risk of hypertension development in those who are overweight.

Kallikrein System and Angiotensin-Converting Enzyme

ACE has a dual effect in controlling blood pressure. It can convert angiotensin I to angiotensin II and can inactivate bradykinin. ACE is a more potent factor in the kallikrein–kinin system than in the renin–angiotensin system since bradykinin has a very low K_m (254). Bradykinin is a powerful vasodilator formed by the action of kallikrein on kininogen and stimulates prostaglandin formation. Higher ACE levels increase inactivation of bradykinin while increasing angiotensin II formation. ACE blockers decrease angiotensin II formation and increase the total bradykinin activity. Decreased kallikrein levels have been associated with hypertension (255–259). A major gene has been shown in segregation analyses to be responsible for a large portion of the phenotypic variability of urinary kallikrein excretion (260,261). It was found that inheritance followed a codominant pattern after the interactive effects of dietary potassium (as measured by urinary potassium excretion) were modeled. Increased potassium intake in persons who had high kallikrein levels (from the inferred high-kallikrein genotype which would protect one from hypertension) did not affect kallikrein levels. However, in persons inferred to be heterozygous at the kallikrein locus urinary kallikrein excretion had a very strong relationship with dietary potassium. Increased intake of potassium was related to increased kallikrein excretion and theoretically could protect the heterozygotes if there is a direct cause and effect relationship. Persons with the low-kallikrein genotype appeared to be unable to change kallikrein excretion even with increased potassium intake. Since the inferred kallikrein gene is also common and presumed to be a susceptibility gene, it is likely that both AGT and kallikrein genes will interact in some manner on the expression and regulation of two of the main blood pressure control systems: the renin–angiotensin and kallikrein–kinin systems.

Susceptibility loci alone presumably do not account for hypertension in the absence of other risk factors. Defects in the renin–angiotensin vasoconstricting system and the kallikrein–kinin vasodilating system may act synergistically to promote hypertension. Long-term blockade of bradykinin B_2 receptors by Hoe-140 in WKY normotensive rats did not cause an increase in blood pressure (262). However, blockade of the B_2 receptors during a normally nonpressor infusion of A-II caused significant blood pressure elevation. Infusion of low A-II doses into Brown Norway normotensive rats with normal kallikrein levels does not increase blood pressure. If the same dose of A-II is given to Brown Norway Katholiek rats, which have a complete lack of kallikrein, blood pressure rises faster than in control rats (263). Factors leading to hypertension may also change as hypertension develops. In DOCA-salt rats it was suggested that mineralocorticoids increase kallikrein levels to compensate for elevated vasoconstriction (264). As hypertension developed, kallikrein levels fell to low levels, no longer counteracting the vasoconstrictive effects of DOCA-salt.

Salt Sensitivity and Adrenal Nonmodulation

Salt sensitivity appears to be a continuous trait, but using various definitions to dichotomize the distribution, it has been suggested that salt sensitivity exists in approximately 50% of hypertensive subjects (265). One possible determinant of increased sodium sensitivity could be the hypertension susceptibility allele for the angiotensinogen gene. The presence of this allele may increase a person's blood pressure response to elevated dietary sodium intake. The person may either need less dietary sodium to activate the renin–angiotensin system or be overresponsive to fixed levels of sodium intake. Low-renin hypertensives seem to have increased sodium sensitivity. In the face of elevated angiotensinogen and the resulting increased angiotensin II, chronic vasoconstriction and sodium reabsorption would reduce the renin to low levels. The angiotensinogen gene itself is probably not regulated by plasma renin levels and would continue to produce high levels of angiotensinogen. Therefore the AGT gene is a reasonable candidate for the increased prevalence of low renin levels in sodium-sensitive individuals. Kallikrein levels are also reduced by increased sodium intake (255).

Evidence that AGT genotype variation is associated with salt sensitivity is also provided by nonmodulation studies. Nonmodulation has been defined as an abnormal blunted renal or adrenal response to infused angiotensin II, which is significantly more prevalent in the hypertensive population than the normotensive population (266,267). It is a very familial trait and has significant bimodality. Nonmodulators also tend to be salt sensitive. Recent work (PN Hopkins, unpublished results) has shown that variation at the M235 locus is associated with blunted renal-plasma-flow response to A-II infusion—especially in normotensive relatives of hypertensive patients. Change in renal plasma flow on a high sodium (200 mEq) diet to angiotensin II infusion was significantly more blunted in 235T homozygotes (−103 ml/min in 235T homozygotes versus −129 ml/min in those with the other two genotypes, $p = 0.005$). In addition to the effect of the 235T alleles on modulation of the renal/adrenal system, there was an interaction between AGT genotype and BMI. The 235T homozygotes were more susceptible to the blunting effects of obesity on renal plasma flow response than were persons with other genotypes.

CELLULAR ION TRANSPORT SYSTEMS

Ion transport across cell membranes has been the focus of a great deal of research on blood pressure control because of the inferred relationship of the activity of these systems to cellular sodium and calcium homeostasis and vascular smooth muscle contractility. Some of these systems include Na–Li countertransport, Na–K cotransport, Na–K ATPase transport, Na–H antiporter, Na–Ca exchange, Ca ATPase, $Cl–HCO_3$ transport, and the associated intracellular and extracellular levels of the ions these systems exchange. There are multiple mechanisms which control the activity of these cellular transport systems and intracellular ion content, including genetic control of baseline activity, ion concentration, and the number of transporters, cellular pH, cellular membrane lipid composition, and local or systemic circulating factors.

Table 6 shows that there appears to be considerable genetic involvement in the activity or concentration of many of the ionic variables involved with hypertension. These genetic factors combine to give hypertension the appearance of a polygenic trait. The h^2 term is an estimate of polygenic heritability and low estimates do not mean that there is no major-gene effect. Evidence for single major genes has been found for some of these variables. These genes are likely susceptibility genes, since the presence of the gene often does not lead to hypertension. The interaction of multiple genes along with environmental risk factors is likely responsible for the age at onset and severity of hypertension.

TABLE 6. *Heritability, common-household, and shared screening-date effects of biochemical measurements on 2,500 members of 98 Utah pedigrees*

Variables	h^2	c^2	d^2
Cell cation tests			
Na–Li countertransport	0.58	0.02	0.08
Intraerythrocytic Na	0.58	0.14	0.20
Ouabain-binding sites	0.56	0.16	0.12
Na-K-ATPase pump activity	0.22	0.03	0.35
Li–K cotransport	0.30	0.00	0.26
Lithium leak	0.43	0.00	0.40
Intraerythrocytic Mg	0.29	0.00	0.56
Blood tests			
Mg concentration	0.57	0.24	0.00
Na concentration	0.14	0.01	0.52
K concentration	0.23	0.07	0.18
Total Ca concentration	0.14	0.13	0.17
Phosphate concentration	0.30	0.08	0.04
Renin activity	0.07	0.00	0.74
Uric acid concentration	0.31	0.08	0.04
Fasting blood glucose	0.15	0.00	0.09
Total cholesterol	0.42	0.08	0.00

Adapted from Williams et al., ref. 310.

h^2, Polygenic heritability; c^2, common-household effect (chronic shared environment); d^2, same-day screening effect (immediate shared-environment or same-day measurement effects).

Na–Li Countertransport, Na–H Antiporter, and Na–K–Cl Cotransport

Segregation analysis suggests that Na–Li countertransport is a recessive trait with high levels in about 5% of the population (268,269). This system is thought to represent some form of Na–H exchange (270), but has its own unique properties (271). It is clearly familial and increased in hypertensive versus normotensive subjects.

Na–H exchange is an important cellular control system to maintain pH within an optimal range for proper cellular function (272). Na–H antiport units are found in many cells and tissues, including skeletal muscle and the brush border of the kidney proximal tubule. Increased cellular functions which cause greater acidity and lower pH invoke an otherwise silent Na–H antiport system to extrude H, thereby increasing pH. A metabolic shift toward utilization of fats rather than carbohydrates may produce more acid products, promoting more acid intracellular pH. Increased stimulation of sodium–hydrogen exchange increases Na reabsorption, perhaps leading to volume-related blood pressure increases. This may be followed by compensating increased Na–Ca exchange and increased intracellular calcium, fostering increased smooth muscle contractility and hypertension (273). Intracellular calcium may be a mediating factor between transport system abnormalities and vasoconstriction. Increased intracellular free Ca stimulates Na–H exchange across the plasma membrane, while increased cellular calcium in the juxtaglomerular cells in the kidney also has direct effects on renin release and enzyme activity (274).

The activity of the Na–H antiporter or Na–Li countertransport are modulated by other factors as well. Insulin increases activation of the antiporter, as it does with other transport systems (275). Resnick et al. proposed that intracellular cation imbalances may be responsible for an underlying insulin resistance, specifically, decreased cellular pH and Mg and increased Ca (276,277). Metabolic cellular abnormalities reflected by cation and pH imbalances may stimulate insulin production to activate the Na–H exchange system to compensate for these abnormalities. In addition, catecholamines, which reduce the effectiveness of insulin on glucose uptake, increase intracellular levels of calcium (114,115) and may be synergistic with the above mechanisms.

Na–H antiporter activity is affected through both the diacyl glycerol/protein kinase C cascade and the phosphoinositol cascade. The protein kinase C pathway is connected to specific growth factors that may be involved in vessel remodeling (278,279), leading to increased blood pressure and cardiovascular disease. Angiotensin II increases sodium reabsorption (280) probably by G-protein-mediated inhibition of adenylate cyclase. This inhibition increases Na–H exchange and bicarbonate reabsorption. Angiotensin II is itself a growth factor and may act with Na–H exchange mechanisms as a structural as well as physiologic factor in the development of hypertension (281).

In spite of the attractive hypotheses surrounding Na–Li countertransport and the Na–H antiporter, a linkage study of the gene controlling the ubiquitous expression of Na–H exchange to Na–Li countertransport, blood pressure, or hypertension failed to show linkage (282). Other isoforms exist for expression of the antiporter specifically in the kidney which remain as candidate genes for hypertension and ion transport.

Na–K cotransport has also been proposed as having a genetic basis of expression (283). However, segregation analysis using large pedigrees has not yet been able to show evidence for a major gene controlling this phenotype. This transport system probably maintains cellular Cl at appropriate levels (284). Low Na–K cotransport has been especially associated with low-renin hypertension, whereas elevated Na–Li countertransport is more closely associated with high-renin hypertension (285). Similar to the results found for angiotensin, differences in renin control suggest that ion transport and the renin–angiotensin system may share some similar regulatory mechanisms.

Membrane Fluidity and Lipids

Lipids and lipoproteins influence the level of most ion transport systems, with triglycerides or VLDL cholesterol having the strongest correlations (286,287). Triglycerides and VLDL-C are also higher in persons inferred to have the high Na–Li countertransport genotype (268). If triglyceride levels alter ion transport in a causal pathway leading to hypertension, this may be one link between dyslipidemic hypertension and coronary heart disease. The hypothesized mechanism is through alterations in membrane lipid content, changing the membrane fluidity and capability of individual transport units to operate normally. There are mixed findings supporting the relationship of dyslipidemia, ion transport, and hypertension. Changes in membrane fluidity have been associated with increased countertransport levels (288,289). Membrane fluidity is decreased by cellular calcium loading (290) and this decrease is greater in hypertensive than in normotensive patients (291). Low-dietary-salt intake increases membrane fluidity (292), providing another pathway for the development of hypertension.

Persons with familial combined hyperlipidemia have high triglycerides and smaller, denser LDL particles as opposed to persons with familial hypercholesterolemia. The Na–Li countertransport levels in the former group were 0.43 mmol/L red blood cells (RBC)/hr as opposed to the levels in the latter group of 0.16 for hypertensives and 0.23 for normotensives (293). Normolipidemic adults have levels of 0.28 mmol/L RBC/hr. This implies that the particular circulating phospholipid species and cholesterol levels are important in determining the composition of the cell membrane and ion transport activity. Evidence that lipids or lipoproteins may affect blood pressure are provided from both epidemiological studies and cellular studies. Triglycerides predicted the development of hypertension in normotensive persons followed for 7 years (26). Also, after exposure to increasing doses of human LDL cholesterol (range of 1–15 μg/ml), cultured smooth muscle cell and rat aortic ring contraction were increased in a dose-dependent fashion, apparently mediated by LDL-induced changes in intracellular pH and calcium concentration (294). Similar effects might occur for intermediate-density lipoprotein (IDL) or beta-VLDL. However, a recent cholesterol-lowering intervention study casts doubt on the importance of cholesterol levels per se on countertransport, even though membrane cholesterol is reduced (295).

Ouabain-Binding Sites, Na–K ATPase Pump, and Intracellular Na

Studies have identified the presence of natriuretic substances that inhibit the sodium–potassium pump. At least four such inhibitory substances have been identified: ouabain (296), linoleic and oleic acids (297), and lysophosphatidylcholine (298). The last three substances have a common precursor, phosphatidylcholine, a phospholipid in the cell membrane. Population genetic analyses have not shown strong evidence for major-gene determination of the Na–K ATPase pump, but a recent study in rats suggests that further research in humans is required (299). Segregation analysis of the number of ATPase sites, as measured by the amount of ouabain binding, has shown evidence for a recessive inheritance of an increased number of sites in about 2% of the population (300). High intraerythrocytic sodium levels appeared to segregate as a recessive trait, with a four-allele model fitting better than a two-allele model (301). Since we do not yet know cause and effect relationships, it is possible that higher numbers of pump sites are a response to increased intracellular sodium levels and vasoconstriction. It is equally possible that there are no direct relationships among intracellular sodium, the number or activity of the ATPase sites, and blood pressure as a result of genetic abnormalities.

Systems Analysis Approach to Ion Transport

No one gene involved with cellular ionic homeostasis acts independently of other controls of cellular function. For example, a gene with large effects on the number of Na–K ATPase exchange sites may also affect cellular concentrations of sodium, potassium, or calcium or changed activity of other associated transport systems. In addition to multiple effects of a single gene, each transport system likely reflects influences of multiple genetic variants. In order to separate multiple genetic influences on a single variable and allow for correlated secondary effects of other variables, the statistical technique of principal components was used to combine variables into independent linear equations. Variables that had the same genetic source of variance would most likely show high correlations with one of the newly defined equations, and variables that were not closely involved with a particular gene would have low correlations with that equation, but might have high correlations on another equation that represented the greatest control over the expression of that variable. While somewhat complicated, this technique overcomes problems in genetic analysis of a syndrome such as the multiple metabolic syndrome which has multiple abnormal phenotypes. For example, it is not clear how insulin levels, lipid levels, glucose uptake, or obesity should be combined in a genetic analysis of the multiple metabolic syndrome. Using a principal components approach, however, allows these phenotypes to be combined into multiple equations, each equation representing a possible independent risk factor for this syndrome. Genetic analysis of these multivariate equations may proceed as though it were a single quantitative phenotype.

Using this methodology on multiple-ion transport concentrations and transporters, 14 equations from 14 variables were formed. Segregation analysis showed that there was evidence for five common and three rare major genes among these components (302). Table 7 shows the four variables with the highest correlations on the five components suggested to have common major-gene involvement. The first component segregates as a recessive major gene and appears to resemble the characteristics of familial dyslipidemic hypertension or the multiple metabolic syndrome. Persons are more obese, with high triglyceride levels. In addition, their Na–Li countertransport levels are moderately elevated, but not to the level predicted by the segregating major gene suggested for Na–Li countertransport. Urine creatinine, a correlate of weight, is also correlated with this component. Attempts to use different definitions of ratios of lipids, lipoproteins, or insulin levels in segregation analyses of this syndrome have not found evidence for Mendelian segregation even though there was significant bimodality. However, the principal components analysis allowed combination of some of these variables into a factor which did fit a Mendelian inheritance model. Addition of insulin, glucose, HDL-C, and LDL subfraction levels to this model still needs to be done to verify that component 1 represents all of the features of familial dyslipidemic hypertension rather than one of the suggested obesity genes.

The second component with major-gene effects is designated the ouabain-binding component because there are higher intraerythrocytic sodium levels in conjunction with a reduced number of ouabain-binding sites. The activity of the Na–K ATPase pump correlates poorly with this component. However, the reduced number of sites agrees with previous segregation analyses using only the number of sites as a univariate phenotype (300).

It appears that there may be two additional genes affecting Na–Li countertransport levels, one dominant (component 3) and one recessive (component 4). Each of these two independent components with major-gene segregation had high correlations with Na–Li countertransport. The mean countertransport levels in gene carriers were much higher (0.48 and 0.50 mmol/l RBC/h) than found for gene carriers of component 1 (0.39 mmol/l RBC/h). Triglycerides correlated inversely with component 4, so that gene carriers inferred to carry the gene represented by component 4 had below-normal triglycerides, while component 3, without a significant correlation with triglycerides, had normal or slightly elevated triglyceride levels. It appears that the two countertransport components have different biochemical profiles of the measured variables. If there are two genetic components to Na–Li countertransport, this would explain the suggested heterogeneity in other studies, where the genetic

TABLE 7. *Variables with the strongest correlations with five principal components inferred to have major-gene inheritance*

Principal component	1. Familial dyslipidemic HBP	2. Ouabain-binding sites	3. Na–Li countertransport	4. Na–Li countertransport	5. BMI
Variable 1	BMI	RBC Na	Na–Li CNT	Na–Li CNT	BMI
Variable 2	Triglyceride	Number of sites	Urine K	Triglyceride	Urine K
Variable 3	Na–Li CNT	Plasma K	Plasma K	Urine K	Triglyceride
Variable 4	Urine creatinine	Plasma Na	Cell Na leak	Plasma Na	Urine creatinine
Inheritance	Recessive	Recessive	Dominant	Recessive	Recessive
Abnormal genotype	8.6%	7.6%	2.0%	3.1%	2.0%

CNT, Countertransport.

transmission was not according to Mendelian expectations. The moderate correlation of Na–Li countertransport on component 1 will also reduce analytic heterogeneity since the persons with elevated Na–Li countertransport presumably due to increased triglyceride and body mass index levels are separated from those who appear to carry a gene directly related to countertransport independently of triglyceride levels. Separation into three genetic components influencing Na–Li countertransport seems to have resolved the transmission problem and may allow subsetting of the families for more powerful linkage analyses to find the responsible gene.

The fifth genetic component appears to be a gene for moderate obesity, but with normal triglyceride levels. Triglyceride levels are highly correlated with this factor, but the gene carriers do not have elevated levels compared to those without the gene. Therefore, while triglyceride levels correlate with higher body mass index, hypertriglyceridemia is not related to the inferred underlying gene affecting obesity in families segregating for this component.

BLOOD PRESSURE REACTIVITY

In a review of the literature using meta analysis, the majority of 39 studies found increased blood pressure reactivity in hypertensive subjects, but the findings were not entirely consistent across the studies examined (303). There are likely many factors involved in study variability, including heterogeneity of the underlying physiology. One recent study has shown that mental stress was associated with vasoconstriction in obese subjects but vasodilatation in lean subjects, even though both groups increased mean arterial pressure (304). Isometric stress was associated with exaggerated arterial pressure and resistance in both groups. In a 6.5-year prospective study, larger systolic and diastolic blood pressure responses to mental and physical stressors were associated with higher follow-up resting blood pressures (305). A twin study showed that systolic and diastolic blood pressure response to a mental arithmetic test was highly heritable (50%) (306). Another study in pedigrees and twins showed that blood pressure levels during both mental and physical stressor tests had a significant genetic component of about the same magnitude as the resting blood pressure measurements (307).

CAUSAL GENETIC MUTATIONS

Glucocorticoid-remediable aldosteronism (GRA) has been shown to be determined by a single, dominantly inherited genetic defect on chromosome 8 (308). There is an unequal crossing over between the paired chromosomes containing the gene for 11β-hydroxylase with a homologous (95% identical) gene for aldosterone synthase resulting in hypertension. This occurrence can completely explain the observed pathophysiology of this disorder, which causes severe hypertension in youths, very early strokes, and mortality. Diagnosis of this condition is important because it is unresponsive to usual antihypertensive therapies (e.g., diuretics), which greatly decrease serum potassium in this disorder, but it is responsive to glucocorticoid therapy.

Liddle's syndrome is caused by a defect in the β subunit of the sodium channel of the kidney epithelium (309). It is also dominantly inherited and results in early age at onset of hypertension and usually hypokalemia. Plasma renin activity and aldosterone are low even when dietary sodium is low. Four different mutations in a small region of this gene lead to expression of the syndrome.

SUMMARY OF THE FUTURE OF HYPERTENSION GENETICS

With the advent of human genetic maps using highly polymorphic markers, studies in the next few years will be able to identify genes that increase the risk of or cause hypertension. Causal genes have been recently identified. The identification of glucocorticoid-remediable aldosteronism has allowed specific medications to be prescribed which otherwise would not have been used, preventing fruitless and perhaps dangerous treatment by common first-line medications. The angiotensinogen gene is representative of the class of genes that increase susceptibility to hypertension. These types of genes will facilitate division of patients into risk or diagnostic groups so that effects of other identified genes or environmental factors may be determined within homogeneous groups. True gene–environment and gene–gene interactions will be able to be observed and described, allowing better pharmacologic investigation of how to effectively treat hypertension. Molecular genetics of hypertension will identify specific enzymes, receptors, or hormones that can be controlled by the development of new drugs. Controlling one of the major risk factors for cardiovascular disease without aggravating other risk factors, such as lipid or glucose metabolism, by the treatment of hypertension should reduce morbidity and mortality.

REFERENCES

1. Guyton AC. *Textbook of Medical Physiology,* 5th ed. Philadelphia: Saunders; 1976:924.
2. MacMahon S, Peto R, Cutler J, Collins R, Sorlie P, Neaton J, Abbott R, Godwin J, Dyer A, Stamler J. Blood pressure, stroke, and coronary heart disease. Part 1. Prolonged differences in blood pressure: prospective observational studies corrected for the regression dilution bias. *Lancet* 1990;335:765–774.
3. Medical Research Council Working Party. MRC trial of treatment of mild hypertension: principal results. *Br Med J* 1985;291:97–104.
4. SHEP Cooperative Research Group. Prevention of stroke by antihypertensive drug treatment in older persons with isolated systolic hypertension. Final results of the systolic hypertension in the elderly program (SHEP). *JAMA* 1991;265:3255–3264.
5. Collins R, Peto R, MacMahon S, Hebert P, Fiebach NH, Eberlein KA, Godwin J, Qizilbash N, Taylor JO, Hennekens CH. Blood pressure, stroke, and coronary heart disease. Part 2. Short-term reductions in blood pressure: overview of randomised drug trials in their epidemiological context. *Lancet* 1990;335:827–838.

6. Dahlöf B, Lindholm LH, Hansson L, Scherstén B, Ekmon T, Wester P-O. Morbidity and mortality in the Swedish Trial in Old Patients with Hypertension (STOP-Hypertension). *Lancet* 1991;338: 1281–1285.
7. Yusuf S, Lessem J, Jha P, Lonn E. Primary and secondary prevention of myocardial infarction and strokes: An update of randomly allocated, controlled trials. *J Hypertens* 1993;11(Suppl 4):S61–S73.
8. Neaton JD, Wentworth D. Serum cholesterol, blood pressure, cigarette smoking, and death from coronary heart disease. *Arch Intern Med* 1992;152:56–64.
9. Stamler J. Epidemiology, established major risk factors, and the primary prevention of coronary heart disease. In: Parmley WW, Chatterjee K, eds. *Cardiology,* Vol 2. Philadelphia: Lippincott; 1987;1: 1–41.
10. Neaton JD, Kuller LH, Wentworth D, Borhani NO. Total and cardiovascular mortality in relation to cigarette smoking, serum cholesterol concentration, and diastolic blood pressure among black and white males followed up for five years. *Am Heart J* 1984;108:759–769.
11. Joint National Committee. The fifth report of the Joint National Committee on Detection, Evaluation, and Treatment of High Blood Pressure (JNC V). *Arch Intern Med* 1993;153:154–183.
12. Robertson WB, Strong JP. Atherosclerosis in persons with hypertension and diabetes mellitus. *Lab Invest* 1968;18:539–551.
13. Solberg LA, McGarry PA. Cerebral atherosclerosis in persons with selected diseases. *Lab Invest* 1968;18:613–619.
14. Stephens T, Craig CL, Ferris BF. Adult physical fitness and hypertension in Canada: findings from the Canada Fitness Survey II. *Can J Pub Health* 1986;77:291–298.
15. Sprecher DL, Schaefer EJ, Kent KM, Gregg RE, Zech LA, Hoeg JM, McManus B, Roberts WC, Brewer HJ. Cardiovascular features of homozygous familial hypercholesterolemia: Analysis of 16 patients. *Am J Cardiol* 1984;54(1):20–30.
16. Keys A, Menotti A, Aravanis C, Blackburn H, Djordevic BS, Buzina R, Dontas AS, Fidanza F, Karvonen MJ, Kimura N, Mohacek I, Nedeljkovic S, Puddu V, Punsar S, Taylor HL, Conti S, Kromhout D, Toshima H. The Seven Countries Study: 2,289 Deaths in 15 Years. *Prev Med* 1984;13:141–154.
17. Gordon T, Garcia-Palmieri MR, Kapan A. Differences in coronary heart disease in Framingham, Honolulu and Puerto Rico. *J Chron Dis* 1974;27:329–344.
18. Kozarevic D, Pirc D, Dawber TR, Gordon T, Zukel W, Vojvodic N. The Yugoslavia cardiovascular disease study. 1. The incidence of coronary heart disease by area. *J Chron Dis* 1976;29:405–414.
19. Kozarevic D, Pirc B, Racic Z. The Yugoslavia cardiovascular disease study. II. Factors in the incidence of coronary heart disease. *Am J Epidemiol* 1976;104:133–140.
20. Ferrara LA, Mancini M, Celentano A, Galderisi M, Iannuzzi R, Marotta T, Gaeta I. Early changes of the arterial carotid wall in uncomplicated primary hypertensive patients. Study by ultrasound high-resolution B-mode imaging. *Arterioscler Thromb* 1994;14:1290–1296.
21. Suurküla M, Agewall S, Fagerberg B, Wendelhag I, Widgren B, Wikstrand J. Ultrasound evaluation of atherosclerotic manifestations in the carotid artery in high-risk hypertensive patients. *Arterioscler Thromb* 1994;14:1297–1304.
22. Hopkins PN, Williams RR. A survey of 246 suggested coronary risk factors. *Atherosclerosis* 1981;40(1):1–52.
23. Chobanian AV, Lichtenstein AH, Nilakhe V, Haudenschild CC, Drago R, Nickerson C. Influence of hypertension on aortic atherosclerosis in the Watanabe rabbit. *Hypertension* 1989;14:203–209.
24. Xu C, Galgov S, Zatina MA, Zarins CK. Hypertension sustains plaque progresson despite reduction of hypercholesterolemia. *Hypertension* 1991;18:123–129.
25. Friedman GD, Selby JV, Quesenberry CP Jr, Armstrong MA, Klatsky AL. Precursors of essential hypertension: Body weight, alcohol and salt use, and parental history of hypertension. *Prev Med* 1988;17: 387–402.
26. Hunt SC, Stephenson SH, Hopkins PN, Williams RR. Predictors of an increased risk of future hypertension in Utah pedigrees: A screening analysis. *Hypertension* 1991;17:969–976.
27. Lauer RM, Burns TL, Clarke WR, Mahoney LT. Childhood predictors of future blood pressure. *Hypertension* 1991;18(Suppl I):I-74–I-81.
28. Hunt SC, Williams RR. Genetic factors in human hypertension. In: Swales JD, ed. *Textbook of Hypertension.* Oxford: Blackwell; 1994: 519–538.
29. Hunt SC, Williams RR, Barlow GK. A comparison of positive family history definitions for defining risk of future disease. *J Chron Dis* 1986;39:809–821.
30. Carmelli D, Cardon LR, Fabsitz R. Clustering of hypertension, diabetes, and obesity in adult male twins: Same genes or same environments? *Am J Hum Genet* 1994;55:566–573.
31. Buja LM, Kovanen PT, Bilheimer DW. Cellular pathology of homozygous familial hypercholesterolemia. *Am J Pathol* 1979;97(2): 327–357.
32. Glagov S, Ozoa AK. Significance of the relatively low incidence of atherosclerosis in the pulmonary, renal and mesenteric arteries. *Ann NY Acad Sci* 1968;149:940–955.
33. Curmi PA, Juan L, Tedgui A. Effect of transmural pressure on low density lipoprotein and albumin transport and distribution across the intact arterial wall. *Circ Res* 1990;66(6):1692–1702.
34. Fry DL. Mass transport, atherogenesis, and risk. *Arteriosclerosis* 1987;7:88–100.
35. Friedman MH. How hemodynamic forces in the human affect the topography and development of atherosclerosis. In: Glagov S, Newman WP III, Schaffer SA, eds. *Pathobiology of the Human Atherosclerotic Plaque.* New York: Springer-Verlag; 1990:303–315.
36. Ku DN, Giddens DP. Pulsatile flow in a model carotid bifurcation. *Arteriosclerosis* 1983;3(31):31–39.
37. Haudenschild CC, Grunwald J, Chobanian AV. Effects of hypertension on migration and proliferation of smooth muscle in culture. *Hypertension* 1985;7(Suppl I):I-101–I-104.
38. Scannapieco G, Pauletto P, Pagnan A, Mattiello A, Biffanti S, Jori G, Palu CD. Lipoprotein binding to cultured aortic smooth muscle cells from normotensive and hypertensive rats. *J Hypertens* 1988;6: S269–S271.
39. Frangos JA, Eskin SG, McIntire LV, Ives CL. Flow effects on prostacyclin production by cultured human endothelial cells. *Science* 1985; 227:1477–1479.
40. Buga GM, Gold ME, Fukuto JM, Ignarro LJ. Shear stress-induced release of nitric oxide from endothelial cells grown on beads. *Hypertension* 1991;17:187–193.
41. Tsao PS, Lewis NP, Wang B, Cooke JP. Flow-induced nitric oxide inhibits monocyte adhesion to endothelial cells. *Circulation* 1994; 90(Suppl I):I-29(abst).
42. Friedman MH. A biologically plausible model of thickening of arterial intima under shear. *Arteriosclerosis* 1989;9(511):511–522.
43. Glagov S, Zarins C, Giddens DP, Ku DN. Hemodynamics and atherosclerosis. Insights and perspectives gained from studies of human arteries. *Arch Pathol Lab Med* 1988;112(1018):1018–1031.
44. Uematsu M, Kitabatake A, Tanouchi J, Doi Y, Masuyama T, Fujii K, Yoshida Y, Ito H, Ishihara K, Hori M, Inoue M, Kamada T. Reduction of endothelial microfilament bundles in the low-shear region of the canine aorta. Association with intimal plaque formation in hypercholesterolemia. *Arterioscler Thromb* 1991;11:107–115.
45. Gibson CM, Diaz L, Kandarpa K, Sacks FM, Pasternak RC, Sandor T, Feldman C, Stone PH. Relation of vessel wall shear stress to atherosclerosis progression in human coronary arteries. *Arterioscler Thromb* 1993;13:310–315.
46. Berkson DM, Stamler J, Lindberg HA, Miller WA, Stevens EL, Soyugenc R, Tokich TJ, Stamler R. Heart rate: An important risk factor for coronary mortality. Ten-year experience of the Peoples Gas Co. Epidemiologic Study (1958–68). In: Jones RJ, ed. *Atherosclerosis Proceedings of the 2nd international symposium on atherosclerosis.* New York: Springer-Verlag; 1970:382–389.
47. Texon M. Atherosclerosis. Its hemodynamic basis and implication. *Med Clin N Am* 1974;58:257–268.
48. Castelli WP, Garrison RJ, Wilson PWF, Abbott RD, Kalousdian S, Kannel WB. Incidence of coronary heart disease and lipoprotein cholesterol levels. The Framingham Study. *JAMA* 1986;256:2835–2838.
49. Criqui MH, Cowan LD, Heiss G, Haskell WL, Laskarzewski PM, Chambless LE. Frequency and clustering of nonlipid coronary risk factors in dyslipoproteinemia: The Lipid Research Clinic's program prevalence study. *Circulation* 1986;73(Suppl 1):140–150.
50. Williams PT, Fortmann SP, Terry RB, Garay SC, Vranizan KM, Ellsworth N, Wood PD. Associations of dietary fat, regional adiposity, and blood pressure in men. *JAMA* 1987;257:3251–3256.
51. Reaven GM, Hoffman BB. A role for insulin in the aetiology and course of hypertension? *Lancet* 1987;2:435–436.
52. Selby JV, Newman B, Quiroga J, Christian JC, Austin MA, Fabsitz

RR. Concordance for dyslipidemic hypertension in male twins. *JAMA* 1991;265:2079–2084.
53. Williams RR, Hunt SC, Hopkins PN, Stults BM, Wu LL, Hasstedt SJ, Barlow GK, Stephenson SH, Lalouel JM, Kuida H. Familial dyslipidemic hypertension: evidence from 58 Utah families for a syndrome present in approximately 12% of patients with essential hypertension. *JAMA* 1988;259:3579–3586.
54. Williams RR, Hopkins PN, Hunt SC, Wu LL, Hasstedt SJ, Lalouel JM, Ash KO, Stults BM, Kuida H. Population-based frequency of dyslipidemia syndromes in coronary prone families in Utah. *Arch Intern Med* 1990;150:582–588.
55. Hunt SC, Wu LL, Hopkins PN, Stults BM, Kuida H, Ramirez ME, Lalouel J-M, Williams RR. Apolipoprotein, low density lipoprotein subfraction, and insulin associations with familial combined hyperlipidemia: study of Utah patients with familial dyslipidemic hypertension. *Arteriosclerosis* 1989;9:335–344.
56. Genest JJ, Martin-Munley SS, McNamara JR, Ordovas JM, Jenner J, Myers RH, Silberman SR, Wilson PWF, Salem DN, Schaefer EJ. Familial lipoprotein disorders in patients with premature coronary artery disease. *Circulation* 1992;85:2025–2033.
57. Assmann G, Schulte H. Relation of high-density lipoprotein cholesterol and triglycerides to incidence of atherosclerotic coronary artery disease (the PROCAM experience). *Am J Cardiol* 1992;70:733–737.
58. Rohlfing JJ, Brunzel JD. The effects of diuretics and adrenergic-blocking agents on plasma lipids. *West J Med* 1986;145:210–218.
59. Krauss RM. Relationship of intermediate and low-density lipoprotein subspecies to risk of coronary artery disease. *Am Heart J* 1987;113: 578–582.
60. Austin MA, King M-C, Vranizan KM, Newman B, Krauss RM. Inheritance of low-density lipoprotein subclass patterns: results of complex segregation analysis. *Am J Hum Genet* 1988;43:838–846.
61. De Graaf J, Swinkels DW, de Haan AFJ, Demacker PNM, Stalenhoef AFH. Both inherited susceptibility and environmental exposure determine the low-density lipoprotein-subfraction pattern distribution in healthy Dutch families. *Am J Hum Genet* 1992;51:1295–1310.
62. Austin MA, Breslow JL, Hennekens CH, Buring JE, Willett WC, Krauss RM. Low-density lipoprotein subclass patterns and risk of myocardial infarction. *JAMA* 1988;260:1917–1921.
63. McNamara JR, Campos H, Ordovas JM, Peterson J, Wilson PWF, Schaefer EJ. Effect of gender, age and lipid status on low density lipoprotein subfraction distribution: Results from the Framingham Offspring Study. *Arteriosclerosis* 1987;7:483–490.
64. Sachinidis A, Locher R, Vetter W. Generation of intracellular signals by low density lipoprotein is independent of the classical LDL receptor. *Am J Hypertens* 1991;4:274–279.
65. Nishina PM, Johnson JP, Naggert JK, Krauss RM. Linkage of atherogenic lipoprotein phenotype to the low density lipoprotein receptor locus on the short arm of chromosome 19. *Proc Natl Acad Sci USA* 1992;89:708–712.
66. Teng B, Sniderman AD, Soutar AK, Thompson GR. Metabolic basis of hyperapobetalipoproteinemia. Turnover of apolipoprotein B in low density lipoprotein and its precursors and subfractions compared with normal and familial hypercholesterolemia. *J Clin Invest* 1986;77: 663–672.
67. Bu X, Krauss RM, DeMeester C, Lopez R, Daneshma S, Puppione D, Gray R, Lusis AJ, Rotter JI. Multigenic control of LDL particle size in 24 coronary artery disease pedigrees. *Circulation* 1992;86:I-552(abst).
68. Rotter JI, Chen Y-DI, Bu X, Gray R, Brown J, Reaven GM, Krauss R, Lusis AJ. Quantitative fasting insulin levels in coronary artery disease families are linked to the apoA1-C3-A4 complex—identification of a major genetic locus for syndrome X? *Am J Hum Genet* 1992; 51:26(abst).
69. Wojciechowski AP, Farrall M, Cullen P, Wilson TME, Bayliss JD, Farren B, Griffin BA, Caslake MJ, Packard CJ, Shepherd J, Thakker R, Scott J. Familial combined hyperlipidemia linked to the apolipoprotein AI-CIII-AIV gene cluster on chromosome 11q23–q24. *Nature* 1991;349:161–164.
70. Hayden MR, Kirk H, Clark C, Frohlich JJ, Robisin SW, McLeod R, Hewitt J. DNA polymorphisms in and around the apoA-I-CIII gene and genetic hyperlipidemias. *Am J Hum Genet* 1987;40:421–430.
71. Kwiterovich PO Jr. Genetics and molecular biology of familial combined hyperlipidemia. *Curr Opin Lipidol* 1993;4:133–143.
72. Coresh J, Beaty TH, Kwiterovich PO. Pedigree and sib-pair linkage analysis suggest the apolipoprotein B gene is not the major gene influencing plasma apolipoprotein B levels. *Am J Hum Genet* 1992;50: 1038–1045.
73. Williams RR, Hopkins PN, Hunt SC, Schumacher MC, Elbein SC, Wilson DE, Stults BM, Wu LL, Hasstedt SJ, Lalouel JM. Familial-dyslipidaemic hypertension and other multiple metabolic syndromes. *Ann Med* 1992;24:469–475.
74. Wu D-A, Bu X, Jeng C-Y, Sheu WHH, Warden CH, Katsuya T, Dzau VJ, Reaven GM, Lusis AJ, Chen Y-DI, Rotter JI. Evidence for linkage of blood pressure to the lipoprotein lipase and glucose transporter 2 loci: genetic support for syndrome X. *Circulation* 1994;90:I-129(abst).
75. Babirak SP, Brown BG, Brunzell JD. Familial combined hyperlipidemia and abnormal lipoprotein lipase. *Arterioscler Thromb* 1992;12: 1176–1183.
76. Brunzell JD. Familial lipoprotein lipase deficiency and other causes of the chylomicronemia syndrome. In: Scriver CR, Beaudet AL, Sly WS, Valle D, eds. *The Metabolic Basis of Inherited Disease,* 6th ed. New York: McGraw-Hill; 1989:1165–1180.
77. Harlan WR Jr, Winesett PS, Wasserman AJ. Tissue lipoprotein lipase in normal individuals and in individuals with exogenous hypertriglyceridemia and the relationship of this enzyme to assimilation of fat. *J Clin Invest* 1967;46:239–247.
78. Wilson DE, Edwards CQ, Chan IF. Phenotypic heterogeneity in the extended pedigree of a proband with lipoprotein lipase deficiency. *Metab Clin Exp* 1983;32:1107–1114.
79. Wilson DE, Emi M, Iverius PH, Hata A, Wu LL, Hillas E, Williams RR, Lalouel JM. Phenotypic expression of heterozygous LPL deficiency in the extended pedigree of a proband homozygous for a missense mutation. *J Clin Invest* 1990;86:735–750.
80. Wion L, Kirchgessner TG, Lusis AJ, Schotz MC, Lawn RM. Human lipoprotein lipase complementary DNA sequence. *Science* 1987;235: 1638–1641.
81. Deeb SS, Peng R. Structure of the human lipoprotein lipase gene. *Biochemistry* 1989;28:4131–4135.
82. Emi M, Wilson DE, Iverius PH, Wu L, Hata A, Hegele R, Williams RR, Lalouel J-M. Missense mutation (Gly to Glu188) of human lipoprotein lipase imparting functional deficiency. *J Biol Chem* 1990;265: 5910–5916.
83. Dichek HL, Fojo SS, Beg OU, Skarlatos SI, Brunzell JD, Cutler GB Jr, Brewer HB Jr. Identification of two separate allelic mutations in the lipoprotein lipase gene of a patient with the familial hyperchylomicronemia syndrome. *J Biol Chem* 1991;266:473–477.
84. Wilson DE, Hata A, Kwong LK, Lingam A, Shuhua J, Ridinger DN, Yeager C, Kaltenborn KC, Iverius PH, Lalouel J-M. Mutations in exon 3 of the lipoprotein lipase gene segregating in a family with hypertriglyceridemia, pancreatitis, and non-insulin-dependent diabetes. *J Clin Invest* 1993;92:203–211.
85. Garfinkel AS, Nilsson-Ehle P, Schotz MC. Regulation of lipoprotein lipase: induction by insulin. *Biochim Biophys Acta* 1976;424: 264–273.
86. Babirak SP, Iverius PH, Fujimoto WY, Brunzell JD. Detection and characterization of the heterozygote state for lipoprotein lipase deficiency. *Arteriosclerosis* 1989;9:326–334.
87. Reaven G. Role of insulin resistance in human disease. *Diabetes* 1988; 37:1595–1607.
88. Kaplan NM. Upper-body obesity, glucose intolerance, hypertriglyceridemia, and hypertension. *Arch Intern Med* 1989;149:1514–1520.
89. Fuh MM-T, Shieh SM, Wu DA, Chen YDI, Reaven GM. Abnormalities of carbohydrate and lipid metabolism in patients with hypertension. *Arch Intern Med* 1987;147:1035–1038.
90. Welborn TA, Wearne K. Coronary heart disease incidence and cardiovascular mortality in Busselton with reference to glucose and insulin concentrations. *Diabetes Care* 1979;2:154–160.
91. Pyörälä K. Relationship of glucose tolerance and plasma insulin to the incidence of coronary heart disease: Results from two population studies in Finland. *Diabetes Care* 1979;2:131–141.
92. Ducimetiere P, Eschwege L, Papoz JL, Calude RJR, Rosselin G. Relationship of plasma insulin levels to the incidence of myocardial infarction and coronary heart disease mortality in a middle-aged population. *Diabetologia* 1980;19:205–210.
93. Sicree RA, Zimmet PZ, King HOM, Coventry JS. Plasma insulin response among Nauruans: Prediction of deterioration in glucose tolerance over six years. *Diabetes* 1987;36:179–186.
94. Saad MF, Pettitt DJ, Mott DM, Knowler WC, Nelson RG, Bennett

PH. Sequential changes in serum insulin concentration during the development of non-insulin-dependent diabetes. *Lancet* 1989;1: 1356–1358.
95. Haffner SM, Stern MP, Hazuda HP, Mitchell BM, Patterson JK. Cardiovascular risk factors in confirmed prediabetic individuals. *JAMA* 1990;263:2893–2898.
96. Charles MA, Fontbonne A, Thibult N, Warnet JM, Rosselin GE, Eschwege E. Risk factors for NIDDM in a white population: Paris prospective study. *Diabetes* 1991;40:796–799.
97. Skarfors ET, Lithell HO, Selinus I. Risk factors for the development of hypertension: a 10-year longitudinal study in middle-aged men. *J Hypertens* 1991;9:217–223.
98. Niskanen LK, Uusitupa MI, Pyorala K. The relationship of hyperinsulinemia to the development of hypertension in type 2 diabetic patients and in non-diabetic subjects. *J Hum Hypertens* 1991;5:155–159.
99. Haffner SM, Valdez RA, Hazuda HP, Mitchell BD, Morales PA, Stern MP. Prospective analysis of the insulin-resistance syndrome (syndrome X). *Diabetes* 1992;41:715–722.
100. Lissner L, Bengtsson C, Lapidus L, Kristjansson K, Wedel H. Fasting insulin in relation to subsequent blood pressure changes and hypertension in women. *Hypertension* 1992;20:797–801.
101. DeFronzo RA, Cooke CR, Andres R, Faloona GR, Davis PJ. The effect of insulin on renal handling of sodium, potassium, calcium, and phosphate in man. *J Clin Invest* 1975;55:845–855.
102. Baum M. Insulin stimulates volume absorption in the rabbit proximal convoluted tubule. *J Clin Invest* 1987;79:1104–1109.
103. Rowe JW, Young JB, Minaker KL, Stevens AL, Pallotta J, Landsberg L. Effect of insulin and glucose infusions on sympathetic nervous system activity in normal man. *Diabetes* 1981;30:219–225.
104. King GL, Goodman AD, Buzney S, Moses A, Kahn CR. Receptors and growth-promoting effects of insulin and insulinlike growth factors on cells from bovine retinal capillaries and aorta. *J Clin Invest* 1985; 75:1028–1036.
105. Lever AF. Slow pressor mechanisms in hypertension: a role for hypertrophy of resistance vessels? *J Hypertens* 1986;4:515–524.
106. Pershadsingh HA, McDonald JM. Direct addition of insulin inhibits a high affinity Ca2-ATPase in isolated adipocyte plasma membranes. 1979;281:495–497.
107. Draznin B, Kao M, Sussman KE. Insulin and glyburide increase cytosolic free-Ca2 concentration in isolated rat adipocytes. *Diabetes* 1987; 36:174–178.
108. Frederich RC Jr, Kahn BB, Peach MJ, Flier JS. Tissue-specific nutritional regulation of angiotensinogen in adipose tissue. *Hypertension* 1992;19:339–344.
109. Modan M, Halkin H, Almog S, Lusky A, Eshkol A, Shefi M, Shitrit A, Fuchs Z. Hyperinsulinemia: A link between hypertension obesity and glucose intolerance. *J Clin Invest* 1985;75:809–817.
110. Ferrannini E, Buzzigoli G, Bonadonna R, Giorico MA, Oleggini M, Graziadei L, Pedrinellia R, Brandi L, Bevilacqua S. Insulin resistance in essential hypertension. *N Engl J Med* 1987;317:350–356.
111. Reaven GM. Insulin resistance, hyperinsulinemia, and hypertriglyceridemia in the etiology and clinical course of hypertension. *Am J Med* 1991;90(Suppl 2A):7S–12S.
112. Daly PA, Landsberg L. Hypertension in obesity and NIDDM: role of insulin and sympathetic nervous system. *Diabetes Care* 1991;14: 240–248.
113. Cryer PE. Physiology and pathophysiology of the human sympathoadrenal neuroendocrine system. *N Engl J Med* 1980;303:436–444.
114. Roth J, Grunfeld C. Mechanism of action of peptide hormones and catecholamines. In: Wilson JD, Foster DW, eds. *Williams Textbook of Endocrinology,* 7th ed. Philadelphia: Saunders; 1985:76–122.
115. Landsberg L, Young JB. Catecholamines and the adrenal medulla. In: Wilson JD, Foster DW, eds. *Williams Textbook of Endocrinology,* 7th ed. Philadelphia: Saunders; 1985:891–965.
116. Troisi RJ, Weiss ST, Segal MR, Cassano PA, Vokonas PS, Landsberg L. The relationship of body fat distribution to blood pressure in normotensive men: The normative aging study. *Int J Obes* 1990;14:515–525.
117. Peiris AN, Sothmann MS, Hoffmann RG, Hennes MI, Wilson CR, Gustafson AB, Kissebah AH. Adiposity, fat distribution, and cardiovascular risk. *Ann Intern Med* 1989;110:867–872.
118. Thiebaud D, DeFronzo RA, Jacot E, Golay A, Acheson K, Maeder E, Jequier E, Felber JP. Effect of fatty acids on glucose production and utilization in man. *J Clin Invest* 1982;72:1737–1747.
119. Ferrannini E, Barrett EJ, Bevilacqua S, DeFronzo RA. Effect of fatty acids on glucose production and utilization in man. *J Clin Invest* 1983; 72:1737–1747.
120. Berliner JA, Territo M, Almada L, Carter A, Shafonsky E, Fogelman AM. Lipoprotein-induced insulin resistance in aortic endothelium. *Diabetes* 1984;33:1039–1044.
121. Kissebah AH, Adams PW, Wynn V. Interrelationship between insulin secretion and plasma free fatty acid and triglyceride transport kinetics in maturity onset diabetes and the effect of phenethylbiguanide (Phenformin). *Diabetologia* 1974;10:119–130.
122. Greenberg BH, Blackwelder WC, Levy RI. Primary type V hyperlipoproteinemia. A descriptive study in 32 families. *Ann Intern Med* 1977; 87:526–534.
123. Reaven GM, Lerner RL, Stern MP, Farquhar JW, Nakanishi R. Role of insulin in endogenous hypertriglyceridemia. *J Clin Invest* 1967; 46:1756–1767.
124. Reaven GM. Insulin resistance, hyperinsulinemia, hypertriglyceridemia, and hypertension: Parallels between human disease and rodent models. *Diabetes Care* 1991;14:195–202.
125. Olefsky J, Reaven GM, Farquhar HW. Effects of weight reduction on obesity. *J Clin Invest* 1974;53:64–76.
126. Reaven GM, Ho H, Hoffman BB. Somatostatin inhibition of fructose induced hypertension. *Hypertension* 1989;14:117–120.
127. Krotkiewski M, Mandroukas K, Sjostrom L, Sullivan L, Wetterqvist H, Bjorntorp P. Effects of long-term physical training on body fat, metabolism, and blood pressure in obesity. *Metabolism* 1979;28: 650–658.
128. Boden G, Chen X, Ruiz J, White JV, Rossetti L. Mechanisms of fatty acid-induced inhibition of glucose uptake. *J Clin Invest* 1994; 93:2438–2446.
129. Williams RR, Hunt SC, Schumacher MC, Hopkins PN, Wu LL, Barlow GK, Stults BM, Wilson DE, Lalouel JM. Genes, hypertension and coronary heart disease: Evidence for shared metabolic pathophysiology. In: Smith U, Brunn NE, Hedner T, Hokfelt B, eds. *Hypertension: An Insulin-Resistant Disorder. Genetic Factors and Cellular Mechanisms.* Amsterdam: Elsevier; 1991:89–101.
130. Izzo JL, Swislocki ALM. Workshop III—Insulin resistance: is it truly the link? *Am J Med* 1991;90(Suppl 2A):2A-26S–2S-31S.
131. Marigliano A, Tedde R, Sechi LA, Pala A, Pisanu G, Pacifico A. Insulinemia and blood pressure: relationships in patients with primary and secondary hypertension, and with or without glucose metabolism impairment. *Am J Hypertens* 1990;3:512–526.
132. Reaven GM, Ho H. Renal vascular hypertension does not lead to hyperinsulinemia in Sprague-Dawley rats. *Am J Hypertens* 1992;5: 314–317.
133. Bennett PH, Stern MP. Worship VII: patient population and genetics: role in diabetes. *Am J Med* 1991;90(Suppl 2A):2A-76S–2A-79S.
134. Finch D, Davis G, Bower J, Kirchner K. Effect of insulin on renal sodium handling in hypertensive rats. *Hypertension* 1990;14: 514–518.
135. Hall JE, Coleman TG, Mizelle HL. Does chronic hyperinsulinemia cause hypertension? *Am J Hypertens* 1989;2:171–173.
136. Hall JE, Brands MW, Kivlighn SD, Mizelle HL, Hildebrandt DA, Gaillard CA. Chronic hyperinsulinemia and blood pressure. Interaction with catecholamines? *Hypertension* 1990;15:519–527.
137. Hall JE, Summers RL, Brands MW, Keen H, Alonso-Galicia M. Resistance to metabolic actions of insulin and its role in hypertension. *Am J Hypertens* 1994;7:772–788.
138. Meehan WP, Buchanan TA, Hsueh W. Chronic insulin administration elevates blood pressure in rats. *Hypertension* 1994;24(2):1012–1017.
139. Kageyama S, Yamamoto J, Isogai Y, Fujita T. Effect of insulin on sodium reabsorption in hypertensive patients. *Am J Hypertens* 1994; 7:409–415.
140. Schumacher MC, Hasstedt SJ, Hunt SC, Williams RR, Elbein SC. Fasting insulin levels segregate as autosomal recessive trait in familial NIDDM pedigrees. *Diabetes* 1992;41:416–423.
141. Fuller JH. Epidemiology of hypertension associated with diabetes mellitus. *Hypertension* 1985;7(Suppl II):II-3–II-7.
142. Working group report on management of patients with hypertension and high blood cholesterol. U.S. Department of Health and Human Services; 1990. NIH publication no 90-2361.
143. Lüscher TF, Boulanger CM, Dohi Y, Yang Z. Endothelium-derived contracting factors. *Hypertension* 1992;19:117–130.
144. Nishikibe M, Tsuchida S, Okada M, Fukuroda T, Shimamoto K, Yano M, Ishikawa K, Ikemoto F. Antihypertensive effect of a newly synthe-

sized endothelin antagonist, BQ-123, in a genetic hypertensive model. *Life Sci* 1993;52(8):717–724.
145. McMahon EG, Palomo MA, Brown MA, Bertenshaw SR, Carter JS. Effect of phosphoramidon (endothelin converting enzyme inhibitor) and BQ-123 (endothelin receptor subtype A antagonist) on blood pressure in hypertensive rats. *Am J Hypertens* 1993;6(8):667–673.
146. Boulanger CM, Tanner FC, Hahn AWA, Werner A, Lüscher TF. Oxidized low-density lipoproteins induce mRNA expression and release of endothelin from human and porcine endothelium. *Circ Res* 1992; 70:1191–1197.
147. Kourembanas S, Marsden PA, McQuillan LP, Faller DV. Hypoxia induces endothelin gene expression and secretion in cultured human endothelium. *J Clin Invest* 1991;88:1054–1057.
148. Resink TJ, Hahn AWA, Scott-Burden T, Powell J, Weber E, Bühler FR. Angiotensin II induction of PDGF: A-chain expression in cultured rat vascular smooth muscle cells is preceded by thrombospondin gene transcription. *Biochem Biophys Res Commun* 1990;168:1303–1310.
149. Lerman A, Edwards BS, Hallet JW, Heublein DM, Sondberg SM, Burnett JCJ. Circulating and tissue endothelin immunoreactivity in advanced atherosclerosis. *N Engl J Med* 1991;325:997–1001.
150. Bunchman TE, Brookshire CA. Cyclosporine-induced synthesis of endothelin by cultured human endothelial cells. *J Clin Invest* 1991; 88:310–314.
151. Kon V, Badr KF. Biological actions and pathophysiologic significance of endothelin in the kidney. *Kidney Int* 1991;40:1–12.
152. Mortensen LH, Fink GD. Captopril prevents chronic hypertension produced by infusion of endothelin-1 in rats. *Hypertension* 1992;19: 676–680.
153. Berge KE, Berg K. No effect of a *Taq*1 polymorphism in DNA at the endothelin I (EDN1) locus on normal blood pressure level or variability. *Clin Genet* 1992;41:90–95.
154. Furchgott RF, Zawadzki JV. The obligatory role of endothelial cells in the relaxation of arterial smooth muscle by acetylcholine. *Nature* 1980;288:373–376.
155. Scharfstein JS, Keaney JF, Slivka A, Welch GN, Vita JA, Stamler JS, Loscalzo J. *In vivo* transfer of nitric oxide between a plasma protein-bound reservoir and low molecular weight thiols. *J Clin Invest* 1994;94:1423–1439.
156. Chen PY, Sanders PW. Role of nitric oxide synthesis in salt-sensitive hypertension in Dahl/Rapp rats. *Hypertension* 1993;22:812–818.
157. Rees DD, Palmer RMJ, Moncada S. The role of endothelium-derived nitric oxide in the regulation of blood pressure. *Proc Natl Acad Sci USA* 1989;86:3375–3378.
158. Chu A, Chambers DE, Lin C-C, Kuehl WD, Palmer RMJ, Moncada S, Cobb FR. Effects of inhibition of nitric oxide formation on basal vasomotion and endothelium-dependent responses of the coronary arteries in awake dogs. *J Clin Invest* 1991;87:1964–1968.
159. Lacolley PJ, Lewis SJ, Brody MJ. Role of sympathetic nerve activity in the generation of vascular nitric oxide in urethane-anesthetized rats. *Hypertension* 1991;17:881–887.
160. Vallance P, Collier J, Moncada S. Effects of endothelium-derived nitric oxide on peripheral arteriolar tone in man. *Lancet* 1989;2: 997–1000.
161. Linder L, Kiowski W, Buhler FR, Luscher TF. Indirect evidence for release of endothelium-derived relaxing factor in human forearm circulation *in vivo*. Blunted response in essential hypertension. *Circulation* 1990;81:1762–1767.
162. Panza JA, Quyyumi AA, Brush JE, Epstein SE. Abnormal endothelium-dependent vascular relaxation in patients with essential hypertension. *N Engl J Med* 1990;323:22–27.
163. Calver A, Collier J, Moncada S, Vallance P. Effect of local intra-arterial N^G-monomethyl-L-arginine in patients with hypertension: the nitric oxide dilator mechanism appears abnormal. *J Hypertens* 1992; 10:1025–1031.
164. Lüscher TF, Vanhoutte PM, Raij L. Antihypertensive therapy normalizes endothelium-dependent relaxations in salt-induced hypertension of the rat. *Hypertension* 1987;9(Suppl III):III-193–III-197.
165. Dananberg J, Sider RS, Grekin RJ. Sustained hypertension induced by orally administered nitro-L-arginine. *Hypertension* 1993;21:359–363.
166. Baylis C, Mitruka B, Deng A. Chronic blockade of nitric oxide synthesis in the rat produces systemic hypertension and glomerular damage. *J Clin Invest* 1992;90:278–281.
167. Hansen J, Jacobsen TN, Victor RG. Is nitric oxide involved in the tonic inhibition of central sympathetic outflow in humans. *Hypertension* 1994;24:439–444.
168. Steinberg HO, Brechtel G, Johnson A, Fineberg N, Baron AD. Insulin-mediated skeletal muscle vasodilation is nitric oxide dependent. A novel action of insulin to increase nitric oxide release. *J Clin Invest* 1994;94:1172–1179.
169. Salazar FJ, Pinilla JM, Lopez F, Romero JC, Quesada T. Renal effects of prolonged synthesis inhibition of endothelium-derived nitric oxide. *Hypertension* 1992;20:113–117.
170. Sigmon DH, Carretero OA, Beierwaltes WH. Angiotensin dependence of endothelium-mediated renal hemodynamics. *Hypertension* 1992; 20:643–650.
171. Sigmon DH, Beierwaltes WH. Renal nitric oxide and angiotensin II interaction in renovascular hypertension. *Hypertension* 1993;22: 237–242.
172. Mattson DL, Roman RJ, Cowley AW. Role of nitric oxide in renal papillary blood flow and sodium excretion. *Hypertension* 1992;19: 766–769.
173. Alberola A, Pinilla JM, Quesada T, Romero JC, Salom MG, Salazar FJ. Role of nitric oxide in mediating renal response to volume expansion. *Hypertension* 1992;19:780–784.
174. Ito S, Ren Y. Evidence for the role of nitric oxide in macula densa control of glomerular hemodynamics. *J Clin Invest* 1993;92: 1093–1098.
175. Chen PY, Sanders PW. L-Arginine abrogates salt-sensitive hypertension in Dahl/Rapp rats. *J Clin Invest* 1991;88:1559–1567.
176. Patel A, Layne S, Watts D, Kirchner KA. L-Arginine administration normalizes pressure natriuresis in hypertensive Dahl rats. *Hypertension* 1993;22:863–869.
177. Bredt DS, Hwang PM, Glatt CE, Lowenstein C, Reed RR, Snyder SH. Cloned and expressed nitric oxide synthase structurally resembles cytochrome P-450 reductase. *Nature* 1991;351:714–718.
178. Nadaud S, Bonnardeaux A, Lathrop M, Soubrier F. Gene structure, polymorphism and mapping of the human endothelial nitric oxide synthase gene. *Biochem Biophys Res Commun* 1994;198:1027–1033.
179. Bonnardeaux A, Nadaud S, Charru A, Jeunemaitre X, Corvol P, Soubrier F. Lack of evidence for linkage study of the endothelial nitric oxide synthase gene in essential hypertension. *Circulation* 1995;91: 96–102.
180. Ludmer PL, Selwyn AP, Shook TL, Wayne RR, Mudge GH, Alexander RW, Ganz P. Paradoxical vasoconstriction induced by acetylcholine in atherosclerotic coronary arteries. *N Engl J Med* 1986;315: 1046–1051.
181. Förstermann U, Mügge, Alheid U, Haverich A, Frölich JC. Selective attenuation of endothelium-mediated vasodilation in atherosclerotic human coronary arteries. *Circ Res* 1988;62:185–190.
182. Golino P, Piscione F, Willerson JT, Cappelli-Bigazzi M, Focaccio A, Villari B, Indolfi C, Russolillo E, Condorelli M, Chiariello M. Divergent effects of serotonin on coronary-artery dimensions and blood flow in patients with coronary atherosclerosis and control patients. *N Engl J Med* 1991;324:641–648.
183. Kuo L, Davis MJ, Cannon MS, Chilian WM. Pathophysiological consequences of atherosclerosis extend into the coronary microcirculation. Restoration of endothelium-dependent responses by L-arginine. *Circ Res* 1992;70:465–476.
184. Reddy KG, Nair RN, Sheehan HM, Hodgson J. Evidence that selective endothelial dysfunction may occur in the absence of angiographic or ultrasound atherosclerosis in patients with risk factors for atherosclerosis. *J Am Coll Cardiol* 1994;23:833–843.
185. Henry PD. Hyperlipidemic arterial dysfunction [Editorial]. *Circulation* 1990;81:697–699.
186. Sellke FW, Armstrong ML, Harrison DG. Endothelium-dependent vascular relaxation is abnormal in the coronary microcirculation of atherosclerotic primates. *Circulation* 1990;81:1586–1593.
187. Yasue H, Matsuyama K, Matsuyama K, Okumura K, Morikami Y, Ogawa H. Responses of angiographically normal human coronary arteries to intracoronary injection of acetylcholine by age and segment. *Circulation* 1989;81:482–490.
188. Vita JA, Treasure CB, Nabel EG, McLenachan JM, Fish RD, Yeung AC, Vekshtein VI, Selwyn AP, Ganz P. Coronary vasomotor response to acetylcholine relates to risk factors for coronary artery disase. *Circulation* 1990;18:491–497.
189. Egashira K, Inou T, Kirooka Y, Yamada A, Maruoka Y, Kai H, Sugimachi M, Suzuki S, Takeshita A. Impaired coronary blood flow re-

sponse to acetylcholine in patients with coronary risk factors and proximal atherosclerotic lesions. *J Clin Invest* 1993;91:29–37.

190. Kuhn FE, Mohler ER, Satler LF, Reagan K, Lu DY, Rackley CE. Effects of high-density lipoprotein on acetylcholine-induced coronary vasoreactivity. *Am J Cardiol* 1991;68:1425–1430.
191. Sorensen KE, Celermajer DS, Georgakopoulos D, Hatcher G, Betteridge DJ, Deanfield JE. Impairment of endothelium-dependent dilation is an early event in children with familial hypercholesterolemia and is related to the lipoprotein (a) level. *J Clin Invest* 1994;93:50–55.
192. Chin HP, Liu CR, Liu CH, Blankenhorn DH. Very early aortic responses during atherosclerosis induction in rabbits: Measurement by duplex ultrasound. I. Non-invasive study of aortic hyperresponsiveness to serotonin. *Atherosclerosis* 1990;83:1–8.
193. Harrison DG, Armstrong ML, Freiman PC, Heistad DD. Restoration of endothelium-dependent relaxation by dietary treatment of atherosclerosis. *J Clin Invest* 1987;80:1808–1811.
194. Heistad DD, Mark AL, Marcus ML, Piegors DJ, Armstrong ML. Dietary treatment of atherosclerosis abolishes hyperresponsiveness to serotonin: implications for vasospasm. *Circ Res* 1987;61:346–351.
195. Osborne JA, Lento PH, Siegfried MR, Stahl GL, Fusman B, Lefer AM. Cardiovascular effects of acute hypercholesterolemia in rabbits. Reversal with lovastatin treatment. *J Clin Invest* 1989;83:465–473.
196. Benzuly KH, Padgett RC, Kaul S, Piegors DJ, Armstrong ML, Heistad DD. Functional improvement precedes structural regression of atherosclerosis. *Circulation* 1994;89:1810–1818.
197. Creager MA, Cooke JP, Mendelsohn ME, Gallagher SJ, Coleman SM, Loscalzo J, Dzau VJ. Impaired vasodilation of forearm resistance vessels in hypercholesterolemic humans. *J Clin Invest* 1990;86: 228–234.
198. Drexler H, Zeiher AM, Meinzer K, Just H. Correction of endothelial dysfunction in coronary microcirculation of hypercholesterolaemic patients by L-arginine. *Lancet* 1991;338:1546–1550.
199. Drexler H, Zeiher AM. Endothelial function in human coronary arteries *in vivo*. Focus on hypercholesterolemia. *Hypertension* 1991; 18(Suppl II):II-90–II-99.
200. Chowienczyk PJ, Watts GF, Cockcroft JR, Ritter JM. Impaired endothelium-dependent vasodilation of forearm resistance vessels in hypercholesterolaemia. *Lancet* 1992;340:1430–1432.
201. Casino PR, Kilcoyne CM, Quyyumi AA, Hoeg JM, Panza JA. Investigation of decreased availability of nitric oxide precursor as the mechanism responsible for impaired endothelium-dependent vasodilation in hypercholesterolemic patients. *J Am Coll Cardiol* 1994;23:844–850.
202. Leung W-H, Lau C-P, Wong C-K. Beneficial effect of cholesterol-lowering therapy on coronary endothelium-dependent relaxation in hypercholesterolaemic patients. *Lancet* 1993;341:1496–1500.
203. Gould KL, Martucci JP, Goldberg DI, Hess MJ, Edens RP, Latifi R, Dudrick SJ. Short-term cholesterol lowering decreases size and severity of perfusion abnormalities by positron emission tomography after dipyridamole in patients with coronary artery disease. A potential noninvasive marker of healing coronary endothelium. *Circulation* 1994;89:1530–1538.
204. Ornish D, Scherwitz LW, Doody RS, Kesten D, McLanahan SM, Brown SE, DePuey EG, Sonnemaker R, Haynes C, Lester J, McAllister GK, Hall RJ, Burdine JA, Gotto AM. Effects of stress management training and dietary changes in treating ischemic heart disease. *JAMA* 1983;249:54–59.
205. Andrews TC, Selwyn AP, Ganz P, Naimi C, Kadro W, Barry J, Raby KE. The effect of cholesterol lowering on myocardial ischemia. *Circulation* 1994;90(Suppl I):I-27 (abst).
206. Minor RL, Myers PR, Guerra R, Bates JN, Harrison DG. Diet-induced atherosclerosis increases the release of nitrogen oxides from rabbit aorta. *J Clin Invest* 1990;86:2109–2116.
207. Galle J, Mulsch A, Busse R, Bassenge E. Effects of native and oxidized low density lipoproteins on formation and inactivation of endothelium-derived relaxing factor. *Arterioscler Thromb* 1991;11: 198–203.
208. Weisser B, Locher R, Mengden T, Sachinidis A, Vetter W. Oxidation of low-density lipoprotein increases vasoconstriction *in vitro*. *J Hypertens* 1991;9:S172–S173.
209. Chin JH, Azhar S, Hoffman BB. Inactivation of endothelial derived relaxing factor by oxidized lipoproteins. *J Clin Invest* 1992;89:10–18.
210. Mangin EJ, Kugiyama K, Nguy JN, Kerns SA, Henry PD. Effects of lysolipids and oxidatively modified low density lipoprotein on endothelium-dependent relaxation of rabbit aorta. *Circ Res* 1993;72: 161–166.
211. Inoue N, Hirata K, Yamada M, Hamamori Y, Matsuda Y, Akita H, Yokoyama M. Lysophosphatidylcholine inhibits bradykinin-induced phosphoinositide hydrolysis and calcium transients in cultured bovine aortic endothelial cells. *Circ Res* 1992;71:1410–1421.
212. Matsuda Y, Hirata K, Inoue N, Suematsu M, Kawashima S, Akita H, Yokoyama M. High density lipoprotein reverses inhibitory effect of oxidized low density lipoprotein on endothelium-dependent arterial relaxation. *Circ Res* 1993;72:1103–1109.
213. Ohara Y, Peterson TE, Harrison DG. Hypercholesterolemia increases endothelial superoxide anion production. *J Clin Invest* 1993;91: 2546–2551.
214. Reis SE, Gloth ST, Blumenthal RS, Resar JR, Zacur HA. Gerstenblith G, Brinker JA. Ethinyl estradiol acutely attenuates abnormal coronary vasomotor responses to acetylcholine in postmenopausal women. *Circulation* 1994;89(1):52–60.
215. Collins P, Rosano GMC, Adamopoulos S, McNeil J, Ulrich L, Sarrel PM, Poole-Wilson PA. Coronary arterial acetylcholine-induced vasoconstriction is reversed by intracoronary administration of estradiol-17β in menopausal women with coronary artery disease. *J Am Coll Cardiol* 1994;23(Feb Suppl):7A (abst).
216. Gilligan DM, Badar DM, Panza JA, Quyyumi AA, Cannon RO. Acute vascular effects of estrogen in postmenopausal women. *Circulation* 1994;90:786–791.
217. Volterrani M, Rosano GMC, Coats A, Collins P. Effect of estradiol-17b on forearm blood flow in menopausal women. A double blind randomized study. *J Am Coll Cardiol* 1994;23:(Feb Suppl):273A (abst).
218. Chowienczyk PJ, Watts GF, Cockcroft JR, Brett SE, Ritter JM. Sex differences in endothelial function in normal and hypercholesterolaemic subjects. *Lancet* 1994;344:305–306.
219. Cooke JP, Singer AH, Tsao P, Zera P, Rowan RA, Billingham ME. Antiatherogenic effects of L-arginine in the hypercholesterolemic rabbit. *J Clin Invest* 1992;90:1168–1172.
220. Hamon M, Vallet B, Bauters C, Wernert N, McFadden EP, Lablanche J-M, Dupuis B, Betrand ME. Long-term oral administration of L-arginine reduces intimal thickening and enhances neoendothelium-dependent acetylcholine-induced relaxation after arterial injury. *Circulation* 1994;90:1357–1362.
221. Moncada S, Higgs A. The L-arginine–nitric oxide pathway. *N Engl J Med* 1993;329:2002–2012.
222. Naruse K, Shimizu K, Muramatsu M, Toki Y, Miyazaki Y, Okumura K, Hashimoto H, Ito T. Long-term inhibition of NO synthesis promotes atherosclerosis in the hypercholesterolemic rabbit thoracic aorta. PGH_2 does not contribute to impaired endothelium-dependent relaxation. *Arterioscler Thromb* 1994;14:746–752.
223. ACCORD Study Group. Nitric oxide donors reduce restenosis after coronary angioplasty. *J Am Coll Cardiol* 1994;23(Feb Suppl):59A (abst).
224. Jeunemaitre X, Rigat B, Charru A, Houot AM, Soubrier F, Corvol P. Sib pair linkage analysis of renin gene haplotypes in human essential hypertension. *Hum Genet* 1992;88:301–306.
225. Jeunemaitre X, Lifton RP, Hunt SC, Williams RR, Lalouel J-M. Absence of linkage between the angiotensin converting enzyme locus and human essential hypertension. *Nature Genet* 1992;1:72–5.
226. Alderman MH, Madhavan S, Ooi WL, Cohen H, Sealey JE, Laragh JH. Association of the renin-sodium profile with the risk of myocardial infarction in patients with hypertension. *N Engl J Med* 1991;324: 1098–1104.
227. Jeunemaitre X, Soubrier F, Kotelevtsev Y, Lifton RP, Williams CS, Charru A, Hunt SC, Hopkins PN, Williams RR, Lalouel JM, Corvol P. Molecular basis of human hypertension: role of angiotensinogen. *Cell* 1992;71:169–180.
228. Jeunemaitre X, Charru A, Chatellier G, Dumont C, Sassano P, Soubrier F, Menard J, Corvol P. M235T variant of the human angiotensinogen gene in unselected hypertensive patients. *J Hypertens* 1993; 11:S80–S81.
229. Hata A, Namikawa C, Sasaki M, Sato K, Nakamura T, Tamura K, Lalouel J-M. Angiotensinogen as a risk factor for essential hypertension in Japan. *J Clin Invest* 1994;93:1285–1287.
230. Caulfield M, Lavender P, Farrall M, Munroe P, Lawson M, Turner P, Clark AJL. Linkage of the angiotensinogen gene to essential hypertension. *N Engl J Med* 1994;330:1629–1633.

231. Lu S, Pershadsingh H, Purcell T, Wong A, Spence MA, Flodman P, Kurtz TW. Cross-sectional analysis of angiotensinogen genotypes and blood pressures in Mexican Americans. *Hypertension* 1994;24:381 (abst).
232. Grim CE, Lifton RP, Wilson TW, Viswanathan A, Etienne C, Wilson DM, Grim CM, Grell GAC. The angiotensinogen gene MT235 is not associated with blood pressure in blacks in Dominica. *Hypertension* 1994;24:381 (abst).
233. Iwai N, Kinoshita M. Molecular variant of the angiotensinogen gene and essential hypertension in Japanese. *Hypertension* 1994;24:381 (abst).
234. Rotini C, Morrison L, Cooper R, Oyejide C, Effiong E, Ladipo M, Osotemiher B, Ward R. Angiotensinogen gene in human hypertension. Lack of an association of the 235T allele among African Americans. *Hypotension* 1994;24(5):591–594.
235. Gould AB, Green B. Kinetics of the human renin and human renin substrate reaction. *Cardiovasc Res* 1971;5:86–89.
236. Cain MD, Walters WA, Catt KJ. Effects of oral contraceptive therapy on the renin–angiotensin system. *J Clin Endocrinol* 1971;33: 671–676.
237. Menard J, Catt KJ. Effects of estrogen treatment on plasma renin parameters in the rat. *Endocrinology* 1973;92:1382–1388.
238. Klett C, Bader M, Ganten D, Hackenthal E. Mechanism by which angiotensin II stabilizes messenger RNA for angiotensinogen. *Hypertension* 1994;23:I-120–I-125.
239. Blaine EH, Davis JO, Harris PD. A steady-state control analysis of the renin–angiotensin–aldosterone system. *Circ Res* 1972;30:713–730.
240. Brown AJ, Casals-Stenzel J, Gofford S, Lever AF, Morton JJ. Comparison of fast and slow pressor effects of angiotensin II in the conscious rat. *Am J Physiol* 1981;241:H381–H388.
241. Sealey JE, Blumenfeld JD, Bell GM, Pecker MS, Sommers SC, Laragh JH. On the renal basis for essential hypertension: nephron heterogeneity with discordant renin secretion and sodium excretion causing a hypertensive vasoconstriction–volume relationship. In: Laragh JH, Brenner BM, eds. *Hypertension: Pathophysiology, Diagnosis and Management.* New York: Raven Press; 1990:1089–1103.
242. Gahnem F, von Lutterotti N, Camargo MJF, Laragh JH, Sealey JE. Angioternsinogen dependency of blood pressure in two high-renin hypertensive rat models. *Am J Hypertens* 1994;7(10 pt. 1):899–904.
243. Fasola AF, Martz BL, Helmer OM. Plasma renin activity during supine exercise in offspring of hypertensive parents. *J Appl Physiol* 1968;25:410–415.
244. Jeunemaitre X, Charru A, Gyan E, Dumont C, Soubrier F, Corvol P. Association of the human angiotensinogen gene M235T mutation with hypertension in 181 French hypertensive families. *J Hypertens* 1994; 12(Suppl 3):S71.
245. Watt GCM, Harrap SB, Foy CJW, Holton DW, Edwards HV, Davison HR, Connor JM, Lever A, Fraser R. Abnormalities of glucocorticoid metabolism and the renin–angiotensin system: A four-corners approach to the identification of genetic determinants of blood pressure. *J Hypertens* 1992;10:473–482.
246. Walker WG, Whelton PK, Saito H, Russel RP, Hermann J. Relation between blood pressure and renin, renin substrate, angiotensin II, aldosterone and urinary sodium and potassium in 574 ambulatory subjects. *Hypertension* 1979;1:287–291.
247. Ménard J, El Amrani A-IK, Savoie F, Bouhnik J. Angiotensinogen: an attractive and underrated participant in hypertension and inflammation. *Hypertension* 1991;18:705–706.
248. Gardes J, Bouhnik J, Clauser E, Corvol P, Ménard J. Role of angiotensinogen in blood pressure homeostasis. *Hypertension* 1982;4: 185–189.
249. Rakugi H, Jacob HJ, Krieger JE, Ingelfinger JR, Pratt RE. Vascular injury induces angiotensinogen gene expression in the media and neointima. *Circulation* 1993;87:283–290.
250. Kimura S, Mullins JJ, Bunnemann B, Metzger R, Hilgenfeldt U, Zimmermann F, Jacob H, Fuxe K, Ganten D, Kaling M. High blood pressure in transgenic mice carrying the rat angiotensinogen gene. *EMBO J* 1992;11:821–827.
251. Tamura K, Umemura S, Iwamoto T, Yamaguchi S, Kobayashi S, Takeda K, Tokita Y, Takagi N, Murakami K, Fukamizu A, Ishii M. Molecular mechanism of adipogenic activation of the angiotensinogen gene. *Hypertension* 1994;23:364–368.
252. Landsberg L. Obesity and hypertension: experimental data. *J Hypertens* 1992;10(Suppl 7):S195–S201.
253. Edens NK, Leibel RL, Hirsch J. Mechanism of free fatty acid re-esterification in human adipocytes *in vitro. J Lipid Res* 1990;31: 1423–1431.
254. Skidgel RA, Erdös EG. Angiotensin I-converting enzyme. In: Izzo Jr JL, Black HR, eds. *Hypertension Primer.* Dallas: American Heart Association; 1993:12–13.
255. Margolius HS, Horwitz D, Pisano JJ, Keiser HR. Urinary kallikrein excretion in hypertensive man: Relationships to sodium intake and sodium-retaining steroids. *Circ Res* 1974;35:820–825.
256. Ura N, Shimamoto K, Nakao T, Ogasawara A, Tanaka S, Mita T, Nishimiya T, Iimura O. The excretion of human urinary kallikrein quantity and activity in normal and low renin subgroups of essential hypertension. *Clin Exp Hypertens* 1983;A5(3):329–337.
257. Mersey JH, Williams GH, Emanuel R, Dluhy RG, Wong PY, Moore TJ. Plasma bradykinin levels and urinary kallikrein excretion in normal renin essential hypertension. *J Clin Endocrinol Metab* 1979;48: 642–647.
258. Keiser HR. The kallikrein–kinin system in essential hypertension. *Clin Exp Hypertens* 1980;2:675–691.
259. Carretero OA, Oza NB, Schork A. Renal tissue kallikrein, plasma renin, and plasma aldosterone in renal hypertension. *Acta Physiol Lat Am* 1974;24:448–452.
260. Berry TD, Hasstedt SJ, Hunt SC, Wu LL, Smith JB, Ash KO, Kuida H, Williams RR. A gene for high urinary kallikrein may protect against hypertension in Utah kindreds. *Hypertension* 1989;13:3–8.
261. Hunt SC, Hasstedt SJ, Wu LL, Williams RR. A gene–environment interaction between inferred kallikrein genotype and potassium. *Hypertension* 1993;22:161–168.
262. Madeddu P, Parpaglia PP, Demontis MP, Varoni MV, Fattaccio MC, Glorioso N. Chronic inhibition of bradykinin B2-receptors enhances the slow vasopressor response to angiotensin II. *Hypertension* 1994; 23:646–652.
263. Majima M, Mizogami S, Kuribayashi Y, Katori M, Oh-ishi S. Hypertension induced by a nonpressor dose of angiotensin II in kininogen-deficient rats. *Hypertension* 1994;24:111–119.
264. Nolly N, Carretero OA, Lama MC, Miatello R, Scicli AG. Vascular kallikrein in deoxycorticosterone acetate-salt hypertensive rats. *Hypertension* 1994;23(Suppl 1):I185–I1185.
265. Weinberger MH. Clinical studies of the role of dietary sodium in blood pressure. In: Laragh JH, Brenner BM, eds. *Hypertension: Pathophysiology, Diagnosis, and Management.* New York: Raven Press; 1990:1999–2010.
266. Lifton RP, Hopkins PN, Williams RR, Hollenberg NK, Williams GH, Dluhy RG. Evidence for heritability of non-modulation essential hypertension. *Hypertension* 1989;13:884–889.
267. Williams GH, Dluhy RG, Lifton RP, Moore TJ, Gleason R, Williams R, Hunt SC, Hopkins PN, Hollenberg NK. Non-modulation as an intermediate phenotype in essential hypertension. *Hypertension* 1992; 20:788–796.
268. Hasstedt SJ, Wu LL, Ash KO, Kuida H, Williams RR. Hypertension and sodium–lithium countertransport in Utah pedigrees: evidence for major locus inheritance. *Am J Hum Genet* 1988;43:14–22.
269. Rebbeck TR, Turner ST, Michels VV, Moll PP. Genetic and environmental explanations for the distribution of sodium–lithium countertransport in pedigrees from Rochester, MN. *Am J Hum Genet* 1991; 48:1092–1104.
270. Canessa ML, Morgan K, Semplicini A. Genetic differences in lithium–sodium exchange and regulation of the sodium–hydrogen exchanger in essential hypertension. *J Cardiovasc Pharmacol* 1988; 12(Suppl 3):S92–S98.
271. Semplicini A. The Li+/Na+ countertransport in hypertension. In: Coca A, Garay RP, eds. *Ionic Transport in Hypertension: New Perspectives.* Boca Raton, Florida: CRC Press; 1994:89–117.
272. Aviv A, Lasker N. Proposed defects in membrane transport and intracellular ions as pathogenic factors in essential hypertension. In: Laragh JH, Brenner BM, ed. *Hypertension: Pathophysiology, Diagnosis, and Management.* New York: Raven Press; 1990:923–937.
273. Blaustein MP, Hamlyn JM. Sodium transport inhibition, cell calcium, and hypertension. The natriuretic hormone/Na+-Ca2+ exchange/ hypertension hypothesis. *Am J Med* 1984;77:45–59.
274. Fray JCS, Park CS, Valentine AND. Calcium and control of renin secretion. *Endocrine Rev* 1987;8:53–93.
275. Moore RD. Effects of insulin upon ion transport. *Biochim Biophys Acta* 1983;737:1–49.

276. Resnick LM, Gupta RK, Soza RE, Corbett ML, Laragh JH. Intracellular pH in human and experimental hypertension. *Proc Natl Acad Sci USA* 1987;84:7663–7667.
277. Resnick LM, Gupta RK, Gruenspan H, Alderman MH, Laragh JH. Hypertension and peripheral insulin resistance: Possible mediating role of intracellular free magnesium. *Am J Hypertens* 1990;3: 373–379.
278. Berk BC, Brock TA, Webb RC, Taubman MB, Atkinson WJ, Gimbrone MAJ, Alexander RW. Epidermal growth factor, a vascular smooth muscle mitogen, induces rat aortic contraction. *J Clin Invest* 1985;75:1083–1086.
279. Moolenaar WH, Tertoolen LGJ, DeLaat SW. Phorbol ester and diacylglycerol mimic growth factors in raising cytoplasmic pH. *Nature* 1984;312:371–373.
280. Harris PJ, Navar LG. Tubular transport responses to angiotensin: editorial review. *Am J Physiol* 1985;248:F621–F630.
281. Conlin PR, Williams GH, Canessa ML. Angiotensin II-induced activation of Na(+)–H+ exchange in adrenal glomerulosa cells is mediated by protein kinase C. *Endocrinology* 1991;129:1861–1868.
282. Lifton RP, Hunt SC, Williams RR, Lalouel JM. Exclusion of the Na^+/H+ antiporter as a candidate gene in human essential hypertension by genetic linkage analysis. *Hypertension* 1991;17:8–14.
283. Cusi D, Fossali E, Piazza A, Tripodi G, Barlassina C, Pozzoli E, Vezzoli G, Stella P, Soldati L, Bianchi G. Heritability estimate of erythrocyte Na–K–Cl cotransport in normotensive and hypertensive families. *Am J Hypertens* 1991;4:725–34.
284. Garay RP, Cavalier S, Hannaert PA. The [Na+,K+,Cl−] cotransport system: relevance in essential hypertension. In: Coca A, Garay RP, eds. *Ionic Transport in Hypertension: New Perspectives.* Boca Raton, Florida: CRC Press; 1994:45–56.
285. Arrázola A, Diez J. Correspondences between the activity of the renin–angiotensin system and the erythrocyte Na+ transport abnormalities in hypertension. *Am J Hypertens* 1990;3:412–414.
286. Hunt SC, Williams RR, Smith JB, Ash KO. Associations of three erythrocyte cation transport systems with plasma lipids in Utah subjects. *Hypertension* 1986;8:30–36.
287. Hunt SC, Williams RR, Ash KO. Changes in sodium–lithium countertransport correlate with changes in triglyceride levels and body mass index over two and one-half years of followup in Utah. *Cardiovasc Drugs Ther* 1990;4:357–362.
288. Levy R, Paran E, Keynan A, Livne A. Essential hypertension: improved differentiation by the temperature dependence of Li efflux in erythrocytes. *Hypertension* 1983;5:821–827.
289. Engelmann B, Op Den Kamp JAF, Roelofsen B. Replacement of molecular species of phosphatidylcholine: Influence on erythrocyte Na transport. *Am J Physiol* 1990;258(*Cell Physiol* 27):C682–C691.
290. Sauerheber RD, Lewis UJ, Esgate JA, Gordon LM. Effect of calcium, insulin and growth hormones on membrane fluidity: A spin label study of rat adipocytes and human erythrocyte ghosts. *Biochim Biophys Acta* 1980;597:292–304.
291. Tsuda K, Masuyama Y. Age-related changes in membrane fluidity of erythrocytes in essential hypertension. *Am J Hypertens* 1990;3: 714–716.
292. Masuyama Y, Tsuda K, Shima H, Ura M, Takeda J, Kimura K, Nishio I. Membrane abnormality of erythrocytes is highly dependent on salt intake and renin profile in essential hypertension: An electron spin resonance study. *J Hypertens* 1988;6(Suppl 4):S266–S268.
293. Hunt SC, Wu LL, Williams RR. Abnormalities of ion transport in hypercholesterolemia and hypertriglyceridemia: A link with essential hypertension? In: Coca A, Garay RP, eds. *Ionic Transport in Hypertension: New Perspectives.* Boca Raton, Florida: CRC Press; 1994: 273–300.
294. Sachinidis A, Mengden T, Locher R, Brunner C, Vetter W. Novel cellular activities for low density lipoprotein in vascular smooth muscle cells. *Hypertension* 1990;15:704–711.
295. Lijnen P, Celis H, Fagard R, Staessen J, Amery A. Influence of cholesterol lowering on plasma membrane lipids and cationic transport systems. *J Hypertens* 1994;12:59–64.
296. Hamlyn JM, Harris DW, Clark MA, Rogowski AC, White RJ, Ludens JH. Isolation and characterization of a sodium pump inhibitor from human plasma. *Hypertension* 1989;13:681–689.
297. Tamura M, Kuwano H, Kinoshita T, Inagami T. Identification of linoleic and oleic acids as endogenous Na+,K^+,−ATPase inhibitors from acute volume-expanded hog plasma. *J Biol Chem* 1985;260: 9672–9677.
298. Tamura M, Inagami T, Kinoshita T, Kuwano H. A search for endogenous Na^+,K^+−ATPase inhibitor in acutely volume-expanded hog plasma led to lysophosphatidylcholine γ-stearoyl. *J Hypertens* 1987; 5:219–225.
299. Ruiz-Opazo N, Barany F, Hirayama K, Herrera VL. Confirmation of mutant alpha 1 Na,K−ATPase gene and transcript in Dahl salt-sensitive/JR rats. *Hypertension* 1994;24:260–270.
300. Hasstedt SJ, Wu LL, Kuida H, Williams RR. Recessive inheritance of a high number of sodium pump sites. *Am J Med Genet* 1989;34: 332–337.
301. Hasstedt SJ, Hunt SC, Wu LL, Williams RR. The inheritance of intraerythrocytic sodium level. *Am J Med Genet* 1988;29:193–203.
302. Hasstedt SJ, Hunt SC, Wu LL, Williams RR. Evidence for multiple genes determining sodium transport. *Genet Epidemiol* 1994;11: 553–568.
303. Pickering TG, Gerin W. Cardiovascular reactivity and the role of behavioral factors in hypertension: A critical review. *Ann Behav Med* 1990;12:3–16.
304. Rockstroh JK, Schmieder RE, Schächinger H, Messerli FH. Stress response pattern in obesity and systemic hypertension. *Am J Cardiol* 1992;70:1035–1039.
305. Matthews KA, Woodall KL, Allen MT. Cardiovascular reactivity to stress predicts future blood pressure status. *Hypertension* 1993;22: 479–485.
306. Smith TW, Turner CW, Ford MH, Hunt SC, Barlow GK, Stults BM, Williams RR. Blood pressure reactivity in adult male twins. *Health Psychol* 1987;6:209–220.
307. Hunt SC, Hasstedt SJ, Kuida H, Stults BM, Hopkins PH, Williams RR. Genetic heritability and common environmental components of resting and stressed blood pressures, lipids, and body mass index in Utah pedigrees and twins. *Am J Epidemiol* 1989;129:625–638.
308. Lifton RP, Dluhy RG, Powers M, Rich GM, Cook S, Ulick S, Lalouel J-M. A chimaeric 11β-hydroxylase/aldosterone synthase gene causes glucocorticoid-remediable aldosteronism and human hypertension. *Nature* 1992;355:262–265.
309. Shimkets RA, Warnock DG, Bositis CM, Nelson-Williams C, Hansson JH, Schambelan M, Gill JR Jr, Ulick S, Milora RV, Findling JW, Canessa CM, Rossier BC, Lifton RP. Liddle's Syndrome: Heritable human hypertension caused by mutations in the β subunit of the epithelial sodium channel. *Cell* 1994;79:407–414.
310. Williams RR, Hasstedt SJ, Hunt SC, Wu LL, Hopkins PN, Berry TD, Stults BM, Barlow GK, Kuida H. Genetic traits related to hypertension and electrolyte metabolism. *Hypertension* 1991;17(Suppl I):I-69–I-73.

Atherosclerosis and Coronary Artery Disease,
edited by V. Fuster, R. Ross, and E. J. Topol.
Lippincott-Raven Publishers, Philadelphia © 1996.

CHAPTER 14

Renin–Angiotensin System and Atherosclerotic Vascular Disease

Victor J. Dzau and Aram V. Chobanian

Key Words: Angiotensin II; Angiotensin-converting enzyme; Hypertension; Myocardial infarction; Renin–angiotensin system.

INTRODUCTION

The circulating renin–angiotensin system (RAS) plays an important role in circulatory and fluid-electrolyte homeostasis (1). The circulating peptide hormone angiotensin II is the product of two sequential proteolytic cleavages from the prohormone angiotensinogen that is synthesized by the liver and released into the circulation (Fig. 1). The first proteolytic step involves the aspartyl protease renin, secreted by the kidney. The product, angiotensin I, is then cleaved by angiotensin-converting enzyme (ACE) in the pulmonary capillary bed, producing the active octapeptide angiotensin II. The angiotensin II then enters the systemic circulation as a systemic hormone and is carried to target organs, such as blood vessels, kidneys, the adrenal glands, and the heart.

In addition to the angiotensin II formed in the circulation as a hormone, recent evidence has demonstrated the local synthesis of angiotensin II in various tissues (2,3). The production of local angiotensin II occurs due to the existence and action of one or more components of the RAS in these target tissues. In particular, ACE is widely expressed in the endothelium of all blood vessels, and this endothelial membrane-bound enzyme can potentially control local angiotensin II synthesis in specific vascular beds. Local angiotensin II appears to exert autocrine–paracrine effects on local cardiovascular tissue functions (Table 1) and participates in the pathophysiology of cardiovascular diseases. In particular, angiotensin II plays an important role in the development of atherosclerosis and vascular disease.

Victor J. Dzau: Falk Cardiovascular Research Center, Stanford University School of Medicine, Stanford, California 94305.
Aram V. Chobanian: Boston University School of Medicine, Boston, Massachusetts 02118.

ANGIOTENSIN II AND ATHEROSCLEROSIS

Angiotensin II is a potent vasoconstrictor. Angiotensin II binding to its type 1 receptor (AT1) activates a cascade of second messenger systems. The direct effects of angiotensin II binding to target receptors include the activation of phospholipase C, which results in metabolites that modulate calcium-sensitive protein kinase C (PK-C) and cytoplasmic calcium concentrations. Angiotensin II binding also activates receptor-operated calcium channels, giving rise to calcium influx and increased contraction. The raised intracellular free calcium and PK-C-mediated protein phosphorylation activate nuclear elements with long-term effects on gene expression, protein synthesis, mitogenesis, and/or hypertrophy. Based on the various actions of angiotensin II, this peptide can contribute to the pathobiology of atherosclerosis either directly via its cellular growth actions or secondarily via its role in hypertension. In this chapter, we will discuss both effects of angiotensin.

Effects via Hypertension

As a potent vasoconstrictor and stimulus for sodium and water retention, angiotensin II can elevate systemic blood

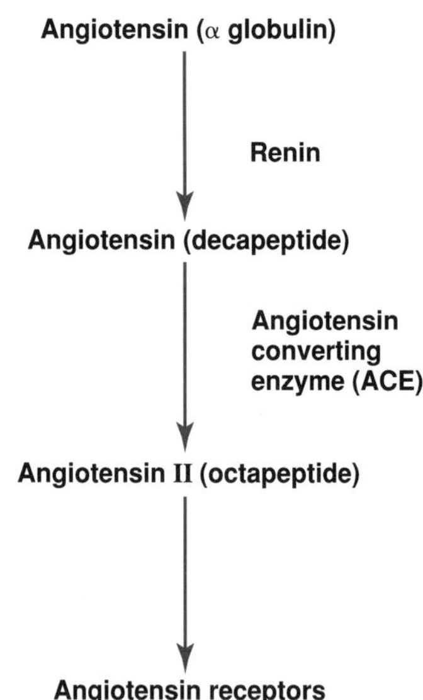

FIG. 1. Biochemical cascade of the renin–angiotensin system.

pressure. Increased blood pressure alters arterial structure and function. In the rat, the earliest arterial changes appear to occur in the endothelium with alterations in shape of aortic endothelial cells and increase in their number within 2 weeks of deoxycorticosterone-salt (DOC-salt) administration (4). A variety of other changes follow, including adherence of leukocytes to the endothelial surface and their penetration into the intima, accumulation of smooth muscle cells and macrophages in the subendothelial space, and increases in extracellular matrix (5). Hypertension also increases arterial permeability (6) and impairs endothelium-dependent relaxation (7).

In the presence of hyperlipidemia, hypertension promotes the development of atherosclerosis, although with low plasma lipids it appears mainly to cause intimal and medial thickening (8). Hypertension may alter the cellular composition of atherosclerotic plaques. Studies in the Watanabe heritable hyperlipidemic (WHHL) rabbit have indicated that hypertension induces a relative increase in intimal smooth muscle cells and decrease in macrophages as compared to the normotensive WHHL rabbit (9).

TABLE 1. *Cardiovascular tissue renin–angiotensin functions*

Tissue	Documented and putative functions
Kidney	Renal blood flow, glomerular filtration rate, glomerular hemodynamics, sodium reabsorption
Blood vessel	Vascular tone, vascular hypertrophy
Heart	Myocardial metabolism, hypertrophy, and contractility
Adrenal	Aldosterone secretion, catecholamine release (?)

Adapted from Dzau, ref. 2.

These studies are consistent with the observations that hypertension alters the phenotypic expression of a subpopulation of arterial smooth muscle cells from the resting to proliferative phase. Increased thymidine synthesis has been observed in both endothelial and smooth muscle cells of spontaneously hypertensive rats, although only a small fraction of such cells appear to undergo such change (10,11). In several forms of chronic hypertension in the rat, aortic smooth muscle cells also exhibit hypertrophy and nuclear polyploidy rather than cellular hyperplasia (12,13).

Hypertension causes increases in arterial connective tissue components, including collagen, elastin, fibronectin, and glycosaminoglycans. In view of the observations that extracellular proteins such as fibronectin may influence the growth of cultured cells, studies have been performed on the relationship between changes in arterial extracellular matrix and cellular growth in response to hypertension. Several forms of hypertension, including that induced by angiotensin II infusion, cause very rapid changes in aortic fibronectin expression, synthesis, and accumulation (14). With angiotensin II infusion, the effects may occur within the first day. The expression of arterial transforming growth factor beta-1 (TGFβ1), which appears to influence the regulation of fibronectin (15), also is increased rapidly by blood pressure elevation (16). Interrelationships between cellular and connective tissue alterations may be important in the remodeling of the arterial wall that occurs with hypertension.

In situ hybridization studies examining the cellular changes in fibronectin and TGFβ1 mRNA in response to hypertension have been of interest. With DOC-salt hypertension, much of the observed increase in arterial expression of both fibronectin and TGFβ1 surprisingly was localized in the periadventitia, whereas in normal controls, the messages for both substances were distributed throughout the vessel wall. These data raise the interesting possibility that the adventitia plays a role in the regulation of arterial changes with hypertension.

Direct Vascular Effects of Angiotensin

Angiotensin II appears to have an important effect on arterial connective tissue that is in part independent of its effect on blood pressure. Periods of angiotensin II infusion as brief as 1 day in the rat caused increases in fibronectin expression and content and the expression of structural collagen components. These actions were inhibited by losartan, therefore indicating that the effects are mediated through the AT1 angiotensin receptor. Interestingly, other antihypertensive drugs such as prazosin and hydralazine failed to influence the connective tissue responses, despite normalization of blood pressure.

Recent studies in smooth muscle cells have shown that angiotensin II has direct growth-stimulating effect on vascular smooth muscle cells. This growth-promoting activity is a result of growth-factor activation by angiotensin. Angiotensin II has been shown to be involved in the activation of three autocrine–paracrine growth factors—fibroblast growth factor (FGF), TGFβ1, and platelet-derived growth factor (PDGF)—in vascular smooth muscle cell (VSMC) (18). A key determinant in the regulation of angiotensin II-induced hypertrophy appears to be TGFβ1. Our data in smooth muscle cells suggest that TGFβ1 is antiproliferative and leads to cellular hypertrophy. In the absence or inhibition of TGFβ1, the principal effect of angiotensin is mitogenesis or hyperplasia resulting from the activation of FGF and PDGF (18,19). The simultaneous activation of TGFβ1 appears to override the proliferative activity of other growth factors and results in smooth muscle cell hypertrophy.

In various diseases such as atherosclerosis and neointimal hyperplasia, there is evidence for increased angiotensin II production in the vascular lesion. For example, it has been reported that 1–2 weeks after balloon angioplasty injury of the rat carotid artery or abdominal aorta, ACE expression is induced in the injured vessel, especially in the neointima (20). The level of vascular ACE and consequently angiotensin II correlated with the size of the neointima. In human atherosclerotic lesions, a marked increase in ACE activity in vascular cells, especially in lipid-laden macrophages within the plaque, has been demonstrated. These data suggest that local ACE and angiotensin II exert a paracrine growth effect in lesion formation. To further examine the importance of local ACE in regulating angiotensin II production and function, the effects of in vitro and in vivo gene transfer of ACE into cultured vascular smooth muscle cells and intact blood vessels were studied. The transfection of ACE cDNA into VSMC (which contain low levels of ACE) resulted in three- to fourfold increases in ACE activity and a parallel angiotensin II-mediated cellular hypertrophy (21). Cotransfection of renin and ACE cDNAs led to a synergistic effect, suggesting that both renin and ACE are rate determining in angiotensin II generation and function.

The in vivo gene transfer study shows convincingly the importance of tissue ACE. We transfected ACE cDNA into intact injured rat common carotid artery in vivo and studied the consequences 3 days and 2 weeks later. A threefold increase in vascular ACE as well as local angiotensin-mediated hypertrophy in the transfected segment of the common carotid was observed, but no increase occurred in the nontransfected control vessel or in the vessel transfected with the control vector (vector without ACE cDNA) (22). Since the transfected segment is exposed to the same blood pressure and neurohormones (including circulating plasma renin activity and plasma ACE levels) as the control segment, these results are strong evidence for a local ACE effect in angiotensin II production and consequently function.

Recent data provide further evidence that angiotensin II plays an important role in the pathophysiology of atherosclerosis and ischemic events (Table 2). As discussed previously, angiotensin has been shown to stimulate vascular cell growth and migration (18), two important processes in atherosclerosis and restenosis. In addition to intimal smooth muscle lesions, the lipid-laden macrophages contribute importantly to the atherosclerotic plaque. Angiotensin II can stimulate the transformation of monocytes to macrophages in the presence of oxidized low-density-lipoprotein (LDL) cholesterol. Simultaneously, the activation of macrophage in the presence of oxidized LDL cholesterol stimulates the cellular expression of ACE and presumably angiotensin II synthesis (23). Thus, a potential local positive feedback process leads to increased ACE and angiotensin II levels in the atherosclerotic lesion. In addition, angiotensin II may participate in the pathophysiology of acute ischemic syndromes. Recent evidence in humans (24) and in cultured cells (25) shows the stimulation of plasminogen-activator inhibitor (PAI) in response to angiotensin II. Thus, angiotensin may attenuate thrombolysis through stimulation of PAI. In addition, angiotensin appears to be involved in platelet activation and aggregation. Thus one of the mechanisms by which ACE inhibitors may prevent recurrent myocardial infarction (MI) is by prevention of atherosclerosis and other processes leading to the precipitation of ischemic events.

TABLE 2. *Direct cellular actions of angiotensin on atherogenesis*

Activation of growth factors and cytokines
Vascular smooth muscle migration and growth
Increased oxidative stress and perioxidation of low-density lipoprotein
Expression of endothelial leukocyte adhesion molecule
Monocyte/macrophage activation
Extracellular matrix production

The clinical relevance of the above vascular effects of angiotensin II may be reflected in the recent studies of Alderman et al. (26) and Cambien et al. (27). First, it has been reported that plasma renin activity predicts MI in patients with hypertension, irrespective of serum cholesterol levels (26,28). The MONICA study by Cambien et al. (27) reported that a deletion polymorphism in the gene for ACE was a potent risk factor for MI. Among patients with normal LDL cholesterol and body mass (low-risk patients), MI was three times more likely in the presence of the ACE polymorphism. Although these findings have not been verified, they may provide additional support for the role of altered RAS in human vascular disease. The importance of ACE and of angiotensin II in atherosclerosis is also supported by studies examining the effects of ACE inhibitors in hypercholesterolemic animals, as discussed subsequently.

ANGIOTENSIN-CONVERTING ENZYME INHIBITOR DRUGS AND ATHEROSCLEROSIS

Several classes of antihypertensive drugs, including beta-adrenergic blockers, alpha-1 receptor antagonists, calcium antagonists, and ACE inhibitors, have been shown to retard atherosclerosis in hypercholesterolemic normotensive animals (28). Species differences exist with respect to the action

TABLE 3. *Antiatherosclerotic effects of selected antihypertensive drugs in hypercholesterolemic animals*

Drug	Animal model	Effect on atherosclerosis
Thiazide diurectic	Cholesterol-fed rabbit	None
Beta-blockers		
Propranolol	Cholesterol-fed rabbit	Inhibition
	WHHL rabbit	None
	Cholesterol-fed monkey	Inhibition
Metoprolol	Cholesterol-fed rabbit	Inhibition
Hydralazine	Cholesterol-fed rabbit	None
Alpha-1-blockers		
Doxazosin	Cholesterol-fed guinea pig	Inhibition
Calcium antagonists		
Dihydropyridines	Cholesterol-fed rabbit	Inhibition
	WHHL rabbit	None
	Cholesterol-fed monkey	Equivocal
Verapamil	Cholesterol-fed rabbit	Inhibition
	WHHL rabbit	None
Diltiazem	Cholesterol-fed rabbit	Inhibition
	WHHL rabbit	None
ACE inhibitors		
Captopril	Cholesterol-fed rabbit	Inhibition
	WHHL rabbit	Inhibition
	Cholesterol-fed monkey	Inhibition
Transdolapril	WHHL rabbit	Inhibition
Enalapril	Cholesterol-fed rabbit	Inhibition
Perindopril	Cholesterol-fed minipig	Inhibition
Fosinopril	Cholesterol-fed hamster	Inhibition

Adapted from Chobanian, ref. 29.
ACE, Angiotensin-converting enzyme. WHHL, Watanabe heritable hyperlipidemic.

of the different drugs. The only antihypertensive class showing antiatherosclerotic effects in all models tested is the ACE inhibitor group (29). Several members of this class, including captopril, enalapril, trandolapril, perindopril, and fosinopril, shared this effect. The range in models studied included the WHHL rabbit, cholesterol-fed rabbit, cholesterol-fed monkey, minipig, and hamster (Table 3).

Various actions of ACE inhibitors could participate in such vasculoprotective effects (Table 4). Inhibition of cellular growth by inhibition of angiotensin II production, as discussed in other sections of this chapter, is an important consideration. Such a hypothesis is supported by the observation that the atherosclerotic plaques of captopril- and trandolapril-treated WHHL rabbits showed marked decreases in cellularity and reduction in intimal and medial thickness compared to untreated WHHL rabbits (30,31). As discussed earlier, other actions of ACE inhibitors could also be involved, including enhancement of bradykinin, nitric oxide, and prostaglandin effects (32), inhibition of leukocyte adherence to the endothelium (33), and improvement in endothelium-dependent functions. Indeed, ACE is known to degrade bradykinin and other peptides (34), and ACE inhibition will lead to increased tissue bradykinin levels, while reducing angiotensin production (35) (Fig. 2). Bradykinin can exert effects on the endothelium by activating the arachidonic acid cascade, which results in prostacyclin biosynthesis, as well as by stimulating the release of endothelium-derived relax-

TABLE 4. *Potential mechanisms for vasculoprotective actions of angiotensin-converting enzyme inhibitors*

Effects on atherosclerotic processes (plaque progression, regression, disruption)
- Blood pressure and other hemodynamic effects
- Reduction in vascular cell proliferation and migration
- Improvement in endothelial functions (including increased nitric oxide production)
- Inhibition of adherence and penetration of monocytes
- Reduction of ACE in modified SMC and/or macrophages
- Reduction of oxidative stress and possible inhibition of LDL oxidation

Effects on ischemic processes (triggering events)
- Hemodynamic effects on blood pressure and local vascular tone
- Microvascular vasodilation (increase coronary reserve)
- Inhibition of platelet aggregation and adhesion
- Reduction in PAI-1 production

SMC, Smooth muscle cells; LDL, low-density lipoprotein; PAI-1, plasminogen-activator inhibitor.

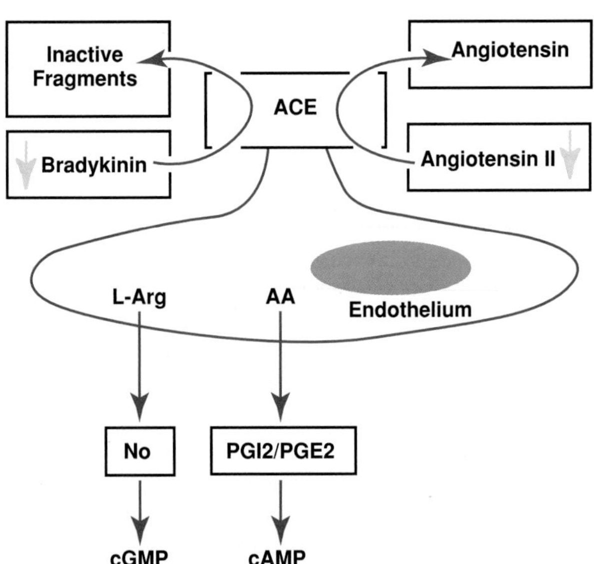

FIG. 2. Angiotensin-converting enzyme *(ACE)* has dual functions on angiotensin II production and bradykinin degradation. The latter influences nitric oxide and prostacyclin production. *L-Arg,* L-arginine; *NO,* nitric oxide; *PGI2,* prostacyclin; *PGE2,* prostaglandin; *cGMP,* cyclic guanosine monophosphate; *cAMP,* cyclic adenosine monophosphate; *AA,* arachidonic acid.

ing factor (EDRF) or nitric oxide (NO). By reducing angiotensin II and increasing NO (or EDRF), ACE inhibitors may cause relaxation and inhibit the remodeling process. Indeed, the recent study of Cooke et al. demonstrated that enhanced NO production by the dietary feeding of the NO substrate L-arginine inhibited atherosclerosis in cholesterol-fed rabbits (36). NO inhibits platelet aggregation and adhesion, blocks VSMC proliferation, and inhibits macrophage adherence to the vessel wall (37,38). All these effects are antiatherosclerotic. Thus ACE inhibitor may exert an antiatherogenic effect in part via increased NO production.

In vitro studies of arteries from cholesterol-fed rabbits with impaired endothelium-dependent relaxation provide supportive evidence. Impairment of endothelial-mediated relaxation in response to acetylcholine is an early marker of endothelial dysfunction and atherosclerosis in rabbits (39). The addition of the ACE inhibitor ramipril restores endothelial relaxation (40). Recently, it has been demonstrated that a significant part of the blockade by ACE inhibitor of neointimal hyperplasia development after vascular injury of the rat carotid artery is due to its bradykinin-NO effect (41). Thus, the vascular protective effect of ACE inhibitor may be due to the combined action of reduced angiotensin II and enhanced endothelial function. These effects, in turn, inhibit VSMC migration and proliferation, modulate extracellular matrix synthesis, increase thrombolysis, and reduce platelet aggregation and monocyte adhesion (Table 4).

The potential role of blood pressure reduction in the antiatherosclerotic action of ACE inhibitors remains unclear. The doses of ACE inhibitors used in the studies involving the WHHL rabbit caused modest reductions in blood pressure, but to levels which were well tolerated and were still within the normal range (30,31). In the cholesterol-fed rabbit, however, a dissociation between the blood pressure and antiatherosclerotic action of perindopril has been reported (42). On the other hand, in very recent studies involving the WHHL rabbit, low doses of trandolapril which were sufficient to reduce serum and arterial ACE activity markedly but were not adequate to lower blood pressure had no effect whatsoever on aortic atherosclerosis (43).

The clinical significance of the antiatherosclerotic action of either ACE inhibitors or other antihypertensive drugs remains to be determined. Indirect evidence which has been interpreted as supporting such effects in humans by ACE inhibition has been obtained in studies of patients with left ventricular dysfunction treated with either captopril or enalapril. In both the SAVE and SOLVE studies, patients who received the ACE inhibitor had an approximately 25% lower incidence of myocardial infarction than did the controls (44). However, although these observations are of interest, their relationship to changes in atherosclerosis remains unknown.

FUTURE DIRECTIONS

The recent studies on the cellular and molecular actions of angiotensin and related molecules (bradykinin, nitric oxide) have increased our understanding of the roles of these substances in atherogenesis and coronary ischemia. The observations that (a) activation of the renin–angiotensin system is associated with coronary artery disease; (b) subjects with DD genotype of the ACE gene are at increased risk for myocardial infarction; and (c) ACE inhibitors reduce recurrent myocardial infarction in patients with left ventricular dysfunction, have raised many intriguing questions which are shaping the direction of future research and clinical applications. For example, will ACE inhibitors prevent myocardial infarction and ischemic events in coronary patients who do not have left ventricular dysfunction? Is this class of drug effective in the primary prevention of coronary heart disease? What are the ''real'' mechanisms of ACE inhibitors' vasculoprotective actions? Will this class of drugs provide selective efficacy to patients with specific genotypes (e.g., ACE gene DD polymorphism)? These questions are being examined actively in many ongoing basic and clinical studies. The outcomes of the major multicenter clinical trials will be available in the next 5 or more years. Their results will undoubtedly exert a major influence on future clinical practice.

REFERENCES

1. Dzau VJ, Pratt RE. Renin–angiotensin system. In: Fozzard HA, et al., eds. *The Heart and Cardiovascular System.* New York: Raven Press; 1991:1817–1850.
2. Dzau VJ. Circulating versus local renin–angiotensin system in cardiovascular homeostasis. *Circulation* 1988;77(Suppl 19):1–4.
3. Paul M, Bachman J, Ganten D. The tissue renin–angiotensin system in cardiovascular disease. *Trends Cardiovasc Med* 1992;2:94.
4. Haudenschild CC, Prescott MF, Chobanian AV. Aortic endothelial and subendothelial cells in experimental hypertension and aging. *Hypertension* 1981;3:I-148–I-153.
5. Haudenschild CC, Prescott MF, Chobanian AV. Effects of hypertension and its reversal on aortic intimal lesions in the rat. *Hypertension* 1980; 2:33–44.
6. Wiener L, Lattes RG, Meltzer BG, Spiro G. The cellular pathology of experimental hypertension. Evidence for increased vascular permeability. *Am J Pathol* 1969;54:187–207.
7. Brush JE, Cannon RO, Schenke WH, Bonow RO, Leon MG, Maron BJ, Epstein SE. Angina due to coronary microvascular disease in hypertensive patients without left ventricular hypertrophy. *N Engl J Med* 1988;319:1302–1307.
8. Chobanian AV, Lichtenstein AH, Nilakhe V, Haudenschild CC, Drago R, Nickerson C. Influence of hypertension on aortic atherosclerosis in the Watanabe rabbit. *Hypertension* 1989;14:203–209.
9. Nickerson CJ, Haudenschild CC, Chobanian AV. Effects of hypertension and hyperlipidemia on the myocardium and coronary vasculature of the WHHL rabbit. *Exp Mol Pathol* 1992;56:173–185.
10. Schwartz SM, Benditt EDP. Aortic endothelial cell replication. Effects of age and hypertension in the rat. *Circ Res* 1977;41:248–255.
11. Schwartz SM, Campbell GR, Campbell JH. Replication of smooth muscle cells in vascular disease. *Circ Res* 1986;41:248–255.
12. Owens GK, Schwartz SM. Vascular smooth muscle cell hypertrophy and hyperploidy in the Goldblatt hypertensive rat. *Circ Res* 1983;53: 491–501.
13. Lichtenstein AH, Brecher P, Chobanian AV. Effects of deoxycorticosterone-salt on cell ploidy in the rat aorta. *Hypertension* 1986;8:II-50–II-54.
14. Takasaki I, Chobanian AV, Sarzani R, Brecher P. Effect of hypertension on fibronectin expression in the rat aorta. *J Biol Chem* 1990;265: 21935–21939.
15. Ignotz RA, Endo T, Massague J. Regulation of fibronectin and type I

collagen on RNA levels by transforming growth factor-β. *J Biol Chem* 1987;262:6443–6446.
16. Sarzani R, Brecher P, Chobanian AV. Growth factor expression in aorta of normotensive and hypertensive rats. *J Clin Invest* 1989;83: 1404–1408.
17. Himeno H, Crawford DH, Hosoi M, Chobanian AV, Brecher P. Angiotensin II alters fibronectin independent of hypertension. *Hypertension* 1994;23:823–826.
18. Itoh H, Mukoyama M, Pratt RE, Gibbons GH, Dzau VJ. Multiple autocrine growth factors modulate vascular smooth muscle cell growth response to angiotensin II. *J Clin Invest* 1993;91:2268–2274.
19. Gibbons GH, Pratt RE, Dzau VJ. Vascular smooth muscle cell hypertrophy vs. hyperplasia: Autocrine transforming growth factor beta 1 expression determines growth response to angiotensin II. *J Clin Invest* 1992;90:456–461.
20. Rakugi H, Kim DK, Krieger JE, Wang DS, Dzau VJ, Pratt RE. Induction of angiotensin converting enzyme in the neointima after vascular injury. Possible role in restenosis. *J Clin Invest* 1994;93:339–346.
21. Morishita R, Gibbons GH, Kaneda Y, Ogihara T, Dzau VJ. Novel and effective gene transfer technique for study of vascular renin angiotensin system. *J Clin Invest* 1993;91:2580–2585.
22. Morishita R, Gibbons GH, Pratt RE, Tomita N, Kaneda Y, Ogihara T, Dzau VJ. Autocrine and paracrine effects of atrial natriuretic peptide gene transfer on vascular smooth muscle and endothelial cellular growth. *J Clin Invest* 1994;94:824–839.
23. Momoso N, Pratt RE, Dzau VJ. Unpublished data.
24. Vaughan DE, Declerck PJ, Vanhoutte P, De Mol M, Collen D. Reactivated recombinant plasminogen activator inhibitor-1 (rPAI-1) effectively prevents thrombolysis *in vivo*. *Thromb Haemostasis* 1992;68: 60–63.
25. Rydzewski B, Zelezna B, Tang W, Sumners C, Raizada MK. Angiotensin II stimulation of plasminogen activator inhibitor-1 gene expression in astroglial cells from the brain. *Endocrinology* 1992;130:1255–1262.
26. Alderman MH, Madhavan S, Ooi WL, Cohen H, Sealey JE, Laragh JH. Association of the renin-sodium profile with the risk of myocardial infarction in patients with hypertension. *N Engl J Med* 1991;324: 1098–1104.
27. Cambien F, Poirier O, Lecerf L, Evans A, Cambou JP, Arveiler D, Luc G, Bard JM, Bara L, Ricard S, et al. Deletion polymorphism in the gene for angiotensin-converting enzyme is a potent risk factor for myocardial infarction. *Nature* 1992;359:641–644.
28. Dzau VJ. Renin and myocardial infarction in hypertension. *N Engl J Med* 1991;324:1128.
29. Chobanian AV. Can antihypertensive drugs reduce atherosclerosis and its clinical complications? *Am J Hypertens* 1994;7(Suppl II): 119S–125S.
30. Chobanian AV, Haudenschild CC, Nickerson C, Drago R. Antiatherogenic effect of captopril in the Watanabe heritable hyperlipidemic rabbit. *Hypertension* 1990;15:327–331.
31. Chobanian AV, Hausenschild CC, Nickerson C, Hope S. Trandolapril inhibits atherosclerosis in the Watanabe heritable hyperlipidemic rabbit. *Hypertension* 1992;20:473–477.
32. Becker RHA, Wiemer G, Linz W. Preservation of endothelial function by ramipril in rabbits on a long-term atherogenic diet. *J Cardiovasc Pharmacol* 1991;18(Suppl 2):S110–S115.
33. Clozel M, Kuhn H, Hefti F, Baumgartner HR. Endothelial dysfunction and subendothelial monocyte macrophages in hypertension. *Hypertension* 1991;18:132–141.
34. Skidgel RA, Defendini R, Erdos EG. Angiotensin I converting enzyme and its role in neuropeptide metabolism. In: Turner AJ, ed. *Neuropeptides and Their Peptidases*. New York: Ellis Horwood-VCH; 1988; 165–188.
35. Carretero OA, Miyazaki S, Scicli AG. Role of kinins in the acute antihypertensive effect of the converting enzyme inhibitor, captopril. *Hypertension* 1981;3:18.
36. Cooke JP, Singer AH, Tsao P, Zera P, Rowan RA, Billingham ME. Antiatherogenic effects of L-arginine in the hypercholesterolemic rabbit. *J Clin Invest* 1992;90:1168–1172.
37. Radomski MW, Palmer RMJ, Moncada S. An L-arginine/nitric oxide pathway present in human platelets regulates aggregation. *Proc Natl Acad Sci USA* 1990;87:5192.
38. Kubes P, Suzuki M, Granger DN. Nitric oxide: An endogenous modulator of leukocyte adhesion. *Proc Natl Acad Sci USA* 1991;88:4651.
39. Jayakody L, Kappagoda T, Senaratne MPJ, et al. Impairment of endothelium-dependent relaxation: An early marker for atherosclerosis in the rabbit. *Br J Pharmacol* 1988;94:335.
40. Webb RC, Finta KM, Fisher M, et al. Ramipril reverses impaired endothelium-dependent relaxation in arteries from rabbits fed an atherogenic diet. *FASEB J* 1992;6(Part I):3022.
41. Farhy RD, Carretero OA, Ho KL, Scicli AG. Role of kinins and nitric oxide in the effects of angiotensin converting enzyme inhibitors on neointima formation. *Circ Res* 1993;72:1202–1210.
42. Schuh JR, Bhehm DJ, Frierdich GE, McMahon EG, Blaine EH. Differential effects of renin–angiotensin system blockade on atherogenesis in cholesterol-fed rabbits. *J Clin Invest* 1993;91:1453–1458.
43. Chobanian AV, Hope S, Brecher P. Dissociation between the anti-atherosclerotic effect of trandolapril and suppression of serum and aortic angiotensin converting enzyme activity in the Watanabe heritable hyperlipidemic rabbit. *Hypertension* 1995 [in press].
44. Pfeffer MA, Braunwald E, Moye LA, Basta L, Brown EJ, Cuddy TE, Davis BR, Geltman EM, Goldman S, Flaker GC, Klein M, Lamas GA, Packer M, Rouleau J, Rouleau JL, Rutherford J, Wertheimer JH, Hawkins CM. Effect of captopril on mortality and morbidity in patients with left ventricular dysfunction after myocardial infarction. *N Engl J Med* 1992;327:669–677.

Atherosclerosis and Coronary Artery Disease,
edited by V. Fuster, R. Ross, and E. J. Topol.
Lippincott-Raven Publishers, Philadelphia © 1996.

CHAPTER 15

Clinical Classifications of Hypertensive Diseases

Edward D. Frohlich

Key Words: Hypertension, pathophysiology; Pressor mechanisms; Essential hypertension; Hypertension, target organ involvement; Left ventricular hypertrophy; Hypertension, diagnostic evaluation; Antihypertensive therapy; Diuretics; β-Adrenergic receptor blockers; Angiotensin converting enzyme inhibitors; Calcium antagonists; α-Adrenergic receptor blockers.

INTRODUCTION

Systemic arterial hypertension is one of the most common cardiovascular diseases in industrialized societies. It is present in over 50 million Americans, and it occurs with increasing prevalence with aging. Furthermore, the disease is a major risk factor underlying occlusive epicardial coronary arterial disease (i.e., coronary heart disease) and is a major factor that exacerbates the atherosclerotic disease process.

In this chapter, a number of hypertensive diseases are discussed in terms of a series of classifications. The large number of pressor and depressor mechanisms that serve to maintain arterial pressure in the normal individual are discussed. This is then extended to an etiological classification of the various primary and secondary forms of hypertensive disease by indicating the interrelationship of the factors that participate pathophysiologically in these diseases and how they are also brought into play with treatment. The discussion continues by considering the classification of hypertensive disease according to severity of arterial pressure elevation as well as with respect to target organ involvement.

The final aspect of the chapter considers a classification of antihypertensive therapy and how this is related to the recent recommendations for antihypertensive therapy by the Joint National Committee's fifth report. This discussion is not restricted to a single algorithm for therapy; it also considers how treatment can be modified when complicating factors of disease (including comorbidity) are considered through an approach to individualization of drug therapy.

HYPERTENSION: A MULTIFACTORIAL DISEASE

As presented in this discussion of the classifications of hypertensive disease the fundamental considerations underlying the hypertensive diseases continue to expand dramatically. Specific genetic mechanisms are now being elucidated in experimental forms of naturally developing hypertension, and the first reports of specific genes that are involved in clinical hypertension are beginning to be identified. In addition to these fundamental factors, recent experimental and clinical studies have identified new biological mechanisms that participate importantly in the various expressions of the hypertensive diseases. These mechanisms involve local growth factors, hormones, and peptides in vessels, heart, kidney, and brain and their roles in controlling or elevating arterial pressure, in producing arteriolar thickening and ventricular hypertrophy, and in promoting glomerular hyperfil-

E. D. Frohlich: Departments of Medicine and Physiology, Louisiana State University; Departments of Medicine and Pharmacology, Tulane University; and Alton Ochsner Medical Foundation, New Orleans, Louisiana 70121.

tration and possibly hypertensive renal disease. Additionally, some of these local growth factors have also been implicated in the atherogenic process and, hence, may open a way to understand the interrelationship between hypertension and atherosclerosis, as one seems to exacerbate the other. Finally, these new considerations no doubt will make possible the consideration of innovative modes of therapy involving some of the new local factors (e.g., endothelin, atrial natriuretic factor, peptides, and their antagonists), agonists and antagonists of membrane channel receptors, intracellular regulators, and even gene therapy in hypertension.

Over the years new concepts of the pathogenesis and treatment of hypertension have provided mind-boggling extrapolations to other cardiovascular diseases. Consider, for examples, the concepts of ''unloading'' the heart with ganglion-blocking therapy and vasodilators, control of intravascular (i.e., plasma) volume, adrenergic receptor blockade, inhibition of the renin–angiotensin system, the development and reversal of ventricular hypertrophy, and prevention of further deterioration of renal function in diabetes mellitus. With this past record of successes and the anticipated innovations suggested above, the future for further understanding of hypertension and its relationships with other cardiovascular diseases is truly exciting.

REGULATION OF BLOOD PRESSURE AND HYPERTENSION

Most workers in the field of hypertension have come to appreciate the concept that the control of arterial pressure is multifactorial (1,2). Thus, elevation of arterial pressure, even when specific causes can be identified, is multiplied through the interplay of physiological pressor and depressor factors (Fig. 1) (3). This is most clearly evidenced in patients with the most common clinical expression of systemic arterial hypertension, essential hypertension. This primary form of hypertension occurs in over 90% of patients with abnormally elevated arterial pressure. Thus, despite the more obvious or apparent participation of perhaps only a few specific pressor mechanisms in certain patients, the interrelationship that exists among those pressor mechanisms means that other possibilities exist whereby the elevated pressure may be expressed clinically in those affected patients. This becomes most evident and important clinically when antihypertensive therapy is prescribed, because reduction of the elevated pressure brings into play a variety of additional physiologically adaptive systemic homeostatic responses, even though pressure was abnormally elevated at the outset.

This ''mosaic'' concept, introduced by Page (1) almost 45 years ago and emphasizing the multifactorial causation of elevated arterial pressure in hypertension, has been supported clinically by observations that the disease is frequently associated with a familial predisposition that may be associated with other abnormalities that also have a familial or genetic predisposition. Among these other comorbid conditions are exogenous obesity, enhanced sodium sensitivity, carbohydrate intolerance and diabetes mellitus, hyperuricemia and gout, hypercholesterolemia and other hyperlipidemias, and, of course, accelerated atherosclerogenesis with occlusive coronary artery disease, stroke, sudden death, and renal functional impairment (4). Still more recently, this pathophysiological multifactorial concept has been reinforced by the demonstration of a number of genetic alterations that have also been associated with hypertension (5). Thus, hypertension does not seem to be based solely on one or even two genetic abnormalities but, rather, is considered to be polygenetic in basis with facilitated expression of cer-

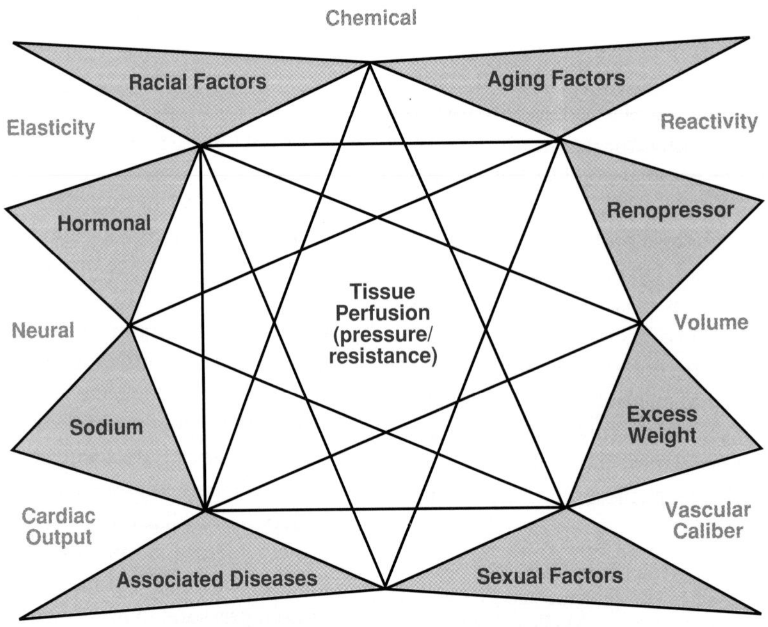

FIG. 1. Mosaic. (From ref. 3, with permission.)

tain alterations of gene function by environmental factors (e.g., excess sodium intake). Moreover, some of these genetic alterations have been associated with specific pressor and depressor mechanisms, so that there is great likelihood of interrelationships between altered genotype and phenotype in patients with hypertension. For example, one recent report relates development of left ventricular hypertrophy to the DD genotype of the angiotensin-converting enzyme (ACE) gene in middle-aged men (6).

PATHOPHYSIOLOGICAL MECHANISMS

Because of the foregoing concept concerning the pathogenesis of hypertensive diseases, in this chapter hypertension is considered from a pathophysiological point of view and then by a more traditional etiological means. This is followed by a more recent approach of staging the severity of hypertensive disease, then by a more pragmatic clinical functional approach, and finally, with a therapeutic classification taking into consideration the ''wedding'' of pathophysiological mechanisms with mechanisms of drug action.

Control of arterial pressure is subserved through a large number of pressor and depressor mechanisms in normotensive as well as hypertensive individuals (Table 1). As indicated above, these were initially described by Page as a ''mosaic'' of factors that interrelate with each other in a more or less kaleidoscopic fashion to maintain normal tissue perfusion in response to systemic arteriolar constriction, but at the ''expense'' of the abnormally elevated pressure (1). In any individual with hypertension, the seeming participation of any single factor naturally impacts on the participation of many others. For example, in what might appear to be a straightforward mechanism for elevating arterial pressure by means of a mechanical obstruction to the forward flow of blood by a coarctation of the aorta, a variety of other factors can also participate in the pathophysiological problem. Thus, if the coarctation is above the renal arteries, renal ischemic changes might result so that the intrarenal angiotensin system is secondarily stimulated through the release of renin from the juxtaglomerular apparatus. Should this be severe enough, secondary hyperaldosteronism may result by means of the generation of angiotensin II, which, in turn, stimulates aldosterone release from the adrenal cortex. This, in turn, would result in the development of hypokalemic alkalosis and with additional associated electrolytic and metabolic changes. Furthermore, even when the coarctation is repaired surgically, during the immediate postoperative period there may be a precipitous rise in arterial pressure, which frequently is controlled by sympathetic blockade. This suggests the possible provocation of an augmented sympathetic discharge as the baroreceptors sense the sudden reduction of arterial pressure that is associated with the repair of the coarctation.

As another example of the participation of a multiplicity of pressor mechanisms in causation of hypertension, consider the patient with occlusive renal arterial disease. In this patient, arterial pressure is elevated by the release of renin from the renal juxtaglomerular apparatus as a consequence of the reduced renal blood flow, renal baroreceptor stimulation, and other intrarenal factors. Additionally, consequences of the increased circulating level of angiotensin II include release of aldosterone from the adrenal cortex, possibly an initial release of catecholamines from the adrenal medulla, enhanced adrenergic outflow from specific cardiovascular medullary centers in the brain, stimulation of specific central thirst-promoting centers, and a contracted plasma volume as a result of postcapillary venoconstriction and, additionally, a pressure natriuresis by the kidney. Accompanying this sec-

TABLE 1. *Pressor and depressor mechanisms involved in hypertension*[a]

1. Mechanical
2. Neural
   a. Adrenergic, parasympathetic
   b. Central, peripheral
3. Catecholamines
   a. Norepinephrine
   b. Epinephrine
   c. Dopamine
4. Renopressor (i.e., renin–angiotensin) system
5. Renal
   a. Sodium
   b. Other ions (e.g., potassium, magnesium, calcium, chloride)
   c. Water and fluid balance
6. Hormonal
   a. Thyroid
   b. Parathyroid
   c. Growth
   d. Adrenal cortical (e.g., cortisol, aldosterone)
   e. Vasopressin
   f. "Third factor" (i.e., ouabain)
   g. Erythropoietin
7. Peptides and growth factors
   a. Atrial natriuretic factor
   b. Endothelin
   c. Insulin
   d. Vasoactive intestinal polypeptide
   e. Protooncogenes
   f. Growth factors (e.g., platelet-derived growth factor, β-transforming growth factor, insulin-derived growth factors)
   g. Endothelial-derived relaxing (nitric oxide, EDRF) and constriction (EDCF) factors
   h. Many others
8. Volume
   a. Renal factors
   b. Electrolytic (e.g., sodium)
   c. Humoral control (e.g., antidiuretic hormone, atrial natriuretic factor, "third" factor)
9. Serotonin
10. Depressor factors
    a. Histamine
    b. Kinins
    c. Prostaglandins
    d. Renal neutral medullary phospholipid

[a] From Frohlich (7), with permission.

ondary hyperaldosteronism are hypokalemic alkalosis, hypomagnesemia, and hypercalemia. Not only do each of these mechanisms interact in the patient with hypertension and with hemodynamically significant renal arterial disease, but local autocrine/paracrine mechanisms (involving the kinin, prostaglandin, and perhaps other systems) come into play within the kidney and elsewhere. These latter factors are extremely important when one considers the management of the patient with bilateral renal arterial disease who had been treated with an ACE inhibitor and who subsequently developed an acceleration of the hypertensive disease process with malignant hypertension and, perhaps, further renal functional impairment (7).

The foregoing clinical examples were selected to demonstrate the importance of the multiplicity of pathophysiological factors that participate in patients with what might otherwise be considered straightforward forms of secondary hypertension from a mechanistic point of view. These very same interrelationships occur, but perhaps more subtly, in patients with primary or essential hypertension. However, in these patients, the underlying disease mechanisms are related to inborn genetic alterations that, in turn, impact on their clinical expressions in primary hypertension (5,8,9). Thus, this ubiquitous disease, essential hypertension, is considered to result from genetic alterations involving abnormal gene expression that may be facilitated through specific environmental factors (e.g., sodium). Among these genetic alterations are those that affect functional expression of the renin–angiotensin system (e.g., angiotensinogen, renin, ACE, the autonomic nervous system (e.g., through catecholamine biosynthesis), endocrine systems (e.g., expression of altered enzymes of steroid hormone biosynthesis), sodium metabolism (e.g., via enzymes that control sodium ionic channel and exchange mechanisms), and control of other humoral and peptide agents. Thus, each of the genetic factors that participate in normal blood pressure regulation may be altered in hypertensive diseases. Furthermore, they also come into play when arterial pressure is reduced therapeutically. In that regard, when arterial pressure is reduced by certain antihypertensive agents (e.g., antiadrenergic agents or direct-acting vascular smooth muscle relaxants), there is an ingress of extravascular water into the circulation that offsets the therapeutic reduction in pressure (10,11). This phenomenon leads to the state of pseudotolerance and may be counteracted by the addition of small doses of diuretics if not already prescribed or by higher doses of diuretics if smaller doses have been employed (12).

ETIOLOGICAL CLASSIFICATION

From a clinical point of view, the various hypertensive diseases have been classified according to whether they result from a known factor or disease (i.e., secondary forms of hypertension) or whether no known specific clinical cause of the hypertension can be identified (i.e., primary or essential hypertension). Actually, 90% to 95% of all patients with hypertension have essential hypertension; only 5% to 10% of patients with persistently elevated arterial pressures have hypertension of a known etiology (Table 2).

Following the concept presented above concerning the mechanisms that participate in elevating arterial pressure, it is logical to relate the various secondary forms of hypertensive disease to specific pressor and depressor mechanism(s) that can be identified clinically (Tables 1 and 2). Thus, a mechanical factor impairing the forward flow of blood in the aorta (e.g., aortic coarctation, mechanical obstruction of the aorta by tumor) will elevate pressure proximal to that aortic obstruction. A number of neurological diseases are complicated by hypertension. They may be central (e.g., brain tumors or trauma, porphyria, diencephalic syndrome) or peripheral (e.g., pheochromocytoma). In either case, the final common pathway explaining the elevated arterial pressure is based on increased adrenergic outflow from the brain, catecholamine release from nerve endings, or adrenergic receptor stimulation (e.g., hyperdynamic β-adrenergic circulatory state). Increased participation of the renin–angiotensin system is classically demonstrated by occlusive renal arterial lesions (e.g., by fibrosis or atherosclerosis) (13), although not all patients with these lesions have an elevated arterial pressure (14). Hemodynamically significant occlusive renal arterial lesions may also be produced by emboli to the kidney, renal cysts or tumors, radiation fibrosis of the kidney, or compression of the renal artery by tumor, and hypertension can be caused by renin-producing tumors within the kidney.

Many patients with parenchymal disease of the kidney will have hypertension, but not all. In those patients who do have parenchymal renal disease and hypertension, the elevated arterial pressure is related primarily to an inability of the kidney to excrete sodium and water, even if renal function is normal clinically; in other patients there may be an additional participation of the renin–angiotensin system (15). In the former group, the arterial pressure is directly related to the intravascular (plasma) volume (15). The impaired renal excretory component of the hypertension has been termed by some workers in the field to be a "renoprival" factor, which may be demonstrated best by the patient with severe renal functional impairment who is able to achieve optimal control of elevated arterial pressure before hemodialysis by increasing the filtration pressures during dialysis (16). A number of hormonal substances, when produced in excess, may elevate arterial pressure; these include thyroid, parathyroid, growth hormone, and several adrenal steroidal hormones (produced by tumor, hyperplasia, or enzymatic deficiencies).

In addition to these better-known clinical entities, hypertension may be produced by an excessive amount of circulating humoral substances. This might be exemplified by the patient with metastatic carcinoid, who produces excessive amounts of serotonin that are inadequately metabolized by metastatic liver disease, or in porphyria, in which participa-

TABLE 2. *Primary and secondary hypertension*[a]

Primary (essential) hypertension (hypertension of undetermined cause)

Borderline (labile) essential hypertension
Essential hypertension (sustained arterial hypertension)
- Diastolic hypertension
- Isolated systolic hypertension

Secondary hypertensions

Coarctation of the aorta
Renal arterial diseases (renal vascular disease with hypertension)
- Nonatherosclerotic (fibrosing) renal arterial disease
- Atherosclerotic renal arterial disease
- Aneurysm(s) of renal artery
- Embolic renal arterial disease
- Extravascular compression (of renal artery): tumor, fibrosis
- Perinephric hull (Page kidney)

Renal parenchymal diseases
- Chronic pyelonephritis
- Acute glomerulonephritis
- Chronic glomerulonephritis
- Polycystic renal disease
- Diabetic nephropathy
- Others: amyloidosis, ureteral obstruction, etc.

Hormonal disease
- Thyroid
  - Hyperthyroidism
  - Hypothyroidism
  - Hashimoto's thyroiditis
- Adrenal
  - Cushing disease or Cushing syndrome
  - Primary hyperaldosteronism
    - Adenoma
    - Bilateral hyperplasia
  - Adrenal enzyme deficiencies
  - Pheochromocytoma
- Others
  - Ectopic production of pressor hormones
  - Growth hormone excess
  - Hypercalcemic disease states (including hyperparathyroidism)

Drugs, chemicals, and foods
- Excessive alcohol intake
- Excessive dietary sodium intake
- Exogenously administered adrenal steroids: birth control pills; adrenal steroids for asthma, malignancies; anabolic steroids
- Licorice excess (imported)
- Over-the-counter preparations (e.g., phenylpropanolamine, nasal decongestants)
- Milk-alkali syndrome; hypervitaminosis D
- Snuff
- Complications from specific therapy
  - Antidepressant therapy (tricyclics; monoamine oxidase inhibitors)
  - Chronic steroid administration
  - Cyclosporine (transplantation and certain diseases requiring immunosuppressive therapy)
  - Beta-adrenergic receptor agonists (e.g., for asthma)
  - Radiation nephritis, arteritis

[a] From Frohlich (2), with permission.

tion of the central nervous system occurs in those patients with essential hypertension who may have impaired endothelial-dependent vasodilating or constricting factors (17–19). It is also possible that arterial pressure might be elevated in the patient with deficient amounts of vasodilating agents (7,17). Finally, secondary hypertension might be produced by any of a variety of ingested over-the-counter medications (e.g., nose drops, oral contraceptives, steroidal substances, aspirin, nonsteroidal antiinflammatory agents, tricyclic antidepressants with guanethidine or guanabenz), foodstuffs (e.g., licorice, tyramine-containing foods, beverages), or diets with excessive amounts of sodium in the patient who is more sensitive to sodium excess (e.g., with renal or cardiac failure) (20).

Primary (or essential) hypertension is, by far, the most common hypertension, occurring in approximately 90–95% of all patients with hypertension. In the United States, the Third National Health and Nutrition Survey, in 1993, estimated that there were approximately 50 million Americans with essential hypertension (21). This reduction of approximately 17% from the prior survey (which estimated 59 million people in the United States with essential hypertension), has been attributed to the broad acceptance of several lifestyle modifications by the general public. These nonpharmacological modifications of personal life style include weight control, sodium restriction, alcohol moderation, adoption of a regular isotonic exercise program, and smoking cessation (21,22). Thus, this 10 million decrease in patients with essential hypertension has been attributed to an unanticipated practice of primary prevention measures that would otherwise predispose the involved individuals to an abnormally elevated arterial pressure.

With the publication of the Joint National Committee's fifth report (JNC-V) in 1992, a new classification of essential hypertension was introduced (Table 3) (22). For the first time this report takes into consideration elevated systolic as well as diastolic pressure. The patient's baseline (or pretreatment) blood pressure is established after at least three indirect pressure measurements are obtained on at least three separate occasions. The measurements should be obtained under well-prescribed resting conditions not influenced by prior smoking, restrictive clothing, etc. (22). However, if the physician believes that the height of arterial pressure is of sufficient concern to warrant immediate treatment, subse-

TABLE 3. *Classification of blood pressure for adults age 18 years and older (22)*

Category	Systolic (mm Hg)	Diastolic (mm Hg)
Normal	<130	<85
High normal	130–139	85–89
Hypertension		
Stage 1	140–159	90–99
Stage 2	160–179	100–109
Stage 3	180–209	110–119
Stage 4	≥210	≥120

quent pressure measurements on other occasions obviously are not warranted.

Elevated systolic and diastolic pressures are defined in this report as 140 and 90 mm Hg or greater, respectively (22). Patients with systolic and diastolic pressures ranging from 130 through 139 and 85 through 89 mm Hg, respectively, are considered to have high normal pressures. Moreover, the heights of the systolic and diastolic pressures are classified according to stages of increasing severity of pressure elevation (1 through 4). Most importantly, the pressure (i.e., systolic or diastolic) that is greatest permits rating of the stage severity (22). This classification, then, accomplishes two major points: (a) it underscores the concept that the elevation of systolic pressure is at least as important as the diastolic pressure elevation, and (b) no longer is any elevation of arterial pressure to be considered "mild," because all levels of severity confer a significantly increased risk of increased (and premature) cardiovascular morbidity and mortality. The concept of "borderline" hypertension areas is also downplayed in this report (22). Nevertheless, this still leaves a major practical controversy, and this "gray" area relates to whether the physician should institute pharmacological treatment for those patients whose systolic and diastolic pressures range from 140 through 159 and 90 through 94 mm Hg, respectively.

TABLE 4. *Laboratory studies that may be of value in the diagnostic evaluation of the patient with hypertension*

Complete blood count
White blood cell count (and differential)
Hemoglobin concentration[a]
Hematocrit[a]
Adequacy of platelets
Blood chemistries
Sugar (fasting, 2 hr postprandial, or tolerance test)[a]
Uric acid[a]
Cholesterol and triglyceride concentrations[a]
Low- and high-density cholesterol concentrations[a]
Renal function (blood urea and/or serum creatinine)[a]
Serum electrolytes (Na[a], K, Cl, CO_2) concentrations
Calcium and phosphate concentrations
Total protein and albumin concentration
Hepatic function (alkaline phosphatase, bilirubin, serum enzymes)
Urine studies
Urinalysis[a]
Urine culture
24-hr collection (protein, Na, K, creatinine)
Electrocardiogram (12-lead)[a]

[a] Those tests currently recommended in the Joint National Committee's fifth report (22).

Functional Classification

Hypertension as a disease is manifested clinically by its effects on its major target organs (i.e., heart, brain, and kidneys). These effects are assessable by means of clinical and laboratory studies. As already indicated, not all patients having hypertension may warrant pharmacological therapy. However, all patients with hypertension should come under close medical management, even if this means that the patient is instructed to institute the various nonpharmacological life-style modifications with instructions to return for further follow-up consultations at regularly prescribed intervals. In order to arrive at an appropriate plan for subsequent management, the patient should be evaluated comprehensively. Thus, to assess target organ involvement, the initial evaluation should include a careful medical history, physical examination, and laboratory evaluation (22).

Inherent in this evaluation is a careful search for a family history of cardiovascular illnesses and premature death as well as for other risk factors predisposing the patient to hypertension, coronary heart disease, stroke, and renal failure. This clinical evaluation should include a number of laboratory studies that will be of value in detecting those comorbid risk factors, clinical evidence of target organ involvement resulting from hypertensive vascular disease, as well as for the detection of secondary causes of hypertensive disease (Tables 4 and 5). In this regard, it is also extremely important to evaluate the patient for hypertensive retinopathy (Table 6) (23,24) and history of transient ischemic attacks or of more severe sensory or motor neurological deficit. Cardiac involvement can be ascertained using electrocardiographic criteria for left atrial abnormality and left ventricular hypertrophy (Table 7) (25–30) or echocardiographic criteria for increased left atrial size, left ventricular mass or wall thicknesses, or ventricular function (31,32). (The reader is referred to Phillips and Diamond, *this volume,* for a complete discussion of the criteria for calculating left ventricular mass, wall thicknesses, and indices of ventricular function.) Renal functional impairment is assessed by quantitative measurement of proteinuria and elevation of serum creatinine or blood urea nitrogen. Clinical evaluation is extremely valuable and includes ascertaining evidence of secondary forms of hypertension (e.g., renal arterial bruits, facial and body habitus and characteristics of Cushing's syndrome or disease, reduction or delay of femoral pulsations for aortic coarctation, hypokalemic alkalosis for indication of primary or secondary hyperaldosteronism, and symptoms presented in the patient's history suggesting pheochromocytoma or ingestion of certain drugs or foods). Each of these considerations, including the patient's age, race, and gender, should provide information that suggests the need for immediacy and intensity of medical treatment.

Therapeutic Classification

It follows, then, from the foregoing discussions concerning these various classifications of hypertension, that a consideration of therapeutic classifications naturally follows. Treatment may be selected on the basis of etiology, func-

TABLE 5. *Classification of known hypertensive diseases according to pressor mechanisms*

Primary pressor mechanisms	Clinical diagnosis	Other implicated pressor mechanisms	Specific tests
Mechanical	Coarctation of aorta	Renopressor	Chest X-ray, angiography
Catecholamines	Pheochromocytoma	Volume, renopressor, neural	Plasma catecholamines, CAT scan
Renopressor	Renal arterial disease	Aldosterone, volume, neural	Renal arteriography; plasma renin activity or angiotensin I level
Hormonal	Thyrotoxicosis	Thyroid, neural	Thyroid function studies
	Hyperparathyroidism	Calcium on vascular smooth muscle	Serum calcium; parathormone level
	Oral contraceptives	Renopressor	Plasma renin activity
	Acromegaly, gigantism	Growth hormone and factors	Growth hormone
	Cushing's syndrome or disease	Compounds D, F	17-OH steroids
	Primary hyperaldosteronism	Volume, electrolytes	Aldosterone, renin
	Adrenal virilism	Volume, electrolytes	Ketosteroids
	Hydroxylase deficiencies	Volume, electrolytes	Corticosteroids
	DOC-tumors	Volume, electrolytes	17-OH steroids
Volume	Renal parenchymal disease	Electrolytes, renopressor	IVP, urine culture, renal biopsy, renal function studies, measurement of body fluid volumes
Neural	Essential hypertension; borderline hypertension	Catecholamines, volume, renopressor	Hemodynamics, plasma renin activity; measurement of fluid volumes; assessment
	β-Adrenergic hypercirculatory state	Adenylate cyclase, cAMP	Hemodynamics; isoproterenol infusion
	Porphyria	Catecholamines	
	Diencephalic syndrome	Renopressor	Porphobilinogen
	Brain tumor		CAT scan, MRI

TABLE 6. *Classification of hypertensive retinopathy*

A. Keith–Wagener–Barker Classification (23)
   Group I: tortuosity, minimal constriction
   Group II: above + arteriovenous nicking
   Group III: above + hemorrhages and exudates
   Group IV: papilledema

B. American Ophthalmological Society Committee Classification (Wagener–Clay–Gipner) (24)
   1. Generalized arteriolar constriction
      Grade 1: arterioles ¾ normal caliber; A/V ratio of 1:2
      Grade 2: arterioles ½ normal caliber; A/V ratio of 1:3
      Grade 3: arterioles ⅓ normal caliber; A/V ratio of 1:4
      Grade 4: arterioles thread-like or invisible
   2. Focal arteriolar constriction or sclerosis
      Grade 1: localized arteriolar narrowing to ⅔ caliber of proximal segment
      Grade 2: localized arteriolar narrowing to ½ caliber of proximal segment
      Grade 3: localized arteriolar narrowing to ⅓ caliber of proximal segment
      Grade 4: arterioles invisible beyond focal constriction
   3. Generalized sclerosis
      Grade 1: increased light-striping; mild AV nicking
      Grade 2: coppery arteriolar color; moderate AV nicking; veins almost completely invisible below arteriolar crossing
      Grade 3: silver arteriolar color; severe AV nicking
      Grade 4: arterioles visible only as fibrous cords without bloodstreams
   4. Hemorrhage and exudates, grades 1 to 4 (based on number of affected quadrants divided by 2)
   5. Papilledema, grades 1 to 4 (based on diopters of elevation)

tional mechanisms, severity of pressure elevation, target organ involvement, or comorbid diseases.

High Normal

Patients with "high normal" levels of arterial pressure (i.e., 130–139/85–89 mm Hg) are more likely predisposed to develop an elevated pressure at some subsequent time. These patients should return for repeated blood pressure measurements at more frequent intervals. This may be facili-

TABLE 7. *Diagnostic electrocardiographic cardiac criteria*

1. Left atrial abnormality (ECG), two of four (25)
   a. P wave in lead II ≥ 0.3 mV and ≥ 0.12 sec (26)
   b. Bipeak interval in notched P wave ≥ 0.04 sec (27)
   c. Ratio of P wave duration to PR segment ≥ 1.6 (lead II) (28)
   d. Terminal atrial forces (in V_1) ≥ 0.04 sec
2. Left ventricular hypertrophy (25)
   a. Ungerleider index ≥ +15% (chest X-ray alone)
   b. Ungerleider index ≥ +10% (chest X-ray + two of the following ECG criteria)
      (1) Sum of tallest R and deepest S waves ≥ 4.5 mV (precordial) (29)
      (2) LV "strain," i.e., QRS and T wave vectors 180° apart (30)
      (3) QRS frontal axis < 0°
   c. All three ECG criteria (above)

TABLE 8. *Life-style modifications for hypertension control and/or overall cardiovascular risk (22)*

Lose weight if overweight.
Limit alcohol intake to no more than 1 oz of ethanol per day (24 oz of beer, 8 oz of wine, or 2 oz of 100-proof whiskey).
Exercise (aerobic) regularly.
Reduce sodium intake to less than 100 mmol per day (<2.3 g of sodium or <6 g of sodium chloride).
Maintain adequate dietary potassium, calcium, and magnesium intake.
Stop smoking and reduce dietary saturated fat and cholesterol intake for overall cardiovascular health.
Reducing fat intake also helps reduce caloric intake—important for control of weight and type II diabetes.

tated with the use of calibratable sphygmomanometers suited for home use. The likelihood for subsequent development of hypertension is enhanced particularly if there is a family history of hypertension and premature death. If blood pressure rises to the lower levels of stage I blood pressure levels (i.e., 140–150/90–95 mm Hg), earlier pharmacological therapy may be indicated, particularly if there is evidence of target organ (i.e., heart, kidneys, brain) involvement from hypertensive disease. In any event, it would be of particular value to instruct these patients who are more predisposed to develop hypertension about the value and feasibility of life-style modifications, including tobacco cessation, weight control (to within 15% of ideal body weight), dietary sodium restriction (to less than 100 mEq or 2.3 g of sodium daily), alcohol moderation (1 oz or less ethanol intake daily), and a regular isotonic exercise program (Table 8). This program not only has been shown to be of value in the primary prevention of hypertension (21) but will significantly reduce the numbers of antihypertensive drugs and their dosages when ultimately prescribed (22).

Stage I Hypertension

At the present time patients with lower levels of diastolic pressure elevation (i.e., 90 through 94 mm Hg) are at definite risk for premature cardiovascular morbidity and mortality (22) and should certainly be considered to be potential beneficiaries of an antihypertensive treatment program. This might be instituted initially, as described above, with life-style modification measures. Each of these measures (with the exception of stopping smoking) has been shown to reduce arterial pressure significantly in a population of patients with hypertension. However, with respect to the smoking issue, several multicenter studies have shown that when smokers who receive propranolol for antihypertensive therapy are treated, and their outcomes are compared with those of a similar group of hypertensive patients who smoke but who are treated with a thiazide diuretic, they achieve similar reductions in arterial pressure, but myocardial infarction and stroke are not prevented (33,34). Patients with stage I isolated systolic hypertension (i.e., 140 through 159 mm Hg) are also at a greater risk for subsequent development of cardiovascular events. In general, however, the recent Joint National Committee's fifth report (JNC-V) recommends that antihypertensive drug therapy be initiated with stage I hypertension, especially if target organ involvement and high risk family history are present (22).

Stage I and II Hypertension

If blood pressure is not controlled within a reasonable time (1 to 3 months) in patients with levels of 140 to 159/90 to 95 mm Hg, institution of antihypertensive drug therapy is a wise option. In these individuals, therapy may be initiated with low initial doses of a diuretic, β-adrenergic receptor blocking agent, an ACE inhibitor, a calcium antagonist, or an α_1- or α/β-adrenergic receptor blocking agent (Fig. 2). The most recent JNC-V report indicates that the diuretic and β-blocker may be considered "preferred" choices because in multicenter controlled clinical trials these agents have been shown to reduce cardiovascular morbidity and mortality. This is in contrast to the ACE inhibitors, calcium antagonists, α_1-adrenergic and α/β-adrenergic receptor blockers, which have been shown to be equally efficacious in controlling arterial pressure but have not yet been demonstrated to reduce cardiovascular morbidity and mortality in controlled trials involving patients with hypertension (22). Recent controlled trials have shown such benefit with ACE inhibitors in patients with coronary heart disease having had prior myocardial infarction or cardiac failure, but these trials did not involve patients with hypertension (22). Should arterial pressure not be controlled with low doses of these various classes of antihypertensive drugs, full doses may then be employed. Alternatively, it may be wise to change to another class of drugs or to add a second antihypertensive agent from the six classes of drugs. A listing of all currently available antihypertensive agents, their usual dosage range, and mechanism(s) of action (5) is presented in Table 9.

Some individuals have interpreted this JNC-V report to state that only the diuretics and β-blockers are recommended for the initial treatment of patients with hypertension. To the contrary, each of the foregoing six classes of antihypertensive agents (diuretics, β-blockers, calcium antagonists, ACE inhibitors, and α_1 and α/β-blockers) is recommended for initial therapy. To this end, certain classes (not necessarily diuretics or β-blockers) of agents are particularly recommended for individualized therapy (Table 10). The report specifically details specific cardiovascular, renal, and other clinical conditions in which certain drug classes (or even specific agents) are particularly preferred, when special monitoring of therapy is required, and which of these agents are relatively or absolutely contraindicated. Thus, in the case of specific cardiovascular problems, the β-blockers and calcium antagonists are both preferred for the hypertensive patient with angina pectoris, coronary heart disease, or prior myocardial infarction; and the diuretics and ACE inhibitors

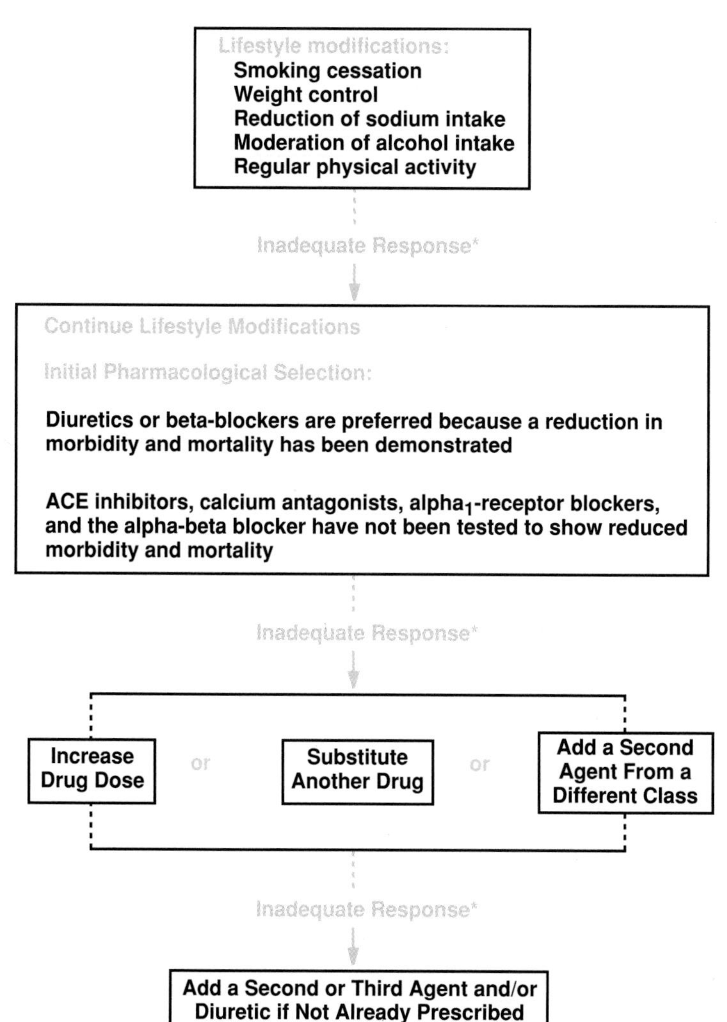

FIG. 2. Treatment algorithm (22).

are preferred for those patients with cardiac failure. (Other examples are detailed in Table 10).

Stage III and IV Hypertension

Therapy should be initiated with any one of the six classes of antihypertensive agents in less than full doses. Patients with stage III or IV hypertension should return for follow-up examination more frequently (perhaps in 2 weeks or earlier), and, if pressure is not optimally controlled, the same alternatives as depicted in Fig. 1 might be pursued. Thus, the dose of the initially prescribed agent might be increased to its full amount, or an alternative agent might be prescribed, or a second agent may be added to the agent that was prescribed initially. In selecting the second agent to be added to the one initially prescribed, it is wise to choose one that will at least add to or potentiate the antihypertensive effectiveness of the first compound. In this regard, the diuretic (in less than full doses, perhaps 12.5 or 25 mg of hydrochlorothiazide or its equivalents) has been found to be particularly effective without significantly exacerbating its intrinsic potential to produce metabolic side effects. This consideration is of particular relevance if the diuretic was not selected initially because of preexisting carbohydrate intolerance, hyperlipidemia, hyperuricemia, or the concern for development of hypokalemia (particularly in those patients with left ventricular hypertrophy or a history of cardiac failure. In selecting an initial agent for antihypertensive therapy, it might be especially worthwhile to consider comorbid diseases, other prescribed drug therapy, or preexisting metabolic alterations. In this regard, a series of additional tables were included in the JNC-V report that may be of particular value to the physician with particular interest in cardiovascular medicine. In addition to those cited above (Tables 9 and 10), Table 11 concerns adverse effects of particular relevance, and Table 12 details important drug interactions. Space does not permit further discussion of those urgent or emergent complications of hypertensive disease, but these are also summarized well and succinctly in that report (22).

TABLE 9. *Antihypertensive agent (22)*

Drug	Usual dosage range (mg/day)[a]	Frequency (qd unless otherwise noted)	Mechanisms of antihypertensive drug action	Comments
Initial Choices				
I. Diuretics				
Thiazides and related agents			Decreased plasma volume, decreased extracellular fluid volume, and decreased cardiac output initially, followed by decreased total peripheral resistance with normalization of cardiac output. Chronic effects include a slight decrease in extracellular fluid volume.	For thiazide and loop diuretics, lower doses and dietary counseling should be used to avoid metabolic changes. Thiazides and related agents are more effective antihypertensives than loop diuretics except in patients with serum creatinine ≥221 μmol/liter (2.5 mg/dl). Hydrochlorothiazide and chlorthalidone are generally the preferred thiazides. They were used most in clinical trials.
• Bendroflumethiazide	2.5–5.0			
• Benzthiazide	12.5–50.0			
• Chlorothiazide	125–500	bid		
• Chlorothalidone	12.5–50.0			
• Cyclothiazide	1–2			
• Hydrochlorothiazide	12.5–50.0			
• Hydroflumethiazide	12.5–50.0			
• Indapamide	2.5–5.0			
• Methyclothiazide	2.5–5.0			
• Metolazone	0.5–5.0			
• Polythiazide	1–4			
• Quinethazone	25–100			
• Trichlormethiazide	1–4			
Loop diuretics			See thiazides.	Higher doses of loop diuretics may be needed for patients with renal impairment or congestive heart failure. Ethacrynic acid is the only alternative for patients with allergy to thiazide and sulfur-containing diuretics.
• Bumetanide	0.5–5.0	bid		
• Ethacrynic acid	25–100	bid		
• Furosemide	20–320	bid		
Potassium-sparing			Increased potassium reabsorption. Aldosterone antagonist.	Weak diuretics. Used mainly in combination with other diuretics to avoid or reverse hypokalemia from other diuretics. Avoid when serum creatinine ≥221 μmol/liter (2.5 mg/dl). May cause hyperkalemia, and this may be exaggerated when combined with angiotensin-converting enzyme (ACE) inhibitors or potassium supplments
• Amiloride HCl	5–10	qd or bid		
• Spironolactone	25–100	qd or bid		
• Triamterene	50–150	qd or bid		
II. Adrenergic Inhibitors				
Beta-blockers			Decreased cardiac output and increased total peripheral resistance. Decreased plasma renin activity. Atenolol, betaxolol, and metoprolol are cardioselective.	Selective agents will also inhibit. β-receptors in higher doses; all may aggravate asthma.
• Atenolol	25–100[b]			
• Betaxolol HCl	5–40			
• Bisoprolol fumarate	5–20			
• Metoprolol tartrate	50–200	qd or bid		
• Metoprolol (extended release)	50–200			
• Nadolol	20–240[b]			
• Propranolol HCl	40–240	bid		
• Propranolol (long acting)	60–240			
• Timolol maleate	20–40	bid		
β-blockers with intrinsic sympathomimetic activity (ISA)			Acebutolol is cardioselective.	No clear advantage for agents with ISA except in patients with bardycardia who must receive β-blocker; these drugs produce fewer or no metabolic side effects.
• Acebutolol HCl	200–1,200[b]	bid		
• Carteolol HCl	2.5–10.0[b]			
• Penbutolol sulfate	20–80[b]			
• Pindolol	10–60[b]	bid		
α/β-blocker			Same as β-blockers plus α_1-blockade.	Possibly more effective in blacks than other β-blockers. May cause postural effects, and titration should be based on standing blood pressure.
• Labetalol HCl	200–1,200	bid		
• Prazosin HCl	1–20			
• Terazosin	1–20			

TABLE 9. *Continued.*

Drug	Usual dosage range (mg/day)[a]	Frequency (qd unless otherwise noted)	Mechanisms of antihypertensive drug action	Comments
III. ACE inhibitors			Block formation of angiotensin II, promoting vasodilation and decreased aldosterone. Also increase bradykinin and vasodilatory prostaglandins.	Diuretic doses should be reduced or discontinued prior to starting ACE inhibitors whenever possible to prevent excessive hypotension. Reduce dose of those drugs marked with a superscript *b* in patients with serum. creatinine ≥221 μmol/liter (2.5 mg/dl). May cause hyperkalemia in patients with renal impairment or in those receiving potassium-sparing agents. Can cause acute renal failure in patients with seven bilateral renal artery stenosis or severe stenosis in an artery to a solitary kidney.
Benazepril HCl	10–40[b]	qd or bid		
Captopril	12.5–150.0[b]	bid		
Cilazapril	2.5–5.0	qd or bid		
Enalapril maleate	2.5–40.0[b]	qd or bid		
Fosinopril sodium	10–40	qd or bid		
Lisinopril	5–40[b]	qd or bid		
Perindopril[c]	1–16[b]	qd or bid		
Quinapril HCl	5–80	qd or bid		
Ramipril	1.25–20.0[b]	qd or bid		
Spirapril[c]	12.5–50.0	qd or bid		
IV. Calcium antagonists				
Diltiazem HCl/verapamil HCl			Block the inward movement of calcium ions across cell membranes and cause smooth-muscle relaxation.	Diltiazem and verapamil also block the slow channels in the heart and may reduce the sinus rate and produce heart block.
• Diltiazem	90–360	tid		
• Diltiazem (sustained release)	120–360	bid		
• Diltiazem (extended release)	180–360			
• Verapamil	80–480	bid		
• Verapamil (long acting)	120–480	qd or bid		
Dihydropyridines				Dihydropyridines are more potent peripheral vasodilators than diltiazem and verapamil and may cause more dizziness, headache, flushing, peripheral edema, and tachycardia.
• Amlodipine besylate	2.5–10.0			
• Felodipine	5–20			
• Isradipine	2.5–10.0	bid		
• Nicardipine HCl	60–120	tid		
• Nifedipine	30–120	tid		
• Nifedipine (GITS)	30–90			
Supplemental choices				
I. Centrally acting α_2-agonists			Stimulate central α_2-receptors that inhibit efferent sympathetic activity.	Clonidine patch is replaced once a week. None of these agents should be withdrawn abruptly. Avoid in nonadherent patients.
• Clonidine HCl	0.1–1.2	bid		
• Clonidine TTS (patch)[d]	0.1–0.3	qw		
• Guanabenz acetate	4–64	bid		
• Guanfacine HCl	1–3			
• Methyldopa	250–2,000	bid		
II. Peripheral-acting adrenergic antagonist			Inhibit catecholamine release from neuronal storage sites.	May cause serious orthostatic and exercise-induced hypotension.
Guanadrel sulfate				
Guanethidine monosulfate	10–75	bid		
Rauwolfia alkaloids	10–100			
• Rauwolfia root	50–200		Deplete tissue stores of catecholamines.	
• Reserpine	0.05[e]–0.25			
III. Direct vasodilators				
• Hydralazine HCl	50–300	bid to qid	Direct smooth-muscle vasodilation (primarily arteriolar).	Hydralazine is subject to phenotypically determined metabolism (acetylation). With each agent, the patient should be given a diuretic and a β-blocker for fluid retention and reflex tachycardia.
• Minoxidil	2.5–80.0	qd or bid		

[a] The lower dose indicated is the preferred initial dose, and the higher dose is the maximum per day. Most agents require 2–4 weks for complete efficacy; more frequent dosage adjustments are not advised except for severe hypertension. The dosage range may differ slightly from what is recommended on the package insert.

[b] These drugs are excreted by the kidney and require dosage reduction in the presence of renal impairment (serum creatinine ≥221 μmol/liter 2.5 mg/dl).

[c] This drug is not approved by the Food and Drug Administration.

[d] Weekly patch is 1,2,3 equivalent to 0.1–0.3 mg/day, respectively.

[e] A 0.1-mg dose may be given qod to achieve this dosage.

TABLE 10. *Guideline for selecting initial antihypertensive drug therapy in the presence of special considerations (22)*

Clinical situation	Preferred	Requires special monitoring	Relatively or absolutely contraindicated
I. Cardiovascular			
Angina pectoris	Beta-blockers, calcium antagonists		Direct vasodilators
Bradycardia/heart block, sick sinus syndrome			β-Blockers, labetalol HCl, diltiazem HCl, verapamil HCl
Cardiac failure	Diuretics, angiotensin-converting enzyme (ACE) inhibitors		β-Blockers, calcium antagonist, labetalol
Hypertrophic cardiomyopathy with severe diastolic dysfunction	β-Blockers, diltiazem, verapamil		Diuretics, ACE inhibitors, α_1-blockers, hydralazine HCl, minoxidil
Hyperdynamic circulation	β-Blockers		Direct vasodilators
Peripheral vascular occlusive disease		β-Blockers	
Postmyocardial infarction	Nonintrinsic sympathomimetically active β-blockers		
II. Renal			ACE inhibitors
Bilateral renal arterial disease or severe stenosis in artery to solitary kidney			
Renal insufficiency			
• Early (serum creatinine 130–221 μmol/liter, 1.5–2.5 mg/dl)			Potassium-sparing agents, potassium supplements
• Advanced (serum creatinine ≥221 μmol/liter (2.5-mg/dl)	Loop diuretics	ACE inhibitors	Potassium-sparing agents, potassium supplements
III. Other			
Asthma/chronic obstructive pulmonary disease			β-Blocker, labetalol
Cyclosporine-associated hypertension	Nifedipine, labetalol	Verapamil, diltiazem, nicardipine HCl	
Depression		α_2-Agonists	Reserpine
Diabetes mellitus			
• Type I (insulin dependent)		β-Blockers	
• Type II		β-Blockers; diuretics	
Dyslipidemia		β-Blockers; diuretics	
Liver disease		Labetalol	Methyldopa
Vascular headache	β-Blockers		
Pregnancy			
• Preeclampsia	Methyldopa; hydralazine		Diuretics; ACE inhibitors
• Chronic hypertension	Methyldopa		ACE inhibitors

Isolated Systolic Hypertension

Until relatively recently, although it was well known that isolated systolic pressure elevation was associated with increased risk, information was not available to indicate whether therapeutic reduction of that pressure elevation would be associated with a reduction in those risks. At least three independent national studies [the Systolic Hypertension in the Elderly Program in the United States (35), the Medical Research Council Trial in Great Britain (36), and the STOP-Hypertension Trial in Sweden (37)] demonstrated that pressure reduction was associated with a significant reduction in risk. Each of these studies employed the diuretic alone or in combination with a β-blocker. Other reports, published earlier, emphasized the efficacy and importance of treating diastolic hypertension in the elderly (Table 13) (38–40). Largely because of these findings, the systolic pressure was included in the newer classification of hypertensive disease severity and in the recommendations of pharmacotherapy in the JNC-V report (22).

SUMMARY

The various hypertensive diseases, with particular emphasis on essential hypertension, have been discussed by means of presenting a sequence of clinically relevant classifications. By discussing initially the means by which arterial pressure is normally controlled through a mechanistic classification, an etiological classification of the variety of hypertensive diseases seemed reasonable. With these concepts taken into consideration, it followed that a classification of

TABLE 11. *Adverse antihypertensive drug effects (22)*

Drug	Selected side effects	Precautions and special considerations
I. Diuretics		
Thiazides and related diuretics	Hypokalemia, hypomagnesemia, hyponatremia, hyperuricemia, hypercholesterolemia, hypertriglyceridemia, dysfunction, weakness.	Except for metolazone and indapamide, ineffective in renal failure (serum creatine ≥221 μmol/liter (2.5 mg/dL); hypokalemia increases digitalis toxicity; may precipitate acute gout.
Loop diuretics	Same as for thiazides except loop diuretics do not cause hypercalcemia.	Effective in chronic renal failure.
Potassium-sparing agents	This group is associated with hyperkalemia. Spironolactone can cause gynecomastia, mastodynia, menstrual irregularities, diminished libido in males.	Danger of hyperkalemia in patients with renal failure, in patients treated with angiotensin-converting enzyme (ACE) inhibitors or with nonsteroidal antiinflammatory agents. Triamterene is associated with the danger of renal calculi.
II. Adrenergic inhibitors β-Blockers	Bronchospasm, may aggravate peripheral arterial insufficiency, fatigue, insomnia, exacerbation of congestive heart failure (CHF), masking of symptoms of hypoglycemia. Also, hypertriglyceridemia, decreased high-density lipoprotein cholesterol (except for those drugs with intrinsic sympathomimetic activity). Reduced exercise tolerance.	Should not be used in patients with asthma, chronic obstructive pulmonary disease (COPD), CHF with systolic dysfunction, heart block (greater than first degree), and sick sinus syndrome; use with caution in insulin-treated diabetics and patients with peripheral vascular disease; should not be discontinued abruptly in patients with ischemic heart disease.
α/β-Blocker	Bronchospasm, may aggravate peripheral vascular insufficiency, orthostatic hypotension.	Should not be used in patients with asthma, COPD, CHF, heart block (greater than first degree), and sick sinus syndrome; use with caution in insulin-treated diabetics and patients with peripheral vascular disease.
α-Receptor blockers	Orthostatic hypotension, syncope, weakness, palpitations, headache.	
III. ACE inhibitors	Cough, rash, angioneurotic edema, hyperkalemia, dysgeusia.	Hyperkalemia can develop, particularly in patients with renal insufficiency; hypotension has been observed with initiation of ACE inhibitors, expecially in patients with high plasma renin activity or in those receiving diuretic therapy; can cause reversible, acute renal failure in patients with bilateral renal artery stenosis or unilateral stenosis in a solitary kidney and in patients with cardiac failure and with volume depletion; rarely can induce neutropenia or proteinuria; absolutely contraindicated in the second and third trimesters of pregnancy.
IV. Calcium antagonists		
Dihydropyridines • Amlodipine besylate • Felodipine • Isradipine • Nicardipine HCl • Nifedipine	Headache, dizziness, peripheral edema, tachycardia, gingival hyperplasia.	Use with caution in patients with congestive heart failure; may aggravate angina and myocardial ischemia.

TABLE 12. *Selected drug interactions with antihypertensive therapy[a] (22)*

Diuretics

Possible situations for decreased antihypertensive effects

- Cholestyramine and colestipol HCl decrease absorption.
- Nonsteroidal antiinflammatory agents (NSAIDs), including aspirin and OTC ibuprofen, may antagonize diuretic effectiveness.

Possible situations for increased antihypertensive effects

- Combinations of thiazides—especially metolazone—with furosemide can produce profound diuresis, natriuresis, and kaliuresis in renal impairment.

Effects of diuretics on other drugs

- Diuretics can raise serum lithium levels and increase toxicity by enhancing proximal tubular reabsorption of lithium.
- Diuretics may make it more difficult to control dyslipidemia and diabetes.

β-Blockers

Possible situations for decreased antihypertensive effects

- NSAIDs may decrease the effects of β-blockers.
- Rifampin, smoking, and phenobarbital decrease serum levels of agents primarily metabolized by the liver through enzyme induction.

Possible situations for increased antihypertensive effects

- Cimetidine may increase serum levels of β-blockers that are primarily metabolized by the liver through enzyme inhibition.
- Quinidine may increase the risk of hypotension.

Effects of β-blockers on other drugs

- Combinations of diltiazem HCl or verapamil HCl with β-blockers may have additive sinoatrial and atrioventricular node depressant effects and may also promote negative inotropic effects on the failing myocardium.
- The combination of β-blockers and reserpine may cause marked bradycardia and syncope.
- β-Blockers may increase serum levels of theophylline, lidocaine HCl, and chlorpromazine through reduced hepatic clearance.
- Nonselective β-blockers prolong insulin-induced hypoglycemia and promote rebound hypertension by unopposed α stimulation. All β-blockers mask the adrenergically mediated symptoms of hypoglycemia and have the potential to aggravate diabetes.
- β-Blockers may make it more difficult to control dyslipidemia.
- Phenylpropanolamine, which can be obtained OTC in cold and diet preparations, pseudoephedrine, ephedrine, and epinephrine can cause elevations in blood pressure by unopposed α-receptor-induced vasoconstriction.

Angiotensin-converting enzyme (ACE) inhibitors

Possible situations for decreased antihypertensive effects

- NSAIDs, including aspirin and OTC ibuprofen, may decrease blood pressure control.
- Antacids may decrease the bioavailability of ACE inhibitors.

Possible situations for increased antihypertensive effects

- Diuretics may lead to excessive hypotensive effects (hypovolemia).

Effects of ACE inhibitors on other drugs

- Hypokalemia may occur with potassium supplements, potassium-sparing agents, and NSAIDs.
- ACE inhibitors may increase serum lithium levels.

Calcium antagonists

Possible situations for decreased antihypertensive effects

- Serum levels and antihypertensive effects of calcium antagonists may be diminished by these interactions—rifampin/verapamil; carbamazepine/diltiazem and verapamil; phenobarbital and phenytoin/verapamil.

Possible situations for increased antihypertensive effects

- Cimetidine may increase pharmacological effects of all calcium antagonists by inhibition of hepatic metabolizing enzymes resulting in increased serum levels.

Effects of calcium antagonists on other drugs

- Digoxin and carbamazepine serum levels and toxicity may be increased by verapamil and possibly diltiazem.
- Serum levels of prazosin HCl, quinidine, and theophylline may be increased by verapamil.
- Serum levels of cyclosporine may be increased by diltiazem, nicardipine HCl, and verapamil. The cyclosporine dose may need to be decreased.

α-Blockers

Possible situations for increased antihypertensive effects

- Concomitant antihypertensive drug therapy, especially diuretics, may increase chance of postural hypotension.

Sympatholytics

Possible situations for decreased antihypertensive effects

- Tricyclic antidepressants may decrease the effects of centrally acting and peripheral norepinephrine depleters.
- Sympathomimetics, including OTC cold and diet preparations, amphetamines, phenothiazines, and cocaine, may interfere with the antihypertensive effects of guanethidine monosulfate and guanadrel sulfate.
- The severity of clonidine HCl withdrawal reaction can be increased with β-blockers.
- Monoamine oxidase inhibitors may prevent degradation and metabolism of norepinephrine released by tyramine-containing foods and may cause hypertension. They may also cause hypertensive reactions when combined with reserpine or guanethidine.

Effects of sympatholytics on other drugs

- Methyldopa may increase lithium levels.

[a] This table does not include all potential drug interactions with antihypertensive drugs.

TABLE 13. *Effects of therapy in older hypertensive patients*

	Clinical trial						
	Australian (38)	EWPHE (39)	Coope and Warrender (40)	STOP-Hypertension (37)	MRC (36)	SHEP (35)	HDFP (41)[a]
Number of patients	582	840	884	1,627	4,396	4,736	2,374
Age range (years)	60–69	>60	60–79	70–84	65–74	60–80[b]	60–69
Mean BP at entry (mm Hg)	165/101	189/101	197/100	195/102	185/91	170/77	170/101
Relative risk of event (treated versus control)							
Stroke	0.67	0.64	0.58[b]	0.53[b]	0.75[b]	0.67[b]	0.56[b]
CAD	0.82	0.80	1.03	0.87[c]	0.81	0.73[b]	0.85[b]
CHF	—	0.78	0.68	0.49[b]	—	0.45[b]	—
All CVD	0.69	0.71[b]	0.76[b]	0.60[b]	0.83[b]	0.68[b]	0.84[b]

[a] Includes data circulated by the HDFP Coordinating Center.
[b] Statistically significant.
[c] Myocardial infarction only; sudden deaths decreased from 13 to 4.

disease by severity of arterial pressure elevation and target organ involvement was offered. This approach was followed by a classification of therapeutic alternatives that took into consideration the severity of pressure elevation, target organ involvement, comorbid diseases, and coexisting therapy for other conditions.

REFERENCES

1. Page IH. Pathogenesis of arterial hypertension. *JAMA* 1949;140: 451–458.
2. Frohlich ED. Pathophysiology of systemic arterial hypertension. In: Schlant RC, Alexander RW, O'Rourke RA, Roberts R, Sonnenblick EH, eds. *Hurst's The Heart,* 8th ed. New York: McGraw-Hill; 1993: 1391–1401.
3. Frohlich ED. The first Irvine H. Page lecture: The mosaic of hypertension; past, present, and future. *J Hypertens* 1988;6(Suppl 4):2–11.
4. Stokes J III. Cardiovascular Risk Factors. In: Frohlich ED, ed. *Preventive Aspects of Coronary Heart Disease.* Philadelphia: F.A. Davis; 1990:3–20.
5. Kurtz TW, Spence MA. Genetics of essential hypertension. *Am J Med* 1993;94:77–84.
6. Schunkert H, Hense HW, Holmer SR, Stender M, Perz S, Keil U, Lorell BH. Association between a deletion polymorphism of the angiotensin-converting-enzyme gene and left ventricular hypertrophy. *N Engl J Med* 1994;330:1634–1638.
7. Frohlich ED. Current approaches in the treatment of hypertension. *Curr Probl Cardiol* 1994;19(7):399–469.
8. Ward R. Familial aggregation and genetic epidemiology of blood pressure. In: Laragh JH, Brenner BM, eds. *Hypertension: Pathophysiology, Diagnosis, and Management.* Vol. 1. New York: Raven Press; 1990: 81–100.
9. Morris BJ. Identification of essential hypertension genes. *J Hypertens* 1993;11:115–120.
10. Tarazi RC, Dustan HP, Frohlich ED. Relation of plasma to interstitial fluid volume in essential hypertension. *Circulation* 1969;40:357–365.
11. Weil JV, Chidsey CA. Plasma volume expansion resulting from interference with adrenergic functions in normal man. *Circulation* 1968; 37:54–61.
12. Dustan HP, Tarazi RC, Bravo EL. Dependence of arterial pressure on intravascular volume in treated hypertensive patients. *N Engl J Med* 1972;286:861–866.
13. McCormack LJ, Poutasse EF, Meaney TF, Noto TJ, Dustan HP. A pathologic–arteriographic correlation of renal arterial disease. *Am Heart J* 1966;72:188–198.
14. Dustan HP, Humphries AW, DeWolfe VG, Page IH. Normal arterial pressure in patients with renal arterial stenosis. *JAMA* 1964;187: 1028–1029.
15. Frohlich Ed, Tarazi RC, Dustan HP. Hemodynamic and functional mechanisms in two renal hypertension: Arterial and pyelonephritis. *Am J Med Sci* 1971;261:189–195.
16. Dustan HP, Page IH. Some factors in renal and renoprival hypertension. *J Lab Clin Med* 1964;64:948–959.
17. Panza JA, Casino PR, Kilcoyne CM, Quyyumi AA. Impaired endothelium-dependent vasodilation in patients with essential hypertension: Evidence that the abnormality is not at the muscarinic receptor level. *J Am Coll Cardiol* 1994;23:1610–1616.
18. Yanagisawa M, Kurihara H, Kimura S, Tomobe Y, Kobayashi M, Mitsui Y, Yazaki Y, Goto K, Masaki T. A novel potent vasoconstrictor peptide produced by vascular endothelial cells. *Nature* 1988;332: 411–415.
19. Sadoshima J, Xu Y, Slayter HS, Izumo S. Autocrine release of angiotensin II mediates stretch-induced hypertrophy of cardiac myocytes *in vitro. Cell* 1993;75:977–984.
20. Oren S, Grossman E, Messerli FH, Frohlich ED. High blood pressure: Side effects of drugs, poisons, and food. *Cardiol Clin North Am* 1988; 6:467–474.
21. Whelton PK (Chairman), National High Blood Pressure Education Program Working Group. National High Blood Pressure Education Program Working Group report on primary prevention of hypertension. *Arch Intern Med* 1993;153:186–208.
22. Joint National Committee on Detection, Evaluation, and Treatment of High Blood Pressure. The Fifth Report of the Joint National Committee on Detection, Evaluation, and Treatment of High Blood Pressure (JNC-V). *Arch Intern Med* 1993;153:154–183.
23. Keith HM, Wagener HP, Barker NN. Some different types of essential hypertension: Their course and prognosis. *Am J Med Sci* 1939;197: 332–343.
24. Wagener HP, Clay GE, Gipner JF. Classification of retinal lesions in presence of vascular hypertension: Report submitted by committee. *Trans Am Ophthalmol Soc* 1947;45:57–73.
25. Frohlich Ed, Tarazi RC, Dustan HP. Clinical–physiological correlations in the development of hypertensive heart disease. Circulation 1971;44:446–455.
26. Thomas P, DeJong D. The P-wave in the electrocardiogram in the diagnosis of heart disease. *Br Heart J* 1967;16:241.
27. Macruz R, Perloff JK, Case RB. Method for the ECG recognition of atrial enlargement. *Circulation* 1958;17:882–889.
28. Morris JJ Jr, Estes HR Jr, Whalen RE, Thompson HK, McIntosh HD. P-wave analysis in valvular heart disease. *Circulation* 1964;29:242–252.
29. McPhie J. Left ventricular hypertrophy: Electrocardiographic diagnosis. *Australas Ann Med* 1958;7:317–327.
30. Grant RP, ed. *The Spatial Vector Approach: Clinical Electrocardiography.* New York: McGraw-Hill; 1957.

31. Dunn FG, Chandraratna PN, de Carvalho JGR, Basta LL, Frohlich ED. Pathophysiologic assessment of hypertensive heart disease by echocardiography. *Am J Cardiol* 1977;39:789–795.
32. Dreslinsk GR, Frohlich ED, Dunn FG, Messerli FH, Suarez DH, Reisin E. Echocardiographic diastolic ventricular abnormality in hypertensive heart disease: Atrial emptying index. *Am J Cardiol* 1981;47: 1087–1090.
33. Greenberg G, Thompson SG, Brennan PJ. The relationship between smoking and the response to antihypertensive treatment in mild hypertensives in the Medical Research Council's Trial of Treatment. *Int J Epidemiol* 1987;16:25–30.
34. Langford HG, Stamler J, Wassertheil-Smoller S, Prineas RJ. All-cause mortality in the Hypertension Detection and Follow-Up Program: Findings in the whole cohort and for persons with less severe hypertension, with and without other traits related to risk of mortality. *Prog Cardiovasc Dis* 1986;29(Suppl 1):29–54.
35. SHEP Cooperative Research Group. Prevention of stroke by antihypertensive drug treatment in older persons with isolated systolic hypertension. *JAMA* 1991;265:3255–3264.
36. MRC Working Party. Medical Research Council trial of treatment of hypertension in older adults: Principal results. *Br Med J* 1992;304: 405–412.
37. Dahlöf B, Lindholm LH, Hansson L, Scherstén B, Ekbom T, Wester P-O. Morbidity and mortality in the Swedish Trial in Old Patients with Hypertension (STOP-Hypertension). *Lancet* 1991;338:1281–1285.
38. Management Committee. Treatment of mild hypertension in the elderly. *Med J Aust* 1981;2:398–402.
39. Amery A, Birkenhäger W, Brixko P, et al. Mortality and morbidity results from the European Working Party on High Blood Pressure in the Elderly trial. *Lancet* 1985;1:1349–1354.
40. Coope J, Warrender TS. Randomized trial of treatment of hypertension in elderly patients in primary care. *Br Med J* 1986;293:1145–1151.
41. Stamler J. Risk factor modification trials: Implications for the elderly. *Eur Heart J* 1988;9(Suppl D):9–53.

Atherosclerosis and Coronary Artery Disease,
edited by V. Fuster, R. Ross, and E. J. Topol.
Lippincott-Raven Publishers, Philadelphia © 1996.

CHAPTER 16

Management of Hypertension

Norman M. Kaplan

Key Words: Hypertension, management of; hypertension, definition of; hypertension, evaluation of; lifestyle modifications; drug therapy.

INTRODUCTION

As the consequence of the confluence of multiple factors, the management of hypertension has become the most common indication for visits to physicians by adults in the United States (1). These factors include (a) the increasing incidence of hypertension with age, in concert with the striking increase in the number of the elderly in the population, (b) widespread recognition of the increase in relative risk for cardiovascular disease from even slightly elevated pressures, (c) the availability of relatively easy to take antihypertensive agents which have been shown to reduce cardiovascular morbidity and mortality and which have been aggressively promoted by multiple pharmaceutical companies, and (d) the underlying therapeutic activism of physicians in the United States, who are more willing to treat lesser degrees of hypertension than are physicians elsewhere (2).

Norman M. Kaplan: Department of Internal Medicine, University of Texas Southwestern Medical Center, Dallas, Texas 75235-8899.

Despite these multiple factors that have pushed hypertension to the forefront of public health awareness, a number of other forces have held back the fulfillment of the goal of adequate control of hypertension. Although more and more Americans have had their hypertension recognized and treated over the past 20 years, the proportion who are adequately controlled remains only slightly above 50% if the blood pressure level for control is liberally defined as below 160/95 mm Hg (3) (Fig. 1). If the more conservative definition of below 140/90 mm Hg is used, the NHANES III (1988–1991) data show only 21% of hypertensives in the United States to be adequately managed (3).

The fundamental reason for this shortfall is the nature of hypertension: a chronic condition that is asymptomatic for its first 15–20 years, whose therapy promises not a cure but only far distant benefits, but which burdens the patient with considerable economic costs and, often, adverse side effects. Beyond these unfavorable fundamental features, a number of problems have surfaced in the management of hypertension in usual clinical practice that interfere with its adequate control (Table 1).

In the course of this chapter, many of these causes will be addressed. As a preview, the steps listed in Table 2 are offered as general guidelines to improve patient adherence

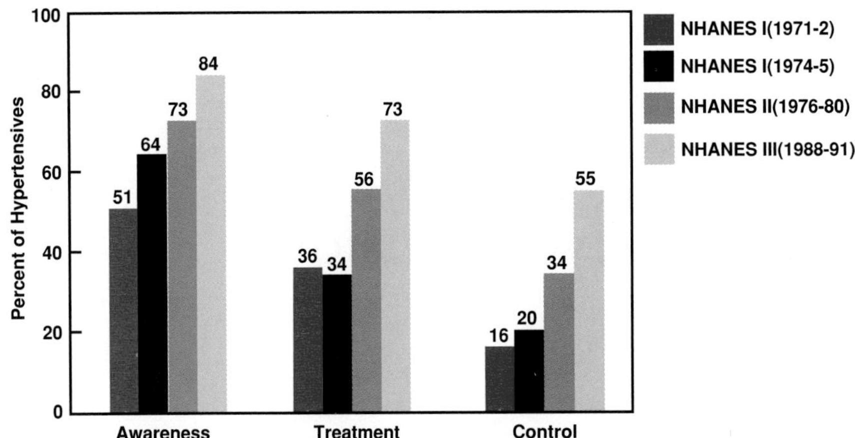

FIG. 1. Hypertension awareness, treatment, and control (threshold, 160/95 mm Hg). Percentages of the National Health and Nutrition Examination Surveys (NHANES) populations with hypertension (defined as a blood pressure of 160/95 mm Hg or more on one or two examinations) who were aware of the condition, who were receiving treatment, and whose hypertension was controlled. (Source: Joint National Committee on Detection, Evaluation, and Treatment of High Blood Press, ref. 3).

to antihypertensive therapy. Rather than following these steps in the order shown in Table 2, this chapter will be divided into three main subheadings that subsume these guidelines: Diagnosis and Evaluation, Lifestyle Modifications, and Drug Therapy.

DIAGNOSIS AND EVALUATION

Blood pressure constantly changes. The changing blood pressure reflects *short-term* variability at rest affected by breathing and heart beating under the influence of the auto-

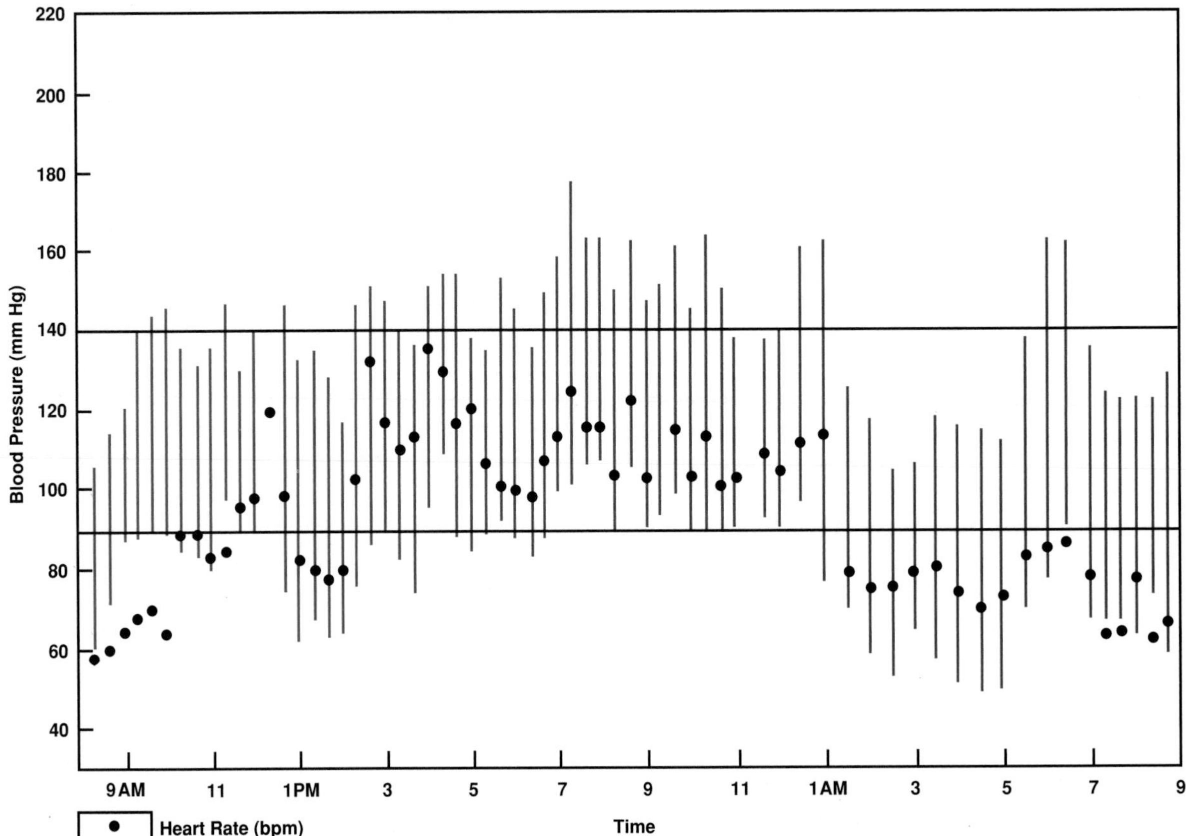

FIG. 2. Computer printout of blood pressures obtained by ambulatory blood pressure monitoring over 24 hr beginning at 9 A.M. in a 50-year-old man with hypertension receiving no therapy. The patient slept from midnight until 6 A.M. *Solid circles,* heart rate. (From Zachariah et al., ref. 59.)

TABLE 1. *Causes for inadequate responsiveness to therapy*

Pseudoresistance
- White-coat or office elevations
- Pseudohypertension in elderly

Nonadherence to therapy
- Lack of consistent and continuous primary care
- Inconvenient and chaotic dosing schedules
- Side effects of medication
- Cost of medication
- Instructions not understood
- Inadequate patient education
- Organic brain syndrome (e.g., memory deficit)

Drug-related causes
- Doses too low
- Inappropriate combinations (e.g., two centrally acting adrenergic inhibitors)
- Rapid inactivation (e.g., hydralazine)
- Drug interactions:

Nonsteroidal antiinflammatory	Oral contraceptives
Sympathomimetics	Adrenal steroids
Nasal decongestants	Licorice (e.g., chewing tobacco)
Appetite suppressants	Cyclosporine
Cocaine	Erythropoietin
Caffeine	Cholestyramine

- Antidepressants (monoamine oxidase inhibitors, tricyclics)
- Excessive volume contraction with stimulation of renin–aldosterone
- Hypokalemia (usually diuretic-induced)
- Rebound after clonidine withdrawal

Associated conditions
- Smoking
- Increasing obesity
- Sleep apnea
- Insulin resistance/hyperinsulinemia
- Ethanol intake more than 1 oz a day (>3 portions)
- Anxiety-induced hyperventilation or panic attacks
- Chronic pain
- Intense vasoconstriction (Raynaud's, arteritis)

Secondary hypertension
- Renal insufficiency
- Renovascular hypertension
- Pheochromocytoma
- Primary aldosteronism

Volume overload
- Excess sodium intake
- Progressive renal damage (nephrosclerosis)
- Fluid retention from reduction of blood pressure
- Inadequate diuretic therapy

Modified from Joint National Committee on Detection, Evaluation, and Treatment of High Blood Pressure, ref. 3.

nomic nervous system, *daytime* variability reflecting mental and physical activity and modulated by baroreceptors, and *diurnal* variability induced by inactivity and sleep (4). The degree of variability is best appreciated by automatically recorded noninvasive ambulatory monitoring (5) (Fig. 2). The tracing shows readings taken every 15 min while awake during the day and readings taken every 30 min while asleep at night in an untreated hypertensive man.

Financial restraints limit the use of ambulatory monitoring, although it would save money if used when indicated, mainly by identifying the 20% or more of patients with only office or white-coat hypertension, most of whom would be treated if diagnosed only by office readings (6).

TABLE 2. *General guidelines to improve patient adherence to antihypertensive therapy*

Be aware of the problem and be alert to signs of patient nonadherence

Establish the goal of therapy: to reduce blood pressure to near normotensive levels with minimal or no side effects

Educate the patient about the disease and its treatment
- Involve the patient in decision making
- Encourage family support

Maintain contact with the patient
- Encourage visits and calls to allied health personnel
- Allow the pharmacist to monitor therapy
- Give feedback to the patient via home blood pressure readings
- Make contact with patients who do not return

Keep care inexpensive and simple
- Do the least workup needed to rule out secondary causes
- Obtain follow-up laboratory data only yearly unless indicated more often
- Use home blood pressure readings
- Use nondrug, no-cost therapies
- Use the fewest daily doses of drugs needed
- Use generic drugs and break larger doses of tablets in half
- If appropriate, use combination tablets
- Tailor medication to daily routines

Prescribe according to pharmacologic principles
- Add one drug at a time
- Start with small doses, aiming for 5- to 10-mm Hg reductions at each step
- Have medication taken immediately upon awakening in the morning or after 4 a.m. if patient awakens to void
- Prevent volume overload with adequate diuretic and sodium restriction

Be willing to stop unsuccessful therapy and try a different approach

Anticipate side effects

Adjust therapy to ameliorate side effects that do not spontaneously disappear

Continue to add effective and tolerated drugs, stepwise, in sufficient doses to achieve the goal of therapy

The Need for Home Recordings

Absent the ready availability of ambulatory monitoring, there is an obvious need for out-of-the-office readings by readily available home blood pressure devices. With these inexpensive (@ $30), generally accurate, easy-to-use devices, multiple readings can be self-recorded (7). For the diagnosis of hypertension, two or more sets a day should be taken with at least two readings on each occasion and more if needed to obtain a stable level. An early-morning and late-afternoon timing is appropriate, but additional readings should be obtained at times of emotional stress or when symptoms occur that might be attributable to hypertension, e.g., headache or dizziness.

Multiple readings should be taken and recorded in a diary for 4–8 weeks. Most patients will show a fall in pressures over the first few weeks, overcoming their own "white-coat" anxiety over self-measurements of blood pressure. The average of all of the subsequent readings can be used to ascertain the presence of hypertension, using the level of 140/90 mm Hg as an appropriate dividing line. The average of home recordings will be 5–10 mm Hg lower than the average of multiple office readings, but most authorities (8) recommend institution of therapy only at office levels above 150/95 mm Hg, comparable to home levels of 140/90 mm Hg.

The Importance of Office Elevations

Even transiently elevated office readings should not, however, be disregarded even if all subsequent readings are normal. Remember that most data on the risks of hypertension are based on one or a few sets of office readings (9). Nonetheless, the risks from hypertension are not uniform; only a minority of those with stage 1 or 2 hypertension (140/90 up to 179/109) will suffer an overt premature cardiovascular event in their lifetime. Increasingly strong evidence supports the logical conclusion that those with less sustained hypertension, i.e., the white-coat hypertensives, will be more likely to escape the increased risks that apply to the overall population at any level of hypertension. Nonetheless, white-coat hypertensives are not as normal as persistently normotensive people (10).

For those with office readings that would support the diagnosis (and treatment) of hypertension but with out-of-the-office readings that are generally considered not to mandate the need for drug therapy, the best course is to continue to monitor closely the patient's pressure while using the presence of an elevated office reading to motivate the patient to modify his or her lifestyle appropriately.

Assessment of Overall Cardiovascular Risk

After careful determination of the patient's usual blood pressure, an assessment of other cardiovascular risk factors and the degree of target organ damage must be made in order to decide upon the need and form of therapy. A group of New Zealand physicians has provided an appropriate list of the features that should be considered (11) (Table 3). They used the Framingham study experience to ascertain the degree of risk, separating men from women (who have a lesser risk at any given level of pressure) and both groups into decades of age. Based upon their interpretation of the benefits of therapy shown in the large clinical trials, they decided to recommend institution of active drug therapy only for those with an expected 20% or higher risk of developing a cardiovascular event over the next 10 years (Fig. 3). Additionally, they recommend therapy for all with pressure above 170/100 mm Hg regardless of their level of risk. They also recommend referral for additional investigation for all patients below age 40 years with pressure above 150/90 mm Hg.

TABLE 3. *Features considered in the decision to treat*

Other risk factors
Cigarette smoking
Total cholesterol/HDL cholesterol ratio > 6
Diabetes
Obesity (body mass index > 30)
Family history of premature cardiovascular disease (in parent or sibling before age 55 years)
Symptomatic cardiovascular disease
Angina or silent ischemia
Myocardial infarction
Coronary angioplasty or bypass surgery
Heart failure
Left ventricular hypertrophy demonstrated by ECG or echocardiography
Transient ischemic attacks
Stroke
Peripheral vascular disease
Familial hyperlipidemia
Other target organ damage such as renal disease

Adapted from Consensus Development Conference Report, ref. 60, and Jackson et al., ref. 11.

These recommendations may be considered to be too conservative, denying some patients valuable protection. For some patients, more aggressive use of drugs is indicated. For example, even mildly hypertensive diabetics with early

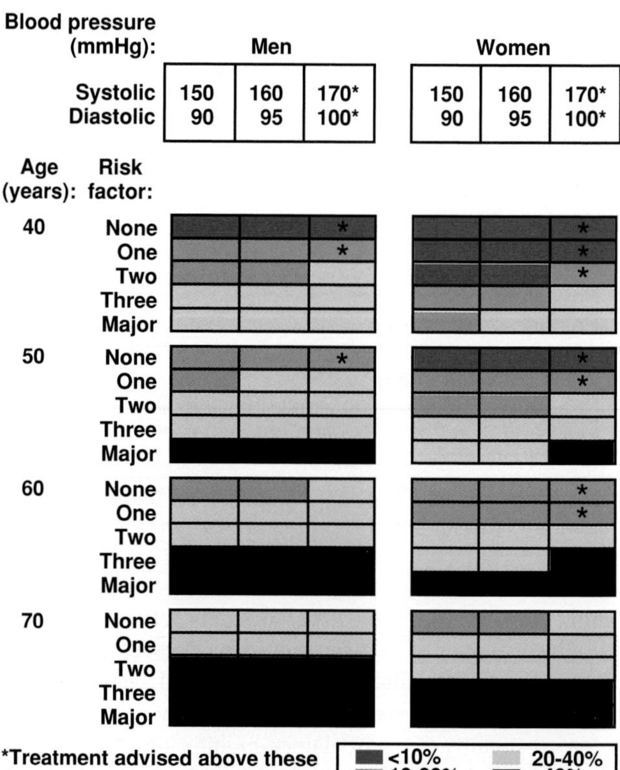

FIG. 3. Approximate 10-year risk of a cardiovascular disease event per 100 patients, by risk factor status. (From Jackson et al., ref. 11.)

evidence of nephropathy clearly benefit from reduction of their blood pressure (12). But, as I have noted (2), this overall strategy is sound:

> The bottom line comes down to this: The majority of hypertensives have fairly mild, asymptomatic hypertension, and the benefits of treatment—measured as the reduction in complications—progressively fall the milder the degree of hypertension. Many patients receive relatively little benefit, yet are exposed both to adverse side effects and to the fairly large financial costs of therapy. Therefore, for maximal patient benefit, a management strategy based on overall risk is rational and appropriate.

Evaluation for Secondary Forms of Hypertension

In addition to the determination of usual blood pressure and an assessment of overall cardiovascular risk status and the degree of target organ damage, a reasonable search for secondary forms of hypertension should be made. The history (Table 4) and physical examination (Table 5) can uncover multiple clues, not only to traditional secondary forms, but to a variety of contributing factors, such as increasing obesity (particularly with sleep apnea), intake of agents that may raise the pressure, and dietary factors that may play a role.

TABLE 4. *Important aspects of patient history*

Duration of the hypertension
Last known normal blood pressure
Course of the blood pressure
Prior treatment of the hypertension
Drugs: types, doses, side effects
Intake of agents that may cause hypertension
Estrogens
Sympathomimetics
Adrenal steroids
Excessive sodium intake
Family history
Hypertension
Premature cardiovascular disease or death
Familial diseases: pheochromocytoma, renal disease, diabetes, gout
Symptoms of secondary causes
Muscle weakness
Spells of tachycardia, sweating, tremor
Thinning of the skin
Flank pain
Symptoms of target organ damage
Headaches
Transient weakness or blindness
Loss of visual acuity
Chest pain
Dyspnea
Claudication
Presence of other risk factors
Smoking
Diabetes
Dyslipidemia
Physical inactivity
Dietary history
Sodium
Alcohol
Saturated fats
Psychosocial factors
Family structure
Work status
Educational level
Sexual function
Features of sleep apnea
Early-morning headaches
Daytime somnolence
Loud snoring
Erratic sleep

TABLE 5. *Important aspects of the physical examination*

Accurate measurement of blood pressure
General appearance: distribution of body fat, skin lesions, muscle strength, alertness
Funduscopy
Neck: palpation and auscultation of carotids, thyroid
Heart: size, rhythm, sounds
Lungs: rhonchi, rales
Abdomen: renal masses, bruits over aorta or renal arteries, femoral pulses
Extremities: peripheral pulses, edema
Neurologic assessment

A simple set of laboratory tests is usually indicated, including a urine analysis, hematocrit, automated blood chemistry (glucose, creatinine, electrolytes), serum total and high-density lipoprotein (HDL) cholesterol and triglycerides, and an electrocardiogram. Only if features suggestive of a specific secondary cause are noted by history, physical exam, and initial lab should additional workup be performed (Table 6). The only important exception is the need to rule out renovascular hypertension in every patient with a high index of clinical suspicion (13) (Table 7). The best noninvasive test for those with a moderate degree of clinical suspicion is the captopril-enhanced isotopic renogram with measurement of simultaneous plasma renin activity (13). For those with features indicating a high index of suspicion, selective renal arteriography is the only way to be sure that renovascular stenoses are not involved.

In the future, echocardiography and assessments of coronary blood flow may be more widely performed in the routine evaluation and management of hypertension. In view of the evidence described by Phillips and Diamond *(this volume)*, the effects of therapy may be best monitored by such techniques. For now, however, they are not cost-effective and will continue to be performed primarily for research.

LIFESTYLE MODIFICATIONS

Once the diagnosis of hypertension is established and the appropriate evaluation performed, attention should be directed at modifying unhealthy lifestyles. These are more common among hypertensive patients than normotensive people and contribute considerably to both the hypertension and the increased risks for premature cardiovascular disease. The prescription should follow that recommended in the 1993 Joint National Committee report (3) (Table 8).

TABLE 6. *Overall guide to workup for secondary causes of hypertension*

Diagnosis	Diagnostic procedure	
	Initial	Additional
Chronic renal disease	Urinalysis, serum creatinine, renal sonography	Isotopic renogram, renal biopsy
Renovascular disease	Plasma renin before and 1 hr after captopril	Aortogram, isotopic renogram 1 hr after captopril
Coarctation	Blood pressure in legs	Aortogram
Primary aldosteronism	Plasma potassium, plasma renin and aldosterone (ratio)	Urinary potassium, plasma or urinary aldosterone after saline load; adrenal computed tomography (CT) and scintiscans
Cushing's syndrome	Morning plasma cortisol after 1 mg of dexamethasone at bedtime	Urinary cortisol after variable doses of dexamethasone; adrenal CT and scintiscans
Pheochromocytoma	Spot urine for metanephrine	Urinary catechols; plasma catechols, basal and after 0.3 mg clonidine; adrenal CT and scintiscans

Cessation of Smoking

Until recently, the contribution of the pressor effects of smoking to the most common causes of premature mortality in smokers, coronary heart disease and stroke, was missed for a very simple reason: The blood pressure was hardly ever measured while the smoker was smoking. Smoking has been forbidden in virtually all health-care facilities for many years. The period from the time the smoker puts out the last cigarette to the time the blood pressure is recorded is far beyond the duration of the pressor effect of the cigarette smoke. Therefore, lower blood pressures have generally been recorded in chronic (nonsmoking) smokers because they weigh 10–20 lb less, on average, than do nonsmokers.

Recently, blood pressures have been recorded during the act of smoking (14). As seen in Fig. 4, a major pressor effect is seen over the 15 min of the tracing. By 30 min, the effect is largely gone. However, the typical smoker smokes 20 cigarettes per day, so that a fairly persistent rise in pressure may be expected.

If, despite all efforts to get the smoker to quit, the patient continues to smoke, the blood pressure should be recorded while the patient is smoking (away from the physician's office). The smoking pressure is the one that must be controlled. A great deal more about the adverse cardiovascular effects of smoking is provided in the chapter by Becker et al. *(this volume).*

TABLE 7. *Testing for renovascular hypertension: clinical index of suspicion as a guide to selecting patients for workup*

Low (should not be tested)
- Borderline, mild or moderate hypertension, in the absence of clinical clues

Moderate (noninvasive tests recommended)
- Severe hypertension (diastolic blood pressure greater than 120 mm Hg)
- Hypertension refractory to standard therapy
- Abrupt onset of sustained, moderate to severe hypertension at age <20 or >50 years
- Hypertension with a suggestive abdominal bruit (long, high-pitched, and localized to the region of the renal artery)
- Moderate hypertension (diastolic blood pressure exceeding 105 mm Hg) in a smoker, a patient with evidence of occlusive vascular disease (cerebrovascular, coronary, peripheral vascular), or a patient with unexplained but stable elevation of serum creatinine
- Normalization of blood pressure by an angiotensin-converting enzyme inhibitor in a patient with moderate or severe hypertension (particularly a smoker or a patient with recent onset of hypertension)

High (may consider proceeding directly to arteriography)
- Severe hypertension (diastolic blood pressure greater than 120 mm Hg with either progressive renal insufficiency or refractoriness to aggressive treatment (particularly in a patient who has been a smoker or has other evidence of occlusive arterial disease)
- Accelerated or malignant hypertension (grade III or IV retinopathy)
- Hypertension with recent elevation of serum creatinine, either unexplained or reversibly induced by an angiotensin-converting enzyme inhibitor
- Moderate to severe hypertension with incidentally detected asymmetry of renal size

From Mann and Pickering, ref. 13.

Reduction of Excess Weight

As noted by Rayfield *(this volume),* obesity is a leading contributor to hypertension (as well as to diabetes). It likely

TABLE 8. *Lifestyle modifications for treatment of hypertension*

Stop smoking (for overall cardiovascular health)

Proven value
- Lose weight, particularly for upper body obesity
- Reduce sodium intake to 110 mmol/day (2.4 g sodium or 6 g of NaCl)
- Moderate alcohol intake to no more than two usual portions per day
- Exercise (isotonic) regularly
- Increase potassium intake from fresh fruits and vegetables

Unproven value
- Relax and relieve stress
- Eat less saturated fat, more fish oils
- Maintain adequate calcium and magnesium intake

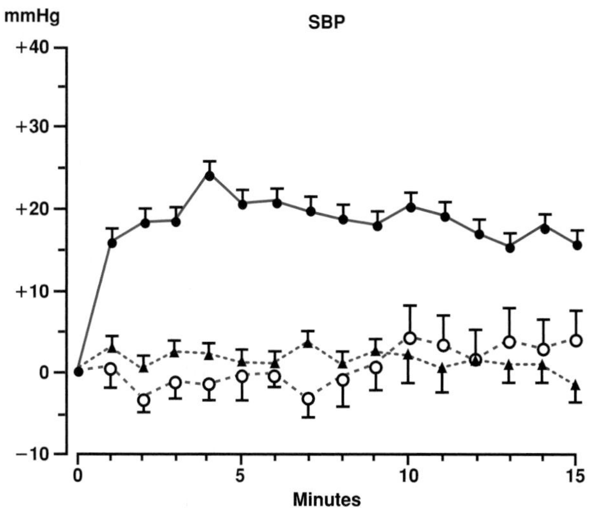

FIG. 4. Changes in systolic blood pressure over 15 min after smoking the first cigarette of the day within the first 5 min *(solid circles),* during no activity *(open circles),* and during sham-smoking *(triangles)* in ten normotensive smokers. (From Groppelli et al., ref. 14.)

does so by inducing insulin resistance that appears to involve an attenuation of the usual vasodilatory effect of insulin in the presence of obesity (15). All obese hypertensives (and about half of nonobese hypertensives) are insulin resistant (16) and the consequent hyperinsulinemia may accentuate hypertension by a number of mechanisms (Fig. 5). As seen in Fig. 5, the presence of upper-body (visceral or abdominal) obesity is particularly pathological, associated with a high likelihood of dyslipidemia, diabetes, and hypertension, which, in concert, markedly accelerate coronary heart disease (17).

Although the hypertension seen with generalized obesity may not be associated with as many cardiovascular complications as seen with hypertension in lean subjects (18), the reduction of excess weight is an effective way to lower blood pressure and is likely, thereby, to reduce cardiovascular risk. Caution is needed in the use of sympathomimetic agents taken to suppress appetite that may raise the blood pressure, but reports of increased weight loss have been reported with serotonin-uptake inhibitors (fluoxetine) that do not have a pressor effect (19).

Sodium Restriction

Despite continual attempts to smear the benefits of achievable moderate sodium restriction with the putative dangers of impractical severe sodium deprivation (20), the evidence continues to grow both for a causal role of dietary sodium excess in the pathogenesis of hypertension (21) and for a significant reduction in blood pressure by reduction of intake by about one-half, to around 100 mmol per day (22). There are no reports of ill effects from such moderate restriction and it should be fairly easily accomplished by avoidance of extra salt in cooking and at the table and of heavily salted processed foods at the market. The return to fresh foods which are low in sodium and high in potassium is more compatible with human physiology that evolved through eons of exposure to this ''natural'' diet. Modern humans appear unable to cope with the recent flood of extra sodium and a population-wide reduction in sodium intake could, by shifting the entire population's pressure downward only a few millimeters, prevent a major portion of premature cardiovascular disease (23).

Moderation of Alcohol Consumption

Too much alcohol is a cause of hypertension and a great amount of morbidity (24), so that those who drink more than two portions daily on average must be advised to reduce

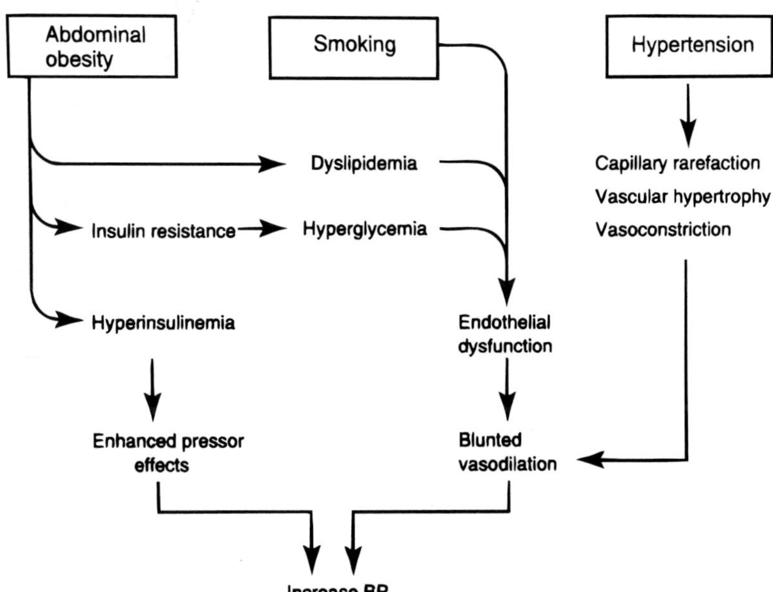

FIG. 5. A scheme for the interactions among abdominal obesity, insulin resistance, and hyperinsulinemia along with smoking and hypertension showing that they may raise blood pressure (BP) by enhanced pressor effects and blunted vasodilation.

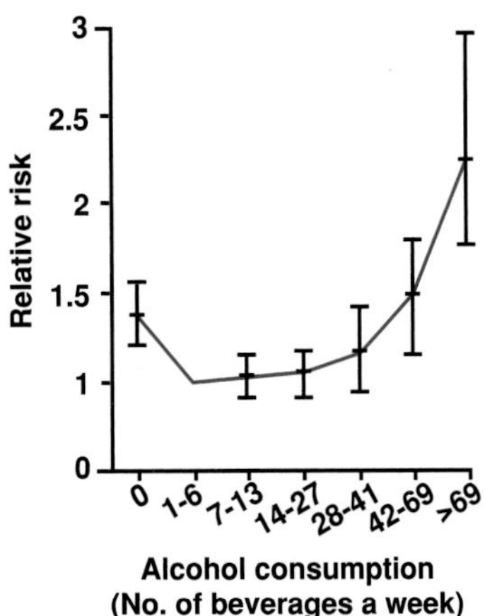

FIG. 6. The relative risk of death over a 12-year followup of 13,285 Danish men and women who were categorized by their initial level of alcohol consumption as determined by questionnaire. (From Grønbæ et al., ref. 25.)

their intake. On the other hand, small amounts of alcohol, up to two drinks daily, do not raise the blood pressure and provide significant protection from coronary disease and thereby a reduction in mortality (25) (Fig. 6). Therefore, the majority of hypertensives, who drink in moderation, should be advised to continue this healthful habit.

Increased Physical Activity

Increased levels of physical activity, easily accomplished even without structured exercise programs, are associated with less coronary disease and a lower incidence of hypertension (see the chapter by Fishman, *this volume*) (26). A reduction of pressures that are already elevated can be accomplished with regularly repeated dynamic exercise (27). Such dynamic (aerobic) exercise modulates sympathetic responsiveness; static (isometric) exercise of a moderate level may also provide an antihypertensive effect (28). These effects are independent of weight loss and both may lower blood pressure by improving insulin sensitivity.

Other Lifestyle Modifications

An increase in potassium intake has been shown usually to lower blood pressure (29), but that should be provided by increasing consumption of high-potassium fresh foods rather than by potassium supplements. Neither calcium supplements (30) nor magnesium supplements (31) have been found to lower blood pressure of patients who are not deficient in these minerals, but adequate intakes of these and other essential elements and vitamins should be provided.

Similarly, reductions of saturated fat intake likely provide little antihypertensive effect, although they may be beneficial for overall cardiovascular health. On the other hand, a meta-analysis of 31 placebo-controlled trials found a dose–response effect of fish oil, reducing pressure by −0.66/−0.35 mm Hg per g of omega-3 fatty acids (32).

Even though stress may contribute, via sympathetic nervous activation, to the pathogenesis of hypertension, most controlled trials of stress reduction by one or another method of relaxation have failed to show a sustained antihypertensive effect (33).

The Additive Effects of Multiple Modifications

In the Treatment of Mild Hypertension Study (TOMHS), 902 patients with stage 1 (diastolic blood pressure, DBP, 90–99) hypertension were instructed in a four-prong program of lifestyle modifications: weight reduction, sodium restriction, increased physical activity, and moderation of alcohol (34). The majority of the patients were then randomly assigned to take one of five antihypertensive drugs, but 234 were given a placebo and all patients were followed for 48 months. By the end of the study, the extent of adherence to the four lifestyle modifications was modest at best (Fig. 7). Nonetheless, the additive effect of these relatively small changes produced an 8.6/8.6 mm Hg fall in blood pressure at the end of the 4 years. This significant antihypertensive effect was accompanied by reductions in left ventricular mass and improvements in the HDL/total cholesterol ratio.

These impressive results should give encouragement to both physicians and patients to use lifestyle modifications as an effective, inexpensive, and broadly protective therapy.

DRUG THERAPY

While lifestyle modifications are continued, those hypertensives, likely the majority, who are not adequately controlled should be started on antihypertensive drugs. The long list of available agents can rationally be divided into three main categories or subclasses (Table 9).

Choice of Initial Drug

As many as half of all hypertensives will have their pressure controlled with any one drug and all but a very few, those with dangerously high levels, should be started only on one drug so as to bring the pressure down gradually and to identify adverse effects from any given agent (see Table 2). Not unexpectedly, all orally taken antihypertensive agents are equally effective in the overall hypertensive population, since the doses chosen are those which provide about a 10% reduction in blood pressure in about 70% of those tested during preapproval trials. Therefore, the choice of agent should not be based on overall efficacy. Nonetheless, caution is needed not to overtreat some who are more sensitive to any given agent by prescribing ''usual'' doses (35). Moreover, as will be noted subsequently, some groups, such as African-Americans and the elderly, may be more or less responsive to certain choices.

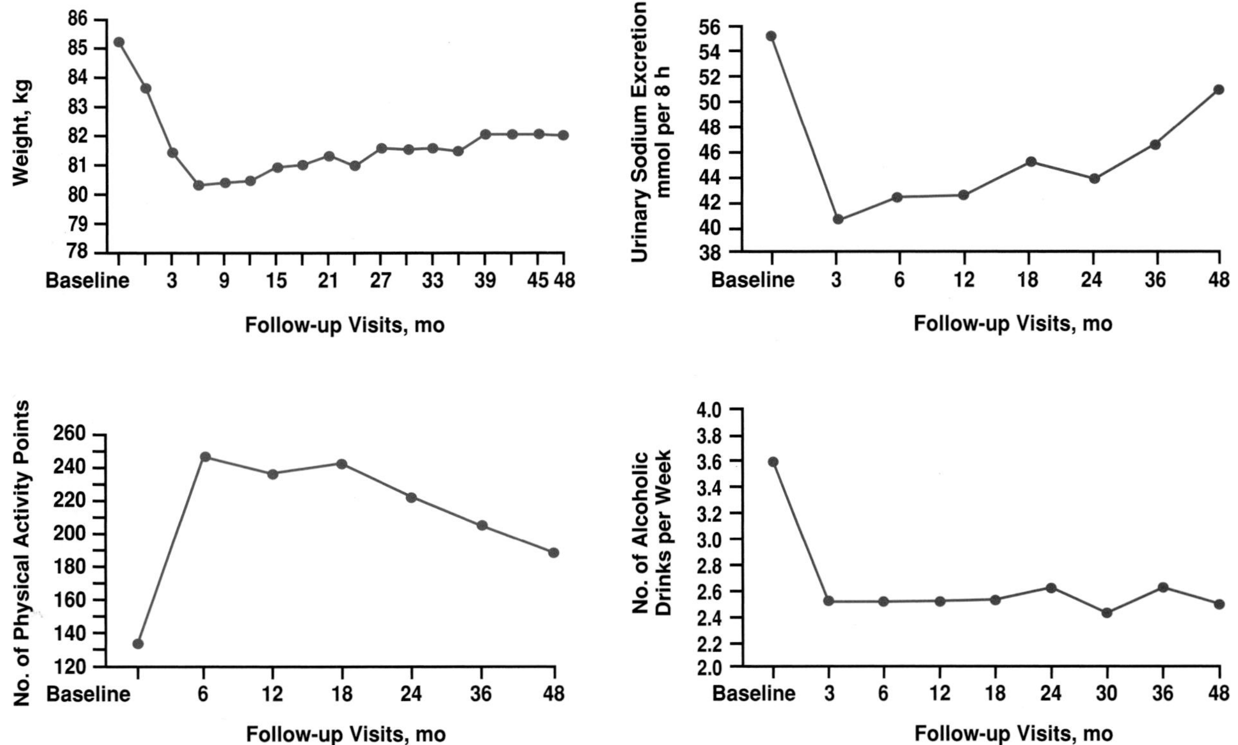

FIG. 7. The changes in the four lifestyle modifications achieved by the 902 participants over the 48 months of the Treatment of Mild Hypertension Study. The results in the 234 patients who took no antihypertensive drug were similar to those in the entire group. (From Neaton et al., ref. 34.)

Current Practice

In the United States and elsewhere, the use of diuretics and beta-blockers, the two most popular classes from the early 1970s until the late 1980s, has been decreasing steadily over the past 5 years, while the use of angiotensin-converting enzyme (ACE) inhibitors and even more so of calcium channel blockers (CCBs) has been rising markedly along with some additional use of the second generation of alpha$_1$-blockers.

These changes in clinical practice have arisen for multiple reasons, including (a) widespread concerns over biochemical aberrations induced by diuretics and beta-blockers, in particular dyslipidemia and insulin resistance, (b) the use of these concerns to explain an apparent shortfall in the extent of reduction in coronary mortality in diuretic- and beta-blocker-based clinical trials from that expected from the degree of blood pressure reduction based upon epidemiological evidence (36), (c) the availability of new vasodilatory agents which lower blood pressure "more physiologically" by reducing peripheral resistance rather than by shrinking fluid volume or reducing cardiac output, and (d) perhaps most

TABLE 9. *Antihypertensive drugs available in the United States*

Diuretics	*Adrenergic inhibitors*		*Sasodilators*	
Thiazides	Peripheral inhibitors	Beta receptor blockers	Direct	ACE inhibitors
Chlorthalidone	Guanadrel	Acebutolol	Hydralazine	Benazepril
Indapamide	Guanethidine	Atenolol	Minoxidil	Captopril
Metolazone	Reserpine	Betaxolol		Enalapril
Thiazides		Bisoprolol	Calcium blockers	Fosinopril
	Central alpha$_2$ agonists	Carteolol	Amlodipine	Lisinopril
Loop diuretics	Clonidine	Metoprolol	Diltiazem	Quinapril
Bumetanide	Guanabenz	Nadolol	Felodipine	Ramipril
Furosemide	Guanfacine	Penbutolol	Isradipine	
Torsemide	Methyldopa	Pindolol	Nicardipine	
Potassium sparers	Alpha$_1$ receptor blockers	Propranolol	Nifedipine	
Amiloride	Doxazosin	Timolol	Verapamil	
Spironolactone	Prazosin	Combined alpha and beta blocker		
Triamterene	Terazosin	Labetalol		

importantly, the effective marketing of these new agents to practitioners who are more than willing to change to newer, presumably better, agents.

The 1993 Joint National Committee Recommendations

On the background of these widespread changes, the 1993 Joint National Committee (JNC) report (3) recommends that diuretics and beta-blockers be given *preference* when drug therapy is initiated (Fig. 8). The report states:

> Because diuretics and beta blockers have been shown to reduce cardiovascular morbidity and mortality in controlled clinical trials, these two classes of drugs are preferred for initial drug therapy. The alternative drugs—calcium antagonists, angiotensin converting enzyme (ACE) inhibitors, $alpha_1$ receptor blockers, and the alpha-beta blocker—are equally effective in reducing blood pressure. Although these alternative drugs have potentially important benefits, they have not been used in long-term controlled trials to demonstrate their efficacy in reducing morbidity and mortality and therefore should be reserved for special indications or when diuretics and beta blockers have proved unacceptable or ineffective.

The report then details a number of other factors to be considered in the choice of initial therapy: ''The cost of medication, metabolic and subjective side effects, and drug–drug interactions . . . also to be considered in the selection of initial therapy are demographic characteristics, concomitant diseases that may be beneficially or adversely affected by the antihypertensive agent chosen and the use of other drugs that may lead to drug interactions.''

Consideration of these additional factors will, I believe, lead to a continuation of current trends: the use of various classes of drugs, the specific choice based upon multiple factors, in particular the presence of concomitant diseases that recommend a specific choice.

Individualized Therapy

The choice of therapy is logically based upon the known features of the various classes of drugs (Table 10) and the needs of the individual patient (Table 11). The preferences noted in Table 11 by two pluses (+ +) are generally supported by multiple clinical trials. However, the words of the 1993 JNC report should not be forgotten: Only ''diuretics and beta blockers have been shown to reduce cardiovascular morbidity and mortality in controlled clinical trials.'' To be sure, the other classes may prove to be equal to or better than diuretics and beta-blockers, but the proper large controlled trials to demonstrate their long-term efficacy are only now beginning and the results from these trials will not be available for 6–10 years.

Therefore, the cautious (some would say the prudent) practitioner may stick only with those agents that have been tested. My attitude and the opinion of almost all students of clinical hypertension are that the use of the newer agents is justifiable and, for most of the concomitant diseases listed in Table 11, preferable.

The Goal of Therapy

Once the initial and, if needed, subsequent choices are made, the goal of therapy needs to be established. Until recently, it was usually stated to be, ''As low as possible with-

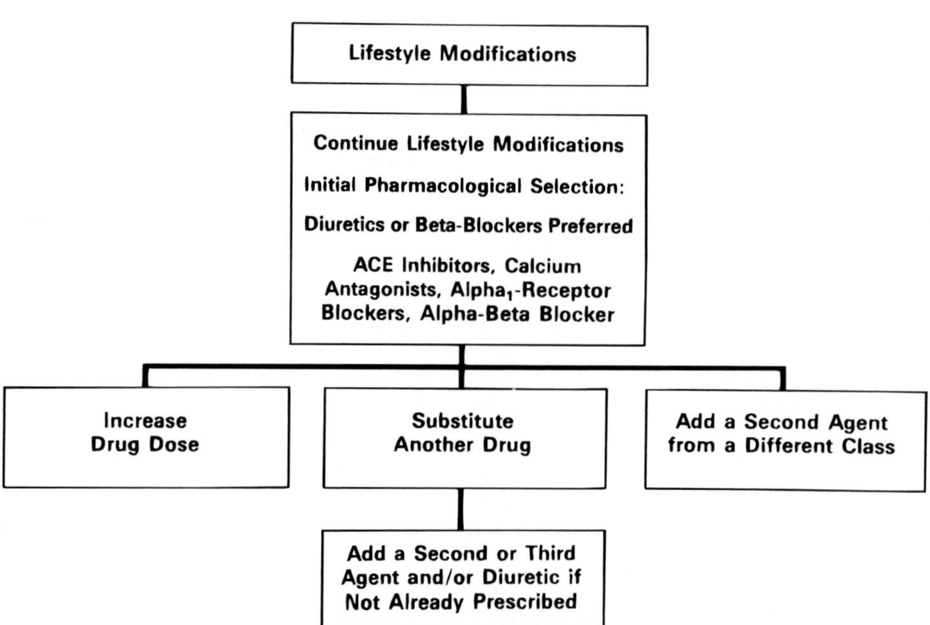

FIG. 8. Simplified algorithm for treatment of hypertension. ACE, Angiotensin-converting enzyme. (From Joint National Committee on Detection, Evaluation, and Treatment of High Blood Pressure, ref. 3.)

TABLE 10. *Characteristics of available choices for initial therapy*

	Diuretics	Centrally acting agents	Alpha-blockers	Beta-blockers	ACE inhibitors	Calcium antagonists
Hemodynamic effect	Initial volume shrinkage Peripheral vasodilation	Reduce cardiac output	Peripheral vasodilation	Reduce cardiac output	Peripheral vasodilation	Peripheral vasodilation
Side effects						
Overt	Weakness Palpitations	Sedation Dry mouth	Postural dizziness	Bronchospasm Fatigue Prolong hypoglycemia	Cough Taste disturbance Rash	Flushing Local edema Constipation (verapamil)
Hidden	Hypokalemia Hypercholesterolemia Glucose intolerance Hyperuricemia	Withdrawal syndrome Autoimmune syndromes (methyldopa)	—	Glucose intolerance Hypertriglyceridemia Decrease HDL cholesterol	Leukopenia Proteinuria	AV conduction (verapamil, diltiazem)
Contraindications	Preexisting volume contraction	Orthostatic hypotension Liver disease (methyldopa)	Orthostatic hypotension	Asthma Heartblock	Pregnancy	—
Cautions	Diabetes mellitus Gout Digitalis toxicity	—	—	Peripheral vascular disease Insulin-requiring diabetes Allergy Coronary spasm Withdrawal angina	Renal insufficiency Renovascular disease	Heart failure
Special advantages	Effective in African-Americans, elderly Enhance effectiveness of all other agents	No alteration in blood lipids No fluid retention (guanabenz)	No decrease in cardiac output No alteration in blood lipids No sedation Relieve symptoms of prostatic hypertrophy	Reduce recurrence of coronary disease Reduce manifestations of anxiety Coexisting angina, migraine, glaucoma	No CNS side effects Treat CHF Reduce recurrences of coronary disease and development of CHF Probable renal protection	Effective in African-Americans, elderly No CNS side effects Coronary vasodilation

out causing bothersome side effects.'' However, two sets of observations have complicated the issue.

First came the recognition of a ''J'' curve, an increased incidence of coronary ischemic events when the diastolic pressure was reduced below 85 mm Hg (37), an observation that has now been amply confirmed (38). The data now include two prospective studies (39,40). In one of the latter, an increase in myocardial infarctions was noted in those whose initial pulse pressure was in the highest tertile (greater than 62 mm Hg) and whose pressures were reduced by 18 mm Hg or more by treatment (40). This finding is particularly ominous since such wide pulse pressures are most common in the elderly with predominately systolic hypertension.

Some argue that the J curve does not reflect the induction of coronary ischemia by reduction of systemic pressure, but rather an epiphenomenon explained by underlying coronary ischemia which leads to reduced cardiac output and lower systemic pressure (41). However, the prospective studies argue against this explanation. Moreover, the hypertensive myocardium is clearly (and uniquely) susceptible to is-

TABLE 11. *Individualized choices of therapy*

Coexisting condition	Diuretic	Beta-blocker	Alpha-blocker	Calcium blocker	ACE inhibitor
Older age	++	+/−	+	+	+
African-American	++	+/−	+	+	+/−
Angina	+/−	++	+	++	+
Postmyocardial infarction	+	++	+	+/−	++
Congestive failure	++	−	+	−	++
Cerebrovascular disease	+	+	+/−	++	+
Renal insufficiency	++	+/−	+	++	++
Diabetes	−	−	++	+	++
Dyslipidemia	−	−	++	+	+
Asthma	+	−	+	+	+
Benign prostatic hypertrophy			++		

++, Preferred. +, Suitable. +/−, Usually not preferred. −, Usually contraindicated.

chemia when systemic pressures and subsequently coronary perfusion pressure are lowered. The hypertrophied myocardium needs more oxygen but cannot be provided more when perfusion pressure is lowered, because of the poor autoregulatory ability of atherosclerotic coronary vessels, i.e., decreased coronary reserve, and the inability to extract more oxygen than is already extracted under normal circumstances. Therefore, I believe a J curve exists and caution should be taken in lowering diastolic pressures below 85 mm Hg, particularly in patients with known preexisting coronary disease.

At the same time as the evidence for a cardiac J curve has surfaced, increasingly convincing data have suggested that much lower pressures than usually are sought may be needed to protect the kidneys from progressive glomerular sclerosis and nephron loss. Both experimental (42) and clinical (43) data show protection from progressive renal damage when systemic diastolic pressures are lowered below 80 mm Hg, particularly with ACE inhibitors, which provide additional efferent arteriolar dilation.

Therefore, for maximal renal protection and likely for maximal cerebrovascular protection, lower pressures may be desirable than for maximal cardiac protection. More aggressive pressure reduction will almost certainly be sought increasingly in the management of diabetics with early nephropathy.

Regression of Left Ventricular Hypertrophy

Left ventricular hypertrophy (LVH) is commonly seen by echocardiography in hypertensive patients. Most drugs as they lower blood pressure will regress LVH (34) with the exception of the direct vasodilators hydralazine and minoxidil (see Phillips and Diamond, *this volume*). If inexpensive, partial echocardiograms are available, they may be a better way to monitor the effectiveness of therapy, rather than depending only upon occasional blood pressure measurements. For most patients, a larger number of home blood pressure recordings likely will provide the needed data.

Resistant Hypertension

Perhaps 10% of patients will not be responsive to full doses of three or more antihypertensive agents, i.e., they will be resistant. Multiple factors may be involved, as noted in Table 1. An even larger number have pseudoresistance, that is, high office readings, but normal out-of-the-office readings (7). Therefore, when patients appear to be resistant, ambulatory or home readings should be obtained to ensure that true resistance is present.

When it is, the most common cause is volume overload from the combination of heavy sodium intake, reduced renal

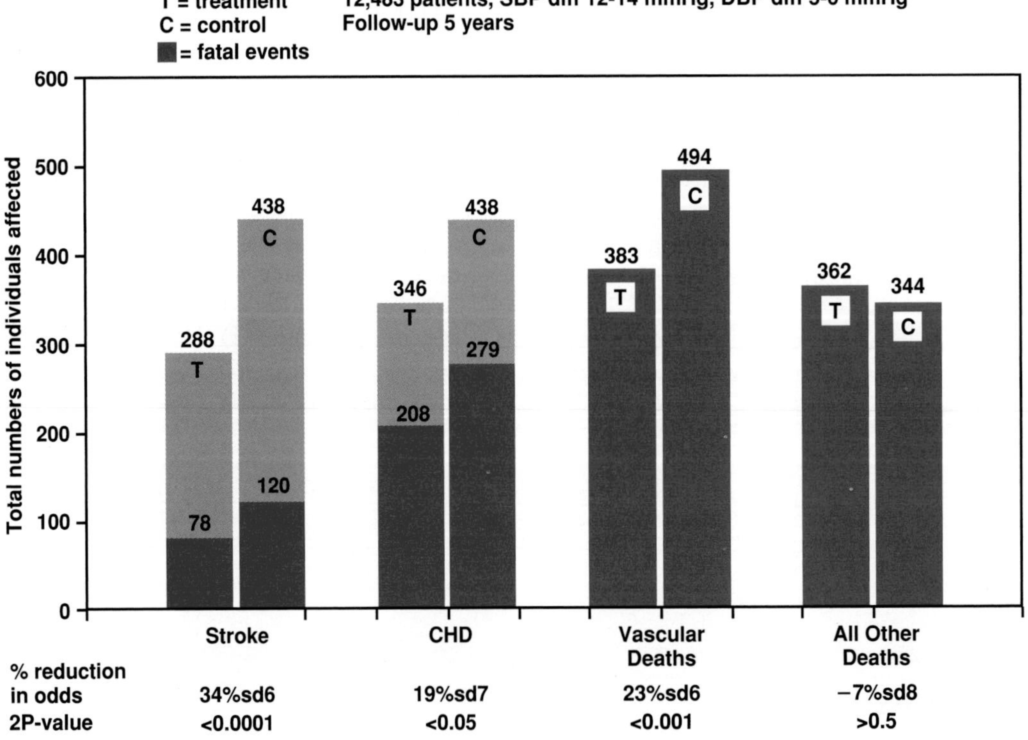

FIG. 9. Effects of blood pressure reduction on stroke, coronary heart disease (CHD), vascular death, and nonvascular death in elderly patients. Combined results of five randomized trials of antihypertensive treatment in patients >60 years of age. T, treatment; C, control; shaded area, number of fatal events. There were 12,483 patients, with systolic blood pressure difference 12–14 mmHg and diastolic blood pressure difference 5–6 mmHg. Follow-up 5 years. (From MacMahon and Rodgers, ref. 49.)

excretory capacity from nephrosclerosis, increased renal avidity for sodium when systemic pressures are lowered, and inadequate diuretic therapy. The last, inadequate diuretic, is commonly attributable to the widespread practice of using once-daily doses of the loop diuretic furosemide. As is well described (44), the duration of action of furosemide (and bumetanide) is only a few hours; for the remaining 21 hr, all of the sodium excreted while the drug works is retained, so the patient ends up no different than before with regard to volume status and blood pressure.

Longer-acting diuretics are able to provide the slight degree of volume contraction needed to maintain lower blood pressures. For patients with good renal function, various thiazides, chlorthalidone, or indapamide are suitable; for patients with renal impairment, metolazone or the recently marketed longer-acting loop diuretic torasemide are appropriate.

If volume overload is not responsible, secondary forms of hypertension should be looked for (Tables 6 and 7). In addition, reasons for nonadherence to therapy and drug-related problems should be sought. Fortunately, when appropriate steps are taken to find and correct the causes, most cases of resistant hypertension can be brought under adequate control (45).

SPECIAL POPULATIONS

Less information is available about the treatment of women with hypertension and that which is available suggests that they may not obtain the same degree of protection as do men (46).

Similarly, African-Americans may not receive the same degree of protection from progressive renal damage as do white hypertensives given similar therapy (47). They also tend to respond less well to renin-suppressing drugs, beta-blockers, and ACE inhibitors (48).

The Elderly

In the past few years, three large clinical trials have added conclusive data to that previously available documenting the benefit of treating elderly hypertensives (49) (Fig. 9). These trials (50–52) treated over 10,000 patients whose average age was 72 years, starting with a low dose of a diuretic in most. The overall cardiac protection observed among the elderly given active therapy was even greater than that noted in the multiple trials involving patients under age 65 years (36).

Despite these documented benefits, caution is needed in treating elderly hypertensives, mainly because of the common presence of factors that may increase their risks from drug therapy (Table 12). The patients in the clinical trials were, by choice and necessity, fairly healthy. Therefore, the benefits they achieved may not be shared by the larger population of elderly, who often have coexisting problems. Particular attention should be given to the common coexistence of postural hypotension which often must be dealt with before supine and seated hypertension can be treated (53).

TABLE 12. *Factors that might contribute to increased risk of pharmacologic treatment of hypertension in the elderly*

Factor	Potential complication
Diminished baroreceptor activity	Orthostatic hypotension
Impaired cerebral autoregulation	Cerebral ischemia with small falls in systemic pressure
Decreased intravascular volume	Orthostatic hypotension Volume depletion, hyponatremia
Sensitivity to hypokalemia	Arrhythmia, muscular weakness
Decreased renal and hepatic function	Drug accumulation
Polypharmacy	Drug interaction
CNS changes	Depression, confusion

Diabetic Hypertensives

As detailed further by Rayfield *(this volume)*, all diabetics are prone to develop hypertension. Type I diabetics often develop nephropathy and, thereafter, hypertension usually

TABLE 13. *Hypertensive emergencies*

Accelerated-malignant hypertension
Cerebrovascular
- Hypertensive encephalopathy
- Atherothrombotic brain infarction with severe hypertension
- Intracerebral hemorrhage
- Subarachnoid hemorrhage

Cardiac
- Acute aortic dissection
- Acute left ventricular failure
- Acute or impending myocardial infarction
- After coronary bypass surgery

Renal
- Acute glomerulonephritis
- Renal crises from collagen vascular diseases
- Renovascular hypertension
- Severe hypertension after kidney transplantation

Excessive circulating catecholamines
- Pheochromocytoma crisis
- Food or drug interactions with monoamine oxidase inhibitors
- Sympathomimetic drug abuse (cocaine)
- Rebound hypertension after sudden cessation of antihypertensive drugs

Eclampsia
Surgical
- Severe hypertension in patients requiring immediate surgery
- Postoperative hypertension
- Postoperative bleeding from vascular suture lines

Severe body burns
Severe epistaxis

Modified from Kaplan, ref. 57, with permission.

appears because of inability to excrete sodium loads. Type II diabetics are likely to have hypertension because of their underlying obesity and insulin resistance.

The therapy of diabetic hypertensives poses additional challenges, but also the potential for additional advantages beyond the therapy of nondiabetic hypertensives. The challenges involve the tendency of both diuretics and beta-blockers to further worsen underlying insulin resistance and dyslipidemia and of the latter agents to increase hazards from insulin-induced hypoglycemia (54). The potential advantages of therapy include the demonstrated slowing of the progression of nephropathy by ACE inhibitors (43) and the ability to improve insulin sensitivity with ACE inhibitors and alpha-blockers (55). In addition, newer antidiabetic agents (metformin, ciglitazone) which improve insulin sensitivity may lower blood pressure, presumably by reducing hyperinsulinemia (56).

THE MANAGEMENT OF HYPERTENSIVE CRISES

Although they occur in only a small percentage of patients, life-threatening hypertensive crises must be effectively managed (57). The crises appear in various guises (Table 13), some demanding immediate reduction of the pressure by a parenteral drug (Table 14), others requiring rapid attention but often manageable with oral agents.

Once the crisis is over, attention should be directed to possible causes. In particular, renovascular hypertension must almost always be ruled out (see Table 7).

CONCLUDING COMMENTS

Hypertension can almost always be effectively managed, but even in carefully monitored clinical trials where all possible ways to ensure adherence to therapy are used, as many as one-third of enrolled patients do not achieve adequate control (58). As noted at the beginning of this chapter, many impediments can interfere with management. It is hoped that the principles elucidated in this chapter will help clinicians achieve the true goal of antihypertensive therapy: protection from premature cardiovascular morbidity and mortality.

The Future Management of Hypertension

As more about the pathogenesis of hypertension is uncovered, more specific therapies should become available. Cur-

TABLE 14. *Parenteral drugs for treatment of hypertensive emergency (in order of rapidity of action)*

Drug	Dosage	Onset of action (min)	Duration of action	Adverse effects
Vasodilators				
Nitroprusside (Nipride, Nitropress)	0.25–10 μg/kg/min as IV infusion	Instantaneous	1–2 min	Nausea, vomiting, muscle twitching, sweating, thiocyanate and cyanide intoxication
Nitroglycerin	5–100 μg/min as IV infusion	2–5	3–5 min	Headache, vomiting, methemoglobinemia, tolerance with prolonged use
Diazoxide (Hyperstat)	50–100 mg IV bolus repeated, or 15–30 mg/min by IV infusion	2–4	6–12 hr	Nausea, hypotension, flushing, tachycardia, chest pain
Hydralazine (Apresoline)	10–20 mg IV 10–50 mg IM	10–20 20–30	3–8 hr	Tachycardia, flushing, headache, vomiting, aggravation of angina
Enalaprilat (Vasotec IV)	1.25–5 mg q 6 hr	15	6 hr	Precipitous fall in blood pressure in high-renin states; response variable
Nicardipine	2–8 mg/hr IV	5–10	30–60 min	Tachycardia, headache, flushing, local phlebitis
Adrenergic inhibitors				
Phentolamine (Regitine)	5–15 mg IV	1–2	3–10 min	Tachycardia, flushing
Trimethaphan (Arfonad)	0.5–5 mg/min as IV infusion	1–5	10 min	Paresis of bowel and bladder, orthostatic hypotension, blurred vision, dry mouth
Esmolol (Brevibloc)	200–500 μg/min for 4 min, then 50–300 μg/kg/min IV	1–2	10–20 min	Hypotension, nausea
Labetalol (Normodyne, Trandate)	20–80 mg IV bolus every 10 min 2 mg/min IV infusion	5–10	3–6 hr	Vomiting, scalp tingling, burning in throat, postural hypotension, dizziness, nausea

IV, Intravenous; IM, intramuscular.

rently, agents which work through some of the more recently described factors (atrial natriuretic factor, endothelin, nitric oxide) are being intensively investigated. They may be found to control hypertension more effectively than currently available agents acting nonspecifically.

Although it will likely never be possible to prevent or relieve hypertension by genetic manipulations, prevention may be possible by appropriate lifestyle changes intensively applied to those who are genetically identified to carry the propensity to hypertension.

In addition to the more focused therapy of hypertension, all of the maneuvers described in this book that decreases the risks of atherosclerosis will need to be applied to the highly vulnerable hypertensive patient with care not to worsen the other risk factors while the hypertension is being treated.

REFERENCES

1. Schappert SM. National ambulatory medical survey: 1991 summary. NCHS Advance Data, No. 230, Vital and Health Statistics of the National Center for Health Statistics. Hyattsville, Maryland: National Center for Health Statistics; 1993; U.S. Department of Health and Human Services Publication (PHS) 93-1250.
2. Kaplan NM. Treatment of hypertension: nondrug therapy. In: *Clinical hypertension,* 6th ed. Baltimore: Williams and Wilkins; 1994:171–190.
3. Joint National Committee on Detection, Evaluation, and Treatment of High Blood Pressure. The fifth report of the Joint National Committee on Detection, Evaluation, and Treatment of High Blood Pressure (JNC V). *Arch Intern Med* 1993;153:154–183.
4. Conway J. Blood pressure and heart rate variability. *J Hypertens* 1986; 4:261–263.
5. Zachariah PK, Summer WE III. The clinical utility of blood pressure load in hypertension. *Am J Hypertens* 1993;6:194S–197S.
6. Krakoff LR. Ambulatory blood pressure monitoring can improve cost-effective management of hypertension. *Am J Hypertens* 1993;6: 220S–224S.
7. Kaplan NM. Measurement of the blood pressure. In: *Clinical hypertension,* 6th ed. Baltimore: Williams and Wilkins; 1994:23–46.
8. Swales JD. Guidelines on guidelines. *J Hypertens* 1993;11:899–903.
9. Kannel WB, Cupples LA, D'Agostino RB, Stokes J III. Hypertension, antihypertensive treatment, and sudden coronary death. The Framingham Study. *Hypertension* 1988;11(Suppl II):II-45–II-50.
10. Julius S, Mejia A, Jones K, et al. "White coat" versus "sustained" borderline hypertension in Tecumseh, Michigan. *Hypertension* 1990; 16:617–623.
11. Jackson R, Barham P, Bills J, Birch T, McLennan L, MacMahon S, Maling T. Management of raised blood pressure in New Zealand: A discussion document. *Br Med J* 1993;307:107–110.
12. Kasiske BL, Kalil RSN, Ma JZ, Liao M, Keane WF. Effect of antihypertensive therapy on the kidney in patients with diabetes: A meta-regression analysis. *Ann Intern Med* 1993;118:129–138.
13. Mann SJ, Pickering TG. Detection of renovascular hypertension. State of the art: 1992. *Ann Intern Med* 1992;117:845–853.
14. Groppelli A, Giorgi DMA, Omboni S, Parati G, Mancia G. Persistent blood pressure increase induced by heavy smoking. *J Hypertens* 1992; 10:495–499.
15. Baron AD, Brechtel-Hook G, Johnson A, Hardin D. Skeletal muscle blood flow. A possible link between insulin resistance and blood pressure. *Hypertension* 1993;21:129–135.
16. DeFronzo RA, Ferrannini E. Insulin resistance. A multifaceted syndrome responsible for NIDDM, obesity, hypertension, dyslipidemia, and atherosclerotic cardiovascular disease. *Diabetes Care* 1991;14: 173–194.
17. McKeigue PM, Ferrie JE, Pierpoint T, Marmot MG. Association of early-onset coronary heart disease in South Asian men with glucose intolerance and hyperinsulinemia. *Circulation* 1993;87:152–161.
18. Carman WJ, Barrett-Connor E, Sowers MF, Khaw K-T. Higher risk of cardiovascular mortality among lean hypertensive individuals in Tecumseh, Michigan. *Circulation* 1994;89:703–711.
19. Goldstein DJ, Rampey AH Jr, Enas GG, Potvin JH, Fludzinski LA, Levine LR. Fluoxetine: a randomized clinical trial in the treatment of obesity. *Int J Obesity* 1994;18:129–135.
20. Muntzel M, Drüeke T. A comprehensive review of the salt and blood pressure relationship. *Am J Hypertens* 1992;5:1S–42S.
21. Kimura G, Brenner BM. A method for distinguishing salt-sensitive from non-salt sensitive forms of human and experimental hypertension. *Curr Opin Nephrol Hypertens* 1993;2:341–349.
22. Law MR, Frost CD, Wald NJ. By how much does dietary salt reduction lower blood pressure? III—Analysis of data from trials of salt reduction. *Br Med J* 1991;302:819–824.
23. Rose G. *The strategy of preventive medicine.* Oxford: Oxford University Press, 1992.
24. World Hypertension League. Alcohol and hypertension. *J Hypertens* 1991;5:227–232.
25. Grønbæ M, Deis A, Sørensen TIA, Becker U, Borch-Johnsen K, Müller C, Schnohr P, Jensen G. Influence of sex, age, body mass index, and smoking on alcohol intake and mortality. *Br Med J* 1994;308:302–306.
26. Paffenbarger RS Jr, Hyde RT, Wing AL, Lee I-M, Jung DL, Kampert JB. The association of changes in physical-activity level and other lifestyle characteristics with mortality among men. *N Engl J Med* 1993; 328:574–576.
27. Arroll B, Beaglehole R. Does physical activity lower blood pressure? A critical review of the clinical trials. *J Clin Epidemiol* 1992;45:439–447.
28. Wiley RL, Dunn CL, Cox RH, Hueppchen NA, Scott MS. Isometric exercise training lowers resting blood pressure. *Med Sci Sports Exerc* 1992;24:749–754.
29. Cappuccio FP, MacGregor GA. Does potassium supplementation lower blood pressure? A meta-analysis of published trials. *J Hypertens* 1991; 9:465–473.
30. Galløe AM, Graudal N, Møller J, Bro H, Jørgensen M, Christensen HR. Effect of oral calcium supplementation on blood pressure in patients with previously untreated hypertension: A randomized double-blind, placebo-controlled, crossover study. *J Hum Hypertens* 1993;7: 43–45.
31. Paolisso G, Di Maro G, Cozzolino D, Salvatore T, D'Amore A, Lama D, Varricchio M, D'Onofrio F. Chronic magnesium administration enhances oxidative glucose metabolism in thiazide treated hypertensive patients. *Am J Hypertens* 1992;5:681–686.
32. Morris MC, Sacks F, Rosner B. Does fish oil lower blood pressure? A metaanalysis of controlled trials. *Circulation* 1993;88:523–533.
33. Trials of Hypertension Prevention Collaborative Research Group. The effects of nonpharmacologic interventions on blood pressure of persons with high normal levels. Results of the Trials of Hypertension Prevention, Phase I. *JAMA* 1992;267:1213–1220.
34. Neaton JD, Grimm RH Jr, Prineas RJ, Stamler J, Grandits GA, Elmer PJ, Cutler JA, Flack JM, Schoenberger JA, McDonald R, Lewis CE, Liebson PF. Treatment of mild hypertension study (TOMHS): Final results. *JAMA* 1993;270:713–724.
35. Kaplan NM. The appropriate goals of antihypertensive therapy: Neither too much nor too little. *Ann Intern Med* 1992;116:686–690.
36. MacMahon S, Peto R, Cutler J, Collins R, Sorlie P, Neaton J, Abbott R, Godwin J, Dyer A, Stamler J. Blood pressure, stroke, and coronary heart disease. Part 1: Prolonged differences in blood pressure: Prospective observational studies corrected for the regression dilution bias. *Lancet* 1990;335:765–774.
37. Cruickshank JM. Coronary flow reserve and the J curve relation between diastolic blood pressure and myocardial infarction. *Br Med J* 1988;297:1227–1230.
38. Farnett L, Mulrow CD, Linn WD, Lucey CR, Tuley MR. The J-curve phenomenon and the treatment of hypertension. Is there a point beyond which pressure reduction is dangerous? *JAMA* 1991;265:489–495.
39. Lindblad U, Råstam L, Rydén L, Ranstam J, Isacsson S-O, Berglund G. Control of blood pressure and risk of first acute myocardial infarction: Skaraborg hypertension project. *Br Med J* 1994;308:681–686.
40. Madhavan S, Ooi WL, Cohen H, Alderman MH. Relation of pulse pressure and blood pressure reduction to the incidence of myocardial infarction. *Hypertension* 1994;23:395–401.
41. Hansson L. How far should blood pressure be lowered? What is the role of the J-curve? *Am J Hypertens* 1990;3:726–729.

42. Anderson S, Brenner BM. Progressive renal disease: A disorder of adaptation. *Q J Med* 1989;70:185–189.
43. Lewis EJ, Hunsicker LG, Bain RP, Rohde RD. The effect of angiotensin-converting-enzyme inhibition on diabetic nephropathy. *N Engl J Med* 1993;329:1456–1462.
44. Kelly RA, Wilcox CS, Mitch WE, Meyer TW, Souney PF, Rayment CM, Friedman PA, Swartz SL. Response of the kidney to furosemide. II. Effect of captopril on sodium balance. *Kidney Int* 1983;24:233–239.
45. Yakovlevitch M, Black HR. Resistant hypertension in a tertiary care clinic. *Arch Intern Med* 1991;151:1786–1792.
46. Anastos K, Charney P, Charon RA, Cohen E, Jones CY, Marte C, Swiderski DM, Wheater ME, Williams S. Hypertension in women: What is really known? *Ann Intern Med* 1991;115:287–293.
47. Walker WG, Neaton JD, Cutler JA, Neuwirth R, Cohen JD. Renal function change in hypertensive members of the multiple risk factor intervention trial. Racial and treatment effects. *JAMA* 1992;268: 3085–3091.
48. Materson BJ, Reda DJ, Cushman WC, Massie BM, Freis ED, Kochar MS, Hamburger RJ, Fye C, Lakshman R, Gottdiener J, Ramirez EA, Henderson WF. Single-drug therapy for hypertension in men. A comparison of six antihypertensive agents with placebo. *N Engl J Med* 1993;328:914–921.
49. MacMahon S, Rodgers A. The effects of blood pressure reduction in older patients: An overview of five randomized controlled trials in elderly hypertensives. *Clin Exp Hypertens* 1993;15:967–978.
50. SHEP Cooperative Research Group. Prevention of stroke by antihypertensive drug treatment in older persons with isolated systolic hypertension. Final results of the Systolic Hypertension in the Elderly Program (SHEP). *JAMA* 1991;266:3255–3264.
51. Dahlöf B, Lindholm LH, Hansson L, Scherstén B, Ekbom T, Wester P-O. Morbidity and mortality in the Swedish Trial in Old Patients with Hypertension (STOP-Hypertension). *Lancet* 1991;338:1281–1285.
52. Medical Research Council Working Party. Medical Research Council trial of treatment of hypertension in older adults: Principal results. *Br Med J* 1992;304:405–412.
53. Kaplan NM. The promises and perils of treating the elderly hypertensive. *Am J Med Sci* 1993;305:183–197.
54. Cristlieb RA. Treatment selection considerations for the hypertensive diabetic patient. *Arch Intern Med* 1990;150:1167–1774.
55. Lithell HOL. Effect of antihypertensive drugs on insulin, glucose, and lipid metabolism. *Diabetes Care* 1991;14:203–209.
56. Giugliano D, Quatraro A, Consoli G, Minei A, Ceriello A, De Rosa N, D'Onofrio F. Metformin for obese, insulin-treated diabetic patients; improvement in glycaemic control and reduction of metabolic risk factors. *Eur J Clin Pharmacol* 1993;44:107–112.
57. Kaplan NM. Hypertensive crises. In: *Clinical hypertension,* 6th ed. Baltimore: Williams and Wilkins; 1994:281–298.
58. Ménard J. Improving hypertension treatment. Where should we put our efforts: New drugs, new concepts, or new management? *Am J Hypertens* 1992;5:252S–258S.
59. Zachariah PK, Sheps SG, Smith RL. Defining the roles of home and ambulatory monitoring. *Diagnosis* 1988;10:39–50.
60. A Consensus Development Conference Report to the National Advisory Committee on Core Health and Disability Support Services. In: The management of raised blood pressure in New Zealand. Wellington, New Zealand: National Advisory Committee on Core Health and Disability Support Services; 1992.

Atherosclerosis and Coronary Artery Disease,
edited by V. Fuster, R. Ross, and E. J. Topol.
Lippincott-Raven Publishers, Philadelphia © 1996.

CHAPTER 17

Hypertensive Heart Disease

Robert A. Phillips and Joseph A. Diamond

Key Words: Left ventricular hypertrophy; Left ventricular mass; Diastolic function; Hypertension; Microcirculation; Autoregulation; Coronary flow reserve; Treatment; Diagnosis.

INTRODUCTION

Hypertensive heart disease is a common disorder associated with a markedly increased risk of cardiovascular morbidity and mortality. The purpose of this chapter is to review (a) the epidemiologic evidence for left ventricular hypertrophy (LVH) as a risk factor for cardiovascular disease, (b) the structural changes in the hypertensive heart that provide the substrate for increased risk, (c) the etiology of LVH, (d) the identification and treatment of LVH in clinical practice, and (e) the abnormalities of diastolic function and coronary circulation that accompany LVH; systolic dysfunction in hypertension has been recently reviewed (1,2) and will not be covered.

R. A. Phillips and J. A. Diamond: Hypertension Section, Division of Cardiology, Mount Sinai Medical Center, New York, New York 10029.

DEFINITION OF HYPERTENSIVE HEART DISEASE AND EPIDEMIOLOGY OF LEFT VENTRICULAR MASS

Hypertensive heart disease occurs in association with elevated arterial blood pressure. Its manifestations include diastolic dysfunction, increased left ventricular mass, and coro-

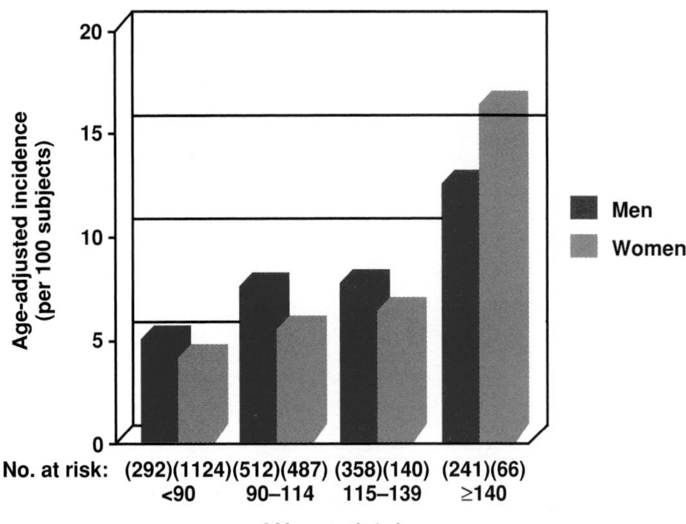

FIG. 1. Effect of LV mass on age-adjusted incidence of cardiovascular disease over a 4-year period in the Framingham Heart Study. (Adapted from Levy et al., ref. 5.)

nary flow abnormalities. Echocardiographically determined left ventricular hypertrophy (LVH) is defined as a left ventricular (LV) mass in the upper 2.5% to 5% of the adult population. It occurs in approximately 15–20% of hypertensive patients (3). When considered as a discrete, categorical variable, LVH significantly increases the risk of coronary artery disease, congestive heart failure, cerebrovascular accidents, ventricular arrhythmia, and sudden death (4–6). Left ventricular hypertrophy increases the relative risk of mortality by twofold in subjects with coronary artery disease and by fourfold in those with normal epicardial coronary arteries (7,8). In addition, when LV mass is considered as a continuous variable, a relatively linear relationship exists between cardiovascular risk and the absolute amount of LV mass. During 4 years of follow-up in the Framingham Heart Study, each 50 g/m increase in LV mass was associated with a 1.49 relative risk of cardiovascular disease for men and 1.57 for women. The effect on cardiovascular mortality was even more striking, with a 1.73 relative risk for each 50 g/m for men and 2.12 for women (5) (Fig. 1).

LEFT VENTRICULAR STRUCTURE

Left Ventricular Geometric Patterns

Subjects with hypertension have different patterns of ventricular shape and geometry that are associated with markedly different risks for cardiovascular disease (Fig. 2). Ventricular structure has commonly been categorized according to one of two ratios: (a) disproportionate septal thickening compared to the posterior wall (ratio ≥1.3), a pattern that may be quite common in subjects with LV wall thickness >15 mm (9), and (b) the ratio of [(2 × posterior wall thickness)/LV internal dimension], which is defined as relative wall thickness (RWT). RWT ≥0.45 is the arbitrary cutoff often used to define concentric hypertrophy, a geometric pattern in which the LV internal dimension remains normal and LV mass increases as a result of increased wall thickness. This is the pattern typically associated with pressure overload. In eccentric hypertrophy, the LV internal dimension dilates, and RWT is <0.45. This is the pattern typically associated with volume overload. Increased relative wall thickness with normal LV mass is termed concentric remodeling (10). In one study of hypertensive subjects followed for 10 years, the incidence of a cardiovascular event was 30% in those with concentric LVH, 25% in those with eccentric LVH, 15% in those with concentric remodeling, and 9% in those with normal LV mass (Fig. 3) (11). Mortality data

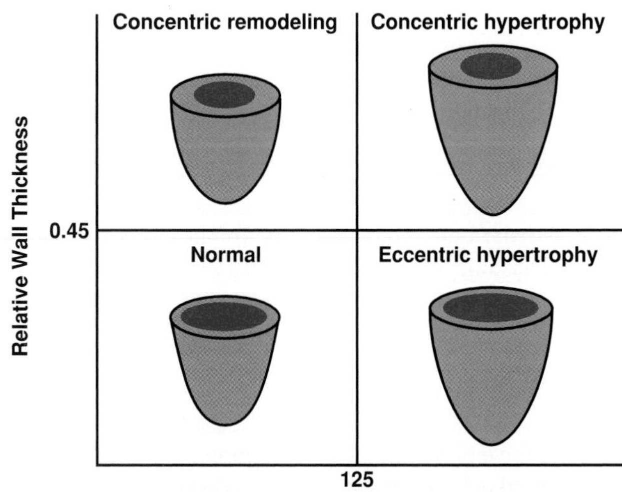

FIG. 2. Various forms of left ventricular geometry associated with hypertensive heart disease. Relative wall thickness is a ratio defined as: (sum of septum and posterior wall/left ventricular internal dimension). LV mass index (mass/body surface area) >125 g/m^2 is approximately the 95th percentile for men. (From Frolich et al.)

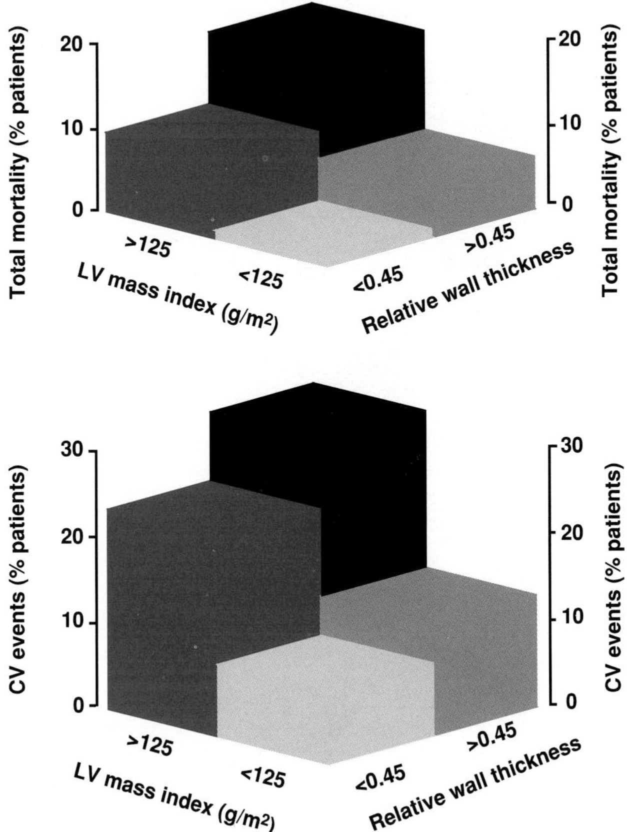

FIG. 3. Relationship among mortality, CV events, and left ventricular geometry in hypertensive subjects followed for 10 years. The incidence of a cardiovascular event and mortality was as follows: concentric LVH *(black rectangle)* > eccentric LVH *(striped rectangle)* > concentric remodeling *(stippled rectangle)* > normal LV mass and geometry *(unshaded rectangle).*

on hypertensive subjects with disproportionate septal thickening and increased LV mass are not available. These subjects have similar degrees of ventricular ectopy and depressed LV diastolic function as, and even more atrial arrhythmias than, those with concentric LVH (12).

Estimates of the prevalence of various forms of ventricular structure vary widely depending on the hemodynamic and demographic characteristics of the population. Greater severity of hypertension, advancing age, and higher peripheral resistance with normal intravascular volume increases the prevalence of concentric hypertrophy. Among subjects with LVH, eccentric hypertrophy is more common in younger subjects and those with relative volume overload (13). The shift from an eccentric to a concentric pattern among subjects with LVH may result from the increase in peripheral vascular resistance that occurs with aging. Compared to Caucasians with the same level of blood pressure, blacks in both the United States and the United Kingdom tend to have increased relative wall thickness and LV mass (14–18). One potential explanation is a blunted nocturnal decline in blood pressure in blacks compared to Caucasians (19). Gender may also influence ventricular geometry. In the Framingham study, 31% of the men and 57% of the women with isolated systolic hypertension (ISH) had increased LV mass (20). Hypertrophy tended to be of the concentric variety in women and the eccentric variety in men. Although it is generally accepted that obesity increases both wall thickness and LV internal dimension, it is controversial if the ultimate effect is a predominance of concentric or eccentric hypertrophy (21–23). In an obese individual, the geometric pattern of the ventricle will most likely be determined by whether obesity-associated volume overload (leading to an eccentric pattern) predominates over afterload (leading to a concentric pattern) (24).

Myocardial Composition

Increases in myocyte and interstitial mass that occur as the heart hypertrophies alter ventricular and vascular performance, creating a substrate for increased cardiovascular morbidity and mortality. The heart is composed of several different cell types and an extracellular matrix. Myocytes constitute approximately 75% of the heart mass (Fig. 4); the remaining 25% is the cardiac interstitium, which is comprised of the coronary vasculature, fibroblasts, macrophages, and mast cells. In hypertensive heart disease, myocytes hypertrophy, and interstitial components undergo hyperplasia, hypertrophy, and remodeling (25,26). Excess collagen production by fibroblasts increases total interstitial and periarteriolar fibrosis. This reduces ventricular compliance. Vascular smooth muscle cells undergo hyperplasia and hypertrophy that result in medial hypertrophy and coronary artery wall remodeling that is characterized by increased wall-to-lumen ratio (27). These structural changes decrease vasodilator capacity.

ETIOLOGY OF LVH

Hemodynamic Factors

Because of its profound effect on cardiovascular morbidity, it is important to determine the factors that initiate LV growth. The effect of blood pressure, as well as virtually every factor known to influence blood pressure, has been investigated for its independent effect on LV mass (Table 1).

There is very strong evidence for a causal relationship between blood pressure and absolute amount of LV mass. This was first reported over 60 years ago (25) and led to the view that myocardial hypertrophy is an adaptive cardiac response that reduces wall stress and allows the ventricle to maintain mechanical efficiency (28,29). In the Framingham Heart Study, 10% of the variation in LV mass among subjects is accounted for by differences in systolic blood pressures averaged over 30 years (30). Similarly, average blood pressure obtained during awake hours in hypertensive sub-

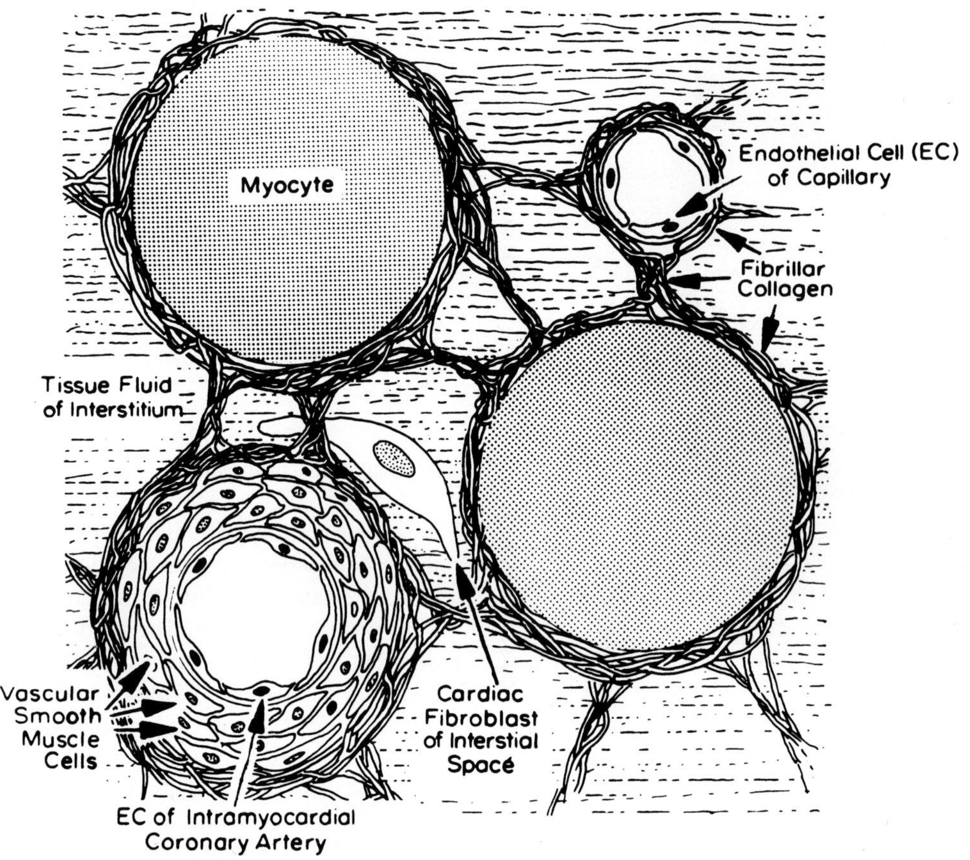

FIG. 4. Schematic representation of the cellular composition of the myocardium. The heart is composed of several different cell types and an extracellular matrix. Myocytes constitute approximately 75% of the heart mass. The remaining 25% is the cardiac interstitium, which is comprised of the coronary vasculature, fibroblasts, macrophages, and mast cells. (From Weber and Brilla, ref. 26, with permission.)

jects accounts for 10–25% of LV mass variation (31–33), whereas blunted nocturnal fall in blood pressure is associated with increased LV mass (34). In hypertensives, approximately 40% ($r = 0.66$, $p < 0.001$) of the variation in LV mass is accounted for by total LV load or peak meridional wall stress (35). In normotensives, enhanced augmentation of systolic pressure by reflected waves, a process associated with aging of the arterial tree, elevates wall stress and is associated with increased LV mass (36). Other hemodynamic factors associated with increased mass are volume, which obviously directly increases LV mass, and intrinsic contractility of the ventricle. An intrinsically hypercontractile ventricle requires less wall thickening to overcome wall stress, and thus an inverse relationship exists between LV mass and intrinsic myocardial contractility (35).

The sequence of events that leads from increased wall stress to cellular hypertrophy is only beginning to be elucidated (37). It is likely that increased wall stress activates a stretch receptor, which, through a series of cellular and subcellular events, activates growth genes, such as c-*myc* and c-*jun,* to up-regulate myocardial cell protein synthesis (28). Myocardial protein degradation may also be suppressed by increased wall tension (39). Heterogeneous cellular, subcellular, and molecular responses to the same degree of wall stress might all modify the degree of LV hypertrophy.

Nonhemodynamic Factors

Clinical studies that suggest a role for ''nonhemodynamic'' influences on LV mass must be interpreted with the knowledge that there may have been incomplete characterization of hemodynamic factors that affect LV mass, such as nocturnal blood pressure. Nevertheless, there is a large body of data indicating that the degree of left ventricular mass may be affected by many nonhemodynamic factors (Table 1). For example, in both normotensive children and adults, the degree of LV mass before blood pressure elevation is a predictor of future blood pressure. This suggests that common factors may influence both processes (40,41) and that LV mass may in some way influence blood pressure (42).

There is evidence to support a role for a genetic influence on LV mass. Perhaps the most interesting is the recent finding that a deletion in a noncoding region of the gene for angiotensin-converting enzyme is associated with electrocardiographic evidence of LVH (43). The association was

TABLE 1. *Association between LV mass and hemodynamic and nonhemodynamic factors*

Factor	Strength of evidence supporting a causal role in LV mass
Blood pressure/wall stress	Very strong (25,30–35)
LV volume	Very strong (35)
Obesity	Very strong (21,23,51,60,61)
Growth hormone and IGF-1	Strong (76,77)
Gender	Strong (54–56)
Race	Strong (14,16–18,48)
Age	Strong (women only?) (49–53)
Alcohol	Needs confirmation (62)
Intrinsic myocardial contractility	Needs confirmation (35)
Blood viscosity	Needs confirmation (334)
Insulin resistance	Needs confirmation (60,79)
Parathyroid hormone	Needs confirmation (67)
Angiotensin II	Needs confirmation (70)
Aldosterone (collagen synthesis)	Needs confirmation (26)
Polymorphism of the ACE gene	Needs confirmation (43)
Sodium intake	Needs confirmation (63)
Na^+/H^+ exchanger and $Na^+–K^+–Cl^-$ cotransport system	Needs confirmation (335)
Intracellular $[Ca^{2+}]$	Needs confirmation (64)
Plasma renin activity	Controversial (66–68)
Norepinephrine	Controversial (47,66,73–75)
Na^+/Li^+ exchanger	Controversial (335,336)

strongest in men who were normotensive, which further supports the concept that this association is independent of hemodynamic factors. The DD genotype may also be associated with concentric remodeling of the LV, a geometric pattern associated with increased cardiovascular risk (44). Epidemiologic evidence for genetic influence on LV mass includes offspring studies that generally, but not uniformly, demonstrate that LV mass in children of hypertensive parents is elevated independently of blood pressure (45,46). However, one twin study in which monozygotic twins had only minimally less intertwin variation in wall thickness than dizygotic twins or sibling pairs indicates that genetic influences on LV mass can be modified by environmental factors (47).

Further evidence for a genetic influence on LV mass is that race appears to be a determinant of ventricular structure. Studies over the past three decades suggest that for equal levels of blood pressure, blacks have greater relative wall thickness and LV mass for equivalent degrees of hypertension than Caucasians. In the Evans County Georgia study conducted between 1960 and 1962, electrocardiographic evidence of LVH was two- to threefold higher in blacks at any given level of pressure (48). In the early 1980s Dunn demonstrated with M-mode echocardiography that, for the same level of blood pressure, blacks had greater left ventricular mass (15). Hammond et al. (16) showed that for the same blood pressure and LV mass, relative wall thickness (concentric remodeling) was greater in blacks. Similarly, in the Trial of Mild Hypertension Study (TOMHS), even though blood pressure and LV mass were the same, blacks had greater wall thickness than whites (14). Similar findings were obtained in a study from London, England, which showed that for equal levels of previously untreated blood pressure, blacks had increased LV mass and RWT compared to whites (17). Even in the absence of hypertension, Hinderliter et al. (18) demonstrated that young adult blacks tend to have greater relative wall thickness than whites, suggesting that differences in ventricular structure may be inherent. Among other factors that could account for increased LV mass and RWT is that blacks have a greater total hemodynamic burden than whites because of a blunted fall in nocturnal blood pressure (19). This altered blood pressure pattern begins in adolescence.

Age and gender, obesity, and other dietary factors affect LV mass. Aging is associated with increased LV mass, but this effect may be more pronounced in women than men (49–53). Women have less LV mass for the same degree of office-determined blood pressure (54). Some of this difference is probably accounted for by reduced lean muscle mass in women compared to men (55). Experimental data suggest that some of the gender difference may be hormonally mediated (56). In addition, at least part of this gender difference may be related to a greater "white coat" effect in women, a phenomenon in which blood pressure obtained in the office is higher than the usual daily pressures. For the same level of office pressure, women have lower 24-h ambulatory blood pressure and thus would be expected to have lower LV mass (57–59).

Some studies have suggested that there are sex-specific determinants of LV mass. In the Tecumseh study of normotensive adults, LVH in men was associated with evidence of increased sympathetic nervous system activity and hyperinsulinemia, whereas in women obesity was the major determinant of LVH (60). In hypertensive women studied by the Cornell group, obesity was the predominant factor determining LV mass, whereas in men, hemodynamic factors, age, and degree of obesity all contributed (23). In Framingham, obesity increased LV mass in elderly men and women (51). Obese subjects have a greater incidence of hypertrophy, which is accounted for by increased wall thickness and oftentimes by increased left ventricular internal dimension (21,23,61). These changes are reversible with weight loss (61). Excessive alcohol intake is directly related to increased LV mass (62), and excess sodium intake may be a signal for hypertrophy (63).

Several hormones have been related to the hypertrophic process (37,64,65). The role of the plasma renin–angiotensin–aldosterone axis in hypertensive end-organ pathophysiology has been extensively explored. Some experimental and human studies (66,67) have linked plasma renin activity to degree of left ventricular hypertrophy, but this is not universally accepted (68). The product of renin activity, angiotensin I, is the substrate for angiotensin-converting enzyme. Approximately 50% of the variation in angiotensin-converting enzyme (ACE) levels can be explained by genetic factors, one of which is a deletion polymorphism in the gene that encodes for ACE. This deletion polymorphism is associated with an increased incidence of electrocardiographic LVH (43), concentric LV geometry (44), and greater risk of myocardial infarction (69). Expression and/or regulation of the ACE gene, and thus ultimately angiotensin II levels, may modulate development of LVH. This is supported by in vitro studies in which local release of angiotensin II in response to mechanical stretch is a necessary permissive factor for induction of the hypertrophic growth response (70). Aldosterone, whose synthesis is partially controlled by angiotensin II levels, appears to regulate cardiac fibroblast metabolism and growth (26). These observations may explain why elevated plasma renin levels confer a greater risk for myocardial infarction in patients with hypertension (71).

Several lines of evidence suggest that norepinephrine may influence LV mass. Regression of LVH in spontaneously hypertensive rats is enhanced by drugs that inhibit adrenergic stimuli (66). Elevated plasma norepinephrine levels in the absence of hypertension cause LVH in dogs (72), and significant increases in LV mass are induced by several weeks of diet-induced elevated endogenous catecholamine levels in normotensive offspring of hypertensive parents (73). These observations may be explained by the stimulatory role of norepinephrine on the plasma renin–angiotensin–aldosterone axis and by evidence in cell culture that, through α_1-receptors, norepinephrine can activate growth-promoting oncogenes (74). However, although it is theoretically appealing, a significant body of experimental literature questions the importance of the adrenergic stimuli in LVH development (68). Furthermore, only a minority of patients with pheochromocytoma have LVH despite the fact that this disease is characterized by extraordinarily high levels of norepinephrine (75).

Hormones and factors that regulate general growth may also be involved in myocardial hypertrophy. For example, marked increases in LV mass occur in acromegalics as a result of elevated growth hormone and insulin-like growth factor 1 (IGF-1) (76). The IGF-1 levels are higher in hypertensives with LVH (77). In utero, insulin is a trophic factor that causes macrosomia (78). Insulin levels and the degree of insulin resistance may independently modulate LV mass in normotensives and borderline hypertensive subjects (60,79). One explanation for this finding is that insulin resistance leads to increased levels of intracellular calcium, possibly as a result of decreased Na^+,K^+-ATPase activity (80). Elevated intracellular calcium may be an important stimulus for myocardial actin and myosin protein synthesis (64). This ionic hypothesis (81) may also explain the association between parathyroid hormone levels and LV mass in hypertensives (67).

DETECTION AND MEASUREMENT OF LVH

M-Mode Echocardiography

M-mode echocardiography is the most widely used anatomically validated method for determining left ventricular mass (82). Most laboratories currently obtain M-mode tracings with two-dimensional directed imaging (83). To obtain a technically adequate study, the patient is imaged in the parasternal short-axis view from the highest possible interspace. This increases the likelihood of achieving an image plane orthogonal to the LV anatomic long axis, yielding a "round" LV image in the parasternal view. The M-mode cursor is then directed through the center of the two-dimensional parasternal short axis, just distal to the mitral valve leaflets, and the M-mode gains are adjusted to optimize endocardial and epicardial interfaces. To properly measure walls and to prevent inclusion of right- and left-sided chordal echos in the septal and posterior wall, several guidelines are helpful. These include recording of the M-mode tracing with simultaneous viewing of the two-dimensional image, measurement of interfaces that show continuous motion throughout the cardiac cycle, and discarding of tracings that show abrupt posterior motion of septum in midsystole. The latter finding reflects an incorrect beam angle from a low parasternal window. In research studies, measurements of the interfaces is usually performed with the Penn convention, which excludes endocardial and epicardial surfaces in measurement of wall thickness and includes endocardial surfaces in the LV dimension measurement (82). Measurements are made in diastole on the R wave of the QRS complex. The LV mass is then calculated according to the formula:

$$1.04[(\text{ivs} + \text{pwd} + \text{lvid})^3 - \text{lvid}^3] - 13.6$$

Comparable LV mass values can be obtained with measurements made according to the American Society of Echocardiography (ASE) convention using the following formula (84):

$$0.8\ (\text{ASE mass}) + 0.6\ \text{g}$$

The ASE measurements are made at the onset of the QRS and are based on the leading-edge method (85).

There is currently no uniform method for indexing LV mass measurements for body size. The majority of published literature indexes mass by the subject's body surface area (BSA), expressed as grams per square meter (55). De Simone et al. (86) suggested that indexing LV mass by height to the 2.7 power avoids underestimation of LV hypertrophy in obese subjects (86). Until late 1994, most publications from The Framingham Heart Study indexed LV mass by the subject's height in meters (3), but recently that study has recommended indexing mass by the subject's height to the second power (87). Cutoff values for LVH based on different indexing methods are listed in Table 2.

Despite careful attention to the technical points noted above, several studies indicate that there is considerable vari-

TABLE 2. *Criteria for defining LVH based on various indexing methods*[a]

	LVM/height$^{2.7}$ (g/m$^{2.7}$) (87)	LVM/BSA (g/m^2) (4,55)	LVM/height (g/m) (87,337)	LVM/height^2 (g/m^2) (87)
95th percentile				
Men	52	125	138	78
Women	41	100	95	58
97th percentile				
Men		134		
Women		110		
2 SD above mean				
Men			143	
Women			102	

[a] BSA, body surface area; LVM, LV mass, Penn Convetion; SD, standard deviation.

ability in an individual measurement of LV mass (88,89). In the TOMHS study, the width of the 95% confidence interval for a single replicate measurement of LV mass was 60 g, or approximately 35 g/m^2 (90). Using these estimates, it can be calculated that unless LV mass index is >152 g/m^2 in a man or >128 g/m^2 in a woman, then LVH cannot be definitely diagnosed. Conversely, unless LV mass index is <116 g/m^2 in a man and <92 g/m^2 in a woman, absence of LVH cannot be definitively confirmed. Furthermore, because most studies show only a 20- to 30-g decrease in LV mass with antihypertensive treatment, a value well within the range of error of the test, routine measurement of LV mass in clinical practice is not recommended (89,91). Two-dimensional directed M-mode can be used to evaluate the effect of two different treatments on LV mass in clinical trials. The TOMHS investigators (90) calculated that approximately 109 subjects are needed per treatment group to detect a 20-g difference in treatment effect. These calculations assume a 5% possibility that such a difference is only a chance event and a 90% chance that a statistically significant difference will be detected if it exists (α of 0.05 and a power of 0.90). With these caveats in mind, cautious application of echocardiography in order to determine LV mass is reasonable in the following situations: (a) the elderly patient with resistant hypertension and significant drug side effects, in whom the presence of normal LV mass could be used to justify less aggressive treatment; (b) the young (age <40) hypertensive with mild hypertension, in whom the detection of LV hypertrophy would accelerate the initiation and acceptance of treatment; (c) the patient in whom ambulatory or home blood pressure monitoring demonstrates a significant white coat effect, because confirmation of a normal LV mass would bolster the argument against therapy.

Two-Dimensional Measurements, MRI, CT, and Three-Dimensional Imaging

Other techniques are being evaluated for their ability to measure LV mass accurately with less variability of the measurement. Two-dimensional measurements using Simpson's rule and the area–length method have been standardized and may be reproducible (92,93). However, acceptance of these measurements has been limited by several factors. These include lack of anatomic validation of the technique, which may be a result of incorrect assumptions about ventricular geometry in unusually shaped ventricles, and technical difficulties in obtaining endocardial and epicardial interfaces, especially of the lateral wall (84). These problems may be resolved by nuclear magnetic resonance imaging, which can give highly reliable and anatomically validated LV mass measurements (94,95). Three-dimensional echocardiography may also resolve these difficulties (96–98).

LEFT VENTRICULAR MASS REGRESSION

Regression of LV mass with effective blood pressure reduction has been demonstrated in over 400 clinical studies, but fewer than 10% have been double-blind placebo-controlled studies (99). Since few of these studies have been long term, it has not been determined if regression of LVH increases survival (100). It is unlikely, however, that LV mass regression will prove detrimental because LV function is not adversely affected, and diastolic function often improves (101–106). In addition, in the TOMHS trial, in which there was LV mass regression, total cardiovascular events were reduced (107).

Blood pressure reduction with all classes of antihypertensive agents reduces LV mass, with the possible exception of pure vasodilators such as minoxidil and hydralazine (66). Meta-analysis of over 100 studies demonstrates a moderately strong relationship between blood pressure reduction and LV mass regression (108). This confirms the hemodynamic contribution to LV mass and demonstrates that greater blood pressure reduction is associated with greater mass regression.

It is controversial, however, if antihypertensive agents can regress LV mass independently of their effect on blood pressure. For example, in animal studies, converting enzyme inhibitors can reduce LV mass without lowering blood pressure (109). However, one meta-analysis of human studies suggested that for equal levels of blood pressure reduction, β-blockers, converting enzyme inhibitors, and calcium channel blockers regress LVH to the same degree, whereas diuretics reduce chamber dimension but do not lead to regression of hypertrophied muscle.

This conclusion, however, has been challenged in two recent randomized trials, which suggest that diuretics are as effective as, if not more effective than, other drug classes for reducing LV mass. In the TOMHS trial, blood pressure was reduced by a combination of weight loss plus either placebo or one of five antihypertensive drug classes (β-blocker, α-blocker, calcium channel blocker, converting enzyme inhibitor, and diuretic) (107). At 1 and 4 years, all groups demonstrated LV mass regression, confirming that weight loss in conjunction with blood pressure reduction reduces LV mass. Surprisingly, only the chlorthalidone group had greater LV mass regression than the weight loss/placebo group. This was accounted for by reduced internal dimension as well as reduced wall thickness. Similar results were recently reported by the VA Cooperative Study Group, where, for equal levels of blood pressure reduction, hydrochlorothiazine had a greater effect on LV mass regression than other antihypertensive agents (110).

DIASTOLIC FUNCTION IN HYPERTENSION

Clinical Presentation

The clinical presentation of diastolic dysfunction in hypertensive heart disease is highly variable, ranging from asymptomatic findings on noninvasive testing to overt congestive heart failure despite normal systolic function (111–116). It has been estimated that 30% of patients with congestive heart failure have normal systolic function but abnormal diastolic function (116). The 7-year cardiovascular mortality approaches 50% in patients with this presentation, and many of these patients are hypertensive (117). Symptoms are accounted for by prolonged left ventricular relaxation and/or decreased compliance, which lead to either early or late diastolic shifts in the pressure–volume relationship (118) (Fig. 5).

Asymptomatic diastolic abnormalities may also occur early in the course of hypertension and precede detectable hypertrophy (33,112,119–121). Prevalence in adults without hypertrophy and with ambulatory awake blood pressure ≥130/85 mm Hg may be as high as 33% (33). Once LVH develops, however, these asymptomatic abnormalities may cause decreased exercise ejection fraction and blunt the expected rise in exercise cardiac output (122). This latter finding is probably the precursor to exertional dyspnea and fatigue associated with hypertension and normal systolic function.

Factors Affecting Diastolic Function

Genetic, structural, metabolic, and hemodynamic factors can affect diastolic function in resting conditions and during states of increased demand or ischemia. Young adult offspring of hypertensive parents demonstrate a tendency toward abnormal LV filling even before a detectable rise in blood pressure, suggesting that the factors that lead to these abnormalities may be inherited (123). In general, diastolic function is inversely related to LV mass in patients with hypertension (112,133,124–126), and regression of LV mass with calcium channel blockers, β-adrenergic blockers, and converting enzyme inhibitors is often (101,105,106, 127–129) but not uniformly (130) associated with improved LV diastolic function. Finding of a diastolic abnormality in the absence of hypertrophy may indicate that the heart is beginning to hypertrophy in response to hemodynamic or nonhemodynamic stimuli. This is suggested by evidence from the canine model of renal artery stenosis, where LV filling becomes progressively more abnormal in response to increasing LV mass (131). This early change appears to be dependent on increased myocyte size rather than increased fibrosis (132). However, there is also strong evidence that abnormal filling is partially accounted for by interstitial collagen deposition that occurs with LVH and aging, leading to passive structural changes that result in increased chamber stiffness (26,133,134).

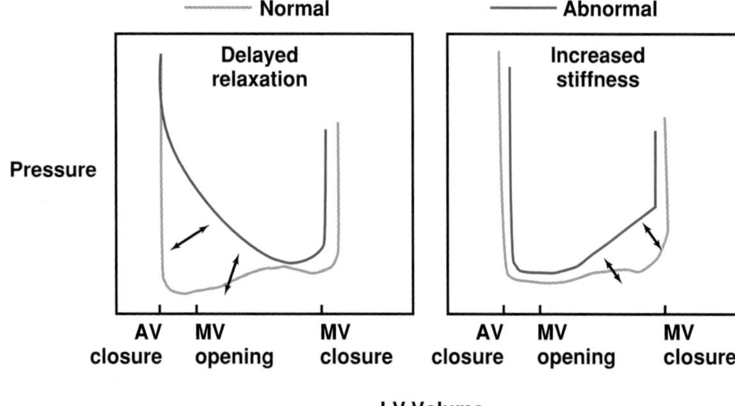

FIG. 5. In hypertensive heart disease, two types of shifts in diastolic pressure–volume relationship result in diastolic dysfunction. Patients may manifest one or both types of abnormalities. In the **left panel,** slow relaxation leads to reduced rate of LV pressure decay, which causes LV diastolic pressure to be elevated during early diastole, reducing early LV filling (see Fig. 6). In the **right panel,** increased myocardial or chamber stiffness leads to elevated left ventricular end-diastolic pressure. (Adapted from Carroll et al.)

Ischemia has a pronounced effect on diastolic function, and this is exacerbated even in the minimally hypertrophied heart (135). Several metabolic/biochemical factors that are not fully elucidated are probably involved to slow inactivation of the actin–myosin complex and delay relaxation. Baseline ATP levels in the pressure-overload hypertrophied heart are either similar to controls or slightly lower (136,137). Although it may be normal in the resting state (138), the rate of sarcoplasmic uptake of calcium, an energy-dependent and ATP-requiring step, is markedly reduced by hypoxia (139). However, diastolic dysfunction in the hypertrophied ventricle may not be fully explained by depletion of high-energy phosphates. When the isolated buffer-perfused rat heart was subjected to conditions of hypoxia, despite similar rates of ATP depletion as control hearts, hypertrophied hearts developed significantly more ischemia than controls at equivalent rates of coronary flow (136). This led the authors of that study to conclude that hypertrophy-induced alterations in calcium handling, such as changes in the calcium transient, that are abnormal even under resting conditions (140), might contribute to ischemia-induced diastolic dysfunction in LVH. In the intact dog, however, under conditions of increased oxygen demand, there was decreased conversion of phosphocreatinine to ATP in the hypertrophied heart (137), suggesting that high-energy phosphate metabolism is unfavorably altered by hypertrophy. Perhaps differences in results between the isolated heart and the intact heart are caused by failure of the intact heart to deliver adequate blood flow because of decreased coronary flow reserve.

Increased hemodynamic load and systolic function affect diastolic performance. In isolated hearts, increases in afterload early in systole impair relaxation (141). Wall stress in untreated hypertensives is inversely related to diastolic function (126). When studied with ambulatory monitoring, previously untreated borderline and mild hypertensive patients demonstrate a linear relationship between blood pressure and abnormal left ventricular filling (33,142). The degree to which acute reduction in blood pressure per se improves LV diastolic performance has not been adequately evaluated, and studies are difficult to interpret because the agents used can themselves affect performance (143,144).

Enhanced systolic performance is associated with improved diastolic function (126,145). The apparent mechanism is that systolic function directly affects the efficiency of elastic recoil (145). Increased recoil, in turn, augments the ability of the heart to generate negative pressure during early diastole, a "suction" phenomenon which increases LV filling. Catecholamines enhance diastolic function and improve LV filling through enhancement of myocardial restoring forces and recoil during isovolumic relaxation (146).

Aging has profound effects on diastolic function, which are reflected in reduced rate of LV relaxation and increased diastolic stiffness. This effect has been confirmed by various noninvasive measurements of diastolic function (33,50, 147–152). Among normal subjects in the Framingham Heart Study, age was the predominant factor affecting Doppler indices of diastolic function, with a Pearson correlation coefficient of −0.80 between age and the ratio of early to late peak filling velocity (E/A ratio) (153). Hypertension, including isolated systolic hypertension, further depresses diastolic function in older subjects (120,154,155). Exercise may reverse depressed LV diastolic function associated with aging (156).

Noninvasive Measurement of Diastolic Function

Diastolic function can be evaluated by several methods. The rate of isovolumic pressure decay, early and late LV filling, and pressure–volume relationships can be derived from cardiac catheterization (157–159). Although these measurements are the most accurate indices of diastolic function, they require an invasive procedure. Inferences regarding the diastolic properties of the ventricle can be obtained noninvasively with several techniques, such as radionuclide angiography (160) and echocardiographic techniques including M-mode (161), Doppler echocardiography (162), and acoustic quantification (163). These techniques yield information on all phases of diastole, including isovolumic relaxation, early and late LV filling (33,120,164), and temporal differences in regional filling (regional nonuniformity) (165).

Doppler echocardiographic evaluation of LV inflow is the most widely used noninvasive measure of diastolic function (166). In the setting of normal ventricular relaxation, immediately after mitral valve opening LV pressure is significantly lower than left atrial (LA) pressure, and therefore the gradient between the LA and LV is relatively high (Fig. 6). This results in a high peak velocity of early filling (E) and significant emptying of the blood in the left atrium in early diastole. As a result, the peak velocity of the late filling wave

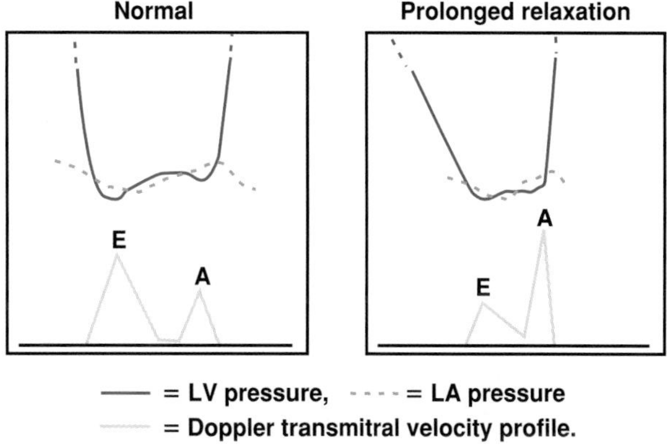

FIG. 6. Left ventricular and left atrial pressure contour and corresponding Doppler transmitral velocity profile in normal subjects **(left).** Prolonged left ventricular relaxation leads to reduced LV filling in early diastole and increased late diastolic filling **(right).** (Modified from Nishimura et al.)

(A) is low. If LV relaxation prolongs, LV pressure decline after mitral valve opening is delayed, so that the gradient between the left atrium and left ventricle in early diastole is reduced, and equilibration of pressure between the two chambers may be delayed. In the setting of normal LV function, this is reflected on the Doppler recording as a reduced E and higher A/E ratio and/or a prolonged deceleration time of the early filling wave (167,168). One mechanism for the enhanced A wave is a result of a combination of two factors: (a) as a result of decreased LV filling, LV pressure is lower than normal just prior to the atrial contraction; and (b) the delayed atrial emptying causes a rise in atrial pressure. These two factors lead to a higher gradient between the left atrium and left ventricle at atrial systole and hence to an enhanced peak A wave.

Using Doppler echocardiography, one group studied normal subjects between the ages of 20 and 50 (mean 35 $\pm$ 9), with heart rates $\leq$90 beats/min and no evidence of coronary artery disease. The average value for the peak A to peak E ratio (A/E ratio) was 0.67 $\pm$ 0.16; an A/E ratio of 0.99 was two standard deviations above this mean value (33). These data have been corroborated by others, who have similarly shown that an A/E ratio $\geq$1 in subjects under 50 years of age is significantly higher than the range for normal subjects (150). Framingham Heart Study data, however, suggest that an A/E of 1 may be in the upper range of normal for a 40- to 50-year-old and only clearly abnormal if the subject is under age 40 (Fig. 7) (169). Using Doppler echocardiography, several groups have demonstrated that approximately 20% of untreated borderline or mild hypertensives demonstrate diastolic filling abnormalities in the absence of LVH (33,170). In addition, there may be a threshold of average awake ambulatory blood pressure, 130/85 mm Hg, below which neither diastolic abnormalities nor LVH is detected (Fig. 8) (33).

Pitfalls in Interpretation of Noninvasive Measurements

Interpretation of the information derived from Doppler echocardiography should be viewed in the context of the many dynamic factors that can affect Doppler variables. These include changes in afterload, systolic performance, heart rate, and cardiac filling pressures (167,171). For example, the peak velocity of late LV filling (peak A) is directly related to heart rate (172). Therefore, a beneficial pharmacological intervention that simultaneously increases heart rate and the height of the A wave could be incorrectly interpreted as adversely affecting diastolic function. Conversely, a pharmacological intervention that raises left ventricular end-diastolic pressure could be incorrectly interpreted as beneficial if it simultaneously lowers the A wave and raises the E wave, i.e., ''pseudonormalization'' of the Doppler profile. This was demonstrated in a study in which verapamil was given to patients with coronary artery disease (173). This intervention resulted in an increased velocity of the early filling velocity (E wave) and a shortening of isovolumic relaxation. Invasive studies, however, showed that these seemingly beneficial changes were in fact associated with a prolongation of the time constant of relaxation and an increase in left ventricular end-diastolic pressure (LVEDP). Thus, increased LVEDP and LA filling pressures, not improved LV relaxation, caused a pattern of Doppler ''pseudonormalization'' characterized by a higher E wave, lower A wave, and shortened isovolumic relaxation time.

Emerging Techniques to Measure Diastolic Function

One of the challenges facing noninvasive evaluation of diastolic function is to devise methods by which LVEDP can be serially evaluated. One group has suggested that atrial natriuretic peptide, a measure of LV filling pressures, be

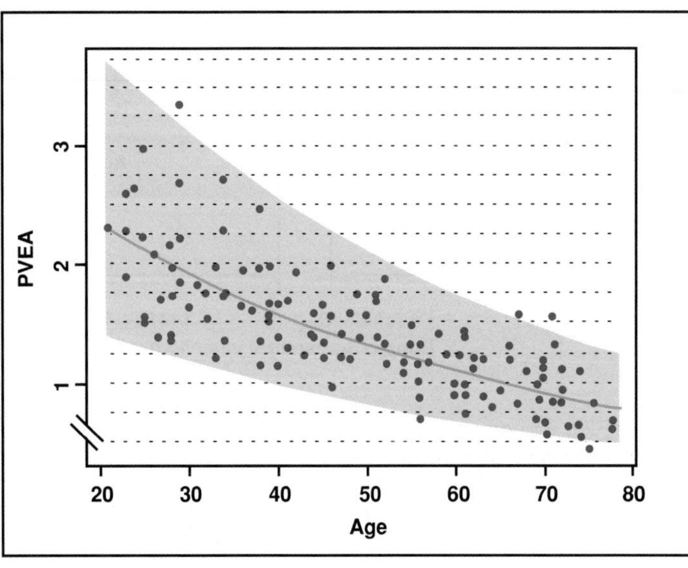

FIG. 7. Plot of predicted value of ratio of peak velocity of early filling/late filling (E/A) ratio in normal subjects studied in the Framingham Heart Study. *Solid curvilinear lines* represent the 95% confidence intervals. At approximately age 40, an E/A ratio below 1 is outside of the 95% confidence interval. (From Benjamin et al., ref. 169, with permission.)

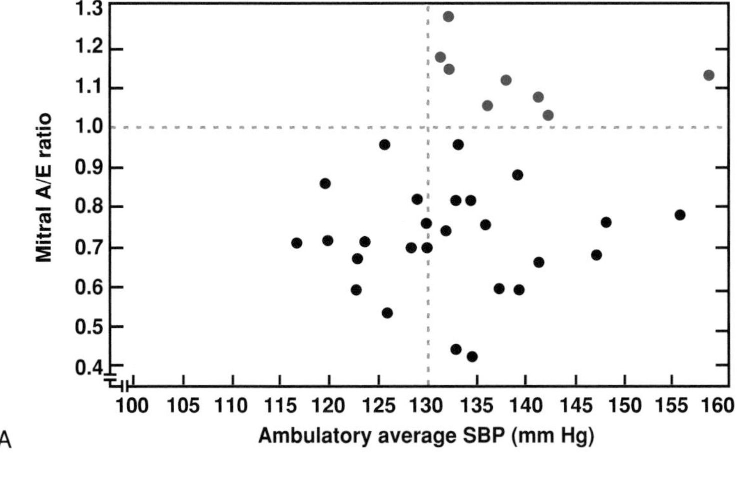

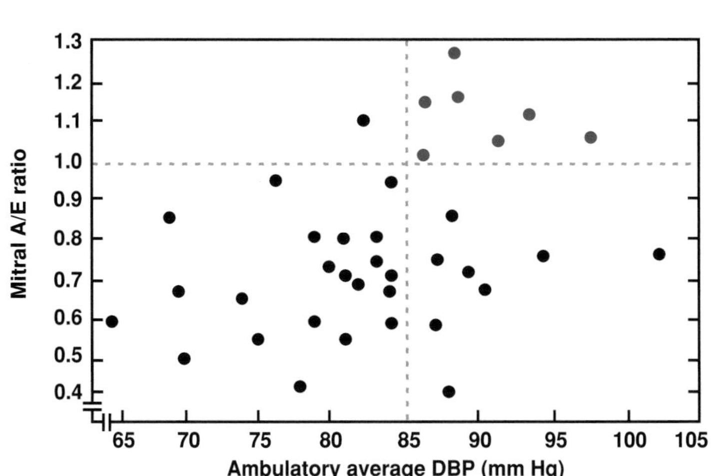

FIG. 8. Ratio of late (A) to early (E) left ventricular inflow velocity (A/E ratio) in 37 subjects (<50 years old) plotted against **(left panel)** average ambulatory awake systolic blood pressure (SBP) and **(right panel)** average awake ambulatory diastolic blood pressure (DBP). All subjects were untreated, without evidence of coronary disease, and were referred for evaluation borderline hypertension. *Horizontal hatched line* indicates A/E ratio ≥1 is abnormal in this population; *vertical hatched line* indicates blood pressure above which abnormal A/E ratio was detected. All subjects (eight, *open circles*) had SBP > 130 mm Hg. In **right panel,** only one of 22 subjects *(closed circles)* with diastolic pressure <85 mm Hg had abnormal A/E ratio, and this subject had SBP > 130; all other subjects with abnormal A/E ratio (seven, *open circles*) had DBP >85. (Reprinted with permission from the American College of Cardiology from Phillips et al., ref. 33.)

used to interpret changes in noninvasively derived LV filling parameters. Plasma levels of atrial natriuretic peptide (ANP) increase when the atria are stretched as a result of increased filling pressures (174–176). Conversely, ANP levels fall as LVEDP decreases. This physiology was exploited to interpret a Doppler evaluation of diastolic function in severely hypertensive subjects treated for 1 year with nifedipine (106). Over the year, the Doppler early filling (E wave) increased while the A wave decreased. Atrial natriuretic peptide levels fell over the year, suggesting that LVEDP had decreased. The authors concluded it was likely that the increased velocity of early filling and decreased A wave resulted from improved left ventricular relaxation.

Several new Doppler techniques are emerging that may allow for serial noninvasive interpretation of LVEDP. Among these is measurement of pulmonary venous inflow (177–179). Its usefulness rests on the fact that during atrial contraction, flow into the pulmonary vein reverses as the pulmonary veins become a ''low-pressure sink'' for the contracting atrium. Increased LVEDP creates more ''afterload'' for the atrium, leading to increased height and duration of the ''reverse flow'' wave. Furthermore, the difference in pulmonary venous and mitral flow velocity duration at atrial contraction is related to the increase in LVEDP (178). Therefore, prolonged pulmonary venous velocity duration at atrial contraction, coupled with a shortened duration of the mitral A wave, suggests increasing LVEDP. Conversely, a shorter pulmonary venous velocity duration coupled with a lengthened transmitral A wave at atrial contraction suggests decreased LVEDP.

Another promising Doppler technique to assess LVEDP rests on the observation that diastolic flow is initially directed toward the ventricular apex (transmitral A wave) and then wraps around and enters the left ventricular outflow tract just before ejection (180,181). This ''preejection wave,'' termed the Ar wave, can be identified on recordings of the left ventricular outflow tract. The time from peak of the transmitral A wave to the peak of the Ar wave (A–Ar interval) is inversely related to left ventricular chamber stiffness and LVEDP (180); i.e., the stiffer the ventricular or the higher the LVEDP, the shorter the A–Ar interval.

Color M-mode assessment of left ventricular filling is based on the interval from color M-mode peak velocity at the mitral tip to peak velocity in the apical region of the left ventricle. The interval is directly related to the time constant of isovolumic relaxation. Prolongation of the time constant, which indicates delayed LV relaxation, is associated with prolongation of the color M-mode time interval of filling.

This interval may be independent of heart rate and LVEDP. If these properties are confirmed, this technique would become extremely useful in the serial assessment of LV relaxation (182,183).

Effect of Antihypertensive Treatment on Diastolic Dysfunction

Treatment of hypertensive patients with symptoms of congestive heart failure secondary to diastolic dysfunction is guided by relatively few studies. Topol et al. (115) analyzed morbidity and mortality in 21 elderly hypertensive patients with marked concentric hypertrophy, supernormal LV systolic function, and depressed LV diastolic function. These patients were treated with a variety of antihypertensive and cardioactive agents because of heart failure, angina, stroke, or syncope. Of the 12 patients who received vasodilators (nitrates, hydralazine, prazosin, or captopril), six had a severe hypotensive reaction, and one died. By contrast, all nine patients who received β-blockers or calcium antagonists improved, and four subjects had less dyspnea after discontinuation of digoxin and furosemide. In a prospective study of 20 patients (15 hypertensive) treated in a 5-week crossover design in which verapamil and placebo were compared, verapamil treatment significantly decreased symptoms and improved exercise time (184). Compared to baseline, verapamil significantly improved LV filling, whereas placebo had no significant effect. However, probably because of a ''carryover'' effect of verapamil-induced improvement into the placebo phase of the crossover design, there was no difference between verapamil and placebo in LV filling. In six severely hypertensive patients followed for 4 months, in whom four received concomitant diuretic, nifedipine treatment was associated with symptomatic improvement (185). In another study, ten subjects with hypertension, LVH, and congestive heart failure (CHF) secondary to diastolic dysfunction were treated in a nonrandomized, uncontrolled study with the converting enzyme inhibitor enalapril and a low-sodium diet (129). After an average of 9 months of treatment, heart failure symptoms resolved in all subjects without diuretics. Diastolic function as measured by Doppler did not change after an initial decrease in blood pressure but significantly improved (decreased A/E ratio and deceleration time) after LV mass regression.

Although these studies are small, they have led to the recommendation that diuretics and pure vasodilators should be avoided in patients with congestive heart failure secondary to diastolic dysfunction and that the first line of treatment include β-blockers or calcium antagonists (186,187). Despite these recommendations, management of symptoms in these patients often requires use of diuretics (118).

The effect of antihypertensive treatment on noninvasively derived LV filling abnormalities in asymptomatic subjects has been studied with a variety of agents. Virtually no study has reported conversion from asymptomatic to symptomatic status with treatment. Thus, analysis of therapy relies on serial measurements of noninvasively derived measures of LV filling. As noted above, these studies are extremely difficult to evaluate without data on filling pressures, which are rarely provided. For example, one 8-week study comparing verapamil to lisinopril suggested that verapamil was superior because of treatment-induced shorter time to peak LV filling, reduced isovolumic relaxation time, and greater first-half filling. In that study, lisinopril actually prolonged resting isovolumic relaxation time (188). An equally compelling alternative explanation, however, is that verapamil's effect was a result of increased filling pressures (173) and lisinopril's were from decreased filling pressures.

Although one should keep this caveat in mind, many studies done over the past several years suggest that verapamil and dihydropyridine calcium channel blockers improve diastolic function (101,105,106,188,189). It is likely that some of these salubrious effects are pharmacological, but some of these studies suggest that improved filling is dependent on coincident LV mass regression (101,105,106). Studies with diltiazem showed no significant benefit, but these were flawed by either short duration of treatment (113) or by inclusion of patients whose LV diastolic function was nearly normal at baseline (190).

The effect of β-blocker therapy on diastolic function has been variable, with some studies demonstrating improved filling (in association with, but possibly independent of LV mass regression) (101,127,128) and others showing no effect (105,191). Because β-blockade antagonizes catecholamine-mediated LV relaxation, it has been suggested that β-blockade can improve diastolic function only if accompanied by blood pressure reduction, relief of ischemia, and prolongation of the time for LV filling (114,192).

Studies on the effect of converting enzyme inhibitors on diastolic function in asymptomatic hypertensives have had variable effects. Because angiotensin II (A-II) has a direct negative effect on myocardial relaxation (193), inhibition of A-II would be expected to improve LV filling. In one study in which captopril induced significant LV mass regression, Doppler indices of LV filling did not change (130). However, LV filling was normal at baseline, and thus it would not be expected that LV filling would improve. Both lisinopril (194) and enalapril have been shown to improve Doppler- or M-mode-derived indices of diastolic function (103).

DETERMINANTS OF CORONARY BLOOD FLOW ABNORMALITIES IN THE PRESENCE OF LVH

The predominant mechanism regulating coronary blood flow is the effect of oxygen demand on coronary vascular resistance. In hypertensive patients with LVH, structural and functional alterations in the small coronary vessels, increasing ventricular wall stress, and alterations in the rheologic properties of blood (e.g., increased viscosity) inhibit the ability of the coronary microcirculation to regulate overall coronary blood flow (195). This may be a major influence on the early natural history of hypertensive and nonhypertensive ischemic syndromes. These include the predisposition of hypertensive patients to heart failure and myocardial infarction and the morbidity and mortality of patients with epicardial coronary disease. Abnormalities of the coronary microcirculation may be responsible for angina pectoris in patients with normal coronary arteries (syndrome X), aortic stenosis, dilated cardiomyopathy, and cardiac allograft vasculopathy in heart transplant recipients.

Coronary Vessel Pathology in LVH

Various vascular abnormalities result in a reduction in the total maximal cross-sectional area of the coronary microvasculature. These include inadequate vascular growth in response to increasing muscle mass, changes in vessel wall composition, vascular remodeling, and vascular endothelial dysfunction.

Rarefaction of Arterioles

Morphometric studies in various animal models suggest that inadequate growth of the coronary microvascular bed is one factor limiting myocardial perfusion in the presence of pressure-overload myocardial hypertrophy (196–203). The capacity for coronary angiogenesis decreases over time. Between the ages of 9 and 14 years, heart weight increases fourfold while capillary density decreases by 28%. Capillary density in the hypertrophied heart is also age dependent. Adults with acquired aortic stenosis have decreased capillary density, whereas children with congenital aortic stenosis maintain capillary density by increasing capillary supply in proportion to myocyte volume (201,204,205). As hypertrophy progresses in the adult with hypertension, there is an insufficient angiogenesis to compensate for the increasing myocardial mass. The mechanisms for angiogenesis are complex. Factors released with increased vascular wall tension that influence cell-to-cell interactions, extracellular matrix molecules, and the inhibition and stimulation of endothelial growth factors may be important (206,207).

Medial Wall Thickening

Pressure overload with coronary arterial hypertension causes vascular medial hypertrophy with decreased lumen diameter and increased ratio of media thickness to lumen diameter (media–lumen ratio) (208–211). Comparisons of coronary vascular morphology and coronary resistance in normotensive Wistar–Kyoto (WKY) and spontaneously hypertensive rats (SHR) showed a nearly twofold increase in medial layer thickness in the coronary arterioles of the hypertensive rats (195). There was also a significantly increased ratio of medial thickness to vessel radius and increased minimal coronary resistance in the SHRs. The cellular basis for this increase in medial layer thickness is predominantly rearrangement of smooth muscle cells within the medial layers of the arterial wall and not an increase in individual myocyte cell size (212).

Perivascular and Interstitial Fibrosis

In addition to medial layer hypertrophy, pressure-overloaded cardiac hypertrophy with hypertension causes increased vascular and perivascular deposition of collagen (213–215). Inhibition of collagen deposition in vascular and extravascular myocardial tissue in the Wistar rat shows that coronary flow reserve is mostly determined by medial thickening, independent of collagen deposition. Nevertheless, collagen deposition does affect coronary blood flow because there is more reversal of coronary flow abnormalities after removing the pressure load on the heart (aortic banding) in the rats with less collagen deposition (215).

Increased Vascular Water Content

A 10% to 15% increase in the water content of arterial walls occurs in hypertensive patients. A high concentration of vascular water produces thickening of the vascular walls (even in the absence of hypertrophy) and may also cause a reduction in coronary flow reserve (195).

Endothelial Dysfunction

Vascular endothelium is an important modulator of vascular smooth muscle tone. Furchgott and Zawadzki first demonstrated that acetylcholine and other endothelial-dependent vasodilators lose their vasodilator effect when the endothelium is damaged. These vasodilators exert their effect by causing the endothelial cells to release an endogenous potent vasodilator, endothelium-derived relaxing factor (EDRF), now known to be nitric oxide (NO) (216). Impairment of endothelial function is an early vascular abnormality resulting in abnormal myocardial blood flow in patients with coronary artery disease, angina pectoris with normal coronary arteriograms, and hypertension with LVH. Although hypertensive patients have appropriate responses to the endothelial-independent vasodilators, most studies demonstrate a blunted response to acetylcholine-stimulated endothelial-dependent vasodilatation (217–221). Imbalance between endothelial-mediated vasodilatation and vasoconstriction may be an early lesion in hypertension. In spontaneously hypertensive rats (SHRs), impaired endothelial-dependent relaxation occurred before the development of overt hypertension (222). This was caused by increased production of an endothelium-derived, cyclooxygenase-dependent vasoconstrictor(s) that may be the superoxide anion.

Myocardial Hypertrophy and Wall Stress

Increased wall stress (which is one factor initiating the development of LVH in hypertensive patients) may directly moderate coronary flow reserve by causing physical compression of blood vessels. Elevated wall stress may stimulate the release of vasoactive substances that alter vascular function and growth (195). Patients with nonhypertensive left ventricular hypertrophy without ventricular dilatation and increased wall tension (i.e., some cases of aortic stenosis, hypertrophic obstructive and hypertrophic nonobstructive cardiomyopathy with no ventricular dilatation) do not have decreased coronary flow reserve. Those with hypertension with similar degrees of left ventricular hypertrophy, or aortic stenosis with ventricular dilation and increased left ventricular end diastolic pressures, however, show abnormally decreased flow reserve (223,224). This effect is also seen in patients with dilated cardiomyopathy (225) and dilated ventricles caused by aortic regurgitation (226,227).

ALTERATIONS OF CORONARY AUTOREGULATION AND FLOW RESERVE WITH LVH

The coronary circulation is able to maintain a relatively stable blood flow supply over a wide range of perfusion pressures (228–231). This range varies in different experiments but is generally between 70 and 130 mm Hg in humans (232). Coronary flow decreases markedly when perfusion pressure drops below the lower limit of autoregulation.

Proposed Mechanisms of Autoregulation

Both metabolic and myogenic mechanisms may produce autoregulation of coronary flow. Different sites in the microvascular may have different dominant mechanisms of control (233). The smallest coronary arterioles are predominantly sensitive to metabolic factors, whereas larger arterioles are more reactive to myogenic stimuli. According to the metabolic theory, a decrease in coronary artery perfusion pressure results in decreased blood flow. Subsequent decreases in myocardial substrate availability or increases in production of metabolites produce vasodilatation (234). Potential mediators include oxygen (myocardial oxygen tension), potassium and calcium ion concentrations (transmembrane potentials), osmolality, adenosine, prostaglandins, carbon dioxide, and hydrogen ion concentrations (235–237). Myogenic regulation is an intrinsic mechanism: application of force to vascular smooth muscle results in contraction (238–240). In the coronary circulation, there are difficulties in demonstrating myogenic responses because they are closely integrated with metabolic factors (241).

Relationship Between Autoregulated Coronary Flow and Maximal Coronary Flow

Coronary flow reserve is, for any given perfusion pressure, the decrease in coronary resistance over the resting state that occurs after maximal coronary vasodilatation. A normal human heart can increase coronary flow by a factor of four to five times over the resting state (223). Coronary flow increases above resting autoregulated levels after transient coronary arterial occlusion (reactive hyperemia), exercise, pacing, or injection of agents such as dipyridamole, adenosine, papaverine, or hyperosmolar iodinated contrast media (242). Loss of autoregulation occurs during these events. Coronary flow reserve is a dynamic value that is dependent on coronary perfusion pressure. Because there is no autoregulation during states that produce maximal coronary flow, the relationship between coronary flow and coronary perfusion pressure is linear. Relatively small changes in perfusion pressure produce large changes in coronary flow reserve.

Factors That Confound the Measurement of CFR

Increased heart rate, contractility, and afterload all decrease CFR, and therefore all confound measurement of coronary flow reserve. It is not clear if they increase baseline flow, decrease maximal flow, or both (243,244). In humans, Doppler measurements of coronary blood flow during pacemaker-induced tachycardia show increased resting coronary flow velocity but not peak velocity with papaverine administration (244). The use of potent vasodilators to quantify coronary flow reserve may result in a blunted measurement, if there is any significant increase in heart rate. Body size may also influence absolute values of maximal coronary blood flow (245). Elevations in aortic pressure increase myocardial oxygen consumption and blood flow. Consequently, shifts in mean aortic pressure produce alterations in autoregulated (resting) blood flow. By using the relationship among mean aortic pressure, coronary flow reserve, and coronary vascular resistance (coronary flow = mean aortic pressure/coronary resistance), one may calculate a coronary resistance ratio (246). The resistance ratio may be less sensitive than a flow ratio to changes in arterial pressure (242).

In addition to external confounding factors, there are intrinsic factors in the definition and measurement of CFR that produce confusion. Coronary flow reserve can be measured either as the difference of maximal and resting flow (absolute CFR) or the ratio of maximal flow to resting flow (relative CFR). It is not clear which measurement is clinically more relevant. In hypertensive patients with left ventricular hypertrophy, it is possible to have a normal or mildly increased absolute coronary flow reserve with a reduced relative coronary flow reserve (242).

Many current methods of measuring coronary flow reserve are not sensitive to changes in coronary flow reserve over different layers of myocardium. Coronary flow reserve is lower in subendocardial muscle for all perfusion pressures. Some of the newer noninvasive techniques such as cine-CT and NMR may be able to measure CFR in the different layers of myocardium; however, data are still very preliminary.

Effect of Hypertension and LVH on CFR

Coronary flow reserve can be measured as absolute flow or as flow per unit muscle mass (Fig. 9) (247). Although resting absolute coronary blood flow of the entire left ventricle increases with LVH, resting coronary blood flow per gram of myocardium is unchanged. Total maximal ventricular flow does not significantly change with acquired LVH, whereas total flow per gram of myocardium decreases. This is because of the lack of vascular growth in response to increasing muscle mass. Thus, when absolute flow is measured, resting flow is high, and maximal flow is normal (panel A, Fig. 9). If flow per gram is measured, resting flow per gram myocardium is normal, but maximal flow per gram myocardium is reduced (panel B, Fig. 9). Consequently, CFR is less than normal whether measured as absolute flow or flow per gram of myocardium.

In the presence of hypertension, absolute coronary flow reserve may theoretically be normal or increased despite higher resting absolute coronary blood flow. This is because of the higher coronary perfusion pressure (shift to the right side of the curve) as shown by R_3 in Fig. 9. Nevertheless, in most cases of hypertensive heart disease, vascular abnormalities and increased LVEDP result in reduced maximal flow and thus a decrease in coronary flow reserve (224,248–250). Most (226,249,251), but not all (252,253), studies show an inverse linear relationship between the extent of LVH and coronary flow reserve.

Other factors (e.g., race, gender, diabetes, cigarette smoking, prior therapies) also influence coronary flow reserve (254–258). In a recent evaluation of endothelial-dependent vasodilatation of the brachial artery, reduced flow-mediated dilation was related to age. Noticeable decline began in men after age 40 years, but function was preserved in women until their 50s (259). This delay in women may reflect protective effects of estrogen because their decline appeared to correlate with the onset of menopause. In a study of the coronary circulation, age and total serum cholesterol were found to be independent predictors of a blunted vasodilatory response to acetylcholine (260). Analysis of spontaneously hypertensive rat (SHR) strains and normotensive rats showed that hypertension and aging independently result in structural alterations in coronary resistance vasculature with a decrease in the ratio of lumen diameter to wall thickness. Arteriolar density was not decreased by aging (261). Racial differences were demonstrated in a study showing that blacks have decreased CFR compared to Caucasians, independent of LVH (254).

Hypertension may alter coronary flow reserve prior to the development of LVH. This was suggested by a cross-sectional analysis of hypertensive and nonhypertensive pa-

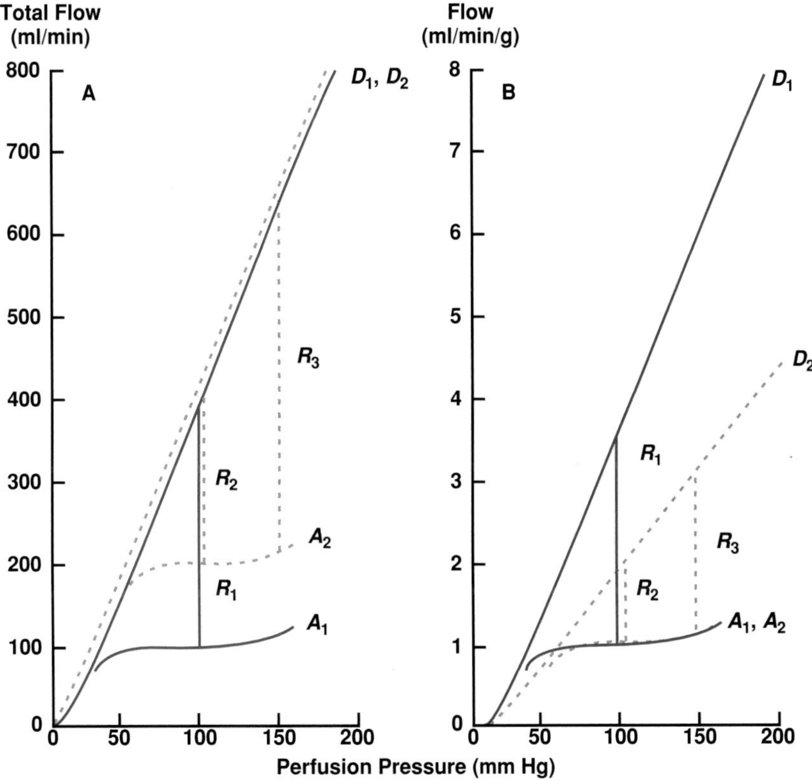

FIG. 9. Diagram of coronary flow reserve in the presence of hypertrophy. In **panel A,** absolute flow is measured (ml/min). In **panel B,** flow per unit mass (ml/min per g) is measured. A, autoregulated flows; D, pressure flow line during maximal vasodilatation; R, flow reserve. Normal are A_1, D_1, R_1, and *solid lines.* Hypertrophied are A_2, D_2, R_2, R_3, and *dashed lines.* In both scenarios, coronary flow reserve is diminished. R_3 represents coronary flow reserve when perfusion pressures are elevated. (From Hoffman, ref. 232, with permission.)

tients. Although coronary flow reserve was lowest in untreated hypertensive patients with increased LV mass, patients with hypertension and normal LV mass had lower CFR than normotensive patients (262). This must be viewed with caution, however, because cross-sectional studies do not allow one to analyze other factors that may influence coronary blood flow such as duration of hypertension and prior antihypertensive therapies. Whether or not linearly related, most studies suggest that LVH is strongly associated with reduced coronary flow reserve. Thus, abnormalities of coronary flow reserve may partially explain why patients with hypertension and LVH are at increased risk for myocardial ischemia and infarction (5).

Effect of BP Reduction on Autoregulated Blood Flow and CFR

Experimental and clinical studies demonstrate that blood pressure reduction in hypertensive patients with LVH may result in increased myocardial ischemia. Resting absolute coronary flow is high in these patients, and loss of autoregulated flow occurs at higher perfusion pressures (the autoregulatory curve is shifted upward and to the right). In experimentally induced LVH, although marked reductions in coronary perfusion pressure from 100 to 40 mm Hg have minimal effect on autoregulation in the subepicardium, the ability of the subendocardium to autoregulate is reduced by more than 50% (263). This may account for the increased size of myocardial infarction associated with experimentally induced coronary ligation in hypertrophied hearts (264,265). Recovery of stunned myocardium (systolic thickening and regional myocardial blood flow) in the period immediately following transient coronary occlusion is delayed in the presence of LVH, and even more so when blood pressure is lowered during this early reperfusion period (266).

Blood pressure reduction in hypertensive human subjects without LVH does not significantly change resting coronary blood flow when perfusion pressure is acutely lowered with nitroprusside from 120 to 70 mm Hg. However, when hypertrophy is present with hypertension, there is a marked decline in flow as perfusion pressure decreases from 90 to 70 mm Hg (Fig. 10) (267). This suggests that a reduction of blood pressure to less than 90 mm Hg in patients with LVH could cause ischemia. This observation may in part explain the limited impact that blood pressure reduction has on reducing mortality from coronary artery disease as compared to reducing the incidence of nonfatal and fatal stroke in studies in which patients had both systolic and diastolic hypertension. Analysis of several large prospective observational studies suggests that a 5 to 6 mm Hg decrease in diastolic blood pressure would cause a 20% to 25% reduction in coronary events. However, this degree of reduction in blood pressure has resulted in only a 14% decrease in coronary events (268,269).

A J-curve may describe the relationship between mortality rate from myocardial infarction and treated diastolic blood pressure (270). The J-curve implies that hypertensive subjects without coronary disease may benefit from decreasing blood pressure as much as possible; however, those with ischemic disease and a treated diastolic blood pressure of <85–95 mm Hg may have an upturn in coronary events. This is presumably a result of inadequate perfusion of coronary arteries. Support for and against this relationship is based on differing interpretations and results of retrospective analyses of several large treatment trials or programs (271–275). For example, in one retrospective analysis, men with LVH or ischemic patterns on ECG had an increased

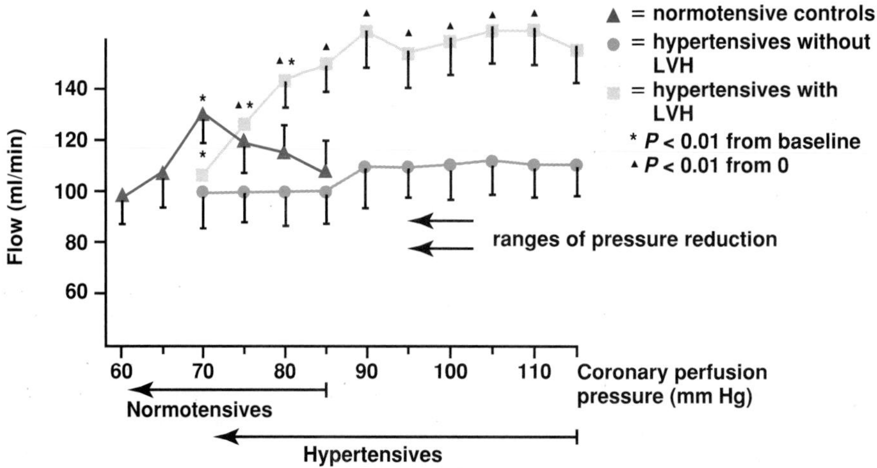

FIG. 10. Effect of acute reduction in coronary perfusion pressure on coronary autoregulation in controls with normotension, patients with hypertension without LVH, and patients with hypertension and LVH. Autoregulatory curves for hypertension with LVH is shifted upward and to the right. At coronary perfusion pressure <90 mm Hg, patients with hypertension and LVH have marked loss of coronary autoregulation. (Adapted from Polese et al., ref. 267, with permission.)

incidence of MI when treated diastolic blood pressures were below 95 mm Hg (276). By contrast, in the Systolic Hypertension in the Elderly (SHEP) trial, coronary events were decreased in subjects with evidence of LVH by ECG criteria and low treatment diastolic blood pressures (277). Although this may argue against a J-curve, it is important to realize that these patients had low diastolic pressures before treatment, and hence their autoregulatory curve was already adjusted to lower pressure.

The possibility of a J-curve poses obvious treatment dilemmas for the physician. For example, although the hypertrophied heart may suffer deleterious effects from "excessively" low blood pressure, the rate of progression of kidney disease may be blunted by significantly lower pressure (278), a hypothesis that is being tested in the African American Study of Kidney Disease and Hypertension (projected completion in year 2001). Because subjects with LVH often have renal dysfunction, the point to which BP is lowered may be a tradeoff between renal and cardiovascular complications.

Recommendations for the safest level of blood pressure reduction in patients with LVH can be only speculative at this point. In patients with isolated systolic hypertension, in which the pretreatment diastolic BP is already low, SHEP trial data indicate that further reduction of diastolic BP is safe. On the other hand, patients with diastolic hypertension and LVH (without renal disease) may suffer complications of reduced coronary blood flow when blood pressure is lowered below 85–90 mm Hg, particularly in the presence of CAD. Whether or not lowering blood pressure below 85–90 mm Hg is warranted in the presence of renal disease and LVH will require further study. The presence of systolic dysfunction, particularly in association with CAD, adds more controversial variables to this dilemma and will require more investigation.

EFFECT OF EPICARDIAL CORONARY ARTERY DISEASE ON CFR

Current research is focusing on the alterations of CFR that occur in the presence of CAD. At the site of coronary stenoses, autoregulation maintains normal resting flow with as much as 85% stenosis. In more severe stenoses, there is a large pressure gradient between the aorta and coronary artery with a drop in coronary flow from loss of autoregulation (279). The ability to augment flow with maximal vasodilatation is also hampered by severe coronary obstructions. Thus, coronary flow reserve decreases.

After acute myocardial infarction, the coronary vasodilator response in the infarcted myocardial region remains severely impaired despite successful recanalization of the infarct-related artery by thrombolysis (280). This has been attributed to dysfunction of resistance vessels in the infarcted zone. Recent studies using PET quantification of coronary flow reserve show that patients with either chronic stable angina or recent myocardial infarction have reduced coronary flow reserve in regions supplied by normal arteries remote from ischemic or infarcted myocardium (281,282). The reasons for this are not yet clear. The impairment in CFR may be a manifestation of microvascular endothelial dysfunction, an early phase of angiographically undetectable coronary atherosclerosis. These abnormalities may play a crucial role in the natural history of coronary artery disease and the ventricular remodeling that occurs after myocardial infarction.

EFFECT OF ANTIHYPERTENSIVE TREATMENT ON CFR

In order to reduce the risk of coronary events in arterial hypertension, therapy should be geared at reversing the chief cardiac manifestations: left ventricular hypertrophy and coronary microcirculatory abnormalities.

Studies in hypertensive rodent and canine models show that reduction of wall stress results in regression of LVH, reversal of coronary vascular abnormalities, and improved overall coronary blood flow (215,283–286). The effects of antihypertensive therapy on vascular pathology in humans, however, are not well understood. Heagerty, Bund, and Aalkjaer (287) obtained serial skin biopsies of subcutaneous resistance arterioles in hypertensive patients. After long-term treatment with various combinations of β-blockers, calcium channel blockers, diuretics and ACE inhibitors, they demonstrated partial regression of the medial layer of these vessels (287). It is not known if parallel changes occur in coronary vessels.

There are few human studies on the effects of antihypertensive therapy on coronary blood flow reserve. Preliminary data using the gas chromatographic argon method of quantifying coronary flow reserve showed improved flow reserve in hypertensive patients after 12 months of therapy with enalapril (288). By blocking the production of angiotensin II, angiotensin-converting enzyme inhibitors may be effective in improving coronary flow reserve. This may be related to a reduction in perivascular and interstitial fibrosis (289).

The effect of calcium channel blockers on coronary flow reserve is even less clear. Although they produce favorable hemodynamic effects with reversal of pressure overload and regression of LVH, several studies suggest that certain calcium channel blockers do not significantly change, or may even reduce, coronary flow reserve (290–292). Theoretically, calcium channel blockers may reduce coronary flow reserve by blocking the effect of endogenous vasodilators such as adenosine (293).

METHODS OF MEASUREMENT OF CFR

Radionuclide-Labeled Microspheres

Since the first studies utilizing particles to study the circulation by Pohlman in the early 1900s, various materials (e.g., glass, ceramic, carnauba wax) were developed as microspheres (294,295). Macroaggregates of albumin can be radiolabeled and can be used in humans because they are metabolizable and release the nuclide label for excretion. The lack of uniformity of size is a disadvantage for measuring organ blood flow (296–299). Insoluble inert plastic microspheres are made in uniform spherical sizes. They are the most commonly used nuclide-labeled microsphere and are considered the ''gold standard'' for measuring blood flow (300). Because the microspheres are permanently lodged in tissues and are quantified by counting dissected tissue samples in a well counter, this technique is only suitable for animal research studies. The particles injected into the systemic circulation cannot recirculate because of capillary entrapment. The distribution in body organs will be proportional to organ blood flow provided that certain criteria be met: (a) an adequate number of spheres must be injected, but not so many as to produce hemodynamic alterations; (b) the spheres must be well mixed at the site of the injection; and (c) all microspheres must be entrapped in the peripheral microcirculation during the first circulation, so the sphere size must be large enough to prevent them from passing through the organs into the venous system (300–303). Under these conditions, blood flow to any organ may be calculated using Heymann's formula (300).

Invasive Techniques

Coronary sinus thermodilution is accomplished by cannulating the coronary sinus via percutaneous right heart catheterization (304). This method is inexpensive, widely available, and safe; however, there are important limitations (305). The region of the left ventricle that is assessed is dependent on the position of the catheter within the coronary sinus and is unpredictable. This problem can be partially solved by placing the catheter in the great cardiac vein, thus limiting flow predominantly to the distribution of the left anterior descending artery (306).

Gas clearance methods use several nonradioactive gases (nitrous oxide, hydrogen, helium, and argon) and radioactive xenon-133. In this technique, simultaneous arterial and coronary sinus blood samples are obtained for measurements of gas concentration during the saturation or destruction phase of gas administration. These techniques are time consuming and require special equipment for sample analysis. Very stable conditions are required for accurate measurements. As with thermodilution, spatial resolution is limited. The use of radioactive ^{133}Xe has increased the spatial resolution of the gas clearance approach. However, this gas must be introduced directly into the coronary arteries and requires a multicrystal γ camera and computer for data acquisition and analysis. In both thermodilution and gas clearance techniques, the long time constant of the method (seconds to minutes) limits their use in rapid serial assessment of coronary flow (i.e., before and after drug infusion or exercise). Gas clearance techniques are reasonably accurate; however, this is limited to flow rates <200 mg/100 g.

Videodensitometry measures the contrast transit time from videodensitometric data. This requires intraarterial injection of contrast. This method is accurate over a wide range of coronary flow, and rapid serial measurements may be obtained. This approach is used to measure flow in bypass grafts (307). New advances have allowed ultrafast CT to replace conventional angiography in videodensitometry. The increased density resolution with computed tomography allows for intravenous injection of the contrast (308). Spatial resolution has improved with videodensitometry by the addition of digital subtraction angiography (309). Regional flow reserve is calculated by comparing appearance time and maximum contrast concentration at baseline and during maximal coronary vasodilatation. Various color- and intensity-coded images are used to depict timing and density of contrast medium as it travels through the coronary circulation. This technique is accurate over a wide range of coronary flow reserve; however, it is technically demanding and requires specialized imaging equipment. Furthermore, this technique is subject to motion artifact.

The development of an intracoronary 3 French Doppler catheter has made it possible to record changes in phasic flow velocity in individual coronary arteries in conscious humans. This is accomplished during cardiac catheterization (310). Although absolute flows cannot be measured, changes in coronary blood flow velocity accurately reflect coronary flow reserve over a wide range of flows. This accuracy is lost, however, if the cross-sectional area of the artery at the site of the Doppler crystal does not change. This is achieved by pretreating the coronary arteries with nitrates. On the whole, Doppler measurement of coronary flow reserve is accurate and has been validated against the microsphere, thermodilution, and other methods (310,311).

Noninvasive Techniques

Noninvasive imaging techniques used to quantify coronary flow reserve include positron emission tomography (PET), ultrafast computed tomography, contrast echocardiography, transesophageal Doppler techniques, magnetic resonance imaging, and single-photon emission computed tomography.

The most accurate noninvasive measure of regional myocardial blood flow noninvasively was made by the measurement of positron-emitting flow tracers such as ^{13}N-ammonia ($^{13}NH_3$) and rubidium-82 (^{82}Rb) (312–318). Limitations of these tracers, such as the dependence of metabolism as well as perfusion on uptake, are overcome by freely diffusable tracers such as ^{15}O-water ($H_2{}^{15}O$) and ^{11}C-butanol (319,320). However, these tracers must be produced in an on-site cyclotron, and they label the myocardium and blood pool simultaneously. Although ^{82}Rb can be produced in an inexpensive generator, the overall cost effectiveness and availability of PET scanning remain important issues. Other limitations include the limited resolution of positron cameras and imaging motion artifacts.

Analysis of time–video-intensity curves after injection of ultrasonic contrast microbubbles allows assessment of coronary flow reserve by two-dimensional echocardiography (321,322). This technique shows promise; however, there are limitations. Changes in intramyocardial blood volume with coronary vasodilators affect the time–intensity curve, often resulting in underestimation of coronary flow reserve. The size and type of ultrasonic contrast microbubbles may also influence the time–video-intensity curves. Finally, this technique requires sophisticated ultrasound systems.

Transesophageal Doppler echocardiography is a seminoninvasive method of determining coronary flow reserve that does not require as much specialized technical equipment as does PET imaging. It is safe and may be used for serial measurements. Adequate Doppler images are obtained in approximately 70% of patients, however, and the angle between the exploring ultrasound beam and vessel direction often causes underestimation of blood flow velocities (323).

Thallium-201 imaging perfusion defects are associated with depressed coronary vasodilator reserve in hypertensive patients with chest pain who do not have obstructive coronary artery disease (244,324). After intravenous injection, the early myocardial uptake of radionuclide imaging agents such as thallium-201 and technetium-99m teboroxime is proportional to regional myocardial blood flow over a wide range of coronary flow. With high coronary flow, however, there is a flattening of the uptake curve, thus limiting the resolution. In the canine model, uptake of these agents significantly correlated with a wide range of regional flow as determined by the radioactive microsphere technique (325–327). Studies are currently being conducted with these agents to see if single-photon emission tomography accurately quantifies coronary flow reserve. This technique may provide a more widely available and less costly alternative to PET (328,329).

There are other noninvasive tools that are in early stages of investigation. Intravenous contrast injection followed by in vivo analysis of regional contrast clearance by ultrafast CT quantitates blood flow and volume. There is a curvilinear relationship with microsphere measurement of coronary blood flow in the canine model (330). A major limitation of this technique is inaccuracy of measurement at high myocardial flow rates. This has been overcome by injection of the contrast directly into the aortic root (331). This modification, however, makes the technique invasive and thus not suited to routine clinical evaluations. More investigation of less invasive means of administering contrast will be needed.

Indirect quantification of coronary flow reserve by velocity mapping of diastolic ascending aortic blood flow by magnetic resonance imaging (MRI) is under study (332). According to this technique, retrograde flow in the ascending aorta during systole and diastole minus the antegrade flow during diastole equals the coronary diastolic flow. Direct measure of coronary flow by MRI is hampered by motion of the coronary arteries during cardiac contraction and respiration and the small size of the coronary arteries. New mathematical models are being developed to allow intracoronary analysis of blood flow velocity by MRI (333). Thus, MRI is a promising noninvasive technique for accurate assessment of coronary blood flow. Although it has been validated against phantom models of blood flow, future research will require comparison with invasive methods.

THE FUTURE OF EVALUATION AND TREATMENT OF HYPERTENSIVE HEART DISEASE

Over the next several years, many developments are likely to occur. Positive results on the effect of LV mass regression on mortality may emerge. Better methods for reproducible measurements of LV mass, such as three-dimensional echocardiographic imaging and MRI, may become more widespread, allowing accurate serial measurements of LV mass. Increased understanding of the cellular and biochemical basis of abnormal myocardial contraction and relaxation associated with myocardial hypertrophy and interstitial fibrosis will occur. For example, studies of human biopsy material may delineate subcellular changes in the myocyte that account for altered handling of intracellular calcium, which results in diastolic and eventually systolic dysfunction. Genes and growth factors that control myocardial growth will be determined. This will include clarification of the molecular mechanism by which hemodynamic stimuli initiate LVH of the genotypes that predispose to LVH. Identifying these genes may allow design of agents that can turn off vascular and myocardial hypertrophy. The role of hormonal, dietary, and other nonhemodynamic factors that influence LV mass will be clarified.

The link between abnormalities of the coronary microcirculation and increased cardiovascular morbidity and mortality associated with hypertensive heart disease will be further clarified in the near future. New imaging techniques and refinements in existing techniques such as PET imaging, MRI, and ultrafast CT will allow for more accurate and serial quantification of myocardial blood flow and flow reserve. Animal models will be developed to study the biochemical and genetic factors controlling angiogenesis, endothelial secretion of regulatory factors, and vascular smooth muscle changes in these disease states.

REFERENCES

1. Schwartzkopff B, Motz W, Vogt M, Strauer B. Heart failure on the basis of hypertension. *Circulation* 1993;87(Suppl IV):IV-66–IV-72.
2. Katz AM. The cardiomyopathy of overload: An unnatural growth response in the hypertrophied heart. *Ann Intern Med* 1994;121: 363–371.
3. Levy D, Anderson KM, Savage D, Kannel WB, Christiansen JC, Castelli WP. Echocardiographically detected left ventricular hypertro-

phy: Prevalence and risk factors. The Framingham Heart Study. *Ann Intern Med* 1988;108:7–13.

4. Casale PN, Devereux RB, Milner M, Zullo G, Harshfield GA, Pickering TG, Laragh JH. Value of echocardiographic measurement of left ventricular mass in predicting cardiovascular morbid events in hypertensive men. *Ann Intern Med* 1986;105:173–178.
5. Levy D, Garrison RJ, Savage DD, Kannel WB, Castelli WP. Prognostic implications of echocardiographically determined left ventricular mass in the Framingham Heart Study. *N Engl J Med* 1990;322: 1561–1566.
6. Bikkina M, Larson MG, Levy D. Asymptomatic ventricular arrhythmias and mortality risk in subjects with left ventricular hypertrophy. *J Am Coll Cardiol* 1993;22:1111–1116.
7. Cooper RS, Simmons BE, Castaner A, Santhanam V, Ghali J, Mar M. Left ventricular hypertrophy is associated with worse survival independent of ventricular function and number of coronary arteries severely narrowed. *Am J Cardiol* 1990;65:441–445.
8. Ghali JK, Liao Y, Simmons B, Castaner A, Cao G, Cooper RS. The prognostic role of left ventricular hypertrophy in patients with or without coronary artery disease. *Ann Intern Med* 1992;117:831–836.
9. Lewis JF, Maron BJ. Diversity of patterns of hypertrophy in patients with systemic hypertension and marked left ventricular wall thickening. *Am J Cardiol* 1990;65:874–881.
10. Ganau A, Devereux RB, Roman MJ, De Simone G, Pickering TG, Saba PS, Vargiu P, Simongini I, Laragh JH. Patterns of left ventricular hypertrophy and geometric remodeling in essential hypertension. *J Am Coll Cardiol* 1992;19:1550–1158.
11. Koren MJ, Devereux RB, Casale PN, Savage DD, Laragh JH. Relation of left ventricular mass and geometry to morbidity and mortality in uncomplicated essential hypertension. *Ann Intern Med* 1991;114: 345–352.
12. Nunez BD, Lavie CJ, Messerli FH, Schmieder RE, Garavaglia GE, Nunez M. Comparison of diastolic left ventricular filling and cardiac dysrhythmias in hypertensive patients with and without isolated septal hypertrophy. *Am J Cardiol* 1994;74:585–589.
13. Savage DD, Garrison RJ, Kannel WB, Levy D, Anderson SJ, Stokes J, Feinleib M, Castelli WP. The spectrum of left ventricular hypertrophy in a general population sample: The Framingham Study. *Circulation* 1987;75(Suppl I):I-26–I-33.
14. Liebson PR, Grandits G, Prineas R, Dianzumba S, Flack JM, Cutler JA, Grimm R, Stamler J. Echocardiographic correlates of left ventricular structure among 844 mildly hypertensive men and women in the treatment of mild hypertension study (TOMHS). *Circulation* 1993; 87:476–486.
15. Dunn FG, Oigman W, Sungard-Rise K, Messerli FH, Ventura H, Reisen E, Frohlich ED. Racial differences in cardiac adaptation to essential hypertension determined by echocardiographic indexes. *J Am Coll Cardiol* 1983;5:1348–1351.
16. Hammond IW, Alderman MH, Devereux RB, Lutas EM, Laragh JH. Contrast in cardiac anatomy and function between black and white patients with hypertension. *J Natl Med Assoc* 1984;76:247–255.
17. Mayet J, Shahi M, Foale RA, Poulter NR, Sever PS, McG Thom SA. Racial differences in cardiac structure and function in essential hypertension. *Br Med J* 1994;308:1011–1014.
18. Hinderliter AL, Light KC, Willis PW. Racial differences in left ventricular structure in healthy young adults. *Am J Cardiol* 1992;69: 1196–1199.
19. Harshfield GA, Alpert BS, Willey ES, Somes GW, Murphy JK, Dupaul LM. Race and gender influence ambulatory blood pressure patterns of adolescents. *Hypertension* 1989;14:598–603.
20. Krumholz HM, Larson M, Levy D. Sex differences in cardiac adaptation to isolated systolic hypertension. *Am J Cardiol* 1993;72:310–313.
21. Lauer MS, Anderson KM, Levy D. Separate and joint influences of obesity and mild hypertension on left ventricular mass and geometry: The Framingham Heart Study. *J Am Coll Cardiol* 1992;19,1:130–134.
22. Schmieder RE, Messerli FH. Does obesity influence early target organ damage in hypertensive patients. *Circulation* 1993;87:1482–1488.
23. De Simone G, Devereux RB, Roman MJ, Alderman MH, Laragh JH. Relation of obesity and gender to left ventricular hypertrophy in normotensive and hypertensive adults. *Hypertension* 1994;23: 600–606.
24. Messerli FH. Clinical determinants and consequences of left ventricular hypertrophy. *Am J Med* 1983;(September 26):51–56.
25. Chantin A, Barksdale EE. Experimental renal insufficiency produced by partial nephrectomy. II. Relationship of left ventricular hypertrophy, the width of the cardiac muscle fiber and hypertension in the rat. *Arch Intern Med* 1933;52:739.
26. Weber KT, Brilla CG. Pathological hypertrophy and cardiac interstitium. Fibrosis and renin–angiotensin–aldosterone system. *Circulation* 1991;83:1849–1865.
27. Schwartzkopff B, Motz W, Frenzel H, Vogt M, Knauer S, Eckehard Strauer B. Structural and functional alterations of the intramyocardial coronary arterioles in patients with arterial hypertension. *Circulation* 1993;88:993–1003.
28. Grossman W, Jones D, McLaurin LP. Wall stress and patterns of hypertrophy in the human left ventricle. *J Clin Invest* 1975;56:56–64.
29. Badeer HS. Biological significance of cardiac hypertrophy. *Am J Cardiol* 1964;14:133–137.
30. Lauer MS, Anderson KM, Levy D. Influence of contemporary versus 30-year blood pressure levels on left ventricular mass and geometry: The Framingham Heart Study. *J Am Coll Cardiol* 1991;18,5: 1287–1294.
31. Rowlands DB, Glover DR, Ireland MA, McLeay RAB, Stallard TJ, Watson RDS, Littler WA. Assessment of left-ventricular mass and its response to antihypertensive treatment. *Lancet* 1982;1:467–470.
32. Devereux RB, Pickering TG, Harshfield GA. Left ventricular hypertrophy in patients with hypertension: Importance of blood pressure response to regular recurring stress. *Circulation* 1983;68:470–476.
33. Phillips RA, Goldman ME, Ardeljan M, Arora R, Eison HB, Buyan Y, Krakoff LR. Determinants of abnormal left ventricular filling in early hypertension. *J Am Coll Cardiol* 1989;14:979–985.
34. Guerrier M, Schillaci G, Verdecchia P, Gatteschi C, Guglielmo B, Boldrini F, Porcellati C. Circadian blood pressure changes and left ventricular hypertrophy in essential hypertension. *Circulation* 1990; 81:528–536.
35. Genau A, Devereux RB, Pickering TG, Roman MJ, Schnall PL, Santucci S, Spitzer MC, Laragh JH. Relation of left ventricular hemodynamic load and contractile performance to left ventricular mass in hypertension. *Circulation* 1990;81:25–36.
36. Saba PS, Roman MJ, Pini R, Ganau A, Devereux RB. Relation of carotid pressure waveform to left ventricular anatomy in normotensive subjects. *J Am Coll Cardiol* 1993;22:1873–1880.
37. Morgan HE, Baker KM. Cardiac hypertrophy. Mechanical, neural and endocrine dependence. *Circulation* 1991;83:13–25.
38. Schunkert H, Jahn L, Izumo S, Apstein CS, Lorell BH. Localization and regulation of *c-fos* and *c-jun* protooncogene induction by systolic wall stress in normal and hypertrophied rat hearts. *Proc Natl Acad Sci USA* 1991;88:11480–11484.
39. Magid NM, Borer JS, Young MS, Wallerson DC, DeMonteiro C. Suppression of protein degradation in progressive cardiac hypertrophy of chronic aortic regurgitation. *Circulation* 1993;87:1249–1257.
40. Mahoney LT, Schieken RM, Clarke WR, Lauer RM. Left ventricular mass and exercise response predict future blood pressure. The Muscatine study. *Hypertension* 1988;12:206–213.
41. De Simone G, Devereux RB, Roman MJ, Schlussel Y, Alderman MH, Laragh JH. Echocardiographic left ventricular mass and electrolyte intake predict arterial hypertension. *Ann Intern Med* 1991;114: 202–209.
42. Devereux RB. Does increased blood pressure cause left ventricular hypertrophy or vice versa? *Ann Intern Med* 1990;112:157–159.
43. Schunkert H, Hense H, Holmer SR, Stender M, Perz S, Keil U, Lorell BH, Riegger GAJ. Association between a deletion polymorphism of the angiotensin converting-enzyme gene and left ventricular hypertrophy. *N Engl J Med* 1994;330:1634–1638.
44. Gharavi AG, Phillips RA, Diamond JA, et al. Deletion polymorphism of the angiotensin-converting enzyme gene is associated with concentric remodeling of the left ventricle. *J Am Coll Cardiol* 1995;25:136A (abstr).
45. Himmelmann A, Svensson A, Hansson L. Blood pressure and left ventricular mass in children with different maternal histories of hypertension: The Hypertension in Pregnancy Offspring Study. *J Hypertens* 1993;11:263–268.
46. van Hooft IMS, Grobbee DE, Waal-Manning HJ, Hofman A. Hemodynamic characteristics of the early phase of primary hypertension: The Dutch Hypertension and Offspring study. *Circulation* 1993;87: 1100–1106.
47. Adams TD, Yanowitz FG, Fisher AG, et al. Heritability of cardiac

size: An echocardiographic and electrocardiographic study of monozygotic and dizygotic twins. *Circulation* 1985;71:39–44.
48. Beaglehole R, Tyroler HA, Cassell JC, Deubner DC, Bartel AG, Hames CG. An epidemiological study of left ventricular hypertrophy in the biracial population of Evans County, Georgia. *J Chronic Dis* 1974;28:549–559.
49. Savage DD, Drayer JIM, Henry WL, et al. Echocardiographic assessment of cardiac anatomy and function in hypertensive patients. *Circulation* 1979;59:623–632.
50. Gerstenblith G, Frederiksen J, Yin FCP, Fortuin NJ, Lakatta EG, Weisfeldt ML. Echocardiographic assessment of a normal adult aging population. *Circulation* 1977;56:273–278.
51. Levy D, Garrison RJ, Savage DD, Kannel WB, Castelli WP. Left ventricular mass and incidence of coronary heart disease in an elderly cohort: the Framingham heart study. *Ann Intern Med* 1989;110: 101–107.
52. Shub C, Klein AL, Zachariah PK, Bailey KR, Tajik AJ. Determination of left ventricular mass by echocardiography in a normal population: Effect of age and sex in addition to body size. *Mayo Clin Proc* 1994; 69:205–211.
53. De Simone G, Devereux RB, Roman MJ, Ganau A, Chien S, Alderman MH, et al. Gender differences in left ventricular anatomy, blood viscosity and volume regulatory hormones in normal adults. *Am J Cardiol* 1991;68:1704–1708.
54. Hinderliter AL, Light KC, Park WWI. Gender differences in left ventricular structure and function in young adults with normal or marginally elevated blood pressure. *Am J Hypertens* 1992;5:33–36.
55. Devereux RB, Lutas EM, Casale PN, et al. Standardization of M-mode echocardiographic left ventricular anatomic measurements. *J Am Coll Cardiol* 1984;4:1222–1230.
56. Cabral AM, Vasquez EC, Moyses MR, Antonio A. Sex hormone modulation of ventricular hypertrophy in sino-aortic denervated rats. *Hypertension* 1988;11(Suppl 1):93–97.
57. Diamond JA, Ardeljan M, Travis A, et al. Are moderately and severely hypertensive women misclassified and overtreated? *J Am Coll Cardiol* 1993;21(Suppl A):471A (abstr).
58. Eison H, Phillips RA, Ardeljan M, Krakoff LR. Differences in ambulatory blood pressure between men and women with mild hypertension. *J Hum Hypertens* 1990;4:400–404.
59. Pickering TG, James GD, Boddie C, Harshfield GA, Blank S, Laragh JH. How common is white coat hypertension? *JAMA* 1988;259: 225–228.
60. Marcus R, Krause L, Weder AB, Dominguez-Mejia A, Schork NJ, Julius S. Sex-specific determinants of increased left ventricular mass in the Tecumseh blood pressure study. *Circulation* 1994;90:928–936.
61. MacMahon SW, Wilcken DEL, MacDonald GJ. The effect of weight reduction on left ventricular mass. *N Engl J Med* 1986;314:334–339.
62. Manolio TA, Levy D, Garrison RJ, Castelli WP, Kannel WB. Relation of alcohol intake to left ventricular mass: The Framingham Heart Study. *J Am Coll Cardiol* 1991;17:717–721.
63. Schmeider RE, Messerli FH, Garavaglia GE, Nunez BE. Dietary salt intake: A determinant of cardiac involvement in essential hypertension. *Circulation* 1988;78:951–956.
64. Marban E, Koretsune Y. Cell calcium, oncogenes, and hypertrophy. *Hypertension* 1990;15:652–658.
65. Dubus I. Origin and mechanisms of heart failure in hypertensive patients: Left ventricular remodelling in hypertensive heart disease. *Eur Heart J* 1993;14(Suppl J):76–81.
66. Sen S, Tarazi RC, Khairallah PA, Bumpus FM. Cardiac hypertrophy in spontaneously hypertensive rats. *Circ Res* 1974;35:775–781.
67. Bauwens FR, Duprez DA, De Buyzere ML, De Backer TL, Kaufman JM, Van Hoecke JV, Vermeulen A, Clement DL. Influence of the arterial blood pressure and nonhemodynamic factors on left ventricular hypertrophy in moderate essential hypertension. *Am J Cardiol* 1991;68:925–929.
68. Devereux RB, Pickering TG, Cody RJ, Cody RJ, Laragh JH. Relation of renin–angiotensin system activity to left ventricular hypertrophy and function in experimental and human hypertension. *J Clin Hypertens* 1987;3:87–103.
69. Cambien F, Poirier O, Lecerf L, Evans A, Cambou J-P, Arveiler D, Luc G, Bard J-M, Bara L, Ricard S, et al. Deletion polymorphism in the gene for angiotensin-converting enzyme is a potent risk factor for myocardial infarction. *Nature* 1992;359:641–644.
70. Sadoshima J, Xu Y, Slayter HS, Izumo S. Autocrine release of angiotensin II mediates stretch-induced hypertrophy of cardiac myocytes in vitro. *Cell* 1993;75:977–984.
71. Alderman MH, Madhavan S, Ooi WL, Cohen H, Sealey JE, Laragh JH. Association of the renin–sodium profile with the risk of myocardial infarction in patients with hypertension. *N Engl J Med* 1991;324: 1098–1104.
72. Laks MM, Morady F, Swan HJC. Myocardial hypertrophy produced by chronic infusion of subhypertensive doses of norepinephrine in the dog. *Chest* 1973;64:75–78.
73. Trimarco B, Ricciardelli B, De Luca N, De Simone A, Cuocolo A, Galva MD, Picotti GB, Condorelli M. Participation of endogenous catecholamines in the regulation of left ventricular mass in progeny of hypertensive parents. *Circulation* 1985;72(1):38–46.
74. Simpson P. Role of proto-oncogenes in myocardial hypertrophy. *Am J Cardiol* 1988;62:13G–19G.
75. Shub C, Cueto-Garcia L, Sheps S, Ilstrup DM, Tajik AJ. Echocardiographic findings in pheochromocytoma. *Am J Cardiol* 1986;57: 971–975.
76. Lim MJ, Barkan AL, Buda AJ. Rapid reduction of left ventricular hypertrophy in acromegaly after suppression of growth hormone hypersecretion. *Ann Intern Med* 1992;117:719–726.
77. Andronico G, Mangano M-T, Nardi E, Mulè G, Piazza G, Cerasola G. Insulin-like growth factor 1 and sodium–lithium countertransport in essential hypertension and in hypertensive left ventricular hypertrophy. *J Hypertens* 1993;11:1097–1011.
78. Geffner ME, Golde DW. Selective insulin action on skin, ovary and heart in insulin-resistant states. *Diabetes Care* 1988;11:500–505.
79. Phillips RA, Krakoff LR, Ardeljan M, et al. Relation of left ventricular mass to insulin resistance and blood pressure in non-obese subjects. *J Am Coll Cardiol* 1994;23:48A (abstr).
80. Prakash TR, MacKenzie SJ, Ram JL, et al. Insulin stimulates gene transcription and activity of $Na^{+}K^{+}$ ATPase in vascular smooth muscle cells. *Hypertension* 1992;20:443 (abstr).
81. Resnick LM. Ionic basis of hypertension, insulin resistance, vascular disease, and related disorders: The mechanism of "syndrome X." *Am J Hypertens* 1993;6:123S–134S.
82. Devereux RB, Reichek N. Echocardiographic determination of left ventricular mass in man: Anatomic validation of the method. *Circulation* 1977;55:613–618.
83. Feigenbaum H. *Echocardiography,* 4th ed. Philadelphia: Lea & Febiger; 1986:50–187.
84. Devereux RB, Alonso DR, Lutas EM, et al. Echocardiographic assessment of left ventricular hypertrophy: Comparison to necropsy findings. *Am J Cardiol* 1986;57:450–458.
85. Sahn DJ, DeMaria A, Kisslo J, Weyman A. The Committee on M-Mode Standardization of Echocardiography: Recommendations regarding quantitation in M-mode echocardiography: Results of a survey of echocardiographic measurements. *Circulation* 1978;58: 1073–1078.
86. De Simone G, Daniels SR, Devereux RB, Meyer RA, Roman MJ, De Divitiis O, Alderman MH. Left ventricular mass and body size in normotensive children and adults: Assessment of allometric relations and impact of overweight. *J Am Coll Cardiol* 1992;20:1251–1260.
87. Lauer MS, Anderson KM, Larson M, Levy D. A new method for indexing left ventricular mass for differences in body size. *Am J Cardiol* 1994;74:487–491.
88. Devereux RB. Detection of left ventricular hypertrophy by M-mode echocardiography. Anatomic validation, standardization, and comparison to other methods. *Hypertension* 1987;9(Suppl II):II-19–II-26.
89. Gottdiener JS, Livengood SV, Meyer PS, Chase GA. Should echocardiography be performed to assess effects of antihypertensive therapy? Test–retest reliability of echocardiography for assessment of left ventricular mass and function. *J Am Coll Cardiol* 1995;25(2):424–430.
90. Grandits GA, Liebson PR, Dianzumba S, Prineas RJ. Echocardiography in multicenter clinical trials: Experience from the treatment of the mild hypertension study. *Contr Clin Trials* 1994;15:395–410.
91. Haynes RB, Lacourciere Y, Rabkin SW, Leenen FHH, Logan AG, Wright N, Evans CE. Report of the Canadian Hypertension Society Consensus Conference: 2. Diagnosis of hypertension in adults. *Can Med Assoc J* 1993;149(4):409–418.
92. American Society of Echocardiography Committee on Standards, Schiller NB, Shah PM, Crawford M, DeMaria A, Devereux RB, Feigenbaum H, Gutsgesell H, Reichek N, Sahn D, et al. Recommenda-

tions for quantitation of the left ventricle by two-dimensional echocardiography. *J Am Soc Echo* 1989;2(5):358–367.
93. Collins HW, Kronenberg MW, Byrd BF. Reproducibility of left ventricular mass measurements by two-dimensional and M-mode echocardiography. *J Am Coll Cardiol* 1989;14:672–676.
94. Keller AM, Peschock RM, Malloy CR, et al. In vivo measurement of myocardial mass using nuclear magnetic resonance imaging. *J Am Coll Cardiol* 1986;8:113–117.
95. Riley-Hagan M, Peshock RM, Stray-Gundersen J, Katz J, Ryschon TW, Mitchell JH. Left ventricular dimensions and mass using magnetic resonance imaging in female endurance athletes. *Am J Cardiol* 1992;69:1067–1074.
96. King DL, Harrison MR, King DL Jr, Gopal AS, Martin RP, DeMaria AN. Improved reproducibility of left atrial and left ventricular measurements by guided three-dimensional echocardiography. *J Am Coll Cardiol* 1992;20:1238–1245.
97. Siu SC, Rivera JM, Guerrero JL, Handschumacher MD, Lethor JP, Weyman AE, Levine RA, Picard MH. Three-dimensional echocardiography: In vivo validation for left ventricular volume and function. *Circulation* 1993;88:1715–1723.
98. Gopal AS, Keller AM, Rigling R, King DLJ, King DL. Left ventricular volume and endocardial surface area by three-dimensional echocardiography: Comparison with two-dimensional echocardiography and nuclear magnetic resonance imaging in normal subjects. *J Am Coll Cardiol* 1993;22:258–270.
99. Schmieder RE. Reversal of left ventricular hypertrophy: Analysis of 412 published studies. *Am J Hypertens* 1994;7:25A (abstr).
100. Messerli FH, Soria F. Does a reduction in left ventricular hypertrophy reduce cardiovascular morbidity and mortality. *Drugs* 1992;44(Suppl 1):141–146.
101. Smith VE, White WB, Meeran MK, Karimeddini MK. Improved left ventricular filling accompanies reduced left ventricular mass during therapy of essential hypertension. *J Am Coll Card* 1986;8:1449–1454.
102. Schmieder RE, Messerli FH, Sturgill D, Garavaglia GE, Nunez BD. Cardiac performance after reduction of myocardial hypertrophy. *Am J Med* 1989;87:22–27.
103. Grandi AM, Venco A, Barzizza F, Casadei B, Marchesi E, Finardi G. Effect of enalapril on left ventricular mass and performance in essential hypertension. *Am J Cardiol* 1989;63:1093–1097.
104. Trimarco B, DeLuca N, Ricciardelli B. Cardiac function in systemic hypertension before and after reversal of left ventricular hypertrophy. *Am J Cardiol* 1988;62:745–750.
105. Schulman SP, Weiss JL, Becher LC, Gottlieb SO, Woodruff KM, Weisfeldt ML, Gerstenblith G. The effects of antihypertensive therapy on left ventricular mass in elderly patients. *N Engl J Med* 1990;322:1350–1356.
106. Phillips RA, Ardeljan M, Shimabukuro S, Goldman ME, Garbowit DL, Eison HB, Krakoff LR. Normalization of left ventricular mass and associated changes in neurohormones and atrial natriuretic peptide after one year of sustained nifedipine therapy for severe hypertension. *J Am Coll Cardiol* 1991;17:1595–1602.
107. Neaton JD, Grimm RH Jr, Prineas RJ, Stamler J, Grandits GA, Elmer PJ, Cutler JA, Flack JM, Schoenberger JA, McDonald R, et al. Treatment of mild hypertension study: Final results. *JAMA* 1993;270:713–724.
108. Dahlof B, Pennert K, Hansson L. Reversal of left ventricular hypertrophy in hypertensive patients. A metaanalysis of 109 treatment studies. *Am J Hypertens* 1992;5:95–110.
109. Linz W, Schaper J, Wiemer G, Albus U, Schölkens BA. Ramipril prevents left ventricular hypertrophy with myocardial fibrosis without blood pressure reduction: A one year study in rats. *Br J Pharmacol* 1992;107:970–975.
110. Gottdiener JS, Reda DJ, Williams DW, et al. Regression of left ventricular mass with monotherapy in mild-moderate hypertension: Interaction of drug with systolic blood pressure, age, race and weight. *Circulation* 1994;90:I-565 (abstr).
111. Fouad FM, Slominiski JM, Tarazi RC. Left ventricular diastolic function in hypertension: Relation to left ventricular mass and systolic function. *J Am Coll Cardiol* 1984;3:1500–1506.
112. Smith VE, Schulman P, Karimeddini M, White WB, Meeran MK, Katz AM. Rapid left ventricular filling in left ventricular hypertrophy II. Pathological hypertrophy. *J Am Coll Cardiol* 1985;5:869–874.
113. Inouye I, Massie B, Loge D, Topic N, Silverstein D, Simpson P, Tubau J. Abnormal left ventricular filling: An early finding in mild to moderate systemic hypertension. *Am J Cardiol* 1984;53:120–126.
114. Bonow RO, Udelson JE. Left ventricular diastolic dysfunction as a cause of congestive heart failure: Mechanisms and management. *Ann Intern Med* 1992;117:502–510.
115. Topol EJ, Traill GV, Fortuin NJ. Hypertensive cardiomyopathy of the elderly. *N Engl J Med* 1985;312:277–282.
116. Soufer R, Wohlgelernter D, Vita N, et al. Intact systolic left ventricular function in clinical congestive heart failure. *Am J Cardiol* 1985;55:1032–1036.
117. Setaro JF, Soufer R, Remetz MS, Perlmutter RA, Zaret BL. Long-term outcome in patients with congestive heart failure and intact systolic left ventricular performance. *Am J Cardiol* 1992;69:1212–1216.
118. Brutsaert DL, Sys SU, Gillebert TC. Diastolic failure: Pathophysiology and therapeutic implications. *J Am Coll Cardiol* 1993;22:318–325.
119. Snider AR, Gidding SS, Rocchini AP, et al. Doppler evaluation of left ventricular diastolic filling in children with systemic hypertension. *Am J Cardiol* 1985;56:921–926.
120. Phillips RA, Coplan NL, Krakoff LR, Yeager K, Ross R, Gorlin R, Goldman ME. Doppler echocardiographic analysis of left ventricular filling in treated hypertensive patients. *J Am Coll Cardiol* 1987;9:317–322.
121. Dianzumba SB, DiPette DJ, Cornman C, Weber E, Joyner CR. Left ventricular filling characteristics in mild untreated hypertension. *Hypertension* 1986;8(Suppl I):I-156–I-160.
122. Cuocolo A, Sax FL, Brush JE, Maron BJ, Bacharach SL, Bonow RO. Left ventricular hypertrophy and impaired diastolic filling in essential hypertension. Diastolic mechanisms for systolic dysfunction during exercise. *Circulation* 1990;81:978–986.
123. Graettinger WF, Neutel JM, Smith DHG, Weber MA. Left ventricular diastolic filling alterations in normotensive young adults with a family history of systemic hypertension. *Am J Cardiol* 1991;68:51–56.
124. Shapiro LM, McKenna WJ. Left ventricular hypertrophy: Relationship of structure to diastolic function in hypertension. *Br Heart J* 1984;51:637–642.
125. Hartford M, Wikstrand J, Wallentin I, Ljungman S, Wilhelmsen L, Berglund G. Diastolic function of the heart in untreated primary hypertension. *Hypertension* 1984;6:329–338.
126. Fouad FM, Slominski JM, Tarazi RC. Left ventricular diastolic function in hypertension: Relation to left ventricular mass and systolic function. *J Am Coll Cardiol* 1984;3:1500–1506.
127. White WB, Schulman P, Karimeddini MK, Smith VE. Regression of left ventricular mass is accompanied by improvement in rapid left ventricular filling following antihypertensive therapy with metoprolol. *Am Heart J* 1989;117:145–150.
128. Trimarco B, DeLuca N, Rosiello G. Improvement of diastolic function after reversal of left ventricular hypertrophy induced long-term antihypertensive treatment with tertatolol. *Am J Cardiol* 1989;64:745–751.
129. Gonzalez-Fernandez RB, Altieri PI, Diaz LM, Rodriguez PJ, Fernandez J, Miranda JG, Baez J, Cantellops D, Lugo JE. Effects of enalapril on heart failure in hypertensive patients with diastolic dysfunction. *Am J Hypertens* 1992;5:480–483.
130. Shahi M, Thorn S, Poulter N, Sever PS, Foale RA. Regression of hypertensive left ventricular hypertrophy and left ventricular diastolic dysfunction. *Lancet* 1990;336:458–461.
131. Douglas PS, Berko B, Lesh M, Reichek N. Alterations in diastolic function in response to progressive left ventricular hypertrophy. *J Am Coll Cardiol* 1989;13:461–467.
132. Douglas PS, Tallant B. Hypertrophy, fibrosis and diastolic dysfunction in early canine experimental hypertension. *J Am Coll Cardiol* 1991;17:530–536.
133. Brilla CG, Janicki JS, Weber KT. Cardioreparative effects of lisinopril in rats with genetic hypertension and left ventricular hypertrophy. *Circulation* 1991;83:1771–1779.
134. Villari B, Campbell SE, Hess OM, Mall G, Vassalli G, Weber KT, Krayenbuehl HP. Influence of collagen network on left ventricular systolic and diastolic function in aortic valve disease. *J Am Coll Cardiol* 1993;22:1477–1484.
135. Lorell BH, Grice WN, Apstein CS. Influence of hypertension with minimal hypertrophy on diastolic function during demand ischemia. *Hypertension* 1989;13:361–370.
136. Wexler LF, Lorell BH, Momomura S, Weinberg EO, Ingwall JS, Apstein CS. Enhanced sensitivity to hypoxia-induced diastolic dys-

function in pressure-overload left ventricular hypertrophy in the rat: Role of high-energy phosphate depletion. *Circ Res* 1988;62:766–775.
137. Osbakken M, Douglas PS, Ivanics T, Zhang D, Van Winkle T. Creatinine kinase kinetics studied by phosphorus-31 nuclear magnetic resonance in a canine model of chronic hypertension-induced cardiac hypertrophy. *J Am Coll Cardiol* 1992;19:223–228.
138. Ito Y, Suko J, Chidsey CA. Intracalcium and myocardial contractility. V. Calcium uptake of sarcoplasmic reticulum fractions in hypertrophied and failing rabbit hearts. *J Mol Cell Cardiol* 1974;6:237–247.
139. Harding DP, Poole-Wilson PA. Calcium exchange in rabbit myocardium during and after hypoxia: Effect of temperature and substrate. *Cardiovasc Res* 1980;14:435–445.
140. Gwathmey JK, Morgan JP. Altered calcium handling in experimental pressure-overload hypertrophy in the ferret. *Circ Res* 1985;57: 836–843.
141. Brutsaert DL, Rademakers FE, Sys SU, Gillebert TC, Housmans PR. Analysis of relaxation in the evaluation of ventricular function of the heart. *Prog Cardiovasc Dis* 1985;28:143–163.
142. White WB, Schulman P, Dey HM, Katz AM. Effects of age and 24-hour ambulatory blood pressure on rapid left ventricular filling. *Am J Cardiol* 1989;63:1341–1347.
143. Franchi F, Fabbri G, Monopoli A, Rossi D, Matassi L, Strazzulla G, Bisi G. Left ventricular diastolic filling improvement obtained by intravenous verapamil in mild to moderate essential hypertension: A complex effect. *Cardiology* 1989;76:32–41.
144. Betocchi S, Cuocolo A, Pace L, Chiariello M, Trimarco B, Alfano B, Ricciardelli B, Salvatore M, Condorelli M. Effect of intravenous verapamil administration of left ventricular diastolic function in systemic hypertension. *Am J Cardiol* 1987;59:624–629.
145. Udelson JE, Bacharach SL, Cannon RO, Bonow RO. Minimum left ventricular pressure during b-adrenergic stimulation in human subjects. Evidence for elastic recoil and diastolic ''suction'' in the normal heart. *Circulation* 1990;82:1174–1182.
146. Rademakers FE, Buchalter MB, Rogers WJ, Zerhouni EA, Weisfeldt ML, Weiss JL, Shapiro EP. Dissociation between left ventricular untwisting and filling. Accentuation by catecholamines. *Circulation* 1992;85:1672–1581.
147. Harrison TR, Dixon K, Russell RO, Bidwai PS, Coleman HN. The relation of age to the duration of contraction, ejection, and relaxation of the normal human heart. *Am Heart J* 1964;67:189–199.
148. Miyatake K, Okamoto M, Kinoshita N, et al. Augmentation of atrial contribution to left ventricular inflow with aging as assessed by intracardiac Doppler flowmetry. *Am J Cardiol* 1984;64:315–323.
149. Phillips RA, Krakoff LR, Coplin NL, Yeager K, Ross R, Gorlin R, Goldman ME. Normal aging produces left ventricular diastolic abnormalities detectable by Doppler echocardiography. *Clin Res* 1986; 34(2):336A.
150. Van Dam I, Fast T, DeBoo J, et al. Normal diastolic filling patterns of the left ventricle. *Eur Heart J* 1988;9:165–171.
151. Spirito P, Maron BJ. Influence of aging on Doppler echocardiographic indices of left ventricular diastolic function. *Br Heart J* 1988;59: 672–679.
152. Arora RR, Machac J, Goldman ME, Butler RN, Gorlin R, Horowitz SF. Atrial kinetics and left ventricular diastolic filling in the healthy elderly. *J Am Coll Cardiol* 1987;9:1255–1260.
153. Benjamin EJ, Plehn JF, D'Agostino RB, Belanger AJ, Comai K, Fuller DL, Wolf PA, Levy D. Mitral annular calcification and the risk of stroke in an elderly cohort. *N Engl J Med* 1992;327:374–379.
154. Psaty BM, Furberg CD, Kuller LH, Borhani NO, Rautaharju PM, O'Leary DH, Bild DE, Robbins J, Fried LP, Reid C. Isolated systolic hypertension and subclinical cardiovascular disease in the elderly: Initial findings from the Cardiovascular Health Study. *JAMA* 1992; 268:1287–1291.
155. Sagie A, Benjamin EJ, Galderisi M, Larson MG, Evans JC, Fuller DL, Lehman B, Levy D. Echocardiographic assessment of left ventricular structure and diastolic filling in elderly subjects with borderline isolated systolic hypertension (the Framingham Heart Study). *Am J Cardiol* 1993;72:662–665.
156. Levy WC, Cerqueira MD, Abrass IB, Schwartz RS, Stratton JR. Endurance exercise training augments diastolic filling at rest and during exercise in healthy young and older men. *Circulation* 1993;88: 116–126.
157. Weiss JL, Frederiksen JW, Weisfeldt ML. Hemodynamic determinants of the time-course of fall in canine left ventricular pressure. *J Clin Invest* 1976;58:751–760.
158. Grossman W, McLaurin LP. Diastolic properties of the left ventricle. *Ann Intern Med* 1976;84:316–326.
159. Hess OM, Ritter M, Schneider J, Grimm J, Turina M, Krayenbuehl HP. Diastolic stiffness and myocardial structure in aortic valve disease before and after valve replacement. *Circulation* 1984;69:855–865.
160. Spirito P, Maron BJ, Bonow RO. Noninvasive assessment of left ventricular diastolic function: Comparative analysis of Doppler echocardiographic and radionuclide angiographic techniques. *J Am Coll Cardiol* 1986;7:518–526.
161. Shapiro LM, Mackinnon J, Beevers DG. Echocardiographic features of malignant hypertension. *Br Heart J* 1981;46:374–379.
162. Kitabatake A, Inoue M, Asao M, et al. Transmitral blood flow reflecting diastolic behavior of the left ventricle in health and disease—a study by pulsed Doppler technique. *Jpn Circ J* 1982;46:92–102.
163. Chenzbraun A, Pinto FJ, Popylisen S, Schnittger I, Popp RL. Filling patterns in left ventricular hypertrophy: A combined acoustic quantification and Doppler study. *J Am Coll Cardiol* 1994;23:1179–1185.
164. Hanrath P, Mathey DG, Siegert R, Bleifeld W. Left ventricular relaxation and filling pattern in different forms of left ventricular hypertrophy: An echocardiographic study. *Am J Cardiol* 1980;45:15–23.
165. Nakashima Y, Nii T, Ikeda M, Arakawa K. Role of left ventricular regional nonuniformity in hypertensive diastolic dysfunction. *J Am Coll Cardiol* 1993;22:790–795.
166. Spirito P, Maron BJ. Doppler echocardiography for assessing left ventricular diastolic function. *Ann Intern Med* 1988;109:122–126.
167. Choong CY, Abascal VM, Thomas JD, Guerrero JL, McGlew S, Weyman AE. Combined influence of ventricular loading and relaxation on the transmitral flow velocity profile in dogs measured by Doppler echocardiography. *Circulation* 1988;78:672–683.
168. Himura Y, Kumada T, Kambayashi M, Hayashida W, Ishikawa N, Nakamura Y, Kawai C. Importance of left ventricular systolic function in the assessment of left ventricular diastolic function with Doppler transmitral flow velocity recording. *J Am Coll Cardiol* 1991;18: 753–760.
169. Benjamin EJ, Levy D, Anderson KM, Wolf PA, Plehn JF, Evans JC, Comai K, Fuller DL, St John Sutton M. Determinants of Doppler indexes of left ventricular diastolic function in normal subjects (the Framingham Heart Study). *Am J Cardiol* 1992;70:508–515.
170. Laufer E, Jennings GL, Dewar E. Prevalence of cardiac structural and functional abnormalities in untreated primary hypertension. *Hypertension* 1989;13:151–162.
171. Ishida Y, Meisner JS, Tsujioka K, Gallo JI, Yoran C, Frater RWM, Yellin EJ. Left ventricular filling dynamics: Influence of left ventricular relaxation and left atrial pressure. *Circulation* 1986;74:187–196.
172. Appleton CP, Carucci MJ, Henry CP, Olajos M. Influence of incremental changes in heart rate on mitral flow velocity: Assessment in lightly sedated, conscious dogs. *J Am Coll Cardiol* 1991;17:227–236.
173. Nishimura RA, Schwartz RS, Holmes DR Jr, Tajik AJ. Failure of calcium channel blockers to improve ventricular relaxation in humans. *J Am Coll Cardiol* 1993;21:182–188.
174. Raine AEG, Erne P, Burgisser E, Muller FB, Bolli P, Burkart F, Buhler FR. Atrial natriuretic peptide and atrial pressure in patients with congestive heart failure. *N Engl J Med* 1986;315:533–537.
175. Eison HB, Rosen MJ, Phillips RA, Krakoff LR. Determinants of atrial natriuretic factor in the adult respiratory distress syndrome. *Chest* 1988;95:1040–1045.
176. Rodeheffer RJ, Tanaka I, Imada T, Hollister AS, Robertson, Inagami T. Atrial pressure and secretion of atrial natriuretic factor into the human central circulation. *J Am Coll Cardiol* 1986;8:18–26.
177. Matsuda Y, Toma Y, Matsuzaki M, et al. Change of left atrial systolic pressure waveform in relation to left ventricular end-diastolic pressure. *Circulation* 1990;82:1659–1667.
178. Rossvoll O, Hatle LK. Pulmonary venous flow velocities recorded by transthoracic Doppler ultrasound: Relation to left ventricular diastolic pressures. *J Am Coll Cardiol* 1993;21:1687–1696.
179. Appleton CP, Galloway JM, Gonzales MS, Gaballa M, Basnight MA. Estimation of left ventricular filling pressures using two-dimensional and Doppler echocardiography in adult patients with cardiac disease. Additional value of analyzing left atrial size, left atrial ejection fraction and the difference in duration of pulmonary venous and mitral

flow velocity at atrial contraction. *J Am Coll Cardiol* 1993;22: 1972–1982.
180. Pai RG, Suzuki M, Heywood JT, Ferry DR, Shah PM. Mitral A velocity wave transit time to the outflow tract as a measure of left ventricular diastolic stiffness: Hemodynamic correlations in patients with coronary artery disease. *Circulation* 1994;89:553–557.
181. Pai RG, Shakudo M, Yoganathan AP, Shah PM. Clinical correlates of the rate of transmission of transmitral "A" wave to the left ventricular outflow tract in left ventricular hypertrophy secondary to system hypertension, hypertrophic cardiomyopathy or aortic valve stenosis. *Am J Cardiol* 1994;73:831–834.
182. Stugaard M. Color M-mode Doppler improves the diagnosis of diastolic dysfunction in coronary artery disease. *Circulation* 1993;88: 1170 (abstr).
183. Stugaard M, Smiseth OA, Risöe C, Ihlen H. Intraventricular early diastolic filling during acute myocardial ischemia: Assessment by multigated color M-mode Doppler echocardiography. *Circulation* 1993;88:2705–2713.
184. Setaro JF, Zaret BL, Schulman DS, Black HR, Soufer R. Usefulness of verapamil for congestive heart failure associated with abnormal left ventricular diastolic filling and normal left ventricular systolic performance. *Am J Cardiol* 1990;66:981–986.
185. Given BD, Lee TH, Stone PH, Dzau VJ. Nifedipine in severly hypertensive patients with congestive heart failure and preserved ventricular systolic function. *Arch Intern Med* 1985;145:281–285.
186. The Fifth Report of the Joint National Committee on Detection, Evaluation, and Treatment of High Blood Pressure (JNC V). *Arch Intern Med* 1993;153:154–183.
187. Gaasch WH. Diagnosis and treatment of heart failure based on left ventricular systolic or diastolic function. *JAMA* 1994;271(16): 1276–1280.
188. Clements IP, Bailey KR, Zachariah PK. Effects of exercise and therapy on ventricular emptying and filling in mildly hypertensive patients. *Am J Hypertens* 1994;7:695–702.
189. Zusman RM, Christensen DM, Higgins J, Boucher CA. Nifedipine improves left ventricular function in patients with hypertension. *J Cardiovasc Pharmacol* 1991;18:843–848.
190. Szlachcic J, Tubau JF, Vollmer C, Massie BM. Effects of diltiazem on left ventricular mass and diastolic filling in mild to moderate hypertension. *Am J Cardiol* 1989;63:198–201.
191. Zusman RM, Christensen DM, Federman EB, et al. Nifedipine, but not propranolol, improves left ventricular systolic and diastolic function in patients with hypertension. *Am J Cardiol* 1989;64:51F–61F.
192. Fouad FM, Slominski MJ, Tarazi RC, Gallagher JH. Alterations in left ventricular filling with beta-adrenergic blockade. *Am J Cardiol* 1983;51:161–164.
193. Schunkert H, Dzau VJ, Tang SS, Hirsch AT, Apstein CS, Lorell BH. Increased rat cardiac angiotensin converting enzyme activity and mRNA expression in pressure overload left ventricular hypertrophy. *J Clin Invest* 1990;86:1913–1920.
194. Esper RJ, Burrieza OH, Cacharrón JL, Fábregues G, Baglivo HP. Left ventricular mass regression and diastolic function improvement in mild and moderate hypertensive patients treated with lisinopril. *Cardiology* 1993;83:76–81.
195. Strauer BE. The concept of coronary flow reserve. *J Cardiovasc Pharmacol* 1992;19(Suppl 5):S67–S80.
196. Bache RJ. Effects of hypertrophy on the coronary circulation. *Prog Cardiovasc Dis* 1988;31:403–440.
197. Anversa P, Sonnenblick EH. Ischemic cardiomyopathy: Pathophysiologic mechanisms. *Prog Cardiovasc Dis* 1990;32:1–22.
198. Greene AS, Tonellato PJ, Lui J, Lombard JH, Cowley AW. Microvascular rarefaction and tissue vascular resistance in hypertension. *Am J Physiol* 1989;256:H126–H131.
199. Rakusan K, Legato M, editors. *The Stressed Heart.* Boston: Martinus Nijhoff; 1987:107–123.
200. Marcus ML, Harrison DG, Chilian WM, Koyanagi S, Inou T, Tomanek RJ, Martins JB, Eastham CL, Hiratzka LF. Alterations in the coronary circulation in hypertrophied ventricles. *Circulation* 1987; 75(Suppl I):I-19–I-25.
201. Breisch EA, White FC, Nimmo LE, Bloor CM. Cardiac vasculature and flow during pressure-overload hypertrophy. *Am J Physiol* 1986; 251:H1031–H1037.
202. Rakusan K, Wicker P, Abdul-Samad M, Turek Z. Failure of swimming exercise to improve capillarization in cardiac hypertrophy of renal hypertensive rats. *Circ Res* 1987;61:641–647.
203. Smolich JJ, Walker AM, Campbell GR, Adamson TM. Left and right ventricular myocardial morphometry in fetal, neonatal, and adult sheep. *Am J Physiol* 1989;257:H1–H9.
204. Rakusan K, Flanagan MF, Geva T, Southern J, Van Praagh R. Morphometry of human coronary capillaries during normal growth and the effect of age in left ventricular pressure-overload hypertrophy. *Circulation* 1992;86:38–46.
205. Tomanek RJ. Effects of age and exercise on the extent of the myocardial capillary bed. *Anat Rec* 1970;167:55–62.
206. D'Amore PA, Thompson RW. Mechanisms of angiogenesis. *Annu Rev Physiol* 1987;49:453–464.
207. Hudlicka O. What makes blood vessels grow? *J Physiol* 1991;1–24.
208. Short D. Morphology of the intestinal arterials in chronic human hypertension. *Br Heart J* 1966;28:184–192.
209. James TN. Morphologic characteristics and functional significance of focal fibromuscular dysplasia of small coronary arteries. *Am J Cardiol* 1990;65:126–136.
210. Tomanek RJ, Plamer PY, Pfeiffer GL, et al. Morphologic characteristics and functional significance of focal fibromuscular dysplasia of small coronary arteries, arterioles and capillaries during hypertension and left ventricular hypertrophy. *Circ Res* 1986;58:38–46.
211. Schwartzkopff B, Motz W, Knauer S, et al. Morphometric investigation of intramyocardial arterioles in right septal endomyocardial biopsy of patients with arterial hypertension and left ventricular hypertrophy. *J Cardiovasc Pharmacol* 1992;20:2–7.
212. Korsgaard N, Aalkjaer C, Heagerty AM, Izzard AS, Mulvany MJ. Histology of subcutaneous small arteries from patients with essential hypertension. *Hypertension* 1993;22:523–526.
213. Gilligan JP, Spector S. Synthesis of collagen in cardiac and vascular walls. *Hypertension* 1984;44–49.
214. Iwatsuku K, Cardinale GJ, Spector S, Udenfriend S. Reduction of blood pressure and vascular collagen in hypertensive rats by B-aminoproprionitrile. *Proc Natl Acad Sci USA* 1977;74:360–362.
215. Isoyama S, Ito J, Sato K, Takishima T. Collagen deposition and the reversal of coronary reserve in cardiac hypertrophy. *Hypertension* 1992;20:491–500.
216. Furchgott RF, Zaqadski JV. The obligatory role of endothelial cells in the relaxation of arterial smooth muscle by acetylcholine. *Nature* 1980;288:373–376.
217. Brush JE, Faxon DP, Salmon S, Jacobs AK, Ryan TJ. Abnormal endothelium-dependent coronary vasomotion in hypertensive patients. *J Am Coll Cardiol* 1992;19:809–815.
218. Motz W, Vogt M, Rabenau O, Scheler S, Luckhoff A, Strauer BE. Evidence of endothelial dysfunction in coronary resistance vessels in patients with angina pectoris and normal coronary angiograms. *Am J Cardiol* 1991;68:996–1003.
219. Panza JA, Quyyumi AA, Brush JE, Epstein SE. Abnormal endothelium-dependent vascular relaxation in patients with essential hypertension. *N Engl J Med* 1990;323:22–27.
220. Treasure CB, Klein JL, Vita JA, Manoukian SV, Renwick GH, Selwyn AP, Ganz P, Alexander RW. Hypertension and left ventricular hypertrophy are associated with impaired endothelium-mediated relaxation in human coronary resistance vessels. *Circulation* 1993;87:86–93.
221. Vrints CJ, Bult H, Hilter E, Herman AG, Snoeck JP. Impaired endothelium-dependent cholinergic coronary vasodilation in patients with angina and normal coronary arteriograms. *J Am Coll Cardiol* 1992; 19:21–31.
222. Jameson M, Dai F-X, Lüscher T, Skopec J, Diederich A, Diederich D. Endothelium-derived contracting factors in resistance arteries of young spontaneously hypertensive rats before development of overt hypertension. *Hypertension* 1993;21:280–288.
223. Strauer BE. Coronary hemodynamics in hypertensive heart disease. Basic concepts, clinical consequences, and experimental analysis of regression of hypertensive microangiopathy. *Am J Med* 1988; 84(Suppl 3A):45–54.
224. Strauer BE. Ventricular function and coronary hemodynamics in hypertensive heart disease. *Am J Cardiol* 1979;44:999–1006.
225. Cannon RO III. Dynamic limitation of coronary vasodilator reserve in patients with dilated cardiomyopathy and chest pain. *J Am Coll Cardiol* 1987;10:1190.
226. Pichard AD, Smith H, Holt J, Meller J, Gorlin R. Coronary vascular

reserve in left ventricular hypertrophy secondary to chronic aortic regurgitation. *Am J Cardiol* 1983;51:315–320.
227. Villari B, Hess OM, Moccetti D, Vassalli G, Krayenbuehl HP. Effect of progression of left ventricular hypertrophy on coronary artery dimensions in aortic valve disease. *J Am Coll Cardiol* 1992;20: 1073–1079.
228. Rouleau J, Boerboom LE, Surjadhana A, Hoffman JIE. The role of autoregulation and tissue diastolic pressures in the transmural distribution of left ventricular blood flow in anesthetized dogs. *Circ Res* 1979; 45:804–815.
229. Guyton RA, McClenathan JH, Michaelis LL. Evolution of regional ischemia distal to a proximal coronary stenosis: Self propagation of ischemia. *Am J Cardiol* 1977;40:381–392.
230. Mosher P, Ross J, McFate PA, Shaw RF. Control of coronary blood flow by an autoregulatory mechanism. *Circ Res* 1964;14:250.
231. Driscol TE, Moir TW, Eckstein RW. Autoregulation of coronary blood flow: Effect of intraarterial pressure gradients. *Circ Res* 1964; 15:103–111.
232. Hoffman JI. A critical view of coronary reserve. *Circulation* 1987; 75(Suppl I):I-6–I-11.
233. DeFily DV, Chilian WM. *Cardiology in Review*. Baltimore: Williams & Wilkins; 1994:67–76.
234. Berne RM, Rubio R. Cardiac nucleotides in hypoxia: Possible role in regulation of coronary blood flow. *Am J Physiol* 1963;204:317–322.
235. Marcus ML. *The Coronary Circulation in Health and Disease*. New York: McGraw-Hill; 1983:84–85.
236. Dole WP, Nuno DW. Myocardial oxygen tension determines the degree and pressure range of coronary autoregulation. *Circ Res* 1986; 59:202–215.
237. Samaha FF, Heineman C, Ince J, Fleming J, Balban RS. ATP-sensitive potassium channel is essential to maintain basal coronary vascular tone in vivo. *Am J Physiol* 1992;262:C1220–C1227.
238. Bayliss WM. On the local reaction of the arterial wall to changes in internal pressure. *J Physiol* 1902;28:220–231.
239. Folkow B. Intravascular pressure as a factor regulating the tone of the small vessels. *Acta Physiol Scand* 1949;17:289–310.
240. Marcus ML. *The Coronary Circulation in Health and Disease*. New York: McGraw-Hill; 1983:147–154.
241. Johnson PC, Borh DF, Somylo PA, Sparks HV, eds. *The Cardiovascular System*. 1980:409–442.
242. Hoffman JIE. Maximal coronary flow and the concept of coronary vascular reserve. *Circulation* 1984;70:153–159.
243. Cleary RM, Ayon D, Moore NB, DeBoe SF, Mancini GBJ. Tachycardia, contractility and volume loading alter conventional indexes of coronary flow reserve, but not the instantaneous hyperemic flow versus pressure slope index. *J Am Coll Cardiol* 1992;20:1261–1269.
244. Rossen JD, Winniford MD. Effect of increases in heart rate and arterial pressure on coronary flow reserve in humans. *J Am Coll Cardiol* 1993; 21:343–348.
245. O'Keefe DD, Hoffman JIE, Cheitlin R, O'Neill MJ, Allard RJ, Shapkin E. Coronary blood flow in experimental canine left ventricular hypertrophy. *Circ Res* 1978;43:619.
246. Bretschneider HJ. Parmakotherapie coronarer durch Blutungsstorungen mit kreislaufwirksamen Subtanzen. *Deutsch Ges Med* 1963; 69:583.
247. Wicker P, Tarazi RC. Coronary blood flow in left ventricular hypertrophy: A review of experimental data. *Eur Heart J* 1982;3:111.
248. Opherk D, Mall G, Zebe H, Schwarz F, Weihe E, Manthey J, Kubler W. Reduction of coronary reserve: A mechanism for angina pectoris in patients with arterial hypertension and normal coronary arteries. *Circulation* 1984;69(1):1–7.
249. Prichard AD, Gorlin R, Smith H, Ambrose J, Meller J. Coronary flow studies in patients with left ventricular hypertrophy of the hypertensive type: Evidence for an impaired coronary vascular reserve. *Am J Cardiol* 1981;47:547–554.
250. Goldstein RA, Haynie M. Limited myocardial perfusion reserve in patients with left ventricular hypertrophy. *J Nucl Med* 1990;31: 255–258.
251. Diamond JA, Machac J, Henzlova M, et al. Quantitative Adenosine-Thallium perfusion imaging for assessing coronary flow reserve in arterial hypertension. *J Am Coll Cardiol* 1993;21(Suppl A):288A (abstr).
252. Houghton JL, Frank MJ, Carr AA, von Dohlen TW, Prisant M. Relations among impaired coronary flow reserve, left ventricular hypertrophy and thallium perfusion defects in hypertensive patients without obstructive coronary artery disease. *J Am Coll Cardiol* 1990;15: 43–51.
253. Marcus ML, White CW. Coronary flow reserve in patients with normal coronary angiograms. *J Am Coll Cardiol* 1985;6:1254–1256.
254. Houghton JL, Prisant M, Carr AA, Flowers NC, Frank MJ. Racial differences in myocardial ischemia and coronary flow reserve in hypertension. *J Am Coll Cardiol* 1994;23:1123–1129.
255. Gould LK, Martucci JP, Goldberg DI, Hess MJ, Edens RP, Latifi R, Dudrick SJ. Short-term cholesterol lowering decreases size and severity of perfusion abnormalities by positron emission tomography after dipyridamole in patients with coronary artery disease. A potential noninvasive marker of healing coronary endothelium. *Circulation* 1994;89:1530–1538.
256. Quillen JE, Rossen JD, Oskarsson HJ, Minor Rl, Lopez AG, Winniford MD. Acute effects of cigarette smoking on the coronary circulation: Constriction of epicardial and resistance vessels. *J Am Coll Cardiol* 1993;22:642–647.
257. Celermajer DS, Sorensen KE, Georgakopoulos D, Bull C, Thomas O, Robinson J, Deanfield JE. Cigarette smoking is associated with dose-related and potentially reversible impairment of endothelium-dependent dilation in healthy young adults. *Circulation* 1993;88: 2149–2155.
258. Nasher PJ, Brown RE, Oskarsson H, Winniford MD, Rossen JD. Maximal coronary flow reserve and metabolic coronary vasodilation in patients with diabetes mellitus. *Circulation* 1995;91:635–640.
259. Celermajer DS, Sorensen KE, Spiegelhalter DJ, Georgakopoulos D, Robinson J, Deanfield JE. Aging is associated with endothelial dysfunction in healthy mean years before the age-related decline in women. *J Am Coll Cardiol* 1994;24:471–476.
260. Zeiher AM, Drexler H, Saurbier B, Just H. Endothelium-mediated coronary blood flow modulation in humans. Effects of age, atherosclerosis, hypercholesterolemia, and hypertension. *J Clin Invest* 1993;92: 652–662.
261. Vitullo JC, Penn MS, Rakusan K, Wicker P. Effects of hypertension and aging on coronary arteriolar density. *Hypertension* 1993;21: 406–414.
262. Antony I, Nitenberg A, Foult J-M, Aptecar E. Coronary vasodilator reserve in untreated and treated hypertensive patients with and without left ventricular hypertrophy. *J Am Coll Cardiol* 1993;22:514–520.
263. Harrison DG, Florentine MS, Brooks LA, Cooper SM, Marcus ML. The effect of hypertension and left ventricular hypertrophy on the lower range of coronary autoregulation. *Circulation* 1988;77(5): 1108–1115.
264. Koyanagi S, Eastham CL, Harrison DG, Marcus ML. Increased size of myocardial infarction in dogs with chronic hypertension and left ventricular hypertrophy. *Circ Res* 1982;50:55.
265. Dellsperger KC, Clothier JL, Hartnett JA, Haun LM, Marcus ML. Acceleration of the wavefront of myocardial necrosis by chronic hypertension and left ventricular hypertrophy in dogs. *Circ Res* 1988; 63:87–96.
266. Taylor AL, Murphree S, Buja LM, Villarreal MC, Pastor P, Eckles R. Segmental systolic responses to brief ischemia and reperfusion in the hypertrophied canine left ventricle. *J Am Coll Card* 1992;20: 994–1002.
267. Polese A, DeCesare N, Montorsi P, Fabbiocchi F, Gauzzi M, Loaldi A, Guazzi MD. Upward shift of the lower range of coronary flow autoregulation in hypertensive patients with hypertrophy of the left ventricle. *Circulation* 1991;83:845–853.
268. MacMahon S, Peto R, Cutler J, Collins R, Sorlie P, Neaton J, Abbott R, Godwin J, Dyer A, Stamler J. Blood pressure, stroke, and coronary heart disease. Part 1, prolonged differences in blood pressure: Prospective observational studies corrected for the regression dilution bias. *Lancet* 1990;335:765–774.
269. Collins R, Peto R, MacMahon S, Hebert P, Fiebach NH, Eberlein KA, Godwin J, Qizilbash N, Taylor JO, Hennekens CH. Blood pressure, stroke, and coronary heart disease. Part 2, short-term reductions in blood pressure: Overview of randomized drug trials in their epidemiological context. *Lancet* 1990;335:827–838.
270. Cruickshank JM, Thorp JM, Zacharias FJ. Benefits and potential harm of lowering high blood pressure. *Lancet* 1987;1:581–584.
271. Alderman MH, Ooi WL, Madhavan S, Cohen H. Treatment-induced blood pressure reduction and the risk of myocardial infarction. *JAMA* 1989;262:920–924.

272. Farnett L, Mulrow CD, Linn WD, Lucey CR, Tuley MR. The J-curve phenomenon and the treatment of hypertension. Is there a point beyond which pressure reduction is dangerous? *JAMA* 1991;265: 489–495.
273. Fletcher AE, Bulpitt CJ. How far should blood pressure be lowered? *N Engl J Med* 1992;326:251–254.
274. McCloskey LW, Psaty BM, Koepsell TD, Aagaard GN. Level of blood pressure and risk of myocardial infarction among treated hypertensive patients. *Arch Intern Med* 1992;152:513–520.
275. Weinberger MH. Do no harm. Antihypertensive therapy and the "J" curve. *Arch Intern Med* 1992;152:473–476.
276. Lindblad U, Rastam L, Ryden L, Ranstam J, Isacsson S, Berglund G. Control of blood pressure and risk of first acute myocardial infarction: Skaraborg hypertension project. *Br Med J* 1994;308:681–686.
277. Hansson L. Future goals for the treatment of hypertension in the elderly with reference to STOP-hypertension, SHEP, and the MRC trial in older adults. *Am J Hypertens* 1993;6(Suppl):40S–43S.
278. Walker WG, Neaton JD, Cutler JA, Neuwirth R, Cohen JD. Renal function change in hypertensive members of the Multiple Risk Factor Intervention Trial: Racial and treatment effects. *JAMA* 1992;268: 3085–3091.
279. Klocke FJ, Ellis AK, Canty JM Jr. Interpretation of changes in coronary flow that accompany pharmacologic interventions. *Circulation* 1987;75(Suppl V):V-34–V-38.
280. Jeremy RW, Links JM, Becker LC. Progressive failure of coronary flow during reperfusion of myocardial infarction: Documentation of the no reflow phenomenon with positron emission tomography. *J Am Coll Cardiol* 1990;16:695–704.
281. Uren NG, Marraccini P, Gistri R, De Silva R, Camici PG. Altered coronary vasodilator reserve and metabolism in myocardium subtended by normal arteries in patients with coronary artery disease. *J Am Coll Cardiol* 1993;22:650–658.
282. Uren NG, Crake T, Lefroy DC, De Silva R, Davies GJ, Maseri A. Reduced coronary vasodilator function in infarcted and normal myocardium after myocardial infarction. *N Engl J Med* 1994;331: 222–227.
283. Anderson PG, Bishop SP, Digerness SB. Vascular remodeling and improvement of coronary reserve after hydralazine treatment in spontaneously hypertensive rats. *Circ Res* 1989;64:1127–1136.
284. Canby CA, Tomanek RI. Role of lowering arterial pressure on maximal coronary flow with and without regression of cardiac hypertrophy. *Am J Physiol* 1989;257:H1110–H1118.
285. Ishihara K, Zile MR, Nagatsu M, Nakano K, Tomita M, Kanazawa S, Clamp L, DeFreyte G, CArabello BA. Coronary blood flow after the regression of pressure-overload left ventricular hypertrophy. *Circ Res* 1992;71:1472–1481.
286. Sato F, Isoyama S, Takishima T. Normalization of impaired coronary circulation in hypertrophied rat hearts. *Hypertension* 1990;16:26–34.
287. Heagerty AM, Bund SJ, Aalkjaer C. Effects of drug treatment on human resistance arteriole morphology in essential hypertension: Direct evidence for structural remodelling of resistance vessels. *Lancet* 1988;2:1209–1212.
288. Vogt M, Motz WH, Schwartzkopf B, Strauer BE. Pathophysiology and clinical aspects of hypertensive hypertrophy. *Eur Heart J* 1993; 14(Suppl D):2–7.
289. Yamada H, Fabris B, Allen AM, et al. Localization of angiotensin converting enzyme in the rat heart. *Circ Res* 1991;68:141–149.
290. Rossen JD, Simonetti I, Marcus ML, Braun P, Winniford MD. The effect of diltiazem on coronary flow reserve in humans. *Circulation* 1989;80:1240–1246.
291. Vrolix MC, Sionis D, Piessens J, Van Lierde J, Willems JL, De Geest H. Changes in human coronary flow reserve after administration of intracoronary diltiazem. *J Cardiovasc Pharmacol* 1991;18(Suppl 9): S64–S67.
292. Diamond JA, Machac J, Henzlova MJ, Martin K, Krakoff LR, Ardeljan M, Travis A, Phillips RA. Effect of long term calcium channel blocker antihypertensive therapy on coronary physiology. *J Am Coll Cardiol* 1994;256A.
293. Merrill G, Young M, Dorell S, Krieger L. Coronary interactions between nifedipine and adenosine in the intact dog heart. *Eur J Pharmacol* 1982;81:543–550.
294. Pohlman AG. The course of the blood through the heart of the fetal mammal, with a note on the reptilian and amphibian circulations. *Anat Rec* 1909;3:75–109.
295. Wagner HNJ, Rhodes BA, Sasaki Y, et al. Studies of the circulation with radioactive microspheres. *Invest Radiol* 1969;4:374–386.
296. Wagner HNJ, Sabiston DCJ, Iio M, et al. Regional pulmonary blood flow in man by radioisotope scanning. *JAMA* 1964;187:601–603.
297. Wagner HNJ, Jones E, Tow DE, et al. A method for the study of the peripheral circulation in man. *J Nucl Med* 1965;6:150–154.
298. Rhodes BA, Zolle I, Buchanan JW. Preparation of metabolizable radioactive human serum albumin microspheres for studies of the circulation. *Radiology* 1969;92:1453–1460.
299. Zolle I, Rhodes BA, Wagner NHJ. Preparation of metabolizable radioactive human serum albumin microspheres for studies of the circulation. *Int J Appl Radiat Isot* 1970;21:155–167.
300. Heymann MA, et al. Blood flow measurements with radionuclide-labeled particles. *Prog Cardiovasc Dis* 1977;20:55.
301. Hales JRS. Radioactive microsphere techniques for studies of the circulation. *Clin Exp Pharmacol Physiol* 1974;1:31–46.
302. Skiegekoto K, Van Heerdan PD, Tohru M, Wagner HNJ. Measurement of distribution of cardiac output. *J Appl Physiol* 1968;25: 696–700.
303. Warren DJ, Ledingham JGG. Measurement of cardiac output distribution using microspheres. Some practical and theoretical considerations. *Cardiovasc Res* 1974;8:570–581.
304. Ganz W, Tamura K, Marcus HS, Donoso R, Yoshida D, Swan HJC. Measurement of coronary sinus blood flow by continuous thermodilution in man. *Circulation* 1971;44:181–195.
305. Rossen JD, Oskarsson H, Stenberg RG, Braun P, Talman CL, Winniford MD. Simultaneous measurement of coronary flow reserve by left anterior descending coronary artery Doppler and great cardiac vein thermodilution methods. *J Am Coll Cardiol* 1992;20:402–407.
306. Winniford MD, Rossen JD, Marcus ML. Clinical importance of coronary flow reserve measurements in humans, Part I. *Mod Concepts Cardiovasc Dis* 1989;58:25–29.
307. Smith HC, Frye RI, Donald DE, Davis GE, Pluth JR, Sturm Rek Wood EH. Roentgen videodensitometric measurement of coronary blood flow. Determination from simultaneous indicator-dilution curves to selected sites in the coronary circulation and in coronary artery saphenous vein grafts. *Mayo Clin Proc* 1971;46:800.
308. Rumberger JA, Feiring AJ, Hiratzka LF, Reiter SJ, Stanford W, Marcus ML. Determination of changes in coronary bypass graft flow rate using cine-CT. *J Am Coll Cardiol* 1986;7:155A (abstr).
309. Wilson RF, Vogel R, LeFree M, Bates E, O'Neill W, Foster R, Kirlin P, Smith D, Pitt B. Application of digital techniques to selective coronary arteriography: Use of myocardial contrast appearance time to measure coronary flow reserve. *Am Heart J* 1984;107:153–164.
310. Wilson RF, Laughlin DE, Ackell PH, Chilian WM, Holida MD, Hartley CJ, Armstrong ML, Marcus ML, White CW. Transluminal, subselective measurement of coronary artery blood flow velocity and vasodilator reserve in man. *Circulation* 1985;72:82–92.
311. Wangler RD, Peters KG, Laughlin DE, Tomanek RJ, Marcus ML. A method for continuously assessing coronary velocity in the rat. *Am J Physiol* 1981;10:H816.
312. Gould KL, Schelbert HR, Phelps ME, Hoffman EJ. Noninvasive assessment of coronary stenoses with myocardial perfusion imaging during pharmacologic coronary vasodilation. *Am J Cardiol* 1979;43: 200.
313. Mullani NA, Goldstein RA, Gould KL, Marani SK, Fisher DJ, O'Brien HA, Loberg MD. Myocardial perfusion with rubidium-82 I. Measurement of extraction fraction and flow with external detectors. *J Nucl Med* 1983;24:898.
314. Goldstein RA, Mullani NA, Marani SK, Fisher DJ, Gould KL, O'Brien HA. Myocardial perfusion with rubidium-82 II. Effects of metabolic and pharmacologic interventions. *J Nucl Med* 1983;24:907.
315. Schelbert HR, Phelps ME, Hoffman EJ, Huang D, Selin CE, Kuhl DE. Regional myocardial perfusion assessed with N-13 labeled ammonia and positron emission computerized axial tomography. *Am J Cardiol* 1979;43:209.
316. Schelbert HR, Phelps ME, Huang S, MacDonald NS, Hansen J, Kuhl DE. N-13 labeled ammonia as an indicator of myocardial blood flow. *Circulation* 1981;63:1259.
317. Bellina RC, Parodi O, Camici PA, Salvadori PA, Taddei L, Fusani RG, Klassen GA, Abbate AL, Donato L. Simultaneous in vitro and in vivo validation of nitrogen-13 ammonia for the assessment of regional myocardial blood flow. *J Nucl Med* 1990;31:1335.
318. Hutchins GD, Schwaiger M, Rosenspire KC, Krivokapick J, Schelbert

H, Kuhl DE. Noninvasive quantification of regional blood flow in the human heart using N-13 ammonia and dynamic positron emission tomographic imaging. *J Nucl Med* 1990;31:1335.

319. Parker JA, Beller GA, Hoop B, Holman BL, Smith W. Assessment of regional myocardial blood flow and regional fractional oxygen-extraction in dogs, using O-15 water and O-15 hemoglobin. *Circ Res* 1978;42:511.
320. Merlett P, Mazoyer B, Hittinger L, Valette H, Saal JP, Bendriem B, Crozatier B, Castaigne A, Syrota A, Rande JLD. Assessment of coronary reserve in man: Comparison between positron emission tomography with oxygen-15 labeled water and intracoronary Doppler technique. *J Nucl Med* 1993;34:1899–1904.
321. Porter TR, D'Sa A, Turner C, Jones LA, Minisi AJ, Mohanty PK, Vetrovec GW, Nixon JV. Myocardial contrast echocardiography for the assessment of coronary blood flow reserve: Validation in humans. *J Am Coll Cardiol* 1993;21:349–355.
322. Cheirif J, Zoghbi WA, Raizner AE, Minor ST, Winters WL, Klein MS, DeBauche TL, Lewis JM, Roberts R, Quinones MA. Assessment of myocardial perfusion in humans by contrast echocardiography. I. Evaluation of regional coronary reserve by peak contrast intensity. *J Am Coll Cardiol* 1919;11:735–743.
323. Iliceto S, Marangelli V, Memmola C, Rizzon P. Transesophageal doppler echocardiography evaluation of coronary blood flow velocity in baseline conditions and during dipyridamole-induced coronary vasodilation. *Circulation* 1991;83:61–69.
324. Legrand V, Hodgson JM, Bates ER, Aueron FM, Mancini J, Smith JS, Gross MD, Vogel RA. Abnormal coronary flow reserve and abnormal radionuclide exercise test results in patients with normal coronary angiograms. *J Am Coll Cardiol* 1985;6:1245–1253.
325. Nielson AT, Morris KG, Murdock R, et al. Linear relationship between the distribution of thallium-201 and blood flow in ischemic and non-ischemic myocardium during exercise. *Circulation* 1980;61:797.
326. Beanlands R, Muzik O, Nguyen N, Petry N, Schwaiger M. The relationship between myocardial retention of technetium-99m teboroxime and myocardial blood flow. *J Am Coll Cardiol* 1992;20:712–719.
327. Sinusas AJ, Shi Q, Saltzberg MT, Vitols P, Jain D, Wackers FJT, Zaret BL. Technetium-99m-tetrofosmin to assess myocardial blood flow: Experimental validation in an intact canine model of ischemia. *J Nucl Med* 1994;35:664–671.
328. Machac J, Diamond JA, Vallabhajosula S, Henzlova MJ, Martin K, ALI K, Sadeghi A, Travis A, Mezrow C, Gandses A, et al. Validation of a noninvasive method of measuring coronary blood reserve: A split dose thallium-201 rest/stress imaging. *J Am Coll Cardiol* 1994;256A (abstr).
329. Lien DC, Araujo LI, Budinger T, Alavi A. Quantification of myocardial blood flow can be obtained with technetium-99m-teboroxime and fast dynamic SPECT scanning. *J Am Coll Cardiol* 1993;21:376A (abstr).
330. Rumberger JA, Bell MR, Sheedy PF, Stanson AW. In vivo quantification of intramyocardial blood volume by ultrafast computed tomography. *Circulation* 1988;78:II-398.
331. Weiss RM, Otoadese EA, Noel MP, DeJong SC, Heery SD. Quantitation of absolute regional myocardial perfusion using cine computed tomography. *J Am Coll Cardiol* 1994;23:1186–1193.
332. Bogren HG, Buonocore MH. Measurement of coronary artery flow reserve by magnetic resonance velocity mapping in the aorta. *Lancet* 1993;342:899–900.
333. Poncelet BP, Weisskoff RM, Wedeen VJ, Brady T, Kantro H. Time of flight quantification of coronary flow with echo-planar MRI. *Magnet Reson Med* 1993;447–457.
334. Devereux RB, Drayer JIM, Chien S, Pickering TG, Letcher RL, DeYoung JL, Sealey JE, Laragh JH. Whole blood viscosity as a determinant of cardiac hypertrophy in systemic hypertension. *Am J Cardiol* 1986;54:592–595.
335. De la Sierra A, Coca A, Paré JC, Sánchez M, Valls V, Urbano-Márquez A. Erythrocyte ion fluxes in essential hypertensive patients with left ventricular hypertrophy. *Circulation* 1993;88:1628–1633.
336. Nosadini R, Semplicini A, Fioretto P, et al. Sodium–lithium countertransport and cardiorenal abnormalities in essential hypertension. *Hypertension* 1991;18:191–198.
337. Levy D, Savage DD, Garrison RJ, Anderson KM, Kannell WB, Castelli WP. Echocardiographic criteria for left ventricular hypertrophy: The Framingham Heart Study. *Am J Cardiol* 1987;59:956–960.

Atherosclerosis and Coronary Artery Disease,
edited by V. Fuster, R. Ross, and E. J. Topol.
Lippincott-Raven Publishers, Philadelphia © 1996.

CHAPTER 18

Cigarette Smoking and Atherosclerosis

Randall S. Stafford and Carl G. Becker

Key Words: Addiction; Endothelium; Leukocytes; Neurotransmitter; Nicotine; Plaque; Thrombosis.

INTRODUCTION

Consumption of tobacco products is a potent risk factor for atherosclerosis. Because of the more than 170,000 annual smoking-related cardiovascular deaths in the United States (33), cigarette smoking is a critical public health problem requiring a broad, multifaceted approach.

Cigarette smoke is a complex mixture of constituents with a broad range of biological activities. Synergizing with other risk factors, smoking contributes to atherosclerosis through multiple pathways involving the cellular constituents of blood, the coagulation system, the walls of blood vessels, and the immune system. For most of this century, increasing cardiovascular disease paralleled increasing cigarette smoking. Over the past 25 years, however, a 50% reduction in cardiovascular mortality has followed reductions in cigarette smoking (115,221). Because there appears to be no safe level of exposure to cigarette smoke (159), clinical interventions that focus on smoking cessation are a key strategy in the treatment and prevention of cardiovascular disease. Using a simple, yet systematic approach that focuses on nicotine addiction, physicians can effectively alter the smoking-related biological mechanisms that lead to atherosclerosis and its complications.

The purpose of this chapter is to describe the relationship of tobacco consumption, principally cigarette smoking, to the pathogenesis of arteriosclerotic cardiovascular disease and its complications, review the multiple pathogenic mechanisms that may be involved in this relationship, and review strategies of smoking cessation and overcoming addiction to nicotine in the prevention of cardiovascular disease.

R. S. Stafford: General Internal Medicine Unit, Massachusetts General Hospital, and Department of Medicine, Harvard Medical School, Boston, Massachusetts 02114.

C. G. Becker: Department of Pathology, Medical College of Wisconsin, Milwaukee, Wisconsin 53226.

TOBACCO AND ATHEROSCLEROSIS

Cardiovascular disease is the major cause of disability and death in the United States. It is estimated that in 1987 approximately 1 million people died of various cardiovascular diseases, and of these deaths, 200,000 were directly related to smoking cigarettes (161,162). The increase in cardiovascular disease in this century parallels the trends observed in the prevalence of smoking. There has been a decrease in deaths from cardiovascular disease of approximately 50% over the last 25 years (115,221). Fifty to sixty percent of this decrease is attributed to changes in life style, and it is estimated that 24% of this decrease is related to reduction in cigarette smoking. There appears to be no safe level of exposure to cigarette smoke (159). For each ten cigarettes smoked per day there is an 18% increase in cardiovascular mortality in men and a 31% increase in women (133). Smoking as few as one to four cigarettes a day was associated with a doubling of risk for coronary heart disease in the Nurses' Health Study (244). Younger smokers appear to be at more risk of ischemic heart disease than older smokers. This may suggest that certain individuals are more at risk of developing cardiovascular diseases if they smoke. It may also indicate that with advancing age other diseases have a greater effect on mortality.

Cigarette smoking is a major independent risk factor for arteriosclerotic disease, equivalent to either hypertension or hypercholesterolemia, with which it can synergize in the induction and progression of disease (64). A positive correlation has been established between smoking and the severity of atherosclerosis in coronary and cerebral arteries and the aorta (224). Because of the large number of substances in cigarette smoke, the association between smoking and the development of atherosclerosis and its complications may involve many mechanisms or systems including the nervous system, the immune system and its related mediator pathways, the coagulation system, and the endocrine system as well as the cellular elements of blood and the cells and connective tissue elements of the walls of arteries. These are reviewed below.

The Plant

Tobacco belongs to the genus *Nicotiana,* named for Jean Nicot, a French diplomat who sent tobacco seeds from Portugal to the Court of France at the end of the 16th Century. *Nicotiana* is in the family Solanaceae, which includes the deadly nightshade as well as comestibles such as tomato, eggplant, and peppers, with which tobacco shares antigenic and other chemical determinants (11). These antigenic similarities may in part account for the high degree of immunologic sensitivity to tobacco antigens that will be described later. Although the genus includes some 60 different species, *N. tabacum* and *N. rusticum* are the two species most cultivated for use as tobacco products because they are highly adaptive, being both extremely disease resistant and able to be grown profitably under a wide variety of climatic and soil conditions. Development of tobacco plants resistant to a wide variety of viral, bacterial, fungal, and insect pests has been a major goal of the Department of Agriculture here and in other countries that provide direct or indirect support to the tobacco industry. It is likely that the selection and propagation of disease-resistant cultivars is capable of generating a wide variety of potentially toxic chemicals and has resulted in an increased ability of tobacco to induce disease in users. Tobacco is harvested as green leaves, which are then either flue or heat cured, air cured, or in the case of some oriental tobaccos, sun or fire cured by exposure to wood smoke (248,251). The last is a significant cause of deforestation in developing countries (220). The curing process is also an important step in the generation of oxidized derivatives of plant compounds that may contribute to the development of disease in the user.

The Cigarette

Most American and European cigarettes are made from blends of tobacco differing genetically and in the method of curing. In order to use as much of the tobacco as possible, methods were developed to reconstitute tobacco in sheets in a process analogous to the manufacture of paper. In the production of cigarettes, humectants, sugars, and a variety of flavorings are added. The additives are held to be proprietary, and whether they or their derivatives contribute to health risk is not known. The formulation of sheet tobacco or of "puffed tobacco," which has more filling capacity and burns more rapidly, can affect the amount of particulates and nicotine yield produced consequent to lighting the cigarette. The number of ventilatory holes in cigarette paper is important to cooling of smoke and controlling the rate of burning. More ventilation results in less air drawn through the zone of pyrolysis, leading to a reduction in the level of most mainstream components of smoke, including nicotine, and an increase in the production of sidestream smoke during the smoldering period. The net result of these manufacturing strategies has been to reduce the costs of cigarette manufacture and reduce the yield of tar and nicotine per cigarette. This has resulted in an increase in consumption of cigarettes necessary to satisfy addiction to nicotine (248,249).

Cigarette Smoke

The smoking cigarette is a highly efficient drug delivery system. The temperature of the burning tip of the cigarette during puffing may reach 900°C, yet smoke entering the mouth is nearly body temperature. This is a result of the combined effects of the porosity of the cigarette paper, added humidifying agents like glycerol, and storage conditions. Mainstream smoke is generated during puffing in the burning and hot zones of the cigarette, and sidestream smoke is generated at temperatures of about 600°C in the smoldering period between puffs. The majority of the 4,865 known constituents of smoke are formed behind the burning zone through explosion of tobacco granules in the pyrolysis–distillation zone. Many of these products are created in this zone through alteration of substances originally present. The released and often modified constituents are then carried in a vapor stream, where they form heterogeneous particles measuring between 0.2 and 1.3 mm in diameter, depending on the presence and type of filter. The particulate nature of mainstream smoke may be important relative to their distribution in airways, but the nature of the surface of the particles may be important to the efficiency with which smoke can activate inflammatory pathways following inhalation. When a cigarette is smoked, many of the constituents of tobacco remain unburned, and molecules up to 100 kDa in molecular mass are delivered in mainstream smoke. This is of importance with respect to the immunologic and immunopathological consequences of smoking, which will be described below. The R. J. Reynolds Tobacco Company is introducing a "smokeless cigarette" in which the tobacco does not burn but uses smoldering charcoal to extract the flavor and nicotine (117). This may reduce a number of products of combustion but could actually produce a higher yield of other, unburnt substances with different pathological effects.

One conventional cigarette yields approximately 400 to 500 mg of mainstream smoke, of which 30% is derived from tobacco and the rest from air drawn through the cigarette. Mainstream smoke contains approximately 500 gaseous compounds in the vapor phase including nitrogen (58%), oxygen (12%), carbon dioxide (13%), and carbon monoxide (3.5%). The vapor phase also includes hydrogen, methane, other hydrocarbons, aldehydes and ketones, hydrogen cyanide, nitrogen oxides, volatile nitriles, and several hundred minor constituents (24,120,171). The particulate phase, defined operationally as particles greater than 0.1 μm that are trapped on a glass fiber pad (70), contains the majority of genotoxic and carcinogenic substances in cigarette smoke, polyphenols and phenolic and catechol derivatives thereof, and, at pH 5.5, nicotine (119). At pH 6.5, nicotine follows the vapor phase. Because nicotine is addictive, toxic to endothelial cells, capable of stimulating release of catecholamines, and some of its derivatives are carcinogenic, it can be seen that the conditions of smoking and the nature of the tobacco used can greatly influence biological consequences (118). The particulate phase of smoke also contains free radicals including a quinone–hydroxyquinone complex in the particulate phase and one in the vapor phase that is generated by the oxidation of nitric oxide (NO) to nitrous oxide (NO_2). These may be important in inducing tissue injury through effects on proteins or on lipid peroxidation and/or in modifying other constituents of smoke (41). The particulate phase of cigarette smoke also includes a variety of insecticides and their derivatives as well as aluminum, cadmium, lead, mercury, nickel, and polonium-210 (37,42,120). Compounds generated by reduction reactions are more common in sidestream smoke and include ammonia, aromatic amines, and volatile, carcinogenic amines (120). More detailed compilations of the constituents of the particular phase and vapor phases of mainstream smoke are given by Hoffmann and Wynder (120).

CONSTITUENTS OF CIGARETTE SMOKE AND THE INDUCTION OF CARDIOVASCULAR DISEASE

Many of the multitudes of highly chemically reactive substances in either mainstream or sidestream smoke may participate in the initiation and progression of atherosclerosis and its thrombotic complications. Because many of these are unstudied with respect to their biological effects, what is known may be less important than what is unknown, and the interactions among different constituents of smoke may permit or amplify the activity of any individual component once it comes in contact with blood and tissue components of the smoker. Further, it is conceivable that the mechanisms underlying the relationship between active smoking and the putative relationship between passive smoking and atherosclerosis may, at least in part, be different, given the differences in the constituents and their concentrations in these forms of smoke. Many of the effects of smoking on the cardiovascular system may be related to the lung as a portal of entry for smoke (Fig. 1). The pulmonary epithelium permits the easy passage of even relatively large molecules, which can then react with protein and cellular components of blood. Further, the lung is rich in macrophages, mast cells, and lymphocytes, which, stimulated by smoke constituents, can release a wide variety of pharmacologically active constituents including cytokines. The products of these reactions are generated in or enter pulmonary capillaries and are rapidly delivered into the systemic arterial circulation. It follows that the magnitude of mediator release from these cells would be greater in those individuals who are immunologically sensitized to constituents of tobacco smoke. Finally, some constituents of smoke and their metabolites may have multiple roles with respect to the pathogenesis of cardiovascular disease. Differences in the capacity of different individuals to form metabolites of these substances could modify the effect of these smoke constituents on atherosclerosis.

Cigarette Constituents, Neurotransmitter Release, and Endothelial Damage

Examination of the possible roles of nicotine in the pathogenesis of atherosclerosis illustrates many of the principles stated above. In addition to being responsible for tobacco addiction (18,247), described in detail later, nicotine appears to act presynaptically, leading to the release of acetylcholine, norepinephrine, dopamine, serotonin, vasopressin, growth hormone, adrenocorticotropic hormone, β-endorphin, pro-

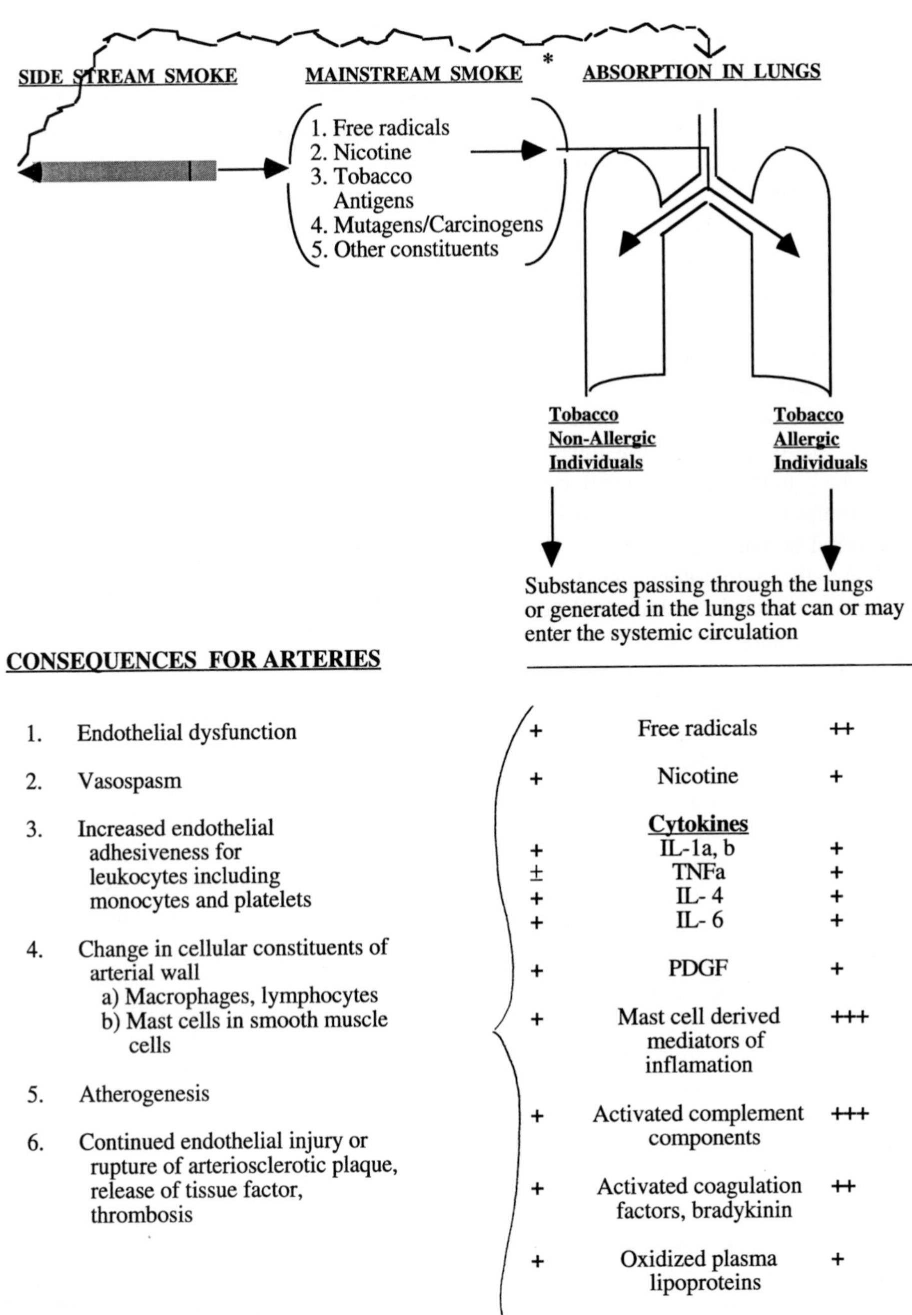

*Some components of sidestream smoke may have similar effects.

FIG. 1. Lung absorption of sidestream and mainstream smoke.

lactin, and cortisol. Nicotine also excites nicotinic receptors in the spinal cord, autonomic ganglia, and adrenal medulla, leading to release of epinephrine. It also stimulates release of catecholamines and facilitates the release of neurotransmitters from sympathetic nerves in blood vessels (17). Release of these catecholamines contributes to the increase in heart rate and blood pressure associated with smoking, and direct and indirect effects on platelets and cellular constituents of the walls of blood vessels may contribute to atherogenesis.

Nicotine has also been reported to be directly cytotoxic for vascular endothelial cells in vitro. Metabolites of nicotine have been demonstrated to be carcinogenic (118), and it may also enhance tumorigenicity by inhibiting apoptosis (250). These latter observations concerning nicotine may be pertinent to the monoclonal hypothesis concerning the development of atherosclerotic plaques. The fact that nicotine may be an inhibitor of apoptosis or programmed cell death may indicate a permissive role in plaque growth irrespective of the mechanisms initiating proliferation of vascular smooth muscle cells. Cotinine, a major metabolite of nicotine, is currently viewed as the best marker of tobacco exposure through either active inhalation or passive smoke exposure (7,106). However, in using this marker it appears that serum cotinine levels are higher in black than in white smokers, implying differences in rate of metabolism (234). These differences may be related to higher rates of some smoking-related cancers in blacks but might also pertain to differences in the rate of progression of atherosclerosis. Thus, even for the most extensively studied substance in cigarette smoke, there are a number of mechanisms through which it or its metabolites could contribute to the pathogenesis of atherosclerosis with varying effects in different individuals.

Many investigators (reviewed by Pittilo, ref. 192) have reported that exposure to tobacco smoke results in endothelial injury or perturbation. This toxicity has been attributed to nicotine and/or carbon monoxide. More recently, however, attention has focused on the multiple roles of oxidants in cigarette smoke in contributing to atherogenesis, including the induction of endothelial dysfunction. The presence of free radicals in smoke has been mentioned previously. Treatment of human umbilical vein endothelial cells with plasma from human volunteer smokers or with plasma exposed to cigarette smoke resulted in activation of the pentose monophosphate pathway, extrusion of glutathione, decreased ATP, and release of angiotensin-converting enzyme, suggesting that endothelial injury was mediated by free radicals in smoke (172). Exposure of hamsters to smoke resulted in increased xanthine oxidase activity in plasma and rolling and subsequent adhesion of leukocytes to endothelium of venules and arteries. These effects were greatly attenuated by treatment with CuZn-superoxide dismutase, confirming the role of oxidants in inducing endothelial dysfunction (150).

Cigarette Smoke and Lipoproteins

Cigarette smoking is associated with significant changes in both the level of lipoproteins and lipids in plasma as well as structural alterations of lipoproteins that may contribute to the association between smoking and the development of atherosclerosis and its complications. Analysis of 54 published studies on the effect of smoking on serum lipid and lipoprotein concentrations indicated that smokers had significantly higher serum concentrations of cholesterol, triglycerides, VLDL cholesterol, and LDL cholesterol and lower serum concentrations of HDL cholesterol and apolipoprotein A-I than nonsmokers, and these changes were greater in heavy smokers than light smokers. It was also observed that these changes occurred in both young and old smokers (46,47). The effect of oxidants in cigarette smoke on plasma low-density lipoprotein (LDL) may be important in the relationship between smoking and the pathogenesis of atherosclerosis. It has been demonstrated that cigarette smoking renders LDL more susceptible to peroxidative modification by cellular elements such as macrophages and vascular smooth muscle cells (110). Peroxidation of LDL is enhanced when the LDL is rich in polyunsaturated fatty acids (197). It has also been reported that HDL inhibits the peroxidation of LDL.

Smoking may also affect other aspects of lipid metabolism. Treatment of plasma in vitro with the vapor phase of cigarette smoke was found to dramatically inhibit lecithin-cholesterol acyltransferase (LCAT) activity and both increase the negative charge on HDL and cross-linking with apolipoproteins A-I and A-II (162). These studies taken together may explain why smoking acts in synergy with LDL as a risk factor for atherosclerosis and its complications. From these data it has been hypothesized that the lower incidence of coronary heart disease in the presence of heavy smoking in Japan and China is because plasma LDL levels are generally lower and HDL levels generally higher in citizens of those countries (221).

These studies also imply that a diet high in polyunsaturated lipids will be helpful in reducing risk of coronary artery disease only if smoking is also discontinued. It could be harmful if smoking is continued. Oxidation of LDL causes it to be taken up by the "scavenger receptor" of macrophages in atherosclerotic plaques in which oxidized LDL can also be demonstrated in association with monocyte chemoattractant protein 1 (252). Oxidized LDL can inhibit release of endothelially derived relaxing factor (EDRF) or response of endothelial cells to EDRF that might augment the response of vessels to vasoconstrictive agents including catecholamines released in response to nicotine (145). It has also been demonstrated that administration of oxidized LDL stimulated adherence of leukocytes to endothelial cells of precapillary venules and arterioles. Adherence could be inhibited by prior administration of either antibodies to integrins on leukocytes or of an inhibitor of leukotriene synthesis (151). Oxidized LDL has been demonstrated to be autoantigenic, and the titer of autoantibodies to malondialdehyde-LDL has been reported to be an independent predictor of the progression of carotid atherosclerosis in Finnish men (210). Further, oxidized LDL can induce expression of granulocyte and macrophage colony-stimulating factors by endothelial cells (55). Overviews of the multiple roles that oxidized LDL may have in the pathogenesis of atherosclerosis can be found in other chapters of this book and in several references (38,186,222,247).

Cigarette Smoke, Leukocytes, and the Complement System

The effect of oxidized LDL stimulating adhesion of leukocytes to endothelium may act synergistically with the effects of tobacco smoke on the complement system. Exposure of serum to cigarette smoke was observed to result in cleavage of the internal thioester bond of the third component of complement (C3), leading to activation of C3 (136,137). Rats exposed to cigarette smoke had increased levels of chemotactic activity for leukocytes and monocytes in alveolar lavage fluid that was inhibited by pretreatment with a cobra venom factor that depletes C3 (138). The nature of the C3-activating substance(s) in smoke is unknown. It has been demonstrated that nicotine is chemotactic for neutrophils and enhances their response to chemotactic peptides (231). It has also recently been shown that tobacco glycoprotein (TGP), a complex of glycoprotein, polyphenols, and iron present in flue-cured tobacco leaves and in cigarette smoke condensate or tar, can activate the classical pathway of complement, activating C1 (1). This effect appears to result from binding of polyphenol moieties to the globular region of the C1 molecule because free chlorogenic acid, a polyphenol constituent of cigarette smoke, can produce the same effect. It is of interest that when C1 is activated by free polyphenols or TGP, its activity is no longer inhibited by C1 inactivator. Neither the TGP nor free polyphenols have any demonstrable direct effect on C4, C2, or C3. These data taken together indicate that components of smoke may activate the complement system directly through at least two mechanisms and generate the anaphylotoxic peptides C3a and C5a, leading to mast cell release (C3a and C5a) and up-regulation (C5a) of expression of integrin molecules on surfaces of polymorphonuclear neutrophils, monocytes, lymphocytes, and natural killer cells (27,219).

Consequences of increased expression of integrin molecules by leukocytes would be enhanced adherence of these cells to vascular endothelial cells that have been induced to express proteins of the selectin family (P and E selectins) and intercellular adhesion molecules (ICAMs) of the immunoglobulin superfamily such as ICAM-1, ICAM-2, and vascular cell adhesion molecule (VCAM) (21,26). Expression of these immunoglobulin superfamily molecules on endothelial cells is regulated by the transcription factor NF-*k*B (nuclear factor *k*B), and, as hypothesized by Collins, the function of this family of nuclear regulatory proteins may be a common pathway in the pathogenesis of atherosclerosis (43). These events are of obvious importance to the pathogenesis of tobacco-associated inflammatory disease of the lung, but they may also contribute to the pathogenesis of atherosclerosis.

Immune responses to tobacco constituents may greatly amplify their pathogenic potential. Tobacco glycoprotein, described earlier, is a complex of glycoprotein, iron, and polyphenols or derivatives thereof that can be isolated from flue-cured tobacco leaves and from cigarette smoke condensate (10,11). The TGP has been shown to stimulate release of IL-1α, IL-1β, and IL-6 and elevate steady-state levels of mRNA of IL-1 and IL-6, PDGF-A, and PDGF in human pulmonary macrophages obtained by bronchoalveolar lavage (87). It has also been shown to stimulate selective expression of IgE in guinea pigs, mice, and rabbits (13,88).

Approximately one-third of human volunteers exhibit immediate cutaneous hypersensitivity when injected intracutaneously with this antigen (11,66). This high incidence of hypersensitivity may result from several factors, including the prevalence of tobacco smoke in the environment, antigens cross-reactive with tobacco antigens among other plants, including some commonly eaten (11,14), and selective stimulation of IgE production by tobacco antigens. The mechanism underlying this selective effect on IgE production by TGP appears to rest with the ability of the polyphenol epitopes to stimulate human peripheral blood Th2 lymphocytes, a subset of T-helper cells, to proliferate and express IL-4, thereby influencing switching of B lymphocytes to production of IgE (9). Interleukin-4 has also been shown to promote adhesion of eosinophils and basophils, but not neutrophils, to endothelium by inducing expression of VCAM-1 (211). Also, because of its polyphenol epitopes, TGP can stimulate polyclonal proliferation in and immunoglobulin synthesis by murine B cells (40) and proliferation of peripheral T cells and differentiation of human B cells as measured by synthesis of IgG, IgA, and IgM (86). Because of polyphenol epitopes, TGP can stimulate proliferation of bovine aortic smooth muscle cells (12) and, as mentioned above, activate factor XII of the intrinsic pathway of coagulation.

Most of these effects of TGP can be reproduced by coupling polyphenol epitopes to other carrier proteins, e.g., bovine serum albumin. Polyphenols, which structurally resemble flavonoids and tannins, are important to plant defenses against viral, bacterial, fungal, and insect parasites and have a wide range of pharmacological activities (112). Some of these effects are immunosuppressive, and some immunostimulatory (167). The proinflammatory effects of cotton bract tannins are thought to be important to the pathogenesis of byssinosis (203) and, like TGP, stimulate IL-1 production by human peripheral blood monocytes (209). Selection of disease-resistant cultivars is often related to their capacity to produce polyphenols (112). Approximately 200 different phenolic compounds, many breakdown products of polyphenols, are present in cigarette smoke (120). A number of intact polyphenols including chlorogenic acid and scopoletin are also present in cigarette smoke. The polyphenols and many of their products, especially when oxidized, are highly reactive and readily haptenize, raising the possibility that coupling of these substances to host proteins may give rise to autoimmune phenomena that may be involved in the pathogenesis of smoking-associated pulmonary and cardiovascular disease.

Smokers have higher serum levels of IgE than nonsmokers (48). The level of IgE correlates better with a history of smoking than with a history of allergy. Further, the level of IgE does not fall with age as it does in nonsmokers. Elevated levels of IgE have been positively associated with myocardial infarction, stroke, and large-vessel peripheral arterial disease in men (49). It has also been reported that increased numbers of mast cells were present in the adventitia, outer media, and intima in raised arteriosclerotic lesions in the aortas and coronary arteries of young people (6).

Conceivably, cytokines from populations of T lymphocytes (109) and other inflammatory cells present in arteriosclerotic plaques might contribute to the growth and differentiation of mast cells in these plaques in addition to contributing to other aspects of the inflammatory milieu of the developing plaques. The development of human mast cells from their progenitors is reviewed in Ishizaka et al. (129).

The above observations may be pertinent to the pathogenesis of atherosclerosis and its complications in several ways. First, inhalation of smoke constituents in sensitized smokers might trigger vasospasm, dysrhythmia, and sudden death with cardiac anaphylaxis (153). Cardiac anaphylaxis, mediated by IgE antibodies reactive with TGP isolated from cured tobacco leaves or cigarette smoke condensate, has been induced in guinea pigs and rabbits (154). Mast cells, in addition to producing acute inflammatory mediators such as histamine following antigenic challenge, can also release IL-1 and TNF-α from preformed stores in addition to being able to synthesize these cytokines (93). It has further been demonstrated that E-selectin is expressed in endothelial cells in organ cultures during the late phase of the allergic response and that this expression can be blocked with antibodies to IL-1 and TNF-α (152).

Combining these various observations permits the construction of the following scenario. Antigenic constituents of cigarette smoke could sensitize certain individuals. If that sensitization occurred early in life, it might be especially likely to stimulate IgE responses to the antigen, as seen in the association between maternal smoking and childhood asthma (175) and in experiments indicating that neonatal sensitization with TGP gives rise to persistent and selective IgE responses (13,154). Later inhalation of these antigens in cigarette smoke would result in enhanced release of inflammatory mediators such as histamine and TNF-α from pulmonary mast cells that, in addition to mediating local effects, would stimulate expression of selectins and intercellular adhesion molecules on endothelium of coronary and systemic arteries. Release of mast cell tryptase (214) might augment these effects by providing another means of activating the complement system. These effects would be amplified by cytokines, described above, released from pulmonary macrophages.

Cigarette Smoke Constituents and Thrombosis

The net effect of the changes described in the preceding paragraph would be to begin the process of adhesion and emigration of inflammatory cells in the walls of arteries and the concomitant process of converting the endothelial surface from antithrombotic to prothrombotic through provoking endothelial injury to release underlying factor VII, downregulate production of thrombomodulin and the anticoagulant and profibrinolytic effects of proteins C and S, decrease expression of tissue plasminogen activator, and increase expression of tissue plasminogen activator inhibitor (193). These changes, in addition to the ability of certain tobacco constituents to activate factor XII, would favor thrombogenesis on a surface with diminished capacity to lyse thrombi (169). Activation of factor XII would also enhance thrombus formation following plaque erosion or rupture. In either of these settings, activated factor XI would drive the intrinsic pathway after the initial reaction among tissue factor, factor VII, and factor X had been modulated by lipoprotein association coagulation inhibitor (LACI) (61).

Elevation of fibrinogen, also found in smokers and a risk factor for coronary artery disease (113,164), might be a consequence of the effect of IL-1 generated by alveolar macrophages in response to smoke constituents on hepatocytes that synthesize fibrinogen (68). That fibrinogen is elevated for several years (164) after stopping smoking may be related to the ability of some tobacco constituents, including polyphenols, to bind to proteins in the lung and persist for long periods of time.

Elevations of factor VII coagulant activity in smokers might reflect continued endothelial perturbation associated with smoking (113). Smoking-associated cardiovascular disease is also increased in a synergistic manner by changes in sex hormonal status such as menopause or the use of oral contraceptives, possibly through changes in levels of various clotting factors and/or activity of regulatory proteins such as antithrombin III (94,95,190,240).

In fact, smoking itself can induce changes in hormonal status. Smoking has been associated with the earlier appearance of menopause, possibly removing the "protective" effect of estrogen with respect to the progression of atherosclerosis and its complications. Also, increased irreversible 2-hydroxylation of estradiol has been demonstrated in female and male smokers, leading to an increase of estrogen metabolites that have minimal peripheral estrogenic activity and are rapidly cleared from the circulation (165,166).

The above hypothesis concerning the role of immune reactions to tobacco products in the pathogenesis of atherosclerosis and its complications suggests that the smoker allergic to tobacco constituents is at greater risk than the nonallergic smoker and that risk might have been increased by maternal and paternal smoking habits and by genetic determinants of allergy. It would also suggest that such individuals might be particularly susceptible to the development of cardiovascular disease consequent to exposure to second-hand smoke.

Alterations induced directly or indirectly by smoking in the endothelium and vessel walls may contribute to altered platelet function in smokers. Decreased platelet survival time, increased numbers of aggregated platelets in the circulation, and release of platelet proteins have been described in smokers (168,212). Increased production of prostacyclin metabolites and excessive production of thromboxane A_2 have also been described in the blood of smokers (174). Alterations of platelet sensitivity to prostacyclin have been described in the blood of active smokers and in individuals passively exposed to cigarette smoke (25).

It is of interest that many of the effects of smoking on

platelets appear to be related to substances other than nicotine (20). These changes in addition to those induced by catechols released in response to nicotine may contribute to atherosclerosis and its complications through effects on vessel tone, platelet reactivity, generation of PDGF and other cytokines, and thrombus formation. Obviously, other conditions might contribute to this process. For example, chronic smokers have been reported to be insulin resistant and hyperinsulinemic, perhaps resulting in amplification of the effects of such mitogens as platelet-derived growth factor, and to have elevated VLDL cholesterol and triglycerides and lower HDL cholesterol than members of a control group of nonsmokers (74).

Cigarette Smoke Constituents and Smooth Muscle Proliferation: The Monoclonal Hypothesis Concerning Plaque Development

The hypothesis that atherosclerotic plaques arise as monoclonal proliferations of smooth muscle cells following a mutational event must also be considered in relation to the association of smoking with atherosclerosis because of both the quantity and number of different mutagens and carcinogens in cigarette smoke and the fact that some constituents can also stimulate the release of a variety of cytokines, thus providing both initiators and promoters of neoplasia. In this connection, it has been demonstrated that overexpression of the tumor suppressor protein p53 occurs in association with the presence of cytomegalovirus infection, possibly as the result of inhibition of p53 function by the viral protein IE84 (218). Overexpression of p53 has also been described in bladder epithelium of smokers with early stages of bladder cancer (253) and in cancers of the lung (243). These observations suggest that smoking might also induce changes leading to overexpression associated with mutational changes in the p53 gene or have effects on viral oncoproteins resulting in enhanced growth of atherosclerotic plaques.

The monoclonal hypothesis, as developed and tested by Benditt and Benditt (16), focused on vascular smooth muscle cells. Further, it has been reported that cockerels injected with 7,12-dimethylbenz(*a*)anthracene, a polynuclear aromatic hydrocarbon, in nontumorigenic doses developed atherosclerotic plaques. DNA extracted from these plaques also induced transformation of NIH 3T3 cells (187). However, in addition to vascular smooth muscle cells, other cellular constituents of the arteriosclerotic plaque may also be altered mutationally by exposure to constituents of tobacco smoke, possibly changing the life expectancy of these cells and, quantitatively or qualitatively, their pattern of production of cytokines and growth factors. In this connection, smoking has been associated with an increased incidence of lymphoma, leukemia, and multiple myeloma (155), and adducts of environmental mutagens/carcinogens and DNA, including those derived from tobacco smoke, have been described in white blood cells and have been proposed as biomarkers for exposure to environmental carcinogens (188). Some of the carcinogens associated with tobacco can also be found in products of combustion of hydrocarbon fuels, raising the question of whether contaminants in addition to tobacco constituents in the external environment may contribute to the pathogenesis of atherosclerosis through effects on DNA and RNA. If this is the case, then the monoclonal hypothesis concerning the origin of atherosclerotic plaques greatly expands the role of the environmental factors that need to be considered in any evaluation of risk.

PROMOTING TOBACCO CESSATION IN CLINICAL PRACTICE

Clinical interventions aimed at tobacco cessation are a key strategy in the prevention and treatment of coronary artery disease and atherosclerosis. However, current practices are inadequate, in part because of physician barriers to more extensive efforts (163,176). Physicians may feel uncomfortable confronting behavioral risk factors, may be discouraged by the relatively few patients who take their advice to quit, and may feel that they lack sufficient skills or resources in smoking cessation. The remainder of this chapter will focus on providing guidance to physicians in (a) acquiring a basic knowledge about smoking, nicotine addiction, and clinical interventions; (b) developing clinical skills in counseling, health education, and nicotine replacement therapy; and (c) translating information and skills into practice.

DEMOGRAPHICS AND EPIDEMIOLOGY OF SMOKING

Although smoking is decreasing in prevalence, more than a quarter of adult Americans smoke cigarettes. As physicians confront the habits of these individual smokers, their efforts are affected by the demographics and epidemiology of cigarette initiation, maintenance, and cessation.

Cigarette smoking in the United States is a relatively recent phenomenon. Before the early 1900s most tobacco was consumed in the form of snuff, followed by cigars and pipe tobacco. Cigarettes accounting for less than 5% of tobacco products. Cigarette smoking quickly came to dominate by the 1940s and then reached a plateau in the 1950s and early 1960s. Per capita consumption of cigarettes peaked in 1963 (Fig. 2), but smoking prevalence peaked in 1965 with 40% of adults smoking (80). Since 1965, there has been a steady, gradual decline in cigarette consumption. This decrease in prevalence has been four times more rapid for men (0.84 percentage points per year on average) compared to women (0.21 percentage points per year). Based on trends through 1989, Fiore (80) estimated that in the year 2000, 22% of American adults would still be smoking cigarettes. Centers for Disease Control estimates for the prevalence of adult, regular smokers for 1990 (25.5%), 1991 (25.6%), and 1992

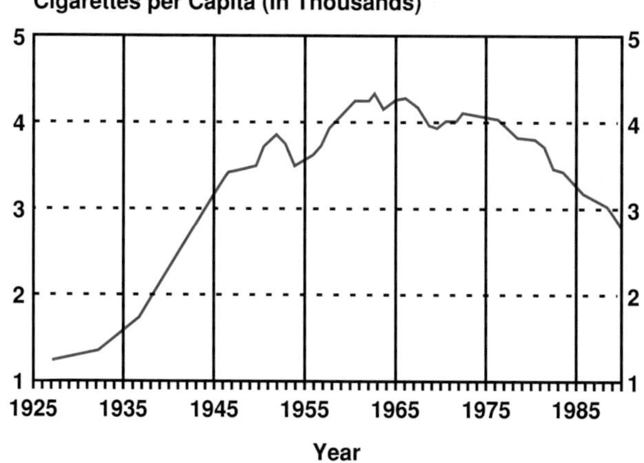

FIG. 2. Adult per capital consumption of cigarettes, United States, 1925–1990.

(25.6%) suggest a temporary plateau in declining rates of smoking (32,35,36). Recent redefinition to include those smoking only on some days brings the prevalence of smoking in 1992 to 26.5% of all adults. This translates to the consumption of half a trillion cigarettes.

Tobacco consumption in the United States is comparable to that in many other developed nations but exceeds that of several western European countries (29). As in the United States, cigarette consumption is declining in other developed nations (191). Consumption in less-developed nations is generally lower, but it has been increasing as U.S. exports increase to offset declining domestic sales (156).

The cigarettes smoked by Americans have changed over the past 50 years. In 1950, filtered cigarettes accounted for less than 1% of total consumption, compared to 95% in 1988 (80). In addition, the average nicotine and tar content of cigarettes has declined. Cigarette smoking continues to be the dominant form of tobacco consumption, although smokeless tobacco use is rising, especially among teen-age boys (81).

A majority of cigarette smokers begin smoking before reaching adulthood. Ninety percent of regular smokers report starting smoking before the age of 21; 50% start before 18 years of age (81). Between 1950 and 1980, rates of smoking initiation for men decreased dramatically at all ages except for 12- to 15-year-olds (149). For women, however, slightly decreased initiation in 18- to 24-year-olds was offset by increased initiation in 12- to 15-year-olds. By 1980, patterns of initiation for young men and women had converged and have remained unchanged for the past decade (149). The combined effects of initiation, cessation, and attrition through death result in a peak prevalence of smoking in early adulthood (25 to 44 years of age) (28). Fewer women (25%) than men (29%) smoke (36), a narrower difference than in 1965 [32% for women versus 50% for men (35)]. This convergence is explained by the fact that smoking initiation has fallen less rapidly in women than men, not by gender differences in cessation.

Race and ethnicity also predict the prevalence of cigarette smoking. In 1992, blacks (28%) and whites (27%) had similar smoking prevalence rates that were higher than those of either Hispanics (21%) or Asians (15%) (36). Since 1965, absolute differences between black (43%) and white (40%) smoking prevalence have changed little (36,83). Compared to whites, blacks are less likely to be heavy smokers. Ten percent of black smokers smoked more than 20 cigarettes per day in 1985, compared to 21% in white smokers. Novotny et al. (173) found the black–white difference in smoking to be explained by other demographic and socioeconomic variables. Compared to non-Hispanics, Hispanics smoke less frequently and are less likely to be heavy smokers. For women, the lower rates of smoking for Hispanics (18%) and Asians (4%) are especially pronounced.

Socioeconomic status is the most potent predictor of smoking. Adults below poverty level (35%) have higher smoking prevalence than those at or above poverty level (25%) (36). College graduates (16%) are less likely to smoke than adults with less than high school education (32%) (36). This is a new phenomenon (81,191,235). In 1966, smoking prevalence in college graduates (34%) was similar to that in high school graduates (37%) (80), but educational differences appear to be increasing (191). A similar pattern is seen by occupation, with professional men in 1985 to 1990 (16%) much less likely to smoke than laborers (39%), a difference that has widened since 1977 to 1980 (22% versus 33%) (45).

The ratio of former smokers to current smokers indicates that college graduates are the most likely to have quit smoking, especially compared to those with below high school education. Based on this ratio, men tend to quit more than women, and whites tend to quit more than blacks (80). Lighter smokers are more likely to quit smoking (91). Among all former smokers, 70% have quit on their own without formal intervention (82). Physicians can be most effective when they complement smokers' own efforts to quit. As more smokers become former smokers, however, the remaining smokers may require more intensive efforts to promote cessation.

NICOTINE ADDICTION

Of the substances present in cigarette smoke, nicotine is the most important in defining patterns of cigarette use. Smokers use tobacco primarily for the desirable direct effects of nicotine and to avoid the undesirable symptoms of nicotine withdrawal. Although multiple factors lead to cigarette smoking (85), cigarettes would not produce large numbers of habitual users if they did not contain nicotine (17). Nicotine addiction is critical in physicians' attempts to help their patients stop smoking.

The significance of nicotine addiction has long been underestimated, in part because of the legal use of tobacco products. Nicotine shares many characteristics with other drugs of dependence. Drug dependence or addiction has been variously defined (5,31,71), but most definitions include: (a) highly controlled or compulsive use, (b) psychoactive effects, (c) drug effects that reinforce use, and (d) continued use despite harmful effects. Nicotine use in cigarette and smokeless tobacco meets these criteria. In addition, like many other addictive substances, nicotine is associated with recurrent craving, the development of tolerance, and the presence of withdrawal symptoms with abstinence. Although it is difficult to compare different substances, nicotine, cocaine, and heroin all have relapse rates around 75% within 6 months of abstinence (18).

Nicotine use is compatible with a high level of functioning; unlike many other drugs of dependence, whose use is episodic, daily cigarette smoking is the norm. Because tobacco is associated with compulsive use, substantial craving, and a rapid onset of withdrawal symptoms, it is difficult for most smokers to abstain for more than a few waking hours (18). Several typologies have been developed that differentiate smokers by the degree of their dependence on nicotine (76,77,139,194). The Fagerstrom Tolerance Questionnaire (FTQ) provides an index ranging from 0 to 11 of nicotine dependence based on eight questions with average smokers scoring 5 to 7 with a standard deviation of 2 (77). As a single measure, daily cigarette consumption tends to correlate with dependence measured by the FTQ. The length of time a patient takes between waking up and having his or her first cigarette may be a useful indicator for high (less than 5 min) and low (more than 30 min) levels of nicotine addiction.

Cigarettes are a highly effective system for delivering nicotine. Inhalation of cigarette smoke results in rapid absorption of nicotine in the alveoli with immediate peaking of cerebral arterial nicotine levels (114). Some nicotine also may be absorbed through the buccal mucosa, as with smokeless tobacco. The average nicotine absorption from a single cigarette is 1 mg (17). Brain nicotine levels quickly fall after smoking as nicotine is redistributed to other tissues. However, the 2-h elimination half-life allows trough nicotine levels to rise with subsequently smoked cigarettes (17). Most smokers maintain blood nicotine levels of 10 to 50 ng/ml, with single cigarettes transiently adding 5 to 30 ng/ml to this concentration (17). The rapidity of drug dosing through inhalation allows nicotine to be precisely titrated and controlled. Combined with its psychodynamic effects, this titration makes nicotine highly addictive.

Nicotine has two sets of psychopharmacological effects that are instrumental in its dependence potential: direct effects and withdrawal effects. Nicotine's direct effects occur with inhalation of cigarette smoke. They tend to be perceived as positive and include pleasure, arousal, improved performance with repetitive tasks, relief of anxiety, decreased hunger, and muscle relaxation (18,148). In addition, basal metabolic rate and heart rate are increased by nicotine.

Withdrawal effects occur following abstinence from nicotine. Falling nicotine levels after smoking can generate withdrawal symptoms that eventually lead to the next cigarette. Withdrawal symptoms generally peak during the first 2 days of abstinence and include irritability, impatience, anger, restlessness, hunger, weight gain, anxiety, sleep disturbance, craving for cigarettes, dyspepsia, difficulty concentrating, and impaired performance (30,122,123). These symptoms gradually decline during the first 2 weeks after cessation. At 1 month, difficulty concentrating, hunger, and weight gain remain, although net discomfort scores are no different at 1 month compared to precessation. At 6 months, only weight gain and hunger are increased over precessation levels (122). In some smokers, symptoms of depression may be triggered by cessation (85,96,108). The intensity of these withdrawal symptoms induces resumption of cigarette smoking after short-term abstinence. Relapse after 1 month is more likely to be mediated by social and psychological factors.

Tolerance develops with nicotine use, so that greater and greater levels of nicotine are required for the same direct, positive effects. Tolerance is mediated by the desensitization of nicotinic acetylcholine receptors, both acutely and chronically (204). A daily smoking cycle develops in which cigarettes early in the day induce pleasure, but the development of tolerance through the day makes smokers less able to achieve these pleasurable effects, and later cigarettes are smoked to prevent withdrawal symptoms. Abstinence during sleep allows nicotine levels to diminish with partial reversal of tolerance (18).

Beyond nicotine addiction, a complex set of social and psychological factors also influence cigarette use (85). Cigarette smoking, often initiated prior to adulthood, is a deeply ingrained habit that is an integral part of smokers' daily routines. Smoking tends to become associated with enjoyable activities, such that these activities may trigger a desire to smoke. The routine of manipulating cigarettes may reinforce continued use. Smokers also use cigarettes as a method of coping with stress, anger, anxiety, or loneliness. In addition, the nicotine in cigarettes may be employed to regulate mood. Cigarette smoking takes place in a complex social system that discourages smoking but simultaneously strongly reinforces initiation and maintenance of smoking through family and peer influences, social and cultural norms regarding fashion, cigarette advertisements, and access to relatively inexpensive cigarettes (8,156). The complex interaction of these influences with nicotine addiction must be considered in tobacco cessation strategies. These other forces should not be neglected even with a clinical focus of nicotine addiction.

BENEFITS OF SMOKING CESSATION

Smoking-attributable mortality accounts for over 400,000 annual deaths, a quarter of all deaths in the United States (34). Annually, 180,000 smoking-related deaths are from cardiovascular disease, 27% of all cardiovascular mortality. In addition, smoking contributes to reduced quality of life for those who live with smoking-related conditions. Tobacco cessation can dramatically diminish the likelihood of these adverse outcomes, especially for cardiovascular disease.

Many of the pathophysiological changes produced by cigarette smoke are reversible. The benefits of smoking cessation occur regardless of smoking duration, the age of the smoker, or the presence of smoking-related diseases. The magnitude of this benefit can motivate smokers to consider cessation and should prompt physicians to intervene with their patients who smoke. The benefits of smoking cessation accrue over time: some adverse effects of smoking rapidly reverse following cessation, and others only gradually dissipate.

The earliest benefits of cessation are the respiratory symptoms associated with smoking, including cough, dyspnea, and phlegm production. Relief from these symptoms is more likely to motivate smokers than are statistics regarding reduction in mortality. Cough and phlegm production may increase transiently as respiratory cleansing mechanisms recover but then fall below baseline levels.

The overall mortality rates of former smokers decline rapidly after cessation. However, the excess risk of smoking never returns to the baseline of never smokers (30). Projections based on mortality data indicate that 35-year-old men and women who quit add 2.3 and 2.8 years, respectively, to their life expectancy (232,233). The early benefits of tobacco cessation may not be apparent statistically because newly diagnosed smoking-related illnesses increase the likelihood of both death and cessation. Studies controlling for this effect suggest that cessation has an immediate benefit (134).

The reduction of cardiac events in former smokers has both immediate and delayed components, reflecting the complex relationship of smoking and coronary artery disease (205). Mechanisms such as altered platelet function, vasospasm, and reduced oxygen-carrying capacity are rapidly reversible following cessation. However, the development of atherosclerotic plaques is minimally reversible, and the main benefit of cessation may be to slow the progression of existing lesions. Within 1 to 2 years of quitting, the risk of myocardial infarction falls by 30% in men and by 40% in women (205,206). The risk of myocardial infarction in former smokers approaches that of never smokers within 2 to 4 years after cessation (205).

The greatest benefits of tobacco cessation are in reducing cardiovascular mortality. Five-year mortality rates in a series of studies (3,58,132,217) indicate that the mortality of continuing smokers is approximately double that of those who quit. Krumholz (144) estimates that quitting after a myocardial infarction adds 1.7 years of life compared to patients continuing to smoke.

Smoking cessation also produces a reduction in cerebrovascular accidents. Risk of stroke is reduced within 2 years after cessation, a risk that diminishes to that comparable to never smokers after 5 years. The risk of respiratory cancers declines after cessation. In 6 to 10 years after cessation, the risk of dying from lung cancer falls to about 40% for both men and women (30). Even after 15 years of abstinence, however, the incidence of lung cancer remains 10% to 20% higher than that in never smokers. Other health benefits of smoking cessation include reduction of symptoms from peripheral vascular disease, reduction in aortic aneurysm mortality, reduced peptic ulcer disease, improved blood pressure control, increased high-density lipoprotein (HDL) levels, and better pregnancy outcomes (30,131,132,161).

Fear of weight gain following smoking cessation frequently is used to rationalize the continuation of smoking. Evidence suggests that a variety of mechanisms (189) contribute to an average weight gain following smoking cessation of 6.4 lb (140). The health risks associated with weight gain following smoking cessation are negligible compared to the benefits of cessation (30).

MODELS OF SMOKING CESSATION

Two complementary models guide behavioral scientists' current views of the process of smoking cessation: (a) the incentive/disincentive model and (b) the stages of cessation model.

Incentive/Disincentive Model of Smoking Cessation

The incentive/disincentive model assumes that there is a constant dynamic for smokers between the incentives and disincentives to continue smoking (18). The incentives to continue smoking include pleasure from smoking, cigarette advertising, social pressure from friends or family members who smoke, a coping mechanism for negative emotions, stress reduction from cigarettes, fear of weight gain, and the negative consequence of cessation (withdrawal). The disincentives include the cost of cigarettes, the personal health risks of smoking, the risks to others, the odor of cigarette smoke, the growing stigma of smoking, and antismoking advertisements. A smoker will remain a smoker until the personal disincentives outweigh the incentives to continue smoking. The role of clinical intervention is to enhance the disincentives: to educate the patient about the health effects of smoking and to personalize these risks. The clinician may also work to minimize the incentives to continue smoking through reassurance about the time-limited nature of nicotine withdrawal and by prescribing nicotine replacement.

A complementary model of smoking cessation views cessation as a series of cognitive stages that smokers move through as they prepare to stop. The clinical relevance of these stages is that as smokers move through these stages, they need different interventions. The stages are precontemplation, contemplation, preparation, action, and maintenance (versus relapse) (67,195) (Fig. 3). The precontemplation stage represents smokers not seriously considering cessation and unlikely to respond to information or consider quitting as an option. Smokers in the contemplation stage have begun to consider cessation. They are more open to information,

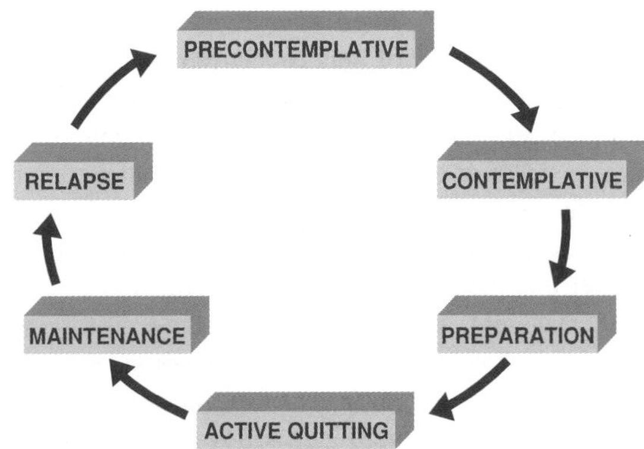

FIG. 3. Stages of smoking cessation.

and physicians can motivate these smokers toward acting on their desires to quit. The incentive/disincentive model applies well to these two stages. Motivated smokers then move into a phase of preparation for quitting. Active quitters are attempting to give up cigarettes and need tools to help them manage the negative social, psychological, and physical consequences of abstinence. Former smokers in the maintenance stage have passed through the acute difficulties of cessation but are always at risk for relapse to smoking.

Stepped-Care Approach to Smoking Cessation Interventions

Clinical intervention in smoking is more effective if particular activities are matched with patient characteristics and if interventions gradually escalate in intensity (179). A stepped-care approach begins by offering the least costly and least intensive intervention to all smokers. Subsequent steps require additional resources and are directed at smokers with particular characteristics, including those who fail previous attempts using less intensive techniques. Although the particular components of a stepped-care approach to smoking cessation is still in evolution, a five-step model includes (a) brief physician advice and counseling with patient self-help, (b) counseling and education in formal programs, (c) nicotine replacement therapy, (d) additional pharmacological agents, and (e) inpatient treatment of nicotine addiction in concert with hospitalization for smoking-related illnesses. Although there is no evidence confirming the effectiveness of a stepped-care approach, there is indirect support. The natural history of smoking cessation suggests that some smokers quit with minimal intervention while other smokers quit only with more intensive intervention. Similar algorithms apply to the treatment of hypertension (130) or hypercholesterolemia (170), where treatment options are simultaneously personalized for clinical characteristics and provided in a stepped-care approach.

Beyond choosing an appropriate level of care for each smoker, the physician must modify this level based on patient characteristics. Treatments aimed at smoking cessation may be more effective if individualized on the basis of smoking motives (216). In addition, differing degrees of pharmacological sensitivity may define levels of dependence in smokers (194). The demographic characteristic of the smoker may also be of use in directing the therapeutic intervention. For example, teen-age smokers are less likely to respond to messages about long-term health effects and more likely to respond to the immediate, negative effects of smoking on athletic performance and bad breath.

Brief Intervention

So-called ''minimal contact'' interventions should apply to all smokers. These activities take little physician time, incorporate flexibility, and yet provide a strong quit-smoking message. Although the quit rate following brief physician interventions is low, over time a substantial number of smokers will quit. This clinical activity may be more cost effective than other well-accepted clinical practices (53).

Effective minimal contact interventions encompass (a) assessing smoking status and smoking history, (b) presenting a strong recommendation to quit smoking at each clinic visit with a cogent rationale, (c) suggesting basic techniques and coping skills for cessation, (d) offering self-help materials, and (e) arranging for follow-up (99,157,180). Although each of these tasks can be easily accomplished by most physicians, current data suggest that physician practices are inadequate (227,239). Physicians frequently fail to determine whether or not their patients smoke and, among their patients who do smoke, infrequently recommend tobacco cessation (52,89,176,239). Specific training in smoking cessation skills appears to enhance the effectiveness of physicians (142,158,178,246).

The first step is to ask a patient whether he or she smokes cigarettes or uses other tobacco products. A focused smoking history also should cover (a) years of smoking, (b) daily cigarette consumption, (c) history of past quitting attempts, (d) degree of nicotine dependence (''How long after waking do you have a cigarette?''), and (e) current level of interest in quitting. These details can help direct physician interventions.

The next step is to advise smokers to quit. The physician should not exhaustively review the extensive medical rationale for quitting. Rather, the physician should attempt to personalize the benefits of smoking cessation to the patient's specific situation. This is particularly true at early stages in the process of quitting (precontemplation and contemplation). Mentioning the probability that future events will be avoided is rarely as convincing as reference to the immediate medical and nonmedical benefits of cessation. Physicians should concentrate on reasons for quitting that are tailored to patient characteristics. Patients are more likely to respond favorably to positive imagery about the challenges of cessation (245). Providing a rationale for quitting should be combined with a strong, succinct recommendation to stop smoking (''As your physician, I must advise you to stop smoking.'') (99).

The next step in brief physician interventions depends on the smoker's readiness to quit. For precontemplative and contemplative smokers, a realistic goal is moving these patients to the next stage. For smokers in the preparation or active quitting phases, the physician should reinforce the rationale for quitting and provide specific assistance to increase the likelihood of success. Providing assistance in quitting involves a range of specific tasks, including promoting self-confidence, providing health education, teaching concrete techniques and coping skills, and anticipating difficulties that may arise in the process of quitting. It is often helpful to acknowledge patients' fears about quitting by reinforcing your professional opinion that they are capable of giving up cigarettes. Two useful educational topics are nicotine addiction and symptoms of nicotine withdrawal. Concrete suggestions that physicians may give to smokers include (a) asking the smoker to set a specific quit date, (b) advising abrupt cessation on this date, with or without a preliminary period of tapering, (c) advising the smoker to avoid specific situations that are linked to smoking (conditioned cues early on during cessation, especially coffee, alcohol, and smoking sections of restaurants), (d) suggest substitution of other activities for smoking, particularly exercise and hobbies involving ''handling,'' and (e) enhancing social support around cessation, such as making the home smoke-free and advising co-workers, family, and friends that the patient is quitting (85,126,180). Establishing a written contract with smokers may be a useful behavioral modification strategy (176). Physicians should reassure patients that past failures at cessation do not necessarily doom them to fail on subsequent attempts. Providing written self-help materials can enhance the message that physicians provide (54). A variety of resources are available that specifically focus on such topics as the health effects of smoking, the health benefits of quitting, nicotine addiction, and coping skills for cessation. As a primary intervention, self-help materials have been shown to be a cost-effective method of achieving cessation (4,54). Davis et al. (62) estimated that combining stop-smoking leaflets with cessation and maintenance manuals cost $399 per quitter at 1 year.

Arranging for follow-up applies to all smokers, whether or not they have an active interest in quitting. At the very least, precontemplative smokers should receive a message that smoking will remain a concern (75,176). For active quitters, follow-up should be scheduled during the acute phase of cessation, when the quitter will benefit from reinforcement.

The effectiveness of brief physician intervention depends on the population of smokers who receive it. In several studies, year-end quit rates up to 15% have been observed. Brief physician interventions may complement efforts that patients have initiated on their own. Smokers appear to quit smoking at a rate of approximately 1% per year without external interventions. The net effect of physician counseling has been estimated at 2.7% (53), although other sources suggest that the net effect of physician counseling may be greater (176). Although relatively few smokers quit on the basis of minimal contact interventions, if such interventions were applied widely, a substantial number of smokers would be helped to quit. If there are a total of 48 million smokers in the United States (36), and average net effectiveness is 2.7%, an additional approximately 1.3 million smokers would quit annually if minimal contact intervention were applied universally.

Simple physician counseling is a cost-effective practice. Cummings et al. (53), assuming a quit rate of 2.7% above the background rate at 1 year following brief physician counseling, estimated a cost of $444 per quitter (in 1984 dollars). Each year of life saved through smoking cessation cost $750. Smoking cessation advice was far more cost-effective than treating moderate hypertension ($11,300 per year of life saved), mild hypertension ($24,400), or hypercholesterolemia ($65,000 to $108,000) (53). For comparison, coronary artery bypass grafting (CABG) for severe angina has been estimated to cost between $3,800 and $30,000 per year of life gained (1981 dollars), depending on anatomic extent of disease (238). β-Adrenergic antagonist therapy after myocardial infarction costs between $3,600 and $23,400 per year of life saved (100).

Formalized Treatment Programs/Use of Ancillary Services

A second, more intensive level of intervention aimed at tobacco cessation includes formal stop-smoking programs, individual services by other health professionals, and medically oriented smoking cessation clinics. Although the criteria for who will benefit from these services is not well established, smokers who have repeatedly failed past serious attempts at cessation may benefit from the additional structure and opportunities for social support provided by these services. Those whose clinical condition or degree of nicotine addiction suggests the need for a more intensive approach to cessation may also benefit from services that complement brief physician interventions by reinforcing and expanding the messages presented by physicians. Smoking cessation programs are widely available that provide health education, ongoing reinforcement of cessation, and group interaction around cessation issues. These programs consist of multiple sessions employing a multidisciplinary approach, often focusing on concrete behavioral goals. The cost of such programs varies depending on the sponsor, but low-cost programs are often available. The American Cancer Society and the American Lung Association sponsor such programs in many communities. The linkage between these groups and physician intervention has been bolstered by health insurers requiring completion of such programs for nicotine patch reimbursement (160).

Smoking cessation programs appear to be cost effective. Altman et al. (4), evaluating an eight-session smoking cessation class, estimated the cost per quitter at the end of the course at $399 (in 1981 dollars). Assuming a 55% relapse between the end of the course and 1 year (73), the cost per quitter at 1 year would be $887.

Brief physician interventions also can be extended by referring patients to other health professionals for follow-up counseling or specific services. Useful services include health educators (to reinforce and expand on physician counseling), dietitians (for weight gain issues), psychologists (for stress reduction and behavioral modification), and physical therapists (for initiating exercise programs). The effectiveness of these specific services has not been evaluated rigorously. A meta-analysis of counseling for smoking cessation in 39 trials indicates that multiple encounters with different health care providers enhances the likelihood of cessation (141).

Although several studies have suggested that hypnosis may be modestly useful (128,213), its success appears to depend on combining it with other interventions (213). Acupuncture has proponents (39), but there are no convincing research studies suggesting an independent benefit (213).

For patients in need of multiple, additional professional services, referral to a multidisciplinary smoking cessation clinic may be an effective method of coordinating services. Such clinics give smokers access to multiple services that augment physician advice while they promote a behavioral approach to cessation (126). Such clinics have the expertise and resources to pursue more intensive interventions, should this be necessary.

Nicotine Replacement

The development of nicotine replacement therapy has drastically altered physicians' approach to smoking cessation. The rationale for short-term nicotine replacement is to prevent or relieve nicotine withdrawal symptoms produced with abstinence (19,124). By allowing patients to overcome the physical addiction to nicotine, attention can be focused on the behavioral aspects of cigarette smoking. Nicotine replacement also is a sanctioned behavior that substitutes for smoking without inducing withdrawal symptoms and can reduce the reinforcing effect of cigarettes during transient relapses that would otherwise lead to a resumption of smoking (19). Within a stepped-care approach, nicotine replacement applies to a large portion of smokers in need of a more aggressive approach. Nicotine replacement should be combined with earlier steps within the stepped-care approach: physician interventions and smoking cessation programs.

Nicotine replacement is available in the United States by prescription as nicotine gum and nicotine transdermal patches. Nicotine gum was first available in 1983, and nicotine patches were first marketed in 1990 (216). A nicotine metered-dose inhaler (229) and a nicotine nasal spray (225) are being developed. Combining forms of nicotine replacement may be advantageous in specific situations.

Nicotine replacement in pregnancy is controversial and should be limited to women whose likelihood of successful cessation will be substantially enhanced. Similar cautions apply to patients with stable coronary artery disease, including stable angina, arrhythmias, and myocardial infarction. Nicotine replacement is contraindicated in patients with recent myocardial infarction, unstable angina, or life-threatening arrhythmias, although the patch appears safe in stable coronary artery disease (69). Nicotine replacement products have been approved by the Food and Drug Administration (FDA) for smoking cessation. Chronic nicotine replacement beyond 1 year is not recommended, given the known toxicity of this drug. However, some patients may develop dependence and may benefit from long-term therapy if the only alternative is resumption of smoking. Although the consequences of long-term replacement are unknown, they are likely to be less than those of continued smoking (20). The use of nicotine replacement to reduce cigarette smoking also may have net benefits but clearly is not as beneficial as outright cessation and is not recommended (19). Smoking while using nicotine replacement should be discouraged.

Nicotine Gum

Nicotine gum is available as 2 or 4 mg of nicotine bound to a buffered resin. Through intermittent slow chewing and resting the gum against the buccal mucosa, a peak plasma concentration less than half that of one cigarette is obtained in 15 to 30 min. Using either fixed dosing every 1 to 2 h or ad lib dosing matched to patient need, the initial daily dose (approximately 10 to 15 pieces of gum) is continued for 2 months and then tapered. Nicotine gum is contraindicated in patients with jaw problems. Common side effects of nicotine gum include gastric irritation, nausea, jaw soreness, hiccups, and anorexia (228). Long-term dependence may develop in approximately 5% to 10% of patients (124).

Nicotine gum has been shown to reduce nicotine withdrawal symptoms (103). One meta-analysis (146) found that in smoking clinics, nicotine gum led to an abstinence rate at 6 months of 27%, compared to 18% for placebo gum. However, no difference was noted in general medical practice settings. More recent studies suggest a benefit in general medical practice settings. However, these results suggest that a behavioral component enhances the effectiveness of nicotine replacement.

Oster et al. (184) estimated that 6.1% of smokers will be abstinent at 1 year with the combination of physician advice and nicotine gum use compared to 4.5% with physician advice alone, a 35% increase. The effectiveness of nicotine gum appears to be enhanced in nicotine-dependent patients (124) and when higher doses are employed (228).

The cost of nicotine gum is approximately $28 to $40 per week or $336 to $480 for 12 weeks of treatment (59). The cost-effectiveness of nicotine gum as an adjunct to physician advice has been estimated at between $4,113 and $9,473 per year of life saved (1984 dollars) (184). Nicotine replacement may be less cost effective in smokers who have failed other interventions.

Transdermal Nicotine Patches

Transdermal nicotine patches have become the dominant form of replacement because of simple once-a-day dosing that produces relatively steady nicotine blood levels. These characteristics are effective in minimizing nicotine withdrawal symptoms and increasing patient adherence. The patches contain a matrix with a fixed dose of nicotine that diffuses through the skin into the bloodstream. Peak plasma concentrations occur after 6 to 8 h. Steady-state nicotine concentrations of 10 to 23 ng/ml are obtained in 2 to 4 days, approximately half that of cigarette smokers. Formulation of the patches varies among the four patch manufacturers, but all involve patches with declining nicotine content (for example 21 mg/day, 14 mg/day, 7 mg/day) for gradual tapering of replacement. Most smokers begin on the highest-dose patch. Lighter smokers with a low degree of nicotine addiction should begin on an intermediate dose, as should smokers weighing less than 100 pounds and those with known coronary artery disease.

Although patch manufacturers recommend a long duration of treatment before discontinuing nicotine replacement, a shorter course of 2 weeks at each of three doses (or three weeks at two doses) appears equally effective (81). Patients at higher risk for relapse may require longer courses of treatment. The patch is applied each morning to a different hairless skin site. Regardless of manufacturer recommendations, each of the four patches available in the United States can be worn either during waking hours (16-h dosing) or for 24 h a day. Patients experiencing insomnia may minimize this side effect with 16-h dosing (185). For highly addicted smokers, 24-h dosing may be more effective in blunting early morning nicotine craving. When these two dosing schemes were compared, no significant differences in short- or long-term quit rates were observed (60). Smoking during the first 2 weeks of patch use predicts ultimate relapse to smoking (135), making it critical for physicians to discourage concomitant smoking, especially during the initial weeks of patch use. A study of patch users in the general population found that 47% smoked while using the nicotine patch (182). Advice to avoid smoking while using transdermal nicotine is especially important for smokers with coronary artery disease.

Nicotine patches are contraindicated in smokers with severe skin breakdown. Transdermal nicotine may be used cautiously in patients with stable coronary artery disease. The most common side effect of patch use is skin irritation caused by nicotine (78). In addition, some patients develop a skin reaction to the patch adhesive and may be able to employ a different brand. Headache, fatigue, dyspepsia, nausea, dizziness, insomnia, and diarrhea have been reported as side effects, although these symptoms overlap with nicotine withdrawal symptoms (2,105). A small portion of former smokers develop dependence on the nicotine patch, although this may be less harmful than continuing to smoke and is less likely than with nicotine gum (114). Failure to maintain abstinence after transdermal nicotine use predicts failure on subsequent attempts using the patch (230).

The use of nicotine patches has been shown to be effective in facilitating smoking cessation. When compared to placebo patches, nicotine patches reduce withdrawal symptoms and approximately double short-term and long-term abstinence (2,60,84,101,104,105,125,127,185,207,208,242). Clinical trials have shown cessation rates of 30% to 41% for nicotine patch users versus 4% to 21% for placebo patches at the end of a 6-week treatment phase (185). Relapse subsequent to patch use is common: cessation rates decline rapidly with time to approximately half of the initial rates after 6 to 12 months. Several predictors of patch effectiveness have been demonstrated. The cessation rates with patches are generally poorer for highly dependent smokers, although the relative benefit over placebo is greater for this group (228). Higher cessation rates have been reported when patches are combined with behavioral support, which appears to increase the absolute benefit of transdermal nicotine over placebo as well (185). This finding stresses the multifactorial influences on tobacco use, with nicotine addiction being one of several important forces. A 50% increase in cessation rates has been noted with the use of 21 mg/day patches versus 14 mg/day (105).

The wholesale price of a single patch is approximately $4 (59). Treatment cost $28 per week or $168 for 6 weeks of treatment. Although the manufacturers discourage cutting the patches to achieve a lower dose, the actual risks of this cost-saving measure are unclear. Health insurance reimbursement for patches is not universal. Many insurers retroactively reimburse for patches after completion of a qualified smoking cessation program (160).

The cost effectiveness of nicotine patches has not been examined formally. However, given the similarity of cost and quit rates, the average cost of a year of life saved is likely to be similar to that of nicotine gum. Based on this assumption, the use of transdermal nicotine for smoking cessation is a cost-effective strategy when compared to many other medical interventions.

Other forms of nicotine replacement are being developed. Nasal nicotine spray reaches peak serum concentrations after 5 min and has been shown to be more effective than placebo spray for short-term cessation (225). The pharmacodynamics of nicotine metered-dose inhalers are similar and also have been shown to be more effective than a placebo (229). The faster delivery of nasal or inhaled nicotine may be more effective than nicotine gum or patch in blunting transient craving but also may have greater liability for abuse and dependence.

Comparing Forms of Nicotine Replacement

Past studies of nicotine gum and nicotine patches show generally similar rates of short-term and longer-term cessation (101). One direct comparison showed no difference between nicotine gum and transdermal nicotine in combination with behavioral therapy (197). Tang et al. (226) suggest on the basis of a meta-analysis that various forms of nicotine replacement have similar effectiveness except for the most highly nicotine dependent smokers, where the 4-mg gum may be more effective. Given the similar costs of gum and patches, the convenience, acceptability, reduced dependence potential, and minimal side effect of transdermal nicotine suggest that it may be best suited for most smokers planning to quit. However, selected smokers may benefit from the ad lib dosing, shorter time to peak concentration, and oral stimulation provided by nicotine gum.

The combination of nicotine gum with transdermal nicotine also may be advantageous in particular patients. By supplementing the steady-state nicotine from the patch, ad lib dosing of nicotine gum may diminish the risk of relapse. Use of the gum may allow improved pharmacological and behavioral control of withdrawal symptoms. Patients failing past cessation attempts using either form of nicotine replacement alone may be candidates for combination therapy. Early reports on inhaled and nasal nicotine suggest that their rapid absorption may make them well suited for combination with transdermal nicotine (18).

Other Pharmacological Adjuncts

Long-term smoking cessation rates are low, even with intensive interventions that combine physician counseling, formal treatment programs, and nicotine replacement. This provides a rationale for other pharmacological approaches to cessation. The most promising agents are antidepressants, clonidine, and anxiolytics, although their role in smoking cessation has yet to be defined. Concurrent use of nicotine replacement may be beneficial.

Depression has a complex relationship to smoking. Smokers may differ from nonsmokers in several psychological dimensions related to depressed mood (107). Smokers with major depression or dysthymia may be difficult to motivate to quit smoking (44,96). In addition, abstinence from nicotine appears to induce or worsen depression in a significant number of smokers (96), placing them at high risk for relapse, perhaps as a form of self-medication. These connections suggest that antidepressant medications may be useful in a sizable subpopulation of smokers. Several small studies suggest that antidepressants enhance quit rates in unselected populations of smokers (72,215). Among antidepressants, serotonin reuptake inhibitors, with their relatively benign side-effect profile, may have a role in smoking cessation. Cognitive–behavioral psychotherapy for depression may also enhance cessation efforts in patients at high risk for depression (107).

Clonidine, a centrally acting α_2-receptor agonist used in alcohol and opiate withdrawal, probably has relatively little benefit in tobacco cessation. Although clonidine reliably reduces craving (97), clonidine-versus-placebo comparisons have yielded ambiguous results. Several studies have noted improved short-term quit rates (97,98,237), but most studies suggest that clonidine provided no prolonged benefit in enhancing smoking cessation (63,90,116,196). Clonidine has high rates of side effects, as high as 92% in one study (63), among them drowsiness, dry mouth, dizziness, altered mental state, hypotension, blurred vision, fatigue, and sexual dysfunction. The clinical use of clonidine cannot be recommended in light of side effects, the preponderance of negative studies, and safer alternatives.

The prominence of withdrawal symptoms related to anxiety, irritability, anger, and restlessness suggests that medications blunting these symptoms could contribute to successful cessation. Anxiolytic medications are frequently prescribed with this goal (51), although adequate clinical trails are lacking. Buspirone, a nonbenzodiazepine anxiolytic, has been shown to increase quit rates in two small studies (202,241). Alprazolam, a benzodiazepine, has been shown to reduce the intensity of withdrawal symptoms (97). Whether this translates into increased rates of smoking cessation has not been demonstrated. Antidepressants with anxiolytic properties, such as the serotonin reuptake inhibitors, may be particularly beneficial in facilitating smoking cessation, although future studies are required to assess the efficacy of these agents.

Hospital-Based Smoking Cessation Treatment

For smokers unsuccessful at quitting with less intensive interventions, or for smokers with underlying medical conditions, inpatient smoking cessation treatment during hospital stays for acute illness may be an effective approach. Several programs have been developed that provide a multidisciplinary approach to smoking cessation among inpatients (144,177,183,199,223,227). A common strategy of these programs is to combine strong physician advice to stop smoking with follow-up education and counseling by nurses. Hospital nonsmoking policies are an important element of this process. Smoking cessation activities begun in the hospital are followed by continued counseling once patients leave the hospital.

Hospital-based cessation services for patients with cardiac events have been advocated (181). Despite their life-threatening nature, many smokers continue to smoke after hospitalization for myocardial infarction and coronary artery bypass grafting (147). Hospital-based programs may have their greatest benefit in the secondary prevention of future cardiac events for these patients. For patients undergoing diagnostic or revascularization procedures, those patients with greater disease generally show higher rates of smoking cessation (50,56,92).

Hospital-based treatment appears to be capable of doubling the short-term quit rates for inpatients who smoke (144), although a lack of such an effect has been reported (199). Inpatient smoking cessation programs appear to be very cost effective when initiated after myocardial infarction. Krumholz et al. (144) estimated that a nurse-managed intervention initiated during hospitalization for a myocardial infarction cost $380 per quitter and $220 per year of life saved.

MATCHING PATIENTS TO SPECIFIC INTERVENTIONS

Matching patients to particular steps of care or personalizing interventions within a step is based on several characteristics of smokers: readiness to quit, degree of nicotine dependence, daily cigarette consumption, patient demographics, clinical characteristics, and history of past cessation attempts (Fig. 4).

Clinical interventions may be tied with the smoker's stage of readiness for smoking cessation. Interventions that are appropriate at one stage may not be appropriate at another. For example, detailed information on health risks may work for contemplative smokers but may be ineffective in precontemplaters and irrelevant to actively quitting smokers.

More aggressive clinical management also should be directed at smokers with a greater degree of dependence on nicotine. As described above, the Fagerstrom Tolerance Questionnaire (FTQ) provides a measure of nicotine dependence (77). The most dependent smokers (FTQ index >7) may derive the greatest benefit from nicotine replacement. Smoking more than two packs per day or spending less than 5 min between waking and the first cigarette could be employed as simplified measures of nicotine dependence.

The clinical characteristics of the smoker may also enable clinical intervention to be directed more effectively. The presence of smoking-related disease should lead to an increase in the intensity of efforts to facilitate cessation. Patients with risk factors for these diseases may also benefit from more intensive efforts to promote cessation. Clinicians also should treat other cardiovascular risk factors more aggressively in their patients who smoke (117,170).

Several clinical situations present unique opportunities to facilitate smoking cessation. The new diagnosis or exacerbation of a smoking-related disease personalizes the health risks of smoking and increases the patient's motivation to quit (200). There is an immediate benefit of smoking cessation following myocardial infarction. Because many of these clinical events involve hospitalization, these events may provide an opportunity for inpatient nicotine treatment programs aimed at smoking cessation (179).

A patient's history of past cessation attempts may guide therapy. A patient who has never tried to quit or who has been temporarily successful with brief physician counseling might be effectively treated with brief counseling. Smokers who have failed these simple interventions should be treated more aggressively in an escalating manner. Nicotine replacement is appropriate in patients who have failed previous attempts with physician counseling or smoking cessation programs.

SMOKING CESSATION IN CORONARY ARTERY DISEASE

Smoking cessation interventions are vital in the clinical management of atherosclerosis. Because of the ubiquitous prevalence of early atherosclerosis among the populations of developed nations, smoking cessation is a key intervention for the primary prevention of cardiac events. Cessation in smokers with known coronary artery disease, with the goal of secondary prevention of future cardiac events, may

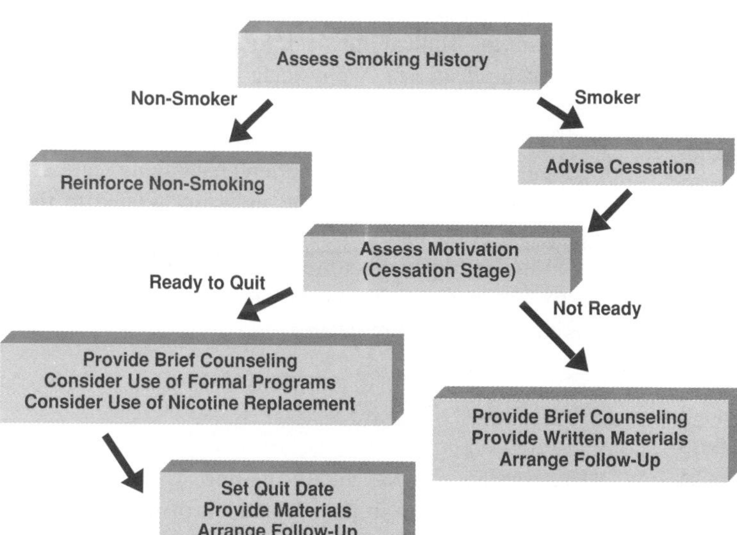

FIG. 4. Physician smoking intervention.

be even more important (201). Compared to the malignant and nonmalignant respiratory effects of smoking, many of the vascular and cardiac effects of smoking are reversible with cessation. Several studies have demonstrated the substantial benefits of cessation and great risks with continued smoking after myocardial infarction. In a typical study, Aberg et al. (3) noted an 8-year mortality of 39% for smokers and 22% for nonsmokers. Smoking cessation also results in a slower progression of angiographically demonstrated coronary atherosclerosis (111). A new diagnosis of symptomatic coronary artery disease, however, often makes smokers more conducive to behavioral changes (200,227). Recent hospitalization and the diagnosis of coronary artery disease are independently predictive of smoking cessation (91).

Traditional approaches to physician-delivered counseling about cigarette smoking appear to apply to smokers with known coronary artery disease. Patients with coronary artery disease appear to follow the same stages in progressing toward tobacco cessation (143). As with other smokers, physicians should provide a forceful message encouraging cessation followed by specific education about nicotine addiction and advice regarding coping mechanisms. Because of the benefits of cessation in smokers with coronary artery disease, more intensive interventions are justified in this population. As suggested above, inpatient intervention with a multidisciplinary focus is well suited to patients who have smoked their way to a cardiac event requiring hospitalization.

Although there have been concerns about nicotine replacement use in coronary artery disease, these fears do not appear to be valid provided that caution is used. Because patients with coronary artery disease have the most to gain from cessation and may be particularly motivated to quit after cardiac events, the cautious use of nicotine replacement should be strongly considered in those patients in whom abstinence is otherwise unlikely (20,102). Three studies have examined the use of nicotine replacement in coronary artery disease patients (47,69,198). No serious adverse cardiac events were associated with nicotine patch use. However, adverse cardiac events have been reported in the setting of heavy smoking with concurrent patch use (46,57,236). The absolute rate of myocardial infarction in patients smoking while using the patch is less than 5 per million transdermal nicotine prescriptions (181). By eliminating the other toxins present in cigarette smoke, nicotine replacement is likely to be safer than smoking (121), especially because total nicotine doses are generally lower with patch use than with smoking (20). However, if successful cessation has a moderate likelihood without nicotine replacement, other less intensive interventions should be exhausted. It is recommended that transdermal nicotine be initiated at an intermediate dose (14 mg/day) rather than at a higher dose (185). Because smoking while wearing the patch appears to occur in as many as 50% of patch users (182), coronary artery disease patients must be strongly warned about the dangers of smoking while wearing the patch and monitored with follow-up visits.

Because cardiac risk factors work in a synergistic manner, efforts at risk factor modification should confront all risk factors simultaneously (65,111). Smoking interventions should be more intensive for patients with known coronary artery disease or with other risk factors for the development of atherosclerosis. Efforts focused on cessation for these patients have the greatest benefits. Similarly, efforts aimed at modifying other risk factors should be more intensive in patients who smoke (170).

PHYSICIAN ACTIVITIES BEYOND INDIVIDUAL PATIENTS

Physicians can facilitate smoking cessation beyond their contact with individual patients by taking broad responsibility for increasing the disincentives for their patients to smoke. Smoking should be discouraged in the office by the posting of nonsmoking signs (157). Efforts may be made to encourage nonsmoking among all members of the office, especially physicians.

Outside the office, physicians can support the activities of private and governmental agencies that encourage smoking prevention and cessation. This may range from promoting work-site and public nonsmoking policies, contributing to community-oriented smoking efforts, supporting restrictions on tobacco advertising, promoting counteradvertising, and advocating increased taxation on cigarettes (8,15,22,23,79, 110,156). These public policy measures complement and extend the gains made through smoking cessation interventions.

SUMMARY

Cigarette smoking plays a dominant role in the etiology of atherosclerosis. Clinical interventions aimed at smoking cessation, although currently underutilized, must be a key strategy in the clinical approach to coronary artery disease and its complications. A physician-centered approach employing increasingly intensive steps that match patients to specific modes of treatment is evolving. The modification of patient behaviors, although often challenging, can effectively reduce the morbidity and mortality related to these behaviors. Simple interventions that appear to have low efficacy in inducing patients to stop smoking are actually cost-effective because of the potent causative linkage between smoking and premature death.

ACKNOWLEDGMENTS

The assistance of Ms. Judith Behling, Ms. Jean Rieman, and Ms. Alice Braun in the preparation of this manuscript is gratefully acknowledged. Special thanks to Nancy Rigotti,

M.D. for her helpful comments on an earlier version of this chapter.

REFERENCES

1. Koethe SM, Nelson KE, Becker CG. Activation of the classical pathway of complement by tobacco glycoprotein (TGP).
2. Abelin T, et al. Controlled trial of transdermal nicotine patch in tobacco withdrawal. *Lancet* 1989;1:7–10.
3. Aberg A, et al. Cessation of smoking after myocardial infarction. Effects on mortality after 10 years. *Br Heart J* 1983;49:416–422.
4. Altman DG, et al. The cost-effectiveness of three smoking cessation programs. *Am J Public Health* 1987;77:162–165.
5. APA. *Diagnostic and Statistical Manual of Mental Disorders* (ed 3, rev). Washington, DC: American Psychiatric Association; 1987.
6. Atkinson JB, et al. The association of mast cells and atherosclerosis: A morphologic study of early atherosclerotic lesions in young people. *Hum Pathol* 1994;25:154–159.
7. Axelrad CM, et al. Biochemical validation of cigarette smoke exposure and tobacco use. In: Sandhu SS, DeMarini DM, eds. *Short-Term Bioassays in the Analysis of Complex Environmental Mixtures.* New York: Plenum Press; 1987:115–126.
8. Bartecchi CE, MacKenzie TD, Schrier RW. The human costs of tobacco use. *N Engl J Med* 1994;330:907–912.
9. Baum CG, et al. Cellular control of IgE induction by a polyphenol-rich compound. *J Immunol* 1990;145:779–784.
10. Becker CG, Dubin T. Activation of factor XII by tobacco glycoprotein. *J Exp Med* 1977;146:457–467.
11. Becker CG, Dubin T, Wiedemann HP. Hypersensitivity to tobacco antigen. *Proc Natl Acad Sci USA* 1976;73:1712–1716.
12. Becker CG, Hajjar DP, Hefton JM. Tobacco constituents are mitogenic for arterial smooth muscle cells. *Am J Pathol* 1985;120:1–5.
13. Becker CG, Levi R, Zavecz JH. Induction of IgE antibodies to antigen isolated from tobacco leaves and from cigarette smoke condensate. *Am J Pathol* 1979;96:249–255.
14. Becker CG, Van Hamont N, Wagner M. Tobacco, cocoa, coffee, and ragweed: Cross reacting allergens that activate factor XII dependent pathways. *Blood* 1981;58:861–867.
15. Becker DM, et al. Setting the policy, education, and research agenda to reduce tobacco use. Workshop I. AHA Prevention Conference III. Behavior change and compliance: Keys to improving cardiovascular health. *Circulation* 1993;88:1381–1386.
16. Benditt E, Benditt JM. Evidence for a monoclonal origin of human atherosclerotic plaques. *Proc Natl Acad Sci USA* 1973;70:1753–1756.
17. Benowitz NL. Pharmacologic aspects of cigarette smoking and nicotine addiction. *N Engl J Med* 1988;319:1318–1330.
18. Benowitz NL. Cigarette smoking and nicotine addiction. *Med Clin North Am* 1992;76:415–438.
19. Benowitz NL. Nicotine replacement therapy: What has been accomplished—can we do better? *Drugs* 1993;45:157–170.
20. Benowitz NL, et al. Nicotine effects on eicosanoid formation and hemostatic function: Comparison of transdermal nicotine and cigarette smoking. *J Am Coll Cardiol* 1993;22:1159–1167.
21. Bevilacqua MP. Endothelial–leukocyte adhesion molecules. *Annu Rev Immunol* 1993;11:767–804.
22. Bierer MF, Rigotti NA. Public Policy for the control of tobacco-related diseases. *Med Clin North Am* 1992;76:515–539.
23. Breslow L, Johnson M. California's Proposition 99 on tobacco and its impact. *Annu Rev Pub Health* 1993;14:585–604.
24. Brunnemann KD, Hoffmann D. Pyrolytic origins of major gas phase constituents of cigarette smoke. *Recent Adv Tobacco Sci* 1982;8: 103–140.
25. Burghuber OC, et al. Platelet sensitivity to prostacyclin in smokers and nonsmokers. *Chest* 1986;90:34–38.
26. Butcher EC. Leukocyte–endothelial cell recognition: Three (or more) steps to specificity and diversity. *Cell* 1991;67:1033–1036.
27. Carlos TM, Harlan JM. Membrane proteins involved in phagocyte adherence to endothelium. *Immunol Rev* 1990;114:5–28.
28. CDC. Cigarette smoking in the United States, 1986. *Morbid Mortal Weekly Rep* 1987;36:581–584.
29. CDC. *Reducing the Health Consequences of Smoking: 25 Years of Progress—A Report of the Surgeon General, 1989.* Rockville, MD: USDHHS, PHS; 1989.
30. CDC. *The Health Benefits of Smoking Cessation: A Report of the Surgeon General, 1990.* Washington DC: USDHHS, PHS; 1990.
31. CDC. Cigarette smoking among adults—United States, 1988. *Morbid Mortal Weekly Rep* 1991;40:757–759.
32. CDC. Cigarette smoking among adults—United States, 1990. *Morbid Mortal Weekly Rep* 1992;41:354–355, 361–362.
33. CDC. Cigarette smoking-attributable mortality and years of potential life lost—United States, 1990. *Morbid Mortal Weekly Rep* 1993;42: 645–649.
34. CDC. Physician and other health-care professional counseling of smokers to quit—United States, 1991. *Morbid Mortal Weekly Rep* 1993;42:845–847.
35. CDC. Cigarette smoking among adults—United States, 1991. *Morbid Mortal Weekly Rep* 1993;42:230–233.
36. CDC. Cigarette smoking among adults—United States, 1992, and changes in the definition of current cigarette smoking. *Morbid Mortal Weekly Rep* 1994;43:342–346.
37. Chiba M, Masironi R. Toxic and trace elements in tobacco and tobacco smoke. *Bull WHO* 1992;70:269–275.
38. Chisholm G. Oxidized lipoproteins and leukocyte-endothelial interactions: Growing evidence for multiple mechanisms. *Lab Invest* 1993; 68:369–371.
39. Choy DSJ, Lutzker B, Meltzer D. Effective treatment for smoking cessation. *Am J Med* 1983;75:1033–1036.
40. Choy JW, et al. Effects of tobacco glycoprotein on the immune system. I. TGP is a T-independent B cell mitogen for murine lymphoid cells. *J Immunol* 1985;134:3193–3198.
41. Church DF, Pryor WA. Free-radical chemistry of cigarette smoke and its toxicological implications. *Environ Health Perspect* 1985;64: 111–126.
42. Cohen BS, Eisenbud M, Harley NH. Alpha radioactivity in cigarette smoke. *Radiat Res* 1979;83:190–196.
43. Collins T. Biology of disease. Endothelial nuclear factor-κB and the initiation of the atherosclerotic lesion. *Lab Invest* 1993;68:499–508.
44. Covey LS, et al. Effect of history of alcoholism or major depression on smoking cessation. *Am J Psychiatry* 1993;150:1546–1547.
45. Covey LS, Zang EA, Wynder EL. Cigarette smoking and occupational status: 1977 to 1990. *Am J Publ Health* 1992;82:1230–1234.
46. Craig WY, Palomaki GE, Haddow JE. Cigarette smoking and serum lipid and lipoprotein concentrations: An analysis of published data. *Br Med J* 1989;298:784–788.
47. Craig WY, et al. Cigarette smoking associated changes in blood lipids and lipoprotein levels in the 8- to 19-year-old age group: A meta-analysis. *Pediatrics* 1990;85:155–158.
48. Criqui MH, et al. IgE and cardiovascular disease. *Am J Med* 1987; 82:964–968.
49. Criqui MH, et al. Epidemiology of immunoglobulin E levels in a defined population. *Ann Allergy* 1990;64:308–313.
50. Crouse JR, Hagaman AP. Smoking cessation in relation to cardiac procedures. *Am J Epidemiol* 1991;134:699–703.
51. Cummings SR, et al. Internist and nicotine gum. *JAMA* 1988;260: 1565–1569.
52. Cummings SR, et al. Smoking counseling and preventive medicine: A survey of internists in private practices and a health maintenance organization. *Arch Intern Med* 1989;149:345–349.
53. Cummings SR, Rubin SM, Oster G. The cost-effectiveness of counseling smokers to quit. *JAMA* 1989;261:75–79.
54. Curry SJ. Self-help interventions for smoking cessation. *J Consult Clin Psychol* 1993;61:790–803.
55. Cushing SD, et al. Minimally modified low density lipoprotein induces monocyte chemotactic protein I in human endothelial cells and smooth muscle cells. *Proc Natl Acad Sci USA* 1990;87:5134–5138.
56. Cutter G, et al. The natural history of smoking cessation among patients undergoing coronary arteriography. *J Cardiopul Rehabil* 1985; 5:332–340.
57. Dacosta A, et al. Myocardial infarction and nicotine patch: A contributing or causative factor. *Eur Heart J* 1993;14:1709–1711.
58. Daly LE, et al. Long-term effect on mortality of stopping smoking after unstable angina and myocardial infarction. *Br Med J* 1983;287: 324–326.
59. Data ME. *Drug Topics 1994 Redbook.* Montvale, NJ: 1994.
60. Daughton DM, et al. Effect of transdermal nicotine delivery as an

adjunct to low-intervention smoking cessation therapy: A randomized, placebo-controlled, double-blind study. *Arch Intern Med* 1991;151: 745–749.

61. Davie EW, Fujikawa K, Kisiel W. The coagulation cascade: Initiation, maintenance and regulation. *Biochemistry* 1991;30:10363–10369.
62. Davis A, Faust R, Ordentlich M. Self-help smoking cessation and maintenance programs: A comparative study with 12-month follow-up by the American Lung Association. *Am J Public Health* 1984;74: 1212–1217.
63. Davison R, et al. The effect of clonidine on the cessation of cigarette smoking. *Clin Pharmacol Ther* 1988;44:265.
64. Dawber TR. *The Framingham Study. The Epidemiology of Atherosclerotic Disease.* Cambridge, MA: Harvard University Press; 1980.
65. DeBusk RF, et al. A case-management sytsem for coronary risk factor modification after acute myocardial infarction. *Ann Intern Med* 1992; 120:721–729.
66. Denburg J, et al. Hypersensitivity to tobacco glycoprotein in human peripheral vascular disease. *Ann Allergy* 1981;47:8–13.
67. DiClemente C, et al. The process of smoking cessation: An analysis of precontemplation, contemplation, and preparation stages of change. *J Consult Clin Psychol* 1991;59:295–304.
68. Dinarello CA. Interleukin-1 and interleukin-1 antagonism. *Blood* 1991;77:1627–1652.
69. Disease WGftSoTNiPwCA. Nicotine replacement therapy for patients with coronary artery disease. *Arch Intern Med* 1994;154:989–995.
70. Dube MF, Green CR. Methods of collection of smoke for analytical purposes. *Recent Adv Tobacco Sci* 1982;8:42–102.
71. Edwards G, Arif A, Hodgson R. Nomenclature and classification of drug- and alcohol-related problems: A shortened version of a WHO memorandum. *Br J Addict* 1982;77:3–20.
72. Edwards NB, et al. Doxepin as an adjunct to smoking cessation: A double-blind pilot study. *Am J Psychiatry* 1989;146:373–376.
73. Evans D, Lane DS. Long-term outcome of smoking cessation workshops. *Am J Public Health* 1980;70:725–727.
74. Facchini FS, et al. Insulin resistance and cigarette smoking. *Lancet* 1992;339:1128–1130.
75. Fagerstrom K. Effects of nicotine chewing gum and follow-up appointments in physician-based smoking cessation. *Prev Med* 1984; 13:517–527.
76. Fagerstrom KO, Heatherton TF, Kozlowski LT. Nicotine addiction and its assessment. *Ear Nose Throat J* 1991;69:763–768.
77. Fagerstrom KO, Schneider NG. Measuring nicotine dependence: A review of the Fagerstrom Tolerance Questionnaire. *J Behav Med* 1989; 12:159–182.
78. Farm G. Contact allergy to nicotine from a nicotine patch. *Contact Derm* 1993;29:214–215.
79. Farquhar JW. Keynote address: How health behavior relates to risk factors. *Circulation* 1993;88:1376–1380.
80. Fiore MC. Trends in cigarette smoking in the United States. *Med Clin North Am* 1992;76:289–303.
81. Fiore MC, Newcombe P, McBride P. Natural history and epidemiology and tobacco addiction. In: Orleans CT, Slade J, eds. *Nicotine Addiction: Principles and Management.* New York: Oxford University Press; 1993:89–104.
82. Fiore MC, et al. Methods used to quit smoking in the United States: Do cessation programs help? *JAMA* 1990;263:2760–2765.
83. Fiore MC, et al. Trends in cigarette smoking in the United States: The changing influence of gender and race. *JAMA* 1989;261:49–55.
84. Fiore MC, et al. The effectiveness of the nicotine patch for smoking cessation: A meta-analysis. *JAMA* 1994;271:1940–1947.
85. Fisher EB, Lichtenstein E, Haire-Joshu D. Multiple determinants of tobacco use and cessation. In: Slade J, ed. *Nicotine Addiction: Principles and Management.* New York: Oxford University Press, 1993; 59–88.
86. Francus T, et al. Effects of tobacco glycoprotein (TGP) on the immune system. II. TGP stimulates the proliferation of human T cells and the differentiation of human B cells in immunoglobulin secreting cells. *J Immunol* 1988;140:1823–1829.
87. Francus T, et al. IL-1, IL-6 and PDGF mRNA expression in alveolar cells following stimulation with a tobacco-derived antigen. *Cell Immunol* 1992;145:156–174.
88. Francus T, Siskind GW, Becker CG. The role of antigen structure in the regulation of IgE isotype expression. *Proc Natl Acad Sci USA* 1983;80:3430–3434.
89. Frank E, et al. Predictors of physicians' smoking cessation advice. *JAMA* 1991;266:3139–3144.
90. Franks P, Harp J, Bell B. Randomized, controlled trial of clonidine for smoking cessation in a primary care setting. *JAMA* 1989;262: 3011–3013.
91. Freund KM, et al. Predictors of smoking cessation: The Framingham Study. *Am J Epidemiol* 1992;135:957–964.
92. Frid D, et al. Severity of angiographically proven coronary artery disease predicts smoking cessation. *Am J Prev Med* 1991;7:131–135.
93. Galli SJ. New concepts about the mast cell. *N Engl J Med* 1993;328: 257–265.
94. Gitel SN, Stephenson RC, Wessler S. The activated factor X–antithrombin III reaction rate: A measure of the increased thrombotic tendency induced by estrogen-containing oral contraceptives in rabbits. *Haemostasis* 1978;7:10–18.
95. Gitel SN, Wessler S. Do natural estrogens pose an increased risk of thrombosis in postmenopausal women. *Thromb Res* 1978;13: 279–283.
96. Glassman AH. Cigarette smoking: Implications for psychiatric illness. *Am J Psychiatry* 1993;150:546–553.
97. Glassman AH, et al. Cigarette craving, smoking withdrawal, and clonidine. *Science* 1984;226:864–866.
98. Glassman AH, et al. Heavy smokers, smoking cessation, and clonidine. *JAMA* 1988;259:2863–2866.
99. Glynn TJ, Manley MW. *How to Help Your Patients Stop Smoking.* Washington DC: USDHSS, NIH Pub No 92-3064; 1991.
100. Goldman L, et al. Costs and effectiveness of routine therapy with long-term beta-adrenergic antagonists after acute myocardial infarction. *N Engl J Med* 1988;319:152–157.
101. Gora ML. Nicotine transdermal systems. *Ann Pharmacother* 1993; 27:742–750.
102. Gourlay S. The pros and cons of transdermal nicotine therapy. *Med J Aust* 1994;160:152–159.
103. Gross J, Stitzer ML. Nicotine replacement: Ten-week effects on tobacco withdrawal symptoms. *Psychopharmacology* 1989;98: 334–341.
104. Group ICRFGPR. Effectiveness of a nicotine patch in helping people stop smoking: Results of a randomized trial in general practice. *Br Med J* 1993;306:1304–1308.
105. Group TNS. Transdermal nicotine for smoking cessation: Six-month results from two multicenter controlled clinical trials. *JAMA* 1991; 266:3133–3138.
106. Haley NJ, Axelrad CM, Tilton KA. Validation of self-reported smoking behavior: Biochemical analysis of cotinine and thiocyanate. *Am J Public Health* 1983;93:1204–1207.
107. Hall SM, et al. Nicotine, negative affect, and depression. *J Consult Clin Psychol* 1993;61:761–767.
108. Hall SM, et al. Nicotine gum and behavioral treatment in smoking cessation. *J Consult Clin Psychol* 1985;53:256–268.
109. Hansson G, Holm J, Jonasson L. Detection of activated T lymphocytes in the human atherosclerotic plaque. *Am J Pathol* 1989;135:169–175.
110. Harats D, et al. Cigarette smoking renders LDL susceptible to peroxidative modification and enhanced metabolism by macrophages. *Atherosclerosis* 1989;79:245–252.
111. Haskell WL, et al. Effects of intensive multiple risk factor reduction on coronary atherosclerosis and clinical cardiac events in men and women with coronary artery disease. The Stanford Coronary Risk Intervention Project (SCRIP). *Circulation* 1994;89:975–990.
112. Havsteen B. Flavonoids, a class of natural products of high pharmacological potency. *Biochem Pharmacol* 1985;32:1141–1148.
113. Heinrich J, et al. Fibrinogen and factor VII in the prediction of coronary risk. Results from the PROCAM study in healthy men. *Arterioscler Thromb* 1994;14:54–59.
114. Henningfield JE, Keenan RM. Nicotine delivery kinetics and abuse liability. *J Consult Clin Psychol* 1993;61:743–750.
115. Higgins M, Thom T. Trends in CHD in the United States. *Int J Epidemiol* 1989;18:S58–S66.
116. Hilleman DE, et al. Randomized, controlled trial of transdermal clonidine for smoking cessation. *Ann Pharmacol* 1993;27:1025–1028.
117. Hilts PJ. Less smoke and less tar, but full dose of nicotine. *The New York Times.* 1994: 1.
118. Hoffmann D, Hecht SS. Perspectives in cancer research. Nicotine-derived N-nitrosamines and tobacco related cancer: Current status and future directions. *Cancer Res* 1985;45:935–944.

119. Hoffmann D, et al. Model studies in tobacco carcinogenesis with the Syrian golden hamster. *Prog Exp Tumor Res* 1979;24:370–390.
120. Hoffmann D, Wynder EL. Chemical constituents and bioactivity of tobacco smoke. *IARC Sci Publ* 1986;74:145–165.
121. Hughes JR. Risk–benefit assessment of nicotine preparations in smoking cessation. *Drug Safety* 1993;8:49–56.
122. Hughes JR, et al. Symptoms of tobacco withdrawal: A replication and extension. *Arch Gen Psychaitry* 1991;48:52–59.
123. Hughes JR, Hatsukami D. Signs and symptoms of tobacco withdrawal. *Arch Gen Psychiatry* 1986;43:289–294.
124. Hughes JR, Miller SA. Nicotine gum to help stop smoking. *JAMA* 1984;252:2855–2858.
125. Hurt RD, et al. Nicotine patch therapy for smoking cessation combined with physician advice and nurse follow-up: One-year outcome and percentage of nicotine replacement. *JAMA* 1994;271:595–600.
126. Hurt RD, et al. A comprehensive model for the treatment of nicotine dependence in a medical setting. *Med Clin North Am* 1992;76: 495–514.
127. Hurt RD, et al. Nicotine replacement therapy with the use of a transdermal nicotine patch: A randomized double-blind, placebo-controlled trial. *Mayo Clin Proc* 1990;65:1529–1537.
128. Hyman GJ, et al. Treatment effectiveness of hypnosis and behavior therapy in smoking cessation: A methodological refinement. *Addict Behav* 1986;11:355–365.
129. Ishizaka T, et al. Development of human mast cells from their progenitors. *Curr Opin Immunol* 1993;5:937–943.
130. JNC. The 1988 report of the Joint National Committee on the detection, evaluation, and treatment of high blood pressure. *Arch Intern Med* 1988;148:1023–1038.
131. Jonas MA, et al. Statement on smoking and cardiovascular disease for health professionals. *Circulation* 1992;86:1664–1669.
132. Jonason T, Bergstrom R. Cessation of smoking in patients with intermittent claudication. Effects on the risk of peripheral vascular complications, myocardial infarction and mortality. *Acta Med Scand* 1987; 221:253–260.
133. Kannel WB, Higgins M. Smoking and hypertension as predictors of cardiovascular risk in population studies. *J Hypertens* 1990;8(5): S3–S8.
134. Kawachi I, et al. Smoking cessation and time course of decreased risks of coronary heart disease in middle-aged women. *Arch Intern Med* 1994;154:169–175.
135. Kenford SL, et al. Predicting smoking cessation: Who will quit with and without the nicotine patch? *JAMA* 1994;271:589–594.
136. Kew RR, Ghebrehiwet B, Janoff A. Cigarette smoke can activate the alternative pathway of complement in vitro by modifying the third component of complement. *J Clin Invest* 1985;75:1000–1007.
137. Kew RR, Ghebrehiwet B, Janoff A. Characterization of the third component of complement after activation by cigarette smoke. *Clin Immunol Immunopathol* 1987;44:248–258.
138. Kew RR, Janoff A, Ghebrehiwet B. Cleavage of the third component of complement (C3) in lung fluids after acute cigarette smoke inhalation. *Am Rev Respir Dis* 1983;127:154.
139. Killen JD, et al. Are heavy smokers different from light smokers?: A comparison after 48 hours without cigarettes. *JAMA* 1988;260: 1581–1585.
140. Klesgas RC, Myers AW, LaVesque ME. Smoking, body weight and their effects of smoking behavior: A comprehensive review of the literature. *Psychol Bull* 1989;106:204–230.
141. Kottke TE, et al. Attributes of successful smoking cessation interventions in medical practice: A meta-analysis of 39 controlled trials. *JAMA* 1988;259:2882–2889.
142. Kottke TE, et al. A randomized trial to increase smoking intervention by physicians: Doctors helping smokers, round one. *JAMA* 1989;261: 2102–2106.
143. Kristeller JL, et al. Smoking intervention for cardiac patients: In search of more effective strategies. *Cardiology* 1993;82:317–324.
144. Krumholz HM, et al. Cost-effectiveness of a smoking cessation program after myocardial infarction. *J Am Coll Cardiol* 1993;22: 1697–1702.
145. Kugiyama K, et al. Impairment of endothelium-dependent arterial relaxation by lysolecithin in modified low density lipoproteins. *Nature* 1990;344:160–162.
146. Lam W, Sacks HS, Sze PC. Meta-analysis of randomized controlled trials of nicotine chewing gum. *Lancet* 1987;2:27–30.
147. Leaman DM, Brower RW, Meester GT. Coronary bypass surgery: A stimulus to modify existing risk factors? *Chest* 1982;81:16–19.
148. Lee EW, DAlonzo GE. Cigarette smoking, nicotine addiction, and its pharmacologic treatment. *Arch Intern Med* 1993;153:34–48.
149. Lee L, Gilpin EA, Pierce JP. Changes in the patterns of initiation of cigarette smoking in the United States: 1950, 1965, and 1980. *Cancer Epidemiol Biomarkers Prevent* 1993;2:593–597.
150. Lehr H-A, et al. Cigarette smoke elicits leukocyte adhesion to endothelium in hamsters: Inhibition by CuZn-SOD. *Free Radical Biol Med* 1993;14:573–81.
151. Lehr H-A, et al. Stimulatiohn of leukocyte/endothelium interaction by oxidized low-density lipoprotein in hairless mice. Involvement of CDIIb/CD18 adhesion receptor complex. *Lab Invest* 1993;68: 388–395.
152. Leung DYM, Pober JS, Cotran RS. Expression of endothelial-leukocyte adhesion molecule-1 in elicited late phase allergic reactions. *J Clin Invest* 1991;87:1805–1809.
153. Levi R. Human inflammatory disease. In: Marone G et al., eds. *Cardiac Anaphylaxis: Models, Mediators, Mechanisms and Clinical Considerations.* Toronto: BC Decker; 1988.
154. Levi R, et al. Cardiac and pulmonary anaphylaxis in guinea pigs and rabbits induced by glycoprotein isolated from tobacco leaves and cigarette smoke condensate. *Am J Pathol* 1982;106:318–325.
155. Linet MS, et al. Is cigarette smoking a risk factor for non-Hodgkin's lymphoma or multiple myeloma? Results from the Lutheran Brotherhood Cohort Study. *Leuk Res* 1992;16:621–624.
156. MacKenzie TD, Bartecchi CE, Schrier RW. The human costs of tobacco use. *N Engl J Med* 1994;330:975–980.
157. Manley M, Epps RP, Glyn T. The clinician's role in promoting smoking cessation among clinic patients. *Med Clin North Am* 1992; 477–494.
158. Manley M, et al. Clinical interventions in tobacco control: A National Cancer Institute training program for physicians. *JAMA* 1991;266: 3172–3173.
159. Maron DJ, Fortmann SP. Nicotine yield and measures of cigarette smoke exposure in a larger population: Are lower yield cigarettes safer. *Am J Public Health* 1987;77:546–549.
160. McAfee T. Transdermal nicotine: Clarifications, side effects, and funding. *JAMA* 1993;269:1939–1940.
161. McBride PE. The health consequences of smoking: Cardiovascular diseases. *Med Clin North Am* 1992;76:333–353.
162. McCall MR, et al. Modification of LCAT activity and HDL activity. *Arterioscler Thromb* 1994;14:248–253.
163. McPhee SJ, Detmer WM. Office-based interventions to imprvoe delivery of cancer prevention services by primary care physicians. *Cancer* 1993;72 (Suppl):1110–1112.
164. Meade TW, Imeson J, Stirling Y. Effects of changes in smoking and other characteristics on clotting factors and the risk of ischemic heart disease. *Lancet* 1987;2:986–988.
165. Michnovicz JJ, et al. Increased 23-hydroxylation of estradiol as a possible mechanism for the anti-estrogenic effect of smoking. *N Engl J Med* 1986;315:1305–1309.
166. Michnovicz JJ, et al. Cigarette smoking alters hepatic estrogen metabolism in men: Implication for atherosclerosis. *Metabolism* 1989;38: 537–541.
167. Middleton EJ, Kandaswami C. Effects of flavonoids on immune and inflammatory cell functions. *Biochem Pharmacol* 1992;43: 1167–1179.
168. Mustard JF, Murphy EA. Effect of smoking on blood coagulation and platelet survival in man. *Br Med J* 1963;1:846–849.
169. Nachman RL. Thrombosis and atherogenesis: Molecular connections. *Blood* 1992;79:1897–1906.
170. NCEP. Summary of the second report of the National Cholesterol Education Program (NCEP) expert panel on the detection, evaluation, and treatment of high blood cholesterol in adults (adult treatment panel II). *JAMA* 1993;269:3015–3023.
171. Norman V. An overview of the vapor phase, semivolatile and nonvolatile components of cigarette smoke. *Recent Adv Tobacco Sci* 1977;3: 28–58.
172. Noronha-Dutra AA, Epperlein MM, Woolf N. Effect of cigarette smoking on cultured human endothelial cells. *Cardiovasc Res* 1993; 27:774–778.
173. Novotny TE, et al. Smoking by blacks and whites: Socioeconomic and demographic differences. *Am J Pub Health* 1988;78:1187–1189.

174. Nowak J, et al. Biochemical evidence of a chronic abnormality in platelet and vascular function in healthy individuals who smoke cigarettes. *Circulation* 1987;76:6–14.
175. O'Connor GT, Sparrow D, Weiss ST. The role of allergy and nonspecific airway hyperresponsiveness in the pathogenesis of chronic obstructive pulmonary disease. *Am Rev Respir Dis* 1989;140:225–252.
176. Ockene JK. Physician-delivered interventions for smoking cessation: Strategies for increasing effectiveness. *Prev Med* 1987;16:723–737.
177. Ockene JK, et al. Smoking cessation and severity of disease: The Coronary Artery Smoking Intervention Study. *Health Psychol* 1992; 11:119–126.
178. Ockene JK, et al. Increasing the efficacy of physician-delivered smoking interventions: A randomized clinical trial. *J Gen Intern Med* 1991; 6:1–6.
179. Orleans CT. Treating nicotine dependence on a medical setting: A stepped-care model. In: Orleans CT, Slade J, eds. *Nicotine Addiction: Principles and Management.* New York: Oxford University Press; 1993:145–161.
180. Orleans CT, et al. Minimal contact quit smoking strategies for a medical setting. In: Orleans CT, Slade J, eds. *Nicotine Addiction: Principles and Management.* New York: Oxford University Press, 1993: 181–220.
181. Orleans CT, Ockene JK. Routine hospital-based quit-smoking treatment for the postmyocardial infarction patient: An idea whose time has come. *J Am Coll Cardiol* 1993;22:1703–1705.
182. Orleans CT, et al. Use of transdermal nicotine in a state-level prescription plan for the elderly: A first look at "real-world" patch users. *JAMA* 1994;271:601–607.
183. Orleans CT, et al. A hospital quit-smoking consult service: Clinical report and intervention guidelines. *Prev Med* 1990;19:198–212.
184. Oster G, et al. Cost-effectiveness of nicotine gum as an adjunct to physician advice against cigarette smoking. *JAMA* 1986;256: 1315–1318.
185. Palmer KJ, Bucklet MM, Foulds D. Transdermal nicotine: A review of the pharmacodynamic and pharmacokinetic properties and therapeutic efficacy as an aid to smoking cessation. *Drugs* 1992;44:498–529.
186. Parthasarathy S, Steinberg D, Witztum JL. The role of oxidized low-density lipoproteins in the pathogenesis of atherosclerosis. *Annu Rev Med* 1992;43:219–225.
187. Penn A, Hubbard FC Jr, Parkes JL. Transforming potential is detectable in arteriosclerotic plaques of young animals. *Arterioscler Thromb* 1991;11:1053–1058.
188. Perera F, et al. Molecular epidemiology and cancer prevention. *Cancer Detect Prev* 1990;14:639–644.
189. Perkins KA. Weight gain following smoking cessation. *J Consult Clin Psychol* 1993;61:768–777.
190. Petitti DB, et al. Risk of vascular disease in women. Smoking, oral contraceptives, noncontraceptive estrogen, and other factors. *JAMA* 1979;242:1150–1154.
191. Pierce JP, et al. Trends in cigarette consumption in the United States: Educational differences are increasing. *JAMA* 1989;261:56–60.
192. Pittilo RM. Cigarette smoking and endothelial injury: A review. In: *Tobacco Smoking and Atherosclerosis.* New York: Plenum Press; 1989.
193. Pober JS, Cotran RS. Cytokines and endothelial biology. *Physiol Rev* 1990;70:427–451.
194. Pomerlau OF, et al. Why some people smoke and others do not: New perspectives. *J Consult Clin Psychol* 1993;61:723–731.
195. Prochazka JO, DiClemente CC. States and processes of self-change of smoking: Towards an integrative model of change. *J Consult Clin Psychol* 1983;51:390–395.
196. Prochazka JO, et al. Transdermal clonidine reduced some withdrawal symptoms but did not increase smoking cessation. *Arch Intern Med* 1992;152:2065–2069.
197. Reaven P, et al. Effects of oleate-rich and linoleate-rich diets on the susceptibility of low density lipoprotein to oxidative modification in mildly hypercholesterolemic subjects. *J Clin Invest* 1993;91:668–676.
198. Rennard S, et al. Transdermal nicotine enhances smoking cessation in coronary artery disease patients [abstract]. *Chest* 1991;100:5S.
199. Rigotti NA, McKool KM, Shiffman S. Predictors of smoking cessation after coronary artery bypass graft surgery. Results of a randomized trial with 5-year follow-up. *Ann Intern Med* 1994;120:287–293.
200. Rigotti NA, et al. Smoking cessation following admission to a coronary care unit. *J Gen Intern Med* 1991;6:305–311.
201. Robinson JG, Leon AS. The prevention of cardiovascular disease. Emphasis on secondary prevention. *Med Clin North Am* 1994;78: 69–98.
202. Robinson MD, et al. Buspirone effect of tobacco withdrawal symptoms: A randomized placebo-controlled trial. *J Am Board Fam Pract* 1992;5:1–9.
203. Rohrbach MS, et al. Plant polyphenols. In: Hemingway RW, Laks PE, eds. New York: Plenum Press; 1992:803–824.
204. Rosecrans JA, Karan LD. Neurobehavioral mechanisms of nicotine action: Role in the initiation and maintenance of tobacco dependence. *J Subst Abuse Treat* 1993;1:161–170.
205. Rosenberg L, et al. The risk of myocardial infarction after quitting smoking in men under 55 years of age. *N Engl J Med* 1985;313: 1511–1514.
206. Rosenberg L, Palmer JR, Shapiro S. Decline in the risk of myocardial infarction in women who stop smoking. *N Engl J Med* 1990;322: 213–217.
207. Russell M, et al. Targeting heavy smokers in general practice: Randomised controlled trial of transdermal nicotine patches. *Br Med J* 1993;306:1308–1312.
208. Sachs DPL, Sawe U, Leischow SJ. Effectiveness of a 16-hour transdermal nicotine patch in a medical practice setting, without intensive group counseling. *Arch Intern Med* 1993;153:1881–1890.
209. Sakagami H, et al. Stimulation of monocyte iodination and IL-1 production by tannins and related compounds. *Anticancer Res* 1992;12: 377–388.
210. Salonen JT, et al. Autoantibody against oxidized LDL and progression of carotid atherosclerosis. *Lancet* 1992;339:883–887.
211. Schleimer RP, et al. IL-4 induces adherence of human eosinophils and basophils but not neutrophils to endothelium. *J Immunol* 1992; 148:1086–1092.
212. Schmidt KG, Rasmussen JW. Acute platelet activation induced by smoking. *Thromb Haemostas* 1984;51:279–282.
213. Schwartz JL. Methods of smoking cessation. *Med Clin North Am* 1992;76:451–476.
214. Schwartz LD, Huff TF. *Biology of Mast Cells and Basophils.* St. Louis: Mosby Year Book; 1993.
215. Sellers EM, Naranjo CA, Kadlec K. Do serotonin uptake inhibitors decrease smoking? Observations in a group of heavy drinkers. *J Clin Psychopharmacol* 1987;7:417–420.
216. Schiffman S. Assessing smoking patterns and motives. *J Consult Clin Psychol* 1993;61:732–742.
217. Sparrow DRR, Colton T. The influence of cigarette smoking on prognosis after a first myocardial infarction. *J Chronic Dis* 1978;31: 425–532.
218. Speir E, et al. Potential role of human cytomegalovirus and p53 interaction in coronary restenosis. *Science* 1994;265:391–395.
219. Springer TA. Adhesion receptors of the immune system. *Nature* 1990; 346:425–434.
220. Stebbins KR. Transnational tobacco companies and health in underdeveloped countries: Recommendations for avoiding a smoking epidemic. *Soc Sci Med* 1990;30:227–235.
221. Stein Y, Harats D, Stein O. Why is smoking a major risk factor for coronary heart disease in hyperlipidemic subjects? *Ann NY Acad Sci* 1993;686:66–69.
222. Steinberg D, et al. Beyond cholesterol. Modifications of low density lipoprotein that increase its atherogenicity. *N Engl J Med* 1989;320: 915–924.
223. Stevens VJ, et al. A smoking-cessation intervention for hospital patients. *Med Care* 1993;31:65–72.
224. Strong JP, Oatman MC. Effects of smoking on the cardiovascular system. In: *Behavioral Interventions for the Cardiologist.* 205–221.
225. Sutherland G, et al. Randomized controlled trial of nasal nicotine spray in smoking cessation. *Lancet* 1992;340:324–329.
226. Tang JI, Law M, Wald N. How effective is nicotine replacement therapy in helping people to stop smoking? *Br Med J* 1994;308(21): 6.
227. Taylor CB, et al. Smoking cessation after acute myocardial infarction: Effects of a nurse-managed intervention. *Ann Intern Med* 1990;113: 118–123.
228. Tonnesen P, et al. Effect of nicotine chewing gum in combination with group counseling on the cessation of smoking. *N Engl J Med* 1988;318:15–18.

229. Tonnesen P, et al. A double-blind trial of a nicotine inhaler for smoking cessation. *JAMA* 1993;269:1268–1271.
230. Tonnesen P, et al. Recycling with nicotine patch in smoking cessation. *Addiction* 1993;88:533–539.
231. Totti N, et al. Nicotine is chemotactic for neutrophiles and enhances neutrophil responses to chemotactic peptides. *Science* 1984;223: 169–171.
232. Tsevat J. Impact and cost-effectiveness of smoking interventions. *Am J Med* 1992;92[S1A]:43S–47S.
233. Tsevat J, et al. Expected gains in life expectancy from various coronary heart disease risk factor modifications. *Circulation* 1991;83: 1194–1201.
234. Wagenknecht LE, et al. Racial differences in serum cotinine levels among smokers in the coronary artery risk development in (young) adults study. *Am J Public Health* 1990;80:1053–1056.
235. Wagenknecht LE, et al. Cigarette smoking behavior is strongly related to educational status: The CARDIA study. *Prev Med* 1990;19: 158–169.
236. Warner JG, Little WC. Myocardial infarction in a patient who smoked while wearing a nicotine patch. *Ann Intern Med* 1994;120:695.
237. Wei H, Young D. Effect of clonidine on cigarette cessation and in the alleviation of withdrawal symptoms. *Br J Addict* 1988;83:1221–1226.
238. Weinstein MC, Stason WB. Cost-effectiveness of interventions to prevent or treat coronary heart disease. *Annu Rev Public Health* 1985; 6:41–63.
239. Wells KB, et al. The practices of general and subspecialty internists in counseling about smoking and exercise. *Am J Public Health* 1986; 76:1009–1013.
240. Wessler S, et al. Estrogen-containing oral contraceptive agents. A basis for their thrombogenicity. *JAMA* 1976;236:2179–2182.
241. West RJ, Hajek P, McNeil A. Effect of buspirone on cigarette withdrawal symptoms and short-term abstinence rates in a smokers clinic. *Psychopharmacology* 1991;104:91–96.
242. Westman EC, Leven ED, Rose JE. The nicotine patch in smoking cessation. A randomized trial with telephone counseling. *Arch Intern Med* 1993;153:1917–1923.
243. Westra W, et al. Overexpression of the p53 tumor suppressor gene product in primary lung adenocarcinoma is associated with cigarette smoking. *Am J Surg Pathol* 1993;17:213–220.
244. Willett WC, et al. Relative and absolute excess risks of coronary heart disease among women who smoke cigarettes. *N Engl J Med* 1987; 317:1303–1309.
245. Willms DG, et al. Patients' perspectives of a physician-delivered smoking cessation intervention. *Am J Prev Med* 1991;7:95–100.
246. Wilson DM, et al. A randomized trial of a family physician intervention for smoking cessation. *JAMA* 1988;260:1570–1574.
247. Wilztum JL. Role of oxidized low density lipoprotein in atherogenesis. *Br Heart J* 1993;69(Suppl):S12–S18.
248. Worldwide uost. *Worldwide Use of Smoking Tobacoo.* 1986.
249. Wright JL, Churg A. Effect of long-term cigarette smoke exposure on pulmonary vascular structure and function in the guinea pig. *Exp Lung Res* 1991;17:997–1009.
250. Wright SC, et al. Nicotine inhibition of apoptosis suggests a role in tumor promotion. *FASEB J* 1993;7:1045–1051.
251. Wynder EL, Hoffman D. *Tobacco and Tobacco Smoke: Studies in Experimental Carcinogenesis.* New York: Academic Press; 1967.
252. Yla-Herttuala S, et al. Expression of monocyte chemoattractant protein 1 in macrophage-rich areas of human and rabbit atherosclerotic lesions. *Proc Natl Acad Sci USA* 1991;88:5252–5256.
253. Zhang ZF, et al. Tobacco smoking occupation and p53 nuclear overexpression in early stage bladder cancer. *Cancer Epidemiol Biomark Prev* 1994;3:19–24.

Atherosclerosis and Coronary Artery Disease,
edited by V. Fuster, R. Ross, and E. J. Topol.
Lippincott-Raven Publishers, Philadelphia © 1996.

CHAPTER 19

Diabetes and Obesity

Doron Aronson and Elliot J. Rayfield

Key Words: Diabetes; Hyperglycemia; Atherosclerosis; Nephropathy; Hypertension; Insulin Resistance; Dyslipidemia; Coagulopathy; Endothelium; Glycosylation; Abdominal obesity.

INTRODUCTION

Both insulin-dependent (IDDM) and non-insulin-dependent diabetes mellitus (NIDDM) are powerful and independent risk factors for cardiovascular disease. Since 1987, diabetes mellitus has been listed as the seventh leading cause of death in the United States. Atherosclerosis is the major cause of premature death in patients with either insulin-dependent or non-insulin dependent diabetes, accounting for virtually 80% of all deaths and 75% of all hospitalizations of diabetic patients.

Diabetes affects atherogenesis through multiplicity of potential mechanisms. The specific effects of hyperglycemia are mediated through the irreversible glycosylation and glycoxidation of structural proteins in the arterial wall and an enhanced potential for oxidative damage. However, diabetes is associated with a number of factors that contribute to the accelerated atherosclerosis. Most of these factors are also recognized as independent risk factors of atherosclerosis and coronary artery disease.

An atherogenic lipoprotein profile including increased very low-density lipoprotein (VLDL) and VLDL remnants, decreased high-density lipoprotein (HDL), and the predominance of the atherogenic small dense low-density lipoproteins (LDL) is characteristic of diabetes. Hypertension is more prevalent in diabetic patients and markedly accelerates the atherosclerotic process. Alterations in endothelial function and the coagulation system play a role in the accelerated atherosclerosis and thrombosis that characterize the diabetic state. These include abnormal endothelial modulation of vasomotor tone, increased levels of fibrinogen, increased platelet aggregability, and impaired fibrinolytic system from decreased activity of plasminogen activator inhibitor type I (PAI-1).

D. Aronson: Mount Sinai Medical School, New York, New York 10029
E.J. Rayfield: Mount Sinai Medical School, New York, New York 10029

Hyperinsulinemia and insulin resistance caused by genetic factors or obesity are an integral part of non-insulin-dependent diabetes. The combination of insulin resistance and compensatory hyperinsulinemia further predisposes these patients to coronary heart disease (CHD). Insulin resistance is associated with other cardiovascular risk factors, including elevated blood pressure, dyslipidemia, impaired fibrinolysis, and a central pattern of fat distribution. In addition, the direct proliferative and mitogenic actions of insulin on vascular smooth muscle cells may contribute to the atherosclerotic process.

ATHEROSCLEROSIS AND DIABETES

Both IDDM and NIDDM are powerful and independent risk factors of atherosclerosis, coronary artery disease (CAD), stroke, and peripheral arterial disease (1,2). Atherosclerosis is a major health problem in patients with diabetes, accounting for virtually 80% of all deaths among North American diabetic patients, compared with one-third of all deaths in the general North American population (3). Three-quarters of these deaths result from coronary heart disease. The remaining one-fourth is the admixture of accelerated cerebral and peripheral vascular disease, each of which is increased approximately fivefold in diabetic patients compared with their nondiabetic counterparts. More than 75% of all hospitalizations for diabetic complications are attributable to cardiovascular disease (4). Diabetes is also the most common cause of heart disease in young persons. In addition, more than 50% of patients newly diagnosed with non-insulin-dependent diabetes mellitus are found to have preexisting CAD at the time of diabetes diagnosis (5). Several autopsy studies have shown that diabetic subjects have more extensive atherosclerosis of both coronary and cerebral vessels than age- and sex-matched nondiabetic controls. In the International Atherosclerosis Project, 23,000 subjects from 14 countries were examined. The severity of coronary atherosclerosis in diabetics varied in parallel with the population from the same country. However, the effect of diabetes was superimposed on any level of average severity of atherosclerosis (6). Other studies confirm that the prevalence of atherosclerosis among diabetic patients varies considerably according to geographic or ethnic origin and in parallel with overall population differences in atherosclerosis frequency (7,8). Thus, diabetes does not appear to be the primary cause of atherosclerosis. However, when present, diabetes accelerates the natural progression of atherosclerosis in all populations (6).

Diabetics have a larger number of coronary vessels involved, more diffuse distribution of atherosclerotic lesions, and a more severe narrowing of the left main coronary artery (9,10,12). There is also an increased prevalence of complicated atheroma, with plaque fissuring (11). Younger individuals with IDDM are not spared. Severe and extensive luminal narrowing of major coronary arteries was found in patients with onset of IDDM before age 15 who died before the age of 40 (12). Angiographic studies comparing diabetics to matched controls indicate that the major differences between the two groups is a significantly higher frequency of multiple-vessel disease in diabetics (13,14).

TABLE 1. *Factors contributing to atherosclerosis in diabetes*

Abnormalities in lipoprotein levels and composition
Hypertension
Insulin resistance and hyperinsulinemia
Advanced glycosylation of proteins in plasma and arterial wall
"Glycoxidation" and oxidation
Procoagulant state
Endothelial dysfunction

Diabetes affects atherogenesis through multiple potential mechanisms (Table 1). Many of the proatherogenic effects of diabetes are related to alterations in lipoprotein concentrations as well as atherogenic lipoprotein compositional changes. These include increased VLDL and VLDL remnants; small, dense LDL; and decreased HDL. Hypertension is more prevalent among individuals with NIDDM and those with IDDM who developed nephropathy. High circulating insulin levels in patients with NIDDM may also be atherogenic. Furthermore, hyperinsulinemia is a marker for other risk factors, such as hypertension and an atherogenic lipoprotein profile, which often coexist. A procoagulant state exists in diabetes as a result of increased levels of clotting factors, increased platelet aggregability, and decreased activity of plasminogen activator inhibitor type I (PAI-1). Altered endothelial cell release of vasoactive mediators results in abnormal modulation of vascular smooth muscle tone. The unique effects of hyperglycemia mediated through the mechanism of protein glycation and glycoxication increase atherogenicity by affecting vessel wall structural proteins and enhancing the potential for oxidative damage. Glycation of the LDL particle impairs its recognition by the LDL receptor and renders it more susceptible to oxidative modification.

Coronary Artery Disease in NIDDM

Coronary heart disease is a major health problem in NIDDM. It is the leading cause of death among patients with NIDDM regardless of duration of diabetes. Several population-based studies have consistently shown that the relative risk ratio of cardiovascular disease in NIDDM compared to the general population is increased twofold to fourfold (2,15, 16,19,25,31). The rather consistent pattern of mortality among diabetics appears surprising, particularly because the duration of prospective observations varies widely. One exception, however, are the Pima Indians, in whom coronary artery disease is absent or rare among nondiabetics with extremely high relative risk for diabetics (17). Although NIDDM patients have an increased atherogenic risk factor profile (older age, hypertension, low HDL), statistical adjustments fail to remove an independent effect of diabetes per se (31). The increased cardiovascular risk is particularly striking in women. Many studies, including the Framingham (15), Rancho Bernardo (18), Bedford (19), and Joslin Clinic (29), reported a disproportionate impact of CAD in diabetic women compared with diabetic men. The usual protection that premenopausal women have against atherosclerosis is lost when diabetes is present (20).

Although the degree and duration of hyperglycemia are the principal risk factors for microvascular complications (21), in NIDDM there is no obvious association between the extent or severity of macrovascular complications and the duration or severity of the diabetes (4,8,31). An increased prevalence of CAD is apparent in newly diagnosed NIDDM subjects (22). Because many years of asymptomatic hyperglycemia may precede the clinical diagnosis of NIDDM, the estimation of duration of diabetes may be biased. In fact, even impaired glucose tolerance has been shown to be associated with increased cardiovascular risk despite minimal hyperglycemia (19,23–25).

Insulin resistance may be the linking factor among impaired glucose tolerance, NIDDM, and CAD. In genetically prone individuals, insulin resistance is the earliest detectable defect and can occur 15–25 years or more before the clinical onset of overt diabetes (26). Moreover, insulin resistance is associated with other atherogenic risk factors such as hypertension, lipid abnormalities, and a procoagulant state (see Hypertension and Insulin Resistance, below). Thus, the factor most likely to be related to CAD among individuals with impaired glucose tolerance and diabetics is the unknown duration of insulin resistance rather than the duration of diabetes per se (31).

However, other studies suggest that the level of chronic hyperglycemia, as determined by measurements of glycosylated hemoglobin, may also be an independent risk factor for coronary heart disease, particularly in women (27,28).

Coronary Artery Disease in IDDM

In contrast to NIDDM, cardiovascular risk can be examined in IDDM patients to determine the extent that pure diabetes-related factors (e.g., hyperglycemia, disease duration, and glycosylation of proteins and lipoproteins) cause the enhanced CAD risk of diabetes. Long-term follow-up of patients with IDDM from the Joslin Diabetes Center demonstrated an excess of cardiovascular mortality as compared to the general population (29). An excess of CAD in patients with IDDM can be observed only after the age of 30. The first cases of clinically manifest CAD occur late in the third decade or in the fourth decade of life regardless of whether diabetes developed early in childhood or in late adolescence. The CAD risk increases rapidly after the age of 40, and by the age of 55 years, 35% of men and women with IDDM die of CAD. This rate of CAD mortality far exceeded that observed in an age-matched nondiabetic cohort from the Framingham Heart Study (8% for nondiabetic men and 4% for nondiabetic women) (29). As with women with NIDDM, the protection from CAD observed in nondiabetic women is lost in women with IDDM (29–31). The fact that a subset of IDDM patients have severe coronary atherosclerosis before the age of 55 regardless of whether diabetes developed in childhood or adolescence suggests that diabetes mainly accelerates the progression of early atherosclerotic lesions that occur, even in the absence of diabetes, at a young age in the general population (29).

Two long-term follow-up studies from the Joslin Clinic and from the Steno Memorial Hospital have demonstrated that when nephropathy is superimposed on diabetes, the prevalence of CAD increases dramatically. Data from the Steno Memorial Hospital indicate that in patients with persistent proteinuria, the relative mortality from cardiovascular disease was 37 times that in the general population, whereas in patients without proteinuria, cardiovascular mortality was only 4.2 times higher (32). In a case-control study of IDDM patients who were followed from the onset of microalbuminuria, coronary heart disease developed eight times more frequently than in a comparable diabetic population (33). In the Joslin Clinic cohort, the risk of development of CAD in patients with persistent proteinuria was 15 times higher than those without this complication (29). Nearly all patients with diabetic nephropathy over the age of 45 have one or more coronary stenoses >50% of the vessel diameter (34). Microalbuminuria in IDDM is, therefore, not only a marker for renal disease but also a potent risk marker of CAD.

Recent prospective studies demonstrated that in NIDDM patients, microalbuminuria is also an independent predictor of increased cardiovascular mortality (11,35,36). Proteinuria in a patient with NIDDM increases the risk of fatal CAD by a factor of only two to four. The mechanisms linking microalbuminuria with increased cardiovascular mortality are largely unknown. However, when nephropathy is superimposed on diabetes, some of the atherogenic mechanisms present in diabetes are accentuated. An aggregation of risk factors for cardiovascular disease, including hypertension, lipid abnormalities, and fibrinolysis and coagulation alterations, are detectable in the early stages of diabetic nephropathy, in which renal function is preserved (37). Hypertension is frequently present in diabetic nephropathy, even when the creatinine concentrations remain normal, and can intensify CAD in IDDM patients. The lipoprotein profile in diabetic patients with microalbuminuria includes elevated LDL and chylomicron remnant levels, decreased HDL levels, and elevated Lp(a) levels (38–40), all of which are atherogenic. In addition, PAI-1 activity, factor VII, and plasma fibrinogen are significantly higher in microalbuminuric IDDM patients (41). Finally, nephropathy results in accelerated accumulation of advanced glycosylation end products (AGE) in the circulation and tissue that parallels the severity of renal functional impairment (42). Accumulation of AGE products in tissue promotes atherosclerosis (see Advanced Glycosylation End Products, below). Although these risk factors undoubtedly contribute to the accelerated development of atherosclerosis in patients with diabetic nephropathy, they may not fully explain the high cardiovascular mortality of microalbuminuric patients (37).

Diabetic nephropathy occurs only in a subset of approximately 30% to 40% of IDDM patients (43). The risk for the development of diabetic nephropathy is only partially determined by glycemic control and is highly influenced by genetic susceptibility (44,45). Familial clustering of cardiovascular disease occurs in diabetic patients with nephropathy. Cardiovascular disease is twice as common a cause of death among parents of diabetic patients with nephropathy than among parents of diabetic patients without nephropathy. Among diabetics with nephropathy, those who had a cardiovascular event are six times more likely to have a familial history of cardiovascular disease than those who had no such event. A history of cardiovascular disease in both parents or in the father of an IDDM patient increases the risk of nephropathy in the offspring ten- or threefold, respectively (46). Parents of diabetic offspring with nephropathy also have higher levels of arterial blood pressure than do parents whose diabetic offspring do not have diabetic nephropathy (47,48). Thus, a subgroup of IDDM subjects have a genetically determined predisposition to renal disease and hypertension, and this predisposition is also linked to enhanced risk of CAD. This inherited susceptibility to CAD would be expected to be expressed in those patients with poor glycemic control.

The red blood cell sodium–lithium countertransport (Na^+,Li^+-CT) activity may be a possible genetic link between hypertension and diabetic nephropathy, both markers of macrovascular disease. An elevated Na^+,Li^+-CT activity is the most consistent marker for essential hypertension (49), and its interindividual variability is largely under genetic control (43). Interestingly, Na^+,Li^+-CT activity is elevated in IDDM patients with albuminuria (47,50) and in parents whose diabetic offspring have nephropathy (51). These observations led to the suggestion that abnormal Na^+,Li^+-CT could be used as a marker for the risk of developing nephropathy and associated complications. However, other studies concluded that the diabetic state per se might be responsible for the elevation in Na^+,Li^+-CT activity (52,53).

Additional genetic factors may contribute to the predisposition of diabetic patients to develop CAD. A variant of the gene encoding angiotensin-converting enzyme (ACE), recognized as an insertion (I) or deletion (D) in intron 16 (the I allele of the ACE gene carries an intronic insertion that is not present in the D allele) has recently been shown to be associated with CAD (54). A deletion polymorphism (DD genotype) in the ACE gene has been shown to confer a high risk of myocardial infarction independently of any of the classical risk factors for CAD (54).

The ACE deletion polymorphism is also a potent cardiovascular risk factor in NIDDM. The D allele of the ACE deletion polymorphism was seen significantly more frequently in patients with NIDDM and established CAD than in patients with NIDDM without clinical or electrocardiographic evidence of CAD (55). Although there is no similar study in patients with IDDM, the II genotype seems to confer a protection against the onset of diabetic nephropathy in patients with IDDM (56,57). The strong association between diabetic nephropathy and CAD in both patients with IDDM and NIDDM and the clustering of diabetic nephropathy in families suggest that a genetic polymorphism affecting ACE gene expression could be associated with susceptibility to vascular complications in diabetic patients. Interestingly, the ACE deletion polymorphism is not associated with hypertension in humans (55) despite the association between the DD genotype and higher ACE levels. The molecular mechanisms of the deleterious effects of the ACE deletion polymorphism are unknown, as is its role in the prevention and detection of CAD in diabetic patients.

SPECIAL CONSIDERATIONS IN DIABETIC PATIENTS WITH CORONARY HEART DISEASE

The clinical expression of CAD in diabetic patients differs from that in nondiabetic patients in several ways, including a higher frequency of silent myocardial infarction and ischemia, greater morbidity and mortality after acute myocardial infarction, decreased reperfusion rates after thrombolytic therapy, and increased restenosis rate following coronary angioplasty.

Silent Myocardial Ischemia in Diabetes

The propensity of diabetic patients to silent myocardial infarction is well established (58,59). In the Framingham study a higher proportion of myocardial infarctions were silent and unrecognized (5). Atypical symptoms such as confusion, dyspnea, fatigue, or nausea and vomiting were the presenting complaint in 32% to 42% of diabetic patients with myocardial infarction compared to 6% to 15% of nondiabetic patients (59,65). In addition, those diabetes who suffered pain with their myocardial infarction characterized their discomfort as less intense compared with nondiabetic patients. These atypical presenting symptoms may lower the clinician's suspicion of infarction and lead to less than optimal care (85).

Recent studies indicate that silent myocardial ischemic episodes also occur with increased frequency in patients with diabetes. Although silent ischemia can be frequently demonstrated in patients with chronic stable angina, these studies indicate that whether assessed by treadmill exercise testing (60,61), ambulatory Holter monitoring (69), or exercise thallium scintigraphy (62–65), silent ischemia is more common in diabetics than in nondiabetics. This finding, however, is not supported by all studies (66,67).

Autonomic neuropathy with involvement of the sensory supply to the heart is a plausible explanation for painless infarction and ischemic episodes in diabetics. Diabetic autonomic neuropathy may involve the afferent fibers running through the cardiac sympathetic nervous system, which is a part of the pain perception pathway from myocardial pain receptors to the cerebral cortex. In autopsies of diabetic patients who died of silent myocardial infarction, typical diabetic neuropathic changes were found in the intracardiac sympathetic and parasympathetic fibers (68).

Several studies documented abnormalities in autonomic function in diabetic patients with silent ischemia (61,62,69). The anginal perceptual threshold—the time from the onset of myocardial ischemia (assessed by ST segment depression) to the onset of chest pain during exercise testing—is prolonged in diabetic patients compared with nondiabetics. This delay in the perception of pain is related to the impairment of autonomic nervous function (70). Autonomic impairment associated with silent ischemia can be detected despite the absence of overt autonomic neuropathy (71) or other microvascular complications (61).

Ischemic episodes with or without angina are associated with similar degrees of left ventricular dysfunction and can be responsible for symptoms of dyspnea or fatigue that in the absence of angina might not be considered ischemic in origin. Therefore, atypical symptoms that cannot be attributed to other causes should encourage the clinician to seek a diagnosis of coronary artery disease in diabetic patients.

Course of Acute Myocardial Infarction

Overall in-hospital mortality for diabetic patients is 1.5 to 2 times higher than for nondiabetic patients experiencing myocardial infarction (76,77). One study analyzing the outcomes of diabetic patients with acute myocardial infarction before the introduction of thrombolysis and coronary angioplasty reported a 28% in-hospital mortality (74). Diabetic women have a particularly poor prognosis, with an almost twofold increase in mortality compared with diabetic men (75,79). The risk conferred by diabetes occurs also among young diabetic patients with a good apparent baseline cardiovascular status (72). Most studies have shown no relationship between duration of known diabetes and in-hospital mortality following myocardial infarction (77,79). Moreover, patients with undiagnosed diabetes but with levels of hemoglobin A_{1C} indicating previous diabetes mellitus also have the same poor outcome after acute myocardial infarction (73).

The excess in-hospital mortality in diabetics is clearly related to an increased incidence of congestive heart failure. The prevalence of congestive heart failure and cardiogenic shock is more common and more severe in diabetic subjects after myocardial infarction than would be predicted from the size of the infarct (74–78). Prognosis after myocardial infarction is related to the residual left ventricular function and thus to the amount of damaged myocardium. However, there is no evidence that diabetic patients sustain more extensive infarctions than nondiabetic patients (74,77,79). Moreover, the increase in congestive heart failure occurs despite a similar left ventricular ejection fraction (assessed by radionuclide ventriculography) in diabetics and nondiabetics, indicating the presence of relatively preserved systolic function despite more manifestations of congestive heart failure (79). This fact strongly implies that additional pathogenic processes compromise myocardial function in diabetic patients and that the congestive symptoms are mainly a result of diastolic dysfunction (79).

Several mechanisms may underlie the increased in-hospital mortality rate in diabetic patients. The higher incidence of pump failure in diabetic patients may be the result of hypocontractility of the noninfarcted myocardium. The MILIS study showed that early after infarction, increased contractility often occurs in noninfarcted areas of the left ventricle and that this compensatory response appears to be blunted in diabetics (79). Early angiography in the TAMI trials also demonstrated worse noninfarct-zone ventricular function in diabetics (80). It is likely that diabetics have more extensive coronary artery disease, which predisposes them to greater dysfunction in areas of noninfarcted myocardium or compromises collateral blood flow. This postulate is supported by necropsy studies demonstrating that patients with IDDM and NIDDM have more extensive coronary obstructions than nondiabetics and by the finding that diabetics suffer more frequent reinfarctions at follow-up. However, left ventricular regional ejection fraction images of the noninfarcted area obtained by radionuclide angiography were found to be significantly lower in NIDDM patients despite a nearly identical extent of necrosis, severity of coronary atherosclerosis, and number of diseased coronary vessels (81). It has been suggested that diabetics tend to develop ischemic cardiomyopathy more frequently than nondiabetic patients because the residual myocardium associated with NIDDM may adversely influence the process of left ventricular remodeling after myocardial infarction.

Diabetes is associated with a cardiomyopathic process that affects left ventricular diastolic function. Arteriolar or capillary involvement by diabetic microangiopathy may lead to more extensive scar formation, diffuse fibrosis, and impaired myocardial relaxation. Clinical or subclinical diabetic cardiomyopathy, characterized by pathological changes in the microvasculature and myocardial interstitium unrelated to large-vessel atherosclerosis, may contribute to the hypocontractility of the noninfarcted myocardium (79,82). Another hypothesis is that the increased mortality in diabetic patients is caused by a disturbance in the autonomic nervous system. Impaired cardiac sympathetic nerve function would reduce the inotropic reserve of the viable muscle.

Diabetic patients surviving the immediate postinfarction complications suffer from recurrent nonfatal and fatal myocardial infarction to a greater degree than do their nondiabetic counterparts (79,83–85). Although immediate postinfarction morbidity and mortality are usually related to congestive heart failure, late mortality tends to be caused by recurrent myocardial infarction, persistent ischemia, or ongoing myocardial damage (85).

Thrombolytic Therapy

It is well established that mortality is significantly reduced among nondiabetic patients with acute myocardial infarction who received thrombolytic therapy such as streptokinase or recombinant tissue-type plasminogen activator (rt-PA). In addition, thrombolytic therapy improves left ventricular function. Although the major studies of these agents after myocardial infarction have included diabetic patients, no study has specifically evaluated the benefit of thrombolytic therapy versus placebo in diabetic patients with acute infarction. The ISIS-II study, which included 1,287 diabetic and 15,694 nondiabetic patients, demonstrated a clear benefit among diabetic patients receiving thrombolytic therapy with streptokinase (86). In the TIMI trial 425 diabetic patients and 2,836 nondiabetic patients were randomized within 4 h of acute myocardial infarction to thrombolytic therapy. The 6-week mortality rates were 8.5% and 3.6%, respectively (87).

In the International Tissue Plasminogen Activator/Streptokinase Mortality Trial the in-hospital mortality rate of patients with diabetes over 10 years was almost double that of all comparable age groups of nondiabetic patients (88). In addition, their postdischarge clinical course was worse, characterized by a greater incidence of reinfarction and stroke and a higher incremental 6-month mortality rate.

In the GISSI-2 study, 1,266 diabetic and 8,096 nondiabetic patients were randomized to receive streptokinase or rt-PA. As determined with a noninvasive index, reperfusion was achieved less frequently in diabetic patients than in nondiabetic patients using streptokinase or rt-PA with or without heparin. In addition, in-hospital mortality rates in patients treated with rt-PA were 7.4% in patients without diabetes, 15.4% in patients with IDDM, and 12.4% in those with NIDDM. In patients treated with streptokinase, the respective mortality rates were 7.2%, 17.4%, and 10.9%. The type of fibrinolytic agent did not affect mortality rates (78).

The TAMI trials were designed to evaluate various reperfusion strategies using rt-PA, urokinase, or a combination of rt-PA and urokinase. In each study, patients underwent two cardiac catheterization procedures, the first at approximately 90 min after initiation of thrombolytic therapy and the second 7 to 10 days later. Despite similar angiographic patency rates 90 min after thrombolytic therapy in patients with and without diabetes, the in-hospital mortality rate was nearly twice as high in patients with diabetes (80).

Thus, although diabetic patients with acute myocardial infarction treated with fibrinolytic therapy benefit by the same mortality reduction as that of nondiabetic patients (88,86,89), the increased in-hospital mortality rates in diabetes remains significant (1.5 to 2.5 times higher than in nondiabetics) (78,80,88,89). Abnormalities in the fibrinolytic system of diabetics may explain the lower reperfusion rates reported in these patients. Both NIDDM and insulin resistance are associated with increased plasminogen activator inhibitor 1 (PAI-1) activity (see Altered Fibrinolysis in Diabetes, below). Elevated PAI-1 activity on admission with acute myocardial infarction reduces the likelihood of a patent infarct-related artery after thrombolytic therapy with rt-PA (90,91). Thus, elevated PAI-1 activity in diabetes may alter the balance between thrombosis and fibrinolysis and account for the lower reperfusion rates and poorer outcome from myocardial infarction in diabetic patients. However, angiographic data from the TAMI trial demonstrate that differences in the effectiveness of thrombolytic therapy are not responsible for the worse outcome in patients with diabetes (80). It appears that the major reason for the higher in-hospital mortality and complication rates in patients with diabetes is primarily related to more extensive coronary artery disease. Patients with diabetes, therefore, should be considered at high risk for a poor outcome and should be treated in a similar fashion to other high-risk groups, with early thrombolytic therapy and perhaps a more aggressive diagnostic and therapeutic approach, and with early revascularization in those with appropriate anatomy.

Percutaneous Transluminal Coronary Angioplasty

Findings in several studies suggest that diabetes is a powerful risk factor for restenosis after percutaneous transluminal coronary angioplasty (PTCA) (92–95). Restenosis is viewed as an intraluminal growth process after a successful angioplasty, and risk factors for restenosis should be risk factors for this growth process. However, classic risk factors for atherosclerosis such as male sex, systemic hypertension, hypercholesterolemia, and continued smoking after the PTCA were not found to be related to luminal narrowing (95). Only diabetes was found to be independently related to the amount of luminal narrowing at follow-up. Diabetics also have an increased incidence of restenosis rates after excimer laser angioplasty (96).

A recent study showed that diabetic patients had a significantly greater restenosis rate after coronary stenting. Restenosis within a stent resulted from smooth muscle cell hyperplasia, which may be the result of the metabolic abnormalities in diabetics (97). However, the factors responsible for increased restenosis in diabetic patients have not as yet been elucidated.

LIPOPROTEIN DISORDERS IN DIABETES

The metabolic abnormalities associated with IDDM and NIDDM result in profound changes in the transport, composition, and metabolism of lipoproteins. Consequently, abnormalities in plasma lipid and lipoprotein concentrations are commonly observed in diabetic individuals, particularly in subjects with uncontrolled IDDM and in many individuals with NIDDM. In the San Antonio Heart Study, a population-based study of diabetes and cardiovascular disease, more than 60% of patients with NIDDM were dyslipidemic, compared with fewer than 25% of nondiabetics (98). However, only 25% were aware of their diagnosis, and fewer than 10% were receiving treatment. Data from the Framingham heart study indicate that elevations of VLDL triglycerides and reductions in HDL levels are about twice as prevalent in diabetic men and women as in nondiabetics. Regardless of geographic or racial origin, NIDDM patients have a two- to threefold excess of dyslipidemia compared with the corresponding nondiabetic population (99,189).

The concentrations and metabolism of plasma lipoproteins in diabetic subjects are influenced by factors specific to the diabetic state, that is, type of diabetes, glycemic control, insulin resistance, the presence of diabetic nephropathy, and the type and method of treatment. Because the two forms of diabetes differ in their basic pathophysiology and other features, including presence or absence of obesity, age, and insulin deficiency versus insulin resistance, it is not surprising that lipoprotein metabolism may differ in IDDM and NIDDM (100,101).

The accelerated atherosclerosis in diabetes is caused, at least in part, by an atherogenic lipoprotein profile. The atherogenic pattern of lipoprotein changes is often present for years before the development of fasting hyperglycemia and the diagnosis of frank diabetes. This may explain why the risk of cardiovascular disease is not related to the duration of diabetes in patients with NIDDM (102). This is in contrast to IDDM, where lipoprotein abnormalities occur in relation to the onset of hyperglycemia. The main factors that influence the concentrations of plasma lipoprotein in IDDM are glycemic control, method of insulin administration, and the presence of nephropathy (see Coronary Artery Disease in IDDM, above).

Triglycerides and VLDL

The most consistent change in lipoproteins associated with both types of diabetes is an increase in very low density lipoprotein (VLDL) levels. Poorly controlled IDDM induces a marked elevation of triglycerides through a combination of overproduction and reduced clearance of VLDL. Increased production is a consequence of an increase in free fatty acid mobilization and high glucose levels. The concentrations of circulating free fatty acids govern the rate of triglyceride esterification in the liver by stimulating both triglyceride synthesis and the assembly and secretion of VLDL particles (103). Maintenance of stored fat in adipose tissue depends on the suppression of hormone-sensitive lipase by insulin. Under conditions of insulin deficiency, the high blood glucose and free fatty acid mobilization provide a substrate for synthesis of triglycerides in the liver with subsequent overproduction of VLDL. Decreased VLDL clearance results from diminished lipoprotein lipase (LPL) activity, as LPL requires insulin for maintenance of normal tissue levels. These abnormalities in VLDL overproduction and clearance are readily reversible with insulin therapy. Thus, the degree of hypertriglyceridemia in IDDM patients is highly dependent on the degree of glycemic control (141). Institution of intensive insulin therapy rapidly restores LPL activity and normalizes hepatic VLDL production, resulting in normal VLDL levels.

In NIDDM, the most common lipoprotein abnormality is hypertriglyceridemia caused by increased VLDL levels (104). Studies of large populations, including the Pima Indians (105), who have virtually no forms of genetic hyperlipidemia, indicate that NIDDM generally produces only a 50–100% elevation of VLDL or total triglycerides when compared with age-, sex-, and weight-matched nondiabetics. Thus, NIDDM subjects with total triglycerides higher than 350–400 mg/dl probably have other genetic disorders in lipoprotein metabolism, which may be exacerbated by the diabetics (106).

The main reason for hypertriglyceridemia in NIDDM is overproduction of triglyceride-rich VLDL in the liver secondary to an increased flow of substrates, particularly glucose and free fatty acids. High rates of free fatty acid transport to the liver are common concomitants of insulin resistance (107). As in IDDM, the presence of hyperglycemia and increased free fatty acid flux to the liver in NIDDM provides an ideal milieu for increased VLDL production. Although a minimal level of insulin is required for secretion of VLDL (108), it remains unclear whether higher than normal insulin levels, in the setting of insulin resistance, contribute to the high VLDL levels by stimulating VLDL production and secretion.

In addition, patients with NIDDM have a defect in clearance of VLDL triglyceride. The LPL activity is depressed in individuals with NIDDM and insulin resistance (122,159). The result is enzymatic activity insufficient to match the overproduction rate, which in turn results in an accumulation of VLDL triglyceride in blood. Improved diabetic control, regardless of the method of treatment, is associated with a decrease in VLDL levels (109,110) because higher insulin concentrations cause lowering of glucose and free fatty acids, the precursors of VLDL production, and stimulate LPL activity. However, several months of treatment may be required to restore tissue LPL activity fully to normal (111). In contrast to the situation in IDDM, where intensive therapy normalizes VLDL levels, therapy in NIDDM only partly corrects VLDL levels in many patients (101).

Very Low-Density Lipoproteins and Atherogenesis

In contrast to the controversy regarding hypertriglyceridemia as an independent risk factor for CAD in the nondiabetic population (Farmer and Gotto, *this volume*), data from the Paris Prospective Study (112) and the World Health Organization multinational trial (113) indicate that elevated triglyc-

TABLE 2. *Atherogenic abnormalities in lipoprotein composition in diabetes*

Lipoprotein	Atherogenic modifications
VLDL	Triglyceride—enriched VLDL
	Cholesteryl-ester-rich VLDL
LDL cholesterol	Glycosylation of apo B
	Small dense LDL
	LDL glycosylation
	LDL susceptible to oxidative modification
HDL cholesterol	HDL glycosylation
	Decreased HDL_2

eride levels are independently associated with increase CAD risk in diabetic patients (114). In both of these studies, the single risk factor that correlated most closely with the occurrence of CAD in diabetic subjects was plasma total triglyceride concentrations. The mechanism for a connection between hypertriglyceridemia and atherosclerosis has not been determined with certainty. However, it is becoming increasingly recognized that the diabetic state is associated with subtle, qualitative changes in the composition of lipoprotein particles that may be relevant to the atherogenic process. These abnormalities can be detected in hyperlipidemic as well as normolipidemic individuals with diabetes (Table 2).

The most consistent observation with regard to VLDL composition in NIDDM is triglyceride enrichment of the particles in association with increased particle size (115). The increased triglyceride levels in diabetes are associated with the presence of large triglyceride-rich particles because the size of VLDL is most likely determined mainly by the amount of triglyceride available. Thus, large triglyceride-rich VLDL are secreted in situations in which excess triglycerides are available for VLDL production, such as in diabetes (159). The VLDL size is an important determinant of its metabolic fate. Large triglyceride-rich VLDL particles may be less efficiently converted to LDL (116), increasing direct removal from the circulation by non-LDL pathways. In addition, overproduction of large triglyceride-rich VLDL is associated with the atherogenic small, dense LDL subclass (see LDL Cholesterol, below) (159).

The VLDL particles in both IDDM and NIDDM can be cholesteryl ester enriched as well as triglyceride enriched and may accumulate despite normal plasma triglyceride levels (117–119). Cholesteryl-ester-enriched VLDL can be taken up by receptors on macrophages and smooth muscle cells, resulting in foam cell formation (120). This lipoprotein closely resembles the VLDL remnant, which is able to produce cholesteryl ester deposition in macrophages and endothelial cells. Thus, the risk of a diabetic individual with hypertriglyceridemia and elevated VLDL levels may be a function of the concentration of cholesteryl-ester-enriched VLDL remnants that are part of the whole plasma VLDL population. The basis of cholesteryl enrichment may be enhanced exchange of cholesteryl ester transfer protein (CETP)-mediated exchange of VLDL triglyceride for HDL cholesteryl ester.

HDL Cholesterol

The antiatherogenic association of HDL is hypothesized to reflect its central role in reverse cholesterol transport (Tall and Breslow, *this volume*), and IDDM patients usually have plasma HDL cholesterol levels within the normal range (121,140). However, in poorly controlled IDDM patients, HDL levels may fall because of reduced LPL activity, as impaired VLDL lypolysis results in reduced formation of HDL (122,142). The major reduction is found in the larger, less dense HDL_2 fraction, while HDL_3 levels are normal (141,142). Both genetic and acquired LPL deficiencies are associated with low HDL because the rate of HDL_2 formation is dependent on the rate of flux of the surface components from triglyceride-rich lipoprotein, which is mediated in part by LPL activity (123). Efficient VLDL catabolism is associated with low plasma triglyceride concentrations and maximal availability of surface components for transfer to HDL. In IDDM patients in excellent glycemic control, LPL activity is increased, and the increased catabolism of VLDL triglycerides increases the HDL compartment. The response of HDL to insulin therapy is slower than that of VLDL, but HDL increases with the degree of glycemic control. In IDDM patients on intensive insulin therapy, HDL levels may be higher than in normal age-, sex-, and weight-matched controls (124,140,142).

In patients with NIDDM, HDL cholesterol levels are typically about 25–30% lower than in nondiabetics (101). Low HDL cholesterol levels are commonly associated with other lipid and lipoprotein abnormalities, particularly high VLDL levels. As in IDDM, decreased HDL in NIDDM usually reflects a preferential decrease in the HDL_2 subfraction. In contrast to IDDM, low plasma HDL levels in NIDDM patients are not related to glycemic control and persist after treatment (125,126). Interestingly, the degree of insulin resistance as measured by euglycemic clamp appears to be inversely related to HDL levels (127). Moreover, subjects with low HDL cholesterol levels are insulin resistant independently of triglyceride levels (128). This explains why HDL levels frequently fail to normalize in response to sulfonylurea or insulin therapy in NIDDM patients.

The mechanism of decreased HDL levels appears to be a consequence of decreased production and increased catabolism of HDL (100). Decreased HDL synthesis is related to impaired clearance of VLDL and decreased LPL activity, as described above. The conversion of HDL_3 to HDL_2 depends on the delipidation action of LPL in plasma. The LPL action is closely linked with the activity of CETP, which simultaneously shuttles cholesteryl ester from HDL to VLDL and LDL and triglycerides from VLDL to HDL. Thus, impaired VLDL clearance and lower LPL activity would be expected to lead to diminished HDL_2 accumulation. Increased catabolism of HDL can occur because in hypertriglyceridemia a high rate of transfer of triglyceride to HDL_3 results in a triglyceride-rich HDL_2, which is highly susceptible to catabolism by hepatic triglyceride lipase (HTGL) (129,130). The HDL triglycerides are hydrolyzed by HTGL, which is an insulin-sensitive enzyme that converts triglyceride-enriched HDL particles to smaller, more dense HDL_3 particles. The HTGL activity has been shown to correlate inversely with HDL_2 in normolipidemic IDDM patients. A positive correlation also exists between HTGL activity and fasting insulin levels in insulin-resistant NIDDM patients (131,132). It is possible that in insulin resistance states, HTGL activity is elevated because the suppression of HTGL by insulin is reduced, resulting in a lower HDL level. Thus, the insulin resistance found in patients with NIDDM may be responsible for the common finding of low HDL in these patients.

Increased CETP activity also contributes to the abnormal HDL metabolism in diabetes, leading to potentially atherogenic lipoprotein modifications. Men with genetically low CETP have a very high HDL and low atherosclerotic risk (133,134). The CETP activity is higher in subjects with sustained hypertriglyceridemia, with net movement of cholesterol ester toward VLDL (134). Facilitated cholesteryl ester transfer may be atherogenic because it pathologically modifies the lipid composition of subpopulations of apo-B-containing lipoproteins to form atherogenic β-VLDL-like particles. Abnormal cholesterol-ester-enriched VLDL particles readily interact with cell surface receptors. An abnormal increase in cholesteryl ester transfer has been reported in both IDDM (135,136) and NIDDM (137,138). In addition, glycation of HDL is thought to interfere with HDL_3 receptor binding (139), thus impairing its ability to promote cholesterol efflux from cells. This might limit the initiation of reverse cholesterol transport.

LDL Cholesterol

The LDL cholesterol levels are generally not elevated in IDDM when compared to age-, sex-, and weight-matched nondiabetics (140). Increased LDL cholesterol levels in patients with IDDM are usually a result of the development of diabetic nephropathy and proteinuria or a result of a coexisting genetic cause of hypercholesterolemia. A positive correlation between glycemic control and cholesterol levels is usually seen only in poorly controlled patients ($HbA_{1c} >$ 11%). In these patients hypercholesterolemia is readily reversible with intensive insulin therapy (141,142). Similarly, LDL cholesterol levels of patients with NIDDM are comparable to those of nondiabetics (143). Improvement of glucose control results in no change or only a modest beneficial effect on LDL cholesterol levels (144,145).

Nonetheless, LDL particles in diabetic patients may be altered in a number of ways that can affect their metabolism and atherogenicity (Table 2). These mainly include alteration in composition, enhanced nonenzymatic glycosylation, and increased susceptibility to oxidative modification.

Glycosylation of LDL apo B (the surface protein of LDL) lysine residues is increased in poorly controlled diabetes, correlating with glucose levels. These residues are essential for the specific recognition of LDL by the LDL receptor. Because approximately 60–70% of LDL clearance is accounted for by the LDL receptor pathway, the result is a decreased catabolism of LDL via the LDL receptor pathway (146). Glycosylation of as few as 2–5% of lysine residues can decrease the in vivo clearance of LDL by 5–25%. In addition, the LDL receptor appears to be regulated to some extent by insulin (147). Thus, a decreased ability to bind the LDL receptor, coupled with down-regulated cellular LDL receptor activity, would lead to reduced LDL clearance, explaining why LDL levels may increase in poorly controlled diabetes and decrease with intensive insulin regimens that achieve near euglycemia (148).

Potentially atherogenic changes in LDL composition have been detected in individuals with diabetes: LDL particles are heterogeneous and differ in lipid composition, density, and size. Different LDL subpopulations may have different atherogenic potential. In normal subjects and in diabetics, two distinct LDL subclass phenotypes, A and B, have been described. Phenotype A is characterized by predominance of large LDL particles, which consist of a major peak of LDL_1 or LDL_2 particles (S_f 6–12 class). The phenotype B consists of a major peak of LDL_3 particles (S_f 3–6) or small dense LDL (149). A predominance of small, dense LDL has been associated with the increased risk of CAD independently of the absolute concentrations of LDL cholesterol (150,151). The mechanism underlying this association is unclear. However, it is possible that small LDL may result in an increased susceptibility to oxidative modification (152) or a lower affinity to the LDL receptor as a result of alterations in the apo B configuration (153).

Although LDL levels may not be significantly elevated in individuals with diabetes, the prevalence of small, dense LDL and the subclass pattern B is higher in individuals with NIDDM (154). Substantial discordance for LDL subclass phenotype B among identical twin pairs indicates that nongenetic factors significantly influence the expression of small, dense LDL and its association with many characteristics of the insulin resistance syndrome (155). In NIDDM the composition of LDL particles is altered, resulting in a preponderance of small, triglyceride-enriched and cholesterol-depleted particles (154,156). Indices of metabolic control do not affect the LDL phenotype pattern (154). However, the presence of small, dense LDL or phenotype B is associated with a lipid profile that includes increased levels of plasma triglycerides, VLDL, and apo B and decreased levels of HDL_2 (149,157,160). A similar lipoprotein profile is associated with insulin resistance (158–160). Moreover, LDL subclass phenotype B is associated with other components of the insulin resistance syndrome, including central obesity, hypertension, glucose intolerance, and hyperinsulinemia (158,160).

Nondiabetic subjects with small, dense LDL (phenotype B) are relatively insulin resistant, glucose intolerant, hyperinsulinemic, hypertensive, and have lower HDL cholesterol concentrations than subjects with LDL phenotype A (160). Thus, LDL subclass phenotype B may be an integral part of the cluster of risk factors that has been termed the insulin resistance syndrome or syndrome X (see Hypertension and Insulin Resistance, below). Hence, whereas LDL cholesterol levels may be relatively normal in NIDDM patients, increased levels of small, dense LDL may contribute to the increased coronary heart disease in normolipidemic patients.

Metabolic abnormalities associated with glycated LDL are also relevant to accelerated atherogenesis in diabetics. Glycosylation enhances uptake of LDL by human aortic intimal cells (161) and monocyte-derived macrophages (162,163), stimulating the formation of foam cells. Glycosylated LDL uptake by endothelial cells and macrophages is probably mediated by a low-affinity, high-capacity surface receptor (called "AGE receptor") and not via the scavenger receptor pathway, which is the usual pathway for heavily modified particles (163–165). Thus, elevation of glucose concentrations may increase the atherogenic potential of LDL particles (166).

Another effect of glycation may be to confer increased susceptibility of LDL to oxidative modification (lipid peroxidation) (167–169). Oxidation of LDL is considered to be a critical step in its atherogenicity (170). This process alters the interaction of LDL with cells, making the LDL a ligand for an alternative, scavenger receptor pathway. This receptor recognizes altered or modified LDL such as oxidized LDL and is able to accumulate cholesterol in an unregulated way. Furthermore, this receptor does not down-regulate de novo synthesis of cholesterol in the cell and is not down-regulated by cellular cholesterol accumulation. Absence of a controlling mechanism accounts for the massive accumulation of cholesterol in the cell, and the transition of the macrophage to a foam cell. Scavenger receptors are active on endothelial cells and macrophages, and oxidatively modified LDL is taken up by monocyte/macrophages more rapidly than native LDL and can therefore generate foam cells. These modifications of LDL may further increase its atherogenic potential in diabetics (171,172). In summary, LDL modified by glycation or oxidation is no longer recognized by the normal LDL receptor but is recognized by the macrophage scavenger receptor or AGE receptor. Unlike the LDL receptor, these receptors do not down-regulate with cellular cholesterol accumulation and thus provide a pathway for the relentless uptake of modified LDL and eventual foam cell formation. In addition, glycosylation and oxidation are closely related and can mutually accelerate each other (173). The combined glycation and oxidation of LDL (glycoxidation) generates a product that is more atherogenic than either glycosylated or oxidized LDL alone (174).

Lipoprotein (a)

Elevated Lp(a) levels have been reported to be associated with an increased risk of coronary heart disease (Scanu and Lawn, *this volume*). A number of studies have examined the possible alterations of Lp(a) in individuals with diabetes. Elevated Lp(a) levels were found in IDDM patients with poor metabolic control and microalbuminuria (175,176). However, in most studies, Lp(a) has failed to show a strong association with vascular complications in IDDM (177,178). Lipoprotein (a) levels are not elevated in NIDDM patients and are not affected by glycemic control (178).

Management of Dyslipidemia in Diabetes

The American Diabetes Association (ADA) recommends an annual fasting measurement of total cholesterol, triglycerides, HDL cholesterol, and calculated LDL cholesterol in all adult diabetic patients (179). If LDL cholesterol or triglyceride levels are elevated, other causes that can affect the lipid profile should be ruled out (e.g., hypothyroidism, nephrotic syndrome, diuretics, β-blockers, estrogen-containing agents). If all values are within acceptable limits, the clinician may consider obtaining this lipid profile less frequently. For triglyceride levels <400 mg/dl, LDL cholesterol is calculated according to the Friedwald formula: LDL = total cholesterol − HDL cholesterol − (triglycerides/5). However, because of altered VLDL composition in individuals with diabetes, the mean differences between calculated (estimated VLDL cholesterol as 20% of total triglyceride) and measured LDL cholesterol concentrations are significantly greater than in control subjects (180). Optimal lipid levels have been proposed by the ADA. These are similar to those recommended by the National Cholesterol Education Program (NCEP) (181) except that the role hypertriglyceridemia may play in the atherosclerotic process in diabetes has been emphasized in the ADA consensus panel recommendations. The ADA consensus development conference on detection

TABLE 3. *American Diabetes Association atherosclerosis risk stratification for diabetic individuals (179)*

Risk for adult diabetic patient	Total cholesterol (mg/dl)	HDL cholesterol (mg/dl)	LDL cholesterol (mg/dl)	Triglycerides (mg/dl)
Acceptable	<200	—	<130	<200
Borderline	200–239	—	130–159	200–399
High	≥240	≤35	≥160	≥400

and management of lipid disorders in diabetes classified patients as shown Table 3.

The NCEP guidelines have specific recommendations for patients with diabetes (see also Farmer and Gotto, *this volume*). The proposed recommendations for premenopausal diabetic women and those for men do not differ because both populations have the same coronary risk. Treatment goals are still based on LDL but advocate a more aggressive treatment for diabetic patients. As a proposed goal, LDL levels in all diabetic individuals should be lowered to <130 mg/dl. In diabetics with established vascular disease, LDL levels should be lowered to <100 mg/dl. Nonpharmacological strategies to treat dyslipidemia and prevent macrovascular complications in diabetes mellitus include dietary modification, weight loss, physical exercise, and improved glycemic control.

Dietary Modifications

Diet is the first therapeutic approach for the management of dyslipidemia as well as hyperglycemia. The diet recommended by the ADA is similar to the diet recommended by the NCEP (Table 4).

Exercise

Regular physical exercise has beneficial effects on glucose levels, insulin sensitivity, and dyslipidemia and complements the diet for weight control (182). To improve glycemic control and insulin sensitivity in patients with NIDDM, exercise is recommended at least 3 days a week for 20 to 45 min at 50% to 70% of maximal oxygen uptake. Before beginning an exercise program, all patients with diabetes should be carefully screened. Patients with IDDM who exercise should be monitored for hyperglycemia, hypoglycemia, ketosis, cardiovascular ischemia, and arrhythmia. Because many patients with NIDDM have preexisting CAD at the time of diabetes diagnosis, all NIDDM patients should be screened for silent ischemia, previously undiagnosed hypertension, neuropathy, retinopathy, and nephropathy before beginning an exercise program.

Glucose Control

In patients with IDDM, intensive insulin therapy is always indicated for the prevention of microvascular disease (21,183). Because the level of glycemic control is the major determinant of lipoprotein levels in IDDM patients, optimal control of plasma glucose should result in normal or below-normal levels of plasma lipids and lipoproteins (184,185). In addition, optimal control should prevent the atherogenic state associated with lipoprotein glycosylation.

TABLE 4. *Dietary guidelines of the American Diabetes Association for the management of dyslipidemia (179)*

1. Caloric restriction to achieve desirable weight.
2. Fat intake <30% of total calories; saturated fat <10%.
3. Cholesterol intake <300 mg/day.
4. Protein intake 0.8 g/kg
5. 50% to 60% of total calories from carbohydrates (preferably complex, unrefined or high in fiber).
6. Alcohol intake limited to <2 equivalents of an alcoholic beverage once or twice a week.

The presence of diabetic nephropathy is a major factor affecting plasma lipoprotein levels in IDDM patients. Patients with diabetic nephropathy tend to have higher levels of plasma triglycerides and LDL cholesterol and lower levels of HDL_2 (185). When significant hyperlipidemia persists in an individual with IDDM and no evidence of diabetic nephropathy, after the achievement of optimal control, the existence of a separately inherited lipid disorder should be suspected.

Unlike IDDM, improved diabetic control in NIDDM may or may not be associated with favorable changes in the lipid profile (186). Improved glycemic control using sulfonylurea (111,187,188) or insulin (111,126) therapy often causes a significant reduction in VLDL triglyceride levels. However, HDL levels frequently will not return to the normal range (126). Despite less than optimal response in lipids, optimal control of plasma glucose levels should be attempted before lipid-lowering agents are added to a patient's therapeutic regimen. However, the physician should not wait too long to initiate concomitant lipid-lowering therapy because the significantly increased risk of macrovascular disease in NIDDM has probably been present for many years before overt diabetes. In addition, "perfect" control of plasma glucose levels is not attained in most NIDDM patients. If 3 to 6 months of nonpharmacological therapy, including dietary modifications, physical exercise, and glycemic control, fails to improve lipid levels, drug therapy is warranted (179).

Drug Therapy

For patients with diabetes and no other CAD risk factors, hygienic measures are followed for 6 months. If LDL or triglyceride levels remain in the high-risk range (LDL $\geq$ 160 mg/dl, triglycerides $\geq$ 400 mg/dl), pharmacological therapy should be considered, with the goal of achieving "acceptable" LDL cholesterol and triglyceride levels (LDL $\leq$ 130 mg/dl, triglycerides $\leq$ 200 mg/dl). For patients with any other risk factors in addition to the diabetes (hypertension, smoking, family history of premature CAD, HDL < 35 mg/dl), drug therapy should be considered even if LDL and triglyceride levels are borderline. Finally, diabetic patients with evidence of macrovascular disease should receive aggressive therapy with treatment goals of LDL $\leq$ 100 mg/dl and triglycerides $\leq$ 150 mg/dl, based on the results of intervention trails in patients without diabetes (179).

Because of the high risk for CAD resulting from NIDDM, some investigators feel that aggressive lowering of LDL cholesterol to less than 100 mg/dl (similar to that recommended for established CAD) should be applied for all of these patients (189). The recent NCEP report has suggested that the stringent goals of therapy recommended for individuals with established CAD (i.e., LDL cholesterol < 100 mg/dl) should also be applied to diabetic patients (181).

Sufficient data are not available for establishing specific target values for raising HDL cholesterol. For low HDL levels the first line of treatment includes increased physical activity, smoking cessation, and weight loss in obesity (181). If drug therapy is needed to lower LDL or triglyceride levels in a patient who also has a low HDL, agents that raise HDL should be considered. Nicotinic acid is more efficacious in increasing HDL levels than fibric acid drugs and HMG-CoA reductase inhibitors, which in turn have similar efficacies (190).

Nicotinic Acid

Nicotinic acid (niacin) is a powerful lipid-lowering agent that reduces the hepatic production of VLDL, which results in a significant reduction of triglycerides and LDL cholesterol. It also increases HDL cholesterol significantly, primarily the HDL_2 fraction. Hence, nicotinic acid exerts favorable effects on plasma concentration of all lipoproteins. Because it is the most inexpensive of all hypolipidemic drugs, nicotinic acid is recommended by the NCEP as first-line therapy for hypertriglyceridemia. Modest doses of nicotinic acid (1 to 3 g/day) produce near-maximal increments in HDL, but larger doses are required for optimal reductions of triglyceride and LDL (190). Unfortunately, although nicotinic acid is effective in diabetics, it frequently causes a deterioration in glycemic control. In one study of patients with NIDDM, a niacin dose of 4.5 g/day reduced plasma cholesterol levels by 24% and triglyceride levels by 45% and raised HDL cholesterol by 34%. However, the glycosylated hemoglobin level increased by 21% (191). The mechanism of the adverse effect of nicotinic acid on glucose metabolism appears to be the induction of insulin resistance (192), which may have particularly undesirable effects in NIDDM patients. Thus, the use of nicotinic acid in any form as first line therapy in dyslipidemic diabetic patients is not recommended. These agents should be reserved for selected patients with refractory dyslipidemias, and only after careful consideration and follow-up evaluation (179). The inability to maintain acceptable glycemic control mandates a discontinuation of this agent.

Fibric Acid Derivatives

The fibric acid derivatives were studied extensively in patients with diabetic dyslipidemia. They lower triglyceride levels by 20% to 50%, elevate HDL cholesterol by 10% to 25%, and have a variable effect of HDL cholesterol levels (193,194). The full effect on lipid levels may require a minimum of 3 to 6 months.

The effect on LDL cholesterol is variable. In patients with normal triglyceride levels, these drugs lower LDL cholesterol by 5% to 15%. However, in hypertriglyceridemic patients, the fall in triglyceride levels is frequently accompanied by an increase in LDL cholesterol levels (194). This increase probably reflects the elimination of small, dense LDL particles characteristic of the hypertriglyceridemic patients, resulting in a less atherogenic LDL cholesterol (195,196). Thus, the adverse LDL particle composition in diabetes can be reversed with fibric acid derivatives.

Gemfibrozil has been used effectively as primary prevention for CAD in the Helsinki Heart Study, in which 135 diabetic men were included. The greatest benefit in CAD reduction was noted in patients with mixed dyslipidemias, including high triglycerides, high LDL cholesterol, and low HDL cholesterol (197). The incidence of cardiovascular events was also lower in patients with NIDDM in the gemfibrozil-treated group. However, because of small number of events, this difference did not reach statistical significance (199). These drugs do not adversely affect glucose metabolism (198,199). Because of these effects, fibric acid derivatives appear to be appropriate treatment for the common lipoprotein abnormalities in diabetics and are probably the drugs of choice for the treatment of hypertriglyceridemia in these patients. Fibric acid derivatives increase the risk for cholesterol gallstones. Because patients with NIDDM are already predisposed to cholelithiasis, this may be a disadvantage.

Bile-Acid-Binding Resin

Cholestyramine is efficacious in decreasing LDL cholesterol levels in patients with NIDDM. In one study, LDL cholesterol levels decreased by an average of 28% with cholestyramine therapy (200). Bile acid resins can increase VLDL triglycerides significantly, particularly if they are already elevated above 250 to 300 mg/dl. Extreme elevations in triglyceride level occur mainly in patients who already had marked hypertriglyceridemia and, in some cases, poorly controlled diabetes. This tendency to increase serum triglyceride levels makes these agents unsuitable as first-line therapy in many diabetic patients who are already significantly hypertriglyceridemic (plasma triglyceride level > 250 to 300 mg/dl) and for those in poor glycemic control.

These agents can be useful in cases of mixed dyslipidemias consisting of both LDL cholesterol and VLDL triglyceride elevations. In such cases, bile acid resins can be used in small doses, particularly in combination with fibric acid derivatives (179). In addition, these agents are the only drug therapy recommended for children and adolescents (185). Because constipation is the major side effect of resin therapy, bile acids resins should be used with great care in patients with diabetic autonomic neuropathy.

HMG-CoA Reductase Inhibitors

HMG-CoA reductase inhibitors are highly effective in lowering cholesterol levels in NIDDM patients in whom the principal finding is elevated LDL cholesterol levels and do not adversely affect glycemic control (201). Usually these drugs do not change the composition of VLDL or LDL particles. They can be recommended for diabetics with high LDL cholesterol concentrations and normal or mildly elevated triglycerides. The HMG-CoA reductase inhibitors reduce the lithogenicity of bile and thus can be advantageous in diabetics with autonomic neuropathy and impaired gallbladder motility causing a predisposition to cholesterol gallstones. The risk of drug-induced myopathy is particularly high in patients with moderately severe renal failure or those concomitantly taking cyclosporine, gemfibrozil, or nicotinic acid. Patients should be instructed to report any muscle pain, tenderness, or weakness and should be monitored with serial measurements of creatine phosphokinase and liver function. A theoretical possibility exists that prolonged therapy with HMG-CoA reductase inhibitors may increase the risk for cataract development in diabetic patients who are already predisposed to cataract formation.

HYPERTENSION AND INSULIN RESISTANCE

Hypertension occurs about twice as frequently in patients with diabetes as in the general population (202,203). An estimated 3 million Americans have both diabetes and hypertension (204). Up to 50% of diabetic patients ultimately become hypertensive. Likewise, patients with essential hypertension are prone to develop NIDDM (205). The prevalence of coexistent hypertension and diabetes is almost twice as great among African-Americans as among whites and is three times greater among Mexican-Americans than among non-Hispanic whites (204). Isolated systolic hypertension is considerably more common in diabetics. Supine hypertension with orthostatic hypotension sometimes occurs in patients with autonomic neuropathy.

The combined presence of hypertension and diabetes considerably accelerates the development of both macrovascular and microvascular diabetic complications. Diabetic individuals with coexisting hypertension have a greater prevalence of ischemic heart disease, stroke, and peripheral vascular disease (202–204). Hypertension also accelerates the progression of diabetic nephropathy (206,216) and diabetic retinopathy (207), which are the leading causes of renal replacement therapy and newly diagnosed blindness in the United States, respectively. However, the most significant manifestation of this combination of diseases is that they confer a greater risk of macrovascular disease in affected individuals.

The time course and natural history of hypertension differ markedly between patients with IDDM and those with NIDDM. The prevalence of hypertension associated with IDDM patients without microalbuminuria is comparable to that of nondiabetic individuals of the same age and sex (208,209). Blood pressure is usually normal at presentation and remains so in nearly all long-term survivors with IDDM who have not developed diabetic nephropathy (210). In the majority of IDDM patients, the onset of hypertension typically occurs during the stage of incipient diabetic nephropathy, as defined by the presence of microalbuminuria (urinary albumin excretion rate of 20–200 μg/min) (211–213). Blood pressure increases gradually, often within the normal range, during the microalbuminuria stage and continues to rise progressively with the development of macroalbuminuria and clinically overt nephropathy (214,215). Hypertension is present in many patients with overt diabetic nephropathy and markedly accelerates the progression of the disease (206,216).

In contrast to IDDM, patients with newly diagnosed NIDDM are frequently hypertensive at the time of diagnosis (202,203,217,218). The excess prevalence of hypertension also occurs in individuals with impaired glucose tolerance and insulin resistance that precedes the development of overt NIDDM. The association between essential hypertension and NIDDM is independent of age, obesity, and renal function (219,220). However, there is a progressive increase in blood pressure with age and with increasing degree of obesity. Isolated systolic hypertension is particularly common in NIDDM and is generally attributed to the loss of elastic compliance in large arteries. In patients with NIDDM the risk of cardiovascular disease is doubled in the presence of hypertension (221).

In NIDDM hypertension usually occurs in association with a cluster of metabolic and cardiovascular features. Epidemiologic data and clinical experience indicate a striking degree of overlap among NIDDM, essential hypertension, and obesity. Analysis of data from the 2,930 participants of the San Antonio Heart Study suggests that by the fifth decade, 85% of diabetics are hypertensive and obese, and 80% of obese subjects have abnormal glucose tolerance and are hypertensive (222). Many of these patients also have dyslipidemia, including high serum VLDL triglyceride levels, low serum HDL, higher proportion of small, dense LDL particles, and possibly impaired fibrinolysis (Table 5). This congregation of cardiovascular risk factors is frequently found in patients with NIDDM.

Several studies have demonstrated a positive correlation between blood pressure and plasma insulin levels or the degree of insulin resistance in obese and lean hypertensive subjects (224,231). It has been proposed that either the insu-

TABLE 5. *The cardiovascular risk factors cluster associated with insulin resistance*

Hyperinsulinemia
Impaired glucose tolerance
Diabetes mellitus
Hypertension
Abdominal obesity
Dyslipidemia
Increased VLDL—triglyceride
Decreased HDL_2
Small, dense atherogenic LDL particles
Elevated PAI-1 activity

TABLE 6. *Quantitative changes of lipoproteins in IDDM*

Lipoprotein	Conventional therapy	Intensive therapy
VLDL	Normal or increased (markedly increased in ketoacidosis)	Decreased
LDL cholesterol	Normal or increased	Normal or decreased
HDL cholesterol	Normal	Increased

lin resistance itself or the accompanying compensatory hyperinsulinemia are the linking pathophysiological mechanisms among glucose intolerance, obesity, hypertension, dyslipidemia, and macrovascular disease. Insulin resistance is characteristic not only of the obese and diabetic state. Essential hypertension, in contrast to secondary forms of hypertension (223), is also an insulin resistance state associated with hyperinsulinemia and glucose intolerance in both obese and nonobese individuals (205,224,225). Insulin resistance is also associated with an abnormal lipoprotein pattern including higher triglycerides and lower HDL levels (Tables 6,7) (225–227). Increasing evidence for the association among insulin resistance, hypertension, dyslipidemia, and CAD led to the description of the insulin resistance syndrome or "syndrome X" in nonobese subjects (205). All of the elements of syndrome X can be seen in obese individuals, although, as previously indicated, they have long been recognized to coexist with obesity.

It is now recognized that insulin resistance is also associated with an increased proportion of small, dense LDL particles (158,160). In contrast, nongenetic, polygenic, and environmental hypercholesterolemia (type IIa) are associated with increased concentrations of large, buoyant LDL particles and are not accompanied by insulin resistance (228,229). The characteristic hyperlipidemia associated with insulin resistance is associated with marked increase in CAD risk (see Lipoprotein Disorders in Diabetes, above). Insulin resistance appears to be related to the regional distribution of body fat, specifically to visceral abdominal obesity rather than subcutaneous or lower body obesity (see Obesity and Atherosclerosis, below) (230). There is evidence that high PAI-1 activity is associated with insulin resistance and compensatory hyperinsulinemia (see Altered Fibrinolysis in Diabetes, below). This abnormality in the fibrinolytic system has recently been added to the cluster of abnormalities comprising syndrome X.

TABLE 7. *Quantitative changes of lipoproteins in NIDDM*

Lipoprotein	Poor control	Good control
VLDL	Markedly increased	Normal or increased
LDL cholesterol	Normal	Normal
HDL cholesterol	Decreased	Normal or decreased

Data both supporting and refuting the association between hyperinsulinemia and hypertension have been reported (231–233). Although the association between hypertension and insulin resistance appears to be widespread, the magnitude of the association may vary according to gender, ethnicity and age (232,234). A strong association between insulin and blood pressure has been documented among some (224,231) but not all Caucasian populations (233). Conversely, studies in Pima Indians (235), African-Americans (232), Pacific Island populations (236), Indians, Creoles and Chinese Mauritians (237) have shown either no correlation or a weak relationship between blood pressure and plasma insulin concentrations. Moreover, in Pima Indians and Mexican-Americans, insulin resistance and hyperinsulinemia are common, but hypertension is rare (232,235). Hence, hyperinsulinemia is not consistently associated with hypertension, indicating that differences in the sensitivity to the postulated effects of insulin among different individuals or ethnic groups determine the interaction among hyperinsulinemia, insulin resistance, and blood pressure.

Pathogenesis of Hypertension in Hyperinsulinemic States

Obesity, NIDDM, and hypertension are insulin resistance states that frequently occur in the same individual. There are several putative mechanisms by which insulin resistance and compensatory hyperinsulinemia could contribute to the pathogenesis of hypertension. These include increased renal sodium retention, stimulation of sympathetic activity, effects on membrane ion-transport systems, and proliferative effects on vascular smooth muscle cells (Fig. 1).

Role of Sodium

Sodium is thought to play an important role in the hypertension associated with diabetes. Even in the absence of renal disease, sodium handling is abnormal in diabetics. The total body exchangeable sodium pool is increased by approximately 10% in diabetic patients compared to nondiabetic subjects. This abnormality has been consistently demonstrated in IDDM and NIDDM patients even with good metabolic control and no complications of diabetes (238,239). The excess in body sodium is also common in normotensive diabetics. In addition, blood pressure in diabetics is salt sensitive (240,241) and tends to correlate positively with exchangeable sodium (239). Removal of excess sodium with a diuretic can effectively improve high blood pressure in diabetes. The fact that an increased pool of total exchangeable sodium occurs both in hypertensive and nonhypertensive individuals suggests differences in cardiovascular sensitivity. Thus, changing from a low- to high-sodium diet increases blood pressure in hypertensive but not in normotensive diabetics (240).

Several factors may contribute to the sodium retention in diabetes. Insulin has a direct stimulatory effect on renal tubu-

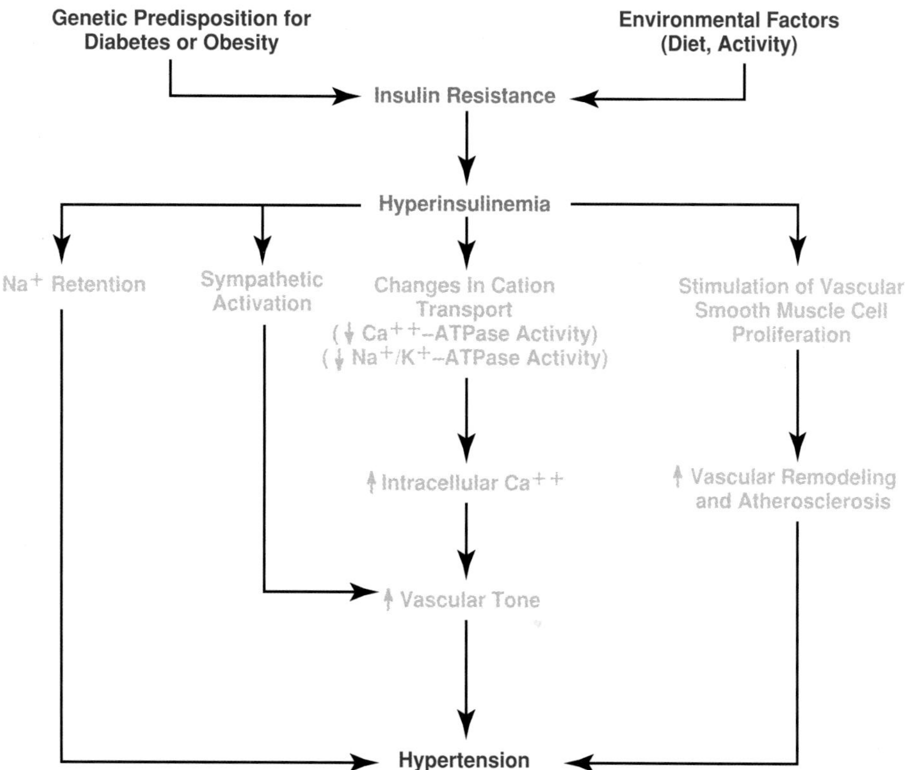

FIG. 1. Mechanisms of hypertension in insulin resistance.

lar sodium reabsorption. The exact tubular site of the insulin antinatriuretic action is controversial, and evidence exists that insulin acts on both the proximal and distal convoluted tubules as well as the loop of Henle (242). Thus, the expansion of total exchangeable sodium in diabetics can be the result of a sodium-retaining action of chronic hyperinsulinemia in NIDDM patients. This postulate assumes the presence of a differential insulin resistance; i.e., there may be resistance to the action of insulin for glucose disposal in muscle while sensitivity to its antinatriuretic effect is maintained.

Increased glomerular filtration of glucose is another mechanism that may contribute to the renal antidiuresis and volume expansion. The increase in the filtered load of glucose can lead to enhanced proximal tubular sodium reabsorption via the glucose–sodium cotransporter, which becomes active in the presence of glycosuria (243). Hence, moderate increases in blood glucose concentrations will cause enhanced reabsorption of sodium salts, resulting in sodium retention (202,238).

Activity of the Sympathetic System

Insulin administered exogenously (247) or stimulated by nutrient ingestion increases sympathetic nervous system activity. The sympathetic actions of insulin have been attributed to its effect on the medial hypothalamus (246). Insulin infusion in humans while euglycemia is maintained raises plasma norepinephrine levels (244,247), and direct recording of sympathetic nervous system activity with microneurography indicates a direct stimulatory effect of insulin at both physiological and supraphysiological levels (245,247). This increase in sympathetic nervous system activity can augment cardiac contractility and cause vasoconstriction in peripheral arterioles with subsequent development of hypertension. Whether this increase persists in the presence of chronic hyperinsulinemia is unclear.

On the other hand, insulin also has an acute vasodilator effect that tends to lower blood pressure (246). In healthy human volunteers, acute insulin infusion produces a decrease in peripheral vascular resistance despite increased sympathetic nerve activity, with a slight drop in diastolic blood pressure (247,248). Hence, insulin fails to increase arterial blood pressure because the sympathetic vasoconstrictor activation is opposed by vasodilation (245). Even long-term hyperinsulinemia associated with insulinoma does not result in elevated blood pressure, and blood pressure does not fall in these patients after tumor resection (249–252). However, the vasodilator effect of insulin does not necessarily negate its possible contribution to the pathogenesis of hypertension. Although under normal conditions the sympathomimetic effect of insulin is balanced by its vasodilator action, the latter effect can be blunted in the presence of insulin resistance (253,254). Therefore, the pressor action of hyperinsulinemia could depend critically on the presence of insulin resistance, a predisposition to hypertension, or both, which can tip the balance between the pressor and depressor actions of insulin in favor of hypertensive actions.

Modulation of Cation Transport

Increased peripheral vascular resistance and enhanced smooth muscle contractile response to agonists are characteristic of hypertension in diabetes (202). The sensitivity of blood pressure responses to pressor hormones such as angiotensin II and norepinephrine is already enhanced in the early, uncomplicated stages of diabetes (239,255). Vascular hyperactivity occurs in patients with both IDDM and NIDDM and in the presence or absence of hypertension. The increased peripheral resistance and vascular reactivity may be related to changes in insulin-mediated Ca^{2+} transport. Increased intracellular calcium is a common finding in both IDDM and NIDDM as well as in obesity and essential hypertension (256). It has been suggested that abnormal cellular calcium homeostasis links insulin resistance and hypertension. Evidence that insulin can regulate vascular smooth muscle contractility by changing intracellular ionized calcium levels comes from a number of observations, including a strong correlation between the level of blood pressure and intracellular ionized calcium levels in hypertensive subjects (257,258). Several abnormalities in cation transport may explain these observations.

Many cell membrane transport systems are influenced by insulin. Insulin affects cation homeostasis through its stimulatory effects on Ca^{2+}-ATPase, Na^+,K^+-ATPase, and the Na^+–H^+ exchanger. The first two ATPase-related cation pumps are essential for maintaining low physiological levels of intracellular calcium. The Ca^{2+}-ATPase is an enzyme that extrudes calcium from cells and is also stimulated by insulin in heart, kidney, liver, and adipocytes (259). Thus, decreased insulin activity caused by insulin resistance can result in decreased Ca^{2+}-ATPase activity, raising intracellular ionized calcium. Decreased activity of erythrocyte membrane Ca^{2+}-ATPase has been observed in NIDDM patients (260). A similar reduction in Ca^{2+}-ATPase activity in vascular smooth muscle of diabetics might provide the basis by which insulin resistance can lead to increased peripheral resistance and hypertension. Because elevated intracellular calcium levels in vascular smooth muscle cells play a key role in establishing and maintaining a state of enhanced vascular resistance, insulin resistance at the level of vascular smooth muscle tissue may lead directly to increased intracellular ionized calcium with activation of smooth muscle contraction and increased peripheral vascular resistance (261). This mechanism can also explain the exaggerated agonist responses, because changes in intracellular ionized calcium are strongly linked to pressor-induced contraction in vascular smooth muscle cells.

The Na^+,K^+-ATPase affects intracellular calcium levels by changing the level of intracellular sodium and thus modulating the Na^+–Ca^{2+} exchanger, which also extrudes calcium out of the cell. This enzyme is also activated by insulin. The effect of insulin on the Na^+,K^+-ATPase is mediated by increasing the affinity of the inwardly facing Na^+-loading site of the membrane-bound Na^+,K^+-ATPase and is obligatorily coupled with increased Na^+ efflux (242). In the absence of insulin, or in the absence of adequate insulin action because of insulin resistance, cells would not be able to extrude Na^+, resulting in inappropriate accumulation of sodium. Indeed, various clinical settings characterized by insulin resistance (glucose intolerance, obesity, hypertension, and their combinations) are associated with reduced Na^+,K^+-ATPase and high intracellular sodium (231,262,263). In IDDM patients, RBC Na^+,K^+-ATPase activity is related to the degree of glycemic control. In such insulinopenic patients, RBC Na^+,K^+-ATPase activity is stimulated by administration of insulin (264). The accumulation of intracellular sodium increases Na^+–Ca^{2+} exchange, resulting in increased intracellular calcium (265). When this coexists with the decreased membrane Ca^{2+}-ATPase activity noted previously, a significant increase in intracellular calcium may ensue. Thus, insulin resistance at the level of vascular smooth muscle tissue could interfere with the normal activity of the Ca^{2+}-ATPase and Na^+,K^+-ATPase pumps, resulting in increased intracellular ionized calcium and increased vascular tone.

Finally, insulin is known to stimulate the activity of the Na^+–H^+ exchanger, which exchanges intracellular H^+ for extracellular Na^+. This ubiquitous transport system is involved in the control of intracellular pH and sodium concentration and of cell growth and proliferation and in proximal renal tubular sodium reabsorption. Thus, if the Na^+–H^+ exchanger retains normal sensitivity to insulin, overactivity of this system as a result of hyperinsulinemia could lead to hypertension through several mechanisms (266). As discussed above, increased intracellular Na^+ is associated with increased intracellular calcium and would be expected to increase vascular tone and to enhance the sensitivity of the vascular smooth muscle cells to the pressor effects of norepinephrine and angiotensin II. The alkalization of the cytoplasm stimulates cellular growth (267), leading to smooth muscle proliferation in the walls of resistance vessels and increased vascular resistance. Overactivity of this system in the renal tubule causes sodium retention.

Several clinical findings support the role of the Na^+–H^+ exchanger in the pathogenesis of hypertension. Increased erythrocyte Na^+–H^+ exchanger activity has been demonstrated in hypertensive individuals (268). The Na^+–H^+ exchanger is the only known genetic marker for essential hypertension (269). Considerable experimental evidence suggests that red cell Li^+–Na^+ exchanger is a functional mode of the red cell Na^{+-H+} exchanger. The RBC Li^+–Na^+ activity is strongly correlated with a heritable predisposition to hypertension as well as to diabetic nephropathy in IDDM patients (see Coronary Artery Disease, above).

Direct Action of Insulin on Arteries

There is evidence that insulin itself may be a risk factor for cardiovascular disease by acting directly as a growth factor or indirectly through stimulation of other growth factors. Insulin can induce proliferation of components of arterial walls to initiate or aggravate macrovascular disease and, if arterioles are affected, could also result in hypertension. Long-term treatment with insulin results in lipid-containing lesions and arterial wall thickening in experimental animals (270). Chronic insulin infusion into one femoral artery of a dog resulted in marked intimal and medial proliferation and the accumulation of cholesterol and fatty acids on the insulin-infused side but not on the contralateral side (271). Receptors for insulin and insulin-like growth factor I (IGF-I) have been identified in blood vessels. Physiological concentrations of insulin stimulate proliferation of cultured smooth muscle cells and fibroblasts (270,272,273). There is evidence that this effect is produced through stimulating IGF-I rather than insulin receptors (274). Similarities of the β-subunit of the insulin receptor to that of the IGF-I receptor enable insulin to stimulate IGF-I receptors. Thus, in the presence of insulin resistance, where the metabolic action of insulin is ineffective, the proliferative response may still occur. Insulin also stimulates cholesterol synthesis and LDL binding in arterial smooth muscle cells and monocyte/macrophages (270).

In summary, although hyperinsulinemia, insulin resistance, and blood pressure may be correlated in some individuals, a cause-and-effect relationship among these variables has not been clearly established. Insulin has been shown in acute studies to have multiple effects on the kidney, sympathetic nervous system, and cardiovascular system that, if sustained, could lead to hypertension. However, it is still uncertain whether the acute effects of insulin can be sustained sufficiently to influence long-term blood pressure regulation. Data regarding the effect of chronic, exogenous hyperinsulinemia on blood pressures are controversial. Hypertension can be induced with chronic administration of insulin in rats (275). Conversely, insulin failed to increase blood pressure in dogs (276). In humans, there have been no reported studies on the long-term renal and cardiovascular responses to insulin infusions. The few long-term studies that have been conducted in animals and the chronic hyperinsulinemia associated with insulinomas do not support the concept that hyperinsulinemia is a major cause of hypertension (277).

Treatment

In view of the adverse effects of hypertension on diabetic macrovascular and microvascular complications, its early diagnosis and effective treatment should have a major impact on morbidity and mortality. Although no randomized clinical trial has tested the effect of antihypertensive therapy on cardiovascular risk in diabetes, by extrapolation from essential and isolated systolic hypertension, aggressive treatment of hypertension in diabetic patients is indicated.

Life-Style Modifications

Life-style modifications include weight management, nutritional modifications, increased physical activity, moderation of alcohol ingestion, and smoking cessation. Obesity is a major contributor to hypertension associated with NIDDM. Because of the strong association among obesity, hypertension, insulin resistance, and dyslipidemia, of all life-style modifications, weight reduction has been shown most clearly to be effective in lowering blood pressure (278). Even a modest reduction in body weight can improve blood pressure and glycemic control. Reduction in weight results in blood pressure reductions through several mechanisms including decreased insulin levels, decreased sympathetic nervous system activity, and correction of cellular cation metabolism, which lead to a fall in vascular resistance (204,278). As discussed previously, sodium retention is present in hypertensive diabetics. Therefore, a moderate restriction of salt intake to a level of less than 100 mmol/day (2.3 g sodium or 6 g sodium chloride) should be recommended (278,279).

Pharmacotherapy

The American Working Group on Hypertension in Diabetes suggests that diabetic patients with blood pressure of 140/90 or above should be considered for pharmacological therapy if a 3-month trial period of nonpharmacological treatment of mild hypertension is not effective in lowering blood pressure. The treatment goal for patients with diabetes is to maintain blood pressure at less than 130/85 (204). Antihypertensive therapy should not worsen glucose control, lipid levels, or concomitant disorders such as peripheral vascular disease or gout.

Isolated systolic hypertension is defined as a systolic blood pressure >140 mm Hg with a diastolic blood pressure <90 mm Hg. The initial goal of therapy is to reduce systolic blood pressure to <160 mm Hg for those with systolic blood pressure ≥180 mm Hg and to lower blood pressure by 20 mm Hg for those with systolic blood pressure between 160 and 179 mm Hg. At isolated systolic blood pressure levels of 140 to 160 mm Hg, life-style modifications may be adjunctive or definitive therapy (203).

Although the general approach to the pharmacological treatment of patients with diabetes and hypertension is similar to that used in hypertensive patients without diabetes, the choice of treatment must rely on data derived from current understanding of the pathophysiology of hypertension in diabetes. In addition, the accompanying insulin resistance and the increased likelihood of dyslipidemia, renal disease, and autonomic neuropathy complicates the decision-making process regarding the selection of pharmacological agents for the management of hypertension in the diabetic patient

TABLE 8. *Drug therapy in hypertensive diabetics*

Drug class	Glucose tolerance	Lipid profile	Other considerations
ACE inhibitors	Increased	Unchanged	Improved insulin sensitivity Reduced intraglomerular pressure
Calcium antagonists	Unchanged	Unchanged	
Thiazide diuretics	Decreased	Increased LDL cholesterol Increased triglycerides Decreased HDL	
β—Blockers (selective)	Decreased	Increased triglycerides Decreased HDL	Masking of hypoglycemic symptoms Delayed recovery from hypoglycemia Severe catecholamine-induced hypertension during hypoglycemic episodes Claudication may be worsened Effective in CAD
α_1—Blockers	Increased	Decreased LDL Increased HDL	Improved insulin sensitivity

(Table 8). Antihypertensive drugs can adversely affect glycemic control or lipid metabolism and potentially alter the efficacy of pharmacological therapy. Autonomic dysfunction is common in diabetics and predisposes them to postural hypotension. These patients may have supine hypertension. In this case, short-acting vasodilators (i.e., angiotensin-converting enzyme inhibitors or calcium antagonists) can be taken shortly before bedtime to reduce nocturnal supine pressures.

Controlling systemic blood pressure is the single most important factor that has been shown to retard the progression of diabetic nephropathy (280,281). However, the induction of normal intraglomerular pressure offers greater protection against glomerular injury. Angiotensin-converting enzyme (ACE) inhibition has the additional benefit of lowering the increased glomerular capillary pressure to normal by eliminating the constricting effect of angiotensin II on efferent arteriolar resistance (282–284). Clinical trials have shown that ACE inhibitors retard the progression from incipient to clinical nephropathy and decrease the rate of progression of overt diabetic nephropathy (284–286). Thus, in the presence of renal disease, ACE inhibitors are probably the antihypertensive therapy of choice (203).

The ideal antihypertensive agent should not have adverse effects on glucose and lipoprotein metabolism and should have a beneficial effect on the complications of diabetes in addition to its antihypertensive effects. Currently, there is no consensus on the initial drug therapy for hypertension in diabetics in the absence of nephropathy. The five major classes of drugs that are generally effective for single-agent therapy are discussed below.

Angiotensin-Converting Enzyme Inhibitors

The ACE inhibitors are effective in diabetics despite the fact that plasma renin activity and serum angiotensin concentrations tend to be low in hypertensive diabetics (287). These drugs are becoming the primary agents of choice for the treatment of hypertension associated with diabetes mellitus because they do not adversely affect the glycemic control and lipid profile (287). In fact, ACE inhibitors may actually enhance insulin sensitivity in NIDDM patients with or without hypertension (288–291). As discussed above, ACE inhibitors are especially desirable in patients with evidence of diabetic nephropathy. A rapid decline in renal function can occur in patients with bilateral renal artery stenosis, which is more common in diabetics. Hyporeninemic hypoaldosteronism is frequently associated with diabetes and predisposes the patients to clinically significant hyperkalemia when ACE inhibitors are initiated.

Calcium Channel Blockers

As noted above, abnormalities in cellular calcium metabolism have been identified in both diabetes and essential hypertension. Based on the previous discussion on the disturbances of cellular calcium metabolism in diabetes and hypertension, there is a rationale for the use of calcium channel blockers in hypertensive diabetics. Indeed, calcium channel antagonists have been shown to reduce blood pressure and restore pressor hyperresponsiveness to normal in diabetic patients. These drugs do not have an adverse effect on glycemic control, lipid metabolism, or renal function (203,204,287). However they have the potential to induce postural hypotension.

α_1-Blockers

α_1-Receptor-blocking agents, particularly those that have a 24-h duration of action (e.g., doxazosin), are effective antihypertensive agents in patients with hypertension and diabetes (204,287). Several studies suggest that these agents may improve insulin resistance (288,292–294) and lipid metabolism (292,295). Specifically, α_1-blockers lower LDL cholesterol and triglycerides and increase HDL cholesterol. These agents should be used with caution because they may cause persistent postural hypotension in diabetics.

Thiazides

Thiazides are often effective antihypertensive agents in diabetes, in which the total body sodium is increased and the extracellular volume is expanded (239). However, these agents can impair glucose tolerance and worsen preexisting insulin resistance (296). Mechanisms that contribute to impaired glucose tolerance include decreased insulin secretion as a result of hypokalemia, decreased insulin sensitivity, and increased hepatic glucose production (297,299). In addition, the lipid profile is adversely affected, with increases in LDL cholesterol and total triglyceride levels and a decrease in HDL levels. The negative metabolic effects of thiazides are dose dependent, and at low doses (i.e., 12.5 to 25 mg or less hydrochlorothiazide), adverse effects on carbohydrate metabolism are uncommon (204,298). Correction of hypokalemia by replacement with potassium salts or concomitant use of potassium-sparing diuretics can prevent the deterioration in glucose tolerance and may restore insulin sensitivity (299). Because insulin resistance, hyperinsulinemia, and dyslipidemia represent major cardiovascular risk factors, these drugs should not be used as first-line agents in the treatment of hypertensive diabetics unless sodium retention is clinically manifested by edema. Once the GFR is substantially reduced (GFR < 30 ml/min), loop diuretics are superior agents. This is a common problem in patients with diabetes and hypertension. In this setting, in which an increased total-body sodium content exists, loop diuretics may be a reasonable choice as antihypertensive agents, especially because other metabolic side effects may not be as prominent as those of the thiazides (287).

β-Blockers

These agents lower the blood pressure mainly by reducing cardiac output and thus do not specifically impact on the underlying mechanisms thought to be important in diabetic hypertension. Several other concerns limit the usefulness of β-blockers in treating patients with diabetes. Like thiazides, β-blockers may aggravate both hyperglycemia and hyperlipidemia. β-Blockers inhibit insulin release, especially when nonselective agents are used (299), and increase insulin resistance and hyperinsulinemia (300). These agents also tend to increase the level of triglycerides and decrease that of HDL cholesterol because of their action to decrease LPL and LACT activity (301). β-Blockers also interfere with the counterregulatory response to catecholamine secretion during hypoglycemia, blunting perception of anxiety, tachycardia, and tremor and delaying recovery from hypoglycemia. However, this is rarely a serious clinical problem, especially when cardioselective β_1-blockers are used. β-Blockers may alter the hemodynamic response to hypoglycemia, resulting in severe hypertension (302). Epinephrine release in response to hypoglycemia normally raises the systolic blood pressure. β-Blockade can result in unopposed α-mediated vasoconstriction and severe hypertensive episodes.

PROPENSITY TO THROMBOSIS

The coagulation and fibrinolytic systems are especially important in atherosclerosis because of the substantial contribution that mural thrombosis may make to the later stages of plaque progression and because thrombotic occlusion plays a vital role in the development of clinical events (303). Diabetes is characterized by a series of alterations in the coagulation and fibrinolytic systems, resulting in a state of thrombophilia. These alterations include increased platelet aggregation, increased levels of coagulation factors, and impaired fibrinolysis (Table 9).

Alterations in Coagulation Factors

Elevated levels of factors VII, IX, X, and XII have been found in diabetes (304). The plasma levels of certain coagulation factors are under acute control of plasma glucose or insulin levels. In nondiabetic individuals, plasma levels of factor VII rise during glucose infusion and return to normal when the infusion is discontinued. In diabetic patients the elevated factor VII levels fall with improved glycemic control (304).

A decrease in the biological activity of antithrombin III (AT-III) occurs in diabetes in the presence of normal antigenic concentrations as a result of nonenzymatic glycosylation of the lysine residue that binds the AT-III to its natural cofactor, heparin (305). Improved glycemic control can restore the normal activity of this molecule. The concentrations and activity of protein C, another important coagulation inhibitor, are decreased in diabetics and rise in response to insulin-induced normoglycemia (306).

Von Willebrand Factor

Plasma concentrations of von Willebrand factor (vWF) are elevated in diabetic patients with or without vascular complications (307,308). The vWF is produced in the endo-

TABLE 9. *Procoagulant state in diabetes*

Increased levles of clotting factors
Decreased coagulation inhibitors
Decreased AT-III activity
Decreased protein C
Platelet function
Increased platelet aggregability
Increased platelet adhesiveness
Increased thromboxane A_2 formation
Impaired fibrinolytic activity
Increased concentrations of PAI-1
Glycosylation of plasminogen

thelium and megakaryocytes and is involved in platelet adherence to the subendothelium. Thus, its increased concentration may contribute to increased platelet adhesion in diabetes (322).

Fibrinogen

Epidemiologic studies have demonstrated a strong and often independent direct correlation between high fibrinogen plasma levels and an increased risk of ischemic heart disease (309). A similar association has been demonstrated in diabetics (310). Fibrinogen levels are often increased in uncontrolled diabetes (311). Levels correlate with glycemic control and fall with intensive insulin therapy (312).

Altered Fibrinolysis in Diabetes

The intensity of endogenous fibrinolysis depends on competing processes in dynamic equilibrium involving circulating activators of plasminogen, primarily tissue-type plasminogen activator (t-PA) and its principal physiological inhibitor, plasminogen activator inhibitor type 1 (PAI-1). Reduced plasma fibrinolytic activity may shift the balance between thrombosis and fibrinolysis toward thrombosis. Such an imbalance creates increased exposure of luminal surfaces of vessel walls to clot-associated mitogens that can potentiate the migration and proliferation of vascular smooth muscle cells, chemotaxis and activation of macrophages, and consequently, accelerated atherosclerosis. Attenuated fibrinolysis as a result of increased of PAI-1 activity is a risk factor for premature coronary artery disease and acute myocardial infarction (313,314).

Fibrinolytic activity is decreased in IDDM and NIDDM patients without coronary artery disease in the presence of a normal or increased t-PA antigen levels and increased PAI-1 activity. Although plasma concentrations of t-PA antigen are normal or elevated, t-PA is biologically inactive because it is bound to its inhibitor (315). The decreased fibrinolytic activity is secondary to increased PAI-1 activity, which often occurs in the presence of insulin resistance and hyperinsulinemia (316,317).

Impaired fibrinolysis may be an important biological link between hyperinsulinemia and atherosclerosis in NIDDM. Elevated concentrations of PAI-1 have been recognized consistently in the plasma of patients with hyperinsulinemia (315–319). In vitro studies have elucidated the mechanism by which insulin could regulate plasma PAI-1 activity. The PAI-1 is synthesized by endothelial cells and hepatocytes. Insulin stimulates PAI-1 production by the hepatoma cell line Hep G2 and in cultures of human hepatocytes. In addition, the increase in PAI-1 in hyperinsulinemic NIDDM patients may be attributable, in part, to the effect of precursors of insulin such as proinsulin on PAI-1 synthesis (313). Improved glycemic control normalizes both t-PA and plasmin levels.

Platelets

Platelets from diabetic subjects exhibit an enhanced adhesiveness, hyperaggregability to various agonists, such as ADP, collagen, and arachidonic acid, as well as increased generation of thromboxane (320). Platelet hypersensitivity is more evident in diabetic patients with vascular complications. However, it is also observed in newly diagnosed diabetic patients, suggesting that altered platelet function may be a consequence of metabolic changes secondary to the diabetic state (321–323).

Thromboxane A_2 (TxA_2), which is synthesized in platelets from arachidonic acid during platelet activation, is a potent platelet activator and vasoconstrictor. Enhanced activity of the arachidonic acid pathway with increased prostaglandin and TxA_2 formation occurs in diabetic individuals (324). There is a significant correlation between TxA_2 production and fasting plasma glucose or HbA_{1C}, and TxA_2 production can be restored by strict glycemic control with continuous subcutaneous insulin infusion (322).

Platelet hyperaggregability is likely to accelerate plaque development by promoting thrombosis and the release of platelet-derived growth factors. In established plaques, such changes may contribute to an acute event. Indeed, spontaneous platelet aggregation has been shown to predict recurrent infarctions following acute myocardial infarction (325) and correlates with increased cardiovascular events in diabetes (326).

ABNORMALITIES IN THE VASCULAR ENDOTHELIUM IN DIABETES

The vascular endothelium participates in a number of important homeostatic cellular functions, including regulation of coagulation, platelet reactivity, control of cell growth, and of vascular tone (327). The vascular endothelium exerts its effect on vascular tone by synthesizing and secreting biologically active substances, which include vasorelaxing agents such as endothelium-derived relaxing factor (EDRF) and prostacyclin (PGI_2), and the vasoconstrictors TxA_2 and endothelin (Wight, *this volume*). Endothelial dysfunction occurs in diabetes mellitus and can potentially contribute accelerated atherosclerosis.

Important among these vasoactive substances is EDRF, now known to be nitric oxide. Endothelial cells stimulated mechanically or by certain hormones, including acetylcholine and serotonin, release EDRF, which diffuses into the underlying smooth muscle and result in vascular relaxation. Endothelium-dependent relaxation of resistance vessels is abnormal in animal models (328) and human diabetes (329–331). The mechanism of diabetes-induced alteration of endothelium-dependent relaxation is unclear. Advanced glycosylation end products (AGEs) have been shown to inactivate nitric oxide rapidly via a direct chemical reaction (332). There is evidence that free radicals may play an important role in the impaired endothelium-dependent relaxation caused by elevated glucose concentrations by inactivating EDRF before it can exert its action on smooth muscle cells. Free radical scavengers such as superoxide dismutase can normalize endothelium-dependent relaxation in diabetic arteries (333).

Nitric oxide protects against the development of vascular disease because it inhibits platelet aggregation and adhesion, circulating monocyte adhesion to endothelial cells, and vascular smooth muscle proliferation. Thus, decreased EDRF may contribute to atherogenesis in diabetes.

Prostacyclin is an inhibitor of platelet aggregation and adhesion to the endothelium and a potent vasodilator, released from endothelium cells. The synthesis of PGI_2 by the vasculature in diabetic patients is reduced (334,335).

Endothelin 1 (ET-1) is a potent vasoconstrictor produced in endothelial cells. It is also a strong mitogen for vascular smooth muscle cells and, thus, may contribute to the atherosclerotic process. Plasma endothelin concentrations are significantly increased in patients with diabetes mellitus in comparison with healthy subjects (336). Physiological concentrations of insulin enhance the secretion of the ET-1 protein and the transcription rate of ET-1 mRNA in endothelial cells (337,338) and stimulate an increase in ET-1 receptor number expressed on vascular target tissues (339). Hence, in the setting of chronic hyperinsulinemia, the continual stimulation of ET-1 production and secretion might increase its mitogenic and vasoconstrictor actions.

ADVANCED GLYCOSYLATION END PRODUCTS

The mechanisms responsible for the complications of diabetes, including coronary artery disease, are poorly understood. Although the initial report of the Diabetes Control and Complications Trial (DCCT) conclusively showed that the greater the average blood glucose in patients with type 1 diabetes (as assessed by hemoglobin A1c), the greater the risk of developing retinopathy, neuropathy, and nephropathy, large-vessel disease missed being statistically significant (21). It is very likely that macroangiopathy (including coronary artery disease) would have been statistically significant had a larger group of patients been studied over a longer period of time.

The U.K. prospective diabetes study (UKPDS) is a multicenter, prospective, randomized intervention trial of 5,100 newly diagnosed patients with NIDDM that aims to determine whether improved glycemic control will prevent complications and reduce the associated morbidity and mortality (340). The endpoints of this study are major clinical events, which, as already mentioned, are mainly secondary to macrovascular disease. The results of this study are expected to be available in 1995.

One of the ascribed mechanisms responsible for the accelerated atherosclerosis in diabetes is advanced glycosylation of lipoproteins and proteins in arterial walls (341). Chronic hyperglycemia leads to the excessive accumulation of nonenzymatic glycosylation products. Initially, glucose is covalently and nonenzymatically attached to reactive amino groups of circulating proteins such as hemoglobin and LDL and of structural proteins including arterial wall collagen (342). A series of chemical reactions occurs in which these early glycosylation products are slowly converted to irreversible advanced glycosylation end products (AGEs) (Fig. 2), which continue to accumulate on proteins over time in vivo (342). The formation of AGEs on structural proteins is irreversible, results in cross-linking of adjacent proteins, and in coronary arteries can act as a nidus for plaque formation (343). Thus, AGE formation on collagen covalently binds to circulating plasma proteins, such as glycosylated LDL and IgG, which participate in the occlusion of diabetic vessels (344–346). Factors that influence the degree of AGE formation are the glucose concentration and the duration of exposure to it (347). However, genetic variations in the ability to detoxify AGE intermediates (e.g., 3-deoxyglucosone) enzymatically may explain why the consequences of a specific level of hyperglycemia may cause variable degrees of coronary artery disease in the diabetic population (348). Specific receptors for proteins modified by AGEs have been identified on both monocyte/macrophages and endothelial cells (349). These receptors are thought to facilitate the ingestion and degradation of AGE-modified proteins, which accumulate more rapidly in diabetic tissues (350). The binding of AGE to its receptors on the macrophage results in the secretion of interleukin I, insulin-like growth factor 1, and tumor necrosis factor (351).

It has been determined that arterial wall collagen from diabetic patients has a fourfold greater content of AGE (by radioreceptor assay) than that from nondiabetic patients (42). Also, arterial wall samples from end-stage renal disease (ESRD) patients with and without diabetes have increased levels of AGE (42). Indeed, the increased mortality noted in patients with ESRD is believed to be a consequence of the increased circulating AGE levels, which result in vascular events involving the coronary, cerebrovascular, and peripheral vascular arteries (119). Immunohistochemical staining utilizing AGE antibodies reveals that the atherosclerotic plaque within coronary arteries of four patients with NIDDM was almost entirely stained with AGE (343). In contrast, vascular lesions in the coronary arteries of 14 nondiabetic patients did not exhibit positive AGE reactivity.

Following the glycation of susceptible amino acids of circulating and structural proteins, further chemical reactions with oxygen free radicals result in glyco-oxidation products that are atherogenic (171). Oxidation of proteins such as LDL can occur without glycosylation. These compounds are also atherogenic (1).

In addition to modified (glycosylated) LDL being deposited on vessel collagen, other means have been described by which glycosylation has been related to smooth muscle cell proliferation. These include platelet-derived growth factor

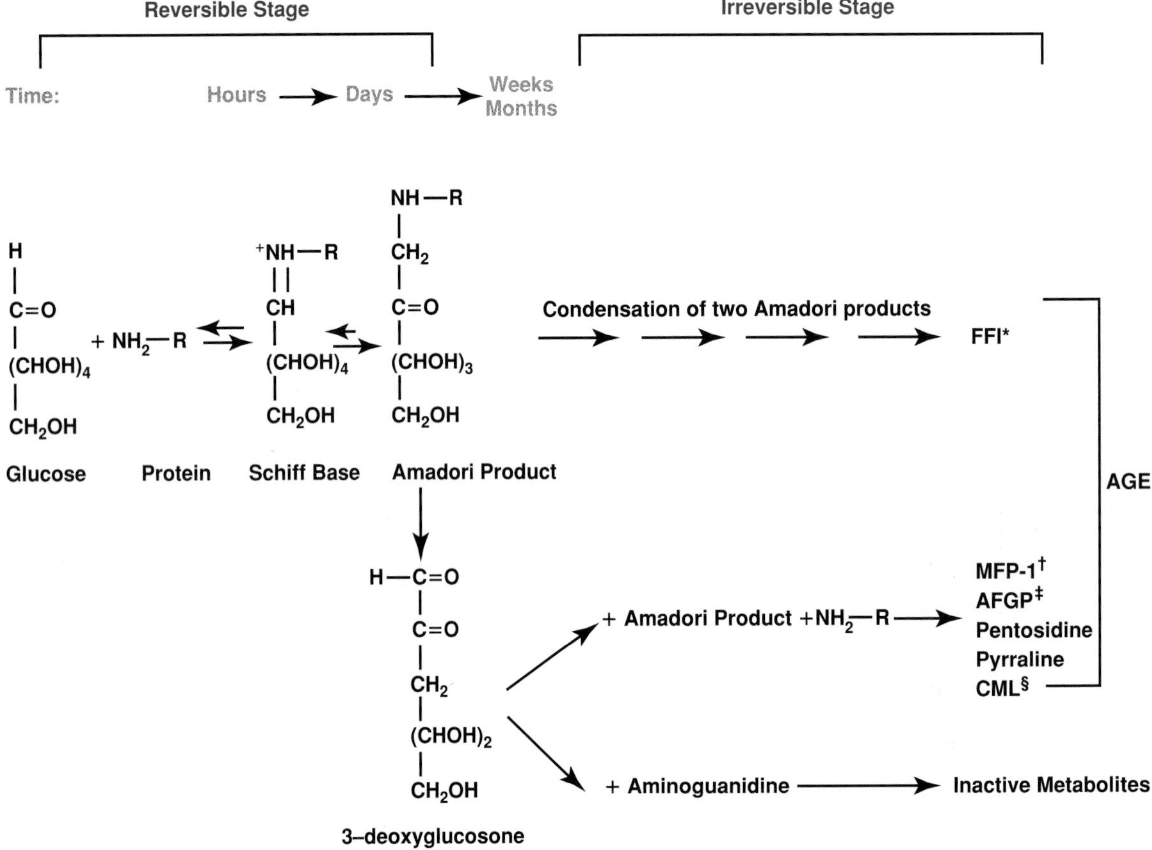

FIG. 2. Formation of reversible, early nonenzymatic glycosylation products and irreversible advanced glycosylation end products (AGE).

and possible mutations promoted by AGE in smooth muscle cell DNA (352).

The various mechanism by which AGEs can participate in the atherogenic process are listed in Table 10. Formation of AGEs in the matrix of vessels can affect the normal functioning of these vessels. The endothelium-derived relaxing factor and antiproliferative factor nitric oxide is quenched by AGEs in direct proportion to their level (332). Abnormalities in the vasodilatory response in diabetic animals correlate with the level of AGEs present and can be abrogated by inhibition of AGE formation.

TABLE 10. *Potential role of AGE in atherogenesis*[a]

AGE accumulation in artery wall
LDL trapping
Increased LDL oxidation
Endothelial cell changes
Permeability is increased by AGE accumulation
Cell adhesion
Procoagulant state
Monocytes/macrophages (contains receptor for AGE-modified proteins)
Chemotaxis and activation
Cytokine/growth factor (IL-1, TNF, PDGF) secretion
Smooth muscle cell proliferation

[a] Modified from Schwartz et al. (1) and Bierman (119).

If an agent could inhibit AGE formation and also large vessel disease in the diabetic state, the connection between AGEs and atherogenesis would be strengthened. Aminoguanidine, a hydrazine compound, was found to reduce the vascular leakage and arterial wall protein cross-linking associated with diabetes (353). It appears that aminoguanidine reacts mainly with non-protein-bound derivatives of early glycosylation products such as 3-deoxyglucosone (354). It is clear that clinical studies in patients with IDDM and NIDDM using aminoguanidine or a derivative compound will be important in attempting to prevent the progression of coronary artery disease despite the best efforts at metabolic control.

OBESITY AND ATHEROSCLEROSIS

The proportion of overweight adults in the United States has been steadily increasing in the past several decades. Presently, approximately one in five adult Americans, or 34 million people, are obese as defined by a weight that is 20% or more above the desirable level (355). Thus, the effects of obesity on the risk of CAD have major implications for public health.

There is no doubt that obesity is associated with increased prevalence of cardiovascular risk factors such as hypertension, diabetes, and dyslipidemia. However, the exact relationship of obesity as an independent risk factor for CAD is controversial (356). The importance of relative weight, body mass index (BMI), skinfold thickness, waist-to-hip ratio, and other measures of adiposity in the prediction CAD has been the subject of long-standing debate because of considerable inconsistencies that were reported for the relationship of obesity to the incidence of CAD (358,361). In the Framingham study, obesity was related to cardiovascular mortality and morbidity even after controlling for other risk factors (357). Judged traditionally, obesity was thus an independent cardiovascular risk factor.

However, autopsy studies show no consistent relationship between previous or current weight and coronary atherosclerosis (361). Evidence for a connection between obesity and atherosclerosis therefore rests on epidemiologic studies. Obesity has been implicated as an independent cardiovascular risk factor in some but not all studies (357–360). According to some authorities, obesity itself is not a significant contributor to CAD (361). In the recent National Cholesterol Education Program expert panel report, obesity was not listed as a positive risk factor (181).

As mentioned previously, obesity exerts much of its effect through the enhancement of other cardiovascular risk factors such as hypertension, insulin resistance, diabetes, and dyslipidemia. These cardiovascular risk factors are closely related to the pattern of distribution of adipose tissue throughout the body. A predominantly abdominal or visceral distribution of body fat is associated with insulin resistance, hypertriglyceridemia, low HDL cholesterol, and elevated blood pressure and correlates better with CAD risk than total adipose tissue mass. This form of fat distribution is an independent predictor of atherogenic metabolic aberrations and of cardiovascular morbidity and mortality (362–365).

People differ with respect to the location of fat. Men tend to have more abdominal fat, giving them the android or "apple" pattern of fat distribution. Women, on the other hand, manifest overweight with greater amounts of gluteal fat and thus have larger hip circumferences, giving them the so-called gynoid or "pear" pattern of fat distribution. Although a predominant abdominal fat distribution is more common in men, both men and women show an increased risk of heart disease when their abdominal fat is increased.

Because body fat distribution is more important than obesity per se with regard to its effect on cardiovascular risk, methods of accurate measurement of the amount and distribution of body fat have become an important clinical consideration. The waist-to-hip circumference ratio (WHR) is by far the most widely used index of regional adipose tissue distribution. The WHR is obtained by measuring the circumference of the abdomen at the smallest part below the rib cage and above the umbilicus, and the gluteal region or hip at the largest circumference at the posterior extension of the buttocks, and taking the ratio (366). The calculation of WHR has proven useful as a measure of fat distribution and associated metabolic and cardiovascular complications of obesity. Men are considered at increased risk if the WHR is >0.95, and women if the WHR is >0.8 (367). In a recent study, a waist circumference over about 100 cm appeared to be most closely associated with disturbances in lipoprotein and carbohydrate metabolism (368).

Computed tomography is an alternative approach that allows the precise measurement of adipose tissue areas at any site of the body and particularly the delineation of the amounts of visceral and subcutaneous fat (388). Although computed tomography is considered the best technique available for measurement of regional adipose tissue distribution, it is expensive and requires irradiation of subjects, therefore limiting its use for clinical and epidemiologic purposes.

Body fat distribution is more important than obesity per se with regard to its effect on glucose and insulin metabolism (365,369). Peripheral hyperinsulinemia and insulin resistance are characteristic features of abdominal obesity because of increased pancreatic secretion and diminished hepatic insulin extraction (364,370). Tumor necrosis factor-α (TNF-α) may have a direct role in the development of insulin resistance in obesity: TNF-α can impair insulin-stimulated glucose uptake in muscle and adipose cells and suppress the expression of the insulin-responsive glucose transporter (GLUT-4) that mediates insulin-dependent glucose uptake in these cells (371). Adipose tissue of several animal models of obesity overexpress TNF-α. Neutralization of TNF-α with a chimeric TNF-α receptor IgG protein in genetically obese Zucker rats increases peripheral disposal of glucose in response to insulin, thus partially reversing insulin resistance (372).

Obesity is a significant, independent risk factor for hypertension (373). The prevalence of hypertension in obese individuals is 25% to 50%, much higher than that of the general population. The risk of hypertension appears to parallel the degree of increased body weight (373–375). Weight gain is also responsible for much of the age-related increases in blood pressure that occur in many societies.

The hypertension associated with obesity is reversible by weight loss and exercise (375,376). Modest weight losses (i.e., 10% of body weight) improve blood pressure and in many patients lower arterial pressure to normal (377,378). Insulin resistance and hyperinsulinemia are well-known metabolic derangements in obesity, and several observations indicate that they may play an important role in the pathogenesis of obesity-induced hypertension (376,379). Obese hypertensive patients tend to be hyperinsulinemic when compared to normotensive control subjects. Fasting plasma insulin concentrations are closely related to the elevation in blood pressure in obese subjects (225,380). In addition, the drop in plasma insulin that occurs with diet or exercise in obese subjects correlates with the drop in blood pressure resulting from these interventions and not with body weight (381). Blood pressure reduction in response to chronic physical conditioning in obese individuals is greatest in patients with the highest circulating insulin levels. The mechanisms by which insulin resistance and hyperinsulinemia have been most frequently postulated to elevate blood pressure have already been discussed.

Obesity is often associated with an atherogenic lipid profile, which is more prominent in persons with abdominal obesity (382). Excessive deposition of abdominal fat is associated with decreased HDL levels (364,383,384). Neither total body fat mass nor regional fat distribution is associated with cholesterol concentrations (364,385). However, abdominal obesity correlates positively with a preponderance of the small, dense LDL subfraction (384). Hence, the dyslipidemia associated with abdominal adiposity appears to be similar to the dyslipidemia seen in patients with NIDDM and insulin resistance, i.e., increased concentrations of small VLDL, presence of the more atherogenic small, dense LDL, and decreased concentrations of HDL_2 (386).

The mechanisms underlying the association between abdominal adiposity and this lipoprotein profile have been elucidated to some extent, although much is still unknown. Adipose tissue is functionally heterogeneous, and marked regional differences can be found in cell number and size, lipoprotein lipase activity, and basal and catecholamine-stimulated lipolytic (hormone-sensitive lipase) activities. The intraabdominal adipose tissue has some metabolic characteristics that are unique in comparison with other adipose tissue. These special features seem to be most pronounced in the regions that are drained by the portal circulation (omental and mesenteric adipose tissue). Thus, portal adipose tissue has an exceedingly sensitive system for the mobilization of free fatty acids (FFA) because of a preponderance of β-adrenergic receptors, little α-adrenergic inhibition, and low density of insulin receptors. Human adipocytes contain catecholamine receptors able to stimulate (β) and inhibit (α_2) the hormone-sensitive lipase through their effects on adenylate cyclase. The higher lipolytic response to catecholamines in omental compared to subcutaneous or femoral adipose cells is in part related to reduced α_2- and increased β-adrenergic receptor density in the former. In addition, subcutaneous abdominal adipocytes are more sensitive than omental adipocytes to the inhibitory action of insulin on the lipolytic process. The high lipolytic activity of omental adipocytes results in a greater flux of FFA to the liver through the portal circulation. Increased portal FFA concentrations stimulate hepatic triglyceride production and VLDL secretion and reduce the hepatic extraction of insulin, contributing to the systemic hyperinsulinemia and resulting in hepatic insulin resistance (387,388).

In summary, in abdominal visceral obesity an insulin-resistant state is consistently observed and is a central component of the relationship among body fat distribution, plasma lipid abnormalities, hypertension, and coronary artery disease (388). The metabolic alterations observed in abdominal obesity are analogous to those observed in the "insulin resistance syndrome" described above. Assessment of visceral adiposity is more relevant than obesity alone in the evaluation of cardiovascular risk. Visceral fat accumulation in subjects with normal body weight may also be significant. Thus, it is possible that nonobese individuals (as determined by BMI) who have excess of intraabdominal mass are at a high risk for CAD. These metabolically obese, normal-weight individuals, although not overweight, have the same metabolic profile of risk factors associated with the insulin resistance syndrome (389,390). However, visceral obesity is a heterogeneous condition, and not every viscerally obese individual will be at high risk of developing diabetes and cardiovascular disease. Abdominal visceral obesity appears to exacerbate existing and probably genetically determined sensitivity to diabetes, dyslipidemia, and atherosclerosis (388), accounting for the observed heterogeneous outcome.

Weight loss has the potential to improve the metabolic conditions of the abdominal obese patient (391). Interestingly, subjects with abdominal obesity may show a preferential mobilization of visceral fat in response to weight loss (392).

FUTURE DIRECTIONS

Basic and clinical research should be directed to elucidate the unique mechanisms causing accelerated atherosclerosis in IDDM, NIDDM, and impaired glucose tolerance. Recent research has focused on the role of glycosylation of arterial wall and microalbuminuria. The use of aminoguanidine and related compounds has yet to be evaluated in humans.

Dyslipidemia is an important contributor to the accelerated atherosclerosis in diabetes. However, the determination of serum lipid and lipoprotein levels in diabetics has not yielded an adequate explanation of the increased risk for CHD. Further insight into the abnormal lipoprotein composition and the metabolic mechanisms that modify lipoprotein particles (glycosylation, oxidation) and determine these changes may offer the answer.

An important clinical problem in diabetes not yet explored through intervention trials is the relationship between diabetic dyslipidemia and vascular disease. Although there is good epidemiologic evidence of the link between plasma lipid and lipoprotein concentrations and macrovascular disease, whether modification of lipid levels reduces disease has not yet been tested in the diabetic population. Although primary and secondary trials of lipid lowering have not been performed in diabetics, it is highly likely that lipid lowering will reduce vascular risk in this high-risk group. Intervention trials are required in diabetics to confirm this proposition.

Clinical trials are required to assess the impact of antihypertensive drug class on microvascular and macrovascular complications in the major endpoints of morbidity and mortality. Such investigation should focus on identifying antihypertensive agents that not only lower blood pressure but also reduce cardiovascular risk. The determination of genetic markers for individual susceptibility of patients with diabetes to hypertension, diabetic nephropathy, and CHD may help to develop strategies for the prevention of these complications.

Research should also evaluate the relevance of hyperinsulinemia and insulin resistance for hypertension and atherosclerosis risk as well as better modes of therapy. Defining the mechanisms responsible for insulin resistance may lead to the development of new "insulin-sensitizing" agents that can improve insulin action, resulting in a wide spectrum of beneficial metabolic effects and a reduced cardiovascular risk.

Further work is needed to clarify the role of insulin as a modulator of PAI-1 synthesis in the setting of insulin resistance and the role of abnormal fibrinolysis in the development of macrovascular complications of diabetes.

The study of the various processes involved in hemostasis in the diabetic setting will lead to a better understanding of the mechanisms involved in the vascular complications of diabetes. Research is also necessary to determine the possible reversal of the hypercoagulable state by improved glycemic control or pharmacological interventions.

There is now increasing evidence that diabetes is associated with abnormalities in endothelial function that contribute to cardiovascular pathology. Understanding the pathophysiology of the abnormal endothelial function in diabetes may lead to the development of new agents that act on this system. Such agents may retard the early lesions of atherosclerosis. The clinical significance of abnormal endothelial function in diabetes remains to be determined.

REFERENCES

1. Schwartz CJ, Valente AJ, Sprague EA, Kelley JL, Cayatte AJ, Rozek MM. Pathogenesis of the atherosclerotic lesion. Implications for diabetes mellitus. *Diabetes Care* 1992;15:1156–1167.
2. Stamler J, Vaccaro O, Neaton JD, Wentworth D. Diabetes, other risk factors and 12-year cardiovascular mortality for men screened in the multiple risk factor intervention trial. *Diabetes Care* 1993;16: 434–444.
3. Barrett-Connor E, Orchard T. Diabetes and heart disease. In: *National Diabetes Data Group, Diabetes Data Compiled 1984* (NIH publication no. 85-1468). Washington, DC: US Dept. of Health and Human Services; 1985:XVI-1–XVI-41.
4. American Diabetes Association. Consensus Statement: Role of cardiovascular risk factors in prevention and treatment of macrovascular disease in diabetes. *Diabetes Care* 1993;16:72–78.
5. Margolis JR, Kannel WB, Feinleib M, Dawber TR, McNamara PM. Clinical features of unrecognized myocardial infarction: Silent and symptomatic. Eighteen year follow up: The Framingham Study. *Am J Cardiol* 1973;32:1–7.
6. Robertson WB, Strong JP. Atherosclerosis in persons with hypertension and diabetes mellitus. *Lab Invest* 1968;18:538–551.
7. Kawate R, Yamakido M, Nishimoto Y, Bennett PH, Harriman RF, Knowler W. Diabetes mellitus and its vascular complications in Japanese migrants on the Island of Hawaii. *Diabetes Care* 1979;2: 161–170.
8. Head J, Fuller JH. International variations in mortality among diabetic patients. The WHO Multinational Study of Vascular Disease in Diabetics. *Diabetologia* 1990;33:447–481.
9. Vigorita VJ, Morre GW, Hutchens GM. Absence of correlation between coronary arterial atherosclerosis and severity or duration of diabetes mellitus of adult onset. *Am J Cardiol* 1980;46:535–542.
10. Waller BF, Palumbo PJ, Lie JT, Roberts WC. Status of the coronary arteries at necropsy in diabetes mellitus with onset after age 30 years. Analysis of 229 diabetic patients with and without evidence of coronary heart disease and comparison to 183 control subjects. *Am J Med* 1980;69:498–506.
11. Mogensen CE. Microalbuminuria predicts clinical proteinuria and early mortality in maturity-onset diabetes. *N Engl J Med* 1984;310: 356–360.
12. Crall FV Jr, Roberts WC. The extramural and intramural coronary arteries in juvenile diabetes mellitus: Analysis of nine necropsy patients aged 19 to 38 with onset of diabetes before age 15 years. *Am J Med* 1978;64:221–230.
13. Vigorito C, Betocchi S, Bonzani G, Guidice P, Miceli D, Piscione F, Condorelli M. Severity of coronary artery disease in patients with diabetes mellitus. Angiographic study of 34 diabetic and 120 nondiabetic patients. *Am Heart J* 1980;100:782–787.
14. Dortimer AC, Shenoy PN, Shrioff RA, Leaman DM, Babb JD, Liedtke AJ, Zelis R. Diffuse coronary artery disease in diabetic patients. Fact or fiction? *Circulation* 1978;57:133–136.
15. Kannel W, McGee D. Diabetes and glucose tolerance as risk factors for cardiovascular disease: The Framingham Study. *Diabetes Care* 1979;2:120–126.
16. Jarrett RJ, Shipley MJ. Type 2 (non-insulin-dependent) diabetes mellitus and cardiovascular disease—putative association via common antecedents; further evidence from the Whitehall Study. *Diabetologia* 1988;31:737–740.
17. Nelson RG, Sievers ML, Knowler WC, Swinburn BA, Pettitt DJ, Saad MF, Liebow IM, Howard BV, Bennett PH. Low incidence of fatal coronary heart disease in Pima Indians despite high prevalence of non-insulin-dependent diabetes. *Circulation* 1990;81:987–995.
18. Barrett-Connor E, Cohn B, Wingard D, Edelstein SL. Why is diabetes mellitus a strong risk factor for fatal ischemic heart disease in women than in men. The Rancho Bernardo Study. *JAMA* 1991;265:627–631.
19. Jarrett RJ, McCarthney P, Keen H. The Bedford Study: Ten year mortality rates in newly diagnosed diabetics, borderline diabetics and normoglycemic controls and the risk indices for coronary heart disease in borderline diabetics. *Diabetologia* 1982;22:79–84.
20. Nathan DM. Long-term complications of diabetes mellitus. *N Engl J Med* 1993;328:1676–1685.
21. The Diabetes Control and Complication Trial Research Group. The effect of intensive treatment of diabetes on the development and progression of long-term complications in insulin-dependent diabetes mellitus. *N Engl J Med* 1993;329:977–986.
22. Unsitupa M, Siitonen O, Pyörälä K, Aro A, Hersio K, Penttilä I, Voutilainen E. The relationship of cardiovascular risk factors to the prevalence of coronary heart disease in newly diagnosed type II (non-insulin dependent) diabetes. *Diabetologia* 1985;28:653–659.
23. Herman JB, Medalie JH, Goldbourt U. Differences in cardiovascular morbidity and mortality between previously known and newly diagnosed adult diabetics. *Diabetologia* 1977;13:229–234.
24. Fuller JH, Shipley MJ, Rose G, Jarrett RJ, Keen H. Coronary heart disease risk and impaired glucose tolerance. The Whitehall Study. *Lancet* 1980;1:1373–1376.
25. Fontbonne A, Eschwege E, Cambien F, Richard JL, Ducimetiere P, Thibult N, Warnet JM, Claude JR, Rosselin GE. Hypertriglyceridemia as a risk factor for coronary heart disease mortality in subjects with impaired glucose tolerance or diabetes: Results from the 11-year follow up of the Paris Prospective Study. *Diabetologia* 1989;32: 300–304.
26. Kahn CR. Insulin action, diabetogenes, and the cause of type II diabetes. *Diabetes* 1994;43:1066–1084.
27. Singer DE, Nathan DM, Anderson KM, Wilson PWF, Evans JC. Association of Hb_{A1c} with prevalent cardiovascular disease in the original cohort of the Framingham Heart Study. *Diabetes* 1992;41:202–208.
28. Kuusisto J, Makkänen L, Pyörälä K, Laakso M. NIDDM and its metabolic control predicts coronary heart disease in elderly subjects. *Diabetes* 1994;43:960–967.
29. Krolewski AS, Kosinski EJ, Warram JH, Leland OS, Busick EJ, Asmal AC, Rand LI, Christlieb AR, Bradley RF, Kahn CR. Magnitude and determinants of coronary artery disease in juvenile-onset, insulin-dependent diabetes mellitus. *Am J Cardiol* 1987;59:750–755.
30. Maser RE, Wolfson SK Jr, Ellis D, Stein EA, Drash AL, Becher DJ, Dorman JS, Orchard TJ. Cardiovascular disease and arterial calcifications in insulin-dependent diabetes mellitus: Interrelation and risk factor profiles. *Arterioscler Thromb* 1991;11:958–965.
31. Donahue RP, Orchard TG. Diabetes mellitus and macrovascular com-

plications. An epidemiological perspective. *Diabetes Care* 1992;15: 1141–1155.

32. Borch-Johnsen K, Kreiner S. Proteinuria: Value as predictor of cardiovascular mortality in insulin-dependent diabetes mellitus. *Br Med J* 1987;294:1651–1654.
33. Jensen T, Borch-Johnsen K, Kofoed-Enevoldsen A, Deckert T. Coronary heart disease in young type I (insulin-dependent) diabetic patients with and without diabetic nephropathy: Incidence and risk factors. *Diabetologia* 1987;30:144–148.
34. Manske CL, Wilson RF, Wang Y, Thomas W. Prevalence of, and risk factors for, angiographically determined coronary artery disease in type I diabetic patients with nephropathy. *Arch Intern Med* 1992; 152:2450–2455.
35. Mattock MB, Morrish NJ, Viberti G, Keen H, Fitzgerald AP, Jackson G. Prospective study of microalbuminuria as predictor of mortality in NIDDM. *Diabetes* 1992;41:736–741.
36. Neil A, Hawkins M, Potok M, Thorogood M, Cohen D, Mann J. A prospective population-based study of microalbuminuria as a predictor of mortality in NIDDM. *Diabetes Care* 1993;16:996–1003.
37. Deckert T, Kofoed-Enevoldsen A, Borch-Johnsen K, Feldt-Rasmussen B, Jensen T. Microalbuminuria: Implications for micro- and macrovascular disease. *Diabetes Care* 1992;15:1181–1191.
38. Jensen T, Stender S, Deckert T. Abnormalities in plasma concentrations of lipoproteins and fibrinogen in type I (insulin-dependent) diabetic patients with increased urinary albumin excretion. *Diabetologia* 1988;31:142–145.
39. Jones SL, Close CF, Mattock MB, Jarrett RJ, Keen H, Viberti GC. Plasma lipid and coagulation factor concentrations in insulin dependent diabetics with microalbuminuria. *Br Med J* 298:487–490.
40. Winocour PH, Durrington PN, Bhatnagar D, Ishola M, Mackness M, Arrol S. Influence of early diabetic nephropathy on very low density lipoprotein (VLDL), intermediate density lipoprotein (IDL), and low density lipoprotein (LDL) composition. *Atherosclerosis* 1991;89: 49–57.
41. Gruden G, Cavallo-Perin P, Bazzan M, Stella S, Vuolo A, Pagano G. PAI-1 and factor VII activity are higher in IDDM patients with microalbuminuria. *Diabetes Care* 1994;43:426–429.
42. Makita Z, Radoff S, Rayfield EJ, Yang Z, Skolnik E, Delaney V, Friedman EA, Cerami A, Vlassara H, et al. Advanced glycosylation end-products in patients with diabetic nephropathy. *N Engl J Med* 1991;325:836–842.
43. Earle K, Viberti C. Familial, hemodynamic and metabolic factors in the predisposition to diabetic kidney disease. *Kidney Int* 1994;45: 434–437.
44. Seaquist ER, Goetz FC, Rich S, Barbosa J. Familial clustering of diabetic kidney disease: Evidence for genetic susceptibility to diabetic nephropathy. *N Engl J Med* 1989;320:1161–1165.
45. Borch-Johnsen K, Nørgaard K, Hommel E, Mathiesen ER, Jensen JS, Deckert T, Parving H-H. Is diabetic nephropathy an inherited complication? *Kidney Int* 1992;41:719–722.
46. Earle K, Walker J, Hill C, Viberti GC. Familial clustering of cardiovascular disease in patients with insulin-dependent diabetes with nephropathy. *N Engl J Med* 1992;326:673–677.
47. Krolewski AS, Canessa M, Warram JH, Laffel LMB, Christlieb AR, Knowler WC, Rand LI. Predisposition to hypertension and susceptibility to renal disease in insulin dependent diabetes mellitus. *N Engl J Med* 1988;318:140–145.
48. Viberti GC, Keen H, Wiseman MJ. Raised arterial pressure in parents of proteinuric insulin-dependent diabetics. *Br Med J* 1987;295: 515–517.
49. Canessa M, Andragna N, Solomon HS, Connolly TM, Tosteson DC. Increased sodium–lithium countertransport in red cells of patients with essential hypertension. *N Engl J Med* 1980;302:772–776.
50. Mangili R, Bending JJ, Scott G, Li K, Gupta A, Viberti GC. Increased sodium–lithium countertransport activity in red blood cells of patients with insulin-dependent diabetes and nephropathy. *N Engl J Med* 1988; 318:146–150.
51. Walker JD, Tariq T, Viberti GC. Sodium-lithium countertransport activity in red cells of patients with insulin-dependent diabetes and nephropathy and their parents. *Br Med J* 1990;301:635–638.
52. Jensen JS, Mathieson ER, Nørgaard K, Hommel E, Borch-Johnsen K, Funder J, Brahm J, Parving H-H, Deckert T. Increased blood pressure and erythrocyte Na^+–Li^+ countertransport activity are not inherited in diabetic nephropathy. *Diabetologia* 1990;33:619–624.
53. Crompton CH, Balfe JW, Balfe JA, Chatzilias A, Daneman D. Sodium–lithium transport in adolescents with IDDM. *Diabetes Care* 1994;17:704–710.
54. Cambien F, Poirier O, Lecerf L, Evans A, Cambou JP, Arveiler D, Luc D, Bard JM, Bara L, Ricard S, Tiret L, Amouyel P, Alhenc-Gelas F, Soubrier F. Deletion polymorphism in the gene for angiotensin-converting enzyme is a potent risk factor for myocardial infarction. *Nature* 1992;359:641–644.
55. Ruiz J, Blanche H, Cohen N, Velho G, Cambien F, Cohen D, Passa P, Froguel P. Insertion/deletion polymorphism of the angiotensin-converting-enzyme gene is strongly associated with coronary heart disease in non-insulin-dependent diabetes mellitus. *Proc Natl Acad Sci USA* 1994;91:3662–3665.
56. Marre M, Bernadet P, Gallois Y, Savagner F, Guyene T-T, Hallab M, Cambien F, Passa P, Alhenc-Gelas F. Relationships between angiotensin I converting enzyme gene polymorphism, plasma levels, and diabetic retinal and renal complications. *Diabetes* 1994;43:384–388.
57. Doria A, Warram JH, Krolewski AS. Genetic predisposition to diabetic nephropathy: Evidence for a role of the angiotensin I-converting enzyme gene. *Diabetes* 1994;43:690–695.
58. Margolis JR, Kannel WS, Feinleib M, Dawber TR, McNamara PM. Clinical features of unrecognized myocardial infarction—silent and asymptomatic. Eighteen year follow-up: The Framingham study. *Am J Cardiol* 1973;32:1–7.
59. Soler NG, Bennett MA, Pentecost BL, Fitzgerald MG, Malins JM. Myocardial infarction in diabetes. *Q J Med* 1975;44:125–132.
60. Nesto RW, Phillips RT, Kett KG, Hill T, Perper E, Young E, Leland OS Jr. Angina and exertional myocardial ischemia in diabetic and nondiabetic patients: Assessment by exercise thallium scintigraphy. *Ann Intern Med* 1988;108:170–175.
61. Marchant B, Umachandran V, Stevenson R, Kopelman PG, Timmis A. Silent myocardial ischemia: Role of subclinical neuropathy in patients with and without diabetes. *J Am Coll Cardiol* 1993;22:1433–1437.
62. Abenavoli T, Rubler S, Fisher VJ, Axelrod HI, Zuckerman KP. Exercise testing with myocardial scintigraphy in asymptomatic diabetic males. *Circulation* 1981;63:54–64.
63. Rubler S, Fisher VJ. The significance of repeated exercise testing with thallium-201 scanning in asymptomatic diabetic males. *Clin Cardiol* 1985;8:621–628.
64. Langer A, Freeman MR, Josse RG, Steiner G, Armstrong PW. Detection of silent myocardial ischemia in diabetes mellitus. *Am J Cardiol* 1991;67:1073–1078.
65. Nesto RW, Phillips RT. Asymptomatic myocardial ischemia in diabetic patients. *Am J Med* 1986;80(Suppl 4C):40–47.
66. Chipkin SR, Frid D, Alpert JS, Baker SP, Dalen JE, Aronin N. Frequency of painless myocardial ischemia in patients with and without diabetes mellitus. *Am J Cardiol* 1987;59:61–65.
67. Callaham PR, Froelicher VF, Klein J, Risch M, Dubach P, Friis R. Exercise-induced silent ischemia: Age, diabetes mellitus, previous myocardial infarction and prognosis. *J Am Coll Cardiol* 1989;14: 1175–1180.
68. Faerman I, Faccio E, Milei J, Nunez R, Jadzinsky M, Fox D, Rapaport M. Autonomic neuropathy and painless myocardial infarction in diabetic patients. *Diabetes* 1977;26:1147–1158.
69. O'Sullivan JJ, Conroy RM, MacDonald K, McKenna TJ, Maurer BJ. Silent ischemia in men with autonomic neuropathy. *Br Heart J* 1991; 66:313–315.
70. Ambepityia G, Kopelman PG, Ingram D, Swash M, Millis PG, Timmis AD. Exertional myocardial ischemia in diabetes: A quantitative analysis of anginal perceptual threshold and the influence of autonomic function. *J Am Coll Cardiol* 1990;15:72–77.
71. Hume L, Oakley GD, Boulton JM, Hardisty C, Ward JD. Asymptomatic myocardial ischemia in diabetes and its relationship to diabetic neuropathy: An exercise electrocardiography study in middle-aged diabetic man. *Diabetes Care* 1986;9:384–388.
72. Singer DE, Moulton AW, Nathan DM. Diabetic myocardial infarction: Interaction of diabetics with other preinfarction risk factors. *Diabetes* 1989;38:350–357.
73. Oswald GA, Corcoran S, Yudkin JS. Prevalence and risks of hyperglycemia and undiagnosed diabetes in patients with acute myocardial infarction. *Lancet* 1984;1:1264–1267.
74. Jaffe AS, Spadaro JJ, Schechtman K, Roberts R, Geltman EM, Sobel BE. Increased congestive heart failure after myocardial infarction of

modest extent in patients with diabetes mellitus. *Am Heart J* 1984; 108:31–37.

75. Savage MP, Korlewski AS, Kenien GG, Lebeis MP, Christlieb AR, Lewis SM. Acute myocardial infarction in diabetes mellitus and significance of congestive heart failure as a prognostic factor. *Am J Cardiol* 1988;62:665–669.
76. Fava S, Azzopardi J, Muscat HA, Fenech FF. Factors that influence outcome in diabetic subjects with myocardial infarction. *Diabetes Care* 1993;16:1615–1618.
77. Yudkin JS, Oswald GA. Determinants of hospital admission and case fatality in diabetic patients with myocardial infarction. *Diabetes Care* 1988;11:351–358.
78. Zuanetti G, Latini R, Maggioni AP, Santoro L, Franzosi MG. Influence of diabetes on mortality in acute myocardial infarction: Data from the GISSI-2 study. *J Am Coll Cardiol* 1993;22:1788–1794.
79. Stone PH, Muller JE, Hartwell T, York BJ, Rutherford JD, Parker CB, Turi ZG, Strauss HW, Willerson JT, Robertson T, Braunwald E, Jaffe A, and The MILIS Study Group. The effect of diabetes mellitus on prognosis and serial left ventricular function after acute myocardial infarction: Contribution of both coronary disease and left ventricular dysfunction to the adverse prognosis. *J Am Coll Cardiol* 1989;14: 49–57.
80. Granger CB, Califf RM, Young S, Candela R, Samaha J, Worley S, Kereiakes DJ, Topol EJ. Outcome of patients with diabetes mellitus and acute myocardial infarction treated with thrombolytic agents. The Thrombolysis and Angioplasty in Myocardial Infarction (TAMI) Study Group. *J Am Coll Cardiol* 1993;21:920–925.
81. Iwasaka T, Takahashi N, Nakamura S, Sugiura T, Tarumi N, Kimura Y. Residual left ventricular pump function after acute myocardial infarction in NIDDM patients. *Diabetes Care* 1992;15:1522–1526.
82. Zarich S, Nesto R. Diabetic cardiomyopathy. *Am Heart J* 1989;118: 1000–1012.
83. Ulvenstam G, Aberg A, Bergstrand R, et al. Long term prognosis after myocardial infarction in man with diabetes. *Diabetes* 1985;34: 787–792.
84. Gilpin E, Ricon F, Dittrich H, Nicod P, Henning H, Ross J. Factors associated with recurrent myocardial infarction within one year after acute myocardial infarction. *Am Heart J* 1991;121:457–465.
85. Jacoby RM, Nesto RW. Acute myocardial infarction in the diabetic patient: Pathophysiology, clinical course and prognosis. *J Am Coll Cardiol* 1992;20:736–744.
86. ISIS-2 (Second International Study of Infarct Survival) Collaborative Group. Randomized trail of intravenous streptokinase, oral aspirin, both, or neither among 17,187 cases of suspected acute myocardial infarction: ISIS-2. *Lancet* 1988;2:349–360.
87. Hillis LD, Forman S, Braunwald E, and The Thrombolysis in Myocardial Infarction (TIMI) Phase II Investigators. Risk stratification before thrombolytic therapy in patients with acute myocardial infarction. *J Am Coll Cardiol* 1990;16:313–315.
88. Barbash GI, White HD, Modan M, Van de Werf F, for the Investigators of the International Tissue Plasminogen Activator/Streptokinase Mortality Trial. Significance of diabetes mellitus in patients with acute myocardial infarction receiving thrombolytic therapy. *J Am Coll Cardiol* 1993;22:707–713.
89. Lynch M, Gammage P, Lamb M, Nattrass M, Pentecost BL. Acute myocardial infarction in diabetic patients in the thrombolytic era. *Diabetic Med* 1994;11:162–165.
90. Barbash GI, Hod H, Roth A, Miller HI, Rath S, Har Zahav Y, Modan M, Zivelin A. Correlation of baseline plasminogen activator inhibitor activity with patency of the infarct related artery after thrombolytic therapy in acute myocardial infarction. *Am J Cardiol* 1989;64: 1231–1235.
91. Gray RP, Yudkin JS, Patterson DL. Enzymatic evidence of impaired reperfusion in diabetic patients after thrombolytic therapy for acute myocardial infarction: A role for plasminogen activator inhibitor? *Br Heart J* 1993;70:530–536.
92. Holmes DR Jr, Vietstra RE, Smith HC, Vetrovec GW, Kent KM, Cowley MJ, Faxon DP, Gruentzig AR, Kelsey SF, Detre KM, Van Raden MJ, Mock MB. Restenosis after percutaneous transluminal coronary angioplasty (PTCA): A report from the PTCA Registry of the National Heart, Lung, and Blood Institute. *Am J Cardiol* 1984; 53:77C–81C.
93. Weintraub WS, Kosinski AS, Brown CL, King SB. Can restenosis after coronary angioplasty be predicted from clinical variables. *J Am Coll Cardiol* 1993;21:6–14.
94. Quigley PJ, Hlatky MA, Hinohara T, Rendall DS, Perez JA, Phillips HR, Califf RM, Stack RS. Repeat percutaneous transluminal coronary angioplasty and predictors of recurrent restenosis. *Am J Cardiol* 1989; 63:409–413.
95. Rensing BJ, Hermans RM, Vos J, Tijssen JGP, Rutch W, Danchin N, Heyndrickx GR, Mast G, Wijns W, Serruys PW, and The CARPORT Study Group. Luminal narrowing after percutaneous transluminal coronary angioplasty. *Circulation* 1993;88:975–985.
96. Rabbani LE, Edelman ER, Ganz P, Selwyn AP, Loscalzo J, Bitti JA. Relation of restenosis after excimer laser angioplasty to fasting insulin levels. *Am J Cardiol* 1994;73:323–327.
97. Carrozza JP, Kuntz RE, Fishman RF, Baim DS. Restenosis after arterial injury caused by coronary stenting in patients with diabetes mellitus. *Ann Intern Med* 1993;118:344–349.
98. Stern MP, Peterson JK, Haffner SM, Hazuda HP, Mitchell BD. Lack of awareness and treatment of hyperlipidemia in type II diabetes in a community survey. *JAMA* 1989;262:360–364.
99. Assmann G, Schulte H. The Prospective Cardiovascular Munster (PROCAM) study: Prevalence of hyperlipidemia in persons with hypertension and/or diabetes mellitus and the relationship to coronary heart disease. *Am Heart J* 1993;116:1713–1724.
100. Ginsberg NH. Lipoprotein physiology in nondiabetic and diabetic states: Relationship to atherosclerosis. *Diabetes Care* 1991;14: 839–855.
101. Howard BV. Lipoprotein metabolism in diabetes mellitus. *J Lipid Res* 1987;28:613–628.
102. Haffner SM, Stern MP, Hazuda HP, Mitchell BD, Patterson JK. Cardiovascular risk factors in confirmed prediabetic individuals. Does the clock for coronary heart disease start ticking before the onset of clinical diabetes? *JAMA* 1990;263:2893–2898.
103. Byrne CD, Brindle NPJ, Wang TWM, Hales CN. Interaction of non-esterified fatty acid and insulin in control of triacylglycerol secretion by Hep G2 cells. *J Biochem* 1991;280:99–104.
104. Howard BV, Howard WJ. Dyslipidemia in non-insulin-dependent diabetes mellitus. *Endocrinol Rev* 1994;15:263–274.
105. Howard BV, Davis M, Pettitt DJ, Knowler WC, Bennett PH. Plasma and lipoprotein cholesterol and triglyceride concentrations in Pima Indians: Distributions differing from those of Caucasians. *Circulation* 1983;68:214–222.
106. Brunzell JD, Hazzard WR, Motulsky AG, Bierman EL. Evidence for diabetes mellitus and genetic forms of hypertriglyceridemia as independent entities. *Metabolism* 1975;24:1115–1121.
107. Reaven GM, Chen YD. Roll of insulin in regulation of lipoprotein metabolism in diabetes. *Diabetes Metab Rev* 1988;4:639–652.
108. Reaven EP, Reaven GM. Mechanisms for development of diabetic hypertriglyceridemia in streptozotocin treated rats: Effect of diet and duration of insulin deficiency. *J Clin Invest* 1974;54:1167–1178.
109. Taskinen MR. Quantitative and qualitative lipoprotein abnormalities in diabetes mellitus. *Diabetes* 1992;41(Suppl 2):12–17.
110. Orchard TJ. Dyslipoproteinemia and diabetes. *Endocrinol Metab Clin North Am* 1990;19:361–380.
111. Pfeifer MA, Brunzell JD, Best JD, Judzewitsch RG, Halter JB, Porte D. The response of plasma triglycerides, cholesterol and lipoprotein lipase activity to treatment in non-insulin-dependent diabetic subjects without familial hypertriglyceridemia. *Diabetes* 1983;32:525–531.
112. Fontbonne A, Eschwege E, Cambien F, Richard JL, Ducimetiere P, Thibult N, Warmet JM, Claude JR, Rosselin GE. Hypertriglyceridemia as a risk factor for coronary heart disease mortality in subjects with impaired glucose tolerance or diabetes: Results from the 11-year follow up of the Paris Prospective Study. *Diabetologia* 1989;32: 300–304.
113. West KM, Ahuja MMS, Bennett PH, Czyczk A, de Acosta OM, Fuller JH, Garb B, Grabauskas V, Jarrett RJ, Koska K, Keen H, Krowlewski AS, Miki E, Schliack V, Teuscher A, Watkins P, Stober JA. The role of circulating glucose and triglyceride concentration and their interaction with other "risk factors" as determinants of arterial disease in nine diabetic population samples from the WHO multinational study. *Diabetes Care* 1983;6:361–369.
114. Goldschmid MG, Barrett-Connor E, Edelstein SL, Wingard DL, Cohn BA, Herman WH. Dyslipidemia and ischemic heart disease mortality among men and women with diabetes. *Circulation* 1994;89:991–997.
115. Howard BV, Abbott WF, Beltz WF, Harper I, Fields RM, Grundy

SM, Taskinen MR. The effect of non-insulin dependent diabetes on very low density lipoprotein and low density lipoprotein metabolism in men. *Metabolism* 1987;36:870–877.
116. Packard CJ, Munro A, Lorimer AR, Gotto AM, Shepherd J. Metabolism of apolipoprotein B in large triglyceride-rich very low density lipoproteins of normal and hypertriglyceridemic subjects. *J Clin Invest* 1984;84:2178–2192.
117. Rivellese A, Riccardi G, Romano R, Giacco L, Petti G, Annuzzi G, Mancini M. Presence of very low density lipoprotein compositional abnormalities in Type I (insulin dependent) diabetic patients; effect of blood glucose optimization. *Diabetologia* 1988;31:844–888.
118. Patti L, Swinburn B, Riccardi G, Rivellese AA, Howard BV. Alternations in very-low-density lipoprotein subfractions in normotriglyceridemic non-insulin-dependent diabetics. *Atherosclerosis* 1991;91: 15–23.
119. Bierman EL. Atherogenesis in diabetes. *Arterioscler Thromb* 1992; 12:647–656.
120. Ginsberg HN. Lipoprotein metabolism and its relationship to atherosclerosis. *Med Clin North Am* 1994;78:1–20.
121. Mattock MB, Salter AM, Fuller JH, Omer T, Gohari R-EI, Sharon D, Keen RH. High density lipoprotein subfractions in insulin-dependent diabetic and normal subjects. *Atherosclerosis* 1982;45:67–79.
122. Eckel RH. Lipoprotein lipase. A multifunctional enzyme relevant to common metabolic diseases. *N Engl J Med* 1989;320:1060–1068.
123. Nikkilä EA, Taskinen MR, Sane T. Plasma high-density lipoprotein concentrations and subfraction distribution in relation to triglyceride metabolism. *Am Heart J* 1987;113:543–548.
124. Nikkilä EA, Hormila P. Serum lipids and lipoproteins in insulin-treated diabetes: Demonstration of increased high-density lipoprotein concentrations. *Diabetes* 1987;27:1078–1086.
125. Kennedy AL, Lappin TRJ, Lavery TD, Hadden DR, Weaver JA, Montgomery DAD. Relation of high-density lipoprotein cholesterol concentration to type of diabetes and its control. *Br Med J* 1978;2: 1191–1194.
126. Hollenbeck CB, Chen YD, Greenfield MS, Lardinois CK, Reaven GM. Reduced plasma high density lipoprotein–cholesterol concentrations need not increase when hyperglycemia is controlled with insulin in non-insulin-dependent diabetes mellitus. *J Clin Endocrinol Metab* 1986;62:605–608.
127. Laakso M, Sarlund H, Mykkanen L. Insulin resistance is associated with lipid and lipoprotein abnormalities in subjects with varying degrees of glucose tolerance. *Arteriosclerosis* 1990;10:223–231.
128. Karhapää P, Malkki M, Laakso M. Isolated low HDL cholesterol: An insulin-resistant state. *Diabetes* 1994;43:411–417.
129. Patsch JR, Prasad S, Gotto AM, et al. High density lipoprotein 2: Relationship of the plasma levels of this lipoprotein species to its composition, to the magnitude of postprandial lipemia, and to the activities of lipoprotein lipase and hepatic lipase. *J Clin Invest* 1984; 80:341–347.
130. Nestel PJ. High density lipoprotein turnover. *Am Heart J* 1987;113: 518–521.
131. Baynes C, Henderson V, Richmond W, Johnston DG, Elkeles RS. The response of hepatic lipase and serum lipoproteins to acute hyperinsulinemia in type II diabetes. *Eur J Clin Invest* 1992;22:341–346.
132. Baynes C, Henderson V, Anyaoku V, Richmond W, Hughes CL, Johnston DG, Elkeles RS. The role of insulin sensitivity and hepatic lipase in the dyslipidemia of type 2 diabetes. *Diabetic Med* 1991;8: 560–566.
133. Inazu A, Brown ML, Hesler CB, Agellon LB, Koizumi J, Takata K, Maruhama Y, Mabuchi H, Hall AR. Increased high-density lipoprotein levels caused by a common cholesteryl–ester transfer protein gene mutation. *N Engl J Med* 1990;323:1234–1238.
134. Sparks D, Frolich JJ, Pritchard PH. Lipid transfer proteins, hypertriglyceridemia, and reduced high-density lipoprotein cholesterol. *Am Heart J* 1991;122:601–607.
135. Bagdade JD, Ritter MC, Subaaiah PV. Accelerated cholesterol ester transfer in patients with insulin-dependent diabetes mellitus. *Eur J Clin Invest* 1991;21:161–167.
136. Dullaart RP, Groener EM, Dickeschei BD, Erkelens W, Doorenbos H. Increased cholesterol ester transfer activity in complicated type I diabetes mellitus: Its relationship with serum lipids. *Diabetologia* 1989;32:14–19.
137. Fielding JC, Reaven GM, Liu G, Fielding PE. Increased free cholesterol in plasma low and very low density lipoproteins in non-insulin-dependent diabetes mellitus: Its role in the inhibition of cholesteryl ester transfer. *Proc Natl Acad Sci USA* 1984;81:2512–2516.
138. Bagdade JD, Lane JT, Subbaiah PV, Otto ME, Ritter MC. Accelerated cholesteryl ester transfer in noninsulin-dependent diabetes mellitus. *Atherosclerosis* 1993;104:69–77.
139. Duell PB, Oram JF, Bierman EL. Nonenzymatic glycosylation of HDL and impaired HDL-receptor mediated cholesterol efflux. *Diabetes* 1991;40:377–384.
140. The DCCT Research Group: Lipid and lipoprotein levels in patients with insulin-dependent diabetes mellitus: The Diabetes Control and Complication Trail (DCCT) experience. *Diabetes Care* 1992;15: 886–894.
141. Sosenko JM, Breslow JL, Mittinen OS, Gabbay KH. Hyperglycemia and plasma lipid levels: A prospective study of young insulin-dependent diabetic patients. *N Engl J Med* 1980;302:650–654.
142. Lopez-Virella MF, Wohltmann HJ, Loadholt CB, Buse MG. Plasma lipids and lipoproteins in young insulin-dependent diabetic patients: Relationship with control. *Diabetologia* 1981;21:216–233.
143. Barrett-Connor E, Witztum JL, Holdbrook M. A community study of high density lipoproteins in adult noninsulin-dependent diabetics. *Am J Epidemiol* 1983;117:186–192.
144. Hughes TA, Clements TS, Fairclough PK, Bell DS, Segrest JP. Effect of insulin therapy on lipoproteins in non-insulin-dependent diabetes mellitus (NIDDM). *Atherosclerosis* 1987;67:105–114.
145. Billingham MS, Milles JJ, Bailey CJ, Hall RA. Lipoprotein subfraction composition in non-insulin-dependent diabetes treated by diet, sulfonylurea, and insulin. *Metabolism* 1989;38:850–857.
146. Steinbrecher UP, Witztum JL. Glycosylation of low density lipoproteins to an extent comparable to that seen in diabetics slows their catabolism. *Diabetes* 1984;33:130–134.
147. Chait A, Bierman EL, Alberts JJ. Low density lipoprotein receptor activity in cultured human skin fibroblasts: Mechanisms of insulin-induced stimulation. *J Clin Invest* 1979;64:1309–1319.
148. Kissebah AH. Low density lipoprotein metabolism in non-insulin-dependent diabetes mellitus. *Diabetes Metab Rev* 1987;3:619–651.
149. Austin MA, King MC, Vranizan KM, Krauss RM. Atherogenic lipoprotein phenotype: A proposed genetic marker for coronary heart disease risk. *Circulation* 1990;82:495–506.
150. Austin MA, Breslow JL, Hennekens CH, Buring JE, Willett WC, Krauss RM. Low-density lipoprotein subclass patterns and risk of myocardial infarction. *JAMA* 1988;260:1917–1921.
151. Campos H, Genest JJ, Blijlevens E, McNamara JR, Jenner JL, Ordovas JM, Wilson PW, Schaefer EJ. Low density lipoprotein particle size and coronary artery disease. *Arterioscler Thromb* 1992;12:187–195.
152. Tribble DL, Vandenberg JJM, Motchnik PA, Ames BN, Lewis DM, Chait A, Krauss RM. Oxidative susceptibility of low-density lipoprotein subfractions is related to their ubiquinol-10 and α-tocopherol content. *Proc Natl Acad Sci USA* 1994;91:1183–1187.
153. Galeano NF, Milne R, Marcel YL, Walsh MT, Levy E, Nguyen TD, Gleeson A, Arad Y, Witte L, Alhaiderі M, Runsey SC, Deckelbaum RJ. Apolipoprotein-B structure and receptor recognition of triglyceride-rich low-density lipoprotein (LDL) is modified in small LDL but not in triglyceride-rich LDL of normal size. *J Biol Chem* 1994;269: 511–519.
154. Fiengold KR, Grunfeld C, Pang M, Doerrler W, Krauss RM. LDL subclass phenotype and triglyceride metabolism in non-insulin-dependent diabetes. *Arterioscler Thromb* 1992;12:1496–1502.
155. Austin MA, Newman B, Selby JV, Edwards K, Mayer EJ, Krauss RM. Genetics of LDL subclass phenotype in women twins. *Arterioscler Thromb* 1993;13:687–695.
156. Stewart MW, Laker MF, Dyer RG, Game F, Mitcheson J, Winocour PH, Alberti KG. Lipoprotein compositional abnormalities and insulin resistance in type II diabetic patients with mild hyperlipidemia. *Arterioscler Thromb* 1993;13:1046–1052.
157. McNamara JR, Jenner JL, Li Z, Wilson PWF, Schaefer EJ. Changes in LDL particle size is associated with changes in plasma triglycerides concentration. *Arterioscler Thromb* 1992;12:1284–1290.
158. Selby JV, Austin MA, Newman B, Zhang D, Quesenberry CP, Mayer EJ, Krauss RM. LDL subclass phenotype and insulin resistance syndrome in women. *Circulation* 1993;88:381–387.
159. Frayn KN. Insulin resistance and lipid metabolism. *Curr Opin Lipidol* 1993;4:197–204.
160. Reaven GM, Chen YDI, Jeppesen J, Maheux P, Krauss RM. Insulin

resistance and hyperinsulinemia in individuals with small, dense low density lipoprotein particles. *J Clin Invest* 1993;92:141–146.
161. Sobenin IA, Tertov VV, Koschinsky T, Bunting CE, Slavina ES, Dedov II, Orekhov AN. Modified low-density lipoprotein from diabetic patients causes cholesterol accumulation in human intimal aortic cells. *Atherosclerosis* 1993;100:41–54.
162. Lyons TJ, Klein R, Baynes JW, Stevenson HC, Lopes-Virella MF. Stimulation of cholesteryl ester synthesis in human monocyte-derived macrophages by low-density lipoproteins from type I (insulin-dependent) diabetic patients: The influence of nonenzymatic glycosylation of low-density lipoprotein. *Diabetologia* 1987;30:916–923.
163. Lopez-Virella MF, Klein RL, Lyons TJ, Stevenson HC, Witztum JL. Glycosylation of low-density lipoprotein enhances cholesteryl ester synthesis in human monocyte-derived macrophages. *Diabetes* 1988; 37:550–557.
164. Vlassara H, Brownlee M, Cerami A. Nodal macrophage receptor for glucose-modified proteins is distinct from previously described scavenger receptor. *J Exp Med* 1986;164:1301–1309.
165. Schmidt AM, Hori O, Brett J, Yan SD, Wautier JL, Stern D. Cellular receptors for advanced glycation end products. Implications for induction of oxidant stress and cellular dysfunction in the pathogenesis of vascular lesions. *Arterioscler Thromb* 1994;14:1521–1528.
166. Lyons TJ. Lipoprotein glycation and its metabolic consequences. *Diabetes* 1992;41(Suppl 2):67–73.
167. Hunt J, Smith CCT, Wolff SP. Autoxidative glycosylation and possible involvement of peroxides and free radicals in LDL modification by glucose. *Diabetes* 1990;39:1420–1425.
168. Bowie A, Owens D, Collins P, Johnson A, Tomkin GH. Glycosylated low density lipoprotein is more sensitive to oxidation: Implications for the diabetic patient? *Atherosclerosis* 1993;102:63–67.
169. Bucala R, Makita Z, Koschinsky T, Cerami A, Vlassara H. Lipid advanced glycosylation: Pathway for lipid oxidation in vivo. *Proc Natl Acad Sci USA* 1993;90:6434–6438.
170. Steinberg D, Parthasarathy S, Carew TE, Khoo JC, Witztum JL. Beyond cholesterol: Modifications of low-density lipoprotein that increase its atherogenicity. *N Engl J Med* 1989;320:915–923.
171. Lyons TJ. Glycation and oxidation: A role in the pathogenesis of atherosclerosis. *Am J Cardiol* 1993;71:26B–31B.
172. Steinberg D, Witztum JL. Lipoproteins and atherogenesis: Current concepts. *JAMA* 1990;264:3047–3052.
173. Bucala R, Makita Z, Koschinsky T, Cerami A, Vlassara H. Lipid advanced glycosylation: Pathway for lipid oxidation in vivo. *Proc Natl Acad Sci USA* 1993;90:6434–6438.
174. Baynes JW. Role of oxidative stress in development of complications in diabetes. *Diabetes* 1991;40:405–412.
175. Jenkins AJ, Steele JS, Janus ED, et al. Increased plasma apolipoprotein(a) levels in IDDM patients with microalbuminuria. *Diabetes Care* 1991;40:787–790.
176. Kapelrud H, Bangstad HJ, Dahl-Jorgensen K, Hanssen KF. Serum Lp(a) lipoprotein concentrations in insulin-dependent diabetic patients with microalbuminuria. *Br Med J* 1991;303:675–678.
177. Maser RE, Usher D, Becker DJ. Lipoprotein(a) concentrations show little relationship to IDDM complications in the Pittsburgh epidemiology of diabetes complications study cohort. *Diabetes Care* 1993;16: 755–758.
178. Haffner SM. Lipoprotein(a) and diabetes. An update. *Diabetes Care* 1993;16:835–840.
179. American Diabetes Association. Consensus statement: Detection and management of lipid disorders in diabetes. *Diabetes Care* 1993;16: 828–839.
180. Rubies-Part J, Reverter JL, Senti M, Pedre-Botet J, Salinas I, Lucas A, Nogues X, Sanmarti A. Calculated low-density lipoprotein cholesterol should not be used for management of lipoprotein abnormalities in patients with diabetes mellitus. *Diabetes Care* 1993;16:1081–1086.
181. The Expert Panel II. Summary of the second report of the National Cholesterol Education Program (NCEP) Expert Panel on detection, evaluation, and treatment of high blood cholesterol in adults. *JAMA* 1993;269:3015–3023.
182. American Diabetes Association. Exercise and NIDDM: Technical review. *Diabetes Care* 1990;13:785–789.
183. Reichard P, Nilsson BY, Rosenqvist U. The effect of long-term intensified insulin treatment on the development of microvascular complications of diabetes mellitus. *N Engl J Med* 1993;329:304–309.
184. Rosenstock J, Strowig S, Cercone S, Raskin P. Reduction in cardiovascular risk factors with intensive diabetes treatment in insulin-dependent diabetes mellitus. *Diabetes Care* 1987;10:729–734.
185. Garg A. Management of dyslipidemia in IDDM patients. *Diabetes Care* 1994;17:224–234.
186. Stern MP, Mitchell BD, Haffner SM, Hazuda HP. Does glycemic control of type II diabetes suffice to control diabetic dyslipidemia? A community perspective. *Diabetes Care* 1991;15:638–644.
187. Greenfield MS, Doberne L, Rosenthal M, Vreman HJ, Reaven GM. Lipid metabolism in non-insulin-dependent diabetes mellitus: Effect of glipizide therapy. *Arch Intern Med* 1982;142:1498–1500.
188. Taskinen MR, Beltz WF, Harper I, Fields RM, Schonfeld G, Grundy SM, Howard BV. Effects of NIDDM on very low density lipoprotein triglyceride and apolipoprotein B metabolism: Studies before and after sulfonylurea therapy. *Diabetes* 1986;35:1268–1277.
189. Garg A, Grundy SM. Management of dyslipidemia in NIDDM. *Diabetes Care* 1990;13:153–169.
190. Kreisberg RA. Low high-density lipoprotein cholesterol: What does it mean, what can we do about it, and what should we do about it? *Am J Med* 1993;94:1–5.
191. Garg A, Grundy SM. Nicotinic acid as therapy for dyslipidemia in non-insulin-dependent diabetes mellitus. *JAMA* 1990;264:723–726.
192. Kahn SE, Beard JC, Schwartz MW, Ward WK, Ding HL, Bergman RN, Taborsky GJ, Porte D. Increased beta-cell secretory capacity as mechanism for islet adaptation to nicotinic acid-induced insulin resistance. *Diabetes* 1989;38:562–568.
193. Vinik AI, Colwell JA. Effects of gemfibrozil on triglyceride levels in patients with NIDDM. *Diabetes Care* 1993;16:37–44.
194. Vega GL, Grundy SM. Gemfibrozil therapy in primary hypertriglyceridemia associated with coronary heart disease. Effect on metabolism of low-density lipoproteins. *JAMA* 1985;253:2398–2403.
195. Lahdenperä S, Tilly-Kiesi M, Vuorinen-Markkola H, Kuusi T, Taskinen MR. Effects of gemfibrozil on low-density lipoprotein particle size, density distribution, and composition in patients with type II diabetes. *Diabetes Care* 1993;16:584–592.
196. Tasi Y, Yuan J, Hunninghake DB. Effect of gemfibrozil on composition of lipoproteins and distribution of LDL subspecies. *Atherosclerosis* 1992;95:35–42.
197. Frick MH, Elo O, Happa K, et al. Helsinki Heart Study: Primary-prevention trial with gemfibrozil in middle-aged men with dyslipidemia. Safety of treatment, changes in risk factors, and incidence of coronary heart disease. *N Engl J Med* 1987;317:1237–1245.
198. Goldberg R, La Belle P, Zupkis R, Ronca P. Comparison of the effects of lovastatin and gemfibrozil on lipids and glucose control in non-insulin-dependent diabetes mellitus. *Am J Cardiol* 1990;66:16B–21B.
199. Koskinen P, Manttari M, Manninen V, Huttunen JK, Heinonen OP, Frick MH. Coronary heart disease incidence in NIDDM patients in the Helsinki Heart Study. *Diabetes Care* 1992;15:820–825.
200. Garg A, Grundy SM. Cholestyramine therapy for dyslipidemia in non-insulin-dependent diabetes mellitus. *Ann Intern Med* 1994;121: 416–422.
201. Garg A, Grundy SM. Lovastatin for lowering cholesterol levels in non-insulin-dependent diabetes mellitus. *N Engl J Med* 1988;318: 81–86.
202. Epstein M, Sowers JR. Diabetes mellitus and hypertension. *Hypertension* 1992;19:403–418.
203. American Diabetes Association. Consensus statement on the treatment of hypertension in diabetes. *Diabetes Care* 1993;16:1394–1401.
204. National High Blood Pressure Education Program Working Group. Report on hypertension and diabetes. *Hypertension* 1994;23:145–158.
205. Reaven GM. Role of insulin resistance in human disease. *Diabetes* 1988;37:1595–1607.
206. Krolewski AS. Predisposition to hypertension and susceptibility to renal disease in insulin dependent diabetes mellitus. *N Engl J Med* 1988;318:140–145.
207. Cignarelli M, De Cicco ML, Damato A, Paternostro A, Pagliarini S, Santoro S, Cardia L, De Pergola G, Giorgino R. High systolic BP increases prevalence and severity of retinopathy in NIDDM patients. *Diabetes Care* 1992;15:1002–1008.
208. Kelleher C, Kingstone SM, Barry DG, Cole MM, Ferriss JB, Grealy G, Joyce C, O'Sullivan DJ. Hypertension in diabetic clinic patients and their siblings. *Diabetologia* 1988;31:76–81.
209. Nørgaard K, Feldt-Rasmussen B, Borch-Johnsen K, Saelan H, Deckert T. Prevalence of hypertension in type 1 (insulin-dependent) diabetes mellitus. *Diabetologia* 1990;33:407–410.

210. Oakley WG, Pyke DA, Tattersall RB, Watkins PJ. Long term diabetes: A clinical study of 92 patients after 40 years. *Q J Med* 1974;43: 145–156.
211. Mogensen CE, Christensen CK. Blood pressure changes and renal function changes in incipient and overt diabetic nephropathy. *Hypertension* 1985;7[Suppl II]:II-64–II-73.
212. Krolewski AS, Warram JH, Christlieb AR, Busick EJ, Kahn CR. The changing natural history of nephropathy in type I diabetes. *Am J Med* 1985;78:785–790.
213. Mathiesen ER, Øxenboll B, Johansen K, Svendsen PA, Deckert T. Incipient nephropathy in type 1 (insulin dependent) diabetes. *Diabetologia* 1984;26:406–410.
214. Feldt-Rasmussen B, Borch-Johnsen K, Mathiesen ER. Hypertension in diabetes as related to nephropathy: Early blood pressure changes. *Hypertension* 1985;7[Suppl II]:II-18–II-20.
215. Mogensen CE, Østerby R, Hansen KW, Damsgaard EM. Blood Pressure elevation versus abnormal albuminuria in the genesis and prediction of diabetic nephropathy. *Diabetes Care* 1992;15:1192–1204.
216. Hasslacher C, Stech W, Wahl P, Ritz E. Blood pressure and metabolic control as risk factors for nephropathy in type 1 (insulin-dependent) diabetes. *Diabetologia* 1985;28:6–11.
217. Lundgren H, Bjorkman, Keiding P, Lundmark S, Bengtsson C. Diabetes in patients with hypertension receiving pharmacological treatment. *Br Med J* 1988;297:1512.
218. Hypertension in Diabetes Study (HDS). I. Prevalence of hypertension in newly presenting type 2 diabetic patients and the association with risk factors for cardiovascular and diabetic complications. *J Hypertens* 1993;11:309–317.
219. Teuscher A, Egger M, Herman JB. Diabetes and hypertension: Blood pressure in clinical diabetic patients and a control population. *Arch Intern Med* 1989;149:1942–1945.
220. Kannell WB, Wilson PWF, Zhang TJ. The epidemiology of impaired glucose tolerance and hypertension. *Am Heart J* 1991;121: 1268–1273.
221. Hypertension in Diabetes Study (HDS). II. Increased risk of cardiovascular complications in hypertensive type 2 diabetic patients. *J Hypertens* 1993;11:319–325.
222. Mitchell BD, Stern MP, Haffner SM, Hazuda HP, Patterson JK. Risk factors for cardiovascular mortality in Mexican Americans and non-Hispanic whites: The San Antonio Heart Study. *Am J Epidemiol* 1990; 131:423–433.
223. Shamiss A, Carroll J, Rosental T. Insulin resistance in secondary hypertension. *Am J Hypertens* 1992;5:26–28.
224. Ferrannini E, Buzzigoli G, Bonadonna R, Giorico MA, Oleggini M, Graziadei L, Pedrenilli R, Brandi L, Bevilacqua S. Insulin resistance in essential hypertension. *N Engl J Med* 1987;317:350–357.
225. Zavaroni I, Bonora E, Pagliara M, Dall'Aglio E, Luchetti L, Buonanno G, Bonati PA, Bergonzani M, Gnudi L, Passeri M, et al. Risk factors for coronary artery disease in healthy persons with hyperinsulinemia and normal glucose tolerance. *N Engl J Med* 1989;320:702–706.
226. Modan M, Halkin H, Luskyn A, Segal P, Fuchs Z, Chetrit A. Hyperinsulinemia is characterized by jointly disturbed plasma VLDL, LDL and HDL levels. *Arteriosclerosis* 1988;8:227–236.
227. Laws A, King AC, Haskell WL, Reaven GM. Relation to fasting plasma insulin concentrations to high density lipoprotein cholesterol and triglyceride concentration in men. *Arterioscler Thromb* 1991;11: 1636–1642.
228. Karhapää P, Voutilainen E, Kovanen PT, Laakso M. Insulin resistance in familial and nonfamilial hypercholesterolemia. *Arterioscler Thromb* 1993;13:41–47.
229. Sheu WHH, Shieh SM, Fih MMT, Shen DDC, Jeng CY, Chen YDI, Reaven GM. Insulin resistance, glucose intolerance, and hyperinsulinemia. Hypertriglyceridemia versus hypercholesterolemia. *Arterioscler Thromb* 1993;13:367–370.
230. Björntorp P. 'Portal' adipose tissue as a generator of risk factors for cardiovascular disease and diabetes. *Arteriosclerosis* 1990;10: 493–496.
231. Modan M, Halkin H, Almog S, Luski A, Eshkol A, Shefi M, Shitrit A, Fuchs Z. Hyperinsulinemia. A link between hypertension obesity and glucose intolerance. *J Clin Invest* 1985;75:809–817.
232. Saad MF, Lillioja S, Nyomba BL, Castillo C, Ferraro R, De Gregdrio M, Ravussin E, Knowler WC, Bennett PH, Haward BV, Bogardus C. Racial differences in the relation between blood pressure and insulin resistance. *N Engl J Med* 1991;324:733–739.
233. Muller DC, Elahi D, Pratley RE, Tobin JD, Andres R. An epidemiological test of the hyperinsulinemia–hypertension hypothesis. *J Clin Endocrinol Metab* 1993;76:544–548.
234. Ferrannini E, Haffner SM, Stern MP, Mitchell BD, Natali A, Hazuda HP, Patterson JK. High blood pressure and insulin resistance: Influence of ethnic background. *Eur J Clin Invest* 1991;21:280–287.
235. Saad MK, Knowler WC, Pettitt DJ, Nelson RG, Mott DM, Bennett PH. Insulin and hypertension: Relationship to obesity and glucose intolerance in Pima Indians. *Diabetes* 1990;39:1430–1435.
236. Collins VR, Dowse GK, Finch CF, Zimmet PZ. An inconsistent relationship between insulin and blood pressure in three Pacific Island populations. *J Clin Epidemiol* 1990;43:1365–1378.
237. Dowse GK, Collins VR, Alberti KG, Zimmet PZ, Tuomilehto J, Chitson P, Gareeboo H. Insulin and blood pressure levels are not related in Mauritians of Asian Indian, Creole or Chinese origin. *J Hypertens* 1993;11:297–307.
238. Weidmann P, Ferrari P. Central role of sodium in hypertension in the diabetic subjects. *Diabetes Care* 1991;14:220–232.
239. Weidmann P, Beretta-Piccoli C, Trost BN. Pressor factors and responsiveness in hypertension accompanying diabetes mellitus. *Hypertension* 1987;7(Suppl II):33–42.
240. Tuck M, Corry D, Trujillo A. Salt-sensitive blood pressure and exaggerated vascular reactivity in the hypertension of diabetes mellitus. *Am J Med* 1990;88:210–216.
241. Dodson PM, Beevers M, Hallworth R, Webberley MJ, Fletcher RF, Taylor KG. Sodium restriction and blood pressure in hypertensive type II diabetes: Randomised blind controlled and crossover studies of moderate sodium restriction and sodium supplementation. *Br Med J* 1989;298:227–230.
242. Weder AB. Sodium metabolism, hypertension, and diabetes. *Am J Med Sci* 1994;307(Suppl 1):S53–S59.
243. Harris RC, Brenner BM, Seifert JL. Sodium–hydrogen exchange and glucose transport in renal microvillus membrane vessels from rats with diabetes mellitus. *J Clin Invest* 1987;77:724–733.
244. Rowe JW, Young JB, Mimaker KL, Stevens AL, Pallotta J, Landsberg L. Effect of insulin and glucose infusions on sympathetic nervous system activity in normal men. *Diabetes* 1981;30:219–225.
245. Berne C, Fagius J, Pollare T, Hjemdahl P. The sympathetic response to euglycemic hyperinsulinemia: Evidence microelectrode nerve recordings in health subjects. *Diabetologia* 1992;35:873–879.
246. Anderson EA, Mark AL. The vasodilator action of insulin: Implications for the insulin hypothesis of hypertension. *Hypertension* 1993; 21:136–141.
247. Anderson EA, Hoffman PR, Balon TW, Sinkey CA, Mark AL. Hyperinsulinemia produces both sympathetic neural activation and vasodilation in normal humans. *J Clin Invest* 1991;87:2246–2252.
248. Anderson EA, Balon TW, Hoffman RP, Sinkey CA, Mark AL. Insulin increases sympathetic activity but not blood pressure in borderline hypertensive humans. *Hypertension* 1992;19:621–627.
249. Tsutsu N, Nunoi K, Kodama T, Nomiyama R, Iwase M, Fujishima M. Lack of association between blood pressure and insulin in patients with insulinoma. *J Hypertens* 1990;8:479–482.
250. O'Brien T, Young WF, Palumbo PJ, O'Brien PC, Service FJ. Hypertension and dyslipidemia in patients with insulinoma. *Mayo Clin Proc* 1993;68:141–146.
251. Pontiroli AE, Alberetto M, Pozza G. Patients with insulinoma show insulin resistance in the absence of arterial hypertension. *Diabetologia* 1992;35:294–295.
252. Leonetti F, Iozzo P, Giaccari A, Sbraccia P, Buongiorno A, Tamburrano G, Andreani D. Absence of clinically overt atherosclerotic vascular disease and adverse changes in cardiovascular risk factors in 70 patients with insulinoma. *J Endocrinol Invest* 1993;16:875–880.
253. Laakso M, Edelman SV, Brechel G, Baron AD. Decreased effect of insulin to stimulate skeletal muscle blood flow in obese men: A novel mechanism for insulin resistance. *J Clin Invest* 1990;1844–1852.
254. Baron AD, Brechtel-Hook G, Johnson A, Hardin D. Skeletal muscle blood flow: A possible link between insulin resistance and blood pressure. *Hypertension* 1993;21:129–135.
255. Beretta-Picolli C, Weidmann P. Exaggerated pressor responsiveness to norepinephrine in non-enzymatic diabetes mellitus. *Am J Med* 1981; 71:829–835.
256. Levy J, Gavin JR, Sowers JR. Diabetes mellitus: A disease of abnormal calcium metabolism? *Am J Med* 1994;96:260–273.
257. Erne P, Bolli P, Burgisser E, et al. Correlation of platelet calcium

with blood pressure: Effect of antihypertensive therapy. *N Engl J Med* 1984;310:1084–1088.

258. Resnick L, Gupta R, Bhargava K, et al. Cellular ions in hypertension, diabetes, and obesity: A nuclear magnetic resonance spectroscopic study. *Hypertension* 1991;17:951–957.
259. Levy J, Zemel MB, Sowers JR. Role of cellular calcium metabolism in abnormal glucose metabolism and diabetic hypertension. *Am J Med* 1989;87(Suppl 6A):7S–16S.
260. Zemel MB, Bedford BA, Zemel PC, Marwah O, Sowers JR. Altered cation transport in non-insulin-dependent diabetic hypertension: Effects of dietary calcium. *J Hypertens* 1988;6:S228–S230.
261. Sowers JR, Standley PR, Ram JL, Jacober S, Simpson L, Rose K. Hyperinsulinemia, insulin resistance, and hyperglycemia: Contributing factors in the pathogenesis of hypertension and atherosclerosis. *Am J Hypertens* 1993;6:260S–270S.
262. Halkin H, Modan M, Shefi M, Almog S. Altered erythrocyte and plasma sodium or potassium in hypertension, a facet of hyperinsulinemia. *Hypertension* 1988;11:71–77.
263. DeLuise M, Blackburn GL, Flier JS. Reduced activity of red-cell sodium–potassium pump in human obesity. *N Engl J Med* 1980;303: 1017–1022.
264. Rahmani-Jourdheuil D, Mourayre Y, Vague P, Boyer J, Juhan-Vague I. In-vivo insulin effect on ATPase activities in erythrocyte membrane from insulin-dependent diabetics. *Diabetes* 1987;36:991–995.
265. Blaustein MP. Sodium ions, calcium ions, blood pressure regulation and hypertension: A reassessment of hypothesis. *Am J Physiol* 1977; 323:C165–C173.
266. Aviv L, Livne A. The Na^+/H^+ antiport, cytosolic free Ca^{2+} and essential hypertension: A hypothesis. *Am J Hypertens* 1988;1: 410–413.
267. Moolenaar WH. Effects of growth factors on intracellular pH regulation. *Annu Rev Physiol* 1986;48:363–376.
268. Adragna NC, Canessa ML, Solomon H, Connolly TM, Tosteson DC. Increased sodium–lithium countertransport in red cells of patients with essential hypertension. *N Engl J Med* 1980;302:772–776.
269. Woods JW, Falk RJ, Pittman AW, Klemmer PJ, Watson BS, Namboodiri K. Increased red-cell sodium–lithium countertransport in normotensive sons of hypertensive patients. *N Engl J Med* 1982;306: 593–595.
270. Stout RW. Insulin and atheroma: 20-year perspective. *Diabetes Care* 1990;13:631–654.
271. Cruz AB, Amatuzio DS, Grande F, Hay LJ. Effect of intraarterial insulin on tissue cholesterol and fatty acids in alloxan-diabetic dogs. *Circ Res* 1961;9:39–43.
272. King GL, Kahn CR, Rechler MM, Nissley SP. Direct demonstration of separate receptors for growth and metabolic activities of insulin and multiplication-stimulating activity (an insulin like growth factor) using antibodies to the insulin receptor. *J Clin Invest* 1980;66: 130–140.
273. Pfefile B, Ditschuneit H. Effects of insulin on growth of cultured human arterial smooth muscle cells. *Diabetologia* 1981;20:155–158.
274. King GL, Goodman D, Buzney S, Moses A, Kahn CR. Receptors and growth promoting effects of insulin and insulin-like growth factors on cells from bovine retinal capillaries and aorta. *J Clin Invest* 1985; 75:1028–1035.
275. Brands MW, Hildebrandt DA, Mizelle HL, Hall JE. Sustained hyperinsulinemia increases arterial pressure in conscious rats. *Am J Physiol* 1991;260:R764–R768.
276. Hall JE, Coleman TG, Mizelle HL, Smith MJ. Chronic hyperinsulinemia and blood pressure regulation. *Am J Physiol* 1990;258: F722–F731.
277. Hall JE, Summers RL, Brands MW, Keen H, Alonso-Galicia M. Resistance to the metabolic action of insulin and its role in hypertension. *Am J Hypertens* 1994;7:772–788.
278. Tjoa HI, Kaplan NM. Nonpharmacological treatment of hypertension in diabetes mellitus. *Diabetes Care* 1991;14:449–460.
279. Dawson KG, McKenzie JK, Ross SA, Chiasson JL, Hamwt P. Report of the Canadian Hypertension Society Consensus Conference: 5. Hypertension and diabetes. *Can Med Assoc J* 1993;149:821–826.
280. Parving HH, Andersen AR, Smidt UM, Hommel E, Mathiesen ER, Svendsen PA. Effect of antihypertensive treatment on kidney function in diabetic nephropathy. *Br Med J* 1987;294:1443–1447.
281. Tuttle KR, DeFronzo RA, Stein JH. Treatment of diabetic nephropathy: A rational approach based on its pathophysiology. *Semin Nephrol* 1991;11:220–235.
282. Zatz R, Dunn BR, Meyer TW, Anderson S, Rennke HG, Brenner BM. Prevention of diabetic glomerulopathy by pharmacologic amelioration of glomerular capillary hypertension. *J Clin Invest* 1986;77: 1925–1930.
283. Hostetter TH. Diabetic nephropathy: Metabolic vs. hemodynamic considerations. *Diabetes Care* 1992;15:1205–1215.
284. Kasiske BL, Kalil RSN, Ma JZ, Liao M. Effect of antihypertensive therapy on the kidney in patients with diabetes. A meta-regression analysis. *Ann Intern Med* 1993;118:129–138.
285. Lewis EJ, Hunsicker LG, Bain RP, Rhode RD. The effect of angiotensin converting enzyme inhibition in diabetic nephropathy. *N Engl J Med* 1993;323:1456–1462.
286. Ravid M, Savin H, Jutrin I, Bental T, Katz B, Lishner M. Long-term stabilizing effect of angiotensin-converting enzyme inhibition on plasma creatinine and on proteinuria in normotensive type II diabetic patients. *Ann Intern Med* 1993;118:577–581.
287. Stein PP, Black HR. Drug treatment of hypertension in patients with diabetes mellitus. *Diabetes Care* 1991;14:425–428.
288. Lithell HO. Effect of antihypertensive therapy on insulin, glucose, and lipid metabolism. *Diabetes Care* 1991;16:203–209.
289. Torlone E, Rambotti AM, Perriello G, Botta G, Santeusanio F, Brunetti P, Bolli GB. ACE-inhibition increases hepatic and extrahepatic sensitivity to insulin in patients with type 2 (non-insulin-dependent) diabetes mellitus and arterial hypertension. *Diabetologia* 1991;34: 119–125.
290. Bak JF, Gerdes LU, Sørensen N, Pedersen O. Effects of perindopril on insulin sensitivity and plasma lipid profile in hypertensive non-insulin-dependent diabetes mellitus. *Am J Med* 1992;92(Suppl 4B): 69S–72S.
291. Arauz-Pacheco C, Ramirez LC, Rios JM, Rashkin P. Hypoglycemia induced by angiotensin converting enzyme inhibitors in patients with non-insulin-dependent diabetes receiving sulphonylurea therapy. *Am J Med* 1990;89:811–813.
292. Swislocki ALM, Hoffman BB, Sheu WH, Chen YD, Reaven GM. Effect of prazosin treatment on carbohydrate and lipoprotein metabolism in patients with hypertension. *Am J Med* 1989;86(Suppl 1B): 14–18.
293. Feher MD, Henderson AD, Wadsworth J, Poulter C, Gelding S, Richmond W, Sever PS, Elkeles RS. Alpha-blocker therapy, a possible advance in the treatment of diabetic hypertension—results of a cross over study of doxazocin and atenolol monotherapy in hypertensive non-insulin dependent diabetic subjects. *J Hum Hypertens* 1990;4: 571–577.
294. Lehtonen A. Doxazocin effects on insulin and glucose in hypertensive patients. *Am Heart J* 1991;121:1307–1311.
295. Ferrari P, Rosman J, Weidmann P. Antihypertensive agents, serum lipoproteins and glucose metabolism. *Am J Cardiol* 1991;67: 26B–35B.
296. Pool PE, Seagren SC, Salel AF. Metabolic consequences of treating hypertension. *Am J Hypertens* 1991;4(Suppl):494S–502S.
297. Moser M, Ross H. The treatment of hypertension in diabetic patients. *Diabetes Care* 1993;16:542–547.
298. Gurwitz JH, Bohn RL, Glynn RJ, Monane M, Mogun H, Avorn J. Antihypertensive drug therapy and the initiation of treatment for diabetes mellitus. *Ann Intern Med* 1993;118:273–278.
299. Pandit MK, Burke J, Gustafson AB, Minocha A, Peiris AN. Drug induced disorders of glucose tolerance. *Ann Intern Med* 1993;118: 529–539.
300. Pollare T, Lithell H, Selinus I. Sensitivity to insulin during treatment with atenolol and metoprolol: A randomised double blind study of the effects on carbohydrate and lipoprotein metabolism in hypertensive patients. *Br Med J* 1989;289:1152–1157.
301. Lijnen P. Biochemical mechanisms involved in the β-blockers-induced changes in serum lipoproteins. *Am Heart J* 1992;124:459–556.
302. Shepherd AMM, et al. Hypoglycemia-induced hypertension in diabetic patients on metoprolol. *Ann Intern Med* 1981;94:357.
303. Schwartz CJ, Valente AJ, Sprague EA, Kelley JL, Cayatte AJ, Rozek MM. Pathogenesis of the atherosclerotic lesion. Implications for diabetes mellitus. *Diabetes Care* 1992;15:1156–1167.
304. Ceriello A, Giugliano D, Quatraro A, Dello Russo P, Torella R. Blood glucose may condition factor VII levels in diabetic and normal subjects. *Diabetologia* 1988;31:889–891.
305. Ceriello A. Coagulation activation in diabetes mellitus: A role of hy-

perglycemia and therapeutic prospects. *Diabetologia* 1993;36: 1119–1125.
306. Ceriello A, Quatraro A, Dello Russo P, Marchi E, Barbanti M, Milani MR, Giugliano D. Protein C deficiency in insulin dependent diabetes: A hyperglycemia related phenomenon. *Thromb Hemostas* 1990;65: 104–107.
307. Banga JD, Sixma JJ. Diabetes mellitus, vascular disease and thrombosis. *Clin Hematol* 1986;15:465–492.
308. Breddin K. Detection of prethrombotic states in patients with atherosclerotic lesions. *Semin Thromb Hemostasis* 1986;12:110–123.
309. Wilhelmsen L, Svardsudd K, Korsan-Bengtsen K, Larsson B, Welin L, Tibblin G. Fibrinogen as a risk factor for stroke and myocardial infarction. *N Engl J Med* 1984;311:501–505.
310. Ganda OP, Arkin CF. Hyperfibrinogenemia: An important risk factor for vascular complications in diabetes. *Diabetes Care* 1992;15: 1245–1250.
311. Jones RL, Peterson CM. Hematologic alterations in diabetes mellitus. *Am J Med* 1981;70:339–352.
312. De Feo P, Gaisano MG, Haymond MW. Differential effects of insulin deficiency on albumin and fibrinogen synthesis in humans. *J Clin Invest* 1991;88:833–840.
313. Hamsten A, de Faire U, Walldius G, Dahlen G, Szamosi A, Landou C, Blomback M, Wiman B. Plasminogen activator inhibitor in plasma: Risk factor for recurrent myocardial infarction. *Lancet* 1987;2:3–9.
314. Nordet TK, Schneider DJ, Sobel BE. Augmentation of the synthesis of plasminogen activator inhibitor type-I by precursors of insulin. A potential risk factor for vascular disease. *Circulation* 1994;89: 321–330.
315. Auwerx J, Bouillon R, Collen D, Geboers J. Tissue-type plasminogen activator antigen and plasminogen activator inhibitor in diabetes. *Arteriosclerosis* 1988;8:68–72.
316. Juhan-Vague I, Alessi M, Vague P. Increased plasma plasminogen activator inhibitor I levels. A possible link between insulin resistance and atherothrombosis. *Diabetologia* 1991;34:475–462.
317. Schneider DJ, Nordt TK, Sobel DE. Attenuated fibrinolysis and accelerated atherogenesis in type II diabetic patients. *Diabetes* 1993;42: 1–7.
318. McGill JB, Schneider CL, Arfken CL, Lucore CL, Sobel BE. Factors responsible for impaired fibrinolysis in obese subjects and NIDDM patients. *Diabetes* 1994;43:104–109.
319. Gray RP, Patterson DHL, Yudkin JS. Plasminogen activator inhibitor activity in diabetic and nondiabetic survivors of myocardial infarction. *Arterioscler Thromb* 1993;113:415–420.
320. Colwell JA, Lopez-Virella MF. A review on the development of large-vessel disease in diabetes mellitus. *Am J Med* 1988;85(Suppl 5A): 113–118.
321. Winocour PD. Platelet abnormalities in diabetes mellitus. *Diabetes* 1992;41(Suppl 2):26–31.
322. Ishii H, Umeda F, Nawata H. Platelet function in diabetes mellitus. *Diabetes Metab Rev* 1992;8:53–66.
323. El Khawand C, Jamart J, Donckier J, Chatelain B, Lavenne E, Moriau M, Buysschaert M. Hemostasis variables in type I diabetic patients without demonstrable vascular disease. *Diabetes Care* 1993;16: 1137–1145.
324. Davì G, Catalano I, Averna M, Notarbartolo A, Sterno A, Ciabattoni G, Patrono C. Thromboxane biosynthesis and platelets function in type II diabetes mellitus. *N Engl J Med* 1990;332:1769–1774.
325. Trip MD, Cats VM, Van Capelle FJL, Vreeken J. Platelet hyperactivity and prognosis in survivors of myocardial infarction. *N Engl J Med* 1990;332:1549–1554.
326. Breddin H, Krzywanek H, Althoff P, Schoffing K, Ubeila K. PARD: Platelet aggregation as a risk factor in diabetes.
327. Vallance P, Calver A, Collier J. The vascular endothelium in diabetes and hypertension. *J Hypertens* 1992;10(Suppl 1):S25–S29.
328. Cohen RA. Dysfunction of vascular endothelium in diabetes mellitus. *Circulation* 1993;87[Suppl V]:V-67–V-76.
329. Calver AC, Collier JG, Vallance PJT. Inhibition and stimulation of nitric oxide synthesis in the human forearm arterial bed of patients with insulin-dependent diabetes. *J Clin Invest* 1992;90:2548–2554.
330. Saenz de Tejada IS, Goldstein I, Azadzoi K, Krane RJ, Cohen RA. Impaired neurogenic and endothelium-mediated relaxation of penile smooth muscle from diabetic men with impotence. *N Engl J Med* 1989;320:1025–1030.
331. Johnstone MT, Creager SJ, Scales KM, Cusco JA, Lee BK, Creager MA. Impaired endothelium-dependent vasodilation in patients with insulin-dependent diabetes mellitus. *Circulation* 1993;88:2510–2516.
332. Bucala R, Tracey KJ, Cerami A. Advanced glycosylation products quench nitric oxide and mediate defective endothelium-dependent vasodilation in experimental diabetes. *J Clin Invest* 1991;87:432–438.
333. Tesfamariam B, Cohen RA. Free radicals mediate endothelial cell dysfunction caused by elevated glucose. *Am J Physiol* 1992;263: H321–H326.
334. Inoguchi T, Umeda F, Ono H, Junisaki M, Watanabe J, Nawata H. Abnormality in prostacyclin stimulatory activity in sera from diabetics. *Metabolism* 1989;38:837–842.
335. Umeda F, Inoguchi T, Nawata H. Reduced stimulatory activity on prostacyclin production by cultured endothelium cells in serum from aged diabetic patients. *Atherosclerosis* 1989;75:61–66.
336. Takahashi K, Ghatei MA, Lam HC, Bloom SR. Elevated plasma endothelin in patients with diabetes mellitus. *Diabetologia* 1990;33: 306–310.
337. Oliver FJ, de la Rubia G, Feener EP, Lee ME, Loeken MR, Shiba T, Quertermous T, King GL. Stimulation of endothelin-1 gene expression by insulin in endothelial cells. *J Biol Chem* 1991;266: 23251–23256.
338. Ren-Ming HU, Levin ER, Pedram A, Frank HJL. Insulin stimulates production and secretion of endothelin from bovine endothelial cells. *Diabetes* 1993;42:351–358.
339. Frank HJL, Levin ER, Ren-Ming HU, Pedram A. Insulin stimulates endothelin binding and action on cultured vascular smooth muscle cells. *Endocrinology* 1993;133:1092–1097.
340. UK Prospective Diabetes Study Group. UK Prospective Diabetes Study (UKPDS). VIII. Study design, progress and performance. *Diabetologia* 1991;34:877–890.
341. Cerami A, Stevens VJ, Monnier VM. Role of nonenzymatic glycosylation in the development of the sequelae of diabetes mellitus. *Metabolism* 1979;28:431–439.
342. Bucala R, Cerami A. Advanced glycosylation: Chemistry, biology, and implications for diabetes and aging. *Adv Pharmacol* 1992;23: 1–34.
343. Nakamura Y, Horii Y, Nishino T, Shiiki H, Sakaguchi Y, Kagoshima T, Dohi K, Makita Z, Vlassara H, Bucala R. Immunohistochemical localization of advanced glycosylation endproducts in coronary atheroma and cardiac tissue in diabetes mellitus. *Am J Pathol* 1993;143: 1649–1656.
344. Brownlee M, Pongor S, Cerami A. Covalent attachment of soluble protein by nonenzymatically glycosylated collagen: Role of the in situ formation of immune complexes. *J Exp Med* 1983;158:1739–1744.
345. Sensi M, Tanzi P, Bruno MR, Mancuso M, Andriani D. Human glomerular basement membrane: Altered binding characteristics following in vitro non-enzymatic glycosylation. *Ann NY Acad Sci USA* 1986; 488:549–552.
346. Brownlee M, Vlassara H, Cerami A. Non-enzymatic glycosylation products on collagen covalently trap low-density lipoprotein. *Diabetes* 1985;34:938–941.
347. Monnier VM, Cerami A. Nonenzymatic glycosylation and browning of proteins in vivo. In: Waller GR, Feather MS, eds. *The Maillard Reaction in Foods and Nutrition.* Washington, DC: American Chemical Society.
348. Brownlee M. Lilly lecture 1993: Glycation and diabetic complications. *Diabetes* 1994;43:836–841.
349. Vlassara H, Brownlee M, Cerami A. Novel macrophage receptor for glucose-modified proteins is distinct from previously described scavenger receptors. *J Exp Med* 1986;164:1301–1309.
350. Vlassara H, Brownlee M, Cerami A. High-affinity-receptor-mediated uptake and degradation of glucose-modified proteins: A potential mechanism for the removal of senescent macromolecules. *Proc Natl Acad Sci USA* 1985;82:5588–5592.
351. Vlassara H, Brownlee M, Manogue KR, Dinarello CA, Pasagian A. Cachectin/TNF and IL-1 induced by glucose-modified proteins: Role in the normal tissue remodeling. *Science* 1988;240:1546–1548.
352. Pamplona R, Bellmunt MJ, Portero M, Prat J. Mechanisms of glycation in atherogenesis. *Med Hypotheses* 1993;40:174–181.
353. Brownlee M, Vlassara H, Kooney T, Ulrich P, Cerami A. Aminoguanidine prevents diabetes-induced arterial wall protein cross-linking. Science 1986;232:1629–1632.
354. Edelstein D, Brownlee M. Mechanic studies of advanced glycosyla-

tion end product inhibition by aminoguanidine. *Diabetes* 1992;41: 26–29.
355. National Institute of Health Consensus Development Panel on the Health Implications of Obesity. Health implications of obesity. National Institute of Health consensus development conference statement. *Ann Intern Med* 1985;103:1073–1077.
356. Pi-Sunyer FX. Medical hazards of obesity. *Ann Intern Med* 1993;119: 665.
357. Hubert HB, Feinleib M, McNamara PM, Castelli WP. Obesity as an independent risk factor for cardiovascular disease: A 26-year follow-up on participants in the Framingham Heart Study. *Circulation* 1983; 67:968–977.
358. Manson JE, Colditz GA, Stampfer MJ, Willett WC, Rosner B, Monson RR, Speizer FE, Hennekens CH. A prospective study of obesity and risk of coronary heart disease in women. *N Engl J Med* 1990;322: 882–889.
359. Feinleib M. Epidemiology of obesity in relation to health hazards. *Ann Intern Med* 1985;103:1019–1024.
360. Manson JE, Stampfer MJ, Hennekens CH, Willett WC. Body weight and longevity. A reassessment. *JAMA* 1987;257:353–358.
361. Barrett-Connor EL. Obesity, atherosclerosis, and coronary artery disease. *Ann Intern Med* 1985;103:1010–1019.
362. Lapidus L, Bengtsson C, Larsson B, et al. Distribution of adipose tissue and risk of cardiovascular disease and death: A 12-year follow up of participants in the population study of women in Gothenburg, Sweden. *Br Med J* 1984;289:1261–1263.
363. Casassus P, Fontbonne A, Thibult N, et al. Upper body fat distribution: A hyperinsulinemia-independent predictor of coronary heart disease mortality—The Paris Prospective study. *Arterioscler Thromb* 1992; 12:1387–1392.
364. Peiris AN, Sothmann MS, Hoffman RG, Hennes MI, Wilson OR, Gustafson AB, Kissebah AH. Adiposity, fat distribution and cardiovascular risk. *Ann Intern Med* 1989;110:867–872.
365. Folsom AR, Kaye SA, Sellers TA, et al. Body fat distribution and 5-year risk of death in older women. *JAMA* 1993;269:483–487.
366. Caro JF. Insulin resistance in obese and nonobese man. *J Clin Endocrinol Metab* 1991;73:691–695.
367. Bary GA. Pathophysiology of obesity. *Am J Clin Nutr* 1992;55: 448S–494S.
368. Pouliot MC, Després JP, Lemieux S, Moorjani S, Bouchard C, Tremblay A, Nadeau A, Lupien PJ. Waist circumference and abdominal sagittal diameter: Best simple anthropometric indexes for abdominal visceral adipose tissue accumulation and related cardiovascular risk in men and women. *Am J Cardiol* 1994;73:460–468.
369. Kissebah AH, Vydelingum M, Murray R, et al. Relation of body fat distribution to metabolic complications of obesity. *J Clin Endocrinol Metab* 1982;54:254–260.
370. Peiris AN, Mueller RA, Smith GA, Struve MF, Kissebah AH. Splanchnic insulin metabolism in obesity. Influence of body fat distribution. *J Clin Invest* 1986;78:1648–1657.
371. Spiegelman BM, Choy L, Hotamisligil GS, Graves RA, Tontonoz P. Regulation of adipocyte gene expression in differentiation and syndromes of obesity/diabetes. *J Biol Chem* 1993;268:6823–6826.
372. Hotamisligil GS, Shargill NS, Spiegelman BM. Adipose expression of tumor necrosis factor—α: Direct role in obesity linked insulin resistance. *Science* 1993;259:87–90.
373. Stamler R, Stamler J, Riedlinger WF, Algera G, Roberts RH. Weight and blood pressure. Findings in hypertension screening of 1 million Americans. *JAMA* 1978;240:1607–1610.
374. Kannel WB, Brand M, Skinner JJ Jr, Dawber TR, McNamara PM. The relation of adiposity to blood pressure and development of hypertension. *Ann Intern Med* 1967;67:48–59.
375. Tuck ML, Sowers J, Dornfeld L, et al. The effect of weight reduction on blood pressure, plasma renin activity, and plasma aldosterone levels in obese patients. *N Engl J Med* 1981;304:930–933.
376. Hall JE. Renal and cardiovascular mechanisms of hypertension in obesity. *Hypertension* 1994;23:381–394.
377. Rocchini AP, Key J, Bordie D, Chico R, Moorehead C, Katch V, Martin M. The effect of weight loss on the sensitivity of blood pressure to sodium in obese adolescents. *N Engl J Med* 1989;321:580–585.
378. Hsueh WA, Buchanan TA. Obesity and hypertension. *Endocrinol Metab Clin North Am* 1994;23:405–427.
379. Kaplan NM. The deadly quartet: Upper body obesity, glucose intolerance, hypertriglyceridemia, and hypertension. *Arch Intern Med* 1989; 149:1514–1520.
380. Manicardi V, Camellini L, Bellodi G, Coscelli C, Ferrannini E. Evidence for an association of high blood pressure and hyperinsulinemia in obese men. *J Clin Endocrinol Metab* 1986;62:1302–1304.
381. Krotkiewski M, Mandroukas K, Sjostrom L, Sullivan L, Wetterqvist H, Bjorntorp P. Effects of long term physical training on body fat, metabolism, and blood pressure in obesity. *Metabolism* 1979;28: 650–658.
382. Ostlund RE, Staten M, Kohrt WM, Schultz J, Malley M. The ratio of waist-to-hip circumference, plasma insulin levels, and glucose intolerance as independent predictors of the HDL_2 cholesterol level in older adults. *N Engl J Med* 1990;322:229–234.
383. Després JP, Moorjani S, Ferland M, et al. Adipose tissue distribution and plasma lipoprotein levels in obese women: Importance of intra-abdominal fat. *Arteriosclerosis* 1989;9:203–210.
384. Terry RB, Wood PD, Haskell WL, Stefanick ML, Krauss RM. Regional adiposity patterns in relation to lipids, lipoprotein cholesterol, and lipoprotein subfraction mass in men. *J Clin Endocrinol Metab* 1989;68:191–199.
385. Haffner SM, Stern MP, Hazuda HP, Pugh J, Patterson JK. Do upper-body and centralized adiposity measure different aspects of regional body-fat distribution? Relationship to non-insulin-dependent diabetes mellitus, lipids, and lipoproteins. *Diabetes* 1987;36:43–51.
386. Terry RB, Wood PD, Haskell WL, Stefanick ML, Krauss RM. Regional adiposity patterns in relation to lipids, lipoproteins cholesterol, and lipoprotein subfraction mass in men. *J Clin Endocrinol Metab* 1989;68:191–199.
387. Bjorntorp P. "Portal" adipose tissue as a generator of risk factors for cardiovascular disease and diabetes. *Arteriosclerosis* 1990;10: 493–496.
388. Bouchard C, Després JP, Mauriège P. Genetic and nongenetic determinants of regional fat distribution. *Endocrinol Rev* 1993;14:72–93.
389. Bjorntorp P. Metabolic implications of body fat distribution. *Diabetes Care* 1991;14:1132–1143.
390. Ruderman NB, Schneider SH, Berchtold P. The "metabolically-obese," normal-weight individual. *Am J Clin Nutr* 1981;34: 1617–1621.
391. Dennis KE, Goldberg AP. Differential effects of body fatness and body fat distribution on risk factors for cardiovascular disease in women. Impact of weight loss. *Arterioscler Thromb* 1993;13: 1487–1494.
392. Leenen R, van der Kooy, Deurenberg P, Seidell JC, Weststrate JA, Schovien FJM, Hautvast JGAJ. Visceral fat accumulation in obesity subjects: Relation to energy expenditure and response to weight loss. *Am J Phsyiol* 1992;263:E913–E919.

PART II

Pathogenesis of Atherosclerosis

General Principles

Atherosclerosis and Coronary Artery Disease,
edited by V. Fuster, R. Ross, and E. J. Topol.
Lippincott-Raven Publishers, Philadelphia © 1996.

CHAPTER 20

New Mouse Models of Lipoprotein Disorders and Atherosclerosis

Jan L. Breslow, Andrew Plump, and Marilyn Dammerman

Key Words: High-density lipoproteins (HDL); Intermediate-density lipoproteins (IDL); Low-density lipoproteins (LDL); Lipoprotein (a); Very-low-density lipoproteins (VLDL).

INTRODUCTION

In humans lipoprotein disorders are strongly associated with coronary heart disease susceptibility. Several types of abnormal lipoprotein patterns are commonly observed in heart attack victims, including elevated LDL cholesterol, reduced HDL cholesterol, usually with increased triglycerides, elevated chylomicron remnant and IDL cholesterol levels, and elevated levels of lipoprotein (a) [Lp(a)]. These patterns are caused by environmental and genetic factors that alter the synthesis, processing, or catabolism of lipoprotein particles. Over the last decade genes have been isolated that code for proteins that interact directly with plasma lipids. There are approximately 17 such lipoprotein transport proteins, including apolipoproteins that coat lipoprotein particles, lipoprotein-processing proteins, and lipoprotein receptors. The genes coding for these proteins have all turned out to be present as single copies in the human genome. They have been sequenced, mapped, and used as candidate genes to identify mutations underlying lipoprotein phenotypes associated with coronary heart disease susceptibility (1). Their role in lipoprotein transport is described in part in Fig. 1.

The lipoprotein transport genes have also been used to make transgenic and knockout animals, principally mice, that have provided new insights into how these genes are expressed and the functions they serve in an intact organism (2–4). Either singly or combined through cross breeding, these genetically altered mice are now being used to make animal models of human lipoprotein disorders associated with coronary heart disease susceptibility (Table 1). In at least one instance a mouse has been produced that develops diffuse fibroproliferative atherosclerotic lesions very much like those seen in humans.

J. L. Breslow, A. Plump, and M. Dammerman: Laboratory of Biochemical Genetics and Metabolism, The Rockefeller University, New York, New York 10021-6399.

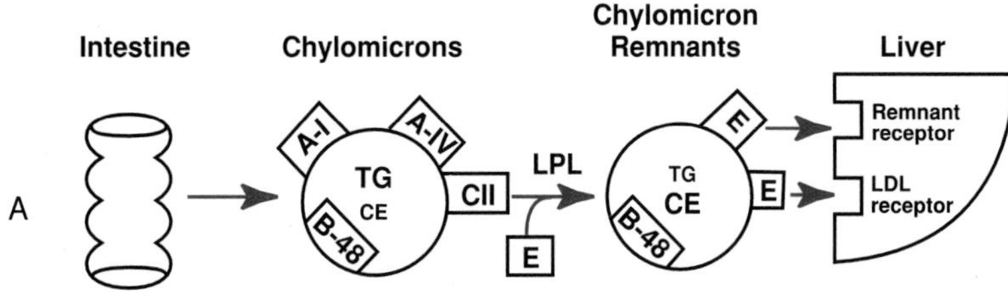

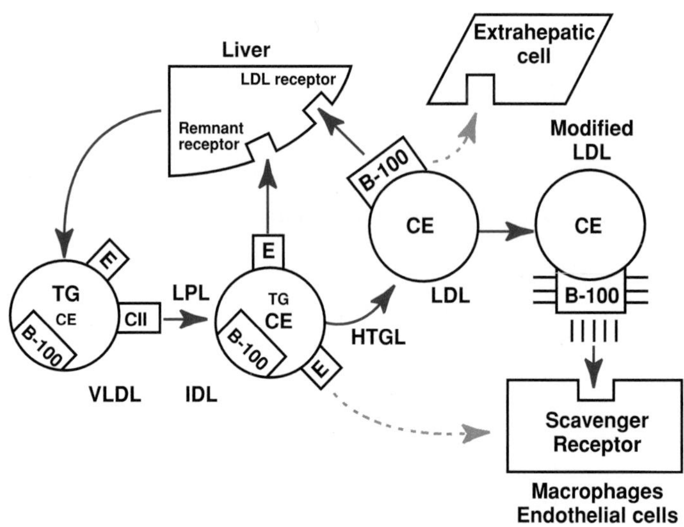

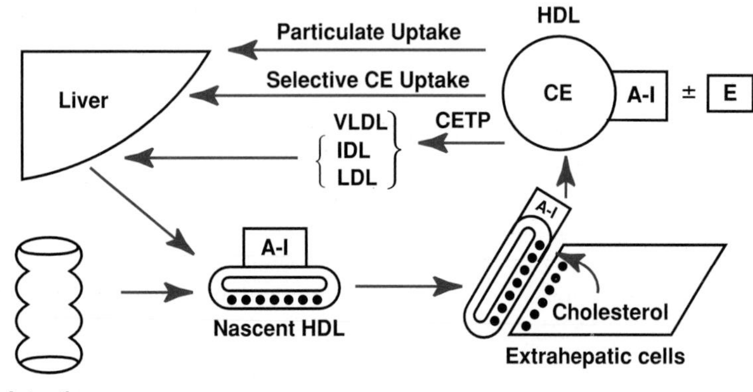

FIG. 1. The major lipoprotein metabolic pathways. See text for details.

INCREASED LDL CHOLESTEROL LEVELS

Increased levels of LDL cholesterol are a significant risk factor for coronary heart disease in humans (5). There is a 2% to 3% change in the risk of heart disease for each 1 mg/dl change in LDL cholesterol levels. The LDL particles are a constituent of the endogenous (nondietary) fat transport pathway and are formed via the action of lipases on precursor particles (Fig. 1). Dietary carbohydrate or fat reaching the liver that is not required for energy or synthetic purposes is converted into triglycerides, packaged with apolipoproteins, and secreted as VLDL particles. Lipoprotein lipase (LPL) present on the capillary endothelium, mainly in adipose tissue and skeletal muscle, hydrolyzes VLDL core triglycerides, using apo C-II on the particle surface as a cofactor. This results in the conversion of VLDL to IDL. The fatty acids thus liberated are reesterified to form triglycerides in adipose tissue or are oxidized to generate energy in muscle. The IDL is cleared from plasma by the LDL receptor, which binds apo E on the IDL surface. The IDL particles that escape

TABLE 1. *Mouse models of lipoprotein disorders associated with coronary artery disease*

Lipoprotein pattern	Mouse	Reference
↑ LDL cholesterol	LDL receptor-deficient	12
	Apo B transgenic	18–20
↓ HDL cholesterol and ↑ VLDL triglyceride	Apo A-I-deficient	39–41
	Apo C-III transgenic	46,47
	Apo C-I transgenic	48
	Apo C-II transgenic	49
	CETP transgenic	53,56,57,78
	Apo A-I, CETP transgenic	54
	Apo A-I, apo C-III, CETP transgenic	55
↑ IDL and chylomicron remnant cholesterol	Apo E-deficient	67–69,80,81
	Apo $E_{3\text{-Leiden}}$ transgenic	66a
	Apo $E_{4\text{-Arg}^{142}\text{Cys}}$ transgenic	66b
↑ Apolipoprotein(a)	Apo(a) transgenic	71
	Apo(a), apo B transgenic	19,20

clearance by this route are subject to further triglyceride hydrolysis by hepatic lipase to form cholesterol-ester-enriched LDL particles. The LDL surface contains a single molecule of apo B, which is recognized by LDL receptors. Approximately 70% of LDL is cleared by the LDL receptor, which is expressed primarily in the liver.

Mouse lipoprotein metabolism differs from that in humans in several respects (Table 2). The mouse is a poor model for elevated LDL cholesterol levels. On a chow diet, mouse LDL cholesterol levels are under 10 mg/dl, and this can only be doubled by feeding a Western-type diet. This contrasts with average human LDL cholesterol levels of 140 mg/dl, with the 95th percentile of the human LDL cholesterol distribution at 250 mg/dl. Several inherited disorders are recognized in humans that cause high levels of LDL cholesterol, and these have suggested genetic manipulations in the mouse that could be used to produce animals with elevated LDL cholesterol levels.

The first of these conditions is familial hypercholesterolemia (FH) (6,7). This is an autosomal dominant disorder caused by a defective LDL receptor gene on human chromosome 19, characterized by elevated plasma LDL. Two phenomena contribute to elevated LDL levels: decreased degradation and increased synthesis. Reduction in functional cell surface LDL receptor molecules impairs LDL catabolism, and failure to carry out receptor-mediated IDL uptake results in enhanced conversion of IDL to LDL, increasing LDL synthesis. Heterozygotes for FH have LDL cholesterol levels approximately double those in unaffected family members. They suffer from premature coronary heart disease, with 25% of men dying of myocardial infarction by the age of 50, compared to less than 5% in the general population. Approximately 75% of heterozygous familial hypercholesterolemics also develop tendon xanthomas. Homozygotes for FH have sixfold elevations in LDL cholesterol levels, with total cholesterol levels in the 600 to 1,000 mg/dl range. Coronary heart disease is often apparent before age 10, and most untreated homozygotes suffer fatal myocardial infarction before age 20. In addition to tendon xanthomas, homozygotes develop planar cutaneous xanthomas. Clearly, genetic modifications changing the number of functional LDL receptors should provide a powerful means of altering mouse LDL cholesterol levels.

TABLE 2. *Critical differences in lipoprotein physiology between humans and mice*

Parameter	Human	Mouse
HDL	50 mg/dl	50 mg/dl
LDL	150 mg/dl	10 mg/dl
CETP	Present	Absent
Lp(a)	Present	Absent
Apo B editing	Intestine	Liver, intestine
Atherosclerosis	Susceptible	Resistant

LDL Receptor Transgenic Mice

Two lines of LDL receptor transgenic mice have been created: the first containing a human LDL receptor cDNA driven by an inducible metallothionein-I promoter (8), and the second containing a human LDL receptor minigene driven by the constitutively expressed transferrin receptor promoter (9). Mice with the LDL receptor under control of the inducible promoter expressed low levels of hepatic LDL receptor in the uninduced state but increased expression twofold when induced with cadmium, a heavy metal known to up-regulate the metallothionein promoter. After heavy metal induction, transgenic mice cleared injected radiolabeled LDL eight to ten times faster than control mice, and the plasma concentrations of LDL receptor ligands, apo B and apo E, declined by more than 90%. Unfortunately, when administered over extended periods of time, cadmium has significant hepatotoxicity, thus precluding long-term studies. To overcome this setback the transferrin-receptor-driven LDL receptor transgenic mice were generated. In these mice high levels of hepatic LDL receptor activity could be achieved without cadmium induction. When these transgenic mice were challenged with a high-cholesterol-containing diet, a diet that normally leads to substantial increases in IDL and LDL in mice, IDL and LDL levels were unaffected. Thus, it appears that unregulated expression of LDL receptors can affect the response of plasma IDL and LDL levels to diet. By extension, variability in LDL receptor expression in humans may help to explain the differences in diet-induced IDL and LDL levels seen from person to person. The LDL receptor transgenic mice have been of further use in assessing a possible role for the LDL receptor in Lp(a) clearance (10) as well as in localizing a domain in the receptor that may influence its appropriate intracellular sorting (11).

LDL Receptor-Deficient Mice

LDL receptor knockout mice have also been created (12). These mice develop an eightfold increase in IDL and LDL cholesterol levels as a result of decreased clearance of these particles. The LDL receptor typically acts to remove lipoproteins that contain the largest apolipoprotein, apo B, using either apo B or apo E as a ligand (13). Metabolic studies in the LDL receptor-deficient mice suggest that the elevation in apo B-containing IDL and LDL results primarily from decreased particle clearance. Studies in these mice further support a role for LDL receptor variation in determining the response of plasma cholesterol to dietary fat and cholesterol intake. When fed a high-fat, 0.2% cholesterol, 10% coconut oil diet, the LDL receptor-deficient mice had a further threefold increase in the IDL cholesterol plus LDL cholesterol level, but this diet did not increase the levels of these lipoproteins in control mice.

The LDL receptor knockout mice have also been used as a model for gene replacement therapy. Intravenous administration of an adenovirus vector containing a human LDL receptor cDNA driven by the cytomegalovirus promoter caused high levels of hepatic LDL receptor expression, increased clearance of apo B-containing lipoproteins, and reduced IDL and LDL lipoproteins. These data support similar experiments in LDL-receptor-deficient humans (familial hypercholesterolemics) (14) and LDL-receptor-deficient rabbits (Watanabe heritable hyperlipidemic rabbits, WHHL) (15,15a,16) in which various viral delivery systems have been used to ameliorate at least temporarily the hypercholesterolemia found in the LDL receptor-deficient state.

The LDL receptor-deficient mouse is a faithful model for the human disorder FH. Although a full report on atherosclerosis susceptibility in the LDL receptor-deficient mice has not yet appeared, one would expect them to develop lesions, if not on chow then on a high-cholesterol and/or high-fat diet. For some types of studies, particularly those involving genetics or the requirement for a large number of animals, the LDL receptor-deficient mouse would be preferable to the previously described animal models of FH, the WHHL rabbit or the LDL receptor-deficient rhesus monkey.

Apo B Transgenic Mice

There are two other inherited conditions in humans characterized by increased LDL cholesterol levels that suggest an alternate approach to making a mouse with high levels of LDL cholesterol. The first of these is familial defective apo B, which is caused by a missense mutation in the apo B gene on human chromosome 2 (1,16). The resulting amino acid substitution, which replaces an arginine at amino acid 3,500 of the 4,536-amino-acid-long apo B polypeptide, disrupts apo B binding to the LDL receptor and impairs LDL uptake. Heterozygosity for this disorder increases LDL cholesterol levels by at least 50% relative to unaffected family members. In general, familial defective apo B may be milder than familial hypercholesterolemia, but patients can present with premature coronary heart disease and tendon xanthomas. The second condition is familial combined hyperlipidemia (FCHL), a complex disorder of unknown etiology, which is the most common genetic hypercholesterolemia and a frequent cause of premature coronary heart disease (1,16,18). This disorder is characterized by elevations of LDL cholesterol and VLDL triglyceride. Affected subjects may have one or both abnormalities, and the lipid profile may vary over time. Xanthomas are uncommon. Metabolic studies have shown overproduction of VLDL apo B. This leads to elevated VLDL and hypertriglyceridemia in some affected family members, although in other family members who have more efficient lipolysis, the consequence is elevated LDL. Familial defective apo B and FCHL suggest that production of a receptor-binding defective form of apo B or overproduction of apo B in mouse liver would elevate mouse LDL cholesterol levels. Because human apo B is recognized poorly by mouse LDL receptors, both strategies can be realized by creating transgenic mice that overproduce human apo B in the liver.

In humans full-length apo B, B100, is produced in the liver, whereas truncated apo B, B48, is produced in the intestine by an mRNA-editing mechanism. In rodent liver apo B mRNA editing also occurs, so mouse liver produces both B48 and B100. Transgenic mice expressing a human apo B minigene driven by the mouse transthyretin promoter have been made (19). These mice have very low levels of human apo B in plasma ($<1\%$ of normal), but the human apo B mRNA transcripts produced in the transgenic mouse liver undergo editing at an efficiency comparable to endogenous mouse apo B mRNA. This indicates that the apo B mRNA editing process can occur across species. Recently, human apo B transgenic mice have been made by microinjecting a large genomic piece of DNA derived from a phagemid vector containing the entire 43-kb gene and 15 to 20 kb of 5′ and 3′ flanking sequence (20,21). Transgenic lines were obtained with varying amounts of human apo B in plasma, from low levels to human physiological levels, without diminution of mouse apo B. Human apo B mRNA was found only in the liver, and mRNA editing occurred. Transgenic lines with high levels of human apo B had a high ratio of B100 to B48 in plasma, whereas the opposite was true for lines with low levels. High-expression human apo B transgenic mice had increased total cholesterol with an increase in LDL cholesterol. The LDL was relatively enriched in triglycerides compared to human LDL, perhaps because of the lack of cholesterol ester transfer protein (CETP) in mouse plasma. A major difference between mouse and human lipoprotein patterns is the low LDL cholesterol level in the mouse. The human apo B transgenic mice are more similar to humans in this respect, although the absolute levels of LDL cholesterol are still low compared to those in hypercholesterolemic humans.

Gene targeting has been used to alter the endogenous mouse apo B gene, and a mouse was created that expressed a truncated protein that is 70% of the wild-type size (22). This mimics human hypobetalipoproteinemia, a disorder associated with a variety of truncated apo B mutations and characterized by low plasma cholesterol and triglyceride levels. Mice homozygous for the mutant apo B70 allele had reduced VLDL, IDL, and LDL cholesterol as well as reduced triglyceride levels. These mice are an excellent model of hypobetalipoproteinemia; however, they also displayed findings not associated with human hypobetalipoproteinemia such as low HDL cholesterol levels and central nervous system abnormalities, exencephalus and hydrocephalus, which have yet to be explained.

REDUCED HDL CHOLESTEROL AND ELEVATED TRIGLYCERIDES

Reduced HDL cholesterol is the most common lipoprotein abnormality associated with coronary heart disease (23). Each 1 mg/dl decrease in HDL cholesterol is associated with a 4% increase in coronary artery disease (CAD) risk. Low HDL cholesterol is often found along with other lipoprotein abnormalities, including high levels of triglycerides in VLDL, increased levels of IDL and dense LDL. There are two major HDL particle size classes in plasma, small HDL_3 and large HDL_2 (24). Nascent HDL particles produced by the liver and small intestine consist primarily of complexes of phospholipid and apo A-I, and remodeling of these particles occurs as they circulate in plasma. The HDL particles attract excess free cholesterol from extrahepatic tissues and from other types of lipoprotein particles. The cholesterol is esterified by the enzyme lecithin:cholesterol acyl transferase (LCAT), using apo A-I and to a lesser extent other apolipoproteins as cofactors, and the resulting cholesterol ester enters the HDL core, enlarging the particle. The HDL particles may also become smaller as a result of the action of CETP, which exchanges the cholesterol ester in HDL for triglyceride in VLDL and IDL. Hepatic lipase can then hydrolyze HDL triglycerides, reducing HDL size. Excess cholesterol in peripheral tissues can thus be transferred from HDL to other lipoprotein particles, which are cleared from plasma primarily by hepatic receptors. This process, termed reverse cholesterol transport, may account in part for the protective effect of HDL on atherosclerosis susceptibility.

Apo A-I Transgenic Mice

Levels of HDL cholesterol are strongly correlated with the levels of its major apolipoprotein, apo A-I (25). Transgenic animals have been made with the human apo A-I gene under the control of its natural flanking sequences (26–28). The apo A-I gene is in a cluster of apolipoprotein genes on human chromosome 11q23 consisting in order of apo A-I, apo C-III, and apo A-IV (Fig. 2). The apo C-III gene is transcribed in the opposite orientation from the other two genes. The apo A-I gene is expressed primarily in liver and intestine and human apo A-I transgenes extending from as little as 256 bp 5′ to 80 bp 3′ of the gene achieved high-level liver expression, whereas this construction and others extending from 5 kb 5′ to 4 kb 3′ of the gene failed to give intestinal expression. Experiments in the transgenic mice have revealed a region approximately 6 kb 3′ to the apo A-I gene, located between −0.2 kb and −1.4 kb 5′ of the apo C-III gene required for apo A-I intestinal expression (Fig. 2). Whether expressed from the liver alone or liver plus intestine, in several transgenic mouse lines and a line of transgenic rats, apo A-I overexpression was found to increase HDL cholesterol levels selectively in a manner proportional to the level of plasma apo A-I. Human apo A-I expression in the mouse also resulted in decreased levels of mouse apo A-I (28–30) as well as changes in the physical properties of HDL. Mouse HDL normally consists of a single major size distribution of particles approximately 10 nm in diameter. In human apo A-I transgenic mice there are two major size distributions of particles, with diameters of approximately 10.3 and 8.8 nm. This corresponds to the two major size distributions of HDL particles in human plasma, HDL_{2b} and HDL_{3a}, respectively. The transgenic mouse studies show that the structure of apo A-I is an important determinant of HDL particle size distribution and, for the first time, suggest an explanation for HDL subspeciation in humans.

Human apo A-I transgenic mice have served as a model system to examine the mechanisms whereby diet and drugs alter HDL cholesterol and apo A-I levels. A high-fat Western-type diet increases HDL cholesterol and apo A-I levels in humans, and this effect has been mimicked in transgenic mice (31). In these animals the main metabolic effect was an increase in HDL cholesterol ester and apo A-I synthetic rates without an increase in apo A-I mRNA levels. In con-

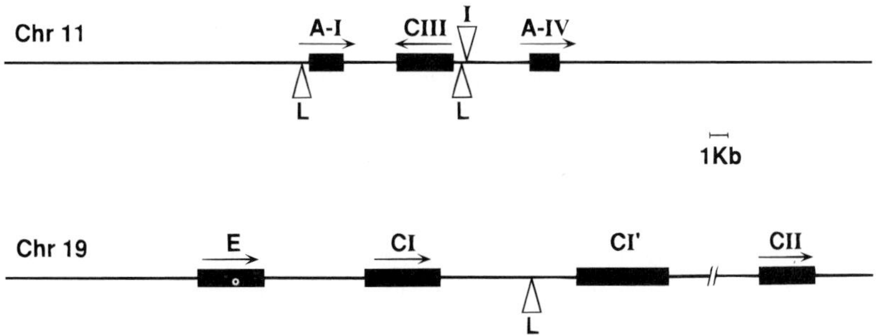

FIG. 2. Tissue-specific enhancer elements in the apo A-I, C-III, A-IV and the apo E, C-I, C-I′, C-II gene clusters. (From Breslow, ref. 4, with permission.)

trast, the lipid-lowering and antioxidant drug probucol decreases HDL cholesterol and apo A-I levels, and this effect could also be reproduced in transgenic mice (32). In probucol-treated mice HDL cholesterol ester fractional catabolic rate increased, and apo A-I synthetic rate decreased. The latter was not accompanied by a change in apo A-I mRNA levels. Thus, over the wide range of apo A-I levels observed in the high-fat-feeding and probucol experiments, there were no changes observed in apo A-I fractional catabolic rates or in apo A-I mRNA levels. Two interesting implications can be drawn from these studies. The first is that over the physiological range of apo A-I levels there is no saturable apo A-I or HDL receptor. The second is that previously unrecognized, potent, post-mRNA levels of regulation exist that regulate apo A-I production in relevant clinical situations.

Human apo A-I transgenic mice have been used to test possible non-lipid-transport functions of HDL. *Trypanosoma brucei* fatally infect livestock, but humans are resistant, apparently because human HDL lyse the organism. Human apo A-I is fully trypanolytic, whereas cattle and sheep apo A-I are not. Plasma from human apo A-I transgenic mice was found to be less trypanolytic than human plasma in vitro, and the transgenic mice were fully susceptible to infection with this organism (33). The difference between the lytic activity of human apo A-I in human and mouse plasma was shown to result from inhibition by mouse HDL apolipoproteins. Thus, it appears that even at low levels mouse apo A-I can antagonize the trypanolytic effect of human apo A-I. In another study, human apo A-I transgenic mice were used to confirm an in vitro observation suggesting that HDL might be an endotoxin-neutralizing component of plasma (34). In this study, after injection of lipopolysaccharide, transgenic mice with twofold more HDL cholesterol had better survival than control mice. This was accompanied by an increased transfer of lipopolysaccharide from the peritoneum to plasma and a marked reduction in endotoxin-induced increase in plasma tumor necrosis factor (TNF-α) levels. Thus, HDL may indeed provide natural protection against endotoxin, and protection may vary with plasma HDL concentration.

Apo-A-I-Deficient Mice

Although it is clear that low HDL cholesterol levels are an important risk factor for coronary heart disease in the general population, there is little understanding of mechanism. Three theories have been proposed: low HDL reflects decreased reverse cholesterol transport from peripheral tissues including the artery wall to the liver, where it can be excreted; low HDL results in decreased direct protection of the blood vessel wall; and low HDL is merely reflective of elevated levels of atherogenic lipoproteins such as VLDL, IDL and dense LDL. Further studies of the physiologic consequences of low HDL would be aided by the creation of an animal model. One method for accomplishing this is suggested by the existence of a small number of patients with mutations of the apo A-I gene that preclude synthesis of the protein. In the homozygous state these patients are characterized by very low to undetectable HDL cholesterol levels, and most of them develop planar xanthomas and coronary heart disease between the ages of 25 and 50 (35–38a).

To mimic these patients and cause a low-HDL state, apo A-I gene knockout mice have been created by gene targeting in embryonic stem cells (39,40). Apo A-I-deficient mice maintained on a chow diet had a 75% reduction in total and HDL cholesterol levels. These mice have been used to study the effect of low HDL on the amount of cholesterol that passes from the peripheral tissues through HDL to the liver. Kinetic studies first demonstrated that the amount of cholesterol ester flux through HDL was diminished by over sevenfold in apo A-I-deficient mice, a decrease consistent with the approximately tenfold decrease in HDL cholesterol ester levels. One might anticipate that these mice have accumulated cholesterol in peripheral tissues and have depleted hepatic cholesterol stores. Despite this large decrease in cholesterol flux, however, peripheral tissues did not accumulate cholesterol or cholesterol ester, and these mice did not develop atherosclerosis (40,41). These two observations suggest that the amount of non-HDL cholesterol in these mice was not sufficient to load peripheral tissues and macrophages of the arterial intima. Alternatively, homeostatic mechanisms were being invoked in peripheral tissues to compensate for the diminished flux (i.e., decreased LDL receptor and HMG-CoA reductase activity). The likelihood is that a combination of decreased loading capacity from decreased non-HDL cholesterol and reduced LDL receptor activity as well as decreased peripheral biosynthesis contributed to the absence of peripheral cholesterol accumulation.

At the opposite end of the cascade, the liver was found to have normal cholesterol and cholesterol ester stores, also suggesting cholesterol homeostasis. Although levels of hepatic LDL receptor and HMG-CoA reductase mRNA were normal, 7α-hydroxylase mRNA was decreased by over 60%. These data suggest that in response to diminished HDL cholesterol flux to the liver, apo A-I-deficient mice are not regulating intrahepatic cholesterol levels by increasing LDL receptor activity or de novo biosynthesis but by decreasing cholesterol excretion in the form of bile acids. In spite of the marked effects on HDL cholesterol levels and HDL cholesterol ester flux, it remains to be determined directly whether apo A-I deficiency causes a decrease in the reverse cholesterol transport of peripheral tissue cholesterol to the liver. The data furthermore suggest that apo A-I deficiency and low HDL cholesterol levels are not sufficient to cause atherosclerosis in mice, which are normally atherosclerosis resistant. To determine whether apo A-I deficiency can modify susceptibility to atherosclerosis, it will be necessary to breed the trait of apo A-I deficiency onto mice with a more atherogenic lipoprotein profile such as the LDL receptor-deficient mice, the human apo B transgenic mice, or the apo E-deficient mice (discussed below).

Apo A-II Transgenic Mice

The second most abundant HDL protein is apo A-II, and transgenic mice expressing human apo A-II have been produced (42). Unlike the human apo A-I transgenics, these animals do not have elevated HDL cholesterol levels, nor do they have diminished levels of mouse apo A-I or apo A-II. The human apo A-II transgenic mice had normal levels of VLDL, IDL and LDL cholesterol and total triglycerides. The lack of effect of excess apo A-II production on HDL cholesterol levels is compatible with clinical studies that fail to show a correlation between plasma apo A-II and HDL cholesterol levels (25) and the relatively normal HDL cholesterol levels reported in an apoA-II-deficient patient (43). The human apo A-II transgenics did show an alteration of HDL particle size with the appearance of a population of 8.0-nm-diameter particles along with the normal-sized mouse HDL particles. The protein composition of the smaller HDL consisted almost entirely of human apo A-II, whereas the larger particles consisted of mouse apo A-I and either mouse or human apo A-II. Thus, human apo A-II appears to affect the quality of HDL particles.

Recently, a transgenic mouse line expressing mouse apo A-II was derived with a two- to threefold elevation of apo A-II levels (44). In contrast to human apo A-II transgenic mice, these animals had a twofold increase in HDL cholesterol levels and a two- to threefold increase in non-HDL cholesterol and triglyceride levels. Mouse apo A-II transgenics also had larger HDL particles. The marked differences in the lipoprotein profiles between mouse and human apo A-II transgenices may be caused by the different physical properties of the two proteins. For example, in plasma, mouse apo A-II is monomeric, whereas human apo A-II is homodimeric. In addition, the two proteins are only about 60% identical in their amino acid sequences. As with apo A-I, apo A-II provides another example of how species differences can affect apolipoprotein behavior in vivo and offers a unique perspective on apolipoprotein function.

LPL Transgenic Mice

As previously noted, low HDL cholesterol levels are often found together with high triglycerides. The principal triglyceride-rich lipoproteins are VLDL and chylomicrons. The initial step in the metabolism of these particles is triglyceride hydrolysis, which is carried out by LPL, a molecule that resides on endothelial surfaces, principally in muscle and adipose tissue. LPL requires apo C-II as a cofactor. Elevated triglycerides are common in the population, with 10% of middle aged men having triglycerides over 250 mg/dl, yet the known genetic causes homozygosity for mutations in LPL or its cofactor apo C-II, are quite rare, with each frequency less than one in a million.

Transgenic mice have been made that overexpress LPL in a tissue-nonspecific manner utilizing a human LPL cDNA driven by the chicken β-actin promoter (45). These mice expressed high levels of the human LPL mRNA in tissues that express endogenous LPL—heart, skeletal muscle, and adipose tissue—as well as in tissues that do not express endogenous LPL, such as lungs, brain, spleen, and aorta. Transgenic mice had fivefold higher LPL activity in adipose tissue and 1.7-fold higher activity in postheparin plasma than controls. The overexpression of LPL activity resulted in a 75% reduction of triglyceride levels and a 1.4-fold increase in HDL_2 cholesterol. Metabolic studies indicated rapid clearance of VLDL triglyceride, and a vitamin A–fat tolerance test suggested rapid clearance of dietary fat from the circulation. When challenged with sucrose, which is known to stimulate VLDL production, LPL transgenic mice did not have elevated plasma VLDL. Finally, the development of hypercholesterolemia was suppressed after high-cholesterol feeding. The LPL transgenic mice confirm that LPL has a strong influence on triglyceride levels in vivo. These transgenic studies also suggest that LPL genetic variation may influence responsiveness to dietary cholesterol in humans.

Apo C Transgenic Mice

Although the mouse normally has low levels of triglycerides and relatively high levels of HDL as compared to humans, LPL overexpression was further able to decrease triglyceride and increase HDL levels. However, it would be more useful to create a mouse with high triglyceride and low HDL. In the course of making transgenic mice to study the *cis*-acting regions responsible for the tissue-specific expression of the apo A-I gene, a DNA construction was used that contained the apo A-I gene plus the neighboring apo C-III gene, which codes for a protein found in VLDL and HDL (3). These mice were found to have massive hypertriglyceridemia, whereas mice made with the apo A-I gene alone had normal triglyceride levels. Several transgenic mouse lines were subsequently made with only the apo C-III gene, and triglyceride levels were found to be proportional to apo C-III gene expression and human apo C-III plasma concentrations (46). In one transgenic line there was a single copy of the transgene and 30–40% extra apo C-III in plasma. These mice had 2.5-fold greater than normal triglyceride levels.

The human apo C-III transgenic mice were the first animal model of primary hypertriglyceridemia. In addition to suggesting a role for apo C-III in primary hypertriglyceridemia, they have offered an avenue for understanding the pathophysiology of the disease. The mechanism of primary hypertriglyceridemia has been extensively studied in these transgenic mice (47). These animals accumulate VLDL that is slightly larger than normal. The VLDL composition is appropriately triglyceride-rich, but there is altered apolipoprotein content with increased apo C-III and diminished apo E. The transgenic mice also have increased plasma free fatty acid levels. Metabolic studies indicate the primary abnormality to be decreased VLDL fractional catabolic rate with a small increase in the VLDL triglyceride but not the apo B production rate. In vitro the transgenic VLDL showed decreased LDL-receptor-mediated uptake by tissue culture cells but normal lipolysis by purified lipoprotein lipase. Thus, the hypertriglyceridemia appears to result from a prolonged VLDL residence time because of a combination of slightly increased production and delayed clearance, a process that, interestingly, does not lead to the accumulation of cholesterol-ester-enriched remnant particles. This implies decreased in vivo lipolysis and tissue uptake, presumably secondary to altered surface apolipoprotein composition.

There are two other C apolipoproteins in VLDL and HDL, apo C-I and apo C-II. Transgenic mouse models of hypertriglyceridemia have been made with both of them. Human apo C-I transgenics (48) are mildly hypertriglyceridemic and have not been extensively studied. The human apo C-II transgenic mice are as hypertriglyceridemic as the apo C-III transgenics, a surprising result when one considers that apo C-II is an activator of LPL (49). As with the human apo C-III transgenics, the human apo C-II transgenic mice accumulated VLDL of almost normal size but with an increased apo C/apo E ratio. These mice also had delayed VLDL clearance but did not have increased production. The human apo C-II transgenic mouse VLDL had markedly decreased binding to heparin-sepharose, suggesting that apo C-II-rich, apo E-poor VLDL may be less accessible to cell surface lipases or receptors within capillary-associated glycosaminoglycan matrices. The human apo C-II transgenic mice are a model of primary hypertriglyceridemia and suggest a more complex role for apo C-II in the metabolism of triglycerides than previously thought. Apo C-II deficiency is known to cause hypertriglyceridemia by decreasing LPL activity. It now appears that overproduction of apo C-II might do this as well, probably by preventing association of VLDL with matrix-bound LPL.

Hypertriglyceridemia is common in humans, but the known genetic abnormalities are quite rare. These transgenic mouse experiments prove that apo C-III and apo C-II overexpression can cause hypertriglyceridemia and suggest that apo C-III and apo C-II gene expression could regulate triglyceride levels in humans. Further evidence for the involvement of the apo C-III gene in hypertriglyceridemia has come from association studies in humans. Population studies have repeatedly shown that apo C-III alleles with an SstI restriction fragment length polymorphism in the 3′ untranslated region are more common in affected Caucasian hypertriglyceridemics than in controls. More recently, five new sites of genetic variation have been identified in the apo C-III gene promoter, and haplotyping utilizing these and the SstI site has revealed three classes of apo C-III alleles, susceptible, neutral, and protective with regard to hypertriglyceridemia (50). Further efforts are under way to identify the causative mutations and prove that apo C-III expression influences human triglyceride levels. In addition, a polymorphism of the apo C-II gene has recently been associated with hypertriglyceridemia (51). Although the association between apo C-II and apo C-III polymorphisms and hypertriglyceridemia may not necessarily be causative, transgenic animals have been critical in suggesting a role for these genes in primary hypertriglyceridemia. These studies demonstrate the utility of transgenic animals in unraveling clues to the genes underlying complex human traits, a process that may become an important paradigm in human genetics.

CETP Transgenic Mice

In the transgenic mouse models thus far described, HDL cholesterol and triglyceride levels have been altered relatively independently of one another. This is because the mouse lacks CETP activity in plasma. In humans it is thought that hypertriglyceridemia actually causes low HDL cholesterol levels through the CETP-mediated exchange of HDL cholesterol esters for triglycerides with subsequent HDL triglyceride hydrolysis by hepatic lipase. CETP deficiency has been described in humans as causing elevated HDL cholesterol levels and reduced levels of non-HDL cholesterol (52). CETP mutations occur frequently among Japanese and in this population are a common cause of high HDL cholesterol levels.

Transgenic techniques have been used to induce CETP activity in mouse plasma. A human CETP minigene driven by the inducible mouse metallothionein-I promoter was used to make a transgenic line with human-like levels of activity in plasma, which could be doubled by feeding zinc (53). After zinc induction, compared to control mice, these mice had 35% and 24% lower levels of HDL cholesterol and apo A-I, respectively, and a smaller HDL particle size (10 nm compared to 9.7 nm mean particle diameter).

These effects of CETP were less than expected based on studies comparing normal and CETP-deficient humans. One possibility for this difference is that mouse and human HDL are significantly different. In order to create mice with a more human-like HDL in the setting of CETP, the human CETP transgenic mice were crossed with human apo A-I transgenic mice. CETP was found to be more potent in mice expressing the human apo A-I transgene (54). After zinc induction, compared to the human apo A-I transgenic mice, the doubly transgenic mice had a more pronounced reduction in HDL cholesterol and apo A-I levels—66% and 42%, respectively—with smaller HDL particles (mean particle diameter of 10.4, 8.8, and 7.4 nm as compared to 9.7, 8.5, and 7.3 nm). In the doubly transgenic mice it was also found that 100% of the CETP was HDL associated, compared with 22% in the singly transgenic animals. Thus, CETP overexpression can reduce HDL cholesterol levels and particle size, an effect that is more dramatic in the setting of human apo A-I-containing HDL. This implies a specific interaction of human CETP with human apo A-I or the particles it produces.

Not only is the activity of human CETP in mouse plasma enhanced by HDL containing human apo A-I, but the CETP-mediated exchange of triglycerides for HDL cholesterol ester is driven by the level of VLDL triglyceride, which is quite low in the mouse. In order to study the relationship between high triglycerides and low HDL cholesterol, a CETP transgene was introduced into the hypertriglyceridemic human apo C-III transgenic mice that coexpressed human apo A-I (55). In these mice, human CETP gene expression reduced HDL cholesterol and apo A-I to very low levels with a dramatic reduction in HDL particle size. This mimics the high-triglyceride–low-HDL-cholesterol phenotype in humans, which is the most common lipoprotein disorder associated with susceptibility to coronary heart disease. The human apo A-I, apo C-III, CETP transgenic mice are the first animal model of this disorder. These animals provide insights into which genes may cause this abnormal phenotype in humans and present opportunities to study the mechanisms of the relationship between this lipoprotein abnormality and atherosclerosis susceptibility.

A cynomologus monkey CETP cDNA driven by the mouse metallothionein-I promoter has also been used to make mice with very high levels of CETP (56). The monkey CETP transgenic mice showed a strong inverse correlation of CETP activity with HDL cholesterol, apo A-I levels, and HDL size and a positive correlation of CETP activity with apo B levels and the size of apo-B-containing lipoproteins. The monkey CETP transgenic mice were also more diet responsive than control animals. Recently, human CETP transgenic mice were also found to show a gene-dosage-dependent effect on apo B levels (57). The experiments with human and monkey CETP transgenic mice confirm the proposed role of CETP in lipoprotein metabolism deduced from other systems and will make it possible to test the effect of CETP on cholesterol homeostasis, particularly reverse cholesterol transport, and atherosclerosis.

ELEVATED CHYLOMICRON REMNANTS AND IDL CHOLESTEROL

Although not normally present in large amounts in fasting plasma, nor commonly measured in coronary heart disease risk factor assessment, chylomicron remnants and IDL are cholesterol-ester-rich particles that are quite atherogenic. Chylomicron remnants and IDL particles are normally cleared from plasma by hepatic chylomicron remnant and LDL receptors, which recognize apo E on the surface of these particles (58). There are three common apo E alleles: E_3 (Caucasian frequency 77%), E_4 (15%), and E_2 (8%). These specify six common apo E phenotypes: $E_{3/3}$ (frequency 59%), $E_{4/4}$ (2%), $E_{2/2}$ (1%), $E_{4/3}$ (23%), $E_{3/2}$ (12%), and $E_{4/2}$ (2%). Mature apo E is 299 amino acids long, and E_4 differs from E_3 by a Cys^{112} Arg substitution, and E_2 differs from E_3 by an Arg^{158} Cys substitution. Apo E_2 is defective in receptor binding, whereas apo E_3 and E_4 bind receptors normally. Individuals with type III hyperlipoproteinemia, who have increased plasma levels of chylomicron remnants and IDL particles as a result of impaired catabolism, generally have the $E_{2/2}$ phenotype. These patients are susceptible to premature coronary heart disease, strokes, and peripheral vascular disease. Type III hyperlipoproteinemia can also be caused by heterozygosity for other rare mutations of apo E.

In addition to type III hyperlipoproteinemia, the apo E phenotype can affect LDL cholesterol levels, atherosclerosis susceptibility, longevity, and predisposition to Alzheimer's disease. Individuals with the $E_{4/3}$ genotype have mean LDL cholesterol levels 5 to 10 mg/dl higher than subjects with the $E_{3/3}$ genotype, and individuals with $E_{3/2}$ have LDL cholesterol levels 10 to 20 mg/dl lower than $E_{3/3}$ subjects (59). In an autopsy study of more than 500 young male trauma victims, $E_{3/2}$ was associated with reduced atherosclerosis relative to $E_{3/3}$ (60). Recently, studies of the elderly have revealed a decreased frequency of the E_4 allele, suggesting that this locus influences longevity (61). In a surprising finding, the E_4 allele has been found to be a risk factor for familial late-onset and sporadic Alzheimer's disease (62,62a). Clearly, mice with genetically altered apo E should provide interesting models for human disease.

Apo E Transgenic Mice

Human apo E transgenic mice have been made utilizing gene constructions containing natural flanking sequences (63,64). The apo E gene is in a cluster with two other apolipoprotein genes on human chromosome 19q13 (Fig. 2). The cluster consists, in order, of the apo E, apo C-I, and apo C-II genes. The genes are transcribed in the same orientation, and there is an apo C-I pseudogene between the apo C-I and apo C-II genes. The endogenous apo E gene is expressed primarily in the liver, with expression at lower levels in most body tissues. Human apo E transgenes extending from 5 kb 5′ to 2 kb 3′ of the gene gave low-level liver expression but high-level kidney expression. Studies have localized a region 11 kb 3′ to the apo E gene, between the apo C-I gene and the apo C-I pseudogene, that is required for high-level liver expression. This region also suppresses kidney expression and may also control the liver expression of the other two apolipoprotein genes in this cluster, apo C-I and apo C-II.

The initial human apo E transgenic mice were made with constructions that lacked the liver control element, and, as a result, the animals produced had relatively low levels of apo E expression with no significant effect of transgene expression on lipoprotein levels. Recently, transgenic mice have been made with the rat apo E gene driven by the metallothionein-I promoter (65,66). After zinc induction, these animals had a fourfold increase in apo E levels accompanied by a significant decrease in VLDL and LDL cholesterol levels. Metabolic studies indicated a severalfold increase in the clearance rate of radiolabeled VLDL and LDL, consistent with the established role for apo E in mediating lipoprotein uptake via the LDL receptor. In addition, these animals were resistant to diet-induced hypercholesterolemia. These studies indicate that apo E overexpression lowers fasting levels of atherogenic lipoproteins and can decrease the response of these lipoprotein fractions to a high-cholesterol diet.

Transgenic mice have also been made with mutant forms of apo E that can cause dominantly inherited type III hyperlipoproteinemia, including $E_{3\text{-Leiden}}$ (tandem duplication of apo E amino acids 120 to 126) (66a) and $E_{4\text{-Arg}^{142}\text{Cys}}$ (66b). In both cases the phenotype was similar, with increased levels of cholesterol and triglyceride in the VLDL and IDL lipoprotein fractions. The $E_{3\text{-Leiden}}$ mice were shown to be extremely responsive to dietary cholesterol. The $E_{3\text{-Leiden}}$ and the $E_{4\text{-Arg}^{142}\text{Cys}}$ mice appear to be reasonable phenocopies of human type III hyperlipoproteinemia and will be useful models to study the genetic and environmental factors which influence the expression of this disease.

Apo E-Deficient Mice

Apo E knockout mice with a true null mutation have also been created (67–69). Homozygous deficient animals are viable and fertile. On a chow diet, which is very low in cholesterol, 0.01% (w:w), and low in fat, 4.5%, they have cholesterol levels of 400 to 500 mg/dl (Table 3). Most of this is in the VLDL plus IDL lipoprotein fractions. When the homozygous apo E knockout mice are fed a Western-type diet (WTD), which has moderate amounts of cholesterol, 0.15%, and fat, 20%, they respond with cholesterol levels of approximately 1,800 mg/dl, also mostly in the VLDL plus IDL lipoprotein fractions (69). On both diets triglyceride levels are minimally elevated. The lipoprotein particles that accumulate in the apo E-deficient mice are similar in size to normal VLDL but are cholesterol ester enriched, similar to β-VLDL (70). Metabolic studies indicate a severe defect in lipoprotein clearance from plasma, as predicted from the known function of apo E as a ligand for lipoprotein receptors. The β-VLDL in the apo E-deficient mice are probably remnants of intestinally derived lipoproteins. Heterozygous apo E knockout mice have diminished plasma apo E levels, normal fasting lipoprotein levels, and slightly delayed postprandial lipoprotein clearance. Thus, half-normal apo E expression in the mouse is nearly sufficient for normal lipoprotein metabolism. As discussed below, the accumulation of atherogenic β-VLDL in the apo E knockout mice is sufficient to produce human-like atherosclerotic lesions.

TABLE 3. *Plasma lipoprotein levels in apo-E–deficient mice and humans[a]*

	TC (mg/dl)	VLDL-C (mg/dl)	HDL-C (mg/dl)
Mouse			
Apo E +/+	100	20	65
Apo E −/−	600	400	50
Apo E −/−, hApo A-I	600	400	100
Human			
Apo E +/+	200	15	50
Apo E −/−	500	250	50

[a] Values in this table represent approximate total plasma cholesterol (TC), VLDL cholesterol (VLDL-C), and HDL cholesterol (HDL-C) levels in control, apo E-deficient, and apo E-deficient mice that overexpress a human apo A-I (LApo A-I) transgene (from ref. 84). For comparison, approximate plasma cholesterol and lipoprotein levels are given for normal and apo E–deficient humans (from ref. 84).

ELEVATED LIPOPROTEIN (a)

In case-control studies, elevated levels of Lp(a) have been found to be an independent risk factor for coronary heart disease. Lipoprotein(a) consists of a large glycoprotein, apo (a), disulfide bonded to the apo B moiety of LDL. In humans levels of Lp(a) vary greatly from less than 0.1 to more than 200 mg/dl. Ninety percent of this variability is genetically determined by the apo (a) gene locus on human chromosome 6q25. Apo (a) resembles plasminogen, containing domains of plasminogen-like kringle IV in multiple copies and of plasminogen-like kringle V and protease in single copies. The protease domain of apo (a) is unable to degrade fibrin. Apo (a) alleles specify proteins that differ in size because of variation in the number of kringle-IV-like domains. The larger apo (a) size forms are associated with lower plasma Lp(a) levels and vice versa. Perhaps because of its resemblance to LDL, Lp(a) is a tightly bound constituent of the atherosclerotic plaque. In addition, through its plasminogen-like properties, Lp(a) may also participate in thrombogenic processes. In vitro it has been shown that Lp(a) can compete with plasminogen for binding to endothelial surfaces and in this manner interfere with the assembly of the fibrinolytic system on vascular surfaces. The physiological function of Lp(a) is unknown.

APO (a) Transgenic Mice

Lipoprotein(a) has a limited phylogenetic distribution and is found only in humans, Old World primates, and hedgehogs. Mice do not express apo (a), but transgenic animals have been made with a human apo (a) gene construction consisting of a cDNA containing 17 kringle IVs, one kringle V, and one protease-coding region driven by the transferrin promoter (71). In these mice expression was achieved in all tissues analyzed, whereas in humans the endogenous gene is normally expressed only in liver. Mean plasma levels equivalent to 9 mg/dl of Lp(a) were achieved, but, in contrast to humans, apo (a) was found in the lipoprotein-free fraction. Infusion of human LDL into these transgenic mice resulted in binding of apo (a) to these lipoproteins, indicating the formation of Lp(a). In addition, when apo (a) transgenic mice were cross-bred with human apo B transgenic mice Lp(a) was also formed (20,21). These experiments suggest that human apo (a) can bind to human apo B but not mouse apo B, perhaps because of the lack of conservation of a crucial cysteine in the mouse protein. These animals and others with higher levels of Lp(a) will be useful in defining the metabolism and function of this protein, eliciting how it participates in the atherosclerotic process, and designing effective pharmacological means for lowering Lp(a).

MOUSE MODELS OF ATHEROSCLEROSIS

The mouse is the best mammalian system for the study of genetic contributions to disease. This is because of easy breeding, the short generation time, and availability of inbred strains, many of which have interesting heritable phenotypes. Additionally, groups in the United States and England have created a refined genetic map of the mouse genome using polymorphic simple sequence repeats that can be assessed relatively easily with PCR (72,73). These markers can be used to map genetic elements associated with specific phenotypes, elements known as quantitative trait loci (QTLs). If a phenotype is well defined the associated QTL can be mapped on average to less than 4 centimorgans. In addition to the existence of interesting lines and the ability to map QTLs, the mouse is the only organism in which gene targeting can be performed. Unfortunately, the mouse is highly resistant to atherosclerosis (Table 2). The benefits of the mouse as a system for studying complex genetic diseases have, nevertheless, prompted substantial efforts directed at altering environment and genes in order to create an atherosclerosis-sensitive species. To date, these efforts have focused on altering the mouse's lipoprotein profile to create more atherogenic lipoprotein patterns (Table 4).

The C57BL/6 Mouse Model of Atherosclerosis

The first attempts at creating an atherosclerosis-sensitive mouse involved dietary interventions. Mice have been fed an unphysiological diet consisting of 1.25% cholesterol, 15% fat, and 0.5% cholic acid. This diet contains 10 to 20 times the amount of cholesterol of a human diet and an unnatural dietary constituent, cholic acid. Although this diet is toxic to mice when fed over a long time period, it does produce a cholesterol level of 200 to 300 mg/dl with increased non-HDL lipoproteins. This is in contrast to a standard chow diet, which produces cholesterol levels of 60 to 80 mg/dl, mostly in HDL. Although the majority of mice do not respond to the high-cholesterol diet, a handful of inbred mouse strains develop foam cell lesions at the base of the aorta in the region of the aortic valves when fed the diet for 4 to 5 months. In this model crosses between resistant and susceptible mouse strains have been used to identify three atherosclerosis susceptibility loci (74).

Transgenic Mouse Models of Atherosclerosis

Transgenic techniques have been used to further exploit this model. Studies in transgenic mice have been used to assess the role of apolipoprotein genes in determining atherosclerosis susceptibility by their ability to elevate HDL levels or alter its composition, to elevate non-HDL levels, or to do both. In these studies two approaches have been used: lipoprotein transport genes have been overexpressed in one of the susceptible strains, C57BL/6, and their effect on diet-induced atherosclerosis studied; and gene targeting has been used to assess the effect of deficiencies in two critical genes, apo A-I and apo E.

In the first study examining susceptibility to diet-induced fatty streaks, human apo A-I gene expression was found to reduce dramatically aortic sinus foam cell lesion area (75). These results suggest that apo A-I expression with its attendant increase in HDL cholesterol levels can protect against early events in atherogenesis. In a second study, human apo A-I and human apo A-II transgenic mice were crossed, and substantially less protection was seen when both genes were expressed than when only human apo A-I was expressed (76). In this study apo A-I only and apo A-I, A-II transgenic

TABLE 4. *Mouse models of atherosclerosis and the effect of lipoprotein-modifying genes on lesion formation*

Mouse model[a]	Transgene	non-HDL-C[b]	HDL-C[b]	Atherosclerosis
C57BL/6 diet-induced	None	↑↑	↓	Aortic root foam cells
	Apo A-I	↑↑	↑↑	↓↓↓↓[c]
	Apo A-II (human)	↑↑	↓	—[c]
	Apo A-I, apo A-II	↑↑	↑↑	↓[c]
	CETP	↑↑↑	↓↓	↑[c]
Hybrid diet-induced	None	↑↑	↓	No lesions
	Apo (a)	↑↑	↓	Aortic root foam cells
Apo E-deficient	None	↑↑↑↑	↓	Diffuse fibroproliferative atherosclerosis
	Apo A-I	↑↑↑↑	↑↑	↓↓↓↓[d]

[a] C57BL/6 are inbred mice fed an atherogenic high-cholesterol, high-fat, cholic acid-containing diet; the hybrid genetic mice are mixtures of C57BL/6 and a resistant strain also fed the atherogenic diet; apo E-deficient mice were fed a low-fat, mouse chow diet.

[b] As compared to chow-fed mice. C, cholesterol.

[c] As compared to C57BL/6 diet-induced mice.

[d] As compared to apo E-deficient mice.

mice had similarly elevated levels of HDL cholesterol; however, human apo A-II expression led to a decrease in the subpopulation of HDL that contained only apo A-I and an increase in the HDL population that contained both apo A-I and apo A-II. Because human apo A-II gene expression did not decrease HDL cholesterol levels but rather altered the composition of the existing HDL, this experiment suggests that not all HDL particles are equally antiatherogenic. Studies have likewise demonstrated that overexpression of mouse apo A-II leads to similar conclusions concerning the role of HDL protein composition in determining atherosclerosis susceptibility (77). Mice that express mouse apo A-II at two- to threefold higher levels than control mice have elevated HDL cholesterol. On a chow diet these mice develop small but detectable fatty streak lesions at the base of the aorta. Although other changes occur in these animals, such as the appearance of an unusual α-migrating apoB-containing particle and hypertriglyceridemia, the results question whether HDL levels alone are sufficient to predict individuals at risk for developing atherosclerotic heart disease.

In addition to HDL levels and HDL protein composition, other factors can determine the ability of HDL to influence atherosclerosis susceptibility. The ratio of non-HDL to HDL cholesterol in humans is an excellent predictor of CAD and suggests that the combination of elevated non-HDL cholesterol and decreased HDL cholesterol may create an atherogenic environment. This profile was created in a line of simian CETP transgenic mice made in the C57BL/6 inbred strain (78). The CETP activity was almost 20-fold greater in these mice than in humans. With this high level of CETP activity, a reciprocal increase in non-HDL and decrease in HDL cholesterol was observed. When challenged with the atherogenic high-cholesterol diet, these mice developed slightly more fatty streaks than control C57BL/6 animals. Of greatest interest to this study was that the degree of atherosclerosis could be correlated with the ratio of non-HDL to HDL cholesterol.

The fact that HDL levels alone are not sufficient to determine one's susceptibility to atherosclerosis was further demonstrated in apo A-I-deficient mice. These mice had an 80% reduction in HDL cholesterol but did not develop atherosclerosis on a chow, high-fat, or high-cholesterol diet (40,41). The suggestion is that elevated non-HDL cholesterol is necessary to create a susceptible environment and that increased or decreased HDL cholesterol acts primarily as a modifier.

The use of a high-cholesterol diet to induce fatty streaks has offered insight into the mechanism by which apo (a) is atherogenic. When fed the high-cholesterol diet, mice expressing a human apo (a) transgene develop fatty streak lesions at the base of the aorta (79). This result is striking in light of the observation that the majority of apo (a) in the plasma of these mice is free and not lipid associated. The conclusion from this study is that the atherogenicity of Lp(a) does not rely fully on the association of apo (a) with the lipoprotein particle. In future studies it will be important to determine whether the transgenic mice that overexpress human apo B and human apo (a) and have Lp(a) are more susceptible to diet-induced fatty streaks than the apo (a)-only mice.

The Apo-E–Deficient Mouse Model of Atherosclerosis

The apo E knockout mouse has provided a new model of atherosclerosis (68,69). Although these animals are outbred, representing a mixture of C67BL/6 and 129 strain genetic backgrounds, they develop widespread fibroproliferative atherosclerotic lesions when fed a chow diet (Fig. 3; see Colorplate 11 for 3C) (80,81). This is in contrast to the diet-induced C57BL/6 model, which requires an extremely high-cholesterol cholic acid diet to produce foam cells localized to the base of the aorta (74). In the apo E-deficient mice, lesions are widespread, developing at the base of the aorta and at the proximal coronaries as well as at the branch points of the major vessels coming off the aorta, including the ca-

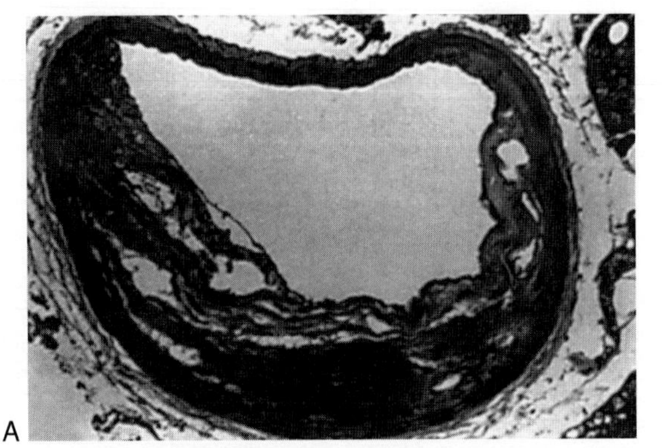

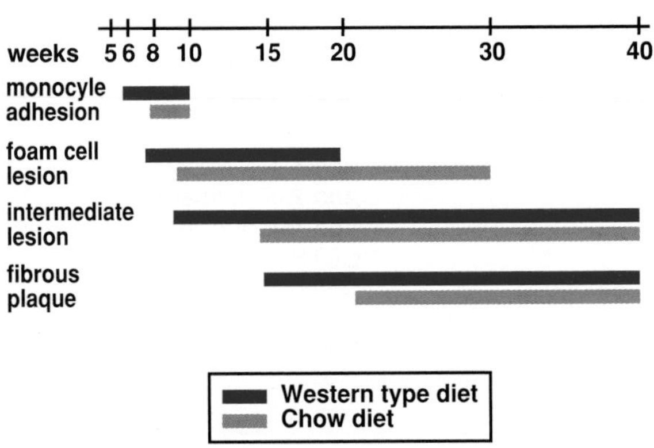

FIG. 3. Atherosclerosis in the apo E-deficient mouse. **A:** An advanced atherosclerotic fibrous plaque from the carotid artery of an apo E-deficient mouse. **B:** The progression of lesion formation in chow and Western-type diet fed apo E-deficient mice. **C:** An aorta from an apo E-deficient mouse stained for lipid with oil red O (see Colorplate section). **C,** from Palinski et al., ref. 82; (**A** and **B,** from Nakashima et al., ref. 80, with permission.)

rotid, intercostal, mesenteric, renal, and femoral arteries (80). Electron microscopy has demonstrated that these lesions probably begin by endothelial cell–monocyte adhesions that progresses to fatty streaks comprised of subintimal foam cells at 6 to 10 weeks of age. Unlike the other mouse models, these lesions rapidly progress to advanced lesions that contain muscular fibrous caps with extracellular matrix deposition and necrotic cores by 15 to 20 weeks of age (Fig. 3). Some lesions show fibrous plaques flanked by foam cells at the shoulder areas. Other lesions have medial necrosis with occasional aneurysm formation. Thus, the single genetic lesion causing apo E absence and severe hypercholesterolemia is sufficient to convert the mouse from a species that is highly resistant to one that is highly susceptible to atherosclerosis.

The apo E-deficient mouse model has proved valuable in assessing several issues concerning the role of environment and genes in atherosclerosis susceptibility. Initial experiments have demonstrated that the apo E-deficient mouse responds appropriately to a human-like Western-type diet containing 0.15% cholesterol and 20% fat. On this diet the progression of atherosclerotic lesions from monocytic adhesions to advanced plaques is accelerated, and the size of these lesions is much greater (69,80). This observation was important because it demonstrated that this model responds in the manner expected to the physiological high-fat diet, and suggests, in addition to the histological similarity to humans, a similarity in response to environmental cues. Other studies in this mouse have begun to address a pressing and controversial question in lipoprotein and vascular biology, the role of oxidized lipoproteins in atherosclerosis. In the apo E-deficient mouse, foam cell lesions are enriched in oxidized epitopes of lipoproteins, and the plasma of these mice contains very high levels of autoantibodies to oxidized lipoproteins (82). As in other systems, it remains to be determined whether the oxidation of lipoproteins in this mouse is cause or effect with respect to lesion development.

A more recent study has demonstrated that overexpression of human apo A-I can elevate HDL cholesterol levels, which can reduce the size and delay the onset of atherosclerotic lesions in the apoE-deficient mouse. The decrease in lesion size in the apo E-deficient, human apo A-I transgenic mouse was inversely proportional to the increase in HDL. Regression analysis indicated that variability in HDL could explain more than 75% of the variability of lesion size in the apo-E–deficient mouse (Fig. 4). This latter observation is remarkable because a very large degree of variability from no lesions to large lesions that occlude over 50% of the aorta can occur in this model. In light of this study and those mentioned above, further work in this model should be of great assistance in assessing the role of diet, genes, and drugs in atherosclerosis susceptibility and greatly accelerate research in this field.

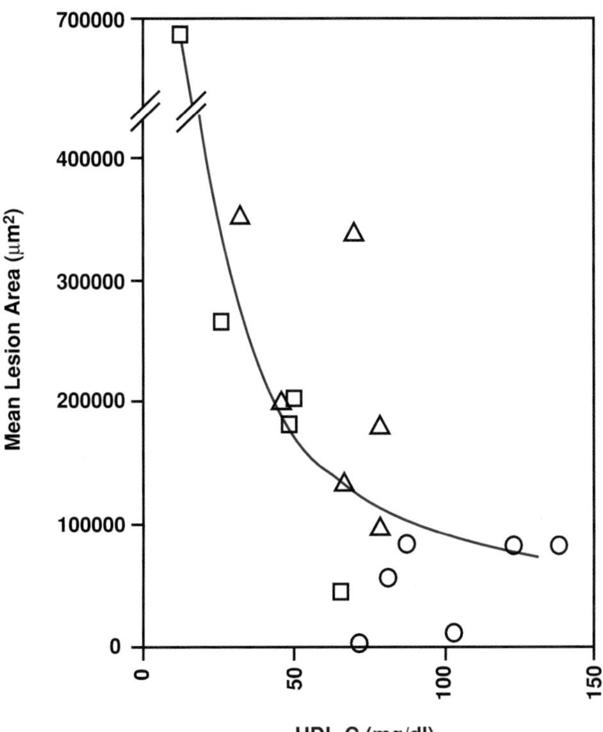

FIG. 4. Correlation of mean lesion area and HDL cholesterol levels in apo E-deficient and apo E-deficient, human apo A-I transgenic mice. *Squares,* apo E -/- mice; *triangles,* apo E -/-, low-expressing human apo A-I mice; *circles,* apo E -/-, high-expressing human apo A-I mice. (From Plump et al., ref. 83, with permission.)

SUMMARY

In humans, lipoprotein disorders are found in the majority of individuals with atherosclerotic heart disease. Four lipoprotein patterns are commonly recognized, including increased LDL cholesterol, reduced HDL cholesterol in association with elevated triglycerides, increased levels of IDL cholesterol and chylomicrons, and increased Lp(a). Conversely, increased HDL cholesterol, low LDL cholesterol, IDL cholesterol and chylomicron remnants, and absent or diminished Lp(a) are associated with resistance to atherosclerosis. Each of the protective profiles and each of the aberrant lipoprotein profiles either exists naturally or has been created in transgenic mice by overexpressing one or a combination of human lipoprotein transport genes or by disrupting endogenous mouse genes. The use of quantitative assays of fatty streak formation in the C57BL/6 diet-induced mouse model and of atherosclerosis in the apo-E–deficient mouse model has provided concrete evidence for involvement of several lipoprotein transport genes in the determination of atherosclerosis susceptibility.

REFERENCES

1. Breslow JL. Lipoprotein transport gene abnormalities underlying coronary heart disease susceptibility. *Annu Rev Med* 1991;42:357–371.

2. Breslow JL. Transgenic mouse models of lipoprotein metabolism and atherosclerosis. *Proc Natl Acad Sci USA* 1993;90:8314–8318.
3. Breslow JL. Insights into lipoprotein metabolism from studies in transgenic mice. *Annu Rev Physiol* 1994;56:797–810.
4. Breslow JL. Lipoprotein metabolism and atherosclerosis susceptibility in transgenic mice. *Curr Opin Lipidol* 1994;5:175–184.
5. Bierman EL. Atherosclerosis and other forms of arteriosclerosis. In: Wilson JD, Braunwald E, Isselbacher KJ, et al, eds. *Harrison's Principles of Internal Medicine,* 12th ed. New York: McGraw-Hill; 1991: 992–1001.
6. Brown MS, Goldstein JL. The hyperlipoproteinemias and other disorders of lipid metabolism. In: Wilson JD, Braunwald E, Isselbacher KJ, et al, eds. *Harrison's Principles of Internal Medicine,* 12th ed. New York: McGraw-Hill; 1991:1814–1825.
7. Goldstein JL, Brown MS. Familial hypercholesterolemia. In: Scrivner CR, Beaudet AL, Sly WS, Valle D, eds. *The Metabolic Basis of Inherited Disease,* Vol I, 6th ed. New York: McGraw-Hill; 1989:1215–1250.
8. Hofmann SL, Russell DW, Brown MS, Goldstein JL, Hammer RE. Overexpression of low density lipoprotein (LDL) receptor eliminates LDL from plasma in transgenic mice. *Science* 1988;239:1277–1281.
9. Yokode M, Hammer RE, Ishibashi S, Brown MS, Goldstein JL. Diet-induced hypercholesterolemia in mice: Prevention by overexpression of LDL receptors. *Science* 1990;250:1273–1275.
10. Hofmann SL, Eaton DL, Brown MS, McConathy WJ, Goldstein JL, Hammer RE. Overexpression of human low density lipoprotein receptors leads to accelerated catabolism of Lp(a) lipoprotein in transgenic mice. *J Clin Invest* 1990;85:1542–1547.
11. Pathak RK, Yokode M, Hammer RE, Hofmann SL, Brown MS, Goldstein JL, Anderson RGW. Tissue-specific sorting of the human LDL receptor in polarized epithelia of transgenic mice. *J Cell Biol* 1990; 111:347–359.
12. Ishibashi S, Brown MS, Goldstein JL, Gerard RD, Hammer RE, Herz J. Hypercholesterolemia in low density lipoprotein receptor knockout mice and its reversal by adenovirus-mediated gene delivery. *J Clin Invest* 1993;92:883–893.
13. Myant N. *Cholesterol Metabolism, LDL, and the LDL Receptor.* San Diego: Academic Press; 1990.
14. Grossman M, Raper SE, Kozarsky K, et al. Successful *ex vivo* gene therapy directed to liver in a patient with familial hypercholesterolemia. *Nature Genet* 1994;6:335–341.
15. Wilson JM, Chowdhury NR, Grossman M, Wajsman R, Epstein A, Mulligan RC, Chowdhury JR. Temporary amelioration of hyperlipidemia in low density lipoprotein receptor-deficient rabbits transplanted with genetically modified hepatocytes. *Proc Natl Acad Sci USA* 1990; 87:8437–8441.
15a. Chowdhury JR, Grossman M, Gupta S, Chowdhury NR, Baker JR Jr, Wilson JM. Long-term improvement of hypercholesterolemia after *ex vivo* gene therapy in LDLR-deficient rabbits. *Science* 1991;254: 1802–1805.
16. Wilson JM, Grossman M, Wu CH, Chowdhury NR, Wu GY, Chowdhury JR. Hepatocyte-directed gene transfer in vivo leads to transient improvement of hypercholesterolemia in low density lipoprotein receptor-deficient rabbits. *J Biol Chem* 1992;267:963–967.
17. Zannis VI, Kardassis D, Zanni EE. Genetic mutations affecting human lipoproteins, their receptors, and their enzymes. In: Harris H, Hirschhorn K, eds. *Advances in Human Genetics,* Vol 21. New York: Plenum Press; 1993:145–319.
18. Kane JP, Havel RJ. Disorders of the biogenesis and secretion of lipoproteins containing the B apolipoproteins. In: Scrivner CR, Beaudet AL, Sly WS, Valle D, eds. *The Metabolic Basis of Inherited Disease,* Vol. I, 6th ed. New York: McGraw-Hill; 1989:1139–1164.
19. Chiesa G, Johnson DF, Yao Z, Innerarity TL, Mahley RW, Young SG, Hammer RH, Hobbs HH. Expression of human apolipoprotein B100 in transgenic mice. *J Biol Chem* 1993;268:23747–23750.
20. Linton MF, Farese RV Jr, Chiesa G, Grass DS, Chin P, Hammer RE, Hobbs HH, Young SG. Transgenic mice expressing high plasma concentrations of human apolipoprotein B100 and lipoprotein(a). *J Clin Invest* 1993;92:3029–3037.
21. Callow MJ, Stoltzfus LJ, Lawn RM, Rubin EM. Expression of human apolipoprotein B and assembly of lipoprotein(a) in transgenic mice. *Proc Natl Acad Sci USA* 1994;91:2130–2134.
22. Homanics GE, Smith TJ, Zhang SH, Lee D, Young SG, Maeda N. Targeted modification of the apolipoprotein B gene results in hypobetalipoproteinemia and developmental abnormalities in mice. *Proc Natl Acad Sci USA* 1993;90:2389–2393.
23. Genest JJ Jr, Martin-Munley SS, McNamara JR, et al. Familial lipoprotein disorders in patients with premature coronary artery disease. *Circulation* 1992;85:2025–2033.
24. Eisenberg S. High density lipoprotein metabolism. *J Lipid Res* 1984; 25:1017–1058.
25. Brinton EA, Eisenberg S, Breslow JL. Human HDL cholesterol levels are determined by apo A-I fractional catabolic rate which correlates inversely with estimates of HDL particle size. Effects of gender, hepatic and lipoprotein lipases, triglyceride and insulin levels, and body fat distribution. *Artheroscler Thromb* 1994;14:707–720.
26. Walsh A, Ito Y, Breslow JL. High levels of human apolipoprotein A-I in transgenic mice result in increased plasma levels of small high density lipoprotein (HDL) particles comparable to human HDL_3. *J Biol Chem* 1989;264:6488–6494.
27. Walsh A, Azrolan N, Wang K, Marcigliano A, O'Connell A, Breslow JL. Intestinal expression of the human apo A-I gene in transgenic mice is controlled by a DNA region 3′ to the gene in the promoter of the adjacent convergently transcribed apo C-III gene. *J Lipid Res* 1993; 34:617–623.
28. Rubin EM, Ishida BY, Clift SM, Krauss RM. Expression of human apolipoprotein A-I in transgenic mice results in reduced plasma levels of murine apolipoprotein A-I and the appearance of two new high density lipoprotein size subclasses. *Proc Natl Acad Sci USA* 1991;88: 434–438.
29. Swanson ME, Hughes TE, St Denny I, France DS, Paterniti JR JR, Tapparelli C, Gfeller P, Burki K. High level expression of human apolipoprotein A-I in transgenic rats raises total serum high density lipoprotein cholesterol and lowers rat apolipoprotein A-I. *Transgen Res* 1992; 1:142–147.
30. Chajek-Shaul T, Hayek T, Walsh A, Breslow JL. Expression of the human apolipoprotein A-I gene in transgenic mice alters high density lipoprotein (HDL) particle size distribution and diminishes selective uptake of HDL cholesteryl esters. *Proc Natl Acad Sci USA* 1991;88: 6731–6735.
31. Hayek T, Ito Y, Azrolan N, Verdery RB, Aalto-Setälä K, Walsh A, Breslow JL. Dietary fat increases high density lipoprotein (HDL) levels both by increasing the transport rates and decreasing the fractional catabolic rates of HDL cholesterol ester and apolipoprotein (apo) A-I. *J Clin Invest* 1993;91:1665–1671.
32. Hayek T, Chajek-Shaul T, Walsh A, Azrolan N, Breslow JL. Probucol decreases apolipoprotein A-I transport rate in control and human apolipoprotein A-I transgenic mice. *Arterioscler Thromb* 1991;11: 1295–1302.
33. Owen JS, Gillett MPT, Hughes TE. Transgenic mice expressing human apolipoprotein A-I have sera with modest trypanolytic activity *in vitro* but remain susceptible to infection by *Trypanosoma brucei. J Lipid Res* 1992;33:1629–1646.
34. Levine DM, Parker TS, Donnelly TM, Walsh A, Rubin AL. *In vivo* protection against endotoxin by plasma high density lipoprotein. *Proc Natl Acad Sci USA* 1993;90:12040–12044.
35. Breslow JL. Familial disorders of high density lipoprotein metabolism. In: Scrivner CR, Beaudet AL, Sly WS, Valle D, eds. *The Metabolic Basis of Inherited Disease,* Vol I, 6th ed. New York: McGraw-Hill; 1251–1266.
36. Schaefer EJ, Heaton WH, Wetzel MG, Brewer HB Jr. Plasma apolipoprotein A-I absence associated with a marked reduction of high density lipoproteins and premature coronary artery disease. *Arteriosclerosis* 1982;2:16–26.
37. Hiasa Y, Maeda T, Mori H. Deficiency of apolipoproteins A-I and C-III and severe coronary heart disease. *Clin Cardiol* 1986;9:349–352.
38. Matsunga T, Hiasa Y, Yanagi Y, Maeda T, Hattori N, Yamakawa K, Yamanouchi Y, Tanaka I, Obara T, Hamaguchi H. Apolipoprotein A-I deficiency due to a codon 84 nonsense mutation of the apolipoprotein A-I gene. *Proc Natl Acad Sci USA* 1991;88:2793–2797.
38a. Lackner KJ, Dieplinger H, Nowicka G, Schmitz G. High density lipoprotein deficiency with xanthomas. *J Clin Invest* 1993;92:2262–2273.
39. Williamson R, Lee D, Hagaman J, Maeda N. Marked reduction of high density lipoprotein cholesterol in mice genetically modified to lack apolipoprotein A-I. *Proc Natl Acad Sci USA* 1992;89:7134–7138.
40. Plump AS, Hayek T, Walsh A, Breslow JL. Diminished HDL cholesterol ester flux in apo A-I deficient mice. *Circulation* 1993;88:I-422.
41. Li H, Reddick RL, Maeda N. Lack of apo A-I is not associated with

increased susceptibility to atherosclerosis in mice. *Arterioscler Thromb* 1993;13:1814–1821.

42. Schultz JR, Gong EL, McCall MR, Nichols AV, Clift SM, Rubin EM. Expression of human apolipoprotein A-II and its effect on high density lipoproteins in transgenic mice. *J Biol Chem* 1993;267:21630–21636.
43. Deeb SS, Takata K, Peng RL, Kajiyama G, Albers JJ. A splice-junction mutation responsible for familial apolipoprotein A-II deficiency. *Am J Hum Genet* 1990;46:822–827.
44. Hedrick CC, Castellani LW, Warden CH, Puppione DL, Lusis AJ. Influence of mouse apolipoprotein A-II on plasma lipoproteins in transgenic mice. *J Biol Chem* 1993;268:20676–20682.
45. Shimada M, Shimano H, Gotoda T, Yamamoto K, Kawamura M, Inaba T, Yazaki Y, Yamada N. Overexpression of human lipoprotein lipase in transgenic mice. *J Biol Chem* 1993;268:17924–17929.
46. Ito Y, Azrolan N, O'Connell A, Walsh A, Breslow JL. Hypertriglyceridemia as a result of human apolipoprotein CIII gene expression in transgenic mice. *Science* 1990;249:790–793.
47. Aalto-Setälä K, Fisher EA, Chen X, Chajek-Shaul T, Hayek T, Zechner R, Walsh A, Ramakrishnan R, Ginsberg HN, Breslow JL. Mechanism of hypertriglyceridemia in human apo CIII transgenic mice: Diminished VLDL fractional catabolic rate associated with increased apo CIII and reduced apo E on the particles. *J Clin Invest* 1992;90:1889–1900.
48. Simonet WS, Bucay N, Pitas RE, Lauer SJ, Taylor JM. Multiple tissue-specific elements control the apolipoprotein E/C-I gene locus in transgenic mice. *J Biol Chem* 1991;265:8651–8654.
49. Shachter NS, Hayek T, Leff T, Smith JD, Rosenberg DW, Walsh A, Ramakrishnan R, Ginsberg HN, Breslow JL. Overexpression of apolipoprotein CII causes hypertriglyceridemia in transgenic mice. *J Clin Invest* 1994;93:1683–1690.
50. Dammerman M, Sandkuijl LA, Halaas J, Chung W, Breslow JL. An apo CIII haplotype protective against hypertriglyceridemia is specified by novel promoter polymorphisms and a known 3′ untranslated region polymorphism. *Proc Natl Acad Sci USA* 1993;92:2262–2273.
51. Hegele RA, Connelly PW, Maguire GF, et al. An apolipoprotein CII mutation, CIILys19-Thr identified in patients with hyperlipidemia. *Disease Markers* 1991;9:73–80.
52. Tall AR. Plasma cholesteryl ester transfer protein. *J Lipid Res* 1993; 34:1255–1274.
53. Agellon LB, Walsh A, Hayek T, Moulin P, Jiang XC, Shelanski SA, Breslow JL, Tall AR. Reduced high density lipoprotein cholesterol in human cholesteryl ester transfer protein transgenic mice. *J Biol Chem* 1991;266:10796–10801.
54. Hayek T, Chajek-Shaul T, Walsh A, Agellon LB, Moulin P, Tall AR, Breslow JL. An interaction between the human cholesteryl ester transfer protein (CETP) and apolipoprotein A-I genes in transgenic mice results in a profound CETP-mediated depression of high density lipoprotein cholesterol levels. *J Clin Invest* 1992;90:505–510.
55. Hayek T, Azrolan N, Verdery RB, Walsh A, Chajek-Shaul T, Agellon LB, Tall AR, Breslow JL. Hypertriglyceridemia and cholesteryl ester transfer protein interact to dramatically alter high density lipoprotein levels, particle sizes, and metabolism. *J Clin Invest* 1993;92: 1143–1152.
56. Marotti KR, Castle CK, Murray RW, Rehberg EF, Polites HG, Melchior GW. The role of cholesteryl ester transfer protein in primate apolipoprotein A-I metabolism. Insights from studies with transgenic mice. *Arterioscler Thromb* 1992;12:736–744.
57. Jiang XC, Masucci-Magoulas L, Ma J, Lin M, Walsh A, Breslow JL, Tall A. Down regulation of LDL receptor mRNA in CETP transgenic mice: Mechanism to explain accumulation of lipoprotein B particle. *Circulation* 1993;88:I-421.
58. Mahley R. Apolipoprotein E: Cholesterol transport protein with an expanding role in cell biology. *Science* 1988;240:622–630.
59. Davignon J, Gregg R, Sing C. Apolipoprotein E polymorphism and atherosclerosis. *Arteriosclerosis* 1988;8:1–21.
60. Hixon J, and the PDAY Research Group. Apolipoprotein E polymorphisms affect atherosclerosis in young males. *Arterioscler Thromb* 1991;11:1237–1244.
61. Kervinen K, Savolainen MJ, Salokannel J, Hynninen A, Heikkinen J, Ehnholm C, Koistinen MJ, Kesaniemi YA. Apolipoprotein E and B polymorphisms—longevity factors assessed in nonagenarians. *Atherosclerosis* 1994;105:89–95.
62. Strittmatter WJ, Saunders AM, Schmechel D, Pericak-Vance M, Enqhild J, Salvesen GS, Roses AD. Apolipoprotein E: High-avidity binding to beta-amyloid and increased frequency of type 4 allele in late-onset familial Alzheimer disease. *Proc Natl Acad Sci USA* 1993;90: 1977–1981.

62a. Corder EH, Saunders AM, Strittmatter WJ, Schmechel DE, Gaskell PC, Small GW, Roses AD, Haines JL, Pericak-Vance MA. Gene dose of apolipoprotein E type 4 allele and the risk of Alzheimer's disease in late onset families. *Science* 1993;261:921–923.

63. Simonet WS, Bucay N, Lauer SJ, Wirak DO, Stevens ME, Weisgraber KH, Pitas RE, Taylor JM. In the absence of a downstream element, the apolipoprotein E gene is expressed at high levels in kidneys of transgenic mice. *J Biol Chem* 1990;265:10809–10812.
64. Smith JD, Plump AS, Hayek T, Walsh A, Breslow JL. Accumulation of human apolipoprotein E in the plasma of transgenic mice. *J Biol Chem* 1990;265:14709–14712.
65. Shimano H, Yamada N, Katsuki M, Shimada M, Gotoda T, Harada K, Murase T, Fukazawa C, Takaku F, Yazaki Y. Overexpression of apolipoprotein E in transgenic mice: Marked reduction in plasma lipoproteins except high density lipoprotein and resistance against diet-induced hypercholesterolemia. *Proc Natal Acad Sci USA* 1992;89: 1750–1754.
66. Shimano H, Yamada N, Katsuki M, Yamamoto K, Gotoda T, Harada K, Shimada M, Yazaki Y. Plasma lipoprotein metabolism in transgenic mice overexpressing apolipoprotein E. *J Clin Invest* 1992;90: 2084–2091.

66a. van der Maagdenberg AMJ, Hofker MH, Krimpenfort PJA, De Brujin I, van Vlijmen B, van der Boom H, Havekes LM, Frants RR. Transgenic mice carrying the apolipoprotein $E_{3\text{-Leiden}}$ gene exhibit hypercholesterolemia. *J Biol Chem* 1993;268:10540–10545.

66b. Fazio S, Lee Y, Sheng Z, Rall SC Jr. Type III hyperlipoproteinemic phenotype in transgenic mice expressing dysfunctional apolipoprotein E. *J Clin Invest* 1993;92:1497–1503.

67. Piedrahita JA, Zhang SH, Hagaman JR, Oliver PM, Maeda N. Generation of mice carrying a mutant apolipoprotein E gene inactivated by gene targeting in embryonic stem cells. *Proc Natl Acad Sci USA* 1992; 89:4471–4475.
68. Zhang SH, Reddick RL, Piedrahita JA, Maeda N. Spontaneous hypercholesterolemia and arterial lesions in mice lacking apolipoprotein E. *Science* 1992;258:468–471.
69. Plump AS, Smith JD, Hayek T, Aalto-Setälä K, Walsh A, Verstuyft JG, Rubin EM, Breslow JL. Severe hypercholesterolemia and atherosclerosis in apolipoprotein E-deficient mice created by homologous recombination in ES cells. *Cell* 1992;71:343–353.
70. Plump AS, Forte TM, Eisenberg S, Breslow JL. Atherogenic β-VLDL in the apo E-deficient mouse: Composition, origin, and fate. *Circulation* 1993;88:I-2.
71. Chiesa G, Hobbs HH, Koschinsky ML, Lawn RM, Maika SD, Hammer RE. Reconstitution of lipoprotein(a) by infusion of human low density lipoprotein into transgenic mice expressing human apolipoprotein(a). *J Biol Chem* 1992;267:24369–24374.
72. Dietrich W, Katz H, Lincoln SE, Shin H-S, Friedman F, Dracopoli NC, Lander ES. Genetic map of the mouse suitable for typing intraspecific crosses. *Genetics* 1992;131:423–427.
73. Copeland NG, Jenkins NA, Gilbert DJ, et al. A genetic linkage map of the mouse: Current applications and future prospects. *Science* 1993; 262:57–66.
74. Paigen B, Mitchell D, Reue K, Morrow A, Lusis A, LeBoeuf RC. Ath-1, a gene determining atherosclerosis susceptibility and high density lipoprotein levels in mice. *Proc Natl Acad Sci USA* 1987;84: 3763–3767.
75. Rubin EM, Krauss RM, Spangler EA, Verstuyft JF, Clift SM. Inhibition of early atherogenesis in transgenic mice by human apolipoprotein AI. *Nature* 1991;353:265–267.
76. Schultz JR, Verstuyft JG, Gong EL, Nichols AV, Rubin EM. Protein composition determines the anti-atherogenic properties of HDL in transgenic mice. *Nature* 1993;365:762–764.
77. Warden CH, Hedrick CC, Qiao J-H, Castellani LW, Lusis AJ. Atherosclerosis in transgenic mice overexpressing apolipoprotein A-II. *Science* 1993;261:469–472.
78. Marotti KR, Castle CK, Boyle TP, Lin AH, Murray RW, Melchior GW. Severe atherosclerosis in transgenic mice expressing simian cholesteryl ester transfer protein. *Nature* 1993;364:73–74.
79. Lawn RM, Wade DP, Hammer RE, Chiesa G, Verstuyft JG, Rubin EM. Atherogenesis in transgenic mice expressing human apolipoprotein(a). *Nature* 1992;360:670–671.

80. Nakashima Y, Plump AS, Raines EW, Breslow JL, Ross R. Apo E-deficient mice develop lesions of all phases of atherosclerosis throughout the arterial tree. *Arterioscler Thromb* 1994;14:133–140.
81. Reddick RL, Zhang SH, Maeda N. Atherosclerosis in mice lacking ApoE. *Arterioscler Thromb* 1994;14:141–147.
82. Palinski W, Ord VA, Plump AS, Breslow JL, Steinberg D, Witztum JL. Apolipoprotein E-deficient mice are a model of lipoprotein oxidation in atherogenesis: Demonstration of oxidation-specific epitopes in lesions and high titers of autoantibodies to malondialdehyde-lysine in serum. *Arterioscler Thromb* 1994;14:606–616.
83. Plump AS, Scott CJ, Breslow JL. Human apolipoprotein A-I gene expression increases high density lipoproteins and suppresses atherosclerosis in the apolipoprotein E-deficient mouse. *Proc Natl Acad Sci USA* 1994;91:9607–9611.
84. Schaefer EJ, Gregg RE, Ghiselli G, Forte TM, Ordovas JM, Zech LA, Brewer H Jr. Familial apolipoprotein E deficiency. *J Clin Invest* 1986; 78:1206–1219.

Atherosclerosis and Coronary Artery Disease, edited by V. Fuster, R. Ross, and E. J. Topol. Lippincott-Raven Publishers, Philadelphia © 1996.

CHAPTER 21

Assembly of Blood Vessels in the Embryo

Mark C. Fishman

Key Words: Angioblasts; Angiogenesis; Neural Crest; Vasculogenesis; VEGF

INTRODUCTION

The development of the vascular tree in the normal embryo is a field well trodden by classical anatomists but not yet by cell or molecular biologists. Future growth will be predictably robust, as exemplified by investigations in the related field of tumor angiogenesis (1), which illustrate the molecular richness to be anticipated, although many of the issues will differ. This chapter serves, therefore, more to outline the questions and current working theories for future work than to delineate a neatly packaged and completed opus.

ENDOTHELIAL ASSEMBLY: VASCULOGENESIS AND ANGIOGENESIS

In many species the first blood vessels are extraembryonic. These form from cellular aggregates on the yolk and include hemoglobin-synthesizing cells surrounded by endothelial cells. Neighboring blood islands fuse during development, generating vascular channels that grow toward and into the embryo. However, the vast majority of intraembryonic blood vessels develop even if the embryo is surgically separated from the extraembryonic source of vessels. Along with other evidence (2), this demonstrates that intraembryonic vessels arise primarily from intraembryonic angioblasts. Two mechanisms of blood vessel formation within the embryo have been distinguished (3). *Vasculogenesis* (4) refers to vessels formed de novo by in situ aggregation of individual angioblasts. *Angiogenesis* (5) refers to vessels generated by sprouting from preexisting vessels. One approach to tracking these processes has been transplantation between species, using markers specific for host or donor cells. With this method the origin of cells can be ascribed to transplanted or host tissue. This work shows that precursors for angioblasts are widely distributed throughout mesodermal tissue (the middle of the three germ layers). These angioblasts appear to be quite migratory and invasive (6).

The assembly of vessels proceeds in different manners in different regions (7–10). It appears that angioblasts are directed to form particular vessels in particular locations by information in the local environment rather than by their lineage or site of origin. The dorsal aortae, the first major intraembryonic vessels, appear to form by vasculogenesis, as angioblasts assemble into small vesicles along the axis of the embryo that then fuse to form a continuous system. The endocardium and posterior cardinal veins also appear to form by vasculogenesis but, in distinction to the dorsal aorta, may do so from angioblasts that migrate to the vessel site (11). Whether there really are populations of angioblasts that, autonomously, have different properties, or whether they are so guided by local cues, remains unknown. Sprouting from preexisting vessels (angiogenesis) appears to be the basis for formation of the intersomitic and vertebral arteries.

M. C. Fishman: Developmental Biology Laboratory and Cardiovascular Research Center, Massachusetts General Hospital, Charlestown, Massachusetts 02129; and Department of Medicine, Harvard Medical School, Boston, Massachusetts 02115.

The brain (12,13), kidney (14), thymus, and limb bud are vascularized by angiogenesis. In the case of the brain, for example, the neuroectoderm does not contain angioblasts, and capillaries first surround the brain and then, at specific times, form sprouts that grow and ramify within the neural tissue. Some internal organs, including lung, pancreas, spleen, and stomach, appear to contain their own angioblasts that assemble locally by vasculogenesis (8).

The embryonic heart functions for many days before it is vascularized. In the human, the heart beats by 3 weeks of gestation, but the coronary orifices are not present until after 5 weeks (15,16). The chick heart initiates contractions at stage 10 (about 1 day), but the myocardium is not vascularized until about 6 days (17). Presumably diffusion through the endocardium suffices for these early stages of development. The coronary progenitor cells are not intrinsic to the heart but rather arrive with the epicardial layer as it encloses the myocardium. They assemble in situ by vasculogenesis, the proximal portion of the tubes growing toward and eventually penetrating the aortic root at multiple sites, only two of which persist as the origins of the left and right coronary arteries. Single-cell tracking has proved that there are different progenitor cells for endothelial and for smooth muscle cells of the coronary arteries (18).

THE TRANSIENCE OF EMBRYONIC VESSELS

The anatomic embryology of the vasculature is well covered in textbooks (19,20). The embryonic circulation is very different from that of the adult. Many vessels are laid down later to be resorbed. A good example is the progressive changes in the aortic arch system, shown in Fig. 1. The bilateral aortic arches branch off of the aortic sac (the continuation of the truncus arteriosus) and extend through the mesenchyme to the bilateral dorsal aortae. These arches are formed during the fourth and fifth weeks of development. All six arches are not present simultaneously, and most disappear completely as development proceeds or leave only a small residu, for example, the maxillary artery from the former arch 1. A similar arch system is present in all vertebrates and is retained as the gill system in fish. In man, the truncus

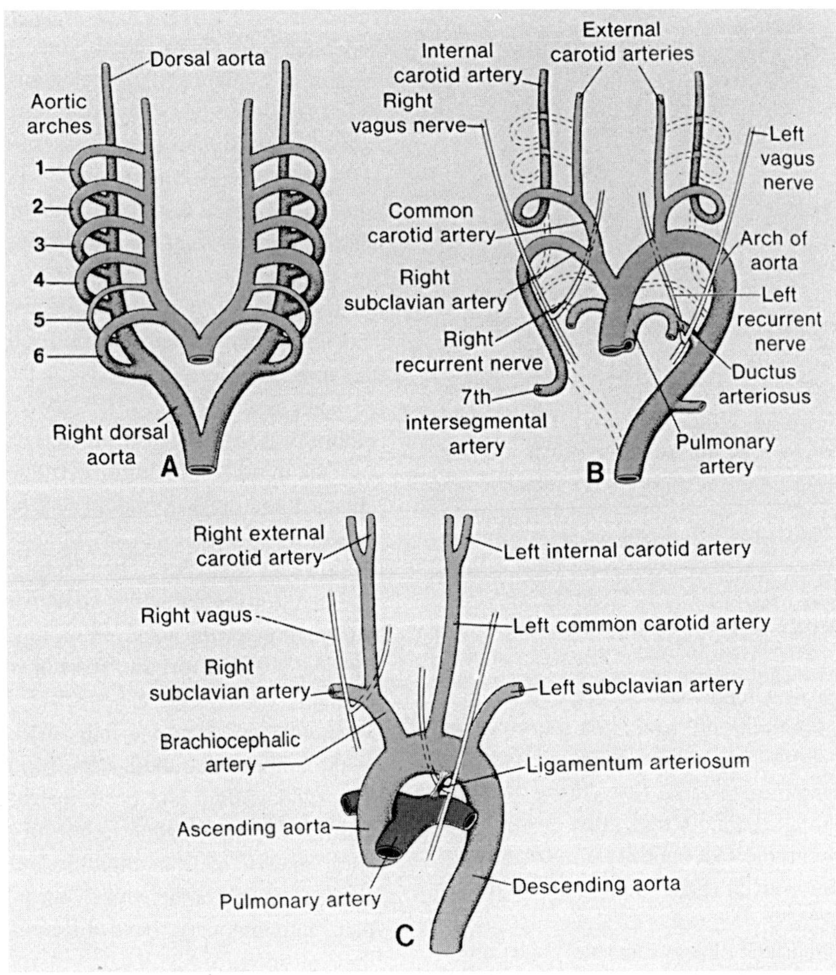

FIG. 1. (A) The idealized aortic arch system. In reality all six arches are not present simultaneously. **(B, C)** The maturation of the aortic arch system. (From Langman, ref. 43, with permission.)

arteriosus and aortic sac also develop a midline septum which will separate outflow from the left and right ventricles. The septation continues to the mouth of the sixth arches, which become the pulmonary arteries. Other arches become incorporated into the mature aortic arch itself or form other vessels to the head and neck, as shown in Fig. 1. The signals that guide these transformations are unknown.

MOLECULAR DETERMINANTS: GROWTH AND TUBULOGENESIS

Many factors have been described that enhance or retard angiogenesis, directed primarily at tumor angiogenesis (for recent review see ref. 1 as well as chapters in this volume). However, little is known about which of these function normally to guide formation of the vasculature during embryogenesis.

Vascular endothelial growth factor (VEGF) and its receptor are expressed in regions of the embryo that suggest that they do play a biological role in development (21). VEGF is a protein (actually several proteins generated by differential RNA splicing) that has mitogenic effects primarily on endothelial cells. It also promotes angiogenesis in test systems, such as the chick chorioallantoic membrane and collagen gels, and induces expression of other genes believed crucial to angiogenesis, such as urokinase and tissue-type plasminogen activators. Some VEGF isoforms are basic in charge and can bind to heparin, meaning that they could remain bound to the extracellular matrix.

VEGF binds to high-affinity sites on the endothelium (22–24). There are several VEGF receptor genes, including *flk-1* and *flt-1,* both of which encode single transmembrane-spanning receptors with a tyrosine kinase sequence intracellularly. In situ hybridization reveals *flk-1* transcripts in endothelia of developing capillaries and large vessels and in the perineural vascular plexus as vascular sprouts begin to invade the brain. It seems that *flk-1* may be expressed even prior to angioblast assembly into tubes (23). *flt* also is expressed in an endothelium-restricted manner in the developing embryo (24). This in vivo expression in the correct place and time is unlike that for the *bek* and *flg* receptors for FGF, which are expressed throughout many organs and only rarely on developing endothelia themselves. Where studied, the pattern of VEGF expression appears appropriate for activating the receptor. For example, in the developing brain, VEGF mRNA is in the ventricular layer of the neuroectoderm, toward which vessels grow and where they branch (25). It is, of course, likely that other ligand–receptor pairs function, perhaps differentially in different regions of the developing vasculature. For example, another presumptive tyrosine kinase receptor, *tie-2* (26), without known ligand, is expressed in developing endothelia throughout the body.

It is likely that assembly of the developing angioblasts into tubes is very dependent on particular cell adhesion molecules and on the extracellular matrix. The basement membrane of vessels, as for other tissues, includes laminin, type IV collagen, and proteoglycans, and, where studied, their secretion accompanies the earliest phases of blood vessel assembly (27). Evidence that adhesion molecules are involved derives from experiments showing, for example, that blocking of cellular integrins blocks the generation of a tube from angioblasts (28), as do antibodies to E-selectin (29). How such adhesion causes tubes is not clear, although if localized to opposite extremities of an endothelial cell, adhesion could serve to generate a tube. This role for E-selectin may be quite different from that induced during inflammation, which enhances leukocyte adhesion.

SMOOTH MUSCLE

As development proceeds, flattened endothelial cells continue as the lining, or *tunica intima,* of the vessels. Less is known about what generates the other, outer layers of blood vessels, i.e., the *tunica media,* which is populated by smooth muscle cells and an extracellular matrix rich in collagen and elastin, and the *tunica adventitia,* the outer layer, which includes blood vessels, nerves, fibroblasts, and collagen fibers. During embryonic mammalian development, the first indications of tunica media are mesenchymal condensation around the dorsal aorta, in the rat appearing 10 days after conception (with a 21-day gestation) (30). Even before this, loose mesenchymal cells in the vicinity of the aorta begin to express muscle actin, suggesting that they have begun to differentiate. These cells coalesce and begin to synthesize actin, desmin, and myosin, as the cells begin to generate the myofilaments that characterize the mature smooth muscle cell (31). The process begins in the cranial region of the aorta, and the tunica media subsequently envelopes the entire vascular system. There is a progressive relative decrease in cellularity and increase in connective tissue (32), presumably contributing to increased strength as blood pressure rises. Cell number increases by mitosis, even through the early postnatal period (33), after which the mitotic rate becomes very low in the absence of injury. It has been noted that regions of the vasculature from which new vessels originate lack a pronounced tunica media until the sprout has occurred (30).

The cellular phenotype of cells of the developing tunica media is of interest, in part because of a potential relationship to the neointima of the atherosclerotic plaque or to the restenotic injury generated by angioplasty. In the perinatal rat the cells are mitotically active and appear secretory rather than contractile, evidencing more prominent Golgi and rough endoplasmic reticulum. This activity is presumably responsible for the relative increase in extracellular matrix with development. Later in development, the cells become quiescent and generate myofibrils and become contractile (31). What drives withdrawal from the cell cycle is unknown, although a homeobox-containing transcription factor, *Gax,* has been proposed because *Gax* expression is almost entirely restricted to vascular smooth muscle in the adult and is down-regulated by growth factors (34). With development, actin, vimentin, desmin, and tropomyosin levels increase, and there is a shift in actin isoforms from β to α (35) and in the smooth muscle myosin heavy chain isoforms (36). The properties of cultured smooth muscle cells (obviously selected and altered in vitro) are different when obtained from embryos or neonates, the latter evidencing lower mitotic rates and sensitivity to certain growth factors (37). Cells with similar "embryonic" properties can be cultured from adult vessels of the rat (38). The resemblance between postnatal smooth muscle cells and those of injured vessels or neointimal lesions has suggested that there is at least a phenotypic similarity of the two cell types (38) or even that a subpopulation of relatively undifferentiated cells might persist and clonally expand under conditions of injury, or that there is a capacity for adult smooth muscle cells to dedifferentiate in the vicinity of injury. However, these studies in the rat may not extrapolate to the human vessel, and it will be very important to examine human atherosclerotic lesions to determine the nature of the smooth muscle cell populations.

THE NEURAL CREST

The musculoconnective tissues (including smooth muscle) of the large vessels that arise from the heart are unusual in that they are of neural crest rather than mesodermal origin (39). The neural crest is a transient structure containing neuroectodermal cells from the neural tube that migrate throughout the body, also giving rise to the sympathetic and parasympathetic nervous systems, the adrenal medulla, thyroid C cells, and melanocytes, among others. The neural crest has been studied extensively by quail/chick transplantation, because the two species do not reject each others' tissues and quail cells bear a characteristic histological marker. Some anterior neural crest cells migrate through the pharyngeal arches and give rise to mesenchymal tissues of the heart and vessels of the head. This domain of the neural crest is referred to as the "cardiac neural crest" and extends from the otic vesicle rostrally to somite 3 caudally. Those neural crest cells that remain in the arches form the nonendothelial supporting structures of the arches and eventually the tunica media of the great vessels that derive from them; those that continue toward the heart form the septum between the aorta and pulmonary artery. Disruption of this area causes a variety of cardiac malformations, including persistent truncus arteriosus and ventricular septal defect (VSD) or single outflow vessel as well as abnormalities of the aortic arch and great vessels (39). In some animals, removal of cardiac neural crest leaves regions of naked endothelium apposed to the pharyngeal endoderm.

How far into the heart the crest cells migrate is unsettled, although it appears that they do not contribute to the coronary arteries. The neural crest cells are committed to specific phenotypes even before they reach their cardiovascular destination. For example, persistent truncus arteriosus results not only from removal of the "cardiac" neural crest but if this region is replaced by neural crest tissue from other locations (40). This contrasts with the dramatic plasticity of neural crest cells in other locations. In other words, it seems that cardiac neural crest tissue is determined prior to arrival at its terminal destination.

FUTURE DIRECTIONS

Fashioning of blood vessels during embryogenesis could be a canonical system for understanding organogenesis. Although we know a great deal about single-cell fate decision making and differentiation, more obscure are the decisions that guide assembly into organ systems. For example, what determines size and limitations in cell number? How do tubes form and maintain their integrity? How are their diameters maintained and smooth interfaces generated between vessels? Because only a few distinct cell types are involved in the earliest blood vessels, at least as distinguished by current markers, the vascular system may be approached with more facility than some other organs, although the lessons may be transferable, because tubulogenesis is a nearly universal feature of organ formation. Clearly it will be crucial to understand inductive interactions between endothelial and smooth muscle cells as well as the tissue-specific signals that promote the particular types of vessel formation that characterize individual organs.

Many approaches might be taken to answer these questions, and different organisms may be more appropriate for different ones. For example, testing of angiogenic factors has been fruitfully studied using the chick chorioallantoic membrane or similar tissues (1). How cell fate decisions are made and the nature of the lineage relationship between blood and blood vessels will either require genetic marking of clonal progeny by inserted genes, such as for β-galactosidase (18), or single-cell tracking by use of injected dye (41). Ultimately, the function of relevant genes needs to be examined in their normal context in the intact animal, i.e., by genetics (42), perturbing either by overexpression or ablation in mice. Another powerful genetic approach is the genetic screen, in which the genome is "saturated" by mutagenesis in order to find most, or potentially all, genes involved in any given process. This has been used to great success in *D. melanogaster* and *C. elegans* but has been infeasible in vertebrates. The zebrafish holds great promise as a vertebrate amenable to largescale screens and to the study of cardiovascular development (42) because it can be raised and bred in the large numbers needed for such efforts, and its embryo is transparent, and the entire vascular tree is microscopically visible.

It will also be crucial to translate these molecular and cellular discoveries of developmental decisions to the study of vascular disease. The postinjury change in phenotype of smooth muscle cells and reendothelialization processes, as discussed in detail elsewhere in this volume, involve some of the same type of discrete phenotypic cellular changes that occur developmentally. It may be that in the embryo it is more feasible to dissect the responsible molecules than it is in the inhomogeneous injured tissue. Finally, it is at least worth speculating that banks of progenitor cells could be established to generate new vessels in their entirety.

REFERENCES

1. Folkman J, Shing Y. Angiogenesis. *J Biol Chem* 1992;267: 10931–10934.
2. Poole TJ, Coffin JD. Vasculogenesis and angiogensis: Two distinct morphogenetic mechanisms establish embryonic vascular pattern. *J Exp Zool* 1989;251:224–231.
3. Risau W, Sariola H, Zerwes HG, Sasse J, Ekblom P, Kemler R, Doetschman T. Vasculogenesis and angiogenesis in embryonic-stem-cell-derived embryoid bodies. *Development* 1988;102:471–478.
4. Gonzalez-Crussi F. Vasculogenesis in the chick embryo. An ultrastructural study. *Am J Anat* 1971;130:441–460.
5. Hertig AT. Angiogenesis in the early human chorion and in the primary placenta of the macaque monkey. *Contrib Embryol Carnegie Inst Washington* 1935;25:37–81.
6. Noden DM. Origins and assembly of avian embryonic blood vessels. *Ann NY Acad Sci* 1990;588:236–249.
7. Pardanaud L, Altmann C, Kitos P, Dieterlen-Lievre F, Buck CA. Vasculogenesis in the early quail blastodisc as studied with a monoclonal antibody recognizing endothelial cells. *Development* 1987;100: 339–349.
8. Pardanaud L, Yassine F, Dieterlen-Lievre F. Relationship between vasculogenesis, angiogenesis and haemopoiesis during avian ontogeny. *Development* 1989;105:473–485.
9. Coffin JD, Poole TJ. Endothelial cell origin and migration in embryonic heart and cranial blood vessel development. *Anat Rec* 1991;231: 383–395.
10. DeRuiter MC, Poelmann RE, Mentink MMT, Vaniperen L, Gittenberger-De Groot AC. Early formation of the vascular system in quail embryos. *Anat Rec* 1992;235:261–274.
11. Poole TJ, Coffin JD. Morphogenetic mechanisms in avian vascular development. *Dev Vasc Syst* 1991;14:25–36.
12. Stewart PA, Wiley MJ. Developing nervous tissue induces formation of blood–brain barrier characteristics in invading endothelial cells: A study using quail–chick transplantation chimeras. *Dev Biol* 1981;84: 183–192.
13. Risau W. Developing brain produces an angiogenesis factor. *Proc Natl Acad Sci USA* 1986;83:3855–3859.
14. Sariola H, Ekblom P, Lehtonen E, Saxen L. Differentiation and vascularization of the metanephric kidney grafted on the chorioallantoic membrane. *Dev Biol* 1983;96:427–435.
15. Bogers AJJC, Gittenberger-de Groot AC, Dubbeldam JA, Huysmans HA. The inadequacy of existing theories on the development of the proximal coronary arteries and their connexions with the arterial trunks. *Int J Cardiol* 1988;20:117–123.
16. Hutchins GM, Kessler-Hanna A, Moore GW. Development of the coronary arteries in the embryonic human heart. *Circulation* 1988;77: 1250–1257.
17. Rychter Z, Ostadal B. Mechanism of the development of coronary arteries in chick embryo. *Fol Morphol* 1971;XIX:113–124.
18. Mikawa T, Fischman DA. Retroviral analysis of cardiac morphogenesis: Discontinuous formation of coronary vessels. *Proc Natl Acad Sci USA* 1992;89:9504–9508.
19. Arey LB. *Developmental Anatomy*. Philadelphia: WB Saunders; 1934.
20. Sadler TW. *Langman's Medical Embryology*. Baltimore: Williams & Wilkins; 1990.
21. Ferrara N. Vascular endothelial growth factor. *Trends Cardiovasc Med* 1993;3:244–250.
22. Eichmann A, Marcelle C, Breant C, Le Douarin NM. Two molecules related to the VEGF receptor are expressed in early endothelial cells during avian embryonic development. *Mech Dev* 1993;42:33–48.
23. Millauer B, Wizigmann-Voos S, Schnurch H, Martinez R, Moller NPH, Risau W, Ullrich A. High affinity VEGF binding and developmental expression suggest *Flk-1* as a major regulator of vasculogenesis and angiogenesis. *Cell* 1993;72:835–846.
24. Peters KG, De Vries C, Williams LT. Vascular endothelial growth factor receptor expression during embryogenesis and tissue repair suggests a role in endothelial differentiation and blood vessel growth. *Dev Biol* 1993;90:8915–8919.
25. Breier G, Albrecht U, Sterrer S, Risau W. Expression of vascular endothelial growth factor during embryonic angiogenesis and endothelial cell differentiation. *Development* 1992;114:521–532.
26. Schnurch H, Risau W. Expression of *tie-2*, a member of a novel family of receptor tyrosine kinases, in the endothelial cell lineage. *Development* 1993;119:957–968.
27. Ekblom P, Klein G, Ekblom M, Sorokin L. The basement membrane of embryonic blood vessels. In: Feinberg RN, Sherer GK, Auerbach R, eds. *The Development of the Vascular System*. 1991;81–92.
28. Drake CJ, Davis LA, Little CD. Antibodies to β_1-integrins cause alterations of aortic vasculogenesis, in vivo. *Dev Dynam* 1992;193:83–91.
29. Nguyen M, Strubel NA, Bischoff J. A role for sialyl Lewis-X/A glycoconjugates in capillary morphogenesis. *Nature* 1993;365:267–270.
30. DeRuiter MC, Poelmann RE, Van Iperen L, Gittenberger-de Groot AC. The early development of the tunica media in the vascular system of rat embryos. *Anat Embryol* 1990;181:341–349.
31. Cliff WJ. The aortic tunica media in growing rats studied with the electron microscope. *Lab Invest* 1967;17:599–615.
32. Gerrity RG, Cliff WJ. The aortic tunica media of the developing rat. I. Quantitative stereologic and biochemical analysis. *Lab Invest* 1975; 32:585–600.
33. Berry CL, Looker T, Germain J. The growth and development of the rat aorta. I. Morphological aspects. *J Anat* 1972;113:1–16.
34. Gorski DH, Patel CV, Walsh K. Homeobox transcription factor regulation in the cardiovascular system. *Trends Cardiovasc Med* 1993;3: 184–190.
35. Kocher O, Skalli O, Cerutti K, Gabbiani F, Gabbiani G. Cytoskeletal features of rat aortic cells during development. *Circ Res* 1985;56: 829–838.
36. Aikawa M, Sivam PN, Kuro-o M, Kimura K, Nakahara K, Takewaki S, Ueda M, Yamaguchi H, Yazaki Y, Periasamy M, Nagai R. Human smooth muscle myosin heavy chain isoforms as molecular markers for vascular development and atherosclerosis. *Circ Res* 1993;73: 1000–1012.
37. Cook CL, Weiser MCM, Schwartz PE, Jones CL, Majack RA. Developmentally timed expression of an embryonic growth phenotype in vascular smooth muscle cells. *Circ Res* 1994;74:189–196.
38. Schwartz SM, Foy L, Bowen-Pope DF, Ross R. Derivation and properties of platelet-derived growth factor-independent rat smooth muscle cells. *Am Pathol* 1990;136:1417–1428.
39. Kirby ML, Waldo KL. Role of neural crest in congenital heart disease. *Circulation* 1990;82:332–340.
40. Kirby ML. Plasticity and predetermination of mesencephalic and trunk neural crest transplanted into the region of the cardiac neural crest. *Dev Biol* 1989;134:402–412.
41. Stainier DYR, Lee RK, Fishman MC. Cardiovascular development in the zebrafish: I. Myocardial fate map and heart tube formation. *Development* 1993;119:31–40.
42. Fishman MC, Stainier DYR. Cardiovascular development: Prospects for a genetic approach. *Circ Res* 1994;74:757–763.

The Normal Artery

Atherosclerosis and Coronary Artery Disease,
edited by V. Fuster, R. Ross, and E. J. Topol.
Lippincott-Raven Publishers, Philadelphia © 1996.

CHAPTER 22

Vascular Endothelium

Paul E. DiCorleto and Michael A. Gimbrone, Jr.

Key words: Adhesion molecules; Cytokines; Endothelial dysfunction; Endothelium-derived relaxing factor; Platelet-derived growth factor; Transforming growth factor-β; Vascular endothelium.

INTRODUCTION

The entire circulatory system is lined by a continuous, single-cell-thick membrane—the vascular endothelium. In the aorta and its main branches (e.g., the coronary arteries), this transparent tissue, together with a modest amount of extracellular matrix, constitutes the normal tunica intima. It is this inner concentric layer of the artery wall that is the primary locus of the atherosclerotic disease process. More than a century ago, anatomic pathologists began to catalog the gross and microscopic changes involving the intima that mark the progression from the early fatty streak lesion to the clinically important complicated plaque (1). However, an appreciation of the pathogenetic mechanisms underlying these changes has developed only recently, largely through the application of modern cellular and molecular biological techniques (2). During the course of these studies, the working concept of the role of vascular endothelium in health and disease has undergone a dramatic evolution. Originally viewed simply as a passive barrier or insulation, the endothelial lining is now considered to be a multifunctional organ whose health is essential to normal vascular physiology, and whose dysfunction can be a critical factor in the pathogenesis of vascular disease (3–8).

In health, vascular endothelium comprises a ''container'' for blood, and forms the biologic interface between circulating blood components and all of the various tissues of the body. It is strategically situated to monitor systemic as well as locally generated stimuli and to alter its functional state (Fig. 1). This adaptive process typically proceeds without notice, contributing to normal homeostasis. However, nonadaptive changes in endothelial structure and function, provoked by pathophysiologic stimuli, can result in localized, acute and chronic, alterations in the interactions of endothelium with the cellular and macromolecular components of circulating blood and of the blood vessel wall (Fig. 2). These alterations include enhanced permeability to (and subsequent oxidative modification of) plasma lipoproteins, hyperadhesiveness for blood leukocytes, and functional imbalances in local pro- and antithrombotic factors, growth stimulators and inhibitors, and vasoactive (dilator, constrictor) substances. These manifestations, collectively termed *endothelial dysfunction,* play an important role in the initiation, progression, and clinical complications of various forms of inflammatory and degenerative vascular diseases.

P. E. DiCorleto: Department of Cell Biology-NC10, Cleveland Clinic Research Institute, Cleveland, Ohio 44195.
M. A. Gimbrone, Jr.: Vascular Research Division, Department of Pathology, Harvard Medical School and Brigham and Women's Hospital, Boston, Massachusetts 02115-5817.

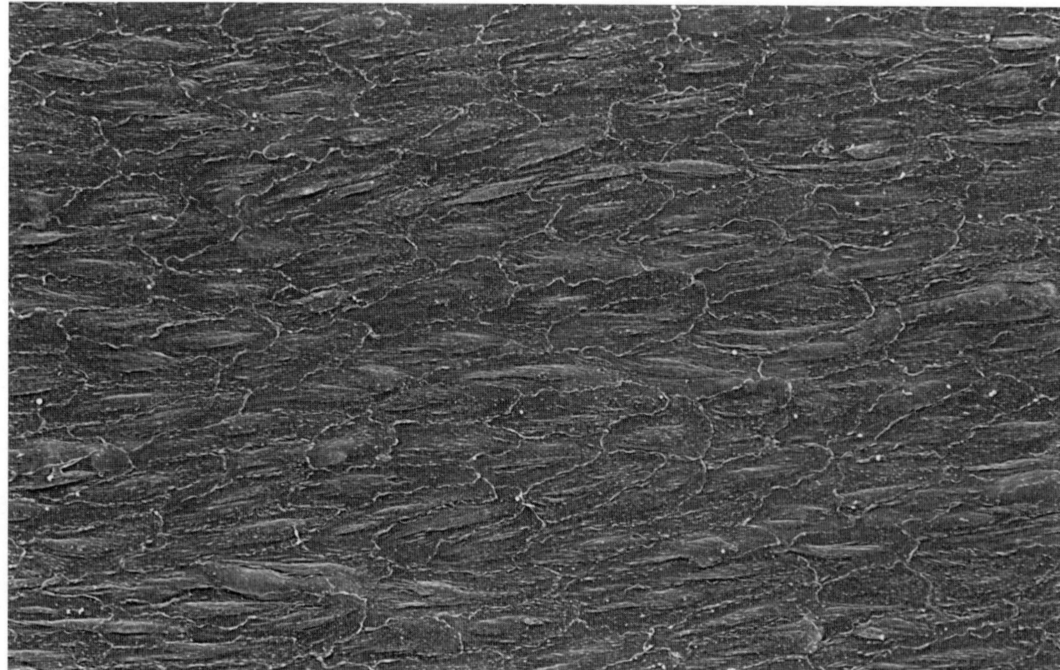

FIG. 1. An *en face* view of arterial endothelium in a normal monkey thoracic aorta. The outlines of the individual endothelial cells can be readily determined. In addition, the location of the nucleus can be seen by the area that is slightly raised over the nuclear prominence in many of the cells. The circulation runs longitudinally from left to right or right to left.

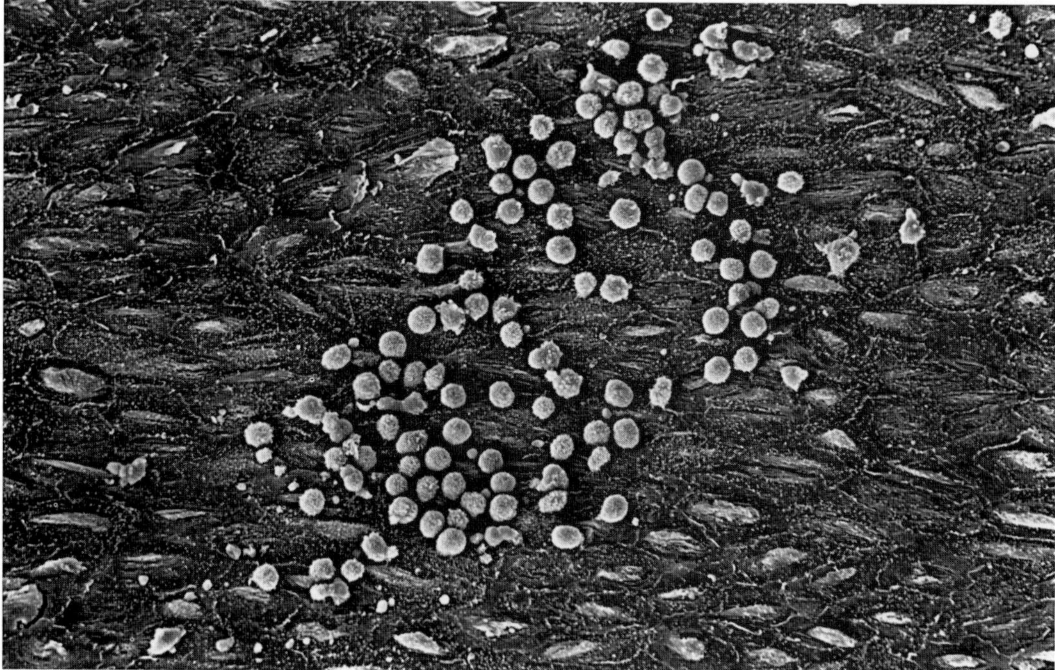

FIG. 2. An *en face* view of a thoracic aorta near a branch point from a hyperlipidemic nonhuman primate where a cluster of leukocytes (both monocytes and T lymphocytes) has adhered to the surface of the endothelium. The endothelium is more cuboidal in shape than that seen in Fig. 1. Presumably, adhesion molecules such as vascular cell adhesion molecule-1 and intercellular adhesion molecule-1 may have formed on the surface to induce the leukocyte adherence in this scanning electron micrograph. This figure represents one of the earliest phases of functional alteration of endothelium in the arterial tree.

This chapter will briefly summarize our current understanding of normal endothelial biology, thus providing a background for discussion of its role in the pathogenesis of atherosclerotic lesions and their thrombotic, inflammatory, and vasospastic complications. We will also consider how insights gained from basic research in endothelial biology and pathobiology may help direct the development of novel diagnostic and therapeutic strategies in coronary artery disease.

NORMAL VASCULAR ENDOTHELIUM

Anatomic and Functional Organization

Interface Location

By virtue of its *anatomic location,* vascular endothelium is a biologically significant interface: it defines intra- and extravascular compartments, serves as a selectively permeable barrier, and provides a continuous nonthrombogenic lining for the cardiovascular system. Its location is also a key factor in its dynamic, reciprocal interactions with other cells, both in the circulating blood and within the vessel wall proper. Thus, endothelial cells, situated at the vessel wall–blood interface, can speak outward to platelets and leukocytes, or inward to smooth muscle cells. This intercellular communication can occur at close range (e.g., endothelial-derived vasorelaxor substances acting on adjacent vascular smooth muscle cells) or at a distance (e.g., endothelial-derived colony-stimulating factors acting on hematopoietic precursors in the bone marrow). In addition, each of the cellular components in these interactions may be subject to modulating influences exerted by extracellular matrix components, many of which are biosynthesized by vascular endothelium. Another functionally important consequence of endothelium's location is its ability to monitor, integrate, and transduce blood-borne signals, thus making it a form of "sensory organ." As will be considered in more detail below, this property extends beyond the realm of soluble stimuli (e.g., hormones, cytokines, bacterial products) to the biotransduction of various types of mechanical forces generated by pulsatile blood flow (e.g., fluid shear stresses, wall tension, intraluminal pressure).

Surface Area

A second important aspect of the structural organization of endothelium is its broad luminal *surface area.* Endothelium is the body's most extensive simple epithelium, its aggregate area totaling several thousand square meters (9). This essentially continuous expanse of living cell membrane can function as a vast solid-phase reactor, a highly selective affinity chromatography "column," or a relatively nonspecific adsorptive "sponge." These surface-related activities are especially enhanced in the microcirculation, where the ratio of the surface of the endothelial container to the volume of contained blood reaches a maximum. The realization that the walls of this *in vivo* blood container can actively participate in the biochemical reactions of blood constituents represents a significant conceptual advance (3,4). Equally important from the pathophysiologic standpoint, is the fact that key surface-related functions of vascular endothelium can be dynamically modulated, thus making the luminal endothelial surface a locus of physiologic regulation and pathologic alteration (10–12).

Regional Specialization

Another relevant aspect of endothelial organization is its *regional specialization.* Despite its apparent morphologic simplicity and relative homogeneity, there is increasing evidence that the vascular endothelial lining does exhibit site-to-site variations that may have important physiologic and pathophysiologic implications. These differences are manifested in properties such as permeability to macromolecules, secretion of biosynthetic products, and responsiveness to various exogenous mediators (13). Interestingly, the question of regional specialization extends down to the level of the individual endothelial cell. For example, ultrastructural techniques have demonstrated the existence of "microdomains" in the luminal surface membrane of endothelial cells that appear to have characteristic patterns in different tissues (14). In addition, despite its thin configuration, each vascular endothelial cell appears to have a clearly definable "apical" or luminal surface, which faces the bloodstream, and a "basal" or abluminal surface, which is in contact with the subendothelial connective tissues, each outfitted with its own distinct complement of intrinsic proteins (15).

Taken together, these basic principles of endothelial organization—its interface location, dynamic surface properties, and regional specialization—have important implications for the vital functions of this tissue in health and disease.

Vital Functions of Endothelium

Selective Permeability Barrier

Endothelium is the primary anatomic site for restriction of macromolecular flux between the blood and the extravascular space. When viewed with the electron microscope, the endothelial lining of the heart and large arteries is of the continuous type. In distinction to the fenestrated and discontinuous varieties found in other settings, continuous endothelium is characterized by tight junctions at the lateral borders of each cell, which restrict the movement of macromolecules such as albumin, and a complex microvesicular system, which has been implicated in macromolecular transport. The latter consists of simple vesicles or caveolae, branched surface-connected canaliculi, and beaded transcellular channels (16,17). In addition, the endothelial surface-associated glycocalyx contains sulfated glycosaminoglycans and other charged species that can selectively adsorb certain macromolecules, for example, growth factors and cytokines.

Dramatic changes can occur in endothelial permeability to blood-borne molecules, acutely and chronically, in response to various physiologic and pathophysiologic stimuli. For example, histamine and other acute inflammatory mediators can act directly on microvascular (primarily postcapillary venular) endothelial cells to stimulate opening of their intercellular junctions, thus permitting rapid exudation of protein-rich fluid into the extravascular space (18). This gap formation is accompanied by endothelial shape change, presumably reflecting an energy-dependent, calcium-mediated cellular contraction process. Thrombin and certain other mediators also appear to induce a pericellular leak via a similar mechanism. It has been suggested that macrovascular endothelium (arterial and venous) can respond acutely to certain soluble mediators with a similar type of permeability change, and that transient gap formation may contribute to the trapping of the relatively large lipoprotein particles in the subendothelial space.

Detailed studies of atherosclerosis lesion-prone areas in hypercholesterolemic rabbits and other animal models have documented enhanced lipoprotein permeability, manifested by the accumulation of plasma-derived low-density lipoprotein (LDL) and β very low density lipoprotein (β-VLDL), primarily via the transcytotic route (19). Normal LDL particles also can enter endothelial cells via the standard LDL receptor-mediated endocytic route, and are then subject to hydrolysis with reesterification of their cholesterol contents, analogous to this process in other cell types. However, in response to elevated plasma levels of lipoproteins, this receptor-mediated pathway usually is downregulated. Lipoproteins delivered to the subendothelial space in hypercholesterolemic animals appear to undergo a complex process of oxidative and physicochemical modification, and can accumulate in relatively large quantities extracellularly in association with newly synthesized, proteoglycan-rich matrix material (20). Endothelial cells, as well as other cells in developing atherosclerotic plaques, can contribute to the oxidative modification of LDL, which results in its endocytic uptake via so-called "scavenger receptors," as discussed elsewhere in this book. In addition, components of oxidized lipoproteins, such as lysophosphatidylcholine, can act on endothelial cells to modify their expression of growth factors, cytokines, and adhesion molecules (21,22). The multiple potential interactions of lipoproteins with endothelium and other cellular components of developing atherosclerotic lesions are considered in more detail below and elsewhere in this book.

The Hemostatic/Thrombotic Balance

Blood normally does not clot inside of its endothelial "container." This failure of endothelium to activate the coagulation cascade or to promote platelet adhesion has been termed "nonthrombogenicity." For many years, this vital function was considered simply as a passive form of insulation, attributable to ill-defined physicochemical properties of the luminal endothelial surface. With the discovery that the vascular wall and, in particular, endothelial cells (23) could synthesize the unique arachidonate metabolite prostacyclin (PGI_2), which proved to be an extraordinarily potent inhibitor of platelet aggregation, a more active "antithrombotic" role for endothelium became apparent. In addition to its major influence on platelet function, endothelium also plays a pivotal role in the coagulation and fibrinolytic system (24). Many of these functions appear to be antithrombotic in nature. For example, several of the body's natural anticoagulant mechanisms (25), including the heparin–antithrombin mechanism, the protein C–thrombomodulin mechanism, and the tissue plasminogen activator mechanism, are endothelial-associated. The molecular components of various of these antithrombotic mechanisms are considered in detail elsewhere in this book.

In contrast to these antithrombotic functions, the endothelial cell also appears capable of active "prothrombotic" behavior. It synthesizes adhesive cofactors for platelets, such as von Willebrand factor, fibronectin, and thrombospondin; procoagulant components, such as factor V; and, as discussed below, can be activated by various pathophysiologic stimuli to express tissue factor, a trigger for the fibrin-generating coagulation cascade (26). Endothelium also generates an inhibitor of the fibrinolytic pathway (plasminogen activator inhibitor-1, PAI-1), which can reduce the rate of fibrin breakdown. Thus, the endothelial cell appears capable of playing a number of roles, both "pro-" and "anti-" hemostatic/thrombotic, that are relevant to maintaining normal blood fluidity, stopping hemorrhage at sites of vascular injury, and affecting pathologic thrombosis. As schematically illustrated in Fig. 3, these endothelial-dependent mechanisms contribute to a dynamic physiologic antagonism or "balance" which can significantly influence the status of local hemostatic/thrombotic activity.

The Vasoconstrictor/Vasodilator Balance

The maintenance of cardiovascular tone traditionally has been viewed as a function of the vascular smooth muscle cell, responding primarily to sympathetic/parasympathetic nerve stimulation or circulating hormones (e.g., products of the renin–angiotensin system). In 1980, the discovery by Furchgott and Zawadzki (27) of a potent endothelium-derived relaxing factor (EDRF) pointed to a significant role for the vascular endothelial cell in the *local* regulation of vascular tone. The elucidation of the chemical nature of EDRF as endogenous nitric oxide, its metabolic pathway of generation via (one or more) nitric oxide synthases, and the cellular mechanisms of its action that result in vasodilatation has added a new dimension to our understanding of the role

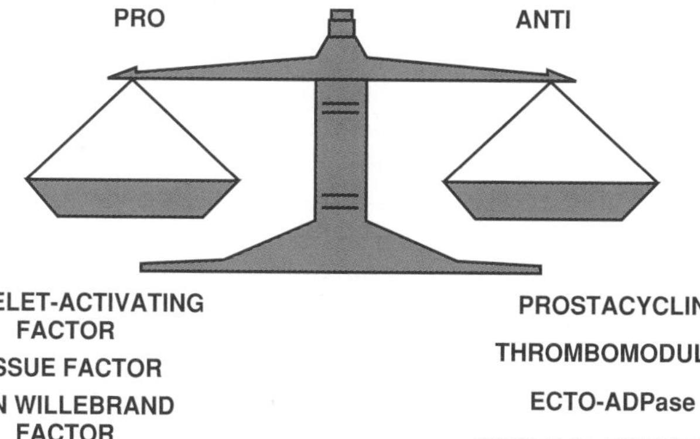

FIG. 3. The vascular endothelial hemostatic–thrombotic balance. Various endothelial-associated factors and functions contribute to a dynamic physiologic antagonism or "balance" which determines the status of local hemostatic or thrombotic activity.

of cell–cell interactions in the regulation of vascular functions (28). Together with prostacyclin, which also has a potent vasorelaxor effect (via different mechanisms of generation and target cell action), nitric oxide and other related compounds thus constitute a class of "natural" endothelial-derived antihypertensive substances.

Balancing the action of these endothelial-derived vasorelaxors are a number of endothelial-derived substances that have vasoconstrictor activity (Fig. 4). These include angiotensin II, generated at the luminal endothelial surface by angiotensin-converting enzyme; platelet-derived growth factor, which is secreted by endothelial cells and can act as a smooth muscle contractile agonist; and the novel vasoconstrictor substance endothelin-1 (29). The latter 18-amino acid peptide is generated by the proteolytic cleavage of a larger precursor, "big endothelin," and resembles the lethal toxin in the venom of certain snakes whose bite can induce coronary vasospasm. Endothelin-1 is reported to be the most potent vasoconstrictor known. Understanding the production of these endothelial-derived vasoconstrictor substances and their mechanisms of target cell action may help provide valuable insights into the normal regulation of vascular tone, as well as new strategies for antihypertensive therapies.

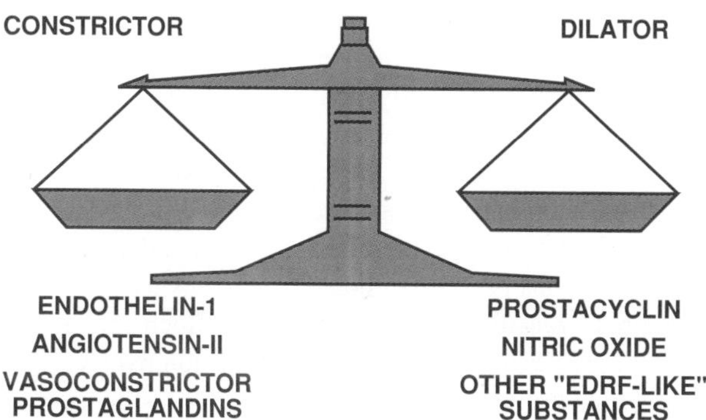

FIG. 4. The vascular endothelial vasoconstrictor–vasodilator balance. Various endothelial products contribute to the local regulation of vascular tone through their effects on smooth muscle contractility. *EDRF:* Endothelium-derived relaxation factor.

Cytokines and Growth Regulatory Molecules

The vascular endothelial lining is also the source of a wide variety of cytokines, growth factors, and growth inhibitors that can act locally, within a given segment of the circulatory tree, to influence the behavior of adjacent vascular cells and interacting blood elements (Table 1). This makes the endothelium a special kind of endocrine organ that can secrete its hormones in a paracrine (acting on neighbors) or even autocrine (acting on self) fashion.

Analogous to the physiologic antagonism of pro- and antithrombotic agents and vasoconstrictor/vasodilators described above, a similar balance also is evident in certain of the endothelial-derived cytokines and growth regulatory molecules with regard to their effects on vascular smooth muscle migration and proliferation. Further details concerning the regulation of the production of these endothelial products, their primary cellular targets, and the pathophysiologic implications of their actions are discussed below, in the context of endothelial dysfunction, and also in other chapters in this book.

TABLE 1. *Endothelial-derived biologic response modifiers*

Cytokines	Growth factors
Interleukin-1(alpha)	Platelet-derived growth factor (PDGF-A, B)
Interleukin-1(beta)	Insulin-like growth factor (IGF-1)
Interleukin-6	Basic fibroblast growth factor (bFGF)
Interleukin-8	Heparin-binding EGF-like growth factor
Monocyte chemotactic protein (MCP-1)	Transforming growth factor-beta
Colony stimulating factors (GM-/M-CSF)	

Transducer of Biomechanical Forces

By virtue of its unique position, in direct contact with flowing blood, the endothelium is constantly exposed to a variety of biomechanical stimuli. These stimuli take the form of specialized types of mechanical forces generated by pulsatile blood flow (e.g., fluid shear stresses, wall tension, intraluminal pressure). Some of these forces appear to be passively transduced across the endothelial layer to other components—cells and extracellular matrix—of the vessel wall, while other forces act directly upon the endothelial cell to modify its metabolic state and even regulate (positively or negatively) gene expression. Certain of these biomechanically induced effects, which include changes in growth factors, vasoconstrictors, vasodilators, and fibrinolytic components, appear to involve transcriptional modulation (30). Recently, a "shear-stress-response element (SSRE)" has been described in the platelet-derived growth factor (PDGF) B-chain gene promoter that appears to be involved in these processes. This *cis*-acting element has been shown by deletional analysis to be necessary for shear-induced transcription of the PDGF B-chain gene, and, interestingly, is also present in the promoters of several other shear-inducible endothelial genes (31), including certain leukocyte adhesion molecules, such as intercellular adhesion molecule-1 (ICAM-1) (32). Experimental analysis of the transduction mechanisms that link externally applied forces to genetic regulatory events within the nucleus (33) may provide new insights into the endothelial activation process.

In addition to its intrinsic cell biological interest, the question of the role of the endothelium as a transducer of biomechanical forces is of particular interest in the context of atherogenesis. It has long been appreciated that the early lesions of atherosclerosis arise in a nonrandom pattern, showing a predilection for branch points and regions of curvature, areas characterized by disturbed blood flow (34). The topic of hemodynamics and atherogenesis is considered in greater detail in another chapter.

THE DYSFUNCTIONAL OR ACTIVATED ENDOTHELIUM

Endothelial Cell Activation: Stimuli and Consequences

As discussed in detail elsewhere in this book, a proposed mechanism for the development of the atherosclerotic plaque, referred to as the "response-to-injury" hypothesis, has had a marked influence during the past two decades on atherosclerosis research. A basic tenet of the original model was that the initiating event in blood vessel disease was an undefined injury to the endothelium which led to endothelial cell loss and exposure of the underlying thrombogenic basement membrane (35). Platelet adherence to this surface and subsequent degranulation would result in the release of multiple bioactive molecules, including platelet-derived growth factor, a potent chemoattractant and mitogen for vascular smooth muscle cells. Intimal proliferation of smooth muscle cells, lipid accumulation, and monocyte infiltration then generated the early atherosclerotic plaque. In this model, the sole "function" of the endothelial cell in the disease process was its susceptibility to injury leading to cell death and sloughing. However, frank denudation of endothelium does not occur as an early event in atherogenesis; only in advanced atherosclerotic plaques have regions of vessel wall lacking intact endothelium been identified morphologically.

The presence of an intact endothelium over lesion-prone areas of artery raises the possibility that the endothelial cell may play an active role in atherogenesis (5,36). Injury to, or activation of, the endothelium may lead to the induction of genes which are suppressed under physiologic rather than pathologic conditions and/or the halting of expression of "beneficial" genes. As depicted in Fig. 5, specific endothelial cell functions that may be directly relevant to atherosclerosis and its clinical sequelae include the expression of leukocyte binding sites on the endothelial cell surface, the altered production of paracrine growth factors, chemoattractants, and vasoreactive molecules, the ability to oxidize LDL and to respond to oxidized lipids and lipoproteins, the ability to express pro- rather than anticoagulant activities, and the modulation of plasma component levels within the vessel wall through changes in permeability function (for recent review, see ref. 37).

An important question that remains unanswered is the source of injury, i.e., causative factor, that leads to altered endothelial cell gene expression during atherogenesis. Multiple candidates for the atherogenic agent have been proposed; however, rigorous identification of the molecule(s) responsible for the initial changes in endothelial cell function that potentially lead to vascular disease has not been achieved. Candidates include local cytokines or proteases (12), viral infection (38,39), variations in shear (30), free radicals and oxidized lipids (40,41), and homocysteine (42) (see Fig. 5). It was proposed recently that these various injury agents may act through a common transcriptional factor(s), nuclear factor-kappa B (NF-κB), which is responsible for the inappropriate gene expression by endothelial cells (43). Multiple other injury-induced signaling pathways may also be involved, as has been recently reviewed (44,45).

It is worthy of note that the concept of an altered endothelium has left the realm of the laboratory and is currently under discussion in the clinical arena. Articles are beginning to appear in the medical literature in which endothelial cell "activation" has been quantitated in humans using various indicators of vascular dysfunction (44,46). Such studies will most certainly grow in number as novel, noninvasive tests are developed to quantitate endothelial cell dysfunction.

Expression of Leukocyte Adhesion Molecules

The past decade has been a very active period for the study of the molecular interactions between blood-borne leu-

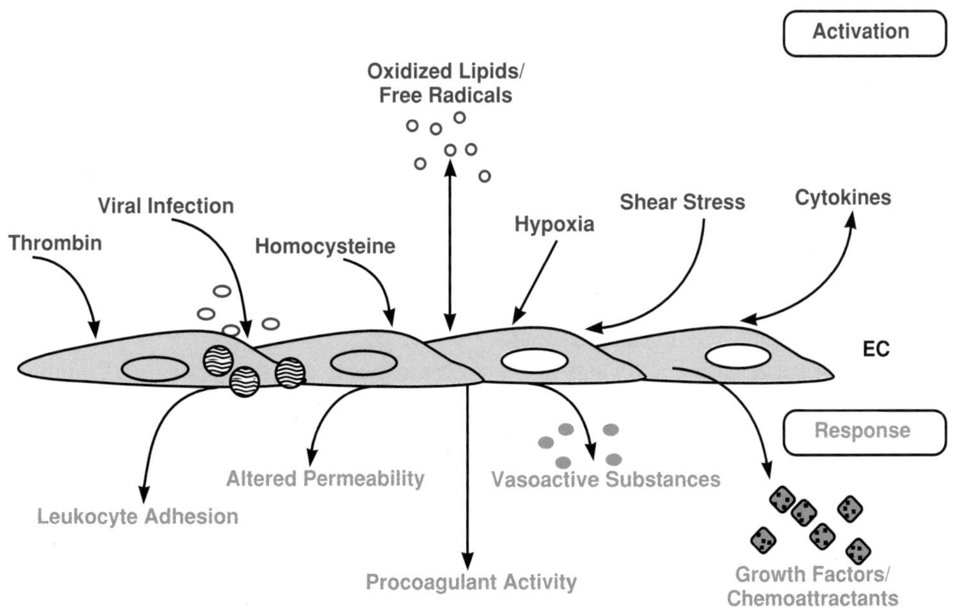

FIG. 5. Generation of a dysfunctional endothelium. A variety of stimulatory or "injury-provoking" agents have been implicated in the process of endothelial cell *(EC)* activation. Many of the responses of the endothelium are associated with the progression of vascular disease (37).

kocytes and the endothelium. This process is of great interest to atherosclerosis researchers due to the well-recognized involvement of both monocytes and T lymphocytes in the developing lesion. The monocyte-derived macrophage has been implicated in multiple aspects of atherosclerotic plaque development (47). These cells contribute to the formation of fatty streak lesions by ingesting massive amounts of lipid and thus developing into foam cells. They also produce growth factors for vascular smooth muscle cells, generate cytotoxic factors for neighboring cells, and emigrate as foam cells from the vessel wall leading to physical damage to the endothelium.

The first step in monocyte recruitment into the subendothelial space is the attachment of this blood-borne cell to the endothelium. The focal adherence of mononuclear cells to lesion-prone regions of large vessels is one of the earliest readily detectable events that occurs in experimentally induced atherosclerosis in various animal models. Topics that are currently under investigation in multiple laboratories include the nature of the underlying mechanisms regulating the expression of leukocyte adhesion proteins on the endothelial cell surface following cellular activation, the mechanism underlying the induction of adhesion by hypercholesterolemia, the specificity of this monocyte adhesion with little if any involvement of neutrophils, and finally the reason monocytes adhere only to specific regions of the vasculature. A now well-accepted model to describe the process of leukocyte attachment to the endothelium and subsequent diapedesis involves the sequential involvement of various adhesion molecules and chemokines (48,49). Both cell types play an active role in the process, which includes an initial rolling or tethering event (selectins), a signaling process (chemokines), and a strong attachment step (the immunoglobulin family members). It must be kept in mind that *in vivo* data supporting this model have been limited to the microvasculature and that leukocyte adhesion to large vessels which develop atherosclerosis may not occur in the same way.

Many recent studies have implicated lipoproteins and their components in inducing leukocyte adhesion to endothelial cells. Minimally modified (oxidized) low-density lipoprotein (LDL), but not native LDL, has been shown to specifically increase monocyte adhesion to cultured endothelial cells (50). Very low density lipoprotein (VLDL) that has been hydrolyzed by lipoprotein lipase was also found to induce increased monocyte adhesion to cultured aortic endothelial cells (51). The underlying mechanism of action of lipoproteins and the specific components responsible for the effects of oxidized LDL and hydrolyzed VLDL on endothelial cells remain unknown. One advance in this direction has been recently provided by Kume et al., who observed that lysophosphatidylcholine, a major component of oxidized LDL, increased mononuclear cell adhesion to cultured human and rabbit arterial endothelial cells (21). This lipid was found to induce the adhesion molecules vascular cell adhesion molecule-1 (VCAM-1) and ICAM-1, but not E-selectin, on the endothelial cell surface, thus distinguishing this stimulus from many other agonists of leukocyte adhesion.

The specific leukocyte adhesion molecules responsible for monocyte adhesion in the absence of neutrophil adhesion in models of atherogenesis remain to be defined. Characteristics of the known endothelial cell/leukocyte adhesion molecules have been recently reviewed in detail (47,52). The primary candidate for the "atherogenic" leukocyte adhesion molecule is VCAM-1 (53). The kinetics of expression of this cytokine-inducible leukocyte adhesion molecule is consistent with its involvement in monocyte adhesion to rabbit aorta following the feeding of a high-cholesterol diet (54). Other adhesion molecules for which some evidence exists, albeit mostly *in vitro,* for their involvement in monocyte adhesion include E-selectin, ICAM-1 and P-selectin (47).

Mechanisms for suppressing increased leukocyte adhesion to EC have also been uncovered recently. Transforming growth factor-β (TGF-β) has been found to inhibit cytokine-induced E-selectin expression in endothelial cells (55), and the antiinflammatory agent deazaadenosine abrogates agonist-induced E-selectin expression and adhesion of monocytes to cultured human aortic endothelial cells (56). Pober and co-workers demonstrated that by elevating cyclic adenosine monophosphate in endothelial cells, using multiple pharmacologic approaches, they could markedly suppress the cytokine-induced expression of E-selectin and VCAM-1 (57). Some of the above approaches to inhibiting this activated endothelial cell function may be generally applicable in causing a dysfunctional endothelium to revert to a more physiologic, ''resting state,'' phenotype.

Prothrombotic Properties of the Activated Endothelium

As discussed above, a healthy physiologic endothelium presents a nonthrombogenic surface to blood cells; however, multiple pathways may be induced in dysfunctional endothelial cells which render these cells thrombogenic. The anticoagulant properties of the endothelium include the production of prostaglandin derivatives and other lipids which inhibit platelet aggregation and the elaboration of antithrombotic proteoglycans and proteins, such as thrombomodulin. Mechanisms by which the procoagulant state develops in large-vessel endothelial cells have been studied principally *in vitro* (58). Activated endothelial cells express tissue factor, which initiates blood coagulation via the extrinsic pathway. Tissue factor activity has been shown to be induced in endothelial cells in response to various agonists, such as endotoxin, interleukin-1 (IL-1), tumor necrosis factor, and thrombin, and altered flow conditions (59–63). The tissue factor expressed by cultured endothelial cells in response to IL-1β has been found to be localized principally to the luminal or apical surface of the cell (59). The cytokine induction of tissue factor expression in endothelial cells is inhibited by retinoic acid (62) or by IL-4 (63). The *in vivo* relevance of these observations remains to be established.

In both native and activated states, the endothelium participates actively in the process of fibrinolysis as it relates to both clot dissolution and tissue repair (64). Activated endothelial cells can inhibit fibrin degradation by reducing the expression of plasminogen activators while increasing expression of plasminogen activator inhibitor-1 (PAI-1). Oxidized lipoproteins, as well as native lipoproteins, were shown recently to cause increased synthesis of PAI-1 by cultured human endothelial cells (65). Multiple proteases, including cathepsin-G, play a role in the fibrinolytic system by regulating the release of PAI-1 as well as plasminogen activator from the endothelial cell surface (66). Finally, a link exists between vasoreactivity and the fibrinolytic activity of endothelial cells, since endothelin (see below) has been found to augment release of both tissue plasminogen activator and PAI-1 from cultured endothelial cells (67).

Vasospasm and the Activated Endothelium

The ability of blood vessels to contract in response to humoral as well as paracrine vasoactive substances is affected by the diseased state of the vessel under study (45,68). Understanding the regulation of endothelial cell production of vasoreactive molecules is therefore of direct relevance to clinical situations and endpoints, such as occlusion of blood flow. A key paracrine modulator of vascular reactivity is endothelin-1, a highly potent vasoconstrictive agent, which has been recently shown to be regulated both by oxidized lipoproteins (69,70) and by shear stress (71). Endothelin-1 is secreted by endothelial cells into the basolateral compartment (72) and its secretion is suppressed by lysophosphatidylcholine (lysoPC), a major component of oxidized LDL (69). LysoPC may act through selective inhibition of a G_i protein-dependent pathway by disrupting receptor–G protein interaction (73). Other modulators of endothelin-1 production by vascular endothelial cells include interferon-gamma (74), interleukin-1β (75), and thrombin (76).

The endothelium also controls vascular tone, depending on the physiologic state of the blood vessel, by secreting vasorelaxants such as nitric oxide. Multiple studies have examined the interrelationships between endothelium-dependent relaxation and hypercholesterolemia both *in vitro* and *in vivo* (77–79). Recent results suggest that oxidized LDL may act directly to inhibit endothelium-dependent arterial relaxation (79) and that this effect is reversible by high-density lipoprotein (80). Regardless of the mechanism, all of the studies, including those in humans, have demonstrated an inverse relationship between atherosclerotic plaque development and vasorelaxation. In an *ex vivo* rabbit model of hypercholesterolemia, increased neutrophil adherence to coronary artery endothelium was found to be due to a reduction in nitric oxide release in the hypercholesterolemia state (78). Hypoxia also causes abnormal contractile responses in the atherosclerotic rabbit aorta, potentially through reduced nitric oxide and cyclic guanosine monophosphate production (81). In the same rabbit model, L-arginine administration, which would provide increased substrate for nitric oxide synthase, overcame the proatherogenic effects of hypercholesterolemia, further implicating nitric oxide production as an antiatherosclerotic event (82). In humans, impaired endothelium-dependent vasodilatation of forearm resistance vessels has been shown in hypercholesterolemic patients (77). Also, patients with coronary risk factors and proximal atherosclerotic lesions were demonstrated to exhibit impaired responsiveness of their coronary vessels to acetylcholine (83). These studies were further reinforced by those in hypercholesterolemic patients in which cholesterol-lowering therapy improved coronary endothelium-dependent relaxation (84).

Growth Factor Production by the Activated Endothelium

As discussed earlier, the endothelium is a potential source of the growth factor(s) responsible for smooth muscle cell migration and proliferation that is a hallmark of the atherosclerotic lesion. The regulation of production of platelet-derived growth factor (PDGF), a mitogen that has been implicated in atherosclerotic plaque development, by endothelial cells and evidence correlating PDGF expression by endothelial cells with dysfunction and vascular disease has been reviewed recently (85). Recent studies have suggested novel ways in which PDGF production may be regulated within endothelial cells. Increasing the osmolarity or the glucose concentration of endothelial cells culture media caused a significant increase in the amount of PDGF produced by the cells (86). These results may have relevance to the well-established association of atherosclerosis with diabetes. Other modulators of PDGF production that have been recently discovered include interleukin-6 (87), hydrogen peroxide (88), and low-molecular-weight fibrinogen degradation products (89). The most efficacious inducer of PDGF production by endothelial cells remains the coagulation system protease α-thrombin, which acts both transcriptionally and posttranscriptionally to cause release of PDGF (90). Of great interest is the recent finding that the promoter of the PDGF B-chain gene contains an element that confers shear-stress responsiveness to this gene (31). As discussed earlier in this chapter, this observation, as well as previous studies reporting modulation of PDGF production by mechanical/physical activation, support a potential mechanistic link between regions of altered shear stress and susceptibility to atherosclerotic plaque development. The above studies highlight the multitude of factors which may modulate the level of growth factors produced by the endothelium under various pathophysiologic conditions.

The endothelium is also known to produce other growth factors in addition to PDGF, for example, insulin-like growth factor-1 (IGF-1), which can act to modulate gene expression and augment proliferation of neighboring smooth muscle cells (91,92). Release of this growth factor by endothelial cells has been found to occur in a polarized manner (91). Basic fibroblast growth factor (FGF), a ubiquitous mitogen, also exhibits regulated expression by the endothelium. Thrombin has been recently shown to cause release of active basic FGF from glycosaminoglycans in the subendothelial matrix (93). The endothelium is also a well-recognized source of the pluripotent growth factor/growth inhibitor transforming growth factor-β (TGF-β). Basic FGF has been found to induce activation of latent TGF-β in endothelial cell cultures by increasing plasminogen activator activity (94,95). Endothelial cells also respond to TGF-β as a growth inhibitor and a recent report has suggested that this protein may alter the differentiated state of endothelium, causing expression of genes by endothelial cells in culture previously thought to be smooth muscle cell-specific (96). Endothelial cells are unique in their ability to distinguish between the isoforms of TGF-β. Specifically, it has been observed that the ability of TGF-β to suppress endothelial cell migration is highly specific for the type-1 and not the type-2 isoform of this growth factor (97).

Inhibiting the Generation of Dysfunctional Endothelium

Two functional classes of compounds—antiinflammatory agents and antioxidants—have been tested *in vitro* for their ability to prevent endothelial cell activation in the presence of stimulators, such as cytokines. The antiinflammatory agent 3-deazaadenosine was found to inhibit thrombin-induced expression of PDGF and leukocyte adhesion molecules in cultured endothelial cells (56). The inhibition was at the level of transcription and did not reflect a general toxic response of the cells, since transcription of "house-keeping" genes was unaffected. In a human endothelial cell–smooth muscle cell coculture system, the antiinflammatory compound leumedin was found to prevent LDL-induced monocyte transmigration (98).

As discussed elsewhere in this book, the results of multiple animal studies using various vascular disease models has led to much excitement regarding the possible antiatherosclerotic properties of antioxidants such as vitamin E (α-tocopherol) or Probucol. It has been hypothesized that the beneficial effects of these agents is due to their ability to inhibit the generation of oxidized LDL—a putative triggering molecule in the atherosclerotic process. Recent results from several investigators point to a novel alternative mechanism of action of antioxidants, that is, through the scavenging of intracellular reactive oxygen intermediates that serve as second messengers in cytokine-induced gene activation in endothelial cells (99–103). Vitamin E has also been demonstrated to enhance prostacyclin production by cultured endothelial cells (104), suggesting a third mechanism by which this antioxidant may alter the progression of atherosclerosis.

Regenerated Endothelium and Collateral Circulation

A continuous endothelial monolayer is required for the maintenance and control of normal vessel wall properties. This continuity may be challenged by pathologic damage induced by one or more of the agents depicted in Fig. 5 or by physical damage due, for example, to a passing catheter or an angioplasty procedure. Much of what is known about the regeneration of endothelium derives from studies of gross denudation, mostly in animal models of vessel wall hyperplasia. Early studies showed that deendothelialization of the rat aorta with a balloon catheter is followed by a reproducible series of events beginning with rapid platelet aggregation, followed by slow reendothelialization, and culminating in marked intimal thickening due to smooth muscle cell migration and proliferation that is apparent within a few weeks. A strong correlation between the duration of denudation and the degree of intimal thickening has been demonstrated (105). Injured regions that are covered by regenerated endothelium within 7 days after injury are completely spared from intimal thickening (106). Rat carotid arteries that are entirely, but gently, denuded are capable of complete endothelial regrowth (107). In contrast to balloon denudation, this method does not cause significant medial damage. These data suggest that the intensity of the vessel trauma is also a critical determinant of endothelial regeneration. The mechanism(s) by which confluent endothelium reduces or prevents intimal thickening has not been resolved. It may be due to the secretion of growth inhibitory substances, or by limiting the exposure of the subendothelial tissue to blood-borne elements, e.g., lipoproteins, growth factors, or elements of the coagulation cascade.

Endothelial regeneration proceeds from the uninjured luminal surface and from the intercostal arteries at approximately 0.1–0.4 mm/day (106). Both endothelial cell migration and proliferation contribute to the reendothelialization process. Migration may in fact be responsible for subsequent proliferation, by formation of regions of low cell density, or by removal of inhibitory mechanisms due to contact. Endothelial regeneration after balloon catheter injury is limited in duration and extent in most animal species. Total axial ingrowth in the rabbit and rat is limited to approximately 3 and 10 mm, respectively (108). The minimal ingrowth of endothelial cells from vessel anastomoses onto impermeable synthetic vascular grafts suggests that a similar limitation exists in humans.

The cause of the incomplete regeneration of endothelium remains unknown, though several explanatory mechanisms have been proposed. The smooth muscle cell pseudointima that forms adjacent to the regenerating endothelium has been suggested as a barrier, but at least one study suggests that this is unlikely (109). Growth factors are likely to have a role in endothelial regeneration, since several, including transforming growth factors, angiogenin, vascular endothelial growth factor, tumor promoters, and acidic and basic FGF, are known to influence endothelial cell migration and proliferation *in vitro* (see refs. 110 and 111 for review). Recent experiments have shown that injection of either acidic or basic FGF stimulates endothelial cell repair after denuding injury (112,113). These data clearly demonstrate the importance of FGF in vascular repair, but do not explain why regenerating cells reach a point where exogenous growth factors are required for further repair. In addition to stimulatory molecules, inhibitors of endothelial cell migration have been identified; TGF-β1 and fibronectin are particularly potent and may regulate repair *in vivo* (114).

The development of collateral circulation, a form of angiogenesis, is another process that requires the migration and proliferation of endothelial cells. The formation of new vessels involves multiple steps, including (a) receipt of angiogenic signals by large-vessel endothelial cells, (b) degradation of the extracellular matrix surrounding the existing vascular bed by secretion of proteases, (c) formation of a capillary ''bud'' by migrating endothelial cells, (d) capillary extension by proliferation of endothelial cells at the distal tip of the vessel, and (e) anastomosis of newly formed tubes to form a continuous microvessel (115). Migration, rather than proliferation, appears to be the controlling step in capillary growth, since angiogenic factors have been identified that stimulate endothelial cell migration but not proliferation *in vitro* (116), and since irradiation of tumors grafted into corneal tissues completely blocks endothelial cell proliferation without altering rates of angiogenesis (117,118). FGF may be an important physiologic regulator of angiogenesis, since continuous delivery of basic FGF in solid-phase pellets increases both collateral circulation (119) and formation of vasa vasorum (120) following arterial injury. Delivery of acidic FGF by gene transfer also stimulates angiogenesis within the intima of blood vessels (121).

SUMMARY

The endothelium, though only a single layer thick at any vascular site, is now understood to be a massive, regionally specific, multifunctional organ, the health of which is essential to normal vascular physiology, and whose dysfunction can be a critical factor in the pathogenesis of multiple vascular diseases. The vascular endothelium is strategically situated to monitor systemic as well as locally generated stimuli and to alter its functional state. This adaptive process typically proceeds without notice, contributing to normal homeostasis. However, nonadaptive changes in endothelial structure and function, provoked by pathophysiologic stimuli, can result in localized, acute and chronic, alterations in the interactions of endothelium with the cellular and macromolecular components of circulating blood and of the blood vessel wall. These alterations include enhanced permeability to (and subsequent oxidative modification of) plasma lipoproteins, hyperadhesiveness for blood leukocytes, and functional imbalances in local pro- and antithrombotic factors, growth stimulators and inhibitors, and vasoactive (dilator, constrictor) substances. These manifestations, collectively termed endothelial dysfunction, play an important role in the initiation, progression, and clinical complications of various forms of inflammatory and degenerative vascular diseases. Further challenges include identification of the triggering agents responsible for endothelial dysfunction in specific vascular diseases and the design of therapeutic regimens that will serve to either prevent the genesis of the dysfunctional endothelium or cause such endothelium to revert to a more physiologic phenotype.

ACKNOWLEDGMENTS

The authors thank Alice Callahan, Carol de la Motte, and Dr. Paul L. Fox for their assistance in the preparation of this chapter, and Masayuki Yoshida and Carol de la Motte for assistance with illustrations. Original research in the authors' laboratories is supported by grants from the National Health Lung and Blood Institute (P01-HL36028, RO1-HL51150-01, and P01-HL48743 to M.A.G.; and P01-HL29582 and R01-HL34727 to P.E.D.). M.A.G. is a recipient of an unrestricted grant for cardiovascular research from the Bristol Myers-Squibb Institute.

REFERENCES

1. Virchow R. Der ateromatose Prozess der Arterien. *Wien Med Wochenschr* 1856;6:825–841.
2. Ross R. The pathogenesis of atherosclerosis: a perspective for the 1990's. *Nature* 1993;362:801–809.
3. Gimbrone MA Jr, ed. *Vascular endothelium in hemostasis and thrombosis.* Edinburgh: Churchill Livingstone; 1986.
4. Gimbrone MA Jr. Vascular endothelium: nature's blood-compatible container. *Ann N Y Acad Sci* 1987;516:5–11.
5. Gimbrone MA Jr. Endothelial dysfunction and atherosclerosis. *J Card Surg* 1989;4:180–183.
6. Simionescu N, Simionescu M, eds. *Endothelial cell biology in health and disease.* New York: Plenum Press; 1988.
7. Simionescu N, Simionescu M, eds. *Endothelial cell dysfunctions.* New York: Plenum Press; 1992.
8. Gimbrone MA Jr. Vascular endothelium in health and disease. In: Haber E, ed. *Molecular cardiovascular medicine.* New York: Scientific American Medicine; 1995: *[in press].*
9. Krogh A. *The anatomy and physiology of capillaries.* New Haven, Connecticut: Yale University Press; 1929:22.
10. Gimbrone MA Jr, Bevilacqua MP. Vascular endothelium: functional modulation at the blood interface. In: Simionescu N, Simionescu M, eds. *Endothelial cell biology in health and disease.* New York: Plenum Press; 1988;255–273.
11. Pober JS. Cytokine-mediated activation of vascular endothelium: physiology and pathology. *Am J Pathol* 1988;133:426–431.
12. Pober JS, Cotran RC. Cytokines and endothelial cell biology. *Physiol Rev* 1990;70:427–451.
13. Fishman AP. Endothelium: a distributed organ of diverse capabilities. In: Fishman AP, ed. Endothelium. *Ann N Y Acad Sci* 1982;401:1–8.
14. Simionescu M, Simionescu N, Palade GE. Differentiated microdomains on the luminal surface of the capillary endothelium. I. Partial characterization of their anionic sites. *J Cell Biol* 1981;90:614–621.
15. Muller WA, Gimbrone MA Jr. Plasmalemmal proteins of cultured vascular endothelial cells exhibit apical-basal polarity: analysis by surface-selective iodination. *J Cell Biol* 1986;103(6):2389–2402.
16. Majno G. Ultrastructure of the vascular membrane. In: Hamilton WF, ed. *Handbook of physiology.* Section 2, Vol II. *Circulation.* Washington, D.C.: American Physiological Society; 1965:2293–2375.
17. Wagner R, Chen S-C. Transcapillary transport of solute by the endothelial vesicular system: evidence from thin serial section analysis. *Microvasc Res* 1991;42:139–150.
18. Svensjo E, Joyner WL. The effects of intermittent and continuous stimulation of microvessels in the cheek pouch of hamsters with histamine and bradykinin on the development of venular leaky sites. *Microcirc Endothelium Lymphatics* 1984;1:381–396.
19. Simionescu N, Simionescu M. Cellular interactions of lipoproteins with the vascular endothelium: endocytosis and transcytosis. In: Shaw JM, ed. *Lipoproteins as carriers of pharmacological agents,* New York: Dekker; 1991:45–95.
20. Witztum JL, Steinberg D. Role of oxidized low density lipoproteins in atherogenesis. *J Clin Invest* 1991;88:1785–1789.
21. Kume N, Cybulsky MI, Gimbrone MA Jr. Lysophosphatidylcholine, a component of atherogenic lipoproteins, induces mononuclear leukocyte adhesion molecules in cultured human and rabbit arterial endothelial cells. *J Clin Invest* 1992;90:1138–1144.
22. Kume N, Gimbrone MA Jr. Lysophosphatidylcholine transcriptionally induces growth factor gene expression in cultured human endothelial cells. *J Clin Invest* 1994;93:907–911.
23. Weksler BB, Marcus AJ, Jaffe EA. Synthesis of prostaglandin I2 (prostacyclin) by cultured human and bovine endothelial cells. *Proc Natl Acad Sci USA* 1977;74:3922–3928.
24. Rosenberg RD, Rosenberg JS. Natural anticoagulant mechanisms. *J Clin Invest* 1984;74:1–6.
25. Esmon CT. The regulation of natural anticoagulant pathways. *Science* 1987;235:1348–1352.
26. Bevilacqua MP, Pober JS, Wheeler ME, et al. Interleukin I (IL-1) activation of vascular endothelium: effects on procoagulant activity and leukocyte adhesion. *Am J Pathol* 1985;121:394–401.
27. Furchgott RF, Zawadzki JV. The obligatory role of endothelial cells in the relaxation of arterial smooth muscle by acetylcholine. *Nature* 1980;288:373–379.
28. Dinerman JL, Lowenstein CJ, Snyder SH. Molecular mechanisms of nitric oxide regulation: potential relevance to cardiovascular disease (Mini-review). *Circ Res* 1993;73:217.
29. Masaki T. Role of endothelin in mechanisms of local blood pressure control. *J Hypertens* 1990;8(Suppl 7):S107.
30. Davies PF, Tripathi SC. Mechanical stress mechanisms and the cell: an endothelial paradigm (Mini review). *Circ Res* 1993;72:239–244.
31. Resnick N, Collins T, Atkinson W, Bonthron DT, Dewey CF Jr, Gimbrone MA Jr. Platelet-derived growth factor B chain promoter contains a *cis*-acting fluid shear-stress-responsive element. *Proc Natl Acad Sci USA* 1993;90:4591–4595.
32. Nagel T, Resnick N, Atkinson WJ, Dewey CF Jr, Gimbrone MA Jr. Shear stress selectively upregulates intercellular adhesion molecule-1 expression in cultured human vascular endothelial cells. *J Clin Invest* 1994;94:885–891.
33. Khachigian LM, Resnick N, Gimbrone MA Jr, Collins T. NF-κB links fluid mechanical forces with vascular endothelial gene expression. Submitted (1994).
34. Glagov S, Zarins C, Giddens DPG, Ku DN. Hemodynamics and atherosclerosis, insights and perspectives gained from studies of human arteries. *Arch Pathol Lab Med* 1988;112:1018–1031.
35. Ross R, Glomset JA. The pathogenesis of atherosclerosis. *N Engl J Med* 1976;295:377; 420–425.
36. DiCorleto PE, Chisolm GM. Participation of the endothelium in the development of the atherosclerotic plaque. *Prog Lipid Res* 1986;25: 365–374.
37. DiCorleto PE, Soyombo AA. The role of the endothelium in atherogenesis. *Curr Opin Lipidol* 1993;4:364–372.
38. Etingin OR, Silverstein RL, Friedman HM, Hajjar DP. Viral activation of the coagulation cascade: molecular interactions at the surface of infected endothelial cells. *Cell* 1990;61:657–662.
39. Etingin OR, Silverstein RL, Hajjar DP. Identification of a monocyte receptor on herpes virus-infected endothelial cells. *Proc Natl Acad Sci USA* 1991;88:7200–7203.
40. Berliner JA, Haberland ME. Role of oxidized low density lipoprotein in atherogenesis. *Curr Opin Lipidol* 1993;4:373–381.
41. Chisolm GM. The oxidation of lipoproteins: implications for atherosclerosis. In: Spatz L, Bloom AD, eds. *Mechanisms and consequences of oxidative damage.* Oxford: Oxford University Press; 1992:78–106.
42. Murphy-Chutorian D, Alderman EL. The case that hyperhomocysteinenemia is a risk factor for coronary artery disease. *Am J Cardiol* 1994;73:705–707.
43. Collins T. Endothelial nuclear factor-kappa B and the initiation of the atherosclerotic lesion. *Lab Invest* 1993;68:499–508.
44. Luscher TF, Tanner FC, Tschudi MR, Noll G. Endothelial dysfunction in coronary artery disease. *Annu Rev Med* 1993;44:395–418.
45. Gerritsen ME, Bloor CM. Endothelial cell gene expression in response to injury. *FASEB J* 1993;7:523–532.
46. Celermajer DS, Sorensen KE, Gooch VM, Spiegelhalter DJ, Miller OI, Sullivan ID, Lloyd JK, Deanfield JE. Non-invasive detection of endothelial dysfunction in children and adults at risk of atherosclerosis. *Lancet* 1992;340:1111–1115.

47. Faruqi RM, DiCorleto PE. Mechanisms of monocyte recruitment and accumulation. *Br Heart J* 1993;69:S19–S29.
48. Springer TA. Traffic signals for lymphocytes recirculation and leukocyte emigration: the multistep paradigm. *Cell* 1994;76:301–314.
49. Butcher EC. Leukocyte-endothelial cell recognition: Three (or more) steps to specificity and diversity. *Cell* 1991;67:1033–1036.
50. Berliner JA, Territo MC. Sevanian A, Ramin S, Kim JA, Bamshad B, et al. Minimally modified low density lipoprotein stimulates monocyte endothelial interactions. *J Clin Invest* 1990;85:1260–1266.
51. Saxena U, Kulkarni NM, Ferguson E, Newton RS. Lipoprotein lipase-mediated lipolysis of very low density lipoproteins increases monocyte adhesion to aortic endothelial cells. *Biochem Biophys Res Commun* 1992;189:1653–1658.
52. Bevilacqua MP. Endothelial-leukocyte adhesion molecules. *Annu Rev Immunol* 1993;11:767–804.
53. Cybulsky MI, Gimbrone MA Jr. Endothelial expression of a mononuclear leukocyte adhesion molecule during atherogenesis. *Science* 1991;251:788–791.
54. Li H, Cybulsky MI, Gimbrone MA Jr, Libby P. An atherogenic diet rapidly induces VCAM-1, a cytokine-regulatable mononuclear leukocyte adhesion molecule, in rabbit aortic endothelium. *Arterioscler Thromb* 1993;13:197–204.
55. Gamble JR, Khew-Goodall Y, Vadas MA. Transforming growth factor-β inhibits E-selectin expression on human endothelial cells. *J Immunol* 1993;150:4494–4503.
56. Shankar R, de la Motte CA, DiCorleto PE. 3-Deazaadenosine inhibits thrombin-stimulated platelet-derived growth factor production and endothelial-leukocyte adhesion molecule-1-mediated monocytic cell adhesion in human aortic endothelial cells. *J Biol Chem* 1992;267: 9376–9382.
57. Pober JS, Slowik MR, De Luca LG, Ritchie AJ. Elevated cyclic-AMP inhibits endothelial cell synthesis and expression of TNF-induced endothelial leukocyte adhesion molecule-1, and vascular cell adhesion molecule-1, but not intercellular adhesion molecule-1. *J Immunol* 1993;150:5114–5123.
58. Antonov AS, Key NS, Smirnov MD, Jacob HS, Vercellotti GM, Smirnov VN. Prothrombotic phenotype diversity of human aortic endothelial cells in culture. *Thromb Res* 1992;67:135–145.
59. Narahara N, Enden T, Wiiger M, Prydz H. Polar expression of tissue factor in human umbilical vein endothelial cells. *Arterioscler Thromb* 1994;14:1815–1820.
60. Bartha K, Brisson C, Archipoff G, De la Salle C, Lanza F, Cazenave JP, Beretz A. Thrombin regulates tissue factor and thrombomodulin mRNA levels and activities in human saphenous vein endothelial cells by distinct mechanisms. *J Biol Chem* 1993;268:421–429.
61. Grabowski EF, Zuckerman DB, Nemerson Y. The functional expression of tissue factor by fibroblasts and endothelial cells under flow conditions. *Blood* 1993;81:3265–3270.
62. Ishii H, Horie S, Kizaki K, Kazama M. Retinoic acid counteracts both the downregulation of thrombomodulin and the induction of tissue factor in cultured human endothelial cells exposed to tumor necrosis factor. *Blood* 1992;80:2556–2562.
63. Herbert JM, Savi P, Laplace MC, Lale A. IL-4 inhibits LPS-, IL-1β- and TNFα-induced expression of tissue factor in endothelial cells and monocytes. *FEBS Lett* 1992;310:31–33.
64. Van Hinsbergh VWM. Impact of endothelial activation on fibrinolysis and local proteolysis in tissue repair. *Ann NY Acad Sci* 1992;667: 151–162.
65. Tremoli E, Camera M, Maderna P, Sironi L, Prati L, Colli S, Piovella F, Bernini F, Corsini A, Mussoni L. Increased synthesis of plasminogen activator inhibitor-1 by cultured human endothelial cells exposed to native and modified LDL: an LDL receptor-independent phenomenon. *Arterioscler Thromb* 1993;13:338–346.
66. Pintucci G, Iacoviello L, Amore C, Evangelista V, Cerietti C, Donati MB. Cathepsin G, a polymorphonuclear cell protease, affects the fibrinolytic system by releasing PAI-1 from endothelial cells and platelets. *Ann N Y Acad Sci* 1992;667:286–288.
67. Yamamoto C, Kaji T, Sakamoto M, Koizumi F. Effect of endothelin on the release of tissue plasminogen activator and plasminogen activator inhibitor-1 from cultured human endothelial cells and interaction with thrombin. *Thromb Res* 1992;67:619–624.
68. Kisanuki A, Asada Y, Hatakeyama K, Hayashi T, Sumiyoshi A. Contribution of the endothelium to intimal thickening in normocholesterolemic and hypercholesterolemic rabbits. *Arterioscler Thromb* 1992; 12:1198–1205.
69. Jougasaki M, Kugiyama K, Saito Y, Nakao K, Imura H, Yasue H. Suppression of endothelin-1 secretion by lysophosphatidylcholine in oxidized low density lipoprotein in cultured vascular endothelial cells. *Circ Res* 1992;71:614–619.
70. Boulager CM, Tanner FC, Bea ML, Hahn AWA, Werner A, Luscher TF. Oxidized low density lipoproteins induce messenger RNA expression and release of endothelin from human and porcine endothelium. *Circ Res* 1992;70:1191–1197.
71. Kuchan MI, Frangos JA. Shear stress regulates endothelin-1 release via protein kinase C and cGMP in cultured endothelial cells. *Am J Physiol* 1993;264:H150–H156.
72. Wagner OF, Christ G, Wojta J, Vierhapper H, Parzer S, Nowotny PJ, Schneider B, Waldhausl W, Binder BR. Polar secretion of endothelin-1 by cultured endothelial cells. *J Biol Chem* 1992;267:16066–16068.
73. Flavahan NA. Lysophosphatidylcholine modifies G protein-dependent signaling in porcine endothelial cells. *Am J Physiol* 1993;264: H722–H727.
74. Lamas S, Michel T, Collins T, Brenner BM, Marsden PA. Effects of interferon-gamma on nitric oxide synthase activity and endothelin-1 production by vascular endothelial cells. *J Clin Invest* 1992;90: 879–887.
75. Katabami T, Shimizu M, Okano K, Yano Y, Nemoto K, Ogura M, Tsukamoto T, Suzuki S, Ohira K, Yamada Y, Sekita N, Yoshida A, Someya K. Intracellular signal transduction for interleukin-1β-induced endothelin production in human umbilical vein endothelial cells. *Biochem Biophys Res Commun* 1992;188:565–570.
76. Emori T, Hirata Y, Imai T, Ohta K, Kanno K, Eguchi S, Marumo F. Cellular mechanism of thrombin on endothelin-1 biosynthesis and release in bovine endothelial cells. *Biochem Pharmacol* 1992;44: 2409–2411.
77. Chowienczyk PJ, Watts GF, Cockcroft JR, Ritter JM. Impaired endothelium-dependent vasodilation of forearm resistance vessels in hypercholesterolaemia. *Lancet* 1992;340:1430–1432.
78. Lefer AM, Ma X. Decreased basal nitric oxide release in hypercholesterolemia increases neutrophil adherence to rabbit coronary artery endothelium. *Arterioscler Thromb* 1993;13:771–776.
79. Galle J, Schenck I, Schollmeyer P, Wanner C. Cyclosporine and oxidized lipoproteins affect vascular reactivity: influence of the endothelium. *Hypertension* 1993;21:315–321.
80. Matsuda Y, Hirata K, Inoue N, Suematsu M, Kawashima S, Akita H, Yokoyama M. High density lipoprotein reverses inhibitory effect of oxidized low density lipoprotein on endothelium-dependent arterial relaxation. *Circ Res* 1993;72:1103–1109.
81. Simonet S, De Bailliencourt JP, Descombes J-J, Mennecier P, Laubie M, Verbeuren TJ. Hypoxia causes an abnormal contractile response in the atherosclerotic rabbit aorta: implication of reduced nitric oxide and cGMP production. *Circ Res* 1993;72:616–630.
82. Cooke JP, Singer AH, Tsao P, Zera P, Rowan RA, Billingham ME. Antiatherogenic effects of L-arginine in the hypercholesterolemic rabbit. *J Clin Invest* 1992;90:1168–1172.
83. Egashira K, Inou T, Hirooka Y, Yamada A, Maruoka Y, Kai H, Sugimachi M, Suzuki S, Takeshita A. Impaired coronary blood flow response to acetylcholine in patients with coronary risk factors and proximal atherosclerotic lesions. *J Clin Invest* 1993;91:29–37.
84. Leung W-H, Lau C-P, Wong C-K. Beneficial effect of cholesterol-lowering therapy on coronary endothelium-dependent relaxation in hypercholesterolaemic patients. *Lancet* 1993;341:1496–1500.
85. DiCorleto PE, Fox PL. Growth factor production by endothelial cells. In: Ryan U, ed. *Endothelial cells,* Vol II. Boca Raton, Florida: CRC Press; 1988:51–61.
86. Mizutani M, Okuda Y, Yamaoka T, Tsukahara K, Isaka M, Bannai C, Yamashita K. High glucose and hyperosmolarity increase platelet-derived growth factor mRNA levels in cultured human vascular endothelial cells. *Biochem Biophys Res Commun* 1992;187:664–669.
87. Calderon TM, Sherman J, Wilkerson H, Hatcher VB, Berman JW. Interleukin-6 modulates c-*sis* gene expression in cultured human endothelial cells. *Cell Immunol* 1992;143:118–126.
88. Montisano DF, Mann T, Spragg RG. H_2O_2 increases expression of pulmonary artery endothelial cell platelet-derived growth factor mRNA. *J Appl Physiol* 1992;73:2255–2262.
89. Lorenzet R, Sobel JH, Bini A, Witte LD. Low molecular weight fibrin-

ogen degradation products stimulate the release of growth factors from endothelial cells. *Thromb Haemostasis* 1992;68:357–363.
90. Soyombo AA, DiCorleto PE. Stable expression of human platelet-derived growth factor B chain by bovine aortic endothelial cells: cell-association and selective proteolytic cleavage by thrombin. *J Biol Chem* 1994;269:17734–17740.
91. Taylor WR, Nerem RM, Alexander RW. Polarized secretion of IGF-I and IGF-I binding protein activity by cultured aortic endothelial cells. *J Cell Physiol* 1993;154:139–142.
92. Gajdusek CM, Luo Z, Mayberg MR. Sequestration and secretion of insulin-like growth factor-I by bovine aortic endothelial cells. *J Cell Physiol* 1993;154:192–198.
93. Benezra M, Vlodavsky I, Ishai-Michaeli R, Neufeld G, Bar-Shavit R. Thrombin-induced release of active basic fibroblast growth factor-heparan sulfate complexes from subendothelial extracellular matrix. *Blood* 1993;83:3324–3331.
94. Flaumenhaft R, Abe M, Mignatti P, Rifkin DB. Basic fibroblast growth factor-induced activation of latent transforming growth factor-β in endothelial cells: regulation of plasminogen activator activity. *J Cell Biol* 1992;118:901–909.
95. Kojima S, Nara K, Rifkin DB. Requirement for transglutaminase in the activation of latent transforming growth factor-β in bovine endothelial cells. *J Cell Biol* 1993;121:439–448.
96. Arciniegas E, Sutton AB, Allen TD, Schor AM. Transforming growth factor beta-1 promotes the differentiation of endothelial cells into smooth muscle-like cells. *J Cell Sci* 1992;103:521–529.
97. Qian SW, Burmester JK, Merwin JR, Madri JA, Sporn MB, Roberts AB. Identification of a structural domain that distinguishes the actions of the type 1 and 2 isoforms of transforming growth factor-β on endothelial cells. *Proc Natl Acad Sci USA* 1992;89:6290–6294.
98. Navab M, Hama SY, Van Lenten BJ, Drinkwater DC, Laks H, Fogelman AM. A new antiinflammatory compound, leumedin, inhibits modification of low density lipoprotein and the resulting transmigration into the subendothelial space of cocultures of human aortic wall cells. *J Clin Invest* 1993;91:1225–1230.
99. Faruqi R, de la Motte CA, DiCorleto PE. α-Tocopherol inhibits agonist-induced monocytic cell adhesion to cultured human endothelial cells. *J Clin Invest* 1994;91:592–600.
100. Schreck R, Baeuerle PA. A role for oxygen radicals as second messengers. *Trends Cell Biol* 1991;1:39–42.
101. Marui N, Offermann MK, Swerlick R, Kunsch C, Rosen CA, Ahmad M, Alexander RW, Medford RM. Vascular cell adhesion molecule-1 (VCAM-1) gene transcription and expression are regulated through an antioxidant-sensitive mechanism in human vascular endothelial cells. *J Clin Invest* 1993;92:1866–1874.
102. Yang J, Xu Y, Hagan MK, Lawley T, Offermann MK. Regulation of adhesion molecule expression in Kaposi's sarcoma cells. *J Immunol* 1994;152:361–373.
103. Schreck R, Rieber P, Baeuerle PA. Reactive oxygen intermediates as apparently widely used messengers in the activation of the NF-kB transcription factor and HIV-1. *EMBO J* 1991;10:2247–2258.
104. Kunisaki M, Umeda F, Inoguchi T, Nawata H. Vitamin E binds to specific binding sites and enhances prostacyclin production by cultured aortic endothelial cells. *Thromb Haemostasis* 1992;68:744–751.
105. Fishman JA, Ryan GB, Karnovsky MJ. Endothelial regeneration in the rat carotid artery and the significance of endothelial denudation in the pathogenesis of myointimal thickening. *Lab Invest* 1975;32:339–351.
106. Haudenschild CC, Schwartz SM. Endothelial regeneration. II. Restitution of endothelial continuity. *Lab Invest* 1979;41:407–418.
107. Lindner V, Reidy MA, Fingerle J. Regrowth of arterial endothelium. Denudation with minimal trauma leads to complete endothelial cell regrowth. *Lab Invest* 1989;61:556–563.
108. Reidy MA, Clowes AW, Schwartz SM. Endothelial regeneration. V. Inhibition of endothelial regrowth in arteries of rat and rabbit. *Lab Invest* 1983;49:569–575.
109. Reidy MA. Endothelial regeneration. VIII. Interaction of smooth muscle cells with endothelial regrowth. *Lab Invest* 1988;59:36–43.
110. Montesano R. Regulation of angiogenesis *in vitro*. *Eur J Clin Invest* 1992;22:504–515.
111. Folkman J, Shing Y. Angiogenesis. *J Biol Chem* 1992;267:10931–10934.
112. Lindner V, Majack RA, Reidy MA. Basic fibroblast growth factor stimulates endothelial regrowth and proliferation in denuded arteries. *J Clin Invest* 1990;85:2004–2008.
113. Bjornsson TD, Dryjski M, Tluczek J, et al. Acidic fibroblast growth factor promotes vascular repair. *Proc Natl Acad Sci USA* 1991;88:8651–8655.
114. Madri JA, Reidy MA, Kocher O, Bell L. Endothelial cell behavior after denudation injury is modulated by transforming growth factor-β1 and fibronectin. *Lab Invest* 1989;60:755–764.
115. Ausprunk DH, Folkman J. Migration and proliferation of endothelial cells in preformed and newly formed blood vessels during tumor angiogenesis. *Microvasc Res* 1977;14:53–65.
116. Folkman J, Klagsbrun M. Angiogenic factors. *Science* 1987;235:442–447.
117. Auerbach R, Arensman R, Kubai L, Folkman J. Tumor-induced angiogenesis: lack of inhibition by irradiation. *Int J Cancer* 1975;15:241–245.
118. Sholley MM, Ferguson GP, Seibel HR, Montour JL, Wilson JD. Mechanisms of neovascularization. Vascular sprouting can occur without proliferation of endothelial cells. *Lab Invest* 1984;51:624–634.
119. Chleboun JO, Martins RN, Mitchell CA, Chirila TV. bFGF enhances the development of the collateral circulation after acute arterial occlusion. *Biochem Biophys Res Commun* 1992;185:510–516.
120. Edelman ER, Nugent MA, Smith LT, Karnovsky MJ. Basic fibroblast growth factor enhances the coupling of intimal hyperplasia and proliferation of vasa vasorum in injured rat arteries. *J Clin Invest* 1992;89:465–473.
121. Nabel EG, Yang Z, Plautz G, et al. Recombinant fibroblast growth factor-1 promotes intimal hyperplasia and angiogenesis in arteries *in vivo*. *Nature* 1993;362:844–846.

Atherosclerosis and Coronary Artery Disease, edited by V. Fuster, R. Ross, and E. J. Topol. Lippincott-Raven Publishers, Philadelphia © 1996.

CHAPTER 23

Role of Alterations in the Differentiated State of Vascular Smooth Muscle Cells in Atherogenesis

Gary K. Owens

Key Words: Myosin heavy chain; Myosin light chain(s); Smooth muscle cells(s).

INTRODUCTION

Intimal migration and proliferation of smooth muscle cells (SMC) is known to play an integral role in development of atherosclerotic disease (1,2). As such, there has been keen interest in identifying factors that have growth-promoting and chemotactic activity for vascular SMC and in determining whether these factors play a role in the atherogenic process (see elsewhere in this text). An additional feature of SMC within atherosclerotic lesions which has been known for many years is that cells exhibit marked differences in morphology and protein expression patterns as compared to normal medial SMC (3–6) (Figs. 1–3). This is characterized by decreased expression of proteins that are characteristic of differentiated smooth muscle (SM), including SM isoforms of contractile proteins, as well as altered growth regulation, lipid metabolism, and decreased contractility (reviewed in ref. 7). These phenotypic changes in the differentiated state of intimal SMC are not simply a function of the growth state of the SMC, since alterations persist even when growth rates return to normal (8–10). Indeed there is considerable evidence to suggest that the alterations in differentiated state of intimal SMC include changes in growth factor receptor expression and growth responsiveness (11–13). Thus, alterations in the differentiated state of intimal SMC are likely to play a key role in the atherogenic process, and there has been considerable interest in identifying the factors and mechanisms responsible for these changes. Before considering this issue, however, we need

G. K. Owens: Department of Molecular Physiology and Biological Physics, University of Virginia School of Medicine, Charlottesville, Virginia 22908.

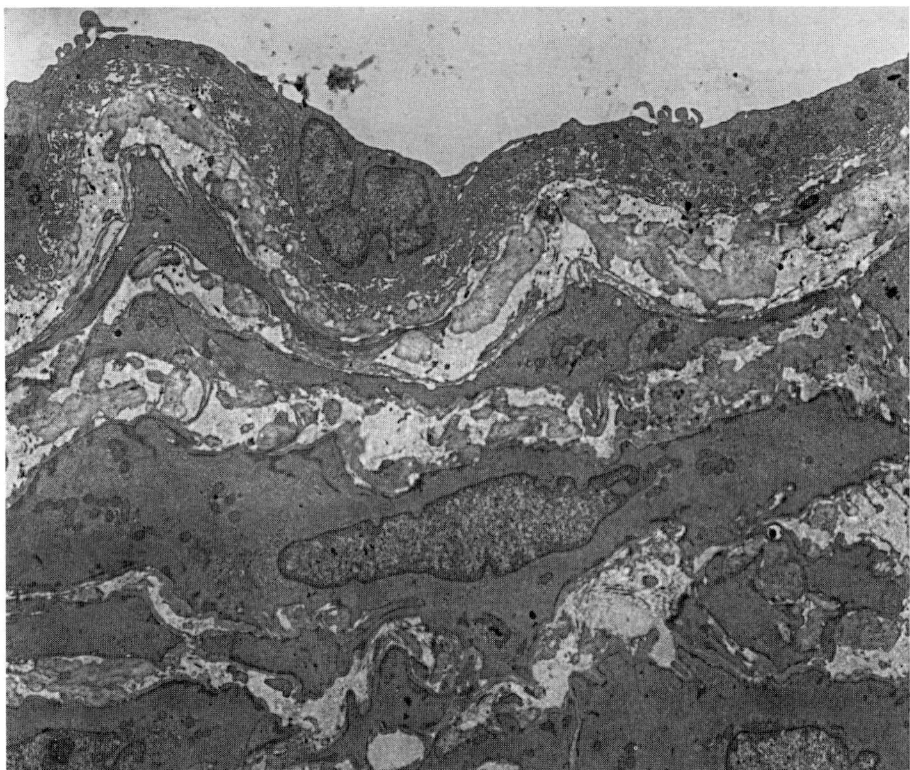

FIG. 1. A transmission electron micrograph of a segment from a normal monkey artery. The endothelial cells lie very close to the internal elastic lamina, beneath which are seen several smooth muscle cells. These cells contain a large complement of myofilaments that surrounds the nucleus. Very few cellular organelles can be seen in this micrograph. (Courtesy of Russell Ross, University of Washington, Seattle, Washington.)

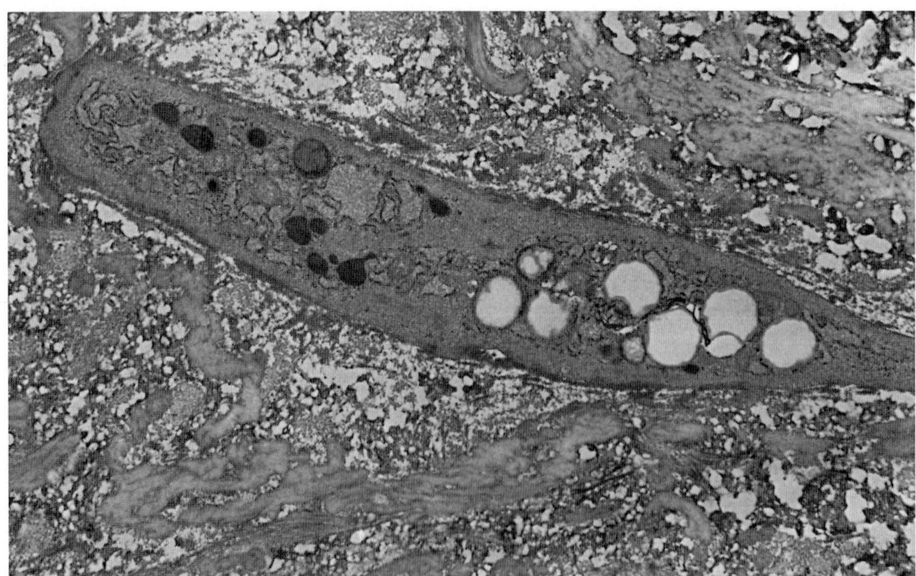

FIG. 2. A portion of a smooth muscle cell in the intima of a lesion of atherosclerosis. This cell is surrounded by large amounts of connective tissue matrix, including collagen fibrils cut transversely, as well as elastic fibers and proteoglycans. The smooth muscle cell is surrounded by an irregular basement membrane. Within the cell can be seen numerous cisternae of rough endoplasmic reticulum and numerous lipid droplets, some of which are dense and others of which have been extracted, suggesting they represent different forms of lipid. Mitochondria are visible as well as some myofilaments. This cell is typical of a "synthetic state" cell usually seen in lesions of atherosclerosis deep within the intima. (Courtesy of Russell Ross, University of Washington, Seattle, Washington.)

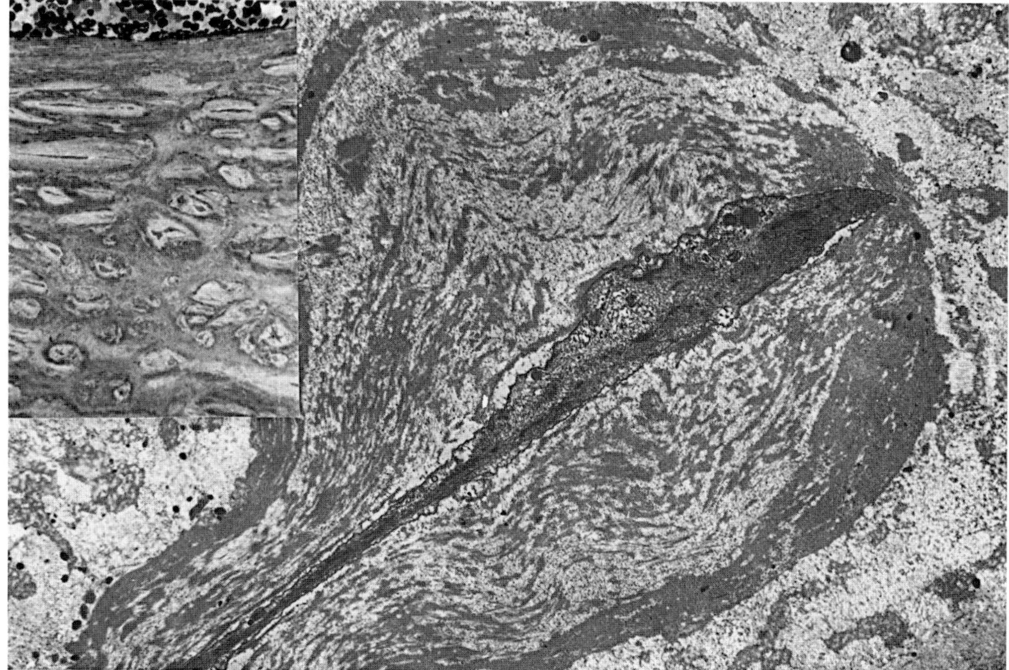

FIG. 3. A smooth muscle cell located in a "lacunar-like space" that often is disrupted when the lesions are fixed and embedded in paraffin. The cells drop out during sectioning because of the relative differences in density between the matrix and the cell. Here the smooth muscle cell can be recognized by the myofilaments within the cell. The cell is surrounded by multiple "onion-skin-like" layers of basement membrane, proteoglycan, and collagen. This is typical of smooth muscle cells in the dense portion of the fibrous cap that overlies a fibrous plaque, an advanced lesion of atherosclerosis. (Courtesy of Russell Ross, University of Washington, Seattle, Washington.)

to first examine the features of normal (fully differentiated) vascular SMC, and how differentiation/maturation is regulated in these cells. I will not review the developmental biology of the SMC since this is covered elsewhere in this text (see refs. 7 and 14 for reviews).

CHARACTERISTICS OF DIFFERENTIATED VASCULAR SMOOTH MUSCLE CELLS

Vascular SMC Are Multifunctional

The primary function of the vascular SMC in mature animals is contraction, and the SMC has evolved a repertoire of appropriate contractile proteins, agonist receptors, ion channels, signal-transducing molecules, etc., to carry out this specialized function. Morphologically, differentiated vascular SM in mature animals is virtually packed with contractile myofilaments and associated structures (15) and is a cell nearly completely geared for contraction (see ref. 7 for a review). Although the principal function of the mature SMC is contraction, this cell is also capable of a multitude of other functions that vary at different developmental stages, during vascular repair, and in vascular disease (see refs. 7 and 16 for reviews). For example, fully differentiated SMC in mature blood vessels proliferate at extremely low rates and produce only small amounts of extracellular matrix proteins. In contrast, these processes are greatly accelerated during development of the vascular system, during vessel remodeling, following vessel injury, and in atherogenesis. The remarkable plasticity of the vascular SMC must be considered a necessary part of the SMC differentiation program that has evolved because it conferred a survival advantage to the organism. That is, a given SMC can exhibit a broad spectrum of different phenotypes in response to different physiologic or pathologic stimuli. If an artery is injured, some SMC must be recruited to repair that injury, while at the same time the contractile function of the blood vessel must be maintained for normal cardiovascular homeostasis.

The plasticity/multiplicity of the SMC has confounded efforts to understand the cellular and molecular processes that control differentiation. Moreover, each of the different phenotypic states of the SMC has somewhat different marker proteins that are characteristic of that state, and presumably differences in the mechanisms that regulate that particular differentiation program. This differs considerably from cardiac and skeletal muscle, which undergo terminal, and essentially irreversible, differentiation and which exhibit much more restricted cellular plasticity (17,18). Control of differentiation in these cell types, while proving to be extremely complex, is nevertheless easier to study because of the stability associated with the terminally differentiated state. Key considerations in studying SMC differentiation are (a) to first determine which (biologically relevant) SMC phenotype is being studied, (b) to identify a repertoire of marker proteins and cellular functions that characterize that phenotypic state and their temporal pattern of expression, and (c) to develop appropriate experimental systems with which to determine the cellular and molecular mechanisms and extrinsic factors that control that process.

It is important to distinguish proteins that are characteristic of a given stage (or state) of SMC differentiation/maturation versus proteins that alone can serve as definitive markers for identification of SMC lineages to the exclusion of all other cell types. While it has been the goal of many investigators to identify the latter, at this time no marker strictly meets these criteria, with the possible exception of SM myosin heavy-chain isoforms SM-1 and SM-2 (19–22). Given the multifunctionality of the SMC and the fact that many of its functions are common to other cell types, the SMC may express few if any cell-specific lineage markers. Clear identification of the SMC and assessment of its state of differentiation must rely on multiple criteria, including expression of multiple SMC selective proteins, the morphologic and functional characteristics of the cell, and, in the case of *in vivo* studies, the cell's anatomic location.

Contractile Proteins as Markers of Differentiated Vascular SMC

The contractile proteins represent logical candidates for use in studying differentiation of SMC. Indeed, mature vascular SM has been shown to express unique isoforms of a variety of contractile proteins that are important for their differentiated function. This includes SM α-actin (23,24), SM myosin heavy chains (19,20), SM myosin light chains (25,26), and SM α-tropomyosin (27–29). In addition, differentiated SMC also express a number of proteins that are part of the cytoskeleton and/or purported to be involved in regulation of contraction, such as calponin (30), SM-22α (30), h-caldesmon (31), gamma-vinculin (32), (α- and β-) metavinculin (32,33), and desmin (24,34), which show at least some degree of SMC specificity/selectivity (reviewed in ref. 7).

SM α-actin is one of six isoactins expressed in mammalian cells (35). Each is a product of a separate gene, although they share an extremely high degree of homology in the protein coding regions (35). Mature, fully differentiated SMC express four actin isoforms, including SM α-actin, nonmuscle β-actin, nonmuscle gamma actin, and SM gamma actin (23,24). The most abundant of the actin isoforms in mature vascular SM is SM α-actin. It is also the single most abundant protein in SMC, making up 40% of total cell protein (36). The high SM α-actin content is required for the high force-generating capabilities of the SMC (23,37).

Results of early studies indicated that SM α-actin was expressed exclusively by SMC and SMC-related cells, such as pericytes (38) and juxtaglomerular cells (39). However, it is now known that it is transiently expressed by a variety of mesodermally derived cells during development, tissue repair, and neoplastic growth (40–42). For example, SM α-actin is transiently expressed in the early stages of differentiation of both cardiac and skeletal myocytes (43,44), as well as in myofibroblasts in healing wounds (40) and in tumors (41). Its expression can also be induced in a number of non-SMC in culture (45,46). Thus SM α-actin expression alone does not provide definitive evidence for SMC lineage. However, its expression in adult animals is highly tissue specific under normal circumstances (24,47). Moreover, there is clear evidence for cell-type-specific regulation of transcription of this gene, thus making it a very useful gene with which to study the molecular regulation of the differentiation program in vascular SM (48–50). SM α-actin is also the first known marker of differentiated SMC that is expressed during vasculogenesis (34,51,52). It is first detected in the presumptive SMC that initially envelope the dorsal aortae at stage 12 (day 2 of development) in chicken (51), and quail (52) embryos. Significantly, at this stage SM α-actin expression was limited to those presumptive SMC that were in direct proximity to dorsal aortic endothelial cells and was not observed in surrounding mesodermal cells.

Thus, SM α-actin is a useful marker of differentiated vascular SMC. It is particularly useful for recognizing the early stages of SMC differentiation, and, as will be discussed later, is one of the last markers of differentiated SMC to be lost when cells undergo phenotypic modulation. However, it alone cannot be used for identification of the SMC lineage to the exclusion of other cell types, since under some circumstances it can be expressed by other cell types.

Mature vascular SMC also express a number of cell-specific/selective isoforms of myosin (19–21,53–55). Myosin is an essential component of the contractile system that is present in all muscle and nonmuscle cells. It is a hexamer consisting of two myosin heavy chains (MHC), a pair of 17-kDa nonphosphorylatable alkali light chains (also designated MLC-1 and MLC-3), and a pair of regulatory (phosphorylatable) 20-kDa light chains (MLC-2). Myosin regulatory light chain from vertebrate SM as well as nonmuscle cells plays a key role in the regulation of SM contraction and nonmuscle cell motility via Ca^{2+}-calmodulin-dependent phosphorylation catalyzed by myosin light-chain kinase (see references 56 and 57 for review). Multiple isoforms of all of these subunits of myosin have been found, and the expression of the isoforms is differentially regulated in a tissue-specific- and developmental-stage-related manner (55,56).

Vascular SMC express at least three SM variants as well as two nonmuscle variants of the heavy chain (19,21,53,54). Kawamoto and Adelstein (58) have classified the 196-kDa nonmuscle-type MHC as NMHC-A and the 198-kDa nonmuscle MHC as NMHC-B. The NMHC-B appears to be identical to the 198-kDa MHC designated SMemb that is expressed in developing rabbit embryonic aortas, intimal SMC of animals with experimental atherogenesis, human atherosclerotic lesions, and cultured SMC (55,59–61). The SMC variants were originally identified on the basis of their differential migration on porous sodium dodecyl sulfate (SDS)–polyacrylamide gels as well as their reactivity with myosin antibodies on Western blots (19,20,61). Results of these studies demonstrated the presence of 204-kDa and 200-kDa MHC proteins which have been identified as SM-1 and SM-2, respectively. Subsequent studies by Periasamy and co-workers (54) demonstrated that the SM variants SM-1 and SM-2 are produced by alternative splicing of a gene that is distinct from the genes encoding nonmuscle, skeletal, or cardiac MHC isoforms. The SM-2 isoform contains 9 amino acids not contained in SM-1 that are encoded by a unique 39-nucleotide exon at the carboxy terminus, whereas the SM-1 isoform contains a longer carboxyl end containing 43 amino acids. The functional significance of these differences in the myosin heavy-chain tail are not known.

More recent studies have identified additional isoform diversity of SM-1 in the S1 head region (53,62,63). These isoforms have been designated SM-1A and SM-1B. Their mRNAs are completely identical in their coding regions except that the SM-1B isoform contains an insert of 21 nucleotides, encoding seven amino acids in a region near the adenosine triphosphate (ATP) binding site in the myosin head. S1 nuclease protection assays demonstrated that SM-1A and SM-1B mRNAs are coexpressed in all SM tissues, although the proportion of the two mRNA differs markedly between tissues. The SM-1A form predominates in most SM tissues, including vascular SMC, whereas SM-1B predominates in intestinal and urinary bladder SMC. Kelley et al. (63) found that the presence of the seven-amino acid insert in SM-1B correlated with a higher velocity of movement of actin filaments *in vitro* and a higher actin-activated Mg^{2+} ATPase activity compared with SM-1A myosin, suggesting that the presence of the insert in SM-1B may be of functional importance and may contribute to differences in contractile properties between different SMC tissues [for a comprehensive review of this area see a recent review by Somlyo (56)].

Expression of SM MHC isoforms has been extensively scrutinized, and shows a high degree of SMC specificity in both mature and developing organisms (19,21,22,55,60, 64,65). Indeed, at this time SM-1 and SM-2 myosin heavy chains may be the most rigorous markers for identification of differentiated SMC. Borrione et al. (66) suggested that SM MHC are expressed at low levels in subconfluent bovine aortic endothelial cells in culture, although not by endothelial cells *in vivo*. However, we have found that the principal antibody employed in these studies (which is now commercially available from Sigma, hSM-V, cat. #M7754) shows cross-reactivity with a 198- to 200-kDa nonmuscle MHC (presumably nonmuscle MHC B or SMEMB; see refs. 58 and 59) that is present in endothelial cells and migrates very closely with SM-2, but is not recognized by our SM MHC-specific monoclonal antibodies (ref. 67, and Thompson and G. K. Owens, *unpublished observations*).

Expression of the various MHC isoforms in SMC shows extensive developmental regulation (21,60). Based on immunocytochemical studies and Western blot analysis with SM-1- and SM-2-specific antibodies as well as S1 nuclease protection assays to distinguish SM-1 versus SM-2 mRNAs, Kuro-o et al. (60) demonstrated that vascular SMC from adult rabbits expressed both SM-1 and SM-2 MHC. In contrast, fetal SMC expressed the 200-kDa nonmuscle and SM-1 MHC isoforms, but not SM-2. Aikawa et al. (21) found that similar developmental changes in MHC expression occur in humans. They reported that SM-1 as well as nonmuscle MHC were expressed in fetal arteries at an early gestational stage, whereas SM-2 was upregulated during late fetal and postnatal development. Miano et al. (22) utilized *in situ* hybridization and RNAase protection assays to assess the temporal and spatial pattern of SMC differentiation during mouse development. Although their assays did not distinguish between SM-1 and SM-2, their results demonstrated that SM MHC expression was completely restricted to SM tissues, and was first evident in the early developing aorta at 10.5 days postcoitum (p.c.). No expression was demonstrated beyond the aorta and its arches until 12.5–13.5 days p.c., when SM MHC mRNA appeared in SMC of the developing gut as well as in peripheral blood vessels. No SM MHC transcripts were ever detected in developing brain, heart, or skeletal muscle, except within blood vessels within these tissues. Taken together, the preceding results establish that SM MHC is a highly specific marker of the SMC lineage. SM-1 appears to be a relatively early SMC differentiation marker, whereas SM-2 appears relatively late in SMC development.

Multiple isoforms of the phosphorylatable 20-kDa regulatory MLC have been described in arterial SM (reviewed in ref. 56). This includes an "SM" regulatory LC (also designated $L_{20\text{-}A}$) and a "nonmuscle" isoform (also designated $L_{20\text{-}B}$). Despite names that imply cell-specific expression, both are expressed in multiple SM as well as nonmuscle cells and tissues (56,68). For example, platelets contain approximately equal amounts of the SM and nonmuscle MLC_{20} isoforms. There are no reports of there being isoformic variants that affect function.

Tropomyosins are rodlike proteins that are usually found in tight association with actin filaments in muscle and nonmuscle cells (27–29). In skeletal and cardiac muscle, tropomyosins play a central role in regulation of contraction through mediation of the calcium response of the troponin complex to actin filaments (69). In contrast, the physiologic role of tropomyosins in SM and nonmuscle cells is poorly understood, due in part to the fact that these cells lack troponin (27,28). Multiple isoforms of tropomyosin have been detected in muscle and nonmuscle cells at both the protein and mRNA levels (70–72). These are the products of an extremely complex (and often confusing) regulatory system involving at least four different genes, each encoding multiple muscle and nonmuscle isoforms through alternative splicing (see ref. 73 for a review). Vascular SMC express several nonmuscle as well as SM tropomyosin isoforms (36,70,72,74). SM α-tropomyosin is a product of differential mRNA splicing from a single α-tropomyosin gene and is distinct from striated and nonmuscle α-tropomyosin isoforms by virtue of expression of exon 2, which encodes for amino acids 39–80 of the protein (72,74). Expression of the SM α-tropomyosin isoform appears to be limited to SMC, at least in adult organisms (72). However, the tissue distribution of SM α-tropomyosin has not been extensively scrutinized due in part to the lack of isoform-specific antibodies. SM α-tropomyosin transcripts are first detectable 4.5–6 days p.c. in extracts of whole-mouse embryos and then increase with developmental age (75). SM α-tropomyosin transcripts are also detectable in undifferentiated embryonic stem cells, and at all stages of embryoid body development *in vitro*. As such, SM α-tropomyosin is not useful as SMC lineage marker for developmental studies. However, the fact that its expression in adult animals is restricted to SMC and is developmentally regulated indicates that it is useful for assessing the relative state of differentiation/maturation of vascular SMC.

Other Markers of Differentiated Vascular SMC

Calponin is a 34-kDa protein that interacts with F-actin and tropomyosin in a Ca^{2+}-independent manner and with calmodulin in a Ca^{2+}-dependent manner, and has also been found to inhibit actin activated MgATPase activity of myosin *in vitro* (reviewed in ref. 30). On the basis of these properties it has been postulated to function as a regulator of SMC contraction. However, the mechanism of actin-linked regulation via calponin is not clear, either with regard to the possible role of phosphorylation or with respect to the reported additional involvement of caldesmon (31,76). Two isoforms of calponin have been identified by molecular cloning (77,78). The encoded isoforms, denoted α and β, have 292 and 252 amino acids and M_r 32,333 and 28,127, respectively. They appear to be derived by alternative splicing, in that the nucleotide sequences are identical except for a 120-base pair insert in calponin α that encodes a 40-amino acid segment corresponding to residues 217–256. A related 22-kDa protein, designated SM-22α, has also been identified in SMC which contains sequence motifs that are homologous to calponin (78). However, unlike calponin, there is no evidence for binding to any contractile protein. At present its function is unknown.

In adult organisms, calponin and SM-22α expression appear to be restricted almost exclusively to SM. Shanahan et al. (79) found high levels of calponin and SM-22α mRNA in aorta, bladder, vas deferens, and uterus, but not in kidney or brain in adult rats. Gimona et al. (80) observed no calponin immunoreactivity in extracts of chicken skeletal muscle, kidney, liver, and spleen. Takahashi et al. (81) found no evidence for expression of calponin in bovine atria, ventricles, or brain cortex, but did observe a 36-kDa immunoreactive protein in bovine adrenal medulla and cortex. Calponin-immunoreactive proteins have also been detected in bovine platelets, human umbilical-vein endothelial cells, and fibroblasts (82,83), although it remains to be established unequivocally that these are indeed calponins.

Calponin and SM-22α expression have been shown to be altered in association with differentiation of SMC. Calponin and SM-22α expression are first detectable in the dorsal aortae of the chick on days 4–6 of embryonic development (51), thus making it one of the earliest markers of differentiated SMC. Likewise, Frid et al. (65) found evidence for developmental regulation of calponin in vascular SMC in humans. They observed that major increases in calponin expression occurred relatively late in development (i.e., >22–24 weeks of gestation). However, consistent with observations of Duband et al. (51), low levels of calponin were also detectable in the 8- to 10-week-old fetus, the earliest developmental time point studied.

Caldesmon is a major calmodulin and actin-binding protein that is found in SM and nonmuscle cells (31). It has been suggested that caldesmon plays a role in regulation of contraction. However, direct evidence for this in intact SM tissues is lacking. Two isoforms of caldesmon can be discerned by their mobility upon SDS–PAGE: h-caldesmon (M_r of 120–150 kDa) and l-caldesmon (M_r of 70–80 kDa) (31) which are generated from a single gene via alternative splicing (31,84). The two isoforms show markedly different cell and tissue distributions. The h-caldesmon isoform is abundantly expressed in differentiated SM, whereas l-caldesmon is found in nonmuscle tissue and cells as well as immature SMC (31,85). Neither caldesmon isoform is detectable in adult skeletal and cardiac muscle. However, h-caldesmon is expressed in the fusion-defective BC_3Hl skeletal myoblast line following serum-depletion and density-dependent differentiation (85). Whereas further studies are needed to determine whether h-caldesmon is also transiently expressed by skeletal myoblasts *in vivo,* it is clear that h-caldesmon expression, like that of SM α-actin, SM MLC, and (possibly) calponin, is not strictly limited to SMC. As such, it cannot be used as an unambiguous marker for identification of SMC lineages to the exclusion of all other cell types.

Expression of caldesmon is developmentally regulated in vascular as well as nonvascular SM. Duband et al. (51) first detected h-caldesmon in the dorsal aorta on embryonic day 6 in the chick. Koteliansky and co-workers (64,65) examined changes in l- and h-caldesmon in human aortic SMC during development based on immunohistochemical staining with monoclonal antibodies for each of these proteins, as well as by gel electrophoretic analyses. Results demonstrated that aortic SMC from 8- to 10-week-old fetuses expressed very low levels of h-caldesmon relative to l-caldesmon. Major increases in h-caldesmon expression in aortic SMC occurred relatively late in development, including a nearly sixfold increase in the ratio of h- to l-caldesmon between 10-week-old fetuses and 24-week-old fetuses. Results indicate that h-caldesmon may be a marker of a later SMC differentiation/maturation stage than SM α-actin, but an earlier marker than SM-2 MHC.

Vinculin is a 117-kDa cytoskeletal protein associated with membrane actin-filament-attachment sites of cell–cell and cell–matrix adherens-type junctions (32,33). There is remarkable heterogeneity of vinculin in the form of antigenically indistinguishable isoelectrophoretic variants, some which show tissue-selective expression (86,87). These include three isoforms designated α, α', and β isoforms that are found in all cell types, and a gamma form that shows selective expression in cardiac and SM (86). In addition to these isovinculins, smooth, cardiac, and skeletal muscle tissues were found to express a protein of 150 kDa that was antigenically related to vinculin, denoted metavinculin (88,89). Two isoforms of metavinculin have been described, denoted α- and β-metavinculin. In SM, both vinculin and metavinculin are located in F-actin-membrane attachment sites of dense plaques (32,33). Both α- and β-metavinculin show tissue-selective expression, with reports thus far showing expression only in smooth and cardiac muscle (86). No information is available as to when gamma-vinculin and α- and β-metavinculin are first expressed during differentiation of vascular SMC. However, developmental increases in expression of vinculin have been shown to occur postnatally in the human aorta (90). As such, the α- and β-metavinculins and gamma-vinculin may be useful markers with which to study differentiation/maturation, although they are clearly not specific for the SMC lineage.

The principal intermediate filament (i.e., 7- to 11-nm filaments) proteins expressed by vascular SM are desmin and vimentin (24,34,91). Cytokeratin has also been detected in immature SMC during development as well as in intimal atherosclerotic lesions (92). The proportion of desmin versus vimentin varies among different SM tissues and among different blood vessels within the vasculature. There also appear to be some species differences in the relative proportions and/or the distribution of these two proteins. Vascular SM in the aorta and other large conduit vessels contains predominantly vimentin rather than desmin (24), whereas the intermediate filaments in SMC of smaller arteries and arterioles as well as gastrointestinal and uterine SMC contain predominantly desmin (24,34,93). Gabbiani and co-workers (24,94) have also presented evidence for heterogeneity in expression of desmin and vimentin within individual SMC within the normal aortic media, with some cells expressing exclusively vimentin and others expressing both of these intermediate filament proteins.

Vimentin is expressed in a wide variety of muscle and nonmuscle cell types, and is expressed very early in the developing embryo prior to the formation of the vasculature (95,96). As such, it is of limited usefulness as either a marker of SMC lineage or for assessing the differentiation/maturation state of the SMC. Desmin is largely, but not exclusively, expressed in muscle cells, including cardiac and skeletal muscle, as well as SM (95,96). Desmin expression is developmentally regulated in skeletal and cardiac muscle, showing marked increases in expression during myogenesis (97). Similarly, desmin expression is developmentally regulated in the SMC of the gut and urogenital tracts of the chicken (95) and mammals (98). However, surprisingly, there is a relative paucity of information regarding whether desmin expression is developmentally regulated in vascular SM, although it does not appear to be expressed early in development of the great vessels in the mouse (96). However, it should be noted that in rodents, desmin is also expressed at low levels in these vessels in mature animals (24). Taken together, studies indicate that desmin is clearly not a specific marker of the SMC lineage, but may be useful in assessing the relative state of differentiation/maturation of vascular SMC within certain, but probably not all blood vessels.

Vascular SMC express a large repertoire of ion channels and membrane receptors that are critical in influencing a cells contractile behavior through effects on its electrical activities and sensitivity to stimulation by hormones, neurotransmitters, and contractile agonists (see refs. 99 and 100 for review). The specific repertoire of ion channels and receptors that are expressed varies widely among different vascular beds, and is a key determinant of the contractile responsiveness of the SMC. Most of these receptors and ion channels are not expressed in multipotential cells that give rise to SMC, but rather appear during differentiation/maturation of the SMC (101,102). For example, there is evidence for developmental regulation of a number of contractile agonist receptors in vascular SMC, including the angiotensin II receptor subtypes (103,104), muscarinic M1, M2, and M3 receptors (105), vasopressin V1a and V2 receptors (106), α_1-adrenergic receptors (107), and β-adrenergic receptors (108). With just a few possible exceptions, the ion channels and receptors expressed by vascular SM are also expressed by many other cell types (99,100,109). As such, they cannot be used as SMC lineage markers, although they are appropriate candidates for use in assessing the relative state of differentiation of SMC.

Summary of SMC Differentiation/Maturation Markers

In summary, at present, the best differentiation/maturation markers for vascular SM would appear to be SM α-actin, the SM myosin heavy chains SM-1 and SM-2, calponin, SM-22α, h-caldesmon, gamma-vinculin, and α- and β-metavinculin. Of these, only the SM myosin heavy chains, and perhaps calponin, appear to be specific for the SMC lineage and capable of identifying SMC to the exclusion of other cell types. However, further scrutiny of these markers may identify exceptions. As such, for now clear identification of SMC as well as assessment of the relative stage of differentiation/maturation of the SMC should rely on use of multiple markers.

REGULATION OF DIFFERENTIATION/ MATURATION IN VASCULAR SMOOTH MUSCLE CELLS

General Principles of Control of Cellular Differentiation

Cellular differentiation is the process by which multipotential cells in the developing organism acquire those cell-specific functions and properties that distinguish them from other cell types (see ref. 110 for a review). Whereas the SMC, like the majority of somatic cells, contains a complete set of genetic material, it expresses only a small number of the genes present. Indeed the essence of understanding the control of differentiation is to determine how a cell coordinately regulates the expression of those families of genes necessary for its specialized function. How is it determined which genes will be expressed, when, and at what levels?

The processes whereby multipotential cells acquire those cell-specific characteristics exhibited in mature animals has conventionally been subdivided into three stages, determination, differentiation, and maturation. Determination is the process by which multipotential cells in the developing embryo become committed to a particular cell lineage. Differentiation is the process by which cells that are committed to a particular cell lineage first manifest those cell-specific characteristics that distinguish that cell type. Maturation refers to the later stages of differentiation and is characterized by acquisition of further cell-specific properties ultimately resulting in the cellular phenotype characteristic of the mature organism. Although these are often considered to be distinct stages, they really form a continuum, with our ability to distinguish the stages being dependent on the extent of our knowledge of the cellular markers that characterize that stage and the molecular processes that control progression from one stage to another. Indeed in most cases the determination event can only be identified retrospectively from cell labeling studies, since by definition cells in this stage have not yet acquired cell-specific characteristics that allow them to be recognized. For purposes of simplicity in this review, we will use the term differentiation to refer to the entire process by which committed but undifferentiated SMC acquire their cell-specific phenotypes, recognizing that the immediate precursor to the differentiated SMC (i.e., SMC myoblast) and the precise embryologic origins of that cell have not been clearly identified (see ref. 7 for review).

Studies in other cells, principally skeletal muscle, have established a number of general principles of differentiation control that are likely to be applicable to differentiation control in multiple cell systems, including vascular SM. One principle that has been established is that differentiation involves continuous regulation, not simply permanent activation or inactivation of genes, and several families of master regulatory genes have been identified that control skeletal muscle differentiation (see refs. 17, 111, and 112 for review). The first of these, MyoD, was isolated by subtractive hybridization approaches using an inducible differentiation system in which multipotential 10T1/2 mouse fibroblasts were converted to skeletal muscle through treatment with the DNA hypomethylating agent 5-azacytidine (113,114). MyoD and the related factors myogenin (115,116), myf-5 (117), and MRF/herculin/myf-6 (118) encode transcriptional regulatory factors that are capable of converting a variety of cell lines, including SM (119), to skeletal myoblasts. The actions of these factors are mediated, at least in part, via the direct activation of a number of muscle-specific genes, including muscle creatine kinase, cardiac α-actin, myosin light chain, and troponin I (see refs. 17 and 111 for review). They are part of a larger family of eukaryotic transcriptional regulators that contain a basic helix–loop–helix (HLH) motif that is involved in protein dimerization and DNA binding. Members of the MyoD family dimerize with ubiquitously expressed members of the HLH family such as E12, E47, and ITF, and subsequently bind a consensus sequence (CANNTG), referred to as an E-box, found in the promoters of many skeletal muscle genes, and activate gene transcription. Another group of transcription factors referred to as the MEF2 proteins have also been shown to play a significant role in the myogenic cascade triggered by the MyoD family (120). Tontonoz et al. (121) recently identified a novel HLH transcription factor, ADD1, that appears to play a role in the regulation of determination- and differentiation-specific gene expression in adipocytes. The preceding studies have thus established the presence of master regulatory genes that are involved in the continuous control of the differentiation program in skeletal muscle, and adipocytes. It must be noted, however, that there is some controversy as to whether the MyoD family should be considered true "lineage control genes" as opposed to "master differentiation control genes," since (a) MyoD and related family members directly activate a large number of differentiation-specific genes in skeletal muscle (17), and (b) a number of putative upstream regulators of the MyoD family have been identified through gene knockout experiments which are expressed prior MyoD in committed but undifferentiated myoblasts (122,123).

Given that contractile function in SM is extremely complex and is dependent on a large number of proteins being expressed at the right time and at the appropriate levels, it seems highly likely that differentiation control in SM will involve at least some "master differentiation" control genes that coordinately regulate expression of those genes necessary for the differentiated function of SMC. However, not all proteins characteristic of differentiated SMC appear to be coordinately regulated at least at the protein level either during development or in disease. As such, if master differentiation control genes exist in SM, they are presumably much more restrictive in the number of target genes that they effect as compared to the MyoD family. Note that the alternative explanation is that the entire family of genes necessary for differentiated function in SM is independently regulated. Whereas this is possible, it seems improbable based on studies in other cell systems. Clearly much more work is needed in this important area, and no master differentiation control genes have been identified in SM, nor has a single transcription factor been identified that is either selective or specific for one of the SM differentiation marker genes. Surprisingly very little work has been done in this important area (see ref. 7 for a review).

Extrinsic Factors that Influence the Differentiated State of Vascular SMC

Consideration of the factors and mechanisms that regulate the differentiated state of SMC is complicated by the extreme plasticity of this cell type which enables it to undergo rapid and reversible changes in its phenotype in response to environmental influences. Indeed, maintenance of the differentiated state of the SMC is likely to be dependent on continuous regulation, rather than more permanent regulatory controls, to a much greater extent than cells with less cellular plasticity such as skeletal muscle (112). This, coupled with evidence that SMC are derived from multiple lineages (as discussed in the chapter by Fishman), suggests that SMC differentiation is under control of complex local cues. These are not well understood. However, a summary of our current understanding of some of these factors is presented in the following sections and in Fig. 4.

Influence of Growth State

A theme that has dominated the field for many years is that growth and differentiation are mutually exclusive processes in SMC, and that the differentiated state of the SMC is largely controlled by factors that regulate its growth. This hypothesis was originally proposed in a series of pioneering studies by Chamley-Campbell et al. (124,125) which demonstrated that loss of myosin- and actin-containing filaments preceded onset of cell proliferation in primary cultures of SMC. These investigators hypothesized that SMC normally exist in a nonproliferating "contractile state" and must modulate to a "synthetic state" as a prerequisite for cellular proliferation. Indeed there is overwhelming evidence showing that SMC in culture show increased growth factor receptor expression and responsiveness, diminished expression of markers of SMC differentiation (as discussed in an earlier section), alterations in lipid metabolism, increased abundance of synthetic cellular organelles, diminished myofilaments, and a host of other features that distinguish them from their *in vivo* counterparts (19,80,124,126–132). However, a

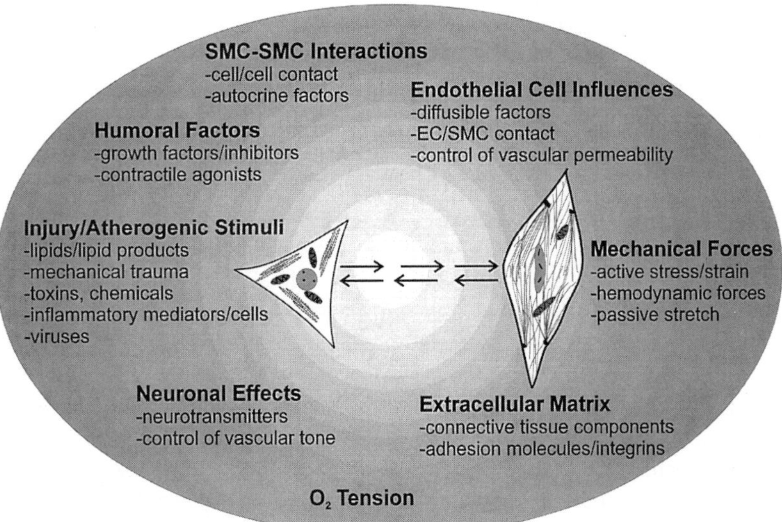

FIG. 4. A summary of some of the extrinsic factors or local environmental cues that are either known or believed to be important in controlling the differentiation/maturation state of the vascular smooth muscle cell *(SMC)*. This figure emphasizes the point that differentiation/maturation of vascular smooth muscle cells is dependent on the complex interaction of a multitude of local environmental cues, not any single factor, and that a change in any one of these may lead to alterations in the differentiated state of the SMC (i.e., "phenotypic modulation"). Importantly, there appear to be a broad range of different phenotypes that can be exhibited by the SMC, depending on the nature of those environmental changes. This includes a spectrum of phenotypes ranging from the highly synthetic proliferative SMC **(left)** to the highly contractile fully differentiated/mature SMC **(right).** The multiple arrows connecting the two cell types are meant to illustrate the multiplicity of phenotypes that are available between these two extremes and the fact that changes appear to be reversible. It should be noted that it cannot be assumed that changes that occur during development are necessarily recapitulated during phenotypic modulation in response to injury, atherogenic stimuli, etc., and for this reason two separate pathways are shown between the two representative cell types rather than simply a single reversible pathway.

weakness has been the inability to distinguish between changes that were truly growth-related and those which merely represented an adaptation to growth/survival in culture. Data were also strictly correlative in nature, and it is unclear whether there was a cause–effect relationship between alterations in SMC phenotype and onset of proliferation. Most importantly, studies have not distinguished whether "phenotypic modulation" was secondary to growth or vice versa. Other groups (133–136), including our own (126), have not observed a prolonged lag period (5–7 days) prior to onset of cell proliferation in culture, and onset of proliferation clearly preceded complete loss of SMC differentiation markers such as actin and myosin. Moreover, such lag times have not been observed in organ culture systems in which cells are not enzymatically dissociated (137,138). Significantly, DeMey et al. (137) showed that loss of contractility in vascular SM organ culture occurred independent of onset of cell proliferation. The time course for SMC modulation proposed based on experiments in primary cultures of SMC (124) is also inconsistent with the kinetics of initiation of SMC proliferation *in vivo* following vascular injury (139). This raises the possibility that the delayed onset of proliferation observed may have been due to the cell culture methods employed rather than to a requirement for phenotypic modulation. Consistent with this, electron microscopic studies have clearly shown that mitotic SMC in intact SM tissues *in vivo* express many characteristics of differentiated SMC (140,141). Thus, whereas the hypothesis that the differentiated state of SMC is a critical determinant of its growth responsiveness is attractive, and is supported by an abundance of circumstantial evidence, a number of critical issues remain to be clearly resolved. Among the central issues that need to be addressed are the following. (a) How distinctive are the various differentiated states that are available to the SMC? (b) What extent of SMC differentiation/maturation is compatible with proliferation? (c) What changes in growth potential are associated with each state? (d) How reversible are transitions from one state to the other? (e) What controls these transitions?

Studies in our laboratory and others have demonstrated that the effect of growth stimulation on expression of SM differentiation markers varies depending on the means of growth stimulation and the SMC differentiation marker examined (19,70,142,143). For example, in early studies we observed that the fractional expression of SM isoforms of actin (126,144) relative to the nonmuscle forms was markedly reduced at the protein level in logarithmically growing subconfluent SMC as compared to postconfluent contact-inhibited SMC (both in 10% fetal bovine serum, FBS) or subconfluent SMC growth arrested in a defined serum-free medium. However, subsequent studies showed that this was due primarily to growth-induced increases in expression of nonmuscle β-actin rather than a reduction in the expression of SM α-actin (142,143). Indeed the accumulation of SM α-actin in postconfluent SMC was not accompanied by corresponding increases in SM α-actin mRNA levels or synthesis per cell, indicating that the SM α-actin gene is constitutively active under these conditions, and that accumulation of α-actin in postconfluent cells was mediated posttranslationally (142,145). In contrast, synthesis of SM myosin isoforms SM-1 and SM-2 was increased in growth-arrested cells as compared to growing cells (19,70).

We also compared the effects of platelet-derived growth factor (PDGF)- (isolated from human platelets) or serum-induced growth on actin expression in postconfluent, quiescent cultures maintained in a defined serum-free medium (142,143,145). Whereas both factors elicited a potent proliferative response, and decreased *fractional* SM α-actin synthesis, their effects on actin isoform expression were quite different. PDGF induced a rapid drop in SM α-actin steady-state mRNA level, as well as in the absolute rate of synthesis of SM α-actin, but had no effect on either nonmuscle β-actin mRNA levels or synthesis (142,145). In contrast, serum stimulated a marked increase in nonmuscle β-actin mRNA levels and synthesis, but had no effect on SM α-actin expression. Additional studies demonstrated that chronic PDGF treatment was capable of repressing SM α-actin expression in the absence of sustained mitogenesis, that PDGF-induced repression of SM α-actin expression was fully reversible, that the A chain of PDGF was not required for these effects, and that the ED_{50} for PDGF-induced mitogenesis was two- to fourfold higher than that for repression of SM α-actin expression (143). Other purified growth factors, including basic fibroblast growth factor (bFGF), epidermal growth factor, insulin-like growth factor, or combinations of these had little or no effect on either SM α-actin expression or SMC growth (143). Additional studies demonstrated that effects of PDGF were not limited to SM α-actin, in that it also markedly suppressed the expression of SM MHC and SM α-tropomyosin at both the protein and mRNA levels (70). These effects, like those on actin, were highly selective, in that PDGF BB nearly abolished expression of the SM variants of these proteins without affecting the nonmuscle variants. In contrast to the effects of PDGF BB, 10% FBS, which stimulated a mitogenic response equal to or greater than that of PDGF BB, increased, rather than decreased, SM α-tropomyosin expression, and induced only very modest decreases in expression of SM MHC. In recent studies, we demonstrated that thrombin, which induces a mitogenic response equivalent to that of PDGF BB (146), stimulated increased, not decreased, expression of both SM α-actin and SM MHC (147). Taken together, results indicate that (a) a drop in expression of a number of SMC differentiation marker proteins is clearly not obligatory for cell cycle entry in cultured vascular SMC, (b) continued expression of at least some SM differentiation markers is compatible with proliferation, (c) the level of expression of SM differentiation proteins is not necessarily a direct function of the proliferative activity of the cell, but rather appears to be dependent on the specific means of growth stimulation, and (d) PDGF BB is unique among the SMC mitogens tested thus far in its ability to selectively suppress the expression of multiple

SMC differentiation markers, and that this activity of PDGF does not directly correlate with its proliferative potential (70,142–144,148). Taken together, our results and those of Thyberg et al. (149) suggest that PDGF BB may play an important role in control of SMC differentiation, and that this role may be distinct from its role as SMC mitogen.

Role of Cell–Cell Interactions in Regulation of SMC Differentiation

As discussed in the chapter by Fishman, vasculogenesis is initiated by formation of capillaries consisting of a single layer of endothelial cells (14,150). During arterialization, presumptive SMC are recruited from the mesenchyme, surround the endothelium, and subsequently differentiate into SM. It is thus reasonable to suggest that endothelial cells might play an important role in the arterialization process. Indeed, cultured endothelial cells have been shown to secrete a variety growth factors for SM, including PDGF and bFGF (151–155), as well as growth inhibitors such as heparin and transforming growth factor-β (TGF-β) (156–158), which can either stimulate or inhibit growth of cultured SMC, depending on the experimental conditions (159–161). Many of these endothelial-derived factors also have chemotactic activity for SMC and may play a role in recruitment and migration of SMC or SMC precursors from primitive mesenchyme during vasculogenesis (151–153). As summarized in the chapter by DiCorletto and Gimbrone, increased production of growth and chemotactic factors by endothelial cells in response to atherogenic stimuli may also play a key role in the initiation of atherosclerosis. There is also evidence that endothelial cells may also play a role in control of SMC differentiation. Campbell and Campbell (158) reported that endothelial cell-conditioned medium, or coculture of primary cultures of SMC with confluent, but not subconfluent endothelial cells, inhibited growth and prevented or delayed at least some of the phenotypic changes that occur in SMC when placed in culture. Addition of heparin to the culture media had similar effects, raising the possibility that effects may be mediated by heparin or heparin-like compounds. Both cultured endothelial cells and SMC are known to secrete a heparin-like molecule that inhibits SMC growth (156,162), with that isolated from postconfluent cells being much more potent than that from subconfluent cells in inhibiting SMC growth. Heparin has also been shown to inhibit myointimal proliferation of SMC *in vivo* following vascular injury (8,163), although it did not prevent injury-induced decreases in SM α-actin expression. Heparin has been reported to increase SM α-actin expression in cultured SMC, but only under conditions in which it had an antiproliferative effect (164). These results suggest that the effects of heparin on SMC differentiation may be secondary to growth inhibition rather than a direct effect on SMC differentiation per se.

Endothelial cells are also known to secrete PDGF BB, which is a potent suppressor of SMC differentiation (142,143). Moreover, numerous investigators have found that endothelial cell coculture as well as endothelial cell-conditioned media promote rather than inhibit SMC growth (16,154). Consistent with these observations, we recently demonstrated that conditioned media from rat aortic endothelial cells stimulated rather than inhibited growth of rat aortic SMC, and potently and selectively suppressed expression of SM α-actin, SM myosin heavy chains, and SM α-tropomyosin (147). This activity was sensitive to heat and protease treatment, was not inhibited by neutralizing antibodies to PDGF or bFGF, bound weakly to heparin sepharose, and had an estimated molecular size of 45 kDa based on gel filtration. The identity of this factor (or factors) has not yet been established.

There is thus evidence that endothelial cells secrete both positive and negative differentiation factors. However, relatively little is known regarding what regulates the balance between these opposing activities. Barrett et al. (165) demonstrated that endothelial cells in culture produce much higher levels of PDGF transcripts than do their *in vivo* counterparts. One possibility is that the effect of endothelial cells on SMC differentiation varies as a function of the growth/differentiated state of the endothelial cell. Key questions that remain to be adequately addressed include: Which endothelial cell-derived factors regulate the differentiation of vascular SMC? What regulates endothelial cell production of both positive and negative SMC differentiation factors? Do SMC influence the differentiated state of the endothelial cell? What is the effect of atherogenic stimuli on endothelial cell expression of factors that influence SMC differentiation?

Neuronal Influences

Interruption of neuronal input has been shown to result in decreased growth and loss of contractility in various SM tissues (166), thus implying a role for the nervous system in regulation of growth and differentiation of SMC. As such, loss of neuronal innervation may contribute to phenotypic modulation of SMC within atherosclerotic lesions. Chamley et al. (124,167) reported that the presence of extrinsic sympathetic neurons delayed phenotypic modulation and growth in primary cultures of pig vas deferens and rabbit aorta and ear artery. Conditioned media from nerve cells did not have similar effects, suggesting that the factors produced are labile or that physical proximity is important for the observed effect. These studies involved morphologic assessment of the differentiated state of SMC on the basis of the relative abundance of actin filaments, and no further studies have been reported in this important area using more definitive indices to assess the differentiated state of the SMC. It is also not clear whether effects of neuronal innervation might be secondary to stimulation of SMC contraction, and further studies are clearly needed in this important area.

Role of Hemodynamic and/or Mechanical Factors in Control of SMC Differentiation

There is considerable circumstantial evidence that mechanical factors or hemodynamic forces such as shear stress and tangential wall stress may play an important role in development of the vascular system as well as in control of SMC differentiation/maturation (168–170). Girard (170) found that incorporation of SMC into developing avian arteries coincided with establishment of blood flow and an increase in luminal hydrostatic pressure. Hu and Clark (168) characterized the hemodynamic forces in stage 12 through stage 29 chicken embryos and found that systolic blood pressure increased from 0.32 torr at stage 12 to 2.0 torr at stage 29, during which time there are marked increases in expression of many SMC differentiation marker proteins. In adult animals, cessation of blood flow and a decrease in hydrostatic pressure are associated with vessel atrophy and/or remodeling (171). Mechanical stretching of cultured SMC has a variety of effects, including induced reorientation of cells (172,173), increased protein and DNA synthesis (174), and increased production of extracellular matrix components (175). Of particular interest, Kanda et al. (172) found that cyclic stretching of bovine aortic SMC within a three-dimensional matrix of type 1 collagen induced reorientation of cells parallel to the direction of stretch and increased the relative abundance of myofilaments and dense bodies as compared to nonstretched cultures. In contrast, Dartsch et al. (173) found that cyclic stretching of SMC monolayer cultures resulted in reorientation of cells nearly perpendicular to the direction of stretch. Recent preliminary studies by Reusch et al. (176) demonstrated that mechanical stretch of cultured rat aortic SMC increased expression of SM myosin heavy chains. We have demonstrated that contractile agonists such as angiotensin II and arginine vasopressin induce selective increases in the expression of SM α-actin and SM MHC in cultured SMC (148). Since these agonists also stimulate increased myosin light chain phosphorylation and shape changes consistent with cell contraction (ref. 177, and G. K. Owens and A. A. Geisterfer, *unpublished observations*), it is possible that the effects observed are secondary to active stress development. Whereas results of these studies suggest that mechanical factors play a role in vascular growth and development, the precise stimuli that are important for these effects and the signal transduction pathways involved are not known. In contrast to normal medial SMC, which are arranged circumferentially (37), SMC within atherosclerotic lesions are randomly oriented. Thus, alterations in the mechanical loading of SMC could be a major factor contributing to phenotypic modulation during atherogenesis.

Role of the Extracellular Matrix in SMC Differentiation

The extracellular matrix has profound effects on cell behavior, including cell migration, proliferation, and differentiation, and undoubtedly plays a key role in vasculogenesis (see refs. 178 and 179 for review). There is abundant evidence that the matrix composition within atherosclerotic lesions is altered as compared to normal medial SMC (ref. 180, and the chapter in this book by Wight).

Growth of cultured SMC on various extracellular matrices such as collagen, matrigel (a basement-membrane-rich matrix material isolated from EHS tumor cells), laminin, and fibronectin (181–184) has been shown to evoke changes in SMC morphology consistent with a change in the differentiated phenotype of the cell. Relatively few studies, however, have examined the effects of specific extracellular matrix components on expression of SMC differentiation marker genes. Hedin et al. (184) found that growth of cultured SMC on fibronectin resulted in decreased expression of SM α-actin. We (M. M. Thompson and G. K. Owens, *unpublished observations*) and Pauly et al. (183) found that SMC grown on matrigel exhibited a much more spindlelike morphology and a greater density of actin filaments than did SMC grown on standard tissue culture plastic. However, we found no changes in the expression of SM α-actin or SM MHC under these conditions. These results should not be interpreted as evidence that these factors are not important in control of SMC differentiation. Rather, results may reflect limitations of the *in vitro* culture system, and/or the specific experimental conditions and matrices that we examined. Clearly, further studies are needed in this important area.

Use of Cultured SMC as Model Systems for Studying Atherogenesis

From the preceding, it is evident that differentiation/maturation of vascular SMC is highly dependent on environmental cues. This, coupled with the fact that even fully mature SMC exhibit a high degree of cellular plasticity, has a number of extremely important implications with regard to understanding changes in the differentiated state of SMC that occur in disease, or in any case where the normal environment of the SMC is altered in any significant way. A prime example of this occurs when SMC are placed in cell culture in which environmental cues are drastically altered as compared to what exists *in vivo*. Not surprisingly, the cultured SMC undergoes extensive changes in its differentiated phenotype (19,80,124,126–132). This is characterized by gradual loss of morphologically and immunocytologically identifiable myofilaments as well as decreased expression of a number of SM contractile proteins, including SM α-actin (126,128), SM myosin heavy chain (19,130), calponin (79,80), SM-22 (79,80), h-caldesmon (80), vinculin/metavinculin (86), and 20-kDa myosin light chains (68,177), and increased expression of the nonmuscle variants of these proteins. Importantly, although we (19,126), like Chamley-Campbell et al. (124), found that alterations in actin and myosin content occurred relatively slowly when SMC were placed in culture, changes in the synthesis of these contractile proteins occurred immediately (19,126). This indicates that the SMC rapidly alters its gene expression patterns in response to cell isolation procedure and placement in culture, and that the slow kinetics of changes in contractile protein content is likely a function of the relatively long half-lives of these proteins.

Whereas there is some evidence that cultured SMC undergo modulation to a phenotype resembling that of the intimal SMC (see refs. 16 and 7 for review), this is no doubt an oversimplification, since there are many environmental cues that exist within a human atherosclerotic lesion that might effect SMC differentiation that are not present in most SMC culture systems, e.g., the presence of lipids and lipid peroxidation products, activated immune cells, altered matrix components and cell adhesion molecules, etc. This being the case, it is important that data obtained in cultured SMC be interpreted with caution, and that results ultimately be tested using *in vivo* model systems.

The extent of phenotypic modulation and its reversibility appears to be dependent on many factors, and this has undoubtedly contributed to many of the controversies that exist in the literature regarding the biology of the vascular SMC. Critical factors include the methods of cell isolation and cell passaging, the initial plating density, the presence or absence of serum or mitogens, the specific lot of serum used, the age of the animal from which cells are derived, and the substrate on which cells are grown (124,125,127,142,144,149, 184,185). Whereas cultured SMC are undoubtedly modulated as compared to their *in vivo* counterparts, much progress has been made in recent years to improve the SMC cultures that are available with respect to retention of differentiated properties, as well as the criteria utilized to evaluate their identity and differentiated state (19,126,128–131, 185). Numerous investigators have shown that SMC derived from a variety of blood vessels and species can be grown under conditions in which they continue to express SM contractile proteins (8,19,124,126–131) as well as contractile responsiveness (177,185–187) for many passages, if not indefinitely in culture. For example, the rat aortic SMC used extensively in our laboratory undergo agonist-induced Ca^{2+} transients and myosin light-chain phosphorylation in response to a variety of different contractile agonists, including angiotensin II, norepinephrine, endothelin, and arginine vasopressin (177). These SMC also continue to express all of the known SMC differentiation markers thus far examined, including SM α-actin, SM MHC, h-caldesmon, SM α-tropomyosin, and SM MLC, albeit at reduced levels relative to expression of the non-SM variants of these proteins (19,70,126,177). We have found that a key to retaining expression of these differentiation markers is to optimize for the intimal yield of viable cells and to passage cells at subconfluency so as to avoid selection for cells that show loss of contact inhibition of growth. Other investigators have reported methods whereby SMC retain contractile capabilities through multiple passages in cell culture (185,186). In most of these cases, SMC contraction was assessed on cells grown on deformable substrates rather than directly on nondeformable plastic culture dishes, thus permitting cell shortening without cells having to disengage from the underlying matrix. Indeed in many cases the ability to show contractile ability in cultured SMC may be due to a detection problem rather than inherent differences in contractile capability of SMC primary lines derived using different cell culture methods. However, this is not to undermine the critical importance of culture methodologies in determining the extent to which cultured SMC express characteristics of differentiated SMC.

Given that cultured SMC are undoubtedly modified as compared to their *in vivo* counterparts, it is important to consider why we use them, and what are appropriate versus inappropriate questions to address using them. Two principal advantages of using cultured cells are (a) to allow better control of experimental variables, that is, identical replicate plates of a single cell type can be exposed to a single experimental variable, something which is almost never possible in intact tissue or whole-animal experiments due to genetic diversity between animals, cell–cell interactions, indirect or unknown effects of your experimental test variable, etc., and (b) to provide a more reliable, manipulatable, and/or consistent source of relatively large amounts of biologic material that is often needed for biochemical or molecular studies. Cultured cell systems provide a very powerful means to study key regulatory pathways that are of interest based on *in vivo* studies, and in particular a means to identify the key components and regulatory controls in that pathway that would not be possible with any other experimental approach. This information can then be tested in a variety of *in vivo* animal model systems, including use, at least in the mouse, of rapidly improving technologies for making transgenic and/or gene knockout/replacement animals (see refs. 188–190 for review).

A very common practice in the vascular biology field has been to try to identify possible *in vivo* differences between vascular SMC on the basis of comparison of the properties of cultured cells derived from different animal models or different vascular sources (e.g., intima versus medial cells). Whereas this has yielded some useful information, results obtained with such an approach must be viewed with caution. A major problem is that there is clear evidence that SMC derived from a different original source, including a different species, different strains of the same species, different ages of animals of the same strain, or even different blood vessels within an individual animal, can undergo *differential* phenotypic modulation under identical culture conditions (191). That is, differences that existed *in vivo* result in the cells responding differently to a given set of culture conditions.

This is not to say that such an experimental approach cannot be a productive means of investigation. Indeed studies from a number of laboratories have identified potentially interesting SMC genes on the basis of qualitative comparisons between SMC derived from different sources. For example, Schwartz and co-workers (192–194) and others (79,195) have identified a number of genes that show altered expression during development, including osteopoitin, elastin, insulin-like growth factor II, F-31, and SM-22, by comparing gene expression patterns between cultured aortic SMC derived from newborn versus adult rats. Similarly, several genes which show altered expression in intimal lesions of atherosclerotic plaques were first identified based on differential expression in cultured SMC derived from intimal versus medial blood vessel segments (196). Results of these studies have shown that SMC derived from different sources can show markedly different phenotypes in culture. Importantly, in some cases, the phenotypes exhibited appear to be consistent between different independent primary cultures from a given source and stable for many passages in culture. An example are the ''pup-'' versus the ''adult-'' derived SMC cultures described by Schwartz and colleagues (192–194). The ''adult'' SMC, which are derived from aortae of 3- to 5-month-old Sprague-Dawley rats, show the typical hill-and-valley morphology that is characteristic of most SMC cultures and their growth is dependent on exogenous growth factors. In contrast, the ''pup''-derived SMC, which are derived from aorta of 3- to 4-day-old Sprague-Dawley rats, show an ''endothelial''-like cobblestone morphology and are capable of growing in the absence of exogenous growth factors (194). The reason for these different phenotypes is not known. Some of the differences observed could represent differential phenotypic modulation of cells derived from different sources to the particular culture conditions employed. However, some of the differences in gene expression found in cultured SMC derived from different sources, such as alterations in elastin, osteopontin, and SM-22 expression (79,192,195), have also been found to exist *in vivo*. As such, use of these SMC culture systems may be valuable in identifying the cellular and molecular processes that control some of the many ''alternative phenotypes'' of the vascular SMC. However, it is of key importance to prove that the phenotype studied is biologically relevant and not an artifact of *in vitro* culture.

ALTERATIONS IN SMOOTH MUSCLE CELL DIFFERENTIATION IN ATHEROSCLEROSIS

Characterization of SMC Within Atherosclerotic Lesions of Humans and Experimental Animal Models

There is unequivocal evidence demonstrating that SMC within human atherosclerotic lesions and myointimal lesions of experimental animals following vascular injury show an altered differentiated phenotype as compared to normal medial SMC (3–6) (Figs. 1–3). This process is characterized by extensive alterations in the morphologic appearance of the cells, including a reduction in myofilaments and an increase in synthetic cellular organelles such as Golgi and rough endoplasmic reticulum. In addition, intimal SMC show reduced levels of a variety of proteins characteristic of differentiated SMC, including SM α-actin, SM myosin heavy chain, h-caldesmon, vinculin, and desmin (3–6,197,198). Based on studies in vascular injury models in animals, the changes in myointimal SMC are at least partially reversible in that expression of SM contractile proteins increases in SMC within chronic lesions (3,8). Thus the changes may be a requisite part of the repair process, with early decreases reflecting a shift to a less differentiated state with an increased growth capacity (8) and later redifferentiation of the cells and return of contractile capabilities.

A key question is: What controls the changes in the differentiated phenotype of the SMC within intimal lesions? Results of studies in cultured SMC showing that growth and differentiation are not necessarily mutually exclusive suggest that phenotypic modulation of intimal SMC cannot be attributed solely to increased growth. Consistent with this, there is a very poor correlation between proliferation rates in intimal SMC and their modified differentiated phenotype in that studies in both humans and experimental animal models have shown that alterations in the differentiated properties of intimal SMC persist even in cases where proliferation rates have returned to normal values (8–10). A likely possibility is that the altered phenotype of lesion SMC is at least in part a consequence of changes in the cellular environment that occur within the intima versus the media, including well-documented changes in the extracellular matrix, growth factor expression, lipid composition, hemodynamic/mechanical forces, etc. (see refs. 199 and 200 for review, and Fig. 4).

Contribution of the Altered Phenotype of Intimal SMC to Atherogenesis

An extremely important question is: Are the changes in the SMC differentiated state within intimal lesions the cause or the consequence of the disease process? Although additional studies are needed, it seems likely that both are correct. That is, the SMC is likely to change its phenotype in response to altered environmental cues that initiate the disease process. This could include many of the known atherogenic risk factors, such as lipid peroxidation products, hypertension, cellular toxins resulting from cigarette smoke, endothelial injury or dysfunction, etc., that are as yet poorly understood (see refs. 199–202 and elsewhere in this book for review). The altered SMC in turn exhibits characteristics that are likely to exacerbate lesion development. For example, there is an abundance of evidence showing altered lipid metabolism, growth factor production, and extracellular matrix production in intimal versus medial SMC both *in vivo* as well as in cultured SMC derived from these two sources (refs. 199, 201, and 202 for review). As such, the failure to regulate appropriately the differentiated phenotype of the vascular SMC is likely a major contributing factor to lesion development and progression. A key question is: What are the critical signals that are necessary for maintenance of the differentiated phenotype of the SMC? As is evident at this late point in this review, these are not well understood, and much remains to be done in this important area.

Origin of Intimal SMC in Atherosclerotic Lesions

Additional key questions are: What is the origin of the SMC that gives rise to the intimal lesion? Does it involve modification of medial SMC that were fully differentiated, or is there a subpopulation of relatively undifferentiated SMC that preexist in the normal blood vessel? Note that the demonstration of the monoclonality of some human atherosclerotic lesions in studies by Benditt and Benditt (203) is not incompatible with either of these possibilities, since their data addressed whether lesion SMC were derived from single versus multiple foci, but did not address the differentiated properties of the SMC of origin. The issue as to whether relatively undifferentiated SMC exist within the normal media and give rise to lesion cells is not totally resolved. However, there is an abundance of morphologic and immunocytologic evidence that indicates that there is not a distinct subpopulation of SMC in the media of normal adult human arteries, as well as in other mammalian species, that could be categorized as an undifferentiated SMC stem cell (21,55). Moreover, studies by Clowes and Schwartz in a rat carotid artery injury model (204) have demonstrated that up to 40–50% of medial SMC proliferate following injury of the rat carotid artery. These results indicate that a major portion of the medial SMC are capable of contributing to intimal lesion formation. This is clearly incompatible with the hypothesis that intimal SMC must be derived from a rare and relatively undifferentiated SMC stem-cell population, at least in this animal model.

There is, however, clear evidence for heterogeneity between SMC in expression of SMC differentiation markers during vascular development (23,55,205,206) (reviewed in ref. 7). There is also evidence for development of heterogeneity in mature animals following induction of experimental atherosclerosis or vascular injury (197,207). For example, Zanellato et al. (197) found evidence for altered expression of MHC isoforms in medial SMC of cholesterol-fed rabbits. Whereas medial SMC in control rabbits stained exclusively with antibodies specific for SM-1 MHC and SM-2 MHC, a subpopulation of medial SMC in the innermost layers of the aorta was observed in cholesterol-fed rabbits that showed loss of staining with an SM-2 MHC antibody but stained with a nonmuscle MHC antibody. Similarly, heterogeneity in vimentin and desmin expression within intimal SMC has been reported following balloon injury of the rat aorta (208). These data are all consistent with the hypothesis that intimal SMC are derived from fully differentiated SMC which undergo changes in their differentiated state in response to injury or atherogenic stimuli, rather than selective recruitment from a preexisting undifferentiated SMC stem-cell population. However, it remains to be determined whether this is also the case for SMC within human atherosclerotic lesions.

Evolution of Atherosclerosis: Implications for Understanding the Response of Differentiated SMC to Atherogenic Stimuli

Whereas the precise nature of the initiating event for atherosclerosis is not known, it is clear that the failure of the SMC to maintain its normal differentiated phenotypic state becomes a key contributing factor in the progression of atherosclerotic disease. Intriguing questions are: Why or how did the response of the SMC to atherogenic stimuli evolve? Is it necessary for survival of the organism or is it purely pathologic? There are a number of issues that must be considered. First, it must be remembered that atherosclerosis is a disease that rarely manifests its effects until late in life, i.e., beyond the normal reproductive years. Moreover, whereas humans have evolved over several million years, atherosclerosis has only been a major health problem relatively recently as the average human lifespan increased to the point where individuals died of it as opposed to other causes. In addition, many atherosclerotic risk factors related to diet, lifestyle, etc., are the consequences of modern civilization. The net consequence is that there has not been and there is unlikely to be significant genetic selection pressure against the disease. As such, from a teological point of view, the nature of the response of the SMC to atherosclerotic stimuli presumably evolved as a consequence of other selection pressures that affect survival of the organism prior to sexual maturity. The most logical candidate is the ability of the SMC to carry out vascular repair. From this perspective, atherogenic stimuli may be viewed of as a relatively recent challenge to the system. The SMC responds using mechanisms that evolved to combat quite different forms of injury. The net consequence is that the outcome is not ideal—some responses are beneficial, while others are not. For example, formation of a stable fibrous cap is beneficial, while luminal encroachment is not. Thus, whereas atherosclerosis has been present in the human species for a very long time, from an evolutionary standpoint it represents a relatively new challenge.

SUMMARY, CONCLUSIONS, AND FUTURE DIRECTIONS

In this chapter I have attempted to summarize our current understanding of how changes in the differentiated state of SMC might contribute to development of atherosclerosis. It is clearly established that the differentiated state of the SMC is altered within atherosclerotic lesions. Moreover, it is clear that these alterations in the differentiated state of the SMC, which include altered lipid metabolism and growth characteristics, cannot be viewed merely as a consequence of the disease, but rather are likely to play a key role in the initiation and progression of the disease process. As such, an understanding of how SMC differentiation/maturation is controlled is likely to be critical to understanding the pathogenesis of this disease. Studies have established (a) that the mature differentiated SMC retains remarkable plasticity such that it can undergo relatively rapid and reversible changes in its phenotype in response to injurious stimuli, and (b) that differentiation/maturation of the SMC appears to be more highly dependent on environmental cues than in cells such as skeletal muscle which undergo terminal differentiation and which exhibit a much more restrictive differentiated phenotype. It is also clear that our understanding of SMC differentiation/maturation is in its infancy and that much remains to be learned regarding the specific environmental cues that control it and the cellular and the molecular mechanisms whereby these environmental stimuli influence expression of genes necessary for the normal differentiated function of vascular SMC. Only when we better understand how SMC differentiation/maturation is normally regulated are we likely to understand how these control processes are altered in atherosclerosis and how the resulting changes in the phenotype of the SMC contribute to lesion development and progression.

ACKNOWLEDGMENTS

This work was supported by grants RO1 HL38854 and PO1 HL19242 from the National Institutes of Health.

REFERENCES

1. Schwartz SM, Ross R. Cellular proliferation in atherosclerosis and hypertension. *Prog Cardiovasc Dis* 1984;26:355–372.
2. Ross R, Glomset JA. The pathogenesis of atherosclerosis. *N Engl J Med* 1976;295:369–377, 420–425.
3. Kocher O, Gabbiani F, Gabbiani G, et al. Phenotypic features of smooth muscle cells during the evolution of experimental carotid artery intimal thickening. Biochemical and morphologic studies. *Lab Invest* 1991;65:459–470.
4. Kocher O, Gabbiani G. Cytoskeletal features of normal and atheromatous human arterial smooth muscle cells. *Hum Pathol* 1986;17: 875–880.
5. Mosse PR, Campbell GR, Campbell JH. Smooth muscle phenotypic expression in human carotid arteries. II. Atherosclerosis-free diffuse intimal thickenings compared with the media. *Arteriosclerosis* 1986; 6:664–669.
6. Glukhova MA, Kabakov AE, Frid MG, et al. Modulation of human aorta smooth muscle cell phenotype: a study of muscle-specific variants of vinculin, caldesmon, and actin expression. *Proc Natl Acad Sci USA* 1988;85:9542–9546.
7. Owens GK. Regulation of differentiation of vascular smooth muscle cells. *Physiol Rev* 1995;*[in press]*.
8. Clowes AW, Clowes MM, Kocher O, Ropraz P, Chaponnier C, Gabbiani G. Arterial smooth muscle cells *in vivo:* relationship between actin isoform expression and mitogenesis and their modulation by heparin. *J Cell Biol* 1988;107:1939–1945.
9. Gordon D, Reidy MA, Benditt EP, Schwartz SM. Cell proliferation in human coronary arteries. *Proc Natl Acad Sci USA* 1990;87: 4600–4604.
10. OBrien ER, Alpers CE, Stewart DK, et al. Proliferation in primary and restenotic coronary atherectomy tissue. Implications for antiproliferative therapy. *Circ Res* 1993;73:223–231.
11. Lindner V, Reidy MA. Expression of basic fibroblast growth factor and its receptor by smooth muscle cells and endothelium in injured rat arteries. An en face study. *Circ Res* 1993;73:589–595.
12. Casscells W, Lappi DA, Olwin BB, et al. Elimination of smooth muscle cells in experimental restenosis: targeting of fibroblast growth factor receptors. *Proc Natl Acad Sci USA* 1992;89:7159–7163.
13. Okazaki H, Majesky MW, Harker LA, Schwartz SM. Regulation of platelet-derived growth factor ligand and receptor gene expression by alpha-thrombin in vascular smooth muscle cells. *Circ Res* 1992;71(6): 1285–1293.
14. Noden DM. Embryonic origins and assembly of blood vessels. *Am Rev Respir Dis* 1993;140:1097–1103.
15. Gerrity RG, Cliff WJ. Aortic tunica media of the developing rat. *Lab Invest* 1975;32:585.
16. Schwartz SM, Campbell GR, Campbell JH. Replication of smooth muscle cells in vascular disease [Review]. *Circ Res* 1986;58:427–444.
17. Olson EN. Regulation of muscle transcription by the MyoD family. The heart of the matter. *Circ Res* 1993;72:1–6.
18. Blau H, Pavlath G, Hardeman E, et al. Plasticity of the differentiated state. *Science* 1985;230:758–766.
19. Rovner AS, Murphy RA, Owens GK. Expression of smooth muscle and nonmuscle myosin heavy chains in cultured vascular smooth muscle cells. *J Biol Chem* 1986;261:14740–14745.
20. Rovner AS, Thompson MM, Murphy RA. Two different heavy chains are found in smooth muscle myosin. *Am J Physiol* 1986;c861–c870.
21. Aikawa M, Sivam PN, Kuro-o M, et al. Human smooth myosin heavy chain isoforms as molecular markers for vascular development and atherosclerosis. *Circ Res* 1993;73:1000–1012.
22. Miano J, Cserjesi P, Ligon K, Perisamy M, Olson EN. Smooth muscle myosin heavy chain marks exclusively the smooth muscle lineage during mouse embryogenesis. *Circ Res* 1994;75:803–812.
23. Owens GK, Thompson MM. Developmental changes in isoactin expression in rat aortic smooth muscle cells *in vivo*. Relationship between growth and cytodifferentiation. *J Biol Chem* 1986;261: 13373–13380.
24. Gabbiani G, Schmid E, Winter S, et al. Vascular smooth muscle cells differ from other smooth muscle cells: predominance of vimentin filaments and a specific-type actin. *Proc Natl Acad Sci USA* 1981; 78:298–300.
25. Hasegawa Y, Ueda Y, Watanabe M, Morita F. Studies on amino acid sequences of two isoforms of 17-kDa essential light chain of smooth muscle myosin from porcine aorta media. *J Biochem* 1992;111: 798–803.
26. Helper DJ, Lash JA, Hathaway DR. Distribution of isoelectric variants of the 17,000-dalton myosin light chain in mammalian smooth muscle. *J Biol Chem* 1988;263:15748–15753.
27. Bretscher A. Thin filament regulatory proteins of smooth muscle and nonmuscle cells. *Nature* 1986;321:726–727.
28. Marston SB, Smith CJW. The thin filaments of smooth muscle. *J Muscle Res Cell Motility* 1985;6:669–708.
29. Lees-Miller JP, Helfman DM. The molecular basis for tropomyosin isoform diversity. *Bioessays* 1991;13:429–437.
30. Winder SJ, Sutherland C, Walsh MP. Biochemical and functional characterization of smooth muscle calponin [Review]. *Adv Exp Med Biol* 1991;304:37–51.
31. Sobue K, Sellers JR. Caldesmon, a novel regulatory protein in smooth muscle and nonmuscle actomyosin systems. *J Biol Chem* 1991;266: 12115–12118.
32. Geiger B, Tokuyasu KT, Dutton AH, Singer SJ. Vinculin, an intracellular protein localized at specialized sites where microfilament bundles terminate at cell membranes. *Proc Natl Acad Sci USA* 1980;77: 4127–4131.
33. Pardo JV, Siliciano JD, Craig SW. Vinculin is a component of an extensive network of myofibril-sarcolemma attachment regions in cardiac muscle fibers. *J Cell Biol* 1983;97:1081–1088.
34. Mitchell JJ, Reynolds SE, Leslie KO, Low RB, Woodcock-Mitchell J. Smooth muscle cell markers in developing rat lung. *Am J Respir Cell Mol Biol* 1990;3:515–523.
35. Vandekerckhove J, Weber K. The complete amino acid sequence of actins from bovine aorta, bovine heart, bovine fast skeletal muscle, and rabbit slow skeletal muscle. *Differentiation* 1979;14:123–133.
36. Fatigati V, Murphy RA. Actin and tropomyosin variants in smooth

muscles. Dependence on tissue type. *J Biol Chem* 1984;259: 14383–14388.
37. Murphy R. Muscle cells of hollow organs. *News Physiol* 1988;3: 124–128.
38. Newcomb PM, Herman IM. Pericyte growth and contractile phenotype: modulation by endothelial-synthesized matrix and comparison with aortic smooth muscle. *J Cell Physiol* 1993;155:385–393.
39. Gomez RA, Lynch KR, Sturgill BC, et al. Distribution of renin mRNA and its protein in the developing kidney. *Am J Physiol* 1989;257: F850–F858.
40. Darby I, Skalli O, Gabbiani G. Alpha-smooth muscle actin is transiently expressed by myofibroblasts during experimental wound healing. *Lab Invest* 1990;63:21–29.
41. Cintorino M, Bellizzi de Marco E, Leoncini P, et al. Expression of alpha-smooth-muscle actin in stromal cells of the uterine cervix during epithelial neoplastic changes. *Int J Cancer* 1991;47:843–846.
42. Sappino AP, Masouye I, Saurat JH, Gabbiani G. Smooth muscle differentiation in scleroderma fibroblastic cells. *Am J Pathol* 1990;137: 585–591.
43. Ruzicka DL, Schwartz RJ. Sequential activation of alpha-actin genes during avian cardiogenesis: vascular smooth muscle alpha-actin gene transcripts mark the onset of cardiomyocyte differentiation. *J Cell Biol* 1988;107:2575–2586.
44. Woodcock-Mitchell J, Mitchell JJ, Low RB, et al. α-Smooth muscle actin is transiently expressed in embryonic rat cardiac and skeletal muscles. *Differentiation* 1988;39:161–166.
45. Marotti KR, Castle CK, Boyle TP, Lin AH, Murray RW, Melchior GW. Severe atherosclerosis in transgenic mice expressing simian cholesteryl ester transfer protein. *Nature* 1993;364:73–75.
46. Arciniegas E, Sutton AB, Allen TD, Schor AM. Transforming growth factor beta 1 promotes the differentiation of endothelial cells into smooth muscle-like cells *in vitro*. *J Cell Sci* 1992;103:521–529.
47. Woodcock Mitchell J, Mitchell JJ, Low RB, et al. Alpha-smooth muscle actin is transiently expressed in embryonic rat cardiac and skeletal muscles. *Differentiation* 1988;39:161–166.
48. Carroll SL, Bergsma DJ, Schwartz RJ. A 29-nucleotide DNA segment containing an evolutionarily conserved motif is required in *cis* for cell-type restricted repression of the chicken alpha-smooth muscle actin gene core promoter. *Mol Cell Biol* 1988;8:241–250.
49. Blank RS, McQuinn TC, Yin KC, et al. Elements of the smooth muscle alpha-actin promoter required in *cis* for transcriptional activation in smooth muscle. Evidence for cell type-specific regulation. *J Biol Chem* 1992;267:984–989.
50. Foster DN, Min B, Foster LK, et al. Positive and negative *cis*-acting regulatory elements mediate expression of the mouse vascular smooth muscle alpha-actin gene. *J Biol Chem* 1992;267:11995–12003.
51. Duband JL, Gimona M, Scatena M, Sartore S, Small JV. Calponin and SM 22 as differentiation markers of smooth muscle: spatiotemporal distribution during avian embryonic development. *Differentiation* 1993;55:1–11.
52. Hungerford JE, Little CD. The developmental biology of vascular smooth muscle as studies with a new monoclonal antibody directed against an embryonic quail vascular smooth muscle antigen. *J Cell Biochem* 1993;17D:198.
53. White S, Martin AF, Periasamy M. Identification of a novel smooth muscle myosin heavy chain cDNA: isoform diversity in the S1 head region. *Am J Physiol* 1993;264:C1252–C1258.
54. Nagai R, Kuro-o M, Babij P, Periasamy M. Identification of two types of smooth muscle myosin heavy chain isoforms by cDNA cloning and immunoblot analysis. *J Biol Chem* 1989;264:9734–9737.
55. Frid MG, Printesva OY, Chiavegato A, et al. Myosin heavy-chain isoform composition and distribution in developing and adult human aortic smooth muscle. *J Vasc Res* 1993;30:279–292.
56. Somlyo AP. Myosin isoforms in smooth muscle: how may they affect function and structure [Review]. *J Muscle Res Cell Motility* 1993;14: 557–563.
57. Murphy RA, Rembold CM, Hai CM. Contraction in smooth muscle: what is latch? *Prog Clin Biol Res* 1990;327:39–50.
58. Kawamoto S, Adelstein RS. Chicken nonmuscle myosin heavy chains: differential expression of two mRNAs and evidence for two different polypeptides. *J Cell Biol* 1991;112:915–924.
59. Kuro-o M, Nagai R, Nakahara K, et al. cDNA cloning of a myosin heavy chain isoform in embryonic smooth muscle and its expression during vascular development and in arteriosclerosis. *J Biol Chem* 1991;266:3768–3773.
60. Kuro-o M, Nagai R, Tsuchimochi H, et al. Developmentally regulated expression of vascular smooth muscle myosin heavy chain isoforms. *J Biol Chem* 1989;264:18272–18275.
61. Babij P, Kawamoto S, White S, Adelstein RS, Periasamy M. Differential expression of SM-1 and SM-2 myosin isoforms in cultured vascular smooth muscle. *Am J Physiol* 1992;262:C607–C613.
62. Babij P. Tissue-specific and developmentally regulated alternative splicing of a visceral isoform of smooth muscle myosin heavy chain. *Nucleic Acids Res* 1993;21:1467–1471.
63. Kelley CA, Takahashi M, Yu JH, Adelstein RS. An insert of seven amino acids confers functional differences between smooth muscle myosins from the intestines and vasculature. *J Biol Chem* 1993;268: 12848–12854.
64. Glukhova MA, Frid MG, Koteliansky VE. Developmental changes in expression of contractile and cytoskeletal proteins in human aortic smooth muscle. *J Biol Chem* 1990;265:13042–13046.
65. Frid MG, Shekhonin BV, Koteliansky VE, Glukhova MA. Phenotypic changes of human smooth muscle cells during development: late expression of heavy caldesmon and calponin. *Dev Biol* 1992;153: 185–193.
66. Borrione AC, Zanellato AM, Giuriato L, Scannapieco G, Pauletto P, Sartore S. Nonmuscle and smooth muscle myosin isoforms in bovine endothelial cells. *Exp Cell Res* 1990;190:1–10.
67. Price RJ, Owens GK, Skalak TC. Immunohistochemical identification of arteriolar development using markers of smooth muscle differentiation: evidence that capillary arterialization proceeds from terminal arterioles. *Circ Res* 1994;75:520–527.
68. Taubman MB, Grant JW, Nadal Ginard B. Cloning and characterization of mammalian myosin regulatory light chain (RLC) cDNA: the RLC gene is expressed in smooth, sarcomeric, and nonmuscle tissues. *J Cell Biol* 1987;104:1505–1513.
69. Ebashi, Ebashi F. A new protein component participating in the superprecipitation of myosin B. *J Biochem* 1964;55:604–613.
70. Holycross BJ, Blank RS, Thompson MM, Peach MJ, Owens GK. Platelet-derived growth factor-BB-induced suppression of smooth muscle cell differentiation. *Circ Res* 1992;71:1525–1532.
71. Hosoya M, Miyazaki J-I, Hirabayashi T. Tropomyosin isoforms in developing chicken gizzard smooth muscle. *J Biochem* 1989;105: 712–717.
72. Wieczorek DF, Smith CW, Nadal Ginard B. The rat alpha-tropomyosin gene generates a minimum of six different mRNAs coding for striated, smooth, and nonmuscle isoforms by alternative splicing. *Mol Cell Biol* 1988;8:679–694.
73. Gunning P, Gordon M, Wade R, Gahlmann R, Lin C-S, Hardeman E. Differential control of tropomyosin mRNA levels during myogenesis suggests the existence of an isoform competition-autoregulatory compensation control mechanism. *Dev Biol* 1990;138:443–453.
74. Ruiz Opazo N, Nadal Ginard B. Alpha-tropomyosin gene organization. Alternative splicing of duplicated isotype-specific exons accounts for the production of smooth and striated muscle isoforms. *J Biol Chem* 1987;262:4755–4765.
75. Muthuchamy M, Pajak L, Howles P, Doetschman T, Wieczorek DF. Developmental analysis of tropomyosin gene expression in embryonic stem cells and mouse embryos. *Mol Cell Biol* 1993;13:3311–3323.
76. Winder SJ, Sutherland C, Walsh MP. A comparison of the effects of calponin on smooth and skeletal muscle actomyosin systems in the presence and absence of caldesmon. *Biochem J* 1992;288:733–739.
77. Takahashi K, Nadal-Ginard B. Molecular cloning and sequence analysis of smooth muscle calponin. *J Biol Chem* 1991;266:13284–13288.
78. Nishida W, Kitami Y, Hiwada K. cDNA cloning and mRNA expression of calponin and SM22 in rat aorta smooth muscle cells. *Gene* 1993;130:297–302.
79. Shanahan CM, Weissberg PL, Metcalfe JC. Isolation of gene markers of differentiated and proliferating vascular smooth muscle cells. *Circ Res* 1993;73:193–204.
80. Gimona M, Sparrow MP, Strasser P, Herzog M, Small JV. Calponin and SM 22 isoforms in avian and mammalian smooth muscle: absence of phosphorylation *in vivo*. *Eur J Biochem* 1992;205:1067–1075.
81. Takahashi K, Hiwada K, Kokubu T. Occurrence of anti-gizzard P34K antibody cross-reactive components in bovine smooth muscles and non-smooth muscle tissues. *Life Sci* 1987;41:291–296.
82. Birukov KG, Stepanova OV, Nanaev AK, Shirinsky VP. Expression

of calponin in rabbit and human aortic smooth muscle cells. *Cell Tiss Res* 1991;266:579–584.

83. Takeuchi K, Takahashi K, Abe M, et al. Co-localization of immunoreactive forms of calponin with actin cytoskeleton in platelets, fibroblasts, and vascular smooth muscle. *J Biochem* 1991;109:311–316.
84. Humphrey MB, Herrera Sosa H, Gonzalez G, Lee R, Bryan J. Cloning of cDNAs encoding human caldesmons. *Gene* 1992;112:197–204.
85. Ueki N, Sobue K, Kanda K, Hada T, Higashino K. Expression of high and low molecular weight caldesmons during phenotypic modulation of smooth muscle cells. *Proc Natl Acad Sci USA* 1987;84:9049–9053.
86. Belkin AM, Ornatsky OI, Kabakov AE, Glukhova MA, Koteliansky VE. Diversity of vinculin/meta-vinculin in human tissues and cultivated cells. Expression of muscle specific variants of vinculin in human aorta smooth muscle cells. *J Biol Chem* 1988;263:6631–6635.
87. Koteliansky VE, Ogryzko EP, Zhidkova NI, et al. An additional exon in the human vinculin gene specifically encodes meta-vinculin-specific difference peptide. Cross-species comparison reveals variable and conserved motifs in the meta-vinculin insert. *Eur J Biochem* 1992;204:767–772.
88. Glukhova MA, Kabakov AE, Belkin AM, et al. Meta-vinculin distribution in adult human tissues and cultured cells. *FEBS Lett* 1986;207:139–141.
89. Siliciano JD, Craig SW. Properties of smooth muscle meta-vinculin. *J Cell Biol* 1987;104:473–482.
90. Glukhova MA, Frid MG, Koteliansky VE. Developmental changes in expression of contractile and cytoskeletal proteins in human aortic smooth muscle. *J Biol Chem* 1990;265:13042–13046.
91. Small JV, Sobieszek A. Studies on the function and composition of the 10-NM (100-A) filaments of vertebrate smooth muscle. *J Cell Sci* 1977;23:243–268.
92. Bader BL, Jahn L, Franke WW. Low level expression of cytokeratins 8, 18 and 19 in vascular smooth muscle cells of human umbilical cord and in cultured cells derived therefrom, with an analysis of the chromosomal locus containing the cytokeratin 19 gene. *Eur J Cell Biol* 1988;47:300–319.
93. Nanaev AK, Shirinsky VP, Birukov KG. Immunofluorescent study of heterogeneity in smooth muscle cells of human fetal vessels using antibodies to myosin, desmin, and vimentin. *Cell Tiss Res* 1991;266:535–540.
94. Rubbia L, Gabbiani G. The cytoskeleton of arterial smooth muscle cells during development, atheromatosis, and tissue culture. *J Cardiovasc Pharmacol* 1989;14(Suppl 6):S9–S11.
95. Bennett GS, Fellini SA, Croop JM, Otto JJ, Bryan J, Holtzer H. Differences among 100-angstrom filament subunits from different cell types. *Proc Natl Acad Sci USA* 1978;75:4364–4368.
96. Schaart G, Viebahn C, Langmann W, Ramaekers F. Desmin and titin expression in early postimplantation mouse embryos. *Development* 1989;107:585–596.
97. Li ZL, Lilienbaum A, Butler-Browne G, Paulin D. Human desmin-coding gene: complete nucleotide sequence, characterization and regulation of expression during myogenesis and development. *Gene* 1989;78:243–254.
98. Franke WW, Schmid E, Freudenstein C, et al. Intermediate-sized filaments of prekeratin type in myoepithelial cells. *J Cell Biol* 1980;84:633–654.
99. Isenberg G. Nonselective cation channels in cardiac and smooth muscle cells [Review]. *EXS* 1993;66:247–260.
100. Smith JB. Angiotensin-receptor signaling in cultured vascular smooth muscle cells [Review]. *Am J Physiol* 1986;250:F759–F769.
101. Blank RS, Swartz EA, Thompson MM, Olson EN, Owens GK. A retinoic acid-induced clonal cell line from multipotential P19 embryonal carcinoma cells expresses smooth muscle characteristics. *Circ Res* 1995;76:742–749.
102. Duckles SP, Banner W. Changes in vascular smooth muscle reactivity during development. *Annu Rev Pharmacol Toxicol* 1984;24:65–83.
103. Viswanathan M, Tsutsumi K, Correa FM, Saavedra JM. Changes in expression of angiotensin receptor subtypes in the rat aorta during development. *Biochem Biophys Res Commun* 1991;179:1361–1367.
104. Grone HJ, Simon M, Fuchs E. Autoradiographic characterization of angiotensin receptor subtypes in fetal and adult human kidney. *Am J Physiol* 1992;262:F326–F331.
105. Caulfield MP. Muscarinic receptors—characterization, coupling and function [Review]. *Pharmacol Ther* 1993;58:319–379.
106. Ostrowski NL, Young WS, Knepper MA, Lolait SJ. Expression of vasopressin V1a and V2 receptor messenger ribonucleic acid in the liver and kidney of embryonic, developing, and adult rats. *Endocrinology* 1993;133:1849–1859.
107. Shaul PW, Magness RR, Muntz KH, DeBeltz D, Buja LM. Alpha 1-adrenergic receptors in pulmonary and systemic vascular smooth muscle. Alterations with development and pregnancy. *Circ Res* 1990;67:1193–1200.
108. Schell DN, Durham D, Murphree SS, Muntz KH, Shaul PW. Ontogeny of beta-adrenergic receptors in pulmonary arterial smooth muscle, bronchial smooth muscle, and alveolar lining cells in the rat. *Am J Respir Cell Mol Biol* 1992;7:317–324.
109. Bean BP, Friel DD. ATP-activated channels in excitable cells [Review]. *Ion Channels* 1990;2:169–203.
110. Darnell J, Lodish H, Baltimore D. *Molecular cell biology*. New York: Freeman; 1986:987–1035.
111. Weintraub H, Davis R, Tapscott S, et al. The myoD gene family: nodal point during specification of the muscle cell lineage. *Science* 1991;251:761–766.
112. Blau H, Baltimore D. Differentiation requires continuous regulation. *J Cell Biol* 1991;112:781–783.
113. Davis RL, Weintraub H, Lassar AB. Expression of a single transfected cDNA converts fibroblasts to myoblasts. *Cell* 1987;51:987–1000.
114. Tapscott SJ, Davis RL, Thayer MJ, Cheng PF, Weintraub H, Lassar AB. MyoD1: a nuclear phosphoprotein requiring a Myc homology region to convert fibroblasts to myoblasts. *Science* 1988;242:405–411.
115. Wright WE, Sassoon DA, Lin VK. Myogenin, a factor regulating myogenesis, has a domain homologous to MyoD. *Cell* 1989;56:607–617.
116. Edmondson DG, Olson EN. A gene with homology to the myc similarity region of MyoD1 is expressed during myogenesis and is sufficient to activate the muscle differentiation program. *Genes Dev* 1989;3:628–640.
117. Braun T, Buschhausen-Denker G, Bober E, Tannich E, Arnold HH. A novel human muscle factor related to but distinct from MyoD1 induces myogenic conversion in 10T1/2 fibroblasts. *EMBO J* 1989;8:701–709.
118. Rhodes SJ, Konieczny SF. Identification of MRF4: a new member of the muscle regulatory factor gene family. *Genes Dev* 1989;3:2050–2061.
119. Van Neck JW, Medina JJ, Onnekink C, van der Ven PF, Bloemers HP, Schwartz SM. Basic fibroblast growth factor has a differential effect on MyoD conversion of cultured aortic smooth muscle cells from newborn and adult rats. *Am J Pathol* 1993;143:269–282.
120. Cserjesi P, Olson EN. Myogenin induces the myocyte-specific enhancer binding factor MEF-2 independently of other muscle-specific gene products. *Mol Cell Biol* 1991;11:4854–4862.
121. Tontonoz P, Kim JB, Graves RA, Spiegelman BM. ADD1: a novel helix–loop–helix transcription factor associated with adipocyte determination and differentiation. *Mol Cell Biol* 1993;13:4753–4759.
122. Olson EN. Signal transduction pathways that regulate skeletal muscle gene expression. *Mol Endocrinol* 1993;7:1369–1378.
123. Lilly B, Galewsky S, Firulli AB, Schulz RA, Olson EN. D-MEF2: a MADS box transcription factor expressed in differentiating mesoderm and muscle cell lineages during *Drosophila* embryogenesis. *Proc Natl Acad Sci USA* 1994;91:5662–5666.
124. Chamley-Campbell J, Campbell GR, Ross R. The smooth muscle cell in culture. *Physiol Rev* 1979;59:1–6.
125. Thyberg J, Hedin U, Sjolund M, Palmberg L, Bottger B. Regulation of differentiated properties and proliferation of arterial smooth muscle cells. *Arteriosclerosis* 1990;10:966–990.
126. Owens GK, Loeb A, Gordon D, Thompson MM. Expression of smooth muscle-specific alpha-isoactin in cultured vascular smooth muscle cells: relationship between growth and cytodifferentiation. *J Cell Biol* 1986;102:343–352.
127. Schwartz SM, Ross R. Cellular proliferation in atherosclerosis and hypertension. *Prog Cardiovasc Dis* 1984;26:355–372.
128. Campbell JH, Kocher O, Skalli O, Gabbiani G, Campbell GR. Cytodifferentiation and expression of alpha-smooth muscle actin mRNA and protein during primary culture of aortic smooth muscle cells. Correlation with cell density and proliferative state. *Arteriosclerosis* 1989;9:633–643.
129. Kocher O, Gabbiani G. Expression of actin mRNAs in rat aortic

smooth muscle cells during deveopment, experimental intimal thickening, and culture. *Differentiation* 1986;32:245–251.
130. Kawamoto S, Adelstein RS. Characterization of myosin heavy chains in cultured smooth muscle cells. *J Biol Chem* 1987;262:7282–7288.
131. Rothman A, Kulik TJ, Taubman MB, Berk BC, Smith CW, Nadal Ginard B. Development and characterization of a cloned rat pulmonary arterial smooth muscle cell line that maintains differentiated properties through multiple subcultures. *Circulation* 1992;86: 1977–1986.
132. Seidel CL, Wallace CL, Dennison DK, Allen JC. Vascular myosin expression during cytokinesis, attachment, and hypertrophy. *Am J Physiol* 1989;256:C793–C798.
133. Haudenschild CC, Grunwald J. Proliferative heterogeneity of vascular smooth muscle cells and its alteration by injury. *Exp Cell Res* 1985; 157:364–370.
134. Schwartz SM, Reidy MA. Common mechanisms of proliferation of smooth muscle in atherosclerosis and hypertension [Review]. *Hum Pathol* 1987;18:240–247.
135. Grunwald J, Chobanian AV, Haudenschild CC. Smooth muscle cell migration and proliferation: atherogenic mechanisms in hypertension. *Atherosclerosis* 1987;67:215–221.
136. Berk BC, Vekshtein V, Gordon H, Tsuda T. Angiotensin II stimulated protein synthesis in cultured vascular smooth muscle cells. *Hypertension* 1989;13:305–314.
137. De Mey JG, Uitendaal MP, Boonen HC, Vrijdag MJ, Daemen MJ, Struyker-Boudier HA. Acute and long-term effects of tissue culture on contractile reactivity in renal arteries of the rat. *Circ Res* 1989;65: 1125–1135.
138. Holycross BJ, Peach MJ, Owens GK. Angiotensin II stimulates increased protein synthesis, not increased DNA synthesis, in intact rat aortic segments, *in vitro*. *J Vasc Res* 1993;30(2):80–86.
139. Clowes AW, Clowes MM, Reidy MA. Kinetics of cellular proliferation after arterial injury. III. Endothelial and smooth muscle growth in chronically denuded vessels. *Lab Invest* 1986;54:295–303.
140. Cobb JLS, Bennett T. An ultrastructural study of mitotic division in differentiated gastric smooth muscle cells. *Z Zellforsch* 1970;103: 177–189.
141. Imai H, Lee KJ, Lee SK, Lee KT, Oneal RM, Thomas WA. Ultrastructural features of aortic cell in mitosis in control and cholesterol-fed swine. *Lab Invest* 1979;23:401–415.
142. Corjay MH, Thompson MM, Lynch KR, Owens GK. Differential effect of platelet-derived growth factor- versus serum-induced growth on smooth muscle alpha-actin and nonmuscle beta-actin mRNA expression in cultured rat aortic smooth muscle cells. *J Biol Chem* 1989;264:10501–10506.
143. Blank RS, Owens GK. Platelet-derived growth factor regulates actin isoform expression and growth state in cultured rat aortic smooth muscle cells. *J Cell Physiol* 1990;142:635–642.
144. Blank RS, Thompson MM, Owens GK. Cell cycle versus density dependence of smooth muscle alpha actin expression in cultured rat aortic smooth muscle cells. *J Cell Biol* 1988;107:299–306.
145. Corjay MH, Blank RS, Owens GK. Platelet-derived growth factor-induced destabilization of smooth muscle α-actin mRNA. *J Cell Physiol* 1990;145:391–397.
146. McNamara CA, Sarembock IJ, Gimple LW, Fenton JW, Coughlin SR, Owens GK. Thrombin stimulates proliferation of cultured rat aortic smooth muscle cells by a proteolytically activated receptor. *J Clin Invest* 1993;91:94–98.
147. Vernon SM, Sarembock IJ, Owens GK. Thrombin-induced proliferation in cultured smooth muscle cells is not associated with downregulation of smooth muscle α-actin gene expression. *Circulation* 1993; 88:I-189(abst).
148. Turla MB, Thompson MM, Corjay MH, Owens GK. Mechanisms of angiotensin II- and arginine vasopressin-induced increases in protein synthesis and content in cultured rat aortic smooth muscle cells. Evidence for selective increases in smooth muscle isoactin expression. *Circ Res* 1991;68:288–299.
149. Thyberg J, Palmberg L, Nilsson J, Ksiazek T, Sjolund M. Phenotypic modulation in primary cultures of arterial smooth muscle cells: on the role of platelet-derived growth factor. *Differentiation* 1983;25: 156–167.
150. Poole TJ, Coffin JD. Vasculogenesis and angiogenesis: two distinct morphogenetic mechanisms establish embryonic vascular pattern. *J Exp Zool* 1989;251:224–231.
151. Silverstein J, Rifkin DB. Endothelial cell growth factors and the vessel wall. *Semin Thromb Hemostasis* 1987;13:504–513.
152. Hannan RL, Kourembanas S, Flanders KC, et al. Endothelial cells synthesize basic fibroblast growth factor and transforming growth factor beta. *Growth Factors* 1988;1:7–17.
153. Collins T, Pober JS, Gimbrone MA Jr, et al. Cultured human endothelial cells express platelet-derived growth factor A chain. *Am J Pathol* 1987;126:7–12.
154. Gajdusek CM, Schwartz SM. Ability of endothelial cells to condition culture medium. *J Cell Physiol* 1982;110:35–42.
155. Risau W, Gautschi Sova P, Bohlen P. Endothelial cell growth factors in embryonic and adult chick brain are related to human acidic fibroblast growth factor. *EMBO J* 1988;7:959–962.
156. Castellot JJ, Favreau LV, Karnovsky MJ, Rosenberg RD. Inhibition of vascular smooth muscle cell growth by endothelial cell-derived heparin. Possible role of a platelet endoglycosidase. *J Biol Chem* 1982; 257:11256–11260.
157. Sato Y, Tsuboi R, Lyons R, Moses H, Rifkin DB. Characterization of the activation of latent TGF-beta by co-cultures of endothelial cells and pericytes or smooth muscle cells: a self-regulating system. *J Cell Biol* 1990;111:757–763.
158. Campbell JH, Campbell GR. Endothelial cell influences on vascular smooth muscle phenotype [Review]. *Ann Rev Physiol* 1986;48: 295–306.
159. Stouffer GA, Owens GK. TGF-beta promotes proliferation of cultured SMC via both PDGF-AA-dependent and PDGF-independent mechanisms. *J Clin Invest* 1994;93:2048–2055.
160. Assoian RK, Sporn MB. Type beta transforming growth factor in human platelets: release during platelet degranulation and action on vascular smooth muscle cells. *J Cell Biol* 1986;102:1217–1223.
161. Owens GK, Geisterfer AA, Yang YW, Komoriya A. Transforming growth factor-beta-induced growth inhibition and cellular hypertrophy in cultured vascular smooth muscle cells. *J Cell Biol* 1988;107: 771–780.
162. Fritze LM, Reilly CF, Rosenberg RD. An antiproliferative heparan sulfate species produced by postconfluent smooth muscle cells. *J Cell Biol* 1985;100:1041–1049.
163. Clowes AW, Clowes MM, Fingerle J, Reidy MA. Regulation of smooth muscle cell growth in injured artery [Review]. *J Cardiovasc Pharmacol* 1989;14(Suppl 6):S12–S15.
164. Desmouliere A, Rubbia Brandt L, Gabbiani G. Modulation of actin isoform expression in cultured arterial smooth muscle cells by heparin and culture conditions. *Arterioscler Thromb* 1991;11:244–253.
165. Barrett TB, Gajdusek CM, Schwartz SM, McDougall JK, Benditt EP. Expression of the *sis* gene by endothelial cells in culture and *in vivo*. *Proc Natl Acad Sci USA* 1984;81:6772–6774.
166. Bevan RD, Tsuru H. Functional and structural changes in the rabbit ear artery after sympathetic denervation. *Circ Res* 1981;49:478–485.
167. Chamley JH, Campbell GR, Burnstock G. Dedifferentiation, redifferentiation and bundle formation of smooth muscle cells in tissue culture: the influence of cell number and nerve fibres. *J Embryol Exp Morphol* 1974;32:297–323.
168. Hu N, Clark EB. Hemodynamics of the stage 12 to stage 29 chick embryo. *Circ Res* 1989;65:1665–1670.
169. Sterpetti AV, Cucina A, D'Angelo LS, Cardillo B, Cavallaro A. Shear stress modulates the proliferation rate, protein synthesis, and mitogenic activity of arterial smooth muscle cells. *Surgery* 1993;113: 691–699.
170. Girard H. Arterial pressure in the chick embryo. *Am J Physiol* 1973; 224:454–460.
171. Langille BL. Remodeling of developing and mature arteries: endothelium, smooth muscle, and matrix [Review]. *J Cardiovasc Pharmacol* 1993;21(Suppl 1):S11–S17.
172. Kanda K, Matsuda T, Oka T. Mechanical stress induced cellular orientation and phenotypic modulation of 3-D cultured smooth muscle cells. *Am Soc Artificial Intern Organs J* 1994;39:M686–M690.
173. Dartsch PC, Hammerle H, Betz E. Orientation of cultured arterial smooth muscle cells growing on cyclically stretched substrates. *Acta Anat* 1986;125:108–113.
174. Wilson E, Mai Q, Sudhir K, Weiss RH, Ives HE. Mechanical strain induces growth of vascular smooth muscle cells via autocrine action of PDGF. *J Cell Biol* 1993;123:741–747.
175. Leung D, Glagov S, Mathews M. A new *in vitro* method for studying cell responses to mechanical stimulation: different effects of cyclic

stretching and agitation on smooth muscle cell biosynthesis. *Exp Cell Res* 1977;109:285–298.
176. Reusch HP, Wagdy H, Ives HE. Mechanical strain induces expression of smooth muscle myosin in cultured vascular smooth muscle cells. *J Cell Biol* 1994;404a.
177. Monical PL, Owens GK, Murphy RA. Expression of myosin regulatory light-chain isoforms and regulation of phosphorylation in smooth muscle. *Am J Physiol* 1993;264:C1466–C1472.
178. Risau W, Lemmon V. Changes in the vascular extracellular matrix during embryonic vasculogenesis and angiogenesis. *Dev Biol* 1988; 125:441–450.
179. Carey DJ. Control of growth and differentiation of vascular cells by extracellular matrix proteins. *Annu Rev Physiol* 1991;53:161–177.
180. Liau G, Winkles JA, Cannon MS, Kuo L, Chilian WM. Dietary-induced atherosclerotic lesions have increased levels of acidic FGF mRNA and altered cytoskeletal and extracellular matrix mRNA expression. *J Vasc Res* 1993;30:327–332.
181. Clyman RI, McDonald KA, Kramer RH. Integrin receptors on aortic smooth muscle cells mediate adhesion to fibronectin, laminin, and collagen. *Circ Res* 1990;67:175–186.
182. Glukhova M, Koteliansky V, Fondacci C, Marotte F, Rappaport L. Laminin variants and integrin laminin receptors in developing and adult human smooth muscle. *Dev Biol* 1993;157:437–447.
183. Pauly RR, Passaniti A, Crow M, et al. Experimental models that mimic the differentiation and dedifferentiation of vascular cells. *Circulation* 1992;86:III-68–III-73.
184. Hedin U, Bottger BA, Luthman J, Johansson S, Thyberg J. A substrate of the cell-attachment sequence of fibronectin (Arg-Gly-Asp-Ser) is sufficient to promote transition of arterial smooth muscle cells from a contractile to a synthetic phenotype. *Dev Biol* 1989;133:489–501.
185. Murray TR, Marshall BE, Macarak EJ. Contraction of vascular smooth muscle in cell culture. *J Cell Physiol* 1990;143:26–38.
186. Bodin P, Richard S, Travo C, et al. Responses of subcultured rat aortic smooth muscle myocytes to vasoactive agents and KCl-induced depolarization. *Am J Physiol* 1991;260:C151–C158.
187. Tagami M, Nara Y, Kubota A, et al. Morphological and functional differentiation of cultured vascular smooth muscle cells. *Cell Tiss Res* 1986;245:261–266.
188. Barinaga M. Knockout mice: round two. *Science* 1994;265:26–28.
189. Gu H, Marth JD, Orban PC, Mossman H, Rajewsky K. Deletion of a DNA polymerase β gene segment in T cells using cell type-specific gene targeting. *Science* 1994;265:103–106.
190. Robbins J. Gene targeting. The precise manipulation of the mammalian genome. *Circ Res* 1993;73:3–9.
191. Rosen EM, Goldberg ID, Shapiro HM, Levenson SE, Halpin PA, Faraggi D. Strain and site dependence of polyploidization of cultured rat smooth muscle. *J Cell Physiol* 1986;128:337–344.
192. Giachelli CM, Majesky MW, Schwartz SM. Developmentally regulated cytochrome P-450IA1 expression in cultured rat vascular smooth muscle cells. *J Biol Chem* 1991;266:3981–3986.
193. Lemire JM, Covin CW, White S, Giachelli CM, Schwartz SM. Characterization of cloned aortic smooth muscle cells from young rats. *Am J Pathol* 1994;144:1068–1081.
194. Schwartz SM, Foy L, Bowen-Pope DF, Ross R. Derivation and properties of platelet-derived growth factor-independent rat smooth muscle cells. *Am J Pathol* 1990;136:1417–1428.
195. Han DK, Liau G. Identification and characterization of developmentally regulated genes in vascular smooth muscle cells. *Circ Res* 1992;71:711–719.
196. Walker LN, Bowen Pope DF, Ross R, Reidy MA. Production of platelet-derived growth factor-like molecules by cultured arterial smooth muscle cells accompanies proliferation after arterial injury. *Proc Natl Acad Sci USA* 1986;83:7311–7315.
197. Zanellato AMC, Borrione AC, Tonello M, Scannapieco G, Pauletto P, Sartore S. Myosin isoform expression in smooth muscle cell heterogeneity in normal and atherosclerotic rabbit aorta. *Arteriosclerosis* 1990;10:996–1009.
198. Giuriato L, Scatena M, Chiavegato A, et al. Localization and smooth muscle cell composition of atherosclerotic lesions in Watanabe heritable hyperlipidemic rabbits. *Arterioscler Thromb* 1993;13:347–359.
199. Campbell GR, Campbell JH. Smooth muscle phenotypic changes in arterial wall hemostasis: implications for the pathogenesis of atherosclerosis. *Exp Mol Pathol* 1985;42:139–162.
200. Gordon D, Schwartz SM. Replication of arterial smooth muscle cells in hypertension and atherosclerosis [Review]. *Am J Cardiol* 1987;59: 44A–48A.
201. Ross R. Rous-Whipple Award Lecture. Atherosclerosis: a defense mechanism gone awry. *Am J Pathol* 1993;143:987–1002.
202. Ross R. The pathogenesis of atherosclerosis–an update [Review]. *N Engl J Med* 1986;314:488–500.
203. Benditt EP, Benditt JM. Evidence for the monoclonal origin of human atherosclerotic plaques. *Proc Natl Acad Sci USA* 1973;70:1753–1756.
204. Clowes AW, Schwartz SM. Significance of quiescent smooth muscle migration in the injured rat carotid artery. *Circ Res* 1985;56:139–145.
205. Barja F, Coughlin C, Belin D, Gabbiani G. Actin isoform synthesis and mRNA levels in quiescent and proliferating rat aortic smooth muscle cells *in vivo* and *in vitro*. *Lab Invest* 1986;55:226–233.
206. Giuriato L, Scatena M, Chiavegato A, et al. Non-muscle myosin isoforms and cell heterogeneity in developing rabbit vascular smooth muscle. *J Cell Sci* 1992;101:233–246.
207. Sartore S, Scatena M, Chiavegato A, Faggin E, Giuriato L, Pauletto P. Myosin isoform expression in smooth muscle cells during physiological and pathological vascular remodeling. *J Vasc Res* 1994;31: 61–81.
208. Gabbiani G, Rungger-Brandle E, De Chastonay C, Franke WW. Vimentin-containing smooth muscle cells in aortic intimal thickening after endothelial injury. *Lab Invest* 1982;265:262–269.

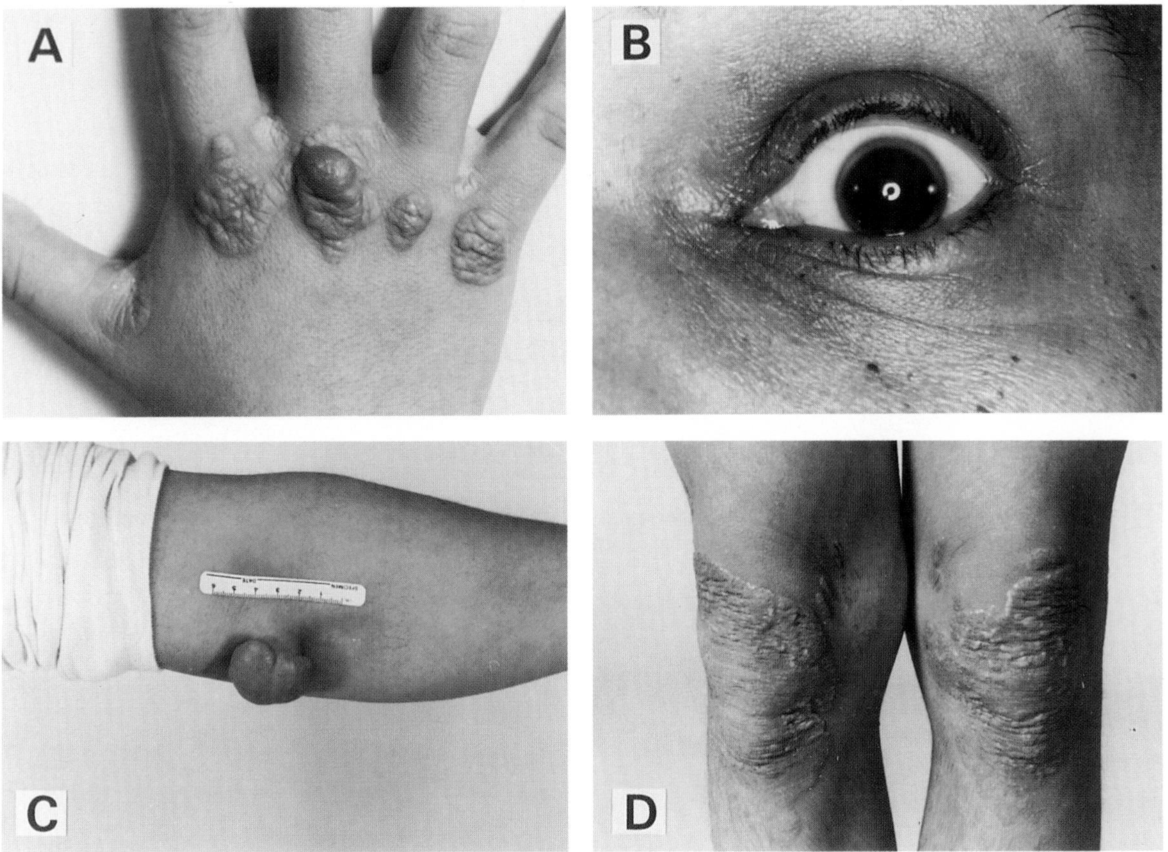

COLORPLATE 1 (Fig. 3, Ch. 5) The clinical manifestations of homozygous familial hypercholesterolemia include interdigital xanthomas **(A),** arcus corneae **(B),** tuberous xanthomas on the elbows **(C),** and planar xanthomas on the posterior thighs, buttocks, and as illustrated here, on the knees **(D).**

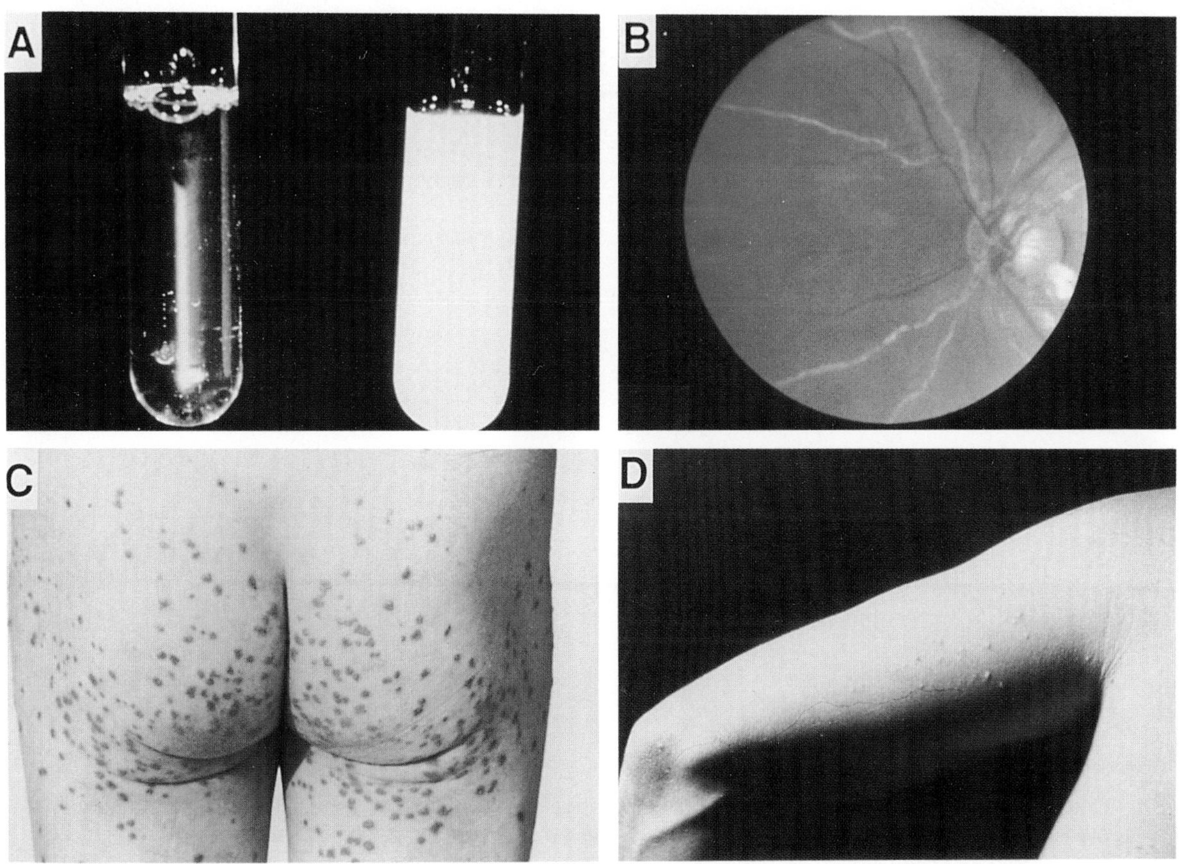

COLORPLATE 2 (Fig. 6, Ch. 5) The major clinical features of patients with the familial hyperchlyomicronemia syndrome. **A:** Examples of a normal fasting plasma sample **(left)** and a lipemic plasma sample **(right)** from a patient after a 24-hr fast. **B–D:** Lipemia retinalis and eruptive xanthomas.

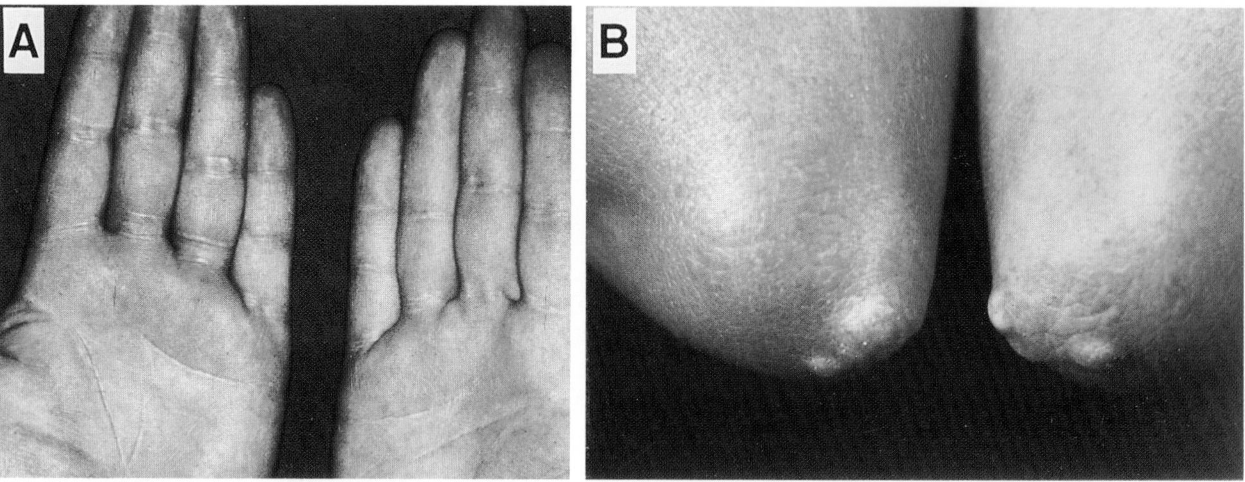

COLORPLATE 3 (Fig. 9, Ch. 5) Clinical features of familial dysbetalipoproteinemia include **(A)** palmar xanthomas, which are virtually pathnomonic for this disease, and **(B)** tuberous xanthomas.

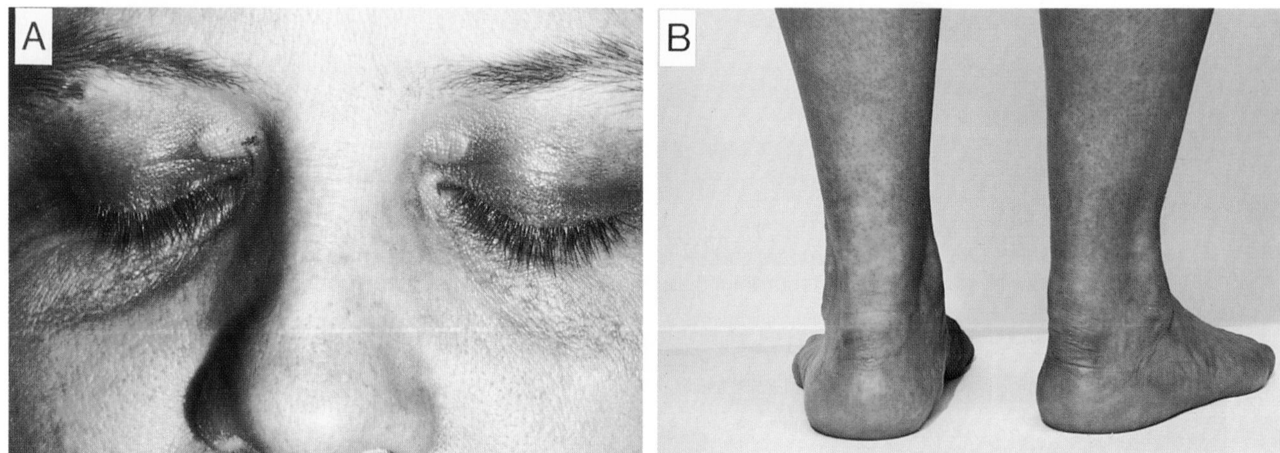

COLORPLATE 4 (Fig. 10, Ch. 5) **(A)** Xanthelasma and **(B)** tendon xanthomas are frequent clinical features of β-sitosterolemia.

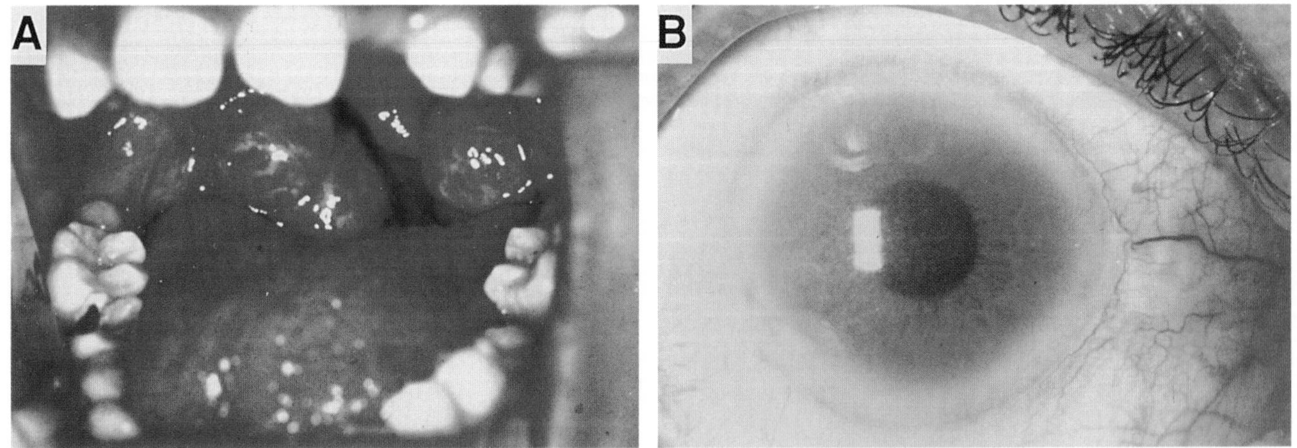

COLORPLATE 5 (Fig. 11, Ch. 5) **A:** Lobulated orange tonsils in Tangier disease are virtually pathgnomonic for this dyslipoproteinemia. **B:** Cloudy corneas are present in Tangier disease patients, but may require slit-lamp examination for detection.

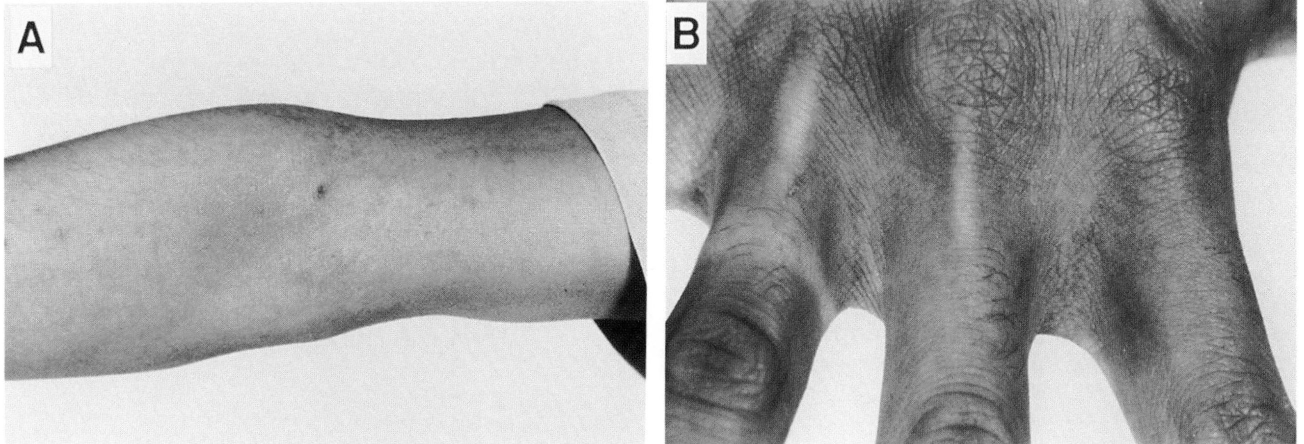

COLORPLATE 6 (Fig. 12, Ch. 5) A,B: Flat, planar xanthomas on the arms and trunk are characteristic clinical features present in patients with apoA-I deficiency.

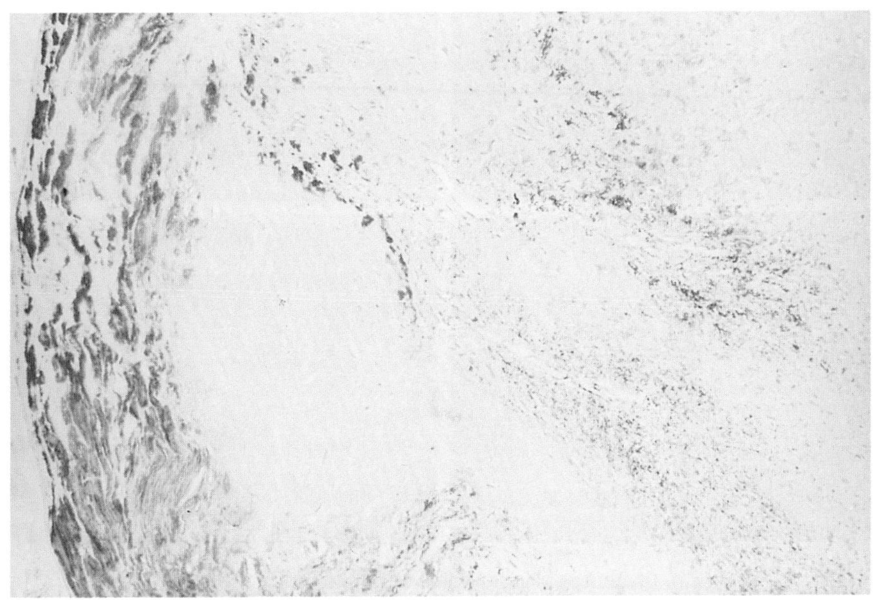

COLORPLATE 7 (Fig. 5, Ch. 9) Lp(a) in an atherosclerotic plaque of human coronary artery. Immunostaining for apo(a) can detect the presence of Lp(a) in the arteries of individuals with elevated plasma concentrations. (Courtesy of Prof. Dr. Axel Niendorf.)

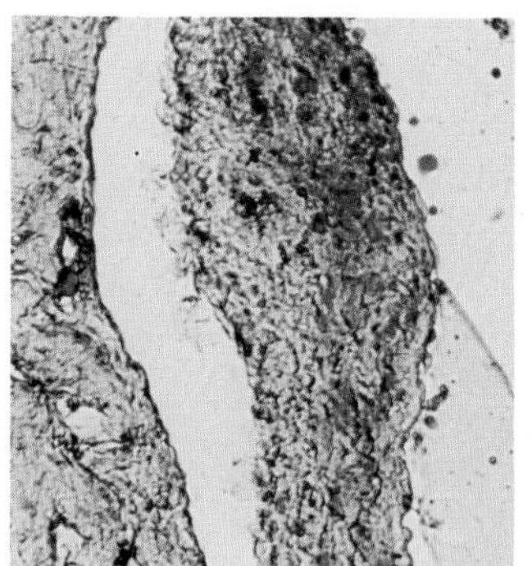

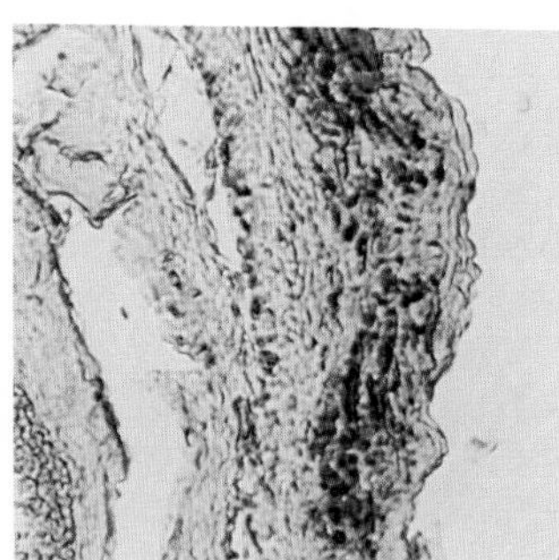

COLORPLATE 8 (Fig. 7, Ch. 9) Transgenic mice expressing human apo(a) develop fatty lesions which co-localize with deposits of the protein. Serial sections are stained for neutral lipids with oil red-O (left panel) or antibody to apo(a) (right panel). Clot lysis and activation of TGF-β are also impaired in these mice. Reprinted from Lawn et al. (107).

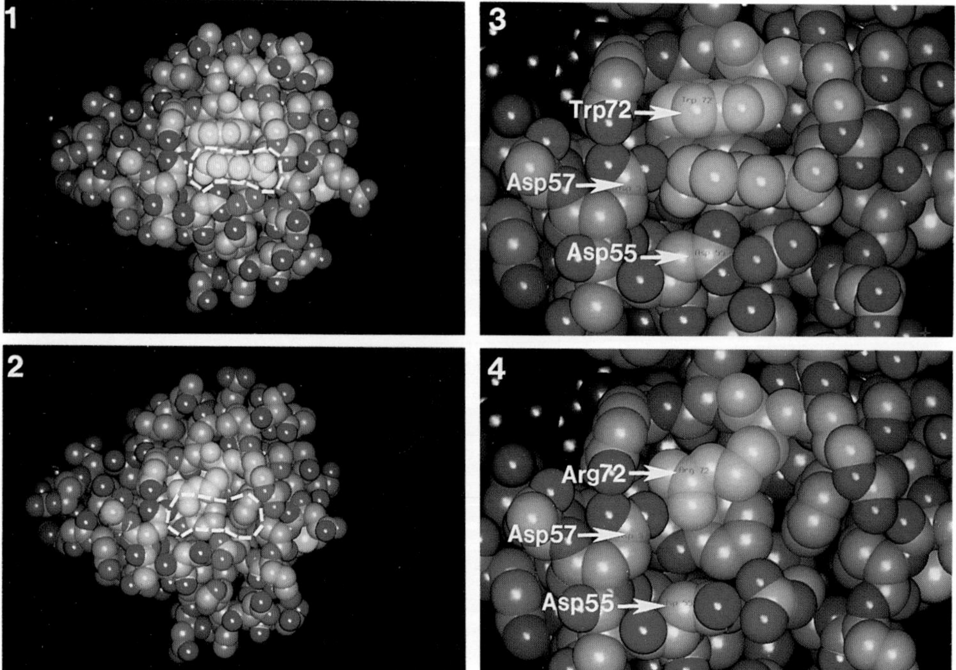

COLORPLATE 9 (Fig. 8, Ch. 9) Space filling models of human and rhesus monkey apo(a) kringle 4_{37}. The models were constructed based upon atomic coordinates derived from the crystal structure of kringle 4 of human plasminogen as described in the methods. Panels 1 (human) and 2 (rhesus) are models of the full kringles, and panels 3 and 4 are close-ups of the vicinity of the functional lysine binding site in the case of the human kringle 4_{37} (panel 3) and the dysfunctional lysine binding site in rhesus kringle 4_{37} (panel 4). In all panels, the atoms in the space filling models are colored by atom type (green, carbon; red, oxygen; blue nitrogen; yellow, sulphur) except for the residue at position 72. The residue at position 72 (Trp, human; Arg, rhesus) is colored cyan. The EACA ligand in human kringle 4_{37} is colored magenta. The dotted line in panel 2 is the position at which the EACA ligand would be placed if it could fit into the rhesus structure. In addition to residue 72, the Asp residues at positions 55 and 57, which are critical components of the lysine-binding site, are also identified. Reprinted from Scanu et al. (78).

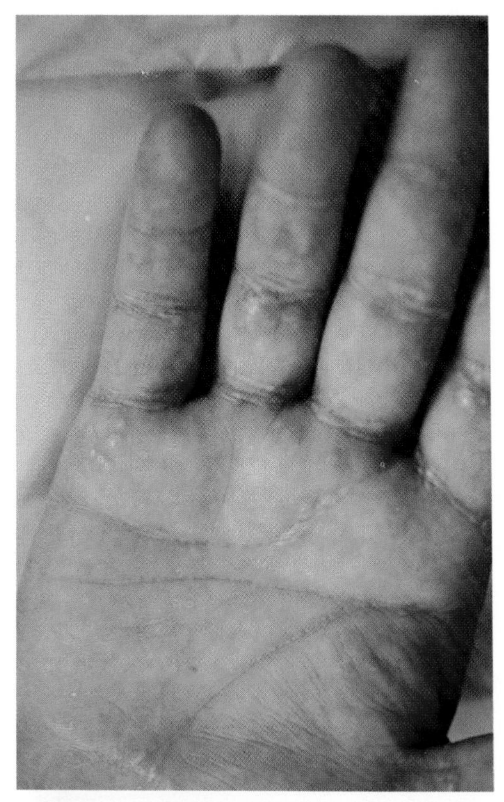

A

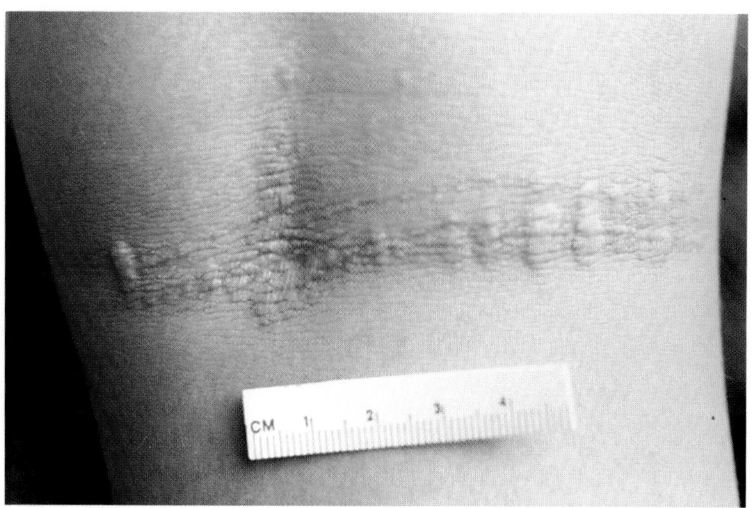

B

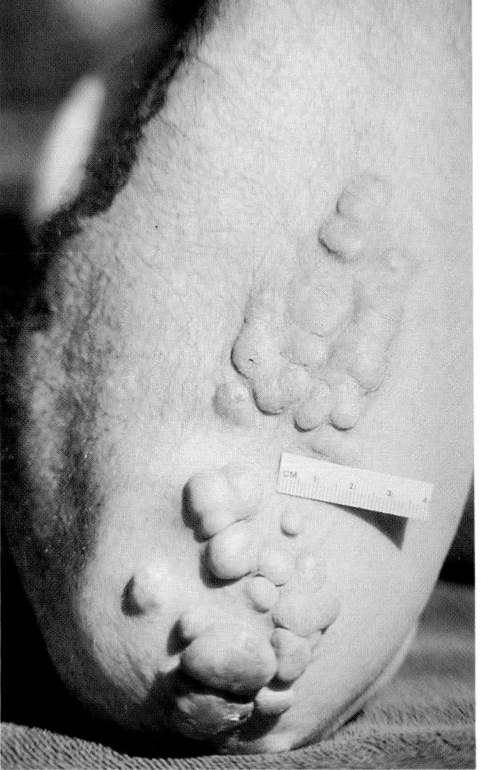

C

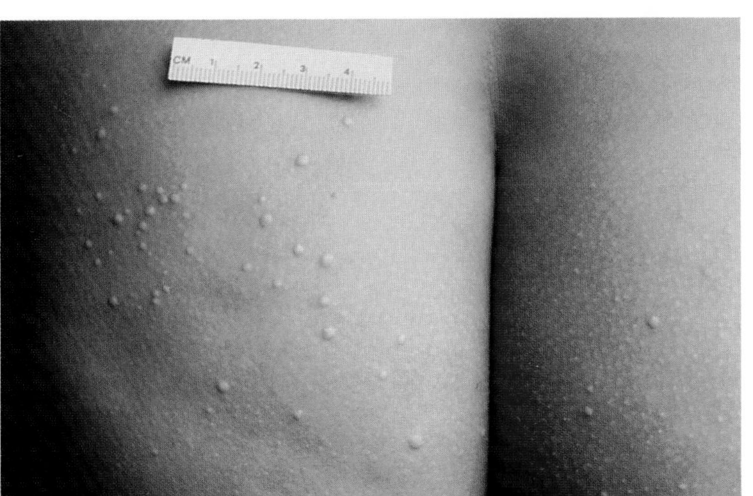

D

COLORPLATE 10 (Fig. 1, Ch. 10) Xanthomas associated with hyperlipidemia. Xanthomas **(A–H)** are associated with disorders predominantly causing hypercholesterolemia while xanthomas J and K are found in patients with severe hypertriglyceridemia. Shown are planar xanthomas of the creases of the palm **(A)** and of the popliteal fossa **(B)** of untreated patients with type III hyperlipoproteinemia. Also apparent are tuberous xanthomas **(A)** (raised above the surface of the skin) of the digits. Planar xanthomas also may occur secondary to biliary obstruction, hypothyroidism, or paraproteinemia. Pictured are tuberoeruptive xanthomas of the forearm **(C)** and buttocks **(D)** of patients with type III hyperlipoproteinemia.

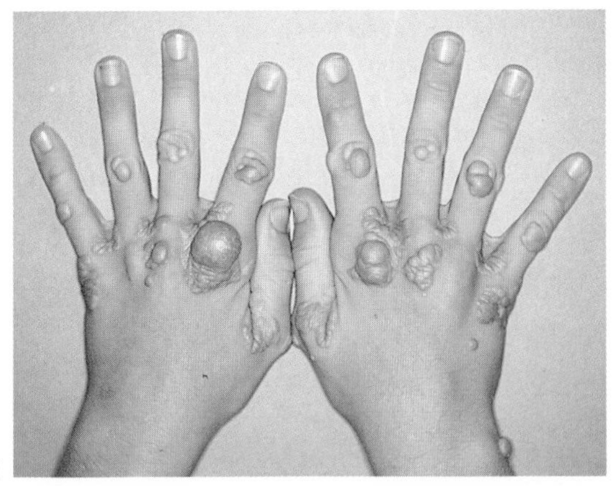
E

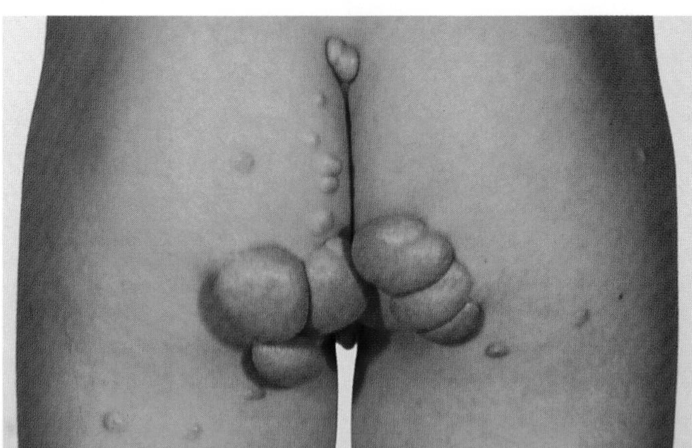
F

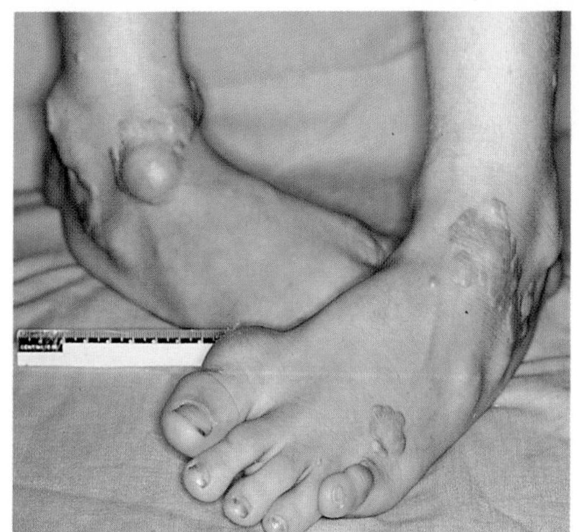
G

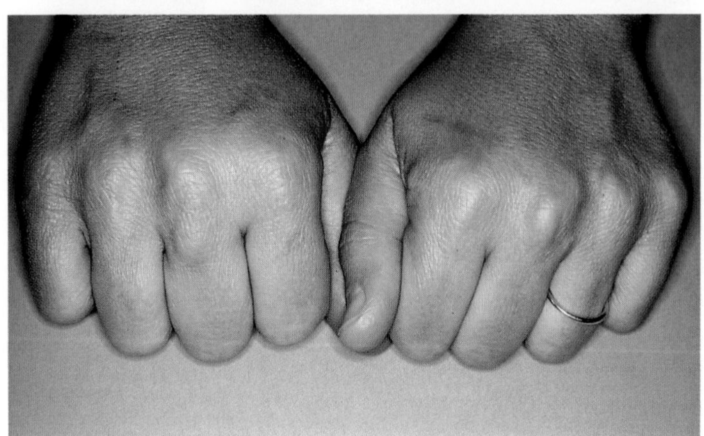
H

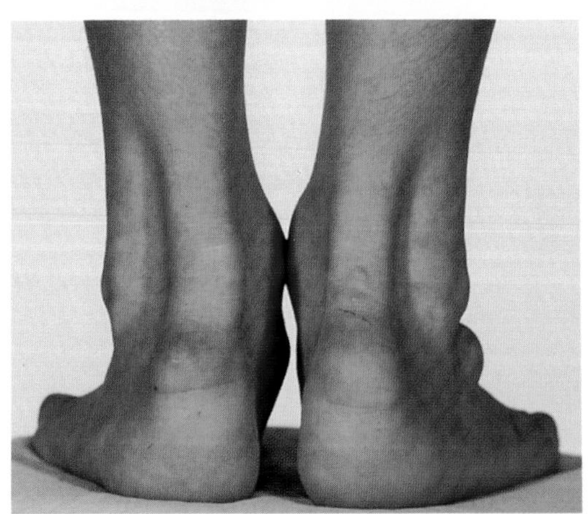
I

COLORPLATE 10 (Fig. 1, Ch. 10) *Continued.* Tuberous xanthomas of the hands **(E),** buttocks **(F),** and feet **(G)** of a patient with homozygous familial hypercholesterolemia are shown. Xanthomas of the extensor tendons of the hands **(H)** and the Achilles tendon **(I)** of a patient with heterozygous familial hypercholesterolemia are seen. Tendon xanthomas are also present occasionally in patients with type III hyperlipoproteinemia. Eruptive xanthomas associated with severe hypertriglyceridemia are shown.

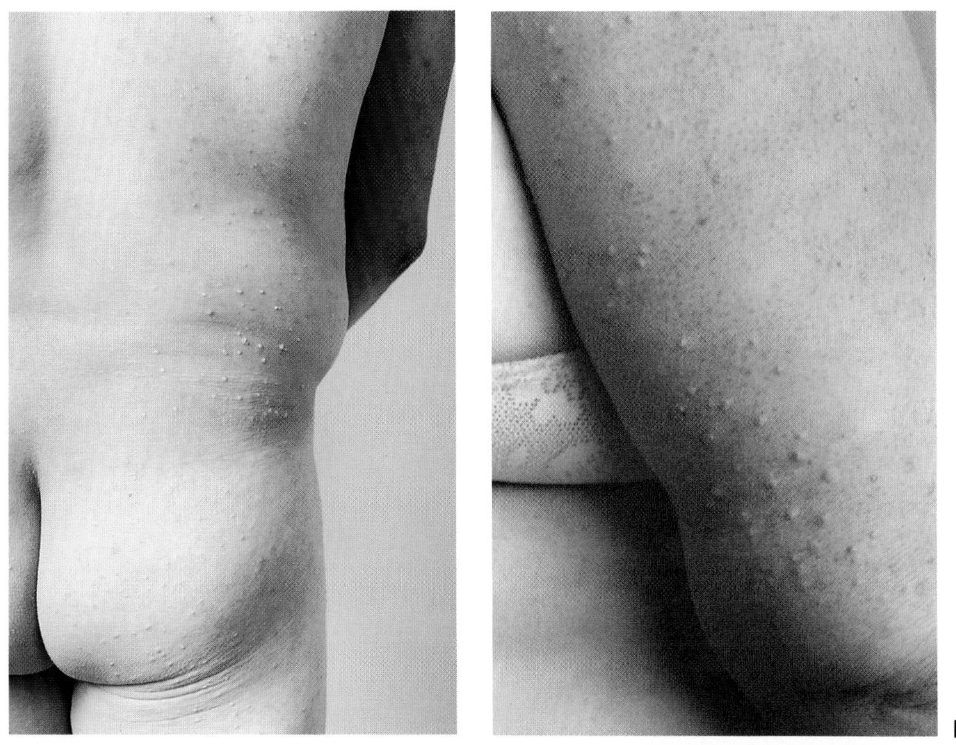

COLORPLATE 10 (Fig. 1, Ch. 10) *Continued.* Back and buttocks **(J)** and posterolateral arm **(K)** of patients with severe chylomicronemia (triglyceride levels above 3,000 mg/dl) are pictured.

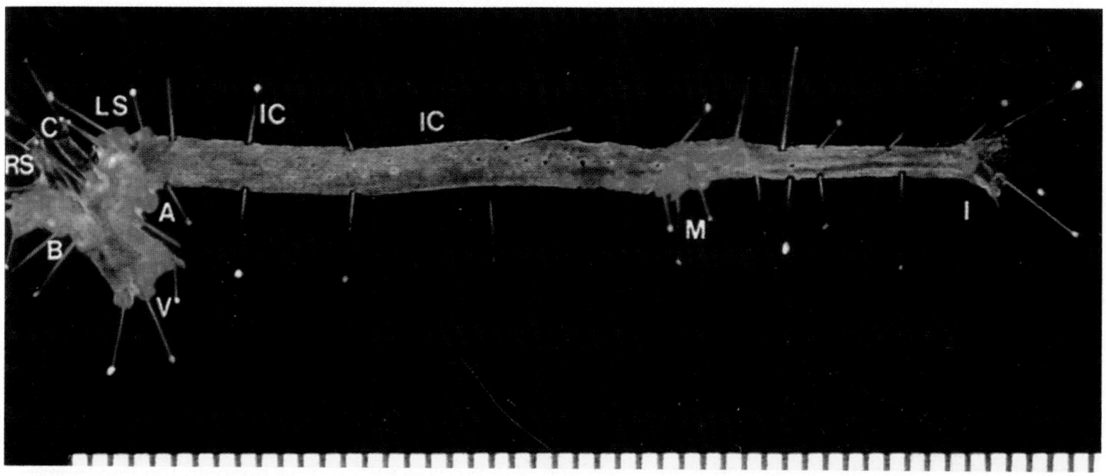

COLORPLATE 11 (Fig. 3C, Ch. 20) An aorta from an apo-E–deficient mouse stained for lipid with oil red O. (From Nakashima et al., ref. 81 with permission.)

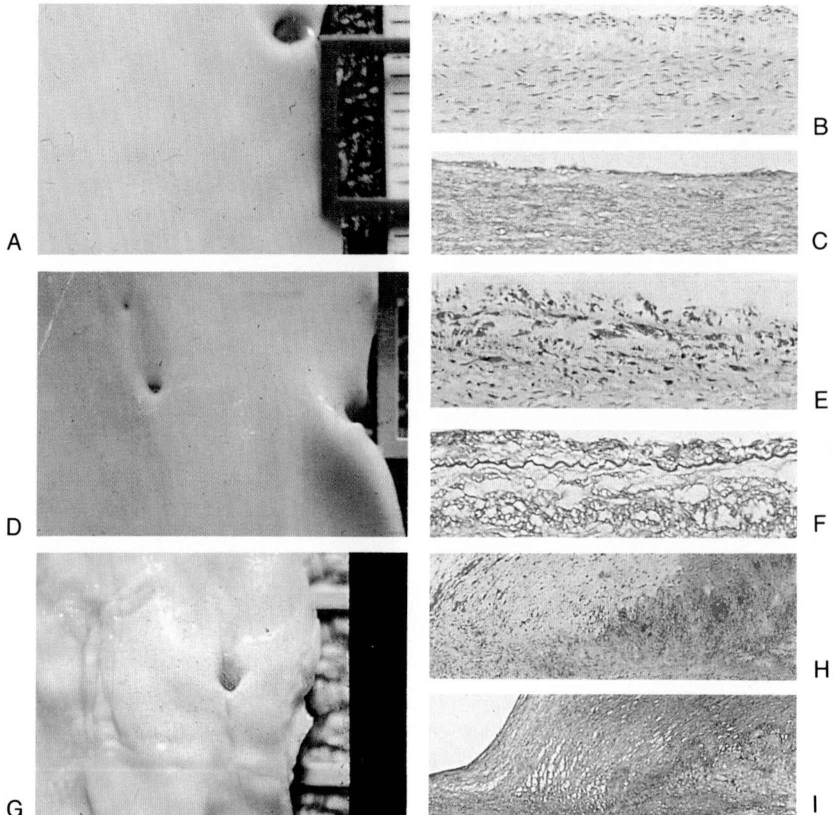

COLORPLATE 12 (Fig. 1, Ch. 27) A: Gross Kodachrome 40 close-up transparency of Sample #O1 from the thoracic aorta showing no apparent gross lesions and a perfectly smooth intimal surface. **B:** Oil Red O (ORO) stain of the 20μ formalin fixed frozen section reveals no discernible microscopic lipid. **C:** Gomori trichrome aldehyde fuchsin (GTAF) stain of 8μ formalin fixed, paraffin embedded, Bouin's mordanted section taken through the center of the illustrated gross sample shown in Fig. 1a and showing only slight diffuse fibrous thickening with no evidence of pathological change in the intima. **D:** Gross picture of standardized Sample #18 of the mid-abdominal aorta with the same film and lighting conditions as above. The light blue color-coded frame indicates that the gross evaluator could discern fatty streaks within the area outlined by the frame. **E:** ORO fat stain of the 20μ frozen section taken through the center of the Sample outlined by the light blue frame and showing multiple monocyte/macrophage (MØ) foam cells as well as a few smooth muscle cells filled with lipid droplets. Note the slight thickening of the intima by this early fatty streak. **F:** Here it is apparent with the GTAF stain that there has been an increase both in elastin (deep purple) and collagen (light blue-green) both above and below the original internal elastic membrane, and that the intima is definitely thickened. Some of the empty spaces in the intima probably represent areas where the lipid has been dissolved by the solvents used for processing these paraffin blocks. **G:** Gross picture of a standardized Sample #16, from a 31 year old male, showing a typical fibrous plaque with relatively advanced disease in the adjacent artery. **H:** The microscopic picture shows a typical fibrous plaque with a large acellular area deep in the thickened intima. This stains deeply with ORO and there is an abundance of smooth muscle cells over this area. Most of the deep red monocyte/macrophages (MØ) are near the shoulder of this necrotic core. **I:** This trichrome stain (GTAF) shows the developing fibrous cap and also a collagen-rich area beneath the impending necrotic core. The clear spaces denote MØ foam cell-rich areas near the edge of the necrotic core.

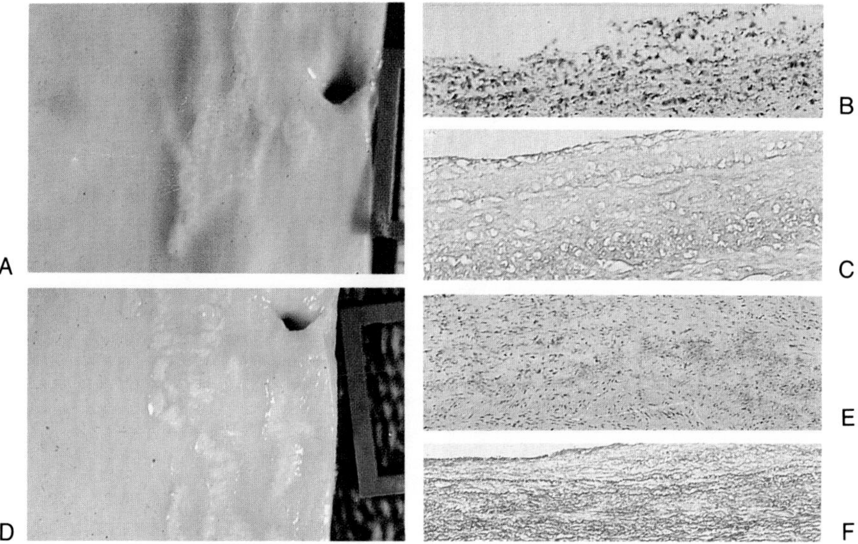

COLORPLATE 13 (Fig. 2, Ch. 27) A: This is a gross picture of typical fatty plaques, the most frequent intermediate lesion type which we found. Here it is shown in Sample #1. In general, these smooth muscle cell-rich type #1 fatty plaques were more frequent in the thoracic aorta. Note the relatively sharp edges of these obviously raised lesions which cast a shadow and which have been classified by the collecting team as a fatty plaque. **B:** This photomicrograph shows a fairly typical macrophage—poor and smooth muscle cell-rich type #1 lesion demonstrated in a formalin-fixed frozen section taken through the center of the fatty plaque shown in Fig. 2a. Notice that many of the smooth muscle cells in the pre-existing media under the area where they have proliferated also contain abundant lipid in their cytoplasm. The only macrophages present are probably represented by the open spaces near the luminal side of the developing plaque. The ORO-stained lipid is almost completely confined to the cytoplasm of smooth muscle cells with very little extracellular lipid apparent. **C:** This paraffin-embedded section through the center of the lesion shown in Fig. 2a is from a "facing" side of the same sample after it has been divided down the center. The 8μ sections have been stained with GTAF. Note the relatively slight indication of blue-green staining collagen and very little evidence of purple-staining elastic tissue in this early lesion which is composed mostly of proliferating smooth muscle cells. **D:** The gross photograph of typical fatty plaque #2 shows the same features of raised lesions with discrete borders as figure 2a. It is from mid-abdominal Sample #18. **E:** This is a microscopic section from the same lesion after formol sucrose fixation and staining as a frozen section with ORO. Note that the lipid is largely extracellular, and even though there has been substantial smooth muscle cell proliferation, the great majority of the ORO staining is of the areas between these very abundant smooth muscle cells in the thickened intima. This is typical of type #1. **F:** The GTAF stain of this lesion demonstrates that there is a very rich smooth muscle cell population with very little evidence of MØ foam cells, and that the intimal thickening is largely composed of collagen-poor and elastin-poor smooth muscle cells. In the paraffin blocks taken through the distal half of Sample #16, these smooth muscle cells stained with GTAF are very evident, and there is no evidence of foam cells or of lipid within smooth muscle cells in the vividly stained cytoplasm.

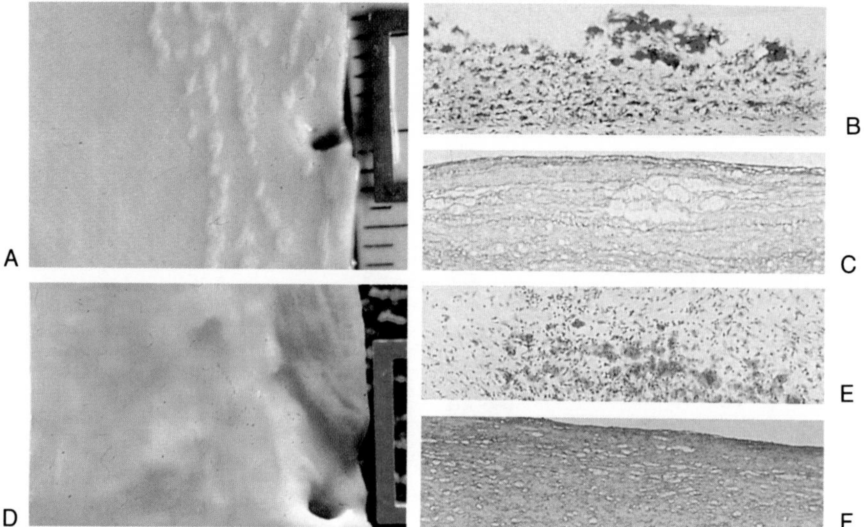

COLORPLATE 14 (Fig. 3, Ch. 27) A: This group of fatty plaques is also located in Sample #1 and has many of the same characteristics that describe the gross appearance of Figure 1a. The location of the sample includes the fifth intercostal ostium counting cephalad from the ostium opposite the coeliac artery. **B:** This photomicrograph of the ORO-stained section from the proximal side of the half-centimeter sample is included within the color-coded frame. It includes many lipid-rich MØ foam cells. These stain very deep red and are much larger than the smooth muscle cells filled with lipid seen at the same magnification. These make up much more than 20% of the ORO positive staining in the section and therefore this is a typical fatty plaque type #3. **C:** This is the GTAF stain of the same sample taken from the paraffin-embedded opposing blot. It demonstrates many MØ foam cells in a confluent area near the center of the developing plaque, so that these cells probably make up more than 20% of the space occupied by the usual cellular and lipid components of the thickened intima. In this stain, the fat-filled macrophages are largely identifiable by the large, open, rounded spaces they leave when the lipid is dissolved during processing. The surrounding tissues are composed mostly of smooth muscle cells which have not synthesized very much collagen or elastin as judged by the trichrome stain. **D:** This is a gross picture of standardized Sample #18 taken near the third ostium below the coeliac artery ostium. It is quite evident that this fatty plaque is almost confluent with the usual lesion-prone area in the middle of the ventral luminal surface of the aorta. The margins are not well shown, but otherwise the lesion has the usual appearance of a typical fatty plaque. Notice the discolored and somewhat roughened intimal surface and the elevated lesions which are especially well demonstrated in the photomicrographs to follow. **E.** This is a fat stain of the lesion shown grossly on the left. It demonstrates a typical type #4 fatty plaque with a very abundant macrophage foam cell-rich and small lymphocyte-rich lesion. The smooth muscle cells shown superficially probably make up less than half of the total cell population. Their cytoplasm is not particularly rich in lipid, but the fat-filled MØ foam cells are prominent. **F:** This GTAF stain of the same lesion, sectioned from the distal paraffin-embedded half of the Sample #18 shown in Fig. 3d, shows a large smooth muscle cell population. The other major feature of this photomicrograph is the numerous open spaces in the more severe portion of the plaque, which is evidence of the prevalence of foam cells that populate this area. Lymphocytes do not stain well with this type of the GTAF stain.

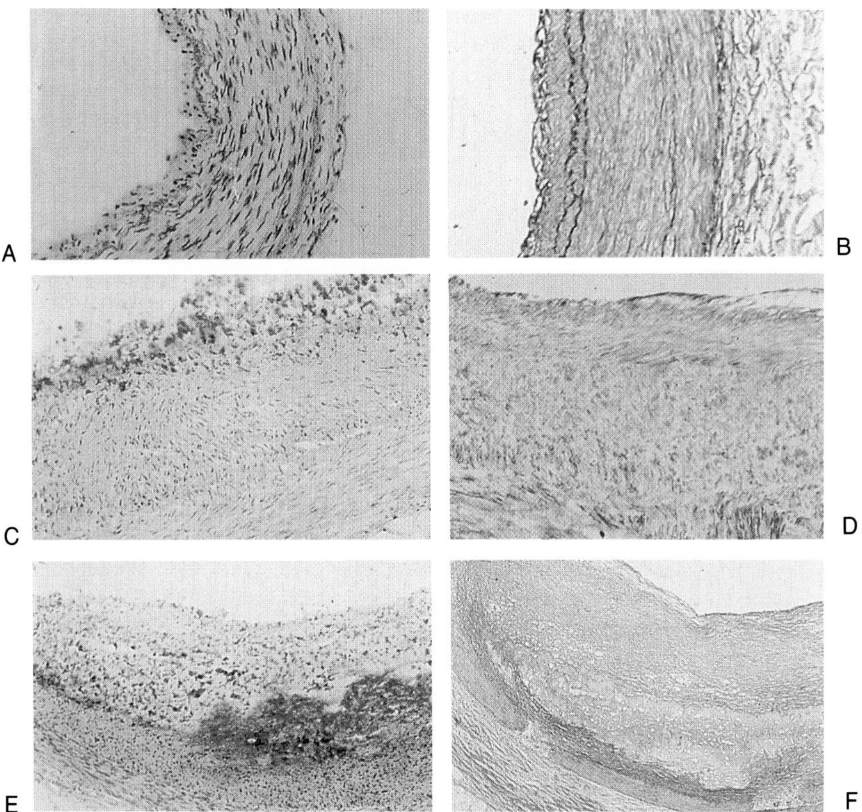

COLORPLATE 15 (Fig. 4, Ch. 27) A: This ORO stain for lipid of the proximal Sample #45 of the left anterior descending (LAD) coronary artery shows a complete absence of stainable lipid and a very thin intimal layer, one or two cells thick. **B:** This is a section through the facing, paraffin-embedded block from the same coronary artery. It shows a slightly thickened intima and a little diffuse fibrous thickening of the intima. Here the internal elastic membrane is duplicated. No evidence of focal fatty streak or fatty plaque formation is seen. **C:** This formol sucrose fixed frozen section stained with ORO shows a typical fatty streak in the LAD Sample #45 which is only elevated 3 or 4 cell widths above the internal elastic lamina (IEL), but which shows abundant lipid-rich MØ foam cells, probably outnumbering the few lipid-containing smooth muscle cells which are also evident. **D:** This is a vividly stained GTAF preparation of the facing distal half of Sample #45 from which the fatty streak was demonstrated in the opposing photograph, 4c. Note the relatively thin and certainly not focally elevated lesion. A number of empty spaces on the luminal side show where lipid has been dissolved from foam cells during the solvent treatment prior to paraffin embedding. The collagen-rich (blue-green) adventitia is also well demonstrated. **E:** This photomicrograph stained with ORO and hematoxylin illustrates a fibrous plaque in the LAD with a developing lipid rich acellular core, some deep blue foci of calcification and an early fibrous cap. The cap contains more lipid filled SMC and MØ than the more advanced ones do. There are a few large deep red lipid-rich MØ foam cells in the region of the area of necrosis. **F:** This GTAF preparation of the same fibrous plaque shows all the features apparent in the fat stain, including the early fibrous cap, which has a rather rich concentration of purple-staining elastin and light blue/green-staining collagen, the latter extending fairly deep into the total plaque depth. The deeper areas demonstrate both the foam cells and the areas of early necrosis by means of large, clear, circular areas and a fairly large acellular area in which one sees a diffuse, pink coloration. The media beneath the fibrous plaque shows two bands, the more superficial one of which is very rich in characteristically-staining smooth muscle cells which have a larger component of deep purple elastin than one usually sees in the media, and a more usual medial layer along with the green adventitial band forming the base of this plaque. No evidence of thrombosis on the luminal side is seen on multiple sections.

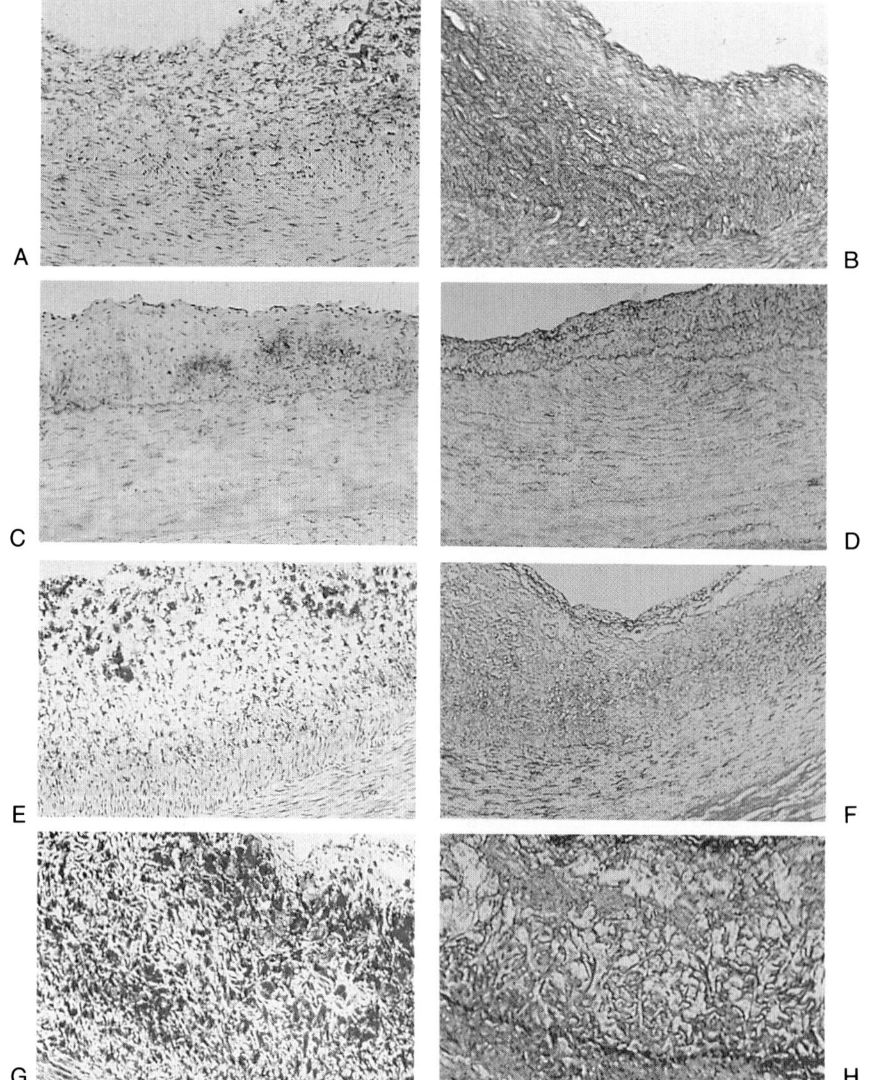

COLORPLATE 16 (Fig. 5, Ch. 27) A: This fatty plaque shows abundant smooth muscle cells whose cytoplasms are filled with lipid and with relatively few MØ foam cells. They are present most numerously on the right side of the section. It is evident that the vast majority of the lipid is intracellular, and that most of the fat filled cells have the appearance of smooth muscle cells. This is typical of fatty plaque type #1. **B:** This same fatty plaque shows a highly cellular, largely smooth muscle cell population, when the lesion shown in 5a is stained with GTAF. There is only evidence of three or four MØ foam cells. The deeper part of the plaque demonstrates a somewhat more elastin dense area, which probably also contains considerable intracellular lipid. **C:** This fatty plaque type #2 demonstrates, almost exclusively, intercellular, i.e. extracellular diffusely dispersed ORO staining with very little evidence of intracellular lipid. The thickened intima is well demarcated from the underlying media and appears to represent an elevated fatty plaque with some areas in which the smooth muscle cells have proliferated but do not retain very much lipid in their cytoplasm. **D:** This GTAF stained section of the same fatty plaque shows a cell-rich, elevated lesion, which reveals essentially no evidence of lipid having been dissolved out of the cytoplasm of cells. The underlying media is apparently almost equal in collagen density to the intimal plaque. **E:** This is an excellent example of a type #3 lesion in the LAD Sample #45. It shows that at least 20% of the cells are deep-staining, lipid-rich, MØ foam cells located mostly in the superficial half of the lesion with some foam cell drop-out, while the deeper area is composed primarily of lipid-laden smooth muscle cells overlying a poorly demarcated, somewhat collagen-rich media. **F:** Here the same fatty plaque is shown stained with GTAF. The more superficial part of the plaque not only shows many ghosts of the ORO staining MØ foam cells, but also shows an elastin-rich luminal edge and a more collagen-rich, deeper structure near the remains of the IEL. **G:** This is an example of the rare type #4 fatty plaque, which in this case is rich in both small lymphocytes, particularly notable in the middle zone of the plaque, and intermixed with a very large population of MØ foam cells which stain deep red and which tend to mask the small, dark lymphocyte population. The other cells are almost exclusively lipid-filled smooth muscle cells. The impression is that about half of the cell population is an almost 50/50 mixture of MØ foam cells and small lymphocytes, while the other half is an approximately half-and-half mixture of smooth muscle cells with and without abundant lipid in their cytoplasm. The underlying media shows some evidence of lipid invasion and is relatively poor in collagen. **H:** The same fatty plaque seen in 5g is composed partially of a mixture of empty spaces where the MØ foam cells have been freed of their lipid during the preparation of the stain. The remaining cells in the intima which are demonstrated by this GTAF are mostly smooth muscle cells, since lymphocytes do not stain well with this type of preparation. The superficial intima shows a thin, elastin-rich, intimal, luminal border, and the deeper layers bordering the IEL show some evidence of lesion extension into the media, perhaps indicating a previous IEL which is not very well preserved.

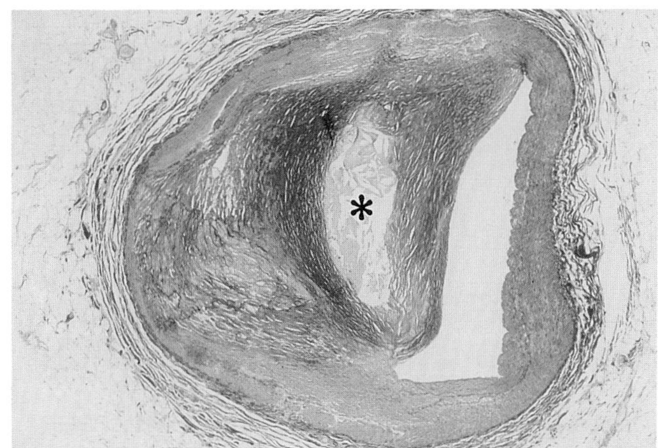

COLORPLATE 17 (Fig. 1, Ch. 28) Atherosclerosis: atherosis and sclerosis. Histologic cross-section of coronary artery illustrating the two main components of mature atherosclerotic plaques: soft, lipid-rich atheromatous "gruel" *(asterisk)* and hard, collagen-rich sclerotic tissue *(blue)*. The sclerotic component usually is, like here, by far the most voluminous plaque component, but the atheromatous component is most dangerous because it may destabilize a plaque, making it vulnerable to rupture. This plaque is probably relatively stable because the soft "gruel" is separated from the vascular lumen by a thick cap of fibrous tissue. Trichrome, staining collagen blue.

A

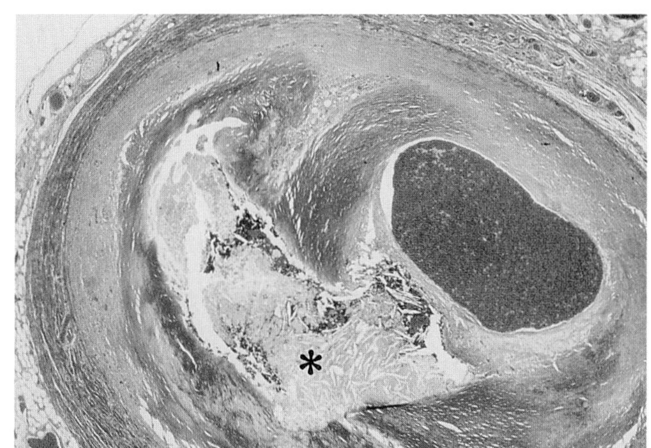

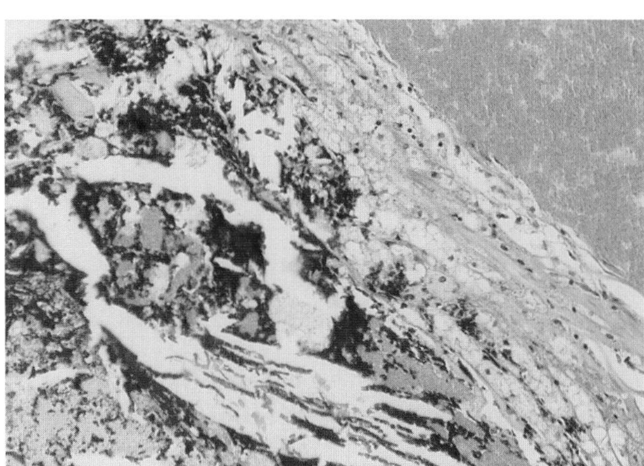

B

COLORPLATE 18 (Fig. 2, Ch. 28) Vulnerable plaque. **A:** Histologic cross-section of coronary artery illustrating a mature plaque containing a large pool of soft atheromatous "gruel" *(asterisk)* that is separated from the vascular lumen only by a thin and foam cell infiltrated cap of fibrous tissue. Such a plaque is probably very unstable and prone to rupture whereby the highly thrombogenic gruel is exposed to the flowing blood. The lumen contains contrast medium injected postmorten. **B:** The foam cell infiltrated fibrous cap at higher magnification. Blood (erythrocytes) and contrast medium are seen in the lipid-rich "gruel" just beneath the fibrous cap, indicating that the cap is ruptured nearby. Trichrome, staining collagen blue and hemorrhage red.

A

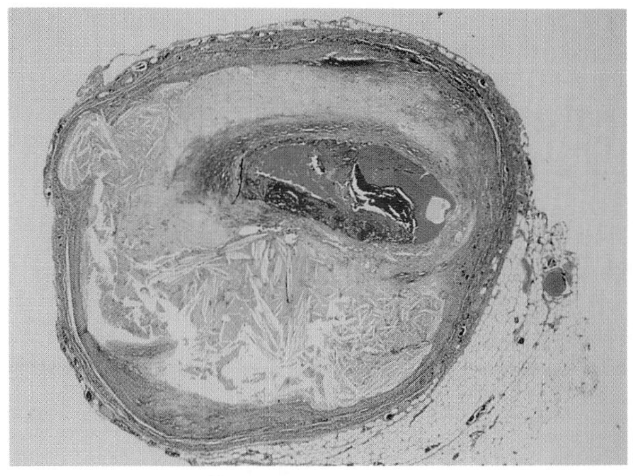

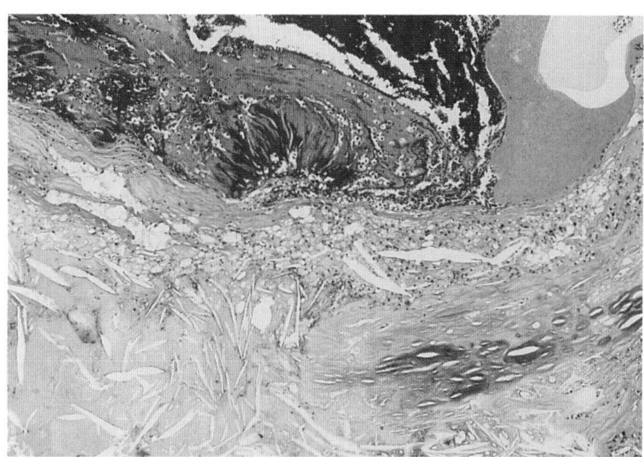

B

COLORPLATE 19 (Fig. 3, Ch. 28) Disrupted plaque with superimposed thrombosis. **A:** Severely stenotic coronary plaque with disrupted surface and nonocclusive thrombosis superimposed. **B:** Higher magnification of the plaque-thrombus interface. Focally, the fibrous cap beneath the thrombus is very thin and heavily infiltrated by foam cells (probably of macrophage origin), indicating ongoing disease activity. Such a fibrous cap is probably very weak and vulnerable and the cap was indeed disrupted nearby, explaining why a luminal thrombus has evolved. Trichrome, staining collagen blue and thrombus red.

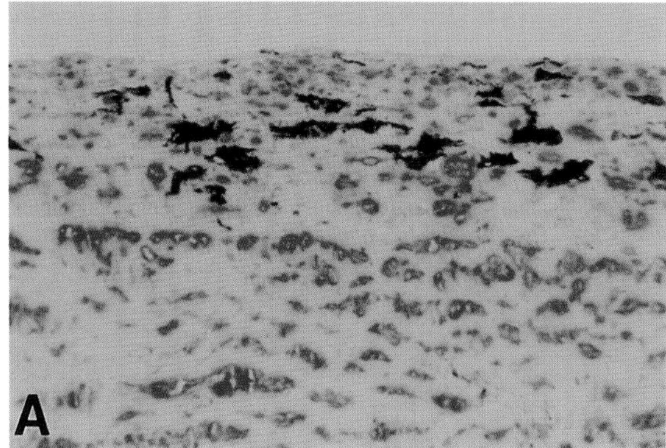

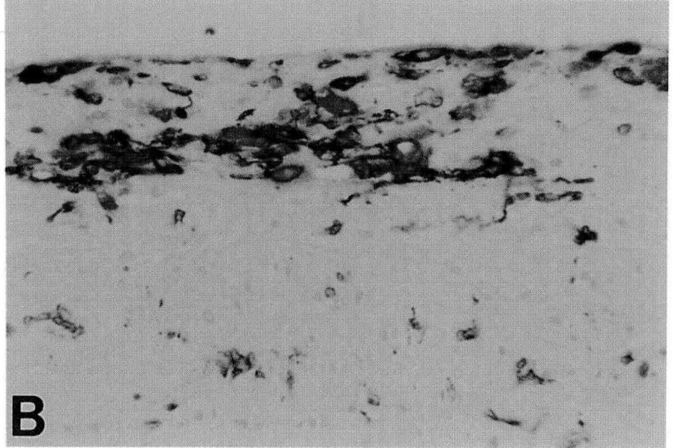

COLORPLATE 20 (Fig. 5, Ch. 30) Varying numbers of monocytes/macrophages are positive for PDGF B-chain in lesions of atherosclerosis. Both the fatty streak from a hypercholesterolemic nonhuman primate **(A)** and the advanced human lesion **(B)** contain cells that stain with an antibody specific for the B-chain of PDGF. In A, the anti-PDGF antibody was detected with an immunoalkaline phosphatase system (red), while in B, the red immunoalkaline phosphatase system was used to develop cells that stained with the anti-macrophage antibody, and cells stained with anti-PDGF B-chain were detected with sequential silver-enhanced immunogold that gives a black granular reaction product. Thus, only a portion of the monocytes/macrophages in the advanced human lesion in (B) contain PDGF B-chain. Magnification ×80 (A) and ×100 (B).

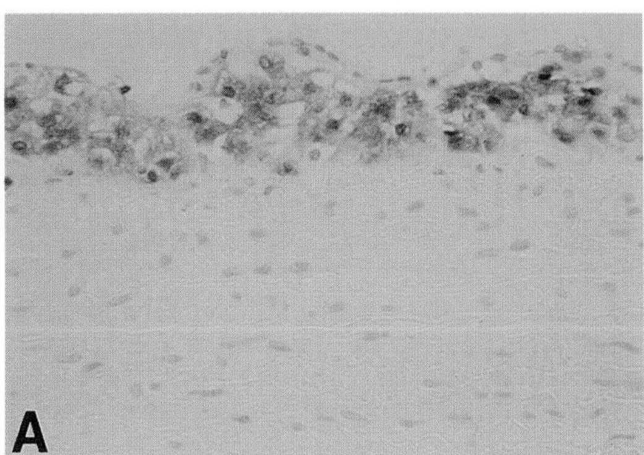

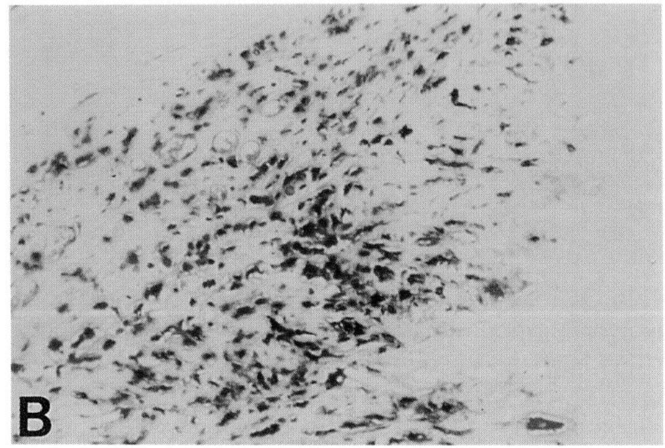

COLORPLATE 21 (Fig. 6, Ch. 30) Both macrophages and smooth muscle cells in lesions of atherosclerosis stain for the proliferating cell nuclear antigen. Within the same section, either smooth muscle cells **(A)** or monocytes/macrophages **(B)** were identified with specific monoclonal antibodies and detected with immunoperoxidase (brown reaction product), while nuclei stained with the proliferating cell nuclear antigen (PCNA) were enhanced with nickel chloride and appear black. Within this nonhuman primate fibrofatty lesion induced with a hypercholesterolemic diet, both macrophages and smooth muscle cells are PCNA positive. Magnification ×80 (A) and ×200 (B).

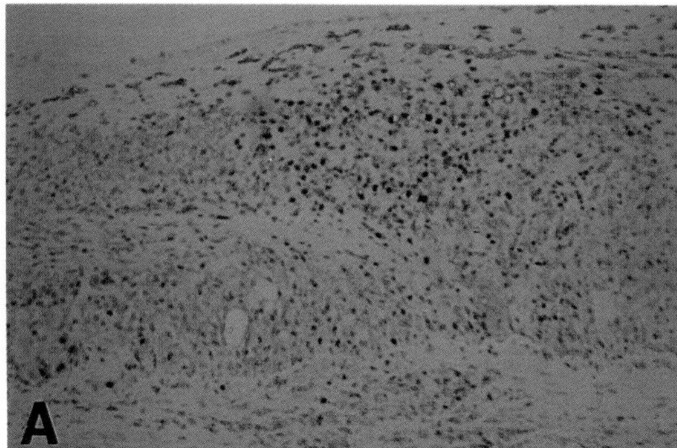

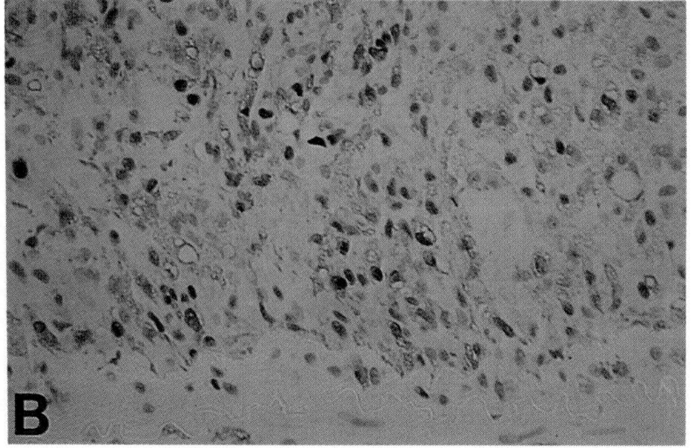

COLORPLATE 22 (Fig. 7, Ch. 30) The monocyte/macrophage is a phagocytic effector cell. This transmission electron micrograph shows a lipid-filled macrophage that appears to have engulfed another cell in an early atherosclerotic lesion from the thoracic aorta of a 6-week-old WHHL rabbit. Magnification ×24,000.

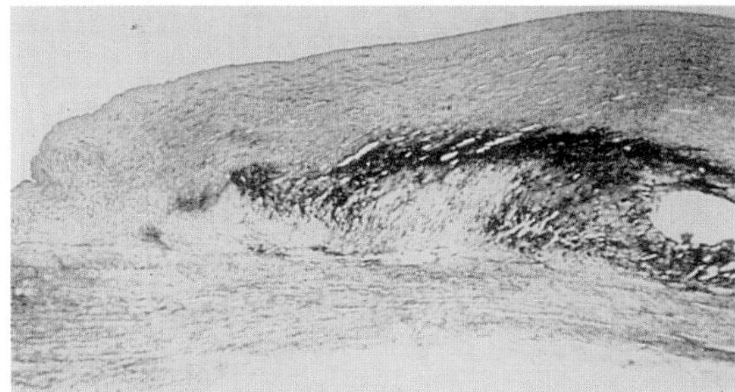

COLORPLATE 23 (Fig. 8, Ch. 30) Cell debris within the core of fibrous plaques contain antigens recognized by anti-macrophage antibodies. This advanced human lesion was stained with antibodies to monocytes/macrophages, and macrophage-specific antigens were detected within the necrotic core of the lesion. Magnification ×50.

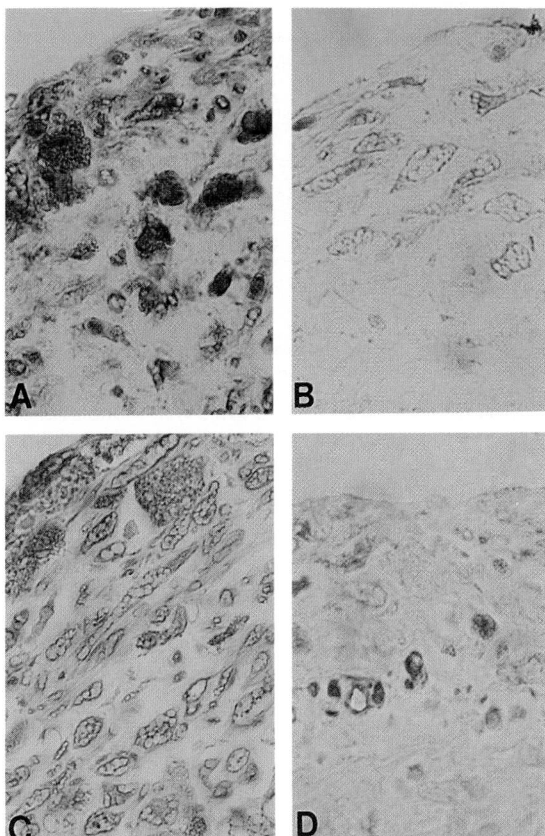

COLORPLATE 24 (Fig. 10, Ch. 30) Evidence for oxidation-specific epitopes and products of macrophage activation in macrophages from human lesions of atherosclerosis. Serial sections of a human fatty streak from the abdominal aorta were immunostained to evaluate the distribution of oxidation-specific epitopes **(A),** 15-lipoxygenase **(B),** monocyte-colony stimulating factor **(C),** and monocyte-chemotactic protein-1 **(D).** Magnification ×2,000.

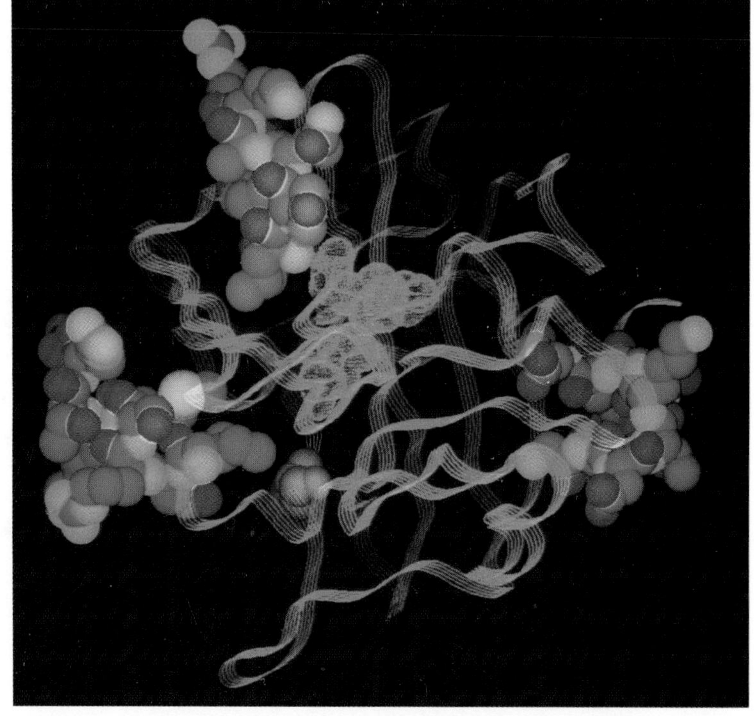

COLORPLATE 25 (Fig. 5, Ch. 32) Structural model of the Factor X catalytic domain. Homology model building techniques were used to construct a model of the catalytic domain of factor X from a crystal structure of trypsinogen. Structurally conversed regions were identified by visual inspection of the structures of trypsin, chymotrypsin, elastase and kallikrein, and the Factor X sequence was aligned manually with the sequence of these proteases. Atomic coordinates for backbone and conserved side chairs of Factor X were assigned directly from trypsinogen for the structurally conserved regions. Coordinates of non-conserved side chains within structurally conserved regions were computed for minimal overlap with other atoms. Atomic coordinates for structurally variable (loop) regions were taken from a prior, unpublished model of Factor Xa (T. Edgington et al.). The initial model structure was energy minimized in stages, first allowing all side chains to relax, and the relaxing all side chains together with the backbone atoms of the loop regions. Blackbone of Factor X catalytic domain, (ribbon diagram). Catalytic triad, blue van der Waal surface (center). Loop peptide 1 (GYDTKQED) [115] CPK surface (right). Loop peptide 2 (IDRSMKTRG) [115], CPK surface left. Loop peptide 3 (LYQAKRFKV) [115], CPK surface (top); Cys residue link to light chain, yellow CPK (lower center). The N-terminus of the catalytic domain is located just above peptide 1, the substrate binding groove is approximately vertical and to the right of the triad, and the C-terminus of the model (lacking 18 residues of Factor X sequences for which no structural information is available) is the C-terminus of peptide 2. Reprinted with permission [115].

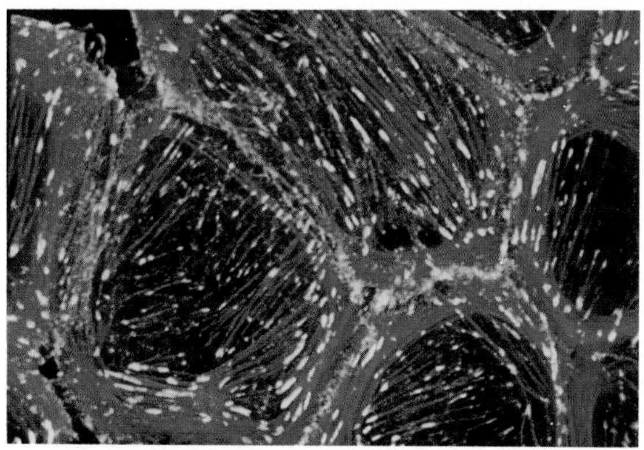

COLORPLATE 26 (Fig. 2, Ch. 34) A monolayer of porcine aortic endothelial cells double-labeled with rhodamine phalloidin and an antibody to vinculin to localize actin microfilaments and vinculin. Note central microfilaments and the dense peripheral band (DPB) of microfilaments. Vinculin is localized to the ends of the central microfilaments and focally along the DPB and is involved in cell adhesion. The central microfilaments are thought to modulate cell–substratum interactions and the DPB to modulate cell–cell adhesion. (Bar, 25 μm).

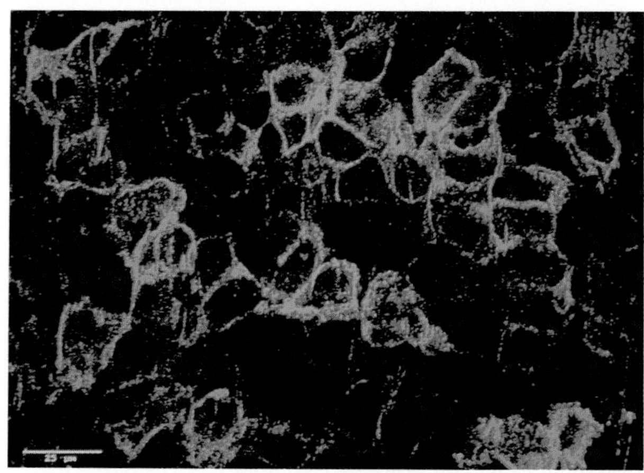

COLORPLATE 27 (Fig. 4, Ch. 34) *In situ* immunofluorescence staining of a carotid artery with an antibody to vascular adhesion molecule-1 (VCAM-1). An artery exposed to 5 days of low shear stress (70% of normal) shows an upregulation of immunofluorescent staining for VCAM-1 in many endothelial cells. This upregulation is associated with monocyte adhesion to the endothelium. Carotid arteries exposed to normal flow show only occasional endothelial staining for VCAM-1 (75). (Bar, 25 μm).

A

IEL

M

B

C

D

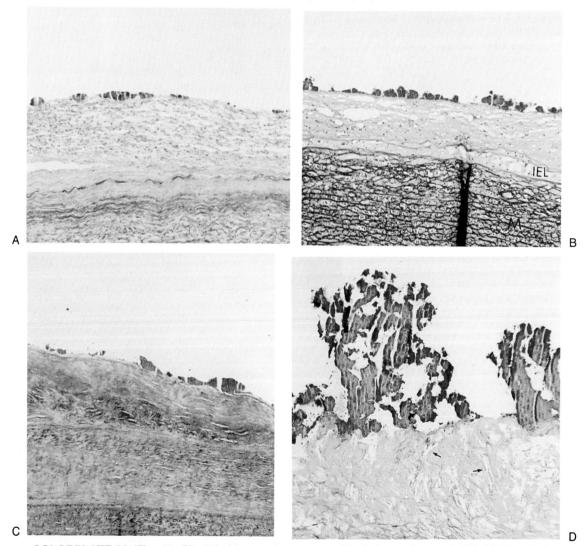

COLORPLATE 28 (Fig. 11, Ch. 36) Atheromatous cores with cholesterol crystals **(A),** highly cellular (hyperplasia) plaques **(B),** collagen-rich plaques **(C),** and fibrolipid plaques **(D)** from human aorta perfused for 5 min at high shear rate (1,690). Platelet deposition was maximal when the atheromatous core was perfused. (From Fernández-Ortiz et al., ref. 78).

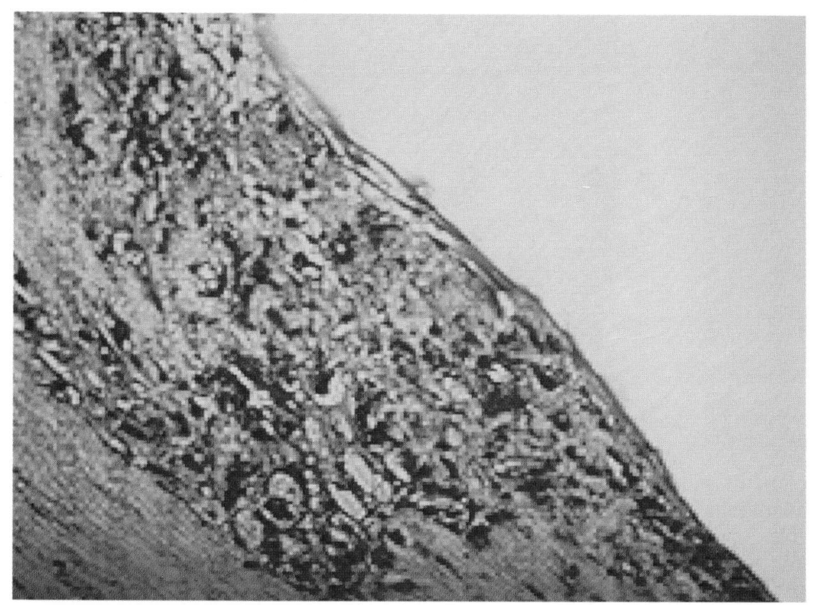

COLORPLATE 29 (Fig. 17, Ch. 37) Endothelin in patients with arteriosclerosis. Plasma levels of endothelin-1 are significantly higher in patients with arteriosclerosis. Endothelin-1 can be detected immunohistochemically in endothelial cells as well as in the intima and media of arteries of patients with arteriosclerosis (Modified from Lerman et al., ref. 147, by permission.)

A

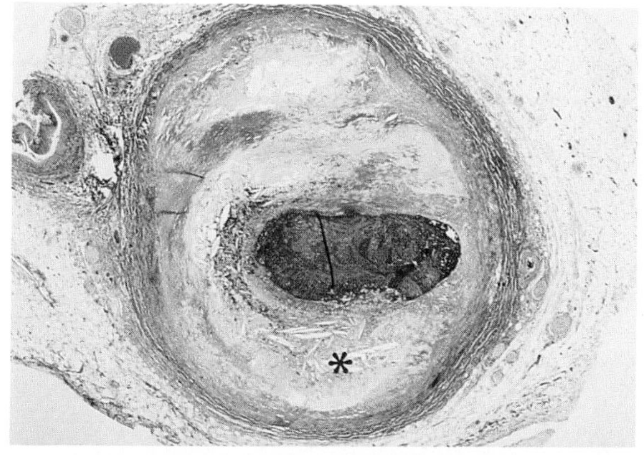

B

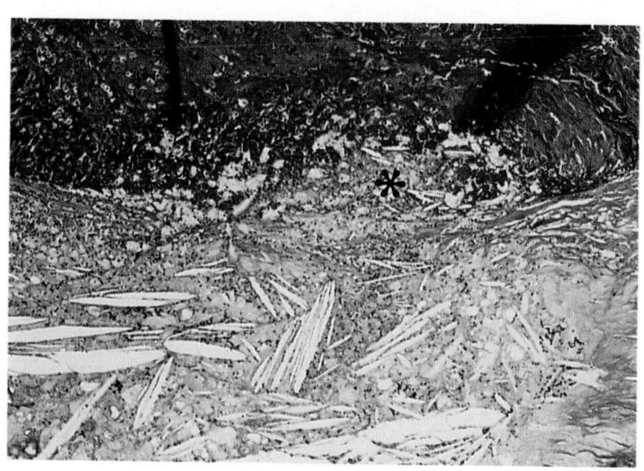

COLORPLATE 30 (Fig. 1, Ch. 38) Atherosclerosis. Histologic cross section of thrombosed coronary artery illustrating the complex nature of atherosclerosis. **A:** The plaque is predominantly sclerotic with a less prominent but dangerous lipid-rich and soft atheromatous component *(asterisk).* The narrowed lumen is occluded by thrombus. **B:** Higher magnification of the plaque–thrombus interface reveals a very thin, foam-cell-infiltrated and disrupted fibrous cap. At the rupture site, thrombogenic substances have been exposed (collagen and lipid-rich atheromatous gruel), and some of the gruel containing cholesterol crystals has been extruded through the ruptured surface into the lumen *(asterisk),* where it is seen buried within the luminal thrombus. (Trichrome, staining collagen blue and thrombus red.)

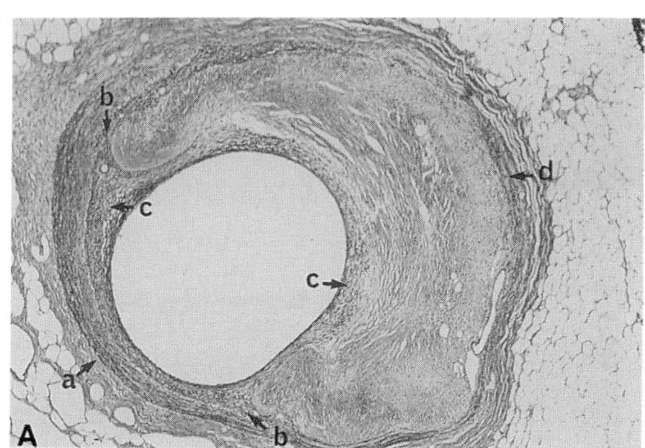

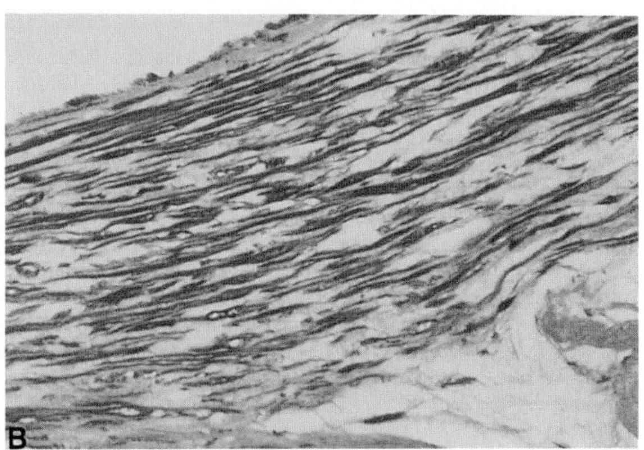

COLORPLATE 31 (Fig. 2, Ch. 38) Neointima. Histologic cross section of coronary artery that was successfully dilated 11 months before death, illustrating the monomorphous nature of neointima. **A:** The lumen is well preserved, the plaque-free segment *(arrow a)* appears stretched, and a healed tear extends into the media at the junction between the plaque and the plaque-free segment *(arrow b).* Newly formed monomorphous tissue *(arrows c)* is seen around the circumference of the lumen and in the tear between the intima and the media. *(Arrow d)* Medial SMCs. **B:** The neointima contains SMCs of contractile phenotype (similar to the medial SMCs at arrow d in A) embedded in a relatively collagen-rich matrix; no atheromatous components (foam cells, cellular debris, extracellular lipid deposits) are seen. (PTHA, staining SMCs black.) (From Nobuyoshi et al., ref. 96, with permission.)

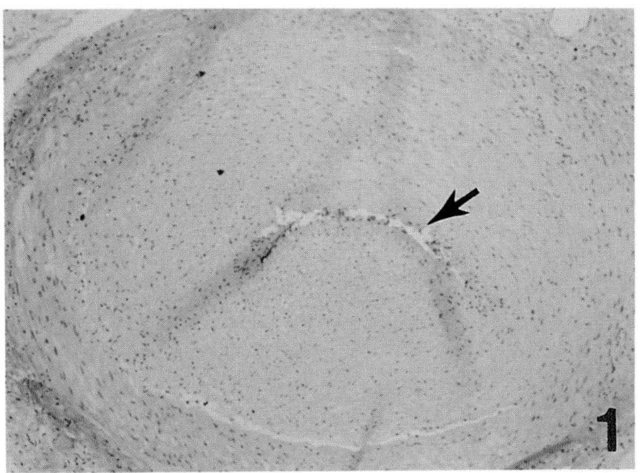

COLORPLATE 32 (Fig. 1, Ch. 40) Cross section of a human coronary artery 11 months after heart transplantation. The prominent diffuse and concentric intimal thickening has narrowed the lumen to a central slit *(arrow)*. Hematoxylin and eosin stain, 60× magnification.

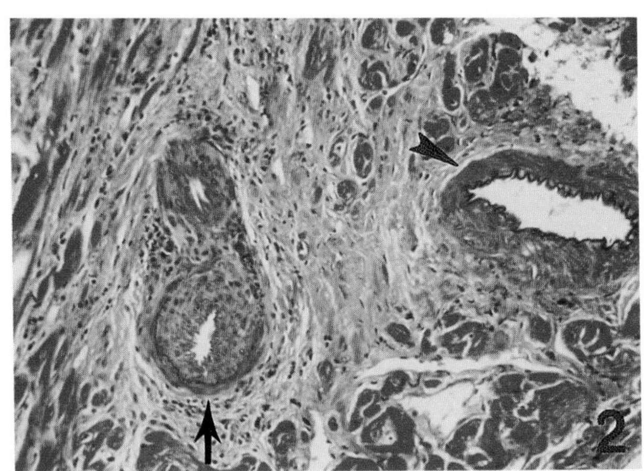

COLORPLATE 33 (Fig. 2, Ch. 40) Rat heart allograft obtained approximately 70 days after transplantation, showing one artery affected by transplant arterioslcerosis *(arrow)* and a nearby artery profile that is normal in appearance *(arrowhead)*. Hematoxylin and eosin stain, 115× magnification.

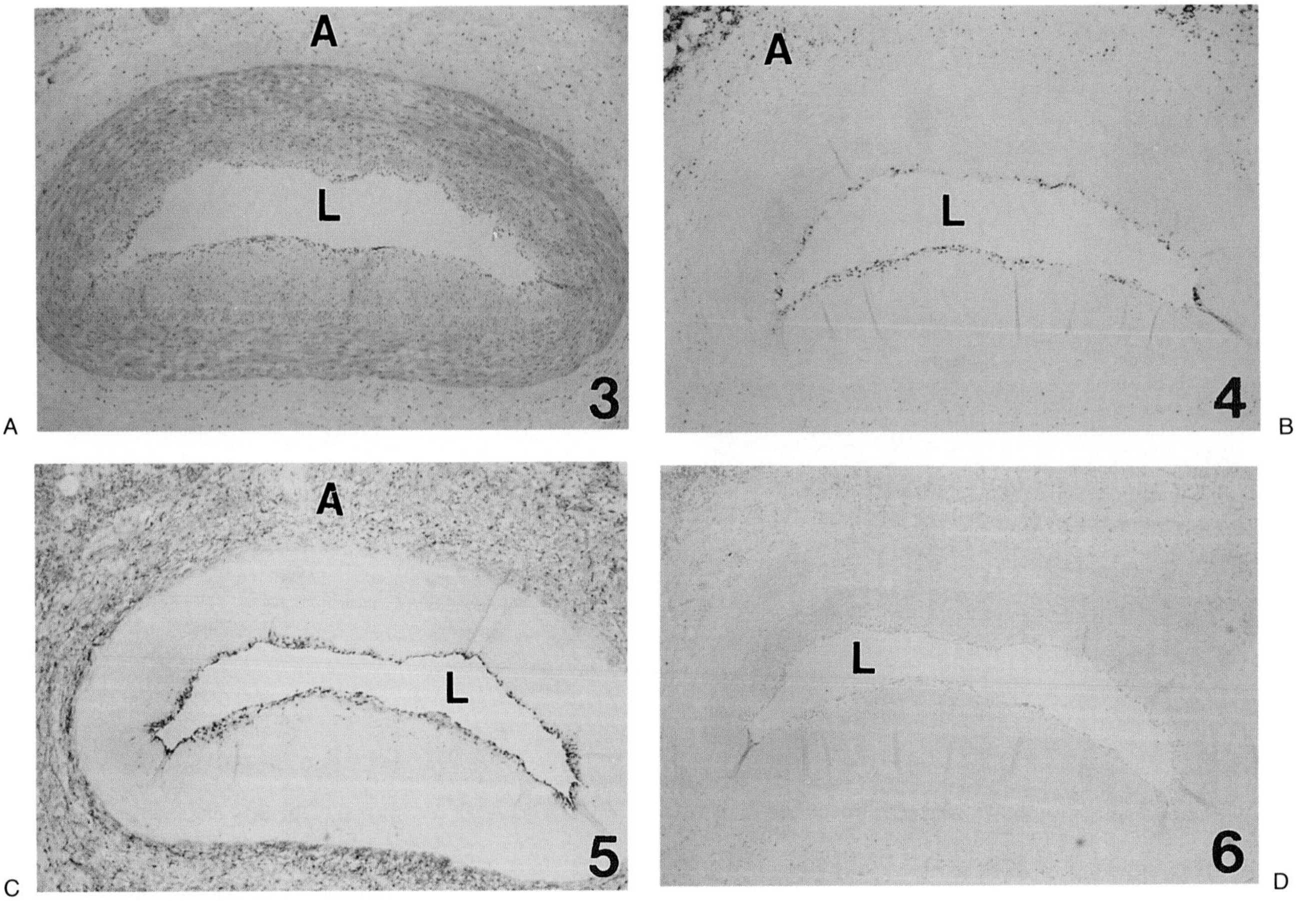

COLORPLATE 34 (Fig. 3, Ch. 40) Serial sections of an affected human coronary artery taken a few months after transplantation. **A:** Hematoxylin- and eosin-stained section showing some diffuse intimal thickening but a noncompromised lumen (L). A fibrotic adventita (A) with some inflammation is present. Methyl green nuclear counterstain, 24× magnification. **B:** CD45 antibody reaction for lymphocytes and monocytes showing a thin periluminal accumulation of inflammatory cells just underneath the endothelium (L, lumen). Scattered lymphocytes in adventitia (A) are also seen. This pattern has been termed "endothelialitis" by some investigators. Methyl green nuclear counterstain, 24× magnification. **C:** HAM56 antibody reaction for macrophages showing a similar perilumenal collection (L, lumen). Scattered macrophages in the adventitia (A) are also seen. Methyl green nuclear counterstain, 24× magnification. **D:** CD20 antibody for B cells showing no appreciable number of B lymphocytes in this tissue (L, lumen). Methyl green nuclear counterstain, 24× magnification.

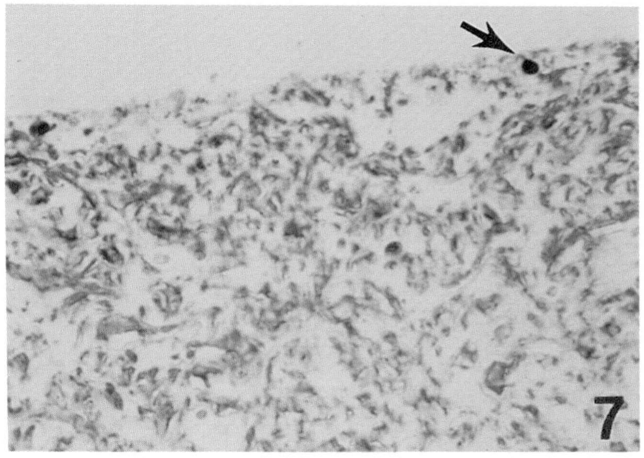

COLORPLATE 35 (Fig. 4, Ch. 40) Human transplant arteriosclerosis lesion from heart 3 years after transplantation, here stained for smooth muscle cells (anti-smooth-muscle α-actin as blue reaction) and the proliferating cell nuclear antigen (PCNA, brown reaction product, see *arrow).* The artery lumen (L) is at the top. Neutral red nuclear counterstain, 370× magnification.

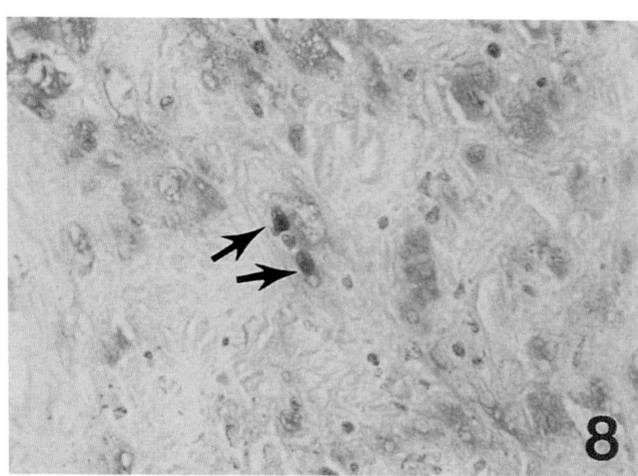

COLORPLATE 36 (Fig. 5, Ch. 40) Human transplant arteriosclerosis lesion from a heart 2 years after transplantation. Here a double-immunolabeling for CD68-positive macrophages (blue reaction product) and the proliferating cell nuclear antigen (PCNA, brown reaction product, see *arrow*) has been performed, indicating several intimal macrophages in this area, two of which show proliferative activity *(arrow).* Neutral red nuclear counterstain, 370× magnification.

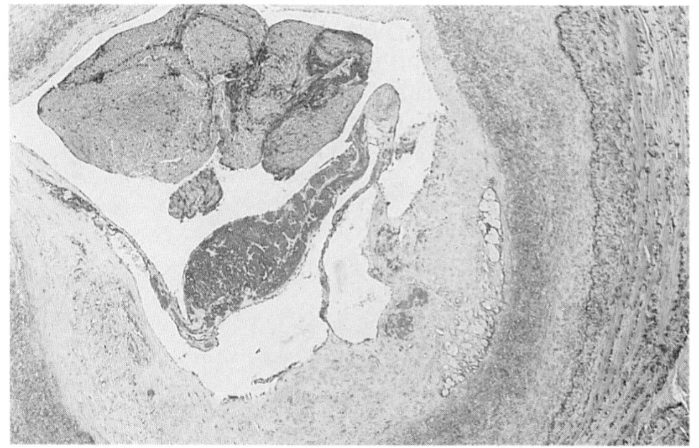

COLORPLATE 37 (Fig. 2, Ch. 41) Photomicrograph of a thrombosed saphenous vein graft to a coronary artery. The section is taken through a vein valve. The lumen contains thrombus. There are several distinct layers of thickening in the graft wall between the lumen and the internal elastic lamina. The luminal layer is composed of material consistent with atherosclerotic plaque and contains areas of foam cell accumulation. (Movat stain; original magnification ×12.8.) (Courtesy Russell Ross, University of Washington, Seattle, Washington.)

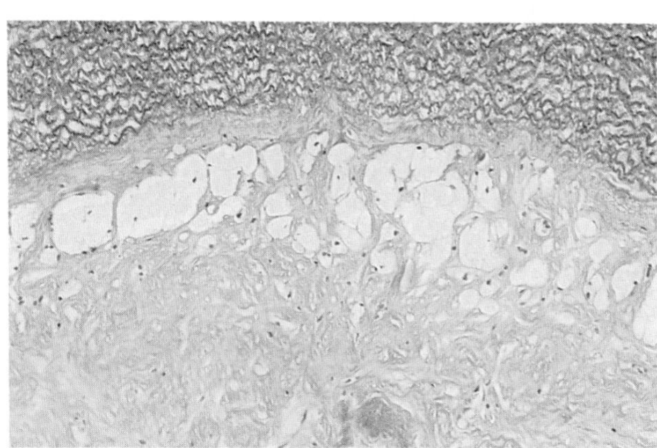

COLORPLATE 38 (Fig. 3, Ch. 41) Higher-power view of the foam cell deposit described in Fig. 2. (Verhoeff–van Gieson stain; original magnification ×51.2.) (Courtesy Russell Ross, University of Washington, Seattle, Washington.)

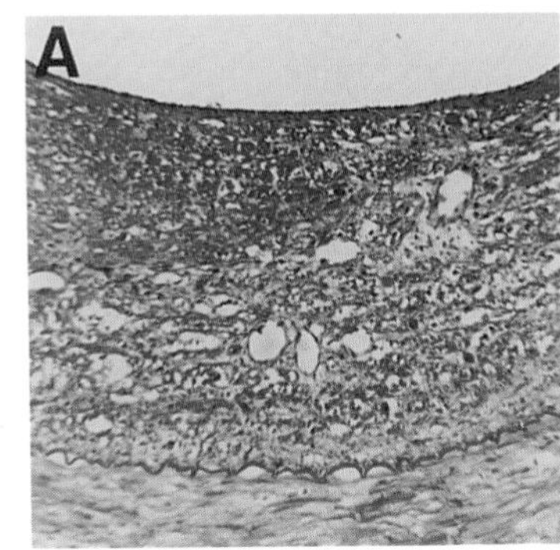

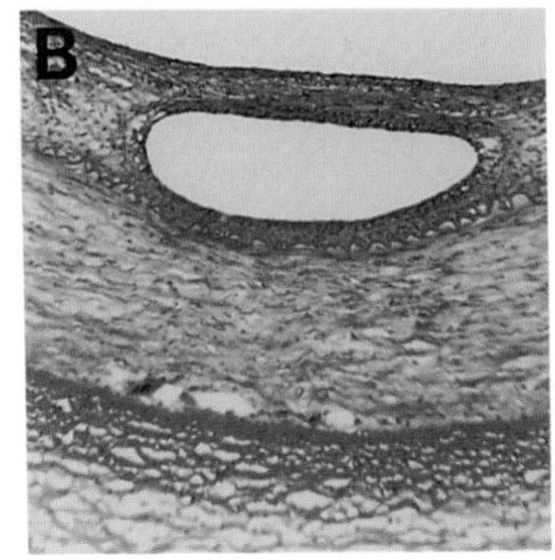

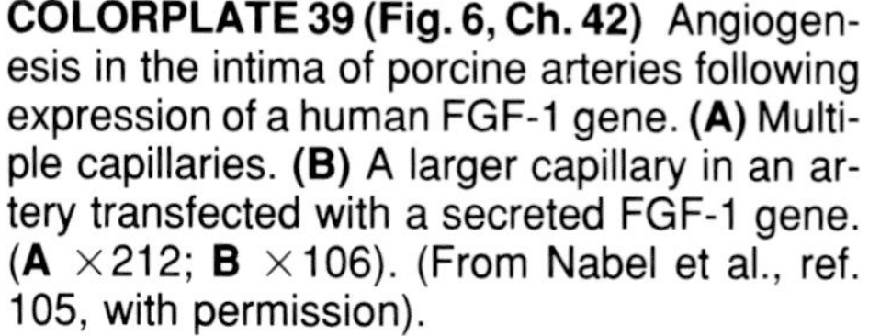

COLORPLATE 39 (Fig. 6, Ch. 42) Angiogenesis in the intima of porcine arteries following expression of a human FGF-1 gene. **(A)** Multiple capillaries. **(B)** A larger capillary in an artery transfected with a secreted FGF-1 gene. (**A** ×212; **B** ×106). (From Nabel et al., ref. 105, with permission).

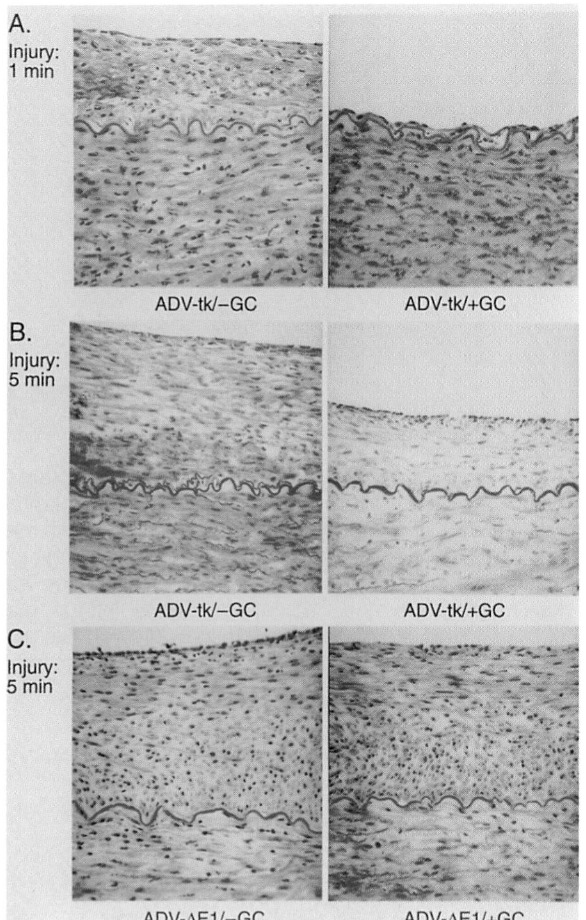

COLORPLATE 40 (Fig. 7, Ch. 42) Effect of ganciclovir treatment on intimal cell proliferation following balloon injury and adenoviral infection with herpes virus thymidine kinase gene. Representative cross sections from pig femoral arteries are shown **(A)** injured for 1 min (mild injury), or **(B,C)** injured for 5 min (severe injury). Arteries were infected with an adenoviral vector encoding for herpes virus thymidine kinase (ADV-*tk*) or a control adenoviral vector without cDNA insert (ADV-ΔE1) and treated with ganciclovir (+GC) or saline (−GC). Arteries were evaluated 3 weeks following balloon injury and adenoviral infection. (Magnification ×200). (From Ohno et al., ref. 191, with permission).

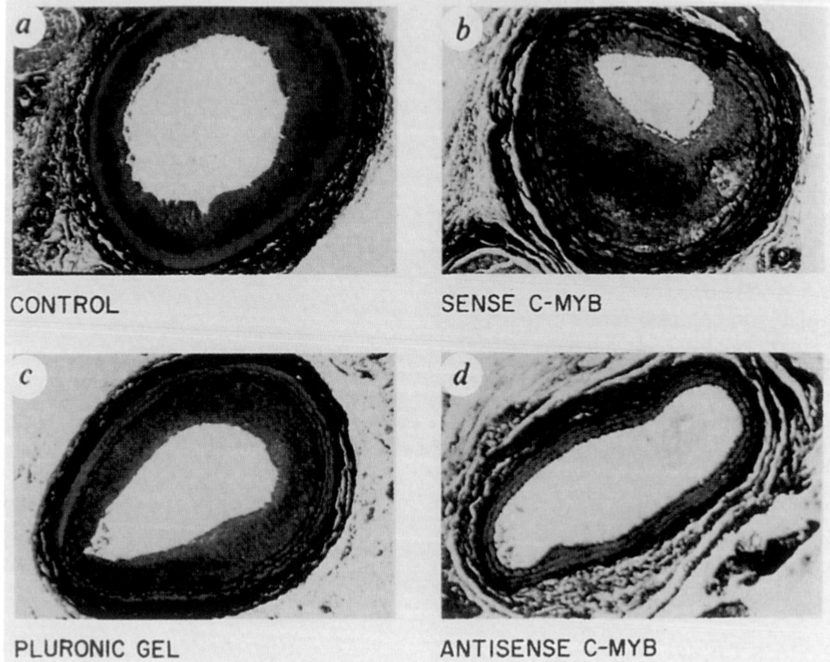

COLORPLATE 41 (Fig. 8, Ch. 42) Effect of *c-myb* oligonucleotides on intimal cell proliferation in rat carotid arteries following balloon injury. Representative cross sections from rat carotid arteries are shown from **(A)** an untreated rat, **(B)** a rat treated with a pluronic gel and sense oligonucleotide, **(C)** a rat treated with pluronic gel and no oligonucleotide, and **(D)** rat treated with pluronic gel containing antisense oligonucleotide. (Magnification ×80). (From Simons et al., ref. 93, with permission.)

Atherosclerosis and Coronary Artery Disease,
edited by V. Fuster, R. Ross, and E. J. Topol.
Lippincott-Raven Publishers, Philadelphia © 1996.

CHAPTER 24

The Vascular Extracellular Matrix

Thomas N. Wight

Key Words: Collagen; Elastic fibers; Extracellular matrix; Glycoproteins; Glycosaminoglycans; Hyaluronan; Low-density lipoproteins; Proteoglycans.

INTRODUCTION

The vascular extracellular matrix (ECM) is a reinforced composite of collagen and elastic fibers embedded in a viscoelastic gel consisting of proteoglycans, hyaluronan, glycoproteins, and water (Table 1). These components interact through entanglement and cross-linking to form a biomechanically active polymer network that imparts tensile strength, elastic recoil, compressibility, and viscoelasticity to the vascular wall. In addition, this network interacts with vascular cells and participates in the regulation of cell adhesion, migration, and proliferation during vascular development and disease. This regulation involves molecular interactions that govern the attachment of vascular cells to specific ECM components, detachment of cells from these components, and molecular rearrangements in the ECM that allow cells to change their shape during division and migration. Furthermore, components of the ECM bind plasma proteins, growth factors, cytokines, and enzymes, and these interactions modulate arterial wall metabolism. Thus, the vascular ECM not only maintains vascular wall structure, it also regulates key events in vascular physiology.

The composition of the ECM is controlled by the coordinate and differential regulation of synthesis and turnover of each of the components. Such differential regulation creates differences in the composition of the vascular ECM during vascular development, between different vascular beds, and in different forms of vascular disease. For example, each layer of the vessel wall (i.e., intima, media, and adventitia) has a different ECM composition. An ECM rich in fibrillar collagen, as is found in the adventitia, will impart stiffness and rigidity, whereas a layer enriched in proteoglycans and hyaluronan, as found in the intima, is more viscoelastic and compressible. Maintaining the appropriate balance of the components in each layer is critical for maintaining vascular wall integrity and resisting rupture and hemorrhage. Additionally, an ECM composition that forms a ''loose'' and hydrated network enriched in attachment proteins promotes vascular cell adhesion, proliferation, and migration in development and early stages of vascular disease, whereas a ''dense'' and fibrous ECM typifies more differentiated vascular tissue and advanced vascular lesions. This review covers the major components of the vascular ECM and discusses the role these molecules play in the normal physiology and pathology of the vascular wall.

T. N. Wight: Department of Pathology, University of Washington School of Medicine, Seattle, Washington 98195.

TABLE 1. *Some of the components of the vascular ECM*

Collagen fibrils	Basement membranes
Type I collagen	Type IV collagen
Type III collagen	Type VIII collagen
Type V collagen	Laminin
Type VI collagen	Entactin
Glycoproteins	Perlecan (HSPG)
Fibronectin	Proteoglycans and associated molecules
Thrombospondin	Hyaluronan
Tenascin	Link protein(s)
Osteopontin	Versican (CSPG)
Elastic fibers	Decorin (DSPG)
Elastin	Biglycan (DSPG)
Fibrillin	Lumican (KSPG)
Emilin	Perlecan (HSPG)
Lysl oxidase	

COLLAGENS

Types and Distribution

Collagens are proteins that consist of a triple helix of polypeptide chains, in which each chain contains at least one stretch of the repeating amino acid sequence Gly-X-Y. Collagens comprise a family of proteins of at least 19 genetically distinct types classified by differences in their amino acid composition and the proportion of the molecule forming the triple helix (1,2). Six of these collagen types have been identified in blood vessels and are types I, III, IV, V, VI, and VIII (3–5). The predominant vascular collagens are type I and III, which comprise up to 80–90% of the total blood vessel wall collagens. These collagens are assembled into cross-banded fibrils and are prominent throughout the ECM of all vascular layers (Figs. 1 and 2). In the normal arterial wall, types I and III collagens are organized into distinct fibrillar bundles, either wedged between elastic fibers in elastic arteries or organized into ''nests'' surrounding medial arterial smooth muscle cells in muscular arteries (6,7). It is unclear whether these fibrillar collagens align to form a distinct network in vascular tissue, because most images demonstrate a wavy-fiber random orientation. Wavy collagen fibers are generally found in ''soft'' tissues and align during loading or pressure changes to prevent tissue failure (8). These collagens provide tensile strength to the vascular wall.

In addition to type I and III interstitial collagens, there are minor amounts of other collagens that provide important properties to vascular tissue. Type IV and VIII collagens are present within vascular basement membranes beneath endothelial cells and surrounding arterial smooth muscle cells (9–12). These molecules self-associate and interact with other molecules to form lattice-like supramolecular networks that serve as an anchoring substrate for vascular cells and as a permeability barrier to plasma proteins (10).

Also present in small amounts in vascular tissue is type V collagen (3–5,13). This collagen codistributes with type I collagen and may participate in the formation of collagen heteropolymers (1,8). A recent survey of type V collagen in human vascular tissue indicates its presence in thickened arterial intimas and in atherosclerotic fibrous plaques (13). The role of this collagen in the arterial wall is not fully understood, but physicochemical studies indicate that this minor collagen may interact with type I collagen to regulate collagen fibril diameter.

Type VI collagen is another minor vascular collagen that forms high-molecular weight aggregates from small collagen monomers by self-association and disulfide bonding (1,8). This collagen appears in all vascular layers between

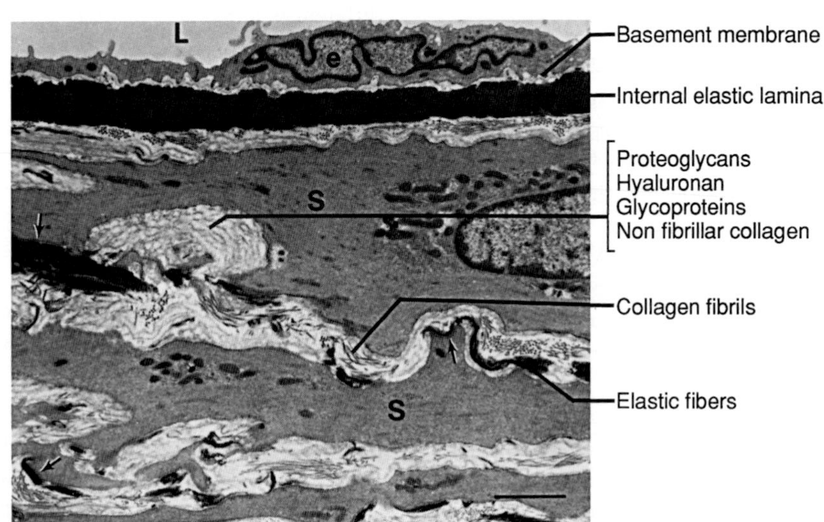

FIG. 1. An electron micrograph of a cross section of a rat superior mesenteric artery. This low-power view demonstrates location of specific ECM components in relation to vascular cells. L, Lumen; e, endothelial cell; s, smooth muscle cell. *Arrows* point to areas of the cell that are closely apposed to elastic fibers. *Bar,* 2 μm. (From Walker-Caprioglio et al., ref. 7, with permission.)

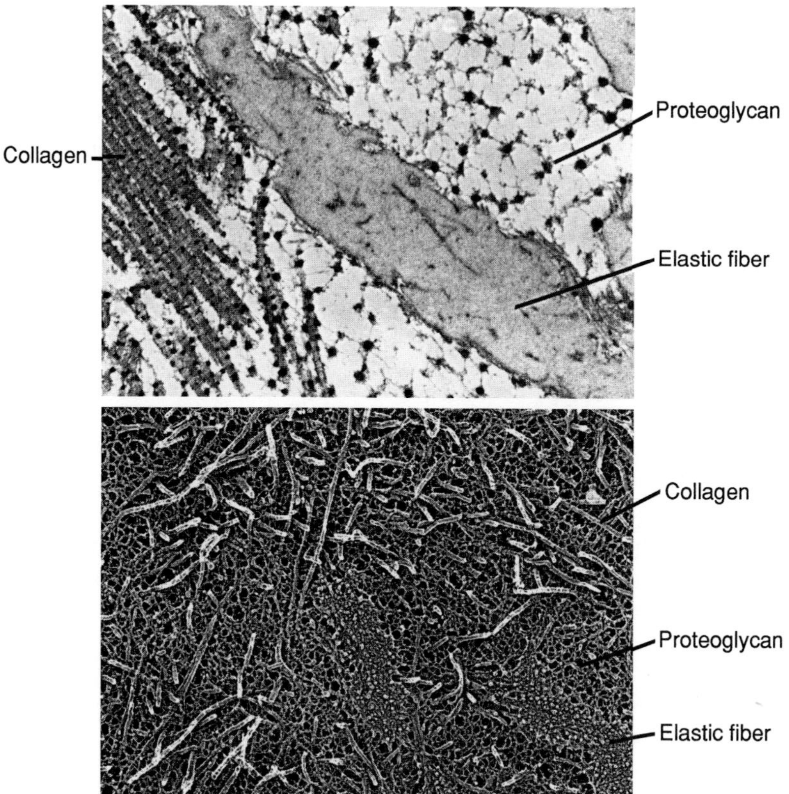

FIG. 2. A: Electron micrograph of vascular ECM demonstrating organization of collagen, elastic fiber, and proteoglycans. The proteoglycans have been preserved with ruthenium red and can be visualized as large granules filling the extracellular space and small granules attached to collagen fibrils. ×86,000. **B:** Electron micrograph of a similar ECM prepared using a quick-freeze–deep-etch procedure without chemical fixation. The ECM consists of a finely woven meshwork of proteoglycan-containing elastic fibers and collagen fibrils. *Bar,* 0.2 μm. (From Mecham, ref. 47, with permission.)

types I and III collagen (3–5). Recent studies suggest that the type VI collagen fibril may not be composed entirely of collagen but is bound together with other ECM molecules such as proteoglycans (14). Type VI collagen appears to constitute a collagen fiber system separate from types I and III, and, because of its numerous Arg-Gly-Asp (RGD) cell binding motifs, may serve as an adhesive substrate for vascular cells (15).

Biosynthesis

The principal source of collagens in the arterial intima and media is the smooth muscle cell. Modulation of collagen synthesis by these cells frequently accompanies phenotypic changes associated with altered cellular behavior. For example, as arterial smooth muscle cells modulate from a quiescent or "contractile state" typical of the normal vessel phenotype to a proliferative or "synthetic state" characteristic of the atherosclerotic phenotype, type I collagen synthesis increases (16). Similar collagen changes occur in phenotypically altered smooth muscle cells in hypertension (17).

A number of factors regulate collagen synthesis by arterial smooth muscle cells. For example, the growth state of the cells (18–21), different growth factors and cytokines (20–23), and the nature of the ECM substrate (22) all influence collagen synthesis by these cells. Cytokines and growth factors generally enhance the synthesis of types I, III, and V collagen, with TGF-β1 exhibiting the most potent effect (21,23). However, TGF-β1-induced type I and III collagen synthesis by human arterial smooth muscle cells is inhibited by interferon γ (21). These studies indicate that factors that regulate vascular cell behavior also affect the collagenous composition of the ECM.

Vascular smooth muscle cells normally reside in the media of the vessel wall surrounded by abundant collagen molecules. Thus, collagens may serve as attachment proteins for arterial smooth muscle cells and influence their behavior. For example, type I collagen substrates promote cultured arterial smooth muscle attachment and proliferation, whereas other ECM components such as elastin maintain these cells in a contractile or nonproliferative phenotype (24). Furthermore, cultured arterial smooth muscle cells express specific type I collagen integrin receptors (i.e., $\alpha_2\beta_1$)

when stimulated to migrate on type I collagen substrates (25). Such studies indicate the importance of arterial smooth muscle cell and type I collagen interaction in determining the migratory cell phenotype.

Endothelial cells also express genes that code for types I, III, IV, and VIII collagens, which influence endothelial cell behavior (26–31). Collagens are known to play a role in the formation of new blood vessels (i.e., angiogenesis). For example, a substrate of type I collagen induces endothelial cells to form capillary tubes in vitro (24), and expression of type I collagen by endothelial cells is characteristic of neovascularization in vivo (30). When endothelial cells "sprout" and form capillary tubes in vitro, type I collagen synthesis is induced (31). Although the role that type I collagen plays in this process is not fully understood, collagen fibrils may serve as a template or cable onto which endothelial cells wrap themselves through tractive restructuring (32). It still remains to be shown whether fibrillar collagen is involved in new vessel formation in vivo.

Vascular Disease

Vascular collagens are critical to vascular wall integrity. Defects in the synthesis and deposition of either type I or type III vascular collagen such as occurs in lethal mutations of the type I collagen gene and in some forms of Ehlers–Danlos syndrome result in aneurysms and rupture of both elastic and muscular arteries (33,34). Vascular collagens also change in amounts and location in different forms of vascular disease (3–5,13,30,35–37). For example, there is topographic variation in the location of types I and III collagen in human atherosclerotic plaques and in restenotic lesions (30,37). Type I collagen expression occurs principally in the fibrous caps and vascularized regions of primary plaques, with less type I collagen in the plaque center where lipid is highest (Fig. 3). However, recent studies indicate that both normal and oxidized low-density lipoproteins bind to type I and III collagen by negative-charge-dependent mechanisms (38). In addition, lipoproteins bind to nonenzymatically glycated collagen fibrils in diabetic vascular tissue (see review, 39). These studies indicate that collagens may retain lipid in atherosclerotic disease.

Type IV collagen increases in multilayer basement membranes beneath endothelial cells and around smooth muscle cells in atherosclerotic arteries (40). The functional significance of these hypertrophic basement membranes is still being explored, but they likely affect the permeability of the vascular wall and the metabolism of the resident vascular cells. Excessive amounts of this material may trap and retain plasma proteins, lipoproteins, growth factors, and/or calcium. Type V collagen also increases in advancing atherosclerotic plaques (41) and may play a role in stabilizing the collagen network during fibrosis.

Variations in the distribution of fibrillar collagen throughout vascular lesions may create regions within the plaque that differ in tensile strength and stiffness. These variations can lead to differences in susceptibility to plaque rupture (35,42,43). For example, plaque fissuring and subsequent thrombosis often occur at boundaries between collagen-rich and collagen-poor zones, such as at the base of the fibrous caps and/or near collagen-poor–lipid-rich regions of the plaque. Exposure of collagen fibrils during vascular tearing results in platelet activation and thrombosis (44). Thrombosis associated with plaque fissures is the most common cause of acute myocardial infarction, sudden cardiac death, and unstable angina (45). Thus, although fibrillar collagens provide blood vessels with tensile strength essential for conduits of the circulatory system, they also provide a potential substrate for initiating the events that lead to occlusive arterial disease.

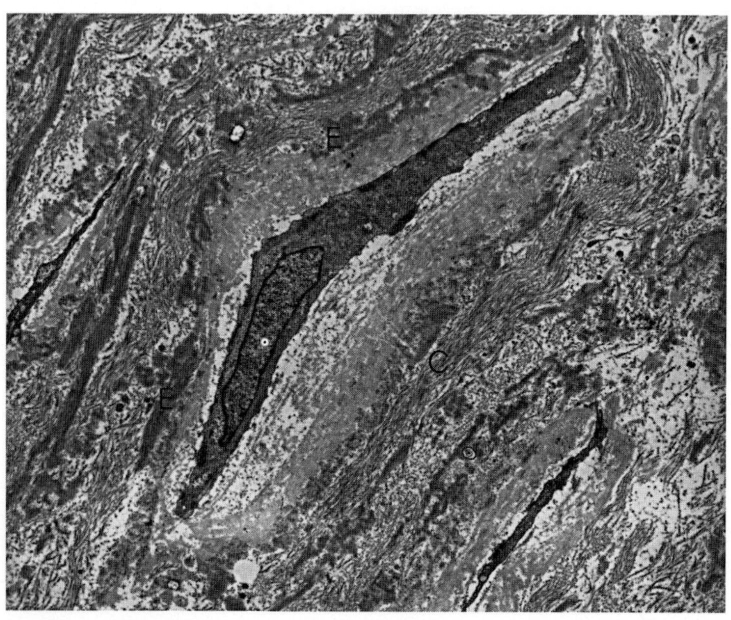

FIG. 3. An electron micrograph of an area of the fibrous cap of a human atherosclerotic lesion demonstrating a smooth muscle cell surrounded by extensive collagen C fibrils. E, elastin. ×10,000. (From Wight TN, ref. 233, with permission.)

ELASTIC FIBERS

Another major structural component of blood vessels is the fibrous protein elastin. Together with collagens, elastin provides mechanical strength and elasticity needed to accommodate pressure changes arising from the pulsatile nature of blood flow as well as the hemodynamic changes created on the wall by the rheology of blood.

Properties and Distribution

Elastic fibers are complex structures that include a hydrophobic 70-kDa elastin protein associated with hydrophilic glycoproteins and enzymes responsible for the internal cross-linking of elastin peptides (46–52). Elastin has an unusual amino acid composition in that it is low in acidic and basic amino acids but rich in hydrophobic amino acids such as valine. Elastin also contains several lysines that serve as sites for complex and unique cross-links between elastin peptides. Such cross-links impart "rubber-like" recoil properties to this protein and render it highly insoluble. Aortic elastin turns over very slowly if at all, and therefore synthesis of elastin occurs principally during perinatal and early growth and decreases to insignificant levels in the adult. In the absence of arterial pathology, arterial elastin is highly stable and long-lasting.

Like the fibrillar collagens, elastic fibers form discrete structures within the ECM that can readily be visualized at the light and electron microscopic level (6,7,53) (Figs. 1, 2, and 4). Elastic fibers are arranged into concentric sheets or lamellae that separate different vascular layers. A thick layer of elastic tissue separates the intima from the media (internal elastic lamina, IEL) and the media from the adventitia (external elastic lamella). In addition, elastic lamellae form boundaries between successive concentric layers of smooth muscle (Fig. 4). Frequently, the elastic lamellae are interconnected by radially oriented elastic fibers that facilitate the transfer of stress throughout the vessel wall (6,7).

The concentration of elastin varies throughout the vascular system. Elastic lamellae are prominent in the larger vessels such as the thoracic aorta, which receives high-pressure pulses of blood from the left ventricle. Elastin concentration decreases in the smaller, more muscular arteries such as the smaller mesenteric arteries (6,7). In large vessels such as the aorta of adult mammals, the number of lamellar units and the radius of the vessel are nearly proportional (54). This allows for tension carried by each lamella to be nearly constant, regardless of the animal's weight, the aortic diameter, or the medial thickness. Thus, elastin acts as a dampening chamber to smooth the pressure wave as it is transmitted down the vessel.

Biosynthesis

The principal source of elastic fibers is the arterial smooth muscle cell, which supports elastic fibrillogenesis in vitro (55–58). Elastin is synthesized as a precursor molecule called tropoelastin (59,60). The human tropoelastin mRNA is transcribed from a single gene and undergoes extensive alternative splicing, resulting in the translation of multiple protein isoforms. Recombinant DNA technology has confirmed earlier predictions that tropoelastin consists of alternating hydrophilic and cross-linking domains, which establish the proper alignment for cross-links to form between adjacent peptides. In addition to these domains, cloning studies have identified a highly basic cysteine-containing sequence at the carboxyl terminus of the tropoelastin molecule, which may mediate the interaction of elastin with the microfibrillar proteins during assembly of the elastic fiber.

The current model for elastic fiber assembly involves the secretion of the precursor tropoelastin together with a 67-kDa elastin-binding protein that associates with the cell surface through a specific membrane protein (61,62). This 67-kDa protein has lectin-binding sites that interact with microfibrillar proteins and a hydrophobic domain that binds hydrophobic sequences within the elastin peptide. Such a "bridging role" implicates this protein and perhaps other

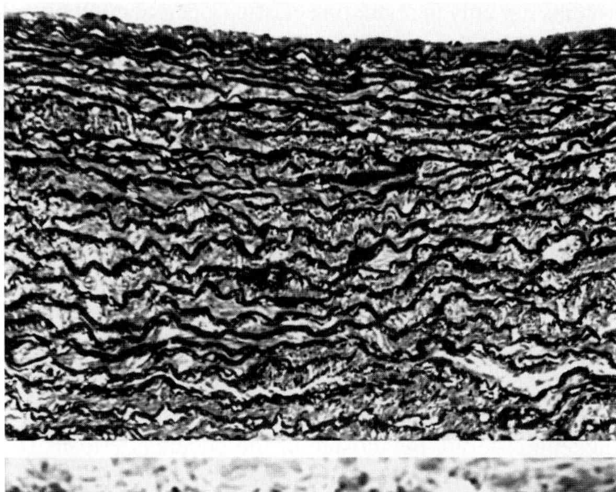

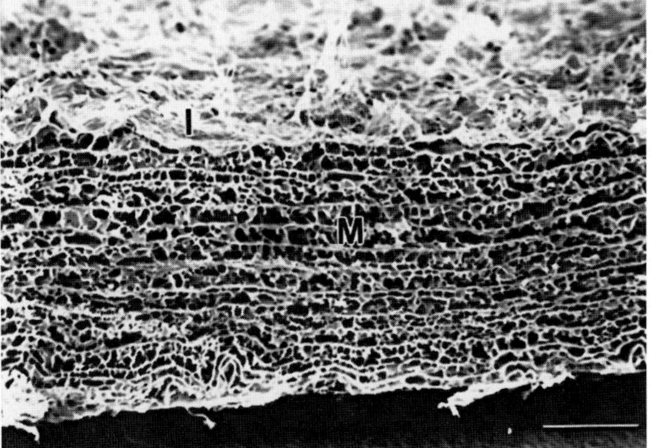

FIG. 4. Organization of elastin in bovine pulmonary artery. **Top:** A cross section of the artery stained with Verheff–Van Gieson elastic stain to demonstrate multiple layers of elastin, ×80. **Bottom:** A scanning electron micrograph of adult rat aorta following removal of nonelastin components. *Bar,* 50 μm. (From Mecham, ref. 47, with permission.)

proteins not only in regulating elastic fiber assembly but also as potential adhesion receptors for arterial smooth muscle cells. For example, additional excess free N-acetylgalactosamine-containing glycosaminoglycans (GAGs) compete for the lectin binding site in the 67-kDa protein and release the 67-kDa protein from the surface of vascular muscle cells (61,62). The release of the 67-kDa protein prevents smooth muscle cell attachment to elastin and promotes their migration. Furthermore, GAGs prevent additional elastic fiber assembly in this system, suggesting a mechanism by which other ECM components regulate elastic fiber assembly. Proteoglycans, for example, have been postulated to inhibit elastic fiber assembly in lathyritic animals (63) and in the intimal thickening during the closure of the ductus arteriosus (61). These studies illustrate how changes in one component of the vascular ECM influence the assembly of other ECM components.

Vascular Disease

Defects in elastic fiber formation or elastic fiber fragmentation leads to "weakening" of the vascular wall, dilation, and aneurysms (63–68). A classic example of the importance of the elastic fiber in arterial wall function is observed in Marfan syndrome (MFS), a connective tissue disease with an incidence of approximately one in 10,000 and a median life expectancy of only 45 years (69,70). The shortened life span of MFS patients is caused primarily by cardiovascular complications, namely dissecting aortic aneurysms. Studies of families of MFS patients have revealed that the principal gene product responsible for this syndrome is the microfibrillar glycoprotein fibrillin, which provides a template for elastin in the formation of the elastic fiber (70). Mutation in the fibrillin gene leads to altered forms of this glycoprotein and impairment of proper elastic fiber assembly in these patients.

Fragmentation or loss of elastic fibers is also frequently seen during atherosclerosis (46,64) and in arteriovenous fistulas (71). The cause of elastic fiber tears in these conditions is not entirely clear but may relate to vascular wall tension brought on by the turbulent flow of blood and to the release of proteases from a variety of cell types including smooth muscle cells (72). Recent studies demonstrate the presence of stromelysin and gelatinase B in atherosclerotic lesions and in aneurysmal aortic wall (73–75). These two metalloproteinases degrade elastin and a number of other ECM com-

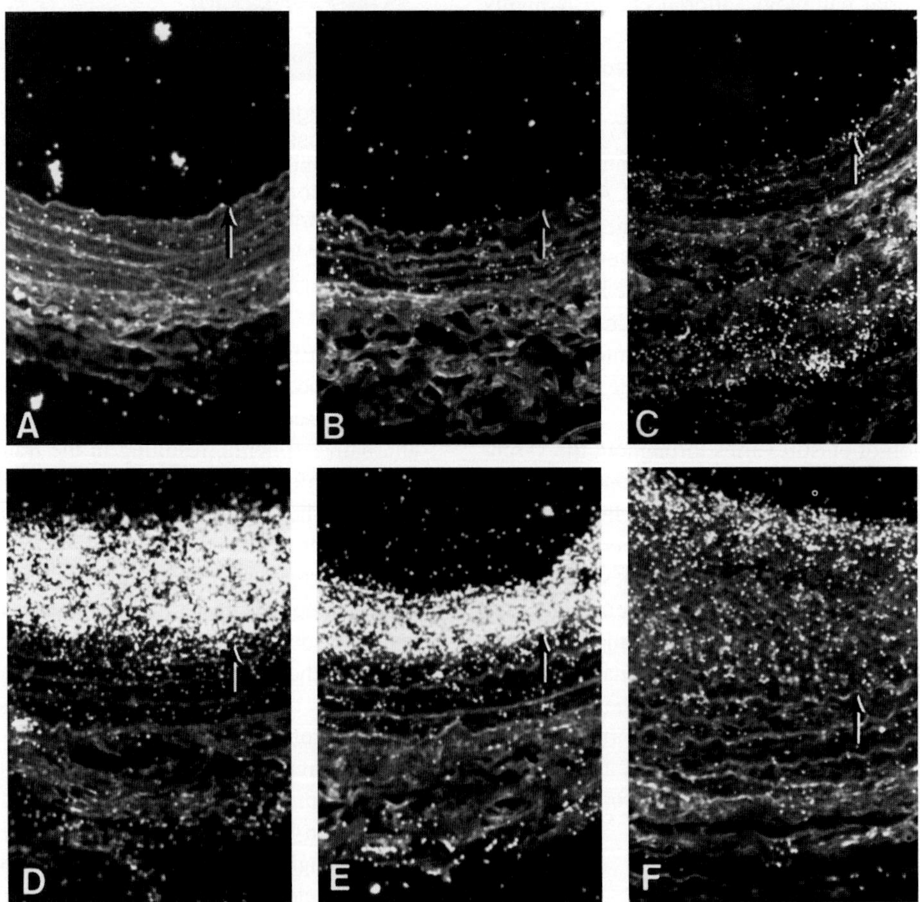

FIG. 5. Dark-field photomicrographs showing time course of tropoelastin transcript induction after rat carotid artery injury by in situ hybridization. **A:** Uninjured. **B:** 2 days. **C:** 1 week. **D:** 2 weeks plus heparin treatment. **F:** 4 weeks after injury. (From Nikkari et al., ref. 78, with permission.)

ponents including proteoglycans, fibronectin, laminin, and many of the collagens. Elastin peptides derived from the degradation of elastic fibers are biologically active as chemoattractants for neutrophils important in arterial remodeling and repair (76). Such studies indicate that components of the elastic fiber are not simply inert structural proteins but are capable of biological activity.

Although elastin turns over very slowly in normal vessels, active elastin synthesis takes place during vascular matrix remodeling associated with vascular injury (Fig. 5). Vascular injury can result from conditions such as hypertension or from physical insults to the blood vessels such as occur during balloon angioplasty or suturing in vascular grafting. It is well established that experimental hypertension in animals leads to increased arterial thickness, resulting principally from increases in elastin and collagen in the vessel wall (77). The deposition of these fibrous proteins in response to hypertension and balloon angioplasty involves accumulation within a thick neointima (78–80), although regional hypertrophy involving increased elastin synthesis occurs in the media of pulmonary arteries in animals subjected to experimental hypertension (81).

Modification of elastic fibers occurs in vascular disease, which can cause loss of normal elastic fiber function. For example, normal aortic elastin appears to consist of a protein–lipid complex with lipids presumably bound by hydrophobic stacking to hydrophobic sites in elastin molecules (46,82). Although the lipid moiety of normal elastin is small, it increases when elastin is isolated from atherosclerotic arteries (83,84). Morphological studies have demonstrated that the "perfibrous lipid" in atherosclerotic plaques (85) is lipid deposited adjacent to and within elastic fibers (86), and lipid–elastin complexes have been isolated from human atherosclerotic vessels (87). Such binding or trapping of lipid in elastin could interfere with normal elastic fiber formation by preventing proper alignment of the peptide monomers during the cross-linking reaction. Lipid associated with elastic fibers may also interfere with elastic recoil because recoil is somewhat dependent on the exposure of lipophilic groups of the native elastin molecule (46). Lipids may also facilitate the breakdown of the elastic fiber because free fatty acids bound to elastin increase the binding of elastolytic enzymes to elastin (88,89).

Elastic fibers may also form a depot for accumulation of calcium in vascular disease (Fig. 6). For example, calcium is a cofactor for several of the elastolytic enzymes, and deposits of calcium are frequently found in elastic fibers (46,47,90,91). Conformational changes induced by organic solvents in elastin promote calcium binding to the fiber (90). Thus, elastin–lipid complexes may promote deposits of calcium in advancing atherosclerosis.

PROTEOGLYCANS/HYALURONAN

Proteoglycans and hyaluronan are hydrophilic molecules and provide the vasculature with viscoelasticity and turgor.

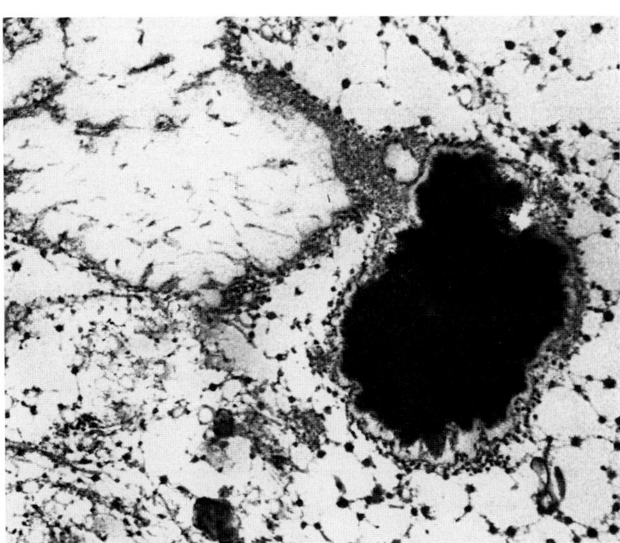

FIG. 6. An electron micrograph of a section of vascular ECM from a patient with idiopathic infantile arterial calcinosis (IIAC) (91). The elastic fiber on the left is extensively calcified, whereas the elastic fiber on the right appears normal. ×43,000.

These molecules also interact with component molecules involved in a number of vascular events and participate in the regulation of vascular permeability, lipid metabolism, hemostasis, and thrombosis (see reviews 92–97). In addition, proteoglycans and hyaluronan interact with vascular cells and with growth factors and cytokines to modify vascular cell adhesion, migration, and proliferation (96).

Types and Distribution

Proteoglycans are protein polysaccharides that share the common structural feature of one or more GAG chains covalently attached to a core glycoprotein backbone. The GAG chains are linear polymers of repeating disaccharides that contain a hexosamine and either a carboxylate or a sulfate ester or both. As a rule, GAGs do not exist "free" in tissue but are attached to core glycoproteins to form distinct families of proteoglycans. However, the GAG hyaluronan, formerly termed hyaluronic acid, is an exception in that it is not covalently linked to a core glycoprotein and exists in the ECM as a high-molecular-weight random-coiled polysaccharide occupying large hydrodynamic domains (98). Hyaluronan polymers self-associate and form regions of ordered helical structures creating continuous networks of pronounced viscoelasticity.

Traditionally, proteoglycans have been classified on the basis of the predominant type of GAG attached to a specific core glycoprotein, e.g., chondroitin sulfate (CSPG), dermatan sulfate (DSPG), heparan sulfate (HSPG), and keratan sulfate (KSPG). However, more recent comparisons of proteoglycan core protein structure by immunochemical and cloning methods have shown that proteoglycans exist as

TABLE 2. *Some of the proteoglycans present in the vascular ECM*

Family (location)	Common name	GAG chain type (number)	Protein core (kDa)	Function
Large interstitial	Versican	CS (15–17)	263	Compressive resilience
Small leucine-rich	Decorin	DS (1)	36	Collagen organization
	Biglycan	DS (2)	38	?
	Lumican	KS (3–4)	35	?
Basement membrane	Perlecan	HS (3)	467	Anionic filtration barrier, binds growth factors
Cell surface (plasma membrane)	Syndecan-1	HS/CS (3–5)	31	ECM receptors, growth factor receptors, binds coagulant enzymes, cytokines, and lipases
	Fibroglycan	HS (3)	20	
	N-Syndecan	HS/CS (3)	35	
	Ryudocan	HS (3)	20	
	Glypican	HS (3)	62	

multigenic families of related core proteins that share common functions within their respective families. A number of different core proteins with variable numbers of GAG chains of different length and composition exist, creating enormous structural diversity in these proteoglycans. A nomenclature has also evolved utilizing trivial names to define specific proteoglycans, and a listing of the common vascular proteoglycans is given in Table 2. Vascular proteoglycan can be found in four locations: (a) in the interstitial ECM; (b) as part of specialized ECM structures such as basement membranes; (c) as part of cell membranes; and (d) intracellularly. Proteoglycans found in each of these locations tend to share common structural features that in part determine their role in these tissue compartments.

The major types of proteoglycans identified in blood vessels include large (~1,000 kDa) CSPGs such as versican (see reviews 92–95,99,100), small (~120–300 kDa) leucine-rich DSPGs such as decorin and biglycan (101–104), KSPGs such as lumican (105), and HSPGs such as perlecan and other basement membrane proteoglycans (106,107). All of these proteoglycans associate with different components of the vascular ECM (Fig. 2) and influence the properties of these components. For example, decorin is located along collagen fibrils and regulates collagen fiber diameter and organization (see review 93). Perlecan inserts into basement membranes and contributes to the permeability characteristics of this structure (10), serves as substrate for vascular cells (108), and retains growth factors involved in vascular remodeling (109). Versican is present throughout the interstitial space of the vascular ECM (93,99,100) and interacts with hyaluronan and link proteins (93,110–112) to fill the ECM space not occupied by the fibrous components of the ECM. These complexes create a reversibly compressible compartment in the vascular ECM and provide a swelling pressure within the ECM that is offset by the collagen fibrils (see review 113). These counterbalancing forces in part allow the blood vessel to resist deformity created by the pulsatile pressures of the circulatory system.

The distribution of proteoglycans throughout the blood vessel wall is variable. For example, the intima is particularly enriched in proteoglycans (see reviews 93,114–116) with lower amounts in the media and adventitia (Fig. 7). Versican/hyaluronan complexes and biglycan are prominent in the intima and media, and decorin is concentrated in the collagen-containing adventitia. Perlecan is present in basement membranes throughout both the intimal and medial layers. The distribution of the KSPG lumican in the vascular wall has not yet been determined.

Proteoglycans are also present on the surface of vascular cells (117–123). These proteoglycans may be inserted directly into vascular cell membranes via hydrophobic sequences in the core proteins, as is the case for the HSPGs of the syndecan family (117,118,121). Other cell surface HSPGs associate with vascular cell membranes by phosphatidylinositol linkages and comprise a separate family of membrane proteoglycans termed glypicans (120). Membrane proteoglycans serve a variety of vascular functions: as attachment proteins for enzymes involved in lipid metabolism (see reviews 95,123) and blood coagulation (see review 124); as binding proteins for the attachment of vascular cells to their ECM (see review 117); and as binding proteins for growth factors and cytokines (see reviews 117,122).

Biosynthesis

The arterial smooth muscle cell is a principal source for vascular proteoglycans and hyaluronan. A number of studies indicate that the synthesis of these molecules is differentially regulated by growth factors and cytokines such as PDGF, TGF-β1, and IL-1 (see reviews 93,125–129). For example, TGF-β1 increases versican and biglycan mRNA expression by arterial smooth muscle cells, and IL-1 increases decorin expression (127–130). The synthesis of proteoglycans is regulated at both the transcription/posttranscription and posttranslation levels. For example, PDGF stimulates the expression of versican mRNA but does not change levels of mRNA for decorin or biglycan (128). On the other hand, PDGF

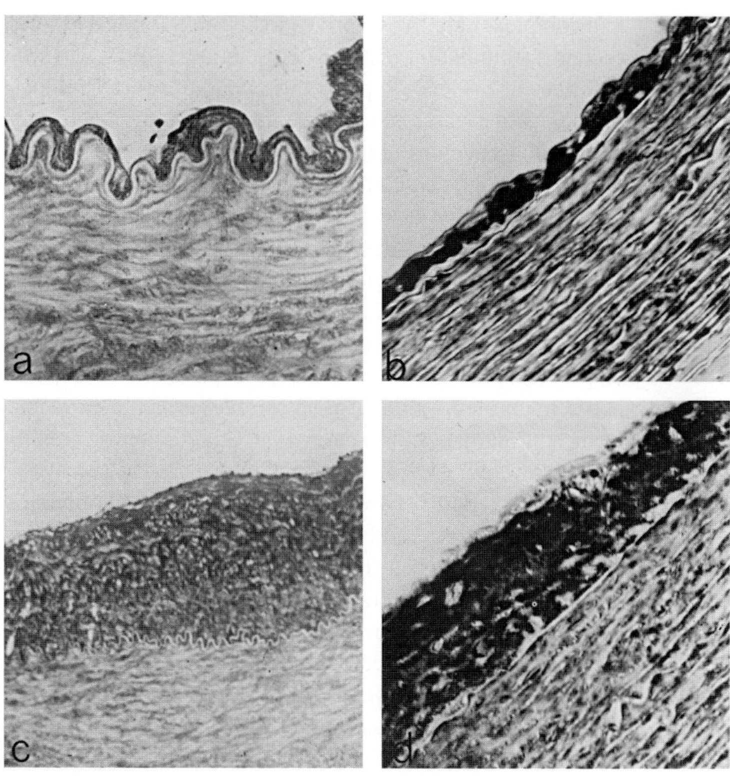

FIG. 7. Light micrographs illustrating that the narrow intima of a normal blood vessel stains more intensely with **(A)** Alcian blue and **(B)** a monoclonal antibody to CSPG than the underlying medial layer. Intimal thickening following injury exhibits intense staining for proteoglycan **(C)** Alcian blue; **(D)** monoclonal antibody to CSPG. *Bar,* 50 μm. (From Wight TN et al., ref. 234, with permission.)

causes lengthening of the GAG chains of all three of these proteoglycans (128,129). Such modifications are likely to influence the biological activity of these molecules. For example, proteoglycans isolated from proliferating arterial smooth muscle cells have longer GAG chains and bind with greater affinity to low-density lipoproteins than proteoglycans isolated from nonproliferating arterial smooth muscle cells (131). Such modifications may have some bearing on the retention of LDL within the vascular ECM that occurs in atherosclerosis (refer to discussion below).

Endothelial cells also synthesize a variety of proteoglycans and hyaluronan and modulate their synthesis in different phenotypic states (see review 93; 132–134). For example, as endothelial cells modulate to a migratory state, they decrease their synthesis of HSPGs and increase the synthesis of DSPGs (see review 93). Recent studies indicate that specific proteoglycans may be involved in this migratory phenotype. For example, decorin is not synthesized by confluent cultures of endothelial cells (132,133) and is absent from the endothelial lining of adult arteries (37). However, when endothelial cells sprout to a migratory angiogenic phenotype and form tubes in vitro, they express decorin as well as type I collagen (31,133). These two ECM molecules may thus provide the appropriate substrate for endothelial cell rearrangement during new vessel formation.

Blood-derived cells that gain access to the arterial wall, such as platelets, mast cells, lymphocytes, and monocytes, also synthesize proteoglycans (135–139). For example, the differentiation of the monocyte into the macrophage is accompanied by increased synthesis of HSPGs and CSPGs that contain oversulfated GAG chains (137). Deposits of these modified proteoglycans within the ECM by macrophages as they invade vascular tissue may have a significant impact on modifying the properties of the ECM during vascular remodeling. Mast cells within the vascular wall synthesize serglycin, a unique proteoglycan that contains highly sulfated heparin and CS chains (138). Serglycin interacts with cationic proteases, histamine, and other components of storage granules and potentially targets these substances to specific vascular locations on release. In addition, proteoglycans released from mast cells interact with lipoproteins and may participate in lipoprotein retention in the vascular ECM (see discussion below) (see review 138). Platelets also may use proteoglycans to target factors such as platelet factor 4 to specific vascular sites during clot formation (139).

The proteoglycan/hyaluronan component of the vascular ECM may also serve as a substrate for vascular cells. For example, hyaluronan associates with the surface of arterial smooth muscle cells through a binding protein termed RHAMM (receptor for hyaluronan-mediated motility). This interaction appears to regulate arterial smooth muscle cell motility because antibodies against this hyaluronan receptor block injury-induced migration of these cells in vitro (140). Furthermore, several types of blood-derived cells that gain access to the arterial wall possess membrane receptors such as CD44 that interact with hyaluronan (141). Therefore, an ECM enriched in hyaluronan may be permissive for the cell recruitment and rearrangement that occur during vascular development and remodeling.

Vascular Disease

The content and distribution of vascular proteoglycans and hyaluronan change as the ECM is remodeled in hypertension (142), diabetes (143–145), atherosclerosis (see reviews 92–94,146–149), and restenosis (37,150,151). Overall, proteoglycans and hyaluronan increase in the early and middle phases of vascular disease and decrease as the lesions become more advanced and fibrotic. However, with the development of more precise probes to examine regional deposits and expression of these molecules, it is clear that there are topographic variations in the distribution of different classes of proteoglycans and hyaluronan as lesions develop. For example, versican is prominent in the ECM of human diffuse intimal thickenings during early stages of human vascular disease, and decorin is localized to the fibrous cap of more advanced atherosclerotic lesions (152). In addition, versican tends to associate with apo-B-containing lipoproteins in atherosclerotic lesions, whereas biglycan colocalizes with lipoproteins enriched in apo E (152). These observations suggest that particular types of proteoglycans may selectively cause the accumulation of specific classes of lipoproteins within the vascular wall (see discussion below).

Proteoglycans and hyaluronan also form a significant part of the ECM as the human vascular wall thickens during restenosis following angioplasty. For example, the fibroproliferative tissue typical of human restenosis contains vascular smooth muscle cells embedded in a loose ECM containing mostly proteoglycan (i.e., versican and biglycan) and hyaluronan (37,151) (Fig. 8). Experimental injury models of restenosis confirm that balloon angioplasty leads to increased expression and deposition of proteoglycans and hyaluronan during the early vascular remodeling phase (see reviews 93,151,153,154). These changes accompany increases in arterial smooth muscle cell proliferation and migration and raise the possibility that proteoglycans and/or hyaluronan contributes to events leading to arterial wall thickening in vascular disease (155). For example, blockage of versican deposits by antibodies or antisense to TGF-β1 significantly retards balloon-injury-induced neointimal expansion in experimental animals (156,157). Such findings indicate the potential importance of targeting these ECM molecules in the prevention of injury-induced restenosis.

Changes in the proteoglycan and hyaluronan content of the ECM in vascular disease dramatically affect the permeability of the vascular wall. For example, increases in proteoglycan and hyaluronan lead to an expansion of the ECM and a network of highly charged and interactive macromolecules. This arrangement creates an ECM that regulates the movement of small and large molecules as they enter the vascular wall from the plasma (158). Macromolecules that encounter this network may be retained through ionic interaction or steric exclusion. The best example underscoring the importance of proteoglycans in the retention of specific macromolecules in the vascular wall is their interactions with plasma lipoproteins (see reviews 92–95,97). Proteoglycan–lipoprotein complexes are hypothesized to be a major cause of lipoprotein accumulation within atherosclerotic lesions, and several lines of evidence support this hypothesis. For example, regions of the vasculature prone to developing atherosclerotic lesions, such as branch points, are characterized by an altered proteoglycan composition (159). Kinetic analysis of LDL permeability at these sites indicate that accumulation of LDL results from selective retention and not increased delivery (160,161). Regions of the vasculature that are enriched in proteoglycans exhibit a propensity to accumulate lipid (see review 93). Furthermore, lipoproteins colocalize to proteoglycan deposits in the vascular ECM (162), and apo B lipoprotein–proteoglycan complexes can be extracted from both human and experimental atherosclerotic lesions (see reviews 92,94,95).

The interaction between proteoglycans and lipoproteins can take many forms and depends on several parameters. For example, proteoglycan–lipoprotein complexes may exist as multiple pools throughout the vascular ECM. Complexes extracted with saline from atherosclerotic lesions contain high amounts of chondroitin sulfate and low amounts of hyaluronan and are cholesterol-ester-enriched (92–95). On the other hand, complexes extracted with proteases have low chondroitin sulfate and high hyaluronan are cholesterol-ester-poor.

The formation of proteoglycan–lipoprotein complexes depends on particular characteristics of the components of the complex. For example, in vitro studies indicate that certain clusters of positively charged peptide sequences within the apo B moiety of LDL interact with negatively charged chondroitin sulfate GAG chains that are part of CSPGs isolated from arterial tissue (see reviews 92–95,97). Although interactions can be demonstrated, the strength of binding is weak, and insoluble complexes can be formed only in the presence of excess calcium. On the other hand, the strength and extent of binding between these two molecules may be influenced by modifications in each of the components, such as the type and/or size of the lipoproteins. For example, binding occurs only with LDL, not HDL, and lipoprotein (a) exhibits increased binding to proteoglycans when compared to LDL (163). Small LDL particles bind proteoglycans to a greater extent than large LDL particles (164). Similarly, changes in the nature of the proteoglycan also affect the interaction. For example, increases in GAG chain length and degree of sulfation increase proteoglycan interaction with lipoproteins (164–167).

Proteoglycan–lipoprotein complexes may also form through intermediate molecules that possess domains able to bind both proteoglycans and lipoproteins. Two such molecules that could function in this way that are expressed in atherosclerotic lesions are lipoprotein lipase and apo E (see review 95; 168). Addition of lipoprotein lipase to vascular ECM dramatically increases the retention of apo-B-containing lipoproteins (reviewed in 95). This retention can be blocked by removing proteoglycans (i.e., HSPGs and CSPGs) from the ECM or by pretreating the ECM with apo-

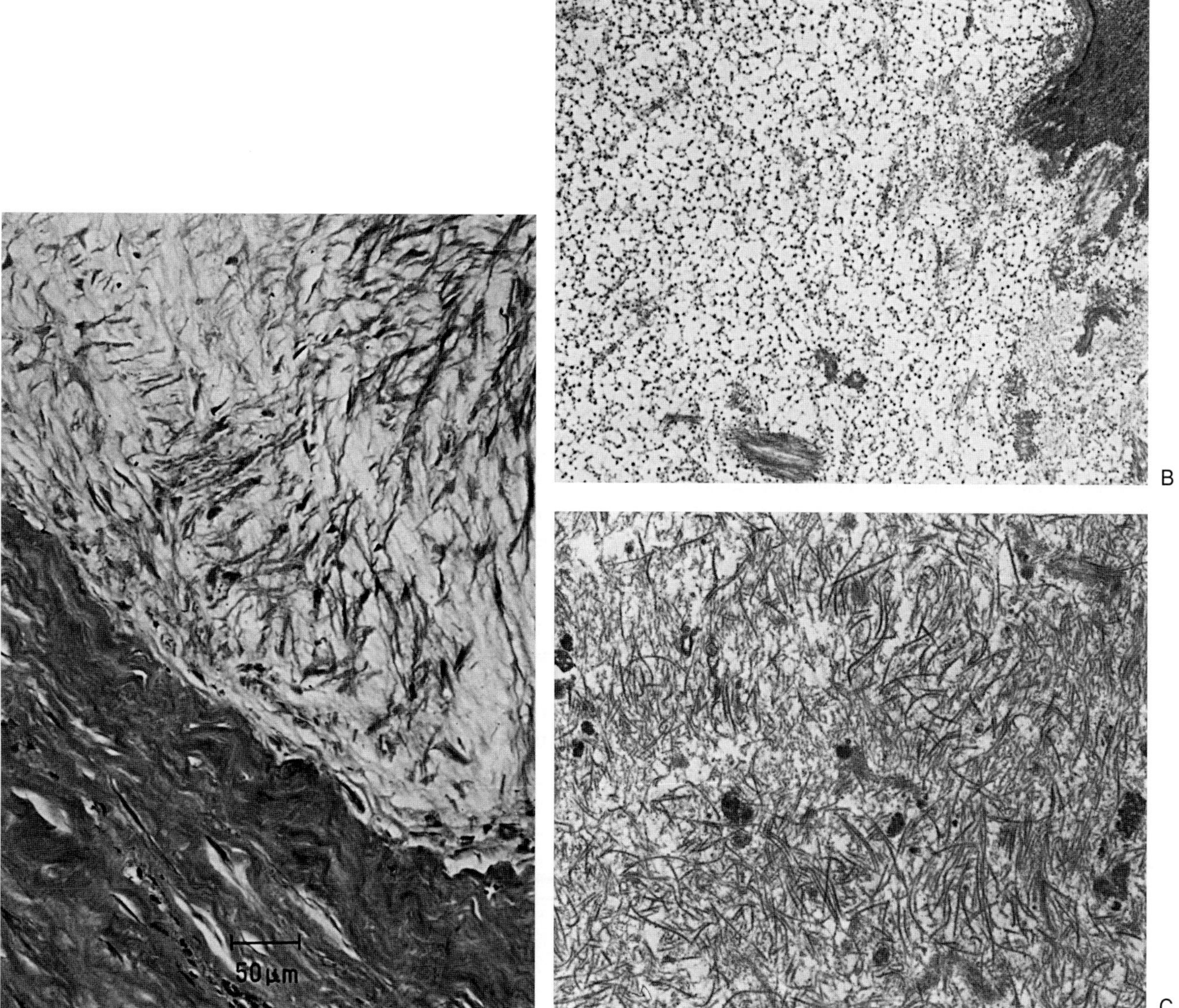

FIG. 8. A: A light microscopic view of typical restenotic tissue exhibiting a loose connective tissue zone and a dense connective zone, ×50. Top panel **(B)** is an electron micrograph of a section of the loose connective tissue zone demonstrating abundant proteoglycan granules. Bottom panel **(C)** is a section from the dense connective tissue zone demonstrating abundant collagen fibrils, ×50,000. (From Riessen et al., ref. 37, with permission.)

E-containing lipoproteins such as apo-E-rich HDL. These data suggest that apo E competes with LDL for proteoglycan binding sites within the vascular ECM and prevents apo B–LDL accumulation. The ability of apo-E–HDL to compete for LDL binding sites within the ECM may be one reason why apo-E-rich HDL is protective against atherosclerosis. The importance of proteoglycan–lipoprotein complexes in the vascular wall is further illustrated by the observations that lipoproteins bound to proteoglycans are more likely to undergo oxidation (reviewed in 94,95).

In addition to promoting deposits of lipid in the vascular ECM, proteoglycans also affect the accumulation of lipid in vascular cells. Complexes of lipoproteins and proteoglycans are rapidly taken up by macrophages via both LDL and scavenger receptors (reviewed in 94,95). Furthermore, catabolism of LDL in these complexes is diminished compared to LDL alone, and this reduced degradation of LDL is accompanied by increased synthesis of cholesterol esters. In addition, lipoprotein lipase enhances the uptake and degradation of LDL by a variety of cells including arterial smooth muscle cells and macrophages (95,169). Removal of cell surface HSPG by heparatinase treatment or the use of mutant cells deficient in cell surface HSPG blocks lipoprotein-lipase-mediated uptake of lipoproteins (170). This pathway may represent a novel LDL-receptor-independent pathway for accumulation of cellular cholesterol-ester-enriched lipoproteins in vascular cells. Intracellular cholesterol deposits also promote proteoglycan synthesis by arterial smooth muscle cells (171).

Although most studies implicate proteoglycans and their associated GAGs in the promotion of arterial disease, a subset of these molecules are protective against atherosclerosis and thrombosis. For example, some forms of heparin, heparan sulfate (HS), and dermatan sulfate are powerful anticoagulants and therefore useful in preventing the generation of fibrin and subsequent thrombosis (reviewed in 124,172). The basis for this activity lies in the ability of these GAGs to interact with serine protease inhibitors (serpins) such as antithrombin III (AT-III) and heparin cofactor II (HC-II) to potentiate the inactivation of clotting enzymes such as factor Xa and thrombin. Heparin and HS principally target the inactivation of thrombin through antithrombin III while dermatan sulfate, in addition to heparin and heparan sulfate, accelerates the inactivation of thrombin by heparin cofactor II.

Heparin and heparan sulfate are related molecules formed from the same building blocks of monosaccharides (see reviews 124,172). Heparin is synthesized only by mast cells in the vascular wall, whereas heparan sulfates are synthesized by all vascular wall cells. Heparin can be distinguished from heparan sulfate in that it contains more sulfate residues and more iduronic acid. However, some forms of heparan sulfate have structural features in common with heparin. For example, some species of heparin and heparan sulfate bind to AT-III at lysl residues, and this binding involves a particular tetrasaccharide sequence present in both heparin and heparan sulfate. This sequence is not present in heparin and heparan sulfate chains that lack anticoagulant activity. Heparan sulfates that possess the ability to bind AT-III are present on the surface of endothelial cells as well as within the vascular ECM. Although these molecules represent a minor portion of the total vascular HSPGs, they have a profound effect on maintaining the nonthrombogenic nature of the endothelial surface and the vascular ECM. Thus, heparin, heparan sulfates, and dermatan sulfates have gained widescale use as therapeutically useful drugs in preventing thrombosis and extension of emboli (124,173,174). Other cell surface proteoglycans such as thrombomodulin also help regulate coagulant activity at the endothelial surface (reviewed in 124). This proteoglycan binds thrombin and also interacts with protein C to inactivate thrombin through an AT-III-independent pathway.

Heparin and heparin-like GAGs also may exhibit antiatherogenic effects by influencing events taking place within the vascular wall itself. For example, heparin (both anticoagulant and nonanticoagulant forms) is effective in blocking the proliferation and migration of arterial smooth muscle cells during neointimal formation following balloon angioplasty in experimental animals (see reviews 175,176). Although the precise mechanism responsible for this protective effect is not known, heparin has a variety of effects that could influence neointimal expansion. Such effects include binding and inactivation of specific growth factors, inhibition of protease activator synthesis and decreased protease activity, modification of intracellular secondary signals associated with the mitogenic response, and alterations to the composition of the ECM (177). One or more of these responses could profoundly affect the behavior of vascular cells as well as the biomechanical properties of the vascular wall. A more thorough understanding of vascular wall ECM changes induced by heparin and related molecules is needed before these molecules can be considered "safe and effective" antagonists of atherosclerosis.

GLYCOPROTEINS

The principal glycoproteins in vascular tissue and synthesized by vascular cells include fibronectin, laminin, thrombospondin, tenascin, and osteopontin (Table 3). These proteins have similar modular structures and contain sequences that allow them to self-associate, interact with other ECM components, and bind to cells through specific cell surface receptors. Through multiple interactions, these macromolecules regulate vascular ECM integrity and provide a variety of substrates for vascular cells.

TABLE 3. *Some vascular ECM components and their cell surface receptors*

Protein	Size (kDa)	Cell surface binding proteins	
		Integrins	Other
Fibronectin	~440	$\alpha_5\beta_1$	
Laminin	~900	$\alpha_6\beta_1$	
		$\alpha_v\beta_3$	
		$\alpha_6\beta_4$	
			32/67 laminin receptor (YIGSR)
			SIKVAV (?)
Thrombospondin	~450		HSPG
Tenascin	~800	$\alpha_2\beta_1$	
Osteopontin	~44–85	$\alpha_v\beta_3$	
		$\alpha_v\beta_1$	
		$\alpha_v\beta_5$	
Hyaluronan	~2–20 × 10^3		RHAMM (receptor for hyaluronan mediated motility), CD 44

Fibronectins

Fibronectins are a family of glycoproteins that are present in blood plasma and the ECM of most tissues. This glycoprotein consists of two similar peptide chains of ~220 kDa held together at one end by disulfide bonds (178). Each chain consists of repeated copies of three distinct types of polypeptide domains (types I, II, III). There are 12 type I repeats, two type II repeats, and 15 to 17 type III repeats in human fibronectin. Approximately 20 different fibronectin chains have been identified in humans, all of which are generated by alternative splicing of the RNA transcript of a single fibronectin gene (179). Many of these variants are expressed in vascular tissue during development and remodeling (180–182).

Fibronectin is present throughout all layers of the vascular ECM and in elevated amounts during development and in the neointima in response to injury and hypertension (180–185). In addition, fibronectin synthesis is increased as smooth muscle cells proliferate and migrate in the intima during closure of the ductus arteriosus during fetal development (186). This glycoprotein also accumulates in intimal thickenings associated with post–cardiac-transplant coronary arteriopathy (187,188) and in restenotic arterial tissue postangioplasty (189) and is deposited in thrombi and plasma clots during thrombus formation. Deposits of this glycoprotein in altered vascular tissue may influence the retention of lipoproteins in the vascular ECM because fibronectin interacts with lipoproteins, possibly through its heparin-binding domain (190).

Fibronectin is a principal attachment protein for vascular cells and serves as a substrate for the migration of vascular cells during development and remodeling (see reviews 191,192). For example, spliced variants of fibronectin are synthesized by vascular endothelial and smooth muscle cells as they migrate (191–195). The principal sites for fibronectin splicing lie on either side of the cell-binding domain of fibronectin, and differential use of these spliced repeats could easily affect the strength of interactions between fibronectin and its cell surface receptor (i.e., $\alpha_5\beta_1$). These results suggest that some aspects of cell behavior are modulated by cues provided by different types and proportions of alternatively spliced fibronectin variants—a theme that is bound to occur for other vascular ECM molecules as well.

Laminin

Laminin is an ~800-kDa trimeric glycoprotein present in vascular basement membranes of endothelial and smooth muscle cells. Like fibronectin, this molecule consists of subunits of polypeptides that contain multiple binding sites for cell surface receptors as well as other ECM molecules (196,197). Laminin also exists as multiple isoforms. These isoforms belong to a family of proteins containing several genetically distinct subunit chains.

Laminin interacts with key basement membrane components such as type IV collagen, nidogen, and HSPG to form the fabric of the basement membrane during embryonic vasculogenesis and vascular wall maturation. Because laminin peptides contain multiple cell-binding sites, this glycoprotein serves as a substrate for vascular cells. For example, the A chain of laminin contains RGD sequences, which can be recognized by multiple integrin receptors, of which $\alpha_6\beta_1$ appears to be the most specific. The B chain of laminin contains the YIGSR sequence, which also serves as a ligand for some cells. Vascular endothelial cells attach to laminin through both β_1 and β_3 integrins and use multiple laminin binding sites, including SIKVAV sequences, to form endothelial tubes in vitro (198,199).

Laminin also interacts with arterial smooth muscle cells through more than one receptor (200,201). This interaction in part maintains these cells in a nonproliferative and contractile phenotype, unlike fibronectin, which promotes modulation of arterial smooth muscle cells to a proliferative and secretory phenotype. The potential importance of laminin in vascular disease is highlighted by studies that demonstrate that the synthetic peptide YIGSR inhibits new blood vessel formation (199) and intimal hyperplasia in experimental animals following balloon angioplasty (202).

Thrombospondin

Thrombospondin (TSP) is a 450-kDa trimeric glycoprotein that consists of three identical 150-kDa chains joined together by disulfide linkages. The glycoprotein exists in more than one form and may constitute a family of related proteins generated by alternative splicing, although more than one TSP gene exists (203). Thrombospondin was first identified in platelet α granules where upon release it promotes platelet aggregation (203–205). Thrombospondin interacts with a number of plasma proteins such as fibrinogen, plasminogen, and histidine-rich glycoprotein and copolymerizes with fibrin in clot formation. However, as is true for many of the other platelet proteins, thrombospondin is synthesized by a variety of cells including vascular endothelial and smooth muscle cells (206–208). Thrombospondin possesses multiple binding sites and interacts with a variety of ECM components such as fibronectin, a number of different collagens, laminin, and HSPGs. Interestingly, TSP also binds to growth factors such as TGF-β1 and may be involved in the activation of this cytokine within the vascular ECM (209). Unlike fibronectin and laminin, which promote cell adhesion, TSP exerts antiadhesive effects that lead to cell rounding and cell detachment (205,210).

Thrombospondin is present in different vascular layers but is elevated in the thickened intima in human vascular disease (211) and in the neointima following experimental balloon angioplasty (208). Increased expression of TSP appears to be linked to a vascular cell growth response (206–208). For example, expression of TSP by arterial smooth muscle cells is regulated by PDGF and angiotensin II. Antibodies to TSP inhibit PDGF-induced proliferation of arterial smooth muscle cells (206). Although TSP appears necessary for arterial smooth muscle cell proliferation, this glycoprotein inhibits endothelial cell proliferation in vitro (213) and angiogenesis in vivo (214). Such opposing actions on two different vascular cell types indicate that this glycoprotein plays a key and somewhat complicated role in regulating vascular cell growth.

Tenascin

Tenascin is a glycoprotein that is transiently present in the vascular ECM. This glycoprotein is a large hexameric protein with disulfide-linked multidomain subunits of 190–240 kDa organized into a six-armed structure. Tenascin is composed of several distinct domains and resembles fibronectin in that a large part of the molecule is composed of fibronectin type III repeats. As is true of other ECM glycoproteins, more than one form of tenascin exists, generated by alternative splicing involving various exons that code for the type III repeats in the molecule (215).

Tenascin is an ECM glycoprotein with a spatially and temporally restricted distribution. It is present in the vascular ECM at early stages of embryonic vasculogenesis (216,217) and, like TSP, is present in increased levels in the neointima following experimental balloon angioplasty (218) and in hypertension (219). In a preliminary study, tenascin was also detected in human restenotic coronary arteries after angioplasty (220).

Tenascin is synthesized by both vascular smooth muscle and endothelial cells and is regulated in part by factors such as PDGF, TGF-β1, and angiotensin II (219,221). Tenascin influences vascular cell adhesion (222,223). For example, there is an RGD cell-binding domain in one of the fibronectin type III repeats within tenascin to which endothelial cells attach by $\alpha_2\beta_1$ and $\alpha_2\beta_3$ integrin receptors. However, tenascin also interferes with endothelial cell adhesion by causing disruption of focal adhesion sites and destabilizing endothelial cell attachment (223). Destabilization of cell contact is accompanied by the expression of tenascin splice variants lacking some of the type III fibronectin repeats, suggesting that different tenascin isoforms may differentially regulate cell attachment. Thus, the expression of vascular tenascin appears to be confined to cellular events associated with embyonic development and remodeling in vascular disease.

Osteopontin

Osteopontin is an acidic, highly phosphorylated glycoprotein first identified in bone but subsequently found in a variety of tissues including blood vessels (see reviews 224,225). Osteopontin is small compared to most ECM molecules and has an average molecular mass ranging from 44 to 85 kDa. The protein contains an RGD cell-binding domain, two potential Ca^{2+} binding sites, and a HSPG binding domain as well. Osteopontin is encoded by a single gene, but alternatively spliced variants exist. However, at this point, it is unknown whether differential splicing of osteopontin leads to altered functions of this molecule.

Osteopontin is not present in the ECM of normal blood vessels but appears in the neointima following experimental balloon angioplasty and is present in human atherosclerotic plaques (224–228). There is a spatial and temporal expression of osteopontin that is coincident with the proliferation and migration of arterial smooth muscle cells during the invasion of the intima following vascular injury and in remodeling (see review 225). The synthesis of osteopontin by arterial smooth muscle cells is partially regulated by cytokines such as bFGF, TGF-β1, and angiotensin II (see reviews 225,229). Osteopontin is also synthesized by macrophages, which may be an important source of this glycoprotein in the reaction to tissue injury (228). These observations suggest a role for osteopontin in the early events associated with vascular disease. Because it contains an RGD cell-binding motif, osteopontin could serve as an adhesive ligand for vascular cells during the early phases of vascular remodeling. In fact, osteopontin supports the adhesion of arterial smooth muscle and endothelial cells through the $\alpha_v\beta_3$ integrin (see review 225), which is an integrin implicated in smooth muscle cell and endothelial migration (230,231). Additionally, recent studies indicate that osteopontin is chemotactic for arterial smooth muscle cells (225).

The finding of osteopontin in advanced atherosclerotic lesions also suggests a role for this molecule in late events of vascular disease. Osteopontin tends to localize around areas of calcification in advanced human atherosclerotic plaques (see review 225,232). These findings, coupled with the fact that osteopontin protein contains specific domains for Ca^{2+} binding, suggest a role for osteopontin in the calcification process involved in human disease. Whether this protein regulates arterial calcification remains to be determined.

SUMMARY

The vascular ECM is a collection of vastly different macromolecules organized into a highly ordered network in close association with the vascular cells that produce them. Each component of the ECM possesses unique structural properties that form the basis for their separate functions within vascular tissue. Together these molecules form the architectural framework of vascular tissue and the mileau for vascular cells. Considerable progress has been made within the past few years identifying specific ECM components that regulate key events in vascular wall physiology and pathology. Thus, it is now clear that the vascular ECM not only serves as a biomechanically active scaffold for blood vessel function but also plays a more complex role in regulating the behavior of vascular cells. Furthermore, because virtually all vascular pathology involves significant and specific changes in the vascular ECM, a more thorough understanding of the properties of this matrix and the factors that regulate synthesis and turnover of individual components of the ECM should hasten a cure for cardiovascular disease—the leading cause of death in the United States and Europe.

ACKNOWLEDGMENTS

This review was prepared with grant support from the National Institutes of Health (HL 18645). I would like to thank Kathleen Braun for preparation of the figures, Anna Lewak Wight for careful editing, and Barbara Kovacich for the typing of the manuscript.

REFERENCES

1. Linsenmeyer T. Collagen. In: Hay ED, ed. *Cell Biology of Extracellular Matrix,* 2nd ed. New York: Plenum Press; 1991:7–44.
2. Mayne R, Brewton RG. New members of the collagen superfamily. *Curr Opin Cell Biol* 1993;5:883–890.
3. Shekhonin BV, Domogatsky SP, Muyzykantov VR, Idelson GL, Rukosuev VS. Distribution of types I, III, IV and V collagen in normal and atherosclerotic human arterial wall: Immunomorphological characteristic. *Collagen Rel Res* 1985;5:355–368.
4. Murata K, Motoyama T. Collagen species in various sized human arteries and their changes with intimal proliferation. *Artery* 1990; 17(2):96–106.
5. Rauterburg J, Jaeger E, Althau M. Collagens in atherosclerotic vessel wall lesions. *Curr Top Pathol* 1993;87:163–192.
6. Clark JM, Glagov S. Transmural organization of the arterial media. The lamellar unit revisited. *Arteriosclerosis* 1985;5:19–34.
7. Walker-Caprioglio HM, Trotter JA, Little SA, McGuffee LJ. Organization of cells and extracellular matrix in mesenteric arteries of spontaneously hypertensive rats. *Cell Tissue Res* 1992;269:141–149.
8. Birk DE, Silver FH, Trelstad RL. Matrix assembly. In: Hay ED, ed. *Cell Biology of Extracellular Matrix,* 2nd ed. New York: Plenum Press; 1991:221–254.
9. Yurchenco PD, Schittny JC. Molecular architecture of basement membranes. *FASEB J* 1990;4:1577–1590.
10. Farquhar MG. The glomerular basement membrane. A selective macromolecular filter. In: Hay ED, ed. *Cell Biology of Extracellular Matrix,* 2nd ed. New York: Plenum Press; 1991:365–418.
11. Kittelberger R, Davis PF, Greenhill NS. Immunolocalization of type VIII collagen in vascular tissue. *Biochem Biophys Res Commun* 1989; 159:414–419.
12. Sage H, Iruela-Arispe ML. Type VIII collagen in murine development. *Ann NY Acad Sci* 1990;580:17–31.
13. Katsuda S, Okada Y, Minamoto T, Oda Y, Matsui Y, Nakanishi I. Collagens in human atherosclerosis: Immunohistochemical analysis using collagen type-specific antibodies. *Arterioscler Thromb* 1992; 12:494–502.
14. Bidanset DJ, Guidry C, Rosenberg LC, Choi HU, Timpl R, Höök M. Binding of the proteoglycan decorin to collagen type VI. *J Biol Chem* 1992;267:5250–5256.
15. Heller-Harrison RA, Carter WG. Pepsin-generated type VI collagen is a degradation product of GP 140. *J Biol Chem* 1984;259:6858–6864.
16. Ang AH, Tachas G, Campbell JH, Bateman JF, Campbell GR. Collagen synthesis by cultured rabbit aortic smooth muscle cells. Alteration with phenotype. *Biochem J* 1990;265:461–469.
17. Crouch EC, Parks WC, Rosenbaum JL, Chang D, Whitehouse L, Wu J, Stenmark KR, Orton EC, Mecham RP. Regulation of collagen production by medial smooth muscle cells in hypoxic pulmonary hypertension. *Am Rev Respir Dis* 1989;140:1045–1051.
18. Kindy MS, Chang CJ, Sonnenshein GE. Serum deprivation of vascular smooth muscle cells enhances collagen gene expression. *J Biol Chem* 1988;263:11426–11430.
19. Liau G, Chan LM. Regulation of extracellular mRNA levels in cultured smooth muscle cells. Relationship to cellular quiescence. *J Biol Chem* 1989;264:10315–10320.
20. Majors AK, Ehrhart LA. Cell density and proliferation modulate collagen synthesis and procollagen mRNA levels in arterial smooth muscle cells. *Exp Cell Res* 1992;200:168–174.
21. Amento EP, Ehsani N, Palmer H, Libby P. Cytokines and growth factors positively and negatively regulate interstitial collagen gene expression in human vascular smooth muscle cells. *Arterioscler Thromb* 1991;11:1223–1230.
22. Thie M, Harrach B, Schönherr E, Kresse H, Robenek H, Rauterberg J. Responsiveness of aortic smooth muscle cells to soluble growth mediators is influenced by cell matrix contact. *Arterioscler Thromb* 1993;13:994–1004.
23. Lawrence R, Hartmann DJ, Sonenshein GE. Transforming growth factor $\beta 1$ stimulates type V collagen expression in bovine vascular smooth muscle cells. *J Biol Chem* 1994;269:9603–9609.
24. Yamamoto M, Yamamoto K, Noumura R. Type I collagen promotes modulation of cultured rabbit arterial smooth muscle cells from a contractile to a synthetic phenotype. *Exp Cell Res* 1993;204:121–129.
25. Skinner MP, Raines EW, Ross R. Dynamic expression of $\alpha_1\beta_1$ and $\alpha_2\beta_1$ integrin receptors by human vascular smooth muscle cells: $\alpha_2\beta_1$ integrin is required for chemotaxis across type I collagen-coated membranes. *Am J Pathol* 1994;145:1070–1081.
26. Tan E, Glassberg E, Olsen DR, Noveral JP, Unger GA, Peltonen J, Li-Chu M, Levine E, Sollberg S. Extracellular matrix gene expression by human endothelial and smooth muscle cells. *Matrix* 1991;11: 380–389.
27. Ingber D, Folkman J. Inhibition of angiogenesis through modulation of collagen metabolism. *Lab Invest* 1988;59:44–51.
28. Nicosia RF, Belser P, Bonanno E, Diven J. Regulation of angiogenesis in vitro by collagen metabolism. *In Vitro Cell Dev Biol* 1991;27A: 961–966.
29. Jackson CJ, Jenkins KL. Type I collagen fibrils promote rapid vascular tube formation upon contact with the apical side of cultured endothelium. *Exp Cell Res* 1991;192:319–323.
30. Rekhter MD, Zhang K, Narayanan AS, Phan S, Schork MA, Gordon D. Type I collagen gene expression in human atherosclerosis. *Am J Pathol* 1993;143:1634–1648.
31. Iruela-Arispe ML, Diglio CA, Sage EH. Modulation of extracellular matrix proteins by endothelial cells undergoing angiogenesis in vitro. *Arterioscler Thromb* 1991;11:805–815.
32. Vernon RB, Lara SL, Iruela-Arispe ML, Angelo JC, Wight TN, Sage EH. Networks of endothelial cells that arise spontaneously in vitro are associated with templates of type I collagen. *In Vitro Cell Dev Biol* 1995;31:120–131.
33. Löhler J, Timpl R, Jaenisch R. Embryonic lethal mutation in mouse collagen 1 gene causes rupture of blood vessels and is associated with erythropoietic and mesenchymal cell death. *Cell* 1984;38:597–607.
34. Pyeritz RE, Stolle CA, Parfrey NA, Myers JC. Ehlers–Danlos syndrome IV due to a novel defect in type III procollagen. *Am J Med Genet* 1984;19:607–622.
35. Burleigh MC, Briggs AD, Lendon CL, Davies MJ, Born GVR, Richardson PD. Collagen types I and III collagen content GAGs and mechanical strength of human atherosclerotic plaque caps: Span-wise variations. *Atherosclerosis* 1992;96:71–81.
36. Jaeger E, Rust S, Roessner A, Kleinhans G, Buchholz B, Althaus M, Rauterberg J, Gerlach U. Joint occurrence of collagen mRNA containing cells and macrophages in human atherosclerotic vessels. *Atherosclerosis* 1991;31:55–68.
37. Riessen R, Isner JM, Blessing E, Loushim C, Nikol S, Wight TN. Regional differences in the distribution of the proteoglycans biglycan and decorin in the extracellular matrix of atherosclerotic and restenotic human coronary arteries. *Am J Pathol* 1994;144:962–974.
38. Jimi S, Sakata N, Matunaga A, Takebayashi S. Low density lipoproteins bind more to type I and III collagens by negative-charge dependent mechanisms than to type IV and V collagens. *Atherosclerosis* 1994;107:109–116.
39. Brownlee M. Glycation products and the pathogenesis of diabetic complications. *Diabetes Care* 1992;15:1835–1843.
40. Ross R, Wight TN, Strandness E, Thiele B. Human atherosclerosis I. Cell constitution and characteristics of advanced lesions of the superficial femoral artery. *Am J Pathol* 1984;114:79–93.
41. Ooshima A. Collagen β chain: Increased proportion in human atherosclerosis. *Science* 1981;213:666–668.
42. Lee RT, Grodzinsky AJ, Frank EH, Kamm RD, Schoen FJ. Structure-

dependent dynamic mechanical behavior of fibrous caps from human atherosclerotic plaques. *Circulation* 1991;83:1764–1770.
43. Falk E. Why do plaques rupture? *Circulation* 1992;86:III-30–III-42.
44. Roald HE, Lyberg T, Dedichen H, Hamers M, Kierulf P, Westvik A-B, Sakariassen KS. Collagen-induced thrombus formation in flowing non anticoagulant human blood from habitual smokers and nonsmoking patients with severe peripheral atherosclerotic disease. *Arterioscler Thromb Vasc Biol* 1995;15:128–132.
45. Davies MJ, Thomas AC. Plaque fissuring—the cause of acute myocardial infarction, sudden ischaemic death and crescendo angina. *Br Heart J* 1985;53:363–373.
46. Sandberg LB, Soskel NT, Leslie JG. Elastin structure, biosynthesis and its relation to disease states. *N Engl J Med* 1981;304:566–579.
47. Mecham RP, Heuser JE. The elastic fiber. In: Hay ED, ed. *Cell Biology of Extracellular Matrix,* 2nd ed. New York: Plenum Press; 1991.
48. Sakai LY, Keene DR, Engvall E. Fibrillin, a new 350-kD glycoprotein, is a component of extracellular matrix microfibrils. *J Cell Biol* 1986; 103:2499–2509.
49. Bressan GM, Dago-Gordini D, Colombatti A, Castellani I, Marigo V, Volpin D. Emilin, a component of elastic fibers preferentially located at the elastin–microfibrils interface. *J Cell Biol* 1993;121: 201–212.
50. Baccaiani-Contri M, Vincenzi D, Cicchetti F, Mori G, Pasquali-Ronchetti I. Immunocytochemical localization of proteoglycans within normal elastic fibers. *Eur J Cell Biol* 1990;53:305–312.
51. Kagan HM, Vaccaro CA, Bronson RE, Tang SS, Brody JS. Ultrastructural immunolocalization of lysl oxidase in vascular connective tissue. *J Cell Biol* 1986;103:1121–1128.
52. Reiser K, McCormick J, Rucker RB. Enzymatic and nonenzymatic cross linking of collagen and elastin. *FASEB J* 1992;6:2439–2449.
53. Roach MR, Song SH. Arterial elastin as seen with scanning electron microscopy. *Scan Microscopy* 1988;2:994–1004.
54. Wolinsky H, Glagov S. A lamellae unit of aortic medial structure and function in mammals. *Circ Res* 1967;20:99–111.
55. Ross R. The smooth muscle cell. II. Growth of smooth muscle in culture and formation of elastic fibers. *J Cell Biol* 1971;50:172–186.
56. Foster J, Miller AML, Benedict MR, Richman RA, Rich CB. Evidence for insulin-like growth factor 1—regulation of chick aortic elastogenesis. *Matrix* 1989;9:328–335.
57. Martin BM, Ritchie AR, Toselli P, Franzblau C. Elastin synthesis and accumulation in irradiated smooth muscle cell cultures. *Connect Tissue Res* 1992;28:181–189.
58. Davidson JM, Zoia O, Liu JM. Modulation of transforming growth factor-beta-1 stimulated elastin and collagen production and proliferation in porcine vascular smooth muscle cells and skin fibroblasts by basic fibroblast growth factor, transforming growth factor β and insulin-like growth factor-1. *J Cell Physiol* 1993;155:149–156.
59. Parks WC, Deak SB. Tropoelastin heterogeneity: Implications for protein function and disease. *Am J Res Cell Mol Biol* 1990;2:399–406.
60. Indik Z, Yeh H, Ornstein-Goldstein N, Rosenbloom J. Structure of the elastin gene and alternative splicing of elastin mRNA. In: Sandell L, Boyd C, eds. *Genes for Extracellular Matrix Proteins.* New York: Academic Press; 1990:221–250.
61. Hinek A, Mecham RP, Keeley F, Okamura-Oho Y, Rabinovitch M. Impaired elastin fiber assembly related to reduced 67kD elastin-binding protein in fetal lamb ductus arteriosus and in cultured aortic smooth muscle cells treated with chondroitin sulfate. *J Clin Invest* 1991;88:2083–2094.
62. Hinek A, Boyle J, Rabinovitch M. Vascular smooth muscle cell detachment from elastin and migration through elastic laminae is promoted by chondroitin sulfate-induced shedding of the 67kDa cell surface elastin binding protein. *Exp Cell Res* 1992;203:344–353.
63. Fornieri C, Baccarani-Contri M, Quaglino D, Pasquali-Ronchetti I. Lysyl oxidase activity and elastin/glycosaminoglycan interactions in growing chick and rat aortas. *J Cell Biol* 1987;105:1464–1469.
64. Robert L, Jacob MP, Frances C, Godeau G, Hornbeck W. Interaction between elastin and elastases and its role in the aging of the arterial wall, skin and other connective tissues, A review. *Mech Ageing Dev* 1984;28:155–166.
65. Tilson MD. Histochemistry of aortic elastin in patients with nonspecific abdominal aortic aneurysmal disease. *Arch Surg* 1988;123: 503–505.
66. Katsuda S, Okada Y, Nakanishi I. Abnormal accumulation of elastin-associated microfibrils during elastolysis in the arterial wall. *Exp Mol Pathol* 1990;52:13–24.
67. Nakashima Y, Sueishi K. Alteration of elastic architecture in the lathyritic rat aorta implies the pathogenesis of aortic dissecting aneurysm. *Am J Pathol* 1992;140:959–969.
68. Lehnert B, Wadouh F, Dwenger A. Relationship between proteolytic enzymes and atherosclerosis in aortic aneurysms. *Surg Gynecol Obstet* 1991;172:345–350.
69. Pyeritz RE. Marfan syndrome. In: Emery AEH, Rimoin DL, eds. *Principles and Practice of Medical Genetics,* 2nd ed. New York: Churchill Livingstone; 1983.
70. Ramirez F, Pereira L, Zhang H, Lee B. The fibrillin–Marfan syndrome connection. *Bioassays* 1993;15:589–594.
71. Davis PF, Ryan PA, Osipowicz J, Anderson MJ, Sweeney A, Stehbens WE. The biochemical composition of hemodynamically stressed vascular tissue: The insoluble elastin of experimental arteriovenous fistulae. *Exp Mol Pathol* 1989;51:103–110.
72. Cohen JR, Sarfatti I, Danna D, Wise L. Smooth muscle cell elastase, atherosclerosis and aortic abdominal aneurysms. *Ann Surg* 1992;216: 327–332.
73. Newman KM, Ogata Y, Malon A, Irizarry E, Gandhi RH, Nagase H, Tilson MD. Identification of matrix metalloproteinases 3 (stromelysin-1) and 9 (gelatinase B) in abdominal aortic aneurysm. *Arterioscler Thromb* 1994;14:1315–1320.
74. Newby AC, Southgate KM, Davies M. Extracellular matrix metalloproteinases in the pathogenesis of arteriosclerosis. *Basic Res Cardiol* 1994;89:59–70.
75. Katsuda S, Okada Y, Okada Y, Imai K, Nakanishi I. Matrix metalloproteinase 9 (92kD gelatinase/type IV collagenase) can degrade arterial elastin. *Am J Pathol* 1994;145:1208–1218.
76. Senior RM, Griffin GL, Mecham RP, Wrenn DS, Prasad KU, Urry DW. Val-Gly-Val-Ala-Pro-Gly, a repeating peptide in elastin is chemotactic for fibroblasts and monocytes. *J Cell Biol* 1994;99:870–874.
77. Keeley FW. Dynamic responses of collagen and elastin to vessel wall perturbation. In: Gotleib A, Langille Lowell B, Fedoroff S, eds. *Atherosclerosis: Cellular and Molecular Interactions in the Artery Wall.* New York: Plenum Press; 1991:101–114.
78. Nikkari ST, Järveläinen HT, Wight TN, Ferguson M, Clowes AW. Smooth muscle cell expression of extracellular matrix genes after arterial injury. *Am J Pathol* 1994;144:1348–1356.
79. Botney MD, Kaiser LR, Cooper JD, Mechan RP, Parghi D, Roby J, Parks WC. Extracellular matrix protein gene expression in atherosclerotic hypertensive pulmonary arteries. *Am J Pathol* 1992;140: 357–364.
80. Liptay MF, Parks WC, Mecham RP, Roby J, Kaiser LR, Cooper JD, Botney. Neointimal macrophages co-localize with extracellular matrix gene expression in human atherosclerotic pulmonary arteries. *J Clin Invest* 1993;91:588–594.
81. Prosser IW, Stenmark KR, Suthar M, Crouch EC, Mecham RP, Parks WC. Regional heterogeneity of elastin and collagen gene expression in intralobar arteries in response to hypoxic pulmonary hypertension as demonstrated by in situ hybridization. *Am J Pathol* 1989;135: 1073–1087.
82. Winlove CP, Parker KH, Ewins AR. Some factors influencing the interactions of plasma lipoproteins with arterial elastin. *Artery* 1988; 15:292–303.
83. Kramsch DM, Hollander W. The interaction of serum and arterial lipoproteins with elastin of the arterial intima and its role in the lipid accumulation in atherosclerotic plaque. *J Clin Invest* 1973;52: 236–247.
84. Saulnier JM, Hauck M. Fulop T Jr, Wallach JM. Human aortic elastin from normal individuals and atherosclerotic patients: Lipid and cation contents; susceptibility to elastolysis. *Clin Chim Acta* 1991;200: 129–136.
85. Smith EB, Evans PH, Downham MD. Lipid in the aortic intima the correlation of morphological and chemical characteristics. *Atherosclerosis* 1967;7:171–186.
86. Guyton JR, Bocon TM, Schifani TA. Quantitative ultrastructural analysis of perifibrous lipid and its association with elastin in non-atherosclerotic human aorta. *Arteriosclerosis.* 1985;5:644–652.
87. Srinvasan SR, Yost C, Radhakrishnamurthy B, Dalferes ER Jr, Berenson GS. Lipoprotein–elastin interactions in human aorta fibrous plaque lesions. *Atherosclerosis* 1981;38:137–147.
88. Jordon RE, Hewitt N, Lewis W, Kagan H, Franzblau C. Regulation

of elastase-catalyzed hydrolysis of insoluble elastin by synthetic and naturally occurring hydropholic ligands. *Biochem J* 1974;13: 3497–3503.

89. Kagan HM, Milbury PE, Kramsch DM. A possible role for elastin ligands in the proteolytic degradation of arterial elastic lamellae in the rabbit. *Circ Res* 1979;44:95–103.
90. Rucker RB, Ford D, Rieman WG, Tom K. Additional evidence for the binding of calcium ions to elastin at neutral sites. *Calcif Tissue Res* 1974;14:317–325.
91. Juul S, Ledbetter D, Wight TN, Woodrum D. New insights into idopathic infantile arterial calcinosis. *Am J Dis Child* 1990;144:229–232.
92. Radhakrishnamurthy B, Srinivasan P, Vijayagopal P, Berenson GS. Arterial wall proteoglycans—biologic properties related to the pathogenesis of atherosclerosis. *Eur Heart J* 1990;11:148–157.
93. Wight TN. Cell biology of arterial proteoglycans. *Arteriosclerosis* 1989;9:1–20.
94. Camejo G, Camejo EH, Olsson U, Bondjers G. Proteoglycans and lipoproteins in atherosclerosis. *Curr Opin Lipidol* 1993;4:385–391.
95. Williams KJ, Tabas I. The response-to-retention hypothesis of early atherogenesis. *Arterioscler Thromb Vasc Biol* 1995;15:551–561.
96. Wight TN, Kinsella MG, Qwarnström. The role of proteoglycans in cell adhesion, migration and proliferation. *Curr Opin Cell Biol* 1992; 4:793–801.
97. Jackson RL, Busch SJ, Cardin AD. Glycosaminoglycans: Molecular properties, protein interaction and role in physiological processes. *Physiol Rev* 1991;71:481–539.
98. Laurent TC, Fraser JRE. Hyaluronan. *FASEB J* 1992;6:2397–2404.
99. Yao LY, Moody C, Schonherr E, Wight TN, Sandell LJ. Identification of the proteoglycan versican in aorta and smooth muscle cells by DNA sequence analysis, in situ hybridization and immunohistochemistry. *Matrix Biol* 1994;4:213–225.
100. Galis ZS, Alavi MZ, Moore S. In situ ultrastructural characterization of chondroitin sulfate proteoglycans in normal rabbit aorta. *J Histochem Cytochem* 1992;40:251–263.
101. Dreher KL, Asundi V, Matzura D, Cowan K. Vascular smooth muscle biglycan represents a highly conserved proteoglycan within the arterial wall. *Eur J Cell Biol* 1990;53:296–304.
102. Stöcker G, Meyer H, Wagener C, Greiling H. Purification and N-terminal amino acid sequence of a chondroitin sulfate/dermatan sulfate proteoglycan isolated from intima/media preparations of human aorta. *Biochem J* 1991;274:415–420.
103. Bianco P, Fisher LW, Young MF, Termine JD, Roby PG. Expression and localization of the small proteoglycans biglycan and decorin in developing human skeletal and nonskeletal tissues. *J Histochem Cytochem* 1990;38:1549–1563.
104. Register TC, Wagner WD, Robbins RA, Lively MO. Structural properties and partial protein sequence analysis of the major dermatan sulfate proteoglycan of pigeon aorta. *Atherosclerosis* 1993;98: 99–111.
105. Funderburgh JL, Funderburgh ML, Mann MM, Conrad GW. Arterial lumican. Properties of a corneal type keratan sulfate proteoglycan from bovine aorta. *J Biol Chem* 1991;266:24773–24777.
106. Couchman JR, Abrahamson DR, McCarthy KJ. Basement membrane proteoglycans and development. *Kidney Int* 1993;43:7984.
107. Murdock AD, Iozzo R. Perlecan: The multidomain heparan sulfate proteoglycan basement membrane and extracellular matrix. *Virchows Arch [A] Pathol Anat* 1993;423:237–242.
108. Hayashi K, Madri JA, Yurchenco PD. Endothelial cells interact with core protein of basement membrane perlecan through β1 and β3 integrins: An adhesion modulated by glycosaminoglycan. *J Cell Biol* 1992;119:945–959.
109. Bashkin P, Doctrow S, Klagsburn M, Svahn MC, Folkman J, Vlodavsky I. Basic fibroblast growth factor binds to subendothelial extracellular matrix and is released by heparatinase and heparin-like molecules. *Biochem* 1989;28:1737–1743.
110. Radhakrishnamurthy B, Jeansonne N, Tracy RE, Berenson GS. A monoclonal antibody that recognizes hyaluronic acid binding region of aorta proteoglycans. *Atherosclerosis* 1993;98:179–192.
111. L'evesque H, Girard N, Maingonnat C, Delpech A, Chauzy C, Tayot J, Courtios H, Delpech B. Localization and solubilization of hyaluronan and of the hyaluronan-binding protein hyaluronectin in human normal and arteriosclerotic arterial walls. *Atherosclerosis* 1994;105: 51–62.
112. Binette F, Cravens J, Kahoussi B, Handenschild DR, Goetinck PF. Link protein is ubiquitously expressed in non-cartilaginous tissues where it enhances and stabilizes the interaction of proteoglycans with hyaluronic acid. *J Biol Chem* 1994;269:19116–19122.
113. Comper WD, Laurent TC. Physiological function of connective tissue polysaccharides. *Physiol Rev* 1979;58:255–315.
114. Stary HC. The sequence of cell and matrix changes in atherosclerotic lesions of coronary arteries in the first 40 years of life. *Eur Heart J* 1990;11:Suppl E 3–19.
115. Merrilees MJ, Beaumont B. Structural heterogeneity of the diffuse intimal thickening and correlation with distribution of TGFβ-1. *J Vasc Res* 1993;30:293–302.
116. Nievelstein P, Fogelman A, Mottino G, Frank JS. Lipid accumulation in the rabbit aortic intima 2 hours after bolus infusion of low density lipoprotein. A deep-etch and immunolocalization study of ultra rapidly frozen tissue. *Arterioscler. Thromb.* 1991;11:1795–1805.
117. Bernfield M, Kokenyeshi R, Kato M, Hinkes MT, Spring J, Gallo RL, Lose EJ. Biology of the syndecans: A family of transmembrane heparan sulfate proteoglycans. *Annu Rev Cell Biol* 1992;8:365–393.
118. Cizmeci-Smith G, Asundi V, Stahl RC, Teichman LJ, Chernousov M, Cowan K, Carey DJ. Regulated expression of syndecan in vascular smooth muscle cells and cloning of rat syndecan core protein cDNA. *J Biol Chem* 1992;267:15729–15736.
119. Edwards IJ, Wagner WD. Cell surface heparan sulfate proteoglycan and chondroitin sulfate proteoglycans of arterial smooth muscle cells. *Am J Pathol* 1992;140:193–205.
120. Mertens G, Cassiman JJ, Van den Berghe H, Vermylen J, David G. Cell surface heparan sulfate proteoglycans from human vascular endothelial cells. Core protein characterization and antithrombin III binding properties. *J Biol Chem* 1992;267:20435–20443.
121. Kojima T, Shworak NW, Rosenberg RD. Molecular cloning and expression of two distinct cDNA-encoding heparan sulfate proteoglycan core proteins from a rat endothelial cell line. *J Biol Chem* 1992; 267:4870–4877.
122. Tanaka Y, Adams DH, Shaw S. Proteoglycans on endothelial cells present adhesion-inducing cytokines to leukocytes. *Immunol Today* 1993;14:111–115.
123. Olivecrona T, Bengtsson-Olivecrona G, Ostergaard P, Liu G, Chevreuil O, Hultin M. New aspects on heparin and lipoprotein metabolism. *Haemostasis* 1993;23:150–160.
124. Bourin M-C, Lindahl U. Glycosaminoglycans and the regulation of blood coagulation. *Biochem J* 1993;289:313–330.
125. Merrilees MJ, Campbell JH, Spanidis E, Campbell GR. Glycosaminoglycan synthesis by smooth muscle cells of differing phenotype and their response to endothelial cell conditioned medium. *Atherosclerosis* 1990;81:245–254.
126. Asundi V, Cowan K, Matzura D, Wagner W, Dreher K. Characterization of extracellular matrix proteoglycan transcripts expressed by vascular smooth muscle cells. *Eur J Cell Biol* 1990;52:98–104.
127. Chen JK, Hoshi H, McKeehan WL. Stimulation of human arterial smooth muscle cell chondroitin sulfate proteoglycan synthesis by transforming growth factor-beta. *In Vitro Cell Dev Biol* 1991;27:6–12.
128. Schönherr E, Järveläinen HT, Sandell LJ, Wight TN. Effects of platelet-derived growth factor and transforming growth factor β1 on the synthesis of a large versican-like chondroitin sulfate proteoglycan by arterial smooth muscle cells. *J Biol Chem* 1991;66:17640–17647.
129. Schönherr E, Järveläinen HT, Kinsella MG, Sandell LJ, Wight TN. Platelet derived growth factor and transforming growth factor-β1 differentially affect the synthesis of biglycan and decorin by monkey arterial smooth muscle cells. *Arterioscler Thromb* 1993;13: 1026–1036.
130. Edwards IJ, Xu H, Wright MJ, Wagner WD. Interleukin-1 upregulates decorin production by arterial smooth muscle cells. *Arterioscler Thromb* 1994;14:1032–1039.
131. Camejo G, Fager B, Rosengren E, Hurt-Camejo E, Bondjers G. Binding of low density lipoproteins by proteoglycans synthesized by proliferating and quiescent human arterial smooth muscle cells. *J Biol Chem* 1993;268:14131–14137.
132. Järveläinen HT, Kinsella MG, Wight TN, Sandell LJ. Differential expression of small chondroitin/dermatan sulfate proteoglycans, PG-I/biglycan and PG-II/decorin, by vascular smooth muscle and endothelial cells in culture. *J Biol Chem* 1991;266:23274–23281.
133. Järveläinen HT, Iruela-Arispe ML, Kinsella MG, Sandell LJ, Sage EH, Wight TN. Expression of decorin by sprouting bovine aortic

endothelial cells exhibiting angiogenesis in vitro. *Exp Cell Res* 1992; 203:395–401.
134. Banerjee SD, Toole BP. Hyaluronan-binding protein in endothelial cell morphogenesis. *J Cell Biol* 1992;119:643–652.
135. Koslet SO, Gallagher JT. Proteoglycans in haemopoietic cells. *Biochim Biophys Acta* 1990;1032:191–211.
136. Owens RT, Wagner WD. Chondroitin sulfate proteoglycan and heparan sulfate proteoglycan production by cultured pigeon peritoneal macrophages. *J Leukocyte Biol* 1992;51:626–633.
137. Edwards IJ, Xu H, Obunike JC, Goldberg IJ, Wagner WD. Differentiated macrophages synthesize a heparan sulfate proteoglycan and an oversulfated chondroitin sulfate proteoglycan that bind lipoprotein lipase. *Arterioscler Thromb Vasc Biol* 1995;15:400–409.
138. Kovanen PT. The mast cell—a potential link between inflammation and cellular cholesterol deposition in atherogenesis. *Eur Heart J* 1993; Suppl. 14:105–117.
139. Nader H. Characterization of a heparan sulfate and a peculiar chondroitin 4-sulfate proteoglycan from platelets. *J Biol Chem* 1991;266: 10518–10523.
140. Savani RC, Wang C, Yang B, Zhang S, Kinsella MG, Wight TN, Stern R, Nance DM, Turley EA. Migration of bovine aortic smooth muscle cells following wounding injury: The role for hyaluronan and RHAMM. *J Clin Invest* 1995;95:1158–1168.
141. Miyake K, Underhill CB, Lesley J, Kincade PW. Hyaluronate can function as a cell adhesion molecule and CD44 participates in hyaluronate recognition. *J Exp Med* 1990;172:69–75.
142. Walker-Caprioglio HM, Koob TJ, McGuffee LJ. Proteoglycan synthesis in normotensive and spontaneously hypertensive rat arteries in vitro. *Matrix* 1992;12:308–320.
143. Wasty F, Alavi MZ, Moore S. Distribution of glycosaminoglycans in the intima of human aortas: Changes in atherosclerosis and diabetes mellitus. *Diabetologia* 1993;36:316–322.
144. Heickendorf L, Ledet T, Rasmussen LM. Glycosaminoglycans in the human aorta in diabetes mellitus: A study of tunica medica from areas with and without atherosclerotic plaque. *Diabetologia* 1994;37: 286–292.
145. Wincour PD, Richardson M. Thrombosis and atherogenesis in diabetes. In: Drazin B, Ecke R. eds. *Diabetes and Atherosclerosis Molecular and Clinical Aspects.* New York: Elsevier; 1993:213–228.
146. Volker W, Schmidt A, Buddecke E. Cytochemical changes in a human arterial proteoglycan related to atherosclerosis. *Atherosclerosis* 1989; 77:117–130.
147. Robbins RA, Wagner WD, Sawyer LM, Caterson B. Immunolocalization of proteoglycan types in aortas of pigeons with spontaneous or diet induced atherosclerosis. *Am J Pathol* 1989;134:615–626.
148. Cherchi GM, Coinu R, Demuro P, Formato M, Sanna G, Tidore M, Tira ME, Deluca G. Structural and functional modifications of proteoglycans in atherosclerosis. *Matrix* 1990;10:362–372.
149. Robbins RA, Wagner WD, Register TC, Caterson B. Demonstration of a keratan sulfate containing proteoglycan in atherosclerotic aorta. *Arterioscler Thromb* 1992;12:83–91.
150. Strauss BH, Chisholm RJ, Keeley FW, Gotlieb AI, Lagan RA, Armstrong P. Extracellular matrix remodeling after balloon angioplasty injury in a rabbit model of restenosis. *Circ Res* 1994;75:650–658.
151. Riessen R, Wight TN, Pastore C, Henley C, Isner JM. Hyaluronan in the extracellular matrix of human restenotic arteries and balloon-injured rat carotid arteries. *Am J Pathol [in press].*
152. O'Brien K, Alpers CE, Ferguson M, Wight TN, Chait A. Colocalization of apolipoprotein E and biglycan in human atherosclerotic plaques. *Am J Pathol [in press].*
153. Richardson M, Hatton MWC. Transient morphological and biochemical alterations of arterial proteoglycan during early wound healing. *Exp Mol Pathol* 1993;58:77–95.
154. Savani RC, Wang C, Shi Y, Kaplan C, Overhiser R, Panek RL, Stern R, Turley EA. Neointimal formation after balloon injury. A role for hyaluronan and the hyaluronan receptor RHAMM. *[in press].*
155. Carey DJ. Control of growth and differentiation of vascular cells by extracellular matrix proteins. *Annu Rev Physiol* 1991;53:161–177.
156. Wolf YG, Rasmussen LM, Ruoslahti E. Antibodies against transforming growth factor-β1 suppress intimal hyperplasia in a rat model. *J Clin Invest* 1994;93:1172–1178.
157. Merrilees MJ, Scott L. Anti sense S-oligonucleotide against transforming growth factor-β1 inhibits proteoglycan synthesis in arterial wall. *J Vasc Res* 1994;31:322–329.
158. Weinbaum S, Chien S. Lipid transport aspects of atherogenesis. *J Biomech Eng* 1993;115(4B):602–610.
159. Curwen KD, Smith SC. Aortic glycosaminoglycans in atherosclerosis-susceptible and -resistant pigeons. *Exp Mol Pathol* 1977;27:121–133.
160. Schwenke DC, Carew TE. Initiation of atherosclerotic lesions in cholesterol fed rabbits. II. Selective retention of LDL vs selective increases in LDL permeability in susceptible sites of arteries. *Arteriosclerosis* 1989;9:908–918.
161. Hermann RA, Malinauskas RA, Truskey GA. Characterization of sites with elevated LDL permeability at intercostal, celiac and iliac branches of normal rabbit aorta. *Arterioscler Thromb* 1994;14: 313–323.
162. Galis ZS, Alavi MZ, Moore S. Co-localization of aortic apoliprotein B and chondroitin sulfate in an injury model from human atherosclerotic lesions. *Am J Pathol* 1993;142:1432–1438.
163. Bihari-Varga M, Gruber E, Rotheneder M, Zechner R, Kostner GM. Interaction of lipoprotein Lp(a) and low density lipoprotein with glycosaminoglycans from human aorta. *Arteriosclerosis* 1988;8: 851–857.
164. Wagner WD, Edwards IJ, St Clair RW, Barakat H. Low density lipoprotein interaction with artery derived proteoglycan: The influence of LDL particle size and the relationship to atherosclerosis susceptibility. *Atherosclerosis* 1989;75:49–59.
165. Alves CS, Mourao PAS. Interaction of high molecular weight chondroitin sulfate from human aorta with plasma low density lipoproteins. *Atherosclerosis* 1988;73:113–124.
166. Cardoso L, Mourao PAS. Glycosaminoglycan fractions from human arteries presenting diverse susceptibilities to atherosclerosis have different binding affinities to plasma LDL. *Arterioscler Thromb* 1994; 14:115–124.
167. Sambandam T, Baker JR, Christner JE, Ekborg SL. Specificity of low density lipoprotein–glycosaminoglycan interaction. *Arterioscler Thromb* 1991;11:561–568.
168. O'Brien KD, Deeb SS, Ferguson M, McDonald TO, Allen MD, Alpers CE, Chait A. Apolipoprotein E localization in human coronary plaques by in situ hybridization and immunohistochemistry and comparison with lipoprotein lipase. *Am J Pathol* 1994;144:538–548.
169. Stein O, Ben-Naim M, Dabach Y, Hollander G, Halperin G, Stein Y. Can lipoprotein lipase be the culprit in cholesterol ester accretion in smooth muscle cells in atheroma? *Atherosclerosis* 1993;99:15–22.
170. Ji Z-S, Brecht WJ, Miranda RD, Hussain MM, Innerarity TL, Mahely RW. Role of heparna sulfate proteoglycans in the binding and uptake of apolipoprotein E-enriched remnant lipoproteins by cultured cells. *J Biol Chem* 1993;268:10160–10167.
171. Vijayagopal P. Enhanced synthesis and accumulation of proteoglycans in cholesterol enriched arterial smooth muscle cells. *Biochem J* 1993;294:603–611.
172. Marcum JA, Rosenberg RD. Anticoagulantly active heparin sulfate proteoglycan and the vascular endothelium. *Semin Thromb Hemostas* 1987;13:464–467.
173. Cadroy Y, Hanson SE, Harker LA. Dermatan sulfate inhibition of fibrin-rich thrombus formation in non human primates. *Arterioscler Thromb* 1993;13:1213–1217.
174. Bendayan P, Boccalon H, Dupauy D, Boneu B. Dermatan sulfate is a more potent inhibitor of clot bound thrombin than unfractionated and low molecular weight heparins. *Thromb Hemostas* 1994;71:576–580.
175. Wright TC, Castellot JJ, Karnovsky MJ. Regulation of cellular proliferation by heparin and heparan sulfate. In: Lane DA, Lindahl U, eds. *Heparin.* London: Edward Arnold; 1989:295–316.
176. Nikkari ST, Clowes AW. Heparin and heparinoids: Control of the intimal hyperplastic response. In: Quinones-Baldrich WJ, ed. *Pharmacologic Suppression of Intimal Hyperplasia.* Austin, TX: RG Landes; 1993:69–79.
177. Snow AD, Bolender RP, Wight TN, Clowes AW. Heparin modulates the composition of the extracellular matrix domain surrounding arterial smooth muscle cells. *Am J Pathol* 1990;137:313–330.
178. Yamada KM. Fibronectin and other cell interactive glycoproteins. In: Hay E, ed. *Cell Biology of Extracellular Matrix,* 2nd ed. New York: Plenum Press; 1991:111–146.
179. Schwarzbauer JE. Alternative splicing of fibronectin—three variants, three functions. *Bioessays* 1991;13:527–533.
180. Risau W, Lemmon V. Changes in vascular extracellular matrix during embryonic vasculogenesis and angiogenesis. *Dev Biol* 1988;125: 441–450.

181. Saouaf R, Takasaki I, Eastman E, Chobanian AV, Brecher P. Fibronectin biosynthesis in the rat aorta in vitro. Changes due to experimental hypertension. *J Clin Invest* 1991;88:1182–1189.
182. Takasaki I, Chobanian AV, Mamuya WS, Brecher P. Hypertension induces alternatively spliced forms of fibronectin in rat aorta. *Hypertension* 1992;20:20–25.
183. Stenman S, Vaheri A. Distribution of a major connective tissue protein fibronectin in normal human tissue. *J Exp Med* 1978;147:1054–1061.
184. Smith EB, Ashall C. Fibronectin distribution in human aortic intima and atherosclerotic lesions, concentration of soluble and collagenase-releasable fractions. *Biochim Biophys Acta* 1986;880:10–15.
185. Rasmussen LH, Garbarsch C, Chemnitz J, Collatz Christnesen B, Lorenzen I. Injury and repair of smaller muscular and elastic arteries. Immunohistochemical demonstration of fibronectin and fibrinogen/fibrin and their degradation products in rabbit femoral and common carotid arteries following a dilatation injury. *Virchows Archiv [A] Pathol Anat* 1989;415:579–585.
186. Boudreau N, Turley E, Rabinovitch M. Fibronectin, Histopath and a hyaluronan binding protein contribute to increased ductus arteriosus smooth muscle cell migration. *Dev Biol* 1991;143:235–247.
187. Molossi S, Clausell N, Rabinovitch M. Coronary artery endothelial interleukin-1 β mediates enhanced fibronectin production related to post-cardiac transplant arteriopathy in piglets. *Circulation* 1993;88: 248–256.
188. Clausell N, Rabinovtich M. Upregulation of fibronectin synthesis by interleuken-1 β in coronary artery smooth muscle cells is associated with the development of the post cardiac transplant arteriopathy in piglets. *J Clin Invest* 1993;92:1850–1858.
189. Clausell N, Correa de Lima V, Molossi S, Liu P, Turley E, Gotlieb AI, Adelman AG, Rabinovitch M. Expression of tumor necrosis factor alpha and accumulation of fibronectin in coronary artery restenotic lesions retrieved by atherectomy. *Br Heart J [in press].*
190. van der Hoek Y, Sangrar W, Côté GP, Kastelein JJP, Koschinsky ML. Binding of recombinant apolipoprotein (a) to extracellular matrix proteins. *Arterioscler Thromb* 1994;14:1792–1798.
191. Madri JA, Basson MD. Extracellular matrix–cell interactions: Dynamic modulators of cell, tissue and organism structure and function. *Lab Invest* 1992;66:519–521.
192. Casscells W. Migration of smooth muscle cells and endothelial cells. Critical events in restenosis. *Circulation* 1992;86:723–729.
193. Clyman RI, McDonald KA, Kramer RH. Integrin receptors on aortic smooth muscle cells mediate adhesion to fibronectin laminin and collagen. *Circ Res* 1990;67:175–186.
194. Glukhova MA, Frid MG, Shekhonin BV, Balabanov YV, Koteliansky VE. Expression of fibronectin variants in vascular and visceral smooth muscle cells in development. *Dev Biol* 1990;141:193–202.
195. Glukhova MA, Frid MG, Shekhonin BV, Vasilevskaya TD, Grunwald J, Saginati M, Koteliansky VE. Expression of extra domain A fibronectin sequence in vascular smooth muscle cells is phenotype dependent. *J Cell Biol* 1989;109:357–366.
196. Tryggvasson K. The laminin family. *Curr Opin Cell Biol* 1993;5: 877–882.
197. Mecham RP. Receptors for laminin on mammalian cells. *FASEB J* 1991;5:2538–2546.
198. Grant DS, Tashiro KI, Sequi-Real B, Yamada Y, Martin GR, Kleinman HK. Two different laminin domains mediate the differentiation of human endothelial cells into capillary like structures in vitro. *Cell* 1989;58:933–943.
199. Schnaper HW, Kleinman HK, Grant DS. Role of laminin in endothelial cell recognition and differentiation. *Kidney Int* 1993;43:20–25.
200. Hedin U, Bottger BA, Forsberg E, Johansson S, Thyberg J. Diverse effects of fibronectin and laminin on phenotypic properties of cultured arterial smooth muscle cells. *J Cell Biol* 1988;107:307–319.
201. Thyberg J, Hultgardh-Nilsson A. Fibronectin and basement membrane components laminin and collagen type IV influence the phenotypic properties of subcultured rat aortic smooth muscle cells differently. *Cell Tissue Res* 1994;276:263–271.
202. Slepian MJ, Massia SP. Local delivery of a YIGSR peptide inhibits neointimal hyperplasia following balloon injury. *Circulation* 1994; 90:(4), pt 2:X-297.
203. Bornstein P. The thrombospondins: Structure and regulation of expression. *FASEB J* 1992;6:3290–3299.
204. Silverstein RL. *Interactions of Thrombospondin with the Fibronolytic System.* Lahau J, ed. Boca Raton, FL: CRC Press; 1993:165–176.
205. Adams JC, Lawler J. Diverse mechanisms for cell attachment to platelet thrombospondin. *J Cell Sci* 1993;104:1061–1071.
206. Majack RA, Goodman LV, Dixit VM. Cell surface thrombospondin is functionally essential for vascular smooth muscle cell proliferation. *J Cell Biol* 1988;106:415–422.
207. Scott-Burden T, Resink TJ, Hahn AW, Buhler FR. Induction of thrombospondin expression in vascular smooth muscle cells by angiotensin II. *J Cardiovasc Pharmacol* 1990;16:S17–S20.
208. Miano JM, Vlasic N, Tota RR, Stemerman MB. Smooth muscle cell immediate early gene and growth factor activation follows vascular injury. A putative in vivo mechanism for autocrine growth. *Arterioscler Thromb* 1993;13:211–219.
209. Schultz-Cherry S, Riberio S, Gentry L, Murphy-Ullrich JE. Thrombospondin binds and activates the small and large forms of latent transforming growth factor-beta in a chemically defined system. *J Biol Chem* 1994;269:26775–26782.
210. Sage H, Bornstein P. Extracellular proteins that modulate cell–matrix interactions. SPARC, tenascin and thrombospondin. *J Biol Chem* 1991;266:24831–14834.
211. Wight TN, Raugi GJ, Mumby SM, Bornstein P. Light microscopic immunolocation of thrombospondin secretion in human tissues. *J Histochem Cytyochem* 1984;33:280–288.
212. Raugi GJ, Mullen JS, Barb DH, Okada T, Mayberg MR. Thrombospondin deposition in rat carotid artery injury. *Am J Pathol* 1990;137: 179–185.
213. Taraboletti G, Roberts D, Liotta LA, Giavazzi R. Platelet thrombospondin modulates endothelial cell adhesion, motility and growth: a potential angiogenesis regulatory factor. *J Cell Biol* 1990;111: 765–772.
214. Good DJ, Polverini PJ, Rastinejad F, Le-Beau MM, Lemons RS, Frazier WA, Bouck NP. A tumor suppressor dependent inhibitor of angiogenesis is immunologically and functionally indistinguishable from a fragment of thrombospondin. *Proc Natl Acad Sci USA* 1990;87: 6624–6628.
215. Erickson HP. Tenascin C, tenascin R, and tenascin X: A family of talented proteins in search of functions. *Curr Opin Cell Biol* 1993;5: 869–876.
216. Hurle JM, Garcia-Martinez V, Ros MA. Immunofluorescent localization of tenascin during the morphogenesis of the outflow tract of the chick embryo heart. *Anat Embryol* 1990;181:149–155.
217. Riou JF, Umbhauer M, Shi DL, Boucaut JC. Tenascin: A potential modulator of cell–extracellular matrix interactions during vertebrate embryogenesis. *Biol Cell* 1992;75:1–9.
218. Hedin U, Holm J, Hansson GK. Induction of tenascin in rat arterial injury, relationship to altered smooth muscle phenotype. *Am J Pathol* 1991;139:649–656.
219. Mackie EJ, Scott-Burden T, Hahn AWA, Kein F, Bernhardt J, Regenass S, Weller A, Buhler FR. Expression of tenascin by vascular smooth muscle cells. Alterations in hypertensive rats and stimulation by Angiotensin II. *Am J Pathol* 1992;141:377–388.
220. Kasayaki N, Ueda M, Lixin W, Teragoki M, Takeuchi I, Tokeda T, Becker AE. Tenascin may serve as a marker for the healing process in human coronary arteries after PCTA. *Circulation* 1993;88:I-656.
221. LaFleur DW, Fagin JA, Forrester JS, Rubin SA, Sharifi BG. Cloning and characterization of alternatively spliced isoforms of rat tenascin. Platelet-derived growth factor-BB markedly stimulates expression of spliced variants of tenascin mRNA in arterial smooth muscle cells. *J Biol Chem* 1994;269:20757–20763.
222. Sriramaroo P, Mendler M, Bourdon MA. Endothelial cell attachment and spreading on human tenascin is mediated by $\alpha2\beta1$ and $\alpha v\beta3$ integrins. *J Cell Sci* 1993;105:1001–1012.
223. Murphy-Ullrich JE, Lightner VA, Aukhil I, Yan YZ, Erickson HP. Focal adhesion integrity is down regulated by the alternatively spliced domain of human tenascin. *J Cell Biol* 1991;115:1127–1136.
224. Denhardt DT, Guo X. Osteopontin: A protein with diverse functions. *FASEB J* 1993;7:1475–1482.
225. Giachelli CC, Schwartz SM, Liaw L. Molecular and cellular biology of osteopontin: Potential role in cardiovascular disease. *Trends Cardiovasc Med* [in press].
226. Hirota S, Imakita M, Kohri K, Ito A, Morri E, Adachi S, Kim H, Kitamura Y, Yutani C, Normura S. Expression of osteopontin messenger RNA by macrophages in atherosclerotic plaques. *Am J Pathol* 1993;143:1003–1008.
227. Ikeda T, Shiraswa T, Esaki Y, Yoshiki S, Hirokawa K. Osteopontin

mRNA is expressed by smooth muscle derived foam cells in human atherosclerotic lesions of the aorta. *J Clin Invest* 1993;92:2814–2820.
228. O'Brien ER, Garvin MR, Stewart DK, Hinohara R, Simpson JB, Schwartz SM, Giachelli CM. Osteopontin is synthesized by macrophage smooth muscle and endothelial cells in primary and restenotic human coronary atherosclerotic plaques. *Arterioscler Thromb* 1994; 14:1648–1656.
229. Gadeau A-P, Campan M, Millet D, Candresse T, Desgranges C. Osteopontin overexpression is associated with arterial smooth muscle cell proliferation in vitro. *Arterioscler Thromb* 1993; 13:120–125.
230. Brooks PC, Clark RAF, Cheresh DA. Requirement of vascular integrin $\alpha v\beta 3$ angiogenesis. *Science* 1994;264:569–572.
231. Choi ET, Engel L, Collow AD, Sun S, Trachtenberg J, Santoro S, Ryan US. Inhibition of neointimal hyperplasia by blocking $\alpha v\beta 3$ integrin with a small peptide antagonist GpenGRGDSPCA. *J Vasc Surg* 1994;19:124–134.
232. Shabahan CM, Cary NR, Metcalfe JC, Weissberg PL. High expression of genes for calcification-regulating proteins in human atherosclerotic plaques. *J Clin Invest* 1994;93:2393–2402.
233. Wight TN. *The extracellular matrix and atherosclerosis in disease of the arterial wall.* In: Camilleri J-P, Berry CL, Riessinger J-N, Bariety J, eds. Flammarion Medical-Sciences, France, 1987;163–173.
234. Wight TN. In: *Biology of Proteoglycan.* Wight TN, Mecham RP, eds. Orlando, FL: Academic Press, 1987;267–300.

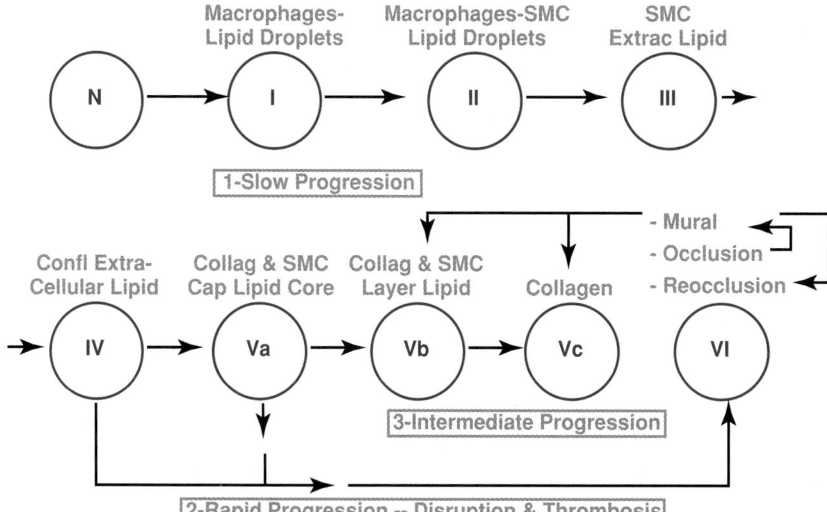

FIG. 2. Schematic of lesion morphology of the progression of coronary atherosclerosis according to the histopathologic findings. (*SMC,* Smooth muscle cells; *Extrac,* extracellular; *Confl,* confluent; *Collag,* collagen. (Reprinted from Fuster, ref. 7, with permission.)

is covered by a thin fibrous cap. Over time types IV and Va can evolve into more stenotic and fibrotic types of lesions, classified as type Vb, which contains increased numbers of smooth muscle cells and connective tissue, as well as lipid; and type Vc, which has still larger amounts of collagen. Both of these types can become increasingly stenotic (Fig. 1). Thus phase 2 can evolve either into phase 3 or phase 4 (Fig. 1). A phase 4 lesion has been classified as having a ''complicated'' type VI lesions (Fig. 2), as a result of lesion rupture or fissure, the formation of a thrombus, and sudden occlusion of the artery with the clinical development of an acute coronary syndrome. The occlusive thrombus may eventually become fibrotic or occlusive phase 5. In contrast, in phase 3, the ''complicated'' type VI lesion can form a mural thrombus, which may not completely occlude the artery and may progress to become a fibrotic, nonocclusive phase 5 (Fig. 1) that may gradually evolve into an occlusive lesion. Because of a more gradual rate of lumen closure, sufficient time may elapse for collateral vessels to form and thus clinical angina may or may not be present (7).

Although this terminology initially appears to be complicated, a perusal of Figs. 1 and 2 demonstrates that this approach takes advantage of both the phases of lesion evolution and the types of lesions, so that investigators and clinicians alike may share a common language and understanding of these processes.

This chapter will emphasize the cellular elements involved in lesion development, including the roles of the monocyte/macrophage, the T-lymphocyte, the smooth muscle cell, and the endothelium, some of their numerous interactions, and many of the molecules for which genes are expressed in these cells that play a role in lesion formation and progression. Chapter 34 deals with the principles associated with the growth-regulatory molecules and cytokines derived from these cells that play a role in the process of atherogenesis.

THE FATTY STREAK AND LESION PROGRESSION

The earliest grossly detectable lesion of atherosclerosis is the fatty streak, which can be found in infants and is ubiquitous in Western society (8–12). The fatty streak consists of an accumulation of lipid within macrophages, or foam cells, in the intima of the artery. The lipid appears to accumulate as a result of active transport of lipoprotein particles by the endothelial cells into the artery wall (13,14). During the process of transcytosis of these lipid (presumably LDL) particles, they may be modified by the endothelial cells, possibly in the form of oxidation (15,16). Simionescu and colleagues have suggested that one of the earliest phases in the process of atherogenesis involves an accumulation of lipid particles beneath the endothelium, sometimes between the basement membrane and the endothelium, and often below the basement membrane. The accumulated lipid has the appearance of LDL particles and of membrane-delimited particles which they have called ''liposomes'' (17). Thus the early entry of lipoprotein particles into the artery wall may result in the deposition of modified LDL (oxLDL) within the intima at early stages of life when intake of lipid is high.

As discussed in Chapter 8, oxLDL may play an important role in inducing the earliest phase of atherogenesis. Because it is injurious to cells, oxLDL can induce a reactive response in the artery wall leading to the inflammatory changes described below. Other forms of modified LDL may behave in a similar manner (18). In diabetics LDL may undergo glycation similar to other substances termed advanced glycation endproducts (AGE), resulting in free radicals similar to those associated with the formation of oxLDL (19,20). Focal accumulation and modification of LDL can have injurious effects that result in changes in the endothelium. The endothelial cells form molecules that result in rolling, attachment, adhesion, and migration of monocytes into the artery, which

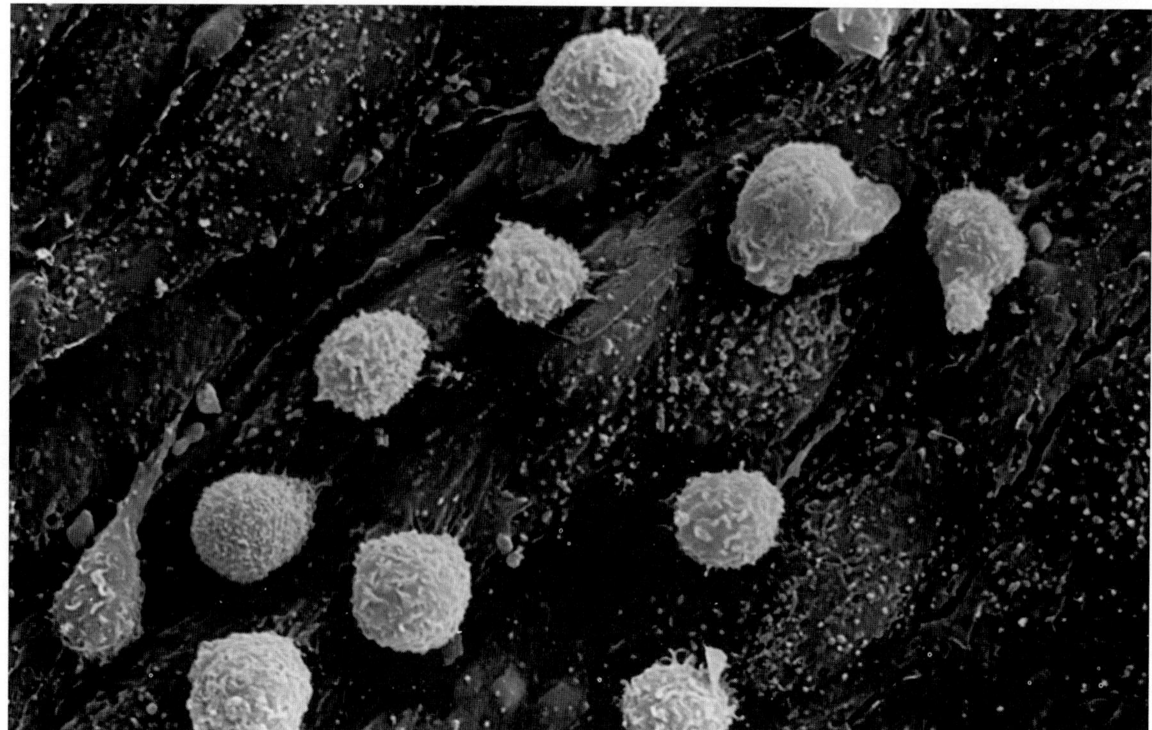

FIG. 3. Scanning electron micrograph showing a number of adherent leukocytes (both monocytes and T cells) on the surface of the endothelium of a hypercholesterolemic nonhuman primate. They demonstrate the first phase of atherogenesis, the formation of adhesion molecules with leukocyte rolling, sticking, adherence, and spreading on the surface of the endothelium.

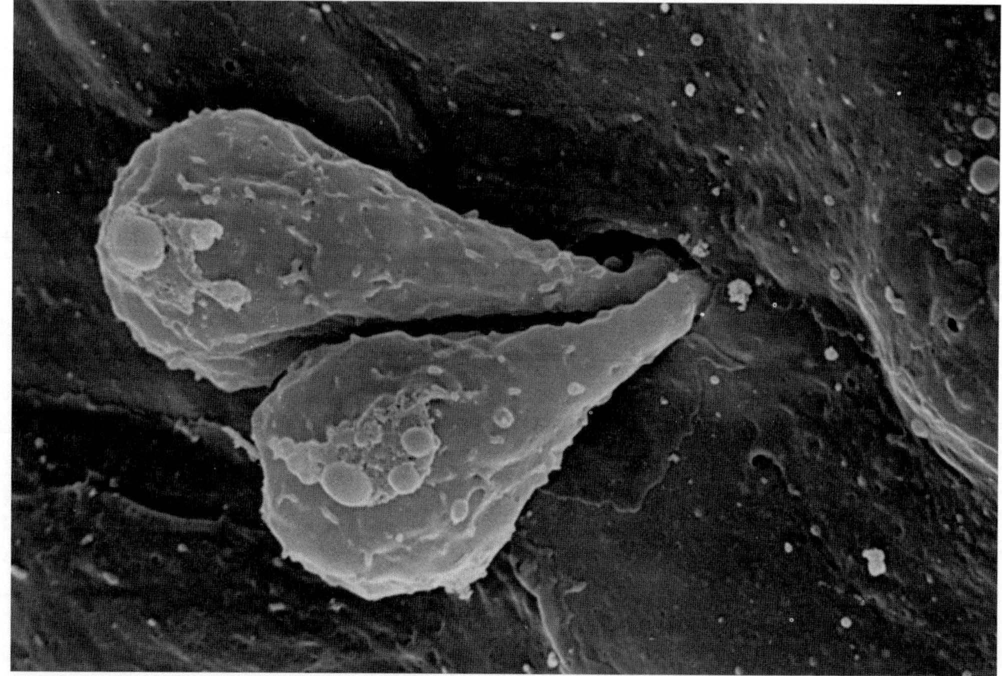

FIG. 4. Scanning electron micrograph demonstrates leukocytes entering into the artery wall between endothelial junctions. Thoracic aorta of nonhuman primate at six months. ×4000. (Reprinted from Masuda and Ross, ref. 47, with permission.)

become activated as macrophages after they enter the intima (21–25). The monocytes adhere as a result of expression by the endothelium of a series of molecules termed selectins (E-, L-, and P-selectin) that can play a role in inducing the monocytes to marginate, roll, and attach on the surface of the endothelium (Fig. 3). The selectins are usually accompanied by formation of vascular cell adhesion molecules (VCAM-1) and intercellular adhesion molecules (ICAM-1) by the endothelium that result in adherence and spreading on the endothelial surface (22). A number of different factors may induce the endothelial cells to express the genes for these molecules. Low shear and turbulent flow characteristics can induce ICAM-1 to form on the endothelium. However, modified LDL has a particular propensity to induce both ICAM-1 and VCAM-1 (22,25,26) and thus may be particularly important in the earliest phases of the inflammatory process (see Chapter 29).

Entry into the artery by the monocytes is generated by the formation of specific chemotactic agents, which form a concentration gradient that leads to the directed migration of the cells from the luminal surface of the endothelium into the artery wall (Fig. 4). Agents such as monocyte chemotactic protein-1 (MCP-1) (27–29), colony-stimulating factors (CSF), and oxLDL (30,31) together with degradation products of the connective tissues can attract the monocytes to enter (32). Once the monocytes have entered the intima and become macrophages, they then take up the modified LDL via scavenger and other receptors and become foam cells (33–35). Together with T-lymphocytes, which appear to accompany the monocytes as they enter the artery wall, the foam cells form the ubiquitous, first, and most common lesion of atherosclerosis, the fatty streak. Grossly, the fatty streak appears as an irregular yellow discoloration on the luminal surface of the artery, due to the accumulation of lipid-filled macrophages (foam cells) that cluster beneath the endothelium. If an individual remains hyperlipidemic, foam cells will continue to accumulate at these sites in large numbers. Fatty streaks can occur throughout the arterial tree. However, they initially form at branches and bifurcations where there is a decrease in blood flow, turbulent flow (see Chapter 34), and an associated focal increase in adhesion molecules (Fig. 5).

With prolonged hyperlipidemia, the fatty streak can become more complicated and take on the appearance of the so-called fibrofatty or intermediate lesion. Thus, it progresses from types I–III to a type IV lesion (Figs. 1 and 2). This lesion may consist of multiple, alternating layers of foam cells and smooth muscle cells, which may be surrounded by some connective tissue in an uneven, complex

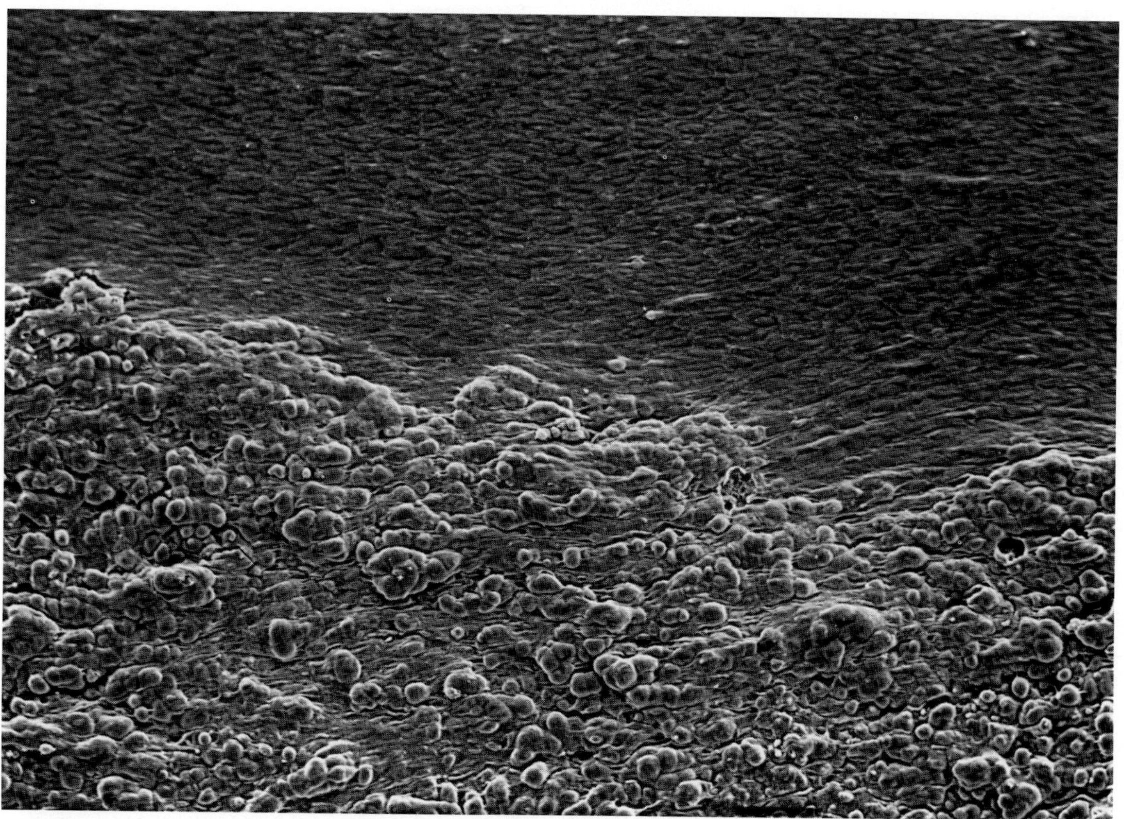

FIG. 5. A fatty streak that has formed in a nonhuman primate, which has been hypercholesterolemic for approximately 1 month. The irregular surface of the endothelium, the deep folds, and bulbous projections demonstrate the presence of foam cells that underlie the endothelium in this fatty streak. A few adherent leukocytes on the surface can be observed. They will enter into the artery wall in the continuing expansion of the fatty streak.

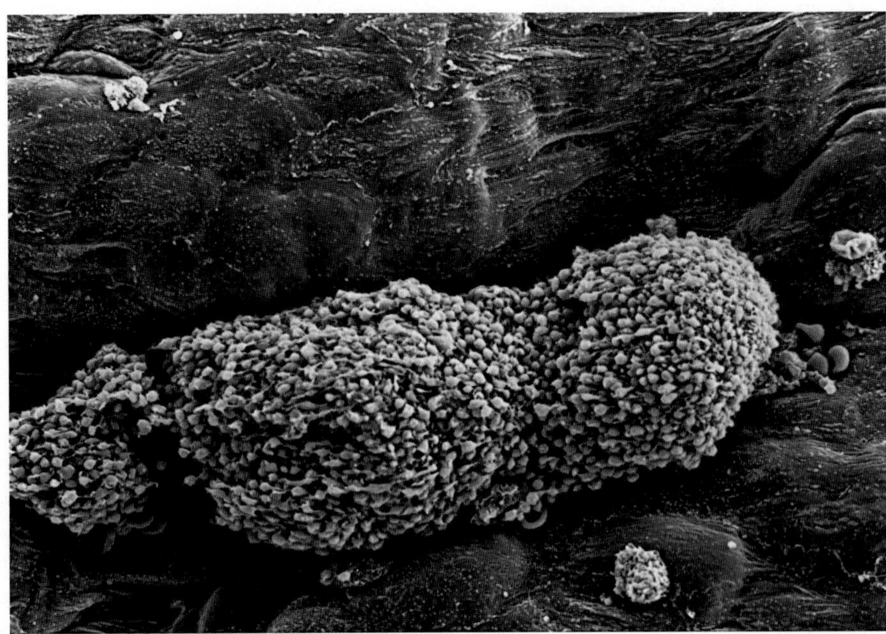

FIG. 6. Numerous platelet aggregates adhere to exposed macrophages associated with a fatty streak. Attached monocytes, presumably in the process of entry into the lesion, are present on the surface of the fatty streak. (Reprinted from Faggiotto and Ross, ref. 46, with permission.)

arrangement. If the lesion increases in size, the intima may become thicker and somewhat raised in its gross appearance as a capsule surrounding a lipid core or type Va lesion. Specifically, the type Va lesion contains a fibrous cap of connective tissue with smooth muscle cells intermixed with monocyte-derived macrophages and T-lymphocytes surrounded by a matrix of varying density consisting of collagen, proteoglycans, and small elastic fibers. When it is sufficiently well formed, the fibrous cap of the type Va lesion overlies accumulations of macrophages, T-lymphocytes, extracellular lipid, necrotic debris, and sometimes calcification and appears to protect the less structured, necrotic elements of the lesion from the blood and thrombus formation (36,37). Eventually, type IV–Va lesions can evolve into the more stenotic and fibrotic type Vb and Vc lesions. However, where the cap is thin or where there are accumulations of macrophages and T-lymphocytes, fissures or erosions may occur for example, at the shoulders of the type Va lesion which can become subject to turbulent rheologic forces. These forces can lead to fissure, tears, ulceration, hemorrhage, and occlusive thrombosis, or the so-called ''complicated'' or type VI lesion of the acute coronary syndromes (see Chapter 31). Most frequently, however, the fissured or ulcerated type VI lesions contain a mural thrombus which, from its organization by connective tissue, can contribute to the rapid and often silent progression of the disease into the most stenotic or occlusive fibrotic type Vb and Vc lesions (Fig. 6).

ANIMAL MODELS OF ATHEROSCLEROSIS

The development of the fatty streak and the progression of the fatty streak to the various intermediate forms and finally to the advanced lesions of atherosclerosis have been observed in a large number of experimental animals, including rabbits (38,39), swine (40–42), pigeons (43,44), nonhuman primates (45–48), and, most recently, in a series of genetically modified transgenic mice (49,50). All of these observations have been confirmed in a series of human lesions obtained from hearts removed for transplant, perfuse fixed, and examined by light and electron microscopy (51).

The genetically modified mice, in particular, the homozygous apoprotein E (ApoE)-deficient and LDL-receptor-deficient mice, offer opportunities to study lesion formation and progression and approaches to intervening in this process in a small murine model that can be genetically modified. These two models, particularly the ApoE-deficient mouse (49) (see Chapter 20), have demonstrated the same cellular involvement observed in the development of human lesions with a sequence of cellular changes at similar sites as those found in both nonhuman primates and humans. It has been possible to demonstrate by *en face* examination in the ApoE-deficient mouse the formation of two adhesion molecules, VCAM-1 and ICAM-1, at sites where fatty streaks are prone to form. These studies show for the first time that ICAM-1 is upregulated at these sites on the basis of the local rheologic properties of the artery. The upregulation of ICAM-1 is related to the formation of the specific adhesion molecule, VCAM-1, which is increased by hyperlipidemia. Together they result in monocyte and lymphocyte adhesion (Y. Nakashima et al., unpublished observations).

Additional approaches using genetically modified mice can include, for example, crossbreeding the ApoE-deficient mouse with the mouse containing the gene for ApoAI that produces increased levels of HDL or with mice containing the transgene for Lp(a), thus studying the effects of combining specific genes upon the incidence of atherosclerosis. Such combinations offer remarkable opportunities to understand the roles of specific molecules in the process of atherogenesis and to develop specific modes of intervention and prevention (see Chapter 20).

THE RESPONSE-TO-INJURY HYPOTHESIS OF ATHEROSCLEROSIS

In 1856, Rudolph Virchow suggested that the lesions of atherosclerosis result from some form of injury to the artery wall (52). His ideas were formulated at about the same time that von Rokitansky suggested that the intimal thickening of the artery resulted from the deposition of fibrin and other blood elements, also associated with some form of injury to the artery (53). Both hypotheses took into account the accumulation of lipid as a primary or secondary phenomenon in association with the injury. In 1946, Duguid suggested that intimal thickening occurred as the result of accumulation of fibrin and platelets (54). Twenty years later, French stressed the inflammatory components of this process as important in the development of the lesions of atherosclerosis (55).

By 1973 (56) it became apparent, based on the work of Wissler and colleagues (57), that smooth muscle accumulation or proliferation was a key element in the development of the lesions of atherosclerosis. Their observations in humans and animals, together with those of Haust (58), led us to suggest that some form of "injury" to the lining endothelium, and possibly to the underlying smooth muscle cells of the artery wall, results in what in its early phases would be considered a protective response (1–4). The injured cells somehow induce a specialized, chronic, inflammatory response followed by a healing or fibroproliferative response. Since the response-to-injury hypothesis was first formulated, it has been tested, modified, retested, and remodified. The most recent formulation suggests that dysfunctional alterations in the overlying endothelium somehow result from the various associated risk factors, resulting in the formation of several adhesive glycoproteins on the surface of the endothelium, which can bind to appropriate receptors on circulating monocytes and T-lymphocytes. These adhesion molecules include E-selectin, P-selectin, VCAM-1, and ICAM-1. After attaching and adhering, the leukocytes are attracted to migrate into the intima of the artery between endothelial cells due to the generation of chemoattractants by the endothelium, by smooth muscle, or both. Once in the intima, the monocytes become activated as macrophages, ingest the modified lipids that precede them into the artery wall, and can also generate molecules that are chemotactic for additional monocytes. Activated macrophages can express genes for a series of growth factors and cytokines (see Chapter 30, Table 2), which can have profound effects upon neighboring macrophages, T-lymphocytes, smooth muscle cells, and the overlying endothelium (1).

Thus three critical processes are involved in the formation of the lesions of atherosclerosis: (a) focal intimal migration, proliferation, and accumulation of macrophages, T-lymphocytes, and smooth muscle cells; (b) formation of connective tissue matrix, including elastic fiber proteins, several forms of collagen, and proteoglycans by the accumulated smooth muscle cells; and (c) accumulation of lipid within macrophages and smooth muscle, as well as the surrounding extracellular matrix.

Studies of the different stages of lesion development in experimental animals described above and in humans support the above description of cellular interactions as key elements in the process of atherogenesis.

The hypothesis proposes that injury to the artery leads to the formation of a specialized, chronic, inflammatory response that involves both monocytes and certain subsets of T-lymphocytes (CD4+ and CD8+). The relative absence of granulocytic cells is notable. This inflammatory response may continue as long as the factors responsible for the endothelial dysfunction remain. Over time, individuals who are chronically hypercholesterolemic, hypertensive, diabetic, are cigarette smokers, have high levels of homocysteine, or have combinations of these factors will continue to have functional injury induced to the lining endothelial cells. As a consequence, this injury will continue to elicit localized, specialized inflammatory responses in the artery wall, which, if sufficiently chronic, may become excessive. In its excess, the inflammation may result in toxic damage to the cells of the artery, as well as an ensuing fibroproliferative response to wall off the inflammation. Taken together, these responses may also become excessive if the stimuli that result in accumulation of smooth muscle and macrophages and formation of connective tissue do not abate. Thus, what begins as a protective, inflammatory-fibroproliferative response can become sufficiently excessive that it, in itself, becomes the disease entity atherosclerosis (1) (Fig. 7).

Recent data have suggested an additional phenomenon that may be partially responsible for leukocyte and smooth muscle accumulation in the lesions of atherosclerosis. This is inhibition of the process of programmed cell death or apoptosis, decreased cell turnover, and toxic cell death. These phenomena are critical in determining whether cells accumulate at a given site. Inhibition of cell turnover and of apoptosis may have an important bearing on the continued accumulation of smooth muscle cells and macrophages in the lesions of atherosclerosis (discussed below).

CELLULAR INTERACTIONS IN ATHEROGENESIS

Endothelium

The response-to-injury hypothesis states that the injurious responses initially occur to the lining endothelium of the

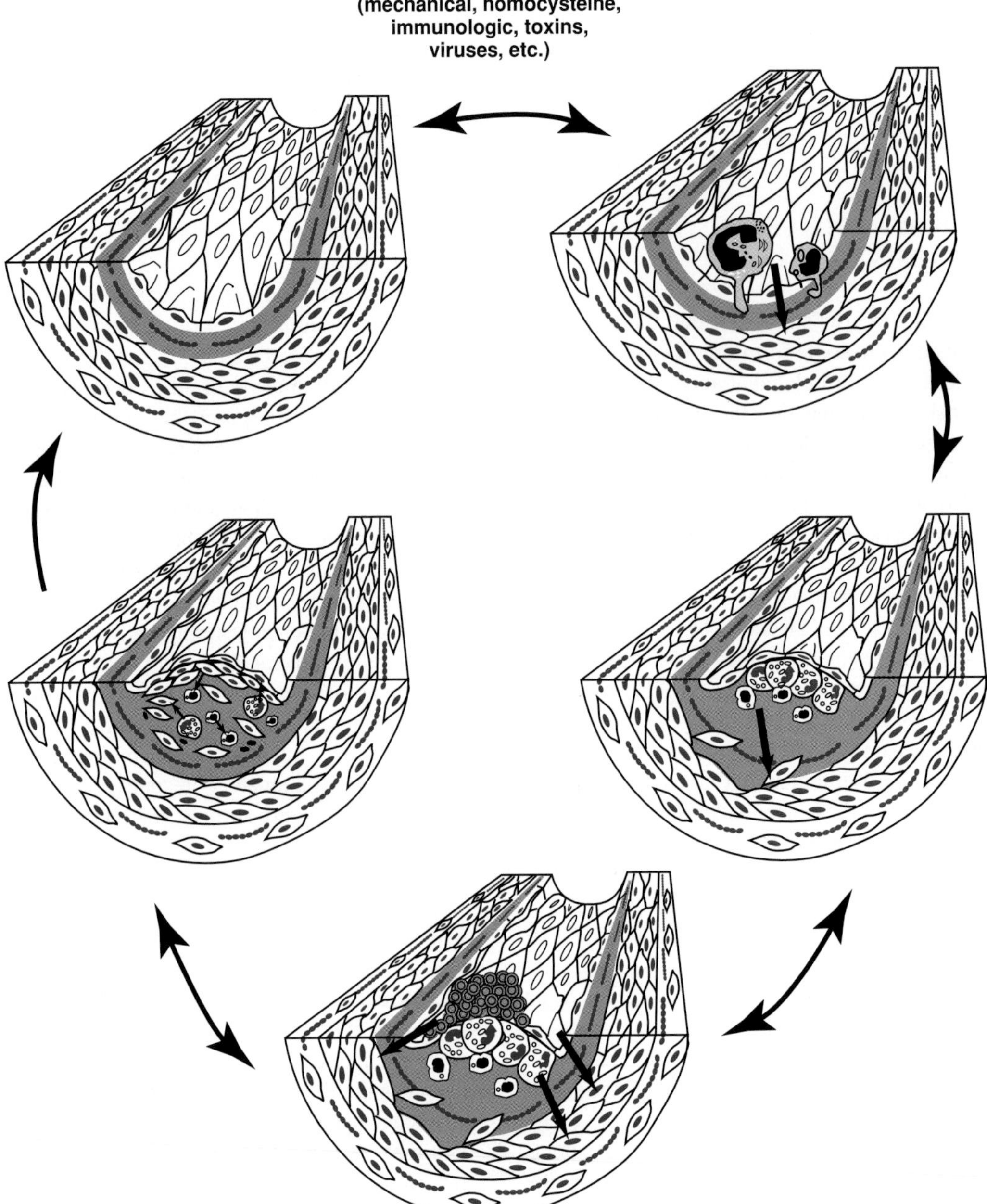

FIG. 7. In the response-to-injury hypothesis of atherosclerosis, several different sources of injury to the endothelium can lead to endothelial cell dysfunction. One of the parameters associated with endothelial cell dysfunction that results from exposure to agents such as oxidized LDL (oxLDL) is increased adherence to monocytes/macrophages and T-lymphocytes. These cells then migrate between the endothelium and localize subendothelially. The macrophages become large foam cells due to lipid accumulation and, with the T cells and smooth muscle, form a fatty streak. The fatty streak can then progress to an intermediate, fibrofatty lesion and ultimately to a fibrous plaque. As the lesions accumulate increasing numbers of cells and the macrophages scavenge the lipid, some of the lipid-laden macrophages may emigrate back into the bloodstream by pushing apart the endothelial cells. Upon doing so, those at sites such as branches and bifurcations where blood flow is irregular with eddy currents and back currents may become thrombogenic sites that lead to formation of platelet mural thrombi. Such thrombi can release many potent growth-regulatory molecules from the platelets that can join with those released by the activated macrophages and possibly by lesion smooth muscle cells into the artery wall. Platelet thrombi can also form at sites where endothelial dysjunction may have occurred. Ultimately, the formation and release of numerous growth-regulatory molecules and cytokines from a network established between cells in the lesion, consisting of activated macrophages, smooth muscle, T cells, and endothelium,

artery, leading to endothelial dysfunction. The endothelium is discussed in detail in Chapter 22. However, it may help to review some of the principal functions of the endothelial cells. They (a) serve as a permeability barrier through which substances from the plasma are transported and solutes are exchanged, (b) provide a nonthrombogenic surface for platelets by the generation of molecules such as prostacyclin (PGI_2), heparan sulfate, and an endothelial ecto-ADPase, (c) maintain vascular tone by the formation of molecules such as nitric oxide (NO), PGI_2, endothelin (ET), and angiotensin II (AII). (NO and PGI_2 can induce vasodilation; ET and AII can induce vasoconstriction), (d) form and secrete growth-regulatory molecules and cytokines, (e) form and maintain a connective tissue matrix including the basement membrane upon which the cells rest, as well as proteoglycans, specific forms of collagen, and other matrix molecules, (f) provide a nonadherent surface for circulating leukocytes, and (g) modify lipoproteins as they are transported into the artery wall (see Chapters 22, 29, and 34).

If some of these functional properties are altered as a result of the effects of hyperlipidemia, hypertension, diabetes, cigarette smoking, or other associated risk factors, then alterations in the homeostatic properties of the endothelium could become important in the genesis of the disease process.

As discussed above, endothelial cells are able to modify substances such as lipoproteins after they bind to receptors and are transcytosed via vesicles from the lumen of the artery to the subendothelial space. In this process they can modify (oxidize) the LDL, and this modified (oxidized) LDL can have profound effects on neighboring cells in the subendothelium. As discussed, oxLDL can induce adhesion molecules on the endothelium and can act as a chemoattractant for monocytes and lymphocytes to help bring them into the artery wall. OxLDL can be phagocytized via scavenger receptors on the monocytes, which become macrophages once they enter into the artery, leading to the formation of foam cells. As noted above, oxLDL can induce the formation of adhesion molecules, including several selectins and VCAM-1 on the surface of the endothelium. Such a cascade of events may result in increasing numbers of adherent leukocytes, which continue to be chemotactically attracted into the artery. After entering the artery, these cells can participate in further modification of the lipoproteins transported into the artery, leading to a vicious cycle of events if the individual remains hyperlipidemic (see Chapters 8 and 30).

Not only can the endothelium provide a nonthrombogenic surface by forming heparan sulfate, NO, and PGI_2, but it can also form a recently discovered ecto-ADPase that can prevent platelet adhesion and thus mural thrombosis (59). The endothelium also balances interactions between the coagulation and fibrinolytic systems by forming both plasminogen activator and urokinase. This balance may be perturbed during atherogenesis by the formation of plasminogen activator inhibitor (PAI-1), which can shift the balance toward thrombosis. Such a change may occur in the endothelium overlying developing lesions of atherosclerosis and thus participate in lesion progression (60–62) (see Chapters 35 and 36).

The endothelium not only lines the surface of the lesions, but is also involved in the process of angiogenesis of advanced thickened lesions, presumably to provide adequate vascularization of cells deep in these large lesions. Barger et al. demonstrated a network of adventitial microvessels that are associated with advanced complicated lesions using postmortem cinematography of silicone polymers and angiography (63). These observations supported early studies that showed a rich vascularization of the adventitia in the vicinity of advanced lesions of atherosclerosis. Apparently, after the intima exceeds a critical thickness, these vessels extend into the intima. O'Brien et al., in a study of atherectomy specimens obtained from advanced lesions of atherosclerosis, demonstrated proliferating cell nuclear antigen (PCNA)-positive endothelium in microvessels associated with advanced lesions both from primary specimens and to a greater degree in specimens from restenotic lesions (64). These sites of increased vascularization were often associated with collections of macrophages within the lesions as well. In addition, the microvasculature in these advanced lesions has been associated with intraplaque hemorrhage of advanced lesions that fissure, ulcerate, and thrombose (65).

Thus not only may the endothelium play a key role in maintaining homeostasis of the vessel by functioning as an intact monolayer over the surface of the lesion, but it may also affect lesion progression by a vascularization of advanced lesions. Alterations in its normal function appear to be critical in inducing both atherosclerosis and its progression.

Monocytes/Macrophages

The usual roles of the macrophage are to present antigen, act as a scavenger cell, and produce bioactive molecules (66). Macrophages are the principal cellular inflammatory mediator in atherogenesis because they are ubiquitous in all stages of the process (1). They act as scavenger cells, which can provide growth-regulatory molecules and cytokines that regulate, in part, the responses of T-lymphocytes, other macrophages, the endothelium, and the smooth muscle cell (67). They may be able to stimulate their own proliferation

lead to progression of the lesions of atherosclerosis to a fibrous plaque or advanced, complicated lesion. Each of the stages of lesion formation is potentially reversible. Thus, lesion regression can occur if the injurious agents are removed or when protective factors intervene to reverse the inflammatory and fibroproliferative processes. (Reprinted from Ross, ref. 1, with permission.)

by production of CSF and that of neighboring smooth muscle cells via platelet-derived growth factor (PDGF), heparin-binding BGF-like growth factor (HB-EGF), and other growth factors (see Chapter 30, Table 2), and lymphocytes via production of interleukin-2 (IL-2). Macrophage replication is a common feature of experimental atherogenesis (68,69). Together with smooth muscle proliferation, the macrophage production represents a key element in the process of cell accumulation in lesions of atherosclerosis (1).

Like endothelium, macrophages are able to modify (oxidize) LDL by a number of pathways, including the generation of NO, lipid peroxidation, and via formation of at least one form of lipoxygenase (70). Via these enzymes, the fatty acids undergo peroxidation, and short-chain aldehydes, ketones, and other substances are formed which can become covalently crosslinked to the apoprotein moiety of the LDL particle, permitting the modified LDL to bind to the scavenger receptor of the macrophage (34,70). If the macrophages form excessive oxLDL, it can be injurious to neighboring cells including smooth muscle and the overlying endothelium (71). To determine whether antioxidants can prevent the injurious effects on cells, clinical studies using vitamins C and E and β-carotene are underway. The pharmacologic agent probucol has been studied in nonhuman primates and in rabbits and produced a significant decrease in lesion size in the rabbit (72,73) and a decrease in fatty streaks and cell turnover in nonhuman primates (74).

The monocyte-derived macrophage can form a number of molecules that can profoundly affect neighboring cells in the lesions of atherosclerosis. Macrophages can form several matrix hydrolytic enzymes such as collagenase, stromelysin, and elastase, all of which may be important in lesion regression, as well as lesion stability (discussed below).

In summary, the monocyte-derived macrophage plays a critical role in inflammation and atherogenesis as a modifier of lipoproteins and as a source of vasoactive substances, of chemotactic, growth-inhibitory, and growth-stimulatory molecules, and of lytic enzymes. The ability to modify and optimize macrophage function, and thus optimize and utilize the protective role of the inflammatory process in order to prevent its excess, may represent a key to controlling the process of atherogenesis.

Smooth Muscle

Smooth muscle accumulation is a key event in the development of the advanced lesions of atherosclerosis—the fibrous plaque and complicated lesion. Normally in humans, there is a gradual concentric increase in the thickness of the intima of most muscular and elastic arteries with increasing age, so that most adults have several layers of circumferential smooth muscle cells in the intima (2). The eccentric, abnormal accumulation of smooth muscle cells in the intima, together with increasing numbers of macrophages and T-lymphocytes, accumulation of necrotic debris, and calcification, as well as the presence of small blood vessels termed vasa vasora, result in the formation of the advanced lesion of atherosclerosis, the fibrous plaque (4). In the past, it was assumed that smooth muscle cells represented a uniform population of cells in the lesion; however, there is increasing evidence to suggest otherwise. There may be diversity in smooth muscle cells in the lesions, such that some may be capable of replicating innumerable times, whereas others may be capable of very few doublings (75). Should such differences exist in smooth muscle cells in the artery wall or in the lesions of atherosclerosis, there is no way at present to distinguish the different types of cells. To complicate, but partially explain, these differences, smooth muscle cells are derived from different embryonic sources at different arterial sites during development (75). Thus some smooth muscle cells may respond differently to agonists than others, and these responses may differ throughout the arterial tree (76). Further, smooth muscle cells may form different phenotypes, two of which have been termed ''synthetic'' and ''contractile'' (77). In the contractile phenotype, cells are rich in myofilaments and contractile apparatus and are able to respond to vasoactive agents. In the synthetic state, they lose contractile elements, become rich in endoplasmic reticulum and Golgi complex, and can respond to a number of growth-regulatory molecules and cytokines. Such factors can be elaborated by the smooth muscle cells themselves as they interact with macrophages, endothelium, platelets, or other smooth muscle cells. Thus the intercellular interactions that occur during lesion formation and progression can profoundly affect the behavior of smooth muscle cells in terms of their migratory and proliferative activities as well as their synthesis of matrix molecules. They are in essence the principal source of connective tissue in the artery and in the lesion of atherosclerosis. Smooth muscle cells may also express more than one phenotype for adhesive molecules on their surfaces, known as integrins, which are important in their adherence to matrix molecules such as collagen, fibronectin, and osteopontin (78). The integrin phenotypic state of the smooth muscle cell may represent an important aspect of the cells' ability to respond to growth-regulatory and migratory signals (see Chapters 23 and 29).

T Cells, Immunity, and Atherosclerosis

Because large numbers of T-lymphocytes and monocyte-derived macrophages coexist within the lesions of atherosclerosis, it is possible that atherogenesis represents both an inflammatory reaction and an immune response (79–81) (see Chapter 31). Both endothelium and smooth muscle, as well as the macrophage, can present antigens to T-lymphocytes present in the lesions, although the nature of the antigen(s) remains unclear. The lesions of common atherosclerosis differ strikingly from those found in rejected transplanted hearts, where massive, concentric lesions form in the coronary arteries. Such immunity-induced lesions are more richly endowed in T-lymphocytes and macrophages than are the lesions of common atherosclerosis (82) (see Chapter 40).

Many T-lymphocytes in the lesions bear CD4 markers for the helper-inducer subclass of T cells, whereas others carry CD8 markers associated with cytolytic T-lymphocytes (82). Hansson and colleagues have determined that many lymphocytes adjacent to smooth muscle cells in the lesions express class II histocompatibility antigens (HLA-DR) (83). Smooth muscle cells can also express the class II histocompatibility complex and can form interferon-γ in the lesions. The lymphocytes in common atherosclerosis appear to be polyclonal (83). However, oxLDL appears to represent at least one source of antigen for the T cells (83). Thus, although immunity appears to play a role in common atherosclerosis, the nature of this role remains to be clarified (discussed in Chapter 31).

RELATIONSHIP OF LESION FORMATION TO FLOW CHARACTERISTICS

Many investigators have noted that the lesions of atherosclerosis begin to form at altered sites of blood flow (see Chapter 34). Lesions initially form at branches and bifurcations associated with outflow tracts where shear forces are decreased and where there is turbulence, back flow, and eddy currents (84). Lesions appear most likely to develop at branch points in an artery and at sites of curvature such as the lesser curvature of the aortic arch. The lateral leading edges of the flow divider at branches appear to be secondarily involved. Areas not associated with a particular outflow tract may be tertiarily involved. Where there is decreased shear, a longer time becomes available for contact between white blood cells, platelets, and the endothelium. If adhesive molecules form on the surface of the endothelium or on the leukocytes, there would be greater opportunity for these cells to stick, adhere, spread, and crawl between the endothleium into the vessel wall. Such interactions could then set the stage for the excessive, inflammatory-fibroproliferative response we call atherosclerosis.

PATHOGENESIS OF VULNERABLE PLAQUES

It is not unreasonable to assume that lipid accumulation, cell proliferation, and extracellular matrix synthesis may be linear with time. However, angiographic studies of the progression of coronary artery disease in humans demonstrate that this may not be so. New high-grade lesions often appear in segments of artery that were normal only months earlier at previous angiographic examination (85). This unpredictable and episodic progression may be caused by plaque disruption followed by thrombosis with changes in plaque geometry that lead to intermittent plaque growth and acute occlusive or ischemic syndromes (86,87). Pathologic studies suggest that small plaque rupture or fissures that result in changes in geometry, or mural thrombosis with fibrous organization, or both, are frequent, and play an important role in both silent and symptomatic progressions of coronary atherosclerosis (36,37). Studies of patients who die suddenly or shortly after the onset of unstable angina or myocardial infarction show that rupture of an atherosclerotic plaque complicated by occlusive thrombus commonly leads to development of an acute ischemic syndrome (88,89). Occlusive thrombi are usually anchored to fissures at the site of disruption. Recent angiographic and angioscopic studies, together with the pathologic studies, have established the association between plaque fissuring or ulceration and development of unstable angina, acute myocardial infarction, and sudden ischemic death (90–93).

Vulnerable or Unstable Mildly Stenotic Lesions

The severity of coronary artery stenosis and the number of diseased vessels are markers of cardiac morbidity and mortality (94). It is important to emphasize that angiographically mild coronary lesions may be associated with progression to severe stenosis or total occlusion, and may account for as many as two-thirds of patients who develop unstable angina or acute myocardial infarction. Ambrose et al. studied patients with unstable angina who underwent two sequential angiograms. Seventy-two percent of the lesions that showed progression had less than 50% stenosis on the first angiogram (95). Such lesions had a narrow neck and overhanging edges or scalloped borders in 71% of cases and are thought to represent plaque disruption with or without a partially occlusive thrombus (95). In fact, several studies showed that an occluded artery with only mild stenosis (less than 50%) on the first angiogram had less than 70% stenosis subsequently (85,96–98). Thus lesions presumably responsible for the acute ischemic event (unstable angina or myocardial infarction) may have only mild to moderate stenosis in a substantial number of patients at the time of the first evaluation. Using highly magnified cineangiographic views, Brown et al. found that the original lesions responsible for an acute myocardial infarction had less than 60% stenosis in two-thirds of patients (99).

Even though angiography is considered the standard means to evaluate coronary anatomy, this method may underestimate the severity of coronary atherosclerosis; consequently, the luminal area, as seen angiographically, may appear preserved despite extensive disease of the vessel (86,100,101). Accordingly, three important issues need to be considered in the evaluation of patients with coronary disease. First, although it is helpful as a determinant of severity of coronary disease, angiography cannot accurately predict the site of future coronary occlusion. Second, in most patients acute ischemic events are not necessarily a complication of severe fibrotic and calcified lesions, but more of the disruption of the associated mildly to moderately stenotic, lipid-rich plaques, often not even visible angiographically. Third, overall angiography may underestimate the extent and severity of atherosclerotic involvement of coronary arteries. Thus it is important to consider that the more severe the coronary disease at angiography, the higher the likelihood of the presence of small plaques prone to disruption (102).

Vulnerable or Unstable Lipid-Rich Plaques

As noted above, recent pathologic studies have revealed that atherosclerotic plaques prone to rupture are commonly composed of a crescentic mass of lipids separated from the vessel lumen by a fibrous cap (103), the so-called types IV and Va lesions (104). Plaques that undergo disruption tend to be relatively soft and have a high concentration of lipids and a thin fibrous cap that overlies the lipid mass (103). A particular configuration of the plaque in which the lipid pool is situated eccentrically is most commonly associated with fissuring (104). The increase in lipid in the pool is believed to result from continued insudation from the plasma. Much of the fibrous tissue between the core and the surface endothelium corresponds to the proteoglycan-rich layer of the intima infiltrated with macrophages and smooth muscle cells. In the fibrous plaque, collagen may have been synthesized as a reaction to the disruption of the intima by the accumulated extracellular lipid. In many cases it may include superimposed microthrombi that were incorporated and became organized (104). Noninvasive imaging of plaques with a high content of lipid is emerging as an important research tool, given the susceptibility of these plaques to rupture. In addition to intravascular ultrasound (100,101), it may soon be possible to detect fatty plaques within the vascular system by high-resolution techniques such as nuclear magnetic resonance imaging with spectroscopy (105–107) (Fig. 8).

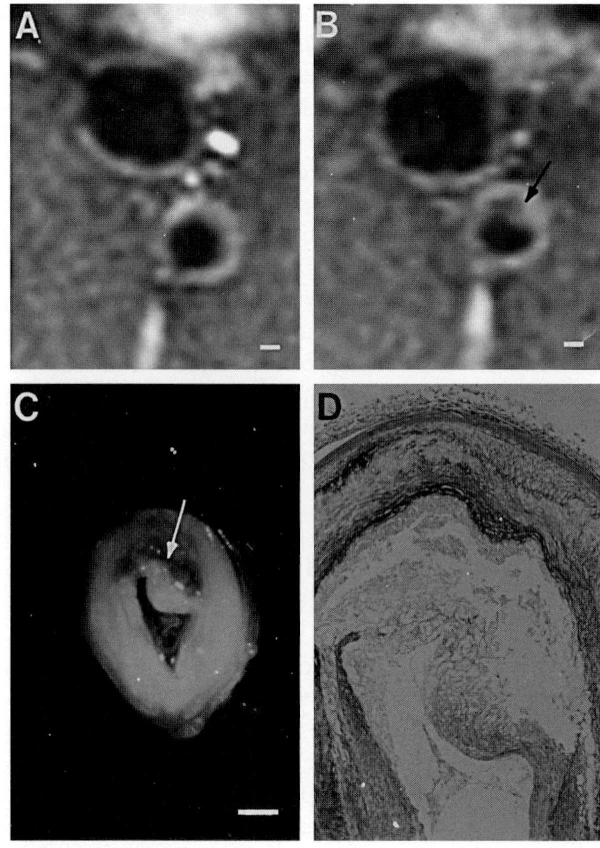

FIG. 8. Detection of plaque fissure by magnetic resonance imaging. The abdominal aortas from two rabbits containing advanced lesions of atherosclerosis were imaged 14 months after injury and initiation of an atherosclerotic diet. They were compared with the abdominal aorta of a control animal of equivalent size fed a normal diet. Serial proton-density weighted (PDW) images were acquired and are an identical distance from the bifurcation in the same animal at two time-points approximately 7 weeks apart. A branch at ~ 7 o'clock provides an internal landmark. These axial sections are derived from a region where clear progression of stenosis was seen in images obtained by time-of-flight angiography (not shown). **A:** PDW image at 12.5 months following diet initiation. **B:** PDW image obtained 7 weeks after the image in A. A dark region (*arrow*) developed spontaneously in the ventral wall of the artery that shows a hemorrhagic defect in a necrotic core, as seen in gross specimen C. **C:** Dissection microscopy of the same vessel segment imaged in B. A hemorrhagic defect in the necrotic core of the fibrous plaque (*arrow*) is apparent in the ventral wall of the artery and corresponds to the opaque region seen when imaged in vivo **(B).** This animal died while being scanned due to an overdose of anesthesia and could not be perfusion fixed. Consequently, the lumen contour was not preserved. **D:** Histology of the vessel segment imaged in B and observed under the dissecting microscope in C. The section is from the area of the defect seen by dissection microscopy in C. The immersion-fixed artery was paraffin embedded, sectioned, and stained with Masson's trichrome. The magnification is 100 ×. (Reprinted with permission from *Nature Medicine*.).

Effects of Local Stress on Plaque Vulnerability

Alterations in stress within the atherosclerotic plaque may be important in the development of plaque rupture. Using computer modeling for the analysis of tensile stress across the artery wall, Richardson et al. (103), Loree et al. (108), and Cheng et al. (109) found high concentrations of stress at the ends of fibrous caps overlying an area of pooled lipid, particularly when the pool exceeds 45% of the vessel circumference (103). In this area, the fibrous cap of the plaque lacks underlying collagen support and tends to be rich in macrophages. Such sites are the most susceptible to rupture (103). Thus the risk of fissuring can be predetermined by at least four factors: circumferential wall stress, localized wall stress or structural configuration, blood flow rheology or external configuration, and lipid density (crystals) as it relates to the process of regression (110–117) (see Chapter 28).

The Role of Macrophages in Vulnerable or Unstable Plaques

As discussed in Chapter 30, macrophages participate in the uptake and metabolism of lipids as well as cellular and metabolic processes during every phase of atherogenesis. In the most advanced stages of the disease, they can release proteases (elastase and collagenase) that, together with toxic products that are generated (free radicals, products of lipid oxidation), may facilitate arterial damage and plaque disruption. Histologic examination of ruptured or nearly ruptured plaques obtained at autopsy has revealed macrophages, and to a lesser extent T-lymphocytes, infiltrating the shoulders of the cap of such plaques (118,119). Atherectomy specimens obtained from patients with acute coronary syndromes revealed significantly greater macrophage-rich areas as compared with patients with stable angina (120). These and other observations (121) suggest that macrophages and, to a lesser degree, T-lymphocytes are markers of unstable plaques and may play a significant role in the pathophysiology of acute coronary syndromes. Macrophages can release metalloproteinases such as interstitial collagenase, gelatinase, and stromalysin, which have been identified in atherosclerotic plaques (122). Shah et al. documented an increase in collagen breakdown when monocyte-derived macrophages were incubated with human aortic plaques, indicating that macrophages could be responsible for plaque disruption (123). Extracts from human and rabbit atherosclerotic plaques revealed macrophages and metalloproteinases, suggesting that macrophages could play an active role in plaque disruption (124,125).

PATHOGENESIS OF DISRUPTED PLAQUES AND THROMBOSIS

Disruption of a vulnerable or unstable plaque with a subsequent change in plaque geometry and thrombosis results in a type VI or complicated lesion. Such a change may result in a sudden increase of stenosis with or without angina, or in acute occlusion with myocardial infarction, unstable angina, or ischemic sudden death. In some cases, plaque disruption may result from rupture of coronary vasa vasora with intraplaque hemorrhage (126).

The plaque fissure or tear may be small, measuring 100–200 nm, allowing blood to enter and expand the plaque without thrombus formation in the arterial lumen (127). Organization of such intraplaque thrombi may contribute to subclinical or clinical progression of the lesions (37,38,86, 87,128). If the tear is large and the thrombus occludes the vessel, the thrombus may be partially lysed (99) or become organized by repair (86). An occlusive thrombus may be invaded by vascular channels and appear partially open at angiography. Table 1 lists the local and systemic factors associated with the thrombotic complications of plaque disruption (87).

TABLE 1. *Thrombotic complications of plaque disruption: local and systemic thrombogenic risk factors*

Local factors
Degree of plaque disruption (fissure, ulcer)
Degree of stenosis (change in geometry)
Tissue substrate (lipid-rich plaque)
Surface of residual thrombus (recurrence)
Vasoconstriction (platelets, thrombin)
Systemic factors
Catecholamines (smoking, stress)
Renin–angiotensin (DD genotype)
Cholesterol, lipoprotein (a), and other metabolic states (homocystinemia, diabetes)
Fibrinogen, impaired fibrinolysis (plasminogen activator inhibitor-1), activated platelets and clotting (factor VII, thrombin generation [fragment 1 + 2], or activity [fibrinopeptide A])

From Fuster, ref. 7, with permission.

High risk indicates labile versus fixed thrombus (unstable angina, non-Q-wave myocardial infarction, Q-wave myocardial infarction); low risk indicates mural thrombus (progressive).

Degree of Plaque Disruption

A computer-assisted nuclear-scintigraphic method using an extracorporeal-perfusion system to study the pattern of platelet and fibrinogen–fibrin deposition in various degrees of vascular injury has been developed by Badimon et al. (127,128). Exposure of a superficially damaged vessel wall (mimicking mild vascular damage) to blood at high shear rates (mimicking a stenosed coronary artery) induced platelet adhesion and aggregation to the exposed vessel within minutes. However, the thrombus could be partially dislodged by the flowing blood, suggesting that the thrombus was labile and left a residual small mural thrombus. As a clinical counterpart, when only the surface of the atherosclerotic plaque is disrupted, the thrombogenic stimulus may be relatively limited, resulting in mural thrombosis with subsequent growth of the plaque.

Exposure of a severely damaged vessel wall (mimicking deep fissuring) to blood may produce a dense platelet thrombus that cannot be easily dislodged (127,128). In patients with unstable angina, aside from the angiographic and angioscopic data showing transient thrombosis close to the time of chest pain at rest (129,130). Complex coronary-artery lesions suggestive of deep fissuring or ulceration are markers of a more persistent coronary occlusion (131). Increases in the transcardiac thromboxane A_2 and serotonin concentrations at sites of such complex lesions probably increase the level of platelet aggregation, promote vasoconstriction, and contribute to neointimal proliferative response (132,133). Very deep ulceration exposes elements of the vessel, leading to persistent thrombotic occlusion and myocardial infarction (134–136).

Degree of Stenosis

Experimentally, Badimon et al. (127,128) found that platelet deposition increased significantly with increased stenosis, indicating shear-induced platelet activation. The apex of a plaque is the segment of greatest platelet accumulation, while the flow recirculation zone distal to the apex is most prone to fibrin deposition (137). These data suggest that the acute thrombotic response to plaque disruption depends in part on sudden geometric changes or degree of stenosis following the disruption—that is, after plaque disruption, a small geometric change with only mild stenosis may result in a small mural thrombus, whereas a larger geometric change or severe stenosis may result in a transient or persistent platelet-rich thrombotic occlusion, causing an acute coronary syndrome (137).

Plaque disruption can produce a rough luminal surface and stimulate the development of an occlusive thrombus. The thrombotic response is influenced by the degree of damage and, more importantly, by the various exposed components of the atherosclerotic plaque. Fernandez-Ortiz et al. (136) studied the thrombogenicity of various human lesions. The lipid core exposed in atheromatous lipid-rich plaques was the most thrombogenic, with thrombus formation four- to sixfold greater than that on all other substrates. The high thrombogenicity of the lipid-rich core may be partly due to high levels of tissue-factor-mediated procoagulant activity (138) or to platelet activators (121), in part released from macrophages. Therefore, the increased propensity of such lipid-rich plaques to lead to acute coronary syndromes may be related both to their vulnerability to disruption and to their increased thrombogenicity.

Vasoconstriction

Although many episodes of unstable angina and acute myocardial infarction are caused by the fissuring or disruption of plaque with superimposed thrombosis, other mechanisms that alter the balance between myocardial oxygen supply and demand must be considered. Maseri et al. (139) used hemodynamic, electrocardiographic, and angiographic monitoring and suggested that coronary vasoconstriction is important in the pathogenesis of ischemic heart disease. Indeed, vasospasm was found to be inducible in a number of patients with anginal syndromes and normal coronary arteries at arteriography (140) and was also found to be an important contributor to intermittent coronary occlusion in patients with acute myocardial infarction who were treated with intracoronary streptokinase. In the acute coronary syndromes, vasoconstriction either may occur as a response to a mildly dysfunctional endothelium near the culprit lesion or, most likely, may be a response to deep arterial damage or plaque disruption of the culprit lesion itself.

The significance of endothelium-dependent modulation of vascular tone has been demonstrated in pathophysiologic studies of arteries (141). Prostacyclin, a prostaglandin derivation, the first such mediator, was described in 1976 by Moncada et al. (142). In 1980, Furchgott and Zawadzki (143) showed that the vasorelaxant effect of acetylcholine depended on the presence of endothelium, specifically on its generation and release of a substance acting on the vascular smooth muscle cells. This endothelium-derived relaxing factor (EDRF) was later characterized as a nitric oxide-containing compound biosynthesized from L-arginine (144). Other causes of the release of EDRF from endothelial cells include shear stress, bradykinin, angiotensin II, histamine, norepinephrine, serotonin, adenosine diphosphate (ADP), and adenosine triphosphate (ATP) (141).

Endothelial cells also release contracting factors. In 1988, Yanagisawa et al. described a potent vasoconstrictor peptide called endothelin (145). Of the various members of the endothelin family, endothelin-1 is the one produced by the endothelium. Cholesterol feeding, thrombin, and local physical factors increase the expression of the preproendothelin gene and thus the release of endothelin-1 (145–147). Thus, the endothelium can profoundly affect vascular tone by releasing relaxing factors such as prostacyclin and EDRF, and contracting factors such as endothelin-1. Under physiologic conditions, EDRF seems to predominate. Alterations in the endothelium, such as occur during atherogenesis or perhaps near the disrupted or culprit plaque in acute coronary syndromes, may cause endothelial cells to generate more mediators that enhance constriction and fewer that enhance dilation (148). Evidence suggests that atherosclerotic arteries have an elevated vascular tone, perhaps related to a deficiency in the production or release of EDRF. Recent coronary arteriographic studies in humans suggest that there is a progressive impairment of endothelial vasoactive function, beginning with selective endothelial dysfunction in angiographically normal arteries in patients with hypercholesterolemia and progressing to vasoconstriction in response to several agonists in atherosclerotic coronary arteries (148). Local secretion of EDRF seems to be diminished and endothelin-1 release seems to be increased in atherosclerotic coronary arteries in humans (149). Based on these observations, chronic atherosclerosis is associated with deficient vasodilation or an exaggerated vasoconstrictor response, perhaps due to endothelial dysfunction. Similarly, atherogenic risk factors such as hypercholesterolemia may increase the likelihood of vasoconstriction. It is also possible that a mildly dysfunctional endothelium in the neighboring area of plaque disruption may contribute to vasoconstriction in the acute coronary syndromes.

Systemic Thrombogenic Risk Factors

High Catecholamines (Smoking, Stress, and Other Factors)

A primary hypercoagulable or thrombogenic state of circulation may favor focal thrombosis (Table 1). Platelet activation and the generation of thrombin may be enhanced by circulating catecholamines (150–152). This catecholamine thrombogenic mechanism and catecholamine-dependent vasoconstriction may be of major importance in humans because they may link emotional stress (153–155), circadian variation (156,157), heavy physical exertion in people who otherwise are sedentary (158), and cigarette smoking (159–163) with the development of arterial thrombosis. A likely explanation is that such hypercatecholamine states which enhance thrombosis and vasoconstriction may trigger an acute coronary syndrome if they coincide with the exact time of plaque disruption (87), which, as previously discussed, is a relatively frequent phenomenon (36,37). However, an alternative explanation is that such hypercatecholamine conditions, by inducing vasoconstriction and ncreasing heart rate, directly trigger plaque disruption (94,109).

Cholesterol Levels, Lipoprotein(a), and Other Metabolic States

Evidence suggests that various dyslipoproteinemias are associated with coronary artery disease in humans, specifically high total serum cholesterol (particularly LDL cholesterol or Apo B) (164) (see Chapter 4), low HDL cholesterol (particularly Apo A1) (164), and high Lp (a) [particularly Apo (a)] (165–167) (see Chapter 9).

Hypercholesterolemia has been associated with hypercoagulability in humans (168) as well as enhanced platelet reactivity manifested at the sites of acute vascular damage induced experimentally (169). Enhanced platelet reactivity has also been documented in young patients with a strong family history of coronary disease, whether or not the coronary disease is related to dyslipoproteinemia (164) (see below for other genetically determined metabolic states). However, the direct effect of high serum cholesterol on thrombus formation in acute myocardial infarction in humans needs further investigation.

Lipoprotein (a) is very similar to LDL cholesterol in its molecular configuration and is an important risk factor for ischemic heart disease, particularly in persons with familial hypercholesterolemia or with a family history of premature coronary disease (165) (see Chapter 4). Apolipoprotein (a) is a glycoprotein present in (a) that has close structural homology with plasminogen (170), with both genes clearly linked on the long arm of chromosome 6 (171). There is evidence to suggest that the close homology of (a) with plasminogen results in competitive inhibition of the fibrinolytic properties of plasminogen (165), predisposing patients to acute thrombotic complications. However, such thrombogenic effect of high Lp(a) has yet to be documented as increasing the incidence of myocardial infarction (167); nevertheless children with high Lp(a) have been shown retrospectively to have increased incidence of parental myocardial infarction at a young age (167).

Other metabolic abnormalities, such as high plasma levels of homocysteine (after methionine loading) and, most importantly, diabetes mellitus, have also been identified as powerful risk factors in patients with coronary disease. Heterozygous homocystinuria or homocystinemia, which is not a rare entity, is now considered to be a possible risk factor for atherosclerotic disease in young people with a strong family history of vascular disease (172,173). However, since endothelial damage with a subsequent proliferative response has been observed in experimental homocystinemia (174), this metabolic condition may be an atherogenic as well as a thrombogenic risk factor. Ongoing studies are focusing on the possible role of heterozygous homocystinuria in myocardial infarction at a young age.

Accelerated atherosclerosis is a major complication of juvenile-onset insulin-dependent diabetes mellitus (IDDM) (175,176) and to a lesser extent of non-insulin-dependent diabetes mellitus (NIDDM) (177). In diabetes mellitus, aside from the role of advanced glycosylation endproducts in IDDM and associated dyslipoproteinemia in NIDDM, it appears that the mechanisms of vascular disease are in part related to an activation of platelets and coagulation factors (177–181). Consistent with the enhancement in thrombogenicity, substantial increase in the incidence of myocardial infarction and microangiopathy have been observed in non-intensively treated diabetics (181,182).

SUMMARY AND FUTURE DIRECTIONS

Coronary atherosclerotic disease, specifically myocardial infarction, is the most frequent cause of mortality in the United States, as well as in most Western countries. In this chapter, the processes leading to myocardial infarction have been described based on the most recent studies of vascular biology. During their development, the lesions of atherosclerosis contain all of the cellular responses that define an inflammatory-fibroproliferative response to "injury." Elements of inflammation are followed by repair in the highly specialized environment of the artery wall. The formation of the different lesions may be modified by the specific local characteristics of the artery wall, including the overlying endothelium and the ability of the smooth muscle cells in the media and intima to respond to causative agents associated with the risk factors that result in lesion formation (1–4). Thus the process of atherogenesis is not a degenerative one, but rather is an active process involving the specialized elements of chronic inflammation associated with those of repair in the artery wall (Fig. 7).

To standardize lesion nomenclature and phases of development, five phases of progression of coronary atherosclerosis (phases 1–5) and eight morphologically different lesions (types I–IV, Va–Vc, and VI) in the various phases have been presented. Our understanding of the pathogenesis of each of the phases of progression and of the various lesion types that precede myocardial infarction, with particular emphasis on the physical, structural, cellular, and chemical characteristics of the "vulnerable or unstable plaques" prone to disruption, is diagrammed in Figs. 1 and 2. The role of plaque disruption in the genesis of the various coronary syndromes and especially acute myocardial infarction has been discussed with particular emphasis on the combination of plaque disruption and a high thrombogenic risk profile—local factors (i.e., degree of plaque disruption, exposure of lipid-macrophage-rich plaque, etc.) and systemic factors (i.e., catecholamines, renin–angiotensin system, [RAS], fibrinogen, etc.)—in the genesis of myocardial infarction.

Recent studies have been fruitful in yielding a better understanding of the processes leading to myocardial infarction, and the near future appears very promising in terms of preventing the number one killer in the Western world.

The processes of atherogenesis involve numerous sources of potential injury to the artery wall and specifically an inflammatory, fibroproliferative, protective response, which in its excess can become a disease process. Numerous molecules have been shown to be potentially important to these responses, including both chains of PDGF, transforming growth factor-β, IL-1, and tumor necrosis factor-α. The possibility of developing specific antagonists to these molecules and of controlling processes of cell adhesion, migration, and proliferation using a number of approaches and more recently developed tools of molecular biology provides opportunities to modify and potentially control these responses. Returning these protective responses to an optimal level and preventing their excess by maintaining homeostasis and control of the local environment may be critical in the prevention and control of the process of atherogenesis. Consequently, optimization of the inflammatory process and its sequelae may be key to the development of approaches to treating and preventing this disease.

REFERENCES

1. Ross R. The pathogenesis of atherosclerosis: a perspective for the 1990s. *Nature* 1993;362:801–809.
2. Ross R, Glomset JA. The pathogenesis of atherosclerosis. *N Engl J Med* 1976;295:369–377, 420–425.
3. Ross R. George Lyman Duff Memorial Lecture. Atherosclerosis—a problem of the biology of arterial wall cells and their interactions with blood components. *Arteriosclerosis* 1981;1:293–311.
4. Ross R. The pathogenesis of atherosclerosis—an update. *N Engl J Med* 1986;14:488–500.
5. Hajjar DP, Fabricant CG, Minick CR, Fabricant J. Virus-induced atherosclerosis. Herpesvirus infection alters arterial cholesterol metabolism and accumulation. *Am J Pathol* 1986;122:62–70.
6. Kuo C, Gown AM, Benditt EP, Grayston JT. Detection of *Chlamydia pneumoniae* in aortic lesions of atherosclerosis by immunocytochemical stain. *Arterioscler Thromb* 1993;13:1501–1504.
7. Fuster V. Lewis A. Conner Memorial Lecture. Mechanisms leading to myocardial infarction: insights from studies of vascular biology. *Circulation* 1994;90:2126–2146.
8. Stary HC. Composition and classification of human atherosclerotic lesions. *Virchows Arch Pathol Anat* 1992;421:277–290.
9. World Health Organization. Report of a study group. Classification of atherosclerotic lesions. *WHO Tech Rep Serv* 1985;143:1–20.
10. Stary HC. Evolution and progression of atherosclerotic lesions in cornary arteries of children and young adults. *Arteriosclerosis* 1989; 9(Suppl I):I19–I32.
11. McGill HC Jr. Persistent problems in the pathogenesis of atherosclerosis. *Arteriosclerosis* 1984;4:443–451.
12. Stary HC, Chandler AB, Glagov S, Guyton JR, Insull W Jr, Rosenfield ME, Schaffer SA, Schwartz CJ, Wagner WD, Wissler RW. A definition of initial, fatty streak and intermediate lesions of atherosclerosis: a report from the Committee on Vascular Lesions of the Council on Arteriosclerosis, American Heart Association. *Circulation* 1994;89: 2462–2478.
13. Simionescu N, Vasile E, Lupu F, Popescu G, Simionescu M. Prelesional events in atherogenesis. Accumulation of extracellular cholesterol-rich liposomes in the arterial intima and cardiac valves of the hyperlipidemic rabbit. *Am J Pathol* 1986;123:109–125.
14. Gimbrone MA Jr. Vascular endothelium in health and disease. In: Haber E, ed. *Molecular Cardiovascular Medicine*. New York: Scientific American Medicine *[in press]*.
15. Steinberg D. Antioxidants and atherosclerosis: a current perspective. *Circulation* 1991;84:1420–1425.
16. Heinecke JW. Cellular mechanisms for the oxidative modification of lipoproteins: implications for atherogenesis. *Coronary Art Dis* 1994; 5:205–510.
17. Mora R, Lupu F, Simionescu N. Prelesional events in atherogenesis. Colocalization of apolipoprotein B, unesterified cholesterol and extracellular phospholipid liposomoes in the aorta of hyperlipidemic rabbit. *Atherosclerosis* 1987;67:143–154.
18. Haberland ME, Fong D, Cheng L. Malondialdehyde-altered protein occurs in atheroma of Watanabe heritable hyperlipidemic rabbits. *Science* 1988;241:215–218.
19. Bucala R, Makita Z, Koschinsky T, Cerami A, Vlassara H. Lipid advanced glycosylation: pathway for lipid oxidation *in vivo*. *Proc Natl Acad Sci USA* 1993;90:6434–6438.
20. Schmidt AM, Hori O, Brett J, Yan SD, Wautier JL, Stern D. Cellular receptors for advanced glycation end products. Implications for induction of oxidant stress and cellular dysfunction in the pathogenesis of vascular lesions. *Arterioscler Thromb* 1993;14:1521–1528.
21. Springer TA. Adhesion receptors of the immune system. *Nature* 1990; 346:425–434.
22. Cybulsky MI, Gimbrone MA Jr. Endothelial expression of a mononuclear leukocyte adhesion molecule during atherogenesis. *Science* 1991;251:788–791.
23. Faruqi RM, DiCorleto PE. Mechanisms of monocyte recruitment and accumulation. *Br Heart J* 1993;69(Suppl):S9–S29.
24. Navab M, Hama SY, Nguyen TB, Fogelman AM. Monocyte adhesion and transmigration in atherosclerosis. *Coronary Art Dis* 1994;5: 198–204.
25. Kim JA, Territo MC, Wayner E, Carlos TM, Parhami F, Smith CW, Haberland ME, Fogelman AM, Berliner JA. Partial characterization of leukocyte binding molecules on endothelial cells induced by minimally oxidized LDL. *Arterioscler Thromb* 1994;24:427–433.
26. Carlos TM, Harlan JM. Membrane proteins involved in phagocyte adherence to endothelium. *Immunol Rev* 1990;114:5–28.
27. Cushing SD, Berliner JA, Valente AJ, Territo MC, Navab M, Parhami F, Gerrity R, Schwartz CJ, Fogelman AM. Minimally modified low density lipoprotein induces monocyte chemotactic protein 1 in human endothelial cells and smooth muscle cells. *Proc Natl Acad Sci USA* 1990;87:5134–5138.
28. Ylä-Herttuala S, Lipton BA, Rosenfeld ME, Sarkioja T, Yoshimura T, Leonard EJ, Witztum JL, Steinberg D. Expression of monocyte chemoattractant protein 1 in macrophage-rich areas of human and rabbit atherosclerotic lesions. *Proc Natl Acad Sci USA* 1991;88: 5252–5256.
29. Leonard EJ, Yoshimura T. Human monocyte chemoattractant protein-1 (MCP-1). *Immunol Today* 1990;11:97–101.
30. Rosenfeld ME, Palinski W, Ylä-Herttuala S, Carew TE. Macrophages, endothelial cells, and lipoprotein oxidation in the pathogenesis of atherosclerosis. *Toxicol Pathol* 1990;18:560–571.
31. Berliner JA, Territo M, Almada L, Carter A, Shafonsky E, Fogelman AM. Monocyte chemotactic factor produced by large vessel endothelial cells *in vitro*. *Arteriosclerosis* 1986;6:254–258.
32. Quinn MT, Parthasarathy S, Steinberg D. Lysophosphatidylcholine: a chemotactic factor for human monocytes and its potential role in atherogenesis. *Proc Natl Acad Sci USA* 1988;85:2805–2809.
33. Goldstein JL, Ho YK, Basu SK, Brown MS. Binding site of macrophages that mediates uptake and degradation of actylated low density lipoprotein, producing massive cholesterol deposition. *Proc Natl Acad Sci USA* 1979;6:333–337.
34. Parthasarathy S, Printz DJ, Boyd, Joy L, Steinberg D. Macrophage

oxidation of low density lipoprotein generates a modified form recognized by the scavenger receptor. *Arteriosclerosis* 1986;6:505–510.

35. Sparrow CP, Parthasarathy S, Steinberg D. A macrophage receptor that recognizes oxidized low density lipoprotein but not acetylated low density lipoprotein. *J Biol Chem* 1989;264:2599–2604.
36. Falk E. Plaque rupture with severe pre-existing stenosis precipitating coronary thrombolysis: characteristics of coronary atherosclerotic plaques underlying fatal occlusion thrombi. *Br Heart J* 1983;50: 127–134.
37. Davies MJ, Bland JM, Hangartner JR, Angelini A, Thomas AC. Factors influencing the presence or absence of acute coronary thrombi in sudden ischemic death. *Eur Heart J* 1989;10:203–208.
38. Rosenfeld ME, Tsukada T, Gown AM, Ross R. Fatty streak initiation in Watanabe heritable hyperlipidemic and comparably hypercholesterolemic fat-fed rabbits. *Arteriosclerosis* 1987;7:9–23.
39. Rosenfeld ME, Tsukada T, Chait A, Bierman EL, Gown AM, Ross R. Fatty streak expansion and maturation in Watanabe heritable hyperlipidemic and comparably hypercholesterolemic fat-fed rabbits. *Arteriosclerosis* 1987;7:24–34.
40. Gerrity RG, Naito HK, Richardson M, Schwartz CJ. Dietary induced atherogenesis in swine. *Am J Pathol* 1979;95:775–792.
41. Gerrity RG. The role of the monocyte in atherogenesis. II. Migration of foam cells from atherosclerotic lesions. *Am J Pathol* 1981;103: 191–200.
42. Gerrity RG, Goss JA, Soby L. Control of monocyte recruitment by chemotactic factor(s) in lesion-prone areas of swine aorta. *Arteriosclerosis* 1985;5:55–66.
43. Jerome WG, Lewis JC. Early atherogenesis in White Carneau pigeons. II. Ultrastructural and cytochemical observations. *Am J Pathol* 1985; 119:210–222.
44. Dehholm EM, Lewis JC. Monocyte chemoattractants in pigeon aortic atherosclerosis. *Am J Pathol* 1987;126:464–475.
45. Faggiotto A, Ross R, Harker L. Studies of hypercholesterolemia in the nonhuman primate. I. Changes that lead to fatty streak formation. *Arteriosclerosis* 1984;4:323–340.
46. Faggiotto A, Ross R. Studies of hypercholesterolemia in the nonhuman primate. II. Fatty streak conversion to fibrous plaque. *Arteriosclerosis* 1984;4:341–356.
47. Masuda J, Ross R. Atherogenesis during low level hypercholesterolemia in the nonhuman primate. I. Fatty streak formation. *Arteriosclerosis* 1990;10:164–177.
48. Masuda J, Ross R. Atherogenesis during low level hypercholesterolemia in the nonhuman primate. II. Fatty streak conversion to fibrous plaque. *Arteriosclerosis* 1990;10:178–187.
49. Nakashima Y, Plump AS, Raines EW, Breslow JL, Ross R. ApoE-deficient mice develop lesions of all phases of atherosclerosis throughout the arterial tree. *Arterioscler Thromb* 1994;14:133–140.
50. Reddick RL, Zhang SH, Maeda N. Atherosclerosis in mice lacking apoE. Evaluation of lesional development and progression. *Arterioscler Thromb* 1994;14:141–147.
51. Davies MJ, Woolf N, Rowles PM, Pepper J. Morphology of the endothelium over atherosclerotic plaques in human coronary arteries. *Br Heart J* 1988;60:459–464.
52. Virchow R. Phlogose und thrombose im gefassystem. In: Virchow R, ed. *Gesammelte Abhandlungen zur Wissenschaftlichen Medicin.* Berlin: Meidinger Sohn and Co.; 1856:458–463.
53. Von Rokitansky C. *A Manual of Pathological Anatomy,* Day GE, transl, Vol 4. London: The Sydenham Society; 1852.
54. Duguid JB. Thrombosis as a factor in the pathogenesis of coronary atherosclerosis. *J Pathol Bacteriol* 1946;58:207–212.
55. French JE. Atherosclerosis in relation to the structure and function of the arterial lumina with special reference to the endothelium. *Int Rev Exp Pathol* 1966;5:253–353.
56. Ross R, Glomset JA. Atherosclerosis and the arterial smooth muscle cell. *Science* 1973;180:1332–1339.
57. Wissler RW, Vesselinovitch D. Atherosclerosis: relationship to coronary blood flow. *Am J Cardiol* 1983;52(2):2A(abst).
58. Haust MD, More RH, Movat HZ. The role of smooth muscle cells in the fibrogenesis of atherosclerosis. *Am J Pathol* 1960;37:377–390.
59. Marcus AJ, Safier LB, Hajjar KA, Ullman HL, Islam N, Broekman MH, Eiroa AM. Inhibition of platelet function by an aspirin-insensitive endothelial cell ADPase. Thromboregulation by endothelial cells. *J Clin Invest* 1991;88:1690–1696.
60. Loskutoff DJ. Regulation of PAI-1 gene expression. *Fibrinolysis* 1991;5:197–206.
61. Loskutoff DJ, Curriden SA. The fibrinolytic system of the vessel wall and its role in the control of thrombosis. *Ann N Y Acad Sci* 1990;598: 238–247.
62. Sawdey MS, Loskutoff DJ. Regulation of murine type I plasminogen activator inhibitor gene expression *in vivo* tissue specificity and induction by lipopolysaccharide tumor necrosis factor-alpha and transforming growth factor-beta. *J Clin Invest* 1991;88:1346–1353.
63. Barger AC, Beeuwkes R III, Lainey LL, Silverman KJ. Hypothesis: vasa vasorum and neovascularization of human coronary arteries. A possible role in the pathophysiology of atherosclerosis. *N Engl J Med* 1984;310:175–177.
64. O'Brien ER, Garvin MR, Stewart DK, Hinohara T, Simpson JB, Schwartz SM, Giachelli CM. Osteopontin is synthesized by macrophage, smooth muscle, and endothelial cells in primary and restenotic human coronary atherosclerotic plaques. *Arterioscler Thromb* 1994; 14:1648–1656.
65. Barger AC, Beeuwkes R III. Rupture of coronary vaso vasorum as a trigger of acute myocardial infarction. *Am J Cardiol* 1990;66: 41G–43G.
66. Van Furth R. Current view on the mononuclear phagocyte system. *Immunobiology* 1982;161:178–185.
67. Nathan CF, Murray HW, Cohn ZA. Current concepts: the macrophage as an effector cell. *N Engl J Med* 1980;303:622–626.
68. Rosenfeld ME, Ross R. Macrophage and smooth muscle cell proliferation in atherosclerotic lesions of WHHL and comparably hypercholesterolemic fat-fed rabbits. *Atherosclerosis* 1990;10:680–687.
69. Gordon D, Reidy M, Benditt EP, Schwartz SM. Cell proliferation of human coronary arteries. *Proc Natl Acad Sci USA* 1990;87: 4600–4604.
70. Rosenfeld ME, Khoo JC, Miller E, Parthasarathy S, Palinski W, Witztum JL. Macrophage-derived foam cells freshly isolated from rabbit atherosclerotic lesions degrade modified lipoproteins, promote oxidation of low-density lipoproteins, and contain oxidation-specific lipid–protein adducts. *J Clin Invest* 1990;87:90–99.
71. Cathcart MK, Morel DW, Chisolm GM. Monocytes and neutrophils oxidize low-density lipoprotein making it cytotoxic. *J Leuk Biol* 1985; 38:341–350.
72. Carew TE, Schwenke DC, Steinberg D. Antiatherogenic effect of probucol unrelated to its hypercholesterolemic effect: evidence that antioxidants *in vivo* can selectively inhibit low-density lipoprotein degradation in macrophage-rich fatty streaks slowing the progression of atherosclerosis in the WHHL rabbit. *Proc Natl Acad Sci USA* 1987; 84:7725–7729.
73. Kita T, Nagano Y, Yokode M, Ishii K, Kume N, Ooshima A, Yoshida H, Kawai C. Probucol prevents the progression of atherosclerosis in Watanabe heritable hyperlipidemic rabbit, an animal model for familial hypercholesterolemia. *Proc Natl Acad Sci USA* 1987;84: 5928–5931.
74. Sasahara M, Raines EW, Chait A, Carew TE, Steinberg D, Wahl PW, Ross R. Inhibition of hypercholesterolemia-induced atherosclerosis in the nonhuman primate by probucol. I. Is the extent of atherosclerosis related to resistance of LDL to oxidation? *J Clin Invest* 1994;94: 155–164.
75. Schwartz SM, Heimark RL, Majesky MW. Developmental mechanisms underlying pathology of arteries. *Physiol Rev* 1990;70: 1177–1209.
76. Thyberg J, Hedin U, Sjolund M, Palmberg L, Bottger BA. Regulation of differentiated properties and proliferation of arterial smooth muscle cells. *Arteriosclerosis* 1990;10:966–990.
77. Campbell GR, Campbell JH, Manderson JA, Horrigan S, Rennick RE. Arterial smooth muscle. A multifunctional mesenchymal cell. *Arch Pathol Lab Med* 1988;112:977–986.
78. Skinner MP, Raines EW, Ross R. Dynamic expression of $\alpha 1\beta 1$ and $\alpha 2\beta 1$ integrin receptors by human vascular smooth muscle cells: $\alpha 2\beta 1$ integrin is required for chemotaxis across type I collagen-coated membranes. *Am J Pathol* 1994;145:1070–1081.
79. Gown AM, Tsukada T, Ross R. Human atherosclerosis. II. Immunocytochemical analysis of the cellular composition of human atherosclerotic lesions. *Am J Pathol* 1986;125:191–207.
80. Munro JM, van der Walt JD, Munro CS, Chalmers JAC, Cox E. An immunohistochemical analysis of human aortic fatty streaks. *Hum Pathol* 1987;18:375–380.

81. Hansson GK, Holm J, Jonasson L. Detection of activated T lymphocytes in the human atherosclerotic plaque. *Am J Pathol* 1989;135: 169–175.
82. Libby P, Hansson GK. Involvement of the immune system in human atherogenesis: current knowledge and unanswered questions. *Lab Invest* 1991;64:5–15.
83. Stemme S, Faber B, Holm J, Wiklund O, Witztum JL, Hannson GK. T lymphocytes from human atherosclerotic plauqes recognize oxidized LDL. *Proc Natl Acad Sci USA [in press].*
84. Davies PF, Robotewskyj A, Griem ML, Dull RO, Polacek DC. Hemodynamic forces and vascular cell communication in arteries. *Arch Pathol Lab Med* 1992;116:1301–1306.
85. Ambrose J, Tannenbaum M, Alexopoulos D, Hjemdahl-Monsen CE, Leavy J, Weiss M, Borrico S, Gorlin R, Fuster V. Angiographic progression of coronary artery disease and the development of myocardial infarction. *J Am Coll Cardiol* 1988;12:56–62.
86. Fuster V, Badimon L, Badimon JJ, Chesebro JH. The pathogenesis of coronary artery disease and the acute coronary syndromes. *N Engl J Med* 1992;326:242–250.
87. Fuster V, Badimon L, Badimon JJ, Chesebro JH. The pathogenesis of coronary artery disease and the acute coronary syndromes (part II). *N Engl J Med* 1992;326:310–318.
88. Davies MJ, Thomas AC. Plaque fissuring: the cause of acute myocardial infarction, sudden ischemic death and crescendo angina. *Br Heart J* 1985;53:363–373.
89. Falk E. Unstable angina with fatal outcome: dynamic coronary thrombosis leading to infarction and/or sudden death: autopsy evidence of recurrent mural thrombosis with peripheral embolization culminating in total vascular occlusion. *Circulation* 1985;71:699–708.
90. Ambrose JA, Winters SL, Stern A, Eng A, Teichholz LE, Gorlin R, Fuster V. Angiographic morphology and the pathogenesis of unstable angina pectoris. *J Am Coll Cardiol* 1985;5:609–616.
91. Sherman CT, Litvack F, Grundfest W, Lee M, Hickey A, Chaux A, Kass R, Blanche C, Matloff J, Morgenstern L. Coronary angioscopy in patients with unstable angina pectoris. *N Engl J Med* 1986;315: 913–919.
92. Ambrose JA, Hjemdahl-Monsen CE, Borrico S, Gorlin R, Fuster V. Angiographic demonstration of a common link between unstable angina pectoris and non-Q wave acute myocardial infarction. *Am J Cardiol* 1988;61:244–247.
93. Levin DC, Fallon JT. Significance of the angiographic morphology of localized coronary stenosis: histopathologic correlations. *Circulation* 1982;66:316–320.
94. Moise A, Lesperance J, Theroux P, Taeymans Y, Goulet C, Bourassa MG. Clinical and angiographic predictors of new total coronary occlusion in coronary artery disease: analysis of 313 nonoperated patients. *Am J Cardiol* 1984;54:1176–1181.
95. Ambrose JA, Winters SL, Arora RR, Eng A, Riccio A, Gorlin R, Fuster V. Angiographic evolution of coronary artery morphology in unstable angina. *J Am Coll Cardiol* 1986;7:472–478.
96. Little WC, Constantinescu M, Applegate RJ, Kutcher MA, Burrows MT, Kahl FR, Santamore WP. Can coronary angiography predict the site of a subsequent myocardial infarction in patients with mild-to-moderate coronary artery disease? *Circulation* 1988;78:1157–1166.
97. Nobuyoshi M, Tanaka M, Mosaka H, Kimura T, Yokoi H, Hamasaki N, Kim K, Shindo T, Kimura K. Progression of coronary atherosclerosis: is coronary spasm related to progression? *J Am Coll Cardiol* 1991; 18:904–910.
98. Giroud D, Li JM, Urban P, Meier B, Rutishauer W. Relation of the site of myocardial infarction to the most severe coronary arterial stenosis at prior angiography. *Am J Cardiol* 1992;69:729–732.
99. Brown BG, Gallery CA, Badger RS, Kennedy JW, Mathey D, Bolson EL, Dodge HT. Incomplete lysis of thrombus in the moderate underlying atherosclerotic lesion during intracoronary infusion of streptokinase for acute myocardial infarction: quantitative angiographic observations. *Circulation* 1986;73:653–661.
100. Nissen SE, Gurley JC, Grines CL, Booth DC, McClure R, Berk M, Fischer C, DeMaria AN. Intravascular ultrasound assessment of lumen size and wall morphology in normal subjects and patients with coronary artery disease. *Circulation* 1991;84:1087–1099.
101. Ge J, Erbel R, Gerber T, Gunter G, Gorge G, Koch L, Haude M, Meyer J. Intravascular ultrasound imaging of angiographically normal coronary arteries: a prospective study *in vivo. Br Heart J* 1994;71: 572–578.
102. Hangartner JRW, Charleston AJ, Davies MJ, Thomas AC. Morphological characteristics of clinically significant coronary artery stenosis in stable angina. *Br Heart J* 1986;56:501–508.
103. Richardson RD, Davies MJ, Born GVR. Influence of plaque configuration and stress distribution on fissuring of coronary atherosclerotic plaques. *Lancet* 1989;2:941–944.
104. A report from the Committee on Vascular Lesions of the Council on Arteriosclerosis, American Heart Association. Definitions of advanced types of atherosclerotic lesions and a historical classification of atherosclerosis. *Circulation [in press].*
105. Toussaint J-F, Southern JF, Falk E, Fuster V, Kantor HL. Atherosclerotic plaque components imaged by nuclear magnetic resonance. *Arterioscler Thromb Vasc Biol [in press].*
106. Toussaint J-F, Southern JF, Fuster V, Kantor HL. ^{13}C-NMR spectroscopy of human atherosclerotic lesions: relation between fatty acid saturation, cholesteryl ester content and luminal obstruction. *Arterioscler Thromb* 1994;14:1951–1957.
107. Skinner MP, Yuan C, Mitsumori L, Hayes CE, Raines EW, Nelson JA, Ross R. Serial magnetic resonance imaging of experimental atherosclerosis detects lesion fine structure, progression and complications *in vivo. Nature Med* 1995;1:69–73.
108. Loree HM, Kamm RD, Stringfellow RG, Lee RT. Effects of fibrous cap thickness on peak circumferential stress in model atherosclerotic vessels. *Circ Res* 1992;71:850–858.
109. Cheng GC, Loree HM, Kamm RD, Fishbein MC, Lee RT. Distribution of circumferential stress in ruptured and stable atherosclerotic lesions. A structural analysis with histopathological correlation. *Circulation* 1993;87:1179–1187.
110. MacIsaac AL, Thomas JD, Topol EJ. Toward the quiescent coronary plaque. *J Am Coll Cardiol* 1993;22:1228–1241.
111. Ku DN, Giddens DP, Zarins CK, Glagov S. Pulsatile flow and atherosclerosis in the human carotid bifurcation: positive correlation between plaque location and low and oscillating shear stress. *Arterioscler Thromb* 1985;5:293–302.
112. Lee RT, Grodzinsky AJ, Frank EH, Kamm RD, Schoen FJ. Structure-dependent dynamic mechanical behavior of fibrous caps from human atherosclerotic plaques. *Circulation* 1991;83:1764–1770.
113. Taeymans Y, Theroux P, Lesperance J, Waters D. Quantitative angiographic morphology of the coronary artery lesions at risk of thrombotic occlusion. *Circulation* 1992;85:78–85.
114. Gibson CM, Diaz L, Kandarpa K, Sacks FM, Pasternak RC, Sandor T, Feldman C, Stone PH. Relation of the vessel wall shear stress to atherosclerosis progression in human coronary arteries. *Arterioscler Thromb* 1993;12:310–315.
115. Gotsman M, Rosenheck S, Nassar H, Welber S, Sapoznikov D, Mosseri M, Weiss A, Lotan C, Rozenman Y. Angiographic findings in the coronary arteries after thrombolysis in acute myocardial infarction. *Am J Cardiol* 1992;70:715–723.
116. Loree HM, Tobias BJ, Gibson LJ, Kamm RD, Small DM, Lee RT. Mechanical properties of model atherosclerotic lesion lipid pools. *Atheroscler Thromb* 1994;14:230–234.
117. Stein PD, Hamid MS, Shivkumar K, Davis TP, Khaja F, Henry JW. Effects of cyclic flexion of coronary arteries on progression of atherosclerosis. *Am J Cardiol* 1994;73:431–437.
118. Van de Wal AC, Becker AE, Van der Loos CM, Das PK. Site of intimal rupture or erosion of thrombosed coronary atherosclerotic plaques is characterized by an inflammatory process irrespective of the dominant plaque morphology. *Circulation* 1994;89:36–44.
119. Davies MJ, Richardson PD, Woolf N, Katz DR, Mann J. Risk of thrombosis in human atherosclerotic plaques: role of extracellular lipid, macrophages, and smooth muscle cell content. *Br Heart J* 1993; 69:377–381.
120. Moreno PR, Falk E, Palacios IF, Newell JB, Fuster V, Fallon JT. Macrophage infiltration in acute coronary syndromes: implications for plaque rupture. *Circulation* 1994;90:775–778.
121. Serneri GGN, Gensini GF, Poggesi L, Modesti PA, Rostagno C, Boddi M, Gori AM, Martini F, Ieri A, Margheri M, Abbate R. The role of extraplatelet thromboxane A_2 in unstable angina investigated with a dual thromboxane A_2 inhibitor: importance of activated monocytes. *Coronary Art Dis* 1994;5:137–145.
122. Henney AM, Wakeley PR, Davies MJ, Foster K, Hembry R, Murphy G, Humphries S. Location of stromelysin gene in atherosclerotic plaques using *in situ* hybridization. *Proc Natl Acad Sci USA* 1991; 88:8154–8158.

123. Shah PK, Falk E, Badimon JJ, Levy G, Fernandez-Ortiz A, Fallon J, Fuster V. Human monocyte-derived macrophages express collagenase and induce collagen breakdown in atherosclerotic fibrous caps: implication for plaque rupture. *Circulation [in press]* .
124. Galis ZS, Sukhova GK, Lark MW, Libby P. Increased expression of matrix metalloproteinases and matrix degrading activity in vulnerable regions of human atherosclerotic plaques. *J Clin Invest* 1994;94: 2493–2503.
125. Galis ZS, Sukhova GK, Kranzhofer R, Clark S, Libby P. Macrophage foam cells from experimental atheroma constitutively produce matrix-degrading proteinases. *Proc Natl Acad Sci USA* 1995;92:402–406.
126. Wilcox JN. Thrombotic mechanisms in atherosclerosis. *Coronary Art Dis* 1994;5:223–229.
127. Badimon L, Badimon JJ, Turitto VT, Vallabhajosula S, Fuster V. Platelet thrombus formation on collagen type 1: a model of deep vessel injury: influence of blood rheology, von Willebrand factor, and blood coagulation. *Circulation* 1988;78:1432–1442.
128. Badimon L, Badimon JJ. Mechanism of arterial thrombosis in nonparallel streamlines: platelet thrombi grow at the apex of stenotic severely injured vessel wall: experimental study in the pig model. *J Clin Invest* 1989;84:1134–1144.
129. Capone G, Wolf NM, Meyer B, Meister SG. Frequency of intracoronary filling defects by angiography in unstable angina pectoris at rest. *Am J Cardiol* 1985;56:403–406.
130. Willerson JT, Golino P, Eidt J, Campbell WB, Buja LM. Specific platelet mediators and unstable coronary artery lesions: experimental evidence and potential clinical implications. *Circulation* 1989;80: 198–205.
131. Richardson SG, Allen DC, Morton P, Murtagh JG, Scott ME, O'Keeffe DB. Pathological changes after intravenous streptokinase treatment in eight patients with acute myocardial infarction. *Br Heart J* 1989;61:390–395.
132. Davies MJ. Successful and unsuccessful coronary thrombolysis. *Br Heart J* 1989;61:381–384.
133. Davies SW, Marchant B, Lyons JP, Timmis AD. Irregular coronary lesion morphology after thrombolysis predicts early clinical instability. *J Am Coll Cardiol* 1991;18:669–674.
134. De Cesare NB, Ellis SG, Williamson PR, Deboe SF, Pitt B, Mancini GB. Early reocclusion after successful thrombolysis is related to lesion length and roughness. *Coronary Art Dis* 1993;4:159–166.
135. Mailhac A, Badimon JJ, Fallon JT, Fernandez-Ortiz A, Meyer B, Chesebro JH, Fuster V, Badimon L. Effect on an eccentric severe stenosis on fibrin(ogen) deposition on severely damaged vessel wall in arterial thrombosis. Relative contribution of fibrin(ogen) and platelets. *Circulation* 1994;90:988–996.
136. Fernandez-Ortiz A, Badimon JJ, Falk E, Fuster V, Meyer B, Mailhac A, Weng D, Shah PK, Badimon L. Characterization of relative thrombogenicity of atherosclerotic plaque components: implications for consequences of plaque rupture. *J Am Coll Cardiol* 1994;23: 1564–1569.
137. Fuster V, Badimon L, Cohen M, Ambrose JA, Badimon JJ, Chesebro J. Insights into the pathogenesis of acute ischemic syndromes. *Circulation* 1988;77:1213–1220.
138. Drake TA, Morrissey JH, Edgington TS. Selective cellular expression of tissue factor in human tissue: implications for disorders of hemostasis and thrombosis. *Am J Pathol* 1989;134:1087–1097.
139. Maseri A, L'Abbate A, Baroldi G, Chierchia S, Marzilli M, Ballestra AM, Severi S, Parodi O, Biagini A, Distante A, Pesola A. Coronary vasospasm as a possible cause of myocardial infarction: a conclusion derived from the study of "preinfarction" angina. *N Engl J Med* 1978; 299:1271–1277.
140. Bertrand ME, LaBlanche JM, Tilmant PY, Thieuleux FA, Delforge MR, Carre AG, Asseman P, Berzin B, Libersa C, Laurent JM. Frequency of provoked coronary arterial spasm in 1089 consecutive patients undergoing coronary arteriography. *Circulation* 1982;65: 1299–1306.
141. Vane JR, Anggaard EE, Botting RM. Regulatory functions of the vascular endothelium. *N Engl J Med* 1990;323:27–36.
142. Moncada S, Gryglewski R, Bunting S, Vane SR. An enzyme isolated from arteries transforms prostaglandin endoperoxides to an unstable substance that inhibits platelet aggregation. *Nature* 1976;263: 663–665.
143. Furchgott RF, Zawadzki JV. The obligatory role of endothelial cells in the relaxation of arterial smooth muscle by acetylcholine. *Nature* 1980;299:372–376.
144. Palmer RMJ, Ashton DS, Moncada S. Vascular endothelial cells synthesize nitric oxide from L-arginine. *Nature* 1988;33:664–666.
145. Yanagisawa M, Kurihara H, Kimura S, Tomobe Y, Kobayashi M, Mitsui Y, Yakzaki Y, Goto K, Masaki T. A novel potent vasoconstrictor peptide produced by vascular endothelial cells. *Nature* 1988;332: 411–415.
146. Lerman A, Webster WMI, Chesebro JH, Edwards WD, Wei C-M, Fuster V, Burnett JC. Circulating and tissue endothelin immunoreactivity in hypercholesterolemic pigs. *Circulation* 1993;88:2923–2928.
147. McClellan G, Weisberg A, Rose D, Winegrad S. Endothelial cell storage and release of endothelin as a cardioregulatory mechanism. *Circ Res* 1994;75:85–96.
148. Zeiher AM, Drexler H, Wollschiager H, Just H. Modulation of coronary vasomotor tone in humans: progressive endothelial dysfunction with different early stages of coronary atherosclerosis. *Circulation* 1991;83:391–401.
149. Vanhoutte PM, Shimokawa H. Endothelium-derived relaxing factor and coronary vasospasm. *Circulation* 1989;80:1–9.
150. Badimon L, Lassila R, Badimon J, Fuster V. An acute stage of epinephrine stimulates platelet deposition to severely damaged vascular wall. *J Am Coll Cardiol* 1990;15(Suppl):181A(abst).
151. Hjemdahl P, Larsson PT, Waller NH. Effects of stress and β-blockade on platelet function. *Circulation* 1991;84(Suppl III):44–61.
152. Larsson PT, Wallen NH, Hjemdahl P. Norepinephrine-induced human platelet activation *in vivo* is only partly counteracted by aspirin. *Circulation* 1994;89:1951–1957.
153. Grignani G, Soffiantino F, Zucchella M, Pacchiarini L, Tacconi F, Bonomi E, Pastoris A, Sbaffi A, Fratino P, Tavazzi L. Platelet activation by emotional stress in patients with coronary artery disease. *Circulation* 1991;83(Suppl II):II-128–II-136.
154. Yeung AC, Vekshtein VI, Krantz DS, Vita JA, Ryan TJ Jr, Ganz P, Selwyn AP. The effect of atherosclerosis on the vasomotor response of coronary arteries to mental stress. *N Engl J Med* 1991;325:1551–1556.
155. Dimsdale JE, Ziegler MG. What do plasma and urinary increases of catecholamines tell us about human response to stressors? *Circulation* 1991;83(Suppl III):36–42.
156. Tofler GH, Brezinski D, Schafer AL, Czeisler CA, Rutherford JD, Willich SN, Gleason RE, Williams GH, Muller JE. Concurrent morning increase in platelet aggregability and the risk of myocardial infarction and sudden cardiac death. *N Engl J Med* 1987;316:1514–1518.
157. Goldberg RJ, Brady P, Muller JE, Chen ZY, de Groot M, Zonneveld P, Dalen JE. Time of onset of symptoms of acute myocardial infarction. *Am J Cardiol* 1990;66:140–144.
158. Mittleman MA, Maclure M, Tofler GH, Sherwood JB, Goldberg RJ, Muller JE. Triggering of acute myocardial infarction by heavy physical exertion. *N Engl J Med* 1993;329:1677–1683.
159. Kimura S, Nishinaga M, Ozawa T, Shimada K. Thrombin generation as an acute effect of cigarette smoking. *Am Heart J* 1994;128:7–11.
160. Cullen JW, McKenna JW, Massey MM. International control of smoking and the US experience. *Chest* 1986;89(Suppl):206S–218S.
161. Buhler FR, Vesanen K, Watters JT, Bolli P. Impact of smoking on heart attacks, strokes, blood pressure control, drug dose, and quality of life aspects in the International Prospective Primary Prevention Study in Hypertension. *Am Heart J* 1988;115:282–288.
162. Fuster V, Chesebro JH, Frye RL, Elveback LR. Platelet survival and the development of coronary artery disease in the young adult: effects of cigarette smoking, strong family history, and medical therapy. *Circulation* 1981;63:546–551.
163. Winniford MD, Wheeland KR, Kremers MS, Ugolini V, van den Berg E Jr, Niggemann EH, Jansen DE, Hillis LD. Smoking-induced coronary vasoconstriction in patients with atherosclerotic coronary artery disease: evidence for adrenergically mediated alterations in coronary artery tone. *Circulation* 1986;73:662–667.
164. Rader DJ, Hoeg JM, Brewer HB Jr. Quantitation of plasma apolipoproteins in the primary and secondary prevention of coronary artery disease. *Ann Intern Med* 1994;120:1012–1025.
165. Loscalzo J. Lipoprotein(a): a unique risk factor for atherothrombotic disease. *Arteriosclerosis* 1990;10:672–679.
166. Ridker PM, Hennekens CH, Stampfer MJ. A prospective study of lipoprotein(a) and the risk of myocardial infarction. *JAMA* 1993;270: 2195–2199.
167. Kostner GM, Czinner A, Pfeiffer KH, Bihari-Varga M. Lipoprotein(a)

concentrations as indicators for atherosclerosis. *Arch Dis Child* 1991; 66:1054–1056.
168. Hunt BJ. The relation between abnormal hemostatic function and the progression of coronary disease. *Curr Opin Cardiol* 1990;5:758–765.
169. Badimon JJ, Badimon L, Turitto VT, Fuster V. Platelet deposition at high shear rates is enhanced by high plasma cholesterol levels: *in vivo* study in the rabbit model. *Arterioscler Thromb* 1991;11:395–402.
170. McLean JW, Tomlinson JE, Kuang WJ, Eaton DL, Chen EY, Fless GM, Scanu AM, Lawn RM. cDNA sequence of human apolipoprotein(a) is homologous to plasminogen. *Nature* 1987;30:132–137.
171. Frank SL, Klisak I, Sparkes RS, Mohandas T, Tomlinson JE, McLean JW, Lawn RM, Lusis AJ. The apoprotein(a) gene resides on human chromosome 6q26–27 in close proximity to the homologous gene for plasminogen. *Hum Genet* 1988;79:352–356.
172. Boers GHJ, Smals AGH, Trijbels FJM, Fowler B, Bakkeren JA, Schoonderwaldt HC, Kleijer WJ, Kloppenborg PW. Heterozygosity for homocystinuria in premature peripheral and cerebral occlusive arterial disease. *N Engl J Med* 1985;33:709–615.
173. Genest JJ Jr, McNamara JR, Upson B, Salem DN, Ordovas JM, Schaefer EJ, Malinow MR. Prevalence of familial hyperhomocyst(e)inemia in men and premature coronary artery disease. *Arterioscler Thromb* 1991;11:1129–1136.
174. Harker LA, Ross R, Slichter SJ, Scott CR. Homocystine-induced atherosclerosis: the role of endothelial cell injury and platelet response in its genesis. *J Clin Invest* 1976;58:731–741.
175. Getz GS. Report on the workshop on diabetes and mechanisms of atherogenesis. *Arterioscler Thromb* 1993;13:459–464.
176. The Diabetes Control and Complications Trial Research Group. The effect of intensive treatment of diabetes on the development and progression of long-term complications in insulin-dependent diabetes mellitus. *N Engl J Med* 1993;329:977–986.
177. Schwartz CJ, Kelley JL, Valente AJ, Cayatte AJ, Sprague EA, Rozek MM. Pathogenesis of the atherosclerotic lesion: implications for diabetes mellitus. *Diabetes Care* 1992;15:1156–1167.
178. Sagel J, Colwell JA, Crook L, Laimins M. Increased platelet aggregation in early diabetes mellitus. *Ann Intern Med* 1975;82:733–738.
179. Schneider DJ, Sobel BE. Effect of diabetes on the coagulation and fibrinolytic systems and its implications for atherogenesis. *Coronary Art Dis* 1992;3:26–32.
180. Colwell JA, Sagel J, Crook L. Correlation of platelet aggregation, plasma factor activity and megathrombocytes in diabetic subjects with and without vascular disease. *Metabolism* 1977;26:279–285.
181. Bensoussan D, Levy-Toledano S, Passa P, Caen J, Caniver J. Platelet hyperaggregation and increased plasma level of von Willebrand factor in diabetics with retinopathy. *Diabetologia* 1975;11:307–312.
182. Jacoby RM, Nesto RW. Acute myocardial infarction in the diabetic patient: pathophysiology, clinical course and prognosis. *J Am Coll Cardiol* 1992;20:736–744.

The Lesions of Atherosclerosis

Atherosclerosis and Coronary Artery Disease,
edited by V. Fuster, R. Ross, and E. J. Topol.
Lippincott-Raven Publishers, Philadelphia © 1996.

CHAPTER 26

The Histological Classification of Atherosclerotic Lesions in Human Coronary Arteries

Herbert C. Stary

Key Words: Atherosclerosis; Histology; Lesion progression; Lesion classification.

INTRODUCTION

This chapter concerns the composition and structure of atherosclerotic lesions in human coronary arteries and the histological classification of the different types of lesions. The classification is derived from the data of many investigators, and it relies in large part on our own study of 691 human subjects aged between birth and 39 years who died, mainly in accidents, and were autopsied within a relatively short interval (1,2). In this study, the coronary arteries were restored to their in vivo dimensions and configurations by perfusion with a fixative (glutaraldehyde) at about physiological pressure. Sequential rather than single cross sections, each only 1 μm thick, were evaluated, and the three-dimensional structure and composition of the artery and of each lesion type was reconstructed. The best-preserved cases were also studied by electron microscopy.

Because it is impossible to follow changes in the histology of a lesion by studying the same lesion over its lifetime, the sequence in the evolution of lesions was deduced by studying the lesions of many persons of different ages. The approach was to characterize the intima and lesions in precisely defined locations of the coronary arteries in infants and children and then to study the same locations in adolescents and adults. The locations chosen for study were known for their predisposition to develop clinical lesions, the so-called progression-prone or advanced lesion-prone regions of the coronary arteries. The contiguous nature of the histology and the time of life at which individual types of lesions occurred and predominated provide strong evidence that each type represents a gradation or stage in a temporal sequence. The characteristic histologies were therefore arranged as a numbered sequence of lesion types. Fig. 1 gives an overview of the histological classification and nomenclature and compares it to nomenclatures that are used when lesions are evaluated with the unaided eye.

In the histological classification, lesions that precede advanced atherosclerotic lesions and may lead to their development are classified as types I, II, and III. They are small lipid deposits that do not disorganize the normal structure of the intima or deform the artery or become clinically overt. The recognition of type III is important because its presence signals the probability of future clinical disease. Advanced atherosclerotic lesions are classified as types IV, V, VI, VII,

H. C. Stary: Department of Pathology, Louisiana State University Medical Center, New Orleans, Louisiana 70112.

Terms for Thick but Histologically Normal Intima Segments Present From Birth	Additional Terms Used for Identical and Probably Identical Intimal Structures
Adaptive intimal thickening	
Eccentric type (eccentric intimal thickening)	Intimal cushion, intimal pad, spindle cell cushion, smooth muscle mass, mucoid fibromuscular plaque, focal intimal hyperplasia
Diffuse type (diffuse intimal thickening)	Musculoelastic intimal thickening, intimal hyperplasia

Histological Classification and Terms Used for Atherosclerotic Lesions		Additional Terms Used and Often Based on Appearance With the Unaided Eye	
Type I lesion	Initial lesion		Early lesions
Type IIa lesion IIb	Progression-prone type II Progression-resistant type II	Fatty streak	
Type III lesion	Preatheroma	Intermediate lesion, transitional lesion	
Type IV lesion	Atheroma	Fibrolipid plaque, fibrous plaque, plaque	Advanced lesions, raised lesions
Type V lesion	Fibroatheroma		
Type VI lesion	Lesion with surface defect, hematoma-hemorrhage, and/or thrombotic deposit	Complicated lesion	
Type VII lesion	Calcific lesion	Calcified plaque	
Type VIII lesion	Fibrotic lesion	Fibrous plaque, plaque	

FIG. 1. Terms used to designate thicker variants of normal intimal structure and different types of human atherosclerotic lesions.

and VIII. By histological criteria, atherosclerotic lesions are considered as advanced when disorganization of the structure of the intima and changes in the outer or inner contour of the arterial segment are present. Such changes are generally associated with accumulations of lipid. Type IV lesions, which begin to appear around the third decade of life, may narrow the arterial lumen only minimally and may not be visible by angiography. However, type IV lesions can quickly become clinically overt by developing a fissure at their surface, a hematoma, and a thrombus.

Up to and including the type IV lesion, lesions increase mainly because lipid accumulates in the intima at a relatively slow and predictable rate in the average susceptible individual. Lesion types that occur from about the fourth decade not only represent chronologically more advanced stages but include pathogenetic mechanisms additional to, and different from, the lipid accumulation that characterizes the first three decades. A main additional mechanism involves collagen formation. Presumably, intimal smooth muscle cells synthesize increased collagen after intimal structure is disorganized by the accumulated lipid. When substantial collagen has been generated, a type V lesion is the result.

Other components that may increase lesion size from about the fourth decade on are the hematoma and thrombus that may follow when a defect develops in the surface of a type IV or type V lesion. We call the resulting lesion type VI. Hematoma and thrombus accelerate lesion growth episodically; lesions revert to slower growth between the episodes. By healing the defect and by converting the thrombotic deposit to extracellular matrix, type VI reverts to the type V morphology, but larger than before.

Minimal lipid accumulations such as type I or type II lesions occur at a young age in almost everyone and in many locations of the coronary arteries, but this is not true of type III or more advanced lesions. Presumably, progression beyond the type II morphology requires an additional or stronger stimulus. There is indication that, in addition to plasma atherogenic lipoprotein levels, relatively small increases in blood pressure may be important for progression.

When advanced coronary lesions are present in young adults or at middle age, the locations at which the lesions are found at autopsy are relatively circumscribed and predictable (1,3,4). The locations at which advanced lesions cause clinical symptoms most often in later life and in which complete occlusions are found at autopsy are the same locations, or they are closely related to them (5–7). These advanced lesion-prone locations are also closely related to the locations at which their minimal precursors are best developed in children and adolescents and at which adaptive intimal thickening is found in everyone (1). The largest advanced lesions extend from the left main bifurcation into the adjacent left anterior descending branch for 1 to 2 cm. Lesions of the same type but generally less thick are closely related to other coronary bifurcations. After middle age, or earlier in persons with very high serum cholesterol levels, advanced lesions may extend out from these typical locations, and the thin peripheries of separate lesions may fuse. The incorporation of a thrombus that may have formed on the periphery of a lesion may also extend a lesion to locations that are not typical. Very high serum cholesterol levels and incorporation of thrombi may also obscure the characteristic eccentric and crescentic configuration around the circumference of the vessel.

Clinical angiographic studies that indicate the possibility of lesion regression in the coronary arteries of human subjects have not to date been clarified by histological studies of these lesions. But the histology of regressing lesions has been investigated in experiments with animals, particularly monkeys, and some extrapolations to the human situation are possible. When risk factors are drastically reduced in man, lesions of types I to III may disappear completely, the size of type IV may be reduced substantially, and types V and VI might decrease somewhat. Type IV, V, and VI lesions might then assume the compositions of type VII or type VIII lesions.

Subsequent sections of this chapter describe the characteristic types (or characteristic developmental stages) of lesions, from the initial, small, and clinically silent lesions to the advanced lesions that cause, or that may suddenly cause, symptoms. But to understand lesions we must first understand the histological structure and composition of arterial intima in locations in which advanced lesions mostly develop.

ADAPTIVE INTIMAL THICKENING

Human coronary arteries normally have both thin and thick intima segments. Differences in thickness are present in everyone from infancy, may develop in the fetus, and are the consequence of physiological variations in shear and tensile forces along the length of the arteries. The thicker intima segments are found at or near branches and are called adaptive intimal thickening. Adaptive thickening is self-limited in growth and does not obstruct blood flow at any age.

After death, as a consequence of vascular collapse and contraction, the thickness of the intima, and particularly of the thicker parts, is greatly emphasized, and adaptive thickening may be pushed into the coronary lumen. When coronary arteries are not redistended to in vivo dimensions before sections for microscopy are prepared, the protrusions may appear as obstructions of the lumen. It is partly to prevent the misdiagnosis of spurious obstructions that a description of the histology of the coronary intima is included in this chapter.

In cross sections of a properly distended coronary artery, an adaptive thickening is an eccentric, crescent-shaped increase in the thickness of the outer wall of a bifurcation (Fig. 2). The thickest part of the crescent may be up to twice the thickness of the media from infancy, although considerable individual variation in degree has been found (8). In an adult, it measures about 15 mm in length, is tapered at its proximal and distal ends, and is thickest at about the level of the apex of the flow divider or just beyond.

Adaptive intimal thickening is composed of two layers. To tell them apart, and to discern their composition, 1-μm-thick sections must be used with light microscopy, or electron microscopy must be used. The inner layer, subjacent to the lumen, is known as the proteoglycan-rich layer because it consists of a connective tissue matrix that is finely reticulated and interpreted as proteoglycan by electron microscopy. Elastic fibers are scarce. Smooth muscle cells are both rough endoplasmic reticulum (RER)-rich (synthetic) and myofilament-rich (contractile) types and occur as widely spaced single cells. The part of the proteoglycan layer near the endothelium contains rare isolated macrophages. The usually much thicker underlying layer has been called the musculoelastic layer because of the abundance of smooth muscle cells and elastic fibers. This layer also contains more collagen. Smooth muscle cells are of the myofilament-rich type and are arranged in close layers. The histological structure is well ordered and typical. Various terms other than adaptive intimal thickening have been used by authors who have observed them in the coronary or in other arteries (9); these terms are listed in Fig. 1. Although the terms and the significance attributed to the thick intima segments have varied, the published descriptions and illustrations of the histology resemble each other closely and doubtless represent adaptive thickening.

The arteries of animal species used in laboratory studies also have adaptive intimal thickening, and in studies of animal arteries adaptive thickening has been found to differ functionally from adjacent thin intima segments. The turnover rates of endothelial cells (10,11), smooth muscle cells (11), and the concentrations of lipoproteins (12) and other plasma components are greater in adaptive thickening. The difference in lipoproteins has also been documented in man (13). These modest increases should not be considered pathological because they remain below the range associated with tissue damage and lipid accumulation.

THE RELATIONSHIP BETWEEN ADAPTIVE INTIMAL THICKENING AND ATHEROSCLEROSIS

Adaptive thickenings of the intima are often mistaken for advanced atherosclerotic lesions because their circumscribed extent, tapered periphery, and eccentric location are identical to the extent, outline, and location of advanced atherosclerotic lesions (Fig. 2). The topographic correspondence between adaptive thickening and advanced lesions is explained

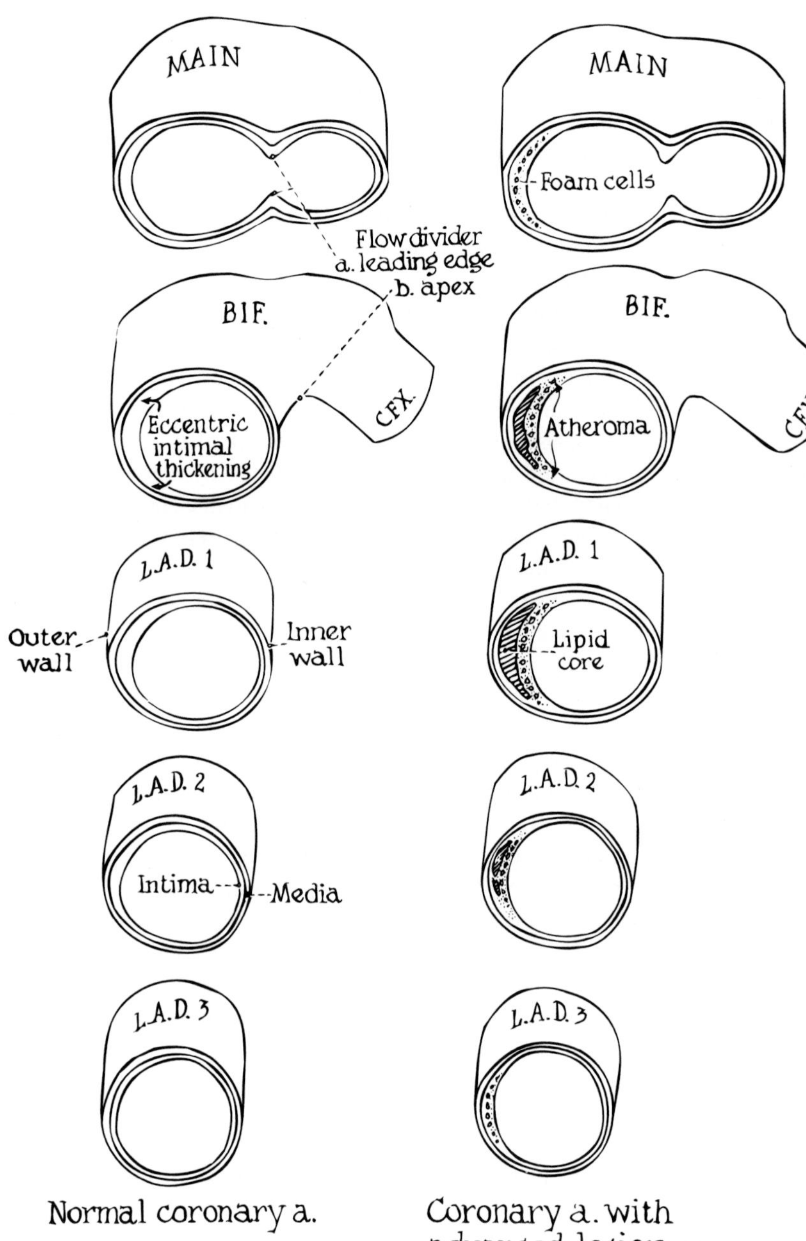

FIG. 2. Drawing of three-dimensional reconstructions of the proximal part of two coronary arteries. A normal coronary artery **(left)** shows the usual location, extent, and form of adaptive (eccentric) intimal thickening. The location, extent, and form of a type IV (atheroma) lesion is shown in the coronary artery to the **right.** Atheroma evolves in adaptive (eccentric) intimal thickening through several earlier lesion types or stages (see text and Figs. 3 and 4). (Reproduced from Stary, ref. 1, with permission.)

by the fluid mechanical forces in these locations. The closely bounded low shear stress that elicits adaptive thickening also increases the time of interaction (the residence time) between blood-borne particles (such as LDL) and the lumen surface, consequently also increasing transendothelial diffusion (14). Therefore, when hyperlipidemia is present, more LDL accumulates in these than in other locations. The frequent presence of even minimal amounts of lipid (such as would be called a fatty streak in locations with a thin intima) within or between the cells of an adaptive thickening has strengthened the belief of many that the entire thickening is atherosclerotic.

Another reason for mistaking adaptive intimal thickening for atherosclerotic ''plaques'' or ''raised lesions'' has already been mentioned. It is the projection of some thicker adaptive thickenings into the lumen of arteries as these collapse after death. Unfortunately, at autopsy, collapsed rather than redistended coronary arteries are most frequently examined, and often only with the unaided eye, which increases the likelihood of misinterpretation.

If adaptive thickening is accepted as a self-limited physiological adjustment to normal differences in fluid mechanical forces along the length of arteries, then atherosclerotic disease constitutes only the superimposed changes. Adaptive intimal thickening is neither a cause nor a prerequisite nor a consequence of lipid accumulation in the same location. This topic is also discussed in the section on the type IIa lesion.

TYPE I LESION

Type I lesions are the very initial and most minimal changes that do not thicken the arterial wall. They consist of only microscopically and chemically detectable lipid deposits in the intima and associated macrophage reactions. Type I lesions are frequent in infants and children and can also be found in some adults, particularly in those with little atherosclerosis or in locations of arteries that are lesion resistant. Because of the more limited technological possibilities early in this century, when many and detailed autopsy studies were performed, little has been written about the initial histological changes. Much of what is known about the initial changes and mechanisms of atherosclerosis has come from studies in animals.

The histological changes in the coronary artery intima consist of small, isolated groups of macrophages and macrophages that contain lipid droplets (macrophage foam cells) (1,8). These cells have been found to accumulate preferentially in regions of the intima with adaptive intimal thickening. In the first 8 months of life, 45% of infants have macrophage foam cells in their coronary arteries. Macrophages without lipid droplets were increased twofold above normal in locations with foam cells (8).

The accumulation of macrophages and macrophage foam cells in the arterial intima is also the initial cellular change in laboratory animals made hypercholesterolemic. Intimal foam cell accumulation is associated with or preceded by an increased adherence of monocytes to the endothelium, particularly over atherosclerosis-prone regions of the intima (15,16). Chemical and immunochemical data from laboratory animals indicate that the intimal macrophage increase and the formation of foam cells are sequels to and cellular markers of pathological accumulations of low-density lipoproteins in the same locations (17,18). The same lipoproteins are always present in the intima, but at lower concentrations. The threshold concentration that induces their accumulation, an increase in macrophages, and the development of foam cells is not known.

TYPE II LESION

The term type II includes all those lesions that are known as fatty streaks. Fatty streaks are visible on the inner surfaces of arteries as relatively flat, yellow-colored streaks or patches. They stain red with Sudan III or Sudan IV, and some become visible only at that time. Sometimes the terms sudanophilic lesion or sudanophilia are used to refer to fatty streaks. However, the determining factor of a type II lesion is its histological composition and not that it is often visible as a fatty streak. The nature of the arterial intima with which a type II lesion is colocalized determines in part whether or not, and how, it is seen on the intimal surface. When colocalized with an adaptive intimal thickening, the macrophage foam cells that generally contain the bulk of the lipid of a type II lesion accumulate some distance below the endothelial surface and may not be visible from the surface as a fatty streak even when stained with a Sudan dye. Type II lesions increase the thickness of the intima by less than a millimeter and do not obstruct arterial blood flow to any degree.

Microscopically, type II lesions are more distinctly defined as lesions than type I and consist primarily of macrophage foam cells stratified in adjacent layers rather than being present as only isolated groups of a few cells. Intimal smooth muscle cells, in addition to macrophages, now also contain lipid droplets. Macrophages without lipid droplets are more numerous than in type I lesions. T lymphocytes have been identified in type II, but they are less numerous than macrophages (19,20). The number of mast cells is greater than in the normal intima, but only isolated mast cells are found, and their number is also much smaller than that of macrophages (2). In laboratory animals the turnover of macrophage foam cells, endothelial cells, and smooth muscle cells is increased in experimentally produced fatty streaks.

Most of the lipid of type II lesions is in cells. The proportions of macrophages and smooth muscle cells containing lipid droplets vary, but in most type II lesions most lipid is in macrophage foam cells. The extracellular space may contain lipid droplets that are smaller than those in the cells, and small vesicular particles. The droplets and particles are large enough to be resolved and distinguished by routine electron microscopy. The derivation of this type of extracellular lipid is discussed in the section on the type IV lesion. Chemically, the lipid of type II lesions consists primarily of cholesterol esters, cholesterol, and phospholipids. The main cholesterol ester fatty acids are cholesteryl oleate and cholesteryl linoleate (21–24).

The arteries of children generally contain type II lesions as the only visible lesions. In spite of many studies, the mode of progression of type II lesions to lesion types that may produce symptoms has not been clear. Therefore, the significance of type II lesions has been questioned. An attempt at the resolution of this controversy is made in the following two sections of this chapter.

TYPE IIa: THE PROGRESSION-PRONE TYPE II LESION

The locations in the arterial tree in which type II lesions can be found are relatively constant. Of the many type II lesions generally present in persons at risk, the subgroup that is colocalized with prominent adaptive thickenings tends to contain somewhat more lipid (more foam cells) and will be first to proceed to type III and then to advanced lesions (Fig. 3). This subgroup of the type II morphology has been called progression-prone, advanced-lesion-prone, or the type IIa lesion. The predictable locations are called progression-prone or advanced-lesion-prone locations. Accumulation of

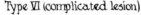

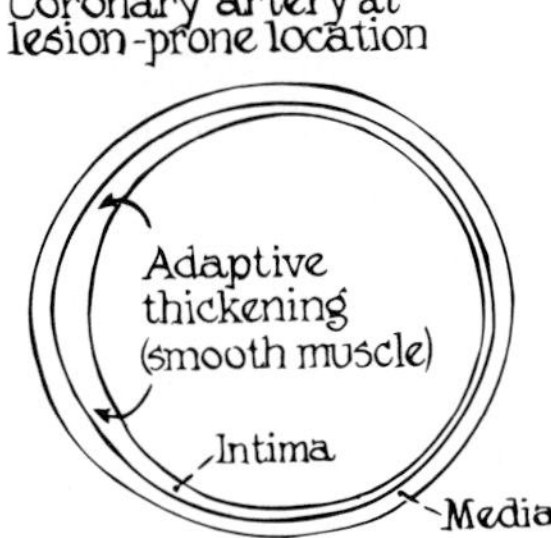

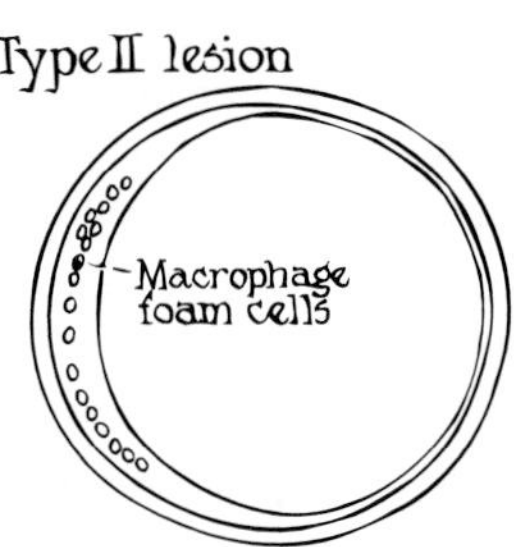

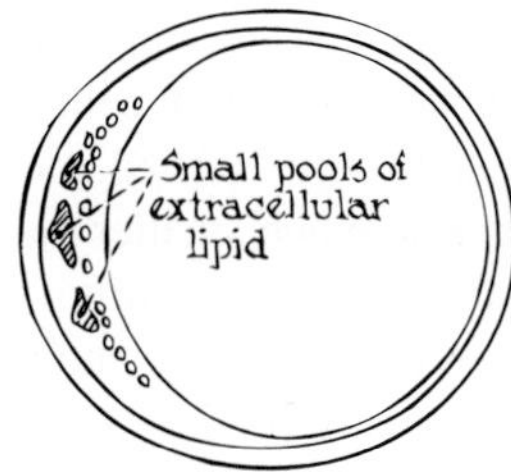

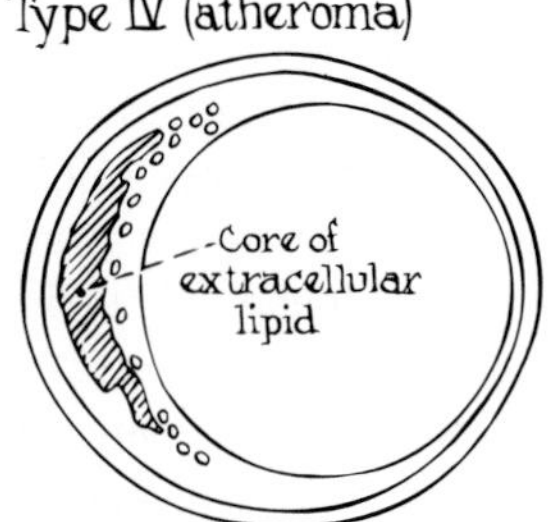

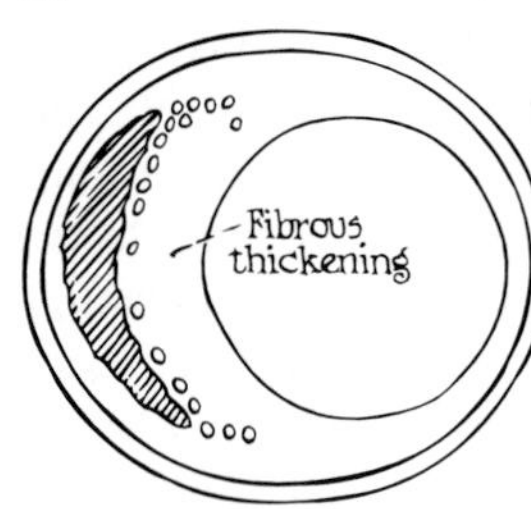

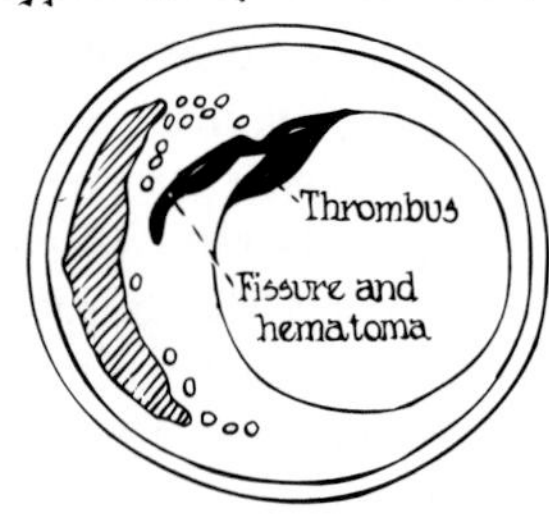

FIG. 3. Drawing of cross sections taken from the identical, most proximal parts of six left anterior descending coronary arteries. The morphology of the intima in this location ranges from adaptive intimal thickening that is always present in this lesion-prone location to a type VI lesion in a case with advanced atherosclerotic disease. The other cross sections show other atherosclerotic lesion types. Identical morphologies may be found in other lesion-prone parts of the coronary and many other arteries.

lipid sufficient to result in the progression of type IIa lesions to advanced lesions appears to occur only in persons with sufficiently high risk factors, that is, with atherogenic plasma lipoproteins and blood pressure above threshold levels. The larger subgroup of type II lesions that either do not progress or progress only slowly or only in persons with very high plasma levels of atherogenic lipoproteins are found in segments with relatively thin intima and may be called progression-resistant or advanced-lesion-resistant or type IIb lesions.

Whether a type II lesion develops at all, and whether it is type IIa or type IIb, is determined in large part by the mechanical forces that act on a particular part of the vessel wall. Fluid mechanical forces that are distinct at some arterial bifurcations and branch vessels enhance the influx of lipoprotein into the intima at those sites. When atherogenic plasma lipoproteins and blood pressure exceed certain threshold levels in an individual, lipid accumulates in the intima, more accumulates at those sites than in other arterial locations, and type IIa lesions develop here. The same mechanical forces cause the self-limited adaptive intimal thickenings that are at those sites from birth in all people regardless of plasma lipoprotein levels. Therefore, type IIa lesions are colocalized with focal intimal thickenings.

In human subjects with very high plasma levels of atherogenic lipoproteins, type II lesions also proceed rapidly to advanced types outside the progression-prone locations. After early middle age, even persons without particularly high plasma cholesterol may also have advanced lesions outside the progression-prone locations.

TYPE III LESION

The designation ''type III lesion'' applies to the stage of development that is, histologically, the bridge between minimal and advanced lesions. The type III lesion is also known as the preatheroma (1,2,25) and as intermediate lesion (26). Type III lesions thicken the intima only slightly more than type II and do not obstruct blood flow. Microscopically, extracellular lipid droplets and particles accumulate to the extent that multiple separate but not sharply defined pools of this material form among the layers of smooth muscle cells of adaptive intimal thickenings with which type III are usually colocalized (Fig. 3). The extracellular droplets and particles are identical to those found only thinly dispersed in some type II lesions and that in much larger amounts constitute the cores of advanced lesions. This extracellular lipid accumulates below the layers of macrophage foam cells, replaces the proteoglycans and fibers that are normally present, and, by increasing the extracellular matrix, drives smooth muscle cells apart. By this definition, collections of extracellular lipid that disrupt the coherence of some structural intimal smooth muscle cells in a circumscribed region of the intima constitute progression beyond a type II lesion. At this stage an extensive, well-delineated accumulation of extracellular lipid (a lipid core) has not developed. Studies of many cases indicate that the lipid core, the characteristic component of most advanced lesions, forms by the increase and confluence of the smaller, separate pools that characterize type III lesions. When human atherosclerotic lesions were studied by lipid physical chemistry, a lesion intermediate between a fatty streak and atheroma, and histologically resembling the type III lesion described above, also became apparent (21,27).

The significance of type III lesions lies in the fact that their presence probably signals future clinical disease in this location. Type I and type II lesions do not have equal predictive significance. In the past, the belief that clinically significant atherosclerotic lesions develop from some type II lesions encountered considerable skepticism (24,28–30). Because type II lesions had been traditionally visualized as fatty streaks, they were considered morphologically too different from atheroma to be its precursor. Nor was the topography of the two lesion types strictly the same, at least not in the aorta (28), and some persons with many fatty streaks lacked advanced lesions, whereas others with advanced lesions had only a few fatty streaks. Moreover, the cholesterol esters of advanced lesions contain a higher proportion of linoleic than oleic acid (24), and the reverse is true for type II lesions (22,24). Nevertheless, some authors were convinced that advanced lesions took their origin in the minimal intimal lipid accumulations of the fatty streak (31,32).

The bridge between the morphologies of the fatty streak and atheroma was found in the progression-prone regions of arteries (i.e., in locations with adaptive intimal thickening). Early in life, progression-prone locations shelter minimal lipid accumulations (type IIa lesions). Later, in young adults, type III lesions and atheromas are found in the same locations. Minimal lipid accumulations in progression-prone locations, because of many layers of smooth muscle cells, are morphologically closer to atheromas than the somewhat more minimal lipid accumulations in regions of the intima that are thin and consist of few smooth muscle cells (IIb lesions). The differences in fatty acids between type II and advanced lesions may be explained by the massive overall increase in lipids and the change from intracellular to predominantly extracellular storage.

TYPE IV LESION

In type IV lesions, a dense accumulation of extracellular lipid occupies the intima in a segment of the artery with an adaptive thickening with which type IV is, at least at first, colocalized (Fig. 3). The accumulation of extracellular lipid is known as the lipid core. The type IV lesion is known as an atheroma. Type IV is the first lesion type to be considered as advanced in this histological classification because of the disruption and disorganization of arterial structure caused by the large accumulation of extracellular lipid. All the features of type II (IIa) lesions are also present, but increased collagen, defects of the lesion surface, and thrombosis are not features of this stage of lesion development.

Type IV lesions are crescent-shaped increases in the thickness of the half of the coronary wall opposite the flow divider of a bifurcation. The greatest thickness of a crescent is generally just beyond a bifurcation (Fig. 2). Location and shape parallel those of the adaptive intimal thickening that is always present in this location and that contributes to the overall thickness of the arterial wall at that point but not to any reduction of the lumen that the superimposed lesion may cause. The accumulated lipid of the lesion may not narrow the arterial lumen much except in persons with very high plasma cholesterol levels. Thus, in many people, the type IV lesion may not be visible by angiography. Disruption of the structural smooth muscle cells by the accumulated lipid may allow an increase in the outer perimeter of the arterial segment involved. However, part of the greater outside dimension, and the oval contour of the artery in segments in which atheroma usually develops, is part of the arterial layout and necessary to accommodate the eccentric adaptive intimal thickening that is present in this location in all people. Although type IV lesions are generally clinically silent, their recognition with intravascular ultrasound or other techniques would be desirable because they have the potential to quickly develop symptom-producing fissures, hematoma, and thrombus (see type VI lesion).

The characteristic core develops from an increase and the consequent confluence of the isolated pools of extracellular lipid that characterize the type III lesion. The increase in lipid results from continued insudation from the plasma. The mechanism and pathway whereby the electron microscopically heterogeneous particles of extracellular lipid form is unclear. The view that a large part is derived from lipid-laden cells is supported by the observation of dead and disintegrated foam cells at the margins of lipid cores, by the extrusion of the residuals of intracytoplasmic lipid droplets from cells, and by the similarity between the extracellular and the intracellular lipid particles (2,33,34). There is also evidence that some extracellular particles may be derived directly from the coalescence of lipoprotein particles derived from the plasma and not previously taken up by cells (35,36).

In the core, clumps of mineral are almost always microscopically visible within the cytoplasm of some dead smooth muscle cells and as components of the extracellular particles of lipid and cell debris. The size of the mineral particles is extremely variable, and they may be too small in many type IV lesions and even in more advanced lesion types to be recognized with any of the current clinical imaging techniques.

The lipid core is in the musculoelastic (deep) part of the intima, and the smooth muscle cells of this layer are dispersed within the entire region of the lipid core including its margins. Dispersed cells have attenuated and elongated cell bodies and may have unusually thick basement membranes. The intima that is between the lipid core and the lumen of the artery contains macrophages and smooth muscle cells with and without lipid droplet inclusions, lymphocytes (37), and mast cells. Capillaries often border the lipid core, particularly at its lateral margins and at the aspect facing the lumen. The core periphery is also a region of dense concentration of macrophages, macrophage foam cells, and lymphocytes. The lipid core emerges before the collagen layers form that may eventually greatly thicken the region above the lipid core. The intima layer above the lipid core of type IV lesions should not be misinterpreted as the collagenous layers that may subsequently develop over the lipid core. This later morphology, if it develops, is then designated as the type V lesion. In the relatively thick histological sections that are used in routine light microscopy, the collagen-poor upper layer of a type IV lesion may be indistinguishable from the same layer changed and thickened by collagen deposition.

TYPE V LESION

Type V lesions are defined as those in which a layer or layers of collagen are added to type IV (Fig. 3). This morphology is also referred to as fibroatheroma. Generally, collagen is synthesized as a reaction to the cell and tissue disruption that result from the accumulation of a core of extracellular lipid. Thus, formation of a lipid core (type IV lesion) precedes collagen formation (type V lesion). Some thick layers of collagen represent the end stage of superimposed thrombi. Such lesions would be classified as type VI if evidence of a thrombus and its remnants had not been erased by the ingrowth of smooth muscle cells into the thrombus and by the formation of collagen. In spite of the layers of smooth muscle cells and newly formed extracellular matrix, type V lesions, like type IV, are susceptible to rupture (or rerupture) and to formation (or reformation) of mural thrombi. That is, they may change, or change again, to type VI lesions. The sequence is explained in the flow diagram in Fig. 4. Multiple episodes may result in multilayered type V lesions. Thus, the artery is increasingly narrowed.

The collagen of type V lesions forms mainly between the lumen and the lipid core, replacing existing proteoglycan-rich matrix. Collagen often becomes the predominant feature, accounting for more of the thickness of the lesion than does the underlying lipid accumulation. Increased collagen is associated with an increase in smooth muscle cells that are rich in rough-surfaced endoplasmic reticulum. Capillaries may be more numerous than in type IV lesions, and microhemorrhages may be present around the capillaries. Lipid may also accumulate in the adjacent media, and medial smooth muscle cells may also be disarranged. The adjacent adventitia may contain accumulations of lymphocytes, macrophages, and macrophage foam cells.

TYPE VI LESION

The morbidity and mortality from coronary atherosclerosis derives largely from lesions classified as type VI and often referred to as complicated lesions. The type VI characteristics consist of disruptions of the lesion surface such as fissures, erosions, or ulcerations, hematoma or hemorrhage, and thrombotic deposits (Fig. 3). Although most type VI lesions have the underlying morphology of type IV or type V, one or more of the additional, complicating components have sometimes been found superimposed on a type II lesion and even on intima without a perceptible lipid accumulation. The superimposed processes accelerate progression, at least temporarily, beyond the gradual rate of growth of type IV and type V lesions. The histological evidence indicates that complicating episodes follow each other at variable and, so far, unpredictable intervals. Sometimes, thrombotic complications appear to be interspersed by months or years without additional episodes. During that time fissures reseal, and hematomas and thrombotic deposits are colonized by smooth muscle cells and converted to collagen. Conversion results in return to a type V morphology, although to a type V lesion that is larger and more obstructive of the arterial lumen than before (see flow diagram in Fig. 4). In other instances, recurrent superimpositions of new layers of thrombus follow in quick succession, and an occlusion builds up within the coronary lumen within hours, days, or weeks (see flow diagram in Fig. 4).

So far, there are no conclusive measures whereby the susceptibility of individual type IV and type V lesions to disruptions of the lesion surface can be measured clinically or histologically, but certain plausible factors are under intensive investigation. Disruptions include fissures, erosions, and ulcerations (38–42). Ulcerations may be extensive and expose and evacuate some of the content of a lipid core. Fissures may occur at the margins of a lesion in regions that generally contain many macrophages and often macrophage foam cells. Factors that could cause or contribute to fissuring and other disruptions include the presence of specific cell types and structural weakness of the intimal lesion at the point of disruption (40), modifications of the shear stress and tensile force to which a lesion is exposed (43,44), spasm (45), and the release of toxic substances and proteolytic enzymes from macrophages within the lesions (32,46). The consequence of a surface disruption is accumulation of blood

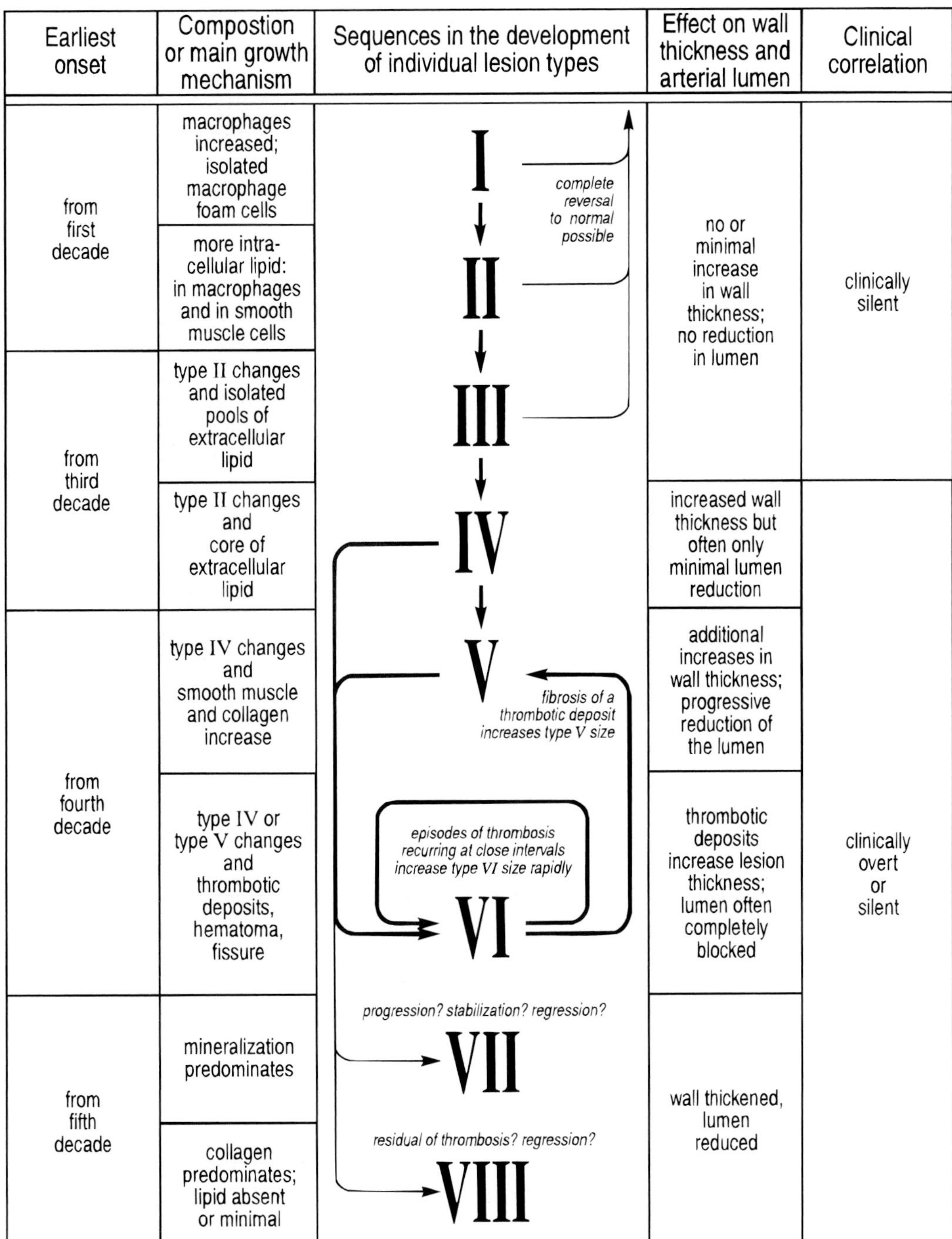

Earliest onset
Compostion or main growth mechanism
Sequences in the development of individual lesion types
Effect on wall thickness and arterial lumen
Clinical correlation
from first decade
macrophages increased; isolated macrophage foam cells
more intra-cellular lipid: in macrophages and in smooth muscle cells
I
II
III
complete reversal to normal possible
no or minimal increase in wall thickness; no reduction in lumen
clinically silent
from third decade
type II changes and isolated pools of extracellular lipid
type II changes and core of extracellular lipid
IV
increased wall thickness but often only minimal lumen reduction
from fourth decade
type IV changes and smooth muscle and collagen increase
V
fibrosis of a thrombotic deposit increases type V size
additional increases in wall thickness; progressive reduction of the lumen
type IV or type V changes and thrombotic deposits, hematoma, fissure
episodes of thrombosis recurring at close intervals increase type VI size rapidly
VI
thrombotic deposits increase lesion thickness; lumen often completely blocked
clinically overt or silent
from fifth decade
mineralization predominates
progression? stabilization? regression?
VII
collagen predominates; lipid absent or minimal
residual of thrombosis? regression?
VIII
wall thickened, lumen reduced

FIG. 4. The flow diagram in the **center column** indicates the pathways in the evolution, progression, and regression of human atherosclerotic lesions. The Roman numerals stand for the histologically characteristic types of lesion enumerated in Fig. 1 and defined in the column to the left of the flow diagram. The direction of the *arrows* indicates the sequence in which the characteristic morphologies may change. From type I to type IV, changes in lesion morphology occur primarily because of increasing accumulation of lipid. Once a type IV lesion has formed, it may change and grow by mechanisms additional to lipid accumulation. The two loops between type IV and type VI illustrate how lesions advance when thrombotic deposits form on their surface. Thrombotic deposits may form many times in the same location and may constitute the principal mechanism for the gradual occlusion of medium-sized arteries.

within the lesion and formation of a thrombus on the surface. Small hemorrhages within lesions may come from newly formed capillaries (47–49). It has been suggested that these could also contribute to the formation of thrombi on the lesion surface.

Although thrombotic deposits and their remnants are the consequence of disruptions of the lesion surface in many or most cases, thrombotic deposits may also form on lesions without an apparent surface defect, hematoma, or hemorrhage. Various systemic thrombogenic risk factors may contribute to the formation of thrombi (50). High plasma fibrinogen levels have been found in persons with clinical ischemic episodes, suggesting that high fibrinogen levels favor thrombus formation (51–54). Lipoprotein Lp(a) may inhibit fibrinolysis by binding to fibrin and/or by interfering with the assembly of fibrinolytic proteins (55,56).

Thrombotic deposits frequently are found superimposed on type IV or type V lesions from the fourth decade of life in the coronary arteries and aortas of populations at autopsy. In a recent study of a population aged 30 to 59 years, 38% of those having advanced lesions in the aorta had thrombi on the surface of the lesions. Immunohistochemistry revealed that an additional 29% of these advanced lesions contained products related to fibrin within the lesions that could represent the remnants of old thrombi (57). These data support other recent studies (58,59).

Some autopsy subjects apparently have long-standing surface defects without thrombus deposition or collagenous thickening. Some depressions in an atherosclerotic lumen surface are endothelialized and appear to be the result of surface defects and evacuated lipid cores. An aneurysmal dilatation of the arterial wall may be another outcome of a surface defect, dissection, and evacuation of accumulated lipid.

TYPE VII AND TYPE VIII LESIONS

Some advanced atherosclerotic lesions do not contain a lipid core nor much or any accumulated lipid of any kind. The intima of such lesions consists of layers of collagen, often hyalinized, or of masses of mineral (calcium) or of a combination of these two components. The term type VII (calcified lesion) applies when a lesion is predominantly mineralized, and the term type VIII (fibrotic lesion) when it consists predominantly of collagen.

Both of these lesion types could, in some cases, represent the histopathological end stages of atherosclerotic lesions that had originally formed through the accumulation of lipid but in which lipid diminished or changed subsequently. The location of the mineral deposits in the intima and observations of many lesions with transitional stages of calcium accumulation indicate that mineral may replace the accumulated remnants of dead cells and extracellular lipid including entire lipid cores. Large accumulations of calcium were found to replace lipid accumulations in the coronary arteries of rhesus monkeys after plasma cholesterol levels that had been very high in the animals for 5 years had been drastically lowered for 2 years or longer (unpublished data).

Some of the type VIII (fibrotic) lesions could be the result of mural thrombi that formed in otherwise undiseased arteries or distal or proximal to atherosclerotic lesions of type IV or V. Furthermore, large lipid accumulations themselves are associated with deposition of collagen, which persists when lipid regresses or is calcified.

SUMMARY AND FUTURE DIRECTIONS

The classification described in this chapter comes from recent autopsy studies in which the natural history of atherosclerotic lesions was studied from their silent inception and evolution to the point when they produce symptoms. Eight histologically characteristic types of lesion were identified, and the Roman numerals with which they were designated give the usual sequence of lesion progression. Lesion types I to IV are formed primarily through the accumulation of lipid in the intima. In types I and II, accumulation is mainly intracellular, in macrophages and smooth muscle cells. Type III lesions contain, in addition, at least as much lipid extracellularly. Type IV is the stage at which so much extracellular lipid has accumulated that the smooth muscle cells at the core of the intima are displaced, atrophic, or dead. Clumps of mineral are now found in dead cells and extracellularly in the lipid core. Although the arterial lumen may not be obstructed much at this stage, the disruption and change of the intima may precipitate events (fissure, hematoma, thrombosis) that will reduce the lumen suddenly. Lesions having developed such complications are designated as type VI.

In response to changes in the intima caused by the accumulated lipid alone, and more so if thrombotic deposits are present, intimal smooth muscle cells generate additional matrix, particularly collagen (type V lesions). Type VII is a lesion that is largely mineralized. The mineral (calcium) replaces earlier accumulations of lipid and dead cells. Similar lesions can be produced in animals by drastically reducing high serum cholesterol. Type VIII lesions consist mainly of layers of collagen, but they lack lipid. Such lesions too could be the end result of lipid regression, or they could be the consequence of a thrombus that had formed in a part of the artery lacking a lipid accumulation.

Besides clarifying the natural history of atherosclerotic lesions in coronary arteries, the classification provides a framework of standard histological morphologies to which images of lesions obtained with all types of clinical techniques can be compared. Matching the clinical images to the corresponding histological lesion types could explain specific clinical manifestations and syndromes and allow individualization of treatment. However, any assumed correspondence between specific clinical images of lesions and specific histological lesion types can be confirmed only when cases that were imaged clinically come to autopsy within a reasonable interval and without having been manipulated in the meantime. To date, such comparative studies are not available in humans. Analysis of atherectomy specimens, although valuable for answering some questions, is unlikely to provide conclusive matching of the established histological lesion types with the clinical images.

The various possible histological outcomes of intravascular therapeutic procedures are not fully understood, and the available descriptions have not been reviewed in this chapter. Nor is the effect of therapeutic lipid lowering on the histology of the various types of human lesion known. Although it requires further study in man, lipid lowering has been studied extensively in animals with some positive results. The histology of the animal lesions indicates that some probably harmful lesion components can regress almost completely (macrophage foam cells and extracellular lipid) and that a small reduction in the size of many advanced lesions (especially type IV) is probably possible in humans, although lipid lowering must be drastic.

ACKNOWLEDGMENTS

The chapter on the histological classification of atherosclerotic lesions in human coronary arteries is based, for the most part, on autopsy studies by the author that have been supported by the National Institutes of Health (grant HL-22739). Data on the compositions and structures of human atherosclerotic lesions were recently compiled, reviewed, coordinated, and published by the American Heart Association's Committee on Vascular Lesions (9,26,60). The classification used in this chapter reflects the conclusions of this committee.

REFERENCES

1. Stary HC. Evolution and progression of atherosclerotic lesions in coronary arteries of children and young adults. *Arteriosclerosis* 1989; 9(Suppl I):19–32.
2. Stary HC. The sequence of cell and matrix changes in atherosclerotic lesions of coronary arteries in the first forty years of life. *Eur Heart J* 1990;11(Suppl E):3–19.
3. Montenegro MR, Eggen DA. Topography of atherosclerosis in the coronary arteries. *Lab Invest* 1968;18:586–593.
4. Fox B, Seed WA. Location of early atheroma in the human coronary arteries. *J Biomech Eng* 1981;103:208–212.
5. Schlesinger MJ, Zoll PM. Incidence and localization of coronary artery occlusions. *Arch Pathol* 1941;32:178–188.
6. Berger RL, Stary HC. Anatomic assessment of operability by the saphenous vein bypass operation in coronary artery disease. *N Engl J Med* 1971;285:248–252.
7. Halon DA, Sapoznikov D, Lewis BS, Gotsman MS. Localization of lesions in the coronary circulation. *Am J Cardiol* 1983;52:921–926.
8. Stary HC. Macrophages, macrophage foam cells, and eccentric intimal thickening in the coronary arteries of young children. *Atherosclerosis* 1987;64:91–108.
9. Stary HC, Blankenhorn DH, Chandler AB, Glagov S, Insull W Jr, Richardson M, Rosenfeld ME, Schaffer SA, Schwartz CJ, Wagner WD, Wissler RW. A definition of the intima of human arteries and of its atherosclerosis-prone regions. *Circulation* 1992;85:391–405.
10. Wright HP. Endothelial mitosis around aortic branches in normal guinea pigs. *Nature* 1968;220:78–79.
11. Stary HC. Proliferation of arterial cells in atherosclerosis. *Adv Exp Med Biol* 1974;43:59–81.
12. Schwenke DC, Carew TE. Quantification in vivo of increased LDL content and rate of LDL degradation in normal rabbit aorta occurring at sites susceptible to early atherosclerotic lesions. *Circ Res* 1988;62: 699–710.
13. Spring PM, Hoff HF. LDL accumulation in the grossly normal human iliac bifurcation and common iliac arteries. *Exp Mol Pathol* 1989;51: 179–185.
14. Glagov S, Zarins CK, Giddens DP, Ku DN. Hemodynamics and atherosclerosis. Insights and perspectives gained from studies of human arteries. *Arch Pathol Lab Med* 1988;112:1018–1031.
15. Gerrity RG. The role of the monocyte in atherogenesis. II. Migration of foam cells from atherosclerotic lesions. *Am J Pathol* 1981;103: 191–200.
16. Lewis JC, Taylor RG, Jerome WG. Foam cell characteristics in coronary arteries and aortas of white Carneau pigeons with moderate hypercholesterolemia. *Ann NY Acad Sci* 1985;454:91–100.
17. Schwenke DC, Carew TE. Initiation of atherosclerotic lesions in cholesterol-fed rabbits I. Focal increases in arterial LDL concentration precede development of fatty streak lesions. *Arteriosclerosis* 1989;9: 895–907.
18. Schwenke DC, Carew TE. Initiation of atherosclerotic lesions in cholesterol-fed rabbits. II. Selective retention of LDL vs. selective increases in LDL permeability in susceptible sites of arteries. *Arteriosclerosis* 1989;9:908–918.
19. Munro JM, Van der Walt JD, Munro CS, Chalmers JA, Cox EL. An immunohistochemial analysis of human aortic fatty streaks. *Hum Pathol* 1987;18:375–380.
20. Katsuda S, Boyd HC, Fligner C, Ross R, Gown AM. Human atherosclerosis. III. Immunocytochemical analysis of the cell composition of lesions of young adults. *Am J Pathol* 1992;140:907–914.
21. Katz SS, Shipley GG, Small DM. Physical chemistry of the lipids of human atherosclerotic lesions. Demonstration of a lesion intermediate between fatty streaks and advanced plaques. *J Clin Invest* 1976;58: 200–211.
22. Geer JC, Malcom GT. Cholesterol ester fatty acid composition of human aorta fatty streaks and normal intima. *Exp Mol Pathol* 1965;4: 500–507.
23. Insull W, Bartsch GE. Cholesterol, triglyceride, and phospholipid content of intima, media, and atherosclerotic fatty streak in human thoracic aorta. *J Clin Invest* 1966;45:513–523.
24. Smith EB, Smith RH. Early changes in aortic intima. *Atheroscler Rev* 1976;1:119–236.
25. Stary HC. Atheroma arises in eccentric intimal thickening from concurrent fatty streak lesions. Electron microscopic study of coronary arteries of 540 persons 1 week to 29 years old. *Fed Proc* 1987;46:418.
26. Stary HC, Chandler AB, Glagov S, Guyton JR, Insull W Jr, Rosenfeld ME, Schaffer A, Schwartz CJ, Wagner WD, Wissler RW. A definition of initial, fatty streak, and intermediate lesions of atherosclerosis. *Circulation* 1994;89:2462–2478.
27. Small DM. Progression and regression of atherosclerotic lesions. Insights from lipid physical biochemistry. *Arteriosclerosis* 1988;8: 103–129.
28. Mitchell JRA, Schwartz CJ. *Arterial Disease*. Philadelphia: FA Davis; 1965.
29. Mauer AM. Risk factors in children and early atherosclerosis (letter to the editor). *N Engl J Med* 1986;314:1579.
30. Mauer AM. Atherosclerosis (letter to the editor). *Pediatrics* 1987;79: 651–653.
31. McGill HC. The lesion. In: Schettler G, Weizel A, eds. *Atherosclerosis III*. Berlin: Springer-Verlag; 1974:27–38.
32. Steinberg D, Witztum JL. Lipoproteins and atherogenesis. Current concepts. *JAMA* 1990;264:3047–3052.
33. Schmitz G, Müller G. Structure and function of lamellar bodies, lipid–protein complexes involved in storage and secretion of cellular lipids. *J Lipid Res* 1991;32:1539–1570.
34. Ball RY, Stowers EC, Burton JH, Cary NRB, Skepper JN, Mitchinson MJ. Evidence that the death of macrophage foam cells contributes to the lipid core of atheroma. *Atherosclerosis* 1995;114:45–54.

35. Guyton JR, Klemp KF, Mims MP. Altered ultrastructural morphology of self-aggregated low density lipoproteins. Coalescence of lipid domains forming droplets and vesicles. *J Lipid Res* 1991;32:953–962.
36. Guyton JR, Klemp KF. Development of the atherosclerotic core region. *Arterioscler Thromb* 1994;14:1305–1314.
37. Jonasson L, Holm J, Skalli O, Bondjers G, Hansson GK. Regional accumulations of T cells, macrophages, and smooth muscle cells in the human atherosclerotic plaque. *Arteriosclerosis* 1986;6:131–138.
38. Constantinides P. Plaque fissuring in human coronary thrombosis. *J Atheroscler Res* 1966;6:1–17.
39. Constantinindes P. Plaque hemorrhages, their genesis and their role in supra-plaque thrombosis and atherogenesis. In: Glagov S, Newman WP, Schaffer SA, eds. *Pathobiology of the Human Atherosclerotic Plaque.* New York: Springer-Verlag; 1990:394–411.
40. Richardson PD, Davies MJ, Born GVR. Influence of plaque configuration and stress distribution on fissuring of coronary atherosclerotic plaques. *Lancet* 1989;2:941–944.
41. Falk E. Why do plaques rupture? *Circulation* 1992;86(Suppl III):30–42.
42. Davies MJ, Woolf N. Atherosclerosis: What is it and why does it occur? *Br Heart J* 1993;69(Suppl):S3–S11.
43. Ku DN, Giddens DP, Zarins CK, Glagov S. Pulsatile flow and atherosclerosis in the human carotid bifurcation. Positive correlation between plaque location and low and oscillating shear stress. *Arteriosclerosis* 1985;5:293–302.
44. Glagov S, Weisenberg E, Zarins CK, Stankunavicius R, Kolettis GJ. Compensatory enlargement of human atherosclerotic coronary arteries. *N Engl J Med* 1987;316:1371–1375.
45. Nobuyoshi M, Tanaka M, Nosaka H, Kimura T, Yokoi H, Hamasaki N, Kim K, Shindo T, Kimura K. Progression of coronary atherosclerosis. Is coronary spasm related to progression? *J Am Coll Cardiol* 1991;18:904–910.
46. Henney AM, Wakeley PR, Davies MJ, Foster K, Hembry R, Murphy G, Humphries S. Localization of stromelysin gene expression in atherosclerotic plaques by in situ hybridization. *Proc Natl Acad Sci USA* 1991;88:8154–8158.
47. Paterson JC. Vascularization and hemorrhage of the intima of arteriosclerotic coronary arteries. *Arch Pathol* 1936;22:313–324.
48. Barger AC, Beeuwkes R III, Lainey LL, Silverman KJ. Hypothesis: Vasa vasorum and neovascularization of human coronary arteries. A possible role in the pathophysiology of atherosclerosis. *N Engl J Med* 1984;310:175–177.
49. Beeuwkes R III, Barger AC, Silverman KJ, Lainey LL. Cinemicrographic studies of the vasa vasorum of human coronary arteries. In: Glagov S, Newman WP, Schaffer SA, eds. *Pathobiology of the Human Atherosclerotic Plaque.* New York: Springer-Verlag; 1990:425–432.
50. Fuster V. Mechanisms leading to myocardial infarction: Insights from studies of vascular biology. *Circulation* 1994;90:2126–2146.
51. Meade TW, North WRS, Chakrabarti R, Stirling Y, Haines AP, Thompson SG. Haemostatic function and cardiovascular death: Early results of a prospective study. *Lancet* 1980;1:1050–1054.
52. Yarnell JWG, Baker IA, Sweetnam PM, Bainton D, O'Brien JR, Whitehead PJ, Elwood PC. Fibrinogen, viscosity, and white blood cell count are major risk factors for ischemic heart disease. *Circulation* 1991;83:836–844.
53. Tracy RP, Bovill EG. Thrombosis and cardiovascular risk in the elderly. *Arch Pathol Lab Med* 1992;116:1307–1312.
54. Ernst E. The role of fibrinogen as a cardiovascular risk factor. *Atherosclerosis* 1993;100:1–12.
55. Loscalzo J. Lipoprotein (a), a unique risk factor for atherothrombotic disease. *Arteriosclerosis* 1990;10:672–679.
56. Scanu AM. Lp(a) as a marker for coronary heart disease risk. *Clin Cardiol* 1991;14(Suppl I):35–39.
57. Yin J, Stary HC. Differences in thrombosis and composition of advanced atherosclerotic lesions between natives and non-natives of Alaska. *FASEB J* 1994;8:A268.
58. Woolf N. *Pathology of Atherosclerosis.* London: Butterworth & Co; 1982.
59. Bini A, Fenoglio JJ, Mesa-Tejada R, Kudryk B, Kaplan KL. Identification and distribution of fibrinogen, fibrin, and fibrin(ogen) degradation products in atherosclerosis. Use of monoclonal antibodies. *Arteriosclerosis* 1989;9:109–121.
60. Stary HC, Chandler AB, Dinsmore RE, Fuster V, Glagov S, Insull W, Rosenfeld ME, Schwartz CJ, Wagner WD, Wissler RW. A definition of advanced types of atherosclerotic lesions and a histological classification of atherosclerosis. *Circulation* 1995;92.

Atherosclerosis and Coronary Artery Disease, edited by V. Fuster, R. Ross, and E. J. Topol. Lippincott-Raven Publishers, Philadelphia © 1996.

CHAPTER 27

The Lesions of Atherosclerosis in the Young

From Fatty Streaks to Intermediate Lesions

Robert W. Wissler, Laura Hiltscher, Toshinori Oinuma, and the PDAY Research Group

Key Words: Fatty streak; fibrous plaque; intermediate lesion.

INTRODUCTION

The commonly used international classification of atherosclerotic lesions has not changed for many years. It was developed from numerous gross observations made in many parts of the world and consisted of a consensus that was acceptable to scholars at a number of centers in the United States of America (1) and by a group of experienced scientists brought together by the World Health Organization (WHO) (2). The main features of this classification were simplicity and definite, easily understood criteria for the classification on which most people could agree:

- A *fatty streak* is defined grossly as any small, often yellowish, often longitudinal, flat or slightly raised area.
- The *fibrous plaque* is usually larger and firmer, and its white or off-white surface usually sets it apart easily from the fatty streak (and, we think, also from the intermediate lesion, the fatty plaque, as we are defining it). Another important difference in the two lesions and between the intermediate lesion and the fibrous plaque is the relative lack of any perceptible increase in collagen microscopically prior to progression to the fibrous plaque. According to a recent article by Miller et al. (3), there appears to be a lack of net collagen increase biochemically in the lesions that precede those with a grossly identifiable fibrous cap.

Time has passed, and starting about 1960, the cellular pathobiology of atherosclerosis has steadily developed into a useful area of investigation (4,5). This development has stimulated increasing interest in the transition of the fatty streak to a fibrous plaque.

Two questions arose in the minds of those investigators—mostly pathologists—who were actively engaged in the study of the pathogenesis of atherosclerosis in humans and in the experimental models whose lesions most resemble those in the human:

R. W. Wissler, L. Hiltscher, and T. Oinuma: Department of Pathology and the PDAY/RFEHA Research Center, University of Chicago Medical Center, Chicago, Illinois 60637.

- Is the fatty streak definition too broad? It includes both ill-defined and barely elevated streaks and quite distinct, well-demarcated, often larger grossly raised lesions that are evident when the artery is opened and flattened.
- Are there easily definable intermediate lesions between the fatty streak and the fibrous plaque that indicate the progression of the plaque? What are their main gross and microscopic features, and how do they vary with age, race, sex, anatomic location, and the various risk factors, including a number of genetic factors?

It has become evident, as we have studied specific designated sites in arteries from over 2,000 cases, that the research protocol developed for the study of the Pathobiological Determinants of Atherosclerosis in Youth (PDAY) (6) offers unique advantages if one hopes to better define and classify the intermediate atherosclerotic lesions.

The Committee on Vascular Lesions of the Council on Arteriosclerosis of the American Heart Association, with which one of the authors has had the privilege of working, has recently published a special report that includes an up-to-date attempt to define the initial fatty streak and intermediate lesions of atherosclerosis (7). This chapter reflects some of the areas that need further definition and further delineation in order to clarify the criteria that can be used to integrate the intermediate lesion and to develop a practical classification of this lesion type. This classification sets the intermediate lesion apart from the classical fatty streak and the classical fibrous plaque, which have been the hallmarks of the current system of organizing the stages of atherosclerosis.

Among the problems posed by this special report are the precise ways of differentiating the fatty streak generally referred to by the AHA committee as a type I lesion, with its abundant macrophages (7), from a type II lesion. These are sometimes also referred to as fatty streaks, but on careful gross/microscopic study in the more than 2,000 PDAY cases, they are quite different from the classical macrophage-rich fatty streaks; they often are almost completely devoid of macrophages and composed almost completely of fat-filled smooth muscle cells. In fact, this type of intermediate lesion, which grossly can be a well-defined and definitely raised plaque, has proven to be the most common of the various subcategories of intermediate lesions that are described and illustrated in detail in this chapter.

At present, it appears that the definition by means of gross/microscopic correlations is one of the major contributions of the PDAY study to the understanding of the developing plaque and to the understanding of progression of this disease process in young individuals from ages 15 through 34.

The sampling strategy (6) that was developed as a result of the computer-assisted mapping of young people's lesion topography by Cornhill et al. (8), has enabled investigators to study the lesion components of well-defined samples of arteries. These have been photographed in the fresh state, close up, with a macro lens, and the investigator has classified them grossly at the time of autopsy and indicated by color-coded frames the type of lesion it appears to be. The choices include no lesion (dark green), fatty streak (bright blue), fatty plaque (burgundy), and fibrous plaque (lilac). We have used the term ''fatty plaque'' to describe most of the intermediate lesions grossly. Because of the generally high quality of the macrophotographs, which permitted these anatomically standardized in situ samples to fill a large proportion of the photographic field, it was possible to define with certainty the gross appearance of the samples from the middle of which the microscopic sections were taken.

This chapter presents in detail for the first time the development and utilization of a new method of defining and classifying intermediate atherosclerotic lesions microscopically, previously presented on slides (9) and as a poster (10). This innovation was made possible because of the unique protocol of PDAY, which specifies classifying developing plaques in the opened artery at the time of autopsy. The lesion components of these same anatomically and diagnostically standardized samples of aorta and coronary arteries, which have been photographed grossly, are then studied and classified microscopically.

SPECIAL APPROACHES EMPLOYED TO DEVELOP THIS NEW CLASSIFICATION

As a part of the painstakingly developed manual of procedures and the training sessions that followed its adoption, high quality and consistency are obtained in the collection, preservation, distribution, and processing of the artery samples. As a result of these efforts, the nine collection centers have been able to achieve a uniform, valuable, and useful centralized file of macrophotographs of the surfaces of the aorta and the right coronary artery. All of these arteries had their grossly visible lesions classified by means of color-coded frames prior to photography, usually accomplished by fine-grain Kodachrome 40 with standardized lighting. Therefore, these gross photographs are now available on more than 2,000 cases as pictures of the unfixed arterial surfaces with an average of seven orientation and close-up views per case.

A collection of microscopic slides on most of these cases has been developed. The sections are through the center of each of the views designated by the color-coded frames and are stained with ''oil red O'' (ORO) and with the Gomori trichrome aldehyde fuchsin (GTAF) connective tissue stain. In order to permit ORO staining for lipid, these facing sections are made from two separate blocks. The sections are within 1 mm of each other and are produced by splitting the standard samples down the middle and preparing half for frozen, fat-stained sections and half for paraffin-embedded sections.

Both of the methods developed in this laboratory are useful for accurate and reproducible computer-assisted quantitation of the location and extent of lipid as well as an immunohistochemically validated evaluation of smooth muscle cells, monocyte-derived Mϕ foam cells, lymphocytes, elastin, and collagen in the developing plaques (11). This methodology makes possible the quantitative evaluation of the microscopically visible aspects of the ventral "lesion-resistant" and dorsal "lesion-prone" areas of each of these standardized samples. One can then compare these results with the gross classification recorded photographically at the time of the autopsy (6).

These gross/microscopic comparisons enabled this laboratory to develop a meaningful method of defining the fatty plaque type of intermediate lesion. Following our observations, which have made it possible to categorize each of these intermediate lesions as belonging to one of the four microscopic variants that were observed, we have then applied the same microscopic classification to the coronary artery lesions observed in the pressure-perfusion-fixed left anterior descending coronary artery (LAD) samples 44 and 45. No gross picture of the intima of the coronary arteries are possible because these LAD arteries are never cut open as a part of the examination procedure. Nevertheless, the cellular distribution of lipid, which is described subsequently, and the characteristics that set the intermediate fatty plaque apart from the fatty streak microscopically appear to be quite applicable to the LAD lesions. The categorization of the LAD coronary artery lesions, as was true in the aorta, can be related to the natural risk factors of age, race, and sex, genetic apolipoprotein phenotypes, and some of the acquired risk factors such as smoking, hypertension, diabetes, and hypercholesterolemia.

A NEW DEFINITION OF THE "INTERMEDIATE" LESION

Some of the preliminary results of the four microscopic variants on 915 cases including both the standardized close-up transparencies and the microscopic study of the central standardized areas shown in the gross photographs of the aorta as well as the pressure-perfusion-fixed LAD coronary arteries have been evaluated and recorded.

The emphasis, so far, is on the development of a data base to permit a new microscopic definition of the intermediate lesion and then establish a larger useful research collection of classified microscopic types of intermediate lesions. Although most "fatty plaques" appear similar on the gross macrophotographs, they are easily distinguishable grossly in the fresh, unstained aorta from the much more indistinct and only slightly raised fatty streaks and from the fibrous plaque (Fig. 1A,D,G; see Colorplate 12A, D, G).

The intermediate coronary lesions we are studying are located in the proximal area of the LAD coronary arteries and are studied only microscopically. The same criteria have been employed to differentiate fatty plaques (intermediate lesions) from fatty streaks and from fibrous plaques (Fig. 4A,C,E; see Colorplate 15A, C, E).

It has become quite evident that in both the aorta and the coronary arteries, the intermediate lesions have a number of rather easily distinguished and categorized microscopic appearances. In both the aorta and the coronary arteries, one can divide the fatty plaques into four types of microscopic lesions.

Microscopically Distinct Types of Intermediate Lesions and Their Frequency in Youth

During the course of classifying and then producing the macrolens photographs, followed by the microscopic study of the same areas, it has become obvious that the usual fatty streak, with its indefinite and indistinct edges and only slightly elevated and discolored appearance, is a frequent lesion. It is often quite rich in fat-filled Mϕ, although a significant number show diffuse intercellular lipid with little stainable lipid inside cells of any kind. However, a more common lesion in these young people is a definite and easily identified raised lesion, even in the fresh unstained artery. Microscopically, this lesion is thicker (8–20 lamellar units) instead of the 3- to 8-unit thickening one usually finds in the fatty streak. Because it always contains abundant lipid microscopically, the term "fatty plaque" is appropriate.

As more experience was gained in the study of the arteries of young people, it became obvious that this lesion is very common (Table 1), but the microscopic components vary greatly from fatty plaque to fatty plaque. Even though the gross appearance is often monotonous, microscopic types are readily discernible, and almost all can be classified as one of the following:

- Type 1. This is a fatty plaque with most of the lipid intracellular. Most of the cells are fat-filled smooth muscle cells (SMC), and very few Mϕ are present.
- Type 2. Most of the mass of the fatty plaque is made up of extracellular lipid. The cells are almost all SMCs, and many contain no lipid; Mϕ are few in number.
- Type 3. This is a very cellular fatty plaque with most of

TABLE 1. *Preliminary survey of gross classification of aortic atheromatous lesions in 100 PDAY cases*

Aortic location	Standard "core" sample	Number of lesions	Fatty streaks	Fatty transitional plaques	Fibrous plaque	Total
Midthoracic	01	20	55	25	0	100
Midabdominal	18	29	33	37	1	100
Lower abdominal	16	30	27	42	1	100
Total		79	115	104	2	300

the lipid intracellular and with many Mϕ foam cells, at least 20% of the total cells.

- Type 4. This type of fatty plaque is quite rare and somewhat similar to type 3, but in addition to the Mϕ there are many lymphocytes. When this type is seen in coronary arteries, the lesions are often concentric rather than eccentric. The mononuclear leukocyte cellular involvement often extends into the media.

Cell Identification and Translation to the Fat Stain Results

We have previously defined the cell populations in a large number of both aortic and coronary artery lesions of PDAY cases immunohistochemically (11,12). This has provided a rich source of information concerning the histomorphological correspondence between the cell types as verified by specific antibodies and their appearance on fat stains, which give an accurate localization of stainable lipid distribution.

In almost all of the Mϕ foam cells in 150 white male subjects, including 750 separate arterial samples, the immunohistochemically identified cells are identical with the fat-stained cells. The large round intensely stained ORO-positive cells are typical in appearance and localization with the HAM56 peroxidase-positive cells in adjacent sections. The SMCs as identified by HHF35, on the other hand, are usually smaller, even when filled with lipid, than those seen with fat stains, which are usually elliptical, with less intense ORO staining. The lymphocytes have been extensively enumerated in immunohistochemical studies previously reported (13). These detailed quantitative cell population results make it plausible that the identification of small lymphocytes with ORO staining can be useful for the purpose of classification of types of intermediate lesions.

The only complications encountered thus far in the use of the above criteria in classifying several hundred cases microscopically has been the occasional lesion that appears to be a mixture of types 1 and 2. Because there is evidence that transition from type 1 to 2 is a usual occurrence, probably signifying progression, the problem is not surprising. Nevertheless, it is a problem, and the advantages and disadvantages of calling them "1.5 lesions" are being explored. If the mixed or paradoxical lesions really are a sign of progression within the intermediate lesion category, that may be a useful refinement, but for the present analysis, we have utilized the prevalent pattern in the most advanced (thickest) part of the developing plaque.

THE PRELIMINARY USE OF THE PROPOSED CLASSIFICATION SYSTEM AND THE VALUE OF THE NEW DEFINITION OF INTERMEDIATE LESION

The value of this way of looking at lesion development in youth is becoming apparent. Studies have established that the various parts of the arterial system react differently at the gross level to the risk factors of age, race, sex, and genetically determined apolipoprotein phenotypes (14,15). It is also evident from the elegant quantitative topographic computer-assisted studies of Cornhill that there are important differences in the distribution and frequency as well as the apparent rate of progression of lesions in the various parts of the arterial tree.

The evaluation of 100 cases selected at random from the PDAY files indicated in a preliminary study that one could indeed define each lesion that is visible in the anatomically standardized core areas of the aorta, both grossly and microscopically, and that one can clearly delineate the fatty plaques (intermediate lesions) from the fatty streaks and the fibrous plaques both grossly and microscopically. Table 1 indicates that the intermediate lesion is the most common lesion encountered in these 300 aortic sections from 100 cases and that it is much more common in the lower abdominal aorta, where the lesions progress most rapidly, than it is in the thoracic aorta. It is also evident that on an overall basis, the classification is valuable for increasing the understanding of progression a little more clearly than has been possible in the past in the study of the pathogenesis of human atherosclerosis. Previously, one simply relied on a definition of fatty streaks, which included a broad spectrum from early, Mϕ-rich lesions to rather highly defined, lipid-containing, SMC-rich, raised lesions. These lesions had no apparent increase in collagenous or other fiber protein content, either histologically by means of trichrome staining or by means of microchemical analysis (3). Under these conditions, many of the details of the pathogenesis, histogenesis, and progression, at the time that one can most readily relate them to risk factors, cannot be distinguished.

The next step in the development of a useful method of classifying the intermediate aortic lesions was demonstrated in a preliminary analysis performed on 140 cases. Those lesions, graded grossly, were also subclassified microscopically and separated into the four types of intermediate lesions by means of the criteria described above. These results are shown in Table 2. Here it becomes apparent that one can gain useful knowledge by means of the simple microscopic delineation of the cell types and the location of the lipid revealed by the ORO fat stains of the aortic common core samples of midthoracic 01, midabdominal 18, and lower abdominal aorta 16. The results obtained by highly reliable and reproducible methods developed in this laboratory indicate the more frequent appearance of Mϕ-rich lesions (type 3) in the thoracic aorta and the more frequent occurrence of lesions with abundant extracellular lipid (type 2) in the lower abdominal aortic area. The table also indicates that the results obtained by evaluation of the midabdominal aortic sample are intermediate between these two contrasting results obtained from the thoracic and the lower abdominal aorta. Some of these phenomena have already been recognized, quantitated by means of micromorphometry, and summarized in previous presentations and publications (11,12,16).

TABLE 2. *Microscopic classification of lesions from 140 cases*

Sample	No microlesions	Micro fatty streak	Fatty plaques: Intracellular lipid predom. 1	Extracellular lipid >50% 2	Mϕ foam cell >20% 3	Rich in lymphocytes 4	Total fatty plaques
01	29	68	18	8	13	0	39
18	37	42	32	18	9	0	59
16	38	32	28	37	4	0	69
44	60	34	9	19	6	2	36
45	58	34	8	15	5	1	29
Total	222	210	95	97	37	3	232

In these reports, the three phenomena that have been most firmly established are those mentioned above:

- The intermediate lesions in the thoracic aorta are largely composed of SMCs filled with lipid and with almost no visible extracellular lipid and very few Mϕ foam cells.
- The intermediate lesions in the abdominal aorta, which are similar to the thoracic aortic lesions in appearance, size, and extent, are most frequently composed largely of extracellular lipid with a more prominent matrix.
- The apo B deposits are somewhat greater in extent, immunohistochemically, in the abdominal aorta than in the thoracic aorta, but there is (in contrast to stainable lipid) very little difference between lesion-prone and lesion-resistant portions of each of the core samples.

ILLUSTRATIONS OF THE SPECTRUM OF AORTIC LESIONS AS CLASSIFIED MICROSCOPICALLY

As can be seen in Fig. 1a, there are typical and representative examples of the normal aortic intimal surface as seen at autopsy that are completely devoid of lesions. There are also intimal sampling sites that have typical fatty streaks (Fig. 1d) and that have typical fibrous plaques (Fig. 1g). The microscopic appearance of each of these time-honored lesions stained with ORO is shown in Fig. 1b after it is applied to precut, floating, frozen sections. The GTAF preparation is shown in Fig. 1c. It readily differentially stains SMC, elastin, and collagen. These representative pictures indicate that in this 20-year age span, the aorta without lesions not only appears grossly normal but usually shows little if any element of diffuse intimal thickening in the standard areas that are always sampled. It is also evident that the fatty streak defined in this manner is a relatively innocuous and thin lesion microscopically and in this typical illustration (Fig. 1d), it is composed largely of fat-filled monocyte-derived macrophages or foam cells (Fig. 1e). At this stage, there is little evidence of increase in SMC numbers in these small, flat, and rather cell-poor lesions, and the GTAF stain (Fig. 1f) shows little increase in collagen or elastin in the intima. The classical fibrous plaque (Fig. 1g), which is encountered relatively infrequently in the PDAY study, has all of the microscopic features of the more or less stabilized advanced plaque that has been described in many publications. It is relatively frequently encountered in the usual autopsy population at academic centers or community hospitals, where most of the cases are beyond middle age. These are likely to be the forerunners of the complicated plaques that can ulcerate and develop overlying mural thrombi as well as other clinically significant complications. Their typical microscopic features as revealed by these two stains are seen in Fig. 1h and 1i. The aortic intermediate lesions as depicted in Fig. 2 (see Colorplate 13) are obviously raised lesions, which can be easily recognized on the close-up photographs of the standardized core areas. These photographs have been obtained for most of the 915 cases included in this study by means of a macrolens attachment to the camera. As can be seen, these developing plaques are classified at the time of autopsy by the investigators by means of color-coded frames. The resulting sections taken through the center of each of these gross lesions are also shown in Fig. 2 and represent the microscopic prototype examples of the four types of intermediate lesions that are defined earlier in this chapter.

Table 1 makes it abundantly clear that the fatty streaks are the most common lesions in the midthoracic aorta (sample 01). The type 2 lesions with predominantly extracellular lipid (Fig. 2d–f; see Colorplate 13, D–F) are much less common in the thoracic aorta than they are in the abdominal aorta, where they represent the predominant type of intermediate lesion (11,12). Tables 1 and 2 also indicate that intermediate lesions are much more common in the abdominal aortic samples than they are in the thoracic aorta samples and that the type 1 lesions, with intracellular lipids (Fig. 2a–c; See Colorplate 13A–C), or the type 3 lesions, with intracellular lipid and a rich population of macrophages (Fig. 3a–3), are much less common in these lower abdominal aortic samples. Figure 3(d–f) (see Colorplate 14, D–F) gives a very graphic view of the relatively rarer type IV lesion. It is much less common in the aorta than in the coronary artery samples. The gross appearance is similar to that of the fatty plaques, but the population of lymphocytes is greatly increased.

The lesions illustrated in Figs. 4 and 5 (see Colorplates

TABLE 3. *Advanced plaques in 1,000 PDAY cases: Aortas and LAD coronary arteries*

Sample	Fibrous cap	Necrosis	Calcium
01	9	2	0
18	42	18	11
16	131	58	18
44	113	96	34
45	106	90	35

15 and 16) are taken from samples 44 and 45 of the pressure perfusion fixed LAD coronary arteries. These samples are located near the origin of the LAD, just distal to the ostium of the left circumflex branch of the main left coronary artery. As can be seen and as described in the legends of these figures, the microscopic lesions of the four types of fatty plaques are very similar to those in the aorta. Even though this artery has never been opened and flattened, it is quite clear that one can identify the intermediate lesion grossly as well as microscopically in the right coronary artery and, in the unopened LAD, almost as readily microscopically, as in the opened and flattened aorta. Our confidence in this statement is strengthened by our having observed and photographed many hundreds of opened and flattened right coronary arteries, which, we have found, have the same variety and spectrum of lesions as we have described in the aorta.

As illustrated in Fig. 1, the fibrous plaques, when present, have a characteristic set of components and a characteristic gross appearance in the unfixed, unstained specimen photographed close up when the aorta is first removed and opened. Although advanced lesions of this type are rare, we have surveyed the fibrous lesions encountered in the various core areas of the aorta and LAD coronary arteries in 1,000 cases, and these results are summarized in Table 3. It is quite evident from these data that, in these same cases, the fibrous lesions with fibrous caps, necrotic centers, and, less commonly, calcification are more prevalent in the lower abdominal aorta and to a lesser extent in the midabdominal aorta. In contrast, the thoracic aorta is rarely the site of this type of advanced lesion in the anatomically standardized area referred to as sample 01.

The results of the microscopic classification of all 915 of the cases, in which we presently have available both macrophotographed and grossly classified lesions as well as the same lesions classified microscopically using the new intermediate lesion designation, are shown in Table 4. These data are derived from 687 men and 228 women between 15 and 34 years (average age 23.5). There were 386 black men, 301 white men, and 121 black women, along with 107 white women. The average age of the males was 22.8 years, and that of the females 27.2.

As Table 4 indicates, there are many samples in each anatomic core site with no gross or microscopic lesions. These did not vary significantly from one sampling site to another. The fatty streaks, on the other hand, are much more numerous in the thoracic aorta than in the abdominal aorta or the proximal LAD coronary artery. Type 1 intermediate lesions with almost all of the lipid in smooth muscle cells are more frequent in the midthoracic aorta, reach a peak in the midabdominal aorta (sample #18), and are still almost three times more frequent in the standardized sample of the lower abdominal aorta than they are in the LAD. In contrast, and as we have emphasized previously (11,12), the type 2 lesions with predominantly extracellular lipid are almost two times as frequent in the lower abdominal aorta samples as in the samples from the thoracic aorta. This corresponds to the notable and often observed slower progression of plaques in the thoracic aorta and the much more frequent progression in the abdominal aorta. Rapid progression in the thoracic aorta usually requires additional stimulatory factors, such as severe hyperlipidemia, coarctation of the aorta, or longstanding hypertension. The especially Mϕ-rich lesions are much more frequent in the thoracic aortic samples. The lesions with numerous lymphocytes are rare, and more of these are found in the proximal LAD coronary artery samples and/or the thoracic aortic samples. The reasons for this are not clear. It is also true that the infrequent concentric atherosclerotic coronary lesions that we have observed in PDAY cases are rich in lymphocytes and, in some instances, are directly related to circulating immune complexes (17,18).

The fibrous plaques in this series with definite necrotic centers and fibrous caps are now included in the new classification proposed by the Committee on Vascular Lesions of the American Heart Association as IV (7) and recently utilized by Fuster in his Conner lecture (19). In this series, these advanced lesions were many times more frequent in the abdominal aortic samples than in the thoracic aorta and,

TABLE 4. *The analysis of all available cases with gross and microscopic lesion classification utilizing the new criteria for intermediate lesion microscopic types*

			Fatty plaques				
Sample no.	No microlesions	Micro fatty streaks	Intracellular lipid predom.: 1	Extracellular lipid >50%: 2	Mϕ foam cell >20%: 3	Rich in lymphocytes: 4	Fibrous plaques
01	235	174	175	117	121	5	2
18	264	128	216	155	102	0	7
16	250	53	164	225	89	1	38
45	388	47	58	206	69	4	102

surprisingly, over twice as frequent in the proximal LAD coronary artery in the lower abdominal aorta. We have no clue as to why this is true of this rather large and systematic study of the arteries of young people who died suddenly or unexpectedly of traumatic causes and who have no evidence of chronic debilitating disease. From the results of analysis of their fatty plaques, it is notable that they have almost as high an incidence of type 2 lesions in the proximal LAD coronary arteries as is seen in the lower abdominal aorta. This proximal coronary artery sample also has the greatest number of cases with no lesions of any of the core sample sites. The proximal LAD coronary core samples have the lowest incidence of fatty streaks and a very low incidence of fatty plaque type 1 or fatty plaque type 3, all of which are usually associated with stabilization of the developing plaque in the thoracic aorta.

THE TYPICAL GROSS AND MICROSCOPIC FEATURES OF EACH TYPE OF INTERMEDIATE LESION IN THE AORTA AND CORONARY ARTERIES

The major distinguishing features of each of the types of lesions we have encountered in this study indicate that the fatty streak is an easily discernible and distinct lesion. The fatty streak accurately fits its descriptive terminology. Its slight elevation is barely perceptible in the fresh gross specimen, and the transition between a completely normal intimal surface and the edges of the lesion is indistinct, as is the slight discoloration of the streak itself compared to the surrounding normal intima (Fig. 1d). In contrast, the fatty plaque is definitely raised, often yellow, and demarcated from the surrounding intima. It presents a distinct difference from the fibrous plaque described below. This fatty plaque is not as firm as a fibrous plaque and presents a comparatively sharply outlined interface with the adjacent intima.

As was previously indicated, the microscopic features of the fatty streak are surprisingly monotonous. One variation is the range of diffuse fibrous thickening in which the lesion arises, as well as the variation in numbers of Mϕ. In general, about half of the fatty streaks have Mϕ foam cells as the major cell type, accompanied by very little additional extracellular lipid. The other half of these lesions have few Mϕ and an abundance of ORO-stainable lipid interstitially, presumably in pools of proteoglycan-rich matrix. There is very little evidence of smooth muscle cell proliferation in either of these two microscopic types of fatty streak. One should also recognize that although grossly "lesion-resistant" areas of the aorta and especially the proximal LAD often show diffuse fibrous thickening, we do not classify these as fatty plaque lesions until there is microscopically detected, ORO-stained intracellular or intercellular lipid.

The fibrous plaque, as recognized and illustrated in this chapter, presents an even more monotonous microscopic appearance. It varies only in the relative proportions of a necrotic lipid/cholesterol and sometimes calcium-rich central core and the dense collagenous fibrous cap, which covers the surface and to some extent encases this advanced lesion.

The fatty plaque, which we have found to be the most frequent of the lesions seen both grossly and microscopically in this study, has a generally monotonous appearance grossly. It can be either elongated or punctate (Fig. 2a,c) or perhaps even a rounded yellow patch grossly, usually with sharp and discrete edges. As seen with the sidelighting we have used in our photographs, it casts a small shadow and thus has to be categorized as a raised plaque (Fig. 2a). On the other hand, its microscopic appearance can be quite variable, and as this study has indicated, the variations in those microscopic forms can be divided into four distinct types.

The new classification is very useful in understanding some of the variables in the pathogenesis of the atherosclerotic plaque. For example, it helps to identify the components of the lesions that are most likely to be associated with progression. It also makes it possible to correlate an individual risk factor with the predominance of a certain type of lesion and with the presence or absence of circulating immune complexes. We have now had the opportunity to utilize this classification for the gross and microscopic study of over 915 cases. Therefore, this chapter represents a summary of the valuable information that the use of this classification has provided so far in two major applications:

- To differentiate the variable nature of the lesions found at the three core sample locations in the aorta and the proximal area of the LAD.
- To study the influence of the most common major risk factors on the microscopic development of intermediate lesions in each part of the arterial system investigated.

Table 4 gives a summary of the data from these cases on which both gross and microscopic classifications were made. It indicates that the same trends that were noted when 100 cases were surveyed (Table 1) are continued when many more cases are included in the analysis. The major value of adding the additional cases has been to extend the numbers sufficiently so that one could study more adequately the influences of the major risk factors.

In this chapter, the major trends are presented that were found in a unifactorial analysis of the influence of the risk factors that are usually measured in these cases. Further work needs to be done in this area, but it is quite evident from the results so far that there may be some very valuable information that can be gained by utilization of the risk factor data in concert with the intermediate lesion classification system.

The major points that can be made from the influence of risk factor analysis and types of intermediate lesions in each of the core sample areas are illustrated in a series of bar graphs (Figs. 6–9), which are derived from microscopic classification of all of the artery samples available from 915 cases. This represents the individual quantitative risk factor analyses on a very large proportion of the samples. The

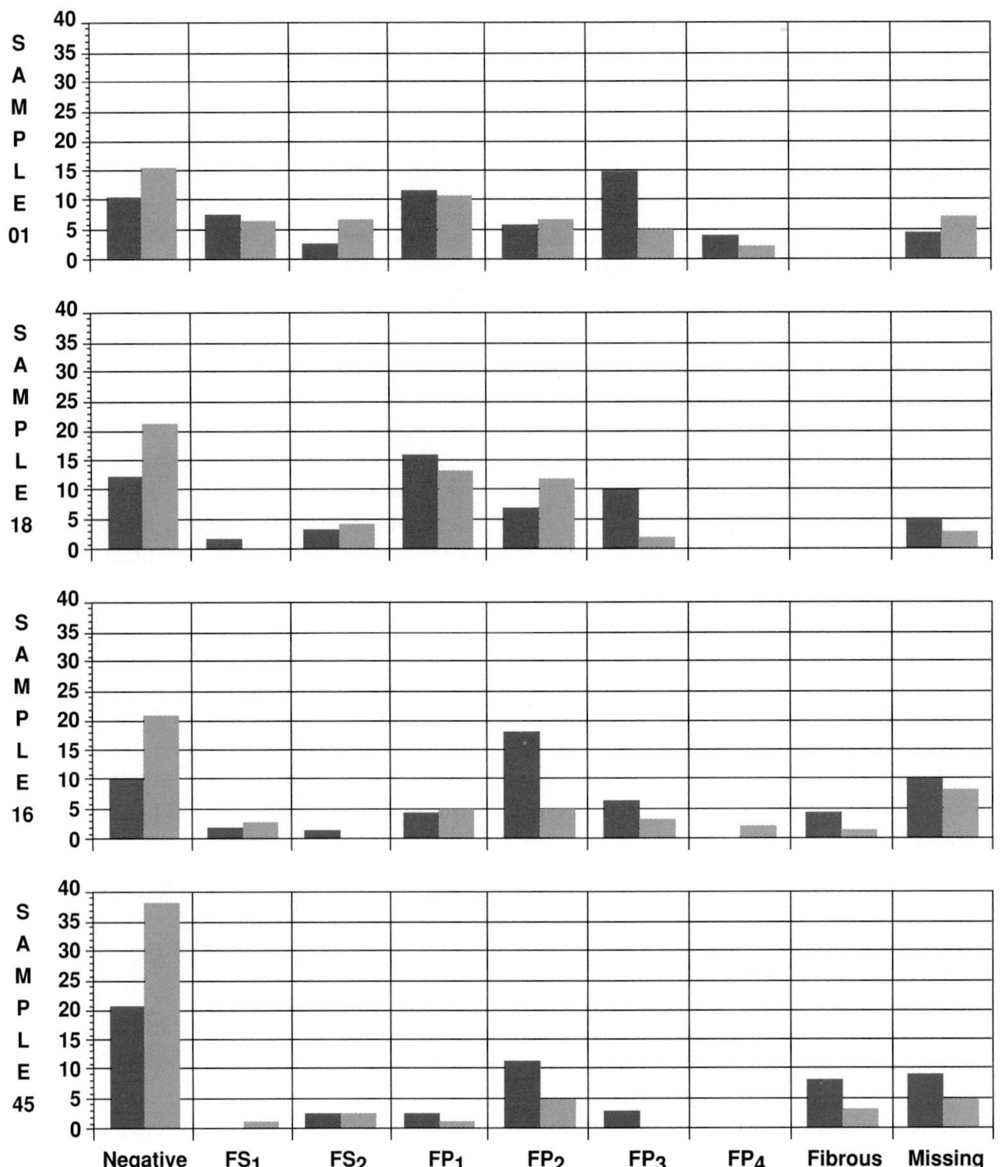

FIG. 6. This family of bar graphs is derived from 550 classified cases with the high extremes and the low extremes of the postmortem serum cholesterol values shown separately. *Solid bars* represent the highest 55 cases, and *light bars* represent the lowest 55 cases. Negatives indicate that no microscopic lesion was seen. FS_1 is a fatty streak in which most of the lipid is intracellular, and in FS_2 it is mostly extracellular. The FP numbers 1 through 4 correspond to the four microscopic types of intermediate lesions, and the term "fibrous" refers to the typical fibrous plaque. "Missing" means that a few microscopic sections were not available.

graphs reveal a number of highly informative associations. These relationships lend themselves to further exploration in relation to the role of each risk factor at the cellular and lesion component level in the histogenesis and pathogenesis of human atherosclerosis during this 20-year age span.

In Fig. 6, the effects of the higher and lower cholesterol values are seen. As with all of these comparisons, the contrast is apparent between the classification of lesions in the top 10% and the bottom 10% on which the risk factor data are available. For cholesterol, this represents 550 cases. The graphic results of the top 55 cases and the bottom 55 cases are shown in this figure. Each microscopic arterial sample has been classified, and the results totaled. It is evident that there are many more negative microscopic sections (no lipid in the intima) in the lower-cholesterol group if the frozen preparations of aortic samples (01, 18, and 16) and the coronary sample (sample 45) are studied after ORO staining. Fatty plaque type 3, as well as type 2, is somewhat more frequent in the thoracic aorta when the postmortem serum cholesterol is high, and this increased frequency for fatty plaque type 3, with its abundant Mϕ foam cells, is found to a greater extent in sample 18 and to a lesser extent in samples

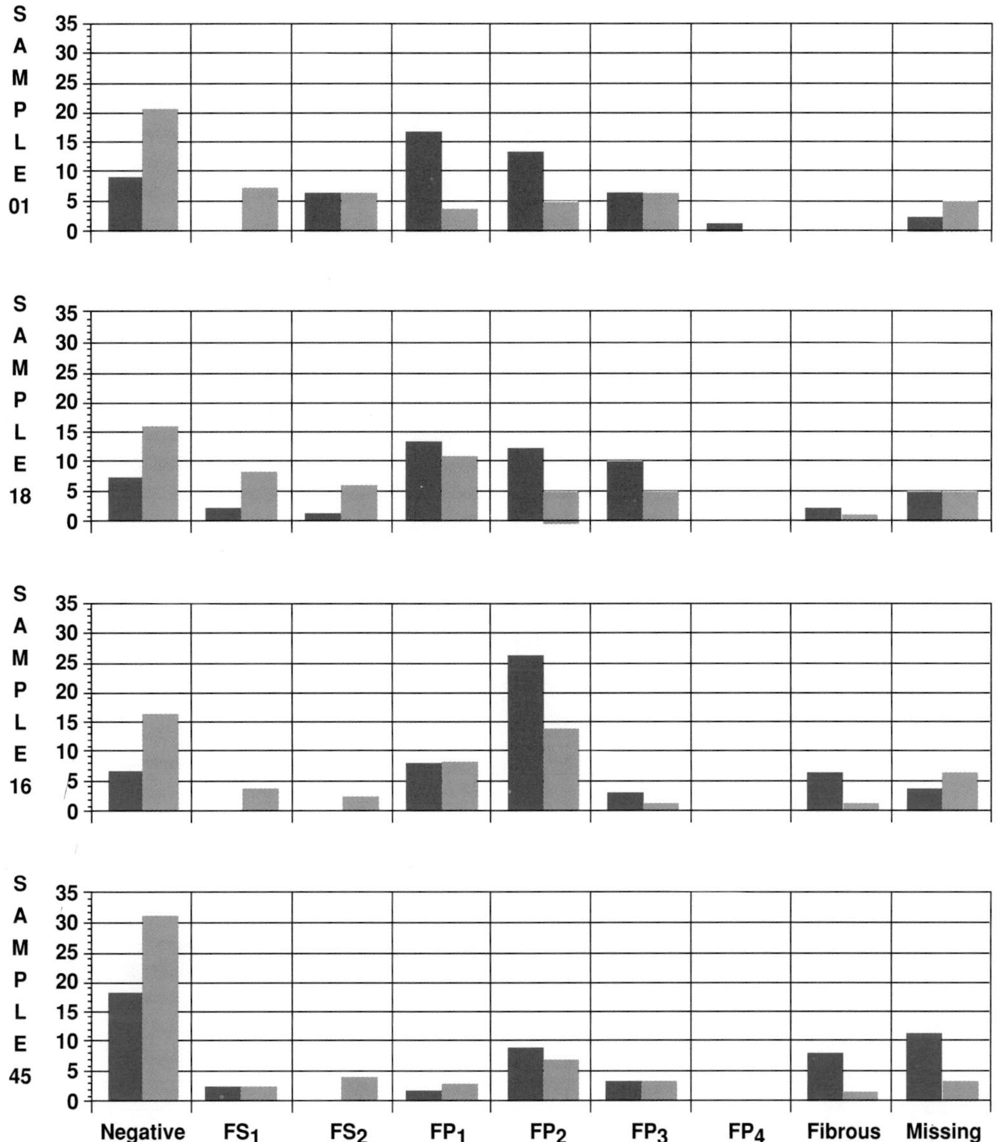

FIG. 7. The 550 classified cases with high extremes and low extremes of the postmortem thiocyanate serum levels are shown. *Solid bars* represent the 55 cases with the highest, and *light bars* the 55 cases with the lowest values. The other symbolic letters, numbers, and abbreviations on the abscissa have the same meanings as in Fig. 6.

16 and 45. This seems to be a consistent effect of hypercholesterolemia. The most consistent effect of high serum cholesterol levels, when evaluated by this method, is a much greater preponderance of fibrous plaques in samples 16 (lower abdominal aorta) and 45 (proximal LAD) in the higher-serum cholesterol group. This seems to indicate that a high serum cholesterol level manifests itself, during this 20-year span, by stimulating and sustaining a higher Mϕ foam cell population in those areas where plaques are not likely to progress—the thoracic aorta and, to a lesser extent, the midabdominal aorta. This is a phenomenon we have documented by actual cell population determination in a smaller group of cases, and these data add to the growing body of evidence that over this 20-year range, the larger Mϕ population appears to be associated with a lack of progression of plaques (11,12). So far, it is not clear why the Mϕ foam cell population becomes more numerous in these relatively "progression-protected, lesion-prone" areas of the aorta and coronary arteries. The other definite association of hypercholesterolemia is with the high incidence of fibrous plaques in hyperlipidemic individuals. This is limited to the areas such as the lower abdominal aorta and proximal LAD coronary artery, where we know that plaques are most likely to progress.

Figure 7 reflects the high and low levels of serum thiocyanate and their association with the intermediate lesion types. Note that with this risk factor, there is a consistent trend in all four arterial samples for more intercellular (i.e., extracel-

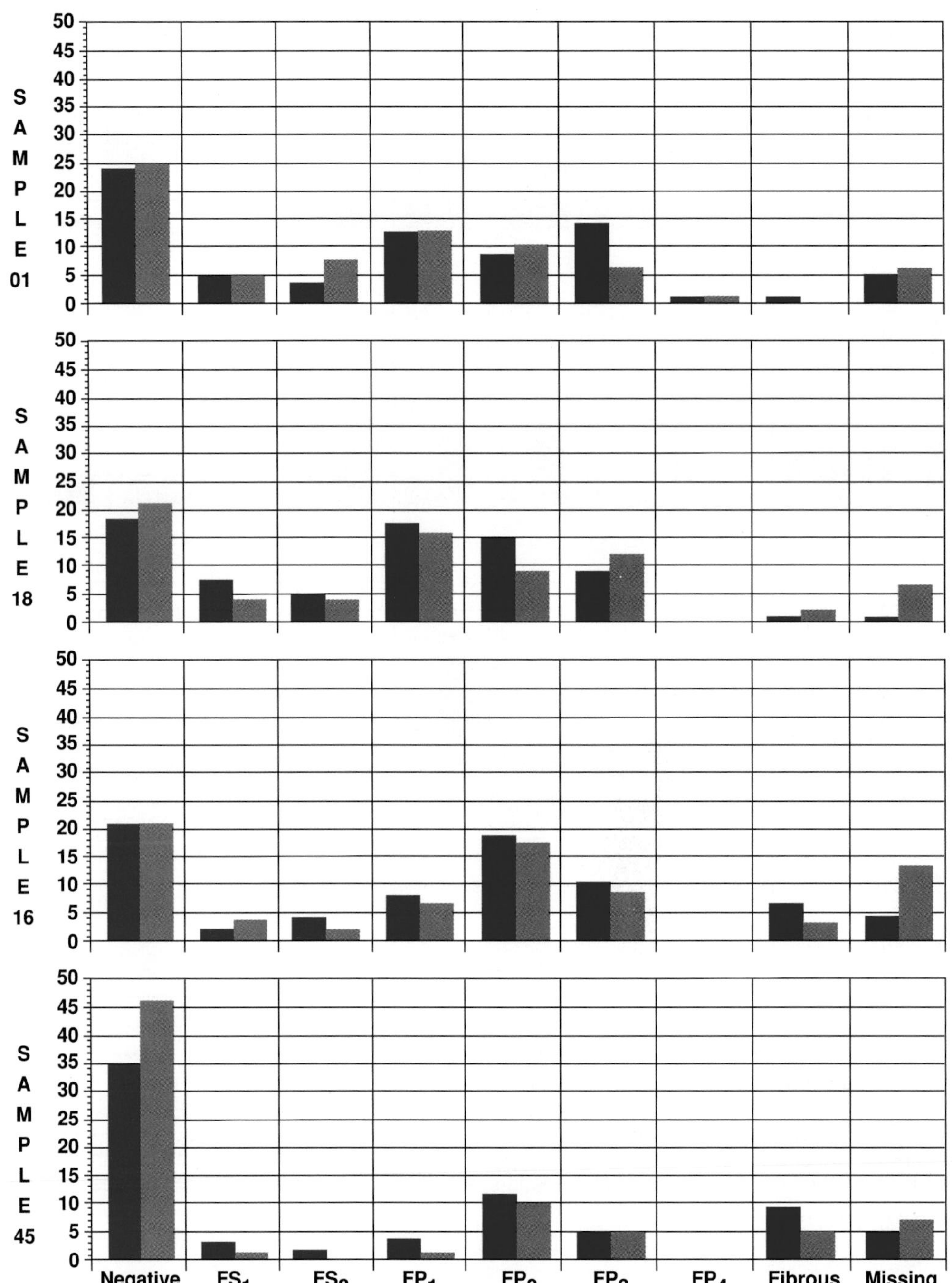

FIG. 8. The 750 classified cases with the high extremes and the low extremes of the glycosylated hemoglobin values are projected. *Solid bars* represent the highest 75 cases, and *light bars* represent the lowest 75 cases. Otherwise, the values are indicated by the same symbols and abbreviations as in the previous two figures.

lular) lipid to be present. This is particularly notable in lower abdominal aortic sample 16, where it is known that aortic lesions progress more consistently and extensively during these 20 years from 15 to and including 34 years of age. The other definite findings are the severalfold higher incidences of fibrous plaques in samples 16 and 45 in smokers. There is also a higher incidence of ORO-negative samples in the lower thiocyanate group, compared to the highest 10% of the 550-case group, in all the core sample sites studied, including the proximal LAD coronary artery.

When glycosylated hemoglobin values at the top and bottom 10% of the 750 cases on which these determinations are available are studied (Fig. 8), there is a tendency for samples with negative lipid staining to be correlated with

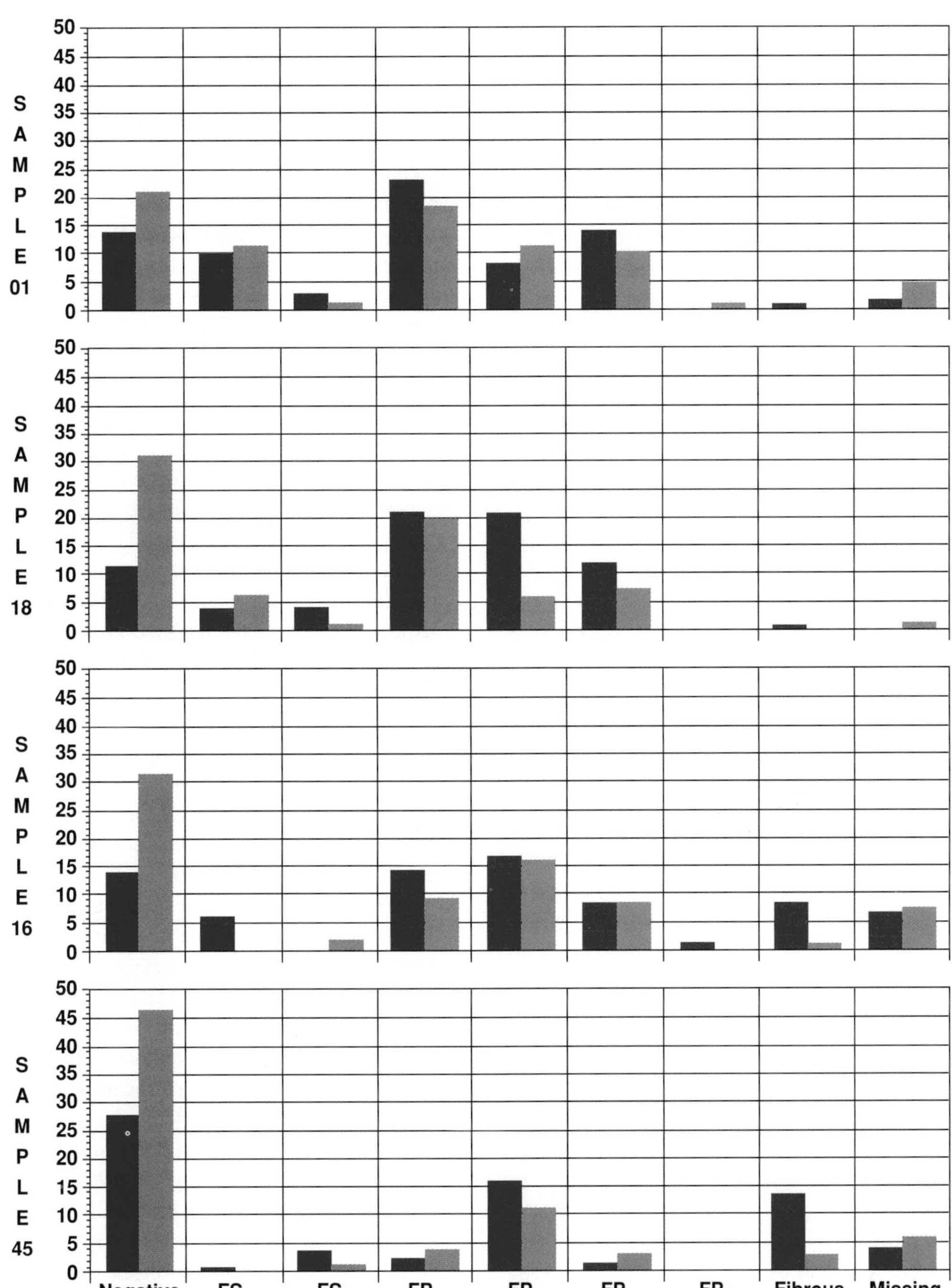

FIG. 9. The 750 classified cases with the high extremes and the low extremes of the renal hypertension indicators are projected. *Solid bars* represent the 75 cases with the highest, and *light bars* the 75 cases with the lowest values. The symbols and abbreviations on the abscissa have the same meaning as in the previous three figures.

the lower values for glycosylated hemoglobin in the proximal LAD sample 45. There was very little indication of a difference in negative samples between the two groups in any standard core sample site of the aorta.

On the other hand, elevated glycosylated hemoglobin values yield a consistently higher incidence of fibrous plaques than those cases that had the lowest glycosylated hemoglobin levels. This indicates that although relatively high glycosylated hemoglobin values apparently are associated microscopically with about twice the incidence of true fibrous plaques, each displaying a lipid-rich acellular core and a definite fibrous cap in the abdominal aorta and in the proximal LAD, the classification system is not helpful in delineating the features or types of the intermediate plaques that result in this increased severity of disease in these young individuals. There are slight trends in the data from sample 16 and sample 45 that suggest that a high glycosylated hemoglobin level may support a somewhat higher incidence of fatty streaks with predominantly extracellular lipid. The numbers so far are so small that the resolution of the problem will have to await additional cases and additional evidence as to how cases with elevated glycosylated hemoglobin postmortem become associated with twice the incidence of fibrous plaques in these highly vulnerable areas.

Figure 9 shows a family of bar graphs reflecting the results of comparing the incidences of the various microscopic types of intermediate lesions with the 10% high and the 10% low values for the hypertension indices in 750 cases (20,21). The results are of interest in three ways:

- Many more samples are completely negative for any pathological lipid deposition in the low end than at the top end of these indices of hypertension, especially in samples 18, 16, and 45.
- There is a severalfold increase in fibrous plaques in the lower abdominal aorta and in the proximal LAD in those cases with a high indication of hypertension.
- There is a trend toward a greater incidence of fatty plaque type 2 in sample 18 when these two extremes of hypertension are compared.

In general, one can summarize the effects of hypertension on plaque development by stating that the individuals with the highest indices for hypertension may be developing more lesions earlier and that the main mechanism may involve the entrance of more lipid and cholesterol into the artery (probably as low-density lipoprotein). This may lead to an earlier predominance of extracellular lipid and ultimately to a greater incidence of advanced fibrous plaques.

All of these early attempts to correlate the microscopic types of intermediate lesions with some of the major individual risk factors will, we believe, ultimately prove to be useful. They are the first step in understanding the various pathogenetic sequences by which the classical risk factors support the accelerated development of fibrous plaques in young people. It is notable that the PDAY data analyzed microscopically indicate that in this age group, from 15 to and including 34, each of these risk factors leads to a two- to sixfold increase in fibrous plaque incidence in samples 16 and 1. There is also a consistent trend for each of these risk factors to support some type of manifestation of plaque development, especially in the lower abdominal aorta or proximal LAD coronary artery.

It is obvious that multifactorial analysis may yield more definitive information when additional cases are available. In fact, there may be a special opportunity, using this grading system, to study early effects of each of these risk factors, singly and in combinations, on some of the highly variable microscopic components of the developing plaques. To that end, efforts are aimed at increasing the numbers of cases available for this type of analysis of the effects of the various major risk factors.

A SUMMARY OF CURRENT FINDINGS EMPHASIZING THE FUTURE VALUE OF THIS METHOD OF CLASSIFYING DEVELOPING ATHEROSCLEROTIC LESIONS

The results of this large-scale study, in which both gross and microscopic evaluation has been possible, reveal the advantages of this new classification system. When the results are compared with the time-honored system of classifying lesions into "fatty streaks" and "fibrous plaques," along with an ill-defined intermediate lesion category, then abundant new information is apparent. It can now be demonstrated clearly that grossly uniform types of raised, intermediate lesions exist. These, we believe, should be regarded as distinct from the fatty streak. For at least 30 years, the fatty plaque has usually been labeled a fatty streak. Now, it is becoming quite easy, without the validation furnished by the gross photographs and the standard samples, to identify the four microscopic types of developing plaques whose gross appearances permit them to fulfill the criteria for fatty plaques. When the standardized gross samples are prepared for microscopic study using a high-resolution fat stain, counterstained with Lilly hematoxylin, it is evident that these gross, clearly defined, raised, yellow fatty plaques can take on at least four different and distinct appearances. If one looks at the newly classified types in relation to the data on anatomic localization or the quantitative data on risk factors determined at the time of postmortem examination, one can develop an understanding of the components of the plaques that are affected by each of these variables. These comparisons are providing new insights into histogenesis and pathogenesis that have not been possible previously. The application of this classification system, incomplete as it is at present, has revealed a number of new and important observations. These include the factors responsible for the development of an abundance of extracellular lipid and the reasons for the persistence of the macrophage component of the lesion far beyond the simple fatty streak. Furthermore, this postmortem study of young people has revealed the unexpected presence of fibrous plaques in relatively large numbers in the coronary arteries as compared to the rather slow and infrequent development in the lower abdominal aorta.

With further study one should be able to utilize the system to get a better understanding of the frequency and a more precise definition of the lesion components that accompany various levels of circulating immune complexes (17,18). Many of the observations that support the special pathogenic mechanisms responsible for this type of accelerated atheroarteritis have been summarized (22).

What are the main contributions of these unifactorial analyses of multiple standardized arterial samples from more than 900 forensic autopsies on young people for which quantitative risk factor data are available? The following emerge as definite findings that need to be placed in apposition to the data presented in the recent report of the AHA Committee on Lesions, of which one of us was a member and coauthor

(7). In fact, it became apparent when the Committee tried to develop a clearly stated gross and microscopic definition of the intermediate lesion that there was a lack of definitive information and some confusion in the published reports on this subject. The reasons for this were largely the lack of a data base in which standard "core" areas of arteries from many individuals could be studied both grossly and microscopically. Furthermore, no other group of scientists had the advantage of close-up photography of grossly classified lesions that could be compared with high-resolution fat stains under conditions in which the cellular and lipid components of the microscopic sections could be clearly defined.

Now that this objective has been attained to a great extent, one can clarify a number of the indefinite bits of information that have been published on the intermediate or transitional lesion.

- It is clear that the late-stage fatty streak or the intermediate lesion (types II or III) in the recent Committee on Lesions report is not always rich in Mϕ (7). The PDAY results indicate that only about half of the 402 classical fatty streaks that have been studied grossly and microscopically in the aorta (Table 4) have more than 20% of their lipid in Mϕ foam cells. The other lesions of this type have most of the stainable lipid interstitially, i.e., extracellularly.
- Both the lower abdominal and the proximal LAD coronary arteries sampled (samples 16 and 45) had definitely higher proportions of the fatty streak with intercellular lipid (fatty streak type 2).
- The fatty plaque types of intermediate lesions in the aorta do not consistently have a large amount of extracellular (i.e., intercellular or interstitial) lipid as implied in the Committee report. In fact, in the 915 cases examined, 1,707 fatty plaques were observed, and of these 613 had most of the lipid in smooth muscle cells with very few Mϕ foam cells visible and almost no visible interstitial lipid. There were 703 fatty plaques that were composed largely of smooth muscle cells with abundant extracellular lipid (Table 4). The remaining 391 fatty plaques were rich in Mϕ foam cells and/or small lymphocytes.
- It is clear from the evaluation of many hundreds of PDAY lesions that both the classical "fatty streaks" and the intermediate lesions may develop in an almost completely normal intima. At this age, diffuse or adaptive fibrous thickening or focal intimal thickening is not a necessary preexisting condition for atheromatous lesion formation in the lesion-prone areas. In fact, the intima adjacent to the gross and microscopic lesions is usually only one or two lamellar units thick. We do believe that the hemodynamic principles established by Glagov et al. (23) and others are important determinants of "lesion-prone" and "lesion-resistant" areas, but they are not always reflected by intimal thickening before lipid is deposited.
- In our experience, the "progression-prone" fatty plaques, which have been classified as type 2 fatty plaques, are among our most frequent microscopic types. They correspond to the type IIA and type III intermediate fatty streaks or intermediate lesions, as defined by the Committee. However, they are definitely raised plaques grossly, and they are indistinguishable grossly from the other three microscopic types of fatty plaques that make up the constellation of intermediate lesions seen microscopically.
- The type III lesions as defined by the Committee really are intermediate lesions microscopically. They have developing pools of intercellular lipid and are much more frequent in the lower abdominal aorta and in the proximal LAD coronary artery than in the other two standardized aortic core samples that have been studied. It must be emphasized that, in the PDAY study, these type 2 lesions are indistinguishable grossly from the other microscopic fatty plaques; in particular, this is true of the fatty plaques types 1 and the fatty plaques type 2 as shown in the illustrations (Fig. 2a,d). This means that microscopic evaluation is necessary in order to learn the most about lesion development.

It is clear that a number of points need further clarification in order to gain the most information from the four microscopic types of fatty plaques represented in this classification of intermediate lesions. These include a further quantitative study of the cell populations in each of the microscopic types, a delineation of the lymphocytes in the lesions, and a more definitive study of the relationships of each lesion type of fatty plaque to the various risk factors, including a number that have not yet been evaluated. The apo E phenotypes, the influence of homocysteine levels, and the paradoxical increase in fatty streaks and fatty plaques in young women, especially young black women, need more attention. A number of previous studies have revealed this association, even though these fatty plaques did not seem to progress nearly as consistently as those in white men.

Obviously, one of the major contributions of this intensive study of developing lesions thus far has been the demonstration of the value of standardization of sampling, careful gross classification according to well-developed criteria, quantitative risk factor data, and efforts to delineate the microscopic components of cells and lipid into an orderly set of microscopically defined types.

ACKNOWLEDGMENTS

The authors are indebted to the following individuals, who contributed greatly to the development of this chapter: Mary C. Gorney, Blanche Berger, Alexander Arguelles, Taryn McFadden, Patti Dickson, Gordon Bowie, Rudolph Banovich, and Robert Skurauskis.

The Pathobiological Determinants of Atherosclerosis in Youth (PDAY) Research Group consists of the following people (and is supported by the following grants from NIH):

Directory. Program Director: R. W. Wissler, PhD, MD, University of Chicago; Associate Directors: A. L. Robertson, Jr., MD, PhD, University of Illinois; J. P. Strong, MD, Louisiana State University.

Steering Committee. J. F. Cornhill, DPhil, Ohio State Univeristy; H. C. McGill, Jr., MD, and C. A. McMahan, PhD, University of Texas Health Science Center at San Antonio; A. L. Robertson, Jr., MD, PhD, University of Illinois; J. P. Strong, MD, Louisiana State University; R. W. Wissler, PhD, MD, University of Chicago.

University of Alabama. Department of Medicine: Principal Investigator: S. Gay, MD; Coinvestigators: R. E. Gay, MD, and C.-Q. Huang, MD (HL-33733); Department of Biochemistry; Principal Investigator: E. J. Miller, PhD; Coinvestigators: D. K. Furuto, PhD; M. S. Vail; A. J. Narkates (HL-33728).

Albany Medical College. Principal Investigator: A. Daoud, MD; Coinvestigators: A. S. Frank, PhD; M. A. Hyer; E. C. McGovern (HL-33765).

Baylor College of Medicine: Principal Investigator: L. C. Smith, PhD; Coinvestigator: F. M. Strickland, PhD (HL-33750).

University of Chicago. Principal Investigator: R. W. Wissler, PhD, MD; Coinvestigators: D. Vesselinovitch, DVM, MS; A. Komatsu, MD, PhD; Y. Kusumi, MD; R. T. Bridenstein, MS; R. J. Stein, MD; R. H. Kirschner, MD; M. Bekermeier, HTASCP; B. Berger, HTASCP; L. Hiltscher, HTASCP (HL-33740).

The University of Illinois. Principal Investigator: A. L. Robertson, Jr., MD, PhD; Coinvestigators: R. J. Stein, MD; E. E. Emeson, MD; L. Ghosh, MD; H. M. Yamashiroya, PhD; R. J. Buschmann, PhD; E. R. Donoghue, Jr., MD; T. L. An, MD; E. Choi, MD; N. Jones, MD; M. J. Jumbelic, MD; M. S. Kalelkar, MD; U. Konakei, MD; Barry Lifschultz, MD; M.-L. Shen, PhD; R. Yang, MS; V. R. Gumidyala, MD; R. Harper, B.S.; F. Norris, HTL, HTASCP (HL-33758).

Louisiana State University. Principal Investigator: J. P. Strong, MD; Coinvestigators: G. T. Malcom, PhD; W. P. Newman, III, MD; M. C. Oalmann, DrPH; P. S. Roheim, MD; A. K. Bhattacharyya, PhD; M. A. Guzman, PhD; A. A. Hatem, MD; C. A. Hornick, PhD; C. D. Restrepo, MD; R. E. Tracy, MD, PhD (HL-33746); C. C. Breaux, MS; S. E. Hubbard; C. S. Zsembik; D. G. Gibbs (HL-33746).

University of Maryland. Principal Investigator: W. J. Mergner, MD, PhD; Coinvestigators: J. H. Resau, PhD; R. D. Vigorito, MS, PA; Q.-C. Yu, MD; J. Smialek (HL-33752).

Medical College of Georgia. Coprincipal Investigators: A. B. Chandler, MD; R. N. Rao, MD; Coinvestigators: D. G. Falls, MD; B. O. Spurlock, BA; Associate Investigators: K. B. Sharma, MD; J. S. Sexton, MD; Research Assistants: K. K. Smith, HTASCP; G. W. Forbes (HL-33772).

University of Nebraska. Principal Investigator: B. M. McManus, MD, PhD; Coinvestigators: J. W. Jones, MD; T. J. Kendall, MS; J. A. Remmenga, BS; W. C. Rogler, BS (HL-33778).

Ohio State University. Principal Investigator: J. F. Cornhill, DPhil; Convestigators: W. R. Adrion, MD; P. M. Fardel, MD; B. Gara, MS; E. Herderick; J. Meimer, MS; L. R. Tare, MD (HL-33760).

Southwest Foundation for Biomedical Research. Principal Investigator: J. E. Hixson, PhD; P. K. Powers (HL-39913).

The University of Texas Health Science Center at San Antonio. Principal Investigator: C. A. McMahan, PhD; Co-investigators: G. M. Barnwell, PhD; H. C. McGill, Jr., MD; Y. N. Marinez, MA; T. J. Prihoda, PhD; H. S. Wigodsky, MD, PhD (HL-33749).

Vanderbilt University. Principal Investigator: R. Virmani, MD; Coinvestigators: J. B. Atkinson, MD, PhD; C. W. Harlan, MD (HL-33770).

West Virginia University. Principal Investigator: S. N. Jagannathan, PhD; Coinvestigators: B. Catherson, PhD; J. L. Frost, MD; K. Murali; K. Rao, MD; S. Jagannathan; P. Johnson; N. F. Rodman, MD (HL-33748).

REFERENCES

1. Holman RH, McGill HC Jr, Strong JP, Geer GC. The natural history of atherosclerosis: The early aortic lesions as seen in New Orleans in the middle of the 20th century. *Am J Pathol* 1958;34:209–235.
2. Uemura K, Sternby N, Vanecek R, et al. Grading atherosclerosis in aorta and coronary arteries obtained at autopsy. *Bull WHO* 1964;31: 297–320.
3. Miller EJ, Malcom GT, McMahan CA, Strong JP. Atherosclerosis in young white males: Arterial collagen and cholesterol. *Matrix* 1993;13: 289–294.
4. Haust MD, More RH, Movat HZ. The role of the smooth muscle cell in the fibrogenesis of atherosclerosis. *Am J Pathol* 1960;37:377–389.
5. Wissler RW, Vesselinovitch D, Komatsu A. The contribution of studies of atherosclerotic lesions in young people to future research. *Ann NY Acad Sci* 1990;264:3018–3024.
6. Wissler RW. USA multicenter study of the pathobiology of atherosclerosis in youth. *Ann NY Acad Sci* 1991;623:26–39.
7. Stary HC, Chandler AB, Glagov S, Guyton JR, Insull W Jr, Rosenfeld ME, Schaffer SA, Schwartz CJ, Wagner WD, Wissler RW. A definition of initial, fatty streak, and intermediate lesions of atherosclerosis. *Arterioscler Thromb* 1994;14:840–856.
8. Cornhill JF, Herderick EE, Stary HC. Topography of human aortic sudanophilic lesions. In: Liepsch DW, ed. *Blood Flow in Larger Arteries: Applications to Atherogenesis and Clinical Medicine*. Basel: Karger; 1990:13–19.
9. Wissler RW, Komatsu A, Curi E, Hiltscher L. Classification of the intermediate atherosclerotic lesions in young people [Abstract]. In: *XI International Symposium on Drugs Affecting Lipid Metabolism*. 1992.
10. Wissler RW, Hiltscher L, Gage A, Bekermeier M. A useful classification of the intermediate atherosclerotic lesion in the aortas of young people (gross and microscopic lesions). Poster presented at the 26th Hugh Lofland Conference on Arterial Wall Metabolism, Bowman-Gray School of Medicine, Winston-Salem, North Carolina, May, 1993.
11. Wissler RW, Komatsu A, Ko C, Kusumi Y, Vesselinovitch D. The cell populations and other components of the atheromatous lesions in young people. In: Hauss WH, Wissler RW, Bauch H-J, eds. *New Aspects of Metabolism and Behavior of Mesenchymal Cells During the Pathogenesis of Atherosclerosis*. Opladen: Westdeutscher Verlag; 1991:49–60.
12. Komatsu A, Wissler RW, Vesselinovitch D. Cell populations in atheromatous lesions in young people. *Arteriosclerosis* 1989;9:709a.
13. Robertson AL Jr, Stein RJ, Katsura Y, Buschmann RJ. Preclinical coronary atherosclerosis in young trauma victims. Summary of a paper presented at the Annual Meeting Society for Cardiovascular Pathology, Atlanta, Georgia, 1992.
14. Glagov S, Rowley DA, Kohout RI. Atherosclerosis of the human aorta and its coronary and renal arteries. *Arch Pathol Lab Med* 1961;72: 558–571.

15. Glagov S. Hemodynamic risk factors: Mechanical stress, mural architecture, medial nutrition and the vulnerability of arteries to atherosclerosis. In: Wissler RW, Geer JC, eds. *The Pathogenesis of Atherosclerosis*. Baltimore: Williams & Wilkins; 1972:164–199.
16. Wissler RW. New insights into the pathogenesis of atherosclerosis as revealed by PDAY. *Atherosclerosis* 1994;108:S3–S20.
17. Wissler RW, Vesselinovitch D, Ko C. The effect of circulating immune complexes on atherosclerotic lesions in experimental animals and in younger and older humans. *Transplant Proc* 1989;21:3707–3708.
18. Wissler R.W. Human transplant atheroarteritis and its relationship to other forms of risk factor engendered injury of the artery wall: Summarizing presentation. In: *New Pathogenic Aspects of Arteriosclerosis Emphasizing Transplantation Atheroarteritis*. Hauss WH, Wissler RW, Bauch HJ, eds. Openladen, Germany: Westdentscher Verlag, 1994; 137–145.
19. Fuster V. Mechanisms leading to myocardial infarction—insights from studies of vascular biology. Lewis A. Conner Memorial Lecture. *Circulation* 1994;90:2126–2146.
20. Tracy RE, Mercante DE, Moncada A, Berensen G. Quantitation of hypertensive nephrosclerosis on an objective rational scale of measure in adult and children. *Am J Clin Pathol* 1986;85:312–318.
21. Tracy RE, MacLean CJ, Reed DM, Hayashi T, Gandia M, Strong JP. Blood pressure, nephrosclerosis, and age: An autopsy study in the Honolulu Heart Project. *Mod Pathol* 1988;1:420–427.
22. Wissler RW, Vesselinovitch D, Davis HR, Lambert PH, Bekermeier M. A new way to look at atherosclerotic involvement of the artery wall and the functional effects. *Ann NY Acad Sci* 1985;454:9–22.
23. Glagov S, Zarins C, Giddens DP, Ku DN. Hemodynamics and atherosclerosis: Insights and perspectives gained from studies of human arteries. *Arch Pathol Lab Med* 1988;112:1018–1031.

Atherosclerosis and Coronary Artery Disease,
edited by V. Fuster, R. Ross, and E. J. Topol.
Lippincott-Raven Publishers, Philadelphia © 1996.

CHAPTER 28

Pathogenesis of Plaque Disruption

Erling Falk, Prediman K. Shah, and Valentin Fuster

Key Words: Atheromatous core; Calcification; Degeneration; Lipoproteins; Necrosis; Ossification; Plaque rupture; Tensile stress; Thrombosis; Vasoconstriction.

INTRODUCTION

Coronary atherosclerosis without thrombosis is in general a benign disease. Coronary lesions are present in most individuals after two decades of life, particularly in Western countries, and mature plaques may narrow the arterial lumen limiting blood flow and myocardial perfusion. Survival is, however, good if thrombotic complications can be prevented (1,2). Therefore, the question as to why the atherosclerotic plaque, after years of indolent growth, suddenly gives rise to life-threatening luminal thrombosis becomes vital. Recent clinical and pathoanatomic observations indicate that plaque type (composition and biology) rather than plaque size (stenosis severity) is most important for development of thrombus-mediated acute coronary syndromes; lipid-rich and soft plaques are more dangerous than collagen-rich and hard plaques because of increased vulnerability and thrombogenicity (1–4).This chapter will explore potential mechanisms responsible for the sudden conversion of a slowly progressing atherosclerotic plaque to a life-threatening atherothrombotic lesion—an event known as plaque rupture, disruption, or fissuring (5–7).

Erling Falk: DHF Cardiovascular Pathology Unit, Skejby University Hospital, 8200 Aarhus N, Denmark.
Prediman K. Shah: Division of Cardiology, Cedars-Sinai Medical Center, Los Angeles, California 90048-0750.
Valentin Fuster: Cardiovascular Institute and Department of Medicine, Mount Sinai Medical Center, New York, New York 10029-6574.

ATHEROGENESIS

Atherosclerosis is the result of a complex interaction between flow, blood, and vessel wall, involving the following pathological processes: (a) *inflammation* with increased endothelial permeability (8,9), endothelial activation (10–14), and monocyte recruitment (15–18); (b) *growth* with smooth muscle cell (SMC) proliferation, migration, and matrix synthesis (19–23); (c) *degeneration* with lipid accumulation (24–27); (d) *necrosis,* possibly due to cytotoxic effects of oxidized lipid (27–30); (e) *calcification/ossification* that may be an active rather than a dystrophic process (31,32);

and finally, (f) *thrombosis* with platelet recruitment and fibrin formation (1–4,33,34). The later process, thrombosis, is usually considered a complication of the atherosclerotic process itself.

Early Lesions

Atherosclerotic plaques tend to develop in areas with preexisting adaptive intimal thickening at sites of oscillating or low shear stress (35,36). In these lesion-prone areas, increased endothelial permeability (8,9,37) and endothelial activation (10–14) lead to insudation of plasma and monocyte recruitment, accompanied or followed by intimal SMC proliferation, migration, and matrix synthesis (19). Insudated lipoproteins may be trapped in intima (22,23,26) and endocytosed by the recruited monocyte-derived macrophages, probably via scavenger receptors after oxidative modification, giving rise to the characteristic lipid-filled foam cells (27). Also, intimal SMC may internalize insudated lipoproteins. Collections of such lipid-filled foam cells may be seen macroscopically as yellow streaks or dots barely raised above the intimal surface, constituting a significant component of the early lesion termed fatty streak (38). Although activated and dysfunctioning, the endothelium is usually intact in lesion-prone areas and over early lesions (39–41).

Mature Plaques

The early lipid-driven inflammation is accompanied or followed by SMC proliferation, matrix synthesis, and extracellular lipid accumulation that may give rise to mature and clinically significant atherosclerotic plaques (28,29). Ongoing inflammation with recruitment of monocyte-derived macrophages, T lymphocytes (11,18), and a few mast cells (42–44) may destroy the adjacent endothelium, and focal denuded areas, often with platelets adhering to the exposed subendothelial tissue, are frequently found over mature plaques (40,41). Platelets and microthrombi may now contribute to plaque growth by stimulating adjacent cells within the plaque and/or being incorporated into the lesion (1,19,45). Platelet degranulation products, thrombin and fibrin(ogen), possess chemotactic and mitogenic properties (33,46), and all key cells in human plaques express receptors for both platelet-derived growth factor and thrombin (19,47). Therefore, platelets and thrombin are probably critical in the evolution of mature plaques by mediating proliferative, migratory, synthetic, and inflammatory processes.

Vulnerable Plaques

In patients with ischemic heart disease, the coronary arteries are diffusely involved with confluent ''plaquing'' (48), but individual plaques vary greatly in composition, consistency, and vulnerability to rupture. As the name ''atherosclerosis'' implies, mature plaques consist typically of two main components: soft, lipid-rich *atheromatous* ''gruel'' and hard, collagen-rich *sclerotic* tissue (Fig. 1; see Colorplate 17). The sclerotic component usually is by far the most voluminous plaque component, constituting >70% of an average stenotic coronary plaque (49,50). Sclerosis is, however, relatively innocuous because the collagen-rich matrix secreted by SMC hardens and stabilizes plaques, protecting them against disruption. In contrast, the less voluminous atheromatous component is most dangerous because it softens and destabilizes plaques, making them vulnerable to rupture whereby the highly thrombogenic gruel is exposed to the flowing blood (51)—a life-threatening event (Fig. 2; see Colorplate 18).

Atheromatous Core Formation

During atherogenesis, plasma macromolecules such as albumin, fibrinogen, and lipoproteins insudate plaques from the lumen and advanced plaques are also insudated from the base via new and fragile capillaries originating from adventitial vasa vasorum (neovascularization) (8,52). Insudated lipid may be trapped within the extracellular matrix, where it may accumulate directly, or the lipid may be endocytosed by macrophages, probably via their scavenger receptors after oxidative modification, giving rise to intracellular lipid accumulation which may be followed by foam cell necrosis and release of the lipid-rich contents into the extracellular space (27–30). The individual significance of direct trapping and foam cell necrosis in extracellular lipid accumulation and the formation of a lipid-rich atheromatous core within a mature plaque is unknown (53,54), but the latter macrophage-related pathway is widely believed to be most important (27–30), which is why the lipid-rich core has also been called ''necrotic core'' (55–57) and ''atheronecrosis'' (58,59). Recent pathoanatomic findings suggest, however, that the lipid-rich core does not originate primarily from the debris of dead foam cells in the superficial intima (fatty streaks), but rather arises from lipids accumulating gradually in the extracellular matrix of the deep intima (26,60) where lipoproteins may be trapped because of complex binding to glycosaminoglycans, collagen, and/or fibrinogen (22,23). Immunohistochemically, a striking extracellular colocalization for fibrinogen, apolipoprotein(a), and apolipoprotein B has been described in atherosclerotic plaques, linking thrombogenic factors and lipoproteins in atherogenesis (61).

The atheromatous core is (a) avascular (62,63), (b) hypocellular except at the periphery, where macrophage foam cells are frequently present (62,64,65), (c) devoid of supporting collagen (66), (d) rich in extracellular lipids, predominantly cholesterol and its esters (56,67), and (e) soft like gruel. The consistency of the ''gruel'' depends on lipid composition (crystalline cholesterol versus liquid esters) and temperature. At room temperature postmortem, the ''gruel'' usually has a consistency like toothpaste and it is even softer at body temperature in vivo (56,66,67).

Atherogenic Risk Factors

Clinical observations indicate that endothelial dysfunction, even evaluated in vessels resistant to atherosclerosis, is an early and reliable marker for the presence of atherogenic risk factors (39,68–72). It is unknown, however, how these various risk factors for clinical disease influence the development, composition, and vulnerability of coronary plaques. Age, male sex, hypercholesterolemia, hypertension, smoking, and diabetes correlate with the extent of coronary ''plaquing'' present postmortem (percentage of surface covered with mature plaques) (73–82), but possible differences in plaque composition have not been reported. On the contrary, fibrous tissue seems to constitute the most voluminous component of mature coronary plaques, irrespective of individual risk factors (49,50,83–86). Preliminary data indicate, however, that smokers may have more extracellular lipids, particularly oxidized low-density lipoprotein, in their plaques than nonsmokers (54).

PLAQUE DISRUPTION

Plaques containing a soft atheromatous core may rupture, i.e., the fibrous cap separating the core from the lumen may disintegrate, tear, or break, whereby the highly thrombogenic gruel is suddenly exposed to the flowing blood (Fig. 3; see Colorplate 19). The tears vary greatly in size, most of them being of microscopic size, but some being extensive and readily seen by the naked eye due to the associated hemorrhage into the plaque [also called intraintimal thrombosis (6,66)] and/or luminal thrombosis (7). The intimal tears run more often longitudinally than transversely (7).

Plaque disruption is very important clinically, underlying about 75% of thrombi responsible for acute coronary syndromes (5,6,87). Superficial macrophage-related intimal erosions without frank disruption, i.e., no deep plaque injury, are found beneath the remaining fatal thrombi (about 25%), usually in combination with a severe atherosclerotic stenosis (5,6,88,89).

Concept of Plaque Disruption: Vulnerability Versus Triggers

The risk of plaque disruption is related to *intrinsic* properties of individual plaques (their vulnerability) and *extrinsic* forces acting on plaques (rupture triggers). The former predispose plaques to rupture, while the latter may precipitate disruption if vulnerable plaques are present.

Intrinsic Vulnerability of Plaques

Plaque disruption most frequently occurs where the fibrous cap is thinnest, most heavily infiltrated by foam cells, and therefore weakest. For eccentric plaques, that is often the junction between the plaque and the adjacent less diseased vessel wall, called the shoulders of the plaque (88). Pathoanatomic examination of intact and disrupted plaques and mechanical testing of isolated fibrous caps indicate that a plaque's vulnerability to rupture depends on the following: (a) size and consistency of the atheromatous core, (b) thickness and collagen content of the fibrous cap, (c) inflammation within the cap, and (d) ''fatigue'' of the cap. Long-term repetitive cyclic stresses may weaken a material and increase its vulnerability to fracture, ultimately leading to sudden and unprovoked (i.e., untriggered) mechanical failure due to ''fatigue.'' Therefore, fatigue is discussed here as one of the determinants of plaque vulnerability rather than being included in the subsequent section on rupture triggers.

Atheromatous Core

The size and consistency of the atheromatous core vary greatly from plaque to plaque and are critical for the stability of individual lesions. Although the average stenotic coronary plaque contains much more hard fibrous tissue than soft atheromatous gruel, a significant atheromatous component is usually present in culprit lesions responsible for acute coronary syndromes (4,66). Gertz and Roberts reported the composition of plaques in 5-mm segments from 17 infarct-related arteries examined postmortem and found much larger atheromatous cores in the 39 segments with plaque disruption than in the 229 segments with intact surface (32% and 5%–12% of plaque area, respectively) (63). By studying aortic plaques, Davies et al. found a similar relation between atheromatous core size and plaque disruption and they identified a critical threshold; intact aortic plaques containing a core occupying more than 40% of the plaque area were considered particularly vulnerable and at high risk of rupture and thrombosis (90).

Regarding consistency of the gruel and plaque stability, lipid in the form of cholesteryl esters softens plaque, whereas crystalline cholesterol has the opposite effect (56,67). Based on animal experiments (56,91), lipid-lowering therapy in humans is expected to deplete plaque lipid with an overall reduction in liquid cholesteryl esters and a relative increase in crystalline cholesterol, theoretically resulting in a stiffer and more stable atheromatous lesion (92).

Fibrous Cap

Cap thinning and reduced collagen content increase a plaque's vulnerability to rupture (93). Fibrous caps vary widely in thickness, cellularity, matrix, strength, and stiffness. Caps of eccentric plaques are often thinnest and infiltrated with foam cells/macrophages at their shoulder regions, where they most frequently rupture (88). Collagen is important for the tensile strength of tissues, and disrupted aortic caps seem to contain less collagen than do intact caps (94).

For fibrous caps of the same tensile strength, caps covering mildly or moderately stenotic plaques are more prone to rupture than caps covering stenotic plaques because the former have to bear a greater circumferential tension (according to Laplace's law; see below) (93). Loss of cells and calcification in fibrous caps are associated with increased stiffness (95), but the significance of cap stiffness for rupture propensity is unknown.

Cap Inflammation

It has been known for a long time that disrupted fibrous caps usually are heavily infiltrated by macrophage foam cells (5,62,96,97) (Fig. 3), and recent observations revealed that rupture-related macrophages are activated, indicating ongoing inflammation at the site of plaque disruption (89,98). For eccentric plaques, the shoulder regions are sites of predilection for both active inflammation (endothelial activation (11,12) and macrophage infiltration (88)) and disruption (88), and mechanical testing of aortic fibrous caps indicates that foam cell infiltration indeed weakens caps locally, reducing their tensile strength (99).

Richardson et al. studied 85 coronary thrombi postmortem and found a disrupted atheromatous plaque beneath 71 (84%) of the thrombi (88). The fibrous cap had ruptured at shoulder regions of eccentric plaques in 42 cases (67% of rupture sites were foam cell infiltrated) and at other locations in the other 29 cases (86% of rupture sites were foam cell infiltrated). Van der Wal et al. identified superficial macrophage infiltration in plaques beneath all 20 coronary thrombi examined, whether or not the underlying plaque was disrupted or just eroded (89). Evaluated by immunohistochemical technique, the macrophages and adjacent T lymphocytes (SMCs were usually lacking at rupture sites) were activated, indicating ongoing disease activity. These postmortem studies of patients dying from coronary thrombosis have recently been expanded by an in vivo study of atherectomy specimens from culprit lesions responsible for stable angina, unstable rest angina, or non-Q-wave myocardial infarction (100). Culprit lesions responsible for the acute coronary syndromes contained significantly more macrophages than did lesions responsible for stable angina pectoris (14% versus 3% of plaque tissue occupied by macrophages) (100). Macrophages are capable of degrading extracellular matrix by phagocytosis or by secreting proteolytic enzymes such as plasminogen activators and metalloproteinases (101), which may weaken the fibrous cap, predisposing it to rupture. Collagen is the main component of caps responsible for their tensile strength, and human monocyte-derived macrophages grown in culture may express collagenase and degrade collagen of aortic fibrous caps during incubation (102). Several studies have identified matrix-degrading proteinases in human coronary plaques (103–105), and lipid-filled macrophages (foam cells) may be particularly active in destabilizing plaques (106), predisposing them to rupture. Furthermore, monocytes/macrophages could also play a detrimental role after plaque disruption, promoting thrombin generation and luminal thrombosis (57,107–113).

Activated mast cells may secrete powerful proteolytic enzymes and mast cells are indeed present in shoulder regions of mature coronary plaques, but at very low density (mast cell to macrophage ratio about 1:20) (43). Neutrophils are also capable of destroying tissue by secreting proteolytic enzymes (114), but neutrophils are rarely found in intact plaques (10,89,115). They may occasionally be found in disrupted plaques beneath coronary thrombi, probably entering these plaques shortly after disruption (89), and neutrophils may also migrate into the arterial wall shortly after reperfusion of occluded arteries in response to ischemia/reperfusion (116).

Fatigue

A steady load that does not fracture a material may weaken it if the load is applied repeatedly. This repetitive stress may ultimately lead to sudden fracture of the tissue due to "fatigue," analogous to the repetitive bending of a paper clip that weakens it until it suddenly breaks (117). Cyclic stretching, compression, bending, flexion, shear, and pressure fluctuations may "fatigue" and weaken a fibrous cap that ultimately may rupture unprovoked, i.e., spontaneously. Lowering the frequency (heart rate) and magnitude (flow and pressure related) of loading should reduce the risk of plaque disruption if fatigue plays a role (118–121).

Extrinsic Triggers of Plaque Disruption

Coronary plaques are constantly stressed by a variety of biomechanical and hemodynamic forces that may precipitate or "trigger" disruption of vulnerable plaques (7,117,122). Stresses imposed on plaques are usually concentrated at the weak points discussed above, namely at points where the fibrous cap is thinnest and tearing most frequently occurs (93,123).

Circumferential Tensile Stress

Blood pressure induces both circumferential tension in and radial compression of the surrounding vessel wall. If blood pressure and plaque disruption are related, it is probably via tensile rather than compressive stresses (95). The circumferential wall tension (tensile stress) caused by the blood pressure is given by Laplace's law, which relates luminal pressure and radius to wall tension: the higher is the blood pressure and the larger is the luminal diameter, the more tension develops in the wall (122). If components within the wall (soft gruel, for example) are unable to bear the imposed load, the stress is redistributed to adjacent structures (fibrous cap over gruel, for example) where it may be critically concentrated (88,93,123). As mentioned, the consistency of the gruel may be important for this stress redistribution because the stiffer is the gruel, the more stress it can bear and correspondingly less is redistributed to the adjacent fibrous cap (92). Richardson et al. computed the distribution of circumferential tensile stress within simulated plaques and found that eccentric pools of soft material concentrated stress on the adjacent fibrous cap, especially near its shoulders, and these computed high-stress points correlated well with sites of rupture found in a necropsy series (88). Cheng et al. computed the stress distribution in plaques that actually had ruptured and confirmed that most fibrous caps (58%) indeed had ruptured where the computed circumferential stress was highest (123). Importantly, the thickness of the fibrous cap is most critical for the peak circumferential stress: the thinner is the fibrous cap, the higher is the stress that develops in it (93). However, weak points not caused by cap thinning but created by focal macrophage activities could explain why rupture does not always occur where the computed (thickness-dependent, circumferential stress is maximal (88,123). Furthermore, mechanical shear stresses may develop in plaques at the interface between tissues of differing stiffness, resulting in shear failure. Calcified plates and adjacent noncalcified tissue may, for example, slide against each other, "shearing" plaques area (122,124), as confirmed by necropsy findings of some tears at such sites (88).

Regarding stenosis severity and plaque rupture, the tension created in fibrous caps of mildly or moderately stenotic plaques is greater than that created in caps of severely stenotic plaques (smaller lumen) with the same cap thickness and exposed to the same blood pressure (Laplace's law) (93,117). Consequently, mildly or moderately stenotic plaques are generally "stressed" more than severely stenotic plaques and may therefore be more prone to rupture.

Compressive Stress

Plaque disruption may occur from the lumen into the plaque due to increase in luminal pressure, or the cap may rupture from the plaque into the lumen due to increase in intraplaque pressure caused by, for example, vasospasm, bleeding from vasa vasorum, plaque edema, and/or collapse of compliant stenoses.

Vasospasm reduces the circumferential tension in fibrous caps by narrowing the lumen (Laplace's law). Nevertheless, spasm could theoretically rupture plaques by compressing the atheromatous core, "blowing" the fibrous cap out into the lumen (96,125–127). Plaque disruption and vasospasm do indeed frequently coexist (128,129), but the former most likely gives rise to the latter rather than vice versa (129–132). Onset of myocardial infarction is uncommon during or shortly after drug-induced spasm of even severely diseased coronary arteries (133,134), indicating that spasm infrequently precipitates spontaneous plaque disruption and/or luminal thrombosis. According to Kaski et al. (134), spasm-prone lesions do not seem to progress more rapidly than do corresponding fixed lesions. Furthermore, spasmolytic drugs (calcium antagonists, for example) have never proven effective in preventing myocardial infarction in patients with vasospastic angina. However, contrary to the result of Kaski et al. (134), Nobuyoshi et al. found a strong positive correlation between ergonovine-induced coronary spasm and subsequent plaque progression, with or without infarct development (135).

Bleeding and/or transudation (edema) into plaques from the thin-walled new vessels originating from vasa vasorum and frequently found at the plaque base (52,136) could theoretically increase the intraplaque pressure with resultant cap rupture from the inside (137). Although tiny bleedings are frequently found at the base of advanced lesions (138), it is difficult to imagine how a small capillary bleeding can disrupt a fibrous cap against the much higher luminal pressure (139).

Collapse of severe but compliant stenoses caused by negative transmural pressures may produce highly concentrated compressive stresses from buckling of the wall with bending deformation, preferentially involving plaque edges (see below) (140), and, theoretically, this might contribute to plaque disruption.

Circumferential Bending Stress

The propagating pulse wave causes cyclic changes in lumen size and shape with deformation and bending of plaques, particularly the "soft" ones (141). For normal compliant arteries, the cyclic diastolic–systolic change in lumen diameter is about 10% (122), but it becomes less with age and during atherogenesis because of increase in stiffness (142,143). Generally, concentric plaques do not change as much during the cardiac cycle as eccentric plaques do. The latter typically bend at their edges, i.e., at the junction between the stiff plaque and the more compliant plaque-free vessel wall. Also, changes in vascular tone cause bending of eccentric plaques at their edges. Cyclic bending may in the long term weaken these points, leading to unprovoked "spontaneous" fatigue disruption, while a sudden accentuated bending may "trigger" rupture of a weakened cap.

Longitudinal Flexion Stress

The coronary arteries tethered to the surface of the beating heart undergo cyclic longitudinal deformations by axial bending (flexion) and stretching, particularly the left anterior descending coronary artery (144). Angiographically, the angle of flexion was recently found to correlate with subsequent lesion progression, but the coefficient of correlation was low (144). Like circumferential bending, a sudden accentuated longitudinal flexion may "trigger" plaque disruption, while long-term cyclic flexion may "fatigue" and weaken the plaque.

Hemodynamic Stress

Low and/or oscillating shear stress may influence endothelial function and promote atherogenesis below intact endothelium (35,145,146). High blood velocity within stenotic lesions may, however, shear the endothelium away (147), but whether high hemodynamic shear alone may disrupt a stenotic plaque is questionable (63). Hemodynamic stresses are usually much smaller than mechanical stresses imposed by blood and pulse pressures (117). Theoretically, fluttering of severe but compliant stenoses between collapse and patency (140,148–150) and turbulent pressure fluctuations distal to severe asymmetric stenoses could "fatigue" the plaque surface, promoting plaque disruption (151). Unfortunately, the exact longitudinal location of plaque disruption (upstream, within, or downstream of the stenosis) is unknown for coronary plaques. Carotid plaques reportedly often tear proximal to or within the most stenotic region (152,153).

Triggering of Disease Onset: Plaque Disruption, Thrombosis, and/or Spasm

Does plaque disruption occur at random, solely due to ongoing intrinsic disease activity and fatigue, or may extrinsic biomechanical and/or hemodynamic factors also play a role in precipitating or "triggering" rupture of vulnerable plaques? It is tempting to speculate so, but we do not know for sure. What we know is that onset of rupture/thrombosis-related clinical events such as unstable rest angina, myocardial infarction, and sudden coronary death does not occur at random; a great fraction appears to be "triggered" by external factors or conditions. Triggering of disease onset is covered by the chapter by Muller et al., *this volume,* and we shall here only briefly summarize what may be deduced about plaque disruption from clinical observations.

Onset of acute coronary syndromes does not occur at random (154–160). Myocardial infarction occurs at increased frequency in the morning (154,161–163), particularly within the first hour after awakening (164), on Mondays (163,165,166), during winter months (167,168) and on colder days the year around (169), and during emotional stress (170–173) and vigorous exercise (174,175). Possible "triggers" of disease onset—also called "acute risk factors" (155)—have been reported by nearly 50% of patients with myocardial infarction (176). The pathophysiologic mechanisms responsible for the nonrandom and apparently often "triggered" onset of infarction are unknown, but probably are related to (155,177) (a) *plaque disruption,* likely caused by surges in sympathetic activity with a sudden increase in blood pressure, pulse rate, heart contraction, and coronary blood flow (178); (b) *thrombosis,* occurring on previously disrupted or intact plaques when the systemic thrombotic tendency is high because of platelet hyperaggregability (179–186), hypercoagulability (187), and/or impaired fibrinolysis (188–191); and (c) *vasoconstriction,* occurring locally around a coronary plaque or generalized (192,193).

The beneficial effect of beta-blockade in the secondary prevention of myocardial infarction provides strong evidence for the theory that plaque disruption may trigger disease onset. Beta-blocker therapy reduces reinfarction by 25% (194,195) without having any proven antiatherogenic (196), antithrombotic (183), fibrinolytic (197,198), or spasmolytic (199,200) effects in humans. On the contrary, beta-blockers may induce or potentiate atherogenic dyslipoproteinemia (201), platelet aggregation (183), and vasoconstriction (200). Nonetheless, beta-blockade blunts the morning peak in onset of infarction probably by blunting the sympathetic surge in the morning (202,203), indicating that mechanical and hemodynamic forces could be critical in triggering plaque disruption and disease onset. Accordingly, the beneficial effect of beta-blockade on reinfarction has been related to the reduction in heart rate (118), and a similar effect on reinfarction has been obtained by the heart-rate-reducing calcium antagonists verapamil and diltiazem (204–206)—in sharp contrast to the results obtained with the heart-rate-increasing nifedipine (206). Activation of the sympathetic nervous system and hypercatecholaminemia associated with arousal, exercise, emotional stress, and smoking could, however, trigger onset of infarction not only via beta-adrenoceptors, but also via alpha-receptors, promoting platelet aggregation and vasoconstriction (179–186,192, 193,207–212). Sudden thrombus growth on previously disrupted or intact plaques due to changes in platelet function, coagulation, and/or fibrinolysis is probably an important mechanism responsible for onset of acute coronary syndromes (2).

IDENTIFICATION OF VULNERABLE AND DISRUPTED PLAQUES

Coronary angiography is suitable for the identification of culprit lesions responsible for myocardial ischemia, but visualization of the arterial wall rather than the lumen is necessary for the identification of early lesions and nonstenotic vulnerable plaques. Intravascular ultrasound (213–218) and angioscopy (87,128,218–221) may reveal important plaque and surface features not seen angiographically, and magnetic resonance imaging (222–226), spectroscopy (227–229), and scintigraphy (230–236) may in the near future improve the in vivo identification and characterization of coronary plaques further. Increased endothelial permeability with insudation of plasma constitutents, lipoprotein accumulation, endothelial activation with expression of adhesion molecules, monocyte recruitment, macrophage retention and cell activation within lesions, denudation and ulceration of plaque surfaces with platelet adhesion, aggregation, and degranulation, activation of coagulation, and ongoing fibrinolysis characterize actively progressing atherosclerosis and vulnerable high-risk plaques—features that might be visualized in living persons by appropriate imaging techniques. Even a simple blood sample may reveal signs of inflammation (237–239) and activation of endothelial cells (240–242), leukocytes (109,110,112,113,243), platelets (244), coagulation (245–247), and fibrinolysis (245,246, 248–252) that may prove to be useful in differentiating between quiescent and progressing atherosclerosis.

PLAQUE DISRUPTION: CLINICAL MANIFESTATIONS

Plaque disruption is common (7,253). It is followed by a variable amount of hemorrhage into the plaque through the disrupted surface and luminal thrombosis causing rapid plaque growth—probably the most important mechanism responsible for the unpredictable, sudden, and nonlinear progression of coronary lesions frequently observed angiographically (254). Another mechanism underlying episodic plaque growth could be accelerated SMC proliferation and matrix synthesis driven by superficial inflammation, endothelial denudation, platelet adhesion/degranulation, and blood-derived growth factors (255).

Silent Plaque Disruption

Plaque disruption itself is asymptomatic, and the associated rapid plaque growth also is usually clinically silent. Autopsy data indicate that 9% of "normal" healthy persons are walking around with disrupted plaques in their coronary arteries, increasing to 22% in persons with diabetes or hypertension (256). Many persons dying of ischemic heart disease harbor both thrombosed and nonthrombosed disrupted plaques in their coronary arteries (138,253,257,258). As many as 103 disrupted plaques were identified in 47 persons dying of coronary artery disease, and only 40 of the ruptures were associated with significant luminal thrombosis—the ones responsible for the final heart attacks (5). The majority of the other 63 ruptured plaques probably represent rapid but silent plaque growth.

Acute Coronary Syndromes

Following plaque disruption, hemorrhage into the plaque, luminal thrombosis, and/or vasospasm may cause sudden flow obstruction, giving rise to new or changing symptoms. There seem to be three major determinants for the thrombotic response to plaque disruption: (a) character and extent of exposed plaque components (local thrombogenic substrates) (51,259); (b) degree of stenosis and surface irregularities activating platelets (local flow disturbances) (5,51, 253,260–262); and (c) thrombotic–thrombolytic equilibrium at the time of plaque disruption (systemic thrombotic tendency) (2,244,245,263–266). The clinical presentation and the outcome depend on the severity and duration of ischemia. A nonocclusive or transiently occlusive thrombus most frequently underlies primary unstable angina with pain at rest and non-Q-wave myocardial infarction, while a more stable and occlusive thrombus is most frequently seen in Q-wave infarction—overall modified by vascular tone and collateral flow (2,267). The lesion responsible for out-of-hospital cardiac arrest or sudden death is often similar to that of unstable angina: a disrupted plaque with superimposed nonocclusive thrombosis (138,268,269).

Acute Myocardial Infarction Versus Occlusion

Myocardial infarction results most frequently from the sudden occlusion of a mildly or moderately stenotic lesion, giving rise to the notion that less severely obstructive plaques rather than severely obstructive plaques are most vulnerable to rupture (1,135,270–275). The more stenotic lesions do, however, most frequently progress to total occlusion, but they often do so silently without infarct development because of well-developed collateral circulation (275–281). Angiographically, coronary atherosclerosis appears to be a focal disease, but most patients with ischemic heart disease have such widespread "plaquing" that virtually no vascular segment is left entirely normal (48). The most severe stenosis at highest risk of occlusion (but relatively low risk of resultant myocardial infarction) is always outnumbered by nonstenotic lesions at lower risk of occlusion (but higher risk of resultant myocardial infarction), overall giving a higher pooled risk of infarction resulting from occlusion of one of the many nonsevere stenoses than from occlusion of the most severe stenosis (279,280). Therefore, although mild-to-moderate stenoses more frequently give rise to acute coronary syndromes than do severe stenoses, an individual mildly to moderately obstructive plaque is not necessarily more vulnerable to rupture than a severely obstructive plaque.

PREVENTION OF PLAQUE DISRUPTION

The risk of plaque disruption is a function of both *plaque vulnerability* (intrinsic disease) and *rupture triggers* (extrinsic forces); the former predisposes the plaque to rupture, while the latter may precipitate it. Therefore, plaque disruption may be prevented by stabilizing plaques against disruption and/or by avoiding or reducing potential trigger activities.

Plaque Stabilization

Experimental animal studies indicate that atherosclerosis is a dynamic process where arterial function, lumen size, plaque size, and plaque composition may change independently. Following diet-induced atherosclerosis in monkeys, lipid lowering results in rapid normalization of endothelial function, disappearance of macrophage foam cells from lesions, depletion of plaque lipid (preferentially cholesterol esters resulting in a smaller and stiffer lipid-rich core), and loss of vasa vasorum (282–288). Furthermore, mature collagen may increase (284,289)—overall resulting in a larger vascular lumen and a modified but not necessarily a smaller plaque (286). Such ''regressive'' changes should stabilize plaques against disruption, but this approach has not been tested because of lack of a suitable animal model of plaque disruption. Experimentally, atherosclerosis may be modified and probably stabilized by a variety of non-lipid-lowering approaches, including elevation of high-density lipoprotein (290), use of antioxidants (291,292), administration of appropriate dietary fatty acids (293), exercise conditioning (294,295), avoidance of psychosocial stress (296–298), angiotensin-converting enzyme (ACE) inhibition (299–301), blood pressure lowering (302), and estrogen replacement therapy (303,304).

Clinical observations indicate that human plaques may be stabilized against disruption by antiatherogenic therapy, including modifications of lifestyle and serum lipids (305–311)—a topic covered in the chapter by Brown and Fuster, *this volume*. It should be stressed, however, that significant clinical benefit may be obtained just by stabilizing plaques, let alone regression (305,306). Three lipid-lowering trials with angiographic follow up have independently shown that stability of coronary plaques over short term is associated with a good long-term prognosis; disease progression on trial predicted posttrial myocardial infarction and cardiac death (312–314). Stabilization of vulnerable rupture-prone coronary plaques converts a potentially fatal disease into a more benign condition.

ACE may contribute to the development of coronary artery disease and myocardial infarction (315–317) and ACE inhibition seems to reduce the risk of major ischemic events (reinfarction and cardiac death) by about 22% in patients with low ejection fractions (318–320), probably via multiple beneficial mechanisms (321). ACE inhibitors may influence both atherogenesis (plaque vulnerability) and trigger mechanisms responsible for disease onset (plaque disruption, thrombosis, and/or vasospasm). The latter is commented on below in the section on trigger reduction. The hypothesis that these drugs are antiatherogenic and prevent or slow the progression of coronary artery disease is now being tested in clinical trials (322).

Preliminary data suggest that antioxidant vitamins may slow the progression of coronary artery disease (323), but contrasting results have recently been reported for femoral artery disease treated with the strong antioxidant probucol (324). Estrogen replacement therapy seems to provide powerful protection against myocardial infarction and cardiovascular death in postmenopausal women, probably mediated via multiple antiischemic mechanisms that include a direct effect of estrogen on the vessel wall (2), but the effect on coronary artery disease progression is still unknown.

Trigger Reduction

Avoiding or reducing trigger activities may prevent plaque disruption. Exercise and the associated sympathetic neurohormonal activation could precipitate onset of myocardial infarction via sudden plaque disruption (178), activation of platelets (2,183,185,186,208,209,325) and coagulation (187), and/or coronary vasoconstriction (326). Nonetheless, only a small fraction of all myocardial infarctions (about 5%) are related to, or triggered by, vigorous exertion such as shoveling snow (178,327), and only sedentary people seem to be at increased risk of exercise-related infarction [relative risk from 7 (175) to 107 (174)]. Although physically unfit people usually are advised to avoid heavy physical exertion, it is unknown whether refraining from such activities reduces myocardial infarction in sedentary people or just postpones it (174). Of more interest for prevention, regular exercise may retard plaque progression (328) and seems to provide protection against myocardial infarction and coronary deaths (329–333), at least in part by eliminating the triggering effect of sudden vigorous exertion (174,175).

Cigarette smoking is the most important preventable cause of morbidity and mortality from coronary artery disease (334,335). Clinical data indicate that smoking accelerates the progression of coronary artery disease (336–338). The increased risk associated with smoking appears to be rapidly reversible by cessation (336,339,340), implicating acute triggering mechanisms (plaque disruption, thrombosis, and/or vasoconstriction) rather than chronic atherogenic mechanisms as being mainly responsible for smoking-related disease progression (207,210–212,341–347). Regarding smoking and atherogenesis, preliminary autopsy data indicate that smokers have more extracellular lipids in their plaques, which should imply greater vulnerability to rupture (54).

Beta-blockers (194,195) and possibly heart-rate-reducing calcium antagonists (204–206) may delay or prevent plaque disruption by reducing the mechanical and hemodynamic load on vulnerable plaques, explaining the beneficial effect of these drugs in the secondary prevention of myocardial infarction (118,119). As mentioned, the protective effect of beta-blockers has been related to their heart-rate-lowering efficacy: the lower is the heart rate, the better is the protection against reinfarction and death (118). The maximum benefit achievable by trigger reduction therapy is, however, limited unless the progression of the disease is also arrested. Coronary plaques are stressed constantly and just reducing peak stresses will probably only postpone the time where a progressive vulnerable plaque inevitably will rupture. Even complete elimination of the morning excess of acute coronary events associated with the morning surge in sympathetic activity will prevent only a small fraction of all clinical events (348) because the vast majority occur ''untriggered'' in the morning or at other times of the day. Successful plaque stabilization eliminates the prerequisite for plaque disruption: the vulnerable plaque. Therefore, to obtain maximum benefit, both approaches, plaque stabilization and trigger reduction, should be pursued.

As mentioned above, ACE inhibition may not only modify atherogenesis and plaque vulnerability, but also trigger mechanisms responsible for disease onset (321). For example, the renin–angiotensin system may interact with fibrinolytic function (349) and ACE inhibition may influence endogenous fibrinolysis resulting in a reduced thrombotic response to plaque disruption (350). Importantly, ACE inhibition seems to reduce mortality and reinfarction also in the presence of beta-blocker therapy, suggesting an independent therapeutic effect (320).

TREATMENT OF PLAQUE DISRUPTION

The most feared consequence of coronary plaque disruption is thrombotic occlusion. The function of the hemostatic and fibrinolytic systems at the time of plaque disruption, i.e., the actual systemic thrombotic tendency, is important for the outcome, documented by the beneficial effect of antithrombotic therapy in patients at risk of plaque disruption (351–356). In case of plaque disruption, antiplatelet agents and/or anticoagulants may limit the thrombotic response and prevent mural thrombosis from progressing to thrombotic occlusion (2,357). If the latter occurs, thrombolysis and/or mechanical intervention may reopen the culprit artery (358–360). Of interest, lipid lowering not only may stabilize plaques against disruption, it may also improve endothelial function (361–363) and reduce the thrombotic response to plaque disruption/erosions via beneficial effects on platelets, coagulation, fibrinolysis, and blood viscosity (364–368).

SUMMARY

Atherosclerosis without thrombosis is in general a benign disease. However, acute thrombosis frequently complicates the course of coronary atherosclerosis, causing unstable angina, myocardial infarction, and sudden death. The mechanism responsible for the sudden conversion of a stable disease to a life-threatening condition is usually plaque disruption with superimposed thrombosis. The risk of plaque disruption depends more on plaque composition and vulnerability (plaque type) than on degree of stenosis (plaque size). Major determinants of a plaque's vulnerability to rupture are (a) the size and consistency of the lipid-rich atheromatous core, (b) the thickness and collagen content of the fibrous cap, and (c) ongoing inflammation within the cap. Plaque disruption tends to occur at points where the plaque surface is weakest and most vulnerable, which coincide with points where stresses, resulting from biomechanical and hemodynamic forces acting on plaques, are concentrated. Therefore, the risk of plaque disruption is a function of both *plaque vulnerability* (intrinsic disease) and *rupture triggers* (extrinsic forces). The former predisposes the plaque to rupture, while the latter may precipitate it. The challenge of today is to identify and treat the dangerous vulnerable plaques responsible for infarction and death—to find and treat only angina-producing stenotic lesions is no longer enough. For prevention and treatment, a systemic approach that addresses all coronary plaques will prove to be most rewarding.

REFERENCES

1. Fuster V, Badimon L, Badimon J, Chesebro JH. The pathogenesis of coronary artery disease and the acute coronary syndromes. *N Engl J Med* 1992;326:242–250,310–318.
2. Fuster V, Lewis A. Conner Memorial Lecture. Mechanisms leading to myocardial infarction: Insights from studies of vascular biology. *Circulation* 1994;90:2126–2146.
3. Shah PK, Forrester JS. Pathophysiology of acute coronary syndromes. *Am J Cardiol* 1991;68(Suppl C):16C–23C.
4. Falk E. Morphologic features of unstable atherothrombotic plaques underlying acute coronary syndromes. *Am J Cardiol* 1989;63(Suppl E):114E–120E.
5. Falk E. Plaque rupture with severe pre-existing stenosis precipitating coronary thrombosis. Characteristics of coronary atherosclerotic plaques underlying fatal occlusive thrombi. *Br Heart J* 1983;50: 127–134.
6. Davies MJ, Thomas AC. Plaque fissuring—the cause of acute myocardial infarction, sudden ischaemic death, and crescendo angina. *Br Heart J* 1985;53:363–373.
7. Falk E. Why do plaques rupture? *Circulation* 1992;86(Suppl III):III-30–III-42.
8. Zhang Y, Cliff WJ, Schoefl GI, Higgins G. Plasma protein insudation as an index of early coronary atherogenesis. *Am J Pathol* 1993;143: 496–506.
9. Valenzuela R, Shainoff JR, DiBello PM, Urbanic DA, Anderson JM, Matsueda GR, Kudryk BJ. Immunoelectrophoretic and immunohistochemical characterizations of fibrinogen derivatives in atherosclerotic aortic intimas and vascular prosthesis pseudointimas. *Am J Pathol* 1992;141:861–880.
10. Van der Wal AC, Das PK, Tigges AJ, Becker AE. Adhesion molecules on the endothelium and mononuclear cells in human atherosclerotic lesions. *Am J Pathol* 1992;141:1427–1433.
11. Poston RN, Haskard DO, Coucher JR, Gall NP, Johnson-Tidey RR. Expression of intercellular adhesion molecule-1 in atherosclerotic plaques. *Am J Pathol* 1992;140:665–673.
12. Johnson-Tidey RR, McGregor JL, Taylor PR, Poston RN. Increase in the adhesion molecule P-selectin in endothelium overlying atherosclerotic plaques. *Am J Pathol* 1994;144:952–961.
13. Davies MJ, Gordon JL, Gearing AJH, Pigott R, Woolf N, Katz D, Kyriakopoulos A. The expression of the adhesion molecules ICAM-1, VCAM-1, PECAM, and E-selectin in human atherosclerosis. *J Pathol* 1993;171:223–229.
14. Wood KM, Cadogan MD, Ramshaw AL, Parums DV. The distribution of adhesion molecules in human atherosclerosis. *Histopathology* 1993;22:437–444.
15. Ylä-Herttuala S, Lipton BA, Rosenfeld ME, Särkioja T, Yoshimura T, Leonard EJ, Witztum JL, Steinberg D. Expression of monocyte chemoattractant protein 1 in macrophage-rich areas of human and rabbit atherosclerotic lesions. *Proc Natl Acad Sci USA* 1991;88: 5252–5256.
16. Nelken NA, Coughlin SR, Gordon D, Wilcox JN. Monocyte chemoattractant protein-1 in human atheromatous plaques. *J Clin Invest* 1991; 88:1121–1127.
17. Faruqi RM, DiCorleto PE. Mechanisms of monocyte recruitment and accumulation. *Br Heart J* 1993;69(Suppl):S19–S29.
18. Hansson GK. Immune and inflammatory mechanisms in the development of atherosclerosis. *Br Heart J* 1993;69(Suppl):S38–S41.
19. Ross R. The pathogenesis of atherosclerosis: A perspective for the 1990s. *Nature* 1993;362:801–809.
20. Benditt EP. Origins of human atherosclerotic plaques. The role of altered gene expression. *Arch Pathol Lab Med* 1988;112:997–1001.
21. Marx J. CMV-p53 interaction may help explain clogged arteries [commentary]. *Science* 1994;265:320.
22. Berenson GS, Radhakrishnamurthy B, Srinivasan R, Vijayagopal P,

Dalferes ER. Arterial wall injury and proteoglycan changes in atherosclerosis. *Atherosclerosis* 1988;112:1002–1010.
23. Wight TN. Cell biology of arterial proteoglycans. *Arteriosclerosis* 1989;9:1–20.
24. Steinberg D, Parthasarathy S, Carew TE, Khoo JC, Witztum JL. Beyond cholesterol. Modications of low-density lipoprotein that increase its atherogenicity. *N Engl J Med* 1989;320:915–924.
25. Ylä-Herttuala S, Rosenfeld ME, Parthasarathy S, Sigal E, Särkioja T, Witztum JL, Steinberg D. Gene expression in macrophage-rich human atherosclerotic lesions. 15-Lipoxygenase and acetyl low density lipoprotein receptor messenger RNA colocalize with oxidation specific lipid–protein adducts. *J Clin Invest* 1991;87:1146–1152.
26. Guyton JR, Klemp KF. Transitional features in human atheroscerosis. Intimal thickening, cholesterol clefts, and cell loss in human aortic fatty streaks. *Am J Pathol* 1993;143:1444–1457.
27. Witztum JL. The oxidation hypothesis of atherosclerosis. *Lancet* 1994;344:793–795.
28. Schwartz CJ, Valente AJ, Sprague EA, Kelley JL, Nerem RM. The pathogenesis of atheroslcerosis: An overview. *Clin Cardiol* 1991; 14(Suppl I):1–16.
29. Davies MJ, Woolf N. Atherosclerosis: What is it and why does it occur? *Br Heart J* 1993;69(Suppl):S3–S11.
30. Mitchinson MJ. The new face of atherosclerosis. *Br J Clin Pract* 1994;48:149–151.
31. Demer LL, Watson KE, Boström K. Mechanism of calcification in atherosclerosis. *Trends Cardiovasc Med* 1994;4:45–49.
32. Shanahan CM, Cary NRB, Metcalfe JC, Weissberg PL. High expression of genes for calcification-regulating proteins in human atherosclerotic plaques. *J Clin Invest* 1994;93:2393–2402.
33. Rabbani LE, Loscalzo J. Recent observations on the role of hemostatic determinants in the development of the atherothrombotic plaque. *Atherosclerosis* 1994;105:1–7.
34. Falk E, Fernández-Ortiz A. Role of thrombosis in atherosclerosis and its complications. *Am J Cardiol* 1995;75:5B–11B.
35. Glagov S, Zarins C, Giddens DP, Ku DN. Hemodynamics and atherosclerosis. Insights and perspectives gained from studies of human arteries. *Arch Pathol Lab Med* 1988;112:1018–1031.
36. Stary HC, Blankenhorn DH, Chandler AB, Glagov S, Insull W, Richardson M, Rosenfeld ME, Schaffer SA, Schwartz CJ, Wagner WD, Wissler RW. A definition of the intima of human arteries and of its atherosclerosis-prone regions. A report from the Committee on Vascular Lesions of the Council on Arteriosclerosis, American Heart Association. *Circulation* 1992;85:391–405.
37. Fry DL, Herderick EE, Johnson DK. Local intimal-medial uptakes of 125I-albumin, 125I-LDL, and parenteral Evans blue dye protein complex along the aortas of normocholesterolemic minipigs as predictors of subsequent hypercholesterolemic atherogenesis. *Arterioscler Thromb* 1993;13:1193–1204.
38. Stary HC, Chandler AB, Glagov S, Guyton JR, Insull W Jr, Rosenfield ME, Schaffer SA, Schwartz CJ, Wagner WD, Wissler RW. A definition of initial, fatty streak, and intermediate lesions of atherosclerosis. A report from the Committee on Vascular Lesions of the Council on Arteriosclerosis, American Heart Association. *Circulation* 1994;89: 2462–2478.
39. Reddy KG, Nair RN, Sheehan HM, Hodgson JM. Evidence that selective endothelial dysfunction may occur in the absence of angiographic or ultrasound atherosclerosis in patients with risk factors for atherosclerosis. *J Am Coll Cardiol* 1994;23:833–843.
40. Davies MJ, Woolf N, Rowles PM, Pepper J. Morphology of the endothelium over atherosclerotic plaques in human coronary arteries. *Br Heart J* 1988;60:459–464.
41. Bürrig K-F. The endothelium of advanced arteriosclerotic plaques in humans. *Arterioscler Thomb* 1991;11:1678–1689.
42. Kaartinen M, Penttilä A, Kovanen PT. Mast cells of two types differing in neutral protease composition in the human aortic intima. Demonstration of tryptase- and tryptase-/chymase-containing mast cells in normal intimas, fatty streaks, and the shoulder region of atheromas. *Arterioscler Thomb* 1994;14:966–972.
43. Kaartinen M, Penttilä A, Kovanen PT. Accumulation of activated mast cells in the shoulder region of human coronary atheroma, the predilection site of atheromatous rupture. *Circulation* 1994;90: 1669–1678.
44. Atkinson JB, Harlan CW, Harlan GC, Virmani R. The association of mast cells and atherosclerosis: A morphologic study of early atherosclerotic lesions in young people. *Hum Pathol* 1994;25:154–159.
45. Spurlock BO, Chandler AB. Adherent platelets and surface microthrombi of the human aorta and left coronary artery: A scanning electron microscopy feasibility study. *Scanning Microsc* 1987;1: 1359–1365 [Erratum. *Scanning Microsc* 1988;2(2):1214].
46. Wilcox JN. Thrombotic mechanisms in atherosclerosis. *Coron Artery Dis* 1994;5:223–229.
47. Nelken NA, Solfer SJ, O'Keefe J, Vu T-KH, Charo IF, Coughlin SR. Thombin receptor expression in normal and atherosclerotic human arteries. *J Clin Invest* 1992;90:1614–1621.
48. Roberts WC. Diffuse extent of coronary atherosclerosis in fatal coronary artery disease. *Am J Cardiol* 1990;65(Suppl F):2F–6F.
49. Kragel AH, Reddy SG, Wittes JT, Roberts WC. Morphometric analysis of the composition of atherosclerotic plaques in the four major epicardial coronary arteries in acute myocardial infarction and in sudden coronary death. *Circulation* 1989;80:1747–1756.
50. Kragel AH, Reddy SG, Wittes JT, Roberts WC. Morphometric analysis of the composition of coronary arterial plaques in isolated unstable angina pectoris with pain at rest. *Am J Cardiol* 1990;66:562–567.
51. Fernández-Ortiz A, Badimon J, Falk E, Fuster V, Meyer B, Mailhac A, Weng D, Shah PK, Badimon L. Characterization of the relative thrombogenicity of atherosclerotic plaque components: Implications for consequences of plaque rupture. *J Am Coll Cardiol* 1994;23: 1562–1569.
52. Zhang Y, Cliff WJ, Schoefl GI, Higgins G. Immunohistochemical study of intimal microvessels in coronary atherosclerosis. *Am J Pathol* 1993;143:164–172.
53. Guyton JR, Klemp KF, Black BL, Bocan TMA. Extracellular lipid deposition in atherosclerosis. *Eur Heart J* 1990;11(Suppl E):20–28.
54. Wissler RW, The PDAY Collaborating Investigators. New insights into the pathogenesis of atherosclerosis as revealed by PDAY. *Atherosclerosis* 1994;108(Suppl):S3–S20.
55. Tracy RE, Devaney K, Kissling G. Characteristics of the plaque under a coronary thrombus. *Virchows Arch [Pathol Anat]* 1985;405: 411–427.
56. Small DM. Progression and regression of atherosclerotic lesions. Insights from lipid physical biochemistry. *Arteriosclerosis* 1988;8: 103–129.
57. Wilcox JN, Smith KM, Schwartz SM, Gordon D. Localization of tissue factor in the normal vessel wall and in the atherosclerotic plaque. *Proc Natl Acad Sci USA* 1989;86:2839–2843.
58. Tracy RE, Kissling GE. Age and fibroplasia as preconditions for atheronecrosis in human coronary arteries. *Arch Pathol Lab Med* 1987; 111:957–963.
59. Tracy RE, Kissling GE. Comparisons of human populations for histologic features of atherosclerosis. A summary of questions and methods for geographic studies. *Arch Pathol Lab Med* 1988;112:1056–1065.
60. Guyton JR, Klemp KF. Development of atherosclerotic core region. Chemical and ultrasturcutral analysis of microdissected atherosclerotic lesions from human aorta. *Arterioscler Thromb* 1994;14: 1305–1314.
61. Beisiegel U, Niendorf A, Wolf K, Reblin T, Rath M. Lipoprotein(a) in the arterial wall. *Eur Heart J* 1990;11(Suppl E):174–183.
62. Friedman M. The coronary thrombus: Its origin and fate. *Hum Pathol* 1971;2:81–128.
63. Gertz SD, Roberts EC. Hemodynamic shear force in rupture of coronary arterial atherosclerotic plaques. *Am J Cardiol* 1990;66: 1368–1372.
64. Stary HC. Evolution and progression of atherosclerotic lesions in coronary arteries of children and young adults. *Arteriosclerosis* 1989; 9(Suppl I):I-19–I-32.
65. Guyton JR, Klemp KF. The lipid-rich core region of human atherosclerotic fibrous plaques. Prevalence of small-lipid droplets and vesicles by electron microscopy. *Am J Pathol* 1989;134:705–717.
66. Davies MJ. A macro and micro view of coronary vascular insult in ischemic heart disease. *Circulation* 1990;82(Suppl II):II-38–II-46.
67. Lundberg B. Chemical composition and physical state of lipid deposits in atherosclerosis. *Atherosclerosis* 1985;56:93–110.
68. Celermajer DS, Sorensen KE, Gooch VM, Spiegelhalter DJ, Miller OI, Sullivan ID, Lloyd JK, Deanfield JE. Non-invasive detection of endothelial dysfunction in children and adults at risk of atherosclerosis. *Lancet* 1992;340:1111–1115.
69. Celermajer DS, Sorensen KE, Georgakopoulos D, Bull C, Thomas

O, Robinson J, Deanfield JE. Cigarette smoking is associated wtih dose-related and potentially reversible impairment of endothelium-dependent dilation in helathy young adults. *Circulation* 1993;88: 2149–2155.
70. Celermajer DS, Sorensen K, Ryalls M, Robinson J, Thomas O, Leonard JV, Deanfield JE. Impaired endothelial function occurs in the systemic arteries of children with homozygous homocystinuria but not in their heterozygous parents. *J Am Coll Cardiol* 1993;22:854–858.
71. Sorensen KE, Celermajer DS, Georgakopoulos D, Hatcher G, Betteridge DJ, Deanfield JE. Impairment of endothelium-dependent dilation is an early event in children with familial hypercholesterolemia and is related to the lipoprotein(a) level. *J Clin Invest* 1994;93:50–55.
72. Celermajer DS, Sorensen KE, Spiegelhalter DJ, Georgakopoulos D, Robinson J, Deanfield JE. Aging is associated with endothelial dysfunction in healthy men years before the age-related decline in women. *J Am Coll Cardiol* 1994;24:471–476.
73. Solberg LA, Strong JP. Risk factors and atherosclerotic lesions. A review of autopsy studies. *Arteriosclerosis* 1983;3:187–198.
74. Holme I, Solberg LA, Weissfeld L, Helgeland A, Hjermann I, Leren P, Strong JP, Williams OD. Coronary risk factors and their pathway of action through coronary raised lesions, coronary stenoses and coronary death. Multivariate statistical analysis of an autopsy series: The Oslo Study. *Am J Cardiol* 1985;55:40–47.
75. Reed DM, MacLean CJ, Hayashi T. Predictors of atherosclerosis in the Honolulu heart program. I. Biologic, dietary, and lifestyle characteristics. *Am J Epidemiol* 1987;126:214–225.
76. Reed DM, Strong JP, Resch J, Hayashi T. Serum lipids and lipoproteins as predictors of atherosclerosis. An autopsy study. *Arteriosclerosis* 1989;9:560–564.
77. Newman WP, Freedman DS, Voors AW, Gard PD, Srinivasan SR, Cresanta JL, Williamson GD, Webber LS, Berenson GS. Relation of serum lipoprotein levels and systolic blood pressure to early atherosclerosis. The Bogalusa Heart Study. *N Engl J Med* 1986;314: 138–144.
78. Robertson WB, Strong JP. Atherosclerosis in persons with hypertension and diabetes mellitus. *Lab Invest* 1968;18:538–551.
79. Crall FV, Roberts WC. The extramural and intramural coronary arteries in juvenile diabetes mellitus. *Am J Med* 1978;64:221–230.
80. McGill HC. The cardiovascular pathology of smoking. *Am Heart J* 1988;115:250–257.
81. Pathobiological Determinants of Atherosclerosis in Youth (PDAY) Research Group. Relationship of atherosclerosis in young men to serum lipoprotein cholesterol concentrations and smoking. A preliminary report. *JAMA* 1990;264:3018–3024.
82. Pathobiological Determinants of Atherosclerosis in Youth (PDAY) Research Group. Natural history of aortic and coronary atherosclerotic lesions in youth. Findings from the PDAY study. *Arterioscler Thromb* 1993;13:1291–1298.
83. Kragel AH, Roberts WC. Composition of atherosclerotic plaques in the coronary arteries in homozygous familial hypercholesterolemia. *Am Heart J* 1991;121:210–211.
84. Gertz SD, Malekzadeh S, Dollar AL, Kragel AH, Roberts WC. Composition of atherosclerotic plaques in the four major epicardial coronary arteries in patients ≥90 years of age. *Am J Cardiol* 1991;67: 1228–1233.
85. Dollar AL, Kragel AH, Fernicola DJ, Waclawiw MA, Roberts WC. Composition of atherosclerotic plaques in coronary arteries in women <40 years of age with fatal coronary artery disease and implications for plaque reversibility. *Am J Cardiol* 1991;67:1223–1227.
86. Mautner SL, Lin F, Roberts WC. Composition of atherosclerotic plaques in the epicardial coronary arteries in juvenile (type I) diabetes mellitus. *Am J Cardiol* 1992;70:1264–1268.
87. Forrester JS, Litvack F, Grundfest W, Hickey A. A perspective of coronary disease seen through the arteries of living man. *Circulation* 1987;75:505–513.
88. Richardson PD, Davies MJ, Born GVR. Influence of plaque configuration and stress distribution on fissuring of coronary atherosclerotic plaques. *Lancet* 1989;ii:941–944.
89. Van der Wal AC, Becker AE, van der Loos CM, Das PK. Site of initimal rupture or erosion of thrombosed coronary atherosclerotic plaques is characterized by an inflammatory process irrespective of the dominant plaque morphology. *Circulation* 1994;89:36–44.
90. Davies MJ, Richardson PD, Woolf N, Katz DR, Mann J. Risk of thrombosis in human atherosclerotic plaques: Role of extracellular lipid, macrophage, and smooth muscle cell content. *Br Heart J* 1993; 69:377–381.
91. Wagner WD, St Clair RW, Clarkson TB, Connor JR. A study of atherosclerosis regression in *Macaca mulatta*: III. Chemical changes in arteries from animals with atherosclerosis induced for 19 months and regressed for 48 months at plasma cholesterol concentratons of 300 or 200 mg/dl. *Am J Pathol* 1980;100:633–650.
92. Loree HM, Tobias BJ, Gibson LJ, Kamm RD, Small DM, Lee RT. Mechanical properties of model atherosclerotic lesion lipid pools. *Arterioscler Thromb* 1994;14:230–234.
93. Loree HM, Kamm RD, Stringfellow RG, Lee RT. Effects of fibrous cap thickness on peak circumferential stress in model atherosclerotic vessels. *Circ Res* 1992;71:850–858.
94. Burleigh MC, Briggs AD, Lendon CL, Davies MJ, Born GV, Richardson PD. Collagen types I and III, collagen content, GAGs and mechanical strength of human atherosclerotic plaque caps: Span-wise variations. *Atherosclerosis* 1992;96:71–81.
95. Lee RT, Grodzinsky AJ, Frank EH, Kamm RD, Schoen FJ. Structure-dependent dynamic mechanical behavior of fibrous caps from human atherosclerotic plaques. *Circulation* 1991;83:1764–1770.
96. Friedman M, Van den Bovenkamp GJ. The pathogenesis of a coronary thrombus. *Am J Pathol* 1966;48:19–44.
97. Constantinides P. Plaque fissures in human coronary thrombosis. *J Atheroscler Res* 1966;6:1–17.
98. Buja LM, Willerson JT. Role of inflammation in coronary plaque disruption [Editorial]. *Circulation* 1994;89:503–505.
99. Lendon CL, Davies MJ, Born GVR, Richardson PD. Atherosclerotic plaque caps are locally weakened when macrophage density is increased. *Atherosclerosis* 1991;87:87–90.
100. Moreno PR, Falk E, Palacios IF, Newell JB, Fuster V, Fallon JT. Macrophage infiltration in acute coronary syndromes: Implications for plaque rupture. *Circulation* 1994;90:775–778.
101. Matrisian LM. The matrix-degrading metalloproteinases. *BioEssays* 1992;14:455–463.
102. Shah PK, Falk E, Badimon JJ, Levy G, Fernandez-Ortiz A, Fallon J, Fuster V. Human monocyte-derived macrophages express collagenase and induce collagen breakdown in atherosclerotic fibrous caps: Implications for plaque rupture. *Circulation* 1993;88(Suppl I):I-254(abst).
103. Henney AM, Wakeley PR, Davies MJ, Foster K, Hembry R, Murphy G, Humphries S. Localization of stromelysin gene expression in atherosclerotic plaques by *in situ* hybridization. *Proc Natl Acad Sci USA* 1991;88:8154–8158.
104. Galis ZS, Sukhova GK, Lark MW, Libby P. Increased expression of matrix-metalloproteinases and matrix degrading activity in vulnerable regions of human atherosclerotic plaques. *J Clin Invest* 1994;94: 2493–2503.
105. Brown DL, Hibbs MS, Kearney M, Topol EJ, Loushin C, Isner JM. Expression and cellular localization of 92 kDa gelatinase in coronary lesions of patients with unstable angina. *J Am Coll Cardiol* 1994; (Suppl A):436A(abst).
106. Rennick RE, Ling KLE, Humphries SE, Henney AM. Effect of acetyl-LDL on monocyte-macrophage expression of matrix metalloproteinases. *Atherosclerosis* 1994;109(Suppl):192(abst).
107. Wilcox JN, Harker LA. Molecular and cellular mechanisms of atherogenesis: Studies of human lesions linked with animal modelling. In: Bloom AL, Forbes CD, Thomas DP, Tuddenham EDG, (eds). *Haemostasis and Thrombosis*. London: Churchill Livingstone; 1994; 1139–1152.
108. Palabrica T, Lobb R, Furie BC, Aronovitz M, Benjamin C, Hsu YM, Sajer SA, Furie B. Leukocyte accumulation promoting fibrin deposition is mediated *in vivo* by P-selectin on adherent platelets. *Nature* 1992;359:848–851.
109. Jude B, Agraou B, McFadden EP, et al. Evidence for time-dependent activation of monocytes in the systemic circulation in unstable angina but not in acute myocardial infarction or in stable angina. *Circulation* 1994;90:1662–1668.
110. Leatham EW, Bath PM, Tooze JA, Tuddenham E, Kaski J-C. Monocytes express increased tissue factor in unstable angina and myocardial infarction. *Circulation* 1993;88(Suppl I):I-128(abst).
111. Mazzone A, De Servi S, Ricevuti G, Mazzucchelli I, Fossati G, Pasotti D, Bramucci E, Angoli L, Marsico F, Specchia G, et al. Increased expression of neutrophil and monocyte adhesion molecules in unstable coronary artery disease. *Circulation* 1993;88:358–363.
112. Neri Serneri GG, Abbate R, Gori AM, Attanasio M, Martini F, Giusti

B, Dabizzi P, Poggesi L, Modesti PA, Trotta F, et al. Transient intermittent lymphocyte activation is responsible for the instability of angina. *Circulation* 1992;86:790–797.

113. Neri Serneri GG, Gensini GF, Poggesi L, Modesti PA, Rostagno C, Boddi M, Gori AM, Martini F, Ieri A, Margheri M, et al. The role of extraplatelet thromboxane A2 in unstable angina investigated with a dual thromboxane A2 inhibitor: Importance of activated monocytes. *Coron Artery Dis* 1994;5:137–145.
114. Weiss SJ. Tissue destruction by neutrophils. *N Engl J Med* 1989;320: 365–376.
115. Jonasson L, Holm J, Skalli O, Bondjers G, Hansson GK. Regional accumulations of T cells, macrophages, and smooth muscle cells in the human atherosclerotic plaque. *Arteriosclerosis* 1986;6:131–138.
116. Kloner RA, Giacomelli F, Alker KJ, Hale SL, Matthews R, Bellows S. Influx of neutrophils into the walls of large epicardial coronary arteries in response to ischemia/reperfusion. *Circulation* 1991;84: 1758–1772.
117. MacIsaac AI, Thomas JD, Topol EJ. Toward the quiescent coronary plaque [Review Article]. *J Am Coll Cardiol* 1993;22:1228–1241.
118. Kjekshus JK. Importance of heart rate in determining beta-blocker efficacy in acute and long-term acute myocardial infarction intervention trials. *Am J Cardiol* 1986;57(Suppl F):43F–49F.
119. Fitzgerald JD. By what means might beta blockers prolong life after acute myocardial infarction? *Eur Heart J* 1987;8:945–951.
120. Gillum RF, Makuc DM, Feldman JJ. Pulse rate, coronary heart disease, and death: The NHANES I Epidemiologic Follow-up Study. *Am Heart J* 1991;121:172–177.
121. Hjalmarson Å, Gilpin EA, Kjekshus J, Schieman G, Nicod P, Henning H, Ross J. Influence of heart rate on mortality after acute myocardial infarction. *Am J Cardiol* 1990;65:547–553.
122. Lee RT, Kamm RD. Vascular mechanics for the cardiologist. *J Am Coll Cardiol* 1994;23:1289–1295.
123. Cheng GC, Loree HM, Kamm RD, Fishbein MC, Lee RT. Distribution of circumferential stress in ruptured and stable atherosclerotic lesions. A structural analysis with histopathological correlation. *Circulation* 1993;87:1179–1187.
124. Vito RP, Whang MC, Giddens DP, Zarins CK, Glagov S. Stress analysis of the diseased arterial cross-section. *Adv Bioeng Proc* 1990: 273–276.
125. Leary T. Coronary spasm as a possible factor in producing sudden death. *Am Heart J* 1934;10:338–344.
126. Chapman I. Morphogenesis of occluding coronary artery thrombosis. *Arch Pathol* 1965;80:256–261.
127. Lin CS, Penha PD, Zak FG, Lin JC. Morphodynamic interpretation of acute coronary thrombosis, with special reference to volcano-like eruption of atheromatous plaque caused by coronary artery spasm. *Angiology* 1988(June):535–547.
128. Etsuda H, Mizuno K, Arakawa K, Satomura K, Shibuya T, Isojima K. Angioscopy in variant angina: Coronary artery spasm and intimal injury. *Lancet* 1993;342:1322–1324.
129. Bogaty P, Hackett D, Davies G, Maseri A. Vasoreactivity of the culprit lesion in unstable angina. *Circulation* 1994;90:5–11.
130. Lam JY, Chesebro JH, Steele PM, Badimon L, Fuster V. Is vasospasm related to platelet deposition? Relationship in a porcine preparation of arterial injury *in vivo*. *Circulation* 1987;76:243–248.
131. Golino P, Ashton JH, Buja LM, Rosolowsky M, Taylor AL, McNatt J, Campbell WB, Willerson JT. Local platelet activation causes vasoconstriction of large epicardial canine coronary arteries *in vivo:* Thromboxane A_2 and serotonin are possible mediators. *Circulation* 1989;79:154–166.
132. Zeiher AM, Schächinger V, Weitzel SH, Wollschläger H, Just H. Intracoronary thrombus formation causes focal vasoconstriction of epicardial arteries in patients with coronary artery disease. *Circulation* 1991;83:1519–1525.
133. Bertrand ME, LaBlanche JM, Tilmant PY, Thieuleux FA, Delforge MR, Carre AG, Asseman P, Berzin B, Libersa C, Laurent JM. Frequency of provoked coronary arterial spasm in 1089 consecutive patients undergoing coronary arteriography. *Circulation* 1982;65: 1299–1306.
134. Kaski JC, Tousoulis D, McFadden E, Crea F, Pereira WI, Maseri A. Variant angina pectoris. Role of coronary spasm in the development of fixed coronary obstructions. *Circulation* 1992;85:619–626.
135. Nobuyoshi M, Tanaka M, Nosaka H, Kimura T, Yokoi H, Hamasaki N, Kim K, Shindo T, Kimura K. Progression of coronary atherosclerosis: Is coronary spasm related to progression? *J Am Coll Cardiol* 1991; 18:904–910.
136. Barger AC, Beeuwkes R, Lainey LL, Silverman KJ. Hypothesis: Vasa vasorum and neovascularization of human coronary arteries. A possible role in the pathophysiology of atherosclerosis. *N Engl J Med* 1984; 310:175–177.
137. Barger AC, Beeuwkes R. Rupture of coronary vasa vasorum as a trigger of acute myocardial infarction. *Am J Cardiol* 1990;66(Suppl G):41G–43G.
138. Davies MJ, Thomas A. Thrombosis and acute coronary-artery lesions in sudden cardiac ischemic death. *N Engl J Med* 1984;310:1137–1140.
139. Constantinides P. Cause of thrombosis in human atherosclerotic arteries. *Am J Cardiol* 1990;66(Suppl G):37G–40G.
140. Aoki T, Ku DN. Collapse of diseased arteries with eccentric cross section. *J Biomech* 1993;26:133–142.
141. Mizushige K, Reisman M, Buchbinder M, Dittrich H, DeMaria AN. Atheroma deformation during the cardiac cycle: Evaluation by intracoronary ultrasound. *Circulation* 1993;88:I-550(abst).
142. Hori M, Inoue M, Shimazu T, Mishima M, Kusuoka H, Abe H, Kodama K, Nanato S. Clinical assessment of coronary arterial elastic properties by the image processing of coronary arteriograms. *Comput Cardiol* 1983;393–395.
143. Alfonso F, Macaya C, Goicolea J, Hernandez R, Segovia J, Zamorano J, Bañuelos C, Zarco P. Determinants of coronary compliance in patients with coronary artery disease: An intravascular ultrasound study. *J Am Coll Cardiol* 1994;23:879–884.
144. Stein PD, Hamid MS, Shivkumar K, Davis TP, Khaja F, Henry JW. Effects of cyclic flexion of coronary arteries on progression of atherosclerosis. *Am J Cardiol* 1994;73:431–437.
145. Gibson CM, Diaz L, Kandarpa K, Sacks FM, Pasternak RC, Sandor T, Feldman C, Stone PH. Relation of vessel wall shear stress to atherosclerosis progression in human coronary arteries. *Arterioscler Thromb* 1993;13:310–315.
146. Davies PF, Tripathi SC. Mechanical stress mechanisms and the cell. An endothelial paradigm. *Circ Res* 1993;72:239–245.
147. Gertz SD, Uretzky G, Wajnberg RS, Navot N, Gotsman MS. Endothelial cell damage and thrombus formation after partial arterial constriction: Relevance to the role of coronary artery spasm in the pathogenesis of myocardial infarction. *Circulation* 1981;63:476–486.
148. Santamore WP, Bove AA, Carey RA. Tachycardia induced reduction in coronary blood flow distal to a stenosis. *Int J Cardiol* 1982;2: 23–37.
149. Gould KL. Collapsing coronary stenosis—a Starling resistor. *Int J Cardiol* 1982;2:39–42.
150. Binns RL, Ku DN. Effect of stenosis on wall motion. A possible mechanism of stroke and transient ischemic attack. *Arteriosclerosis* 1989;9:842–847.
151. Loree HM, Kamm RD, Atkinson CM, Lee RT. Turbulent pressure fluctuations on surface of model vascular stenoses. *Am J Physiol* 1991; 261:H644–H650.
152. Svindland A, Torvik A. Atherosclerotic carotid disease in asymptomatic individuals. A histological study of 53 cases. *Acta Neurol Scand* 1988;78:506–517.
153. Bassiouny HS, Davis H, Massawa N, Gewertz BL, Glagov S, Zarins CK. Critical carotid stenoses: Morphologic and chemical similarity between symptomatic and asymptomatic plaques. *J Vasc Surg* 1989; 9:202–212.
154. Muller JE, Tofler GH, Stone PH. Circadian variation and triggers of onset of acute cardiovascular disease. *Circulation* 1989;79:733–743.
155. Muller JE, Abela GS, Nesto RW, Tofler GH. Triggers, acute risk factors and vulnerable plaques: The lexicon of a new frontier. *J Am Coll Cardiol* 1994;23:809–813.
156. Beard CM, Fuster V, Elveback LR. Daily and seasonal variation in sudden cardiac death, Rochester, Minnesota, 1950–1975. *Mayo Clin Proc* 1982;57:704–706.
157. Willich SN, Maclure M, Mittleman M, Arntz H-R, Muller JE. Sudden cardiac death: Support for a role of triggering in causation. *Circulation* 1993;87:1442–1450.
158. Lampert R, Rosenfeld L, Batsford W, Lee F, McPherson C. Circadian variation of sustained ventricular tachycardia in patients with coronary artery disease and implantable cardioverter-defibrillators. *Circulation* 1994;90:241–247.
159. Figueras J, Lidón RM. Circadian rhythm of angina in patients with

unstable angina: Relationship with extent of coronary disease, coronary reserve and ECG changes during pain. *Eur Heart J* 1994;15: 753–760.

160. Cannon CP, Théroux P, Gibson R, Kufera J, Feldman T, Chaitman B, McCabe CH, Braunwald E, for the TIMI-3 Registry Investigators. Brigham and Women's Hospital B, MA: Clinical profile of 4600 patients with unstable angina and non-Q wave MI: Results of the TIMI-3 Registry. *Circulation* 1992;86(Suppl I):I-387(abst).
161. Hansen O, Johansson BW, Gullberg B. Circadian distribution of onset of acute myocardial infarction in subgroups from analysis of 10,791 patients treated in a single center. *Am J Cardiol* 1992;69:1003–1008.
162. Willich SN, Collins R, Peto R, Linderer T, Sleight P, Schröder R. Morning peak in the incidence of myocardial infarction: Experience in the ISIS-2 trial. ISIS-2 (Second International Study of Infarct Survival) Collaborative Group. *Eur Heart J* 1992;13:594–598.
163. Gnecchi-Ruscone T, Piccaluga E, Guzzetti S, Contini M, Montano N, Nicolis E. Morning and Monday: Critical periods for the onset of acute myocardial infarction. The GISSI 2 Study Experience. *Eur Heart J* 1994;15:882–887.
164. Goldberg RJ, Brady P, Muller JE, Chen ZY, de Groot M, Zonneveld P, Dalen JE. Time of onset of symptoms of acute myocardial infarction. *Am J Cardiol* 1990;66:140–144.
165. Thompson DR, Pohl JE, Sutton TW. Acute myocardial infarction and day of the week. *Am J Cardiol* 1992;69:266–267.
166. Willich SN, Löwel H, Lewis M, Hörmann A, Arntz H, Keil U. Weekly variation of acute myocardial infarction. Increased Monday risk in the working population. *Circulation* 1994;90:87–93.
167. Ornato JP, Siegel L, Craren EJ, Nelson N. Increased incidence of cardiac death attributed to acute myocardial infarction during winter. *Coron Artery Dis* 1990;1:199–203.
168. Douglas AS, al Sayer H, Rawles JM, Allan TM. Seasonality of disease in Kuwait. *Lancet* 1991;337:1393–1397.
169. Marchant B, Ranjadayalan K, Stevenson R, Wilkinson P, Timmis AD. Circadian and seasonal factors in the pathogenesis of acute myocardial infarction: The influence of environmental temperature. *Eur Heart J* 1994;25(Abst Suppl):473(abst).
170. Trichopoulos D, Katsouyanni K, Zavitsanos X, Tzonou A, Dalla Vorgia P. Psychological stress and fatal heart attack: The Athens (1981) earthquake natural experiment. *Lancet* 1983;1:441–444.
171. Meisel SR, Kutz I, Dayan KI, Pauzner H, Chetboun I, Arbel Y, David D. Effect of Iraqi missile war on incidence of acute myocardial infarction and sudden death in Israeli civilians. *Lancet* 1991;338:660–661.
172. Gelernt MD, Hochman JS. Acute myocardial infarction triggered by emotional stress. *Am J Cardiol* 1992;69:1512–1513.
173. Jacobs SC, Friedman R, Mittleman M, Maclure M, Sherwood J, Benson H, Muller JE. 9-Fold increased risk of myocardial infarction following psychological stress as assessed by a case–control study. *Circulation* 1992;86(Suppl I):I-198(abst).
174. Mittleman MA, Maclure M, Tofler GH, Sherwood JB, Goldberg RJ, Muller JE. Triggering of acute myocardial infarction by heavy physical exertion. Protection against triggering by regular exertion. *N Engl J Med* 1993;329:1677–1683.
175. Willich SN, Lewis M, Löwel H, Arntz H-R. Schubert F, Schröder R. Physical exertion as a trigger of acute myocardial infarction. *N Engl J Med* 1993;329:1684–1690.
176. Tofler GH, Stone PH, Maclure M, Edelman E, David VG, Robertson T, Antman EM, Muller JE, and the MILIS Study Group. Analysis of possible triggers of acute myocardial infarction (the MILIS Study). *Am J Cardiol* 1990;66:22–27.
177. Devereux RB, Alderman MH. Role of preclinical cardiovascular disease in the evolution from risk factor exposure to development of morbid events. *Circulation* 1993;88:1444–1455.
178. Curfman GD. Is exercise beneficial—or hazardous—to your heart? [Editorial]. *N Engl J Med* 1993;329:1730–1731.
179. Tofler GH, Brezinski D, Schafer AI, Czeisler CA, Rutherford JD, Willich SN, Gleason RE, Williams G, Muller JE. Concurrent morning increase in platelet aggregability and the risk of myocardial infarction and sudden cardiac death. *N Engl J Med* 1987;316:1514–1518.
180. Brezinski DA, Tofler GH, Muller JE, Pohjola-Sintonen S, Willich SN, Schafer AI, Czeisler CA, Williams GH. Morning increase in platelet aggregability. Association with assumption of the upright posture. *Circulation* 1988;78:35–40.
181. Ridker PM, Manson JE, Buring JE, Muller JE, Hennekens CH. Circadian variation of acute myocardial infarcton and the effect of low-dose aspirin in a randomized trial of physicians. *Circulation* 1990; 82:897–902.
182. Jafri SM, VanRollins M, Ozawa T, Mammen EF, Goldberg AD, Goldstein S. Circadian variation in platelet function in healthy volunteers. *Am J Cardiol* 1992;69:951–954.
183. Hjemdahl P, Larsson PT, Wallen NH. Effects of stress and beta-blockade on platelet function. *Circulation* 1991;84(Suppl VI): V144–V161.
184. Grignani G, Soffiantino F, Zucchella M, Pacchiarini L, Tacconi F, Bonomi E, Pastoris A, Sbaffi A, Fratino P, Tavazzi L. Platelet activation by emotional stress in patients with coronary artery disease. *Circulation* 1991;83(Suppl II):II-128–II-136.
185. Hjemdahl P, Chronos NA, Wilson DJ, Bouloux P, Goodall AH. Epinephrine sensitizes human plateles *in vivo* and *in vitro* as studied by fibrinogen binding and P-selectin expression. *Arterioscler Thromb* 1994;14:77–84.
186. Badimon L, Lassila R, Badimon J, Fuster V. An acute surge of epinephrine stimulates platelet deposition to severely damaged vascular wall. *J Am Coll Cardiol* 1990;15:(Suppl):181A(abst).
187. Prisco D, Paniccia R, Guarnaccia V, Olivo G, Taddei T, Boddi M, Gensini GS. Thrombin generation after physical exercise. *Thromb Res* 1993;69:159–164.
188. Andreotti F, Davies GJ, Hackett DR, Khan MI, DeBart ACW, Aber VR, Maseri A, Kluft C. Major circadian fluctuations in fibrinolytic factors and possible relevance to time of onset of myocardial infarction, sudden cardiac death and stroke. *Am J Cardiol* 1988;62:635–637.
189. Angleton P, Chandler WL, Schmer G. Diurnal variation of tissue-type plasminogen activator and its rapid inhibitor (PAI-1). *Circulation* 1989;79:101–106.
190. Bridges AB, McLaren M, Scott NA, Pringle TH, McNeill GP, Belch JJ. Circadian variation of tissue plasminogen activator and its inhibitor, von Willebrand factor antigen, and prostacyclin stimulating factor in men with ischaemic heart disease. *Br Heart J* 1993;69:121–124.
191. Masuda T, Ogawa H, Miyao Y, Yu Q, Misumi I, Sakamoto T, Okubo H, Okumura K, Yasue H. Circadian variation in fibrinolytic activity in patients with variant angina. *Br Heart J* 1994;71:156–161.
192. Panza JA, Epstein SE, Quyyumi AA. Circadian variation in vascular tone and its relation to alpha-sympathetic vasoconstrictor activity. *N Engl J Med* 1991;325:986–990.
193. Quyyumi AA, Panza JA, Diodati JG, Lakatos E, Epstein SE. Circadian variation in ischemic threshold. A mechanism underlying the circadian variation in ischemic events. *Circulation* 1992;86:22–28.
194. Yusuf S, Peto J, Lewis J, et al. Beta blockade during and after myocardial infarction: An overview of the randomized trials. *Prog Cardiovasc Dis* 1985;27:335–371.
195. Yusuf S, Sleight P, Held P, McMahon S. Routine medical management of acute myocardial infarction. Lessons from overviews of recent randomized controlled trials. *Circulation* 1990;82:II117–II134.
196. Loaldi A, Polese A, Montorsi P, De Cesare N, Fabbiocchi F, Ravagnani P, Guazzi MD. Comparison of nifedipine, propranolol and isosorbide dinitrate on angiographic progression and regression of coronary arterial narrowings in angina pectoris. *Am J Cardiol* 1989;64: 433–439.
197. Hamsten A, Wiman B, deFaire U, Blomback M. Increased plasma levels of a rapid inhibitor of tissue plasminogen activator in young survivors of myocardial infarction. *N Engl J Med* 1985;313: 1557–1563.
198. Wright RA, Perrie AM, Stenhouse F, Alberti KGMM, Riemersma RA, MacGregor IR, Boon NA. The long-term effects of metoprolol and epanolol on tissue-type plasminogen activator and plasminogen activator inhibitor 1 in patients with ischaemic heart disease. *Eur J Clin Pharmacol* 1994;46:279–282.
199. Shimizu H, Lee JD, Ogawa KB, Shimizu K, Yamamoto M, Hara A, Nakamura T. Efficacy of denopamine, a beta 1 adrenoceptor agonist, in preventing coronary artery spasm. *Jpn Cir J* 1993;57:175–182.
200. Heintzen MP, Strauer BE. Peripheral vascular effects of beta-blockers. *Eur Heart J* 1994;15(Suppl C):2–7.
201. Leren P. Ischaemic heart disease: How well are the risk profiles modulated by current beta blockers? *Cardiology* 1993;82(Suppl 3):8–12.
202. Muller JE, Stone PH, Turi ZG, Rutherford JD, Czeisler CA, Parker C, Poole WK, Pasamani E, Roberts R, Robertson T, Sobel BE, Willerson JT, Braunwald E, and the MILIS Study Group. Circadian variation in the frequency of onset of acute myocardial infarction. *N Engl J Med* 1985;313:1315–1322.
203. Willich SN, Linderer T, Wegscheider K, Leizorovicz A, Alamercery

I, Schroder R, and the ISAM Study Group. Increased morning incidence of myocardial infarction in the ISAM Study: Absence with prior β-adrenergic blockade. *Circulation* 1989;80:853–858.
204. The Danish Study Group on Verapamil in Myocardial Infarction. The effect of verapamil on mortality and major events after myocardial infarction. The Danish Verapamil Infarction Trial II (DAVIT II). *Am J Cardiol* 1990;66:779–785.
205. Pahor MP, The CRIS Investigators C, Univ. Cattolica. Secondary prevention of myocardial infarction with verapamil: Calcium Antagonist Reinfarction Italian Study (CRIS). *Eur Heart J* 1994;15(Abst Suppl):134(abst).
206. Held PH, Yusuf S. Calcium antagonists in the treatment of ischemic heart disease: Myocardial infarction. *Coron Artery Dis* 1994;5:21–26.
207. Fuster V, Chesebro JH, Frye RL, Elveback LR. Platelet survival and the development of coronary artery disease in the young adult: Effects of cigarette smoking, strong family history and medical therapy. *Circulation* 1981;63:546–551.
208. Kestin AS, Ellis PA, Barnard MR, Errichetti A, Rosner BA, Michelson AD. Effect of strenuous exercise on platelet activation state and reactivity. *Circulation* 1993;88:1502–1511.
209. Larsson PT, Wallen NH, Hjemdahl P. Norepinephrine-induced human platelet activation *in vivo* is only partly counteracted by aspirin. *Circulation* 1994;89:1951–1957.
210. Kimura S, Nishinaga M, Ozawa T, Shimada K. Thrombin generation as an acute effect of cigarette smoking. *Am Heart J* 1994;128:7–11.
211. Winniford MD, Wheelan KR, Kremers MS, Ugolini V, van den Berg E Jr, Niggemann EH, Jansen DE, Hillis LD. Smoking-induced coronary vasoconstriction in patients with atherosclerotic coronary artery disease: Evidence for adrenergically mediated alterations in coronary artery tone. *Circulation* 1986;73:662–667.
212. Moliterno DJ, Willard JE, Lange RA, Negus BH, Boehrer JD, Glamann DB, Landau C, Rossen JD, Winniford MD, Hillis LD. Coronary-artery vasoconstriction induced by cocaine, cigarette smoking, or both. *N Engl J Med* 1994;330:454–459.
213. Nissen SE, Gurley JC, Grines CL, et al. Intravascular ultrasound assessment of lumen size and wall morphology in normal subjects and patients with coronary artery disease. *Circulation* 1991;84:1087–1099.
214. Hodgson JM, Reddy KG, Suneja R, Nair RN, Lesnefsky EJ, Sheehan HM. Intracoronary ultrasound imaging: Correlation of plaque morphology with angiography, clinical syndrome and procedural results in patients undergoing coronary angioplasty. *J Am Coll Cardiol* 1993;21:35–44.
215. Ge J, Erbel R, Gerber T, Görge G, Koch L, Haude M, Meyer J. Intravascular ultrasound imaging of angiographically normal coronary arteries: A prospective study *in vivo*. *Br Heart J* 1994;71:572–578.
216. Roelandt JRTC, di Mario C, Pandian NG, Wenguang L, Keane D, Slager CJ, de Feyter PJ, Serruys PW. Three dimensional reconstruction of intracoronary ultrasound images. Rationale, approaches, problems, and directions. *Circulation* 1994;90:1044–1055.
217. Escaned J, Serruys PW, di Mario C, Roelandt JRTC, de Feyter PJ. Intracoronary ultrasound and angioscopic imaging facilitating the understanding and treatment of post-infarction angina. *Eur Heart J* 1994;15:997–1001.
218. Baptista J, de Feyter P, di Mario C, Escaned J, Serruys PW. Stable and unstable anginal syndromes: Target lesion morphology prior to coronary interventions using angiography, intra-coronary ultrasound and angioscopy. *Eur Heart J* 1994;15(Abst Suppl):321(abst).
219. Mizuno K. Angioscopic examination of the coronary arteries: What have we learned? *Heart Dis Stroke* 1992;1:320–324.
220. Nesto RW, Sassower MA, Manzo KS, Bymes CM, Friedl SE, Muller JE, Abela GS. Angioscopic differentiation of culprit lesions in unstable versus stable coronary artery disease. *J Am Coll Cardiol* 1993;21(Suppl A):195A(abst).
221. Den Heijer P, Foley DP, Hillege HL, Lablanche JM, van Dijk RB, Franzen D, Morice MC, Serra A, de Scheerder IK, Serruys PW, Lie KI, on behalf of the European Working Group on Coronary Angioscopy. The ''Ermenoville'' classification of observations at coronary angioscopy—evaluation of intra- and inter-observer agreement. *Eur Heart J* 1994;15:815–822.
222. Asdente M, Pavesi L, Oreste PL, Colombo A, Kuhn W, Tremoli E. Evaluation of atherosclerotic lesions using NMR microimaging. *Atherosclerosis* 1990;80:243–253.
223. Pearlman JD, Southern JF, Ackerman JL. Nuclear magnetic resonance microscopy of atheroma in human coronary arteries. *Angiology* 1991;42:726–733.
224. Merickel MB, Berr S, Spetz K, Jackson TR, Snell J, Gillies P, Shimshick E, Hainer J, Brookeman JR, Ayers CR. Noninvasive quantitative evaluation of atherosclerosis using MRI and image analysis. *Arterioscler Thromb* 1993;13:1180–1186.
225. Toussaint J-F, Southern JF, Falk E, Fuster V, Kantor HL. Atherosclerotic plaque components imaged by nuclear magnetic resonance. *Circulation* 1993;88:I-S20(abstr).
226. Kandarpa K, Jakab P, Patz S, Schoen FJ, Jolesz FA. Prototype miniature endoluminal MR imaging catheter. *J Vasc Interv Radiol* 1993;4:419–427.
227. Toussaint J-F, Southern JF, Fuster V, Kantor HL. 13C-NMR spectroscopy of human atherosclerotic lesions: Relation between fatty acid saturation, cholesteryl ester content and luminal obstruction. *Arterioscler Thromb* 1994;14:1951–1957.
228. Baraga JJ, Feld MS, Rava RP. *In situ* optical histochemistry of human artery using near infrared Fourier transform Raman spectroscopy. *Proc Natl Acad Sci USA* 1992;89:3473–3477.
229. Manoharan R, Baraga JJ, Feld MS, Rava RP. Quantitative histochemical analysis of human artery using Raman spectroscopy. *J Photochem Photobiol B* 1992;16:211–233.
230. Vallabhajosula S, Paidi M, Badimon JJ, Le NA, Goldsmith SJ, Fuster V, Ginsberg HN. Radiotracers for low density lipoprotein biodistribution studies *in vivo:* Technetium-99m low density lipoprotein versus radioiodinated low density lipoprotein preparations. *J Nucl Med* 1988;29:1237–1245.
231. Lees AM, Lees RS, Schoen FJ, Isaacsohn JL, Fischman AJ, McKusick KA, Strauss HW. Imaging human atherosclerosis with ^{99m}Tc-labeled low density lipoproteins. *Arteriosclerosis* 1988;8:461–470.
232. Lupattelli G, Fedeli L, Fiacconi M, Ciuffetti G, Deleide G, Palumbo R, Sinzinger H. Scintigraphic detection of atherosclerosis by means of radiolabelled lipoproteins. *Thromb Haemorrh Disorders* 1991;3/2:61–65.
233. Rapp JH, Connor WE, Lin DS, Porter JM. Dietary eicosapentaenoic acid and docosahexaenoic acid from fish oil. Their incorporation into advanced human atherosclerotic plaques. *Arterioscler Thromb* 1991;11:903–911.
234. Miller DD, Rivera FJ, Garcia OJ, Palmaz JC, Berger HJ, Weisman HF. Imaging of vascular injury with ^{99m}Tc-labeled monoclonal antiplatelet antibody S12. Preliminary experience in human percutaneous transluminal angioplasty. *Circulation* 1992;85:1354–1363.
235. Narula J, Ditlow C, Chen F, Khaw B-A. Monoclonal antibodies for the detection of atherosclerotic lesions. In: Khaw B-A, Narula J, Strauss HW, eds. *Monoclonal Antibodies in Cardiovascular Diseases*. Philadelphia: Lea and Febiger; 1994.
236. Lees RS, Lees AM. Radiopharmaceutical imaging of active atherosclerosis. *Atherosclerosis* 1994;109(Suppl):352(abst).
237. Berk BC, Weintraub WS, Alexander RW. Evaluation of C-reactive protein in active coronary disease. *Am J Cardiol* 1990;65:168–172.
238. Liuzzo G, Biasucci LM, Gallimore JR, Grillo RL, Rebuzzi AG, Pepys MB, Maseri A. The prognostic value of C-reactive protein and serum amyloid A protein in severe unstable angina. *N Engl J Med* 1994;331:417–424.
239. Alexander RW. Inflammation and coronary artery disease [Editorial]. *N Engl J Med* 1994;331:468–469.
240. Wada H, Mori Y, Kaneko T, Wakita Y, Nakase T, Minamikawa K, Ohiwa M, Tamaki S, Tanigawa M, Kageyama S, et al. Elevated plasma levels of vascular endothelial cell markers in patients with hypercholesterolemia. *Am J Hematol* 1993;44:112–116.
241. Seigneur M, Dufourcq P, Conri C, Constans J, Mercie P, Pruvost A, Amiral J, Midy D, Baste JC, Boisseau MR. Levels of plasma thrombomodulin are increased in atheromatous arterial disease. *Thromb Res* 1993;71:423–431.
242. Blann AD. von Willebrand factor and atherosclerosis [Letter]. *Circulation* 1993;88:1962–1963.
243. Biasucci LM, D'Onofrio G, Liuzzo G, Zini G, Caligiuri G, Monaco C, Rebuzzi AG, Bizzi RB, Maseri A. Neurophil activation in unstable angina and acute myocardial infarction is a possible marker of inflammation and of disease activity. *Eur Heart J* 1994;15(Abst Suppl):472(abst).
244. Lam JY, Latour JG, Lesperance J, Waters D. Platelet aggregation, coronary artery disease progression and future coronary events. *Am J Cardiol* 1994;73:333–338.

245. Meade TW, Ruddock V, Stirling Y, Chakrabarti R, Miller GJ. Fibrinolytic activity, clotting factors, and long-term incidence of ischaemic heart disease in the Northwick Park Heart Study. *Lancet* 1993;342: 1076–1079.
246. Herren T, Stricker H, Haeberli A, Do DD, Straub PW. Fibrin formation and degradation in patients with arteriosclerotic disease. *Circulation* 1994;90:2679–2686.
247. Merlini PA, Bauer KA, Oltrona L, Ardissino D, Cattaneo M, Belli C, Mannucci PM, Rosenberg RD. Persistent activation of coagulation mechanism in unstable angina and myocardial infarction. *Circulation* 1994;90:61–68.
248. Fowkes FG, Lowe GD, Housley E, Rattray A, Rumley A, Elton RA, MacGregor IR, Dawes J. Cross-linked fibrin degradation products, progression of peripheral arterial disease, and risk of coronary heart disease. *Lancet* 1993;342:84–86.
249. Jansson JH, Olofsson BO, Nilsson TK. Predictive value of tissue plasminogen activator mass concentration on long-term mortality in patients with coronary artery disease. A 7-year follow-up. *Circulation* 1993;88:2030–2034.
250. Ridker PM, Vaughan DE, Stampfer MJ, Manson JE, Hennekens CH. Endogenous tissue-type plaminogen activator and risk of myocardial infarction. *Lancet* 1993;341:1165–1168.
251. Ridker PM, Hennekens CH, Stampfer MJ, Manson JE, Vaughan DE. Prospective study of endogenous tissue plasminogen activator and risk of stroke. *Lancet* 1994;343:940–943.
252. Ridker PM, Hennekens CH, Cerskus A, Stampfer MJ. Plasma concentration of cross-linked fibrin degradation product (D-dimer) and the risk of future myocardial infarction among apparently healthy men. *Circulation* 1994;90:23236–2240.
253. Frink RJ. Chronic ulcerated plaques: New insights into the pathogenesis of acute coronary disease. *J Invasive Cardiol* 1994;6:173–185.
254. Bruschke AVG, Kramer JR, Bal ET, Haque IU, Detrano RC, Goormastic M. The dynamics of progression of coronary atherosclerosis studied in 168 medically treated patients who underwent coronary arteriography three times. *Am Heart J* 1989;117:296–305.
255. Flugelman MY, Virmani R, Correa R, Yu Z-X, Farb A, Leon MB, Elami A, Fu Y-M, Casscells W, Epstein SE. Smooth muscle cell abundance and fibroblast growth factors in coronary lesions of patients with nonfatal unstable angina. A clue to the mechanism of transformation from the stable to the unstable clinical state. *Circulation* 1993; 88:2493–2500.
256. Davies MJ, Bland JM, Hangartner JRW, Angelini A, Thomas AC, Factors influencing the presence or absence of acute coronary artery thrombi in sudden ischaemic death. *Eur Heart J* 1989;10:203–208.
257. ElFawal MA, Berg GA, Wheatley DJ, Harland WA. Sudden coronary death in Glasgow: Nature and frequency of acute coronary lesions. *Br Heart J* 1987;57:329–335.
258. Qiao JH, Fishbein MC. The severity of coronary atherosclerosis at sites of plaque rupture with occlusive thrombosis. *J Am Coll Cardiol* 1991;17:1138–1142.
259. Van Zanten GH, de Graaf S, Slootweg PJ, Heijnen HFG, Connolly TM, de Groot PG, Sixma JJ. Increased platelet deposition on atherosclerotic coronary arteries. *J Clin Invest* 1994;93:615–632.
260. Badimon L, Badimon JJ. Mechanism of arterial thrombosis in nonparallel streamlines: Platelet thrombi grow on the apex of stenotic severely injured vessel wall. *J Clin Invest* 1989;84:1134–1144.
261. Merino A, Cohen M, Badimon JJ, Fuster V, Badimon L. Synergistic action of severe wall injury and shear forces on thrombus formation in arterial stenosis: Definition of a thrombotic shear rate threshold. *J Am Coll Cardiol* 1994;24:1091–1094.
262. Folts J. An *in vivo* model of experimental arterial stenosis, intimal damage, and periodic thrombosis. *Circulation* 1991;83(Suppl IV):IV-3–IV-14.
263. Trip MD, Cats VM, van Capelle FJL, Vreeken J. Platelet hyperreactivity and prognosis in survivors of myocardial infarction. *N Engl J Med* 1990;322:1549–1554.
264. Thaulow E, Erikssen J, Sandvik L, Stormorken H, Cohn PF. Blood platelet count and function are related to total and cardiovascular death in apparently healthy men. *Circulation* 1991;84:613–617.
265. Wilhelmsen L. Thrombocytes and coronary heart disease [Editorial]. *Circulation* 1991;84:936–938.
266. Prins MH, Hirsh J. A critical review of the relationship between impaired fibrinolysis and myocardial infarction. *Am Heart J* 1991;122: 545–551.
267. Fuster V, Frye RL, Kennedy MA, Connolly DC, Mankin HT. The role of collateral circulation in the various coronary syndromes. *Circulation* 1979;59:1137–1144.
268. Fuster V, Badimon L, Cohen M, Ambrose JA, Badimon JJ, Chesebro J. Insights into the pathogenesis of acute ischemic syndromes. *Circulation* 1988;77:1213–1220.
269. Lo Y-SA, Cutler JE, Blake K, Wright AM, Kron J, Swerdlow CD. Angiographic coronary morphology in survivors of cardiac arrest. *Am Heart J* 1988;115:781–785.
270. Ambrose JA, Tannenbaum MA, Alexopoulos D, Hjemdahl-Monsen CE, Leavy J, Weiss M, Borrico S, Gorlin R, Fuster V. Angiographic progression of coronary artery disease and the development of myocardial infarction. *J Am Coll Cardiol* 1988;12:56–62.
271. Little WC, Constantinescu M, Applegate RJ, Kutcher MA, Burrows MT, Kahl FR, Santamore WP. Can coronary angiography predict the site of a subsequent myocardial infarction in patients with mild-to-moderate coronary artery disease? *Circulation* 1988;78:1157–1166.
272. Brown BG, Gallery CA, Badger RS, Kennedy JW, Mathey D, Bolson EL, Dodge HT. Incomplete lysis of thrombus in the moderate underlying atherosclerotic lesion during intracoronary infusion of streptokinase for acute myocardial infarction: Quantitative angiographic observations. *Circulation* 1986;73:653–661.
273. Hackett D, Davies G, Maseri A. Pre-existing coronary stenoses in patients with first myocardial infarction are not necessarily severe. *Eur Heart J* 1988;9:1317–1323.
274. Taeymans Y, Theroux P, Lesperance J, Waters D. Quantitative angiographic morphology of the coronary artery lesions at risk of thrombotic occlusion. *Circulation* 1992;85:78–85.
275. Webster MW, Chesebro JH, Smith HC, Frye RL, Holmes DR, Reeder GS, Bresnahan DR, Nishimura RA, Clements IP, Bardsley WT, Grill DE, Bailey KR, Fuster V. Myocardial infarction and coronary artery occlusion: A prospective 5-year angiographic study. *J Am Coll Cardiol* 1990;15:218A(abst).
276. Danchin N, Oswald T, Voiriot P, Juillière Y, Cherrier F. Significance of spontaneous obstruction of high degree coronary artery stenoses between diagnostic angiography and later percutaneous transluminal coronary angioplasty. *Am J Cardiol* 1989;63:660–662.
277. Bissett JK, Ngo WL, Wyeth RP, Matts JP, and the POSCH Group. Angiographic progression to total coronary occlusion in hyperlipidemic patients after acute myocardial infarction. *Am J Cardiol* 1990; 66:1293–1297.
278. Berder V, Danchin N, Juillière Y, Sadoul N, Cuillière M, Aliot E, Cherrier F. Angiographic study of spontaneous obstruction of coronary artery stenoses: Do the tightest stenoses have the most benign clinical course? *Eur Heart J* 1991;12(Abst Suppl):231(abst).
279. Giroud D, Li JM, Urban P, Meier B, Rutishauser W. Relation of the site of acute myocardial infarction to the most severe coronary arterial stenosis at prior angiography. *Am J Cardiol* 1992;69:729–732.
280. Alderman EL, Corley SD, Fisher LD, Chaitman BR, Faxon DP, Foster ED, Killip T, Sosa JA, Bourassa MG. Five-year angiographic follow-up of factors associated with progression of coronary artery disease in the Coronary Artery Surgery Study (CASS). CASS participating investigators and staff. *J Am Coll Cardiol* 1993;22:1141–1154.
281. Danchin N. Is myocardial revascularisation for tight coronary stenoses always necessary? [Viewpoint]. *Lancet* 1993;342:224–225.
282. Armstrong ML, Megan MB. Lipid depletion in atheromatous coronary arteries in rhesus monkeys after regression diets. *Circ Res* 1972;30: 675–680.
283. Armstrong ML, Megan MB. Arterial fibrous proteins in cynomolgus monkeys after atherogenic and regression diets. *Circ Res* 1975;36: 256–261.
284. Small DM, Bond MG, Waugh D, Prack M, Sawyer JK. Physicochemical and histological changes in the arterail wall of nonhuman primates during progression and regression of atherosclerosis. *J Clin Invest* 1984;73:1590–1605.
285. Williams JK, Armstrong ML, Heistad DD. Vasa vasorum in atherosclerotic coronary arteries: Responses to vasoactive stimuli and regression of atherosclerosis. *Circ Res* 1988;62:515–523.
286. Kaplan JR, Manuck SB, Adams MR, Williams JK, Register TC, Clarkson TB. Plaque changes and arterial enlargement in atherosclerotic monkeys after manipulation of diet and social environment. *Arterioscler Thromb* 1993;13:254–263.
287. Benzuly KH, Padgett RC, Kaul S, Piegors DJ, Armstrong ML, Heistad

DD. Functional improvement precedes structural regression of atherosclerosis. *Circulation* 1994;89:1810–1818.
288. Heistad DD, Armstrong ML. Sick vessel syndrome. Can atherosclerotic arteries recover? [Editorial]. *Circulation* 1998;89:2447–2450.
289. DePalma RG, Klein L, Bellon EM, Koletsky S. Regression of atherosclerotic plaques in rhesus monkeys. Angiographic. morphologic, and angiochemical changes. *Arch Surg* 1980;115:1268–1278.
290. Badimon JJ, Badimon L, Fuster V. Regression of atherosclerotic lesions by high density lipoprotein plasma fraction in the cholesterol-fed rabbit. *J Clin Invest* 1990;85:1234–1241.
291. Carew TE, Schwenke DC, Steinberg D. Antiatherogenic effect of probucol unrelated to its hypocholesterolemic effect: Evidence that antioxidants *in vivo* can selectively inhibit low density lipoprotein degradation in macrophage-rich fatty streaks and slow the progression of atherosclerosis in the Watanabe heritable hyperlipidemic rabbit. *Proc Natl Acad Sci USA* 1987;84:7725–7729.
292. Sasahara M, Raines EW, Chait A, Carew TE, Steinberg D, Wahl PW, et al. Inhibition of hypercholesterolemia-induced atherosclerosis in the nonhuman primate by probucol. *J Clin Invest* 1994;94:155–164.
293. Leth-Espensen P, Stender S, Ravn H, Kjeldsen K. Antiatherogenic effect of olive and corn oils in cholesterol-fed rabbits with the same plasma cholesterol levels. *Arteriosclerosis* 1988;8:281–287.
294. Link RP, Pedersoli WM, Safanie AH. Effect of exercise on development of atherosclerosis in swine. *Atherosclerosis* 1972;15:107–122.
295. Kramsch DM, Aspen AJ, Abramowitz BM, Kreimendahl T, Hood WB. Reduction of coronary atherosclerosis by moderate conditioning exercise in monkeys on an atherogenic diet. *N Engl J Med* 1981;305: 1483–1489.
296. Kaplan JR, Manuck SB, Clarkson TB, Lusso FM, Taub DB, Miller EW. Social stress and atherosclerosis in normocholesterolemic monkeys. *Science* 1983;220:733–735.
297. Kaplan JR, Pettersson K, Manuck SB, Olsson G. Role of sympathoadrenal medullary activation in the initiation and progression of atherosclerosis. *Circulation* 1991;84(Suppl VI):VI-23–VI-32.
298. Shively CA, Clarkson TB. Social status and coronary artery atherosclerosis in female monkeys. *Arterioscler Thomb* 1994;14:721–726.
299. Aberg G, Ferrer P. Effects of captopril on atherosclerosis in cynomolgus monkeys. *J Cardiovasc Pharmacol* 1990;15(Suppl 5):S65–S72.
300. Chobanian AV, Haudenschild CC, Nickerson C, Drago R. Antiatherogenic effect of captopril in the Watanabe heritable hyperlipidemic rabbit. *Hypertension* 1990;15:327–331.
301. Rolland PH, Charpiot P, Friggi A, Piquet P, Barlatier A, Scalbert E, Bodard H, Tranier P, Mercier C, Luccioni R, et al. Effects of angiotensin-converting enzyme inhibition with perindopril on hemodynamics, arterial structure, and wall rheology in the hindquarters of atherosclerotic mini-pigs. *Am J Cardiol* 1993(Suppl E);71:22E–27E.
302. Chobanian AV, Brecher PI, Haudenschild CC. Effects of hypertension and of antihypertensive therapy on atherosclerosis. *Hypertension* 1986;8(Suppl I):I-15–I-21.
303. Williams JK, Adams MR, Klopfenstein HS. Estrogen modulates responses of atherosclerotic coronary arteries. *Circulation* 1990;81: 1680–1687.
304. Williams JK, Adams MR, Herrington DM, Clarkson TB. Short-term administration of estrogen and vascular responses of atherosclerotic coronary arteries. *J Am Coll Cardiol* 1992;20:452–457.
305. Scandinavian Simvastatin Survival Study Group. Randomised trial of cholesterol lowering in 4444 patients with coronary heart disease: The Scandinavian Simvastatin Survival Study (4S). *Lancet* 1994;344: 1383–1389.
306. MAAS Investigators. Effect of simvastatin on coronrary atheroma: The Multicentre Anti-Atheroma Study (MAAS). *Lancet* 1994;344: 633–638.
307. Brown BG, Zhao X-Q, Sacco DE, Albers JJ. Lipid lowering and plaque regression: New insights into prevention of plaque disruption and clinical events in coronary disease. *Circulation* 1993;87: 1781–1791.
308. Waters D, Lespérance J, Craven TE, Hudon G, Gillam LD. Advantages and limitations of serial coronary arteriography for the assessment of progression and regression of coronary atherosclerosis. Implications for clinical trials. *Circulation* 1993;87(Suppl II):II-38–II-47.
309. Blankenhorn DH, Hodis HN. George Lyman Duff Memorial Lecture. Arterial imaging and atherosclerosis reversal. *Arterioscler Thromb* 1994;14:177–192.
310. Superko HR, Krauss RM. Coronary artery disease regression. Convincing evidence for the benefit of aggressive lipoprotein management. *Circulation* 1994;90:1056–1069.
311. Gould KL. Reversal of coronary atherosclerosis. Clinical promise as the basis for noninvasive management of coronary artery disease. *Circulation* 1994;90:1558–1571.
312. Waters D, Draven TE, Lespérance J. Prognostic significance of progression of coronary atherosclerosis. *Circulation* 1993;87: 1067–1075.
313. Buchwald H, Matts JP, Fitch LL, Campos CT, Sanmarco ME, Amplatz K, Castaneda Zuniga WR, Hunter DW, Pearce MB, Bissett JK, et al. Changes in sequential coronary arteriograms and subsequent coronary events. Surgical Control of the Hyperlipidemias (POSCH) Group. *JAMA* 1992;268:1429–1433.
314. Cashin-Hemphill L, Mach W, LaBree L, Hodis HN, Shircore A, Selzer RH, Blankenhorn DH. Coronary progression predicts future cardiac events. *Circulation* 1993;88(Suppl I):I-363(abst).
315. Cambien F, Poirier O, Lecerf L, Evans A, Cambou J-P, Arveiler D, Luc G, Bard J-M, Bara L, Ricard S, Tiret L, Amouyel P, Alhenc-Gelas F, Soubrier F. Deletion polymorphism in the gene for angiotensin-converting enzyme is a potent risk factor for myocardial infarction. *Nature* 1992;359:641–644.
316. Tiret L, Kee F, Poirier O, Nicaud V, Lecerf L, Evans A, Cambou JP, Arveiler D, Luc G, Amouyel P, et al. Deletion polymorphism in angiotensin-converting enzyme gene associated with parental history of myocardial infarction. *Lancet* 1993;341:991–992.
317. Cambien F, Costerousse O, Tiret L, Poirier O, Lecerf L. Gonzales MF, Evans A, Arveiler D, Cambou JP, Luc G, Rakotovao R, Ducimetiere P, Soubrier F, Alhenc-Gelas F. Plasma level and gene polymorphism of angiotensin-converting enzyme in relation to myocardial infarction. *Circulation* 1994;90:669–676.
318. Yusuf S, Pepine CJ, Garces C, Pouleur H, Salem D, Kostis J, Benedict C, Rousseau M, Bourassa M, Pitt B. Effect of enalapril on myocardial infarction and unstable angina in patients with low ejection fractions. *Lancet* 1992;340:1173–1178.
319. Pfeffer MA, Braunwald E, on Behalf of SAVE Investigators. Effect of captopril on mortality and morbidity in patients with left ventricular dysfunction after myocardial infarction. *N Engl J Med* 1992;327: 669–677.
320. Rutherford JD, Pfeffer MA, Moyé LA, Davies BR, Flaker GC, Kowey PR, Lamas GA, Miller HS, Packer M, Rouleau JL, Braunwald E, on Behalf of the SAVE Investigators. Effects of captopril on ischemic events after myocardial infarction. Results of the Survival and Ventricular Enlargement Trial. *Circulation* 1994;90:1731–1738.
321. Lonn EM, Yusuf S, Jha P, Montague TJ, Teo KK, Benedict CR, Pitt B. Emerging role of angiotensin-converting enzyme inhibitors in cardiac and vascular protection. *Circulation* 1994;90:2056–2069.
322. Texter M, Lees RS, Pitt B, Dinsmore RE, Uprichard ACG. The Quinapril Ischemic Event Trial (QUIET) design and methods: Evaluation of chronic ACE inhibitor therapy after coronary artery intervention. *Cardiovasc Drugs Ther* 1993;7:273–282.
323. Hodis HN, Mack WJ, LaBree L, Hemphill LC, Azen SP. Natural antioxidant vitamins reduce coronary artery lesion progression as assessed by sequential coronary angiography. *J Am Coll Cardiol*; 1994; (Suppl A):481A(abst).
324. Walldius G, Erikson U, Olsson AG, Bergstrand L, Hådell K, Johansson J, Kaijser L, Lassvik C, Mölgaard J, Nilsson S, Schäfer-Elinder L, Stenport G, Holme I. The effect of probucol on femoral atherosclerosis: The Probucol Quantitative Regression Swedish Trial (PQRST). *Am J Cardiol* 1994;74:875–883.
325. Wang JS, Jen CJ, Kung HC, Lin LJ, Hsiue TR, Chen HI. Different effects of strenuous exercise and moderate exercise on platelet function in men. *Circulation* 1994;90:2877–2885.
326. Sacknoff DM, Wilentz JR, Schiffer MB, Bush M, Coplan NL. Exercise-induced ST-segment depression: Relationship to nonocclusive coronary artery spasm. *Am Heart J* 1993;125:242–244.
327. Master AM. The role of effort and occupation (including physicians) in coronary occlusion. *JAMA* 1960;174:84–90.
328. Hambrecht R, Niebauer J, Marburger C, Grunze M, Kalberer B, Hauer K, Schlierf G, Kubler W, Schuler G. Various intensities of leisure time physical activity in patients with coronary artery disease: Effects on cardiorespiratory fitness and progression of coronary atherosclerotic lesions. *J Am Coll Cardiol* 1993;22:468–477.
329. Paffenbarger RS Jr, Hyde RT, Wing AL, Lee IM, Jung DL, Kampert JB. The association of changes in physical-activity level and other

lifestyle characteristics with mortality among men. *Engl J Med* 1993; 328:538–545.
330. Lakka TA, Venäläinen JM, Rauramaa R, Salonen R, Tuomilehto J, Salonen JT. Relation of leisure-time physical activity and cardiorespiratory fitness to the risk of acute myocardial infarction. *N Engl J Med* 1994;330:1549–1554.
331. Berlin JA, Colditz GA. A meta-analysis of physical activity in the prevention of coronary heart disease. *Am J Epidemiol* 1990;132: 612–628.
332. O'Connor GT, Buring JE, Yusuf S, Goldhaber SZ, Olmstead EM, Paffenbarger RS Jr, Hennekens CH. An overview of randomized trials of rehabilitation with exercise after myocardial infarction. *Circulation* 1989;80:234–244.
333. Rodriguez BL, Curb JD, Burchfiel CM, Abbott RD, Petrovitch H, Masaki K, Chiu D. Physical activity and 23-year incidence of coronary heart disease morbidity and mortality among middle-aged men. The Honolulu Heart Program. *Circulation* 1994;89:2540–2544.
334. Jonas MA, Oates JA, Ockene JK, Hennekens CH. Statement on smoking and cardiovascular disease for health care professionals. American Heart Association. *Circulation* 1992;86:1664–1669.
335. Deckers JW, Agema WRP, Huijibrechts IPAM, Erdman RAM, Boersma H, Roelandt JRTC. Quitting of smoking in patients with recently established coronary artery disease reduced mortality by over 40%: Results of a meta-analysis. *Eur Heart J* 1994;15(Abst Suppl): 171(abst).
336. Shah PK, Helfant RH. Smoking and coronary artery disease. *Chest* 1988;94(3):449–452.
337. Nikutta P, Lichtlen PR, Wiese B, Jost S, Dekkers J, Rafflenbeul W, Hugenholtz PG. Influence of cigarette smoking on the progression of coronary artery disease within three years. Results of the INTACT study. *J Am Coll Cardiol* 1990;15(Suppl):181A(abst).
338. Waters D, Higginson L, Gladstone P, Boccuzzi S, Cook T, Lespérance J. Smoking accelerates the progression of coronary atherosclerosis as assessed by serial quantitative coronary arteriography. *Circulation* 1993;88(Suppl I):I-344(abst).
339. Rosenberg L, Kaufman DW, Helmrich SP, Shapiro S. The risk of myocardial infarction after quitting smoking in men under 55 years of age. *N Engl J Med* 1985;313:1511–1514.
340. Rosenberg L, Palmer JR, Shapiro S. Decline in the risk of myocardial infarction among women who stop smoking. *N Engl J Med* 1990;322: 213–217.
341. Kannel WB, D'Agostino RB, Belanger AJ. Fibrinogen, cigarette smoking, and risk of cardiovascular disease: Insights from the Framingham Study. *Am Heart J* 1987;113:1006–1010.
342. Wilhelmsen L, Svardsudd K, Korsan Bengtsen K, Larsson B, Welin L, Tibblin G. Fibrinogen as a risk factor for stroke and myocardial infarction. *N Engl J Med* 1984;311:501–505.
343. Hansen EF, Andersen LT, Von Eyben FE. Cigarette smoking and age at first acute myocardial infarction, and influence of gender and extent of smoking. *Am J Cardiol* 1993;71:1439–1442.
344. Gomex MA, Karagounis LA, Allen A, Anderson JL. Effect of cigarette smoking on coronary patency after thrombolytic therapy for myocardial infarction. TEAM-2 investigators. Second multicenter thrombolytic trials of eminase in acute myocardial infarction. *Am J Cardiol* 1993;72:373–378.
345. Khosla S, Laddu A, Ehrenpreis S, Somberg JC. Cardiovascular effects of nicotine: Relation to deleterious effects of cigarette smoking. *Am Heart J* 1994;127:1669–1672.
346. Roald HE, Orvim U, Bakken IJ, Barstad RM, Kierulf P, Sakariassen KS. Modulation of thrombotic responses in moderately stenosed arteries by cigarette smoking and aspirin ingestion. *Arterioscler Thromb* 1994;14:617–621.
347. Grines CL, Topol EJ, O'Neill WW, George BS, Kereiakes D, Phillips HR, Leimberger JD, Woodlief LH, Califf RM. Effect of cigarette smoking on outcome after thrombolytic therapy for myocardial infarction. *Circulation* 1995;91:298–303.
348. Muller JE, Tofler GH. Triggering and hourly variation of onset of arterial thrombosis. *Ann Epidemiol* 1992;2:393–405.
349. Ridker PM, Gaboury CL, Conlin PR, Seely EW, Williams GH, Vaughan DE. Stimulation of plasminogen activator inhibitor *in vivo* by infusion of angiotensin II. Evidence of a potential interaction between the renin–angiotensin system and fibrinolytic function. *Circulation* 1993;87:1969–1973.
350. Wright RA, Flapan AD, Alberti KG, Ludlam CA, Fox KA. Effects of captopril therapy on endogenous fibrinolysis in men with recent, uncomplicated myocardial infarction. *J Am Coll Cardiol* 1994;24: 67–73.
351. Ridker PM, Manson JE, Gaziano JM, Buring JE, Hennekens CH. Low-dose aspirin therapy for chronic stable angina. A randomized, placebo-controlled clinical trial. *Ann Intern Med* 1991;114:835–839.
352. Juul-Moller S, Edvardsson N, Jahnmatz B, Rosen A, Sorensen S, Omblus R. Double-blind trial of aspirin in primary prevention of myocardial infarction in patients with stable chronic angina pectoris. *Lancet* 1992;340:1421–1425.
353. Fuster V, Dyken ML, Vokonas PS, Hennekens C. Aspirin as a therapeutic agent in cardiovascular disease. Special Writing Group. *Circulation* 1993;87:659–675.
354. Antiplatelet Trialists' Collaboration. Collaborative overview of randomised trials of antiplatelet therapy—I: Prevention of death, myocardial infarction, and stroke by prolonged antiplatelet therapy in various categories of patients. *Br Med J* 1994;308:81–106.
355. Hirsh J, Fuster V. Guide to anticoagulant therapy. Part 1: Heparin. American Heart Association. *Circulation* 1994;89:1449–1468.
356. Hirsh J, Fuster V. Guide to anticoagulant therapy. Part 2: Oral anticoagulants. American Heart Association. *Circulation* 1994;89: 1469–1480.
357. Théroux P, Waters D, Qiu S, McCans J, Guise P, Juneau M. Aspirin versus heparin to prevent myocardial infarction during the acute phase of unstable angina. *Circulation* 1993;88:2045–2048.
358. Simoons ML, Arnold AER. Tailored thrombolytic therapy. A perspective. *Circulation* 1993;88:2556–2564.
359. The TIMI IIIB Investigators. Effects of tissue plasminogen activator and a comparison of early invasive and conservative strategies in unstable angina and non-Q-wave myocardial infarction. Results of the TIMI IIIB trial. *Circulation* 1994;89:1545–1556.
360. Brodie BR, Grines CL, Ivanhoe R, Knopf W, Taylor G, O'Keefe J, Weintraub RA, Berdan LG, Tcheng JE, Woodlief LH, Califf RM, O'Neill WW. Six-month clinical and angiographic follow-up after direct angioplasty for acute myocardial infarction. Final results from the Primary Angioplasty Registry. *Circulation* 1994;25:156–162.
361. Leung W-H, Lau C-P, Wong C-K. Beneficial effect of cholesterol-lowering therapy on coronary endothelium-dependent relaxation in hypercholesterolaemic patients. *Lancet* 1993;341:1496–1500.
362. Gould KL, Martucci JP, Goldberg DI, Hess MJ, Edens RP, Latifi R, Dudrick SJ. Short-term cholesterol lowering decreases size and severity of perfusion abnormalities by positron emission tomography after dipyridamole in patients with coronary artery disease. *Circulation* 1994;89:1530–1538.
363. Egashira K, Hirooka Y, Kai H, Sugimachi M, Suzuki S, Inou T, Takeshita A. Reduction in serum cholesterol with pravastatin improves endothelium-dependent coronary vasomotion in patients with hypercholesterolemia. *Circulation* 1994;89:2519–2524.
364. Hunt BJ. The relation between abnormal hemostatic function and the progression of coronary disease. *Curr Opin Cardiol* 1990;5:758–765.
365. Pearson TA, Marx HJ. The rapid reduction in cardiac events with lipid-lowering therapy: Mechanisms and implications. *Am J Cardiol* 1993;72:1072–1073.
366. Badimon JJ, Badimon L, Turitto VT, Fuster V. Platelet deposition at high shear rates is enhanced by high plasma cholesterol levels. *In vivo* study in the rabbit model. *Arterioscler Thromb* 1991;11:395–402.
367. Lam JYT, L-Lacoste L. Hypercholesterolaemia and platelet thrombosis under arterial flow conditions. *Eur Heart J* 1994;15(Abst Suppl): 488(abst).
368. Hoffmann CJ, Lawson WE, Miller RH, Hultin MB. Correlation of vitamin K-dependent clotting factors with cholesterol and triglycerides in healthy young adults. *Arterioscler Thromb* 1994;14: 1737–1740.

Special Pathogenetic Factors: Inflammation and Immunity

Atherosclerosis and Coronary Artery Disease,
edited by V. Fuster, R. Ross, and E. J. Topol.
Lippincott-Raven Publishers, Philadelphia © 1996.

CHAPTER 29

Traffic Signals on Endothelium for Leukocytes in Health, Inflammation, and Atherosclerosis

Timothy A. Springer and Myron I. Cybulsky

Key Words: Eosinophils; Granulocytes; High endothelial venules (HEV); Lipoproteins; Lymphocytes; Monocytes; Mononuclear leukocytes; Neutrophils; Tumor necrosis factor (TNF); Vascular cell adhesion molecule 1 (VCAM-1).

T. A. Springer: The Center for Blood Research, Department of Pathology, Harvard Medical School, Boston, Massachusetts 02115.

M. I. Cybulsky: Department of Pathology, Harvard Medical School and Brigham and Women's Hospital, Boston, Massachusetts 02115.

INTRODUCTION

During atherogenesis, the emigration of mononuclear leukocytes from blood into the arterial intima is a key feature of initiation and progression of atherosclerotic plaques. This process may represent a protective inflammatory response of the host to intimal accumulation of oxidized lipoproteins. The mechanisms of leukocyte recruitment to the arterial wall during atherogenesis are likely shared by a variety of inflammatory and immune processes; however, leukocyte recruitment in the latter occurs primarily through postcapillary venules and veins. Because of differences in hemodynamics of arterial and venous circulations, some of the steps in arterial leukocyte emigration, e.g., rolling, may differ from emigration in veins. In this chapter, we review the pathophysiological mechanisms of leukocyte emigration and lymphocyte recirculation and then, based on observations in animal models and in human specimens, speculate on the mechanisms that may be relevant to atherogenesis.

The circulatory and migratory properties of white blood cells have evolved to allow efficient surveillance of tissues for infectious pathogens and rapid accumulation at sites of injury and infection. Lymphocytes continually patrol the body for foreign antigens by recirculating from blood, through tissue, into lymph, and back to blood. Lymphocytes acquire a predilection, based on the environment in which they first encounter foreign antigen, to home to or recirculate through that same environment (1,2). Granulocytes and monocytes can emigrate from the bloodstream in response to molecular changes on the surface of blood vessels that signal injury or infection. Lymphocytes can similarly accumulate in response to inflammatory stimuli. The nature of the inflammatory stimulus determines whether lymphocytes, monocytes, neutrophils, or eosinophils predominate, and thus exercises specificity in the molecular signals or "area codes" that are displayed on endothelium and control traffic of particular leukocyte classes.

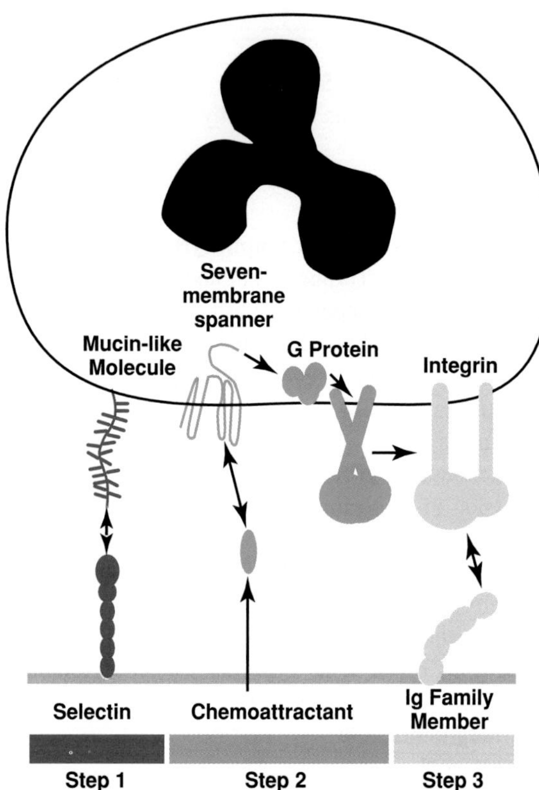

FIG. 1. Three sequential steps provide the traffic signals that regulate leukocyte localization in the vasculature. Selectin molecules that bind carbohydrate ligands, often displayed on mucin-like molecules, are responsible for the initial tethering of a flowing leukocyte to the vessel wall and labile, rolling adhesions (the green light). Tethering brings leukocytes into proximity with chemoattractants that are displayed on or released from the endothelial lining of the vessel wall. Chemoattractants bind to receptors that span the membrane seven times on the surface of leukocytes. These couple to G proteins, which transduce signals that activate integrin adhesiveness (the yellow light). The integrins can then bind to immunoglobulin superfamily (IgSF) members on the endothelium, increasing adhesiveness and resulting in arrest of the rolling leukocyte (the red light). Following directional cues from chemoattractants and using integrins for traction, leukocytes then cross the endothelial lining of the blood vessel and enter the tissue.

Recent findings show that the "traffic signals" for lymphocyte recirculation and for neutrophil and monocyte localization in inflammation are strikingly similar at the molecular level. These "traffic signal" or "area code" molecules are displayed together on endothelium but act on leukocytes in a sequence that was first defined for neutrophils and appears to hold true with slight modification for lymphocyte homing as well (Fig. 1). The selectin or green light allows cells to tether and roll, the chemoattractant or yellow light tells cells to activate integrin adhesiveness and put on the brakes, and the immunoglobulin (Ig) family member or red light binds integrins and causes cells to come to a full stop. These three steps, with multiple molecular choices at each step, provide great combinatorial diversity in signals. Accordingly, the selective responses of different leukocyte classes to inflammatory agents, as well as the preferential recirculation patterns of distinct lymphocyte subpopulations, can be explained by their distinct receptivity to combinations of molecular signals. Following an overview of leukocytes and endothelium, and of the molecules important in their interactions, we review the traffic signals that enable selective emigratory behavior of monocytes and neutrophils and then elaborate how a paradigm of three or four sequential signals can be extended to lymphocyte recirculation. This review updates and extends a previous one (3). (For recent reviews see refs. 4–20.)

THE FUNCTION OF LEUKOCYTE CLASSES CORRELATES WITH CIRCULATORY BEHAVIOR

Neutrophilic granulocytes are among the most abundant leukocytes in the bloodstream and the first to appear at sites of bacterial infection or injury. Neutrophils are produced at the prodigious rate of 10^9 cells/kg body weight per day in the bone marrow and have a half-life in the circulation of 7 h. Their life span after extravasation is hours or less (21). Their primary function is to phagocytose and eliminate foreign microorganisms and damaged tissue.

Monocytes are far less numerous than neutrophils in the blood, where their half-life is about 24 h (22). Like neutrophils, they are phagocytic and accumulate in response to traumatic injury or bacterial infection. However, monocytes differ from neutrophils in that they accumulate at sites where

T lymphocytes have recognized antigen, as in delayed-type hypersensitivity reactions and graft rejection. Monocytes are important effector cells in antigen-specific T-cell immunity, are activated by T-cell products such as interferon-γ (IFN-γ), and can organize around parasites into protective structures called granulomas. After extravasation, monocytes may also differentiate into longer-lived tissue macrophages or mononuclear phagocytes such as the Kupffer cells of the liver, which have a half-life of weeks to months.

In contrast to the neutrophil and monocyte, a lymphocyte may emigrate and recirculate many thousands of times during its life history. Recirculation of lymphocytes correlates with their role as antigen-receptor-bearing surveillance cells. Lymphocytes function as the reservoir of "immunologic memory" and recirculate through tissues to provide systemic memory. Few of the body's lymphocytes are present at any one time in the bloodstream, where their half-life is 2 h. Distinct subsets of lymphocytes extravasate through the microvasculature in tissues such as skin and gut, and through specialized high endothelial venules (HEV) in lymphoid organs (1,6,17). After migrating through tissue, lymphocytes find their way into the lymphatics. They percolate through draining lymph nodes in the lymphatic system and finally enter the thoracic duct, through which they return to the bloodstream. This journey is completed roughly every 1 to 2 days.

ENDOTHELIUM

By displaying specific signals, the endothelium is the most active player in controlling leukocyte traffic. Vascular endothelium is diversified at a number of levels. Large vessels differ from small vessels and capillaries; venular endothelium differs from arterial endothelium; and endothelial phenotype varies between tissues. The preferential migration of leukocytes from postcapillary venules may be related to factors such as shear stress, which is lower there, and hence more favorable for leukocyte attachment, than in capillaries or arterioles, or to events that occur when leukocytes pass through capillaries. However, when flow is controlled so that shear stress is equivalent in arterioles and venules (23), or when the direction of blood flow is reversed (24), attachment and emigration are far greater from venules, suggesting molecular differences in their endothelial surfaces. In agreement with this, P-selectin is much more abundant on postcapillary venules than on large vessels, arterioles, or capillaries (25), and induction of E-selectin and vascular cell adhesion molecule 1 (VCAM-1) expression in inflammation is most prominent on postcapillary venules (9). The mucin-like cluster of differentiation 34 (CD34) molecule is well expressed on capillaries and is absent from most large vessels (26), and CD36 is expressed on microvascular but not large-vessel endothelium (27). The extracellular matrix may exert an influence on endothelial differentiation, as exemplified by modulation of adhesiveness (28). The high endothelium in lymphoid tissue, which expresses addressins for lymphocyte recirculation, is one of the most dramatic examples of endothelial specialization (6).

Inflammatory cytokines dramatically and selectively modulate the transcription and expression of adhesion molecules and chemoattractants in endothelial cells (29). Tumor necrosis factor (TNF) and interleukin-1 (IL-1) increase adhesiveness of endothelium for both neutrophils and lymphocytes and induce ICAM-1, E-selectin, and VCAM-1; IL-4, synergistically with other cytokines, increases adhesion of lymphocytes and induces VCAM-1 (30,31). It is likely that the precise mixture of chemoattractants and cytokines produced at inflammatory sites in vivo determines which types of leukocytes emigrate. Thus, injection into skin of IL-1α induces emigration of neutrophils and monocytes, as do lipopolysaccharide (LPS) and TNF-α, but with more prolonged emigration of the monocytes. IFN-γ induces emigration of monocytes but not neutrophils (22). Interferon-γ and TNF-α, but not IL-1α or LPS, recruit lymphocytes, and IL-4 is ineffective by itself but synergizes with TNF (32–34).

Acting more quickly than cytokines, vasoactive substances such as histamine and thrombin modulate endothelial function in seconds or minutes. They induce secretion of the storage granules of endothelial cells and platelets. Furthermore, they dilate arterioles, increase plasma leakage and thereby raise the hematocrit within microvessels, and thus alter the rheology of blood so as to increase the collision of leukocytes with the vessel wall (35). Furthermore, arteriolar dilation and the ensuing increased blood flow in inflammatory sites are responsible for two of the cardinal signs of inflammation, rubor (redness) and calor (heat), and increased perfusion enhances the discharge and thus accelerates the accumulation of leukocytes.

AREA CODE MOLECULES

Selectins

Multiple protein families, each with a distinct function, provide the traffic signals for leukocytes. The selectin family of adhesion molecules (Fig. 2) has an N-terminal domain homologous to Ca^{2+}-dependent lectins (7,8,9,18,19,36,37). The name selectin capitalizes on the derivation of "lectin" and "select" from the same Latin root, meaning to separate by picking out. Selectins are limited in expression to cells of the vasculature (Fig. 2). L-Selectin is expressed on all circulating leukocytes except for a subpopulation of lymphocytes (38–40). P-Selectin is stored preformed in the Weibel–Palade bodies of endothelial cells and the α granules of platelets. In response to mediators of acute inflammation such as thrombin or histamine, P-selectin is rapidly mobilized to the plasma membrane to bind neutrophils and monocytes (25,41,42). E-Selectin is induced on vascular endothelial cells by cytokines such as IL-1, LPS, or TNF and requires de novo mRNA and protein synthesis (43).

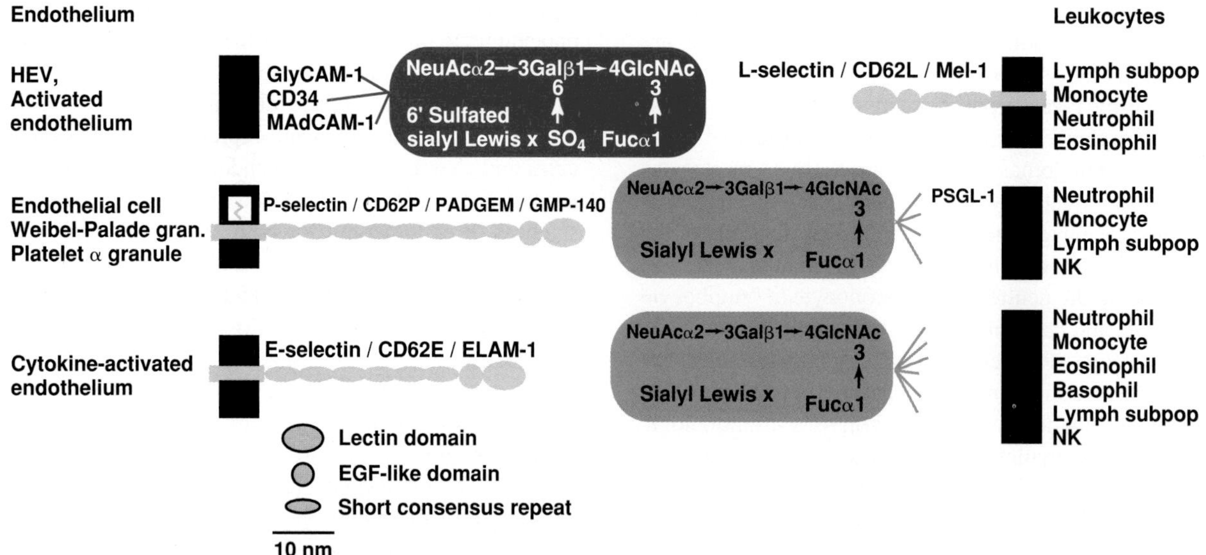

FIG. 2. Selectins and their ligands. The selectins are shown to scale, based on electron micrographs of P-selectin (47), the X-ray structure of E-selectin lectin and EGF domains (49), and estimates of the sizes of the short consensus repeats (SCR) (36). P-Selectin is shown palmitylated on a transmembrane cysteine (291). The carbohydrates are not to scale.

Carbohydrates and Mucin-Like Molecules

All selectins appear to recognize a sialylated carbohydrate determinant on their counterreceptors (7,8,19). E-Selectin and P-selectin recognize carbohydrate structures that are distinct but are both closely related to the tetrasaccharide sialyl Lewis^x and its isomer sialyl Lewis^a (Fig. 2). The actual ligand structures for E- and P-selectin are more complex, as shown by display of the ligand for E-selectin but not P-selectin on fucosyl-transferase-transfected cells that express sialyl Lewis^x (44). The affinity of E-selectin for soluble sialyl Lewis^x is quite low, with $K_d = 0.2–0.8$ mM (45), which suggests that a higher-affinity ligand may yet be identified. P-Selectin is specific for carbohydrate displayed on the P-selectin glycoprotein ligand (PSGL-1), suggesting either that PSGL-1 expresses a specific carbohydrate structure or that PSGL-1 protein forms part of the ligand binding site (46). The affinity of P-selectin for PSGL-1 is high, with a $K_d = 70$ nM (47). Structure–function studies suggest that the Ca^{2+}-binding site and a cluster of basic residues on E-selectin coordinate with the fucosyl and sialic acid carboxylate moieties, respectively, of sialyl Lewis^x (48,49).

The carbohydrate ligands for L- and P-selectin are O-linked to specific mucin-like molecules. Mucins are serine- and threonine-rich proteins that are heavily O-glycosylated and have an extended structure. L-Selectin recognizes at least two mucins in HEV (Fig. 3), glycosylation-dependent cell adhesion molecule 1 (GlyCAM-1), which is secreted (37), and CD34, which is on the cell surface (50). The carbohydrate ligand for L-selectin is related to sialyl Lewis^a and sialyl Lewis^x (51,52), contains sialic acid and sulfate, and is O-linked to mucin-like structures of HEV (19). Structural studies on the carbohydrates of GlyCAM-1 show that 6′-sulfated sialyl Lewis^x (Fig. 2) is a major oligosaccharide capping group, and is a candidate for the ligand structure (53).

The mucin-like P-selectin glycoprotein ligand (PSGL-1) is a disulfide-linked dimer of 120-kDa subunits (46) that is sensitive to O-glycoprotease, which selectively cleaves mucin-like domains (54,55). The PSGL-1 (Fig. 3) was isolated by screening for cDNA that expressed ligand activity (56). COS cells must be transfected with both the PSGL-1 cDNA and *α*-3/4-fucosyl transferase cDNA to express P-selectin ligand activity. By contrast, COS cells cotransfected with cDNA for *α*-3/4-fucosyl transferase and another mucin-like molecule that is expressed by neutrophils, CD43, lack P-selectin ligand activity.

Function of Selectins and Their Ligands

Selectins mediate functions unique to the vasculature, the tethering of flowing leukocytes to the vessel wall and formation of labile adhesions with the wall that permit leukocytes subsequently to roll in the direct of flow. One study demonstrated this with purified P-selectin incorporated into supported planar lipid bilayers on one wall of a flow chamber (57). At wall shear stresses within the range of those found in postcapillary venules, neutrophils formed labile attachments to the P-selectin in the bilayer and rolled in response to fluid drag forces. In other studies, intravascular infusion of a soluble L-selectin/IgG chimera inhibited neutrophil rolling

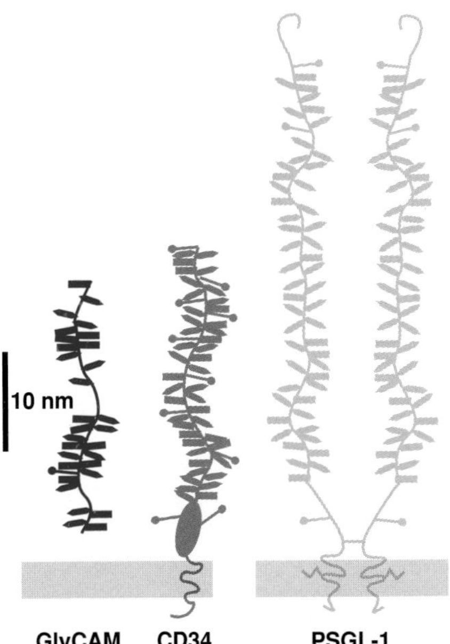

FIG. 3. Mucin-like carriers of selectin ligands. The GlyCAM (37) and CD34 (50,77) molecules synthesized by peripheral lymph node HEV and MAdCAM-1 molecule synthesized by mucosal HEV (see Fig. 5) bear O-linked carbohydrates that bind to L-selectin. CD34 has a globular domain that may be Ig-like (292) and is resistant to O-glycoprotease (293). The PSGL-1 molecule on neutrophils bears O-linked carbohydrates that bind to P-selectin (55,56). A cysteine in the transmembrane region is predicted to be palmitylated. O-Linked sites and N-linked sites are shown as bars and lollipops, respectively. The length of the mucin-like domains and the percentage of serines and threonines that are O-glycosylated are proportioned to measurements for CD43 (45 nm per 224 amino acids and 75% to 90% of O-glycosylation) (72).

attachments in vivo (58), as did infusion of anti-L-selectin monoclonal antibodies (59). More recent studies have shown that neutrophils roll on E-selectin in purified form (60) or on the endothelial cell surface both in vitro (61) and in vivo (62), that monoclonal antibody (mAb) to P-selectin decreases neutrophil rolling in vivo (63), and that neutrophil rolling in the microvasculature of mice genetically deficient in P-selectin is almost completely absent (64).

P- and L-selectin may cooperate with one another, because inhibition of either almost completely inhibits neutrophil rolling in vivo (58,59,64,65). E- and L-selectin also appear to cooperate (60,66–68). A class of ligand that is closely associated with L-selectin on the neutrophil surface is required for the initial tethering during flow to E-selectin bilayers, after which another class of ligands that mediates rolling takes over (69).

Selectins can mediate tethering of a flowing cell in the span of a millisecond. The integrin LFA-1 and the IgSF member CD2 require minutes to develop similar adhesive strength and do not mediate rolling (57,70). It has been hypothesized that selectins differ from other adhesion molecules not in affinity (K_{eq}) but in having much more rapid association (k_{on}) and dissociation (k_{off}) rate constants (57), as has recently been confirmed (Table 1). Rolling is intermittent and appears mediated by random association and dissociation of selectin–ligand bonds, a small number of which tether a leukocyte to the vessel wall at any one time. A rapid association rate facilitates the initial tethering in flow. A rapid dissociation rate ensures that even with multiple selectin–ligand bonds, it will not take long before the bond that is most upstream randomly dissociates, allowing the cell to roll forward a small distance until it is held by the next most upstream bond. (57,71).

The elongated molecular structure of selectins and mucins and their segmental flexibility (47,72) are predicted to enhance their accessibility for binding to counterstructures on closely opposed cells (57). P-Selectin and PSGL-1 are currently the most elongated adhesion molecules known (Figs. 2 and 3) and could bridge together two cells with plasma membranes about 0.1 μm apart. Expression on cytoplasmic protrusions further enhances accessibility. L-Selectin is clustered on microvilli of neutrophils (67,73), which project about 0.3 μm above the surface of a cell with a diameter of 7 μm and contain 90% of the L-selectin (D. Bainton, D. Hammer, and T Springer, *unpublished data*). In keeping with this topographic distribution, rolling in vivo requires the integrity of the L-selectin cytoplasmic domain and is inhibited by cytochalasin B (74). Lymphocytes bind through microvilli to HEV (75,76). Conversely, the mucin-like CD34 molecule (77) is concentrated on filopodia of nonspecialized endothelial cells found in the microvasculature of most tissues (26). These filopodia are concentrated near junctions between endothelial cells, and electron micrographs of granulocytes binding to the microvasculature in inflammatory sites suggest that the earliest binding event is to these filopodia (78).

TABLE 1. *Fast on and off rates of a selectin, and affinity modulation of an integrin*

	k_{on} ($M^{-1}s^{-1}$)	k_{off} (s^{-1})	K_d (μM)
P-Selectin	1.4×10^{7} [a]	1 [b]	0.07 [c]
LFA-1 low affinity [d]	3×10^{2}	0.03	100
LFA-1 high affinity [e]	ND [f]	ND	0.6

[a] Calculated from $k_{on} = k_{off}/K_d$.
[b] At very low P-selectin densities in lipid bilayers, neutrophils attach transiently; i.e., they subsequently detach rather than roll. Measurements of the cellular dissociation rate suggest that the $t_{1/2}$ for dissociation of a single selectin–ligand bond is about 0.7 s (315).
[c] For binding of monomeric, truncated P-selectin to neutrophils (47).
[d] k_{on}, k_{off}, and K_d were measured by competitive inhibition by monomeric, truncated ICAM-1 of binding of Fab to LFA-1 on resting lymphocytes (111).
[e] Same as *d*, but for phorbol-ester-stimulated lymphocytes. Approximately 20% of the cell surface LFA-1 was in the high-affinity state (111).
[f] ND, not determined.

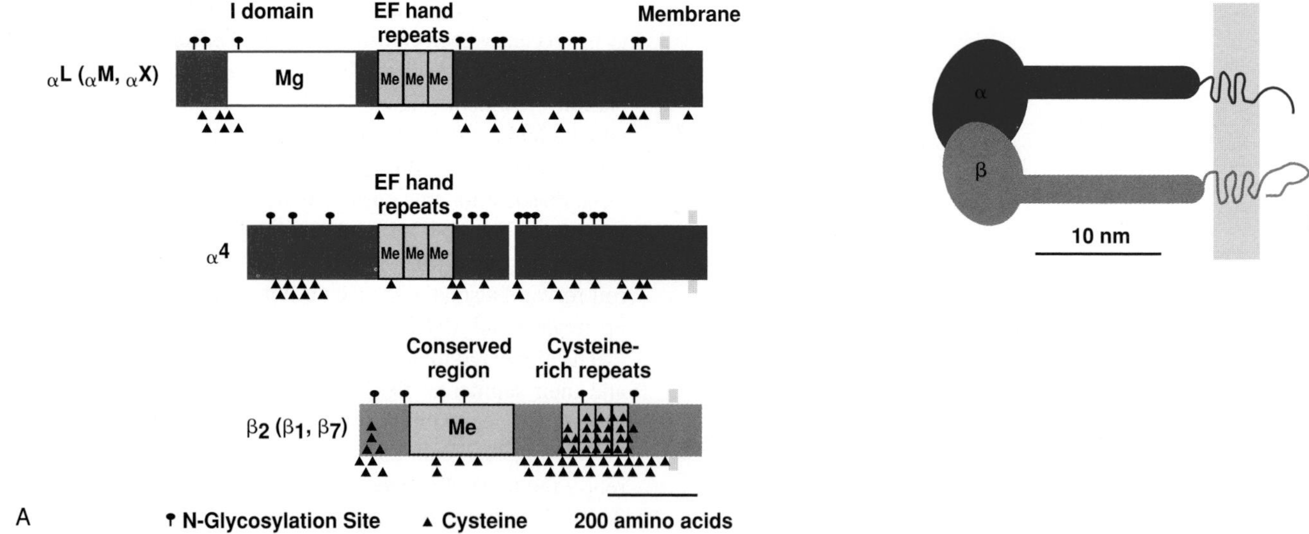

FIG. 4. Integrins that bind endothelial ligands. **A:** Schematics of representative integrin α and β subunits. The structures of α^L (294) and β_2 (295) integrin subunits are shown as representative of α^M and α^X or β_1 and β_7, respectively; cysteines are identical, and glycosylation sites vary but are sparse in the I domain and EF hand repeats. The EF hand repeats are divalent metal-binding motifs that may bind Ca^{2+} or Mg^{2+} (labeled "Me"). A binding site for Mg^{2+} and Mn^{2+} but not Ca^{2+} has been identified in the I domain (110). The α^4 integrin subunit has a posttranslational proteolytic cleavage site (296). A putative divalent cation binding site has been defined in the conserved domain of the integrin β_3 subunit and is shown for β_2 (297). **B:** Scale model of an integrin, based on electron micrographs of the integrins gpIIbIIIa (298) and VLA-5 ($\alpha^5\beta_1$) (299).

Chemoattractants

Chemoattractants are important in activation of integrin adhesiveness and in directing the migration of leukocytes. In chemotaxis, cells move in the direction of increasing concentration of a chemoattractant, which typically is a soluble molecule that can diffuse away from the site of its production, where its concentration is highest (79,80). Leukocytes, which can sense a concentration difference of 1% across their diameter, move steadily in the direction of the chemoattractant. There is much interplay between adhesion molecules and chemoattractants because adhesion to a surface is required to provide the traction necessary for migration directed by chemoattractants, and chemoattractants can activate adhesiveness.

The alternative mechanism to chemotaxis is haptotaxis. In ''haptotaxis,'' cells migrate to the region of highest adhesiveness (81). Thus, on a gradient of an adhesive ligand affixed to the surface of other cells or to the extracellular matrix, and in the absence of a chemotactic gradient, motile cells will tend to accumulate in the region of highest ligand density. Both chemotaxis and haptotaxis can contribute to cell localization, but haptotaxis has yet to be demonstrated in vivo.

Classical leukocyte chemoattractants act broadly, on neutrophils, eosinophils, basophils, and monocytes (Table 2). A recently described family of chemoattractive cytokines, termed chemokines, are 70- to 80-residue polypeptides and have specificity for leukocyte subsets (11,12). Two subfamilies of chemokines have been defined by sequence homology and by the sequence around two cysteine residues (Table 2). The CXC or α chemokines tend to act on neutrophils and nonhematopoietic cells involved in wound healing, whereas the CC or β chemokines tend to act on monocytes and in some cases on eosinophils and lymphocyte subpopulations.

It has long been debated whether chemoattractants can act in the circulation, where they would be rapidly diluted and swept downstream by blood flow. Tethering and rolling of leukocytes through selectins would enhance exposure to chemoattractants by prolonging contact with the vessel wall. However, retention of chemoattractants at their site of production by noncovalent interactions with molecules on the vessel wall and within the inflammatory site may also be important. Heparin-binding sites on chemokines provide a mechanism for retention in the extracellular matrix (82), to enhance concentration gradients, and perhaps to present chemokines on the endothelium to circulating leukocytes (83,84).

Chemoattractant Receptors

Leukocyte chemoattractant receptors have multiple functions. They not only direct migration but also activate integrin adhesiveness and stimulate degranulation, shape change, actin polymerization, and the respiratory burst (85). Chemoattractant receptors are G-protein-coupled receptors that span the membrane seven times. Ligand binding to the

TABLE 2. *Leukocyte chemoattractants*

Chemoattractant	Origin	Responding cells
Classical chemoattractants[a]		
N-Formyl peptides	Bacterial protein processing	Monocyte, neutrophil, eosinophil, basophil
C5a	Complement activation	Monocyte, neutrophil, eosinophil, basophil
Leukotriene B_4	Arachidonate metabolism	Monocyte, neutrophil
Platelet-activating factor (PAF)	Phosphatidylcholine metabolism	Monocyte, neutrophil, eosinophil
CXC chemokines[b]		
IL-8/NAP-1	T lymphocyte, monocyte, endothelial cell, fibroblast, keratinocyte, chondrocyte, mesothelial cell	Neutrophil, basophil
CTAP-III/β-thromboglobulin/ NAP-2	Successive N-terminal cleavage of platelet basic protein released from α-granules	Neutrophil, basophil, fibroblast
gro/MGSA	Fibroblast, melanomas, endothelial cell, monocyte	Neutrophil, melanomas, fibroblast
ENA-78	Epithelium	Neutrophil
CC chemokines[c]		
MCP-1	T lymphocyte, monocyte, fibroblast, endothelial cell, smooth muscle	Monocyte, T lymphocyte subpopulation, basophil
MIP-1α	Monocyte, B and T lymphocyte	Monocyte, T lymphocyte subpopulation, basophil, eosinophil
RANTES	T lymphocyte, platelets	Monocyte, T lymphocyte subpopulation, eosinophil
I-309	T lymphocyte, mast cell	Monocyte

[a] References 80,85.
[b] References 11,12,173,174,255.
[c] References 11,12,84,250–252,255,306–309.

membrane-spanning receptor is coupled to exchange of GTP for GDP bound to the associated G protein heterotrimer and results in activation by the G protein α and $\beta\gamma$ subunits of signaling effectors such as phospholipase $C_{\beta 2}$ (86). This results in release of diacylglycerol and inositol phosphates and mobilization of Ca^{2+}. Neutrophils and lymphocytes express $G\alpha_{i2}$ and $G\alpha_{i3}$ subunits (85,87). The $G\alpha$ subunits of the α_i class are ADP-ribosylated and irreversibly inactivated by pertussis toxin. All of the biological effects of leukocyte chemoattractants are inhibited by pertussis toxin. Coupling through $G\alpha_i$ subunits has been confirmed by reconstitution in transfected cells (86). The lipid mediators LTB_4 and PAF are as active as formylated bacterial peptides, C5a, and IL-8 in stimulating chemotaxis but less active in stimulating the respiratory burst and other functions of neutrophils (85); this correlates with their ability to couple to distinct $G\alpha$ subunits in transfected cells (88).

Cloning of the receptors for formylated bacterial peptides, C5a, and platelet-activating factor (PAF) has shown that they are expressed on both neutrophils and monocytes, whereas the receptor for IL-8 is expressed only on neutrophils (89). The receptor for MCP-1 is expressed on monocytic cells but not on neutrophils (90). Thus, the specificity of chemoattractants is regulated by the cellular distribution of their receptors.

Integrins

Integrins are perhaps the most versatile of the adhesion molecules. Integrin adhesiveness can be rapidly regulated by the cells on which they are expressed. Each integrin contains noncovalently associated α and β subunits with characteristic structural motifs (Fig. 4). Five integrins are important in the interaction of leukocytes with endothelial cells. Their cellular distribution, ligand specificity, and structure are summarized in Table 3 and Fig. 4.

Activation of Integrins

The adhesiveness of LFA-1 and VLA-4 on T lymphocytes is activated by cross-linking of the antigen receptor and other surface molecules (13,20,36). Increased adhesiveness occurs within a few minutes, is not accompanied by any change in quantity of surface expression, and appears to result from both conformational changes that increase affinity for ligand and altered interaction with the cytoskeleton (20,91,92). However, it is unlikely that recognition by T-cell receptors of antigen on endothelial cells (93) is a step in lymphocyte trafficking, because traffic of both lymphocytes that can and cannot recognize specific antigen is increased in antigen-induced inflammation. Although evidence has been presented that binding of neutrophils to selectins can activate adhesiveness of integrins (94), other evidence has failed to confirm this (60,95; T. G. Diacovo and T. A. Springer, *unpublished data*).

Thus far the best candidates for activation of integrin adhesiveness within the vasculature are chemoattractants. Adhesiveness of Mac-1 and LFA-1 on neutrophils and monocytes is activated by N-formylated peptide and IL-8

TABLE 3. *Integrins in leukocyte–endothelial interactions*

Subunits	Names	Distribution	Ligands
Leukocyte integrins[a]			
$\alpha^L\beta_2$	LFA-1, CD11a/CD18	B and T lymphocyte, monocyte, neutrophil	ICAM-1, ICAM-2, ICAM-3
$\alpha^M\beta_2$	Mac-1, CR3, CD11b/CD18	Monocyte, neutrophil	ICAM-1, iC3b, fibrinogen, factor X
$\alpha^X\beta_2$	p150,95, CR4, CD11c/CD18	Monocyte, neutrophil, eosinophil	iC3b, fibrinogen
α^4 Integrins[b]			
$\alpha^4\beta_1$	VLA-4, CD49d/CD29	B and T lymphocyte, monocyte, neural crest-derived cells, fibroblast, muscle	VCAM-1, fibronectin
$\alpha^4\beta_7$	LPAM-1, CD49d/CD$^-$	B and T lymphocyte subpopulations	MAdCAM-1, VCAM-1, fibronectin

[a] References 36,151.
[b] References 36,123,124,131,132,199,310–313.

(96–100). In contrast to LFA-1 on lymphocytes and neutrophils, Mac-1 on neutrophils is increased about tenfold on the surface by chemoattractant-stimulated fusion of secretory granules with the plasma membrane (101); however, this is neither sufficient or necessary for increased adhesiveness (102,103). The transient nature of the activation of integrin adhesiveness (96,104) provides a mechanism for de-adhesion and perhaps for retraction of the trailing edge of a leukocyte from the substrate during cell migration.

Conformational changes in LFA-1 and Mac-1 that are associated with increased adhesiveness are suggested by mAb and Fab that react only with these molecules after cellular activation (105–108). After chemoattractant activation of neutrophils, saturation binding shows that 10% of the surface Mac-1 molecules express an activation epitope, yet mAb to this epitope completely blocks binding to ligands such as ICAM-1 and fibrinogen. This suggests that ligand binding is mediated by a subpopulation of activated Mac-1 molecules (108). The I domain of leukocyte integrins is important in ligand binding (109,110) and expresses activation epitopes (107,108). Recent measurements of the affinity of cell surface LFA-1 for soluble, monomeric ICAM-1 (Table 1) have directly demonstrated that cellular activation increases the affinity of a subpopulation of LFA-1 molecules by approximately 200-fold (111).

Surprisingly, the integrin VLA-4, in contrast to LFA-1 and Mac-1, has recently been found to be capable of supporting rolling. Lymphocytes can tether in flow and subsequently roll on VCAM-1. If activated while rolling by phorbol ester or TS2/16 mAb to the β_1 subunit, the lymphocytes arrest and develop firm adhesion. Activated lymphocytes tether as efficiently as resting lymphocytes but do not roll. Fibronectin can support development of firm adhesion in static conditions but not tethering or rolling in flow. VCAM-1 is less efficient than selectins in mediating tethering and rolling (112).

Immunoglobulin Superfamily Members on Endothelium as Integrin Ligands

In a paradigm first established with ICAM-1 binding to LFA-1, several immunoglobulin superfamily (IgSF) members, expressed on endothelium, bind to integrins expressed on leukocytes (Fig. 5). ICAM-1, ICAM-2, and ICAM-3 are products of distinct and homologous genes and were all initially identified by their ability to interact with LFA-1 (113–115). ICAM-1 has also been found to bind to Mac-1 through a distinct site in its third Ig domain (99,116,117) (Fig. 5). Induction of ICAM-1 on endothelium and other cells by inflammatory cytokines may increase cell–cell in-

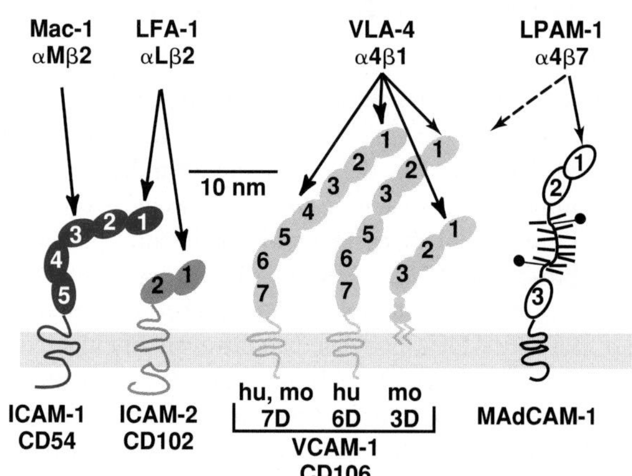

FIG. 5. Immunoglobulin superfamily adhesion receptors on endothelium and their integrin-binding sites. Members of the Ig superfamily share the immunoglobulin domain, composed of 90 to 100 amino acids arranged in a sandwich of two sheets of antiparallel β-strands that is stabilized by one or (in the N-terminal domain of the molecules shown) two disulfide bonds. The immunoglobulins and T-cell receptors are the only known members of this family that undergo somatic diversification. The function of the IgSF in adhesion evolutionarily predates specialization for antigen recognition. The shape and size of the ICAM-1 molecule, with its unpaired Ig domains and bend, were determined by electron microscopy (300,301), as were those of VCAM-1 (128). Immunoglobulin domains are ellipsoids with a length of 4 nm parallel to the β-strands and 2.5 nm in the other dimensions. The mucin-like region of MAdCAM-1 is modeled as described in the legend to Fig. 3; N-linked glycosylation sites in the Ig domains of this and the other molecules are not shown. References for structures (in parentheses) and for localization (in brackets) follow: ICAM-1 (302,303); [117,300]; ICAM-2 (114); VCAM-1 (119,304,305); [125–128]; MAdCAM-1 (130).

teractions and leukocyte extravasation at inflammatory sites, whereas constitutive expression of ICAM-2 may be important for leukocyte trafficking in uninflammed tissues, as in lymphocyte recirculation. ICAM-3 is restricted to leukocytes. All three of the ICAMs contribute to antigen-specific interactions, so that inhibition with mAb to all three is required to completely block LFA-1-dependent antigen-specific T-cell responses (118).

VCAM-1 is inducible by cytokines on endothelial cells and on a more restricted subset of nonvascular cells than ICAM-1 (9). A single VCAM-1 gene gives rise through alternative splicing to a seven-domain isoform and to a second isoform that contains either six domains or three domains and glycosyl phosphatidylinositol membrane anchor (119–121) (Fig. 5). VCAM-1 is a ligand for the integrin $\alpha^4\beta_1$ (VLA-4) and binds weakly to $\alpha^4\beta_7$ (122–124). In contrast to the shorter isoforms, the seven-domain isoform of VCAM-1 has two binding sites for VLA-4, in highly homologous domains 1 and 4 (125–128).

An addressin for lymphocyte recirculation to mucosa is expressed on Peyer's patch HEV and on other venules (129). Now termed mucosal addressin cell adhesion molecule (MAdCAM-1), it contains three Ig-like domains and a mucin-like region interposed between domains 2 and 3 (130) (Fig. 5). The MAdCAM-1 molecule binds the integrin $\alpha^4\beta_7$ but not $\alpha^4\beta_1$ (131,132). Furthermore, carbohydrates attached to the mucin-like domain of MAdCAM-1 bind L-selectin and mediate lymphocyte rolling (133). Thus, MAdCAM-1 has a dual function as an integrin and selectin ligand.

Other Molecules

CD31 is an IgSF member expressed on leukocytes, platelets, and at cell–cell junctions on endothelium (134–140). CD31 can bind homophilically to itself and also heterophilically to an uncharacterized counterreceptor. The mAb crosslinking of CD31, similarly to many but not all other lymphocyte surface molecules, can trigger integrin adhesiveness (140). Interaction between CD31 on endothelial junctions and CD31 on leukocytes appears to be required for transmigration but not for integrin-mediated binding of leukocytes to endothelium (141). CD31–CD31 interaction may represent a fourth step in transendothelial migration that overlaps the integrin-mediated step and may contribute to the maintenance of the permeability barrier function of endothelia during transmigration.

CD44 is a widely distributed molecule in the body that is homologous with cartilage link protein, is extensively alternatively spliced, and can bear heparin sulfate or chondroitin sulfate side chains (142). The best understood function of CD44 is as a major surface receptor for hyaluronate (143,144). Alternatively spliced forms of CD44 are important in tumor metastasis (145) and in localization of antibody-secreting cells (146). CD44 (H-CAM, Hermes) was at one time mistakenly thought to be the human equivalent of murine mel-14 (L-selectin). It participates in vitro in lymphocyte interaction with HEV and activated endothelium (147,148). However, lack of cell surface CD44 has no effect on lymphocyte recirculation in vivo (149).

TOWARD A MULTISTEP MODEL OF NEUTROPHIL EMIGRATION IN INFLAMMATION

Integrins and Selectins

Patients who are genetically deficient in the leukocyte integrins because of mutations in the common β_2 integrin CD18 subunit provided early evidence that adhesion molecules were required for leukocyte extravasation in vivo (150,151). Leukocyte adhesion deficiency I (LAD-I) patients have life-threatening bacterial infections, and neutrophils in these patients fail to cross the endothelium and accumulate at inflammatory sites despite higher than normal levels of neutrophils in the circulation. In vitro, LAD-I neutrophils or normal neutrophils treated with mAb to the leukocyte integrins are deficient in binding to and migrating across resting or activated endothelial monolayers (152,153). Even though capable of binding to activated endothelium through selectins, LAD-I neutrophils fail to transmigrate (153). Monoclonal antibodies to the leukocyte integrin β_2 subunit, and in some cases the integrin α^M subunit, have been found to have profound effects in vivo (15). These mAb prevent the neutrophil-mediated injury that occurs when ischemic tissue is reperfused and thus can prevent death from shock after blood loss, limb necrosis after frostbite or after amputation and replantation, and tissue necrosis from myocardial ischemia and reperfusion. Monoclonal Abs to leukocyte integrins and to ICAM-1 can also inhibit lymphocyte- and monocyte-mediated antigen-specific responses in vivo, including delayed-type hypersensitivity, granuloma formation, and allograft rejection (15).

Whereas mAb to the leukocyte integrin β_2 subunit blocked accumulation of leukocytes in tissue in response to chemoattractants, and stable adhesion of leukocytes in the local vasculature, it had no effect on the number of rolling leukocytes on the vessel wall (154). Furthermore, leukocyte integrins were found to mediate binding of neutrophils to endothelial monolayers in a parallel wall flow chamber at subphysiological but not at physiological shear stresses found in postcapillary venules (153,155).

Parallel studies showed that selectins were required for leukocyte accumulation in vivo and acted at an early step. Antagonists of L-selectin and E-selectin inhibit neutrophil and monocyte influx into skin, peritoneal cavity, and lung in response to inflammatory agents (40,156–159). Monoclonal Ab to L-selectin was shown to inhibit neutrophil accumulation on cytokine-stimulated endothelium at physiological shear stress (100). Stimulation of neutrophils with chemoattractants results within minutes in shedding into the medium of L-selectin, with kinetics similar to up-regulation of surface expression of the integrin Mac-1. Based on this, and the evidence reviewed above, it was hypothesized that selectins might act at a step prior to integrins (160).

Further studies showed that selectins mediate rolling, and function before development of firm adhesion through integrins. At sites of inflammation, leukocytes first attach to the vessel wall in a rolling interaction, then become arrested or firmly adherent at a single location on the vessel wall before diapedesis (161). This process was fully reconstituted with purified components of the endothelial surface (57). At physiological shear stresses, neutrophils attach to and form labile rolling adhesions on phospholipid bilayers containing purified P-selectin but not on bilayers containing ICAM-1. Chemoattractants stimulate strong, integrin-mediated adhesion to bilayers containing ICAM-1 under static conditions but not in shear flow. At physiological shear stresses, if both P-selectin and ICAM-1 are present in the phospholipid bilayer, resting neutrophils attach and roll identically as on bilayers containing P-selectin alone. However, when chemoattractant is added to the buffer flowing through the chamber, the rolling neutrophils arrest, spread, and firmly adhere through the integrin–ICAM-1 interaction. Chemoattractant does not enhance and actually inhibits interactions of neutrophils with bilayers containing P-selectin alone. These findings show that purified adhesion molecules and chemoattractants representing the endothelial signals can reproduce the key events in leukocyte localization in vivo and prove that the selectin-mediated step is a prerequisite for the chemoattractant- and integrin-mediated steps (57). Complementary studies in vivo showed that mAb to L-selectin, or L-selectin/IgG chimeras, decreased both the number of rolling leukocytes (58,59) and the number of leukocytes that subsequently became firmly adherent, whereas mAb to the β_2 integrin subunit only decreased firm adherence of leukocytes. This suggested that L-selectin acts at a step prior to leukocyte integrins (59). In static assays, a factor derived from cytokine-stimulated endothelium induced shedding of L-selectin and, if transmigration was blocked with CD18 mAb, induced release of neutrophils from inverted endothelial monolayers. This also suggested that L-selectin acted before leukocyte integrin-mediated emigration (100). In elegant confirmation of a three-step model in a static assay of neutrophil adhesion to histamine-stimulated endothelium, juxtacrine cooperation between P-selectin and platelet-activating factor (PAF) was found (95). P-selectin tethered neutrophils to endothelium and thereby augmented stimulation by PAF of CD18-dependent neutrophil adhesion. Stimulation of adhesiveness was by PAF and not by P-selectin, as shown with PAF receptor antagonists.

The requirement for the carbohydrate ligands of selectins for leukocyte emigration in vivo has received strong support from studies of two patients with a genetic defect in biosynthesis of fucose and who therefore lack the ligands for E-selectin and P-selectin (162,163). The defect, designated LAD-II, has many clinical similarities to LAD-I, including strikingly depressed neutrophil emigration into inflammatory sites.

Chemoattractants

Chemoattractants appear to be required for transendothelial migration in vitro and in vivo and can induce all steps required for transmigration in vivo. Injection of chemoattractants into skin or muscle leads to robust emigration of neutrophils from the vasculature and accumulation at the injection site (164). Injection of lipopolysaccharide or cytokines that induce IL-8 synthesis also elicits neutrophil emigration. Moreover, mAb to IL-8 markedly inhibits neutrophil emigration into lung and skin in several models of inflammation (165,166).

The effect of pertussis toxin provides further evidence for the importance of $G\alpha_i$-protein-coupled receptors in leukocyte emigration in vivo. Pretreatment of neutrophils with pertussis toxin inhibits emigration into inflammatory sites (167,168).

Chemoattractants impart directionality to leukocyte migration. By contrast to intradermal injection, intravascular injection of IL-8 does not lead to emigration (169). Cytokine-stimulated endothelial monolayers grown on filters secrete IL-8 into the underlying collagen layer. Neutrophils added to the apical compartment emigrate into the basilar compartment, but not when the IL-8 gradient is disrupted by addition of IL-8 to the apical compartment (82). Although IL-8 acts as an adhesion inhibitor in some assays (170), this result may be partially attributable to disruption of a gradient of IL-8 on activated endothelial monolayers when exogenous IL-8 is added on the same side as the neutrophils.

Chemoattractants act on the local tissue as well as on leukocytes. Neutrophil chemoattractants injected into the same skin site hours apart will stimulate neutrophil accumulation the first but not the second time, whereas a second injection into a distant site will stimulate accumulation. Desensitization occurs for homologous chemoattractants only (171,172). Thus, chemoattractants must act on and homologously desensitize a cell type that is localized in tissue. In some cases this localized cell may be the mast cell. Some chemoattractants stimulate the mast cell (which localizes in tissue adjacent to the vasculature) or its better-studied relative, the basophil, to release histamine (173,174) and TNF (175). Histamine induces P-selectin, and TNF induces E-selectin on endothelium. Thus, chemoattractants may indirectly increase selectin expression on endothelium as well as directly activate integrin adhesiveness on leukocytes.

A THREE-STEP AREA CODE FOR SIGNALING NEUTROPHIL AND MONOCYTE TRAFFIC

The above evidence has shown that emigration from the vasculature of neutrophils and monocytes is regulated by at least three distinct molecular signals (Figs. 1 and 6A). A key feature is that selectin–carbohydrate, chemoattractant–receptor, and integrin–Ig family interactions act in sequence, not in parallel. This concept has been confirmed by the observation that inhibition of any one of these steps gives essentially complete, rather than partial inhibition of neutrophil and monocyte emigration. An important consequence of a sequence of steps, at any one of which there are choices of multiple receptors or ligands that have distinct distributions on leukocyte subpopulations or endothelium, is that it provides great combinatorial diversity for regulating the selectivity of leukocyte localization in vivo, as has been emphasized in several reviews (3,7,10,13,14).

''Area code'' models for cell localization in the body (176,177) are particularly apt, because it is now known that at least three sequential steps are involved. The concepts of area codes and traffic signals can be combined by thinking of how telephone traffic is routed by digital signals. Each type of leukocyte responds to a particular set of area code signals. Inflammation alters the expression and location of the signals on vascular endothelium. It is as if leukocytes carry ''cellular phones.'' An example of how this model works is shown in Fig. 6B for the two cell types for which the signals are best understood, neutrophils and monocytes. Chemoattractants provide the greatest number of molecular choices (or ''digits'') and the greatest cellular specificity.

Refinements to the three-step model are in order. First, selectins actually mediate two steps, initial tethering to the vessel wall and rolling (Fig. 6A), which can be distinguished for E-selectin by dependence on different classes of neutrophil ligands (69). Thus, selectins can cooperate, and some selectin–ligand combinations may be more important in tethering and others in rolling. Second, the steps are overlapping rather than strictly sequential (Fig. 6A). Although L-selectin is shed from neutrophils soon after activation (160), the kinetics of shedding by neutrophils in whole blood (minutes) are much slower than the transition from rolling to integrin-mediated attachment (milliseconds to seconds) (59). L-Selectin is shed more slowly from lymphocytes than from neutrophils (178,179). Furthermore, ligands for P-selectin (46) and E-selectin (69) remain on the neutrophil surface after activation. Thus, interactions with selectins will continue after activation of integrins, probably persisting until transendothelial migration is completed. Chemoattractants are required not only for activation of integrin adhesiveness but also for directional cues during the subsequent step of transendothelial migration. Finally, β_1 integrins that bind to extracellular matrix components are undoubtedly required during migration through the subendothelial basement membrane.

LYMPHOCYTE RECIRCULATION: DISTINCT TRAFFIC PATTERNS FOR NAIVE AND MEMORY LYMPHOCYTES

Patrolling the body in search of foreign antigen, lymphocytes follow circuits through both nonlymphoid and lymphoid tissues (Fig. 7). The peripheral lymph nodes draining skin and muscle, and the gut-associated lymphoid tissues such as Peyer's patch, differ in the types of antigens to which lymphocytes are exposed. When collected from lymph draining gut or skin, lymphocytes from adult animals, but not newborns, show a twofold or higher preference to recirculate to the type of organ from which they came and to reappear in the draining lymph (1,2,17,180). This suggests that priming by specific antigen in a particular environment may induce expression of surface receptors that enable preferential recirculation to the type of secondary organ where specific antigen was first encountered. Evidence exists for separate streams of lymphocytes that recirculate through the skin, gut, and lung and that drain into their associated lymphoid tissues (6,17).

Our understanding of the mechanisms of this selectivity has been advanced by the discovery that ''naive'' and ''memory'' lymphocytes prefer different recirculation pathways (181). When naive lymphocytes encounter antigen, those lymphocytes with receptors specific for the antigen are stimulated to expand clonally and are converted to memory lymphocytes that have altered expression of adhesion receptors and circulatory patterns. Lymphocytes that emigrate in the hind leg of a sheep through ''flat'' endothelium in the skin and drain through the afferent lymphatics to the popliteal lymph node are all of the memory phenotype. By contrast, lymphocytes in the efferent lymph from the popliteal lymph node, derived mostly from traffic through HEV, are predominantly of the naive phenotype. Thus, at least for peripheral tissues and lymph nodes, memory lymphocytes emigrate preferentially through tissue endothelium, whereas naive lymphocytes enter the lymph node through HEV (Fig. 7). Memory lymphocytes are more sensitive to specific antigen than naive lymphocytes and thus are better able to respond to antigen in peripheral tissues, which have fewer antigen-presenting cell than lymph nodes (16).

TRAFFIC THROUGH HEV

The ''high'' or cuboidal-shaped endothelial cells found in HEV are specialized for emigration of lymphocytes into peripheral lymph nodes that drain skin and the lymphoid tissues of the mucosa: Peyer's patches, tonsils, and appendix. Emigration into the spleen, by contrast, involves sinusoidal endothelia and molecular mechanisms that are distinct and not yet characterized. About 25% of lymphocytes that circulate through a HEV will bind and emigrate, a much higher percentage than through nonspecialized flat venules (182,183). The HEV phenotype is developmentally regulated. The carbohydrate ligands for L-selectin are absent from peripheral lymph node HEV at birth but are displayed at adult levels by 6 weeks (6). If peripheral lymph nodes are deprived of afferent lymph, the HEV convert from a high to a flat-walled endothelial morphology, lose expression of

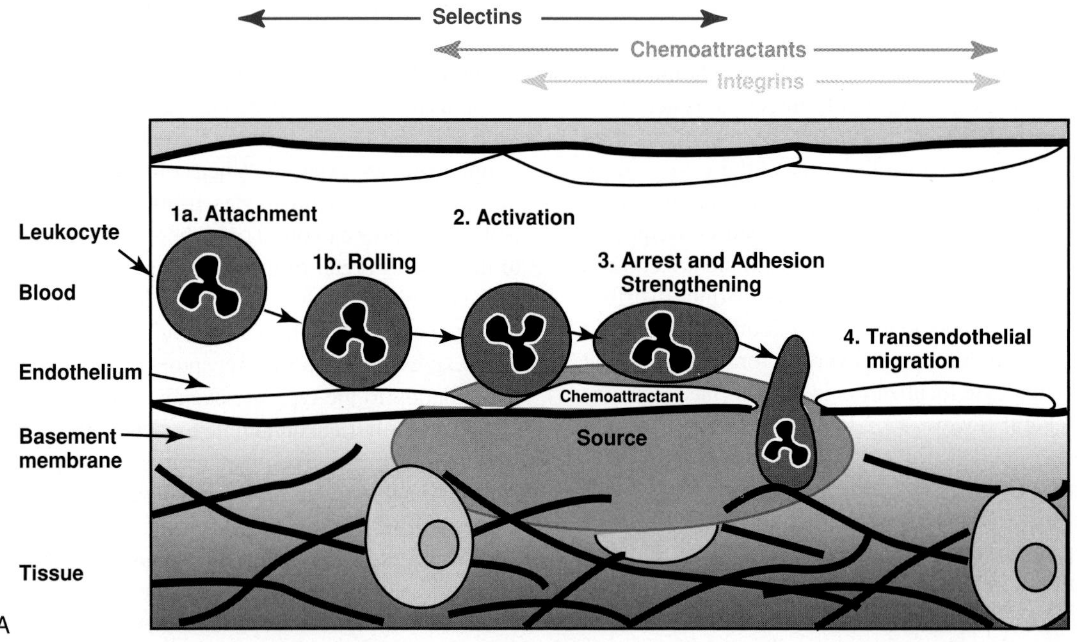

A

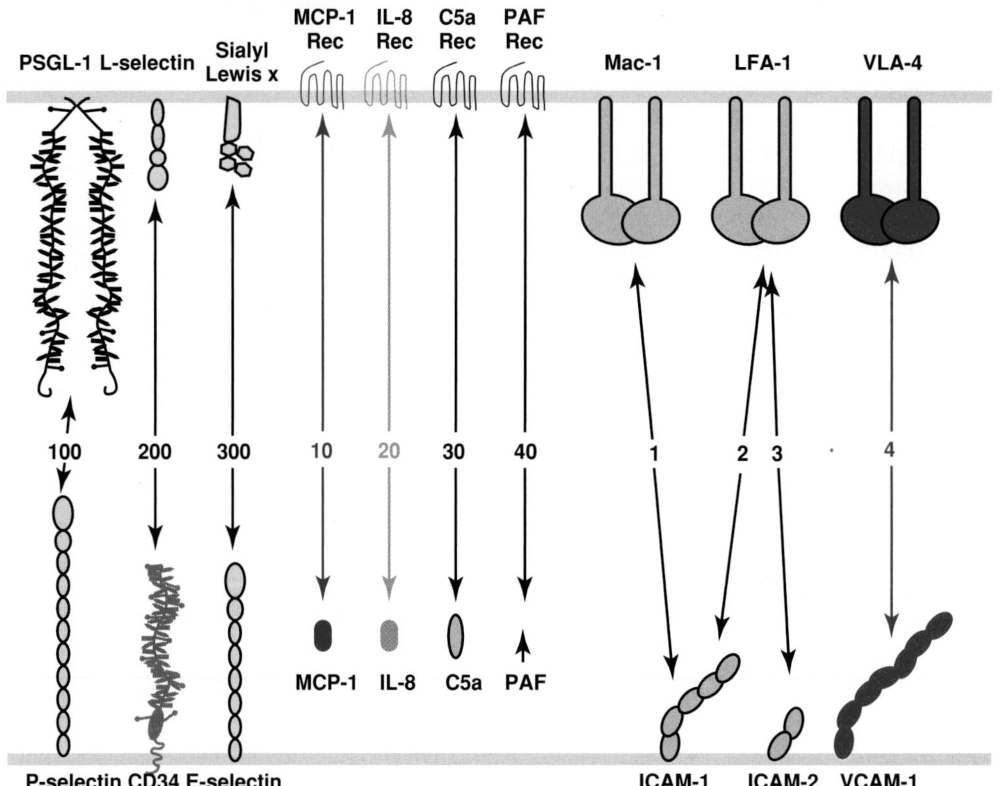

Monocyte Area Codes	111, 211, 311, 112, 212, 312, 113, 213, 313, 114, 214, 314, 134, 234, 334, 144, 244, 344
Neutrophil Area Codes	121, 221, 321, 122, 222, 322, 123, 223, 323
Monocyte and Neutrophil Area Codes	131, 231, 331, 132, 232, 332, 133, 233, 333, 141, 241, 341, 142, 242, 342, 143, 243, 343
Null Area Codes	124, 224, 324

B

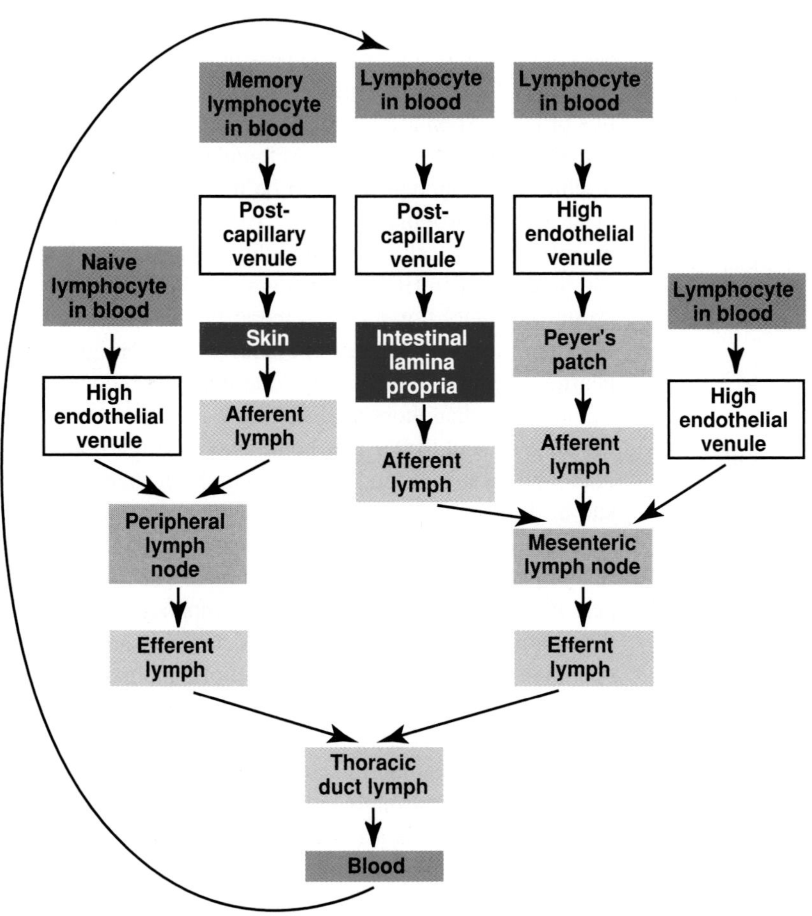

FIG. 7. Lymphocyte recirculation routes.

L-selectin ligands, and lose ability to support lymphocyte traffic (184,185). Introduction of antigen into the node leads to a full restoration of HEV phenotype and function. Furthermore, intense antigenic stimulation can induce formation of HEV in diverse nonlymphoid tissues (6,186).

Molecular Mechanisms Defined by the HEV Binding Assay

When lymphocyte suspensions are overlaid on thin sections cut from frozen lymph nodes, the lymphocytes specifically bind to the morphologically distinct HEV (187). Specific differences have been demonstrated between binding to peripheral lymph node and Peyer's patch HEV (183,188). T lymphocytes bind 1.5-fold better than B lymphocytes to peripheral lymph node HEV in vitro and show a similar preference to recirculate to this site in vivo. B lymphocytes bind two- to threefold better to Peyer's patch than to peripheral lymph node HEV and show similar preference in recirculation in vivo. These preferences are reflected in the preponderance of T cells in peripheral lymph nodes and the preponderance of B lymphocytes in Peyer's patch, where they are important in secretion of IgA and IgM into the mucosa (189). Certain lymphoma cells possess marked preference for binding to Peyer's patch or peripheral lymph node HEV in vitro (188) and for metastasis in vivo to mucosal or peripheral lymphoid tissue, respectively (190). Assay of lymphoma cell binding to HEV in the Stamper–Woodruff assay has led to the identification of two important adhesion pathways.

FIG. 6. The three-step area code model. **A:** Selectins, chemoattractants, and integrins act in sequence, with some overlap. **B:** Combinatorial use of different molecules at each step can generate a large number of different area codes and specificity for distinct leukocyte subpopulations. All of the known selectin and integrin interactions are shown in the hundreds and ones places, respectively; however, only a subset of the chemoattractants is shown in the tens place (see Table 1) because of space limitations. The area codes symbolize how specificity for monocytes, neutrophils, or both can be generated at inflammatory sites. Interactions that are monocyte or neutrophil specific are shown in dark red and light red, respectively.

Molecules Involved in Binding to Peripheral Node HEV

The L-selectin molecule was initially defined in the mouse with the Mel-14 mAb as a molecule on lymphocytes required for binding to peripheral lymph node, but not Peyer's patch, HEV (38). Conversely, the MECA-79 carbohydrate antigen was defined with mAb that bound specifically to peripheral lymph node HEV and blocked lymphocyte binding. The isolated MECA-79 antigen, termed the peripheral node addressin (191), bind to L-selectin on lymphocytes (192). An L-selectin/IgG chimera was also found to bind specifically to HEV in peripheral lymph node and to block lymphocyte binding (193). The L-selectin/IgG chimera was used to isolate two distinct mucin-like ligands, GlyCAM-1, which is secreted by HEV (37), and CD34, a surface molecule on HEV (50). MECA-79 mAb recognizes a carbohydrate determinant that is expressed on multiple protein species in HEV, including GlyCAM-1 and CD34, and compared to L-selectin recognizes an overlapping but distinct set of glycoproteins (37,192). Sialylation and sulfation of the O-linked side chains of the GlyCAM-1 and CD34 molecules are required for activity in binding to L-selectin (19,192,194). The HEV differ from other tissues in carbohydrate processing; GlyCAM-1 and CD34 expressed in transfectants and CD34 in other vascular endothelia do not bind L-selectin chimera under conditions in which binding to HEV is detectable (37). However, an L-selectin ligand with a presumably lower affinity is certainly present on most endothelia, as shown by L-selectin-dependent rolling in vivo and binding in vitro (58,59,68,74,100,195,196).

Molecules Involved in Binding to Peyer's Patch HEV

Elegant screens for mAb with specificity for Peyer's patch HEV and ability to block lymphocyte binding to HEV yielded mAb MECA-367 to the mucosal addressin now termed MAdCAM-1 (129). The MAdCAM-1 molecule is expressed on endothelia in mucosal tissues not only on HEV in Peyer's patch but also on venules in intestinal lamina propria and in the lactating mammary gland (129,197). The MAdCAM-1 molecule has both IgSF domains and a mucin-like domain (130) (Fig. 5).

Similar elegant screens for mAbs with specificity for lymphoma cells that bound to Peyer's patch HEV and with ability to block binding to HEV in the Stamper–Woodruff assay yielded mAbs to the α^4 subunit of the Peyer's patch homing receptor (198). The α^4 subunit was found to be associated with a novel β subunit, β_p (199), which is identical to β_7 (131). The integrin $\alpha^4\beta_7$ but not $\alpha^4\beta_1$ binds to Peyer's patch HEV (131), and $\alpha^4\beta_7$ binds directly to MAdCAM-1 (132).

An Area Code Model for Lymphocyte Migration Through HEV

Peripheral Lymph Node HEV

Although the L-selectin–mucin and $\alpha^4\beta_7$–MAdCAM-1 interactions were identified in parallel assays, recent studies suggest that multiple steps are involved in lymphocyte interaction with HEV and raise the possibility that these interactions may function in distinct, rather than parallel, steps in this process. Soon after its discovery as a lymphocyte homing receptor, L-selectin also was found to be present on neutrophils and eosinophils and to be important in emigration of at least neutrophils (40). As expected from their strong expression of L-selectin, neutrophils and other leukocytes can bind avidly to HEV in the Stamper–Woodruff assay yet do not normally home to peripheral lymph nodes in vivo. Injection of *E. coli* supernatant induces acute emigration of neutrophils through HEV of the draining lymph node. Thus, signals other than those mediated by L-selectin can regulate the class of leukocytes that home into a lymph node (40). Although peripheral node HEV is far richer than any other site in the body in expression of the carbohydrate receptor for L-selectin (200), this is insufficient to explain the specificity of lymphocyte homing to this organ. The findings suggest that L-selectin is required for lymphocyte emigration through peripheral lymph node HEV and may help regulate recirculation of the L-selectin$^+$ subset of lymphocytes; however, L-selectin is insufficient to determine the specificity of the cell types that emigrate, and other, currently undefined molecules are required to achieve specificity.

In vivo studies strongly suggest that lymphocyte emigration through HEV is a multistep process that utilizes area code models similar to those of other leukocytes. Monoclonal Ab to L-selectin almost completely blocks emigration of lymphocytes from blood into peripheral lymph nodes (38,201). However, mAb to the integrin LFA-1 also markedly reduces or almost completely abolishes lymphocyte migration into peripheral lymph nodes (149,202). Thus, molecules of steps 1 and 3 are required for homing to peripheral lymph nodes in vivo. LFA-1 on blood lymphocytes requires activation for binding to its counterstructures ICAM-1 and ICAM-2 (36,104), which are expressed on HEV (203). Binding of L-selectin does not trigger activation of LFA-1 because lymphocytes attach and roll in flow identically on purified peripheral node addressin whether or not purified ICAM-1 is present on the substrate; an additional stimulus is required before lymphocytes will arrest and strengthen adhesion through LFA-1 (316).

G-protein-coupled receptors are required for lymphocyte recirculation and likely provide the signals required to activate the adhesiveness of LFA-1. Pertussis toxin causes lymphocytosis and profoundly depresses lymphocyte recirculation (204). Murine lymphocytes treated with pertussis toxin in vitro and reinfused fail to emigrate into either peripheral lymph nodes or Peyer's patches (205). This suggests that G-protein-coupled receptors of the α_i class are required for lymphocyte emigration through HEV. Results with mice with a transgene for the ADP-ribosylating subunit of pertussis toxin selectively expressed in the T lineage suggest that $G\alpha_i$ proteins are required not only for emigration from the bloodstream but also for emigration from the thymus

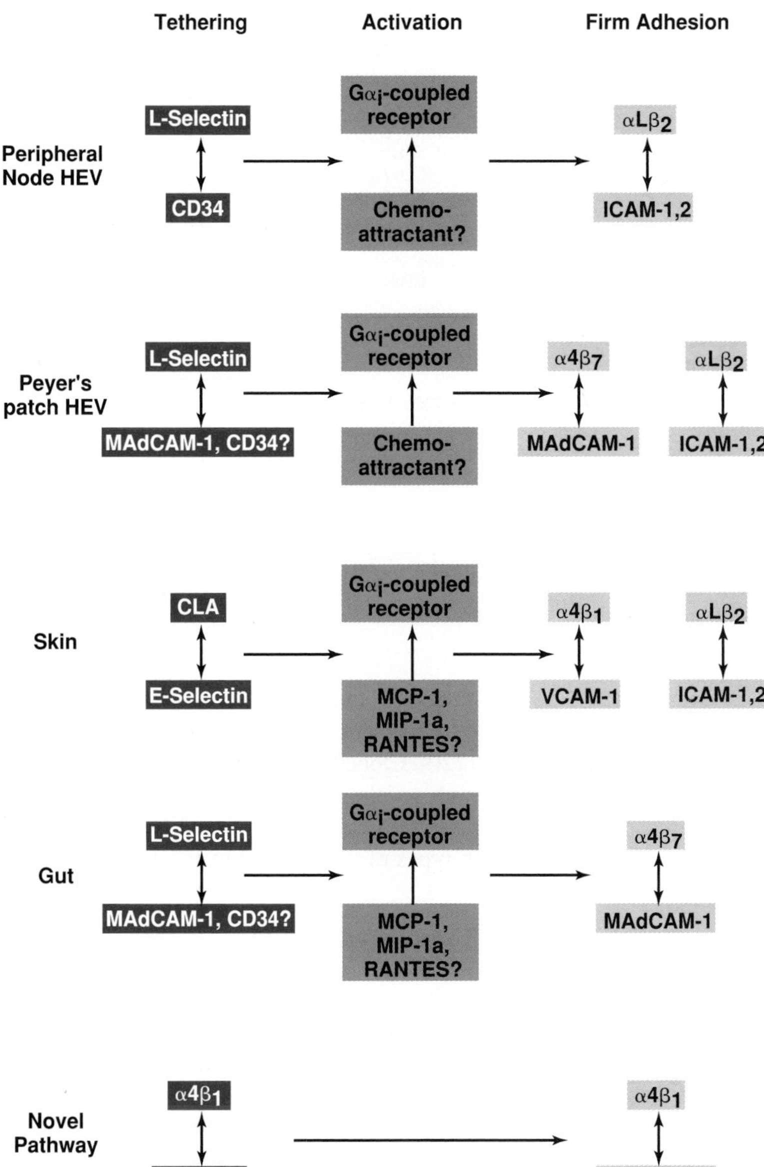

FIG. 8. The three-step or four-step area code paradigm for lymphocytes. For skin and gut, the pathways shown may mediate both recirculation and increased accumulation in inflammation. The novel pathway shown at the bottom may be important when VCAM-1 expression on endothelium is induced by cytokines and may cooperate with the other illustrated pathways. For each organ, the interacting molecules are shown on the top for lymphocytes and on the bottom for endothelia. See text for support for the molecular assignments at each step, based primarily on in vivo data.

(206,207). Despite lack of emigration, pertussis-toxin-treated lymphocytes bind normally to lymph node HEV in vitro. These findings provided the basis for an early proposal for a two-step model in which G-protein-coupled receptors function subsequent to binding of lymphocytes to HEV (208).

Thus, emigration of lymphocytes through peripheral node HEV requires three sequential area code signals that are analogous to those involved in neutrophil emigration from the bloodstream (Fig. 8). Identification of a putative lymphocyte chemoattractant secreted by peripheral lymph node HEV, and a chemoattractant receptor that is predicted to be selectively expressed on the naive subset of lymphocytes that recirculate through peripheral node HEV, will be a subject of intense research interest in coming years.

Peyer's Patch

Monoclonal antibodies to L-selectin block 50% of lymphocyte emigration from blood to Peyer's patch and to the remainder of the intestine (201,209). This is consistent with the lower level of L-selectin ligand in Peyer's patch HEV than in peripheral lymph node HEV (193,210,211). Monoclonal antibodies to certain epitopes on the integrin α^4 and β_7 subunits inhibit by approximately 50% recirculation of lymphocytes to Peyer's patch and intestine but have no effect on recirculation to peripheral lymph node; furthermore, mAb specific for the $\alpha^4\beta_7$ complex are equally effective as mAb to α^4 (209). Moreover, recirculation is inhibited by mAb to MAdCAM-1 (129), implicating $\alpha^4\beta_7$ binding to MAdCAM-1 in recirculation to mucosal tissue. The mAbs to LFA-1 block recirculation to Peyer's patch by 50% to 80% but have no effect on recirculation to the remainder of the intestine (149,202). Thus, both LFA-1 and $\alpha^4\beta_7$ contribute to emigration into mucosal lymphoid tissue.

G-protein-coupled receptors act subsequent to a rolling interaction in Peyer's patch HEV. In contrast with peripheral lymph nodes, Peyer's patches may be visualized by intravital microscopy (182). Normally, lymphocytes roll along Peyer's patch HEV only for a few seconds, then arrest and emigrate. However, prior treatment of lymphocytes with pertussis toxin completely blocks arrest and emigration and prolongs the rolling indefinitely, so that the lymphocytes pass out of the Peyer's patch rather than emigrate (212). It remains to be established, but seems likely, that a chemoattractant presented or secreted by Peyer's patch binds to a $G\alpha_i$-coupled receptor on lymphocytes and activates LFA-1 and $\alpha^4\beta_7$ to mediate arrest and emigration (Fig. 8). Lymphoma cells or lymph node lymphocytes can bind to Peyer's patch HEV or purified MAdCAM-1 without any apparent need for activation; however, activation increases the strength of binding to MAdCAM-1 (131,132). The pertussis toxin studies suggest that activation of blood lymphocytes is required for the last step of arrest and emigration (208,212). Truncation of the cytoplasmic domain of β_7 greatly decreases binding to HEV. Thus, interactions with the cytoplasmic domain can regulate the avidity of $\alpha^4\beta_7$ for MAdCAM-1 (213), similar to regulation of the avidity of LFA-1 for ICAM-1 by the β_2 integrin subunit cytoplasmic domain (214,215).

RECIRCULATION OF MEMORY LYMPHOCYTES

Distinct Pathways Through Skin and Gut

Memory lymphocytes are imprinted so that they are more likely to return to the type of tissue, such as skin or mucosa, where they first encountered antigen (1,2,17). The surface phenotypes of gut- and skin-homing memory cells are distinct (211). Furthermore, staining of lymphocytes in sections of skin and gut with mAb shows distinctive expression of adhesion molecules that may contribute to selective extravasation in these tissues or to subsequent localization within these tissues in specific anatomic compartments (Table 4).

Skin-Homing Lymphocytes

Lymphocytes that extravasate in the skin and appear in afferent lymph have a distinct pattern of expression of adhesion molecules (211) (Table 4). Furthermore, as shown by staining of tissue sections, T lymphocytes localized in the skin but not in the gut express a carbohydrate termed cutaneous lymphocyte-associated antigen (CLA) (216). The CLA antigen is closely related to sialyl Lewis[a] and Lewis[x] (217) and is a ligand for E-selectin (218). Binding of a subpopulation of memory lymphocytes that bears CLA to E-selectin may contribute to the tropism of this subset to the skin (219–221). E-selectin is induced on dermal endothelial cells in delayed type hypersensitivity (222) and in chronically inflamed skin (220). Cloned T cells derived from challenged skin express high levels of CLA and bind to E-selectin, whereas T cell clones derived from blood lymphocytes do not (223). Both types of clones bind to P-selectin.

TABLE 4. *Naive and memory lymphocyte subsets[a]*

Molecule	Naive lymphocytes	Memory lymphocytes
CD45R0	Negative	Positive
CD45RA	High	Low
CD2	Low	High
LFA-3	Negative	Positive
L-selectin	Positive	Positive and negative subsets
α^4	Low	High

	Gut associated	Skin associated
Memory lymphocyte subsets		
CLA	Negative	Positive
$\alpha^E\beta_7$ (HML-1)	Positive	Negative
$\alpha^4\beta_7$[b]	High	Low
$\alpha^4\beta_1$	Low	High
α^6	Low	High

[a] References 211,224,313.
[b] But see ref. 314.

Gut-Homing Lymphocytes

The most organized lymphoid structures in the wall of the gut are the Peyer's patches, which underlie follicle-associated epithelia that contain M cells, which are specialized for uptake of antigen from the gut lumen. Other lymphocytes localize more diffusely in the lamina propria underlying the digestive epithelium and in the epithelial layer. Studies on gut afferent lymph reveal the presence of both memory and naive lymphocytes (211); whether there is differential migration of naive and memory lymphocytes through Peyer's patch HEV and lamina propria postcapillary venules, both of which contribute to gut afferent lymph (Fig. 7), remains unclear. Gut-homing memory lymphocytes display a surface phenotype distinct from skin-homing lymphocytes (Table 4). When injected into the bloodstream, memory lymphocytes from gut afferent lymph display a strong preference to return to gut afferent lymph, whereas naive lymphocytes redistribute randomly (211). Gut afferent memory lymphocytes display an α^4-high, β_1-integrin-low phenotype, suggesting they are $\alpha^4\beta_7^+$ (211) in common with a subpopulation of memory lymphocytes in blood (224). Expression of MAdCAM-1 on both Peyer's patch HEV and postcapillary venules in lamina propria (129), and 50% inhibition by mAb to α^4 and β_7 of migration into both Peyer's patch and intestine (209), suggest a role for $\alpha^4\beta_7$ interaction with MAdCAM-1 in both sites.

A subpopulation of gut lymphocytes distinct from those in lamina propria localize within the epithelium on the external surface of the basement membrane and express the human mucosal lymphocyte (HML-1) integrin $\alpha^E\beta_7$ (224–227). The α^E integrin subunit contains an I domain and a novel proteolytic cleavage site preceded by a stretch of acidic residues, just N-terminal to the I domain (228). Binding of intraepithelial lymphocytes (IEL) to epithelial cell monolayers in vitro is inhibited by mAb to α^E, suggesting that $\alpha^E\beta_7$ may help mediate localization of IEL in epithelia in vivo (229). Intraepithelial T lymphocytes may undergo thymus-independent differentiation in situ, and their recirculation pattern is undefined. The HML-1 integrin is expressed on a subpopulation of 2% to 6% of blood T cells, which are in the memory subset and are CLA^- and L-selectin$^-$ (230). Transforming growth factor β (TGF-β) together with mitogen induces expression of HML-1 on peripheral T cells and increases expression on IEL (226,227). The TGF-β also induces switching of B lymphocytes to production of the IgA class of immunoglobulin (231) the predominant class secreted in the mucosa. These dual effects on differentiation of mucosal lymphocytes suggest the possibility that TGF-β may be an environment-specific cytokine that imprints lymphocytes, when first exposed to antigen, to recirculate selectively to the gut.

ALTERATION OF LYMPHOCYTE TRAFFICKING IN INFLAMMATION

Antigen injected into the tissue of sensitized individuals induces localized accumulation of lymphocytes. These lymphocytes, and those accumulating in tissues in autoimmune disease, are almost all memory cells (232,233). The phenotype of these cells is quite similar to that of lymphocytes trafficking through these sites under basal conditions. This suggests that the signals for lymphocyte trafficking may be qualitatively the same in the basal and inflammatory states and are up-regulated in inflammation. Accumulation of lymphocytes induced by specific antigen or by injection of IFN-γ or TNF-α is significantly inhibited by mAb to either the LFA-1α or the integrin α^4 subunit (234–238). A combination of mAb to LFA-1 and α^4 gives almost complete inhibition of lymphocyte emigration and the resulting induration and plasma leakage (239). Monoclonal Abs to E-selectin and VCAM-1 also inhibit lymphocyte accumulation in delayed-type hypersensitivity in skin (240). Multiple signals are thus required for augmented trafficking of lymphocytes into skin in inflammation (Fig. 8). Both antigen-responsive and -nonresponsive lymphocytes traffic into sites of antigenic stimulation (241). Antigen-specific lymphocytes may accumulate in the site because stimulation through their antigen receptors increases adhesiveness of integrins and causes them to be retained, whereas nonresponsive lymphocytes more rapidly enter the lymphatics and leave the site.

The interaction between VCAM-1 and VLA-4 can mediate both rolling and firm adhesion (112); thus, it does not fit neatly into the three-step paradigm established for neutrophils. The mAbs to LFA-1 or VLA-4 alone do not completely inhibit lymphocyte accumulation in inflammation, and patients with LAD-I show delayed-type hypersensitivity reactions. This suggests that the functions of VLA-4 and LFA-1 are partially overlapping in the step of firm adhesion, but they may also act in series, as in VLA-4-mediated rolling following by LFA-1-mediated firm adhesion. VLA-4 may act together with selectins to augment T-lymphocyte tethering and rolling in the vasculature. All or most memory T lymphocytes lack L-selectin (39,211,242,243). The CLA^+ subset can bind E-selectin, and T lymphocytes can also bind P-selectin (223,244,245). Peripheral blood T lymphocytes are substantially less efficient than neutrophils in tethering in hydrodynamic flow to E-selectin and P-selectin (T. Diacovo, R. Alon, and T. Springer, *unpublished data*); therefore, cooperation of VCAM-1 with E-selectin or P-selectin, or among all three molecules, may be important in enhancing lymphocyte accumulation in inflammation.

Inflammation also affects traffic through HEV. Antigen injected into tissue drains to the regional lymph node and greatly increases blood flow to the node and traffic of naive lymphocytes through HEV (186). Furthermore, memory lymphocytes now appear to enter the node directly; this is associated with induction of VCAM-1 on non-HEV vascular endothelia within the node (186). Entry is inhibited by mAb to α^4, and this suggests a role for interaction of VCAM-1 with $\alpha^4\beta_1$ (186,234).

Lymphocyte chemoattractants are interesting candidates for the step 2 signal for lymphocyte accumulation at inflammatory sites. Pertussis toxin treatment inhibits lymphocyte emigration in response to antigen in delayed-type hypersensitivity (167). Identification of lymphocyte chemoattractants has been hampered by the low motility of lymphocytes compared to monocytes or neutrophils (246) and by the low signal-to-background ratio, typically less than 2 in most chemotaxis assays. Recent interest has focused on chemokines (Table 2). A number of chemokines, all of which were isolated based on chemoattractive activity for neutrophils or monocytes or by cloning genes of unknown function, have subsequently been tested and found to be chemoattractive for lymphocyte subpopulations (11,12). These include IL-8 (247) (but see refs. 248,249), RANTES (250), MIP-1β (84), MIP-1α and β (251,252), and IP-10 (253). There are differences among reports in the subsets found to be chemoattracted, and some reports use lymphocytes preactivated by T-cell receptor cross-linking, which may be relevant to migration within inflammatory sites but not emigration from blood. Of interest, MIP-1β can induce binding of the naive $CD8^+$ subset to VCAM-1, either in solution or when immobilized on a substrate, mimicking presentation by an endothelial cell surface (84,254); the specific effect is modest, equal to background binding. The RANTES cytokine, by contrast to MIP-1β, selectively attracts the memory T lymphocyte subset (250).

Vascular endothelium may function to present chemoattractants to lymphocytes in a functionally relevant way as well as to provide a permeability barrier that stabilizes the chemoattractant gradient. A transendothelial chemotaxis assay more accurately simulates lymphocyte emigration from the bloodstream than filter chemotaxis assays and yields signals over ten times background (255). Because lymphocytes, responding to specific antigen in tissue, signal emigration of further lymphocytes into the site, a chemoattractant was sought in material secreted by mitogen-stimulated mononuclear cells. Purification to homogeneity guided by the transendothelial lymphocyte chemotaxis assay revealed that MCP-1, previously thought to be solely a monocyte chemoattractant, is a major lymphocyte chemoattractant (255). Subsequent studies using the transendothelial chemotaxis assay have confirmed that lymphocytes respond to RANTES and MIP-1α (CC chemokines) but do not respond to IL-8 or IP-10 (CXC chemokines) (256). MCP-1, RANTES, and MIP-1α all selectively attract the memory T-lymphocyte subset and both the CD4 and CD8 subsets. All also attract monocytes but not neutrophils, with MCP-1 being more potent than RANTES or MIP-1α as a monocyte chemoattractant. The physiologically relevant transendothelial assay suggests that CC chemokines tend to attract both monocytes and lymphocytes, in agreement with the long-standing clinical observation that lymphocyte emigration into inflammatory sites is always accompanied by emigration of monocytes. The converse is not true. Monocytes sometimes emigrate in the absence of lymphocytes, correlating with activity of chemoattractants such as C5a and PAF on monocytes but not on lymphocytes. Teleologically, it is important that monocytes accompany lymphocytes into inflammatory sites in order to present antigen and to carry out effector functions in which monocytes are activated by T lymphocytes. MCP-1 is abundantly expressed at sites of antigen challenge and autoimmune disease (12,257,258) and, together with MIP-1α and RANTES, is an excellent candidate to provide the step 2 signal required to activate integrin adhesiveness and emigration of both monocytes and lymphocytes in vivo (Fig. 8).

The finding that resting T lymphocytes that tether and roll on VCAM-1 can spontaneously arrest and develop firm adhesion on VCAM-1 (112) has provocative implications for the multistep model. It suggests that the VLA-4–VCAM-1 interaction not only can mediate the steps of rolling and firm adhesion but may also short-circuit the step of stimulation by chemoattractants of firm adhesion through integrins. This is intriguing, because although a twofold stimulation of adhesiveness of VLA-4 to VCAM-1 has been demonstrated by MIP-1β in one system (84), with the chemoattractant that is most effective in eliciting transendothelial chemotaxis of T lymphocytes, MCP-1, it is difficult to detect stimulation of integrin adhesiveness for ICAM-1 or VCAM-1 on lymphocytes (M. W. Carr, and T. A. Springer, *unpublished data*). Therefore, an alternative pathway may exist in which VCAM-1 can mediate both tethering and arrest of lymphocytes, perhaps in cooperation with other endothelial molecules, before stimulation by chemoattractants. After arrest, chemoattractants would guide transendothelial migration and perhaps stimulate further increases in the adhesiveness of the integrins VLA-4 and LFA-1, important in migration across the endothelium and basement membrane.

ATHEROGENESIS

Introduction

Careful ultrastructural and immunohistochemical studies in various animal models and human tissues have established that the adherence of blood monocytes and lymphocytes to endothelial cells lining large arteries is one of the earliest detectable events in atherosclerosis (259,260). The subsequent transendothelial migration of monocytes and their accumulation in the intima and development into lipid-engorged "foam cells" appear to be important steps in the initiation of atherosclerotic lesions. Monocytes and macrophage foam cells may also contribute to the progression of atherosclerotic lesions by producing cytokines and growth factors (259,260). These, in turn, may amplify mononuclear leukocyte recruitment, induce migration of smooth muscle cells into the intima, and stimulate cell replication. The formation of foam-cell-rich lesions during hypercholesterolemia appears to be a highly regulated process during which the vascular endothelium remains intact and may participate in regulating leukocyte recruitment into the intima by expressing leukocyte adhesion molecules.

Expression of Adhesion Molecules in Animal Models of Atherogenesis

The expression patterns of inducible endothelial leukocyte adhesion molecules have been examined in rabbit hypercholesterolemic models. Initially, VCAM-1 expression was found selectively in arterial endothelial cells covering early foam cell lesions of both dietary and Watanabe heritable hyperlipidemic rabbits (261). VCAM-1 expression in endothelium over foam cell lesions was not uniform but appeared particularly elevated at edges of lesions and extended several cells beyond the edge. In this region, scanning electron microscopy showed that mononuclear leukocyte recruitment through an intact endothelial monolayer was increased and presumably contributed to lateral expansion of lesions (262). The induction of endothelial VCAM-1 expression was an early event, occurring approximately 1 week following the initiation of a hypercholesterolemic diet in rabbits and preceding detectable intimal monocyte/macrophage accumulation (263). Endothelium not involved by foam cell lesions did not express VCAM-1 (261,263). In normocholesterolemic rabbits, VCAM-1 was not expressed by aortic endothelium except at sites that are predilected for foam cell lesion formation—the aortic arch and downstream of arterial ostia.

VCAM-1 was also expressed within neointimal smooth muscle cells near the surface and base of intimal lesions and in the medial smooth muscle cells adjacent to the internal elastic lamina (264,265). In cultured rabbit and human arterial vascular smooth muscle cells, VCAM-1 expression could be induced with appropriate cytokine treatment (265). The pathophysiological function of VCAM-1 in smooth muscle cells remains unknown. One possibility is that VCAM-1 may promote the retention of mononuclear leukocytes within atherosclerotic lesions. Alternatively, smooth muscle cell VCAM-1 may interact with VLA-4 on mononuclear leukocytes, thus activating these cells and initiating cytokine cascades or protease production leading to matrix degradation. Smooth muscle cell VCAM-1 may not have an important biological function and may be a marker of smooth muscle cell migration, activation, or differentiation.

In addition to VCAM-1, ICAM-1 expression was also detected by immunohistochemical staining in rabbit models of atherosclerosis. ICAM-1 was expressed in endothelium over lesions contemporaneously with VCAM-1 (264). Its expression was more uniform than that of VCAM-1, and unlike VCAM-1, ICAM-1 expression extended into noninvolved regions. Extensive ICAM-1 expression was found within intimal foam cell lesions, within macrophages and smooth muscle cells. E-Selectin expression over foam cell lesions was low (264); however, increased expression was found in an alloxan diabetic model (266).

Expression of Adhesion Molecules in Human Atherosclerotic Plaques

Several recent studies utilized immunohistochemistry to examine the expression patterns of leukocyte adhesion molecules in human atherosclerotic plaques obtained at autopsy or from hearts of transplant recipients. Unlike the rabbit models, where early lesions were examined, the human atherosclerotic plaques were generally advanced. In all cases, ICAM-1 expression was found in endothelial cells over plaques and in intimal smooth muscle cells and macrophages (267–271). E-Selectin expression was variable and restricted to vascular endothelium (269–271). Caution should be applied to the interpretation of these data, since some E-selectin antibodies acquired from British Biotechnology have subsequently been shown to cross-react with P-selectin. In advanced human coronary artery plaques, VCAM-1 was expressed focally by luminal endothelial cells, usually in association with inflammatory infiltrates (271,272). Focal endothelial VCAM-1 expression was also found in uninvolved vessels with diffuse intimal thickening. Within plaques, VCAM-1 was expressed by subsets of smooth muscle cells and macrophages and by endothelial cells of neovasculature. The variability of VCAM-1 expression in human atherosclerotic lesions, apart from possible technical difficulties with detection, may reflect states of plaque activity or quiescence with regard to leukocyte recruitment. In contrast to rabbit models, where relatively high levels of hypercholesterolemia are maintained by an atherogenic diet and intimal lesion growth is progressive, humans with atherosclerosis generally have low levels of hypercholesterolemia, and human plaque expansion as a result of leukocyte recruitment may develop at intervals.

Chemoattractants in Atherosclerotic Plaques

Mononuclear leukocytes can respond chemotactically to numerous substances, including peptides, lipids, and modified plasma components. Of particular relevance to atherosclerosis are chemoattractants selective for monocytes and lymphocytes, because these cells and not neutrophils are found in atherosclerotic plaques. Monocyte chemotactic activities have been isolated from atherosclerotic lesions in hypercholesterolemic swine and pigeons (273,274). These activities may result from modification of plasma lipoproteins and from chemokines produced locally in the arterial wall by endothelium, smooth muscle, and infiltrating leukocytes.

The accumulation of LDL in the arterial intima is an early event in atherogenesis and continues in advanced lesions. Its modification in the arterial wall by oxidation (275,276) likely has important pathological consequences. Minimally oxidized LDL can stimulate vascular cells to produce the chemoattractant MCP-1 (277) and cytokine/growth factors (278). Lysophosphatidylcholine, a component of highly oxidized LDL is a monocyte chemoattractant (270) and can induce the expression of VCAM-1 and ICAM-1 on arterial endothelial cells (280).

A number of groups have described chemotactic activity specific for monocytes but not neutrophils produced by cultured vascular endothelial and smooth muscle cells (281,282). This activity was biologically and biochemically characterized, and the bulk was attributed to MCP-1 after its cloning and the development of neutralizing antibody reagents. In an endothelial–smooth muscle cell coculture system, MCP-1 was a key mediator of monocyte transmigration (283), and its expression has been detected in human and rabbit atherosclerotic plaques (284). Another monocyte-specific factor produced in atherosclerotic lesions is M-CSF (CSF-1) (285,286). In addition to acting locally, M-CSF may stimulate increased monocyte production by the bone marrow and account for the monocytosis in hypercholesterolemic animals (287).

Mechanisms of Mononuclear Leukocyte Recruitment to Atherosclerotic Plaques

The induction of leukocyte adhesion molecule expression by arterial endothelium and local production of chemoattractants suggest that these molecules are important in the recruitment of mononuclear leukocytes to an atherosclerotic plaque. The specificity of this process, as in other inflammatory reactions, likely is regulated by the repertoire of adhesion molecules and chemoattractants. Mononuclear leukocytes, but not neutrophils, express VLA-4 and can interact with VCAM-1. Chemokines of the CC family, including MCP-1, whether secreted or bound to proteoglycans on the endothelial surface, can up-regulate mononuclear leukocyte integrins. To date, all of the potential mediators have not been identified, and the in vivo relevance of those that have has not been firmly established.

The initial step in leukocyte emigration, whether in atherosclerosis or inflammation, is the interaction of the circulating leukocyte with the endothelial lining. In venules and veins, this results in leukocyte rolling, mediated by selectins. Although E- and P-selectins can be expressed by arterial endothelium, the rheological factors in these vessels are different. Wall shear stress is significantly higher in arteries. In venules it varies depending on the organ but can be as high as 36 dynes/cm^2 in 30- to 40-μm venules of the cat mesentery (288). Even in venules, hemodynamic parameters that affect leukocyte–endothelial interactions during inflammation are complex (289). Arterial shear stresses depend on the anatomic location and phase of the cardiac cycle, and shear stresses up to 100 dynes/cm^2 can be encountered (290). In experimental settings, arterial segments at different anatomic locations of various animal species will alter their diameters to achieve an average wall shear stress of approximately 15 dynes/cm^2 (290). Atherosclerotic lesions form initially in arterial regions where hemodynamics are complex and shear forces are variable and may even oscillate as a result of flow reversal during different stages of the cardiac cycle. Arterial curvature, branching, and pulsatile blood flow are the main factors generating complex flow patterns (290). Direct visualization of leukocyte–endothelial interactions in large arteries has not been feasible; therefore, it is not known whether leukocyte rolling occurs. An alternative possibility is that firm mononuclear leukocyte adhesion occurs without prior leukocyte rolling, and leukocyte integrins may participate if their functional state is up-regulated in the circulation by hypercholesterolemia and/or circulating monocyte-specific cytokines and growth factors. In vitro interactions between VCAM-1 and VLA-4 can mediate firm adhesion and rolling of leukocytes (112).

When the mechanisms of mononuclear leukocyte recruitment to atherosclerotic plaques are understood, it is likely that clinicians will consider inhibiting this process in order to minimize plaque development. However, in addition to contributing to atherosclerotic plaque initiation, progression, and development of complications, monocytes may have a protective role in the arterial wall. Monocytes engulf lipoproteins and thus prevent excessive extracellular accumulation and oxidation of lipids, which can be toxic to vascular wall cells. This potentially important function should not be overlooked in future therapies for atherosclerosis in which mononuclear leukocyte recruitment to atherosclerotic plaques will be inhibited. In conjunction with these therapies, it may be necessary to utilize lipid-lowering or antioxidant drugs to reduce the accumulation of extracellular lipids in the arterial wall.

ACKNOWLEDGMENTS

We thank the NIH for supporting most of the cited work, and Uli von Andrian for comments on the manuscript.

REFERENCES

1. Cahill RNP, Poskitt DC, Frost H, Trnka Z. Two distinct pools of recirculating T lymphocytes: Migratory characteristics of nodal and intestinal T lymphocytes. *J Exp Med* 1977;145:420–428.
2. Cahill RNP, Poskitt DC, Hay JB, Heron I, Trnka Z. The migration of lymphocytes in the fetal lamb. *Eur J Immunol* 1979;9:251–253.
3. Springer TA. Traffic signals for lymphocyte recirculation and leukocyte emigration: The multi-step paradigm. *Cell* 1994;76:201–314.
4. Carlos TM, Harlan JM. Leukocyte-endothelial adhesion molecules. *Blood* 1994;84:2068–2101.
5. Granger DN, Kubes P. The microcirculation and inflammation: Modulation of leukocyte–endothelial cell adhesion. *J Leukocyte Biol* 1994; 55:662–675.
6. Picker LJ, Butcher EC. Physiological and molecular mechanisms of lymphocyte homing. *Annu Rev Immunol* 1992;10:561–591.
7. Lasky LA. Selectins: Interpreters of cell-specific carbohydrate information during inflammation. *Science* 1992;258:964–969.
8. Bevilacqua MP, Nelson RM. Selectins. *J Clin Invest* 1993;91: 379–387.
9. Bevilacqua MP. Endothelial–leukocyte adhesion molecules. *Annu Rev Immunol* 1993;11:767–804.
10. Butcher EC. Leukocyte-endothelial cell recognition: Three (or more) steps to specificity and diversity. *Cell* 1991;67:1033–1036.
11. Baggiolini M, Dewald B, Moser B. Interleukin-8 and related chemotactic cytokines—CXC and CC chemokines. *Adv Immunol* 1994;55: 97–179.
12. Miller MD, Krangel MS. Biology and biochemistry of the chemokines: A family of chemotactic and inflammatory cytokines. *Crit Rev Immunol* 1992;12:17–46.
13. Shimizu Y, Newman W, Tanaka Y, Shaw S. Lymphocyte interactions with endothelial cells. *Immunol Today* 1992;13:106–112.
14. Zimmerman GA, Prescott SM, McIntyre TM. Endothelial cell interactions with granulocytes: Tethering and signaling molecules. *Immunol Today* 1992;13:93–100.
15. Harlan JM, Winn RK, Vedder NB, et al. *In vivo* models of leukocyte adherence to endothelium. In: Harlan JR, Liu D, eds. *Adhesion: Its Role in Inflammatory Disease*. New York: W.H. Freeman; 1992: 117–150.
16. Mackay CR. Immunological memory. *Adv Immunol* 1993;53: 217–265.
17. Mackay CR. Migration pathways and immunologic memory among T lymphocytes. *Semin Immunol* 1992;4:51–58.
18. McEver RP. Selectins: Novel receptors that mediate leukocyte adhesion during inflammation. *Thromb Haemostas* 1991;65:223–228.
19. Rosen SD. Cell surface lectins in the immune system. *Semin Immunol* 1993;5:237–247.
20. Diamond MS, Springer TA. The dynamic regulation of integrin adhesiveness. *Curr Biol* 1994;4:506–517.
21. Cline MJ. *The White Cell*. Cambridge: Harvard University Press; 1975.
22. Issekutz AC, Issekutz RB. Quantitation and kinetics of blood monocyte migration to acute inflammatory reactions, and IL-1α, TNFα, and IFN-γ. *J Immunol* 1993;151:2105–2115.
23. Ley K, Gaehtgens P. Endothelial, not hemodynamic, differences are responsible for preferential leukocyte rolling in rat mesenteric venules. *Circ Res* 1991;69:1034–1041.
24. Nazziola E, House SD. Effects of hydrodynamics and leukocyte-endo-

thelium specificity on leukocyte–endothelium interactions. *Microvasc Res* 1992;44:127–142.

25. McEver RP, Beckstead JH, Moore KL, Marshall-Carlson L, Bainton DF. GMP-140, a platelet alpha-granule membrane protein, is also synthesized by vascular endothelial cells and is localized in Weibel–Palade bodies. *J Clin Invest* 1989;84:92–99.
26. Fina L, Molgaard HV, Robertson D, Bradley NJ, Monaghan P, Delia D, Sutherland DR, Baker MA, Greaves MF. Expression of the CD34 gene in vascular endothelial cells. *Blood* 1990;75:2417–2426.
27. Swerlick RA, Lee KH, Wick TM, Lawley TJ. Human dermal microvascular endothelial but not human umbilical vein endothelial cells express CD36 *in vivo* and *in vitro*. *J Immunol* 1992;148:78–83.
28. Zhu D, Cheng CF, Pauli BU. Mediation of lung metastasis of murine melanomas by a lung-specific endothelial cell adhesion molecule. *Proc Natl Acad Sci USA* 1991;88:9568–9572.
29. Pober JS, Cotran RS. Cytokines and endothelial cell biology. *Physiol Rev* 1990;70:427–452.
30. Thornhill MH, Wellicome SM, Mahiouz DL, Lanchbury JSS, Kyan-Aung U, Haskard DO. Tumor necrosis factor combines with IL-4 or IFN-gamma to selectively enhance endothelial cell adhesiveness for T cells: The contribution of vascular cell adhesion molecule-1-dependent and -independent binding mechanisms. *J Immunol* 1991;146: 592–598.
31. Masinovsky B, Urdal D, Gallatin WM. IL-4 acts synergistically with IL-1β to promote lymphocyte adhesion to microvascular endothelium by induction of vascular cell adhesion molecule-1. *J Immunol* 1990; 145:2886–2895.
32. Colditz IG, Watson DL. The effect of cytokines and chemotactic agonists on the migration of T lymphocytes into skin. *Immunology* 1992; 272:278.
33. Briscoe DM, Cotran RS, Pober JS. Effects of tumor necrosis factor, lipopolysaccharide, and IL-4 on the expression of vascular cell adhesion molecule-1 in vivo. *J Immunol* 1992;149:2954–2960.
34. Issekutz TB, Stoltz JM, Meide PVD. Lymphocyte recruitment in delayed-type hypersensitivity: The role of IFN-γ. *J Immunol* 1988;140: 2989–2993.
35. Schmid-Schönbein GW, Usami S, Skalak R, Chien S. The interaction of leukocytes and erthrocytes in capillary and postcapillary vessels. *Microvasc Res* 1980;19:45–70.
36. Springer TA. Adhesion receptors of the immune system. *Nature* 1990; 346:425–433.
37. Lasky LA, Singer MS, Dowbenko D, Imai Y, Henzel WJ, Grimley C, Fennie C, Gillett N, Watson SR, Rosen SD. An endothelial ligand for L-selectin is a novel mucin-like molecule. *Cell* 1992;69:927–938.
38. Gallatin WM, Weissman IL, Butcher EC. A cell-surface molecule involved in organ-specific homing of lymphocytes. *Nature* 1983;304: 30–34.
39. Kansas GS, Wood GS, Fishwild DM, Engleman EG. Functional characterization of human T lymphocyte subsets distinguished by monoclonal anti-leu-8. *J Immunol* 1985;134:2995–3002.
40. Lewinsohn DM, Bargatze RF, Butcher EC. Leukocyte-endothelial cell recognition: Evidence of a common molecular mechanism shared by neutrophils, lymphocytes, and other leukocytes. *J Immunol* 1987;138: 4313–4321.
41. Larsen E, Celi A, Gilbert GE, Furie BC, Erban JK, Bonfanti R, Wagner DD, Furie B. PADGEM protein: A receptor that mediates the interaction of activated platelets with neutrophils and monocytes. *Cell* 1989;59:305–312.
42. Geng J-G, Bevilacqua MP, Moore KL, McIntyre TM, Prescott SM, Kim JM, Bliss GA, Zimmerman GA, McEver RP. Rapid neutrophil adhesion to activated endothelium mediated by GMP-140. *Nature* 1990;343:757–760.
43. Bevilacqua MP, Pober JS, Mendrick DL, Cotran RS, Gimbrone MA. Identification of an inducible endothelial–leukocyte adhesion molecule, E-LAM 1. *Proc Natl Acad Sci USA* 1987;84:9238–9242.
44. Larsen GR, Sako D, Ahern TJ, Shaffer M, Erban J, Sajer SA, Gibson RM, Wagner DD, Furie BC, Furie B. P-Selectin and E-selectin: Distinct but overlapping leukocyte ligand specificities. *J Biol Chem* 1992; 267:11104–11110.
45. Nelson RM, Dolich S, Aruffo A, Cecconi O, Bevilacqua MP. Higher-affinity oligosaccharide ligands for E-selectin. *J Clin Invest* 1993;91: 1157–1166.
46. Moore KL, Stults NL, Diaz S, Smith DF, Cummings RD, Varki A, McEver RP. Identification of a specific glycoprotein ligand for P-selectin (CD62) on myeloid cells. *J Cell Biol* 1992;118:445–456.
47. Ushiyama S, Laue TM, Moore KL, Erickson HP, McEver RP. Structural and functional characterization of monomeric soluble P-selectin and comparison with membrane P-selectin. *J Biol Chem* 1993;268: 15229–15237.
48. Erbe DV, Wolitzky BA, Presta LG, Norton CR, Ramos RJ, Burns DK, Rumberger JM, Rao BNN, Foxall C, Brandley BK, Lasky LA. Identification of an E-selectin region critical for carbohydrate recognition and cell adhesion. *J Cell Biol* 1992;119:215–227.
49. Graves BJ, Crowther RL, Chandran C, Rumberger JM, Li S, Huang K-S, Presky DH, Familletti PC, Wolitzky BA, Burns DK. Insight into E-selectin/ligand interaction from the crystal structure and mutagenesis of the lec/EGF domains. *Nature* 1994;367:532–538.
50. Baumhueter S, Singer MS, Henzel W, Hemmerich S, Renz M, Rosen SD, Lasky LA. Binding of L-selectin to the vascular sialomucin, CD34. *Science* 1993;262:436–438.
51. Foxall C, Watson SR, Dowbenko D, Fennie C, Lasky LA, Kiso M, Hasegawa A, Asa D, Brandley BK. The three members of the selectin receptor family recognize a common carbohydrate epitope, the sialyl Lewis^x oligosaccharide. *J Cell Biol* 1992;117:895–902.
52. Berg EL, Magnani J, Warnock RA, Robinson MK, Butcher EC. Comparison of L-selectin and E-selectin ligand specificities: The L-selectin can bind the E-selectin ligands sialyl Le^x and sialyl Le^a. *Biochem Biophys Res Commun* 1992;184:1048–1055.
53. Hemmerich S, Rosen SD. 6′-Sulfated sialyl Lewis x is a major capping group of GlyCAM-1. *Biochemistry* 1994;33:4830–4835.
54. Steininger CN, Eddy CA, Leimgruber RM, Mellors A, Welply JK. The glycoprotease of *Pasteurella haemolytica* A1 eliminates binding of myeloid cells to P-selectin but not to E-selectin. *Biochem Biophys Res Commun* 1992;188:760–766.
55. Norgard KE, Moore KL, Diaz S, Stults NL, Ushiyama S, McEver RP, Cummings RD, Varki A. Characterization of a specific ligand for P-selectin on myeloid cells: A minor glycoprotein with sialylated *O*-linked oligosaccharides. *J Biol Chem* 1993;268:12764–12774.
56. Sako D, Chang XJ, Barone KM, Vachino G, White HM, Shaw G, Veldman GM, Bean KM, Ahern TJ, Furie B, Cumming DA, Larsen GR. Expression cloning of a functional glycoprotein ligand for P-selectin. *Cell* 1993;75:1179–1186.
57. Lawrence MB, Springer TA. Leukocytes roll on a selectin at physiologic flow rates: Distinction from and prerequisite for adhesion through integrins. *Cell* 1991;65:859–873.
58. Ley K, Gaehtgens P, Fennie C, Singer MS, Lasky LA, Rosen SD. Lectin-like cell adhesion molecule 1 mediates leukocyte rolling in mesenteric venules in vivo. *Blood* 1991;77:2553–2555.
59. von Andrian UH, Chambers JD, McEvoy LM, Bargatze RF, Arfors KE, Butcher EC. Two-step model of leukocyte-endothelial cell interaction in inflammation: Distinct roles for LECAM-1 and the leukocyte β_2 integrins *in vivo*. *Proc Natl Acad Sci USA* 1991;88:7538–7542.
60. Lawrence MB, Springer TA. Neutrophils roll on E-selectin. *J Immunol* 1993;151:6338–6346.
61. Abbassi O, Kishimoto TK, McIntire LV, Anderson DC, Smith CW. E-selectin supports neutrophil rolling in vitro under conditions of flow. *J Clin Invest* 1993;92:2719–2730.
62. Olofsson AM, Arfors KE, Ramezani L, Wolitzky BA, Butcher EC, von Andrian UH. E-selectin mediates leukocyte rolling in interleukin-1 treated rabbit mesentery venules. *Blood* 1994;84:2749–2758.
63. Bienvenu K, Granger DN. Molecular determinants of shear rate-dependent leukocyte adhesion in postcapillary venules. *Am J Physiol* 1993;264:H1504–H1508.
64. Mayadas TN, Johnson RC, Rayburn H, Hynes RO, Wagner DD. Leukocyte rolling and extravasation are severely compromised in P-selectin-deficient mice. *Cell* 1993;74:541–554.
65. von Andrian UH, Hansell P, Chambers JD, Berger EM, Filho IT, Butcher EC, Arfors KE. L-selectin function is required for β_2-integrin-mediated neutrophil adhesion at physiological shear rates in vivo. *Am J Physiol* 1992;263:H1034–H1044.
66. Kishimoto TK, Warnock RA, Jutila MA, Butcher EC, Lane C, Anderson DC, Smith CW. Antibodies against human neutrophil LECAM-1 (LAM-1/Leu-8/DREG-56 antigen) and endothelial cell ELAM-1 inhibit a common CD18-independent adhesion pathway in vitro. *Blood* 1991;78:805–811.
67. Picker LJ, Warnock RA, Burns AR, Doerschuk CM, Berg EL, Butcher EC. The neutrophil selectin LECAM-1 presents carbohydrate ligands

to the vascular selectins ELAM-1 and GMP-140. *Cell* 1991;66: 921–933.
68. von Andrian UH, Chambers JD, Berg EL, Michie SA, Brown DA, Karolak D, Ramezani L, Berger EM, Arfors KE, Butcher EC. L-Selectin mediates neutrophil rolling in inflamed venules through sialyl Lewis^x-dependent and -independent recognition pathways. *Blood* 1993;82:182–191.
69. Lawrence MB, Bainton DF, Springer TA. Neutrophil tethering to and rolling on E-selectin are separable by requirement for L-selectin. *Immunity* 1994;1:137–145.
70. Chan P-Y, Lawrence MB, Dustin ML, Ferguson LM, Golan DE, Springer TA. Influence of receptor lateral mobility on adhesion strengthening between membranes containing LFA-3 and CD2. *J Cell Biol* 1991;115:245–255.
71. Hammer DA, Apte SM. Simulation of cell rolling and adhesion on surfaces in shear flow: General results and analysis of selectin-mediated neutrophil adhesion. *Biophys J* 1992;63:35–57.
72. Cyster JG, Shotton DM, Williams AF. The dimensions of the T lymphocyte glycoprotein leukosialin and identification of linear protein epitopes that can be modified by glycosylation. *EMBO J* 1991;10: 893–902.
73. Erlandsen SL, Hasslen SR, Nelson RD. Detection and spatial distribution of the β_2 integrin (Mac-1) and L-selectin (LECAM-1) adherence receptors on human neutrophils by high-resolution field emission SEM. *J Histochem Cytochem* 1993;41:327–333.
74. Kansas GS, Ley K, Munro JM, Tedder TF. Regulation of leukocyte rolling and adhesion to high endothelial venules through the cytoplasmic domain of L-selectin. *J Exp Med* 1993;177:833–838.
75. Van Ewijk W, Brons NHC, Rozing J. Scanning electron microscopy of homing and recirculating lymphocyte populations. *Cell Immunol* 1975;19:245–261.
76. Anderson AO, Anderson ND. Lymphocyte emigration from high endothelial venules in rat lymph nodes. *Immunology* 1976;31:731–748.
77. Simmons DL, Satterthwaite AB, Tenen DG, Seed B. Molecular cloning of a cDNA encoding CD34, a sialomucin of human hematopoietic stem cells. *J Immunol* 1992;148:267–271.
78. Cross AH, Raine CS. Central nervous system endothelial cell–polymorphonuclear cell interactions during autoimmune demyelination. *Am J Pathol* 1992;139:1401–1409.
79. Wilkinson PC. *Chemotaxis and Inflammation.* London: Churchill Livingstone; 1982.
80. Devreotes PN, Zigmond SH. Chemotaxis in eukaryotic cells: A focus on leukocytes and *dictyostelium. Annu Rev Cell Biol* 1988;4:649–686.
81. Carter SB. Haptotaxis and the mechanism of cell motility. *Nature* 1967;213:256–260.
82. Huber AR, Kunkel SL, Todd RF III, Weiss SJ. Regulation of transendothelial neutrophil migration by endogenous interleukin-8. *Science* 1991;254:99–102.
83. Rot A. Endothelial cell binding of NAP-1/IL-8: Role in neutrophil emigration. *Immunol Today* 1992;13:291–294.
84. Tanaka Y, Adams DH, Hubscher S, Hirano H, Siebenlist U, Shaw S. T-cell adhesion induced by proteoglycan-immobilized cytokine MIP-1β. *Nature* 1993;361:79–82.
85. Snyderman R, Uhing RJ. Chemoattractant stimulus-response coupling. In: Gallin JI, Goldstein IM, Snyderman R, eds. *Inflammation: Basic Principles and Clinical Correlates.* New York: Raven Press; 1992:421–439.
86. Wu D, LaRosa GJ, Simon MI. G protein-coupled signal transduction pathways for interleukin-8. *Science* 1993;261:101–103.
87. Beals CR, Wilson CB, Perlmutter RM. A small multigene family encodes G_i signal-transduction proteins. *Proc Natl Acad Sci USA* 1987;84:7886–7890.
88. Amatruda TT, Gerard NP, Gerard C, Simon MI. Specific interactions of chemoattractant factor receptors with G-proteins. *J Biol Chem* 1993;268:10139–10144.
89. Murphy PM. The molecular biology of leukocyte chemoattractant receptors. *Ann Rev Immunol* 1994;12:593–633.
90. Charo IF, Myers SJ, Herman A, Franci C, Connolly AJ, Coughlin SR. Molecular cloning and functional expression of two monocyte chemoattractant protein 1 receptors reveals alternative splicing of the carboxyl-terminal tails. *Proc Natl Acad Sci USA* 1994;91:2752–2756.
91. Faull RJ, Kovach NL, Harlan HM, Ginsberg MH. Stimulation of integrin-mediated adhesion of T lymphocytes and monocytes: Two mechanisms with divergent biological consequences. *J Exp Med* 1994;179: 1307–1316.
92. Ginsberg MH, Du X, Plow EF. Inside-out integrin signalling. *Curr Opin Cell Biol* 1992;4:766–771.
93. Pober JS, Doukas J, Hughes CCW, Savage COS, Munro JM, Cotran RS.The potential roles of vascular endothelium in immune reactions. *Hum Immunol* 1990;28:258–262.
94. Lo SK, Lee S, Ramos RA, Lobb R, Rosa M, Chi-Rosso G, Wright SD. Endothelial–leukocyte adhesion molecule 1 stimulates the adhesive activity of leukocyte integrin CR3 (CD11b/CD18, Mac-1, $\alpha_m\beta_2$) on human neutrophils. *J Exp Med* 1991;173:1493–1500.
95. Lorant DE, Patel KD, McIntyre TM, McEver RP, Prescott SM, Zimmerman GA. Coexpression of GMP-140 and PAF by endothelium stimulated by histamine or thrombin: A juxtacrine system for adhesion and activation of neutrophils. *J Cell Biol* 1991;115:223–234.
96. Lo SK, Detmers PA, Levin SM, Wright SD. Transient adhesion of neutrophils to endothelium. *J Exp Med* 1989;169:1779–1793.
97. Wright SD, Meyer BC. Phorbol esters cause sequential activation and deactivation of complement receptors on polymorphonuclear leukocytes. *J Immunol* 1986;136:1759–1764.
98. Buyon JP, Abramson SB, Philips MR, Slade SG, Ross GD, Weissman G, Winchester RJ. Dissociation between increased surface expression of Gp165/95 and homotypic neutrophil aggregation. *J Immunol* 1988; 140:3156–3160.
99. Diamond MS, Staunton DE, deFougerolles AR, Stacker SA, Garcia-Aguilar J, Hibbs ML, Springer TA. ICAM-1 (CD54): A counter-receptor for Mac-1 (CD11b/CD18). *J Cell Biol* 1990;111:3129–3139.
100. Smith CW, Kishimoto TK, Abbass O, Hughes B, Rothlein R, McIntire LV, Butcher E, Anderson DC. Chemotactic factors regulate lectin adhesion molecule 1 (LECAM-1)-dependent neutrophil adhesion to cytokine-stimulated endothelial cells in vitro. *J Clin Invest* 1991;87: 609–618.
101. Sengelov H, Kjeldsen L, Diamond MS, Springer TA, Borregaard N, Subcellular localization and dynamics of Mac-1 ($\alpha_m\beta_2$) in human neutrophils. *J Clin Invest* 1993;92:1467–1476.
102. Philips MR, Buyon JP, Winchester R, Weissman G, Abramson SB. Up-regulation of the iC3b receptor (CR3) is neither necessary nor sufficient to promote neutrophil aggregation. *J Clin Invest* 1988;82: 495–501.
103. Vedder NB, Harlan JM. Increased surface expression of CD11b/CD18 (Mac-1) is not required for stimulated neutrophil adherence to cultured endothelium. *J Clin Invest* 1988;81:676–682.
104. Dustin ML, Springer TA. T cell receptor cross-linking transiently stimulates adhesiveness through LFA-1. *Nature* 1989;341:619–624.
105. Pircher H, Groscurth P, Baumhutter S, Aguet M, Zinkernagel RM, Hengartner H. A monoclonal antibody against altered LFA-1 induces proliferation and lymphokine release of cloned T cells. *Eur J Immunol* 1986;16:172–181.
106. Keizer GD, Visser W, Vliem M, Figdor CG. A monoclonal antibody (NKI-L16) directed against a unique epitope on the alpha-chain of human leukocyte function-associated antigen 1 induces homotypic cell-cell interactions. *J Immunol* 1988;140:1393–1400.
107. Landis RC, Bennett RI, Hogg N. A novel LFA-1 activation epitope maps to the I domain. *J Cell Biol* 1993;120:1519–1527.
108. Diamond MS, Springer TA. A subpopulation of Mac-1 (CD11b/ CD18) molecules mediates neutrophil adhesion to ICAM-1 and fibrinogen. *J Cell Biol* 1993;120:545–556.
109. Diamond MS, Garcia-Aguilar J, Bickford JK, Corbi AL, Springer TA. The I domain is a major recognition site on the leukocyte integrin Mac-1 (CD11b/CD18) for four distinct adhesion ligands. *J Cell Biol* 1993;120:1031–1043.
110. Michishita M, Videm V, Arnaout MA. A novel divalent cation-binding site in the A domain of the β2 integrin CR3 (CD11b/CD18) is essential for ligand binding. *Cell* 1993;72:857–867.
111. Lollo BA, Chan KWH, Hanson EM, Moy VT, Brian AA. Direct evidence for two affinity states for lymphocyte function-associated antigen 1 on activated T cells. *J Biol Chem* 1993;268:21693–21700.
112. Alon R, Kassner PD, Carr MW, Finger EB, Hemler ME, Springer TA. The integrin VLA-4 supports tethering and rolling in flow on VCAM-1. *J Cell Biol* 1995;128:1243–1253.
113. Rothlein R, Dustin ML, Marlin SD, Springer TA. A human intercellular adhesion molecule (ICAM-1) distinct from LFA-1. *J Immunol* 1986;137:1270–1274.
114. Staunton DE, Dustin ML, Springer TA. Functional cloning of ICAM-

2, a cell adhesion ligand for LFA-1 homologous to ICAM-1. *Nature* 1989;339:61–64.

115. deFougerolles AR, Springer TA. Intercellular adhesion molecule 3, a third adhesion counter-receptor for lymphocyte function-associated molecule 1 on resting lymphocytes. *J Exp Med* 1992;175:185–190.
116. Smith CW, Marlin SD, Rothlein R, Toman C, Anderson DC. Cooperative interactions of LFA-1 and Mac-1 with intercellular adhesion molecule-1 in facilitating adherence and transendothelial migration of human neutrophils in vitro. *J Clin Invest* 1989;83:2008–2017.
117. Diamond MS, Staunton DE, Marlin SD, Springer TA. Binding of the integrin Mac-1 (CD11b/CD18) to the third Ig-like domain of ICAM-1 (CD54) and its regulation by glycosylation. *Cell* 1991;65:961–971.
118. deFougerolles AR, Qin X, Springer TA. Characterization of the function of ICAM-3 and comparison to ICAM-1 and ICAM-2 in immune responses. *J Exp Med* 1994;179:619–629.
119. Moy P, Lobb R, Tizard R, Olson D, Hession C. Cloning of an inflammation-specific phosphatidyl inositol-linked form of murine vascular cell adhesion molecule-1. *J Biol Chem* 1993;268:8835–8841.
120. Terry RW, Kwee L, Levine JF, Labow MA. Cytokine induction of an alternatively spliced murine vascular cell adhesion molecule (VCAM) mRNA encoding a glycosylphosphatidylinositol-anchored VCAM protein. *Proc Natl Acad Sci USA* 1993;90:5919–5923.
121. Kinashi T, St. Pierre Y, Springer TA. Expression of glycophosphatidylinositol (GPI)-anchored and non GPI-anchored isoforms of vascular cell adhesion molecule 1 (VCAM-1) in stromal and endothelial cells. *Blood* 1995;57:168–173.
122. Elices MJ, Osborn L, Takada Y, Crouse C, Luhowskyj S, Hemler ME, Lobb RR. VCAM-1 on activated endothelium interacts with the leukocyte integrin VLA-4 at a site distinct from the VLA-4/fibronectin binding site. *Cell* 1990;60:577–584.
123. Rüegg C, Postigo AS, Sikorski EE, Butcher EC, Pytela R, Erle DJ. Role of integrin $\alpha4\beta7/\alpha4\beta P$ in lymphocyte adherence to fibronectin and VCAM-1 and in homotypic cell clustering. *J Cell Biol* 1992;117: 179–189.
124. Chan BMC, Elices MJ, Murphy E, Hemler ME. Adhesion to vascular cell adhesion molecule 1 and fibronectin: Comparison of $\alpha^4\beta_1$ (VLA-4) and $\alpha^4\beta_7$ on the human B cell line JY. *J Biol Chem* 1992;267: 8366–8370.
125. Osborn L, Vassallo C, Benjamin CD. Activated endothelium binds lymphocytes through a novel binding site in the alternately spliced domain of vascular cell adhesion molecule-1. *J Exp Med* 1992;176: 99–107.
126. Vonderheide RH, Springer TA. Lymphocyte adhesion through VLA-4: Evidence for a novel binding site in the alternatively spliced domain of VCAM-1 and an additional $\alpha4$ integrin counter-receptor on stimulated endothelium. *J Exp Med* 1992;175:1433–1442.
127. Vonderheide RH, Tedder TF, Springer TA, Staunton DE. Residues within a conserved amino acid motif of domains 1 and 4 of VCAM-1 are required for binding to VLA-4. *J Cell Biol* 1994;125:215–222.
128. Osborn L, Vassallo C, Browning BG, Tizard R, Haskard DO, Benjamin CD, Douglas I, Kirchhausen T. Arrangement of domains, and amino acid residues required for binding of vascular cell adhesion molecule-1 to its counter-receptor VLA-4 ($\alpha4\beta1$). *J Cell Biol* 1994; 124(4):601–608.
129. Streeter PR, Lakey-Berg E, Rouse BTN, Bargatze RF, Butcher EC. A tissue-specific endothelial cell molecule involved in lymphocyte homing. *Nature* 1988;331:41–46.
130. Briskin MJ, McEvoy LM, Butcher EC. MAdCAM-1 has homology to immunoglobulin and mucin-like adhesion receptors and to IgA1. *Nature* 1993;363:461–464.
131. Hu MC-T, Crowe DT, Weissman IL, Holzmann B. Cloning and expression of mouse integrin $\beta_p(\beta_7)$: A functional role in Peyer's patch-specific lymphocyte homing. *Proc Natl Acad Sci USA* 1992; 89:8254–8258.
132. Berlin C, Berg EL, Briskin MJ, Andrew DP, Kilshaw PJ, Holzmann B, Weissman IL, Hamann A, Butcher EC. $\alpha4\beta7$ integrin mediates lymphocyte binding to the mucosal vascular addressin MAdCAM-1. *Cell* 1993;74:185–195.
133. Berg EL, McEvoy LM, Berlin C, Bargatze RF, Butcher EC. L-Selectin-mediated lymphocyte rolling on MAdCAM-1. *Nature* 1993;366: 695–698.
134. Muller WA, Ratti CM, McDonnell SL, Cohn ZA. A human endothelial cell-restricted, externally disposed plasmalemmal protein enriched in intercellular junctions. *J Exp Med* 1989;170:399–414.
135. Albelda SM, Muller WA, Buck CA, Newman PJ. Molecular and cellular properties of PECAM-1 (endoCAM/CD31): A novel vascular cell–cell adhesion molecule. *J Cell Biol* 1991;114:1059–1068.
136. Newman PJ, Berndt MC, Gorski J, White GC, Lyman S, Paddock C, Muller WA. PECAM-1 (CD31) cloning and relation to adhesion molecules of the immunoglobulin gene superfamily. *Science* 1990; 247:1219–1222.
137. Simmons DL, Walker C, Power C, Pigott R. Molecular cloning of CD31, a putative intercellular adhesion molecule closely related to carcinoembryonic antigen. *J Exp Med* 1990;171:2147–2152.
138. Albelda SM, Oliver PD, Romer LH, Buck CA. EndoCAM. A novel endothelial cell–cell adhesion molecule. *J Cell Biol* 1990;110: 1227–1237.
139. Stockinger H, Gadd SJ, Eher R, Majdic O, Schreiber W, Kasinrerk W, Strass B, Schnabl E, Knapp W. Molecular characterization and functional analysis of the leukocyte surface protein CD31. *J Immunol* 1990;145:3889–3897.
140. Tanaka Y, Albelda SM, Horgan KJ, Van Seventer GA, Shimizu Y, Newman W, Hallam J, Newman PJ, Buck CA, Shaw S. CD31 expressed on distinctive T cell subsets is a preferential amplifier of $\beta1$ integrin-mediated adhesion. *J Exp Med* 1992;176:245–253.
141. Muller WA, Weigl SA, Deng X, Phillips DM. PECAM-1 is required for transendothelial migration of leukocytes. *J Exp Med* 1993;178: 449–460.
142. Haynes BF, Liao H-X, Patton KL. The transmembrane hyaluronate receptor (CD44): Multiple functions, multiple forms. *Cancer Cell* 1991;3:347–350.
143. Culty M, Miyake K, Kincade PW, Sikorski E, Butcher EC, Underhill C. The hyaluronate receptor is a member of the CD44 (H-CAM) family of cell surface glycoproteins. *J Cell Biol* 1990;111:2765–2774.
144. Aruffo A, Stamenkovic I, Melnick M, Underhill CB, Seed B. CD44 is the principal cell surface receptor for hyaluronate. *Cell* 1990;61: 1303–1313.
145. Günthert U. CD44: A multitude of isoforms with diverse functions. *Curr Top Microbiol Immunol* 1993;184:47–63.
146. Arch R, Wirth K, Hofmann M, Ponta H, Matzku S, Herrlich P, Zöller M. Participation in normal immune responses of a metastasis-inducing splice variant of CD44. *Science* 1992;257:682–685.
147. Jalkanen S, Bargatze RF, de los Toyos J, Butcher EC. Lymphocyte recognition of high endothelium: Antibodies to distinct epitopes of an 85–95 kD glycoprotein antigen differentially inhibit lymphocyte binding to lymph node, mucosal and synovial endothelial cells. *J Cell Biol* 1987;105:983–993.
148. Oppenheimer-Marks N, Davis LS, Lipsky PE. Human T lymphocyte adhesion to endothelial cells and transendothelial migration: Alteration of receptor use relates to the activation status of both the T cell and the endothelial cell. *J Immunol* 1990;145:140–148.
149. Camp RL, Scheynius A, Johansson C, Puré E. CD44 is necessary for optimal contact allergic responses but is not required for normal leukocyte extravasation. *J Exp Med* 1993;178:497–507.
150. Anderson DC, Springer TA. Leukocyte adhesion deficiency: An inherited defect in the Mac-1, LFA-1, and p150,95 glycoproteins. *Annu Rev Med* 1987;38:175–194.
151. Kishimoto TK, Larson RS, Corbi AL, Dustin ML, Staunton DE, Springer TA. The leukocyte integrins: LFA-1, Mac-1, and p150,95. *Adv Immunol* 1989;46:149–182.
152. Buchanan MR, Crowley CA, Rosin RE, Gimbrone MA, Babior BM. Studies on the interaction between GP-180-deficient neutrophils and vascular endothelium. *Blood* 1982;60:160–165.
153. Smith CW, Rothlein R, Hughes BJ, Mariscalco MM, Schmalstieg FC, Anderson DC. Recognition of an endothelial determinant for CD18-dependent neutrophil adherence and transendothelial migration. *J Clin Invest* 1988;82:1746–1756.
154. Arfors KE, Lundberg C, Lindborm L, Lundberg K, Beatty PG, Harlan JM. A monoclonal antibody to the membrane glycoprotein complex CD18 inhibits polymorphonuclear leukocyte accumulation and plasma leakage in vivo. *Blood* 1987;69:338–340.
155. Lawrence MB, Smith CW, Eskin SG, McIntire LV. Effect of venous shear stress on CD18-mediated neutrophil adhesion to cultured endothelium. *Blood* 1990;75:227–237.
156. Jutila MA, Lewinsohn D, Berg EL, et al. Homing receptors in lymphocyte, neutrophil, and monocyte interaction with endothelial cells. In: Springer TA, Anderson DC, Rosenthal AS, et al, eds. *Leukocyte Adhesion Molecules*. New York: Springer-Verlag; 1988:227–235.

157. Jutila MA, Rott L, Berg EL, Butcher EC. Function and regulation of the neutrophil MEL-14 antigen in vivo: Comparison with LFA-1 and MaC-1. *J Immunol* 1989;143:3318–3324.
158. Watson SR, Fennie C, Lasky LA. Neutrophil influx into an inflammatory site inhibited by a soluble homing receptor–IgG chimaera. *Nature* 1991;349:164–167.
159. Mulligan MS, Varani J, Dame MK, Lane CL, Smith CW, Anderson DC, Ward PA. Role of endothelial–leukocyte adhesion molecule 1 (ELAM-1) in neutrophil-mediated lung injury in rats. *J Clin Invest* 1991;88:1396–1406.
160. Kishimoto TK, Jutila MA, Berg EL, Butcher EC. Neutrophil Mac-1 and MEL-14 adhesion proteins inversely regulated by chemotactic factors. *Science* 1989;245:1238–1241.
161. Cohnheim J. *Lectures on General Pathology: A Handbook for Practitioners and Students.* London: The New Sydenham Society; 1889.
162. Etzioni A, Frydman M, Pollack S, Avidor I, Phillips ML, Paulson JC, Gershoni-Baruch R. Recurrent severe infections caused by a novel leukocyte adhesion deficiency. *N Engl J Med* 1992;327:1789–1792.
163. von Andrian UH, Berger EM, Ramezani L, Chambers JD, Ochs HD, Harlan JM, Paulson JC, Etzioni A, Arfors KE. *In vivo* behavior of neutrophils from two patients with distinct inherited leukocyte adhesion deficiency syndromes. *J Clin Invest* 1993;91:2893–2897.
164. Colditz IG. Sites of antigenic stimulation: Role of cytokines and chemotactic agonists in acute inflammation. In: Beh KJ, ed. *Animal Health and Production in the 21st Century.* Melbourne: CSIRO; 1992.
165. Mulligan MS, Jones ML, Bolanowski MA, Baganoff MP, Deppeler CL, Meyers DM, Ryan US, Ward PA. Inhibition of lung inflammatory reactions in rats by an anti-human IL-8 antibody. *J Immunol* 1993; 150:5585–5595.
166. Sekido N, Mukaida N, Harada A, Nakanishi I, Watanabe Y, Matsushima K. Prevention of lung reperfusion injury in rabbits by a monoclonal antibody against interleukin-8. *Nature* 1993;365:654–657.
167. Spangrude GH, Sacchi F, Hill HR, Van Epps DE, Daynes RA. Inhibition of lymphocyte and neutrophil chemotaxis by pertussis toxin. *J Immunol* 1985;135:4135–4143.
168. Nourshargh S, Williams TJ. Evidence that a receptor-operated event on the neutrophil mediates neutrophil accumulation in vivo. *J Immunol* 1990;145:2633–2638.
169. Hechtman DH, Cybulsky MI, Fuchs HJ, Baker JB, Gimbrone MA Jr. Intravascular IL-8: Inhibitor of polymorphonuclear leukocyte accumulation at sites of acute inflammation. *J Immunol* 1991;147: 883–892.
170. Gimbrone MA, Obin MS, Brock AF, Luis EA, Hass PE, Hebert CA, Yip YK, Leung DW, Lowe DG, Kohr WJ, Darbonne WC, Bechtol KB, Baker JB. Endothelial interleukin-8: A novel inhibitor of leukocyte–endothelial interactions. *Science* 1989;246:1601–1603.
171. Colditz IG, Movat HZ. Desensitization of acute inflammatoy lesions to chemotaxins and endotoxin. *J Immunol* 1984;144:2163–2168.
172. Colditz IG. Desensitisation mechanisms regulating plasma leakage and neutrophil emigration. In: Gordon JL, ed. *Vascular Endothelium: Interactions with Circulating Cells.* New York: Elsevier; 1991: 175–187.
173. Kuna P, Reddigari SR, Schall TJ, Rucinski D, Sadick M, Kaplan AP. Characterization of the human basophil response to cytokines, growth factors, and histamine releasing factors of the intercrine/chemokine family. *J Immunol* 1993;150:1932–1943.
174. Bischoff SC, Krieger M, Brunner T, Rot A, Tscharner V, Baggiolini M, Dahinden CA. RANTES and related chemokines activate human basophil granulocytes through different G protein-coupled receptors. *Eur J Immunol* 1993;23:761–767.
175. Walsh LJ, Lavker RM, Murphy GF. Biology of disease. Determinants of immune cell trafficking in the skin. *Lab Invest* 1990;63:592–600.
176. Hood L, Huang HV, Dreyer WJ. The area-code hypothesis: The immune system provides clues to understanding the genetic and molecular basis of cell recognition during development. *J Supramol Struct* 1987;7:531–559.
177. Springer TA. Area code molecules of lymphocytes. In: Burger MM, Sordat B, Zinkernagel RM, eds. *Cell to Cell Interaction: A Karger Symposium.* Basel: S Karger; 1990:16–39.
178. Jung TM, Gallatin WM, Weissman IL, Dailey MO. Down-regulation of homing receptors after T cell activation. *J Immunol* 1988;141: 4110–4117.
179. Spertini O, Kansas GS, Munro JM, Griffin JD, Tedder TF. Regulation of leukocyte migration by activation of the leukocyte adhesion molecule (LAM-1) selectin. *Nature* 1991;349:691–694.
180. Issekutz TB, Chin W, Hay JB. The characterization of lymphocytes migrating through chronically inflamed tissues. *Immunology* 1982; 46:59–66.
181. Mackay CR, Marston WL, Dudler L. Naive and memory T cells show distinct pathways of lymphocyte recirculation. *J Exp Med* 1990;171: 801–817.
182. Bjerknes M, Cheng H, Ottaway CA. Dynamics of lymphocyte–endothelial interactions in vivo. *Science* 1986;231:402–405.
183. Woodruff JJ, Clarke LM, Chin YH. Specific cell-adhesion mechanisms determining migration pathways of recirculating lymphocytes. *Annu Rev Immunol* 1987;5:201–222.
184. Mebius RE, Streeter PR, Breve J, Duijvestijn AM, Kraal G. The influence of afferent lymphatic vessel interruption on vascular addressin expression. *J Cell Biol* 1991;115:85–95.
185. Mebius RE, Dowbenko D, Williams A, Fennie C, Lasky LA, Watson SR. Expression of GlyCAM-1, an endothelial ligand for L-selectin, is affected by afferent lymphatic flow. *J Immunol* 1993;151:6769–6776.
186. Mackay CR, Marston W, Dudler L. Altered patterns of T cell migration through lymph nodes and skin following antigen challenge. *Eur J Immunol* 1992;22:2205–2210.
187. Stamper HB Jr, Woodruff JJ. Lymphocyte homing into lymph nodes: In vitro demonstration of the selective affinity of recirculating lymphocytes for high-endothelial venules. *J Exp Med* 1976;144:828.
188. Butcher EC, Scollay RG, Weissman IL. Organ specificity of lymphocyte migration: Mediation by highly selective lymphocyte interaction with organ-specific determinants on high endothelial venules. *Eur J Immunol* 1980;10:556–561.
189. Stevens SK, Weissman IL, Butcher EC. Differences in the migration of B and T lymphocytes: Organ-selective localization in vivo and the role of lymphocyte–endothelial cell recognition. *J Immunol* 1982;2: 844–851.
190. Bargatze RF, Wu NW, Weissman IL, Butcher EC. High endothelial venule binding as a predictor of the dissemination of passaged murine lymphomas. *J Exp Med* 1987;166:1125–1131.
191. Streeter PR, Rouse BTN, Butcher EC. Immunohistologic and functional characterization of a vascular addressin involved in lymphocyte homing into peripheral lymph nodes. *J Cell Biol* 1988;107: 1853–1862.
192. Berg EL, Robinson MK, Warnock RA, Butcher EC. The human peripheral lymph node vascular addressin is a ligand for LECAM-1, the peripheral lymph node homing receptor. *J Cell Biol* 1991;114: 343–349.
193. Watson S, Imai Y, Fennie C, Geoffroy JS, Rosen SD, Lasky LA. A homing receptor–IgG chimera as a probe for adhesive ligands of lymph node high endothelial venules. *J Cell Biol* 1990;110: 2221–2229.
194. Imai Y, Lasky LA, Rosen SD. Sulphation requirement for GlyCAM-1, an endothelial ligand for L-selectin. *Nature* 1993;361:555–557.
195. Spertini O, Luscinskas FW, Kansas GS, Munro JM, Griffin JD, Gimbrone MA Jr, Tedder TF. Leukocyte adhesion molecule-1 (LAM-1, L-selectin) interacts with an inducible endothelial cell ligand to support leukocyte adhesion. *J Immunol* 1991;147:2565–2573.
196. Spertini O, Luscinskas FW, Gimbrone MA Jr, Tedder TF. Monocyte attachment to activated human vascular endothelium in vitro is mediated by leukocyte adhesion molecule-1 (L-selectin) under nonstatic conditions. *J Exp Med* 1992;175:1789–1792.
197. San Gabriel-Masson C. *Adhesion of lymphocytes to the lactating mammary gland in the mouse.* [Dissertation]. Hershey: Pennsylvania State University; 1992.
198. Holzmann B, McIntyre BW, Weissman IL. Identification of a murine Peyer's patch-specific lymphocyte homing receptor as an integrin molecule with an alpha chain homologous to human VLA-1 alpha. *Cell* 1989;56:37–46.
199. Holzmann B, Weissman IL. Peyer's patch-specific lymphocyte homing receptors consist of a VLA-4-like α chain associated with either of two integrin β chains, one of which is novel. *EMBO J* 1989;8: 1735–1741.
200. Imai Y, Singer MS, Fennie C, Lasky LA, Rosen SD. Identification of a carbohydrate based endothelial ligand for a lymphocyte homing receptor. *J Cell Biol* 1991;113:1213–1221.
201. Hamann A, Jablonski-Westrich D, Jonas P, Thiele HG. Homing receptors reexamined: Mouse LECAM-1 (MEL-14 antigen) is involved

in lymphocyte migration into gut-associated lymphoid tissue. *Eur J Immunol* 1991;21:2925–2929.

202. Hamann A, Westrich DJ, Duijevstijn A, Butcher EC, Baisch H, Harder R, Thiele HG. Evidence for an accessory role of LFA-1 in lymphocyte–high endothelium interaction during homing. *J Immunol* 1988; 140:693–699.
203. deFougerolles AR, Stacker SA, Schwarting R, Springer TA. Characterization of ICAM-2 and evidence for a third counter-receptor for LFA-1. *J Exp Med* 1991;174:253–267.
204. Wardlaw AC, Parton R. *Bordetella pertussis* toxins. *Pharmacol Ther* 1983;19:1–53.
205. Morse SI, Barron BA. Studies on the leukocytosis and lymphocytosis induced by bordetella pertussis. III. The distribution of transfused lymphocytes in pertussis-treated and normal mice. *J Exp Med* 1970; 132:663–672.
206. Chaffin KE, Beals CR, Wilkie TM, Forbush KA, Simon MI, Perlmutter RM. Dissection of thymocyte signaling pathways by *in vivo* expression of pertussis toxin ADP-ribosyltransferase. *EMBO J* 1990;9: 3821–3829.
207. Chaffin KE, Perlmutter RM. A pertussis toxin-sensitive process controls thymocyte emigration. *Eur J Immunol* 1991;21:2565–2573.
208. Spangrude GJ, Braaten BA, Daynes RA. Molecular mechanisms of lymphocyte extravasation. I. Studies of two selective inhibitors of lymphocyte recirculation. *J Immunol* 1984;132:354–362.
209. Hamann A, Andrew DP, Jablonski-Westrich D, Holzmann B, Butcher EC. The role of α4 integrins in lymphocyte homing to mucosal tissues *in vivo*. *J Immunol* 1993;152:3283–3293.
210. Bargatze RF, Streeter PR, Butcher EC. Expression of low levels of peripheral lymph node-associated vascular addressin in mucosal lymphoid tissues: Possible relevance to the dissemination of passaged *akr* lymphomas. *J Cell Biochem* 1990;42:219–227.
211. Mackay CR, Marston WL, Dudler L, Spertini O, Tedder TF, Hein WR. Tissue-specific migration pathways by phenotypically distinct subpopulations of memory T cells. *Eur J Immunol* 1992;22:887–895.
212. Bargatze RF, Butcher EC. Rapid G protein-regulated activation events involved in lymphocyte binding to high endothelial venules. *J Exp Med* 1993;178:367–372.
213. Crowe DT, Chiu H, Fong S, Weissman IL. Regulation of the avidity of integrin $\alpha_4\beta_7$ by the β_7 cytoplasmic domain. *J Cell Biol* 1994; 269:14411–14418.
214. Hibbs ML, Xu H, Stacker SA, Springer TA. Regulation of adhesion to ICAM-1 by the cytoplasmic domain of LFA-1 integrin beta subunit. *Science* 1991;251:1611–1613.
215. Hibbs ML, Jakes S, Stacker SA, Wallace RW, Springer TA. The cytoplasmic domain of the integrin lymphocyte function-associated antigen 1 β subunit: Sites required for binding to intercellular adhesion molecule 1 and the phorbol ester-stimulated phosphorylation site. *J Exp Med* 1991;174:1227–1238.
216. Picker LJ, Michie SA, Rott LS, Butcher EC. A unique phenotype of skin-associated lymphocytes in humans: Preferential expression of the HECA-452 epitope by benign and malignant T cells at cutaneous sites. *Am J Pathol* 1990;136:1053–1068.
217. Berg EL, Robinson MK, Mansson O, Butcher EC, Magnani JL. A carbohydrate domain common to both sialyl Le^a and sialyl Le^x is recognized by the endothelial cell leukocyte adhesion molecule ELAM-1. *J Biol Chem* 1991;266:14869–14872.
218. Berg EL, Yoshino T, Rott LS, Robinson MK, Warnock RA, Kishimoto TK, Picker LJ, Butcher EC. The cutaneous lymphocyte antigen is a skin lymphocyte homing receptor for the vascular lectin endothelial cell-leukocyte adhesion molecule 1. *J Exp Med* 1991;174: 1461–1466.
219. Graber N, Gopal TV, Wilson D, Beall LD, Polte T, Newman W. T cells bind to cytokine-activated endothelial cells via a novel, inducible sialoglycoprotein and endothelial leukocyte adhesion molecule-1. *J Immunol* 1990;145:819–830.
220. Picker LJ, Kishimoto TK, Smith CW, Warnock RA, Butcher EC. ELAM-1 is an adhesion molecule for skin-homing T cells. *Nature* 1991;349:796–798.
221. Shimizu Y, Shaw S, Graber N, Gopal TV, Horgan KJ, Van Seventer GA, Newman W. Activation-independent binding of human memory T cells to adhesion molecule ELAM-1. *Nature* 1991;349:799–802.
222. Cotran RS, Gimbrone MA Jr, Bevilacqua MP, Mendrick DL, Pober JS. Induction and detection of a human endothelial activation antigen in vivo. *J Exp Med* 1986;164:661–666.
223. Alon R, Rossiter H, Springer TA, Kupper TS. Distinct cell surface ligands mediate T lymphocyte attachment and rolling on P- and E-selectin under physiological flow. *J Cell Biol* 1994;127:1485–1495.
224. Schweighoffer T, Tanaka Y, Tidswell M, Erle DJ, Horgan KJ, Luce GEG, Lazarovits AI, Buck D, Shaw S. Selective expression of integrin $\alpha4\beta7$ on a subset of human $CD4^+$ memory T cells with hallmarks of gut-trophism. *J Immunol* 1993;151:717–729.
225. Cerf-Bensussan N, Jarry A, Brousse N, Lisowska-Grospierre B, Guy-Grand D, Griscelli C. A monoclonal antibody (HML-1) defining a novel membrane molecule present on human intestinal lymphocytes. *Eur J Immunol* 1987;17:1279–1285.
226. Kilshaw PJ, Murant SJ. A new surface antigen on intraepithelial lymphocytes in the intestine. *Eur J Immunol* 1990;20:2201–2207.
227. Parker CM, Cepek K, Russell GJ, Shaw SK, Posnett D, Schwarting R, Brenner MB. A family of β_7 integrins on human mucosal lymphocytes. *Proc Natl Acad Sci USA* 1992;89:1924–1928.
228. Shaw SK, Cepek KL, Murphy EA, Russell GJ, Brenner MB, Parker CM. Molecular cloning of the human mucosal lymphocyte integrin α^E subunit. *J Biol Chem* 1994;269:6016–6025.
229. Cepek KL, Parker CM, Madara JL, Brenner MB. Integrin $\alpha^E\beta_7$ mediates adhesion of T lymphocytes to epithelial cells. *J Immunol* 1993; 150:3459–3470.
230. Picker LJ, Terstappen LWMM, Rott LS, Streeter PR, Stein H, Butcher EC. Differential expression of homing-associated adhesion molecules by T cell subsets in man. *J Immunol* 1990;145:3247–3255.
231. Coffman RL, Lebman DA, Shrader B. Transforming growth factor β specifically enhances IgA production by lipopolysaccharide-stimulated murine B lymphocytes. *J Exp Med* 1989;170:1039–1044.
232. Pitzalis C, Kingsley G, Haskard D, Panayi G. The preferential accumulation of helper-inducer T lymphocytes in inflammatory lesions: Evidence for regulation by selective endothelial and homotypic adhesion. *Eur J Immunol* 1988;18:1397–1404.
233. Janossy G, Bofill M, Rowe D, Muir J, Beverley PC. The tissue distribution of T lymphocytes expressing different CD45 polypeptides. *Immunology* 1989;66:517–525.
234. Issekutz TB. Inhibition of *in vivo* lymphocyte migration to inflammation and homing to lymphoid tissues by the TA-2 monoclonal antibody: A likely role for VLA-4 *in vivo*. *J Immunol* 1991;147: 4178–4184.
235. Issekutz TB. Inhibition of lymphocyte endothelial adhesion and in vivo lymphocyte migration to cutaneous inflammation by TA-3, a new monoclonal antibody to rat LFA-1. *J Immunol* 1992;149:3394–3402.
236. Chisholm PL, Williams CA, Lobb RR. Monoclonal antibodies to the integrin α4 subunit inhibit the murine contact hypersensitivity response. *Eur J Immunol* 1993;23:682–688.
237. Yednock TA, Cannon C, Fritz LC, Sanchez-Madrid F, Steinman L, Karin N. Prevention of experimental autoimmune encephalomyelitis by antibodies against $\alpha4\beta1$ integrin. *Nature* 1992;356:63–66.
238. Scheynius A, Camp RL, Puré E. Reduced contact sensitivity reactions in mice treated with monoclonal antibodies to leukocyte function-associated molecule-1 and intercellular adhesion molecule-1. *J Immunol* 1993;150:655–663.
239. Issekutz TB. Dual inhibition of VLA-4 and LFA-1 maximally inhibits cutaneous delayed type hypersensitivity-induced inflammation. *Am J Pathol* 1993;143:1286–1293.
240. Silber A, Newman W, Sasseville VG, Pauley D, Beall D, Walsh DG, Ringler DJ. Recruitment of lymphocytes during cutaneous delayed hypersensitivity in nonhuman primates is dependent on E-selectin and VCAM-1. *J Clin Invest* 1994;93:1554–1563.
241. McCluskey RT, Benacerraf B, McClusky JW. Studies on the specificity of the cellular infiltrate in delayed type hypersensitivity reactions. *J Immunol* 1963;90:466.
242. Tedder TF, Matsuyama T, Rothstein D, Schlossman SF, Morimoto C. Human antigen-specific memory T cells express the homing receptor (LAM-1) necessary for lymphocyte recirculation. *Eur J Immunol* 1990;20:1351–1355.
243. Bradley LM, Atkins GG, Swain SL. Long-term $CD4^+$ memory T cells from the spleen lack MEL-14, the lymph node homing receptor. *J Immunol* 1992;148:324–331.
244. Moore KL, Thompson LF. P-Selectin (CD62) binds to subpopulations of human memory T lymphocytes and natural killer cells. *Biochem Biophys Res Commun* 1992;186:173–181.
245. Damle NK, Klussman K, Dietsch MT, Mohagheghpour N, Aruffo A. GMP-140 (P-selectin/CD62) binds to chronically stimulated but not

resting $CD4^+$ T lymphocytes and regulates their production of proinflammatory cytokines. *Eur J Immunol* 1992;22:1789–1793.
246. Parrott DMV, Wilkinson PC. Lymphocyte locomotion and migration. *Prog Allergy* 1982;18:193–284.
247. Larsen CG, Anderson AO, Appella E, Oppenheim JJ, Matsushima K. The neutrophil-activating protein (NAP-1) is also chemotactic for T lymphocytes. *Science* 1989;241:1464–1466.
248. Kudo C, Araki A, Matsushima K, Sendo F. Inhibition of IL-8 induced $W3/25^+$ ($CD4^+$) T lymphocyte recruitment into subcutaneous tissues of rats by selective depletion of *in vivo* neutrophils with a monoclonal antibody. *J Immunol* 1991;174:2196–2201.
249. Leonard EJ, Yoshimura T, Tanaka S, Raffeld M. Neutrophil recruitment by intradermally injected neutrophil attractant/activation protein-1. *J Invest Dermatol* 1991;96:690–694.
250. Schall TJ, Bacon K, Toy KJ, Goeddel DV. Selective attraction of monocytes and T lymphocytes of the memory phenotype by cytokine RANTES. *Nature* 1990;347:669–671.
251. Taub DD, Conlon K, Lloyd AR, Oppenheim JJ, Kelvin DJ. Preferential migration of activated $CD4^+$ and $CD8^+$ T cells in response to MIP-1α and MIP-1β. *Science* 1993;360:355–358.
252. Schall TJ, Bacon K, Camp RDR, Kaspari JW, Goeddel DV. Human macrophage inflammatory protein α (MIP-1α) and MIP-1β chemokines attract distinct populations of lymphocytes. *J Exp Med* 1993; 177:1821–1825.
253. Taub DD, Lloyd AR, Conlon K, Wang JM, Ortaldo JR, Harada A, Matsushima K, Kelvin DJ, Oppenheim JJ. Recombinant human interferon-inducible protein 10 is a chemoattractant for human monocytes and T lymphocytes and promotes T cell adhesion to endothelial cells. *J Exp Med* 1993;177:1809–1814.
254. Adams DH, Harvath L, Bottaro DP, Interrante R, Catalano G, Tanaka Y, Strain A, Hubscher SG, Shaw S. Hepatocyte growth factor and macrophage inflammatory protein 1β: Structurally distinct cytokines that induce rapid cytoskeletal changes and subset-preferential migration in T cells. *Proc Natl Acad Sci USA* 1994;91:7144–7148.
255. Carr MW, Roth SJ, Luther E, Rose SS, Springer TA. Monocyte chemoattractant protein-1 is a major T lymphocyte chemoattractant. *Proc Natl Acad Sci USA* 1994;91:3652–3656.
256. Roth SJ, Carr MW, Rose SS, Springer TA. Characterization of transendothelial chemotaxis of T lymphocytes. *Am J Pathol [submitted]*.
257. Leonard EJ, Yoshimura T. Human monocyte chemoattractant protein-1 (MCP-1). *Immunol Today* 1990;11:97–101.
258. Villiger PM, Terkeltaub R, Lotz M. Production of monocyte chemoattractant protein-1 by inflamed synovial tissue and cultured synoviocytes. *J Immunol* 1992;149:722–727.
259. Ross R. The pathogenesis of atherosclerosis: A perspective for the 1990s. *Nature* 1993;362:801–809.
260. Munro JM, Cotran RS. Biology of disease. The pathogenesis of atherosclerosis: Atherogenesis and inflammation. *Lab Invest* 1988;58: 249–261.
261. Cybulsky MI, Gimbrone MA Jr. Vascular endothelial cells express a monocyte adhesion molecule during atherogenesis. *Science* 1991;251: 788–791.
262. Walker LN, Reidy MA, Bowyer DE. Morphology and cell kinetics of fatty streak lesion formation in the hypercholesterolemic rabbit. *Am J Pathol* 1986;125:450–459.
263. Li H, Cybulsky MI, Gimbrone MA Jr, Libby P. An atherogenic diet rapidly induces VCAM-1, a cytokine-regulatable mononuclear leukocyte adhesion molecule, in rabbit aortic endothelium. *Arterioscler Thromb* 1993;13:197–204.
264. Cybulsky MI, Allan-Motamed M, Medoff B, Davis V, Collins T, Gimbrone MA Jr. Endothelial expression of leukocyte adhesion molecules during atherogenesis in the rabbit. *FASEB J* 1992;6:1030A.
265. Li H, Cybusky MI, Gimbrone MA Jr, Libby P. Inducible expression of vascular cell adhesion molecule-1 (VCAM-1) by vascular smooth muscle cells in vitro and within rabbit atheroma. *Am J Pathol* 1993; 143:1551–1559.
266. Richardson M, Hadcock SJ, DeReske M, Cybulsky MI. Increased expression in vivo of VCAM-1 and E-selectin by the aortic endothelium of normolipemic and hyperlipemic diabetic rabbits. *Arterioscler Thromb* 1994;14:760–769.
267. Poston RN, Haskard DO, Coucher JR, Gall NP, Johnson-Tidey RR. Expression of intercellular adhesion molecule-1 in atherosclerotic plaques. *Am J Pathol* 1992;140:665–673.
268. Printseva OY, Peclo MM, Gown AM. Various cell types in human atherosclerotic lesions express ICAM-1: Further immunocytochemical and immunochemical studies employing monoclonal antibody 10F3. *Am J Pathol* 1992;140:889–896.
269. Wood KM, Cadogan MD, Ramshaw AL, Parums DV. The distribution of adhesion molecules in human atherosclerosis. *Histopathology* 1993;23:437–444.
270. van der Wal AC, Das PK, Tigges AJ, Becker AE. Adhesion molecules on the endothelium and mononuclear cells in human atherosclerotic lesions. *Am J Pathol* 1992;141:1427–1433.
271. Davis MJ, Gordon JL, Gearing AJH, Pigott R, Woolf N, Katz D, Kyriakopoulos A. The expression of the adhesion molecules ICAM-1, VCAM-1, PECAM, and E-selectin in human atherosclerosis. *J Pathol* 1993;171:223–229.
272. O'Brien KD, Allen MD, McDonald TO, Chait A, Harlan JM, Fishbein D, McCarty J, Ferguson M, Hudkins K, Benjamin CD, Lobb R, Alpers CE. Vascular cell adhesion molecule-1 is expressed in human coronary atherosclerotic plaques. Implications for the mode of progression of advanced coronary atherosclerosis. *J Clin Invest* 1993;92:945–951.
273. Gerrity RG, Goss JA, Soby L. Control of monocyte recruitment by chemotactic factor(s) in lesion-prone areas of swine aorta. *Arteriosclerosis* 1985;5:55–66.
274. Denholm EM, Lewis JC. Monocyte chemoattractants in pigeon aortic atherosclerosis. *Am J Pathol* 1987;126:464–475.
275. Boyd HC, Gown AM, Wolfbauer G, Chait A. Direct evidence for a protein recognized by a monoclonal antibody against oxidatively modified LDL in atherosclerotic lesions from a Watanabe heritable hyperlipidemic rabbit. *Am J Pathol* 1989;135:815–825.
276. Rosenfeld ME, Paklinski W, Yla-Herrtuala S, Butler S, Witztum JL. Distribution of oxidation specific lipid–protein adducts and apolipoprotein B in atherosclerotic lesions of varying severity from WHHL rabbits. *Arteriosclerosis* 1990;10:336–349.
277. Cushing SD, Berliner JA, Valente AJ, Territo MC, Navab M, Parhami F, Gerrity R, Schwartz CJ, Fogelman AM. Minimally modified low density lipoprotein induces monocyte chemotactic protein 1 in human endothelial cells and smooth muscle cells. *Proc Natl Acad Sci USA* 1990;87:5134–5238.
278. Rajavashisth TB, Andalibi A, Territo MC, Berliner JA, Navab M, Fogelman AM, Lusis AJ. Induction of endothelial cell expression of granulocyte and macrophage colony-stimulating factors by modified low-density lipoproteins. *Nature* 1990;344:254–257.
279. Quinn MT, Parthasarathy S, Steinberg D. Lysophosphatidylcholine: A chemotactic factor for human monocytes and its potential role in atherogenesis. *Proc Natl Acad Sci USA* 1988;85:2805–2809.
280. Kume N, Cybulsky MI, Gimbrone MA Jr. Lysophosphatidylcholine, a component of atherogenic lipoproteins, induces mononuclear leukocyte adhesion molecules in cultured human and rabbit arterial endothelial cells. *J Clin Invest* 1992;90:1138–1144.
281. Berliner JA, Territo M, Almada L, Carter A, Shafonsky E, Fogelman AM. Monocyte chemotactic factor produced by large vessel endothelial cells in vitro. *Arteriosclerosis* 1985;6:254–258.
282. Valente AJ, Fowler SR, Sprague EA, Kelley JL, Suenram CA, Schwartz CJ. Initial characterization of a peripheral blood mononuclear cell chemoattractant derived from cultured arterial smooth muscle cells. *Am J Pathol* 1984;117:409–417.
283. Navab M, Hough GP, Stevenson LW, Drinkwater DC, Laks H, Fogelman AM. Monocyte migration into the subendothelial space of a coculture of adult human aortic endothelial and smooth muscle cells. *J Clin Invest* 1988;82:1853–1863.
284. Yla-Herttuala S, Lipton BA, Rosenfeld ME, Sarkioja T, Yoshimura T, Leonard EJ, Witztum JL, Steinberg D. Expression of monocyte chemoattractant protein 1 in macrophage-rich areas of human and rabbit atherosclerotic lesions. *Proc Natl Acad Sci USA* 1991;88: 5252–5256.
285. Rosenfeld ME, Yla-Herttuala S, Lipton BA, Ord VA, Witztum JL, Steinberg D. Macrophage colony-stimulating factor mRNA and protein in atherosclerotic lesion of rabbits and humans. *Am J Pathol* 1992; 140:291–300.
286. Clinton SK, Underwood R, Hayes L. Sherman ML, Kufe DW, Libby P. Macrophage colony-stimulating factor gene expression in vascular cells and in experimental and human atherosclerosis. *Am J Pathol* 1992;140:301–316.
287. Averill LE, Meagher RC, Gerrity RG. Enhanced monocyte progenitor cell proliferation in bone marrow of hyperlipemic swine. *Am J Pathol* 1989;135:369–377.

288. House SD, Lipowsky HH. Leukocyte-endothelium adhesion: Microhemodynamics in the mesentary of the cat. *Microvasc Res* 1987;34:363–379.
289. Nazziola E, House SD. Effects of hydrodynamics and leukocyte–endothelium specificity on leukocyte–endothelium interactions. *Microvasc Res* 1992;44:127–142.
290. Ku DN, Zhu C. The mechanical environment of the artery. In: Sumpio BE, ed. *Hemodynamic Forces and Vascular Cell Biology*. Austin: RG Landes Company; 1993:1–23.
291. Fujimoto T, Stroud E, Whatley RE, Prescott SM, Muszbek L, Laposata M, McEver RP. P-selectin is acylated with palmitic acid and stearic acid at cysteine 766 through a thioester linkage. *J Biol Chem* 1993;268:11394–11400.
292. Barclay AN, Birkeland ML, Brown MH, et al. *The Leucocyte Antigen Facts Book*. London: Academic Press; 1993.
293. Sutherland DR, Marsh JCW, Davidson J, Baker MA, Keating A, Mellors A. Differential sensitivity of CD34 epitopes to cleavage by *Pasteurella haemolytica* glycoprotease: Implications for purification of CD34-positive progenitor cells. *Exp Hematol* 1992;20:590–599.
294. Larson RS, Corbi AL, Berman L, Springer TA. Primary structure of the LFA-1 alpha subunit: An integrin with an embedded domain defining a protein superfamily. *J Cell Biol* 1989;108:703–712.
295. Kishimoto TK, O'Connor K, Lee A, Roberts TM, Springer TA. Cloning of the beta subunit of the leukocyte adhesion proteins: Homology to an extracellular matrix receptor defines a novel supergene family. *Cell* 1987;48:681–690.
296. Takada Y, Elices MJ, Crouse C, Hemler ME. The primary structure of α-4 subunit of VLA-4: Homology to other integrins and possible cell-cell adhesion function. *EMBO J* 1989;8:1361–1368.
297. Loftus JC, O'Toole TE, Plow EF, Glass A, Frelinger AL III, Ginsberg MH. A β_3 integrin mutation abolishes ligand binding and alters divalent cation-dependent conformation. *Science* 1990;249:915–918.
298. Carrell NA, Fitzgerald LA, Steiner B, Erickson HP, Phillips DR. Structure of human platelet membrane glycoproteins IIb and IIIa as determined by electron microscopy. *J Biol Chem* 1985;260:1743–1749.
299. Nermut MV, Green NM, Eason P, Yamada SS, Yamada KM. Electron microscopy and structural model of human fibronectin receptor. *EMBO J* 1988;7:4093–4099.
300. Staunton DE, Dustin ML, Erickson HP, Springer TA. The arrangement of the immunoglobulin-like domains of ICAM-1 and the binding sites for LFA-1 and rhinovirus. *Cell* 1990;61:243–254.
301. Kirchhausen T, Staunton DE, Springer TA. Location of the domains of ICAM-1 by immunolabeling and single-molecule electron microscopy. *J Leukocyte Biol* 1993;53:342–346.
302. Simmons D, Makgoba MW, Seed B. ICAM, an adhesion ligand of LFA-1, is homologous to the neural cell adhesion molecule NCAM. *Nature* 1988;331:624–627.
303. Staunton DE, Marlin SD, Stratowa C, Dustin ML, Springer TA. Primary structure of intercellular adhesion molecule 1 (ICAM-1) demonstrates interaction between members of the immunoglobulin and integrin supergene families. *Cell* 1988;52:925–933.
304. Osborn L, Hession C, Tizard R, Vassallo C, Luhowskyj S, Chi-Rosso G, Lobb R. Direct cloning of vascular cell adhesion molecule 1 (VCAM-1), a cytokine-induced endothelial protein that binds to lymphocytes. *Cell* 1989;59:1203–1211.
305. Polte T, Newman W, Gopal TV. Full length vascular cell adhesion molecule 1 (VCAM-1). *Nucleic Acids Res* 1990;18:5901.
306. Schall TJ. Biology of the RANTES/SIS cytokine family. *Cytokine* 1991;3:165–183.
307. Rot A, Krieger M, Brunner T, Bischoff SC, Schall TJ, Dahinden CA. RANTES and macrophage inflammatory protein 1α induce the migration and activation of normal human eosinophil granulocytes. *J Exp Med* 1992;176:1489–1495.
308. Alam R, Forsythe PA, Stafford S, Lett-Brown MA, Grant JA. Macrophage inflammatory protein-1α activates basophils and mast cells. *J Exp Med* 1992;176:781–786.
309. Kameyoshi Y, Dörschner A, Mallet AI, Christophers E, Schröder JM. Cytokine RANTES released by thrombin-stimulated platelets is a potent attractant for human eosinophils. *J Exp Med* 1992;176:587–592.
310. Hynes RO. Integrins: Versatility, modulation, and signalling in cell adhesion. *Cell* 1992;69:11–25.
311. Hemler ME. VLA proteins in the integrin family: Structures, functions, and their role on leukocytes. *Annu Rev Immunol* 1990;8:365–400.
312. Bochner BS, Luscinskas FW, Gimbrone MA Jr, Newman W, Sterbinsky SA, Derse-Anthony CP, Klunk D, Schleimer RP. Adhesion of human basophils, eosinophils, and neutrophils to interleukin 1-activated human vascular endothelial cells: Contributions of endothelial cell adhesion molecules. *J Exp Med* 1991;173:1553–1556.
313. Horgan KJ, Luce GEG, Tanaka Y, Schweighoffer T, Shimizu Y, Sharrow SO, Shaw S. Differential expression of VLA-α4 and VLA-β1 discriminates multiple subsets of $CD4^{+}CD45RO^{+}$ "memory" T cells. *J Immunol* 1992;149:4082–4087.
314. Kilshaw PJ, Murant SJ. Expression and regulation of $\beta_7(\beta_p)$ integrins on mouse lymphocytes: Relevance to the mucosal immune system. *Eur J Immunol* 1991;21:2591–2597.
315. Alon R, Hammer DA, Springer TA. Lifetime of the P-selectin: carbohydrate bond and its response to tensile force in hydrodynamic flow. *Nature* 1995;374:539–542.
316. Lawrence ML, Berg EL, Butcher EC, Springer TA. Rolling of lymphocytes and neutrophils on peripheral node addressin and subsequent arrest on ICAM-1 in shear flow. *Eur J Immunol* 1995 (*in press*).

Atherosclerosis and Coronary Artery Disease,
edited by V. Fuster, R. Ross, and E. J. Topol.
Lippincott-Raven Publishers, Philadelphia © 1996.

CHAPTER 30

The Role of Macrophages

Elaine W. Raines, Michael E. Rosenfeld, and Russell Ross

Key Words: Atherosclerosis; Lipid; Macrophage; Monocyte; Phagocyte.

INTRODUCTION

A common feature observed in the lesions of atherosclerosis at all stages of lesion development is the presence of monocytes/macrophages. However, other than their ability to accumulate large amounts of lipid, we know relatively little about specific functions of these cells while they are resident in the artery wall. Although the macrophage is capable of secreting a number of mediators that may stimulate lesion progression, an alternative role of these cells, particularly early in lesion development, is most likely a protective response. However, with chronic inflammation and continued monocyte influx, a failure of that protective response may in part be responsible for lesion progression.

In this chapter, we summarize current knowledge of some of the general properties of the monocyte/macrophage with a particular focus on the properties of macrophages in developing lesions. We discuss how these and other capabilities of the monocyte/macrophage may affect cells in the artery wall and alter lesion development. Unresolved questions with particular relevance to the possible role of the monocyte/macrophage are also presented.

E. W. Raines: Department of Pathology, University of Washington School of Medicine, Seattle, Washington 98195.

M. E. Rosenfeld: Pathobiology and Interdisciplinary Program in Nutritional Sciences, University of Washington School of Medicine, Seattle, Washington 98195.

R. Ross: Department of Pathology, Center for Vascular Biology, University of Washington School of Medicine, Seattle, Washington 98195.

THE MONOCYTE/MACROPHAGE: GENERAL PROPERTIES OF A MULTIPOTENT EFFECTOR CELL

The mononuclear phagocyte is known to be an important part of the normal host defense mechanism, principally through its capacities to act as a scavenger cell, an antigen-

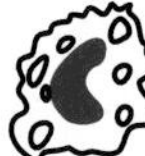
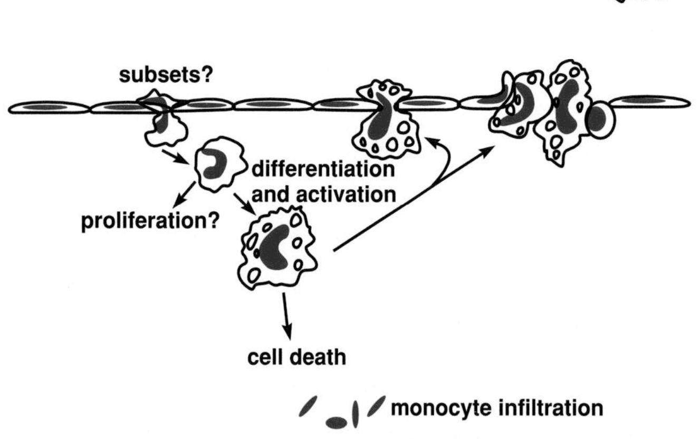

FIG. 1. Monocyte/macrophage influx and turnover in lesions of atherosclerosis. Monocytes adhere to the endothelium at lesion-prone sites (Fig. 2), crawl between the endothelial cells, and localize within the forming intima. Many of these monocytes/macrophages are positive for proliferating cell nuclear antigen (PCNA) (Fig. 7), consistent with cell replication and/or DNA repair. Uptake of lipid with subsequent "foam cell" formation is observed at all stages of lesion development. This uptake may be dependent on monocyte differentiation and may be involved in monocyte/macrophage activation. Lipid-filled macrophages can be observed squeezing between endothelial cells in an apparent exit from the intima (Fig. 3). These foam cells are also seen in areas of endothelial cell denudation and may be involved in promoting the endothelial cell dysfunction associated with endothelial cell loss (Fig. 9). Macrophages in the core of the lesion die but leave cellular antigens that can be detected (Fig. 8). Within more advanced lesions, areas of neovascularization serve as an additional avenue for monocyte infiltration.

presenting cell, and a secretory cell. A hallmark of any chronic inflammatory response is the presence of numerous macrophages together with variable numbers of lymphocytes. In most inflammatory situations, the macrophage contributes to the resolution by scavenging debris from interstitial tissues and then migrating from the site of injury, thereby removing tissue debris (Fig. 1).

Monocytes and probably recently immigrated macrophages are not fully mature cells and can develop further functional competence, as well as undergo further divisions, after they have entered the tissue (1). The transformation into tissue macrophages is presumably a response to developmental as well as tissue-specific stimuli. In the bone marrow, for example, the presence of colony-stimulating factors (CSF) such as GM-CSF and M-CSF have been shown to be important for the subsequent induction of different macrophage phenotypes following migration of the committed bone marrow progenitors (monocytes) into specific tissues (2). Further, there appear to be extensive functional and antigenic variations in tissue macrophages that may reflect both stages of differentiation and/or activation of the macrophages (3) in response to tissue-specific stimuli. These variations exist both among different tissues and in different areas of the same tissue (4,5). For example, within a single tissue such as the spleen, phenotypic subsets of monocytes and macrophages have been defined based on different antigens expressed on their cell surface and based on differences in morphology and function (6). In some instances, the mononuclear phagocytes terminally differentiate into multinucleated giant cells, and their presence characterizes granulomatous inflammatory responses.

Circulating monocytes spontaneously undergo programmed cell death (apoptosis) unless they are stimulated by monocyte colony-stimulating factor (M-CSF) or inflammatory mediators (7). However, as circulating monocytes differentiate into mature macrophages, this requirement is lost, and tissue macrophages have even been found to be resistant to apoptotic stimuli such as ionizing radiation (8). However, recent evidence suggests that differentiated macrophages retain a novel pathway that initiates apoptosis after activation with specific stimuli, such as zymosan (9). Sensitivity to activation-induced apoptosis appears to be determined in part by previous exposure to particular cytokines. The M-CSF exposure prevents apoptosis, whereas even transient exposure to the proinflammatory cytokine interferon-γ (IFN-γ) increases this apoptotic pathway.

The process of monocyte/macrophage activation is complex, as the effect of the activating signals depends on the state of differentiation of the cell and on the other signals it has met (3,10). Among leukocytes, the monocyte/macrophage secretes the most diverse selection of substances in response to stimuli, and these substances may have effects on surrounding tissues and adjacent cells (11). Table 1 lists the different categories of molecules secreted by macrophages, many with potential relevance to the process of atherogenesis.

TABLE 1. *Multipotent molecules secreted by monocytes/macrophages*

Cyclic nucleotides
Cytokines and immune-modulating factors
Cytotoxic substances
Enzymes and enzyme inhibitors involved in:
Coagulation
Hydrolysis of connective tissue
Lipoprotein metabolism
Extracellular matrix proteins
Factors regulating vascular tone
Prostaglandins and leukotrienes
Reactive oxygen intermediates
Regulators of lipoprotein metabolism
Substances regulating the migration and growth of other cells

In granulomatous inflammation, high-turnover lesions are maintained by brisk proliferation of endogenous macrophages as well as an extensive immigration of new mononuclear phagocytes (10). This response is dependent on the nature of the inciting agent and may be promoted by T cells within the lesion. Macrophages taken from sites of active inflammation have greatly increased properties for endocytosis, digestion, and secretion of a number of proteins, including a factor increasing monocytopoiesis (12). Interestingly, terminally differentiated macrophages containing endocytosed material appear to be the most down-regulated in terms of phagocytic and adherent functions (13). In contrast, when macrophages are pushed to their terminal stage of maturation, evidence exists for a 20- to 30-fold increase in their production of oxygen free radicals in response to zymosan and for down-regulation of c-*fms,* the M-CSF receptor (14). These observations are consistent with M-CSF as a negative regulator of the macrophage respiratory burst (15). Because M-CSF appears to be required for the survival of macrophages and is thought to act by suppressing apoptosis (9,16), either terminal differentiation or a failure of the local environment to support macrophage survival by the production of CSFs could lead to an increase in oxygen free radicals and a decrease in viable macrophages capable of continued removal of debris. All of these elements could be part of the mechanism limiting the extent of an inflammatory response.

PROPERTIES OF THE MONOCYTE/ MACROPHAGE IN DEVELOPING LESIONS OF ATHEROSCLEROSIS

Early Attraction and Retention in Lesion-Prone Areas

One of the earliest observable phenomena in the atherogenic process in hypercholesterolemic animal models is monocyte adherence to the endothelium in nonrandom clusters at lesion-prone sites (17–19) (Fig. 2). As described by Springer and Cybulsky *(this volume),* this process appears to be regulated in large part by the induced expression of specific adherence molecules on endothelial cells, such as vascular cell adhesion molecule 1 (VCAM-1), specific for monocytes and lymphocytes. Up-regulation of VCAM-1 on the surface of the endothelial cells of hypercholesterolemic rabbits precedes detectable intimal monocyte/macrophage accumulation by approximately 1 week (20). VCAM-1 is not expressed by aortic endothelium in normocholesterolemic rabbits except at lesion-prone sites that presumably reflect flow-induced expression as has been observed in vitro (21). However, VCAM-1 is not the only endothelial cell adhesion molecule involved in lesion formation. For example, an antibody to the β_2 integrin on monocytes completely blocks monocyte interaction with ICAM-1 on endothelial cells and partially blocks monocyte emigration into the injured carotid artery in a rabbit model of experimental atherosclerosis (22).

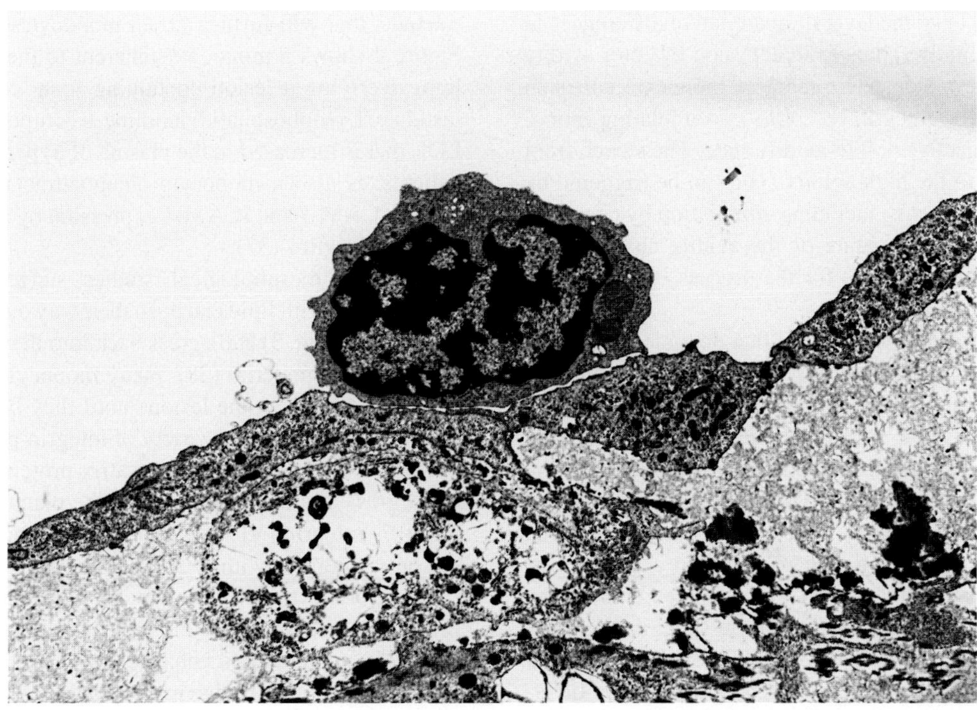

FIG. 2. Monocyte adherence to lesion-prone sites is among the earliest changes seen in developing lesions and persists throughout development of lesions of atherosclerosis. In this transmission electron micrograph, an adherent monocyte is observed attached to the intact endothelium in an early lesion in the thoracic aorta of a 6-week-old WHHL rabbit. (Magnification $\times$34,000.)

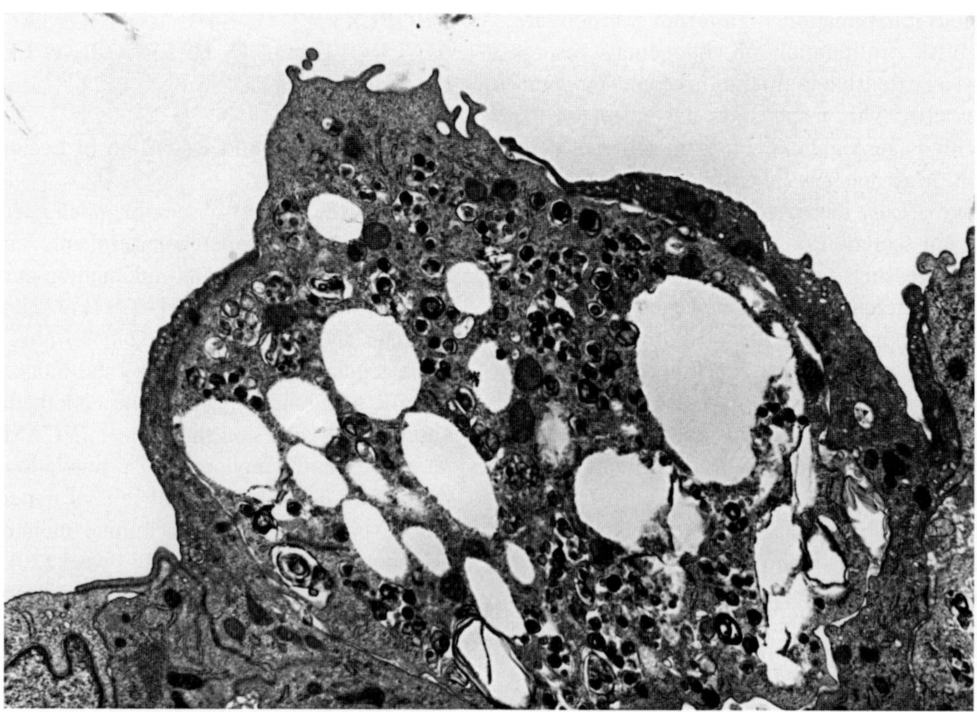

FIG. 3. A lipid-filled foam cell protruding between two endothelial cells. This transmission electron micrograph demonstrates a lipid-filled macrophage that is exposed to the lumen in a transitional lesion from the thoracic aorta of a 9-month-old WHHL rabbit. (Magnification ×40,000.)

A combined blockade of VCAM-1 and ICAM-1 totally prevents monocyte accumulation in the same model (23).

Although the regulation of endothelial cell adhesion molecules appears to be at the level of quantitative differences in expression, qualitative changes in adhesion receptor avidity appear to be the major determinant of monocyte adhesion (24,25). Normally, integrin receptors on circulating monocytes are in an inactive or low-avidity state. The switch from the low-avidity to the high-avidity state can be triggered by a variety of mechanisms, including stimulation by chemoattractants. The transient nature of the avidity changes provides a potential mechanism for the process of deadhesion during cell migration.

The same morphological studies that documented monocyte adherence as the earliest observable cellular event also demonstrated that, following adherence, the monocytes spread, crawl between the endothelial cells, and localize under the endothelium in the intima, where they become foam cells (17–19) Figs. 3 & 4. This demonstration suggests that the monocytes squeeze between the endothelial cells and migrate into the intimas in response to a gradient of chemoattractants situated within the subendothelial space. Expression and production of monocyte-specific chemoattractants MCP-1 (26–30), TNF-α (31,32), IL-1 (32,33), and M-CSF (34,35) appear to be increased in atherosclerotic lesions of both humans and experimental animals. However, based on immunocytochemistry and in situ hybridization at the light microscopic level, it is not clear that endothelial cells are the source of all of these factors in vivo. Rather, it appears that the expression of these factors by smooth muscle cells and monocytes/macrophages already resident within developing lesions may also contribute to chemoattractants that will further attract monocytes into the intima. Figure 2 shows a monocyte adherent to the intact endothelium overlying a lesion containing foam cells and plasma insudate. Lysophosphatidylcholine, a component of oxidized LDL that is increased in the plasma of hypercholesterolemic patients, is also a monocyte chemoattractant (36) and induces VCAM-1 and ICAM-1 expression by arterial endothelial cells in vitro (37).

Although morphological studies suggest that macrophages filled with lipid can push their way out between endothelial cells (Fig. 3) and egress back into the circulation with their ingested material (38), many monocytes/macrophages appear to remain in the lesions until they become necrotic. Macrophages express a variety of integrin proteins that will interact with several different matrix proteins and may prevent egress and movement within the plaque. One example is the β_2 integrin (VLA-4) expressed by monocytes, which not only interacts with VCAM-1 but also with the matrix protein fibronectin (39). In vitro, the chemoattractants MCP-1, MIP-1α, and RANTES increase expression of the β_2 integrins (40), which could enhance both endothelial cell binding and retention of the macrophages within the lesion. Freezing the integrins in the activated state, as has been observed with $\alpha^5\beta_1$ integrin in the human monocyte cell line THP-1 following differentiation (41), could also prevent cell migration out of the lesion. Smooth muscle cell expres-

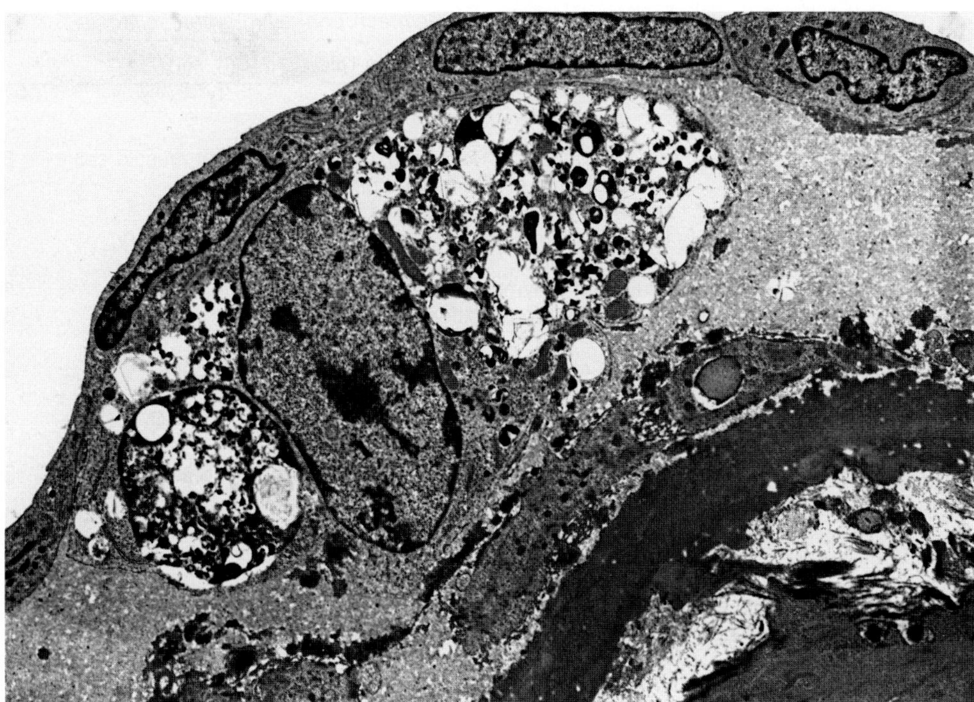

FIG. 4. The monocyte/macrophage is a phagocytic effector cell. This transmission electron micrograph shows a lipid-filled macrophage that appears to have engulfed another cell in an early atherosclerotic lesion from the thoracic aorta of a 6-week-old WHHL rabbit. (Magnification ×24,000.)

sion of VCAM-1 and ICAM-1 in atherosclerotic but not normal vessels (42–45) may further contribute to monocyte/macrophage retention. It is interesting to note that scavenger receptors, in addition to being involved in uptake of modified lipoproteins, can also serve as adhesion receptors (46).

States of Differentiation and Activation

Are All Stages of Macrophage Differentiation Observed in Lesions?

The activation state of monocytes/macrophages within a developing lesion is likely to depend on both the differentiation state of the cell and the local environment. This is suggested by an immunohistochemical study of human aorta and coronary and carotid arteries, in which the differentiation state of monocytes in diffuse intimal thickening, fatty streaks, and atheromatous plaques was evaluated (47). A major phenotype in diffuse intimal thickening, but also observed in subendothelial layers in fatty streaks and more advanced plaques, were cells that stained for MHC class II antigens and CD14 (also referred to as Leu M_3 or gp55, which can function as a receptor for lipopolysaccharide). These same cells were only weakly positive for acid phosphatase and showed no evidence of lipid uptake. Many of these cells were in close apposition with T cells that also stained for MHC class II antigens. Figure 5 (see Colorplate 20) shows a fibrofatty lesion in which immunostaining for HLA-DR is primarily associated with macrophages. These observations would be consistent with the macrophage serving as an antigen-presenting cell in an immune response (see chapter by Hansson, *this volume*). In vitro studies also suggest that HLA-DR expression may be enhanced under hypercholesterolemic conditions (48), with HLA-DR expression most prominent in monocyte-derived macrophages throughout lesion development in hypercholesterolemic models (49).

In contrast, the primary monocytic phenotype seen in fatty streaks and localized to the outer layers of more advanced lesions showed staining for the complement C3bi receptor (OKM1) together with acid phosphatase and oil red O staining for lipid. Finally, large monocytic cells filled with lipid and acid phosphatase in more advanced lesions were immunostained with an antibody to the thrombospondin receptor with little or no expression of the C3bi receptor, especially toward the core of the lesion. These observations are consistent with a gradual shift toward a more differentiated phenotype with presumably longer residence time within the lesion. This interpretation is also supported by staining of fatty streaks with antibodies more specific to circulating monocytes that do not recognize tissue macrophages or foam cells in lesions (50,51). Two proteins that are increased in atherosclerosis and may have functional significance within developing lesions (Table 2), the scavenger receptor and the LDL receptor-related protein (LRP), are also increased during monocyte/macrophage differentiation and foam cell formation in vitro (52,53).

TABLE 2. *Molecules expressed by monocytes/macrophages in atherosclerosis*

Molecule	Possible role	Reference
Secreted proteins		
Cytokines and immune-modulating factors		
Interleukin-1 (IL-1)	Increase adhesion molecule expression, smooth muscle cell migration and proliferation, immune modulation, secondary gene induction	32,33
Interleukin-6 (IL-6)	Activation of coagulation, smooth muscle cell secondary gene induction	129,130
Interleukin-8 (IL-8)	Recruitment of lymphocytes and endothelial cells	29
Leukemia inhibitory factory (LIF)	Differentiation and proliferation of T cells	131
Monocyte chemoattractant protein-1 (MCP-1)	Monocyte chemoattractant, activation of β_2 integrins	26–30
Monocyte colony-stimulating factor (M-CSF)	Monocyte chemoattraction, proliferation, and survival	34,35
Tumor necrosis factor-α (TNF-α)	Increase endothelial cell adhesion molecule expression, monocyte chemoattractant, smooth muscle cell proliferation	31
Enzymes and inhibitors		
Collagenase	Matrix degradation, cell migration, possible plaque rupture, and plaque expansion	117,118
Complement C3b	Prothrombotic and promotion of lipoprotein uptake	132
Factor XIIIa	Prothrombotic	50
Gelatinase	Matrix degradation, cell migration, possible plaque rupture, and plaque expansion	117,118
Lipoprotein lipase	Alteration of lipoprotein metabolism and hydrolysis of core triglycerides of lipoproteins	133–135
15-Lipoxygenase	LDL oxidation and foam cell formation	57
Myeloperoxidase	Formation of cytoxins and reactive oxygen intermediates that oxidize lipoproteins	113
Plasminogen-activator inhibitor	Antifibrinolytic	125,126
Stromelysin	Connective tissue degradation, cell migration, and possible plaque rupture and plaque expansion	116–118
Timp 1 and 2	Prevention of matrix degradation by blocking proteolytic processing of zymogens or blocking substrate binding	117
Extracellular proteins		
Matrix Gla protein (MGP)	Cell adhesion, regulation of calcification	136
Osteopontin	Cell adhesion and migration, neovessel formation, and calcification	137–139
SPARC, osteonectin	Cell migration, proliferation, and neovessel formation	140
Thrombospondin	Cell migration, neovessel formation	122
Regulators of lipoprotein metabolism		
Apolipoprotein E	Modulation of lipoprotein uptake	54,103,134,141–143
27-Hydroxycholesterol	Side-chain degradation in the formation of bile acids from cholesterol	143
Serum amyloid A	Acute phase reactant associated with HDL alteration of lipoprotein metabolism, immune response and platelet function, monocyte chemoattractant	144,145
Substances regulating the migration and growth of other cells		
Acidic fibroblast growth factor (aFGF)	Endothelial cell chemoattractant and proliferation	146,147
Heparin-binding epidermal growth factor (HB-EGF)	Smooth muscle cell chemoattraction and proliferation	148
Platelet-derived growth factor (PDGF)	Smooth muscle cell chemoattraction and proliferation	56
Endothelin-1	Vasoconstriction	149
Cell-Associated Proteins		
Adhesion molecules		
Vascular adhesion molecule-1 (VCAM-1)	Monocyte/macrophage activation and retention	44,150,151
Intercellular cell adhesion molecule (ICAM-1)	Monocyte/macrophage activation and retention	42,150,151
Connexin 43	Gap junctional communication	152

(continued)

TABLE 2. *Continued.*

Molecule	Possible role	Reference
Receptors for		
Advanced glycation end products (AGEs)	Monocyte activation and induction of oxidant stress	153
Complement C3bi	Thrombosis and lipoprotein uptake	131
α_2-Macroglobulin/LDL-receptor-related protein (LRP)	Foam cell formation, uptake of cytokine–α_2-M complexes, protease clearance including plasminogen activator–inhibitor complexes	102,154,155
Modified LDL (scavenger receptor)	Foam cell formation, monocyte recruitment and adhesion	46,57,94,96,156
Thrombin	Monocyte/macrophage activation	157
Urokinase	Pericellular proteolysis facilitate migration	114
Other cell-associated proteins		
70-kDa heat shock protein	Cytoprotective to stress and lethal stimuli	106,158,159
Tissue factor	Coagulation and thrombosis	61

What is the State of Activation of Circulating Cells and Cells within Developing Lesions?

Given the long list of secretory products that the monocyte/macrophage is capable of releasing (Table 1), what do we know about their secretory activity in developing lesions of atherosclerosis? Table 2 lists the molecules expressed by monocytes/macrophages in both experimental models and human lesions, together with their potential roles in atherogenesis. Of particular interest are studies in which combinations of molecules have been evaluated. Some of these studies suggest that there may be selective activation of macrophage functions. For example, increased levels of mRNA for apolipoprotein E and the M-CSF receptor, c-*fms*, are observed in advanced human lesions without elevation of mRNA levels for IL-1 or IL-6 (54). However, such selective activation may depend on the stage of lesion development. Others have reported macrophage foam cells expressing IL-1, TNF-α, and IL-6 in more advanced lesions, but only IL-1 and TNF-α in earlier lesions from young children (55). It is also clear that even within a given lesion, not all macrophages are activated to express the same products. Figure 6B (see Colorplate 21) shows that staining for PDGF-B-chain occurs in only a subset of the macrophages in the human advanced lesion shown. In contrast, PDGF-B chain staining is observed in macrophages throughout the fatty streak from a hypercholesterolemic nonhuman primate (Fig. 6A; see Colorplate 21). Further, immunocytochemical and in situ hybridization studies of macrophage gene expression in human and experimental atherosclerotic lesions have shown that not all macrophages in the lesions are simultaneously induced to express PDGF-BB (56), 15-lipoxygenase (57), MCP-1 (26), and M-CSF (35) or contain oxidation-specific lipid–protein adducts (58). These and other studies raise the possibility that there may be different subsets of monocytes recruited to developing lesions.

There is also accumulating evidence that under some circumstances activation of circulating monocytes may occur prior to entry into the lesions and may be associated with particular risk factors. Monocytes from homozygous familial hypercholesterolemic patients show abnormalities in eicosanoid metabolism (consequently, in the formation of leukotrienes), decreased superoxide anion generation, and increased adhesion (59). Examination of 26 patients with unstable angina demonstrated increased tissue factor expression in isolated monocytes, with and without stimulation, and increased plasma levels of fibrinogen (60). However, the increase in tissue factor expression does not appear to be a consequence of hypercholesterolemia (60,61). Patients with ischemic heart disease have also been reported to have increased secretion of TNF-α in isolated monocytes (62). It is possible that the adhesion process itself may be sufficient to induce activation and the expression of particular monocyte products. Production of the mononuclear chemoattractant protein, MIP-1α, can be inhibited in vitro by blocking ICAM-1-mediated interaction with endothelial cells (63). Both TNF-α and IL-1 release from monocytes can also be induced in vitro by engagement of monocyte proteoglycans (LFA-3, CD44, and CD45) known to be involved in cell–cell adhesion (64).

Is There Evidence for the Presence of Macrophage-Activating Agents in Atherosclerotic Lesions?

The presence of T cells and expression of MHC class II antigens in developing lesions are consistent with an immune response to foreign antigens (see chapter by Hansson, *this volume*). Modified lipoproteins are a particularly probable candidate antigen. Studies have clearly identified the presence of circulating autoantibodies and antibodies within lesions that recognize modified lipoproteins (65) as well as isolation of multiple T-cell clones from human lesions that recognize oxidized LDL (66).

The high prevalence and early onset of cardiovascular disease in patients with diabetes mellitus have focused attention on the potential role of advanced glycosylation end products (AGEs) that accumulate on long-lived extracellular matrix proteins in diabetic individuals (67). From in vitro studies, it appears that AGEs may have the capability within the vascular wall of trapping lipoproteins (68), modifying lipoproteins (69), inactivating nitric oxide activity (70), and interacting with specific cell-surface receptors to induce cytokine and growth factor release from monocytes (71). High levels of AGEs have been observed in lesions in coronary vessels of patients with type II diabetes but not in lesions from nondiabetic individuals (72).

Recent evidence has demonstrated the presence of *Chlamydia pneumoniae* antigens and nucleic acid in coronary atheromas from autopsy patients in South Africa (73). From 25% to 35% of fatty streaks and fibrous plaques stained with antibodies to the *Chlamydia pneumoniae* antigens, and electron micrographs demonstrated their presence within the cytoplasm of both macrophages and smooth muscle cells. As detailed by Kaner and Hajjar *(this volume)*, epidemiologic and pathological evidence exists linking cytomegalovirus and herpes virus infection and atherosclerosis. Particularly intriguing is the in vitro evidence for viral activation of the coagulating cascade and monocyte adhesion to endothelial cells (74).

Thus, a number of examples exist for potential monocyte-activating agents such as AGEs and viral antigens being present in atherosclerotic lesions. Some of these may be particularly prevalent with specific risk factors. More uniformly observed is the association of activated macrophages with lesions containing T cells.

Macrophage Proliferation

As in other inflammatory responses, there is evidence that monocytes/macrophages in lesions of atherosclerosis may be stimulated to proliferate. Early morphological studies by McMillan and Duff (75) demonstrated the presence of mitotic spindles in foam cells within rabbit lesions. Following the development of rabbit macrophage-specific monoclonal antibodies (76), it was demonstrated that up to 40% of the cells that take up thymidine are monocytes/macrophages in atherosclerotic lesions of both cholesterol-fed and Watanabe heritable hyperlipidemic (WHHL) rabbits, using simultaneous immunocytochemistry and ^{3}H-thymidine autoradiography (58). In a fibrofatty lesion from the nonhuman primate (Fig. 7; see Colorplate 22), numerous PCNA-positive macrophages are observed at the base of the lesion. Similar studies by Gordon et al. (77), have demonstrated the presence of proliferating monocytes/macrophages in human coronary and carotid atherosclerotic lesions and in arteriovenous fistulas used for hemodialysis (77,78).

We have observed a distinct spatial variation in the distribution of thymidine-labeled, macrophage-derived foam cells within advanced atherosclerotic lesions in the rabbit (58). In most cases, there are more labeled foam cells situated within the lateral margins of the lesions than in other locations. Because these regions frequently resemble early fatty streaks, this occurrence suggests that macrophages that have newly arrived and are potentially less differentiated and/or activated may exhibit a greater proliferative capacity.

It is still unclear from studies to date on macrophage proliferation in atherosclerotic tissues whether the proliferating cells are monocytes or promonocytes. The fact that many of the proliferating monocytes/macrophages are foam cells suggests that the cells express scavenger receptors and are at least partially differentiated. It is also possible that the very large amount of oxidizable lipid within the foam cells may induce oxidative stress. One result of prolonged oxidative stress in many cell types is DNA fragmentation (79). Thus, the uptake of thymidine or the presence of the proliferating cell nuclear antigen (PCNA) may also be indicative of DNA repair. Interestingly, the chronic administration of the antioxidant probucol to hypercholesterolemic monkeys appears to inhibit macrophage proliferation (80). Further studies are required to differentiate between these two processes and clearly demonstrate that the inflammatory response that occurs in atherosclerotic lesions includes macrophage replication.

Macrophages and Lipid Accumulation

Presence of "Foam Cells" in Atherosclerotic Lesions

It has long been known that macrophages in most tissues function as "scavenger" cells, phagocytose necrotic cell debris, and sometimes appear to engulf whole cells, as shown in Fig. 4. Morphological studies have demonstrated the presence of phagocytic cells containing large numbers of vacuoles and non-membrane-bound lipid droplets in both human and experimental atherosclerotic lesions (81,82). The presence of a large number of lipid droplets gives the cells a "foamy" appearance under light and electron microscopes. Thus, the cells are generally referred to as "foam cells." Immunocytochemical analyses have established that many of these foam cells are of monocyte/macrophage origin (51,76,83) and that macrophage-derived foam cells constitute a significant but variable percentage of the total cells within atherosclerotic plaques at all stages of lesion development (84). This variation likely reflects differences in location within the vascular tree and severity of the plaques, differences in plasma cholesterol levels, as well as the presence of other risk factors.

Biochemical and histological studies of atherosclerotic tissue have demonstrated that lipids deposited in the artery wall during the atherogenic process are predominantly cholesterol esters (with cholesterol oleate being the primary cholesterol ester, especially in fatty streaks) and are likely derived from the direct deposition of lipoproteins in the artery wall (85–88). This demonstration is further supported by immunocytochemical studies with antibodies recognizing apoprotein B and autoradiographic studies using ^{125}I-tyramine-cellobiose-labeled LDL (a nondegradable LDL probe). They have shown that there is preferential trapping and retention of lipoproteins prior to the appearance of monocytes in arteries of cholesterol-fed animals at sites where lesions subsequently form (89–91). Once the monocytes have entered the intima, they appear to become foam cells very rapidly (19). Furthermore, studies with foam-cell-rich fatty streaks in WHHL rabbits have demonstrated that more than 60% of previously injected TC-LDL is found within macrophage-derived foam cells within 48 h (92).

Mechanisms of Lipid Accumulation in Macrophages

The hunt to find the pathways that enable macrophages to accumulate large amounts of lipoprotein-derived cholesterol esters led to the in vitro discovery that rapid lipid loading was dependent on lipoprotein modification and the expression of specific receptors on the plasma membrane of macrophages that bind and internalize the modified lipoproteins (93). Initial in vitro studies of murine peritoneal macrophages showed that these cells take up nonmodified LDL at very slow rates that do not lead to foam cell formation. However, if the LDL particles are modified by being made more cationic or by acetylation, there is rapid uptake and the formation of intracellular lipid droplets (94,95). The process was shown to be saturable and receptor medicated, and the receptor was termed the ''acetyl-LDL'' receptor or, more recently the ''scavenger'' receptor (93,94). There are now known to be at least two isoforms of the macrophage ''scavenger'' receptor (designated types I and II), both of which have been sequenced and cloned from bovine, murine, rabbit, and human macrophages (93). In vitro studies of freshly isolated peripheral blood monocytes show that these cells express low levels of type I and type II scavenger receptors, but there appears to be a selective increase in the level of type I mRNA and protein with differentiation and foam cell formation (52). Immunocytochemical and in situ hybridization studies have demonstrated that many macrophages in human atherosclerotic lesions express both types I and II scavenger receptors (57,96,97), suggesting that these cells have undergone some degree of differentiation following migration into the atherosclerotic lesions and have the capacity to accumulate modified lipoproteins.

Different types of lipoprotein modifications appear to facilitate foam cell formation in vitro, including acetylation, oxidation, aggregation, immune or matrix protein complex formation, and glycation (98). However, it is still unclear whether any of these modifications occur in vivo and lead to recognition by the scavenger receptors or by other macrophage receptors that have high affinities for binding of these variously modified lipoproteins. Immunocytochemical studies suggest that oxidized and glycated lipoproteins may exist in atherosclerotic lesions (58,72,99,100). It has also been shown that macrophages express a specific receptor that recognizes advanced glycosylation end-product proteins (AGE proteins) (101). In addition, macrophages in human atherosclerotic plaques express the LDL receptor-related-protein/α_2-macroglobulin receptor (LRP) (102), a receptor with a very high affinity for lipoproteins containing apoprotein E that is also increased with in vitro differentiation of monocytes (53). Macrophages in human and rabbit atherosclerotic lesions produce and secrete apoprotein E (apo E) (103), and the simultaneous expression of both apo E and the LRP may facilitate further lipid accumulation.

Why Do Foam Cells Form?

Accumulation of large amounts of lipid within macrophages most likely represents a protective phagocytic response to the accumulated and modified lipid. However, it also causes chronic oxidative stress and impairs cellular function. The very large lipid content of foam cells indicates that there is an imbalance between uptake and egress of lipid that may occur for several reasons. First, there appears to be unrestricted uptake of modified lipoproteins, as lipid accumulation does not down-regulate the expression of scavenger receptors (104). Further, if there is any lipid-dependent regulation of the expression of other potentially modified lipoprotein receptors, the continuous deposition and modification of the lipid in the artery wall appear to overwhelm this regulatory capacity.

Coupled with an unrestricted uptake is an apparent inability to generate enough free cholesterol from stored cholesterol esters to allow a balance in the rates of egress and uptake (only free cholesterol can diffuse out of a cell). In vitro studies of foam cells isolated from rabbit lesions indicate that the cells have extremely high levels of acyl-coenzyme A : cholesterol acyl transferase (ACAT) and lysosomal acid cholesterol-ester hydrolase activities but very low levels of cytoplasmic neutral cholesterol-ester hydrolase activity *(unpublished observations)*. This creates a cycle such that the small amount of free cholesterol generated is either utilized for membrane synthesis or rapidly reesterified. This may be further complicated by the absence or reduction of appropriate extracellular acceptors of the free cholesterol such as HDL.

A third possible contributor to the inability of developing foam cells to escape the artery may be the formation of the fibrous cap and/or the inhibition of motility following interactions with oxidized LDL (36). This possibility would prolong the residence time of the cells within the developing lesion and possibly enable foam cells to form even without expression of specific modified lipoprotein receptors.

Macrophage Cell Death and Formation of the Necrotic Core

The necrotic core is a hallmark of an advanced atherosclerotic lesion. It is generally a lipid-rich acellular region at the base of the plaque that contains cell debris and frequently becomes calcified. The presence of a necrotic core can radically alter the structural and contractile properties of the artery (105). However, to date, it is still unclear how the necrotic core is formed. A possibility is that macrophage-derived foam cells become trapped within the lesion by formation of the overlying fibrous cap. These cells must eventually die, either from apoptosis (programmed cell death) or possibly of hypoxia or the cytotoxic effects of oxidized lipids or cytokines secreted by other cells within the lesions. As the macrophages become necrotic, they would release their stored lipid and proteolytic enzymes into the extracellular matrix, leading to the formation of a large pool of lipid and cell debris. Consistent with this possibility is the observation that heat shock protein-70 (HSP-70), a protein elevated in cells under metabolic stress, is elevated in lesions of atherosclerosis, particularly around sites of necrosis and lipid accumulation (106).

To date, there is limited evidence for macrophage apoptosis in atherosclerotic lesions (107). However, there are in vitro studies demonstrating apoptosis in a variety of different types of macrophages, especially following treatment with TNF and other cytokines (108) or oxidized LDL (109). High concentrations of oxidized LDL have also been shown to be cytotoxic to many types of cells in vitro, including macrophages.

Immunocytochemical and biochemical studies of advanced lesions in humans and hypercholesterolemic animals strongly suggest that macrophages are involved in the formation of the necrotic core. These studies have demonstrated that, despite the absence of intact cells within the core, there are still macrophage-specific antigens throughout the core region (76,83), as shown for a human lesion in Fig. 8 (see Colorplate 23). It will be important to determine whether macrophage apoptosis or necrosis predominates in the formation of the necrotic core and if the balance between apoptosis and necrosis is shifted with particular risk factors or with other characteristics of the lesions. It is clear that the possible effectors released by macrophages will differ significantly with these two possibilities. For example, interleukin-1 (IL-1) is processed and released in active form during apoptosis, but not necrosis, of monocytes (110).

POTENTIAL ROLES OF MACROPHAGES IN LESION DEVELOPMENT AND PROGRESSION

The Macrophage as a Phagocytic Effector Cell

The early attraction and retention of monocytes in lesion-prone sites most likely represent the normal inflammatory response to clear the area of foreign or noxious materials that have accumulated locally. Thus, the scavenging of cytotoxic lipids resulting in foam cell formation appears to be a normal protective mechanism with pathological consequences. There is also immunocytochemical and biochemical evidence that lipid hydroperoxides, oxysterols, and other oxidation-specific epitopes characteristic of oxidized LDL exist in atherosclerotic lesions in association with macrophages of both humans and hypercholesterolemic animals (58,99,100). However, this is complicated by the fact that macrophages can themselves induce lipid hydroperoxide formation and the resultant cytotoxic products (111,112). This may potentially occur as a byproduct of the production of reactive oxygen species formed during the respiratory burst or via other cellular mechanisms including the production and secretion of 15-lipoxygenase (15-LO) or myeloperoxidase. The presence of both 15-LO and myeloperoxidase associated predominantly with macrophages has been demonstrated in human atherosclerotic plaques (57,113). The spectrum of oxidant species generated during phagocytic stimulation is highly variable and dependent on the extracellular environment (112).

Another important reason for removing lipid from the artery is its potential effects on the structural properties of the artery. For example, the formation of occlusive thrombi leading to terminal myocardial infarctions occurs following rupture of plaques. Most frequently, plaques rupture through areas of reduced tensile strength, which are usually the areas containing coalesced extracellular lipid (e.g., the lateral margins, where the fibrous cap covering the necrotic core is the thinnest) (105). However, these areas also contain the highest concentrations of macrophages and other inflammatory cells, which themselves appear to contribute to the reduction in tensile strength.

In the normal cycle of the inflammatory response, the cells would take up the foreign substances and reenter the circulation. Although there is evidence suggesting the reentry of some lipid-filled macrophages into the circulation in some experimental models of hypercholesterolemia (38) (Fig. 3), a significant number of macrophages remain within the atherosclerotic lesions. As discussed above, many of the macrophages that remain within the lesions die, through either apoptosis or necrosis. However, as a compensation for the cell death, there appears to be continued recruitment of monocytes into lesions throughout lesion development, primarily at shoulders or within neovascularized areas (Fig. 1). As a result of this continued recruitment of monocytes, a gradient of macrophage differentiation will occur. As has been described, the least mature cells are at the periphery, and the most differentiated are within the core. Because the activation of monocytes/macrophages varies with the state of differentiation and the local stimulants, one would predict a gradient of activation, and the response of adjacent cells to the products of this activation.

Effects of Macrophages on Other Cells Within the Artery Wall

Just as the monocyte/macrophage is dependent on other cells within the artery wall for the provision of M-CSF for survival, it can secrete a number of substances that affect the migration, proliferation, adherence, and metabolic state of other adjacent cells (see Table 2 for specific examples defined within developing lesions). Each of these substances has limited targets. For induction of biological activity, each requires expression of the specific receptor for this substance on the target cell. Some of the products such as MCP-1 and M-CSF would attract more monocytes and support their survival and proliferation. Others such as PDGF would promote smooth muscle cell migration and proliferation (114), and simultaneous expression of urokinase receptor would potentially facilitate migration (115). Matrix degradation induced by stromeylsin (116) and other matrix-degrading enzymes (117,118) could also enhance migration of smooth muscle cells or, alternatively, contribute to plaque rupture to be followed by thrombosis and further cellular infiltration. Still others, such as cytotoxic products like oxidized lipids, may result in endothelial cell dysfunction, suggested in Fig. 9 by the electron-dense endothelial cell overlying the foam cell in a nonhuman primate lesion.

Other macrophage products, such as apo E and lipoprotein lipase, may modulate lipoprotein modification and uptake by surrounding macrophages as well as endothelial cells and smooth muscle cells. Figure 10 (see Colorplate 24) shows immunostaining for some of these products in human lesions. The expression of other growth and metabolic mediators by the endothelial cells and smooth muscle cells in response to lipid uptake may be modulated. Thus, the monocyte/macrophage appears to be the key regulatory cell in amplifying the inflammatory response within the artery wall. Consistent with this are the early and continued presence of monocytes and macrophages throughout lesion development (119) and the association of macrophages with angiogenesis in more advanced lesions (120).

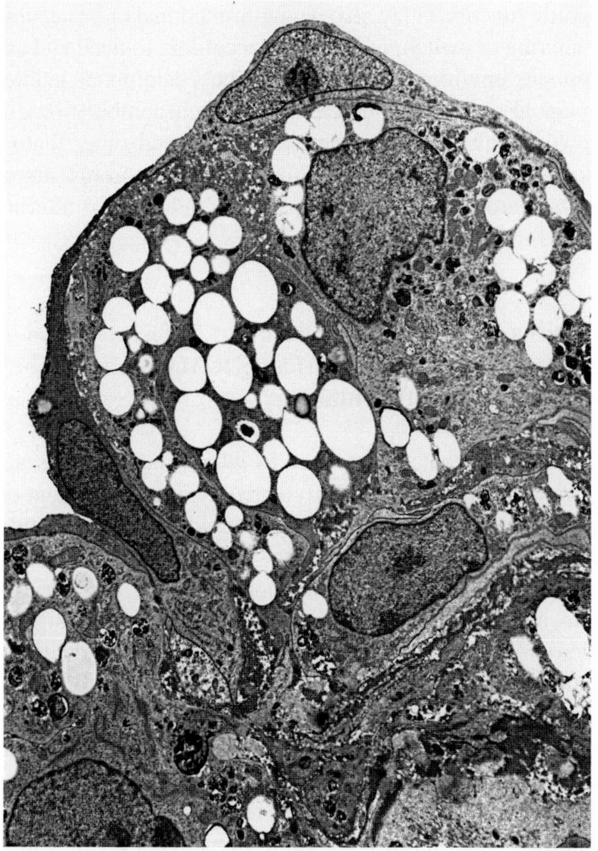

FIG. 9. Numerous examples of electron-dense endothelial cells are observed with endothelial cells stretched over lipid-filled macrophages. In this transmission electron micrograph from a nonhuman primate on a hypercholesterolemic diet for 6 months, the endothelial cell on the left has increased density compared with the endothelial cell on the right. Such changes are observed in cells following injury and cell damage and may reflect local release of toxic substances. (Magnification ×5,550.)

One would also predict that the capacity of the activated macrophage to be an effector cell will depend on its proximity to smooth muscle cells, lymphocytes, endothelial cells, or other macrophages. Electron microscopic evaluation of contacts between macrophages and lymphocytes as well as other macrophages in lesions of atherosclerosis has shown frequent close contacts (121). In contrast, there is an absence of contacts between smooth muscle cells and macrophages, implying more of a paracrine response to macrophage products. This is supported by studies showing that only smooth muscle cells situated adjacent to macrophages in human pulmonary arteries are stimulated to express type I collagen and fibronectin (122). Furthermore, it appears that endothelial cells expressing VCAM-1 in human lesions are frequently located over pockets of subendothelial macrophages (84).

Macrophages and the Fibrinolytic Process

A clear association has been established between an increased volume of monocytes/macrophages in the plaque cap and human aortic plaques undergoing ulceration and thrombosis (123). In these lesions, extracellular lipid pools occupied more than 40% of the cross-sectional area of the plaque. These observations are consistent with studies that indicate decreased tensile properties of monocyte/macrophage-enriched lesions (24). However, monocytes/macrophages may make other contributions that enhance or inhibit thrombosis. Even without the induction of frank endothelial denudation, which could be mediated by macrophage-derived cytotoxic agents, tissue factor expression on lipid laden macrophages could initiate thrombosis as they attempt to leave the lesion (61). Plaque rupture may be promoted by the release of enzymes such as stromelysin that degrade connective tissue (116). In contrast, monocyte/macrophage expression of plasminogen activator inhibitor-1 (PAI-1) within lesions would be expected to be antifibrinolytic (125,126).

UNRESOLVED QUESTIONS

What Attracts and Retains Monocytes in Lesion-Prone Areas?

Although a number of candidate molecules have been identified as discussed above, it is still unclear exactly which molecules support monocyte adherence to large-vessel endothelial cells, what induces the endothelial cells to express these adherence molecules, and what is the temporal expression of specific adhesion molecules during lesion development. Is activation of monocyte adherence molecules critical for endothelial cell binding and transmigration or for retention? In vitro, the endothelial cell adhesion molecules, VCAM-1 and ICAM-1, appear to be induced by alterations in flow-related shear forces (21) and by components of oxidized LDL, such as lysophosphatidylcholine (37). In vivo, does flow initiate the altered adhesion, and do components of oxidized LDL sustain the expression of adhesion molecules and induce the expression of further chemoattractants? There is strong evidence showing a preferential trapping and retention of LDL in lesion-prone sites of rabbit and pigeon aortas prior to the appearance of monocytes in the intima (90,91). If some of the trapped LDL becomes oxidized via either an autoxidation process or cell-mediated pathways, a chemical gradient of oxidized LDL particles could also induce adhesion molecules and attract monocytes into the intima. What other factors are involved, and how do they differ with individual risk factors?

Another unresolved question is what accounts for the retention of the monocytes within the lesions? As noted, there are several possible explanations for why the cells remain. One is that they are continuously bound to matrix proteins within the intima. Further studies are required to determine the nature and extent of monocyte/matrix interactions in vivo and where and when during the development of the lesions specific matrix proteins and their receptors are expressed.

Are There Subsets of Macrophages That Have Differential Effects on Lesion Progression?

The fact that not all macrophages within atherosclerotic lesions simultaneously express the same combination of proteins may simply represent differences in the residence time of the cells within the lesions and thus differences in the degree of differentiation and/or activation within the local microenvironment. On the other hand, as suggested by studies of macrophages in other tissues, it is also possible that there may be predetermined phenotypic subsets of macrophages that are capable of performing different functions. for example, one specific subset of macrophages may be primarily scavenger-type cells that perform house-cleaning functions, and other subsets may be programmed more for immune or inflammatory functions such as antigen presentation and bacteriocidal activities. Additional subsets may be involved with the regulation of vascular tone by virtue of their larger than normal capacity to produce prostanoids, nitric oxide, or vasoconstrictors, and others may function in the structural reorganization of the plaques by producing and secreting cytokines that stimulate smooth muscle cell connective tissue synthesis or secretion of metalloproteinases or their specific inhibitors. Unfortunately, to date, there is no direct evidence for the existence of macrophage subsets in atherosclerotic lesions that exhibit any of these functional differences.

With this in mind, we have performed preliminary immunocytochemical studies designed to determine whether there may be unique scavenger versus immune phenotypes within human lesions. As yet, we have not observed any clear distinction between subsets of macrophages expressing scavenger receptors and those expressing HLA-DR antigens (84). However, we did find macrophages in advanced lesions that were situated in close proximity to the necrotic core that expressed both scavenger receptors and HLA-DR antigens and contained oxidation-specific lipid protein adducts characteristic of oxidized LDL. This finding suggests that some macrophages may be multifunctional and able to accumulate oxidized LDL via the scavenger receptor and potentially present antigenic components of the oxidized LDL particles to T lymphocytes via the HLA-DR complex. A great deal of additional research is required to determine whether there are unique macrophage phenotypes that perform specialized functions. Furthermore, macrophages that appear to perform specific functions may also be multifunctional or be capable of altering or switching functions according to need and appropriate environmental signals. Thus, additional studies should also focus on determining which combinations of growth-regulatory molecules, cytokines, and other factors known to be sequestered within the microenvironments of atherosclerotic lesions are capable of inducing or altering arterial macrophage functions.

Do Different Risk Factors Result in Different Lesion Environments That Alter Monocyte/Macrophage Activation and Differentiation?

It is likely that the manner in which macrophages are activated or stimulated to differentiate will be dependent on the nature of the signals they encounter within the microenvironments of the artery wall. One approach to determining environmental effects on macrophages is to ask whether there are differences in lesion composition and resulting macrophage activity in lesions obtained from individuals exhibiting different, known risk factors for atherosclerosis. Unfortunately, there is a paucity of information concerning correlations between differences in lesion composition with different risk factors as well as any associated differences in the behavior of cells within these lesions. This is partially because of the absence of good animal models in which atherosclerotic lesion development is exacerbated by the presence of additional risk factors (e.g., diabetes, cigarette smoking). However, one possible exception is our knowledge of the effects of hypercholesterolemia. In studies of rabbits consuming large amounts of dietary cholesterol or in humans with homozygous familial hypercholesterolemia, where plasma cholesterol levels are extremely elevated, the resulting atherosclerotic lesions develop much more rapidly and contain a much higher percentage of macrophages than lesions that occur in less responsive animals or in humans with lower plasma cholesterol levels (18,127).

Poorly regulated plasma glucose levels or elevated plasma insulin, both of which occur in diabetes, are very likely to have profound effects on the environments within developing atherosclerotic lesions. Immunocytochemical evidence suggests an increase in AGEs in the arteries of diabetics as compared with lesions from nondiabetic patients. What macrophage products and activation markers are associated with this differential distribution of AGEs? Do AGEs simply represent another mechanism to enhance lipoprotein oxidation, and thus, are there commonalities in the inducing agents with different risk factors?

Is Overamplification of the Normal Macrophage Defensive Role Critical to Lesion Development? To Prevent Lesion Progression, Can This Macrophage-Protective Response Be Regulated?

As outlined in this chapter, the monocyte/macrophage is an important component of the normal host defense mechanism and, within lesions of atherosclerosis, expresses many of the proteins associated with this function (Table 2). However, is overamplification of this macrophage inflammatory response in the artery responsible for lesion progression and ultimately for clinical sequelae associated with heart disease? For example, in the process of phagocytosing lipoproteins that have accumulated in the vessel wall, the macrophage can produce further cytotoxic products and degrade the surrounding matrix, resulting in a substantial alteration of the structural properties of the artery. In addition, many of the molecules produced by macrophages within lesions would be expected to amplify the inflammatory response further, including promotion of macrophage survival and infiltration of more monocytes. Does enhanced survival of macrophages in lesions promote lesion expansion and chronicity of the inflammatory response? A critical component of wound resolution appears to be apoptosis (128), a process for which macrophage function is critical. Is dysregulation of apoptosis a contributor to lesion expansion? As in the wound-healing response, the macrophage is critical to the fibroproliferative response. In the artery, this includes stimulation of smooth muscle cell migration into the intima, proliferation, and connective tissue synthesis. This fibroproliferative response significantly contributes to lesion mass and may prevent the underlying macrophages from leaving the lesion. Does the prolonged retention of macrophages within the lesion further amplify the inflammatory response? Answers to these and other questions related to the regulation of the macrophage inflammatory response will allow us to better define, and possibly modulate, the role of macrophages in the development of lesions of atherosclerosis.

ACKNOWLEDGMENT

This research was supported by grants from the National Heart, Lung and Blood Institutes of Health, grants HL-18645 and HL-47151 to R.R. and E.W.R. and NIH grant RR-00166 to the Northwest Primate Center.

REFERENCES

1. van Furth R. Origin and turnover of monocytes and macrophages. *Curr Top Pathol* 1989;79:125–150.
2. Wijffels JFAM, de Rover Z, Kraal G, Beelen RHJ. Macrophage phenotype regulation by colony-stimulating factors at bone marrow level. *J Leukocyte Biol* 1993;53:249–255.
3. Adams DO, Hamilton TA. The cell biology of macrophage activation. *Annu Rev Immunol* 1984;2:283–318.
4. Van den Oord JJ, de Wolfe-Peeters C, Desmet VJ. The paracortical area in reactive lymph nodes demonstrating sinus histiocytosis. An enzyme and histochemical study. *Virchows Arch [B] Cell Pathol* 1985;48:77–85.
5. Buckley PJ, Smith MR, Braverman MF, Dikson SA. Human spleen contains phenotypic subsets of macrophages and dendritic cells that occupy discrete microanatomic locations. *Am J Pathol* 1987;128:505–520.
6. Rutherford MS, Witsell A, Schook LB. Mechanisms generating functionally heterogenous macrophages: Chaos revisted. *J Leukocyte Biol* 1993;53:602–618.
7. Mangan DF, Wahl SM. Differential regulation of human monocyte programmed cell death (apoptosis) by chemotactic factors and pro-inflammatory cytokines. *J Immunol* 1991;147:3408–3412.
8. van Furth R. Phagocytic cells: Development and distribution of mononuclear phagocytes in normal steady state and inflammation. In: Gallin JI, Goldstein IM, Snyderman R, eds. *Inflammation: Basic Principles and Clinical Correlates.* New York: Raven Press; 1988:218–295.
9. Munn DH, Beall AC, Song D, Wrenn RW, Throckmorton DC. Activation-induced apoptosis in human macrophages: Developmental regulation of a novel cell death pathway by macrophage colony-stimulating factor and interferon γ. *J Exp Med* 1995;181:127–136.
10. Adams DO, Hamilton TA. Molecular transductional mechanisms by which IFNγ and other signals regulate macrophage development. *Immunol Rev* 1987;97:5–27.
11. Nathan CF. Secretory products of macrophages. *J Clin Invest* 1987;79:319–326.
12. Sluiter W, Hulsing-Hesselink E, Elzenga-Claasen I, van Hemsbergen-Oomens LWM, van der Voort van der Kleij-van Andel A, van Furth R. Macrophages as origin of factor increasing monocytopoiesis. *J Exp Med* 1987;166:909–922.
13. Elliott DE, Boros DL. Schistosome egg antigen(s) presentation and regulatory activity by macrophages isolated from vigorous or immunomodulated liver granulomas of *Schistosoma mansoni*-infected mice. *J Immunol* 1984;132:1506–1510.
14. Kreipe H, Radzun HJ, Rudolph P, Barth J, Hansmann ML, Heidorn K, Parawaresch MR. Multinucleated giant cells generated in vitro. Terminally differentiated macrophages with down-regulated c-*fms* expression. Am J Pathol 1988;130:232–243.
15. Phillips WA, Hamilton JA. Colony stimulating factor-1 is a negative regulator of the macrophage respiratory burst. *J Cell Physiol* 1990;144:190–196.
16. Williams GT, Smith CA, Spooncer E, Dexter TM, Taylor DR. Haemopoietic colony stimulating factors promote cell survival by suppressing apoptosis. *Nature* 1990;343:76–79.
17. Gerrity RG. The role of the monocyte in atherogenesis. I. Transition of blood-borne monocytes into foam cells in fatty lesions. *Am J Pathol* 1981;103:181–190.
18. Faggiotto A, Ross R, Harker L. Studies of hypercholesterolemia in the nonhuman primate. I. Changes that lead to fatty streak formation. *Arteriosclerosis* 1984;4:323–340.
19. Rosenfeld ME, Tsukada T, Gown AM, Ross R. Fatty streak initiation in WHHL and comparably hypercholesterolemic fat-fed rabbits. *Arteriosclerosis* 1987;7:9–23.
20. Li H, Cybulsky MI, Gimbrone MA, Libby P. An atherogenic diet

rapidly induces VCAM-1, a cytokine-regulatable mononuclear leukocyte adhesion molecule, in rabbit aortic endothelium. *Arterioscler Thromb* 1993;13:197–204.
21. Nagel T, Resnick N, Atkinson WJ, Dewey CF Jr, Gimbrone MA Jr. Shear stress selectively upregulates intercellular adhesion molecule-1 expression in cultured human vascular endothelial cells. *J Clin Invest* 1994;94:885–891.
22. Kling D, Fingerle J, Harlan JM. Inhibition of leukocyte extravasation with a monoclonal antibody to CD18 during formation of experimental intimal thickening in rabbit carotid arteries. *Arterioscler Thromb* 1992;12:997–1007.
23. Kling D, Fingerle J, Harlan JM, Lobb RR, Lang F. Mononuclear leukocytes invade the arterial intima during thickening formation via CD18- and VLA-4-dependent mechanisms and stimulate smooth muscle migration. *Circ Res [in press]*
24. Hogg N, Harvey J, Cabanas C, Landis RC. Control of leukocyte integrin activation. *Am Rev Respir Dis* 1993;148:S55–59.
25. Smyth SS, Joneckis CC, Parise LV. Regulation of vascular integrins. *Blood* 1993;81:2827–2843.
26. Ylä-Herttuala S, Lipton BA, Rosenfeld ME, Särkioja T, Yoshimura T, Leonard EJ, Witztum JL, Steinberg D. Expression of monocyte chemoattractant protein-1 in macrophage-rich areas of human and rabbit atherosclerotic lesions. *Proc Natl Acad Sci USA* 1991;88: 5252–5256.
27. Yu X, Dluz S, Graves DT, Zhang L, Antoniades HN, Hollander W, Prusty S, Valente AJ, Schwartz CJ, Sonenshein GE. Elevated expression of monocyte chemoattractant protein 1 by vascular smooth muscle cells in hypercholesterolemic primates. *Proc Natl Acad Sci USA* 1992;89:6953–6957.
28. Takeya M, Yoshimura T, Leonard EJ, Takahashi K. Detection of monocyte chemoattractant protein-1 in human atherosclerotic lesions by an anti-monocyte chemoattractant protein-1 monoclonal antibody. *Hum Pathol* 1993;24:534–539.
29. Koch AE, Kunkel SL, Pearce WH, Shah MR, Parikh D, Evanoff HL, Haines GK, Burdick MD, Strieter RM. Enhanced production of the chemotactic cytokines interleukin-8 and monocyte chemoattractant protein-1 in human abdominal aortic aneurysms. *Am J Pathol* 1993; 142:1423–1431.
30. Nelken NA, Coughlin SR, Gordon D, Wilcox JN. Monocyte chemoattractant protein-1 in human atheromatous plaques. *J Clin Invest* 1991; 88:1121–1127.
31. Barath P, Fishbein MC, Cao J, Berenson J, Helfant RH, Forrester JS. Detection and localization of tumor necrosis factor in human atheroma. *Am J Cardiol* 1990;65:297–302.
32. Tipping PG, Hancock WW. Production of tumor necrosis factor and interleukin-1 by macrophages from human atheromatous plaques. *Am J Pathol* 1993;141:1721–1728.
33. Moyer CF, Sajuthi D, Tulli H, Williams JK. Synthesis of IL-1 alpha and IL-1 beta by arterial cells in atherosclerosis. *Am J Pathol* 1991; 138:951–960.
34. Clinton SK, Underwood R, Hayes L, Sherman ML, Kufe DW, Libby P. Macrophage-colony stimulating factor gene expression in vascular cells and in experimental and human atherosclerosis. *Am J Pathol* 1992;140:301–316.
35. Rosenfeld ME, Ylä-Herttuala S. Lipton BA, Ord VA, Witztum JL, Steinberg D. Macrophage colony-stimulating factor mRNA and protein in atherosclerotic lesions of rabbits and man. *Am J Pathol* 1992; 140:291–300.
36. Quinn MT, Parthasarathy S, Fong L, Steinberg D. Oxidatively modified low density lipoproteins: A potential role in the recruitment and retention of monocyte/macrophages during atherogenesis. *Proc Natl Acad Sci USA* 1987;84:2995–2998.
37. Kume N, Cybulsky MI, Gimbrone MA Jr. Lysophosphatidylcholine, a component of atherogenic lipoproteins induces mononuclear leukocyte adhesion molecules in cultured human rabbit endothelial cells. *J Clin Invest* 1992;90:1138–1144.
38. Faggiotto A, Ross R. Studies of hypercholesterolemia in the nonhuman primate. II. Fatty streak conversion to fibrous plaque. *Arteriosclerosis* 1984;4:341–356.
39. Mosesson MW. The role of fibronectin in monocyte/macrophage function. *Prog Clin Biol Res* 1984;154:155–175.
40. Vaddi K, Newton RC. Regulation of monocyte integrin expression by beta-family chemokines. *J Immunol* 1994;153:4721–4732.
41. Faull RJ, Kovach NL, Harlan JM, Ginsberg MH. Stimulation of integrin-mediated adhesion of T lymphocytes and monocytes: two mechanisms with divergent biological consequences. *J Exp Med* 1994;179: 1307–1316.
42. Poston RN, Haskard DO, Coucher JR, Gall NP, Johnson-Tidey RR. Expression of intercellular adhesion molecule-1 in atherosclerotic plaques. *Am J Pathol* 1992;140:665–673.
43. Printseva OY, Peclo MM, Gown AM. Various cell types in human atherosclerotic lesions express ICAM-1. Further immunocytochemical and immunochemical studies employing monoclonal antibody 10F3. *Am J Pathol* 1992;140:889–896.
44. O'Brien KD, Allen MD, McDonald TO, Chait A, Harlan JM, Fishbein D, McCarty J, Ferguson M, Hudkins K, Benjamin CD, Lobb R, Alpers CE. Vascular cell adhesion molecule-1 is expressed in human coronary atherosclerotic plaques. Implications for the mode of progression of advanced coronary atherosclerosis. *J Clin Invest* 1993;92:945–951.
45. Libby P, Li H. Vascular cell adhesion molecule-1 and smooth muscle cell activation during atherogenesis. *J Clin Invest* 1993;93:945–951.
46. Fraser I, Hughes D, Gordon S. Divalent cation-independent macrophage adhesion inhibited by monoclonal antibody to murine scavenger receptor. *Nature* 1993;364:343–346.
47. van der Wal AC, Das PK, Tigges AJ, Becker AE. Macrophage differentiation in atherosclerosis. An in situ immunohistochemical analysis in humans. *Am J Pathol* 1992;141:161–168.
48. Hughes DA, Townsend PJ, Haslam PL. Enhancement of the antigen-presenting function of monocytes by cholesterol: Possible relevance to inflammatory mechanisms in extrinsic allergic alveolitis and atherosclerosis. *Clin Exp Immunol* 1992;87:279–286.
49. Hansson GK, Seifert PS, Olsson G, Bondjers G. Immunohistochemical detection of macrophages and T lymphocytes in atherosclerotic lesions of cholesterol-fed rabbits. *Arterioscler Thromb* 1991;11: 745–750.
50. Poston RN, Hussain IF. The immunohistochemical heterogeneity of atheroma macrophages: Comparison with lymphoid tissues suggests that recently blood-derived macrophages can be distinguished from longer-resident cells. *J Histochem Cytochem* 1993;41:1503–1512.
51. Roessner A, Herrera A, Honing HJ, Vollmer E, Zwadlo G, Schurmann R, Sorg C, Grundmann E. Identification of macrophages and smooth muscle cells with monoclonal antibodies in the human atherosclerotic plaque. *Virchows Arch [A] Pathol Anat* 1987;412:169–174.
52. Geng YJ, Kodama T, Hansson GK. Differential expression of scavenger receptor isoforms during monocyte-macrophage differentiation and foam cell formation. *Arterioscler Thromb* 1994;14:798–806.
53. Watanabe Y, Inaba T, Shimano H, Gotoda T, Yamamoto K, Mokuno H, Sato H, Yazaki Y, Yamada N. Induction of LDL receptor-related protein during the differentiation of monocyte-macrophage. *Arterioscler Thromb* 1994;14:1000–1006.
54. Salomon RN, Underwood R, Doyle MV, Wang A, Libby P. Increased apolipoprotein E and c-*fms* gene expression without elevated interleukin 1 or 6 mRNA levels indicates selective activation of macrophage functions in advanced human atheroma. *Proc Natl Acad Sci USA* 1992;89:2814–2818.
55. Kishikawa H, Shimokama T, Watanbe T. Localization of T lymphocytes and macrophages expressing IL-1, IL-2 receptor, IL-6 and TNF in human aortic intima. Role of cell mediated immunity in human atherogenesis. *Virchows Arch [A] Pathol Anat* 1993;423:433–442.
56. Ross R, Masuda J, Raines EW, Gown AM, Katsuda S, Sasahara M, Malden LT, Masuko H, Sato H. Localization of PDGF-B protein in macrophages in all phases of atherogenesis. *Science* 1990;248: 1009–1012.
57. Ylä-Herttuala S, Rosenfeld ME, Parthasarathy S, Sarkioja T, Sigal E, Witztum JL, Steinberg D. Gene expression in macrophage-rich human atherosclerotic lesions: 15-Lipoxygenase and acetyl-LDL receptor mRNA colocalize with oxidation specific lipid-protein adducts. *J Clin Invest* 1991;87:1146–1152.
58. Rosenfeld ME, Ross R. Macrophage and smooth muscle cell proliferation in atherosclerotic lesions of WHHL and comparably hypercholesterolemic fat-fed rabbits. *Arteriosclerosis* 1990;10:680–687.
59. Stragliotto E, Camera M, Postiglione A, Sirtori M, Di Minno G, Tremoli E. Functionally abnormal monocytes in hypercholesterolemia. *Arterioscler Thromb* 1993;13:944–950.
60. Jude B, Agraou B, McFadden EP, Susen S, Bauters C, Lepelley P, Vanhaesbroucke C, Devos P, Cosson A, Asseman P. Evidence for time-dependent activation of monocytes in the systemic circulation

in unstable angina but not in acute myocardial infarction or in stable angina. *Circulation* 1994;90:1662–1668.
61. Landers SC, Madhu G, Lewis JC. Ultrastructural localization of tissue factor on monocyte-derived macrophages and macrophage foam cells associated with atherosclerotic lesions. *Virchows Arch* 1994;425: 49–54.
62. Vaddi K, Nicolini FA, Mehta P, Mehta JL. Increased secretion of tumor necrosis factor-alpha and interferon-gamma by mononuclear leukocytes in patients with ischemic heart disease. Relevance in superoxide anion generation. *Circulation* 1994;90:694–699.
63. Lukacs NW, Strieter RM, Elner VM, Evanoff HL, Burdick M, Kunkel SL. Intercellular adhesion molecule-1 mediates the expression of monocyte-derived MIP-1 alpha during monocyte-endothelial cell interactions. *Blood* 1994;83:1174–1178.
64. Webb DSA, Shimizu Y, Van Seventer GA, Shaw S, Gerrard TL. LFA-3, CD44, and CD45: Physiologic triggers of human monocyte TNF and IL-1 release. *Science* 1990;249:1295–1297.
65. Ylä-Herttuala S, Palinski W, Butler SW, Picard S, Steinberg D, Witztum JL. Rabbit and human atherosclerotic lesions contain IgG that recognizes epitopes of oxidized LDL. *Arterioscler Thromb* 1994;14: 32–40.
66. Stemme S, Hansson GK. Immune mechanisms in atherogenesis. *Ann Med* 1994;26:141–146.
67. Vlassara H, Bucala R, Striker L. Pathogenic effects of advanced glycosylation: Biochemical, biologic, and clinical implications for diabetes and aging. *Lab Invest* 1994;70:138–151.
68. Brownlee M, Vlassara H, Cerami A. Nonenzymatic glycosylation products on collagen covalently trap low-density lipoprotein. *Diabetes* 1985;34:938–941.
69. Bucala R, Makita Z, Koschinsky T, Cerami A, Vlassara H. Lipid advanced glycosylation: Pathway for lipid oxidation in vivo. *Proc Natl Acad Sci USA* 1993;90:6434–6438.
70. Bucala R, Tracey KJ, Cerami A. Advanced glycosylation products quench nitric oxide and mediate defective endothelium-dependent vasodilatation in experimental diabetes. *J Clin Invest* 1991;87: 432–438.
71. Kirstein M, Brett J, Radoff S, Ogawa S, Stern D, Vlassara H. Advanced protein glycosylation induces transendothelial human monocyte chemotaxis and secretion of platelet-derived growth factor: Role in vascular disease of diabetes and aging. *Proc Natl Acad Sci USA* 1990;87:9010–9014.
72. Nakamura Y, Horii Y, Nishino T, Shiiki H, Sakaguchi Y, Kogoshima T, Dohi K, Makita Z, Vlassara H, Bucala R. Immunohistochemical localization of advanced glycosylation end products in coronary atheroma and cardiac tissue in diabetes mellitus. *Am J Pathol* 1994;143: 1649–1656.
73. Kuo CC, Gown AM, Benditt EP, Grayston JT. Detection of *Chlamydia pneumoniae* in aortic lesions of atherosclerosis by immunocytochemical stain. *Arterioscler Thromb* 1993;13:1501–1504.
74. Etingin OR, Silverstein RL, Friedman HM, Hajjar DP. Viral activation of the coagulation cascade: Molecular interactions at the surface of the infected endothelial cells. *Cell* 1990;61:657–662.
75. McMillan GC, Duff GL. Mitotic activity in the aortic lesions of experimental atherosclerosis in rabbits. *Arch Pathol* 1948;46:179–182.
76. Tsukada T, Rosenfeld ME, Ross R, Gown AM. Immunocytochemical analysis of cellular components in lesions of atherosclerosis in the Watanabe and fat-fed rabbit using monoclonal antibodies. *Arteriosclerosis* 1986;6:601–613.
77. Gordon D, Reidy MA, Benditt EP, Schwartz SM. Cell proliferation in human coronary arteries. *Proc Natl Acad Sci USA* 1990;87: 4600–4604.
78. Rekhter MD, Nicholls SC, Ferguson M, Gordon D. Cell proliferation in human arteriovenous fistulas used for hemodialysis. *Arterioscler Thromb* 1993;13:609–617.
79. Schraufstatter IU, Hinshaw DB, Hyslop PA, Spragg RG, Cochrane CG. Oxidant injury of cells: DNA strand-breaks activate polyadenosine diphosphate-ribose polymerase and lead to depletion of nicotinamide adenine dinucleotide. *J Clin Invest* 1986;77:1312–1320.
80. Chang MY, Sasahara M, Chait A, Raines EW, Ross R. Inhibition of hypercholesterolemia-induced atherosclerosis in *Macaca nemestrina* by probucol: II. Cellular and molecular mechanisms.
81. Poole JC, Florey HW. Changes in the endothelium of the aorta and the behavior of macrophages in experimental atheroma of rabbits. *J Pathol Bacteriol* 1958;75:245–251.
82. Still WJ, Marriott PR. Comparative morphology of the early atherosclerotic lesion in man and cholesterol-atherosclerosis in the rabbit: An electron microscopic study. *J Atheroscler Res* 1964;4:373–386.
83. Gown AM, Tsukada T, Ross R. Human atherosclerosis. II. Immunocytochemical analysis of the cellular composition of human atherosclerotic lesions. *Am J Pathol* 1986;125:191–207.
84. Rosenfeld ME, Pestel E. Cellularity of atherosclerotic lesions. *Coronary Artery Dis* 1994;5:189–197.
85. Smith EB. The influence of age and atherosclerosis on the chemistry of aortic intima, part 1: The lipids. *J Atheroscler Res* 1965;5:224–240.
86. Geer JC, Malcolm GT. Cholesterol ester fatty acid composition of human aorta fatty streaks and normal intima. *Exp Mol Pathol* 1965; 4:500–507.
87. Insull W Jr, Bartsch GE. Cholesterol, triglyceride, and phospholipid content of intima, media, and atherosclerotic fatty streak in human thoracic aorta. *J Clin Invest* 1991;45:513–523.
88. Katz SS, Shipley GG, Small DM. Physical chemistry of the lipids of human atherosclerotic lesions: Demonstration of a lesion intermediate between fatty streaks and advanced plaques. *J Clin Invest* 1976;58: 200-211.
89. Nievelstein PF, Fogelman AM, Mottino G, Frank JS. Lipid accumulation in rabbit aortic intima 2 hours after bolus infusion of low density lipoprotein: A deep etch and immunolocalization study of ultrarapidly frozen tissue. *Arterioscler Thromb* 1991;11:1795–1805.
90. Schwenke DC, Carew TE. Initiation of atherosclerotic lesions in cholesterol-fed rabbits: I. Focal increases in arterial LDL concentration precede development of fatty streak lesions. *Arteriosclerosis* 1989;9: 895–907.
91. Schwenke DC, Carew TE. Initiation of atherosclerotic lesion in cholesterol-fed rabbits. II. Selective retention of LDL vs. selective increases in LDL permeability in susceptible sites of arteries. *Arteriosclerosis* 1989;9:908–918.
92. Rosenfeld ME, Khoo JC, Miller E, Parthasarathy S, Palinski W, Witztum JL. Macrophage-derived foam cells freshly isolated from rabbit atherosclerotic lesions degrade modified lipoproteins, promote oxidation of LDL, and contain oxidation specific lipid–protein adducts. *J Clin Invest* 1991;87:90–99.
93. Krieger M, Herz J. Structure and function of multiligand lipoprotein receptors: Macrophage scavenger receptors and LDL receptor-related protein (LRP). *Annu Rev Biochem* 1994;63:601–637.
94. Goldstein JL, Ho YK, Basu SK, Brown MS. Binding site on macrophages that mediates uptake and degradation of acetylated low density lipoproteins producing massive cholesterol deposition. *Proc Natl Acad Sci USA* 1979;76:333–337.
95. Brown MS, Basu SK, Falck JR, Ho YK, Goldstein JL. The scavenger cell pathway for lipoprotein degradation: Specificity of the binding site that mediates the uptake of negatively-charged LDL by macrophages. *J Supramol Struct* 1980;13:67–81.
96. Matsumoto A, Naito M, Itakura H, Ikemoto S, Asaoka H, Hayakawa I, Kanamori H, Aburatani H, Takaku F, Suzuki H, Kobari Y, Miyai T, Takahashi K, Cohen EH, Wydro R, Housman DE, Kodama T. Human macrophage scavenger receptors: Primary structure, expression, and localization in atherosclerotic lesions. *Proc Natl Acad Sci USA* 1990;87:9133–9137.
97. Naito M, Suzuki H, Mori T, Matsumoto A, Kodama T, Takahashi K. Coexpression of type I and type II human macrophage scavenger receptors in macrophages of various organs and foam cells in atherosclerotic lesions. *Am J Pathol* 1992;141:591–599.
98. Steinberg D, Parthasarathy S, Carew TE, Khoo JC, Witztum JL. Beyond cholesterol. Modifications of low-density lipoprotein that increase its atherogenicity. *N Engl J Med* 1989;320:916–924.
99. Palinski W, Rosenfeld ME, Ylä-Herttuala S, Gurtner GC, Socher SA, Butler SW, Parthasarathy S, Carew TE, Steinberg D, Witztum JL. Low density lipoprotein undergoes oxidative modification in vivo. *Proc Natl Acad Sci USA* 1989;86:1372–1376.
100. Ylä-Herttuala S, Palinski W, Rosenfeld ME, Parthasarathy S, Carew TE, Butler S, Witztum JL, Steinberg D. Evidence for the presence of oxidatively modified low density lipoprotein in atherosclerotic lesions of rabbit and man. *J Clin Invest* 1989;84:1086–1095.
101. Schmidt AM, Hasu M, Popov D, Zhang JH, Chen J, Yan SD, Brett J, Cao R, Kuwabara K, Costache G, Simionescu N, Simionescu M, Stern D. Receptor for advanced glycosylation end products (AGEs) has a central role in vessel wall interactions and gene activation in

response to circulating ACE proteins. *Proc Natl Acad Sci USA* 1994; 91:8807–8811.
102. Luoma J, Hiltunen T, Sarkioja T, Moestrup SK, Gliemann J, Kodama T, Nikkari T, Ylä-Herttuala S. Expression of alpha 2-macroglobulin receptor/low density lipoprotein receptor-related protein and scavenger receptor in human atherosclerotic lesions. *J Clin Invest* 1994;93: 2014–2021.
103. Rosenfeld ME, Butler S, Ord VA, Lipton BA, Dyer CA, Curtiss LK, Palinski W, Witztum JL. Abundant expression of apoprotein E by macrophages in human and rabbit atherosclerotic lesions. *Arterioscler Thromb* 1993;13:1382–1389.
104. Fogelman AM, Haberland ME, Seager J, Hokom M, Edwards PA. Factors regulating the activities of the low density lipoprotein receptor and the scavenger receptor on human monocytes-macrophages. *J Lipid Res* 1981;22:1131–1141.
105. Falk E. Why do plaques rupture? *Circulation* 1992;86:6(Suppl III)30–42.
106. Berberian PA, Jenison MW, Roddick V. Arterial prostaglandins and lysosomal function during atherogenesis. II. Isolated cells of diet-induced atherosclerotic aortas of rabbits. *Exp Mol Pathol* 1985;43: 36–55.
107. Han DKM, Haudenschild CC, Hong MK, Tjurmin A, Liau G, Kent KM. Apoptosis as a determinant of cellularity in advanced atherosclerotic lesions. *Circulation* 1994;90:I291.
108. van de Loosdrecht AA, Ossenkoppele GJ, Beelen RH, Broekhoven MG, Drager AM, Langenhuijsen MM. Apoptosis in tumor necrosis factor-alpha-dependent monocyte-mediated leukemic cell death: A functional, morphologic, and flow cytometric analysis. *Exp Hematol* 1993;21:1628–1639.
109. Reid VC, Mitchinson MJ, Skepper JN. Cytotoxicity of oxidized low density lipoprotein to mouse peritoneal macrophages: An ultrastructural study. *J Pathol* 1993;171:321–328.
110. Hogquist KA, Nett MA, Unanue ER, Chaplin DD. Interleukin 1 is processed and released during apoptosis. *Proc Natl Acad Sci USA* 1991;88:8485–8489.
111. Cathcart MK, Morel DW, Chisolm GM III. Monocytes and neutrophils oxidized low density lipoproteins making it cytotoxic. *J Leukocyte Biol* 1985;38:341–350.
112. Rosen GM, Pou S, Ramos CL, Cohen MS, Britigan BE. Free radicals and phagocytic cells. *FASEB J* 1995;9:200–209.
113. Daugherty A, Dunn JL, Rateri DL, Heinecke JW. Myeloperoxidase, a catalyst for lipoprotein oxidation is expressed in human atherosclerotic lesions. *J Clin Invest* 1994;94:437–444.
114. Raines EW, Ross R. Platelet-derived growth factor in vivo. In: Westermark B, Sorg C, eds. *Cytokines, Vol. 5, The Biology of PDGF.* Basel: S Karger, 1993:74–114.
115. Noda-Heiny H, Daugherty A, Sobel BE. Augmented urokinase receptor expression in atheroma. *Arterioscler Thromb* 1995;15:37–43.
116. Henney AM, Wakeley PR, Davies MJ, Foster K, Hembry R, Murphy G, Humphries S. Localization of stromelysin gene expression in atherosclerotic plaques by in situ hybridization. *Proc Natl Acad Sci USA* 1991;88:8154–8158.
117. Galis ZS, Sukhova GK, Lark MW, Libby P. Increased expression of matrix metalloproteinases and matrix degrading activity in vulnerable regions of human atherosclerotic plaques. *J Clin Invest* 1994;94: 2493–2503.
118. Galis ZS, Sukhova GK, Kranzhöfer R, Clark S, Libby P. Macrophage foam cells from experimental atheroma constitutively produce matrix-degrading proteinases. *Proc Natl Acad Sci USA* 1995;92:402–406.
119. Ross R. The pathogenesis of atherosclerosis: A perspective for the 1990s. *Nature* 1993;362:801–809.
120. Sunderkötter C, Steinbrink K, Goebeler M, Bhardwaj R, Sorg C. Macrophages and angiogenesis. *J Leukocyte Biol* 1994;55:410–422.
121. van der Wal AC, Dingemans KP, van den Bergh Weerman M, Das PK, Becker AE. Specialized membrane contacts between immunocompetent cells in human atherosclerotic plaques. *Cardiovasc Pathol* 1994;3:81–85.
122. Botney MD, Kaiser LR, Cooper JD, Mecham RP, Parghi D, Roby J, Parks WC. Extracellular matrix protein gene expression in atherosclerotic hypertensive pulmonary arteries. *Am J Pathol* 1992;140: 357–364.
123. Davies MJ, Richardson PD, Woolf N, Katz DR, Mann J. Risk of thrombosis in human atherosclerotic plaques: Role of extracellular lipid, macrophage and smooth muscle cell content. *Br Heart J* 1993; 69:377–381.
124. Lendon CL, Davies MJ, Born GV, Richardson PD. Atherosclerotic plaque caps are locally weakened when macrophage density is increased. *Atherosclerosis* 1991;87:87–90.
125. Lupu F, Bergonzelli GE, Heim DA, Cousin E, Genton CY, Bachmann F, Kruithof EK. Localization and production of plasminogen activator inhibitor-1 in human healthy atherosclerotic arteries. *Arterioscler Thromb* 1993;13:1090–1100.
126. Tipping PG, Davenport P, Gallicchio M, Filonzi EL, Apostolopoulos J, Wojta J. Atheromatous plaque macrophages produce plasminogen activator inhibitor type-1 and stimulate its production by endothelial cells and vascular smooth muscle cells. *Am J Pathol* 1993;143: 875–885.
127. Buja LM, Clubb FJ Jr, Bilheimer DW, Willerson JJ. Pathobiology of human familial hypercholesterolemia and related animal model, the Watanabe heritable hyperlipidemic rabbit. *Eur Heart J* 1990;11(Suppl E):41–52.
128. Clark RA. Regulation of fibroplasia in cutaneous wound repair. *Am J Med Sci* 1993;306:42–48.
129. Seino Y, Ikeda U, Ikeda M, Yamamoto K, Misawa Y, Hasegawa T, Kano S, Shimada K. Interluekin 6 gene transcripts are expressed in human atherosclerotic lesions. *Cytokine* 1994;6:87–91.
130. Ikeda U, Ikeda M, Seino Y, Takahashi M, Kano S, Shimada K. Interleukin-6 gene transcripts are expressed in atherosclerotic lesions of genetically hyperlipidemic rabbits. *Atherosclerosis* 1992;92: 213–218.
131. Gillett NA, Lowe D, Lu L, Chan C, Ferrara N. Leukemia inhibitory factor expression in human carotid plaques: Possible mechanism for inhibition of large vessel endothelial regrowth. *Growth Factors* 1993; 9:301–305.
132. Saito E, Fujioka T, Kanno H, Hata E, Ueno T, Matsumoto T, Takahashi Y, Tochihara T, Yasugi T. Completment receptors in atherosclerotic lesions. *Artery* 1992;19:47–62.
133. Ylä-Herttuala S, Lipton BA, Rosenfeld ME, Goldberg IJ, Steinberg D, Witztum JL. Macrophages and smooth muscle cells express lipoprotein lipase in human and rabbit atherosclerotic lesions. *Proc Natl Acad Sci USA* 1991;88:10143–10147.
134. O'Brien KD, Gordon D, Deeb S, Ferguson M, Chait A. Lipoprotein lipase is synthesized by macrophage-derived foam cells in human coronary atherosclerotic plaques. *J Clin Invest* 1992;89:1544–1550.
135. O'Brien KD, Deeb SS, Ferguson M, McDonald TO, Allen MD, Alpers CE, Chait A. Apolipoprotein E localization in human coronary atherosclerotic plaques by in situ hybridization and immunohistochemistry and comparison with lipoprotein lipase. *Am J Pathol* 1994;144: 538–548.
136. Shanahan CM, Cary NR, Metcalfe JC, Weissberg PL. High expression of genes for calcification-regulating proteins in human atherosclerotic plaques. *J Clin Invest* 1994;93:2393–2402.
137. Giachelli CM, Bae N, Almeida M , Denhardt DT, Alpers CE, Schwartz SM. Osteopontin is elevated during neointima formation in rat arteries and is a novel component of human atherosclerotic plaques. *J Clin Invest* 1993;92:1686–1696.
138. Ikeda T, Shirasawa T, Esaki Y, Yoshiki S, Hirokawa K. Osteopontin mRNA is expressed by smooth muscle-derived foam cells in human atherosclerotic lesions of the aorta. *J Clin Invest* 1993;92:2814–2820.
139. Hirota S, Imakita M, Kohri K, Ito A, Morii E, Adachi S, Kim HM, Kitamura Y, Yutani C, Nomura S. Expression of osteopontin messenger RNA by macrophages in atherosclerotic plaques. A possible association with calcification. *Am J Pathol* 1993;143:1003–1008.
140. Raines EW, Lane TF, Iruela-Arispe L, Ross R, Sage EH. The extracellular glycoprotein SPARC interacts with platelet-derived growth factor (PDGF)-AB and -BB and inhibits the binding of PDGF to its receptors. *Proc Natl Acad Sci USA* 1992;89:1281–1285.
141. Babaev VR, Dergunov AD, Chenchik AA, Tararak EM, Yanushevskaya EV, Trakht IN, Sorg C, Smirnov VN. Localization of apolipoprotein E in normal and atherosclerotic human aorta. *Atherosclerosis* 1990;85:239–247.
142. Vollmer E, Roessner A, Bosse A, Bocker W, Kaesberg B, Robenek H, Sorg C, Winde G. Immunohistochemical double labeling of macrophages, smooth muscle cells and apolipoprotein E in the atherosclerotic plaques. *Pathol Res Pract* 1991;187:184–188.
143. Björkhem I, Andersson O, Diczfalusy U, Sevastik B, Xiu RJ, Duan C, Lund E. Atherosclerosis and sterol 27-hydroxylase: Evidence for

a role of this enzyme in elimination of cholesterol from human macrophages. *Proc Natl Acad Sci USA* 1994;91:8592–8596.

144. Meek RL, Urieli-Shoval S, Benditt EP. Expression of apolipoprotein serum amyloid A mRNA in human atherosclerotic lesions and cultured vascular cells: Implications for serum amyloid A function. *Proc Natl Acad Sci USA* 1994;91:3186–3190.
145. Badolato R, Wang JM, Murphy WJ, Lloyd AR, Michiel DF, Bausserman LL, Kelvin DJ, Oppenheim JJ. Serum amyloid A is a chemoattractant: Induction of migration, adhesion, and tissue infiltration of monocytes and polymorphonuclear leukocytes. *J Exp Med* 1994;180: 203–209.
146. Brogi E, Winkles JA, Underwood R, Clinton SK, Alberts GF, Libby P. Distinct patterns of expression of fibroblast growth factors and their receptors in human atheroma and nonatherosclerotic arteries. Association of acidic FGF with plaque microvessels and macrophages. *J Clin Invest* 1993;92:2408–2418.
147. Hughes SE, Crossman D, Hall PA. Expression of basic and acidic fibroblast growth factors and their receptor in normal and atherosclerotic human arteries. *Cardiovasc Res* 1993;28:1214–1219.
148. Miyagawa J, Higashiyama S, Kawata S, Inui Y, Tamura S, Yamamoto K, Nishida M, Nakamura T, Yamashita S, Matsuzawa Y, Taniguchi N. Localization of heparin-binding EGF-like growth factor in the smooth muscle cells and macrophages of human atherosclerotic plaques. *J Clin Invest* 1995;95:404–411.
149. Zeiher AM, Goebel H, Schächinger, Ihling C. Tissue endothelin-1 immunoreactivity in the active coronary atherosclerotic plaque. A clue to the mechanism of increased vasoreactivity of the culprit lesion in unstable angina. *Circulation* 1995;91:941–947.
150. Davies MJ, Gordon JL, Gearing AJ, Pigott R, Woolf N, Katz D, Kyriakopoulos A. The expression of the adhesion molecules ICAM-1, VCAM-1, PECAM, and E-selectin in human atherosclerosis. *J Pathol* 1993;171:223–229.
151. van der Wal AC, Das PK, Tigges AJ, Becker AE. Adhesion molecules on the endothelium and mononuclear cells in human atherosclerotic lesions. *Am J Pathol* 1992;141:1427–1433.
152. Polacek D, Lal R, Volin MV, Davies PF. Gap junctional communication between vascular cells. Induction of connexin 43 messenger RNA in macrophage foam cells of atherosclerotic lesions. *Am J Pathol* 1993;142:593–606.
153. Brett J, Schmidt AM, Yan SD, Zou YS, Weidman E, Pinsky D, Nowygrod R, Neeper M, Przysiecki C, Shaw A, Migheli A, Stern D. Survey of the distribution of a newly characterized receptor for advanced glycation end products in tissues. *Am J Pathol* 1993;143:1699–1712.
154. Lupu F, Heim D, Bachmann F, Kruithof EK. Expression of LDL receptor-related protein/alpha 2-macroglobulin receptor in human normal and atherosclerotic arteries. *Arterioscler Thromb* 1994;14: 1438–1444.
155. Daugherty A, Rateri DL. Presence of LDL receptor-related protein/ α_2-macroglobulin receptors in macrophages of atherosclerotic lesions from cholesterol-fed New Zealand and heterozygous Watanabe heritable hyperlipidemic rabbits. *Arterioscler Thromb* 1994;14:2017–2024.
156. Li H, Freeman MW, Libby P. Regulation of smooth muscle cell scavenger receptor expression in vivo by atherogenic diets and in vitro by cytokines. *J Clin Invest* 1995;95:122–133.
157. Nelken NA, Soifer SJ, O'Keefe J, Vu TK, Charo IF, Coughlin SR. Thrombin receptor expression in normal and atherosclerotic human arteries. *J Clin Invest* 1992;90:1614–1621.
158. Xu Q, Luef G, Weimann S, Gupta RS, Wolf H, Wick G. Staining of endothelial cells and macrophages in atherosclerotic lesions with human heat-shock protein-reactive antisera. *Arterioscler Thromb* 1993;13:1763–1769.
159. Johnson AD, Berberian PA, Tytell M, Bond MG. Differential distribution of 70-kD heat shock protein in arterosclerosis. Its potential role in arterial smooth muscle cell survival. *Arterioscler Thromb* 1995; 15:27–36.

Atherosclerosis and Coronary Artery Disease,
edited by V. Fuster, R. Ross, and E. J. Topol.
Lippincott-Raven Publishers, Philadelphia © 1996.

CHAPTER 31

The Role of the Lymphocyte

Göran K. Hansson and Peter Libby

Key Words: HLA; Interferon-8; Antigen; Heat-shock proteins; Leukocyte adhesion molecules; Macrophages; Oxidized low-density lipoprotein; Tumor necrosis factor (TNF); T lymphocytes; Viral proteins.

INTRODUCTION

It has been known for several decades that mononuclear cells invariably infiltrate the atherosclerotic plaque. This observation led to speculations of a role for immune and inflammatory mechanisms in atherogenesis. The specificity and consequences of these reactions remain, however, obscure. Recent research has elaborated this concept and furnished new evidence that supports a role for immune mechanisms in atherosclerosis. This chapter will consider the possible roles of cell-mediated and humoral immune responses in atherosclerosis, describe the putative triggering antigens, and try to evaluate the effector mechanisms in the context of the atherosclerotic arterial wall. We start with a brief overview of some basic immunologic mechanisms, focusing on the recognition of antigens by T lymphocytes during the initiation of the immune response. Figure 1 depicts this schematically and it is described in further detail in ref. 1 and 2.

Antigen Recognition

An immune response normally starts when a T lymphocyte recognizes a foreign antigen. Once activated, T cells can kill target cells, initiate antibody production by B cells, and activate macrophages. These events may elicit but could also be part of inflammatory reactions. The activation of the T cell is the key to most immune reactions, since T-cell help is required for activation of other immunocompetent cells. It is therefore not surprising that the activation of T cells is strictly regulated.

The T cells are not activated by free, soluble antigen molecules. Instead, they recognize fragments of antigens when presented to them on the surface of antigen-presenting cells. Such fragments can arise during protein synthesis and associate intracellularly with HLA class I proteins (HLA-A, -B, -C). The HLA–peptide fragment complex will appear on the cell surface, where it may be recognized by the T-cell antigen receptor (TCR), an immunoglobulin-like cell surface protein that contains binding sites both for HLA and for the peptide bound to the HLA class I protein. The association between the antigen-presenting cell and the T cell is stabilized by several other receptors, one of which is the CD8 protein on this type of T cell, which binds to the HLA class I molecule on the antigen-presenting cell (Fig. 1A). In the case of a virally infected cell, virus-encoded proteins

G. K. Hansson: Karolinska Institute, Department of Medicine, and King Gustaf V Research Institute, Karolinska Hospital, S-17176 Stockholm, Sweden.

P. Libby: Harvard Medical School, Vascular Medicine and Atherosclerosis Unit, Brigham & Women's Hospital, Boston, Massachusetts 02115.

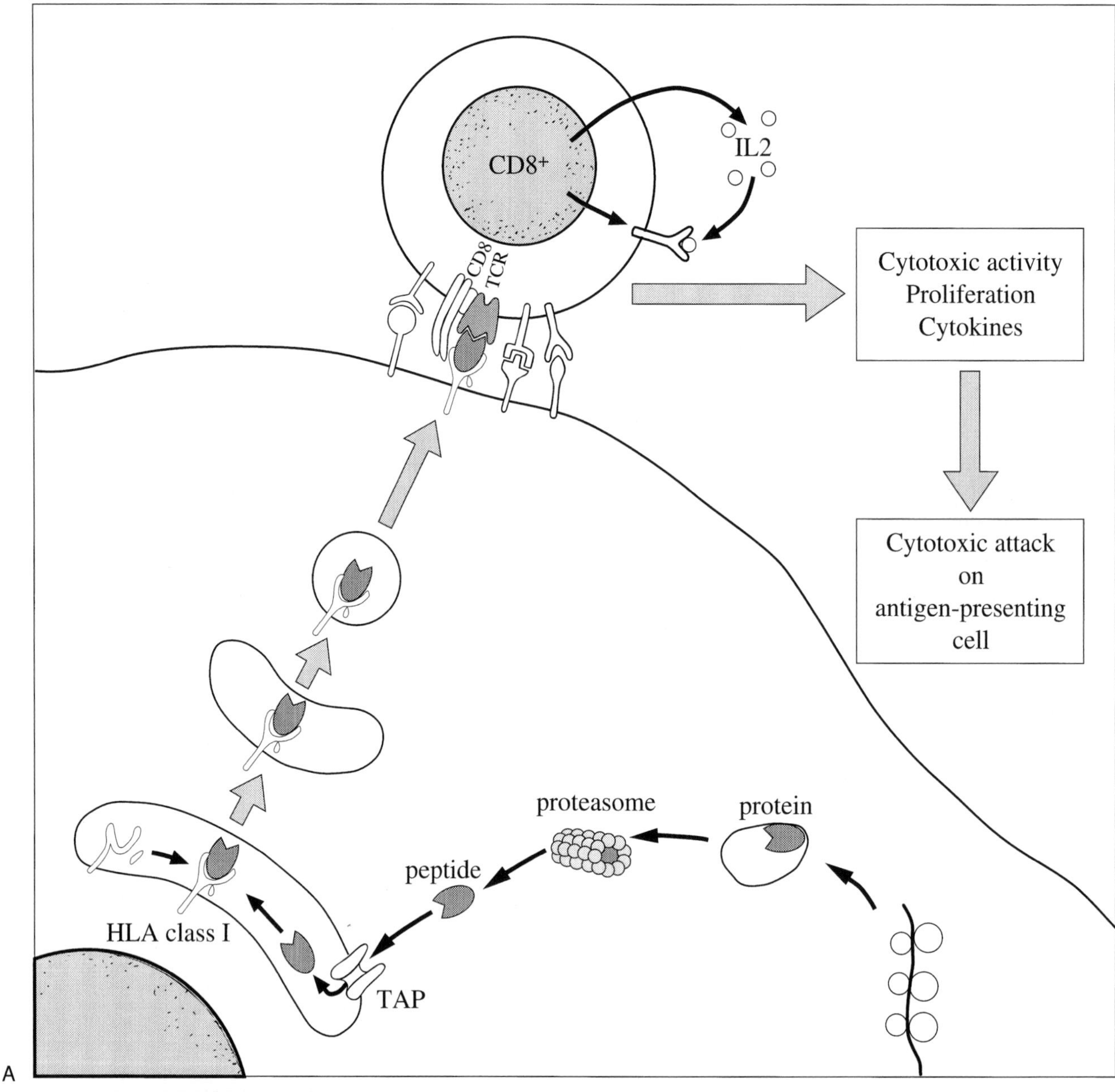

FIG. 1. A: Activation of a CD8+ T lymphocyte. The antigen is a protein that is synthesized by the antigen-presenting cell, typically a viral protein produced on free ribosomes in the cytoplasm. It is partially degraded by a specialized cytoplasmic proteasome complex (not shown) and proteolytic peptide fragments are transported into the endoplasmic reticulum by a transporter complex *(TAP)*. In the endoplasmic reticulum, antigenic peptides bind to newly synthesized HLA-A, -B or -C proteins *(HLA class I)*. The peptide–HLA class I complex is transported to the cell surface, where it can be detected by T cells. The CD8 receptor *(CD8)* binds to the HLA class I protein, while the T-cell antigen receptor *(TCR)* has binding sites both for the antigenic peptide and for HLA. Adhesion receptors on both cells stabilize the interaction and an intracellular signal is generated in the T cell. This results in expression of interleukin-2 receptors *(IL2R)* and autocrine secretion of interleukin-2 *(IL2)*. The T cell proliferates to form a clone with identical TCRs and, thus, identical immunologic specificities. Cytokines are secreted and the cells of the clone develop a cytotoxic capacity. A cytotoxic attack is mounted toward the antigen-presenting cells and in the case of a response to viral antigens, this leads to elimination of virus-infected cells.

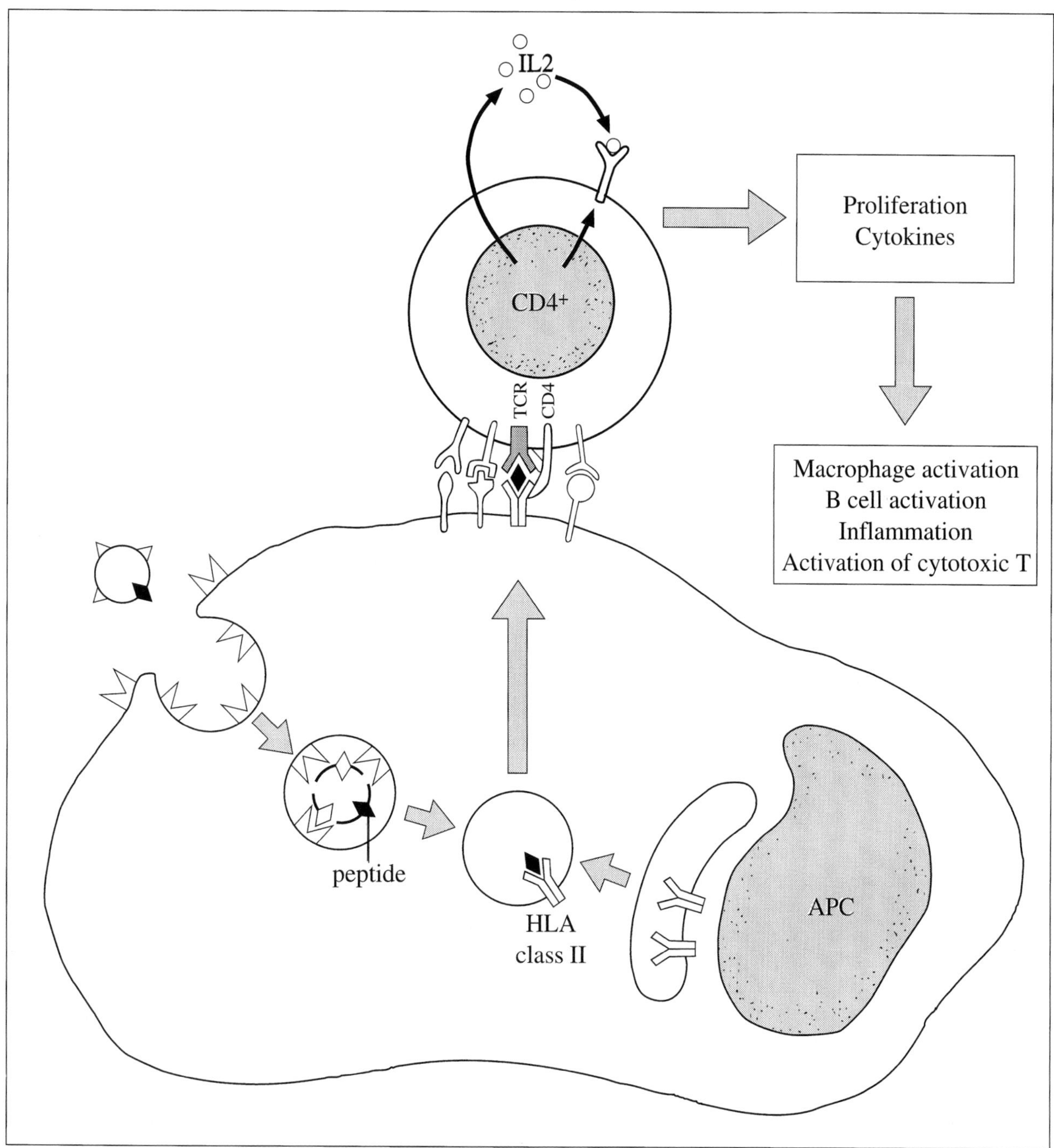

FIG. 1. *Continued.* **B:** Activation of a CD4+ T lymphocyte. The antigen is an exogenous particle or molecule, e.g., a component of a microorganism or an autoantigen. It is taken up by a specialized antigen-presenting cell *(APC)* (e.g., macrophage, endothelial cell, or dendritic cell) through endocytosis and degraded in an endosomal compartment. Antigenic peptides are transported to another endosomal compartment, where they can bind to newly synthesized HLA-DR, -DQ, or -DP *(HLA class II)* proteins. The peptide–HLA class II complex is transported to the cell surface, where it can be detected by CD4+ T cells. The CD4 receptor *(CD4)* binds to HLA class II molecules, while the T-cell antigen receptor *(TCR)* has binding sites both for the antigenic peptide and HLA. Several other receptors on the T cell and the antigen-presenting cell stabilize the cell–cell interaction. An intracellular signal is generated in the T cell, interleukin-2 *(IL2)* and interleukin-2 receptors *(IL2R)* are expressed, and the antigen-specific T cell undergoes clonal expansion. Cytokines are secreted that activate macrophages, B cells, and cytotoxic T cells, initiate inflammatory reactions, and regulate the immune response.

complex with nascent HLA class I proteins, allowing the host immune system to recognize the infected cell.

When the TCR is engaged by an HLA-peptide complex, an activation program ensues and results in cytokine secretion, proliferation, and/or the development of cytotoxic activity. A prerequisite for T-cell activation is, however, that in addition to antigenic peptides, costimulatory factors must be provided by the antigen-presenting cell. These factors include comitogens (interleukin-1) and adhesion molecules that stabilize the binding of the T cell to the antigen-presenting cell. Examples of such adhesion molecules with "accessory" functions in the immune response include intercellular adhesion molecule-1 (ICAM-1) and vascular cell adhesion molecule-1 (VCAM-1).

In the case of the CD8+ subpopulation of T cells, cytotoxic effector functions are prominent and important, for example, when the T-cell response is mounted toward a virus-encoded protein presented in complex with HLA class I by a virally infected cell. These T cells exert cytotoxic activity by the generation of pores in the target cell by synthesis of pore-forming protein complexes, perforins. In addition, oxygen and nitrogen free radicals and enzymes known as granzymes may participate in cell-mediated cytotoxic responses and attack membrane components of the target cell.

The other major subpopulation of T cells carry an HLA receptor called CD4. These cells recognize external antigens that have been taken up and processed by professional antigen-presenting cells (Fig. 1B). B cells can internalize antigens by receptor-mediated endocytosis using their surface antibodies as receptors. Macrophages may use a variety of different receptor-mediated and bulk mechanisms for endocytotic uptake of antigenic material. Vascular endothelial cells are also able to internalize, process, and present foreign antigens to CD4+ T cells (3). The endothelium represents a huge area for antigen presentation since the entire vascular surface is potentially available. The ability of endothelial cells to initiate immune responses also implies that immune mechanisms may preferentially localize to the vessel wall.

After internalization, antigenic proteins are attacked by proteolytic enzymes in an endosomal compartment, resulting in the generation of short (10–20 amino acid residues) oligopeptides that are of suitable size for antigen presentation. These peptides meet HLA class II (HLA-DR, -DQ, and -DP) proteins in a specialized vesicular, intracellular compartment for peptide loading (4). Here, the peptide binds to a groove in the HLA molecule, which is subsequently transported to the cell surface of the antigen-presenting cell. The CD4-bearing T cell will engage the HLA class II protein and the TCR may bind the HLA–peptide complex (Fig. 1B). Again, the result is T-cell activation, provided that the antigen-presenting cell can furnish costimulants such as interleukin-1 and adhesion molecules.

The CD4 activation program includes proliferation, cytokine secretion, and/or T-cell cytotoxic activity (5). In the CD4 cell population, the emphasis is on cytokine secretion rather than on cytotoxic responses. These cytokines initiate antibody production and inflammatory responses. CD4 cells are therefore sometimes called helper cells (although some helper cell activity can be detected also in the CD8 population). The prototypic CD4 response is mounted after phagocytosis of a bacterium by a macrophage. The CD4 cell responds to peptide fragments of the bacterial wall presented on the macrophage surface in conjunction with HLA class II, and initiates antibody production to bacterial antigens via cytokine signals to B lymphocytes.

As mentioned, both B-cell help and induction of inflammation depend on the secretion of cytokines by the CD4 cell. Several different cytokines can induce B-cell growth and differentiation. The particular mix of cytokines determines the type of immunoglobulin that will be secreted (6). Inflammatory responses are elicited by tumor necrosis factors (TNF), lymphotoxin, and interferon-γ, all of which act on vascular endothelial and smooth muscle cells to promote leukocyte adhesion and vasodilation (7–10). In addition, interferon-γ inhibits endothelial and smooth muscle proliferation and activates macrophages, and both interferon-γ and TNF modulate cholesterol metabolism and radical formation by the macrophages (8,11–13). Vascular actions of immune-derived cytokines are discussed in detail in another chapter.

Tolerance and Specificity

The cell surface reactions described above permit highly specific recognition of a myriad of different antigens. Immunologic diversity arises from somatic genetic mechanisms in the lymphoblast and by the selection of T cells capable of "useful" immune responses during T-cell development in the thymus (1,14).

The generation of immune diversity depends on the formation of unique TCR and antibody (Ig) molecules during the development of T and B lymphoblasts. In nonlymphoid cells, both TCR and Ig are encoded by complex genes that contain a large number of alternative segments. These are rearranged, with the deletion of intervening sequences, to form a unique TCR (or immunoglobulin, Ig) gene in each clone of developing lymphoblasts. The protein products of these genes are antigen receptors and antibodies that are unique for each T- and B-cell clone, respectively.

The rearrangement process randomly generates TCR molecules that could bind endogenous as well as exogenous peptides. The former are potentially dangerous since they could be presented "incidentally" on HLA molecules and initiate an autoimmune T-cell attack. Such T cells are therefore sorted out and eliminated during maturation of T cells in the thymus. This process is not yet fully understood, but it involves both positive and negative selection (14). During the former, only those T cells which carry TCR that can bind to HLA molecules present in the thymic microenvironment will receive the stimuli necessary for escaping apoptosis and completing differentiation. The negative selection process eliminates self-reactive T-cell clones, which bind endogenous peptides presented by thymic antigen-presenting cells. Such T cells are killed and only T cells that do not recognize endogenous peptides are permitted to mature and are eventually released into the circulation.

In addition to the thymic "education" of immature T cells, the development of immunologic activity of mature T cells may also involve induction of tolerance to specific antigens. This can be accomplished by presenting antigenic peptides to the T cell without simultaneous costimulatory factors necessary for activation of the T cell. Instead of activation, this form of antigen presentation leads to clonal anergy of the specific T cell. This mechanism probably contributes to the development of tolerance to antigens encountered during adult life.

B-Cell Activation and Antibody Production

The resting B lymphocyte expresses cell surface antibodies that serve as antigen receptors similar to the TCR molecules of the T cell (6). Since antibodies, in contrast to TCR, bind complete antigens such as intact proteins rather than proteolytically processed fragments, B cells can recognize soluble antigens in the extracellular environment. However, activation of naive B cells normally requires not only the recognition of antigen by specific, B-cell surface-bound antibodies, but also "help" in the form of cytokines and adhesion-dependent activation from nearby, activated T cells.

Once activated, the B cell can internalize antigen via its surface antibodies, process it, and present it to T cells. Therefore, T- and B-cell activation occurs in a network of cell–cell contacts involving antibodies, TCRs, HLA molecules, adhesion molecules, and cytokines, all of which are produced by the two cell types. The activation mechanism is well established for protein antigens, but carbohydrate and lipid antigens can elicit B-cell activation and antibody production without involving T cells.

Activated B cells, like T cells, proliferate into clones specific for the initiating antigen. Some of the proliferating B cells differentiate into plasma cells in response to cytokines such as interleukin-6. Plasma cells develop of an excessive rough endoplasmic reticulum and Golgi apparatus and a huge capacity to secrete antibodies. These cells produce most of the circulating antibodies during an infection or after an immunization.

Antigen–Antibody Reactions, Phagocytosis, and Complement Activation

Antibodies recognize antigen, but antibody binding does not by itself eliminate the antigen. This requires the activity of effector mechanisms, the most important of which are Fc receptor-dependent phagocytosis and complement activation (1).

Macrophages, B cells, and several other cell types express Fc receptors for the nonvariable, C-terminal domains of the antibody molecule. These receptors bind aggregated immunoglobulins such as antigen–antibody complexes, comprised of several antibody molecules associated with multivalent antigens. After internalization, lysosomal enzymes can degrade the ingested complexes.

Large, particulate antigens such as cells which cannot be internalized are eliminated in a different way. When antibodies bind to clustered antigens on the surface of the cell, the exposed, clustered Fc domains activate C1, the first component of the complement cascade (1,15). This initiates a cascade reaction similar to coagulation and ends with the formation of polymeric proteins that form pores in the surface membrane of the antigenic particle. This process resembles in many respects the perforin-dependent cytolytic mechanism of cytotoxic T cells.

As by-products, complement activation generates biologically active peptide fragments such as C3a and C5a, which act as chemoattractants and vasodilators. Finally, complement-coated particles can be phagocytized by macrophages and other cells that express C3b receptors. Complement activation therefore accomplishes cytolytic destruction, phagocytic elimination, and inflammatory responses.

To summarize, the immune response can be divided into three different phases: the recognition of antigen, the effectors of the responses, and the regulation of the system. The first depends on unique receptors expressed by T and B cells and their interaction with the antigen. The second phase consists in the generation of cytotoxic cellular and complement-mediated activity as well as the release of hormone-like cytokines that control the inflammatory response of blood vessels and other tissues. The regulatory mechanisms, finally, depend largely on cytokine-mediated and adhesion-dependent signals between immunocompetent cells. We shall now discuss how atherosclerosis may involve these aspects of immune responses.

THE IMMUNE RESPONSE IN HUMAN ATHEROSCLEROSIS

Immunocompetent Cells in Plaques

The cellular events in atherogenesis have been characterized in studies employing a spectrum of morphologic techniques, including light and electron microscopy, histochemistry, immunohistochemistry, and *in situ* hybridization. Together, these studies form the basis for the hypothesis that cellular immune reactions take place in the atherosclerotic plaque.

Poole and Florey, in the 1950s, showed in hypercholesterolemic rabbits that fatty streak-type lesions develop by infiltration of monocyte-like cells in the intima (16). Twenty years later, Fowler et al. (17) and Gerrity (18) used electron microscopy to demonstrate how monocytes develop into foam cells in nascent lesions of experimental animals. Immunohistochemical analysis of human atherosclerotic lesions showed that foam cells express surface antigens specific for the monocyte-macrophage lineage (19–22). A plausible sequence of events in early atherogenesis starts with monocyte adhesion to an intact endothelium, followed by infiltration of these leukocytes into the subendothelial intima, accumulation of cholesterol, and transition into lipid-laden foam cells (23–26). At later stages and in areas of perturbed blood flow, there is also recruitment of monocytes by preferential binding to areas with endothelial injury (27). The existence of scavenger receptors for modified lipoproteins such as oxidized low-density lipoprotein (LDL) on cells of the monocyte-macrophage lineage (28) explains why such a large proportion of foam cells originate from these cells.

The detection of lymphocytes in the atherosclerotic plaque, in contrast to the finding of monocytes, depended entirely on monoclonal antibody technology, as these cells were fairly inconspicuous by morphologic criteria. Using monoclonal antibodies in an immunohistochemical mapping of gene expression in human plaques, it was found (29) that the HLA class II gene HLA-DR is expressed by many smooth muscle cells, although these cells do not normally express this gene. Since HLA-DR is induced by the T-cell cytokine interferon-γ, the obvious conclusion was that T cells present in the lesion induced HLA-DR expression on smooth muscle cells by release of this cytokine (29). Immunohistochemical analysis of the cellular composition of advanced human atherosclerotic plaques supports this interpretation (Fig. 2). Ten to twenty percent of all cells in such lesions express T-cell-specific antigens such as CD3, with approximately two-thirds of the T cells expressing CD4 and one-third the CD8 antigen (21).

The presence of T cells and monocyte-derived macrophages suggests that antigen presentation and immune activation occur in atherosclerotic plaques. One might, however, argue that both cell types accumulate by nonspecific trapping and may be totally inactive. Immunophenotyping and mRNA analysis indicate to the contrary by demonstrating activation of the T cells. Many T cells in atheroma bear interleukin-2 receptors and HLA-DR (30). Flow cytometric analysis of T cells isolated from plaques revealed a total dominance of the memory T-cell phenotype and expression of the VLA-1 (very late activation) antigen (31). Cytokines characteristic of activated T cells have been found in plaques by immunohistochemistry (30) and polymerase chain reaction (32) and the ''aberrant'' expression of HLA-DR in the plaque (29) provides indirect evidence for a local interferon-γ secretion, as discussed earlier.

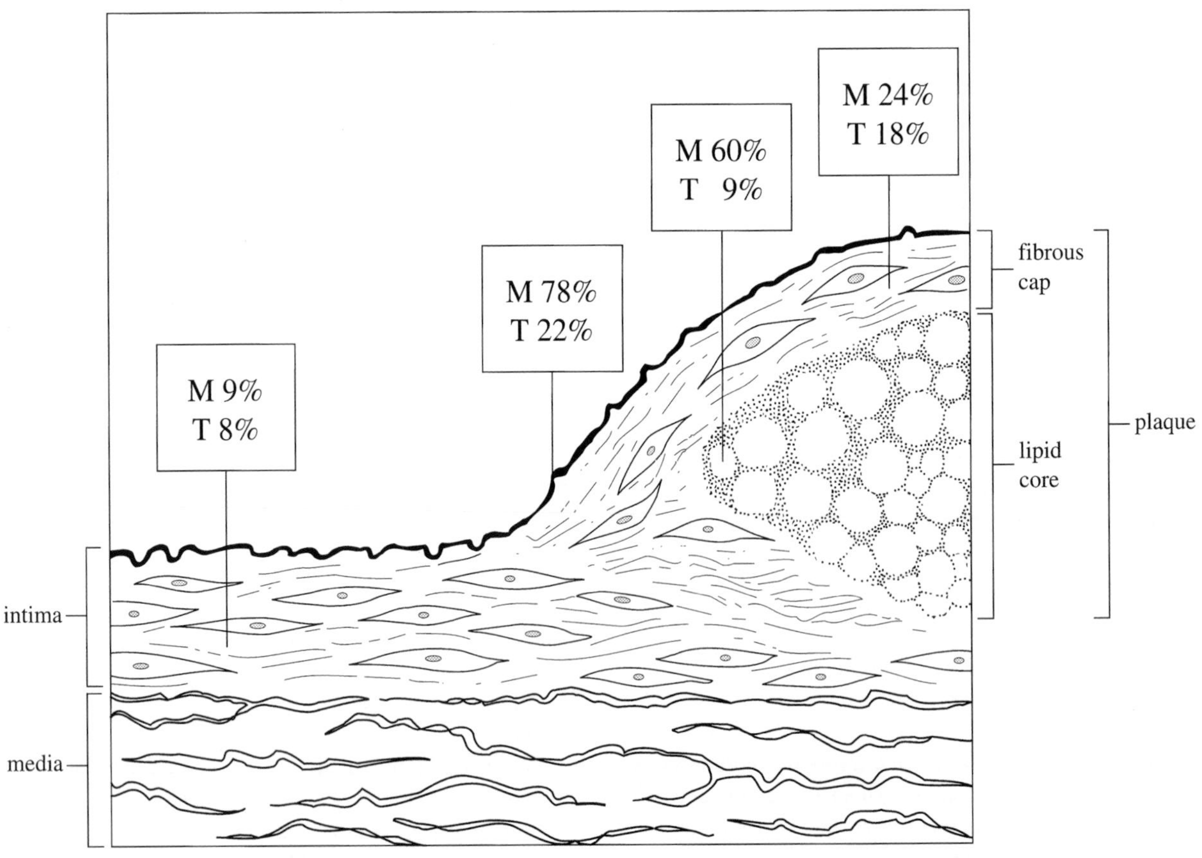

FIG. 2. Monocyte-derived macrophages *(M)* and T lymphocytes *(T)* in an advanced atherosclerotic plaque. Values are expressed as percentages of total cells in different regions of the plaque and are based on immunohistochemical analyses of endarterectomy specimens. (Reprinted from Hansson et al., ref. 69, with permission from the American Heart Association.)

Mechanisms of Lymphocyte Recruitment

As shown above, there is evidence for a local, cell-mediated immune response in the atherosclerotic plaque, although the eliciting antigen(s) remain obscure. Analysis of human lesions and experimental models support the following scenario for the development of the immunopathologic aspect of the disease (Fig. 3).

The T lymphocytes enter the arterial wall at a very early stage of lesion formation and are found in fatty streaks together with macrophages (33,34). The latter, however, always outnumber the T cells, with a ratio of approximately 1:10 to 1:50 between T cells and macrophages. In early lesions, CD8 cells dominate over CD4 with a ratio of approximately 2:1 (33–35). This contrasts with the situation in the advanced plaque (21) and suggests that there may be a switch from a response driven by HLA class I-restricted to HLA class II-restricted antigens during the evolution of the fatty streak into a fibrofatty plaque.

Studies in cholesterol-fed rabbits shed light on the recruitment of T lymphocytes and monocytes to the arterial wall during atherogenesis. The two earliest detectable vascular events after initiation of cholesterol feeding are expression of endothelial adhesion molecules and intimal complement deposition. Focal expression of VCAM-1 (vascular cell adhesion molecule-1) occurs as early as 1 week after the start of the atherogenic diet (36–38), followed by the entry of monocyte-macrophages and other leukocytes during the ensuing weeks (37). VCAM-1 is a ligand for VLA-4, a cell surface protein expressed by lymphocytes and monocytes (39). Granulocytes do not bear VLA-4, providing a possible explanation for the selective recruitment of mononuclear cells to the forming atherosclerotic lesion.

VCAM-1 is not expressed constitutively by endothelial cells, but is inducible by proinflammatory cytokines, including interleukin-1 (IL-1), tumor necrosis factor (TNF), and γ-interferon (37,40). The production of such cytokines in the underlying atheroma likely contributes to the continued expression of VCAM-1 on the surface of the forming plaque. It is uncertain whether nascent lesions contain sufficient local concentrations of IL-1, TNF, or interferon-γ to induce VCAM-1. Surprisingly, VCAM-1 expression is also induced by lysophosphatidylcholine, which may be present in lipoproteins and generated during lipoprotein oxidation and cell membrane injury (41). In the hypercholesterolemic state, lysophosphatidylcholine might therefore perhaps induce VCAM-1 expression on the endothelium. The focal expression of VCAM-1 in lesion-prone areas of hypercholesterolemic animals may result from a combination of local flow alterations that promote influx or retention of lipoproteins and the action of a component of modified lipoprotein, either directly or by inducing a secondary cytokine. It is noteworthy in the context of T-cell activation during atherogenesis (see below) that VCAM-1 not only serves as a leukocyte adhesion molecule, but by engaging VLA-4 on T cells can function as a costimulator or accessory molecule in the T-cell activation pathway.

The vascular reaction in early hypercholesterolemia is characterized not only by *de novo* gene expression in vascular cells, but also by an infiltration and accumulation of plasma proteins. There is a deposition of lipoproteins, but also a prominent infiltration and deposition of immunoglobulins and complement factors. IgG is deposited on intracellular filaments and extracellular collagen fibers due to specific interactions between the Fc part of the immunoglobulin molecule and protein components of these filaments (42). The intracellular accumulation of IgG in injured endothelial cells is particularly striking and can be used to detect damaged endothelial cells (43).

Several complement factors are detectable in the atherosclerotic intima, including C1 and C3b (44). The accumulation of C5b-9 is particularly important since it indicates activation of the complement cascade. C5b-9 deposits are found in the rabbit aorta within 2 weeks after initiation of a cholesterol-rich diet and increase with the progression of the disease process (45). These deposits represent membrane-anchored attack complexes with the capacity to perforate cellular membranes and might cause cytolysis in the atherosclerotic artery. Peptide fragments such as C3a and C5a, which are released during activation of the complement cascade prior to the formation of the C5b-9 complex, exhibit chemotactic and leukocyte-activating properties and could be important for the recruitment of leukocytes to the lesion (46). The initiation of the complement cascade might occur at the IgG deposits at sites of cell injury, but also in regions of cholesterol deposition. Cholesterol may, at least *in vitro,* activate the complement cascade through the alternative pathway in a reaction that is amplified by oxidative modification of the cholesterol molecule (47).

To summarize, early immunologic responses of the atherosclerotic arterial wall include both expression of endothelial leukocyte-adhesion molecules and complement activation. Both of these responses can decisively influence the subsequent formation of the (macrophage-rich) fatty streak. The most comprehensive data on these processes are available in the cholesterol-fed rabbit model, but there is also evidence for their involvement in the human disease (48,49). It will now be important to determine whether the atherosclerotic process can be inhibited by interfering with these phenomena.

ANTIGENS

The presence of activated T cells and macrophages strongly suggest that an immunologic reaction is taking place in the atherosclerotic plaque. The antigens that elicit this response are not yet known and both microorganisms and autoantigens have been proposed to play a role.

In early lesions, the presence of T cells of the CD8 phenotype suggests that an immune response to HLA class I-re-

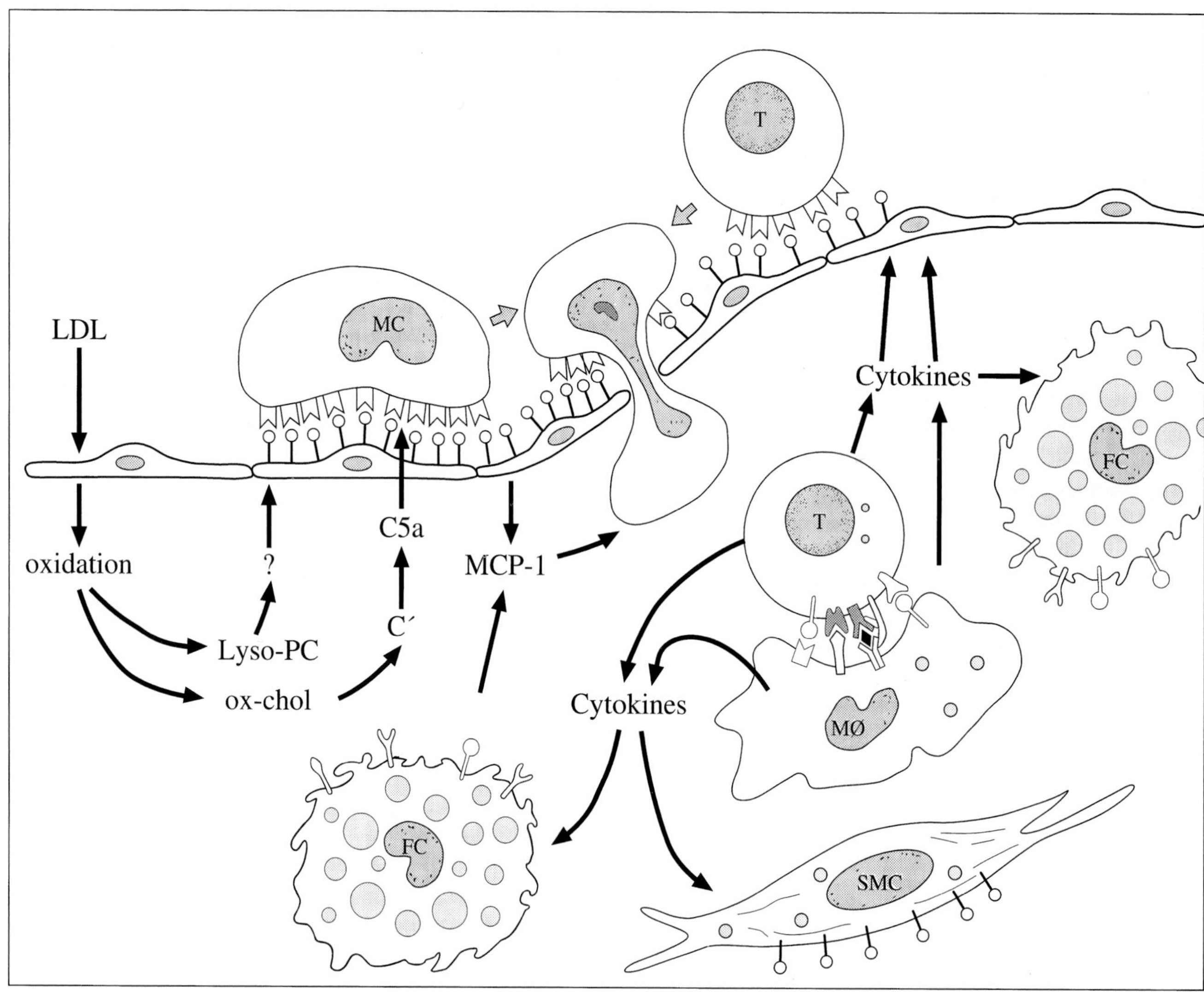

FIG. 3. Postulated recruitment and activation of immunocompetent cells in the early atherosclerotic lesion. Endothelial cells are stimulated to express VCAM-1, possibly by lysophosphatidylcholine *(Lyso-PC)* or other components of LDL oxidized in the intima. Monocytes *(MC)* and T lymphocytes *(T)* adhere to endothelial cells expressing VCAM-1 and other leukocyte adhesion molecules. They are stimulated chemotactically to enter the intima by C5a produced during complement activation (*C′*), which may also be secondary to LDL oxidation *(ox-chol,* oxidized cholesterol*)*. The cytokine, macrophage chemoattractant protein-1 *(MCP-1)* is another potent chemotactic agent that is produced locally in the atherosclerotic plaque. Antigen-specific T cells are activated by monocyte-derived macrophages *(Mø)* in the lesion. Both cell types produce cytokines which act on endothelial cells *(EC),* smooth muscle cells *(SMC),* macrophages, and foam cells *(FC)* to regulate adhesion molecule expression, chemotaxis, procoagulant activity, proliferation, contractility, and cholesterol uptake. In addition, (*EC* and *SMC* release cytokines that act on both inflammatory and vascular cells. For the sake of simplicity, vascular-derived cytokines are not indicated in the figure.

stricted, endogenously synthesized antigens may be taking place. The best-known HLA class I-restricted antigens are **viral proteins,** which are synthesized by the virus-infected cell. It is therefore possible that (at least some of) the CD8+ cells respond to viral antigens in plaque. Antigens of herpes simplex virus type I and cytomegalovirus are present in the arterial wall during atherosclerosis (50). These members of the herpesvirus family are, however, among the most ubiquitous viruses that infect humans. The mere presence of components of such viruses therefore does not prove that they play any pathogenetic role. Further discussion concerning the role of viruses in atherosclerosis can be found in another chapter. Nonviral microorganisms such as *Chlamydia* spp. are other conceivable microbial stimuli for a local immune response during atherogenesis, but there is little information concerning their frequency and distribution in atherosclerotic plaques.

The mature atherosclerotic plaque contains a large number

of CD4+ T cells (21). These cells respond to HLA class II-restricted, exogenous antigens that are taken up from the environment by macrophages, endothelial cells, and other antigen-presenting cells. The ensuing T-cell responses include cytokine secretion and T-cell help for antibody-producing B cells (51). Analysis of antibody responses to plaque components could therefore shed light on the reactivity of the CD4+ T cells.

Autoantibodies to **oxidized LDL** lipoproteins are common in humans (52); their titer appears to correlate with the progression of atherosclerosis (53). Antibodies raised against model antigens such as malondialdehyde (MDA)-conjugated lysine recognize oxidatively modified LDL (54–55). Plaques contain significant amounts of MDA-lysine cross-reactive material (56). It is likely that the B-cell response is dependent on T-cell help and it has therefore been proposed that CD4+ cells in the plaque initiate an autoimmune response to oxidized LDL. The recent observation that CD4+ T cells cloned from human plaques respond to oxidized LDL in an HLA class II-restricted fashion (57) supports this hypothesis. The T-cell epitopes on the oxidized LDL particle, however, have not yet been identified.

Many inflammatory and autoimmune diseases, including atherosclerosis, are associated with antibody production against **heat-shock proteins.** These are intracellular chaperones that stabilize the conformation of other proteins. They are synthesized in increased amounts during cell injury and induce T-cell-dependent antibody production (58). Several heat-shock proteins are found in atherosclerotic lesions (59) and the titer of autoantibodies to heat-shock protein 60 appears to correlate with the extent of carotid atherosclerosis (60). In cholesterol-fed rabbits, immunization with heat-shock protein 60 aggravates atherosclerosis, suggesting that this autoimmune response may be of pathogenic significance (61).

Very few B cells are found in the plaque and it is therefore likely that B-cell activation and antibody production occur in regional lymph nodes. T cells might enter the plaque, respond to antigen, and then migrate through the lymph circulation to regional lymph nodes, where B cells are activated to produce antibodies to the antigen recognized by the T cell. Such a patrolling role of the T cell is known to occur in many other situations (62) and would fit with the phenotypic characteristics of T cells isolated from plaques (31). It probably requires that antigen is present also in the lymph node; this is likely to be the case for oxidized LDL.

Advanced cases of atherosclerosis are sometimes complicated by periadventitial inflammation. In the case of aortic atherosclerosis, this periaortitis can produce huge inflammatory infiltrates. Microscopically, the periaortic lesion is dominated by B lymphocytes and macrophages together with oxidized lipid components and antibodies to oxidized LDL (63,64) and it is possible that the periarterial lesion represents an autoimmune response to oxidized LDL (64). Therefore, although the initial B-cell response probably occurs in lymph nodes, B cells may at later stages localize to and be activated in the periarteritic inflammatory infiltrate.

To conclude, the antigens of atherosclerosis remain obscure, although recent data implicate oxidized LDL and heat-shock proteins as possible targets for CD4+ responses and antibody production associated with atherosclerosis. It still remains to be determined whether such responses are essentially beneficial or detrimental for the artery and the patient.

IMMUNE EFFECTOR MECHANISMS AND THE PATHOGENESIS OF ATHEROSCLEROSIS

It is likely that a local immune reaction occurs in the atherosclerotic plaque, but the pathophysiologic consequences of such reactions remain largely speculative. Humoral immune mechanisms could be involved in elimination of antigenic compounds, but also initiate complement- and macrophage-dependent cytotoxic mechanisms. Cellular immune responses may initiate inflammatory reactions, cell-mediated cytotoxicity, and cytokine-dependent regulatory loops in the atherosclerotic plaque (Table 1).

T-cell-dependent induction of antibody production to plaque antigens such as oxidized LDL could represent a mechanism for antigen elimination. Immune complexes consisting of LDL and anti-LDL antibodies are avidly taken up by Fc receptor-bearing macrophages, which may transform into cholesterol-laden foam cells (65). Antibody binding to cell surfaces may initiate cytotoxic activity. Both the complement cascade and Fc receptor-bearing macrophages and cytotoxic lymphocytes would attack antibody-coated target cells. The presence of membrane-bound C5b-9 complexes in experimental plaques (45) indicates that complement lysis takes place. It is not clear, however, whether this occurs as the result of antibody binding to specific antigens on the surface of cells or is due to an "innocent bystander" attack after alternative complement activation on the extracellular cholesterol deposits (47).

Cellular immune reactions require T-cell activation, and the presence of activated CD4+ and CD8+ T cells suggests that both cytotoxic and immune-regulatory, T-cell-dependent reactions could occur in the plaque. There is little direct evidence for cytotoxic reactions in atherosclerosis. In contrast, several reports demonstrate the presence of immune-regulatory cytokines in the atherosclerotic plaque. Proinflammatory cytokines, including interleukin-1, TNF, interleukin-6, and γ-interferon, are secreted in the plaque (8), probably by T lymphocytes, macrophages, endothelial cells, and smooth muscle cells.

The pathogenetic consequences of such paracrine cytokine secretion could include activation of macrophages and endothelial cells (8), stimulation of immune responses (see above), modulation of cholesterol uptake, and regulation of vascular hemostatic properties. The mechanical and hemodynamic properties of the atherosclerotic arterial wall would be affected by cytokines inhibiting vascular contractility (via

TABLE 1. *Candidate antigens for stimulating cellular immunity in atheroma*

Antigen	Dominating lymphocyte response
Modified lipoprotein constituents	CD4+ T cells
Apolipoprotein B adducts (e.g., malondialdehyde)	B-cell help for antibody production
Apo B fragments	Proinflammatory and immune-regulating cytokines
Cryptic antigens exposed during cell injury	CD4+ T cells
Heat-shock proteins	B-cell help for antibody production
	Proinflammatory and immune-regulating cytokines
Neoantigens expressed in disease	CD8+ T cells
Virus-encoded proteins	Cytotoxic attack on antigen-expressing cells
Cytokine-induced surface antigens?	

induction of nitric oxide synthesis), inhibiting cell proliferation, and inducing matrix-degrading metalloproteinases (10,66,67,68). Most of these mechanisms have been identified and characterized in cell culture studies. There is, however, *in vivo* evidence in experimental animal models for cytokine control of endothelial activation and inhibition of smooth muscle proliferation (38,68,69). It will be important to establish the role of other potential regulatory mechanisms by *in vivo* studies of cytokine action on the vessel wall. Further information regarding cytokine effects on the vessel wall are found in another chapter.

THE SPECIAL CASE OF TRANSPLANT ARTERIOSCLEROSIS

Organ transplantation between histoincompatible individuals elicits a rejection that is largely focused on the blood vessels. Hyperacute rejection is elicited by antibodies reacting with endothelial surface antigens and results in complement-mediated lysis of the endothelium. Acute rejection, in contrast, involves both humoral and cellular reactions against histocompatibility antigens on endothelial and parenchymal cells. The result is a histopathologic pattern of lysis of parenchymal cells and signs of vasculitis, such as perivascular ''cuffing'' by mononuclear leukocytes. Chronic rejection, finally, is characterized by fibrosis of the transplanted organ and intimal hyperplasia of its arteries. The latter process resembles atherosclerosis and has been called transplant arteriosclerosis or graft vascular disease (70). The use of tissue typing and immunosuppressive therapy has reduced the incidence of hyperacute and acute rejection. Currently, chronic rejection/transplant arteriosclerosis represents a major challenge to clinical organ transplantation.

The pathologic process of transplant arteriosclerosis involves the intima of large- and medium-sized arteries. It is usually manifested as a diffuse, concentric, intimal proliferative lesion (70). This contrasts with the focal, eccentric lesions of atherosclerosis. In addition, there is usually much less lipid deposition in the graft lesion. The same cell types are, however, present in both types of lesions: vascular smooth muscle cells, endothelial cells, macrophages, and T lymphocytes. In graft arteriosclerosis, T lymphocytes are more frequent and characteristically accumulate in the subendothelial region (70). HLA class II proteins are expressed in both conditions and there is striking HLA-DR expression in the endothelium covering the transplant lesion (70). The high frequency of T cells and intense HLA-DR staining at the endothelium and subendothelial intima of the graft lesion suggests that an immunologic reaction to allogeneic HLA molecules may occur here.

The pathologic process in transplant arteriosclerosis is likely to involve a T-cell-dependent cellular immune reaction toward allogeneic HLA molecules. This is followed by smooth muscle proliferation, the formation of a neointima, and ischemic organ damage. One could speculate that T cells act similarly in atherosclerosis as in graft arteriosclerosis, stimulating smooth muscle proliferation and enhancing the formation of a neointimal hyperplasia. However, cell culture and animal studies suggest that T cells may inhibit neointimal hyperplasia by releasing growth-inhibitory cytokines (69). The role of T cells in vascular pathology is therefore probably complex and involves indirect as well as direct effects on vascular cells. The exact mixture of cytokines elaborated by local T-cell populations may influence the balance between net cytolytic/cytostatic effects and net promotion of fibrosis and smooth muscle proliferation.

SUMMARY

Morphologic and immunologic studies of human atherosclerosis have established T lymphocytes as an important cellular component of the plaque. They have also provided evidence for a local immune activation in the arterial intima during atherosclerosis. Cell culture studies have identified potential mechanisms of interactions between lymphocytes and other cells involved in the disease process and several crucial aspects of such interactions have been evaluated in animal models of atherosclerosis. The picture that emerges is one of a cellular immune activation involving T cells and macrophages together with an antigen-independent complement activation. Activation of these two systems would activate endothelial cells, inhibit smooth muscle growth, reduce the contractility of the vessel wall, and recruit more lymphocytes and monocytes to the forming lesion. Cytokines released during the cellular immune response might also reduce foam cell formation, but could increase the size of the extracellular cholesterol pool. Acting in concert, the net effect of these various functions would be reduction in the size and mechanical strength of the lesion. Macrophages activated during an immune response might, however, counteract this by releasing growth factors such as platelet-derived growth factor. The relative importance of the various cytokine-modulated event is still unclear and may vary depending on the precise stimulus and phase of the disease process.

Finally, it should be emphasized that the antigen(s) that incite the cellular immune response are not yet identified. Recent studies suggest that heat-shock proteins and oxidized lipoproteins could induce cellular immune reactions, but their role as immunogens in the atherosclerotic plaque remain uncertain. If indeed important local antigens and their T-cell epitopes can be identified, immunologic prevention and/or therapy could be attractive additions to the therapeutic arsenal for the treatment of atherosclerosis.

REFERENCES

1. Abbas AK, Lichtman AH, Pober JS. *Cellular and molecular immunology*, 2nd ed. Philadelphia: Saunders; 1994.
2. Brodsky FM, Guagliardi LE. The cell biology of antigen processing and presentation. *Annu Rev Immunol* 1991;9:707–744.
3. Pober JS, Collins T, Gimbrone MA, et al. Lymphocytes recognize human vascular endothelial and dermal fibroblast Ia antigens induced by recombinant immune interferon. *Nature* 1983;305:726–729.
4. Tulp A, Verwoerd D, Dobberstein B, Ploegh HL, Pieters J. Isolation and characterization of the intracellular MHC class II compartment. *Nature* 1994;369:120–126.
5. Seder RA, Paul WE. Acquisition of lymphokine-producing phenotype by $CD4^+$ T cells. *Annu Rev Immunol* 1994;12:635–673.
6. Banchereau J, Rousset F. Human B lymphocytes: phenotype, proliferation, and differentiation. *Adv Immunol* 1992;52:125–262.
7. Pober JS, Cotran RS. Cytokines and endothelial cell biology. *Physiol Rev* 1990;70:427–456.
8. Libby P, Hansson GK. Involvement of the immune system in human atherogenesis: current knowledge and unanswered questions. *Lab Invest* 1991;64:5–15.
9. Pober JS, Cotran RS. Cytokines and endothelial cell biology. *Physiol Rev* 1990;70:427–456.
10. Hansson GK, Geng YJ, Holm J, Hårdhammar P, Wennmalm Å, Jennische E. Arterial smooth muscle cells express nitric oxide synthase in response to endothelial injury. *J Exp Med* 1994;180:733–738.
11. Hajjar DP, Pomerantz KB. Signal transduction in atherosclerosis: integration of cytokines and the eicosanoid network. *FASEB J* 1992;6:2933–2941.
12. Geng YJ, Hansson GK. Interferon-γ inhibits scavenger receptor expression and foam cell formation in human monocyte-derived macrophages. *J Clin Invest* 1992;89:1322–1330.
13. Li H, Cybulsky MI, Gimbrone MA Jr, Libby P. Inducible expression of vascular cell adhesion molecule-1 by vascular smooth muscle cells *in vitro* and within rabbit atheroma. *Am J Pathol* 1993;143:1551–1559.
14. Robey E, Fowlkes BJ. Selective events in T cell development. *Annu Rev Immunol* 1994;12:675–705.
15. Müller-Eberhard HJ. Molecular organization and function of the complement system. *Annu Rev Biochem* 1988;57:321–347.
16. Poole JCF, Florey HW. Changes in the endothelium of the aorta and the behaviour of macrophages in experimental atheroma of rabbits. *J Pathol Bacteriol* 1958;75:245–252.
17. Fowler S, Shio H, Haley NJ. Characterization of lipid-laden aortic cells from cholesterol-fed rabbits. IV. Investigation of macrophage-like properties of aortic cell populations. *Lab Invest* 1979;41:372–378.
18. Gerrity RG. The role of the monocyte in atherogenesis. I. Transition of blood-borne monocytes into foam cells in fatty lesions. *Am J Pathol* 1981;103:181–190.
19. Vedeler CA, Nyland H, Matre R. *In situ* characterization of the foam cells in early human atherosclerotic lesions. *Acta Pathol Microbiol Immunol Scand* 1984;92C:133–137.
20. Klurfeld DM. Identification of foam cells in human atherosclerotic lesions as macrophages using monoclonal antibodies. *Arch Pathol Lab Med* 1985;109:445–449.
21. Jonasson L, Holm J, Skalli O, Bondjers G, Hansson GK. Regional accumulation of T cells, macrophages, and smooth muscle cells in the human atherosclerotic plaque. *Arteriosclerosis* 1986;6:131–138.
22. Gown AM, Tsukada T, Ross R. Human atherosclerosis. II. Immunocytochemical analysis of the cellular composition of human atherosclerotic lesions. *Am J Pathol* 1986;125:191–207.
23. Faggiotto A, Ross R. Studies of hypercholesterolemia in the nonhuman primate. I. Changes that lead to fatty streak formation. *Arteriosclerosis* 1984;4:323–340.
24. Faggiotto A, Ross R. Studies of hypercholesterolemia in the nonhuman primate. II. Fatty streak conversion to fibrous plaque. *Arteriosclerosis* 1984;4:341–356.
25. Rosenfeld ME, Tsukada T, Gown AM, Ross R. Fatty streak initiation in Watanabe heritable hyperlipemic and comparably hypercholesterolemic fat-fed rabbits. *Arteriosclerosis* 1987;7:9–23.
26. Rosenfeld ME, Tsukada T, Chait A, Bierman EL, Gown AM, Ross R. Fatty streak expansion and maturation in Watanabe heritable hyperlipemic and comparably hypercholesterolemic fat-fed rabbits. *Arteriosclerosis* 1987;7:24–34.
27. Hansson GK, Björnheden T, Bylock A, Bondjers G. Fc-dependent binding of monocytes to areas with endothelial injury in the rabbit aorta. *Exp Mol Pathol* 1981;34:264–280.
28. Brown MS, Goldstein JL. Lipoprotein metabolism in the macrophage: implications for cholesterol deposition in atherosclerosis. *Annu Rev Biochem* 1983;52:223–261.
29. Jonasson L, Holm J, Skalli O, Gabbiani G, Hansson GK. Expression of class II transplantation antigen on vascular smooth muscle cells in human atherosclerosis. *J Clin Invest* 1985;76:125–131.
30. Hansson GK, Holm J, Jonasson L. Detection of activated T lymphocytes in the human atherosclerotic plaque. *Am J Pathol* 1989;135:169–175.
31. Stemme S, Holm J, Hansson GK. T lymphocytes in human atherosclerotic plaques are memory cells expressing CD45RO and the integrin VLA-1. *Arterioscler Thromb* 1992;12:206–211.
32. Geng YJ, Holm J, Nygren S, Bruzelius M, Stemme S, Hansson GK. Expression of macrophage scavenger receptor in atherosclerosis. Relationship between scavenger receptor isoforms, immunocompetent cells, and T cell cytokines. *[Submitted.]*
33. Munro JM, van der Walt JD, Munro CS, Chalmers JAC, Cox EL. An immunohistochemical analysis of human aortic fatty streaks. *Hum Pathol* 1987;18:375–380.
34. Van der Wal AC, Das PK, van de Berg DB, van der Loos CM, Becker AE. Atherosclerotic lesions in humans. *In situ* immunophenotypic analysis suggesting an immune mediated response. *Lab Invest* 1989;61:166–170.
35. Emeson EE, Robertson AL. T lymphocytes in aortic and coronary intimas. Their potential role in atherogenesis. *Am J Pathol* 1988;130:369–376.
36. Cybulsky MI, Gimbrone MA. Endothelial expression of a mononuclear leukocyte adhesion molecule during atherosclerosis. *Science* 1991;251:788–791.
37. Li H, Cybulsky MI, Gimbrone MA, Libby P. An atherogenic diet rapidly induces VCAM-1, a cytokine-regulatable mononuclear leukocyte adhesion molecule, in rabbit aortic endothelium. *Arterioscler Thromb* 1993;13:197–204.
38. Richardson M, Hadcock S, DeReske M, Cybulsky M. Increased expression *in vivo* of VCAM-1 and E-selectin by the aortic endothelium of normolipemic and hyperlipemic diabetic rabbits. *Arterioscler Thromb* 1994;14:760–769.
39. Elices MJ, Osborn L, Takada Y, et al. VCAM-1 on activated endothelium interacts with the leukocyte integrin VLA-4 at a site distinct from the VLA-4/fibronectin binding site. *Cell* 1990;60:577–584.
40. Bevilacqua MP, Pober JS, Mendrick DL, Cotran RS, Gimbrone MA. Identification of an inducible endothelial-leukocyte adhesion molecule. *Proc Natl Acad Sci USA* 1987;84:9238–9242.
41. Kume N, Cybulsky MI, Gimbrone MA. Lysophosphatidylcholine, a component of atherogenic lipoproteins, induces mononuclear leukocyte

adhesion molecules in cultured human and rabbit arterial endothelial cells. *J Clin Invest* 1992;90:1138–1144.

42. Hansson GK, Starkebaum GA, Benditt EP, Schwartz SM. Fc-mediated binding of IgG to vimentin-type intermediate filaments in vascular endothelial cells. *Proc Natl Acad Sci USA* 1984;81:3103–3107.
43. Hansson GK, Schwartz SM. Evidence for cell death in the vascular endothelium *in vivo* and *in vitro*. *Am J Pathol* 1983;112:278–286.
44. Seifert PS, Kazatchkine MD. The complement system in atherosclerosis. *Atherosclerosis* 1988;73:91–104.
45. Seifert PS, Hugo F, Hansson GK, Bhakdi S. Prelesional complement activation in experimental atherosclerosis. Terminal C5b-9 complement deposition coincides with cholesterol accumulation in the aortic intima of hypercholesterolemic rabbits. *Lab Invest* 1989;60:747–754.
46. Hansson GK, Lagerstedt E, Bengtsson A, Heideman M. IgG binding to cytoskeletal intermediate filaments activates the complement cascade. *Exp Cell Res* 1987;170:338–350.
47. Seifert PS, Kazatchkine MD. Generation of complement anaphylatoxins and C5b-9 by crystalline cholesterol oxidation derivatives depends on hydroxyl group number and position. *Mol Immunol* 1987;24: 1303–1308.
48. Poston RN, Haskard DO, Coucher JR, Gall NP, Johnson-Tidey RR. Expression of intercellular adhesion molecule-1 in atherosclerotic plaques. *Am J Pathol* 1992;140:665–673.
49. Seifert PS, Hansson GK. Complement receptors and regulatory proteins in human atherosclerotic lesions. *Arteriosclerosis* 1989;9:802–811.
50. Benditt EP, Barrett T, McDougall JK. Viruses in the etiology of atherosclerosis. *Proc Natl Acad Sci USA* 1983;80:6386–6389.
51. Ehlers S, Smith KA. Differentiation of T cell lymphokine gene expression. The *in vitro* acquisition of T cell memory. *J Exp Med* 1991;173: 25–36.
52. Ylä-Herttuala S, Palinski W, Rosenfeld ME, et al. Evidence for the presence of oxidatively modified low density lipoprotein in atherosclerotic lesions of rabbit and man. *J Clin Invest* 1989;84:1086–1895.
53. Salonen JT, Ylä-Herttuala S, Yamamoto R, et al. Autoantibody against oxidised LDL and progression of carotid atherosclerosis. *Lancet* 1992; 339:883–887.
54. Palinski W, Ylä-Herttuala S, Rosenfeld ME, et al. Antisera and monoclonal antibodies specific for epitopes generated during oxidative modification of low density lipoprotein. *Arterioscler Thromb* 1990;10: 325–335.
55. Palinski W, Rosenfeld ME, Ylä-Herttuala S, et al. Low density lipoprotein undergoes oxidative modification *in vivo*. *Proc Natl Acad Sci USA* 1989;86:1372–1376.
56. Ylä-Herttuala S, Palinski W, Butler SW, Picard S, Steinberg D, Witztum JL. Rabbit and human atherosclerotic lesions cointain IgG that recognizes epitopes of oxidized LDL. *Arterioscler Thromb* 1994;14: 32–40.
57. Stemme S, Faber B, Holm J, Wiklund O, Witztum JL, Hansson GK. T lymphocytes from human atherosclerotic plaques recognize oxidized LDL. *Proc Natl Acad Sci USA [in press]*.
58. Kiessling R, Grönberg A, Ivanyi J, et al. Role of hsp60 during autoimmune and bacterial inflammation. *Immunol Rev* 1991;121:91–111.
59. Xu Q, Kleindienst R, Waitz W, Dietrich H, Wick G. Increased expression of heat shock protein 65 coincides with a population of infiltrating T lymphocytes in atherosclerotic lesions of rabbits specifically responding to heat shock protein 65. *J Clin Invest* 1993;91:2693–2702.
60. Xu Q, Willeit J, Marosi M, et al. Association of serum antibodies to heat-shock protein 65 with carotid atherosclerosis. *Lancet* 1993;341: 255–259.
61. Xu Q, Dietrich H, Steiner HJ, et al. Induction of arteriosclerosis in normocholesterolemic rabbits by immunization with heat shock protein 65. *Arterioscler Thromb* 1992;12:789–799.
62. Mackay CR, Marston WL, Dudler L. Naive and memory T cells show distinct pathways of lymphocyte recirculation. *J Exp Med* 1990;171: 801–817.
63. Parums DV, Chadwick DR, Mitchinson MJ. The localization of immunoglobulin in chronic periaortitis. *Atherosclerosis* 1986;61:117–123.
64. Parums DV, Brown DL, Mitchinson MJ. Serum antibodies to oxidized low-density lipoprotein and ceroid in chronic periaortitis. *Arch Pathol Lab Med* 1990;114:383–387.
65. Griffith RL, Virella GT, Stevenson HC, Lopes-Virella MF. Low density lipoprotein metabolism by human macrophages activated with low density lipoprotein immune complexes. A possible mechanism of foam cell formation. *J Exp Med* 1988;168:1041–1059.
66. Galis Z, Muszynski M, Sukhova G, Simon-Morrissey E, Unemori E, Lark M, Amento E, Libby P. Cytokine-stimulated human vascular smooth muscle cells synthesize a complement of enzymes required for extracellular matrix digestion. *Circ Res* 1994;75:181–189.
67. Wang JM, Sica A, Peri G, Walter S, Padura IM, Libby P, Ceska M, Lindley I, Colotta F, Mantovani A. Expression of monocyte chemotactic protein and interleukin-8 by cytokine-activated human vascular smooth muscle cells. *Arterioscler Thromb* 1991;11:1166–1174.
68. Hansson GK, Holm J. Interferon-γ inhibits arterial stenosis after injury. *Circulation* 1991;84:1266–1272.
69. Hansson GK, Holm J, Holm S, Fotev Z, Hedrich HJ, Fingerle J. T lymphocytes inhibit the vascular response to injury. *Proc Natl Acad Sci USA* 1991;88:10530–10534.
70. Salomon RN, Hughes CCW, Schoen FJ, Payne DD, Pober JS, Libby P. Human coronary transplantation-associated arteriosclerosis. Evidence for a chronic immune reaction to activated graft endothelial cells. *Arterioscler Thromb* 1991;138:791–798.

Atherosclerosis and Coronary Artery Disease,
edited by V. Fuster, R. Ross, and E. J. Topol.
Lippincott-Raven Publishers, Philadelphia

CHAPTER 32

Viral Activation of Thrombo-Atherosclerosis

Robert J. Kaner and David P. Hajjar

Key Words: Colony-stimulating factor 1; Cytomegalovirus; Herpes viruses; Interleukin (1, 1β, 1α, 6); Monocytes; Polymorphonuclear leukocytes; T lymphocytes; Tumor necrosis factor-α.

INTRODUCTION

The pathogenesis of atherosclerosis is a multifactorial process that involves a complex interplay of genetic and environmental factors, as discussed elsewhere in this book. At present, the known risk factors do not account for all cases of human atherosclerosis (1). This suggests that the known risk factors may be synergistic with unidentified initiating factors. This concept, when coupled with the epidemiologic association between viral infection and accelerated atherosclerosis in heart transplant patients (2,3), the observation of viral nucleic acids in the atherosclerotic vessel wall, and the development of animal models of virally induced atherosclerosis under normocholesterolemic conditions (4–7), has led to a resurgence of interest in a possible link between viruses and either the etiology or pathogenesis of atherosclerosis (8). For the past 20 years, studies addressing a viral etiology of atherosclerosis have continued, spurred initially by the early work of Benditt and Benditt (9) and Fabricant et al. (4,10).

Herpes viruses might be capable of inducing atherogenesis by several mechanisms. For example, herpes virus infections may cause an ''initial'' injury event to the endothelium, as in the ''modified response to injury hypothesis'' (11). Alternatively, herpes viruses may induce a monoclonal proliferation of smooth muscle cells in the arterial wall leading to intimal hyperplasia, as hypothesized by Benditt and Benditt (9). Evidence is mounting that early developmental changes in specific vascular beds highly susceptible to the disease predispose certain areas to become the sites for atherogenic changes (12–15). Viruses could be viewed as a potential trigger for this process. This chapter reviews the evidence supporting the hypothesis that herpes viruses, by inducing altered gene function, may be involved as a primary or secondary factor in the pathogenesis of atherosclerosis. The effects of herpes virus infection in vitro on vascular cell metabolism and function are described. Information about candidate viral or transforming genes that might be related to the development of atherosclerosis is also reviewed.

EPIDEMIOLOGIC EVIDENCE LINKING HERPES VIRUS AND ATHEROSCLEROSIS

Seven members of the herpes virus family are now known to infect humans (16). Of these, herpes simplex virus type 1 (HSV-1), herpes simplex virus type 2 (HSV-2), and human

R. J. Kaner: Department of Medicine, Memorial Sloan-Kettering Cancer Center, New York, New York 10021.
D. P. Hajjar: Department of Pathology, Cornell University Medical College, New York, New York 10021.

cytomegalovirus (CMV) have been the primary candidate viruses whose potential relationship to atherosclerosis has been studied. Herpes simplex viral infections are widespread in the general population (17). More than half of children demonstrate antibodies to HSV-1 by 10 years of age (18). The frequency of previous HSV-2 infection is less certain, but various studies cite a prevalence of 0.3% to 22% (19). In the 35- to 44-year-old age group, well over 10% of the general population demonstrates antibodies to HSV-2 (18). A more recent study concluded that the incidence is 16.4% in the population of ages 15 to 74 (20). Antibodies to CMV are even more widespread in the population, indicating previous infection in more than 50% of adults (21).

A seroepidemiologic association between CMV infection and atherosclerosis was originally suggested by Adam et al. (22). This was based on a case-control study of cardiovascular surgery patients who were compared with a control group of subjects who were not undergoing surgery but matched for similar cholesterol levels and other atherosclerosis risk factors. In the 157 pairs evaluated, the incidence of positive CMV antibodies was higher in the surgical group than in the control group (90% and 74%, respectively, $p < 0.001$). A greater percentage of surgical cases than controls had high titers of CMV antibodies (57% and 26%, respectively). There was no correlation between antibody titers and serum cholesterol or triglycerides.

A study in a subgroup of the Framingham patients failed to find an overall association between a history of ever having "fever blisters or cold sores" with the prevalence or 6-year incidence of coronary heart disease (angina pectoris, coronary insufficiency, or myocardial infarction) in patients 58 to 89 years old (23). Previous work in this group of patients had shown a strong correlation of the self-reported history with serologic evidence of previous HSV-1 infection. This study does not completely rule out the possibility of such a relationship, particularly because a subgroup of women with recurrent cold sores had a 1.5-fold relative risk (95% confidence interval 1.0 to 2.1) of developing coronary heart disease.

A recent seroepidemiologic study compared HSV-1, HSV-2, and CMV antibody status to the results of B-mode ultrasonography of the carotid arteries, used as a marker of asymptomatic carotid artery thickening, a manifestation of early atherosclerosis (24); 340 matched case-control pairs from the Atherosclerosis Risk in Communities (ARIC) Study were evaluated. This study found a modest (odds ratio 1.55), though significant ($p = 0.03$), positive association between CMV antibodies and asymptomatic carotid artery thickening.

The strongest epidemiologic link between infection with herpes viruses and atherosclerosis in humans is in the heart transplant population. Several studies have demonstrated a strong correlation between CMV infection and accelerated atherosclerosis in this population. At Stanford University, 300 cardiac transplant patients were treated with immunosuppression and followed prospectively for the occurrence of CMV infection and the development of atherosclerosis. Of those tested, 91 patients developed CMV infections based on (a) positive cultures for CMV, (b) demonstration of characteristic CMV inclusion bodies in tissue samples, and/or (c) a fourfold rise in IgG CMV antibodies. After 5 years of follow-up, the rate of graft loss from accelerated atherosclerosis (with an endpoint of death or retransplantation) was 69% in CMV-infected patients but only 37% in the non-CMV-infected group (2). Furthermore, there was a tenfold greater incidence of patients who died with greater than 50% luminal obstruction in their coronary arteries in the CMV-positive as compared with the non-CMV-infected patients (2). Interestingly, similar results were reported from a somewhat smaller study at the University of Minnesota (25). This study compared rates of cytomegalovirus infection and atherosclerosis in 102 immunosuppressed patients who had received a cardiac transplant and survived for at least 1 year. At 2 years posttransplant, 32% of the CMV-positive patients had coronary artery disease as opposed to 10% of the CMV-negative patients.

These results have been reproduced by investigators from other transplant centers with carefully documented coronary angiography and endomyocardial biopsies (26). Moreover, pathological studies have demonstrated an endothelialitis associated with the accelerated atherosclerosis (27) that correlated with quantitation of the virus in endomyocardial biopsies (28). There are also in vitro data suggesting that CMV infection of endothelial cells up-regulates MHC Class II expression, which may enhance T-cell-mediated inflammatory processes in the vessel wall (29). The studies linking CMV infection to accelerated cardiac allograft atherosclerosis are the strongest data to date in humans linking infection with a herpes virus to atherosclerosis in a specific population.

PATHOBIOLOGICAL EVIDENCE LINKING HERPES VIRUS AND ATHEROSCLEROSIS

In 1984, Gyorkey et al. (30) reported the detection of virions of the herpes virus family in electron microscopic sections from the aortas of 10 of 60 patients with atherosclerosis undergoing cardiovascular surgery. These viral particles were in various stages of viral replication and included empty nucleocapsids and virions with dense cores. They were present in rare smooth muscle and endothelial cells. Of the 1,360 grids that were examined, only 35 showed evidence of virus. Benditt et al. (31) showed evidence of HSV nucleic acids by in situ hybridization in the ascending aorta in tissue removed during coronary bypass surgery. Eleven of 160 tissue samples were positive. In most cases, the tissue was histologically normal. In a second series of experiments examining four tissues that contained abnormally thickened intima, two of the four reacted positively with an HSV-2 probe. The positive staining occurred in cells located in discrete foci of increased cellularity within or adjacent to the intima. Melnick et al. (32) reported the detection of CMV antigen in cells cultured from arterial tissue surgically removed from patients with severe arterial disease. Petrie et al. (33) showed that in situ hybridization techniques would increase the frequency of detection of CMV in cultured smooth muscle cells from arterial plaques relative to immunohistochemical staining. More recently, Hendrix et al. (34) showed that the detection of CMV nucleic acids by polymerase chain reaction (PCR) was possible in 90% of samples obtained from patients with severe atherosclerosis as compared to only 53% in patients with minimal or no atherosclerosis. The presence of the complete viral genome was demonstrated in these samples by both dot–blot DNA hybridization and PCR using probes and primers derived from the immediate early and late genomic regions. Messenger RNA from the immediate early but not the late genomic regions could be demonstrated by in situ DNA hybridization. This suggested to the authors that CMV exists in the vessel wall primarily in a latent state where expression of immediate early messenger RNA transcripts may occur (35) without expression of messenger RNA coding for structural capsid proteins. Indeed, CMV DNA is widely distributed throughout the arterial tree (36), lending credence to the possibility that the vascular system may be the site of latency for this virus. We speculate that this may lead to an alteration in the factors that control growth in the vessel wall predisposing to intimal thickening.

To look for evidence of viral antigens or nucleic acids in the vessel wall at an earlier stage in the formation of the atherosclerotic lesions, Yamashiroya et al. (37) performed immunohistochemical and DNA hybridization studies on the coronary arteries and aortas of young trauma victims using fresh autopsy material. Evidence for HSV or CMV was detected in eight of 20 specimens of coronary arteries. The viral DNA or antigens were found in cells both in the intact luminal surface and in focal clusters of spindle-shaped or foam cells in the intimal layer. This study adds circumstantial evidence to support the hypothesis that viruses might be involved in the early events in atherogenesis.

The development of an animal model for atherosclerosis induced by a herpes virus infection by Fabricant et al. (4–7,38) has provided considerable experimental evidence to support the hypothesis that herpes viruses are involved in the pathogenesis of atherosclerosis. Pathogen-free normocholesterolemic chickens were infected with 100 PFU of Marek's disease virus (MDV), a herpes virus that causes malignant lymphomas of T-cell origin in chickens (39). Uninfected pathogen-free chickens served as a control. At 30 weeks, the virally infected chickens demonstrated grossly visible atherosclerotic lesions in the large coronary arteries, the aorta, and the major aortic branches (4). Detailed histological examination of these atherosclerotic lesions showed a fibroproliferative lesion similar to the proliferative lesions of human atherosclerosis (5). Of interest, the atherosclerotic lesions could be prevented by preimmunizing the animals with a related herpes virus of turkeys (6). Feeding the chickens a high-cholesterol diet produced a synergistic effect on increasing cholesterol accumulation (7). Biochemical analysis of the samples of aortic tissue from the normocholesterolemic, MDV-infected group by Hajjar et al. (7) found a significantly higher content of cholesterol, cholesterol esters (CE), triglycerides, phospholipids, and total lipids than in uninfected controls. The MDV infection also caused an abnormal rise in CE synthesis while reducing CE hydrolase activity, thus causing an alteration in cellular metabolism favoring arterial lipid accumulation (7). Furthermore, the cytoplasmic CE hydrolase could not be activated through the cAMP-dependent protein kinase system following MDV infection (7). These studies conclusively demonstrated that in an animal model, under conditions of normocholesterolemia, a herpes virus can serve as an etiological vector in lesion progression that pathologically and biochemically resembles that of human atherosclerosis and suggests that the virus significantly alters cholesterol metabolism of arteries leading to cholesterol deposition.

The pathogenesis of inflammatory abdominal aortic aneurysms in humans (40) has been linked to CMV (41). In this study PCR was used to detect CMV DNA in 41 aortic lesions excised at surgery and 16 aortic tissues obtained at autopsy. Cytomegalovirus DNA was detected in 88% (7/8) of inflammatory aortic lesions with periaortic fibrosis, including 5/6 aortic aneurysms, 61% (20/33) of atherosclerotic aneurysms, but only 31% (5/16) of autopsy samples without inflammation or atherosclerosis.

This subendothelial inflammation associated with CMV infection can be seen in human hearts as well during atherosclerosis of coronary allografts (42). Of considerable mechanistic interest in this regard is a report of T-lymphocyte activation by CMV-infected allogeneic cultured human endothelial cells (43). In a separate experimental model, CMV infection enhanced smooth muscle cell proliferation and intimal thickening of rat aortic allografts (44), further indicating the potential of this virus to exacerbate vascular disease. Peripheral blood mononuclear cells exhibit enhanced lysis of CMV- or HSV-infected vascular smooth muscle cells, perhaps contributing to cell turnover in an active vascular lesion (45). Finally, different lineages of smooth muscle cells derived from adult versus young animals exhibit differing infectivity for HSV-1 infection in vitro, suggesting age-related differences in susceptibility of vascular smooth muscle cells to herpes viral infection (45a).

BIOCHEMICAL CHANGES ASSOCIATED WITH VIRALLY INDUCED ATHEROSCLEROSIS

Herpes viruses are capable of infecting cells of the vascular wall. The HSV types 1 and 2 can infect bovine and human endothelial cells (46,47) and vascular smooth muscle cells (48). Similarly, human CMV also infects endothelial cells (49) and human vascular smooth muscle cells (50). Infection of cells in vitro with HSV results in an inhibition of host

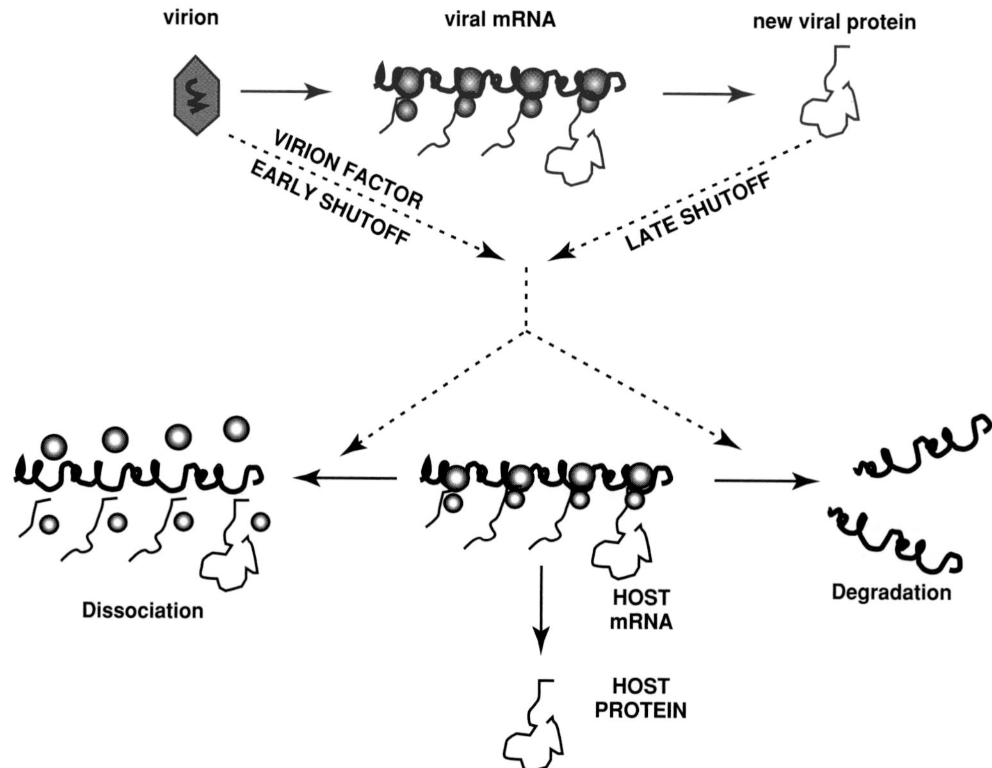

FIG. 1. Infection of cells in vitro with HSV-1 or -2 results in an inhibition of host cellular protein synthesis (51), which occurs in two steps. In the first few hours postinfection, "early shutoff" is mediated by a virion-associated protein and causes dissociation of host cell mRNAs from polysomes, rendering the mRNA nonfunctional and enhancing mRNA degradation (52). Kefalides and colleagues have demonstrated that this mechanism is relevant to the mRNAs encoding extracellular matrix proteins in both human endothelial cells (53) and human arterial smooth muscle cells (54) infected with HSV-1 in vitro. The delayed shutoff of host cell protein synthesis is thought to be mediated by a newly synthesized immediate-early viral gene product, which then causes dissociation of host cell mRNAs from polysomes and degradation of cellular messenger RNAs (55). This shuftoff of host protein synthesis leads to alterations in extracellular matrix, anticoagulant properties, and decreased production of those enzymes involved in lipid catabolic activity, as discussed in the text.

cellular protein synthesis (51) (Fig. 1). This shutoff of host cell protein synthesis occurs in two steps. The first stage, occurring in the first few hours postinfection, ''early shutoff,'' is mediated by a virion-associated protein and causes dissociation of host cell mRNAs from polysomes, rendering the mRNA nonfunctional and enhancing mRNA degradation (52). Kefalides and colleagues have demonstrated that this mechanism is relevant to the mRNAs encoding extracellular matrix proteins in both human endothelial cells (53) and human arterial smooth muscle cells (54) infected with HSV-1 in vitro (Fig. 1). The delayed shutoff of host cell protein synthesis is thought to be mediated by a newly synthesized immediate early viral gene product that then causes degradation of cellular messenger RNAs (55). Some of the viral genes responsible for the inhibition of host cell protein synthesis have been mapped and are discussed below in the molecular biology section.

As mentioned earlier, infection of cells with herpes viruses in vitro produces profound effects on cellular cholesterol metabolism. The concept of herpes virus(es) playing a major role in the etiology and pathogenesis of atherosclerosis was supported by the observation that intracellular and extracellular cholesterol accumulated in cell cultures infected with feline herpes virus (56). Infection of avian smooth muscle cells with MDV in vitro greatly increased the accumulation of cholesterol and CE (57). This type of specific lipid accumulation (which also occurs during the human arteriopathy) was also a result of decreased CE hydrolysis. Detailed analysis of enzyme activation and kinetics showed that the CE cycle is altered, resulting in cytoplasmic CE accumulation (57).

In an attempt to define some of the regulatory mechanisms associated with the control of cytoplasmic cholesteryl esterase in MDV-infected cells, the level of cholesteryl esterase activation in MDV-infected cells was examined in the presence of (a) dibutyryl cAMP, (b) dibutyryl cAMP added together with protein kinase, or (c) agonists of adenylate cyclase. Activation of cytoplasmic cholesteryl esterase activity was blocked in MDV-infected cells but not in uninfected cells and in those infected with a control virus, turkey herpes virus. Furthermore, the rate of cholesterol efflux from arterial smooth muscle cells challenged with dibutyryl cAMP was unresponsive in MDV-infected cells as compared to uninfected or turkey herpes virus-infected cells, in which efflux was increased. Hence, we proposed that the reduced cytoplasmic cholesteryl esterase activity in lipid-laden, herpes-virus-infected cells resulted partly from the inability of the enzyme to be activated by the cAMP–protein kinase mechanism coupled with decreased enzyme synthesis in the infected cell (58). This may contribute to the pathological changes seen in MDV-infected arterial cells, including accumulation of intracellular CEs.

These studies were extended to human arterial smooth muscle cells infected with HSV type 1: HSV also induced accumulation of saturated CE and triacylglycerols in infected cells (59). The infected cells had reductions in the activity of CE hydrolases related to changes in the physical state of the accumulating CE that prevented maximal hydrolytic activity (60) (Fig. 2) and decreased translation of the RNA that encodes the intracellular CE hydrolase (61). In addition, we observed a reduction in both spontaneous and arachidonate-induced release of prostacyclin (PGI_2) (59) in virally infected cells. Hence, we believe that the herpes-virus-induced atherosclerosis results, in part, from an alteration in metabolic control of CE trafficking in the vascular cells, as depicted in Fig. 3.

CYTOKINE INVOLVEMENT IN CHOLESTEROL TRAFFICKING IN VIRALLY INFECTED CELLS

Recent studies have suggested that the immune system may be important in the atherosclerotic lesion because monocytes and T lymphocytes accumulate within the atherosclerotic lesion (62). Viral infection could induce mediator release by immune cells, which might be responsible for phenotypic changes in vascular wall cells such as their ability to bind monocytes or release growth factors. Of interest in this regard are recent studies that show that herpes viruses are capable of inducing messenger RNA expression of monocyte mediator genes. This up-regulation of cytokine gene expression is in contradistinction to the effects on expression of extracellular matrix genes noted above. For example, CMV infection in vitro induces macrophages to increase the expression of specific RNAs for interleukin-1β (IL-1β), tumor necrosis factor-α (TNF-α), and colony-stimulating factor-1 (CSF-1) (63). In a mouse model of her-

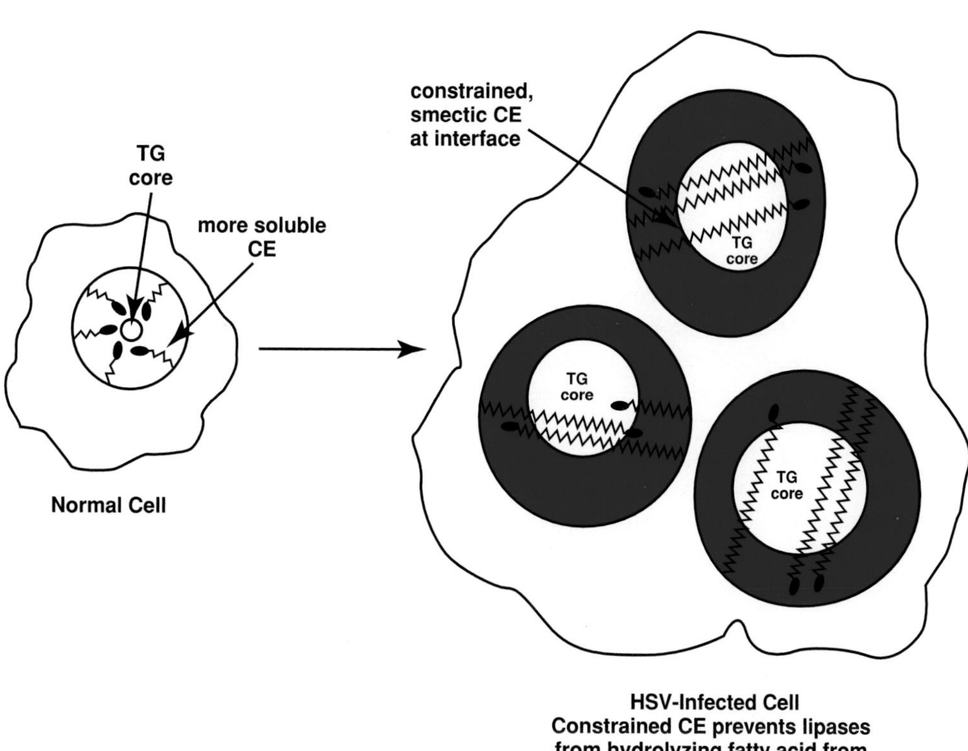

FIG. 2. Proposed model for alterations in TG/CE packing of droplets following HSV infection and its impact on CE hydrolysis. The HSV infection causes retention of monosaturated fatty acids, resulting in "constrained," smectic-like CE at the interface of the TG core of neutral lipid droplets. As a result, CE hydrolytic activity in the HSV-infected cell is reduced because the enzyme has a smaller capacity to catabolize the less fluid substrate (155). (From Hajjar, ref. 156, with permission.)

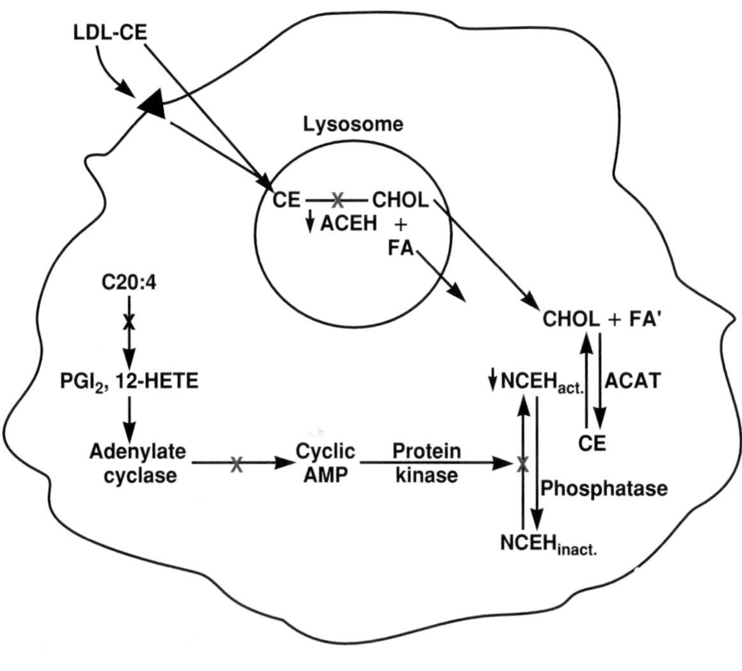

FIG. 3. Herpes virus infection blocks signal transduction pathways in arterial smooth muscle cells. This model shows that HSV infection leads to decreased lysosomal hydrolysis of CE by the ACEH enzyme. In addition, infection leads to decreased conversion of arachadonic acid (C20:4) to PGI_2 and 12-HETE, which in turn can lead to a reduced activation of adenylate cyclase. This results in decreased intracellular cAMP production. Continuing in this altered metabolic sequence of events, decreased cAMP induces less activation of protein kinase A, thus reducing the activation (through phosphorylation) of the cytoplasmic CE hydrolase (NCEH) to the active form from the inactive form. These metabolic events in the cytoplasm, coupled to those in the lysosomes, result in intracellular CE accretion. (From Hajjar, ref. 157, with permission.)

petic keratitis, where function of the corneal endothelium is clearly affected, there is up-regulation of IL-1α and interleukin 6 (IL-6) (63a). The HSV-1 infection of monocytes strongly up-regulates TNF-α release (64); CMV infection of monocytes induces release of TNF-α in vitro and in vivo (65). The role of TNF in the complex cytokine network in mammalian cells is not fully understood, particularly regarding its antiviral activity: TNF-α does appear to play a role in host defense against CMV in vivo (66).

Although TNF is an inducer of interferon messenger RNA transcripts, a well-documented cytokine that has anti-herpesviral activity, others have shown that TNF's antiviral activity is not abolished in the presence of antiserum to interferon (67). Wong and Goeddel (68) have postulated that the antiviral activity of TNF is attributable to lysis of virally infected cells rather than induction of interferon. Other possible mechanisms to explain the action of TNF include eicosanoid metabolism, because TNF's lytic effects can be partially abolished with cyclo-oxygenase inhibitors. Such studies suggest that cytokines, such as TNF, can promote synthesis of eicosanoid product(s) that, in turn, can mediate specific biological effects (69).

Because HSV infection of vascular cells can produce a biochemical and cytopathological effect virtually indistinguishable from atherosclerosis, we hypothesized that these cytokines can prevent CE accretion in arterial smooth muscle cells that is associated with herpes-virus-induced atherosclerosis (69). Both TNF and IL-1, but not interferon, prevented CE accumulation in HSV-infected cells by induction of cAMP-dependent CE hydrolysis. This effect was mediated through the arachidonate 12-lipoxygenase pathway via 12-HETE because pretreatment of cells with a cocktail of lipoxygenase inhibitors abolished the antiviral effect and 12-HETE production in the cell. 12-HETE is the major lipoxygenase metabolite found in arterial smooth muscle cells (69). This overall conclusion is further supported by the data that show that TNF and IL-1 enhance 12-HETE production, which in turn increases both intracellular cAMP levels and CE hydrolysis (69). Collectively, these findings identified for the first time a biochemical mechanism involved in the reduction of lipid accumulation in herpes-virus-infected arterial smooth muscle cells. This is potentially important in terms of cholesterol metabolism, because cytokines are important regulators of intracellular lipid metabolism in both herpes-virus-infected arterial smooth muscle cells (69) and noninfected monocyte-derived macrophages (70). For example, CSF-1 increases the uptake of acetylated low-density lipoproteins by increasing receptor numbers and enhances cholesterol esterification by 24-fold (70).

The immediate-early genes of human CMV are capable of specifically activating transcription of the monocyte–macrophage interleukin 1 β gene as detected in a CAT assay system (71). This is of interest in light of the observation of a 600-fold increase in IL-1β mRNA in atherosclerotic, compared to normal, vessel wall (72). Alternatively, CMV may up-regulate cytokine mRNA expression via activation of specific transcription factors such as NF-κB, AP-1, and CRE/B (73). Pseudorabies virus, another herpes family virus, induces the expression of IL-6 mRNA in infected human fibroblasts (74). Cytomegalovirus up-regulates IL-6 mRNA expression and protein release from human endothelial cells (75). Other members of the herpes virus family, such as Epstein–Barr virus, contain genes that appear to have important regulatory effects on host cell cytokine synthesis (76). This topic is reviewed elsewhere (76).

VIRAL ACTIVATION OF THE COAGULATION CASCADE

Herpes viruses cause a lesion that is characteristic of leukocytoclastic vasculitis with granulocyte infiltration of the artery accompanied by fibrin deposition as well as thrombin formation (77). Hence, this vector has the ability to influence not only atherosclerotic changes but also thrombotic disease. Because the virus causes a fatty-proliferative lesion in animals with the presence of microthrombi (5), such evidence supports the hypothesis that both thrombosis and intimal hyperplasia may be initiated by a virally induced event.

We believe that the surface of an HSV-infected endothelial cell becomes prothrombotic as evidenced by enhanced thrombin generation and enhanced binding of platelets to endothelium (78). Type 1 HSV infection of endothelial cells also up-regulates surface expression of tissue factor, which is not dependent on productive viral infection (79). This prothrombotic state is associated with a decrease in prostacyclin (78) and an inhibition of endothelial cell synthesis of heparan sulfate proteoglycan (80), which is closely related structurally to heparin and has significant anticoagulant activity (81). Moreover, HSV type 1 infection of endothelial cells can also result in quantitative and qualitative changes in the extracellular matrix synthesized and released by these cells (82,83). The matrix proteins synthesized by endothelial cells are inhibited to differing degrees by HSV-1 infection in the order (from most to least inhibition): collagen type IV > fibronectin > thrombospondin (82,83). As noted above, heparan sulfate proteoglycan, as well as chondroitin/dermatan sulfate proteoglycan, is also inhibited by HSV-1 infection (80). Similar inhibition of matrix protein synthesis was also observed in HSV infection of vascular smooth muscle cells (84). In addition to selective effects on matrix protein synthesis, HSV infection of endothelium also has specific effects on receptors for matrix components (85). Alterations in the extracellular matrix and in cell–matrix interactions can have profound effects on vascular cell phenotype and function (86). In conclusion, HSV infection of vascular cells in vitro causes cholesterol accumulation, the induction of a proinflammatory and prothrombotic state on the cell surface, and significant alterations in the extracellular matrix macromolecules synthesized by vascular cells.

Cytomegalovirus infection, although not as well studied as HSV infection of vascular cells, also leads to profound alterations in cellular metabolism (87). Like HSV, CMV induces a procoagulant state on the surface of the endothelial cell (88). The CMV induces expression of MHC class I antigens on the surface of fibroblasts (89) and endothelial cells (90). Cytomegalovirus infection of endothelial cells also markedly enhances the adherence of polymorphonuclear leukocytes (PMN) (91). These effects would be expected to enhance the prothrombotic and proinflammatory milieu of the vascular wall. Both types of processes are implicated in the pathogenesis of atherosclerosis.

A link among the coagulation system, fibrinolysis, and atherosclerosis has been proposed in terms of thrombotic processes at the level of the endothelium. The linkage among lesion development, lipid abnormalities involving lipoprotein(a) [Lp(a)], and the coagulation system is now being broadly defined (92). Early on, studies involving the Eskimos showed that their diet, enriched with polyunsaturated fatty acids, had an impact on platelet function and eicosanoid balance as well as in producing a significantly lower mortality from atherosclerotic heart disease (93). If the vessel wall is injured (or activated), for example, by herpes viruses, the endothelium can become prothrombotic. This includes increased thrombin generation and enhanced binding of platelets to endothelium (78), decreased PGI_2 production (78), enhanced tissue factor production, reduction of thrombomodulin expression (94), and an inhibition of endothelial cell synthesis of heparan sulfate proteoglycan, as noted above.

Abnormalities of fibrinogen metabolism can be linked directly to lipoprotein abnormalities as evident in the recent observation of structural (amino acid) homology between the apoprotein component of human Lp(a) and plasminogen (95), a major protein involved in fibrinolysis (92). This striking example of sequence homology emphasizes how thrombotic processes may be functionally related to atherogenic events.

Raised levels of Lp(a) are associated with an increased incidence of atherosclerosis (92), and the kringle structures common to both proteins are responsible for binding of plasminogen to fibrin. The Lp(a) may bind in this way and block fibrinolysis either by preventing activation of plasminogen to plasmin, as a protease, or by preventing initial access and binding of plasminogen (92).

Herpes simplex virus infection of the endothelium also produces alterations of surface-associated fibrinolysis because the acute infection decreases both plasminogen activator inhibitor-1 activity and the synthesis of tissue plasminogen activator (96).

An important event in the early stages of atherosclerosis is the adhesion of blood cells to the endothelium. Certainly, both platelet (as well as neutrophil) and monocyte adhesion to the endothelium are processes attributable to the pathogenesis of thrombosis and atherosclerosis. Monocytes can migrate into the vessel media and begin accumulating cholesterol, contributing to foam cell formation (14).

An HSV-infected endothelium, similar to endothelium exposed to tumor necrosis factor (TNF) or interleukin-1 (IL-1) (97), binds platelets (78) and granulocytes (98) and expresses tissue factor to a greater extent than noninfected cells (94). The HSV-infected endothelium also expresses glycoproteins encoded by the HSV genome (99) that participate in molecular mimicry as a result of their variable functional role on the endothelium. For example, glycoprotein E (gE) can function as an Fc receptor (99–101) in a complex with glycoprotein I (gI) (102), and glycoprotein C (gC) can also serve as a complement (C3b) receptor (99). A role for these proteins in the pathogenesis of endothelial injury is suggested by the observation that polymorphonuclear (PMN) cell adhesion to HSV-infected endothelium can be blocked by antiviral serum (98).

Central to the pathogenesis of vascular injury is the localized activation of the coagulation cascade and the adhesion of circulating inflammatory cells to the exposed vascular surface. Once adherent, these cells can secrete growth factors, proteolytic enzymes, and cytokines that further perturb the injured vessel surface (14,103). For example, macrophage-derived cytokines such as TNF and IL-1 induce endothelial expression of leukocyte adhesion molecules (104) as well as tissue factor (97), which promote leukocyte accumulation and localized thrombin generation.

IDENTIFICATION OF A MONOCYTE RECEPTOR ON VIRALLY INFECTED ENDOTHELIAL CELLS

An important initiating event in the early stages of atherosclerosis is the binding of circulating monocytes to the endothelium, after which they migrate into the vessel media and begin accumulating cholesterol, contributing to foam cell formation (11). It has been observed that HSV type 1 infection of human umbilical vein endothelial cells produces an increase in the adherence of granulocytes (46). Experiments in our laboratory have demonstrated that infection of endothelial cells with HSV-1 promotes enhanced monocyte–endothelial cell adhesion (105). Enhanced adhesion was blocked by monoclonal antibodies to the virally encoded cell surface glycoprotein gC but not by antibodies to gD or gE. Adhesion was also blocked by treating endothelial cells with specific thrombin inhibitors or by growing cells in prothrombin-depleted serum. Glycoprotein C bound and promoted activation of factor X on infected endothelial cells, thereby contributing to thrombin generation. Factor X also bound to transfected L cells that were induced to express gC by dexamethasone, a hormone that activates the promoter region of the gC gene construct. Cross-linking and immunoprecipitation studies demonstrated factor X–gC complex formation on the surface of these cells, suggesting that gC-dependent thrombin generation by herpes-infected endothelium may be an important mediator of vascular pathology during viral infection.

Thrombin can elicit a variety of cellular events. These include monocyte and neutrophil adhesion and cytokine release. Each of these cytopathological effects is part of the inflammatory response that is thought to be an important aspect of the pathogenesis of atherosclerosis. As summarized in Fig. 4, the molecular mechanism for the increased monocyte adherence was shown to be binding of factor X to HSV glycoprotein C expressed on the cell surface, thereby causing the generation of thrombin (105). The thrombin then led to an increase in monocyte binding, as detailed below.

Endothelial cells express several leukocyte receptors, including GMP-140 (also known as PADGEM or CD-62), ELAM-1, ICAM-1 and -2, and VCAM-1, on their surfaces in response to cytokines or other agonists (106). GMP-140 is a cytoplasmic protein in resting endothelial cells found on the membrane of an intracellular organelle known as the Weibel–Palade body (107). After stimulation by thrombin, histamine, or complement proteins, the Weibel–Palade body is rapidly secreted, and its membrane becomes incorporated into the plasma membrane, causing surface expression of GMP-140 (107). This mechanism of new protein expression, i.e., translocation from a preformed intracellular membrane compartment to the cell surface, does not require de novo

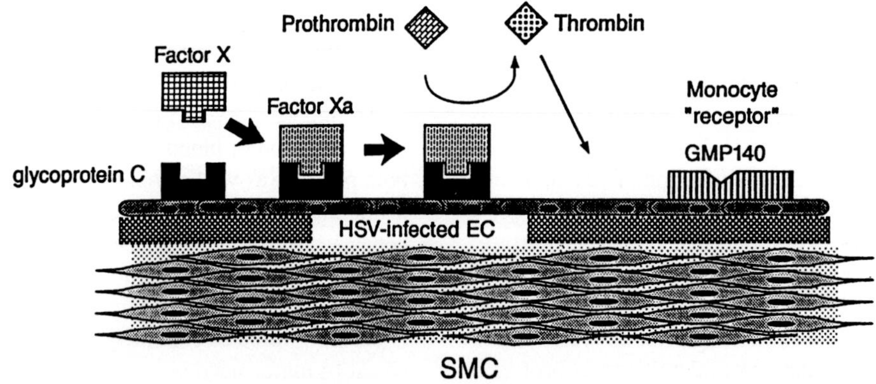

FIG. 4. Viral activation of the coagulation cascade. Hypothetical model depicting how HSV-1 infection can lead to a prothrombotic, proatherosclerotic state on the endothelial surface by inducing the synthesis and expression of glycoprotein (C), which can serve as a binding site for factor X, a key proenzyme of the coagulation cascade. This increased binding of factor X and its subsequent conversion to the active form, factor Xa, can lead to the conversion of prothrombin to thrombin (factor IIa). When thrombin is generated, it can induce surface expression of a monocyte receptor (GMP-140), which in turn can promote monocyte adhesion to the endothelium and induction of an inflammatory response by activation of the cytokine network. (From Hajjar, ref. 157, with permission.)

synthesis of GMP-140 and is consistent with the inhibition of protein synthesis seen in HSV-infected cells. We have also shown that another Weibel–Palade body protein, von Willebrand factor, mediates platelet adhesion to HSV-1-infected endothelial cells (108). As described in the previous section, our recent data support the following model: HSV infection induces endothelial cell surface expression of HSV gC, which acts as a binding site for factor X. The concomitant generation of tissue factor converts bound factor X to an active prothrombinase, leading to the generation of thrombin in the microenvironment of the infection (105).

Recently, we have extended this hypothesis with evidence that thrombin can also act in an autocrine manner to induce expression of the leukocyte receptor GMP-140 (109). Our data are as follows: Monocyte adhesion induced by HSV infection was blocked by anti-GMP-140, suggesting that GMP-140 is a receptor for monocytes on the HSV-infected endothelium (109). These findings are summarized in Fig. 4. This figure shows that HSV-infected endothelial cells generate thrombin, which predisposes to increased monocyte adherence by expressing the monocyte receptor GMP-140. Thrombin generation by these cells was dependent on the expression of HSV gC, which can act as a site for binding of factor X and assembly of the prothrombinase complex. Other receptors do not play a major role in this cell system. For example, the leukocyte integrins (LFA-1, Mac-1, and p150,95) mediate adhesion to ICAM-1 and ICAM-2 on cytokine-stimulated endothelial cells (110) but do not appear to play a role in adhesion to the virally infected cells based on lack of inhibition seen with specific monoclonal antibodies or RGDS peptides (109). Similarly, VCAM-1, which mediates lymphocyte adhesion to stimulated endothelial cells (111), also does not appear to play a role, based on lack of inhibition seen with anti-VCAM antibodies (109). The significance of a procoagulant phenotype of HSV-infected cells is severalfold: local generation of thrombin at the site of infection may activate platelets as well as endothelial cells. It has been reported that thrombin-stimulated platelets adhere to monocytes; thus, platelets may be recruited into the area of injury (11,109,112). The presence of activated platelets and monocytes at the area of infection may further contribute to the development of vascular injury and chronic inflammation by releasing cytokines and lipoxygenase products (109,113,114). Adhesive molecule expression on HSV-infected cells may thus be an initial step in viral-mediated endothelial injury and atherosclerosis.

Most recently, we have analyzed the structural domains of factor X that are involved in the coordination of its binding to membrane receptors that mediate monocyte adhesion (115). Two unrelated surface membrane receptor regions that coordinate this recognition have been identified: CD11b/CD18 on monocytes and glycoprotein C (gC) on HSV-infected endothelium. They recognize a common structural motif in the catalytic domain of factor X (115). This was seen by constituting three spatially distant surface loops that define a unique three-dimensional cell-interacting network in the ligand (Fig. 5; see Colorplate 25). Synthetic peptides recapitulating the three surface loops inhibit factor X binding to monocyte CD11b/CD18 and to endothelial cell herpes virus gC. They block monocyte generation of thrombin and prevent monocyte adhesion to HSV-infected endothelium. Thus, selective interruption of coagulation by such synthetic analogs may impact positively to reduce vascular injury associated with monocyte adherence and HSV infection of endothelium.

MOLECULAR GENETICS OF ATHEROSCLEROSIS

The monoclonal hypothesis of Benditt and Benditt (9) was based on the observation that 75% of atherosclerotic plaques from human tissues removed at surgery or at autopsy demonstrated a monoclonal phenotype of the glucose-6-phosphate dehydrogenase (G-6-PD) enzyme, based on electrophoretic mobility. This technique takes advantage of the fact that the polymorphic forms of this enzyme are expressed in an X-linked fashion. Medial cells from regions adjacent to atherosclerotic plaques and from nonplaque areas display equal amounts of each polymorphic form of the enzyme, as would be expected in an X-linked gene, because one of the two X chromosomes is inactivated early in embryonic development. Similar results were obtained by other laboratories (116,117). Nevertheless, the interpretation of these experiments in supporting the monoclonal hypothesis has been challenged (118), the principal argument being that the G-6-PD marker may be linked to some other gene that gives these cells a selective growth advantage, i.e., a "phenotype-selective advantage hypothesis," without the proliferative lesion being truly monoclonal in origin.

The monoclonal hypothesis suggests that the smooth muscle cell proliferation seen in the atherosclerotic lesion is similar to a benign tumor as, for example, in uterine leiomyomas (119). A logical extension of this hypothesis is to infer that alterations in the smooth muscle cell genome by chemical mutagens or viruses might be involved in the smooth muscle cell proliferation characteristic of human atherosclerosis. Supporting such an idea is the experimental observation of focal smooth cell proliferation induced in the aortic intima of chickens treated with a chemical mutagen initiation–promotion sequence (120). This may be a reasonable explanation that links cigarette smoking with the development of atherosclerosis (121–123), because the urine of smokers is known to contain excessive amounts of mutagenic or premutagenic substances (124).

To extend these observations to the level of the genome, Penn et al. (125) reported the presence of transforming DNA in samples derived from human coronary artery atherosclerotic plaques. Plaque-derived DNA had the capacity to transform NIH 3T3 cells in vitro. The transformed cell lines were capable of forming tumors in nude mice. The original observations regarding the presence of a transforming gene element have been extended into an animal model of early arterial plaques induced by administration of the carcinogen 7,12-dimethylbenz(a)anthracene (DMBA) to cockerels (126). Further studies on vascular smooth muscle derived from human plaques show enhanced expression of the protooncogene *myc* (127), although this could be a marker of enhanced cellular replication without true transformation. Whether the presence of a transforming gene is a generalized phenomenon in atherosclerotic lesions has been challenged by Yew et al., who were unable to detect transforming activity in DNA isolated from atherosclerotic plaques of human carotid arteries (128). Nevertheless, other laboratories have detected evidence of a similar transforming gene in atherosclerotic plaques (129). This study reported the correlation of transformation with the absence of a 140-kDa protein normally secreted by these cells. Interestingly, other studies have identified a 140-kDa antitumorigenic glycoprotein that acts as an antiangiogenesis factor (130,131). The loss of this protein correlates with a transformed phenotype. This study (129) raises the possibility that the transforming gene activity may represent the loss of a normal antioncogene or gene controlling cellular proliferation. The identity of the transforming gene(s) remains elusive.

Although no transforming gene of viral origin has been identified to cause human atherosclerosis, the results of recent studies ''suggest'' that vascular cells, like other cells, have the potential to be transformed by viral genes. Natchtigal and his colleagues have shown that vascular smooth muscle cells were transformed following transfection with a plasmid containing the SV40 early region (132). They also showed that rabbit arterial smooth muscle cells were immortalized following transfection with a plasmid containing the BgI II N fragment (MTRII, Fig. 6B) of HSV-2 (133). Immortalization is probably the most important attribute of transformation, because these cells normally have a finite life span in vitro (133). The transformed cells did not retain the viral DNA sequences, consistent with the findings noted above in HSV-induced transformation. Transformation of rat embryo cells by SV40 can result in marked accumulation of cholesteryl esters, apparently as a result of an alteration in the regulation of low-density lipoprotein receptors (134). Taken together, these studies provide circumstantial evidence that virally induced transformation can predispose to some of the characteristic features of atherogenesis. More studies are necessary to prove that the vessel wall actually contains transformed cells that are part of the foam cell population in atherosclerotic plaque regions. In Fig. 7, we have summarized what we believe to be three cytological alterations induced by herpes virus infection. The atherogenic potential of viruses in acute infection is depicted on the left. The consequences of chronic infection, with ongoing immunologic activation, is depicted on the right. Transformation of vascular smooth muscle cells is depicted in the far right side of the figure, and potential mechanisms of viral transformation are further discussed below.

The transforming potential of herpes viruses (135–137) has been well established in a large number of studies. These studies do not demonstrate a single viral oncogene, a virus-coded transforming protein, or any genomic DNA sequences that directly transform cells by a ''single hit'' kinetic model (137), but they do suggest that the mechanism of transformation is complex. The fact that genomic viral sequences are not retained in the transformed cells makes the elucidation of the transformation mechanism more problematic (138,139). Despite this, the genetic elements involved in transformation have been mapped to specific subsegments of the viral genome (140,141) (see Fig. 5). This was done by cleaving the viral genomic DNA into small fragments, isolating the fragments, and testing which ones retained the capacity to transform target cells into which they were transfected. These experiments led to the designation of specific regions of the viral genome as responsible for this transforming property. There is a single morphological transformation region of HSV-1 (MTRI) (141). Two morphological transforming regions are found in HSV-2: MTRII (129) and MTRIII (142,143). An HSV-1 mutation mediates the degradation of host mRNA responsible in part for the suppression of host protein synthesis noted above (144). Of interest, this fragment overlaps the MTRII of HSV-2 and is within an open reading frame encoding a 1.9-kb RNA leading to synthesis of a 58-kDa protein (145).

The authors proposed two possible interpretations for the comapping of the transforming and host shutoff functions: (a) the two functions could involve different gene products, e.g., if the mechanism of transformation involved a gene insertion into a promoter; or (b) transformation could be an indirect consequence of the inhibition of host protein synthesis (144). This inhibition might lead to transient stress alterations causing rearrangements of genes regulating the cell cycle (144). They also suggested that the more efficient shutoff by HSV-2 (141,146) might explain why this region appears to be transforming only in HSV-2 but not in the homologous region of HSV-1 (141). Because shutoff of host cell protein synthesis is incompatible with long-term survival, the authors also point out (144) that this may explain why viral DNA is not retained in the transformed cells and is lost in daughter generations (138,139).

Very small DNA fragments of a size unable to code for a transforming protein are also capable of inducing morphological transformation (147). As noted above, the DNA used to induce the morphological transformation is not retained within the transformed cell, and there is no evidence for an HSV-coded transforming protein (139).

Human CMV also has two morphological transforming regions (148,149). Viral DNA is not retained in cells transformed by the human CMV strain AD-169; however, there is one report of viral DNA being retained in cells transformed by human CMV strain Towne (150).

The mechanism of transformation by these herpes virus DNA fragments has not been elucidated. Proposals have been made to implicate DNA stem loop structures, ribonucleotide reductase activity, mutagenesis, gene amplification,

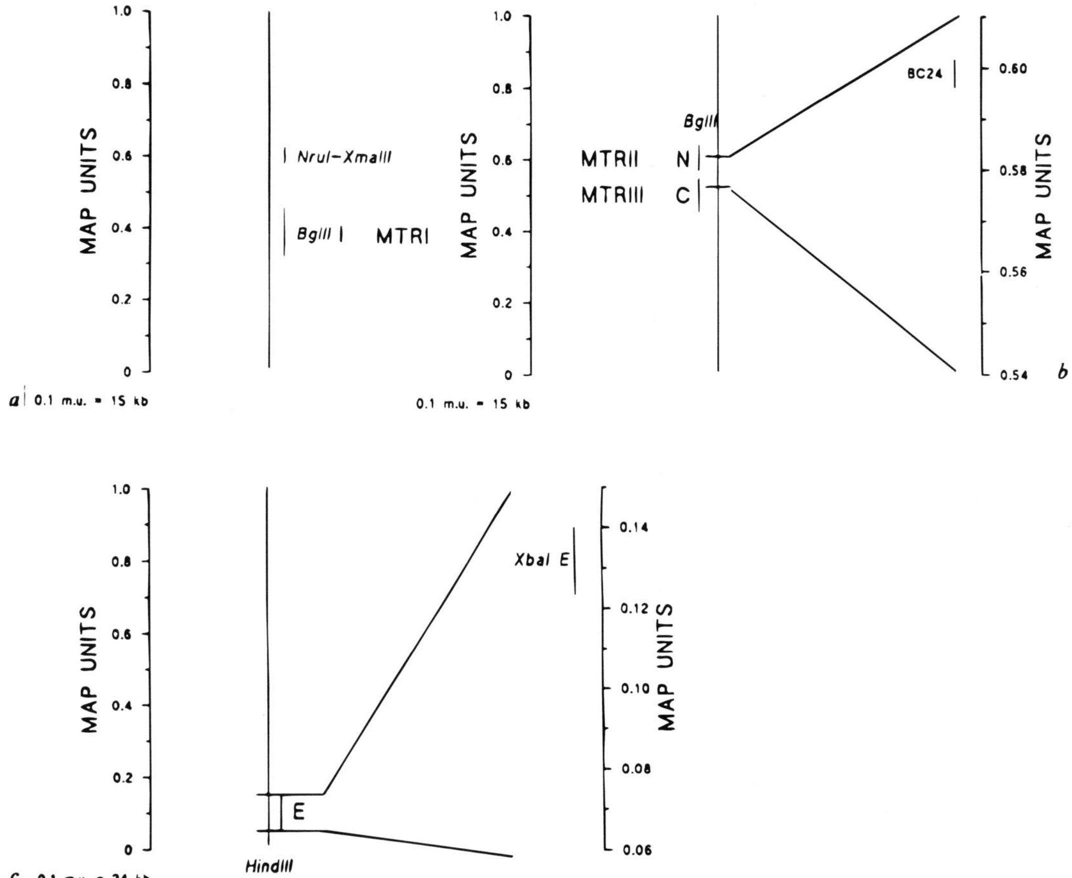

FIG. 6. Genomic organization of herpes virus morphological transforming regions (MTR). Transformation of vascular smooth muscle cells is one mechanism postulated to explain the intimal proliferation seen in the atherosclerotic lesion, as in the "monoclonal hypothesis" (9). These restriction fragments, designated by *capital letters* (prepared from viral genomic DNA by digestion with restriction endonucleases such as BglII, HindIII, XbaI), define viral genomic DNA segments capable of transforming cells in vitro. The location of these gene loci are indicated by arbitrary map units, expressed as the fractional distance in the whole viral genome between 0 and 1.0. **a:** HSV-1 morphologic transforming region I(MTRI) as the BglII I restriction fragment 0.311–0.415 map units. The NruI-XmaIII fragment encodes the virion host shutoff function. **b:** HSV-2 MTRII and MTRIII in BglII restriction fragments N and C, respectively. The BglII N fragment is the only HSV DNA region known to be capable of transforming vascular smooth muscle cells (135) in vitro. The fragment labelled BC24 is a restriction fragment too small to encode an entire protein (147). **c:** Human CMV strain AD-169 restriction fragment HindIII/XbaI E. The XbaI E fragment has significant sequence homology with HSV-2 BglII C (MTRIII). Note that the scale is different in **c** because of the significantly larger size of the human CMV genome. (From Kaner and Hajjar, ref. 158, with permission.)

increased or altered expression of cellular genes, activation of endogenous viruses, protein kinase activity, and the possible interaction between latency of the virus and transformation (reviewed in 135). No conclusive proof exists for any of these mechanisms (135). Recently, shuttle vectors have been employed to study sequence analysis of the mutations induced in cellular DNA by HSV type 1 (151). Of interest, the maximal increase in mutation frequency was noted at 4 h after HSV-1 infection, implicating an immediate-early or early viral protein. Sequence analysis of the chromosomal fragments may lead to information about putative cellular targets for the virally induced mutagenesis. Mutagenesis (151) could be a possible explanation for a "hit-and-run" mechanism (140) of virally induced transformation. Because vascular smooth muscle cells can be transformed by HSV-2 (134), we speculate that herpes-virus-induced transformation may be a contributory mechanism to loss of growth control in the atherosclerotic vessel wall (Fig. 6). The fact that specific regions of viral DNA can be isolated that are consistently capable of transforming targets cells opens the speculative possibility that viruses may transform cells in vivo without even the necessity for viral replication.

In another animal model of viral genes linked to atherosclerosis, Japanese quail genetically susceptible to athero-

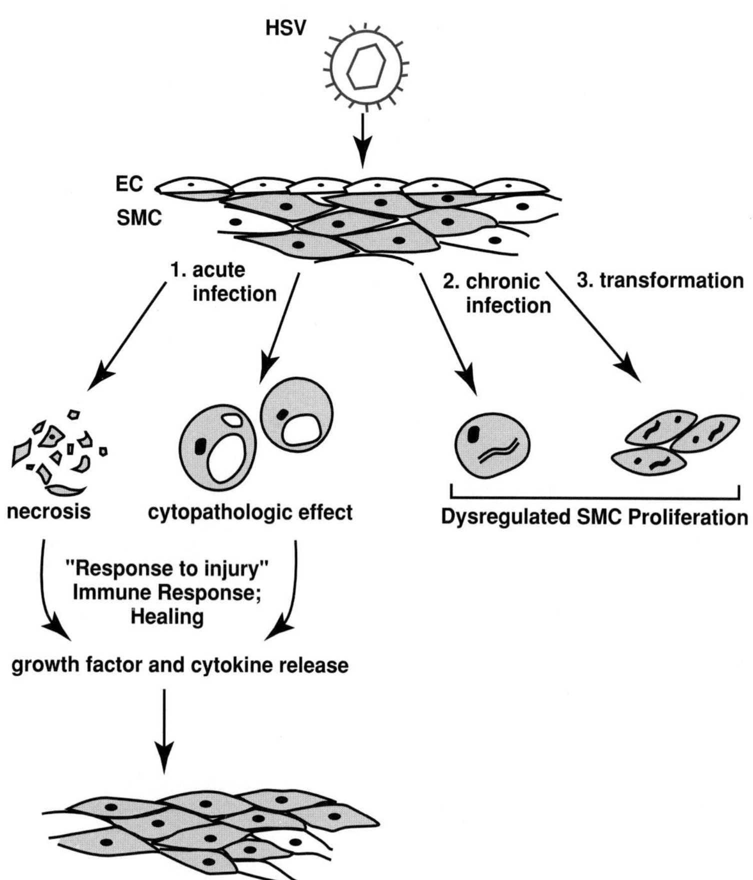

FIG. 7. Three cytological alterations induced by herpes virus infection. A hypothetical model of viral infection of the vessel wall that can induce three cytopathological states is depicted. *Acute infection* can lead to altered cellular morphology, lipid accumulation, altered extracellular matrix, altered functional properties of the vascular cells, and acute inflammation, possibly resulting in smooth muscle cell (SMC) proliferation during the healing process. *Chronic infection* can provide the immunologic stimuli for an ongoing cell-mediated inflammatory response with subsequent cellular infiltration of the vessel wall leading to dysregulated smooth muscle cell proliferation. *Transformation* leads to increased proliferation because the cells lose their capacity to down-regulate growth and cell division appropriately. EC, endothelial cells. (From Kaner and Hajjar, ref. 158, with permission.)

sclerosis were found to have specific DNA segments of Marek's disease herpes virus incorporated into their genome (152). Two lines of Japanese quail, one highly susceptible and the other resistant to atherosclerosis, were developed through genetic selection (153). The susceptible quail developed severe aortic lesions within 9 weeks when fed a high-cholesterol diet. Histological examination showed that their pathology resembled human atherosclerosis (154). When the genomic DNA from these susceptible animals was hybridized with DNA probes prepared by restriction endonuclease digestion of MDV DNA representing about 30% of the total MDV genome, a strong signal was detected in all genetically susceptible animals. In addition, the amount of DNA detected appeared to be proportional to the degree of atherosclerosis in the aortas. Of interest, the restriction patterns developed from endonuclease digestion of the cellular DNA showed that only a limited number of specific endonuclease restriction fragments hybridized to the MDV total probe. These results suggested that a specific part of the MDV genome, but not the total genome, was detectable in atherosclerotic tissue. Functional MDV was not detected by virus isolation, serology, or exposure of other chicks to susceptible quail. Examination of embryos from these different strains suggested that the viral genes were passed through the germ line. The authors concluded that this indicated that either the viral gene or one very closely linked to it was responsible for their susceptibility to atherosclerosis. These conclusions regarding retention of viral DNA in the germ line are quite different from the results observed with HSV-1 transformation in vitro. In addition, vertical transmission of viral DNA in vivo has not been observed previously. It remains to be determined if the MDV probes can cross-hybridize with a normal cellular gene and if the signals detected may be caused by cross-hybridization with a quail gene that exhibits pleomorphism in the DNA of the two strains of quail. If this were the case, the conclusions of the study would have to be altered.

SUMMARY

New data continue to suggest a possible role for viruses in the etiology and/or pathogenesis of atherosclerosis. As outlined above, herpes virus are strong potential candidates as etiologic agents in atherogenesis. This is based on: (a) evidence of widespread infections with these viruses in the general population, and the ability of these viruses to cause systemic infections, implying transmission through the vasculature; (b) the recognition of the association between accelerated atherosclerosis and CMV infection in cardiac allograft recipients; (c) the observation of herpes-virus-induced atherosclerosis occurring in animal models of the disease during normocholesterolemia; (d) profound effects on cholesterol metabolism in human, bovine, and avian arterial smooth muscle cells infected with herpes viruses in vitro, favoring cholesterol accumulation; (e) alterations in extracellular matrix and prothrombotic milieu in vascular cells infected with herpes viruses in vitro; (f) increased monocyte binding of HSV-infected endothelial cells; (g) the transforming potential of herpes viruses; (h) the ability of vascular smooth muscle cells to be transformed by viruses; (i) the recognition of transforming gene elements in atherosclerotic lesions; and (j) the ability of herpes viruses to induce activation of cytokine genes; all of which are potential contributory mechanisms in human atherogenesis.

These data suggest that any etiological or pathophysiological relationship between viruses and atherosclerosis is likely to be complex. Despite all of the progress to date, a cause-and-effect relationship between viruses and atherosclerosis in humans still has not been definitively established. The greatest challenge for future research in this area is to solidify or refute the hypothesis that human viruses cause or contribute to the development of human atherosclerosis.

REFERENCES

1. Gorden T, Garcia-Palmieri MR, Kagen A, Kannel WB, Schiffman J. Differences in coronary heart disease in Framingham, Honolulu and Puerto Rico. *J Chron Dis* 1974;27:329–344.
2. Grattan MT, Moreno-Cabral CE, Starnes VA, Oyer PE, Stinson EB, Shumway NE. Cytomegalovirus infection is associated with cardiac allograft rejection and atherosclerosis. *JAMA* 1989;261:3561–3566.
3. MacDonald K, Rector TS, Braunlan EA, Coubo SH, Olivari MT. Association of coronary artery disease in cardiac transplant recipients with cytomegalovirus infection. *Am J Pathol* 1989;64:359–362.
4. Fabricant CG, Fabricant J, Litrenta MM, Minick CR. Virus-induced atherosclerosis. *J Exp Med* 1978;148:335–340.
5. Minick CR, Fabricant CG, Fabricant J, Litrenta MM. Atheroarteriosclerosis induced by infection with a herpes virus. *Am J Pathol* 1979; 96:673–706.
6. Fabricant CG, Fabricant J, Minick CR. Litrenta MM. Herpes virus induced atherosclerosis in chickens. *Fed Proc* 1983;42:2476–2479.
7. Hajjar DP, Fabricant CG, Minick CR, Fabricant J. Virus induced atherosclerosis: Herpes virus infection alters aortic cholesterol metabolism and accumulation. *Am J Pathol* 1986;122:62.
8. Cunningham MJ, Pasternak RC. The potential role of viruses in the pathogenesis of atherosclerosis. *Circulation* 1988;77:964–966.
9. Benditt EP, Benditt JM. Evidence for a monoclonal origin of human atherosclerotic plaques. *Proc Nat Acad Sci USA* 1973;70:1753–1756.
10. Fabricant CG, Krook L, Gillespie JH. Virus-induced cholestrol crystals. *Science* 1973;181:566–567.
11. Ross R. The pathogenesis of atherosclerosis—an update. *N Engl J Med* 1986;314:488–500.
12. Schwartz SM, Heimark RL, Majesky MW. Developmental mechanisms underlying pathology of arteries. *Physiol Rev* 1990;70: 1177–1209.
13. Schwartz SM, Campbell GR, Campbell JH. Replication of smooth muscle cells in vascular disease. *Circ Res* 1986;58:427–444.
14. Ross R. Atherosclerosis: A problem of the biology of arterial wall cells and their interactions with blood components. *Arteriosclerosis* 1981;1:293–311.
15. Pomerantz KB, Hajjar DP. Eicosanoids in the regulation of arterial smooth muscle cell phenotype, proliferative capacity, and cholestrol metabolism. *Arteriosclerosis* 1989;9:413–429.
16. Frenkel N, Schirmer EC, Wyatt LS, Katsofanas G, Roffman E, Danovich RM, June CH. Isolation of a new herpesvirus from human CD4+ T cells. *Proc Natl Acad Sci USA* 1990;87:748–752.
17. Corey L, Spear PG. Infections with herpes simplex viruses. *N Engl J Med* 1986;314:686–691.
18. Nahmias A, Josey K. Epidemiology of herpes simplex virus 1 and 2. In: Evans AS, ed. *Viral Infections of Humans—Epidemiology and Control.* New York: Plenum Medical Book Co; 1978;253–271.
19. Rooney JF. Epidemiology of herpes simplex. *Ann Intern Med* 1985; 103:404–419.
20. Johnson RE, Nahmias AJ, Magder LS, Lee FK, Brooks CA, Snowden MA. A seroepidemiologic survey of the prevalence of herpes simplex virus type 2 infection in the United States. *N Engl J Med* 1986;321: 7–12.
21. Marshall GS, Rabalais GP, Stewart JA, Dobbins JG. Cytomegalovirus seroprevalence in women bearing children in Jefferson County, Kentucky. *Am J Med Sci* 1993;305(5):292–296.
22. Adam E, Melnick JL, Probesfield JL, Petrie BL, Byrak J, Bailey KR, Accolum CH, Debakey ME. High levels of cytomegalorivus antibody in patients requiring vascular surgery for atherosclerosis. *Lancet* 1987; 2:291–293.
23. Havlik RJ, Blackwelder WC, Kaslow R, Castelli W. Unlikely association between clinically apparent herpesvirus infection and coronary incidence at older ages: The Framingham Heart Study. *Arteriosclerosis* 1989;9:877–880.
24. Sorlie PD, Adam E, Melnick SL, et al. Cytomegalovirus/herpesvirus and carotid atherosclerosis: The ARIC study. *J Med Virol* 1994;42: 33–37.
25. MacDonald K, Rector TS, Braunlin EA, Coubo SH, Olivare MT. Association of coronary artery disease and cardiac transplant recipients with cytomegalovirus infection. *Am J Pathol* 1989;64:359–362.
26. Koskinen PK, Nieminen MS, Krogerus LA, Lemstrom KB, Mattila SP, Hayry PJ, Lautenschlager IT. Cytomegalovirus infection and accelerated cardiac allograft vasculopathy in human cardiac allografts. *J Heart Lung Transplant* 1993;12(5):724–729.
27. Paavonen T, Mennander A, Lautenschlager I, Mattila S, Hayry P. Endothelialitis and accelerated arteriosclerosis in human heart transplant coronaries. *J Heart Lung Transplant* 1993;12(1 Pt 1):117–122.
28. Koskinen PK, Krogerus LA, Nieminen MS, Mattila SP, Hayry PJ, Lautenschlager IT. Quantitation of cytomegalovirus infection-associated histologic findings in endomyocardial biopsies of heart allografts. *J Heart Lung Transplant* 1993;12(3):343–354.
29. Ustinov JA, Loginov RJ, Bruggeman CA, van der Meide PH, Hayry PJ, Lautenschlager IT. Cytomegalovirus induces class II expression in rat heart endothelial cells. *J Heart Lung Transplant* 1993;12(4): 644–651.
30. Gyorkey F, Melnick JL, Guinn GA, Gyorkey P, Debakey ME. Herpes viridae in the endothelial and smooth muscle cells of the proximal aorta of atherosclerotic patients. *Exp Mol Pathol* 1984;40:328–339.
31. Benditt EP, Barrett T, MacDougal JK. Viruses in the etiology of atherosclerosis. *Proc Natl Acad Sci USA* 1983;80:6386–6389.
32. Melnick JL, Petrie BL, Dreisman GR, Burak J, McColam CH, Debakey ME. Cytomegalovirus antigen within human arterial smooth muscle cells. *Lancet* 1983;2:644–647.
33. Petrie BL, Melnick JL, Adam E, Burek J, McCollum CH, DeBakey ME. Nucleic acid sequences of cytomegalovirus in cells cultured from human arterial tissue. *J Infect Dis* 1987;155:158–159.
34. Hendrix MGR, Salimans MMM, VanBoven CPA, Bruggeman CA. High prevalence of latently present cytomegalovirus in arterial walls of patients suffering from grade 3 atherosclerosis. *Am J Pathol* 1990; 136:23–28.
35. Stinski MF, Thomsen DR, Stenberg RM, Goldstein LC. Organization and expression of the immediate early genes of the human cytomegalovirus. *J Virol* 1983;46:1–14.
36. Hendrix MGR, Daemen M, Bruggeman CA. Cytomegalovirus nucleic acid distribution within the human vascular tree. *Am J Pathol* 1991; 138:563–567.
37. Yamashiroya HM, Ghosh L, Yang R, Robertson AL. Herpes viridae in the coronary arteries and aorta of young trauma victims. *Am J Pathol* 1988;130:71–79.
38. Fabricant CG. Atherosclerosis: The consequence of infection with a herpes virus. *Adv Vet Sci Comp Med* 1985;30:39–66.
39. Paterson JC, Cottral GE. Experimental coronary sclerosis III. Lymphomatosis as a cause of coronary sclerosis in chickens. *Arch Pathol* 1950;49:699–707.

40. Walker DI, Bloor K, Williams G, Gillie I. Inflammatrory aneurysms of the abdominal aorta. *Br J Surg* 1972;59:609–614.
41. Tanaka S, Toh Y, Mori R, Komori K, Okadome K, Sugimachi K. Possible role of cytomegalovirus in the pathogenesis of inflammatory aortic diseases: A preliminary report. *J Vasc Surg* 1992;16:274–279.
42. Koskinen P, Lemstrom K, Bruggeman C, Lautenschlager I, Hayry P. Acute cytomegalovirus infection induces a subendothelial inflammation (endothelialitis) in the allograft vascular wall. A possible linkage with enhanced allograft arteriosclerosis. *Am J Pathol* 1994;144(1): 41–50.
43. Waldman WJ, Adams PW, Orosz CG, Sedmak DD. T lymphocyte activation by cytomegalovirus-infected, allogeneic cultured human endothelial cells. *Transplantation* 1992;54:887–896.
44. Lemström KB, Bruning JH, Bruggeman CA, Lautenschlager IT, Häyry PJ. Cytomegalovirus infection enhances smooth muscle cell proliferation and intimal thickening of rat aortic allografts. *J Clin Invest* 1993;92:549–558.
45. Datta SK, Tumilowicz JJ, Trentin JJ. Lysis of human arterial smooth muscle cells infected with herpesviridae by peripheral blood mononuclear cells: Implications for atherosclerosis. *Viral Immunol* 1993;6: 153–160.
45a. Kaner RJ, Medina J, Nicholson AC, Ursea R, Schwartz SM, Hajjar DP. Developmentally regulated herpesvirus plaque formation in arterial smooth muscle cells. *Circ Res* 1993;73:10–14.
46. MacGregor RR, Friedman HM, Macarak EJ, Kefalides NA. Virus infection of endothelial cells increases granulocyte adherence. *J Clin Invest* 1980;65:1469–1477.
47. Friedman HM, Macarak EJ, MacGregor RR, Wolfe J, Kefalides NA. Virus infection of endothelial cells. *J Infect Dis* 1981;143:266–273.
48. Lashgari MS, Friedman HM, Kefalides NA. Suppression of matrix protein synthesis by herpes simplex virus in bovine smooth muscle cells. *Biochem Biophys Res Commun* 1987;143:145–151.
49. Ho DD, Rota TR, Andrews CA, Hirsch MS. Replication of human cytomegalovirus in endothelial cells. *J Infect Dis* 1984;150:956–957.
50. Tumilowicz JJ, Gawlik ME, Powell BB, Trenton JJ. Replication of cytomegalovirus in human arterial smooth muscle cells. *J Virol* 1985; 56:839–845.
51. Sydiskis RJ, Roizman B. Polysomes and protein synthesis in cells infected with a DNA virus. *Science* 1966;153:76–78.
52. Fenwick ML, Clark J. Early and delayed shut off of host protein synthesis in cells infected with herpes simplex virus. *J Gen Virol* 1982;61:121–125.
53. Kefalides NA, Ziaie Z. Herpes simplex virus suppression of human endothelial matrix protein synthesis is independent of viral protein synthesis. *Lab Invest* 1986;55:328–336.
54. London FS, Brinker JM, Ziaie Z, Kefalides NA. Suppression of host mRNA in human smooth muscle cells by a virion competent factor in herpes simplex virus type 1. *Lab Invest* 1990;62:189–195.
55. Nishioka Y, Silverstein S. Degradation of cellular mRNA during infection by herpes simplex virus. *Proc Natl Acad Sci USA* 1977;74: 2370–2374.
56. Fabricant CG, Hajjar DP, Minick CR, Fabricant J. Marek's disease herpes virus infection enhances cholesterol and cholesterol ester accumulation in cultured avian arterial smooth muscle cells. *Am J Pathol* 1981;105:176–184.
57. Hajjar DP, Falcone DJ, Fabricant CJ, Fabricant J. Altered cholesterol ester cycle is associated with lipid accumulation in herpes virus infected avian arterial smooth muscle cells. *J Biol Chem* 1985;260: 6124–6128.
58. Hajjar DP. Herpesvirus infection prevents activation of cytoplasmic cholesteryl esterase in arterial smooth muscle cells. *J Biol Chem* 1986; 261:7611–7614.
59. Hajjar DP, Pomerantz KB, Falcone DJ, Weksler BB, Grant AJ. Herpes simplex virus infection in human arterial cells. *J Clin Invest* 1987; 80:1317–1321.
60. Hajjar DP, Pomerantz KB, Snow JW. Analysis of the physical state of cholesteryl esters in arterial smooth-muscle-derived foam cells by differential scanning calorimetry. *Biochem J* 1990;268:693–697.
61. Hajjar DP, Nicholson AC, Hajjar KA, Sando GN, Summers BD. Decreased messenger RNA translation in herpesvirus-infected arterial cells: Effects on cholesteryl ester hydrolase. *Proc Natl Acad Sci USA* 1989;86:3366–3370.
62. Monroe MJ, Cotran RS. Biology of disease. The pathogenesis of atherosclerosis: Atherogenesis and inflammation. *Lab Invest* 1988;58: 249.
63. Dudding L, Haskel S, Clark BD, Auron PE, Sporn S, Huang ES. Cytomegalovirus infection stimulates expression of monocyte associated mediator genes. *J Immunol* 1989;143:3343–3352.
63a. Staats HF, Lausch RN. Cytokine expression in vivo during murine herpetic stromal keratitis. Effect of protective antibody therapy. *J Immunol* 1993;151(1):277–283.
64. Gosselin J, Flamand L, D'Addario M, Hiscott J, Menezes J. Infection of peripheral blood mononuclear cells by herpes simplex and Epstein–Barr viruses. Differential induction of interleukin 6 and tumor necrosis factor-alpha. *J Clin Invest* 1992;89(6):1849–1856.
65. Smith PD, Saini SS, Raffeld M, Manischewitz JF, Wahl SM. Cytomegalovirus induction of tumor necrosis factor-alpha by human monocytes and mucosal macrophages. *J Clin Invest* 1992;90(5): 1642–1648.
66. Pavic I, Polic B, Crnkovic I, Lucin P, Jonjic S, Koszinowski UH. Participation of endogenous tumour necrosis factor alpha in host resistance to cytomegalovirus infection. *J Gen Virol* 1993;74(Pt 10): 2215–2223.
67. Kohase M, Henriksen-DeStefano D, May T, Vilcek J, Sehgal PB. Induction of β_2-interferon by tumor necrosis factor; a homeostatic mechanism in the control of cell proliferation. *Cell* 1986;45:659–666.
68. Wong GHW, Goeddel DV. Tumor necrosis factors α and β inhibit virus replication and synergize with interferons. *Nature* 1986;323: 819–822.
69. Etingin OR, Hajjar DP. Evidence for cytokine regulation of cholesterol metabolism in herpesvirus-infected arterial cells by the lipoxygenase pathways. *J Lipid Res* 1990;31:299–305.
70. Ishibashi S, Inaba T, Shimano H, Harada K, Inoue I, Mokuno H, Nori N, Gotoda T, Takaku F, Yamada N. Monocyte colony-stimulating factor enhances uptake and degradation of acetylated low density lipoproteins and cholesterol esterification in human monocyte-derived macrophages. *J Biol Chem* 1990;24:14109–14117.
71. Iwamoto GK, Monick MM, Clark BD, Auron PE, Stinsky MF, Hunninghake GW. Modulation of interleukin 1 beta gene expression by the immediate early genes of human cytomegalovirus. *J Clin Invest* 1990;85:1853–1857.
72. Wang AM, Doyle MV, Mark DF. Quantitation of mRNA by the polymerase chain reaction. *Proc Natl Acad Sci USA* 1989;86:9717–9721.
73. Boldogh I, Fons MP, Albrecht T. Increased levels of sequence-specific DNA-binding proteins in human cytomegalovirus-infected cells. *Biochem Biophys Commun* 1993;197(3):1505–1510.
74. Sehgal PB, Helfgott DC, Santhinam U, Tatter SB, Clerick RH, Ghrayeb J, May LT. Regulation of the acute phase and immune responses in viral diseases enhance expression of the beta 2 interferon hepatocyte stimulating factor interleukin 6 gene in virus infected human fibroblasts. *J Exp Med* 1988;167:1951–1956.
75. Almeida GD, Porada CD, St Jeor S, Ascensao JL. Human cytomegalovirus alters interleukin-6 production by endothelial cells. *Blood* 1994; 83(2):370–376.
76. Moore KW, Vieira P, Fiorentino DF, Trounstine ML, Khan TA, Mosmann TR. Homology of cytokine synthesis inhibitory factor (IL-10) to the Epstein–Barr virus gene BCRFI. *Science* 1990;248:1230–1234.
77. Vercellotti GM. Proinflammatory and procoagulant effects of herpes simplex infection on human endothelium. *Blood Cells* 1990;16: 209–216.
78. Visser MR, Tracy PB, Vercellotti GM, Goodman JL, White JG, Jacob HS. Enhanced thrombin generation and platelet binding on herpes simplex virus infected endothelium. *Proc Natl Acad Sci USA* 1988; 85:8227–8230.
79. Key NS, Bach RR, Vercellotti GM, Moldow CF. Herpes simplex virus type I does not require productive infection to induce tissue factor in human umbilical vein endothelial cells. *Lab Invest* 1993; 68(6):645–651.
80. Kaner RJ, Iozzo RV, Ziaie Z, Kefalides NA. Inhibition of proteoglycan synthesis in human endothelial cells after infection with herpes simplex virus type 1 in vitro. *Am J Resp Cell Mol Biol* 1990;2: 423–431.
81. Marcum JA, Atha DH, Fritze LMS, Nawroth P, Stern D, Rosenberg RD. Cloned bovine aortic endothelial cells synthesize anticoagulantly active heparan sulfate proteoglycan. *J Biol Chem* 1986;16: 7505–7517.
82. Macarak EJ, Friedman HM, Kefalides NA. Herpes simplex virus type

1 infection of endothelium reduces collagen and fibronectin synthesis. *Lab Invest* 1985;53:280–286.
83. Ziaie Z, Friedman HM, Kefalides NA. Suppression of matrix protein synthesis by herpes simplex virus type 1 in human endothelial cells. *Coll Rel Res* 1986;6:333–350.
84. Lashgari MS, Friedman HM, Kefalides NA. Suppression of matrix protein synthesis by herpes simplex virus in bovine smooth muscle cells. *Biochem Biophys Res Commun* 1987;143:145–151.
85. Visser MR, Vercellotti GM, McCarthy JB, Goodman JL, Herps TJ, Furcht LT, Jacob HS. Herpes simplex virus inhibits endothelial cell attachment and migration to extracellular matrix proteins. *Am J Pathol* 1989;134:223–230.
86. Thyberg J, Hedin U, Sjolund M, Palmberg L, Bottger BA. Regulation of differentiated properties and proliferation of arterial smooth muscle cells. *Arteriosclerosis* 1990;10:966–990.
87. Albrecht T, Boldogh I, Fons M, AbuBakar S, Deng CZ. Cell activation signals and the pathogenesis of human cytomegalovirus. *Intervirology* 1990;31:68–75.
88. Van Dan-Mieras MCE, Bruggeman CA, Muller AD, Debie WHM, Zwaal RFA. Induction of endothelial cell procoagulant activity by cytomegalovirus infection. *Thromb Res* 1987;47:69–75.
89. Grundy JE, Ayles HM, McKeating JA, Butcher RG, Griffiths PD, Poulter LW. Enhancement of class I HLA antigen expression by cytomegalovirus: Role in amplification of virus infection. *J Med Virol* 1988;25:483–495.
90. Van Dorp WT, Jonges E, Bruggeman CA, Daha MR, Van Es LA, van der Woude FJ. Direct induction of MHC class I, but not class II, expression on endothelial cells by cytomegalovirus infection. *Transplantation* 1989;48:469–472.
91. Span AHM, Vanboven CPA, Bruggeman CA. The effect of cytomegalovirus infection on the adherence of polymorphonuclear leukocytes to endothelial cells. *Eur J Clin Invest* 1989;19:542–548.
92. Thompson WD, Smith EB. Atherosclerosis and the coagulation system. *J Pathol* 1989;159:97–106.
93. Ballard-Barbash R, Callaway CW. Marine fish oils: Role in prevention of coronary artery disease. *Mayo Clinic Proc* 1987;62(2):113–118.
94. Key NS, Vercellotti GM, Winkelmann JC, Moldow CF, Goodman JL, Esmon NL, Esmon CT, Jacob HS. Infection of vascular endothelial cells with herpes simplex virus enhances tissue factor activity and reduces thrombomodulin expression. *Proc Natl Acad Sci USA* 1990; 87:7095–7099.
95. McLean JW, Tomlinson JE, Kuang WJ, et al. cDNA sequence of human apolipoprotein (a) is homologous to plasminogen. *Nature* 1987;300:132–137.
96. Bok RA, Jacob HS, Balla J, Juckett M, Stella T, Shatos MA, Vercellotti GM. Herpes simplex virus decreases endothelial cell plasminogen activator inhibitor. *Thromb Haemosta* 1993;69(3):253–258.
97. Bevilacqua MP, Pober JS, Majeau GR, Fiers W, Cotran RS, Gimbrone MS. Recombinant tumor necrosis factor induces procoagulant activity in cultured human vascular endothelium: Characterization and comparison with the actions of interleukin 1. *Proc Natl Acad Sci USA* 1986;83:4533–4537.
98. Visser MR, Jacob HS, Goodman JL, McCarthy JB, Eurcht LT, Vercellotti GM. Granulocyte mediated injury to herpes simplex virus-infected human endothelium. *Lab Invest* 1989;60:296–304.
99. Friedman HM, Cohen GH, Eisenberg RJ, Sidel CA, Cines DB. Glycoprotein C of herpes simplex virus 1 acts as a receptor for the C3b complement component on infected cells. *Nature* 1984;309:633–635.
100. Cines DB, Lyss AP, Bina M, Corkey R, Kefalides NA, Friedman HM. Fc and C3 receptors induced by herpes simplex virus on cultured human endothelial cells. *J Clin Invest* 1982;69:123–128.
101. Para MF, Baucke RB, Spear PG. Glycoprotein gE of herpes simplex virus type 1: Effects of anti-gE on virion infectivity and on virus-induced Fc-binding receptors. *J Virol* 1982;41:129–136.
102. Johnson DC, Frame MC, Ligas MW, Cross AM, Stow ND. HSV IgG Fc receptor activity depends on a complex of 2 viral glycoproteins gE and gI. *J Virol* 1988;62:1247–1254.
103. Pomerantz KB, Hajjar DP. Eicosanoids in the regulation of arterial smooth muscle cell phenotype, proliferative capacity, and cholesterol metabolism. *Arteriosclerosis* 1989;9:413–429.
104. Bevilacqua MP, Pober JS, Mendrick DL, Cotran RS, Gimbrone MA. Identification of an inducible endothelial–leukocyte adhesion molecule. *Proc Natl Acad Sci USA* 1987;84:9238–9242.
105. Etingin OR, Silverstein RL, Friedman HM, Hajjar DP. Viral activation of the coagulation cascade: Molecular interactions at the surface of infected endothelial cells. *Cell* 1990;61:657–662.
106. McEver RP. GMP-140: A receptor for neutrophils and monocytes on activated platelets and endothelium. *J Cell Biochem* 1991;45: 156–161.
107. Hattori R, Hamilton KK, Fugate RD, McEver RP, Sims PJ. Stimulated secretion of endothelial von Willebrand factor is accompanied by rapid redistribution to the cell surface of the intracellular granule membrane protein GMP-140. *J Biol Chem* 1989;264:7768–7771.
108. Etingin OR, Silverstein RL, Hajjar DP. Von Willebrand factor mediates platelet adhesion to virally infected endothelial cells. *Proc Natl Acad Sci USA* 1993;90:5153–5156.
109. Etingin OR, Silverstein RL, Hajjar DP. Identification of a monocyte receptor on herpesvirus-infected endothelial cells. *Proc Natl Acad Sci USA* 1991;88:7200–7203.
110. Springer TA. Adhesion receptors of the immune system. *Nature* 1990; 346:425–434.
111. Osborn L, Hession C, Tizard R, Vassallo C, Luhowskyj S, Chi-Rosso G, Lobb R. Direct expression cloning of vascular cell adhesion molecule 1, a cytokine-induced endothelial protein that binds to lymphocytes. *Cell* 1989;59:1203–1211.
112. Silverstein RL, Nachman RL. Thrombospondin binds to monocyte–macrophages and mediates platelet–monocyte adhesion. *J Clin Invest* 1987;79:867–874.
113. Bevilacqua MP, Pober JS, Majeau GR, Fiers W, Cotran RS, Gimbrone MS. Recombinant tumor necrosis factor induces procoagulant activity in cultured human vascular endothelium: Characterization and comparison with the actions of interleukin 1. *Proc Natl Acad Sci USA* 1986;83:4533–4537.
114. Etingin OR, Hajjar DP. Evidence for cytokine regulation of cholestrol metabolism in herpesvirus-infected arterial cells by the lipoxygenase pathway. *J Lipid Res* 1990;31:299–305.
115. Altieri DC, Etingin OR, Fair DS, Brunck TK, Geltosky JE, Hajjar DP, Edgington T. Structural motif in factor X mediates binding to monocyte CD11B/CD18 and herpesvirus-infected endothelial glycoprotein C. *Science* 1991;254:1200–1203.
116. Pearson TA, Wang A, Solez K, Heptinstall RH. Clonal characteristics of fibrous plaques and fatty streaks from human aortas. *Am J Pathol* 1975;81:379–385.
117. Thomas WA, Reiner JM, Janakidevi K, Lee KT. Population dynamics of arterial cells during atherogenesis: X. Study of monotypism in atherosclerotic lesions of black women heterozygous for glucose-6 phosphate dehydrogenase (G6PD). *Exp Mol Pathol* 1979;31: 367–386.
118. Thomas WA, Kim DN. Biology of disease: Atherosclerosis as a hyperplastic and/or neoplastic process. *Lab Invest* 1983;48:245–255.
119. Linder D, Gartler SM. Glucose-6 phosphate dehydrogenase mosaicism: Utilization as a cell marker in the study of leiomyomas. *Science* 1965;150:67–68.
120. Majesky MW, Reidy MA, Benditt EP, Juchau MR. Focal smooth muscle proliferation in the aortic intima produced by an initiation promotion sequence. *Proc Natl Acad Sci USA* 1985;82:3450–3454.
121. Strong JP, Richards ML, McGill HC Jr et al. The association of cigarette smoking with coronary and aortic atherosclerosis. *Atherosclerosis* 1969;10:303–317.
122. Albert RE, Vanderlaan M, Burns F, Nishezume M. Effect of carcinogens on chicken atherosclerosis. *Cancer Res* 1977;37:2232–2235.
123. Penn A, Batestini G, Solomon J, Burns F, Albert RE. Dose-dependent size increase of aortic lesions following chronic exposure to 7,12-dimethylbenz(*a*)anthracene. *Cancer Res* 1981;41:588–592.
124. Yamasaki E, Aimes BN. Concentration of mutagens from urine by absorption with a nonpolar resin XID2: Cigarette smokers have mutagenic urine. *Proc Natl Acad Sci USA* 1977;74:3555–3559.
125. Penn A, Garte SJ, Warren L, Nesta D, Mindich B. Transforming gene in human atherosclerotic plaque DNA. *Proc Natl Acad Sci USA* 1986; 83:7951–7955.
126. Penn A, Synder C. Arteriosclerotic plaque development is promoted by polynuclear aromatic hydrocarbons. *Carcinogenesis* 1988;9: 2185–2189.
127. Parkes JL, Cardell RR, Hubbard FC, Hubbard D, Meltzer A, Penn A. Cultured human atherosclerotic plaque smooth muscle cells retain transforming potential and display enhanced expression of the *myc* protooncogene. *Am J Pathol* 1991;138:765–775.
128. Yew PR, Rajavashisth TB, Forrester J, Barath P, Lusis AJ. NIH 3T3

transforming gene not a general feature of atherosclerotic plaque DNA. *Biochem Biophys Res Commun* 1989;165:1067–1071.
129. Ahmed AJ, O'Malley BW, Yatsu FM. Presence of a putative transforming gene in human atherosclerotic plaques. *Circulation* 1990;82: III–35.
130. Rastinejad F, Polverini PJ, Bouck NP. Regulation of the activity of a new inhibitor of angiogenesis by a cancer suppressor gene. *Cell* 1990;56:345–355.
131. Good DJ, Polverini PJ, Rastinejad F, Le-Beau MM, Lemons RS, Frazier WA, Bouck NP. A tumor suppressor-dependent inhibitor of angiogenesis is immunologically and functionally indistinguishable from a fragment of thrombospondin. *Proc Natl Acad Sci USA* 1990; 87:6624–6628.
132. Nachtigal M, Legrand A, Nagpal ML, Nachtigal SA, Greenspan P. Transformation of rabbit vascular smooth muscle cells by transfection with the early region of SV40 DNA. *Am J Pathol* 1990;136:297–306.
133. Nachtigal M, Legrand A, Greenspan P, Nachtigal SA, Nagpal ML. Immortalization of rabbit vascular smooth muscle cells after transfection with a fragment of the BglII N region of herpes simplex virus type 2 DNA. *Intervirology* 1990;31:166–174.
134. Chen JK, Lee J, McClure DB. Altered low density lipoprotein receptor regulation is associated with cholesteryl ester accumulation in simian virus 40 transformed rodent fibroblast cell lines. *In Vitro Cell Dev Biol* 1988;24:353–358.
135. Macnab JCM. Herpes simplex virus and human cytomegalovirus, their roles and morphological transformation in genital cancer. *J Gen Virol* 1987;68:2525–2550.
136. Duff R, Rapp F. Oncogenic transformation of hamster embryo cells after exposure to herpes simplex virus type 2. *Nature* 1971;233:48–50.
137. Duff R, Rapp F. Oncogenic transformation of hamster embryo cells after exposure to inactivated herpes simplex virus type 1. *J Virol* 1973; 12:209–217.
138. Galloway DA, McDougall JK. The oncogenic potential of herpes simplex viruses: Evidence for a "hit and run" mechanism. *Nature* 1983; 302:21–24.
139. Cameron IR, Park M, Dutia BM, Ore A, Macnab JCM. Herpes simplex virus sequences involved in the initiation of oncogenic morphological transformation of rat cells are not required for maintenance of the transformed state. *J Gen Virol* 1985;66:517–527.
140. Camacho A, Spear PG. Transformation of hamster embryo fibroblasts by a specific fragment of the herpes simplex virus genome. *Cell* 1978; 15:993–1002.
141. Reyes GR, Lafemina R, Hayward SD, Hayward GS. Morphological transformation by DNA fragments of human herpes viruses: Evidence for two distinct transforming regions in herpes simplex virus types 1 and 2, and lack of correlation with biochemical transfer of the thymidine kinase gene. *Cold Spring Harbor Symp Quant Biol* 1980;44: 629–641.
142. Peden K, Mounts P, Hayward GS. Homology between mammalian cell DNA sequences and human herpesvirus genomes detected by a hybridisation procedure with high complexity probe. *Cell* 1982;31: 71–80.
143. Jariwalla RJ, Aurelian L, Ts'O POP. Immortalization and neoplastic transformation of normal diploid cells by defined cloned DNA fragments of herpes simplex virus type 2. *Proc Natl Acad Sci USA* 1980; 80:5902–5906.
144. Kwong AD, Kruper JA, Frenkel N. Herpes simplex virus virion host shutoff function. *J Virol* 1988;62:912–921.
145. Frink RJ, Anderson KP, Wagner MJ. Herpes simplex virus type 1 HindIII fragment L encodes spliced and complementary mRNA species. *J Virol* 1981;39:559–572.
146. Powell KL, Courtney RJ. Polypeptides synthesized in herpes simplex virus type 2-infected HEp-2 cells. *Virology* 1975;66:217–228.
147. Galloway DA, Nelson JA, McDougal JK. Small fragments of herpes virus DNA with transforming activity contained insertion sequence like structures. *Proc Natl Acad Sci USA* 1984;81:4736–4740.
148. Oram JD, Downing RG, Akrigg A, Dollery AA, Duggleby CJ, Wilkenson GWG, Greenaway P. Use of recombinant plasmids to investigate the structure of the human cytomegalovirus genome. *J Gen Virol* 1982;59:111–129.
149. Clanton C, Jariwalla RJ, Krejas C, Rosenthal LJ. Neoplastic transformation by cloned human cytomegalovirus DNA fragment uniquely homologies to one of the transforming regions of herpes simplex virus type 2. *Proc Natl Acad Sci USA* 1983;80:3826–3830.
150. El-Beik T, Razzaque A, Jariwalla RJ, Cihlar RL, Rosenthal LJ, Multiple transforming regions of human cytomegalovirus DNA. *J Virol* 1986;60:645–652.
151. Hwang CBC, Shillitoe EJ. DNA sequence of mutations induced in cells by herpes simplex virus type-1. *Virology* 1990;178:180–188.
152. Pyrzak R, Shih JCH. Detection of specific DNA segments of Marek's disease herpesvirus in Japanese quails susceptible to atherosclerosis. *Atherosclerosis* 1987;68:77–85.
153. Shih JCH, Pomen EP, Kao KJ. Genetic selection, general characterization and histology of atherosclerosis-susceptible and resistant Japanese quail. *Atherosclerosis* 1983;49:41.
154. Shih JCH, Pyrzak R, Guy JS. Discovery of noninfectious viral genes complementary to Marek's disease herpes virus in quail susceptible to cholesterol-induced atherosclerosis. *J Nutr* 1989;119:294–298.
155. Hajjar DP, Pomerantz KB. Molecular motions and thermotropic phase behavior of cholesteryl esters: A deuteron nuclear magnetic resonance (NMR) spectroscopy study. *Biophys Chem* 1992;43:255–263.
156. Hajjar DP. Regulation of cholesteryl ester hydrolases. *Adv Enzymol* 1994;69:45–82.
157. Hajjar DP. Viral pathogenesis of atherosclerosis. Impact of molecular mimicry and viral genes. *Am J Pathol* 1991;139:1195–1211.
158. Kaner RJ, Hajjar DP. Viral genes and atherogenesis. In: Lusis AJ, Rotter JI, Sparkes RS, eds. *Monographs in Human Genetics, Vol. 14, Molecular Genetics of Coronary Artery Disease. Candidate Genes and Processes in Atherosclerosis.* Basel: S. Karger; 1992:62–81.

Atherosclerosis and Coronary Artery Disease,
edited by V. Fuster, R. Ross, and E. J. Topol.
Lippincott-Raven Publishers, Philadelphia © 1996.

CHAPTER 33

Cytokines and Growth Regulatory Molecules in Atherosclerosis

Peter Libby and Russell Ross

Key Words: Cytokines; Growth factors; Smooth muscle cells; Endothelium; Macrophages; T cells; Receptors; Autocrine; Paracrine; Apoptosis.

INTRODUCTION

An important theme of contemporary atherosclerosis research concerns the protein molecules that signal changes in cellular functions in the course of lesion formation. The elucidation of signals that stimulate smooth muscle cell mitogenesis provided the initial stimulus for this line of research. More recently the scope has broadened to include functions other than cell division, including directed migration, expression of adhesion molecules, synthesis and breakdown of constituents of the vascular extracellular matrix, and control of vasomotor functions of blood vessels.

The initial focus of smooth muscle cell growth derived from the concept that smooth muscle proliferation must contribute to the accumulation of these cells as documented at various stages of atherosclerosis lesion formation and from the abundance of extracellular matrix molecules elaborated by smooth muscle cells characteristic of advanced atheroma (1–4). The fraction of smooth muscle cells that bear markers of ongoing cell proliferation (e.g., the proliferating cell nuclear antigen, PCNA) appears small (less than 1%) at late stages of lesion evolution (5). Also, long-standing advanced lesions of atherosclerosis contain hypocellular regions densely filled with matrix. Some have interpreted this finding as an indication that smooth muscle cell proliferation does not figure importantly in the genesis of atherosclerosis.

Such analyses of late-stage complicated atheroma usually use specimens derived from autopsy, atherectomy, or at surgical endarterectomy. Lesions of this type, available in a fresh enough state to permit application of contemporary modes of analysis, probably represent a late or "burned out" stage of a long-standing pathological process. The analysis of such a complicated lesion might be likened to the archaeologist's quest for understanding of an ancient civilization based on excavation of ruins, absent the citizens who built the edifices. In this light, the findings of low rates of smooth muscle proliferation and substantial hypocellular regions in advanced atheroma do not necessarily relegate smooth muscle proliferation to the status of an epiphenomenon. Rather, smooth muscle replication may have occurred years earlier in the history of the lesion. This possibility would account

P. Libby: Vascular Medicine and Atherosclerosis Unit, Cardiovascular Division, Department of Medicine, Brigham and Women's Hospital and Harvard Medical School, Boston, Massachusetts 02115.

R. Ross: Center for Vascular Biology, Department of Pathology, University of Washington School of Medicine, Seattle, Washington 98195.

for the relatively low levels of proliferation noted in observations of late-stage lesions. Moreover, hypocellular regions within an atheroma could arise from death or apoptosis of smooth muscle cells during the latter stages of the disease process (see below). Indeed, high indices of smooth muscle cell proliferation would not be expected to occur in an indolent, highly chronic lesion that may require decades to form.

Moreover, the proliferation of smooth muscle cells that occurs during atherogenesis may occur in waves or cycles (6). Angiographic studies of atherosclerotic lesion progression suggest such a discontinuous course for the evolution of occlusive epicardial coronary atheroma (7). Waves of proliferation of smooth muscle cells could arise during crises in the history of the progression of the lesion. For example, rupture of a microvessel within a plaque might lead to local thrombin activation with the ensuing direct and evoked mitogenic responses elicited by this molecule. Thus, measurement of rate of proliferation of smooth muscle cells in end-stage lesions does not negate the importance of smooth muscle cell replication at various times even during the phases of lesion progression and complication.

The study of protein growth regulatory molecules, founded by Levi-Montalcini (8) and Cohen (9) in the 1950s, concentrated on positive regulation of growth control. These protein stimulators of cell proliferation were called "growth factors." In the 1970s, workers in the field of inflammation and immunology discovered that proteins mediated many important aspects of immune and inflammatory responses. As various factors were purified and characterized, they were called cytokines. The cytokines include many nonimmunoglobulin protein mediators of inflammation or immunity. As we have learned more about the molecular structure of cytokines and growth factors and their functions, the distinction seems increasingly artificial. Cytokines and growth factors overlap considerably, such that strict distinction between these families of mediators has become less useful. Hence, the joint consideration in this chapter of both types of growth regulatory molecules.

As noted above, the field of growth control has traditionally accorded great importance to positive growth control, or stimulation of mitogenesis. Equally important but often neglected, negative growth control may also contribute to atherogenesis. Therefore, this discussion of growth regulatory molecules will also consider the actions of protein factors and cytokines that promote cytostasis, cytotoxicity, or programmed cell death (also known as apoptosis).

The regulation of the growth of smooth muscle cells provided the basis of early interest in growth factors in the context of atherogenesis, as previously mentioned. However, we now recognize that replication of at least three other cell types also figures prominently in various phases of atherosclerosis. For example, endothelial repair and neoangiogenesis during plaque evolution require migration and/or proliferation of endothelial cells (10,11). Also, studies such as those alluded to above that measured replicative rates of the various cell types within lesions indicated that macrophages divide as often as, if not more frequently than, smooth muscle cells in experimental and human atherosclerotic lesions (5,12). Recent data also demonstrate that T lymphocytes in the lesion also proliferate. Thus, factors that modulate the proliferation of T cells and macrophages also bear relevance for atherogenesis.

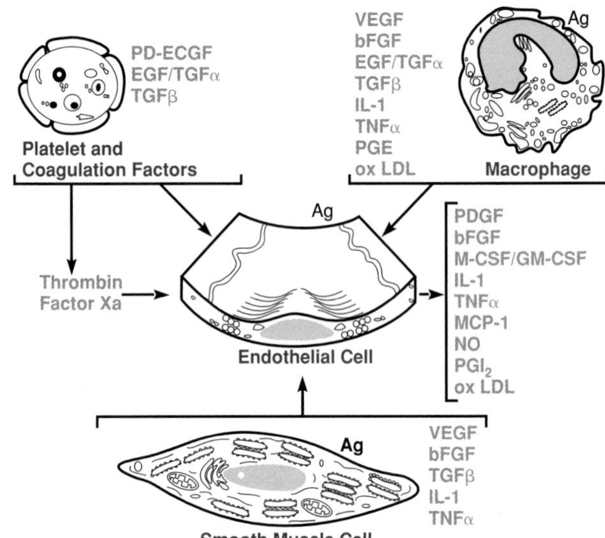

FIG. 1. Endothelium in atherosclerosis. In the genesis of the lesions of atherosclerosis, the endothelium can interact with macrophages, platelets, and smooth muscle as well as T lymphocytes. The principal products of platelets, macrophages, and smooth muscle that may affect the endothelium are shown in this diagram. Endothelial mitogens produced by macrophages include vascular endothelial growth factor (VEGF), FGF, and transforming growth factor-α (TGF-α). TGF-β as well as IL-1 and TNF-α can all inhibit endothelial proliferation. Furthermore, these three molecules can induce secondary gene expression of other growth regulatory molecules, such as PDGF, by the endothelium. TGF-β can also induce endothelial synthesis and secretion of connective tissue matrix. Oxidized LDL produced by endothelium or macrophages can have a profound effect in furthering the injury to the endothelial cells. Similarly, platelets can provide not only PDGF but TGF-α and TGF-β as well. Thrombin and factor Xa from plasma may also stimulate endothelial growth factor production. Several of the molecules expressed by macrophages and platelets can also be generated by smooth muscle cells in the artery wall or in the lesions of atherosclerosis that underlie the endothelium. In turn, the endothelial cells have the capacity to express genes for and synthesize a number of growth regulatory molecules (see box), including molecules that can induce connective tissue proliferation, such as PDGF, bFGF, and TGF-β, or IL-1 and TNF-α, which can induce secondary gene expression for PDGF in endothelium and smooth muscle. The endothelial cells can also be a principal source of mitogenic and activating factors for the underlying macrophages through M-CSF, GM-CSF, or oxidatively modified low-density lipoprotein (oxLDL). Similarly, the endothelial cells can participate in leukocyte chemotaxis by providing chemotactic factors such as oxLDL or MCP-1. Through their capacity to form NO and PGI_2, endothelial cells can profoundly affect the state of dilation or constriction of the artery. The endothelial cell represents the first potential site of oxidation of LDL as it transports the LDL into the artery wall. (From Ross, ref. 62, with permission.)

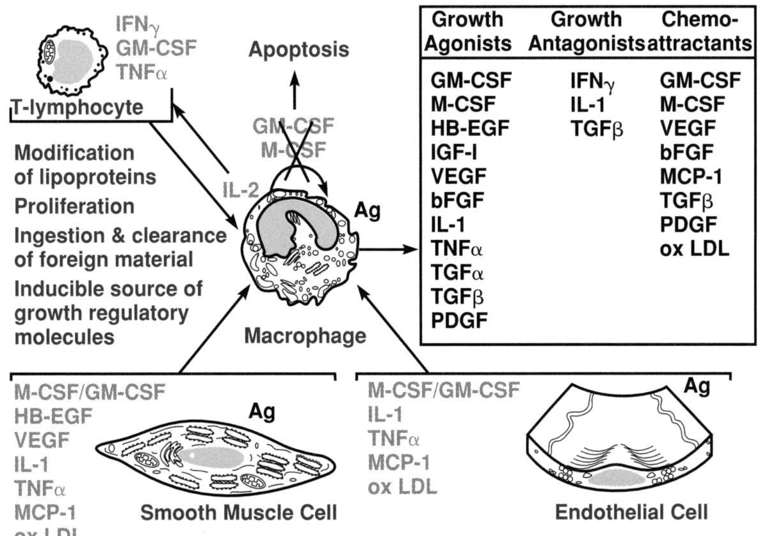

FIG. 2. Macrophages in atherosclerosis. The *antiparallel arrows* between the T lymphocyte and macrophage suggest that some form of immune response may occur during atherogenesis. Interactions between T cells and macrophages can result in proliferation of each of these cell types through IL-2 and CSFs, respectively. All of the cells with which the macrophage can interact, namely, the T lymphocyte, smooth muscle, and endothelium, can furnish M-CSF to the macrophages to maintain cell viability and prevent apoptosis and cell death and participate in further macrophage activation and replication. In addition, smooth muscle and endothelium can present antigens (Ag) at their surfaces and secrete chemoattractants for macrophages, including MCP-1 and oxLDL, as well as factors that can alter macrophage metabolism such as IL-1 or TNF-α. When the macrophages are activated, they can produce an extraordinary number of biologically relevant molecules, some of which are listed in the box in relation to their capacity to induce or inhibit replication of endothelium, smooth muscle, or macrophages themselves, as well as their capacity to make chemoattractants for each of these cell types. (From Ross, ref. 62, with permission.)

The uninitiated may easily become mired in the complexity of the various families of growth regulatory molecules. Therefore, this chapter will not aim or provide an exhaustive compendium or catalog of all of the various factors that may bear relevance to growth control during atherogenesis. Instead, we will outline certain principles of the biology of growth regulatory molecules. Specific discussions of particular growth factors will illustrate the general principles. Figures 1–3 indicate certain factors currently associated with the activities of smooth muscle, macrophages, T cells, and endothelium. Extensive reviews focusing on platelet-derived growth factor (13) and other growth factors (14) are available. These factors may act as intercellular mediators to stimulate or inhibit cell replication, as mediators of cell migration, as stimulators of protein synthesis, and as indirect mediators of cell proliferation. This chapter aims to illustrate these principles by use of selected examples.

A WIDE RANGE OF CELLS PRODUCE GROWTH FACTORS AND CYTOKINES

Growth Factors

One of the first principles encountered in the study of growth factors involves their cells of origin. The first point to bear in mind is that the original names of growth factors, although convenient, have often proven misleading as knowledge of a particular growth regulatory molecule has increased. For example, platelet-derived growth factor (PDGF) was first described as a serum constituent derived from platelets that stimulated the proliferation of mesenchymal cells in vitro (15,16). However, many cells involved in atherogenesis can actually produce PDGF. For example, endothelial cells can elaborate PDGF isoforms that contain both the A and B chains (17,18). (PDGF is a dimeric molecule composed of different assortments of the A and B chains.) Likewise, macrophages can transcribe both the A and B chains of this growth factor and secrete PDGF (19,20).

Interestingly, smooth muscle cells can also produce forms of PDGF. In this case, however, human smooth muscle cells appear capable of expressing principally the A chain of PDGF, which forms dimers that can interact only with the α-receptor for PDGF (21,22). [Two types of receptor subunits interact with PDGF, known as α and β. The α- receptor binds all three possible combinations of the two PDGF isoforms, whereas the β-receptor binds preferentially B-chain-containing dimers of PDGF (23).] The biological effects of the receptor binding isoforms of PDGF may be distinct. The effectiveness of a given form of PDGF as a mitogen depends on the number of relevant receptors on the target cells (24).

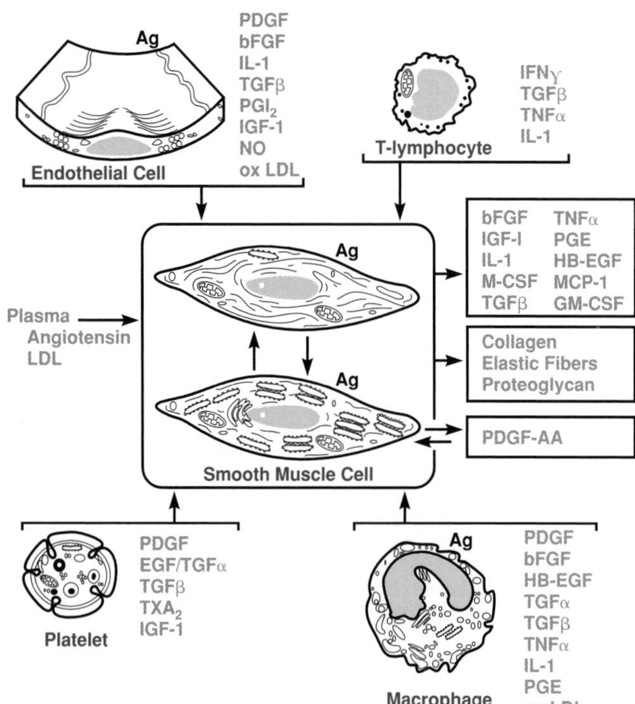

FIG. 3. The two potentially different phenotypic states of the smooth muscle cell. In the modulated phenotype, it is presumed that smooth muscle cells can form connective tissue molecules as well as growth factors such as PDGF-AA and can stimulate themselves as well as their neighbors. In their interactions with the overlying endothelium and neighboring T lymphocytes, platelets, and macrophages, smooth muscle cells can respond to the different cytokines, growth regulatory molecules, and vasodilator and vasoconstrictor substances that can be generated from these cells as well as substances from the plasma such as angiotensin. Thus, the genes that are expressed in the different phenotypic states by the smooth muscle (listed to the right), as well as those expressed by the neighboring cells (listed next to each cell) in the artery wall that result from these cellular interactions, will determine the outcome as to whether a lesion will progress or regress. (From Ross, ref. 62, with permission.)

Different cells vary in the number of such receptors they display, and at least three of the major cell types found in human lesions of atherosclerosis can express various forms of PDGF.

Current understanding of the biology of atherosclerosis accords a potentially important role to PDGF isoforms originating from nonplatelet sources in this process. Finally, although much of the early interest in PDGF focused on its mitogenic effects, current data strongly support an in vitro role for PDGF as a chemoattractant for smooth muscle cells in response to arterial injury (25,26). Its role as a mitogen in human atherosclerosis remains uncertain. These points illustrate how platelet-derived growth factor, originally isolated from platelets by virtue of its mitogenic effect, may derive from endothelium, smooth muscle cells, and macrophages as well as platelets and may be involved in growth stimulation, cell migration, and protein formation in the context of atherosclerosis.

Cytokines

Similar caveats pertain to the cytokines. Consider, for example, the case of the prototypic cytokine interleukin-1 (IL-1). This and the rest of the now multitudinous interleukins bear this name because of the original concept that interleukins mediated communication between leukocytes. As in the case of platelet-derived growth factor, knowledge of the cellular sources of interleukins has expanded markedly. For example, human endothelial cells and smooth muscle cells in addition to macrophages have the capacity to transcribe the genes for both isoforms of interleukin-1 (27,28). (Two separate genes encode IL-1α and -β, which share similar actions despite sharing only 26% sequence similarity at the amino acid level.) In addition, platelets appear capable of expressing IL-1 on their surface (29). Thus, although originally conceived as a messenger between leukocytes, IL-1 can derive from at least three major nonleukocytic cell types involved in atherosclerosis.

GROWTH STIMULATORY MOLECULES CAN ACT DIRECTLY AND INDIRECTLY

Direct Action via Receptors

Most protein stimulators of cell proliferation act primarily through two superfamilies of cell surface receptors that transduce their effects. The first family of receptors have extracellular regions with homology to the immunoglobulin gene while their cytoplasmic portions encode autocatalytic tyrosine kinases. The tyrosine kinase not only can autophosphorylate the receptor but can yield phosphorylation of other substrates involved in distal intracellular signaling events triggered by ligand binding by the extracellular domain. The prototypical example of a tyrosine kinase growth factor receptor of interest in vascular biology is the PDGF receptor mentioned above. Other growth factors that utilize tyrosine kinases for signal transduction include the heparin-binding growth factor family, which includes acidic and basic fibroblast growth factors, vascular endothelial growth factor, insulin and insulin-like growth factor I, and heparin-binding epidermal growth factor.

Another major category of receptor for growth regulatory

molecules spans the cell membrane seven times and interacts with G proteins for intracellular signaling. For example, angiotensin II, a transducer of smooth muscle contraction, also indirectly stimulates smooth muscle cell growth and acts via such a seven-membrane-spanning receptor. [Angiotensin II acts primarily to increase protein within cells rather than stimulate cell division, thus stimulating hypertrophy rather than hyperplasia of vascular smooth muscle cells (30,31).] However, other molecules reported to stimulate growth of smooth muscle cells do not interact with known tyrosine kinase or seven-membrane-domain receptors. For instance, none of the known receptors for IL-1 or TNF resembles these recognized categories of growth factor receptors. The mechanisms of intracellular signaling for the cytokines IL-1 and TNF remain controversial.

A great deal has been learned recently concerning the intracellular signaling pathways that are generated when a specific growth factor binds to its cell surface receptor. For example, PDGF is a potent chemoattractant for arterial smooth muscle as well as a potent mitogen. The intracellular molecules that are generated or phosphorylated and activated that result in chemotaxis have been shown to be clearly different from those that are activated when the cell is induced to traverse the cell cycle and replicate its DNA. By defining these intracellular signals, it may be possible to identify intermediates characteristic for specific cells that may permit modulation of specific cell responses such as chemotaxis or mitogenesis (32). Such information at the cellular and molecular level may prove useful if specific intermediates are found in a given set of signals or in specific cell types such as macrophages or smooth muscle.

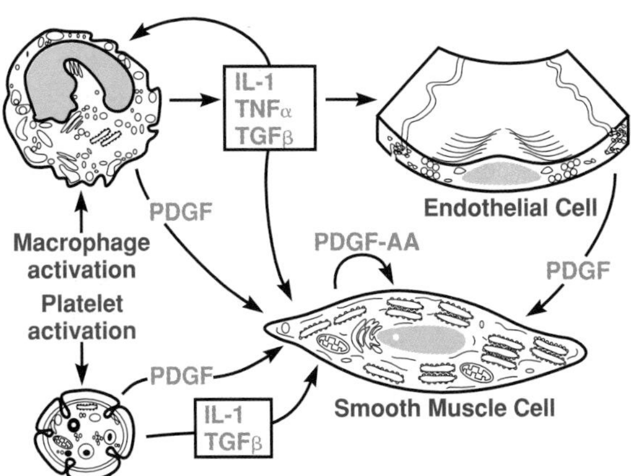

FIG. 4. The common mode of smooth muscle proliferation that can be induced through IL-1, TNF-α, or TGF-β. Each of these molecules can be formed by activated macrophages, and, when they are exposed to endothelial or smooth muscle cells, each of these molecules will induce PDGF B- or A-chain gene expression, respectively. The mitogenic activity induced in endothelium or smooth muscle in vitro by IL-1, TNF-α, or TGF-β can be totally abolished by a neutralizing polyclonal antibody to PDGF. In addition to its capacity to form IL-1, TNF-α, and TGF-β, the macrophage can directly form PDGF and, thus, directly induce smooth muscle cell replication as well. (Modified from Ross, ref. 62.)

INDIRECT ACTION BY INDUCTION OF SECONDARY MEDIATORS

Rather than stimulating smooth muscle cell replication directly, IL-1, TNF-α, and TGF-β each act indirectly by stimulating the local production of autocrine growth stimulants. For example, each factor can induce PDGF A-chain production by human arterial smooth muscle cells and thus stimulate their replication secondarily in an autocrine manner (33). Furthermore, each of these factors can induce PDGF B-chain expression in endothelial cells (34,35). If this should occur, it could then induce a paracrine effect on neighboring smooth muscle cells. Likewise, TNF-α can induce fibroblasts to express PDGF A chain, another example of growth mediation via a secondary growth factor elicited by the first signal (E. J. Battegay et al., *unpublished data*). These examples illustrate the principle of direct and indirect growth stimulation in the context of the vessel wall (Fig. 4).

GROWTH REGULATION CAN INVOLVE BOTH STIMULATION AND INHIBITION

As noted above, traditionally one thinks of growth control as growth stimulation, and as described above, vascular cells, when appropriately activated, can elaborate growth stimulatory molecules that can act on them in an autocrine manner or on neighboring cells in a paracrine fashion. These observations raise the specter of untrammeled growth resulting from an initial stimulus. This view at first appears to be incompatible with what has been interpreted to be the indolent nature of replication within atheroma discussed above. This conundrum highlights the potential importance of not only positive but negative growth control during atherogenesis.

T cells comprise an important component of the leukocytic infiltrate in all phases of atherogenesis (36,37) and may elaborate important cytokine inhibitors of smooth muscle replication (38–40). The T lymphocytes within atheroma exhibit markers of chronic activation (41,42). These cells appear to secrete interferon-γ as shown by two lines of evidence. The first is indirect, namely, the expression of class II histocompatibility antigens on neighboring smooth muscle cells (43). Extensive studies have shown that only interferon-γ among a wide variety of molecules tested can induce the expression of class II histocompatibility molecules on smooth muscle cells (44). Only T lymphocytes and natural killer (NK) cells can elaborate interferon-γ. Because NK cells have not been identified in atherosclerotic plaques, these findings argue for the presence of interferon-γ within advanced atheroma. What is more, advanced atherosclerotic plaques contain immunostainable interferon-γ (41).

Interferon-γ has long been known to exert cytostatic effects on mesenchymal cells. Studies from two laboratories in the 1980s affirmed that this lymphokine can inhibit serum-

or growth-factor-induced proliferation of vascular smooth muscle cells (38–40). Thus, one function of T cells within lesions of atherosclerosis may be inhibition of smooth muscle cell proliferation. In the context of experimental vascular injury, Hansson and colleagues have provided elegant evidence that interferon-γ acts in vivo as an inhibitor of smooth muscle cell replication after injury (39,45).

Transforming growth factor-β (TGF-β) was originally isolated by Todaro and colleagues as a stimulator of growth of cells in soft agar (46,47). At the same time Holley and colleagues sought the biochemical nature of a growth inhibitor present in cultured epithelial cells and converged on the same molecule (48). Thus, from the early days of study of TGF-β, its schizophrenic properties, sometimes a growth stimulator and sometimes an inhibitor, have been evident. Incidentally, the name transforming growth factor-β candidly illustrates the principle that the original name of a growth factor seldom accounts for the spectrum of actions that emerge from subsequent study. For example, transforming growth factor-β neither transforms nor is it a growth factor in general, nor in the context of atherogenesis.

Under most circumstances, in vitro, TGF-β appears to inhibit smooth muscle replication rather than stimulate it. The dual effects of TGF-β as a growth stimulator or growth inhibitor may derive from its effects as a regulator of both PDGF and PDGF receptor expression (24). This concept extends the principle of indirect action of growth factors introduced above.

All of the cell types involved in the formation of the lesions of atherosclerosis can produce TGF-β. When cocultured, endothelial cells and smooth muscle cells (or pericytes in the context of microvascular endothelial cells) can produce activated forms of TGF-β that can inhibit smooth muscle cell proliferation (49,50). Should this occur in vivo, TGF-β may be another pathophysiologically relevant inhibitor of smooth muscle cell replication during atherogenesis. Because cells usually elaborate TGF-β in a latent precursor form that requires activation to gain biological function, simple measurement of TGF-β mRNA or protein may prove misleading (see below).

To add further complexity to the role of TGF-β, although it inhibits smooth muscle cell replication, it is probably the most potent stimulator of the expression of the interstitial collagen gene by smooth muscle cells thus far discovered (51). Smooth muscle cells produce the bulk of the vascular extracellular matrix. The major collagen isoforms that accumulate in complicated atheroma include collagen types I and III. As noted above, advanced lesions contain areas of matrix accumulation that are characterized by a relative paucity of smooth muscle cells. The dual ability of TGF-β to inhibit smooth muscle growth and enhance collagen production may contribute to the appearance of the dense fibrous cap of connective tissue that forms in the late stages of fibrous plaque development.

More recently, programmed cell death in addition to cellular stasis has been considered as a mechanism of negative growth control during atherogenesis. Cells clearly die in the necrotic core of an atheroma. Apoptosis of smooth muscle cells, macrophage-derived foam cells, and possibly other types as well may contribute to this process (52). An appreciation of the mechanisms that control apoptosis has increased remarkably in the last year or so. Recently, inhibition or decrease in factors that prevent apoptosis, such as IGF-1 or PDGF, are being investigated for their possible role in preventing apoptosis of smooth muscle and thus promoting cell accumulation and lesion expansion during atherogenesis. Human atherosclerotic lesions contain apoptotic smooth muscle cells and macrophages. Factors such as the protooncogene *myc,* which normally induce apoptosis, and potential inhibition of *myc* in this process are being investigated. In contrast to plaque cells, there is relatively little apoptosis in normal adult artery. These emerging data suggest that understanding of the accumulation of smooth muscle cells within lesions and the formation of the lipid core require consideration of apoptosis and inhibition of apoptosis in addition to the traditional focus on growth stimulation.

Another novel aspect of negative growth control in the context of atherogenesis involves potential inhibitory effects of nitric oxide on smooth muscle cell replication (53). When produced constitutively by endothelial cells at relatively low levels, nitric oxide, the endogenous endothelial-derived vasodilator, appears to cause chronic vasodilatation in vivo. However, cells within the atherosclerotic plaque, including macrophages and smooth muscle cells, may express a high-capacity cytokine-inducible form of nitric oxide synthase, the enzyme that catalyzes the formation of the nitric oxide radical. If produced in high quantities by activated cells within lesions of atherosclerosis, nitric oxide, by increasing intracellular levels of cGMP, may exert a cytostatic action on smooth muscle cells. Alternatively, if produced in very high levels, or if elaborated together with superoxide radicals yielding the production of peroxynitrite, NO or related radicals might contribute to cell death (54). [NO production by macrophages has long been known to be a microbicidal mechanism utilized by this cell type for intercellular pathogens (55).]

In summary, the aforementioned examples provide insight into the potential role of negative growth control during atherogenesis. Protein mediators may participate in this process directly, as in the case of IL-1, TNF or interferon-γ and may induce the high capacity form of nitric oxide synthase that may promote cytostasis or even cell death.

GROWTH FACTORS FREQUENTLY EXIST IN MULTIPLE FORMS WITH DISTINCT BIOLOGICAL FUNCTIONS

Much discussion of growth factors glibly refers to particular factors as if they were comprised of single entities. In fact, such simplicity virtually never applies. As in the case of the prototypic vascular growth factor PDGF, multiple isoforms exists, as alluded to above. First of all, two genes, each on a separate chromosome, encode the precursors of two distinct proteins for the A chain and the B chain. To function, platelet-derived growth factor must form a covalent dimeric molecule consisting of any of three possible assortments of these two isoforms (AA, AB, or BB). The receptors for PDGF also form three different noncovalent dimers that interact differentially with the three dimeric forms of PDGF. As a consequence, these growth factor isoforms exert different biological actions. For example, the PDGF AA isoform appears to stimulate smooth muscle mitogenesis more weakly than the BB isoform in vitro; however, this results from the decreased number of PDGF β-receptors compared to α-receptors on smooth muscle cells. Other differences relevant to atherogenesis like this also likely exist.

Moreover, the PDGF A chain can undergo differential splicing to yield at least two different translation products. Some biological functions of these splice-variant forms of PDGF appear to be significant. For example, PDGF A can form a truncated version of the A chain, splicing out an amino acid sequence that is coded for by the sixth exon of the PDGF A gene. This sequence specifically binds to a sequence in the proteoglycan heparin sulfate. Thus, the ability to bind cell-surface-associated proteoglycans or to adhere to extracellular proteoglycans may depend on such sequences contained in one isoform but not in others. The same is true for the precursor form of the PDGF B chain. Thus, heterogeneity of PDGF activity exists at the level of the gene and in assembly of the dimers. As discussed below, posttranslational protein processing may also contribute to PDGF heterogeneity. This example illustrates how it is naive to refer merely to "PDGF" without taking into account its multiple isoforms of varying biological potential.

Likewise, interleukin-1, a monomeric mediator, can also arise from two different genes that encode the α or β isoforms of this cytokine. Although the A and B isoforms of PDGF resemble each other remarkably in their biological activities, important aspects of their cell biology are distinct. Notably, the isoform of IL-1 associated with the surface of the cell is usually IL-1α. Yet another member of the IL-1 family encodes an inhibitor of IL-1 action, the IL-1-receptor antagonist. Thus, various members of a complex growth factor family may be expressed at different locales and exert diametrically opposed biological actions, as in the case of IL-1 and the IL-1 receptor antagonist.

We have considered in some detail the heterogeneity of PDGF, the prototypic growth factor, and IL-1, the prototypic cytokine. However, similar considerations apply to virtually all of the other cytokines and growth factors. For example, macrophage colony-stimulating factor exists in membrane-associated and in soluble forms. Similarly, heparin-binding epidermal growth factor exists in membrane-bound and soluble forms (56). Tumor necrosis factor likewise forms trimers that can be either cell-associated or secreted. The fibroblast growth factor family now comprises at least eight members, all with distinct but related structures and varying biological functions. The above examples illustrate how heterogeneity in growth factors is the rule rather than the exception.

POSTTRANSLATIONAL PROCESSING CONTROLS THE FUNCTIONS OF GROWTH FACTORS AND CYTOKINES

The foregoing discussions have alluded to examples of multiple genes encoding members of growth factor families and multiple transcripts arising from a single growth factor or cytokine gene. Another important level of control of the biological effects of growth factors and cytokines resides in posttranslational processing of the protein products. This is an area that has been relatively neglected in growth factor biology, although it may be of paramount importance. Posttranslational processing is most often overlooked in studies of growth factor action in the context of vascular biology. Studies at the level of messenger RNA (e.g., the Northern blot or in situ hybridization) cannot reveal information about the actual posttranslational product of a growth factor that may or may not be expressed in conjunction with RNA if it is indeed translated. Immunocytochemical localization of various growth factors and cytokines most often used as reagents that do not distinguish various products of posttranslational processing, which may exhibit different biological actions. Hence, it is necessary to conclude with some discussion of this important gap area in growth factor and cytokine biology.

The case of TGF-β furnishes a pertinent example. Almost all cell types can express the TGF-β gene and synthesize the precursor of this multipotent mediator. However, the precursor of TGF-β lacks biological activity. Without posttranslational processing involving proteolytic cleavage to release the active form of the molecule, it is devoid of the many biological activities attributed to it. Many in vitro studies have used treatment with acid to activate TGF-β, hardly a physiological stimulus. Indeed, the control of activation of TGF-β appears complex, often requiring interplay among various cell types as discussed above as in the case of cocultures of endothelial and smooth muscle cells (49,50).

Enzymatic mechanisms that may be important in the regulation of TGF-β activity include cell-associated plasmin. The activity of plasmin is further subject to regulation by plasminogen activators and plasminogen activator inhibitors expressed by vascular cells. These examples illustrate the complexities of posttranslational processing and why they should be carefully considered in interpreting experimental results.

SUMMARY

The above discussion highlights certain salient features of the biology of growth factors and cytokines in relation to atherosclerosis. As noted above, we have not attempted to catalog exhaustively the entire canon of known growth factors. Rather, we have aimed to emphasize certain principles that apply to growth factor biology in general, some of which have not been widely considered in the domain of atherosclerosis research.

One point deserving of particular emphasis involves the potential hazard of extrapolating too readily the results of in vitro experiments to the in vivo situation. Cell culture studies have aided immeasurably in the advancement of the growth factor and cytokine field. Nonetheless, investigators must bear in mind that the three-dimensional, multicellular environment within the artery wall differs substantially from the simple single cell type most often studied in monolayer cultures surrounded by unphysiological fluids on an unnatural substrate.

In the case of vascular cells, such caveats apply particularly (57). Vascular smooth muscle cells, when cultured, lose many of the properties they exhibit in situ in the artery wall. Although the modulated phenotype of cultured smooth muscle cells resembles in some aspects those of smooth muscle cells in the intima of atherosclerotic vessels, because of selection during culture and repeated passage, these cells may be quite distant from their in vivo counterparts. Likewise, vascular endothelial cells, which display striking heterogeneity of morphology and function from vascular bed to vascular bed in vivo, often lose their distinct properties when propagated in culture.

Occasionally, the results of in vivo experiments yield major surprises compared to in vitro studies. One such case is the evidence from studies in the rat that PDGF acts primarily as a chemoattractant for smooth muscle cells rather than a mitogen after balloon injury to the carotid artery (26). The precise role of PDGF as a mitogen in vivo in atherogenesis remains to be determined. However, PDGF B chain has been demonstrated by immunohistochemistry in at least 35% of the macrophages present in the lesions of experimental, as well as human, atherosclerosis (58). Also, most smooth muscle cells in these lesions bear immunoreactive PDGF β-receptor, indicating the capability of responding to PDGF-B chain containing isoforms of this growth factor. Thus the potential for PDGF to act as a mitogen, as a chemoattractant, and as a stimulator of protein synthesis is clear. However, there are no data that PDGF acts in these roles during atherogenesis because experiments have not yet been conducted.

Although the effects of growth factors and cytokines are easy to define in vitro, exploring their integrated actions in vivo and assigning to them a distinct role in the pathogenesis of atherosclerosis have proven to be more challenging. Fortunately, the application of molecular genetic technologies should facilitate this task. For example, the ability to perform genetic manipulations that inactivate specific growth factor or cytokine genes should in principle permit the design of experiments to test the specific roles of the different cytokines in the pathogenesis of the lesions. In this regard, the availability of mice genetically modified to produce lesions of atherosclerosis when fed appropriate diets should greatly facilitate the analysis of the actions of growth factors and cytokines (59–61). The creation of compound mutants of mice that have undergone targeted inactivation of specific cytokines or growth factors (when they are not lethal "knockouts") with the various atherosclerosis-susceptible mouse strains should enable an elegant exploration of their roles in the different stages of atherogenesis. The ability to alter locally the expression of growth factor and cytokine genes by vascular gene transfer techniques should also shed light on the in vivo action of these factors. Local genetic modification should prove particularly helpful when somatic genetic alteration is impossible because of a developmental lethality resulting from the mutation in question.

One might find the complexities of the actions of growth factors and cytokines daunting and discouraging. It may be difficult to comprehend and bear in mind the complex multilateral signaling pathways rendered possible by the explosion of knowledge of these factors. One may also despair of controlling a process that contains so many seemingly redundant and overlapping pathways.

A more productive approach would seem to be viewing the very complexity of these signaling pathways that are at play during atherogenesis as an opportunity. Perhaps when we truly understand the pathogenesis of atherosclerosis, the picture will become simpler as we identify a narrower spectrum of signals that actually play causal or primary roles in the process.

REFERENCES

1. Virchow R. *Cellular Pathology*. London: John Churchill; 1858: 342–366.
2. Haust MD, More RH, Movat HZ. The role of smooth muscle cells in the fibrogenesis of arteriosclerosis. *Am J Pathol* 1960;37:377–389.
3. Ross R, Klebanoff SJ. The smooth muscle cell. I. In vivo synthesis of connective tissue proteins. *J Cell Biol* 1971;50(1):159–171.
4. Ross R. Connective tissue cells, cell proliferation and synthesis of extracellular matrix—a review. *Phil Trans R Soc Lond* 1975;271: 247–259.
5. Gordon D, Reidy MA, Benditt EP, Schwartz SM. Cell proliferation in human coronary arteries. *Proc Natl Acad Sci USA* 1990;87(12): 4600–4604.
6. Libby P, Fleet J, Salomon R, Li H, Loppnow H, Clinton S. Possible roles of cytokines in atherogenesis. In: Stein O, Eisenberg S, Stein Y, eds. *Atherosclerosis IX*. Tel Aviv: R&L Creative Communications; 1992:339–350.
7. Bruschke AV, Kramer J Jr, Bal ET, Haque IU, Detrano RC, Goormastic M. The dynamics of progression of coronary atherosclerosis studied in 168 medically treated patients who underwent coronary arteriography three times. *Am Heart J* 1989;117(2):296–305.
8. Levi-Montalcini R. The nerve growth factor: Thirty five years later. In: *Les Prix Nobel—1986*. Stockholm: Almquist & Wiksell; 1987: 279–299.
9. Cohen S. Epidermal growth factor: In: *Les Prix Nobel—1986*. Stockholm: Almquist & Wiksell; 1987:263–275.
10. Brogi E, Winkles J, Underwood R, Clinton S, Alberts G, Libby P. Distinct patterns of expression of fibroblast growth factors and their receptors in human atheroma and non-atherosclerotic arteries: Association of acidic FGF with plaque microvessels and macrophages. *J Clin Invest* 1993;93:2408–2418.
11. O'Brien ER, Garvin MR, Dev R, et al. Angiogenesis in human coronary atherosclerotic plaques. *Am J Pathol* 1994;145(4):883–894.

12. Rosenfeld ME, Ross R. Macrophage and smooth muscle cell proliferation in atherosclerotic lesions of WHHL and comparably hypercholesterolemic fat-fed rabbits. *Arteriosclerosis* 1990;10(5):680–687.
13. Raines E, Bowen-Pope D, Ross R. Platelet-derived growth factor. In: Sporn M, Roberts A, eds. *Handbook of Experimental Pharmacology: Peptide Growth Factors and Their Receptors*. New York: Springer-Verlag; 1990:173–262.
14. Sporn M, Roberts A. *Peptide Growth Factors and Their Receptors*. New York: Springer-Verlag; 1990.
15. Ross R, Glomset JA, Kariya B, Harker L. A platelet-dependent serum factor that stimulates the proliferation of arterial smooth muscle cells in vitro. *Proc Natl Acad Sci USA* 1974;71:1207–1210.
16. Kohler N, Lipton A. Platelets as a source of fibroblast growth-promoting activity. *Exp Cell Res* 1974;87:297–301.
17. Barrett TB, Gajdusek CM, Schwartz SM, McDougall JK, Benditt EP. Expression of the sis gene by endothelial cells in culture and in vivo. *Proc Natl Acad Sci* 1984;81:6772–6774.
18. Collins T, Pober JS, Gimbrone MAJ, et al. Cultured human endothelial cells express platelet-derived growth factor A chain. *Am J Pathol* 1987; 127:7–12.
19. Shimokado K, Raines EW, Madtes DK, Barrett TB, Benditt EP, Ross R. A significant part of macrophage-derived growth factor consists of at least two forms of PDGF. *Cell* 1985;43:277–286.
20. Martinet Y, Bitterman PB, Mornex JF, Grotendorst GR, Martin GR, Crystal RG. Activated human monocytes express the c-*sis* proto-oncogene and release a mediator showing PDGF-like activity. *Nature* 1986; 319:158–160.
21. Sjölund M, Hedin U, Sejersen T, Heldin C-H, Thyberg J. Arterial smooth muscle cells express platelet-derived growth factor (PDGF) A chain mRNA, secrete a PDGF-like mitogen, and bind exogenous PDGF in a phenotype- and growth state-dependent manner. *J Cell Biol* 1988; 106:403–413.
22. Libby P, Warner SJC, Salomon RN, Birinyi LK. Production of platelet-derived growth factor-like mitogen by smooth-muscle cells from human atheromata. *N Engl J Med* 1988;318:1493–1498.
23. Bowen-Pope DF, Hart CE, Seifert RA. Sera and conditioned media contain different isoforms of platelet-derived growth factor (PDGF) which bind to different classes of PDGF receptor. *J Biol Chem* 1989; 264(5):2502–2508.
24. Battegay EJ, Raines EW, Seifert RA, Bowen PDF, Ross R. TGF-beta induces bimodal proliferation of connective tissue cells via complex control of an autocrine PDGF loop. *Cell* 1990;63(3):515–524.
25. Fingerle J, Johnson R, Clowes AW, Majesky MW, Reidy MA. Role of platelets in smooth muscle cell proliferation and migration after vascular injury in rat carotid artery. *Proc Natl Acad Sci USA* 1989; 86(21):8412–8416.
26. Ferns G, Raines E, Sprugel K, Motani A, Reidy M, Ross R. Inhibition of neointimal smooth muscle accumulation after angioplasty by an antibody to PDGF. *Science* 1991;253:1129–1132.
27. Libby P, Ordovàs JM, Auger KR, Robbins H, Birinyi LK, Dinarello CA. Endotoxin and tumor necrosis factor induce interleukin-1 gene expression in adult human vascular endothelial cells. *Am J Pathol* 1986; 124:179–186.
28. Libby P, Ordovas JM, Birinyi LK, Auger KR, Dinarello CA. Inducible interleukin-1 expression in human vascular smooth muscle cells. *J Clin Invest* 1986;78:1432–1438.
29. Hawrylowicz CM, Santoro SA, Platt FM, Unanue ER. Activated platelets express IL-1 activity. *J Immunol* 1989;143(12):4015–4018.
30. Berk BC, Vekshtein V, Gordon HM, Tsuda T. Angiotensin II-stimulated protein synthesis in cultured vascular smooth muscle cells. *Hypertension* 1989;13(4):305–314.
31. Gibbons GH, Pratt RE, Dzau VJ. Vascular smooth muscle cell hypertrophy vs. hyperplasia. Autocrine transforming growth factor-beta 1 expression determines growth response to angiotensin II. *J Clin Invest* 1992;90(2):456–461.
32. Bornfeldt KE, Raines EW, Nakano T, Graves LM, Krebs EG, Ross R. Insulin-like growth factor-I and platelet-derived growth factor-BB induce directed migration of human arterial smooth muscle cells via signaling pathways that are distinct from those of proliferation. *J Clin Invest* 1994;93(3):1266–1274.
33. Raines EW, Dower SK, Ross R. Interleukin-1 mitogenic activity for fibroblasts and smooth muscle cells is due to PDGF-AA. *Science* 1989; 243:393–396.
34. Hajjar KA, Hajjar DP, Silverstein RL, Nachman RL. Tumor necrosis factor-mediated release of platelet-derived growth factor from cultured endothelial cells. *J Exp Med* 1987;166:235–245.
35. Leof EB, Proper JA, Goustin AS, Shipley GD, DiCorleto PE, Moses HL. Induction of c-*sis* mRNA and activity similar to platelet-derived growth factor by transforming growth factor beta: A proposed model for indirect mitogenesis involving autocrine activity. *Proc Natl Acad Sci USA* 1986;83:2453–2457.
36. Jonasson L, Holm J, Skalli O, Bondjers G, Hansson GK. Regional accumulations of T cells, macrophages, and smooth muscle cells in the human atherosclerotic plaque. *Arteriosclerosis* 1986;6:131–138.
37. Tsukada T, Rosenfeld M, Ross R, Gown AM. Immunocytochemical analysis of cellular components in lesions of atherosclerosis in the Watanabe and fat-fed rabbit using monoclonal antibodies. *Arteriosclerosis* 1986;6:601–613.
38. Hansson GK, Jonasson L, Holm J, Clowes MK, Clowes A. Gamma interferon regulates vascular smooth muscle proliferation and Ia expression in vivo and in vitro. *Circ Res* 1988;63:712–719.
39. Hansson GK, Hellstrand M, Rymo L, Rubbia L, Gabbiani G. Interferon-gamma inhibits both proliferation and expression of differentiation-specific alpha-smooth muscle actin in arterial smooth muscle cells. *J Exp Med* 1989;170:1595–1608.
40. Warner SJC, Friedman GB, Libby P. Immune interferon inhibits proliferation and induces 2′,5′-oligoadenylate synthetase gene expression in human vascular smooth muscle cells. *J Clin Invest* 1989;83: 1174–1182.
41. Hansson GK, Holm J, Jonasson L. Detection of activated T lymphocytes in the human atherosclerotic plaque. *Am J Pathol* 1989;315(1): 169–175.
42. Stemme S, Holm J, Hansson GK. T lymphocytes in human atherosclerotic plaques are memory cells expressing CD45RO and the integrin VLA-1. *Arterioscler Thromb* 1992;12(2):206–11.
43. Jonasson L, Holm J, Skalli O, Gabbiani G, Hansson GK. Expression of class II transplantation antigen on vascular smooth muscle cells in human atherosclerosis. *J Clin Invest* 1986;76:125–131.
44. Warner SJC, Friedman GB, Libby P. Regulation of major histocompatibility gene expression in cultured human vascular smooth muscle cells. *Arteriosclerosis* 1989;9:279–288.
45. Hansson GK, Holm J. Interferon-gamma inhibits arterial stenosis after injury. *Circulation* 1991;84(3):1266–1272.
46. Sporn MB, Todaro GJ. Autocrine secretion and malignant transformation of cells. *N Engl J Med* 1980;303:878–880.
47. Todaro GJ, De LJ, Fryling C, Johnson PA, Sporn MB. Transforming growth factors (TGFs): Properties and possible mechanisms of action. *J Supramol Struct Cell Biochem* 1981;15(3):287–301.
48. Tucker RF, Shipley GD, Moses HL, Holley RW. Growth inhibitor from BSC-1 cells closely related to platelet type beta transforming growth factor. *Science* 1984;226:705–707.
49. Antonelli-Orlidge A, Saunders KB, Smith RD, D'Amore PA. An activated form of transforming growth factor beta is produced by cocultures of endothelial cells and pericytes. *Proc Natl Acad Sci USA* 1989;86(2): 4544–4548.
50. Sato Y, Rifkin DB. Inhibition of endothelial cell movement by pericytes and smooth muscle cells: Activation of a latent transforming growth factor-beta 1-like molecule by plasmin during co-culture. *J Cell Biol* 1989;109(1):309–315.
51. Liau G, Chan LM. Regulation of extracellular matrix RNA levels in cultured smooth muscle cells. Relationship to cellular quiescence. *J Biol Chem* 1989;264(17):10315–10320.
52. Libby P, Clinton SK. Cytokines as mediators of vascular pathology. *Nouv Rev Fr Hematol* 1992;34(53):S47–S53.
53. Garg UC, Hassid A. Nitric oxide-generating vasodilators and 8-bromo-cyclic guanosine monophosphate inhibit mitogenesis and proliferation of cultured rat vascular smooth muscle cells. *J Clin Invest* 1989;83(5): 1774–1777.
54. Beckman JS, Chen J, Ischiropoulos H, Crow JP. Oxidative chemistry of peroxynitrite. *Methods Enzymol* 1994;233:229–240.
55. Nathan CF, Hibbs JBJ. Role of nitric oxide synthesis in macrophage antimicrobial activity. *Curr Opin Immunol* 1991;3(1):65–70.
56. Higashiyama S, Lau K, Besner GE, Abraham JA, Klagsbrun M. Structure of heparin-binding EGF-like growth factor. Multiple forms, primary structure, and glycosylation of the mature protein. *J Biol Chem* 1992;267(9):6205–6212.
57. Chamley-Campbell JH, Campbell GR, Ross R. The smooth muscle cell in culture. *Physiol Rev* 1979;58:1–61.

58. Ross R, Masuda J, Raines EW, et al. Localization of PDGF-B protein in macrophages in all phases of atherogenesis. *Science* 1990;248: 1009–1011.
59. Plump AS, Smith JD, Hayek T, et al. Severe hypercholesterolemia and atherosclerosis in apolipoprotein E-deficient mice created by homologous recombination in ES cells. *Cell* 1992;71(2):343–353.
60. Zhang SH, Reddick RL, Piedrahita JA, Maeda N. Spontaneous hypercholesterolemia and arterial lesions in mice lacking apolipoprotein E. *Science* 1992;258:468–471.
61. Nakashima Y, Plump AS, Raines EW, Breslow JL, Ross R. ApoE-deficient mice develop lesions of all phases of atherosclerosis throughout the arterial tree. *Arterioscler Thromb* 1994;14(1):133–140.
62. Ross R. The pathogenesis of atherosclerosis: A perspective for the 1990s. *Nature* 1993;362:801–809.

Atherosclerosis and Coronary Artery Disease,
edited by V. Fuster, R. Ross, and E. J. Topol.
Lippincott-Raven Publishers, Philadelphia © 1996.

CHAPTER 34

The Role of Rheology in Atherosclerotic Coronary Artery Disease

Avrum I. Gotlieb and B. Lowell Langille

Key Words: Endothelium; Mechanical stresses; Hemodynamic shear stress; Atherosclerosis; Centrosomes; Actin microfilaments; Microtubules.

INTRODUCTION

Pulsatile blood flow through coronary arteries is an important regulator of the structure and function of these arteries and has been implicated in the pathogenesis of atherosclerosis (1–4). In the large epicardial coronary arteries, atherosclerosis usually involves the proximal part of the vessel especially at or just beyond branch sites (5). Mechanical stresses of flowing blood on the vessel wall are important stimuli which interact with other endogenous and exogenous factors to regulate endothelial and smooth muscle cell behavior. In this chapter information is presented, within the context of atherogenesis, on the nature of the mechanical stresses to which the vessel wall is exposed. Clinical and experimental evidence is presented to show that these stresses are important modulators of vascular wall function in health and disease. Recent approaches directed at understanding how mechanical forces are transduced to biologic activity are discussed. In addition, exciting new information from the area of large-vessel developmental biology is presented which focuses on the ability of the arterial wall to remodel in the face of changes in hemodynamic shear stress and blood flow. This information is of interest since it is now apparent that the arterial wall and the atherosclerotic plaque undergo considerable remodeling during the initiation and growth of atherosclerotic coronary artery lesions.

MECHANICAL STRESSES ON VASCULAR TISSUE

Forces imposed on vascular tissues are of three types: pressure, tension (stretch), and shear. Pressure represents a force acting inward everywhere on the surface of tissue elements. Tension pulls tissue along one axis, normally without constraining the tissue in other directions. Shear exerts forces in opposite directions on opposite faces of tissue elements. Shear is different from tension in that forces are paral-

Avrum I. Gotlieb and B. Lowell Langille: Vascular Research Laboratory, Department of Pathology, Banting and Best Diabetes Centre, and Toronto Hospital Research Institute, Toronto, Ontario, M5G 2C4, Canada.

lel, not perpendicular, to the surfaces on which they act. Forces exerted on surfaces are expressed as forces per unit area, or stresses. Thus there is tensile stress, shear stress, and pressure.

Larger tissues deform more when under the same stress compared to smaller tissues, so deformation is usually measured in relative terms; stretch is measured as change in length divided by initial length, compression is change in volume divided by initial volume, and shear deformation is the relative displacement of opposite faces of a surface divided by the distance between the faces. When deformations are measured in these relative terms, they are referred to as strains. Thus there is tensile strain, volume strain, and shear strain. When forces and deformations are expressed as stresses and strains, the relationship between the two characterizes the deformability of the arterial tissue per se; it is not affected by the geometry (length, diameter, or curvature) of the vessel.

Shear Stress

Shear stresses are small forces that cause very modest deformation of the full thickness of the artery wall. Even though physiologic shear strains are below 1%, shear stress elicits significant physiologic and pathologic responses from vascular tissues, primarily through an effect on endothelial cells, which are in direct contact with flowing blood.

Plasma in contact with endothelium does not slide along blood vessel walls, so relative motion of adjacent layers of blood is needed to accommodate zero velocities at the endothelial surface and finite flows distant from the artery wall. Shear stresses are produced between fluid layers and are transmitted to the vessel wall. The local shear stress in flowing blood is proportional to blood viscosity (about 0.035 poise in SI units). It also depends on the speed at which adjacent layers of fluid slide past each other, as defined by the *strain rate* dv/dr, the local rate of change of velocity with position:

$$\tau = \mu \cdot dv/dr$$

where τ is shear stress, μ is viscosity, v is velocity, and r is radial position. Often dv/dr is greatest near the vessel wall, so maximal shears are transmitted to wall structures. Average shear stress in major human arteries is between 2 and 20 dyn/cm^2 with very localized increases to 30–200 dyn/cm^2 at branches and wall curvatures. Shear distribution is complex in large vessels because of the pulsatile nature of flow and because secondary flow effects are large near major systemic branch sites.

Secondary flow refers to flow disturbances that result when the momentum of blood entering branch ostia causes flow trajectories (streamlines) to deviate from the direction of the vessel axis. In pulsatile flow, the direction of these streamlines oscillates at the cardiac frequency. These oscillating patterns can be extremely complex; consequently, it is beyond the capacity of current computer analysis to define shear stresses accurately at the sites where they are of greatest interest.

Secondary flows are different from turbulence, which implies that lateral motion of the fluid is random. Turbulence occurs when flow velocities become high enough to destabilize local blood flow patterns.

Pressure

Pressures imposed at the intimal surfaces of arteries equal intravascular blood pressure. The adventitia, however, is normally at near-atmospheric pressures characteristic of most of the extravascular space. Since soft biologic tissues are highly incompressible, direct biologic effects of pressurization may occur only at absolute pressures measured in atmospheres, not those characteristic of the circulation. By contrast, differences in pressure between anatomic sites drive blood flow through the circulation, cause extravasation of fluid and solutes into the artery wall and surrounding tissue, and induce tension in wall tissues.

Arteries, like all pressurized elastic containers, experience circumferential wall tension and stretch by blood pressure. The tensile wall stress is equal to the blood pressure multiplied by the radius of the vessel divided by the wall thickness. Thus if vessels of different radii have the same wall thickness, a given pressure will exert greater stresses on the tissues of the larger vessel.

Tensile Strain

Variations in tensile strain of arteries are 5–10% during the cardiac cycle and can exceed 25% with physiologic adjustments of arterial pressure. Tensile stresses are borne primarily by the media in healthy arteries. Tensile stresses represent an average stress; in some cases, different layers of the media bear significantly different loads, but in large muscular arteries, it is unlikely that stress varies greatly from the intimal to adventitial limits of the media. Similarly, if one considers each lamellar unit (pair of adjacent elastic and muscular layers) in large elastic arteries (6) as a single structural unit, then each probably bears a similar load in healthy arteries.

Diseased large arteries must be given special attention. In early atherosclerosis, for example, intimal lesion tissue accumulates inside a stressed media, but it is not certain that this tissue assumes part of the tensile load on the vessel, at least in the short term. However, there is evidence that the media expands to preserve luminal diameter during early atherogenesis (7). If this medial remodeling occurs, lesion tissues in the intima may assume a tensile load as the vessel expands. Also severe lesions in large arteries may destabilize flow sufficiently to produce turbulence.

Stress concentration, the tendency for tensile forces to become elevated in the vicinity of discontinuities in solid structures, is an important concept when considering atherogenesis. Stress concentration is often associated with holes in structures under tension. Vascular branch sites concentrate tensile stresses. The ostia of side branches of large arteries are surrounded by stressed tissue. Branch geometries yield complex stress patterns, but tension elevation is focused around the ostia and typically yields stresses three to seven times those at distant sites. Consequently, some investigators have implicated tensile stresses in the pathogenesis of atherosclerosis near branch sites; however, at present these studies suffer from an inability to measure tensile stresses at the sites of interest (8,9). Regions of increased stiffness, e.g., sites of calcification, also concentrate stresses and this may contribute to further lesion progression.

HEMODYNAMIC SHEAR STRESS AND ATHEROSCLEROSIS

The localization of fibrofatty plaques at arterial bends and branch points suggests a role for hemodynamics in the pathogenesis of atherosclerosis. It has been proposed that abnormal hemodynamic shear stresses may cause endothelial injury or dysfunction and thereby contribute to atherogenesis. As proposed in Fig. 1, hemodynamic shear stress may affect atherogenesis at several steps. However, the nature of the injurious stress is controversial, and high, low, and fluctuating shears have all been implicated. Relating a specific

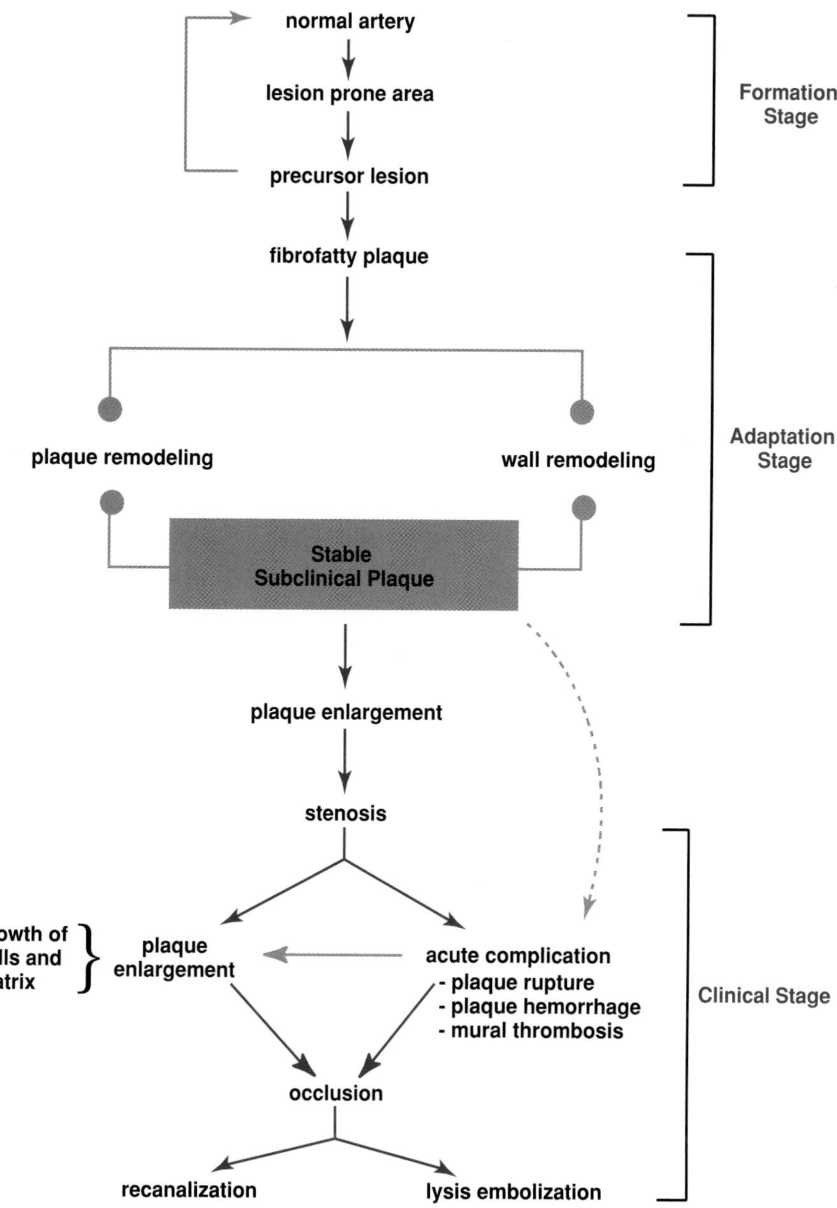

FIG. 1. Hypothesis on the initiation, growth, and complications of an atherosclerotic plaque. Hemodynamic shear stress plays an important role at several steps. **Top:** Shear stress is an important risk factor in the initiation of lesions at lesion-prone areas. **Middle:** Shear stress promotes both atherosclerotic plaque and arterial wall remodeling. **Bottom:** Shear stress promotes plaque enlargement, and is an important factor in plaque rupture; shear stress plays a role in the dislodging of thromboemboli.

change in shear stress to atherogenesis has proved difficult (10) because the lesions arise near arterial bends and branch sites where high, low, and rapidly fluctuating shear occur in close proximity. Here fluctuating shear refers to the directional and temporal fluctuations that are produced by secondary flows (e.g., vortices) near arterial bends, branch sites, and stenoses. Recent attention has focused on low and fluctuating shear stresses, but their effects are difficult to discriminate in vivo since they are often colocalized and tend to occur in small regions that are subjected to complex flow conditions (11,12). More is known about the in vivo responses of endothelium to high shear stress than about responses to low shear stress (13–15).

Current consensus is that lesions in humans occur at sites where shear stresses are low but rapidly fluctuating (11). Exceptions include cholesterol-fed and Watanabe rabbits (hereditary hypercholesterolemia), which get lesions adjacent to the flow dividers of branch sites where shear stresses are high (16,17). In experimental models with complex flows, low-shear regions have been shown to have predilection for the development of atherosclerotic lesions in hypercholesterolemic rabbits (18).

Further studies of flows near branch sites may better define the correlation between shear stress and atherogenesis, but they probably will not elucidate basic mechanisms of the disease because flow patterns are too complex at these sites.

EFFECT OF HEMODYNAMIC SHEAR STRESS ON THE ARTERY WALL

Hemodynamic shear stress affects the structure and function of endothelial cells in the monolayer both in vivo and in vitro. In many instances this results in profound changes in the structure and the function of the arterial wall. Thus, endothelial cells function as signal transducers of shear stress to modulate smooth muscle cell regulation of vasomotor tone in the artery wall. The effect of shear on vascular wall remodeling also occurs through an endothelium-dependent process. Both hemodynamic arguments and available data indicate that vascular responses to altered blood flow (shear stress) are mediated by the endothelium. Hemodynamic arguments are invoked because shear stresses are very small forces that cause minimal deformation of the media (19), whereas the endothelial cells that are in direct contact with flowing blood are exquisitely sensitive to shear (see below). Most data are consistent with this concept and show that responses to altered shear stress require an intact endothelium (19–21).

Shear Stress and Endothelial Cell Shape and Proliferation

Studies of hemodynamic shear stress have shown that the shape and orientation of endothelial cells are determined primarily by blood flow (22–24). The nuclei of arterial endothelial cells are ellipsoid in shape with their major axis aligned in the direction of blood flow (25). Guidance by subendothelial extracellular matrix also contributes to endothelial orientation (26–28).

It has been shown that disturbed flow or turbulent shear stress promotes proliferation, while equivalent laminar shear stress does not (29,30), and that shear stress may even decrease endothelial cell proliferation (31). Mitotic cells in nearly confluent but not quiescent endothelial monolayers were observed under 70 dyn/cm^2 laminar flow. The shear stress did not affect the duration of the different phases of cell division; however, there was an interesting influence on direction of mitosis (32).

Shear Stress and Endothelial Cell Function

Substantial work has documented numerous shear-driven changes in endothelium. These include cell shape changes (33,34) and redistribution of cytoskeleton and organelles (13,35,36), cell proliferation (30,32,37), expression of cell adhesion molecules (76), production of matrix (38), transport of macromolecules (39), and release of vasoactive substances (40,41), growth factors (42–45), and modulators of thrombogenicity (46). The multitude of responses may indicate that multiple signal transduction pathways are activated by shear. Signal transduction appears to involve G proteins (47,48) and the inositol pathway (49,50), and cyclic guanosine monophosphate (cGMP) and cyclic adenosine monophosphate (cAMP) activation have been described. Flow-induced platelet-derived growth factor (PDGF) B-chain expression has been reported to be both dependent (51) and independent of the protein kinase C pathway (45). Shear stimuli have been associated with increases in intracellular Ca^{2+} (52–55), opening of K^+ channels (56,57), and hyperpolarization (58,59), although the latter may be upstream or downstream of signal transduction pathways.

Shear Stress and Motor Tone

Vasomotor responses to altered shear require signaling between endothelium and medial smooth muscle. Vasoactive agents released by endothelium under shear stress include nitric oxide (NO) (60), prostacyclin (PGI2) (61–63), and endothelin (64), and physiologic roles for the first two of these have been demonstrated (60,61).

Shear Stress and the Cytoskeleton

The F-actin microfilament system, a component of the cytoskeleton, is important because of purported roles in the control of cell adhesion, cell migration, maintenance of cell shape, and cell permeability (65). In situ, F-actin is generally

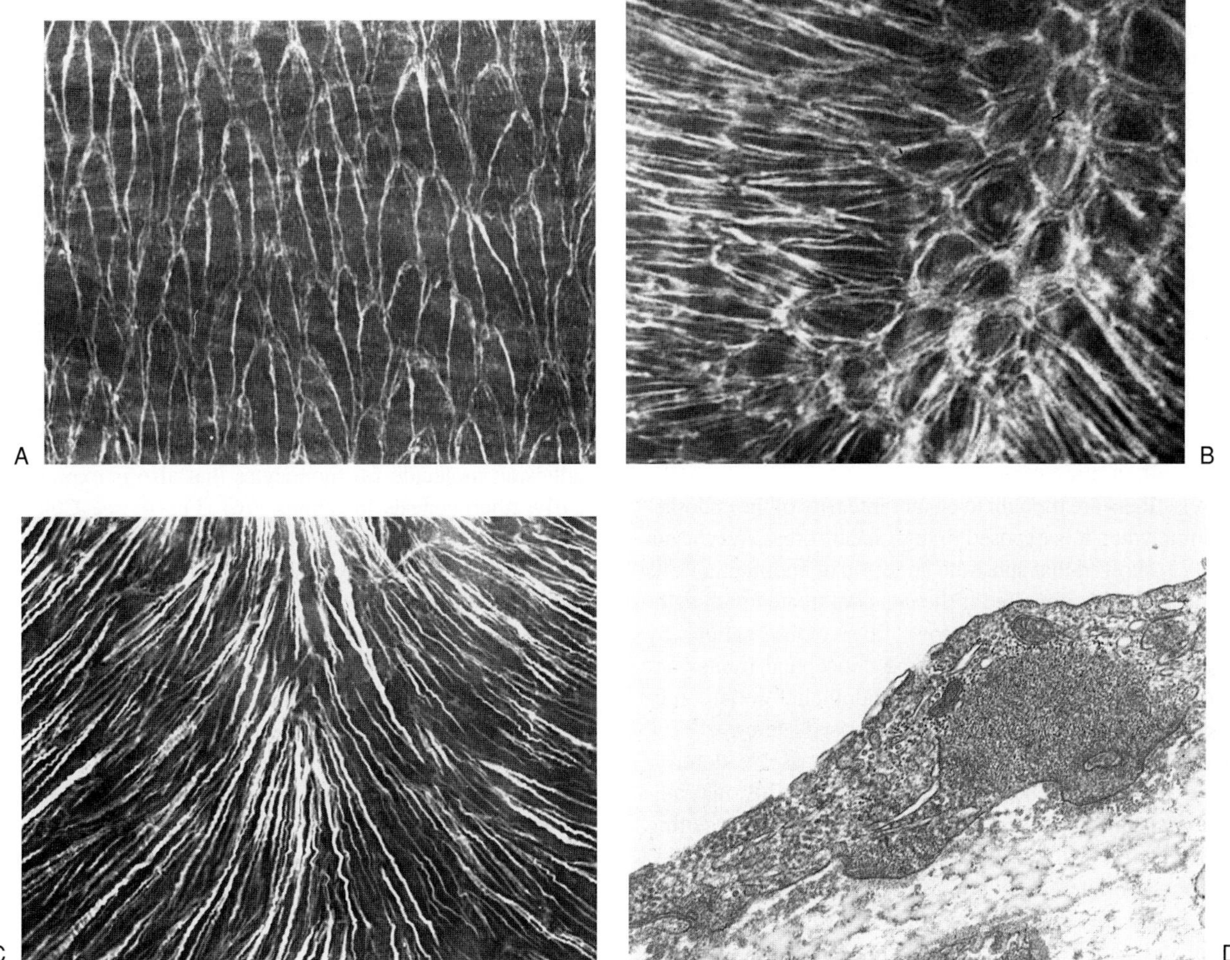

FIG. 3. Endothelium of rabbit aorta labeled in situ with rhodamine phalloidin to localize actin microfilaments (×600). **A:** Thoracic aorta. Note peripheral actin microfilaments and few central microfilaments. **B:** Aortic branch flow divider in area of low shear. Note cobblestone-shaped cells with dense peripheral band on lip of flow divider in area of low shear. Prominent microfilament bundles are seen in area of high shear. **C:** Aortic bifurcation. Note thick prominent microfilament bundles in this area of high shear. **D:** Electron photomicrograph of aortic endothelial cells in area of high shear. Note prominent microfilament bundle (×4,000).

present as a continuous microfilament band around the periphery of cells and in central microfilament bundles, or as "stress fibers," in the central portion of cells (66,67) (Fig. 2; see Colorplate 26) (Fig. 3). A current hypothesis is that central stress fibers are associated with cell substratum adhesion and peripheral fibers with cell–cell adhesion (65).

Stress fibers in endothelial cells are more numerous and prominent in regions of the arterial vasculature exposed to elevated shear stress (68–71). Kim et al. (72) reported profound alterations in F-actin microfilament organization in endothelial cells at sites of elevated shear levels in the normal rabbit aorta. The peripheral microfilament band was disrupted, whereas the central stress fibers were markedly increased in thickness and length. The hypothesis that alterations in hemodynamic shear stress in vivo cause this reorganization of the F-actin microfilament system was supported by studies in which a 60% coarctation was used to alter shear stress in the midabdominal aorta of the rabbit (13). This procedure produces a region of moderately elevated shear downstream from the stenosis, in which peripheral F-actin was dispersed and large central stress fibers were formed. The dynamics of redistribution of F-actin in the period immediately after experimental changes in shear is as follows (14). Within 12–15 h, the number of stress fibers in the central regions of the cells decreased, and some separation of junctional actin in adjacent cells occurred. Long, central stress fibers of variable thickness were evident at 24 h, but the band of actin normally seen at the periphery of the cells could no longer be distinguished. The redistribution of F-actin was completed over the next 24 h by an increase in thickness of central stress fibers. Restoration of normal F-actin distribution after coarctations were removed proceeded more slowly. The long, thick stress fibers that were induced by high shear were replaced by thinner or shorter microfilament bundles 48 h after the coarctations were removed. At 72 h, central stress fibers were primarily long, thin structures. Peripheral F-actin was not fully restored at this time. Peripheral F-actin was restored at 1 week after removal of the coarctation, but there were still more and longer stress fibers at this time than were observed in control aortas. These findings indicate that in vivo actin microfilament distribution can be modulated by experimentally altering flow conditions. Local increases in shear stress induce an orderly, reversible reorganization of cellular actin that is most pronounced and most rapid when shear is most elevated. The process appears to involve an early decrease in the pool of F-actin in the cell, followed by the preferential repolymerization of F-actin. These findings are consistent with evidence of the influence of shear on F-actin distribution in cell culture systems.

Stress fibers are thought to ensure integrity of the endothelial lining when it is exposed to high shear forces. Wechezak et al. (73) showed that substrate adhesion of endothelial cells in a shear field is impaired if the cells are treated with cytochalasin B, which disrupts stress fibers. Observations by Sato and co-workers (74) provide a conceptual framework for this finding. They found that endothelial cells conditioned by shear stress exhibit decreased deformability, whereas microfilament-disrupting agents increase deformability. Presumably, decreased cell deformability may enhance resistance to shear damage, perhaps by distributing stresses more evenly throughout the cell. Satcher et al. (75) raise another interesting possibility. They suggest that if stress fibers are associated with focal contacts at their upstream ends, as Wechezak et al. (73) observed in vitro, then they can serve to "moor" the cells that are exposed to shear forces. Shear forces imposed on the apical surfaces of the cells would then translate into tension in stress fibers that is transmitted to substrate adhesion sites. Early after coarctation, several stress fibers frequently appeared to emanate from a single site located at the upstream limit of the cell. If these stress fibers originate from a common point on the basal surface, then this could be a major site of substrate adhesion (13).

We developed an in vivo model that would allow examination of endothelial cell responses to low shear stresses in the absence of secondary flows and the fluctuation shears they produce (35). We chose to reduce shears in proximal common carotid arteries by ligating the vessel rostral to the thyroid branch, because long and straight arteries are free of secondary flows. In addition, shear stresses are relatively constant along the length of such arteries and Poiseuille flow approximations can provide reasonable estimates of time-averaged shear stress. Thus, well-defined shear stresses are imposed on a large region of endothelium. An additional advantage of the carotid model is that flows approximately doubled in the contralateral carotid, which provided collateral supply to the left carotid circulation, so responses to moderate elevation of shear also could be examined. By contrast, many previous studies of increased shear stress employed arteriovenous anastomoses that increase shear by 4- to 30-fold.

Our most striking observations were made when shear stresses were reduced by 70–80% by ligating distal branches of this vessel. Low shear stress alone caused monocyte emigration across the endothelium, a critical event in early atherogenesis. In addition, there was a reduction in central actin microfilaments, which are thought to regulate cell–substrate adhesion (35). Reduced substrate adhesion may contribute to a loss of endothelial cells that we observed when shear was low. Alternatively, endothelial cell loss may be due to early remodeling of the arteries in response to reduced shear.

We explored the mechanism of leukocyte adhesion and subsequently showed that low shear stress induces expression of vascular cell adhesion molecule-1 (VCAM-1), an adhesion molecule for monocytes that also is expressed in early atherogenesis in rabbits (76) (Fig. 4; see Colorplate 27). Interestingly, increased in shear stress also caused an increase in VCAM-1 expression (77). Thus, both very high and low shear stresses may induce monocyte adherence that is a hallmark of early atherogenesis. The tendency for atherosclerosis to occur at high-shear regions in rabbits may simply reflect more frequent occurrence of such sites in this species. Cybulsky and co-workers found that VCAM-1 is expressed by endothelial cells in the high-shear regions adjacent to flow dividers of branches in normal rabbit arteries (76,77).

We also examined expression of intracellular adhesion molecule-1 (ICAM-1), another leukocyte adhesion molecule, in these vessels. In contrast to VCAM-1, ICAM-1 is downregulated by low shear stress (77). We observed that most endothelial cells normally display ICAM-1 near cell–cell junctions, suggesting that ICAM-1 may mediate endothelial cell–cell adhesion as well. Muller et al. (78) recently showed that platelet/endothelial cell adhesion molecule 1 (PECAM-1) is required for leukocyte transmigration in vitro. It is also possible that this pool of ICAM-1 at cell junctions can be redistributed to the luminal surface when the cells are appropriately stimulated.

Shear-induced modulation of adhesion molecules by cultured endothelium has been reported recently (79), but there are differences between these studies and our in vivo work. First, no VCAM-1 sensitivity to shear is observed in vitro. Second, ICAM-1 sensitivity to shear is only observed at very low shear stresses (<2.5 dyn/cm^2). ICAM-1 distribution is unaffected by shear stresses above this level. The differences between in vitro and in vivo responses to shear may be due to effects of substrate blood constituents or endothelial/smooth muscle cell interactions. The latter may include early vasomotion/remodeling secondary to altered shear, which may substantially affect endothelium.

The insensitivity of ICAM-1 expression to shear above very low levels also has been reported for PDGF B chain (44). Promoter regions of genes for both of these molecules contain so-called shear-stress-responsive elements (42). If the responses driven by this region are ultimately translatable to the in vivo situation, then the responses may be most relevant to repression of gene expression under stasis, rather than modulation over a physiologic range of shear stress.

Shear Stress and Endothelial Repair

In vitro, endothelial cells reendothelialize experimental wounds made in confluent cultures more rapidly if shear stress is perpendicular to the wound edge and thus the cells are aligned in the same direction as the flow (80). In single endothelial cells, shear stress polarized lamellipodia extrusion, which is an important element in cell spreading and cell migration, within 10 min of the onset of flow. This biased lamellipodium development occurred in a direction of flow and was lost within several minutes after flow was reduced (81). During repair of mechanical denudation, fluid shear of 1–4 dyn/cm^2 enhances DNA synthesis compared to static cultures (82). In vivo, endothelial cells are aligned in the direction of flow during repair of large areas of endothelial denudation (83,84). Repair occurs more rapidly in circumferential wounds than in wounds made along the long axis of the vessel. This is because in the latter the cells have to realign in the direction perpendicular to flow. The actin stress fiber content of regenerated endothelial cells correlates with lipid deposition in the injured aorta (85).

Effects of shear stress on endothelial repair in vivo were also dramatic (29,86). When we made narrow, longitudinal denuding injuries to endothelium with a special catheter, a similar redistribution of centrosomes and microtubules which we reported in vitro (87–89) (Figs. 5 and 6) was observed in vivo with normal shear stresses, as was the loss of junctional actin in cells migrating into the wound (86). Upon wound closure, the centrosomes in the center of the closed wound were downstream of the nucleus. In addition, the cells migrated into the wound at an angle that was intermediate between the downstream direction and perpendicular to the wound edge. At wound closure, the cells came together at the midline of the wound in a herringbone fashion. Thus, the orientation of the migrating cells reflected the combined influences of shear stress and the repair stimulus. Very different repair was seen when shear stress was reduced. Large gaps appeared between the endothelial cell at the wound edge, with some cells separating almost entirely from their neighbors. Repair also was slowed, possibly because cells that were losing contact with their neighbors no longer received important cues concerning the appropriate direction of repair. This was manifest in the loss of orientation of the centrosomes toward the wound edge as the cells separated from each other. These studies suggest that cell–cell adhesion is important during endothelial repair. The factors that regulate the essential step of centrosome redistribution are not known in vivo; however, basic fibroblast growth factor (bFGF) has been implicated as an important signal for centrosome redistribution in in vitro studies on wound repair (90).

Shear Stress and Vascular Remodeling

Arteries remodel when shear is changed chronically (19,91,92). Atherosclerotic vessels adapt to lumen narrowing induced by plaque by changing the lumen diameter to restore shear stress toward normal. This compensation is incomplete or does not occur once the lesions occupy more than 45% of the area inside the internal elastic lamina (7). Thus shear stress is an important regulator of vascular remodeling. Studies have been undertaken to understand the processes and mechanisms involved in regulating shear-stress-induced changes in the lumen diameter of the artery wall. This change is biphasic. In the time following the change in shear stress there is a vasomotion of the vessel wall. This is mediated by endothelium-derived relaxing factor (NO) in most cases. Over the next few days to weeks there is a remodeling of the vessel wall leading to a structural entrenchment in the lumen size. Studies have shown that remodeling of collagen and elastin is involved in establishing these chronic changes in neonates but not in adults. The role of elastase has also been explored (93).

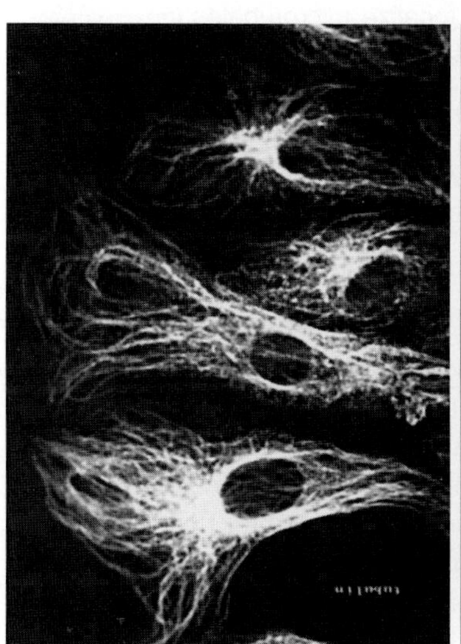

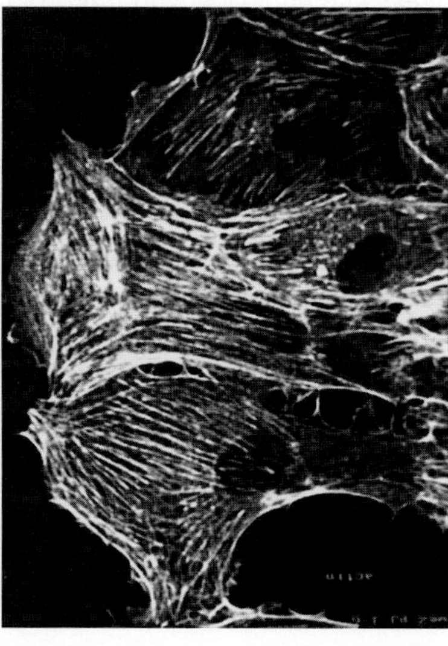

FIG. 5. Porcine aortic endothelial cells double-labeled with rhodamine phalloidin **(right)** and an antibody to tubulin **(left)** to localize actin microfilaments and tubulin. The cells are located at the edge of a denuding wound made in a confluent culture and fixed for staining 8 h after wounding. Note the centrosomes in the front of the cell between the nucleus and the wound edge. The DPB of microfilaments is absent and prominent central microfilaments are oriented in the long axis of the cell (compare to Fig. 2). (Bar, 25 μm.)

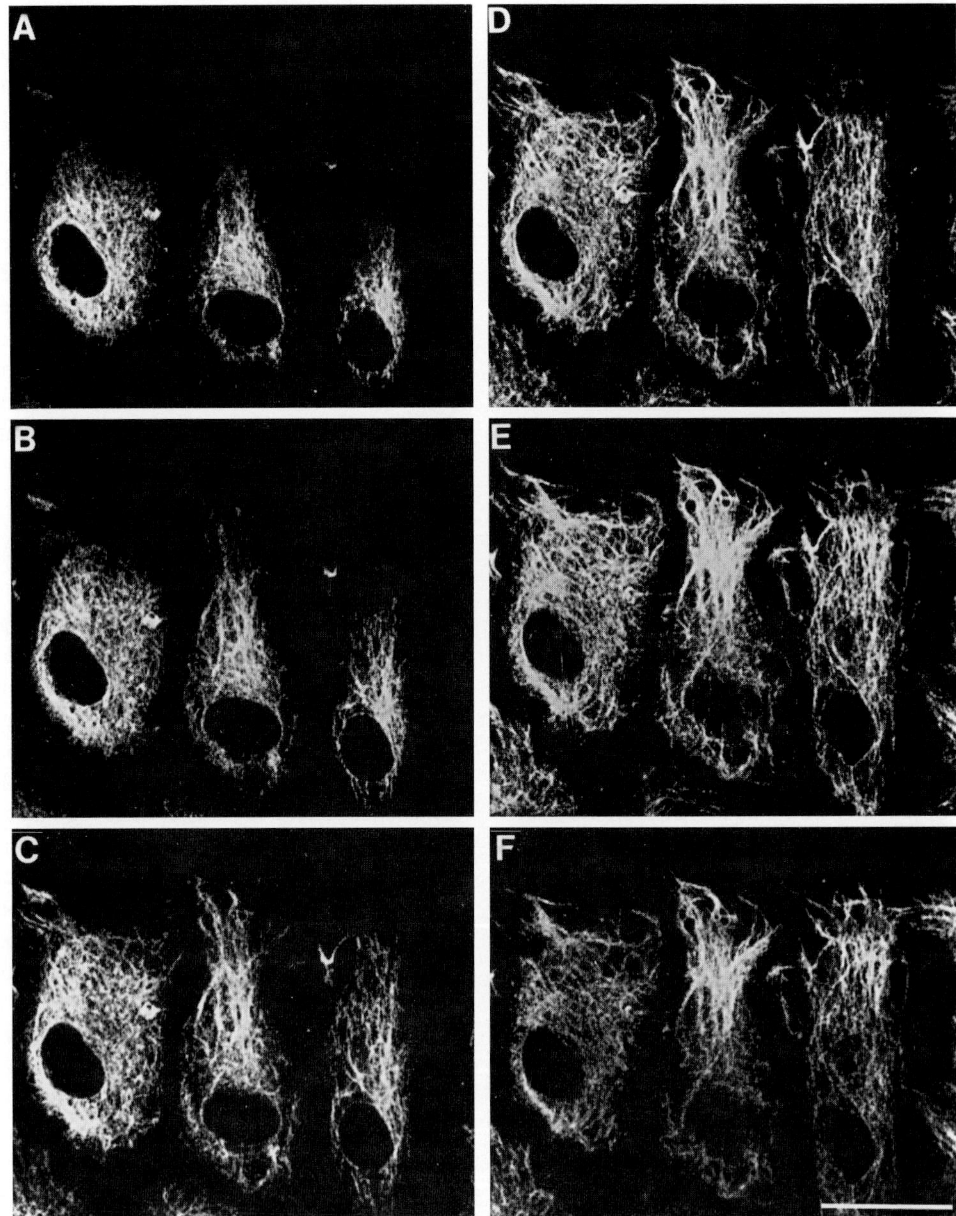

FIG. 6. Porcine aortic endothelial cells stained with an antibody to tubulin to localize microtubules in cells at the edge of a wound (top of each panel) made in a confluent culture. These are confocal images extending from the top of the cell **(A)** to the base **(F)** using 0.5-μm optical sections. Note that the centrosomes are more prominent toward the middle of the cell. This is in contrast to the actin DPB, which is more prominent toward the top and the central microfilaments, which are toward the base of the cell (see Figs. 3, 5). The centrosomes and associated microtubules are involved in the regulation of directed cell migration (89,90). (Bar, 25 μm.)

BIOMECHANICAL FORCES AND GENE EXPRESSION

Laminar shear stress in vitro upregulates transcription of the PDGF-B gene. A *cis*-acting shear stress response element (SSRE) within the promoter region of this gene is required (42,94). The core sequence in this shear stress response element (GAGACC) is also present in other genes that are responsive to shear stress, including those for tissue plasminogen activator (tPA), transforming growth factor beta (TGF-β), and ICAM-1. Studies of other genes have shown that often a rapid induction is seen followed by a downregulation. This has been reported for PDGF-B, bFGF, endothelin-1, and thrombomodulin (45,95–97). The SSRE does not appear to be involved in the downregulation of transcription of endothelin-1 (98).

BLOOD FLOW, VASCULAR DEVELOPMENT, AND REMODELING

Study of vascular development, especially as it relates to blood flow and hemodynamic shear stress, is an expanding area of vascular biology. It is indeed likely that the information gained in vascular development of large vessels will be very important in our understanding of the pathogenesis of atherosclerosis. The common feature that is emerging from the experimental in vivo studies is that vascular remodeling in the large arteries is an important aspect of both development and response to disease processes. Thus a review of some of the important features of developmental vascular biology is in order.

The Embryonic Vasculature

The hypothesis that developmental changes in blood flow are important in controlling the earliest development of the circulation originated with Thoma (99), who examined the developing area vasculosa of the chick embryo. Thoma observed that the channels within the vascular plexus that carried the greatest flows enlarged to become conduit vessels, whereas those that carry modest flows frequently regress. Clark (100) drew similar conclusions based on studies of the vasculature of the developing tadpole tail, and raised the possibility that the "blood flow over the endothelium" may be the stimulus for growth modulation. Forthcoming experimental support for these inferences was largely limited to observations of impaired vascular development following cardiac excision at times when the embryo was considered not to be dependent on circulatory function (100,101). Later, however, Stephan (102) demonstrated that experimental occlusions of the right third aortic arch in chick embryos, which becomes the adult arch in birds, prevented regression of the left arch. The obvious inference is that flow redistribution to the left arch resulted in sustained viability of this vessel. Others have confirmed that manipulating flows influences which aortic arches persist and which regress. However, it is clear that growth versus regression of embryonic vessels cannot be attributed solely to sensitivity to local hemodynamic conditions. For example, it appears inconceivable that the orderly development of the embryonic aortic arches could proceed solely on the basis of hemodynamic cues since large, low-resistance shunts between the ventral and dorsal aorta (e.g., the first aortic arch) regress, while small, high-resistance shunts (e.g., the third arch) enlarge.

The Perinatal Period

The weeks surrounding birth represent a particularly interesting period since it is the only time that very large and abrupt developmental changes in blood flow occur. Furthermore, many vessels exhibit marked decreases in blood flow at birth. These decreases run counter to the gradual increases that prevail throughout most of development, so a flow-dependent discontinuity in vessel growth may be readily discerned. Alternatively, the many metabolic and hormonal changes that characterize this time may elicit quite unique growth modulation that overrides hemodynamic effects.

An approximate halving of perfusion of many arteries, for example, the carotids and iliacs (M. P. Bendeck and B. L. L. Langille, *unpublished data*), probably reflects decreased demands for perfusion since arterial PO2 doubles after lung ventilation is initiated. However, the largest change seen in a major vessel is a more than 90% decrease in blood flow in the subrenal abdominal aorta, which occurs because the majority of fetal abdominal aortic blood flow is delivered to the placenta. In sheep, this dramatic decrease in blood flow is accompanied by a marked reduction in diameter of the vessel and a near arrest of wall tissue accumulation that lasts for at least 3 weeks (104).

In the weeks following birth, arterial growth, and specifically elastin accumulation, correlates with blood flow changes. However, an intriguing, flow-independent modulation of arterial growth occurs in the week surrounding birth (103). This period is characterized by very rapid aortic elastin and collagen accumulation, unrelated to blood flow changes, that produced more than 50% increases in contents of these proteins. The stimulus that drives this rapid connective tissue synthesis is unknown, but it may preadapt arteries to the large increases in pressure that follow parturition (104). Arterial pressures in near-term fetuses are about 45 mm Hg, whereas pressure rises to 65 mm Hg at 3 weeks of age.

Postnatal Arterial Growth

A strong relation between arterial growth and blood flow persists later in development. During postnatal growth and development, experimental changes in blood flow alter developmental changes in vessel diameter. This phenomenon is unlike the remodeling of adult arteries since both increases and decreases in blood flow influence wall tissue contents. Both smooth muscle proliferation and elastin accumulation are affected when flows are manipulated in the subnormal range. When 70% reductions in common carotid blood flows were induced in weanling rabbit by ligating the external carotid, DNA and elastin contents were substantially below those of control vessels 1 month later. However, smooth muscle proliferation becomes relatively insensitive to flows that are above normal levels, whereas elastin accumulation continues to be modulated. Twofold increases in carotid blood flows caused by contralateral common carotid ligation, again in young rabbits, results in 70% elevation in elastin accumulation without a significant influence on DNA or collagen content (di Stefano and Langille, *unpublished data*). These observations that experimental blood flow changes can affect subsequent arterial growth have important implications. They provide strong evidence that normal, developmental changes in tissue perfusion provide hemodynamic cues that modulate growth of the associated vasculature.

Both PDGF-B (43) and bFGF (44) release are shear-sensitive and provide a mechanism for growth modulation by blood flow. Recently, Resnick et al. (42) demonstrated a shear-sensitive response element in the PDGF promoter that also is found in other shear-sensitive genes, including tPA, TGF-β1, and ICAM-1. Recent evidence that PDGF is a survival factor for vascular smooth muscle adds a new twist to the possible role of this molecule is developmental vascular remodeling (105), especially given our current evidence of apoptosis in developmental arterial remodeling (106). Whether these agents exert in vivo control over vessel growth merits further research.

RHEOLOGY AND COMPLICATIONS OF ATHEROSCLEROTIC PLAQUES

Severe atherosclerosis in the coronary artery leads to myocardial ischemia when there is a reduction of the cross-sectional area of the coronary lumen by 75%. In this case, it appears that the coronary circulation cannot meet the demands of an increased requirement of myocardial oxygen above resting levels. The geometric configuration of severe atherosclerotic plaques is generally divided into two types—concentric and eccentric. The latter is the most common. The pathogenesis of further plaque growth is not well understood, nor are the specific influences of hemodynamic factors on eccentric versus concentric lesions. Plaque rupture due to tearing of the fibrous cap at the shoulder of the plaque is thought to be due to hemodynamic stress on the fibrous cap. This rupture often will lead to acute lumen thrombosis and occlusion, which results in an acute myocardial infarction. It is also thought that repeated hemodynamic injury to the endothelium is in part responsible for plaque fissure formation, which may promote mural thrombosis and, in severe cases, acute thrombotic occlusion.

The role of hemodynamic shear stress on the vessel wall distal to a stenotic coronary artery is not well understood. In the area just distal to the plaque, shear is low, while further downstream, shear is elevated (37). Thus one may speculate that these alterations in shear may promote extension of the existing stenotic plaque. Another interesting question is the role of the alteration of shear stress on disease progression following the reduction of coronary artery stenosis post-angioplasty and/or postatherectomy. It is assumed that the distal artery will undergo remodeling once it is exposed to new flows and shear stresses. How this will influence the progress of atherosclerotic disease in the coronary tree is not known.

ACKNOWLEDGMENTS

We acknowledge the secretarial assistance of Sursattie Sarju. This work was supported by Grant MT-6485 from the Medical Research Council of Canada and Grants T-1259 and T-2367 from the Heart and Stroke Foundation of Canada. B.L.L. is supported by a Career Investigator Award from the Heart and Stroke Foundation of Ontario.

REFERENCES

1. McMillan DE. Blood flow and the localization of atherosclerotic plaques. *Stroke* 1985;16:582–587.
2. Nerem RM, Cornhill JF. Hemodynamics and atherogenesis. *Atherosclerosis* 1980;36:151.
3. Sabbah HN, Khaja F, Brymer JF, Hawkins ET, Stein PD. Blood velocity in the right coronary artery: Relation to the distribution of atherosclerotic lesions. *Am J Cardiol* 1984;53:1008–1012.
4. Asakura T, Karino T. Flow patterns and spatial distribution of atherosclerotic lesions in human coronary arteries. *Circ Res* 1990;66: 1045–1066.
5. Stary HC. Macrophages, macrophage foam cells, and eccentric intimal thickening in the coronary arteries of young children. *Atherosclerosis* 1987;64:91–109.
6. Wolinsky H, Glagov S. Lamellar unit of aortic medial structure and function in mammals. *Circ Res* 1967;20:99–111.
7. Glagov S, Weisenberg E, Zarins CK, et al. Compensatory enlargement of human atherosclerotic coronary arteries. *N Engl J Med* 1987;316: 1371–1375.
8. Niimi H. Role of stress concentration in arterial walls in atherogenesis. *Biorheology* 1979;16:223–230.
9. Thubrikar MJ, Baker JW, Nolan SP. Inhibition of atherosclerosis associated with reduction of arterial intraluminal stress in rabbits. *Arteriosclerosis* 1988;8:410–420.
10. Zand T, Majno G, Nunnari JJ, Hoffman AH, Savilonis BJ, MacWilliams B, Joris I. Lipid deposition and intimal stress and strain. *Am J Pathol* 1991;139:101–113.
11. Ku DN, Giddens DP, Zarins CK, Glagov S. Pulsatile flow and atherosclerosis in the human carotid bifurcation: Positive correlation between plaque location and low and oscillating shear stress. *Arteriosclerosis* 1985;5:293.
12. Zarins CK, Giddens DP, Bharadvaj BK, Sottiurai VS, Mabon RF, Glagov S. Carotid bifurcation atherosclerosis: Quantitative correlation of plaque location with flow velocity profiles and wall shear stress. *Circ Res* 1983;53:502–514.
13. Kim DW, Gotlieb AI, Langille BL. *In vivo* modulation of endothelial F-actin microfilaments by experimental alterations in shear stress. *Arteriosclerosis* 1989;9:439–445.
14. Langille BL, Graham JJK, Kim DW, Gotlieb AI. Dynamics of shear-induced redistribution of F-actin in endothelial cells *in vivo*. *Arterioscler Thromb* 1991;II:1814–1820.
15. Zand T, Nunnari JJ, Hoffman AH, Savilonis BJ, MacWilliams B, Majno G, Joris I. Endothelial adaptations in aortic stenosis: Correlation with flow parameters. *Am J Pathol* 1988;133:407–418.
16. Cornhill JF, Roach MR. A quantitative study of the localization of atherosclerotic lesions in the rabbit aorta. *Atherosclerosis* 1976;23: 489–501.
17. Tsukada T, Rosenfeld M, Ross R, Gown AM. Immunocytochemical analysis of cellular components in atherosclerotic lesions. Use of monoclonal antibodies with the Wantanabe and fat fed rabbit. *Arteriosclerosis* 1986;6:601–613.
18. Uematsu M, Kitabatake A, Tanouchi J, Doi Y, Masyama T, Fujii K, Yoshida Y, Ito H, Ishihara K, Hori M, Inoue M, Kamada T. Reduction of endothelial microfilament bundles in the low-shear region of the canine aorta. *Arterioscler Thromb* 1991;11:107–115.
19. Langille BL, O'Donnell F. Reductions in arterial diameter produced by chronic decreases in blood flow are endothelium-dependent. *Science* 1986;231:405–407.
20. Smiesko V, Kozi J, Delezel S. Role of endothelium in the control of arterial diameter by blood flow. *Blood Vessels* 1985;22:247–251.
21. Pohl U, Forstermann U, Busse R. Endothelium-mediated modulation of arterial smooth muscle tone and PGI2-release: Pulsatile versus steady flow. In: Schror K, ed. *Prostaglandins and Other Eicosanoids in the Cardiovascular System.* Basel: Karger; 1985:553–558.
22. Langille BL, Adamson SL. Relationship between blood flow direction and endothelial cell orientation at arterial branch sites in rabbits and mice. *Circ Res* 1981;48:481–488.

23. Ives CL, Eskin SG, McIntire LV, DeBakey ME. The importance of cell origin and substrate in the kinetics of endothelial cell alignment in response to steady flow. *Trans Am Soc Artif Intern Organs* 1983; 29:269–274.
24. Remuzzi A, Dewey CF, Davies PF, Gimbrone A. Orientation of endothelial cells in shear fields *in vitro*. *Biorheology* 1984;21:617–630.
25. Flaherty JT, Pierce JE, Ferrans VJ, Patel DJ, Tucker WK, Fry DL. Endothelial nuclear patterns in the canine arterial tree with particular reference to hemodynamic events. *Circ Res* 1972;30:23–33.
26. Jackman RW. Persistence of axial orientation cues in regenerating intima of cultured aortic explants. *Nature* 1982;296:80–83.
27. Buck RC. Contact guidance in the subendothelial space. Repair of rat aorta in vitro. *Expl Mol Pathol* 1979;31:275–283.
28. Ookawa K, Sato M, Ohshima N. Morphological changes of endothelial cells after exposure to fluid-imposed shear stress; differential responses induced by extracelular matrices. *Biorheology* 1993;30: 131–140.
29. Langille BL, Reidy MA, Kline RL. Injury and repair of endothelium at sites of flow disturbances near abdominal aortic coarctations in rabbits. *Arteriosclerosis* 1986;6:146–154.
30. Davies PF, Remuzzi A, Gordon EJ, Dewey CF Jr, Gimbrone MA Jr. Turbulent fluid shear stress induces vascular endothelial cell turnover *in vitro*. *Proc Natl Acad Sci USA* 1986;83:2114–2117.
31. Levesque MJ, Sprague EA, Schwartz CJ, Nerem RM. The influence of shear stress on cultured vascular endothelial cells: The response of an anchorage-dependent mammalian cell. *Biotechnol Prog* 1989; 5:1–8.
32. Ziegler T, Nerem RM. Effect of flow on the process of endothelial cell division. *Arterioscler Thromb* 1994;14:636–643.
33. Reidy MA, Langille BL. The effect of local blood flow patterns on endothelial cell morphology. *Exp Mol Pathol* 1980;32:276–289.
34. Levesque MJ, Nerem RM. The elongation and orientation of cultured endothelial cells in response to shear stress. *J Biomech Eng* 1985; 107:341–347.
35. Walpola PL, Gotlieb AI, Langille BL. Monocyte adhesion and changes in endothelial cell number, morphology, and F-actin distribution elicited by low shear stress *in vivo*. *Am J Pathol* 1993;142: 1392–1400.
36. Coan DE, Wechezak AR, Viggers RF, Sauvage LR. Effect of shear stress upon localization of the Golgi apparatus and microtubule organizing center in isolated cultured endothelial cells. *J Cell Sci* 1993; 104:1145–1153.
37. Langille BL, Reidy MA, Kline RL. Injury and repair of endothelium at sites of flow disturbances near abdominal aortic coarctations in rabbits. *Arteriosclerosis* 1986;6:146–154.
38. Wechezak AR, Viggers RF, Sauvage LR. Fibronectin and F-actin redistribution in cultured endothelial cells exposed to shear stress. *Lab Invest* 1985;53:639–647.
39. Langille BL. Chronic effects of blood flow on the artery wall. In: Frangos JA, ed. *Physical Forces and the Mammalian Cell*. San Diego: Academic Press; 1993:249–274.
40. Busse R, Pohl U. Chronic effects of blood flow on the artery wall. In: Frangos JA, ed. *Physical Forces and the Mammalian Cell*. San Diego: Academic Press; 1993:223–248.
41. Dewey CF Jr, Bussolari SR, Gimbrone MA Jr, Davies PF. The dynamic response of vascular endothelial cells to fluid shear stress. *J Biomech Eng* 1981;103:177–185.
42. Resnick N, Collins T, Atkinson W, Bonthron DT, Dewey CF Jr, Gimbrone MA Jr. Platelet-derived growth factor B chain promoter contains a *cis*-acting fluid shear-stress-responsive element. *Proc Natl Acad Sci USA* 1993;90:4591–4595.
43. Hsieh H-J, Li N-Q, Frangos JA. Shear stress increases endothelial platelet-derived growth factor mRNA levels. *Am J Physiol* 1991;260: H642–H646.
44. Malek AM, Gibbons GH, Dzau VJ, Izumo S. Fluid shear stress differentially modulates expression of genes encoding basic fibroblast growth factor and platelet-derived growth factor B chain in vascular endothelium. *J Clin Invest* 1993;92:2013–2021.
45. Mitsumata M, Fishel RS, Nerem RM, Alexander RW, Berk BC. Fluid shear stress stimulates platelet derived growth factor expression in endothelial cells. *Am J Physiol* 1993;265(*Heart Circ Physiol*): H3–H8.
46. Diamond SL, Sharefkin JB, Dieffenbach C, Frasier-Scott K, McIntire LV, Eskin SG. Tissue plasminogen activator messenger RNA levels increase in cultured human endothelial cells exposed to laminar shear stress. *J Cell Physiol* 1990;143:364–371.
47. Berthiaume F, Frangos JA. Flow-induced prostacyclin production is mediated by a pertussis toxin-sensitive G protein. *FEBS Lett* 1992; 308:277–279.
48. Ohno M, Gibbons GH, Dzau VJ, Cooke JP. Shear stress elevates endothelial cGMP: Role of a potassium channel and G protein coupling. *Circulation* 1993;88:193–197.
49. Nollert MU, Eskin SG, McIntire LV. Shear stress increases inositol trisphosphate levels in human endothelial cells. *Biochem Biophys Res Commun* 1990;170:281–287.
50. Prasad ARS, Logan SA, Nerem RM, Schwartz CJ, Sprague EA. Flow-related responses of intracellular inositol phosphate levels in cultured aortic endothelial cells. *Circ Res* 1993;72:827–836.
51. Hsieh H-J, Li N-Q, Frangos JA. Shear induced platelet-derived growth factor gene expression in human endothelial cells is mediated by protein kinase C. *J Cell Physiol* 1992;150:552–558.
52. Schilling WP, Mo M, Eskin SG. Effect of shear stress on cytosolic Ca^{2+} of calf pulmonary artery endothelial cells. *Exp Cell Res* 1992; 198:31–35.
53. Shen J, Luscinskas FW, Connolly A, Dewey CF Jr, Gimbrone MA Jr. Fluid shear stress modulates cytosolic free calcium in vascular endothelial cells. *Am J Physiol Cell Physiol* 1992;262:C384–C390.
54. Kuchan MJ, Frangos JA. Role of calcium and calmodulin in flow-induced nitric oxide production in endothelial cells. *Am J Physiol Cell Physiol* 1994;266:C628–C636.
55. Oike M, Droogmans G, Nilius B. Mechanosensitive Ca^{2+} transients in endothelial cells from human umbilical vein. *Proc Natl Acad Sci USA* 1994;91:2940–2944.
56. Olesen SP, Clapham DE, Davies PF. Haemodynamic shear stress activates a K channel current in vascular endothelial cells. *Nature* 1988; 331:168–170.
57. Cooke JP, Rossitch E Jr, Andon NA, Loscalzo J, Dzau VJ. Flow activates an endothelial potassium channel to release an endogenous nitrovasodilator. *J Clin Invest* 1991;88:1663–1671.
58. Schwarz G, Droogmans G, Nilius B. Shear stress induced membrane currents and calcium transients in human vascular endothelial cells. *Pflugers Arch* 1992;421:394–396.
59. Berthiaume F, Frangos JA. Fluid flow increases membrane permeability to merocyanine 540 in human endothelial cells. *Biochim Biophys Acta Bio-Membr* 1994;1191:209–218.
60. Pohl U, Herlan K, Huang A, Bassenge E. EDRF-mediated shear-induced dilation opposes myogenic vasoconstriction in small rabbit arteries. *Am J Physiol Heart Circ Physiol* 1991;261:H2016–H2023.
61. Van Grondelle A, Worthen GS, Ellis D, Mathias MM, Murphy RC, Strife RJ, Reeves JT, Voelkel NF. Increased prostacyclin production in endothelial cells during shear stress and in rat lungs at high flow. *J Appl Physiol* 1984;57:388–395.
62. Frangos JA, Eskin SG, McIntire LV, Ives CL. Flow effects on prostacyclin production by cultured human endothelial cells. *Science* 1985; 227:1477–1479.
63. Koller A, Sun D, Kaley G. Role of shear stress and endothelial prostaglandins in flow- and viscosity-induced dilation of arterioles *in vitro*. *Circ Res* 1993;72:1276–1284.
64. Sharefkin JB, Diamond SL, Eskin SG, McIntire LV, Dieffenbach CW. Fluid flow decreases preproendothelin mRNA levels and suppresses endothelin-1 peptide release in cultured human endothelial cells. *J Vasc Surg* 1991;14:1–9.
65. Gotlieb AI, Langille BL, Wong MKK, Kim DW. The structure and function of the endothelial cytoskeleton. *Lab Invest* 1991;66:123–127.
66. Gotlieb AI, Spector W. Migration into an experimental wound: A comparison of porcine aortic endothelial and smooth muscle cells and the effect of culture irradiation. *Am J Pathol* 1981;103:271–282.
67. Wong MKK, Gotlieb AI. Endothelial monolayer integrity. I. Characterization of dense peripheral band of microfilaments. *Arteriosclerosis* 1986;6:212–219.
68. Colangelo S, Langille BL, Gotlieb AI. Endothelial microfilament distribution in the immediate vicinity of arterial branch sites. *Cell Tissue Res* 1994;278:235–242.
69. White GE, Gimbrone MA Jr, Fujiwara K. Factors influencing the expression of stress fibers in vascular endothelial cells *in situ*. *J Cell Biol* 1983;97:416–424.
70. Wong AJ, Pollard TD, Herman IM. Actin filament stress fibers in vascular endothelial cells *in vivo*. *Science* 1983;219:867–869.

71. Drenckhahn D, Gress T, Franke RP. Endothelial cells under shear stress: Vascular endothelial stress fibers: Their potential role in protecting the vessel wall from rheological damage. *Klin Wochenschr* 1986;64:986–988.
72. Kim DW, Langille BL, Wong MKK, Gotlieb AI. Patterns of endothelial microfilament distribution in the rabbit aorta *in situ*. *Circ Res* 1989;64:21–31.
73. Wechezak AR, Wight TN, Viggers RF, Sauvage LR. Endothelial adherence under shear stress is dependent upon microfilament reorganization. *J Cell Physiol* 1989;139:136–146.
74. Sato M, Levesque MJ, Nerem RM. Micropipette aspiration of cultured bovine aortic endothelial cells exposed to shear stress. *Arteriosclerosis* 1987;7:276–286.
75. Satcher R, De Paolo W, Gimbrone MA, Dewey CF. Endothelial cell structure resulting from shear stress. In: *First World Congress of Biomechanics* 1990;11:243–250.
76. Cybulsky MI, Gimbrone MA Jr. Endothelial expression of a mononuclear leukocyte adhesion molecule during atherogenesis. *Science* 1991;251:788–791.
77. Walpola PL, Gotlieb AI, Cybulsky MI, Langille BL. VCAM-1 expression and monocyte adherence in arteries exposed to altered shear stress. *Arterioscler Thromb Vasc Biol* 1995;15:2–10.
78. Muller WA, Weigl SA, Deng X, Philips DM. PECAM-1 is required for transendothelial migration of leukocytes. *J Exp Med* 1993;178: 449–460.
79. Nagel T, Resnick N, Atkinson WJ, Dewey C Jr, Gombrone MA Jr. Shear stress selectively upregulates intercellular adhesion molecule-1 expression in cultured human vascular endothelial cells. *J Clin Invest* 1994;94:885–891.
80. Ando J, Nomura H, Kamiya A. The effects of fluid shear stress on the migration and proliferation of cultured endothelial cells. *Microvasc Res* 1987;33:62–70.
81. Masuda M, Fujiwara K. The biased lamellipodium development and microtubule organizing center position in vascular endothelial cells migrating under the influence of fluid flow. *Biol Cell* 1993;77: 237–245.
82. Ando J, Komatsuda T, Ishikawa C, Kamiya A. Fluid shear stress enhanced DNA synthesis in cultured endothelial cells during repair of mechanical denudation. *Biorheology* 1990;27:675–684.
83. Schwartz SM, Haudenschild CC, Eddy EM. Endothelial regeneration: I. Quantitative analysis of intimal stages of endothelial regeneration in rat aortic intima. *Lab Invest* 1978;38:568–580.
84. Haudenschild CC, Schwartz SM. Endothelial regeneration. II. Restitution of endothelial continuity. *Lab Invest* 1979;41:407–418.
85. Barja F, Blatter MC, James RW, Pometta D, Gabbiani G. Actin stress fiber content of regenerated endothelial cells correlates with intramural retention of intermediate plus low density lipoproteins in rat aorta after balloon injury. *Atherosclerosis* 1989;76:181–191.
86. Vyalov S, Langille BL, Gotlieb AI. Low shear stress disrupts repair processes and slows *in vivo* reendothelialization. *FASEB J* 1994;8: A661.
87. Gotlieb AI, Subrahmanyan L, Kalnins VI. Microtubule organizing centres and cell migration. Effects of inhibition of migration and microtubules disruption in endothelial cells. *J Cell Biol* 1983;96: 1266–1272.
88. Wong MKK, Gotlieb AI. The reorganization of microfilaments, centrosomes, and microtubules during *in vitro* small wound reendothelialization. *J Cell Biol* 1988;107:1777–1783.
89. Ettenson DS, Gotlieb AI. Centrosome dependent endothelial wound repair requires early transcription following injury. *Arterioscler Thromb* 1993;13:1270–1281.
90. Ettenson DS, Gotlieb AI. Basic fibroblast growth factor is a signal for the initiation of centrosome redistribution to the front of migrating endothelial cells, at the edge of an *in vitro* wound. *Arterioscler Thromb Vasc Biol* 1995;15:2–10.
91. Kamiy A, Togawa T. Adaptive regulation of wall shear stress to flow change in the canine carotid artery. *Am J Physiol* 1980;239:H14–H21.
92. Langille BL, Bendeck MP, Keeley FW. Adaptations of carotid arteries of young and mature rabbits to reduced carotid blood flow. *Am J Physiol* 1989;256:H931–H939.
93. Langille BL, Wong L. Blood flow-induced remodelling of arterial elastin: Role in arterial development. *FASEB J* 1994;8:A1018.
94. Hsieh HJ, Li NQ, Frangos JA. Pulsatile and steady flow induces c-*fos* expression in human endothelial cells. *J Cell Physiol* 154: 143–151.
95. Malek A, Izumo S. Physiological fluid shear stress causes downregulation of endothelin-1 mRNA in bovine aortic endothelium. *Am J Physiol* 263:C389–C396.
96. Malek AM, Green AL, Izumo S. Regulation of endothelin 1 gene fluid shear stress transcriptionally mediated and independent of protein kinase C and cAMP. *Proc Natl Acad Sci USA* 1993;90: 5999–6003.
97. Malek AM, Jackman R, Rosenberg RD, Izumo S. Endothelial expression of thrombomodulin is reversibly regulated by fluid shear stress. *Circ Res* 1994;74:852–860.
98. Ohtsuka A, Ando J, Korenaga R, Kamiya A, Toyama-Sorimachi N, Miyasaka M. The effect of flow on the expression of vascular adhesion molecule-1 by cultured mouse endothelial cells. *Biochem Biophys Res Commun* 1993;193:303–310.
99. Thoma R. *Untersuchagen uber die histogenesis und histomechanik des gefasssytems*. Stuttgart: Enke; 1893.
100. Clark ER. Studies on the growth of blood-vessels in the tail of the frog larva—by observation and experiment on the living animal. *Am J Anat* 1918;23:37–88.
101. Chapman WB. The effect of the heart-beat upon the development of the vascular system in the chick. *Am J Anat* 1918;23:175–203.
102. Stephan F. Les suppléances obtenues expérimentalement dans le système des arcs aortiques de l'embryon d'oiseau. *Comptes Rendu* 1949; 36:647–651.
103. Bendeck MP, Langille BL. Rapid accumulation of elastin and collagen in the aortas of sheep in the immediate perinatal period. *Circ Res* 1991;69:1165–1169.
104. Langille BL, Brownlee RD, Adamson SL. Perinatal aortic growth in lambs: Relation to blood flow changes at birth. *Am J Physiol* 1990; 259:H1247–H1253.
105. Bennett MR, Evan GI, Newby AC. The c-*myc* proto-oncogene mediates vascular smooth muscle cell growth arrest and apoptosis. *FASEB J* 1994;8:A392.
106. Cho A, Courtman DW, Langille BL. Apoptosis (programmed cell death) in arteries of the neonatal lamb. *Circ Res* 1995;76:168–175.

Atherosclerosis and Coronary Artery Disease,
edited by V. Fuster, R. Ross, and E. J. Topol.
Lippincott-Raven Publishers, Philadelphia © 1996.

CHAPTER 35

Platelet Activation

Aaron J. Marcus

Key Words: Eicosanoids; Glycoproteins; Hemostasis; Occlusion; Phospholipids; Platelets.

INTRODUCTION

The role of platelets in the arrest of bleeding (hemostasis) is well understood (1,2). The hemostatic process represents a sequence of biologic events which culminate in spontaneous arrest of hemorrhage from traumatized blood vessels. Hemostasis is accomplished via interactions of at least three biologic systems: components of the vascular wall, platelets, and proteins of the blood coagulation cascade. Under physiologic conditions, platelets function to maintain integrity of the vasculature by preventing increases in vessel fragility and permeability. The substance(s) responsible for this function has not been identified.

Unfortunately, there is a misdirected form of hemostasis which complicates atherosclerosis, leading to 50% of mortal illness in the United States, Europe, and Japan (3–6). This involves sites of pathologic vascular damage consisting of necrotic, fissured atherosclerotic plaques in the coronary or cerebral circulation. Upon ulceration or fissuring, both unpredictable events, these sites become strong agonists for activation of systems which are mainly hemostatic, thereby transforming them into initiators of arterial thrombosis (7,8).

Aaron J. Marcus: Hematology/Oncology, Department of Veterans Affairs Medical Center, New York, New York; Department of Medicine and Pathology, Cornell University Medical College, New York 10021.

These events are discussed in detail by Badimon and Badimon elsewhere in this volume, in connection with the role of platelets and coagulation in the pathogenesis of atherosclerosis. Until recently, platelet activation at the site of a fissured or ruptured atherosclerotic plaque has been virtually unresponsive to currently available therapeutic modalities (5,7,9,10).

INDUCTION OF PRIMARY HEMOSTASIS BY PLATELETS

Unless proven otherwise, arterial thrombosis as now comprehended is primarily a misdirected or amplified form of primary hemostasis and is modulated by blood platelets. Whenever continuity of a blood vessel is interrupted, the immediate response involves participation of platelets and subendothelial matrix, but not proteins of the coagulation system (11,12). Thus, the bleeding time, a clinical test of primary hemostasis, is normal in hemophilia. The damaged vessel elicits a contractile response and simultaneously platelets adhere to subendothelial components—the most important of which is collagen. Von Willebrand factor (vWF) in the subendothelial matrix as well as vWF from plasma rapidly absorb to the injury site, where they induce further platelet adhesion by interacting with the platelet glycoprotein (GP) Ib–IX–V receptor complex (13–15). These initial interactions provoke an increase in platelet reactivity which in turn results in activation of the GPIIb–IIIa receptor complex (integrin $\alpha IIb\beta_3$) (16) on the platelet surface. Adhesiveness of these platelets and their spreading on the injured vessel surface continue in an irreversible manner (17). Activated platelets metabolically produce a releasate which serves as a fluid-phase recruiting modality for other platelets. This recruitment stage leads to an evolving platelet thrombus which gradually occludes the vessel. Clinically, very similar thrombi are responsible for induction of ischemic complications following coronary angioplasty and atherectomy (18,19). Importantly, the initial process is mediated by both circulating vWF and that which was released from activated platelets and endothelial cells. Furthermore, the high shear stress, which occurs in small blood vessels or in larger ones which are partially occluded, necessitates the presence of vWF for the occurrence of platelet adhesion (11,12,20,21). Thus, local accumulation of activated platelets forms an expansile mass of increasing physical size which continues to recruit additional platelets arriving in the microenvironment. Vessel occlusion eventually results. This is beneficial hemostatically, but harmful or even fatal in the setting of atherosclerotic blood vessels (22,23).

Exposed subendothelial collagen to which platelets adhere and spread is one of the strongest agonists for platelet activation (Table 1). Platelet–collagen contact initiates at least four physiologic responses: (a) The platelet release reaction is initiated: biologically active compounds originally stored in intracellular platelet granules are secreted into the fluid phase of the microenvironment. (b) P-selectin, a platelet granule glycoprotein of M_r 140,000, is translocated from granules to the platelet surface, where it mediates adhesion of activated platelets to neutrophils, monocytes, and subsets of lymphocytes. P-selectin belongs to the selectin family of adhesive proteins (24–30). (c) The platelet eicosanoid pathway is initiated, commencing with liberation of arachidonic acid (20:4) from platelet phospholipids by phospholipase(s) (31,32). Free 20:4 is immediately oxygenated to form the labile endoperoxides PGG_2 and PGH_2 (33,34). Simultaneously, 12-hydroxyheptadecatrienoic acid (HHTrE) and malondialdehyde (MDA) are formed. Then PGH_2 is rapidly transformed to thromboxane A_2, as catalyzed by thromboxane synthase (35). Functional implications of MDA and HHTrE are unknown. Cyclooxygenation of arachidonate, which is a prerequisite for formation of further metabolites as catalyzed by PGH synthase-1, is completely blocked by aspirin, which irreversibly acetylates the "active-site" serine residue at position 530 (36). The remainder of the free arachidonate is converted to 12-hydroxyeicosatetraenoic acid (12-HETE) by the aspirin-insensitive cytoplasmic platelet enzyme 12-lipoxygenase (37,38) or is reacylated into the platelet lipid pool. (d) Platelet activation is characterized by a drastic change in morphology from that of a smooth disk to a spiny sphere. This rearrangement of the platelet surface allows for more efficient platelet–platelet contact and adhesion. Shape change also promotes realignment of platelet membrane phospholipoprotein components in a manner which allows them to serve as a highly efficient catalytic procoagulant surface. This promotes firm binding between platelet phospholipoprotein (not phospholipid) and activated coagulation factor X in the presence of active factor V. Furthermore, the phospholipoprotein surface of activated platelets is stimulatory for activation of factor VII from the extrinsic coagulation system (Figs. 1–3).

The above interactions culminate in thrombin formation,

TABLE 1. *Subendothelial matrix proteins that support platelet adhesion*

Matrix constituent	Comment
Collagens	Large family of proteins with certain members supporting platelet adhesion, aggregation, and secretion
Von Willebrand factor	Large multimeric protein critical for the hemostatic function of platelets
Fibronectin	Dimeric or multimeric protein that supports attachment and spreading of platelets
Thrombospondin	Trimeric protein exhibiting both adhesive and antiadhesive properties
Laminin	A protein supporting platelet attachment but not spreading
Microfibrils	A fibular bundle of protein constituents found in certain matrices

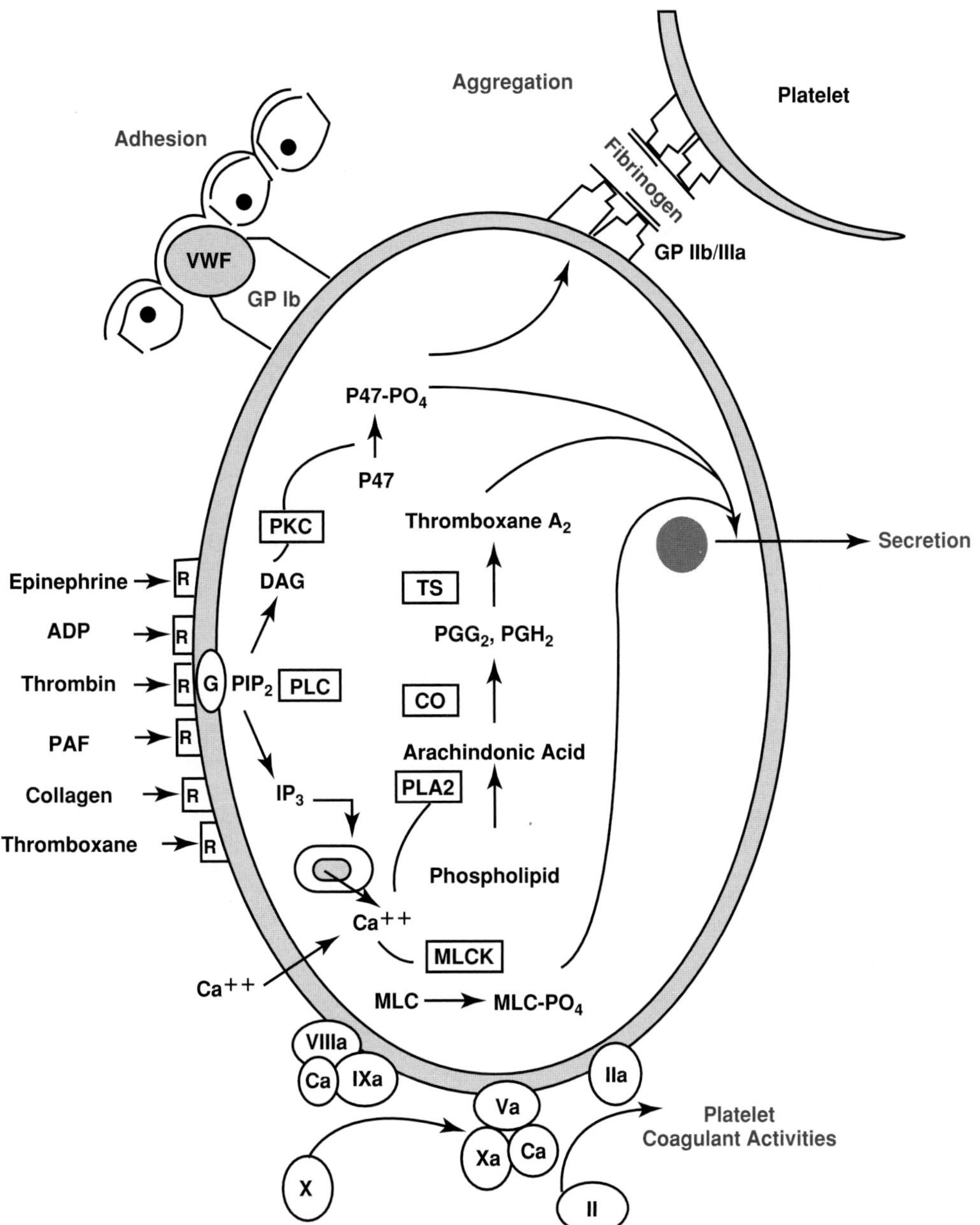

FIG. 1. Mechanisms of platelet activation. Adhesion of platelets to subendothelium beneath an area of injury is mediated by membrane glycoprotein Ib *(GPIb),* which binds von Willebrand factor *(vWF).* Cohesion of platelets into an aggregate is mediated by the glycoprotein IIb/IIIa complex *(GPIIb/IIIa),* which is linked by fibrinogen to GPIIb/IIIa on another platelet in proximity. Platelet agonists such as ADP, collagen, thromboxane, platelet-activating factor *(PAF),* and thrombin interact with specific receptors *(R)* and induce activation of phospholipase C via G proteins (the ADP receptor has not yet been isolated or characterized). Phospholipase C *(PLC)* catalyzes hydrolysis of phosphatidylinositol bis-phosphate *(PIP_2),* with formation of inositol trisphosphate *(IP_3),* which induces calcium *(Ca^{2+})* mobilization from the dense tubular system. Diacylglycerol *(DAG)* is also mobilized and serves to activate protein kinase C *(PKC),* which phosphorylates the cytoplasmic protein P47 (plekstrin). Increased levels of cytoplasmic Ca^{2+} promote phosphorylation of the myosin light chain *(MLC)* by the myosin light-chain kinase *(MLCK).* The Ca^{2+} will also activate phospholipase A_2 *(PLA_2),* which catalyzes release of arachidonic acid from membrane phospholipids. The arachidonate is oxygenated by cyclooxygenase *(CO)* to the transient intermediate endoperoxides PGG_2 and PGH_2, which are subsequently acted upon by thromboxane synthase *(TS)* with formation of thromboxane A_2. The activated platelet phospholipoprotein surface is a catalytic entity for critical enzymatic reactions in the coagulation cascade leading to thrombin formation. These include factor X activation as well as prothrombin (factor II) conversion to thrombin. (From ref. 39, courtesy of Dr. A. Koneti Rao).

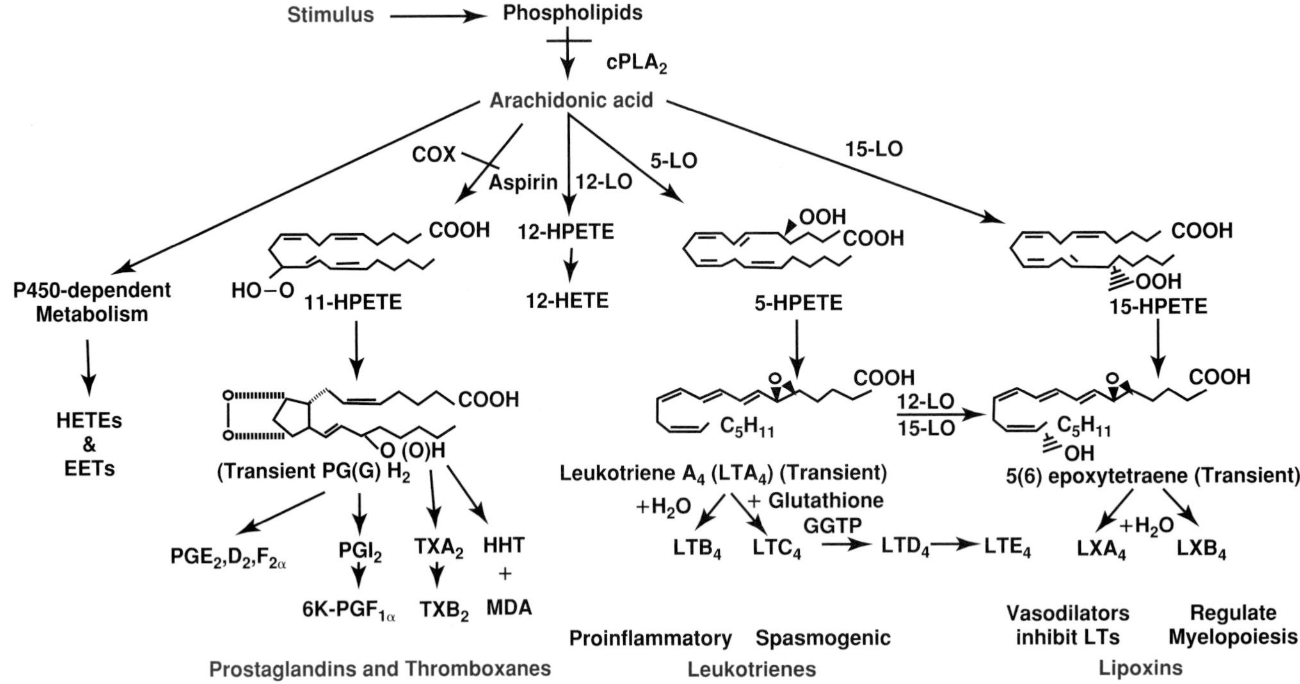

FIG. 2. Eicosanoid metabolism (54–56,62): the major classes and individual species of eicosanoids, including intermediates involved in their biosynthesis. In the pathway from arachidonate to thromboxane, two prostaglandin H *(PGH)* synthase (cyclooxygenase) *(COX)* isozymes have been described: PGH synthase-1 and -2. These isozymes have important functional implications for comprehension of the thrombotic and inflammatory responses (5,33,36,59,60). PGH synthase (a *bis*-oxygenase) catalyzes the insertion of two molecules of oxygen into arachidonate. One is inserted at carbon-11 and the other at carbon-15. Aspirin acetylates homologous serine residues of PGH synthase-1 and -2 (34). The acetyl group of aspirin blocks binding of arachidonate to the active site of PGH synthase (33,36). The transient endoperoxide intermediates *(PGG_2/PGH_2)* are common to several tissues, and therefore their metabolic fate depends upon the specific processing enzyme present in that tissue (thromboxane synthase, prostacyclin synthase). *HETE,* Hydroxyeicosatetraenoic acid; *HPETE,* hydroperoxyeicosatetraenoic acid; *PG,* prostaglandin; *TX,* thromboxane; *HHT,* 12-hydroxyheptadecatrienoic acid; *MDA,* malondialdehyde. **Right:** Reactions involving oxygenation of arachidonate as catalyzed by three cytosolic lipoxygenase *(LO)* enzymes, the 5-, 12-, and 15-lipoxygenases. In leukocytes, the lipoxygenase inserts molecular oxygen into the carbon-5 position (170). The 5-lipoxygenase is responsible for subsequent generation of leukotriene A_4 *(LTA_4)*, a 5,6-epoxide-containing intermediate which is quickly metabolized to leukotriene B_4, the most powerful proinflammatory eicosanoid yet described. In mast cells, basophils, or eosinophils, LTA_4 is conjugated with glutathione, culminating in production of leukotrienes C_4, D_4, and E_4. The latter are also known as the slow-reacting substances of anaphylaxis (SRS-A) (5,54,55,170). *GGTP,* gamma-Glutamyl transpeptidase. **Far right:** Lipoxins *(LX)* (55). These eicosanoids are generated by initial oxygenation at C-15 to form 15-HPETE. The latter is subsequently metabolized to a 5,6-epoxytetraene by 5-lipoxygenase (53,171–173). This 5,6-epoxytetraene or its equivalent can originate from leukotriene A_4 when it is acted upon by either the 12- or 15-lipoxygenase. Lipoxins are also generated during cell–cell interactions or by individual cell types. Lipoxins A_4 and B_4 can induce vasodilatation, inhibit leukotriene activity, and regulate myelopoiesis in the bone marrow (54,173). **Far left:** Metabolism of arachidonate by a cytochrome P-450-dependent enzyme system. In this reaction sequence, arachidonate is oxygenated at each major *cis*-pentadiene site. The cytochrome P-450 can also oxygenate arachidonate and insert alcohol groups with formation of epoxides which are nonallylic. The latter are more stable than leukotriene A_4 or the 5,6-epoxytetraene. The P-450 metabolites of arachidonate are involved in various types of metabolic activities in kidney, the vasculature, platelets, and bone marrow (174,175). *EET.* (Figure kindly provided by Dr. Charles N. Serhan.)

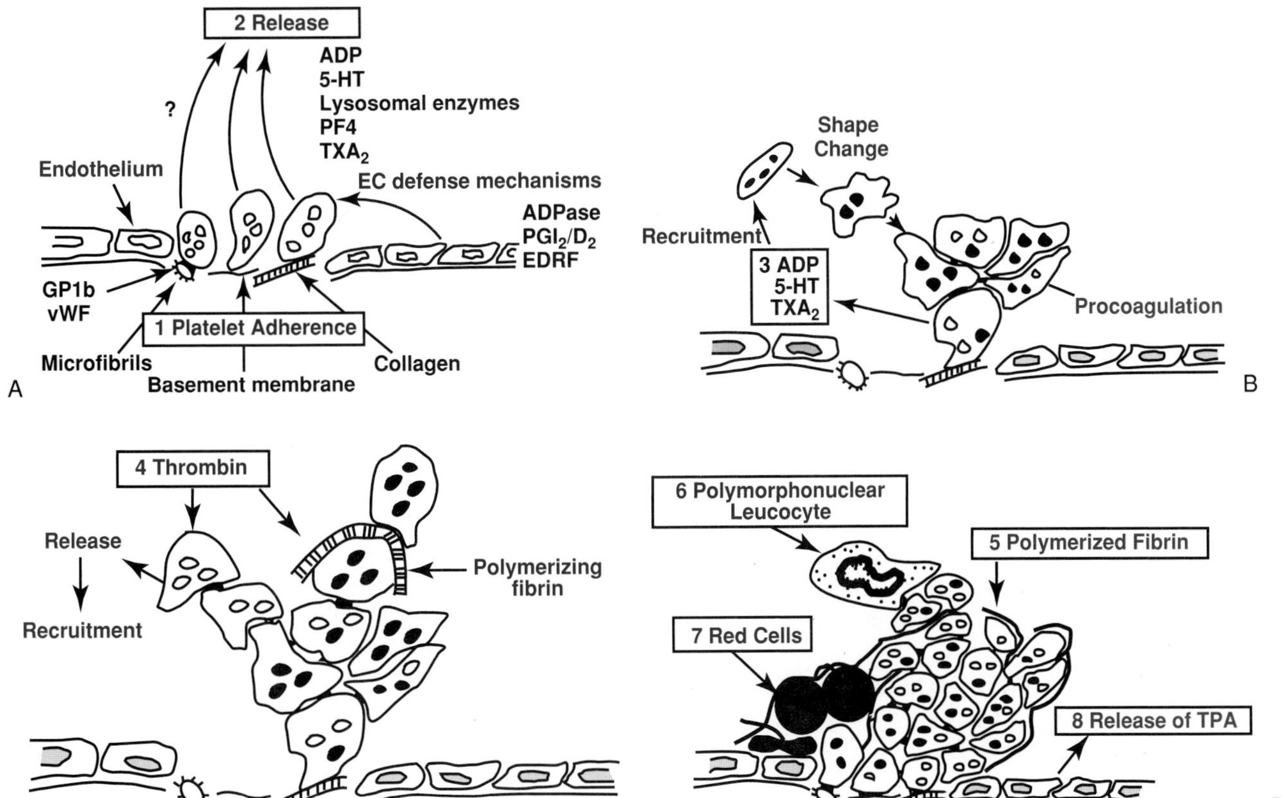

FIG. 3. Stepwise depiction of primary and secondary hemostasis (2,9). **A:** Subendothelial exposure due to vascular injury results in instantaneous platelet adherence to collagen, basement membrane, and microfibrils in the presence of von Willebrand factor *(vWF)* (especially at high shear) and platelet membrane glycoprotein Ib *(GPIb)*. Collagen, which is a major platelet agonist, induces release of ADP and serotonin *(5-HT)* from dense granules as well as several proteins from α-granules. The autacoid thromboxane A_2 *(TXA_2)* is enzymatically formed from arachidonate which has been released from phospholipids. In parallel, endothelial cell defense systems, thromboregulators, function to limit the size of the expanding thrombus. The fluid-phase platelet releasate initiates the recruitment phase of platelet thrombus formation. *PF4,* Platelet factor 4; *EDRF,* endothelium-derived relaxation factor. **B:** ADP, serotonin, and thromboxane are the most important recruiting agents in the platelet releasate. They serve as agonists for additional platelets arriving in the fluid phase. The recruited platelets in turn undergo shape change and aggregate onto the initial layer of activated platelets. Thromboxane and serotonin promote vasoconstriction, which also serves to limit the blood flow and increase cell–cell contact. Phospholipoproteins are now available on the activated platelet surface for catalytic assembly of proteins of the coagulation cascade. **C:** Thrombin formation has important consequences which culminate in the final stages of vascular occlusion. Thrombin promotes further platelet activation, release, and recruitment as well as initiating fibrin formation. Fibrin strands intercalate between activated platelets as the thrombus becomes consolidated (formerly termed "viscous metamorphosis"). Thrombin may also induce activation of intact endothelial cells adjacent to the site of injury. For example, there is increased expression of genes for the platelet-derived growth factor (PDGF), increased monocyte adhesion to endothelium and binding of neutrophils to the endothelial cell surface (66,71). **D:** At this stage, the consolidated platelet thrombus is impermeable and its multicellular composition alters its biochemical properties (6,9). Intact, metabolically viable erythrocytes at the site are prothrombotic in that they increase the reactivity of the releasate from activated platelets, an action which is virtually insensitive to aspirin (51). Neutrophils are also observed in close contact with platelets. The chemotactic activity of the aspirin-insensitive platelet lipoxygenase product 12-HETE may contribute to the arrival of neutrophils. Platelet–neutrophil contact is enhanced by the adhesive platelet glycoprotein P-selectin interacting with its receptor on the neutrophil surface (24,25,27,70). Neutrophils also downregulate reactivity of platelet releasates and these cells may serve an important antithrombotic function (72,176). As the platelet thrombus forms, an unknown signal initiates the fibrinolytic cascade, i.e., release of tissue plasminogen activator *(TPA)* from endothelial cells. (Adapted from Dr. J. F. Mustard with permission.)

which amplifies the initial activating effect of collagen. Platelet activation, release, and recruitment maximally reinforce each other, resulting in additional release, eicosanoid formation, and the appearance of fibrin strands, initially on the outer portion of the platelet thrombus, but also in the interstices between adherent platelets (Fig. 3). These intraplatelet fibrin strands are particularly difficult to ''reach'' therapeutically because of tight consolidation of the mass as induced by thrombin. This is especially true after fibrin has been cross-linked by platelet and plasma factor XIIIa. Finally, total occlusion of the vessel occurs, rendering the hemostatic plug completely impermeable. This postthrombin secondary ''consolidation phase'' completes the hemostatic process under ''physiologic'' circumstances. Unfortunately, this is the same mechanism for formation of thrombi overlying a fissured or ruptured atherosclerotic plaque. These events have been verified by pathologic studies at autopsy, results of thrombolytic therapy, and direct visualization of occlusive thrombi by angioscopy (8). Currently known platelet activation mechanisms are depicted in Fig. 1 (39).

ASPECTS OF PRIMARY HEMOSTASIS OF PERTINENCE TO OCCLUSIVE CARDIOVASCULAR EVENTS

The releasate emerging from activated platelets is responsible for the ''recruitment phase'' of thrombus formation. Several components of platelet releasates are fluid-phase agonists for unstimulated platelets arriving at the site of the developing thrombus. Collagen and thrombin are the principal inducers of platelet secretion, but adenosine diphosphate (ADP) is the most important agonist in the platelet releasate itself (9,40). ADP stimulates platelets directly, but release induced by ADP can only occur when platelets are in direct contact and in motion. Only then will platelets aggregate and form a cohesive mass. This can be verified in vitro by the demonstration that unstirred platelets are unresponsive to exogenously provided ADP unless there is motion and platelet-to-platelet contact (41). The platelet receptor for ADP has not been definitively identified or characterized (42–45). Enzymatic removal of ADP from activated platelet releasates will reverse the platelet aggregation process. As will be discussed, this phenomenon has therapeutic implications, since it can be accomplished prior to thrombin formation and platelet thrombus consolidation (9,46), thus minimizing the total occlusive response.

Released platelet constituents originate from specific intracellular granules, the dense granules. Serotonin (5-hydroxytryptamine, 5-HT), the platelet-derived vasoconstrictor, can also stimulate adrenergic nerve endings in blood vessels. Serotonin receptors are present in coronary arteries, stimulation of which results in vasoconstriction (22). Platelet dense granules are also the site of storage for ADP and calcium. On the other hand, adhesive proteins, such as fibrinogen, fibronectin, vWF, thrombospondin, and vitronectin, are stored in platelet α-granules. The α-granules also contain growth-promoting proteins such as the platelet-derived growth factor (PDGF), transforming growth factor-β (TGF-β), and platelet factor 4 (PF-4) (39,47,48).

Alpha-granules are also the site of coagulation factors. These include factor V, high-molecular-weight kininogen (HMWK), factor XI, protein S, and plasminogen activator inhibitor-1 (PAI-1). Albumin and immunoglobulin G (IgG) are also present. Alpha-granule components are released at lower concentrations of agonists than those required for release of dense-body constituents (16,49).

Recruiting properties of platelet releasates are attributable mainly to ADP and thromboxane A_2. Serotonin may also play a role, possibly in synergy with the latter two components. Importantly, recruitment results in further activation, enhancement of aggregation, and augmentation of the thrombotic process as an occlusive entity. This unfortunately can result in abrupt vessel closure or restenosis of a coronary artery lesion following angioplasty or atherectomy (7,19).

Platelet activation induces structural alterations in platelet glycoproteins IIb/IIIa resulting in a heterodimer complex which expresses fibrinogen receptor activity. The precise biochemical mechanism for this transformation is not known (50). ADP induces exposure of fibrinogen-binding sites on the platelet surface. These serve as cohesive forces between platelets as the thrombus accumulates. Single fibrinogen molecules, which have a dimeric structure, form a ''bridge'' between two GPIIb/IIIa molecules on platelets in proximity. As these reactions proceed toward thrombin formation, the platelet plug becomes consolidated and impermeable. Steps involved in the formation of hemostatic and/or thrombotic platelet plugs are depicted in Fig. 3. As shown in the figure, intact erythrocytes arriving at the site of injury respond to the presence of platelet releasates by increasing production of platelet prothrombotic substances, including free arachidonate and eicosanoids (51,52). Promotion of platelet reactivity by intact erythrocytes may explain the prothrombotic tendency in patients with erythrocytoses due to various causes. This erythrocyte enhancement may also explain why the bleeding time is prolonged in anemic patients but corrected after transfusion. Cell–cell interactions between platelets and erythrocytes are best demonstrated in a system which measures platelet activation and recruitment separately, using cell releasates as agonists (51).

The information cited above would suggest that repeated episodes of or continuing low-level platelet activation may lead to an atheromatous response at specific locations in the vasculature. However, this is a hypothesis which remains to be proven by more definitive tests of platelet activation and its detection in vivo.

ISOFORMS OF CYCLOOXYGENASE (COX-1/PGHS-1 AND COX-2/PGHS-2)

Significance for Aspirin Therapy

As already mentioned, stimulation of platelets with strong agonists results in liberation of arachidonate, which then is enzymatically oxygenated and transformed into biologically important metabolites known as eicosanoids (Fig. 2) (53–55). In platelets, free arachidonate is oxygenated by a particulate cyclooxygenase and a cytoplasmic lipoxygenase. Cyclooxygenation of arachidonate results in formation of transient intermediates—endoxperoxides PGG_2, PGH_2. These are processed by thromboxane synthase to thromboxane A_2 (35,41,56). Thromboxane A_2 is released into the fluid phase, where it induces platelet aggregation, phosphoinositide hydrolysis, protein phosphorylation, and elevation of cytosolic free calcium. Thromboxane does not penetrate cells, but interacts with specific receptor(s) on cell surfaces. These receptors are coupled to adenylyl cyclase via a G_q protein (44,57). Induction of calcium mobilization in platelets by thromboxane A_2 is thought to involve inhibition of adenylyl cyclase, which reduces platelet cyclic adenosine monophosphate (cAMP) (58). Levels of free intracellular calcium in platelets are the final determinant of platelet activation. Novel developments have taken place with regard to the cyclooxygenation step.

PGHS-1 and PGHS-2 (Cox-1 and Cox-2)

An important new development in biochemistry of eicosanoids is the discovery of a second isoform of the cyclooxygenase enzyme (33,34,59–62). The terminology currently in use is PGHS-1 and PGHS-2 (Cox-1 and Cox-2) (63). Both proteins are similar in length, with 604 and 602 amino acids, respectively. The mRNA coding for PGHS-2 is longer than that for PGHS-1, and PGHS-1 contains nucleotide sequences which destabilize the mRNA, thereby promoting degradation. This property is characteristic of early intermediate genes which usually encode transcription factors early in cascade pathways. Expression of the PGHS-2 gene was first demonstrated in fibroblasts, but its induction has been found in macrophages, neurons, bronchial epithelial cells, intestinal epithelial cells, and mast cells. Importantly, PGHS-2 is induced by proinflammatory agonists such as interleukin-1 (IL-1) and tumor necrosis factor. In the absence of serum, cells such as fibroblasts only express PGHS-1, whereas in the presence of serum, cells will express both PGHS-1 and PGHS-2. Glucocorticoids inhibit PGHS-2 synthesis in vitro and in vivo. When PGHS-2 is treated with aspirin, its metabolic product profile is altered: Although formation of PGH_2 is blocked, oxygenation of the 15 position and peroxidase activity persist, resulting in metabolism of arachidonate to 15-hydroxyeicosatetraenoic acid (15-HETE) (33,34). The discovery of PGHS-2 is of particular significance for the inflammatory process. PGHS-2 may be responsible for the proinflammatory effects of eicosanoids, whereas PGHS-1, which is constitutive, leads to production of eicosanoids such as prostacyclin, which has antithrombotic properties and is cytoprotective for gastric mucosa. It is therefore possible that the antiinflammatory effects of aspirin and comparable nonsteroidal inflammatory drugs are due to inhibition of PGHS-2, with the direct toxic effects of aspirin such as gastric irritation being due to inhibition of PGHS-1. Thus, development of selective inhibitors for PGHS-2 may result in a major therapeutic advantage since they do not cause gastric irritation and other side effects (61,62).

SECONDARY HEMOSTASIS: THE PHASE OF CONSOLIDATION

Primary hemostasis represents the interaction between platelets and the vessel wall with formation of a platelet-rich plug. Secondary hemostasis is characterized by formation of an impermeable, consolidated platelet aggregate which has been interlaced and surrounded by a fibrin network induced by the coagulation cascade (Fig. 3). Thrombin formation during secondary hemostasis promotes transformation of fibrinogen to fibrin, thereby conferring permanence to the platelet thrombus. During hemostasis, wherein an interruption in continuity of a normal vessel leads to formation of a hemostatic plug, the entire lumen of the vessel may not be occluded, and the plug may be permeable because thrombin formation may have been less vigorous. In contrast, a thrombus in a coronary artery is induced by a much stronger agonistic force, i.e., the ruptured atherosclerotic plaque at a site of disturbed flow and stenosis (64,65). This gives rise to more thrombin formation, leading to total vessel occlusion and ischemia. These events can also be directly related to reocclusive phenomena occurring after bypass surgery, angioplasty, and endarterectomy (19,64). These concepts can be corroborated by events occurring in clinical disorders of coagulation. For example, in factor VIII or IX deficiency, thrombin formation is markedly reduced and the platelet plug alone cannot sustain hemostasis over a period of time. This gives rise to the "rebleeding" phenomenon so characteristic of patients with defects in the intrinsic coagulation system when a bleeding time is performed for diagnostic purposes, or after surgical procedures, where the diagnosis is not known (8).

As primary hemostasis merges into the second phase, rearranged and reoriented phospholipoprotein on the activated platelet surface catalyzes activation of factor X and prothrombin conversion to thrombin in the presence of factors V and VIII. Thrombin also forms at the site of injury via activation of factor X in the presence of tissue factor and factor VII. As mentioned, the local appearance of thrombin is a critical event because it further amplifies initial reactions initiated by subendothelial collagen (66). Thrombin formation induces a shift in platelet reactivity from adhesion and spreading on the vessel wall as mediated by GPIb–vWF to mechanisms mediated by GPIIb/IIIa which modulate further platelet aggregation and recruitment (17,67).

To summarize: We have discussed primary and secondary hemostasis as it occurs on injured normal or relatively normal vessel surfaces (Fig. 3). In prothrombotic states, the process is initiated by mechanisms which have a much

TABLE 2. *Effects of thrombin on endothelial cells*

Eicosanoid synthesis and release
Synthesis and release of endothelium-dependent relaxing factor (EDRF/NO)
Secretion of von Willebrand factor
Gene and protein expression of tissue factor
Binding of thrombomodulin and activation of protein C
Tissue plasminogen activator and plasminogen-inhibitor-1 (tPA and PAI-1) gene expression and secretion
Release of adenine nucleotides
Neutrophil adhesion via increased P-selectin expression
Synthesis of platelet-activating factor (PAF)
Expression of the platelet-derived growth factor (PDGF) genes
Stimulation of monocyte adhesion

stronger agonistic potential (1,64,68). In atherosclerosis, ruptured or fissured atherosclerotic plaques in regions of disturbed blood flow have a high degree of thrombogenic capacity (64). Furthermore, in stenotic vessels, the shear rate is higher and possibilities for forming mural thrombi due to platelet and fibrin deposition are much greater (69). This explains why arterial thrombosis has been so difficult to prevent and treat (5,70).

Superimposed upon its role as ''keystone of the hemostatic arch,'' thrombin has a broad spectrum of prothrombotic functions, as defined in vitro. Thrombin is chemotactic for monocytes and mitogenic for lymphocytes and vascular smooth muscle cells (3,4,71). Thrombin has also been found to have marked pleiotropic effects on vascular endothelium (71,72). This includes eicosanoid production (73), nitric oxide synthesis (74), vWF secretion, tissue factor expression, and other important responses, as shown in Table 2. The cell–cell interactions induced by thrombin are depicted in Fig. 4 (66,75–77).

THE BLOOD PLATELET

Although sometimes referred to as cells, platelets are actually anuclear fragments derived from bone marrow megakaryocytes. Fragmentation probably occurs via extension of cytoplasmic processes (proplatelets released between endothelial cells in marrow sinuses) (78,79). It has always been assumed hypothetically that there was a hormone or regulatory substance which controlled maturation of stem cells in the marrow to megakaryocytes and subsequently platelet production therefrom. There have been reports of a substance circulating in the plasma of patients with thrombocytopenia which would increase platelet quantities following injection into experimental animals (80). The locution ''thrombopoietin'' was used for such a factor. Newly discovered cytokines were usually tested for their capacity as agonists for megakaryocyte maturation, but their action was slow and side effects were noted.

Very recently, cDNAs for a putative thrombopoietin of

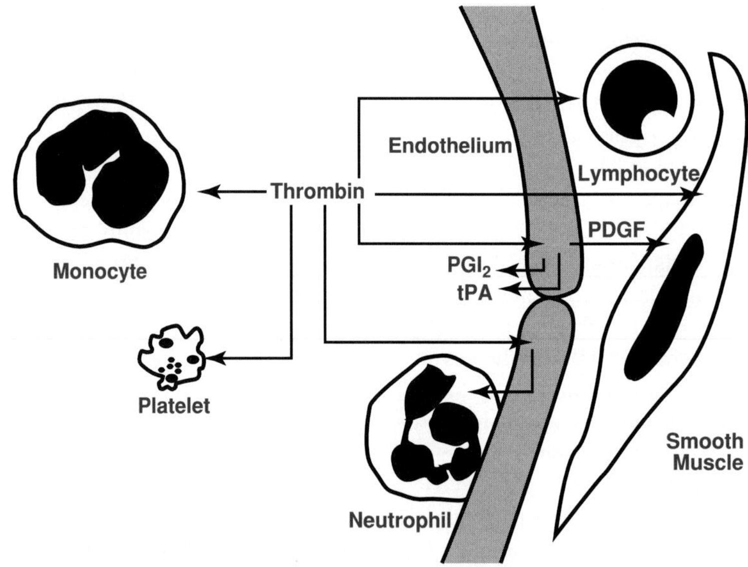

FIG. 4. Composite diagram illustrating putative actions of thrombin as an agonist for various cell types (75). Although it is well recognized that thrombin is the major agonist for platelet activation and recruitment, additional properties of this serine protease continue to be appreciated (31,76,77,116,177). Thrombin induces monocyte chemotactic activity and appears to be mitogenic for lymphocytes and mesenchymal cells. Other functions include induction of eicosanoid metabolism and stimulation of P-selectin activity in endothelial cells. Thrombin initiates release of the smooth muscle cell mitogen platelet-derived growth factor *(PDGF)* from platelets and endothelial cells (3,4). Our comprehension of thrombin action now requires a more global view, which includes participation in hemostasis, thrombosis, the inflammatory response, and proliferative repair mechanisms for vascular injury (66). (From Dr. Shaun R. Coughlin with permission.)

human and murine origin have been cloned and found to encode a glycoprotein with specific activity with regard to megakaryocyte proliferation in vitro. Also, recombinant thrombopoietin can increase platelet quantities in mice and also plays a role in reversing thrombocytopenia. Thrombopoietin was discovered during the observation that a virus capable of inducing a myeloproliferative neoplastic disorder in mice transduced a cellular gene (c-*mpl*), a gene which was homologous to genes encoding a family of hematopoietic growth factor receptors. It was postulated that autonomous transformation of cells by c-*mpl* might activate this hematopoietic growth factor receptor constitutively (81). Using c-*mpl* antisense oligonucleotides, it could be shown that megakaryocyte colony formation, but not other stem-cell colony formation, was inhibited in vitro. Cell lines were generated to express the c-*mpl* receptor, which was then used to identify and clone the c-*mpl* ligand. Porcine plasma from irradiated animals was exposed to c-*mpl* affinity columns. In this way, a porcine genomic clone was obtained and sequenced. A human genomic c-*mpl* ligand clone was produced using the polymerase chain reaction and porcine-based oligonucleotides. A cDNA clone was then isolated from a human fetal liver library. This recombinant c-*mpl* ligand increased platelet levels following injection into animals. In another approach, clones of autonomous mutants of cells expressing c-*mpl* were studied and one was identified wherein transformation was based on c-*mpl* ligand production. A clone was indeed found which was producing c-*mpl* ligand. cDNA libraries were developed from this line and a cDNA for murine c-*mpl* ligand was isolated. The protein could increase platelet levels in mice and stimulate megakaryocyte formation—especially in combination with other growth factors. Thus, c-*mpl* ligand is a thrombopoietin. Northern blotting studies implicate the liver and kidney as principal production sites. The thrombopoietin appears capable of increasing platelet counts (in animals) to levels which have never been obtained before (80,82–85).

Platelets circulate for approximately 10 days at a concentration range of 150,000–440,000/μl. Normal platelets have a diameter of 3.6 $\pm$ 0.7 μm and are 0.9 $\pm$ 0.3 μm in thickness. Platelet volume is 7.06 $\pm$ 4.85 fl. The mean platelet volume (MPV) increases whenever there is a demand for increased thrombopoiesis. This can be directly related to expansion of megakaryocyte size. The MPV is believed to decrease with platelet age, although this is controversial (78). The density of platelets is constant, with a variation of less than 5% in different individuals. A major determinant of platelet density is the platelet α-granule. Seventy percent of platelets are in the circulation and 30% are in the spleen. On a stained blood smear, each oil-immersion field contains approximately 3–10 platelets. Details of platelet morphology are depicted in Fig. 5.

It was initially thought that all platelet α-granule constituents were synthesized in megakaryocytes. This is true for most, but megakaryocytes do endocytose proteins such as fibrinogen, albumin, and IgG from plasma (78,79).

In contrast to other cells, platelets seen to demonstrate a somewhat uncomplicated morphologic appearance. However, this anucleate cell fragment is a very complex functional entity (8,9,86). The unstimulated platelet circulates in a passive manner as a smooth disk, but most, of necessity, possess mechanisms for recognition of injury sites to which it adheres, spreads, and undergoes activation (11,16). Unfortunately, this recognition phenomenon lacks specificity because atheromatous plaques which are fissured or undergoing hemorrhage provide the same message to circulating platelets as do normal vessels which have been traumatized or severed (22,65). Thus, the platelet will adhere, become activated, aggregate, and recruit with formation of a fibrin-platelet thrombus. This, of course, can culminate in coronary or cerebral ischemia. Platelets may possess a regulatory substance for their production, which they release at the end of their lifespan. This putative factor may also be present in the endothelial cell, being released when endothelium "senses" the presence of low quantities of functional platelets. At that point, thrombopoiesis might be enhanced (78). Perhaps this is part of a signal for thrombopoietin production (80,83). In response to mechanical or chemical injury or a roughened, fissured atherosclerotic plaque, platelets rapidly undergo intricate biochemical and physical rearrangements for participating in hemostasis and in host defense systems in general (6,56,66).

In addition to responding to injury, platelets appear to be responsible for maintenance of vascular integrity in the absence of injury and as a protective mechanism against spontaneous hemorrhage. This critical platelet function is poorly understood and controversial. Evidence for such an entity may be summarized as follows: Thrombocytopenia of rapid onset is associated with spontaneous hemorrhage into the skin and mucous membranes. We think of this as due to loss of integrity at the level of vascular endothelium. There is evidence derived from thrombocytopenic animals wherein labeled platelets were adherent to and incorporated into endothelial cells. This phenomenon has rarely been visualized in an experimental setting and it is still postulated that senescent platelets are removed by reticuloendothelial cells in the spleen and liver (78). This is also relevant to the long-standing question of whether platelets are actually deposited in atherosclerotic plaques. This recalls reports in the literature that thrombocytopenia is protective against atherosclerosis (71).

It is well known clinically that patients with chronic thrombocytopenias due to various etiologies develop an ill-defined compensatory mechanism for the absence of "vascular integrity factor(s)." Chronically thrombocytopenic patients rarely bleed spontaneously. Administration of platelet concentrates corrects thrombocytopenic hemorrhage, but frozen and thawed platelets have no such effect. Therefore, factor(s) responsible for maintenance of vascular integrity by platelets are linked to platelet viability. Identification and characterization of a platelet "vascular integrity factor" might eliminate the need for platelet transfusions—which

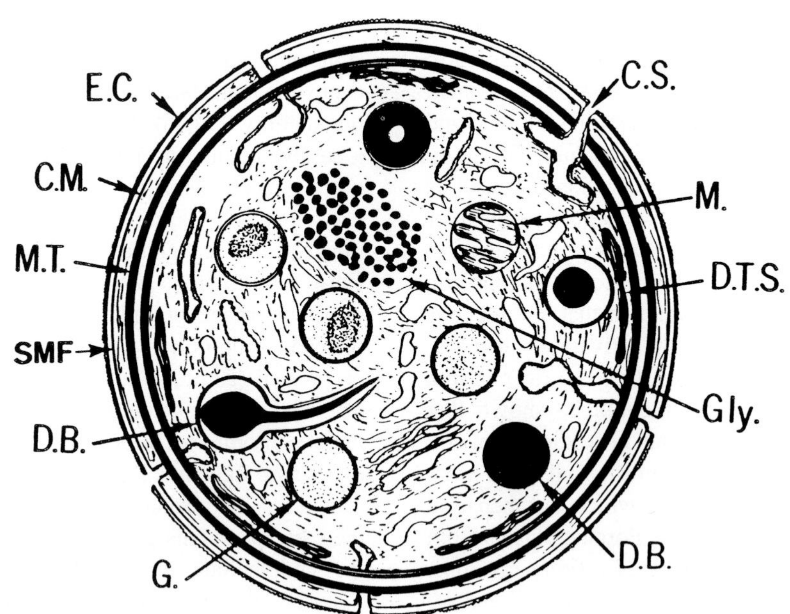

FIG. 5. Platelet ultrastructure as demonstrated in the equatorial plane (178). On the exterior surface of the plasma membrane there is a peripheral zone containing glycoprotein-rich material which is synonymous with glycocalyx *(EC)*. The glycocalyx contains receptors for platelet agonists and inhibitors. Signal transduction mechanisms are thought to originate here. The platelet cell membrane *(CM)* is a classic lipid bilayer, but it is unique in its ability to undergo phospholipoprotein rearrangement in response to activating agents. This rearrangement is responsible for the ability of platelets to bind activated coagulation factors. The cell membrane and submembrane filament area *(SMF)* are characterized by specific invaginations which constitute the lining of channels of the surface-connected open canalicular system *(CS)*. The submembrane filaments are actually the actin filaments of the membrane cytoskeleton. These filaments also form parallel structures which become filopodia when platelets are activated. The circumferential microtubule system *(MT)* also represents the cytoskeleton and is responsible for maintenance of the disk shape of unstimulated platelets. The platelet cytoplasm (sol–gel zone) contains microfilaments, submembrane filaments, the circumferential band of microtubules, and glycogen *(Gly)*. Other formed elements in the sol–gel zone include mitochondria *(M)* and dense bodies *(DB)*, which represent storage sites for ADP, 5-HT, and calcium. In addition to dense bodies, platelet granules are of two types: one is lysosomal and the others (α-granules) *(G)* contain adhesive proteins, some of which are secreted into the fluid phase upon activation (fibrinogen, von Willebrand factor, thrombospondin, and fibronectin). P-selectin translocates to the platelet surface following activation (131), and recently a soluble form has been reported (179). Also present are platelet factor 4, β-thromboglobulin, and platelet-derived growth factor (PDGF) (3,126,127). The dense tubular system *(DTS)* and surface-connected canalicular system are membrane systems within the platelet that represent counterparts of sarcoplasmic reticulum in other cells. (From White, ref. 181, with permission.)

would be a major advance. As the new information on thrombopoietin is brought to clinical fruition, we should have a modality for promoting megakaryocyte maturation and platelet production (80). However, when there is marrow aplasia due to chemotherapy or other toxicities, there are no megakaryocytic stem cells to be stimulated. Thus, if there is indeed a platelet "vascular integrity factor," it would have definite clinical utility.

COAGULATION AND CLOT RETRACTION

Activated platelets strongly promote activity of the intrinsic coagulation system. This was formerly termed "platelet factor 3." As mentioned, the rearranged, activated phospholipoprotein component of the platelet membrane provides the catalytic site for assembly of the "tenase" and "prothrombinase" complexes which activate factor X and prothrombin. The "tenase" and "prothrombinase" complexes can be assembled in vitro on phospholipid vesicles containing anionic phospholipids (87). However, the plasma membrane of the platelet does not contain significant quantities of anionic phospholipid on its outer leaflet (88). Thus, platelet agonists such as thrombin or collagen actually reorient the membrane phospholipoprotein so that anionic phospholipids are thereby exposed. Isolated platelet membranes, on a quantitative basis, contain 20 times more procoagulant activity than that inducible by phospholipid vesicles (89). The efficiency of such membrane procoagulant activity is attested to by the fact that clinical deficiencies in platelet procoagulant activity are extremely rare. It is also important to remember that phospholipid vesicles or subcellular fractions prepared from platelets have no effect whatsoever on the arrest of bleeding.

Another important platelet function is mediation of clot retraction. This phenomenon can be observed in vivo and in vitro (32,79). Clot retraction in vitro requires glucose, ATP, and a strongly consolidated clot resulting from thrombin formation. Retraction of the clot is mediated through an interaction between platelet glycoproteins GPIIb/IIIa and actin in the cytoskeleton. The ATPase activity of myosin acts on actin filaments. The latter are attached to glycoproteins IIb/IIIa in platelet filopodia which in turn have been linked to fibrin strands in the clot. Talin and vinculin, proteins in the cytoskeleton, have also been implicated in clot retraction. Clot retraction is defective in thrombocytopenia and may be absent in thromboasthenia. A retracted clot is a highly permanent structure. Among the goals of fibrinolytic therapy is liquefaction of retracted clots in vivo (90).

THE PLATELET GLYCOPROTEINS

Functional and therapeutic concepts of platelet reactivity were revolutionized by the ability to separate and identify solubilized platelet proteins electrophoretically on polyacrylamide gels (91). For reasons which are unclear, platelet disruption followed by centrifugation of the homogenate results in a pellet which can be studied as if it were a purified membrane preparation. Nomenclature of platelet glycoproteins is based on electrophoretic mobility, with proteins of higher molecular weight demonstrating lower mobility. However, new nomenclature systems are now necessary because proteins identical to those in platelets have been found in other cell types. Other designations include VLA (very late antigens), ECM (extracellular matrix), and CD (clusters of differentiation). Adhesive proteins such as collagen, fibrinogen, and vWF, are ligands for cell-surface receptors. Several adhesive proteins on the platelet membrane belong to the integrin supergene family of adhesive receptors (8,16, 92,94) (Tables 3–5).

TABLE 3. *Adhesive protein receptors on platelets*

Ligand	Receptor(s)	Additional designations
Collagen	GPIa–IIa	VLA-2, $\alpha_2\beta_1$
	GPIIb–IIIa	$\alpha_P\beta_3$
	GPIV	GPIIIb
Fibrinogen	GPIIb–IIIa	$\alpha IIb\beta_3$
Fibronectin	GPIc–IIa	VLA-5, $\alpha_5\beta_1$
	GPIIb–IIIa	$\alpha IIb\beta_3$
Thrombospondin	Vitronectin receptor	$\alpha_V\beta_3$
	GPIV	GPIIIb
Vitronectin	Vitronectin receptor	$\alpha_V\beta_3$
	GPIIb–IIIa	$\alpha IIb\beta_3$
Von Willebrand factor	GPIb–IX	
	GPIIb–IIIa	$\alpha IIb\beta_3$
Laminin	GPIc–IIa region	VLA-6, $\alpha_6\beta_1$

GP, Glycoprotein; VLA, very late antigen.

TABLE 4. *Platelet integrin family*

Integrin	Ligand
GPIa–IIa (VLA-2, $\alpha_2\beta_1$)	Collagen
GPIc–IIa (VLA-5, $\alpha_5\beta_1$)	Fibronectin
GPIIb–IIIa ($\alpha IIb\beta_3$)	Fibrinogen, fibronectin, vitronectin, von Willebrand factor
Vitronectin receptor ($v_2\beta_3$)	—
VLA-6 ($\alpha_6\beta_1$) (mobility similar to that of GPIc–IIa)	Laminin

Platelet Glycoprotein IB

Glycoprotein Ib (GPIb or GPIb–IX) is mainly responsible for the negative surface charge of platelets. This is because GPIb is rich in sialic acid and carbohydrate. There are two disulfide-linked subunits in GPIb (GPIbα, 143 kDa; and GPIbβ, 22 kDa). Glycoprotein Ib is a heterodimer, but is not part of the integrin family of adhesive protein receptors in platelets (16). There are approximately 25,000 molecules of GPIb per platelet. The fact that the α and β chains react with carbohydrate stains suggests that they are located on the outer surface of the platelet membrane. A large segment of the GPIb α chain is located outside the lipid bilayer. This is known as glycocalicin and was originally identified as a proteolytic fragment of GPIbα (94). Glycocalicin is often lost during platelet subcellular fractionation procedures. The proteolysis is probably due to a calcium-dependent platelet protease. Glycocalicin is important for thrombosis because it comprises the main part of the binding site for vWF during platelet adhesion to subendothelium. Interestingly, the carbohydrate portion of GPIb is analogous to the erythrocyte membrane glycoprotein' glycophorin A, the site of expression of MN blood groups. During thrombotic events, the GPIb–IX complex is a receptor for vWF. The vWF also contains functional domains which bind GPIb as well as collagen and microfibrils. Adherence of platelets to subendothelium is therefore mediated in an important way by vWF which adsorbs to subendothelium during thrombotic events (12).

Ristocetin is an antibiotic no longer used because it induces thrombocytopenia. Subsequently, it was learned that this antibiotic promotes platelet agglutination (not aggregation) in the presence of normal concentrations of plasma vWF. Unless ristocetin is present, no interaction will occur between vWF and GPIb on platelets. An interesting unanswered question is whether there is an "in vivo ristocetin" counterpart in human plasma. The ability of vWF to interact with GPIb is known as its ristocetin cofactor activity. In the serious clinical disorder Bernard–Soulier syndrome, GPIb–IX is congenitally absent from platelets. Thus, in vitro vWF cannot bind to Bernard–Soulier platelets, even when ristocetin is added to the patient's platelet-rich plasma. Platelets from the patients do not agglutinate, although plasma levels of vWF are normal.

TABLE 5. *The integrin supergene family of adhesion receptors*

Classification and synonyms				Ligand specificity	Tissue distribution
β_1	VLA_β	α_1	VLA1, CD49a	Ln, Fn, coll	Ws
	Platelet GPIIa	α_2	$VLA2_\alpha$, platelet GPIa, CD49b	Coll, LN	Ws (including platelets)
		α_3	$VLA3_\alpha$, CD49c	Fn, Ln, Coll, epiligrin	Ws
		α_4	$VLA4_\alpha$, CD49d	Fn, VCAM-1	Leukocytes, neural crest
		α_5	$VLA5_\alpha$, platelet GPIc, CD49e	Fn	Ws (including platelets)
		α_6	$VLA6_\alpha$, platelet GPIc′, CD49f	Ln	Ws (including platelets)
		α_7	$VLA7_\alpha$	Ln	Epithelial cells
		α_8	$VLA8_\alpha$	?	Epithelial cells, neurons
		α_9	α_A	?	Epithelial cells
		α_V	CD51	Vn, Fn	Epithelial cells
β_2	LFA-I_β	α_L	LFA-1_α, CD11a	ICAM-1, ICAM-2	Leukocytes
	MAC-I_β	α_M	MAC-1_α, CD11b	C3bi, Fb, factor X, ICAM-1	Leukocytes
	p150, 95_β	α_X	p150, 95_α, CD11c	C3bi, Fb	Leukocytes
	CD18				
β_3	Platelet GPIIIa	α_{IIb}	Platelet GPIIb, CD41	Fb, Fn, Vn, vWf, TSP	Platelets
	VNR_β	α_V	VnR, CD51	Fb, Vn, vWf, Fn, Coll, TSP, osteopontin	Ws (endothelial cells, platelets)
	CD61				
β_4	CD104	α_6	Epithelioid cell receptor, CD49f	Ln	Epithelial cells
β_7		α_4	Lymphocyte receptor, CD49d	Fn, VCAM-1	Leukocytes
		α_E			Epithelial cells
β_5		α_V	Carcinoma cell receptor, CD51	Vn	Carcinoma cells
β_6		α_V	CD51	Fn	Epithelial cells, carcinoma cells
β_8		α_V	CD51	—	—

Coll, collagen; Fb, fibrinogen; Fn, fibronectin; ICAM, intracellular adhesion molecule; Ln, laminin; TSP, thrombospondin; Vn, vitronectin; vWf, von Willebrand factor; VCAM, vascular cell adhesion molecule; VLA, very late activation (antigen); VnR, vitronectin receptor; Ws, widespread.

Mild proteolysis in vitro removes GPIb from the platelet surface. Thus, addition of ristocetin will no longer result in vWF binding. This indicates that the terminal portion of the GPIb α chain is the actual vWF receptor. The GPIX portion of the complex is a single polypeptide with a molecular weight of 20 kDa. How GPIb contributes to the function of the entire complex is not known (17,95). Using cDNA cloning procedures, the primary structures of GPIb and GPIX have been elucidated (13). A leucine-rich motif constitutes the main structural component of the GPIb–IX–V complex. This component is required for platelet participation in hemostasis and thrombosis (13,15,96,97). Glycoprotein Ib can act as a thrombin receptor and has also been identified as a target site for drug-induced platelet antibodies. The immune complex receptor is located in proximity to GPIb on the platelet membrane. Recently, high-affinity α-thrombin binding to platelet glycoprotein Ibα has been demonstrated (94). The glycoprotein Ibα binding site was of high affinity, whereas the seven-transmembrane-domain site was of moderate affinity. Thrombin-induced platelet activation may be initiated at the GPIb site and this information serves to amplify our concepts of the thrombin receptor as originally described (75,98).

In summary, the platelet GPIb–IX complex belongs to a family of leucine-rich glycoproteins and serves as receptor for vWF. The complex has four different subunits (GPIbα, GPIbβ, GPIX, and GPV) and links the plasma membrane with the cytoskeleton. The GPIb–IX complex is functionally defective in the Bernard–Soulier syndrome, resulting in the inability of the patients' platelets to bind vWF and adhere to subendothelium. This gives rise to a severe bleeding disorder, characterized by thrombocytopenia, "giant" platelets, and mucocutaneous bleeding. The disorder is inherited as an autosomal recessive trait. Normal expression of GPIb–IX on the plasma membrane requires synthesis and assembly of all subunits of the complex. Genetic mutations in the GPIb–IX complex have recently been summarized (99).

THE PLATELET GLYCOPROTEIN IIB/IIIA COMPLEX: BIOCHEMICAL PROPERTIES AND THERAPEUTIC IMPLICATIONS

Platelet glycoprotein IIb/IIIa (GPIIb/IIIa) is heterodimeric, and accounts for 2% of total platelet protein. The complex belongs to the integrin superfamily of adhesion receptors (Tables 3–5). The integrin designation of this transmembrane protein complex is $\alpha IIb\beta_3$. Interestingly, the

α subunit (αIIb or GPIIb) and the β subunit (β_3 or GPIIIa) are products of separate genes. The surface of resting platelets contains approximately 80,000 $\alpha IIb\beta_3$ complexes and there are also GPIIb/IIIa complexes on the membranes of platelet α-granules. Additional complexes are located in the open canalicular system, which extends to the platelet plasma membrane (Fig. 5). This distribution suggests that additional GPIIb/IIIa complexes appear on the surface of platelets following agonist exposure. This is probably important for the evolution of a thrombus.

The heavy chain of GPIIb (125 kDa) is disulfide-linked to the light chain (22 kDa). The heavy chain contains four repeating segments which bind calcium and are externally oriented. These segments bear homology to calcium-binding segments of calmodulin. The light chain of GPIIb contains a 91-amino acid-containing extracellular domain, a 26-amino acid transmembrane domain, and a 20-amino acid-containing carboxy-terminal cytoplasmic tail.

The GPIIIa portion of the complex is a single-chain protein (95 kDa) with a 29-amino acid transmembrane portion and a 41-amino acid carboxy-terminal cytoplasmic tail. The extracellular domain contains 56 disulfide-linked cysteine residues (100,101). The $\alpha IIb\beta_3$ complex will dissociate and lose function if calcium is removed by chelation. The platelet alloantigen Bak^a is localized to GPIIb and the alloantigen known as PI^{A1} has been localized to GPIIIa (102).

The GPIIb/IIIa complex functions as a receptor only after platelet activation. Under those conditions the complex will bind its major adhesive ligand, fibrinogen, as well as vWF. This event occurs after stimulation by collagen, thrombin, or epinephrine. Agonists in the platelet releasate such as ADP and thromboxane A_2 will also promote the receptor function of GPIIb/IIIa (2). Since there are also intraplatelet reactions which control ligand binding to the extracellular components of GPIIb/IIIa, the process has also been referred to as ''inside-out'' signaling (100). There is more than one signaling pathway which couples agonist reception to GPIIb/IIIa. Thrombin exposure evokes participation of protein kinase C. In contrast, ADP and epinephrine induce fibrinogen receptor expression in the absence of protein kinase C activity. Platelet aggregation (cohesion) has an absolute requirement for fibrinogen binding. As shown in Table 3, GPIIb/IIIa on the activated platelet surface also binds fibronectin, vWF, and vitronectin, but fibrinogen is by far the most important ligand because it critically cross-links GPIIb/IIIa on adjacent platelets, thus promoting strong cohesion.

One of the most important developments in our comprehension of platelet thrombus formation was elucidation of the specificity of the interaction between fibrinogen and GPIIb/IIIa as determined by amino acid sequences. Fibrinogen is a dimeric ligand, consisting of three pairs of polypeptide chains—alpha, beta, and gamma (103). Each fibrinogen dimer contains three recognition sites for $\alpha IIb\beta_3$. One peptide site is located at the carboxy terminus of the gamma chain of fibrinogen. Interestingly, only six amino acid residues are sufficient for recognition of the sequence. In fact, a peptide with four amino acids is also recognizable. This sequence is arginyl–glycyl–aspartic in addition to one of several other amino acids which are capable of recognition by GPIIb/IIIa (''RGD'' sequences).

Specifically, RGD sequences are found in two portions of the alpha chain of fibrinogen. As might have been anticipated, a large group of proteins contain RGD sequences, several of which bind to GPIIb/IIIa. Thus, the RGD amino acid sequence is ubiquitous and involved in many types of cell adhesion interactions (101,104,105). The gamma-chain sequence is unique to fibrinogen. Peptides containing either the gamma-chain sequence or the RGD sequence inhibit fibrinogen binding to GPIIb/IIIa and therefore platelet aggregation (cohesion).

Table 3 lists other adhesive proteins in the hemostatic system which are ligands for GPIIb/IIIa. All contain at least one RGD sequence, which is involved in binding of fibronectin, vWF, and vitronectin to the platelet surface. However, fibrinogen is by far the most important ligand for GPIIb/IIIa, probably because it is present in high concentrations in plasma. However, in the microcirculation, binding parameters may differ because the aforementioned ligands are present in the subendothelial matrix, but fibrinogen is not (16,100) (Table 1). Thrombospondin, a trimeric adhesive protein, does not directly bind to GPIIb/IIIa. This protein probably functions as a reinforcing moiety by induction of stabilization of a formed platelet thrombus. This may be related to the ability of thrombospondin to bind fibrinogen (106).

It is therefore evident that the absence of platelet–fibrinogen adhesion as induced by the integrin glycoprotein IIb/IIIa receptor on the activated platelet surface presents a therapeutic potential for the prothrombotic state. A monoclonal antibody directed toward platelet glycoprotein IIb/IIIa has entered clinical trials and has been shown to reduce ischemic complications of procedures such as coronary angioplasty and atherectomy (20). Proof of effectiveness of the antibody was at the other end of the spectrum, wherein the risk of bleeding was increased in these patients (7,17–19,107,108). This will be discussed further.

To summarize, the platelet glycoprotein GPIIb/IIIa complex is the receptor for fibrinogen and is essential for adhesion of platelets to each other during the hemostatic (and thrombotic) process. Information as to its functional importance was derived from studies of platelets from patients with the most common inherited platelet disorder: Glanzmann's thrombasthenia. The critical contribution of the GPIIb/IIIa complex to normal hemostasis is evidenced by the fact that the severity of hemorrhage correlates with the quantities of immunologically detectable GPIIb/IIIa (99).

IMPORTANCE OF THE INTEGRIN GROUP OF ADHESION RECEPTORS

Adhesive protein receptors on mammalian and avian cells fall into the classification of integrins (92,104,105,109). Proteins in this group consist of noncovalently associated α and β subunits in the form of α/β heterodimers. There is also a subfamily of integrins—"cytoadhesins"—which include GPIIb/IIIa and the vitronectin receptor. Cytoadhesins contain identical β subunits, but they are complexed with different α subunits.

Because we regard thrombosis and inflammation as parallel events during vascular occlusion, it is pertinent to discuss the other subfamilies in the integrin group. This should become obvious as the discussion of this supergene family evolves (5,6,9,110,111).

The fibronectin receptor and the very late activation (VLA) antigens comprise another subfamily in the integrin group. When surfaces are coated with fibronectin, adhesion of cells to these surfaces is mediated via the fibronectin receptor. The VLA antigens were initially encountered in activated T lymphocytes, but actually have a wider distribution. The β subunit in VLA antigens is identical to the β subunit in the fibronectin receptor (91). The term "integrin" refers to the ability of these receptor complexes to "integrate" biochemical activities of cell surface and cytoplasmic cell components. As shown in Table 5 (kindly provided by Dr. Thomas Kunicki), other leukocyte α-/β-subunit receptors in the integrin family have been identified in a large variety of tissues. This includes the Mac-1 (macrophage-1) and p150,95_{β} complexes, which mediate binding of the complement protein C3bi to monocytes (93). Mac-1 also binds coagulation factor X. Binding of complement is a prerequisite for the phagocytic process as well as granulocyte adherence. Interestingly, the primary amino acid sequence of C3bi contains the RGD sequence. As part of the inflammatory response, opsonized particles are coated with C3bi. The lymphocyte function-associated antigen (LFA-1_{β}) complex plays a role in the adhesive and killer functions of T lymphocytes. Leukocyte adhesion receptors have a distinct α subunit, but the 95-kDa β subunit is common to all leukocyte adhesion receptors. The clinical impact of leukocyte adhesion receptors is clearly delineated in an inherited defect characterized by deficiency or structural alteration in the β subunit of the receptor. This disorder, known as leukocyte adhesion deficiency (LAD), involves development of serious infections which are a direct consequence of defective to absent leukocyte adhesion at sites of inflammation. All three components of the β_2 integrin family are involved (CD11/CD18) (Table 5) (93).

To summarize: The platelet GPIIb/IIIa/αIIbβ_3 complex is a member of the integrin family of adhesive protein receptors (Tables 3–5), more specifically a member of the cytoadhesin subfamily of integrins. In fact, the complex is now classified as an integrin subfamily, i.e., cytoadhesins. As described above, these receptors are highly homologous with and bind to comparable segments on other adhesive proteins which modulate cell–cell interactions (105). The integrin supergene family (Table 5) is involved in a large variety of events involving multiple cells. These include contact-dependent cell growth, monocyte migration through the vasculature, cell motility and migration during embryonic development, and tumor cell metastases. With regard to hemostasis and thrombosis, the receptor function of the GPIIb/IIIa complex is only expressed when the cell is activated. In addition to binding fibrinogen for mediation of the final common pathway of platelet cohesion, GPIIb/IIIa also binds vWF (12). From the latter, it can be inferred that the complex plays a role in platelet adhesion to subendothelium. The ability to bind fibronectin may be related to spreading of platelets on vascular surfaces. As in the case of the platelet release reaction, several agonists are involved and there is a reinforcement system for platelet adhesion in the maintenance of hemostasis. This is also true for the development of thrombosis and atherosclerosis. One system or agonist may predominate or substitute for another as part of multiple pathophysiologic circumstances (9,11).

CONTRACTILE SYSTEMS IN PLATELET SECRETION AND COHESION

It is readily apparent that a consolidated, retracted platelet thrombus, of necessity, must possess marked tensile strength. It resists backpressure of the circulation and tightly adheres to vascular surfaces to which it is attached. This probably explains, in a major way, why it is so difficult to prevent expansion of or dislodge an occlusive platelet-rich thrombus. The contractile systems in platelets are probably the most important modulators of the physical structure of an arterial thrombus. New developments in our comprehension of these systems merit discussion.

If we compare alterations in physical morphology between circulating platelets and erythrocytes, the differences are striking. Erythrocytes in the vasculature can undergo enormous alterations in morphology. These are controlled and altered by their cytoskeleton through interactions with membrane proteins (2). Erythrocyte shape change is rapidly restored by membrane proteins such as spectrin, which maintain their biconcave shape. Such properties differ markedly from those in circulating platelets, which remain as symmetric disks unless activated. Agonists will drastically alter the platelet disk arrangement with a transition to a sphiny sphere. An unstimulated platelet contains a peripheral coil of microtubules which traverse the periphery several times. The microtubule coil and the actin membrane skeleton beneath the plasmalemma maintain the discoid shape of unstimulated platelets. These microtubules are just beneath the plasma membrane and its surface invagination, i.e., the surface-connected canalicular system (Fig. 5). The glycocalyx, comprised of platelet glycoprotein(s), forms a matrix which passes into and through the plasma membrane into the extracellular space.

Upon activation, platelets instantly develop filopodial projections which constitute the spiny portion of the sphere. The rearranged platelet plasma membrane offers more opportunities for surface interactions with other platelets and adjacent cells (transcellular metabolism) (5,9,112). We have already mentioned implications of the rearranged platelet surface phospholipoprotein for coagulation. Shape change is controlled by the actin cytoskeleton, but not the microtubular coil, since the latter is still intact after filopodia have formed. Profiles of microtubules can still be seen in filopodia after thrombin stimulation (79,86).

About 20% of total platelet protein is actin. This is a globular protein with a molecular weight of 42 kDa consisting of two single chains (β- and γ-actin). In resting platelets, 40–50% of actin is filamentous (F-actin). Monomeric actin (G-actin) accounts for the remainder. After platelet activation, F-actin increases to 70–80%, with a corresponding decrease in G-actin. The filopodia extending from the activated platelet surface actually contain polymerized actin. Polymerization of G-actin to F-actin is controlled by platelet profilin. Also, as G-actin monomers polymerize to form F-actin filaments, troponin and tropomyosin are incorporated. Interestingly, these proteins also control actin–myosin interactions in skeletal muscle. Additional possibilities relevant to thrombosis have recently been described (113,114). Following tissue injury, actin can gain access to the circulation. If a consequence of the injury was depletion of the two actin-binding proteins in plasma (vitamin D-binding protein and gelsolin), free actin can induce platelet aggregation in a manner similar to ADP (113).

Another important platelet protein is filamin. Filamin binds actin and is responsible for producing bundles from organizing actin filaments. Filamin phosphorylation is catalyzed by a protein kinase which is controlled by platelet cAMP. Actin filaments in platelets are anchored to the plasma membrane via α-actinin. A major consequence of platelet activation is reorganization of the actin superstructure. This is depicted in Figs. 6 and 7.

Platelet myosin contains six polypeptide chains. Although platelet myosin has properties similar to skeletal muscle myosin, their immunologic properties are different. Platelet myosin has a molecular weight of 46 kDa and each of the six chains contains sites for both actin binding and ATP hydrolysis. One myosin light chain (20 kDa) is phosphorylated by the myosin light-chain kinase (MLCK) (Fig. 1). In addition, myosin can also be phosphorylated by protein kinase C. Activity of MLCK increases in the presence of calcium-calmodulin and is decreased by cAMP-dependent kinase. Phosphorylation is the major determinant of actin–myosin ATPase activity and thereby the platelet contractile process. Increases in cytosolic platelet calcium activate MLCK, induce phosphorylation of myosin, and result in platelet contraction. Dephosphorylation of the myosin light chain by a phosphatase also modulates the contractile process. There is superficial resemblance between contractile phenomena in platelets and in skeletal muscle. However, details of the process are dissimilar.

THE PLATELET CYTOSKELETON

Basically, the platelet cytoskeleton consists of a group of proteins which remain insoluble after platelet exposure to a nonionic detergent followed by ultracentrifugation. The sediment produced by this procedure demonstrates ultrastructural morphology classified as endoplasmic reticulum. Proteins in this sediment can be further defined by gel electrophoresis. It is thought that platelet shape and plasticity

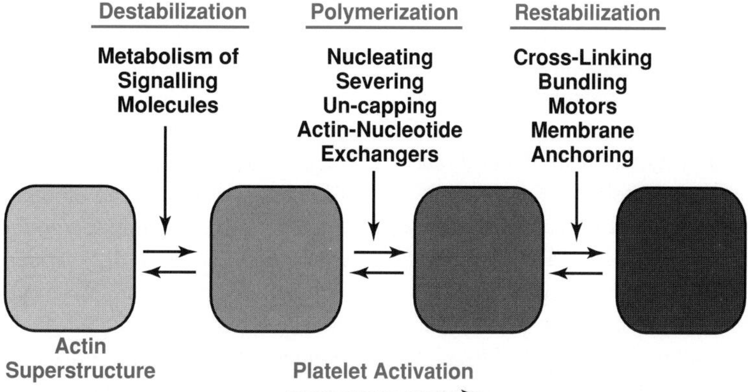

FIG. 6. The actin superstructure of platelets undergoes reorganization when they are activated. Actin is stable in resting platelets, but components of signaling pathways destabilize it. These components include membrane polyphosphoinositides, diacylglycerol, calcium, kinases, phosphatases, and guanosine triphosphate (GTP)-binding proteins (180). Within seconds, actin subunits shift from monomeric to filamentous forms. This polymerization step is under control of actin-binding proteins (capping proteins), severing proteins, nucleating proteins, and proteins which regulate actin nucleotide exchange. In this way, the activated conformation of actin structure becomes stabilized. This involves more actin-binding proteins which cross-link, bundle, anchor, and serve as "motors." Actin is anchored at specific sites on the membrane. Signaling molecules which were originally involved in actin reorganization also play a role in regulation of additional cytoskeletal changes. (From Furman et al., ref. 50, with permission.)

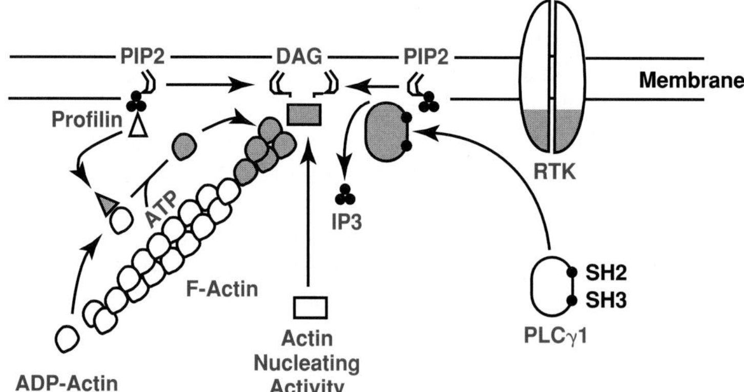

FIG. 7. Cortical actin is regulated by receptor tyrosine kinase. A receptor with tyrosine kinase activity *(RTK)* regulates actin polymerization at the periphery of the cell (*dark areas:* activated forms of the proteins illustrated). After ligand binding, the receptor tyrosine kinase phosphorylates itself. In this form, it binds and phosphorylates specific tyrosine residues of phospholipase C-gamma$_1$ *(PLCγ1)*. The tyrosine-phosphorylated PLCγ1 hydrolyzes phosphatidylinositol bis-phosphate *(PIP_2)*, which in turn releases the second messengers inositol trisphosphate *(IP_3)*, the soluble head group of PIP_2, and diacylglycerol *(DAG)*. DAG remains in the membrane and in this location activates a nucleating protein. This process results in formation of new actin filaments. In addition, PIP_2 releases profilin, which promotes re-formation of ATP from the ADP–actin subunits which have come off the ends of actin filaments **(lower left)**. Therefore, hydrolysis of PIP_2, promotion of nucleation of new actin filaments, and their elongation by subunits to re-form ATP as promoted by profilin are all triggered by the initial activation of the receptor tyrosine kinase. (From Furman et al., ref. 50, with permission.)

are maintained via interactions between the lipid bilayer of the plasma membrane and the cytoskeleton. At least 14 proteins have been identified in the platelet cytoskeletal compartment (42,86).

Platelet activation induces reorganization of the actin cytoskeleton. New information has evolved as to how signaling pathways regulate the extent of actin polymerization. As with almost all other hemostatic and thrombotic systems, the actin superstructure is now conceived as a dynamic entity resulting from the action of several regulatory systems and controlled by specific signaling mechanisms. The prime regulatory mechanism for the actin cytoskeleton was once thought to be an increase in cytosolic calcium as induced by inositol triphosphate formation. We now know that a variety of messengers produced by metabolism of membrane phospholipids regulate the actin cytoskeleton. For example, phosphatidylinositol-4,5-bisphosphate (PIP_2), which is hydrolyzed by phospholipase C gamma-1 (PLC-gamma$_1$), binds to actin-regulating proteins in vitro (Fig. 1). This blocks their interaction with actin. An example of an actin-binding protein is profilin. The latter binds to PIP_2, blocking activity of unphosphorylated PLC-gamma$_1$. Tyrosine phosphorylation activates PLC-gamma$_1$, and the activated phospholipase overcomes profilin inhibition, allowing for hydrolysis of PIP_2. In the setting of PIP_2 hydrolysis, profilin is released from its membrane binding site and diacylglycerol (DAG) is produced (Fig. 7). DAG, via protein kinase C activation, regulates the actin-binding and cross-linking activity of the myristoylated alanine-rich C-kinase substrates (MARCKS). The latter represent a group of protein kinase C substrates (50,115). These steps promote reorganization of the actin superstructure. The isoform of PLC-gamma$_1$, PLC-gamma$_2$, also becomes tyrosine-phosphorylated in platelets stimulated by thrombin (116).

In activated, shape-changed platelets, the response of the actin cytoskeleton is characterized by a shift from monomeric G-actin to filamentous F-actin. Mechanisms of induction of actin polymerization have been further clarified. The affinity of actin monomers for ends of actin filaments is governed by the concentration of free actin in the cell. Affinity is higher when critical concentration is lower. When platelets are activated and the critical concentration of actin decreases, the affinity of actin monomers for the ends of actin filaments increases. Therefore, actin monomers will dissociate from proteins which have transiently sequestered these monomers and they will move to the ends of actin filaments, producing an elongation (114).

In platelets, monomeric actin subunits are bound to their monomeric sequestering protein—thymosin β_4. In resting platelets, the thymosin β_4–monomeric actin complex is associated with the pointed end of the actin filament. The pointed end is the slow-growing end. The critical concentration of actin at the barbed end—the high-affinity, fast-growing end of actin filaments—is one order of magnitude lower than the dissociation constant of the actin–thymosin β_4 complex. In the resting platelet, 60% of actin is monomeric. In activated platelets, less than 10% of actin is monomeric. A consequence of platelet activation is polymerization of actin subunits at the barbed, fast-growing end of its filaments (Fig. 7).

Availability of actin-filament barbed, high-affinity (fast-growing) ends in platelets is regulated in four ways: (a)

Barbed ends are covered by capping proteins which are uncapped during activation, leaving barbed ends accessible for accepting new actin subunits. (b) Actin filaments are severed into smaller filaments, thereby creating new barbed ends. (c) New filaments are generated by compounds known as nucleating proteins. An example is ponticulin, which nucleates actin filaments, thereby generating new actin filaments. (d) If the filaments contain ADP–actin subunits, the high-affinity character of the barbed ends in activated cells will be restored.

Therefore, the main consequence of platelet activation in thrombus formation is to move the actin monomer/filament equilibrium toward formation of new filaments. Mechanisms for regulation of capping proteins and elucidation of modes of action of severing and nucleating proteins are topics for future investigation. Also, it is not known which factors are responsible for the presence of ADP–actin subunits at the barbed end of actin filaments. A major candidate for the ability to sever actin filaments into smaller units, thereby creating new barbed ends, is the protein gelsolin. This is a protein which is calcium and phospholipid regulated in the binding of actin and is associated with the barbed ends (50,117). Profilin, the polyphosphoinositide-regulated actin-binding protein, can increase nucleotide exchange when bound to monomeric actin. ADP–actin subunits are released from the ends of actin filaments and profilin may play a role in exchange of ADP bound to actin subunits for ATP. Therefore, profilin is important for reformation of an active ATP–actin monomer when actin filament turnover is rapid (Fig. 7).

Interestingly, polymerization of actin filaments is only one of several cytoskeletal responses during platelet activation. Arrangement of actin filaments is also controlled by cross-linking, bundling, membrane attachment proteins, and motors (Fig. 6). An important newly comprehended mechanism involves a phenomenon known as "focal adhesion" (50) (Fig. 7). Focal adhesion occurs at a specialized membrane domain where the actin skeleton is attached to a transmembrane integrin (Fig. 8). The transmembrane integrin itself binds to extracellular matrix proteins (100,118). This

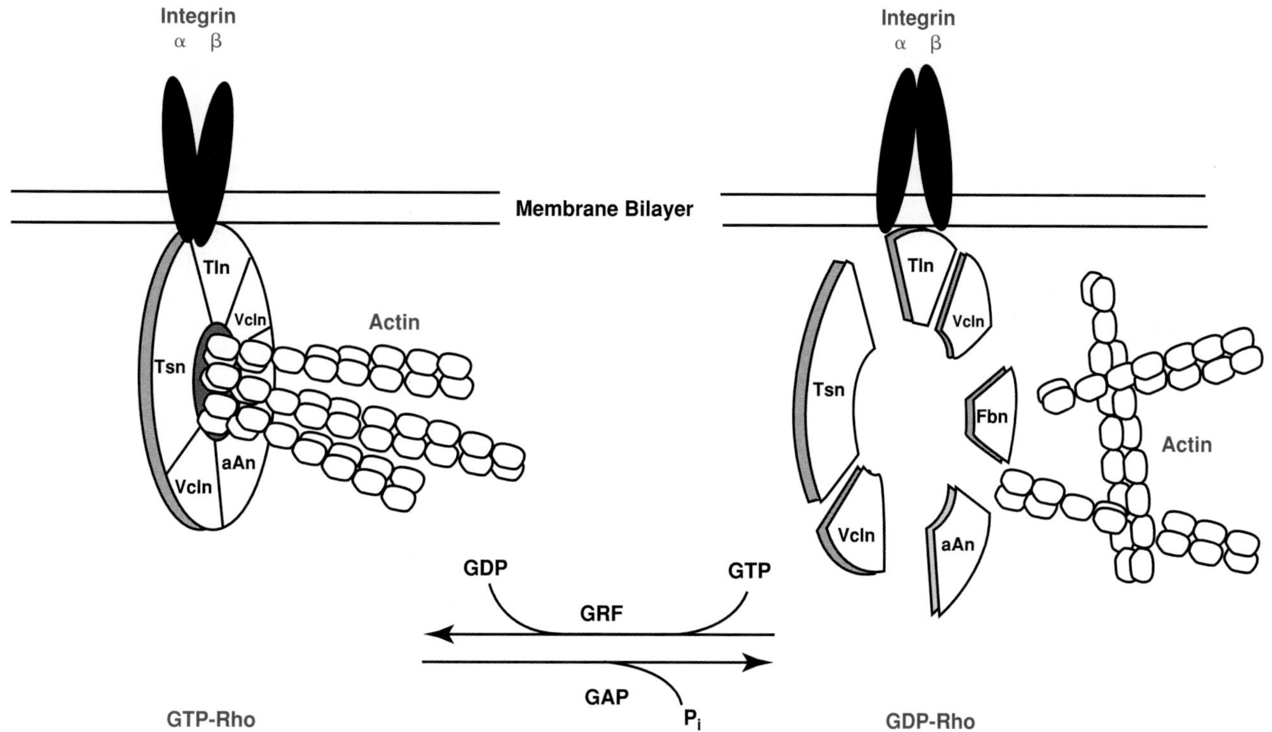

FIG. 8. The focal adhesion. This is a complex protein/lipid structure which forms a bridge between the extracellular matrix and the intracellular actin network. Thus, the focal adhesion represents a specialized domain in the membrane where the actin cytoskeleton is anchored to a transmembrane integrin complex such as platelet glycoproteins IIb/IIIa. As described, the latter functions as a receptor for fibrinogen. Guanosine triphosphate–Rho *(GTP-Rho)* stabilizes the focal adhesion. Proteins which activate GTPase *(GAP)* can initiate disruption of focal adhesions. The focal adhesions per se are stabilized by activation of guanine nucleotide releasing factor *(GRF)*. This factor produces "recharging" of Rho with GTP. This figure demonstrates examples of proteins which can be found in focal adhesions. Included are heterodimeric integrins with α and β subunits, such as platelet glycoproteins (IIb/IIIa), talin *(Tin)*, tensin *(Tsn)*, vinculin *(Vcln)*, fimbrin *(Fbn)*, α-actinin *(αAn)*, and actin filaments. Several other proteins can be associated with focal adhesions, including the two tyrosinases p125^{FAK} and c-Src. (From Furman et al., ref. 50, with permission.)

is especially applicable to our previous discussions of the glycoprotein IIb/IIIa complex and fibrinogen (100). As previously mentioned, fibrinogen is the most important extracellular ligand for GPIIb/IIIa. Activation of GPIIb/IIIa and subsequent binding of fibrinogen are prerequisites for tyrosine phosphorylation of substrates in activated platelets. A platelet tyrosine kinase, pb125^{FAK}, is localized at a focal adhesion site. When platelets are activated, activity of pb125^{FAK} as a tyrosine kinase is increased (119,120).

Rho is a GTP-binding protein. When Rho binds to GTP the structure of focal adhesions is stabilized. If GTP is hydrolyzed, the focal adhesion is disrupted. GTP-binding proteins in the Ras family such as Rho and Rac are involved in regulation of the actin cytoskeleton. The GTP-binding proteins in the Ras family are nucleotide triphosphatases like actin. Activity of GTP-binding proteins is increased by the GAP proteins, which activate GTPases. There are also exchanger-type proteins which interact with GAP proteins in conversion of GDP to GTP. These reactions are controlled by membrane receptor molecules and signaling pathways which are triggered by these receptors. Precise interactions between Ras-like proteins and the actin cytoskeleton remain to be defined (50,100,121).

Recently, a Ras-related, low-molecular-weight GTP-binding protein known as Rap2B was found to associate with the cytoskeleton in activated platelets which have aggregated. Agonist-induced actin polymerization was a requirement for translocation of Rap2B to the cytoskeleton. This suggested that Rap2B interacted with newly formed actin filaments (121). The association of Rap2B with the cytoskeleton could be blocked by a monoclonal antibody to GPIIb/IIIa. Furthermore, platelets from patients with Glanzmann's thrombasthenia (whose platelet membranes do not contain GPIIb/IIIa) did not incorporate Rap2B into the cytoskeleton following thrombin activation. Thus, Rap2B only associates with the platelet cytoskeleton when a functional GPIIb/IIIa complex is present on the platelet membrane. Translocation of Rap2B to the cytoskeleton is also paralleled by translocation of comparable quantities of GPIIb/IIIa (122).

In summary, multiple signaling pathways are activated by agonists such as thrombin and these are involved in regulation of the actin superstructure. Platelet membrane phospholipid metabolism and activation of GTP-binding proteins are critical for modulating actin-dependent events. The actin cytoskeleton itself, in addition to its satellite proteins, controls signaling pathways in activated platelets. These phenomena support the premise that in platelets (as well as vascular cells) there are multiple interacting systems which control responsiveness of a critical platelet component such as actin during the activation process (50). The reason for discussing these systems in such detail is that one or more of these crucial steps may present an opportunity for therapeutics aimed at reduction of platelet reactivity. An induced defect in platelet contractility might eventually represent a novel approach toward reduction of the prothrombotic activities of platelets.

PLATELET GRANULES AND THE PLATELET SECRETORY PROCESS

Relevance for Platelet Recruitment

Very early during primary hemostasis, platelets adhere to subendothelial matrix, achieve attachment, initiate spreading, and become activated (5,9,123). The consequence of platelet activation is production of a releasate which interacts with other platelets in the fluid phase and with vascular cells (48) (Figs. 1 and 3). Additional adhesion interactions follow sequentially and the activated platelet surfaces themselves catalyze thrombin formation. Components of the platelet releasate originate from several varieties of storage granules or appear as a consequence of de novo synthesis from platelet membrane phospholipids (Fig. 2). Platelet dense granules (Figs. 1 and 4) release their contents with great rapidity. Dense granule components act as secondary agonists to control responsiveness of other platelets as well as cells of the vessel wall. A very important dense-body constituent is ADP, which emerges in parallel with ATP. Although ATP can inhibit platelet reactivity, it does not influence the recruiting activity of the platelet releasate. Serotonin (5-hydroxytryptamine, 5-HT) is a powerful vasoconstrictor and may synergize with ADP in platelet activation and recruitment. However, 5-HT itself serves as an agonist for thrombocytes in avian and reptile species, but not in mammals. Calcium secretion from dense granules plays a role in one or more of the calcium-dependent processes occurring in the fluid milieu of the thrombus. This includes coagulation and several prothrombotic metabolic events (49,96,124).

Lysosomes are not morphologically identifiable in platelets, and their function is not comparable to lysosomes in other tissues or blood cells (89,125). Lysosomal activity can be detected in platelet homogenates, but this activity is not measurable in releasates from activated platelets. This is a surface-connected activity which can be increased threefold by treatment with a detergent such as Triton X-100. However, the increment remains particle-bound. This also agrees with the concept that platelets are not truly phagocytic and cannot form phagocytic vacuoles. These properties distinguish platelet lysosomal activity from that associated with neutrophils and macrophages (89). Thus, platelets per se do not play a proinflammatory role upon arrival at sites of fissured or ruptured atherosclerotic plaques. They are proinflammatory with neutrophils via transcellular metabolism (5,112). Platelets contain an endoglycosidase (heparatinase) which is of lysosomal origin. This enzyme cleaves glycosaminoglycans on the endothelial cell surface. However, the fragment resulting does not have proliferative properties (16). Factor XIII is a platelet cytosolic enzyme which nevertheless escapes in a nonmetabolic fashion during platelet activation. The transglutaminase activity of factor XIII is responsible for covalently cross-linking fibrin strands. This confers a high degree of stabilization to the coagulum formed during secondary hemostasis. This stabilizing activity is superimposed upon that of the platelet contractile proteins toward reinforcing the occlusive lesion. Furthermore, factor XIII also cross-links fibronectin and α_2-antiplasmin to fibrin (8).

Platelet α-granules are a major storage modality for proteins which play important roles as growth factors, adhesive moieties, and coagulation factors (126,127). The platelet-derived growth factor (PDGF) promotes smooth muscle proliferation, indicating a possible role in the atherosclerotic process (3,4). PDGF has three isoforms and receptors on smooth muscle and fibroblasts. Importantly, PDGF receptors are of the transmembrane tyrosine kinase type. Signal transduction via PDGF receptors resembles that of other tyrosine kinase receptors such as epidermal growth factor and insulin. Another α-granule-associated growth factor is the connective tissue-activating peptide III (CTAPIII). Actually, this may be the precursor of another secreted platelet protein, β-thromboglobulin, and also bears a relationship to platelet factor 4, which is an antiheparin substance (128). CTAPIII also induces fibroblast proliferation (16).

The versatility of growth factor secretion by cells participating in the inflammatory/fibroproliferative response characteristic of advanced atherosclerosis is demonstrated by the recent description of growth factor secretion by T lymphocytes (111). Thus, it was unanticipated that T cells could produce a heparin-binding epidermal growth factor-like molecule and also basic fibroblast growth factor (111).

Thrombospondin (TSP) is a 450-kDa glycoprotein, also released from activated platelet α-granules. TSP is associated with cell surfaces, which suggests existence of receptors for this protein. Thrombospondin is also synthesized, secreted, and incorporated into the extracellular matrix by endothelial and smooth muscle cells. This molecule can associate with fibrinogen, fibronectin, collagen, laminin, and vWF (129).

The platelet-derived endothelial cell growth factor (PDECGF) is another cytosolic platelet component and therefore is not metabolically released. Promotion of endothelial cell growth by PDECGF is logical because endothelial cells do not have receptors for PDGF. We suggest that PDECGF as well as platelet-derived factor XIII may appear during the latter stages of thrombus formation via nonmetabolic leakage from platelets which have been maximally stimulated, consolidated, and retracted.

The unexpectedly large quantity of coagulation proteins present in platelet α-granules is of interest (8,16,79). As megakaryocytes in the marrow mature, they take up plasma proteins and store them in α-granules, utilizing a transport system which has not been clearly defined. This includes plasma albumin, IgG, and fibrinogen. Megakaryocytes can actually synthesize coagulation factor V.

Protein S, the cofactor for activated protein C, is a platelet α-granule component. This may be related to enhancement of the natural anticoagulant properties of protein C, since factor V is one of its targets (130). Platelet α-granules contain plasminogen activator inhibitor-1 (PAI-1). Release of PAI-1 may prevent excessive fibrinolytic activity from inducing premature dissolution of a clot. Additional platelet α-granule components include adhesive proteins such as fibrinogen, fibronectin, vWF, and vitronectin. The form of vWF found in platelets as compared to megakaryocytes contains the very large multimers which are more effective as hemostatic agents. Vitronectin enters platelets from plasma in a passive manner (16).

The α-granules of unstimulated platelets contain a 140-kDa transmembrane glycoprotein which, upon activation, translocates and fuses with the plasma membrane. A portion of this glycoprotein is then exposed to the platelet microenvironment. This glycoprotein, referred to as P-selectin (CD62), was simultaneously discovered in several laboratories (24,25,131,132). P-selectin is also present in endothelial cells, where it is stored in the Weibel–Palade bodies (30,133). P-selectin antibodies generated to the surface of activated platelets do not react with the surface of resting platelets. This verifies that the mechanism of translocation of P-selectin is platelet activation-dependent. Thus far, there is no uniquely specified function for platelet P-selectin. It would appear to mediate adhesive interactions between platelets, neutrophils, and subsets of lymphocytes (28,29). There are two other selectin families: (a) L-selectins, found in lymphocytes, monocytes, and neutrophils. L-selectins are expressed constitutively and separate from the cells after activation. (b) The E-selectins (ELAM-1, endothelial-leukocyte adhesion molecule-1). The E-selectins are associated with endothelium and require several hours of cytokine exposure prior to induction. RNA and protein synthesis are involved in E-selectin expression. P-selectin-deficient "knock-out" mice have recently been bred. In these animals, leukocyte rolling and extravasation is defective and they also develop a leukocytosis. However, these defects are not fatal (30).

With regard to the other intracellular platelet components, the dense tubular system functions in calcium sequestration. This system in platelets is analogous to sarcoplasmic reticulum in muscle.

THE UNIQUE ADENINE NUCLEOTIDE SYSTEM IN PLATELETS

Platelet ADP is extremely important in thrombosis and atherosclerosis. As we have pointed out, platelets become functionless if release of ADP is blocked or if it is metabolized upon release (9,46). Our comprehension of platelet nucleotide metabolism was clarified mainly through the work of Holmsen (49,134,135). Platelets contain two distinct nucleotide pools. One is known as the "metabolic pool" and is located in the cytosol. The "storage pool" is located in the dense granules. Importantly, these two systems do not interact biochemically. Furthermore, the storage pool cannot synthesize adenine nucleotides de novo when adenine or adenosine is incubated with platelets. In contrast, they are taken up and metabolized to ADP and ATP in the metabolic pool. Upon platelet activation, the storage pool of adenine nucleotides, but not the metabolic pool, is released from dense granules and cannot be replenished.

About 40% of platelet ATP and 50% of ADP is present in the storage pool. As previously discussed, conversion of monomeric actin to its filamentous configuration requires ATP hydrolysis. The ADP resulting from this hydrolytic step will complex with filamentous actin. These metabolic processes involving adenine nucleotides of the metabolic pool verify association of these nucleotides with the cytoskeletal system (49).

PLATELET AGGREGATION (COHESION): SIGNIFICANCE FOR THROMBOSIS

For clinical and research purposes, aggregometry has permitted studies of platelet–platelet interactions as induced by physiologic and model agonists. These reactions can be evaluated with reasonable qualitative and quantitative accuracy, but all studies of aggregation should be accompanied by measurements of dense granule release, such as serotonin and/or ADP (41,73). The size of graphically produced aggregation curves can be deceptive with regard to the quantity of release. Aggregation curves induced by a synthetic eicosanoid endoperoxide may resemble that obtained by collagen, but the endoperoxide produces about 28% serotonin release and collagen produces 66% serotonin release. Thus, the endoperoxide is a relatively weak agonist. The final response to a true platelet agonist is shape change, followed by aggregation (cohesion). Induction of the process and the response evoked vary with the individual stimulus (58,136).

True platelet aggregation is a biochemical event, requiring energy and platelet motion. This is not identical with the platelet clumping or agglutination promoted by ristocetin in the presence of vWF or by antibodies directed toward sensitized platelets which results in thrombocytopenia. As mentioned, measurements of secretion will provide information concerning the degree of platelet activation and the ''recruiting'' capabilities of the platelet releasate (41,51,73).

The basic requirement for platelet cohesion involves addition of an agonist in sufficient concentration to induce shape change, activation, and recruitment. Calcium is needed, although magnesium will suffice, if traces of calcium are available (16). Plasma fibrinogen, in addition to that which is secreted from platelets, is mandatory and at high shear rates, vWF is of critical importance (11,12). Although there is a wide variety of receptors and ligands for participation in platelet adhesion to damaged vessel walls, there is only one receptor for aggregation, GPIIb/IIIa (αIIbβ_3). The latter complex interacts only with fibrinogen or, under conditions of high shear, with vWF (11,12,100,101).

RECRUITMENT IN THROMBOSIS VIA THE PLATELET RELEASE REACTION

The platelet release reaction occurs in response to agonists which have been exogenously added *in vitro* or which appeared in the releasate from activated platelets in proximity *in vivo*. Depending upon strength of the agonist, varying quantities of α-granule and dense-body components are measurable in the releasate. The most important function of the release reaction in hemostasis and thrombosis is recruitment of additional platelets into the aggregate until such time as the vessel lumen is occluded and the thrombus undergoes consolidation and retraction.

As already mentioned, several agonists can be identified in the releasate from activated platelets. These include ADP, 5-HT, arachidonic acid and its cyclooxygenase and lipoxygenase metabolites, as well as α-granule components. These agonists play a critical role in platelet recruitment, which is the main platelet participation mechanism in thrombosis (137).

THE BASIC PLATELET REACTION

Platelet agonists induce the sequence of events described above and shown in Fig. 1: shape change, aggregation, and secretion. Biochemically, secretion is accompanied by elevations in cytoplasmic calcium, protein phosphorylation, and activation of the phosphoinositide pathway (Fig. 1).

Most receptors for platelet agonists consist of proteins which traverse the plasma membrane once or several times

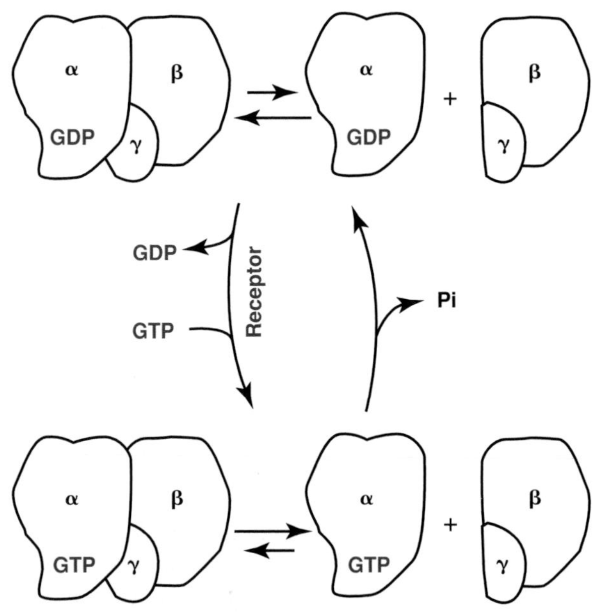

FIG. 9. Working model for activation of guanine nucleotide-binding regulatory proteins (G-proteins) (180). The functional state of a G-protein is determined by the nature of the bound nucleotide. With bound guanosine diphosphate *(GDP),* the G-protein is inactive. This condition favors subunit association **(top).** When guanosine triphosphate *(GTP)* is bound, the G-protein is active. Therefore, the affinity between its α and $\beta\gamma$ subunits is reduced. This promotes subunit dissociation **(bottom).** Activation of receptors has a stimulatory effect on G-proteins by favoring exchange of GTP for GDP. (From Sternweis and Smrcka, ref. 146, with permission.)

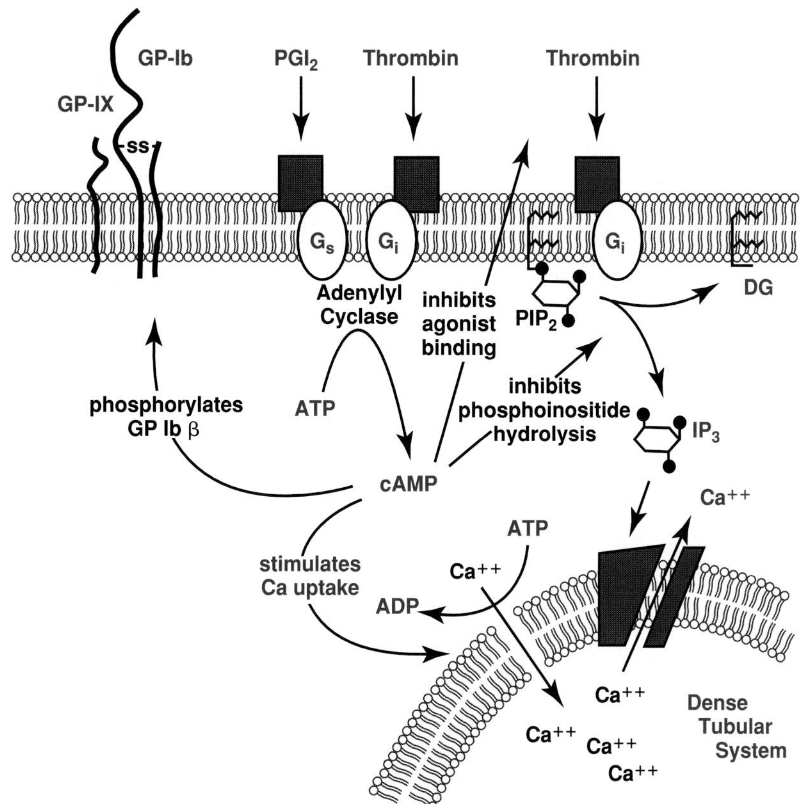

FIG. 10. The role of cyclic AMP *(cAMP)* in platelet activation (43,57). Agents such as PGI_2 whose receptors are coupled to G_s promote synthesis of cAMP by adenylyl cyclase. Production of cAMP is inhibited by agonists such as thrombin with receptors coupled to G_i. Increases in platelet cAMP result in decreases in platelet activation, aggregation, and secretion. These effects are due to inhibition of both agonist binding and inhibition of phosphoinositide hydrolysis induced by the agonist. The inhibition of phosphoinositide hydrolysis leads to a decrease in IP_3 formation and a consequent fall in calcium release from the dense tubular system. Uptake of calcium into the dense tubular system of platelets is increased by cAMP. This results in a reduction in platelet cytosolic calcium, the consequence of which is decreased platelet reactivity. An increase in cAMP also promotes phosphorylation by cAMP-dependent protein kinase(s) of a variety of substrates. These include platelet membrane glycoprotein Ib-β and the low-molecular-weight GTP-binding protein Rap 1B (not shown) (121). Phosphorylation of membrane glycoprotein 1b-β promotes its interaction with the platelet cytoskeleton. Phosphorylation of Rap 1B stimulates its translocation from the membrane to the cytosol (121). *DG,* Diacylglycerol. (From Dr. Lawrence F. Brass with permission.)

(75,98,138,139). The extracellular and transmembrane portions of the receptor constitute the site for agonist binding. The cytosolic domain is involved in activating enzymes inducing second messengers and ion channels in response to receptor occupation. As will be discussed, at least one G-protein is required for completion of the activation process. These proteins mediate interactions between receptors and effectors. An individual G-protein can be stimulatory or inhibitory for the effector (42–44,57) (Fig. 9).

Two intraplatelet metabolic pathways are involved in activation by most agonists (Fig. 10). Both are initiated by enzymatic hydrolysis of membrane phospholipids. When phosphatidylinositol-4,5-bisphosphate (PIP_2) is cleaved by phospholipase C, the phosphoinositide pathway is activated. Products of the reaction are inositol-1,4,5-trisphosphate (IP_3) and diacylglycerol. These metabolites serve as second messengers in the platelet. Thus, IP_3 will release calcium from the dense tubular system, resulting in an increase in cytosolic free calcium—a prerequisite for platelet activation. The elevated calcium levels activate enzymes which were not originally functional at the low calcium concentrations of resting platelets (140). Diacylglycerol activates protein kinase C, which in turn leads to protein phosphorylation on serine and threonine residues. This is accompanied by secretion from platelet granules and expression of the fibrinogen receptor (GPIIb/IIIa). Calcium elevations also activate phospholipase A_2 with liberation of free arachidonate from membrane phospholipids. This occurs via direct action of the enzyme. Thromboxane A_2, the cyclooxygenase-catalyzed eicosanoid metabolite, is detectable in the fluid phase of activated platelets within 6 (56,141).

Platelet activation is inhibited whenever levels of platelet cAMP are elevated. This is the mechanism of action of inhibitors of platelet function such as prostacyclin (PGI_2). In a comparable manner, endothelium-derived relaxing factor or nitric oxide (EDRF/NO) inhibits platelet function by activating cytosolic guanylate cyclase, which increases intracellular levels of cyclic GMP (142–144).

Elevations in platelet cAMP activate cAMP-dependent protein kinases. There are several known substrates for protein kinases. These include glycoprotein Ib-β, actin-binding protein, myosin light chain, and Rap1b. It is not known how phosphorylation of any of these substrates promotes inhibition of platelet activation. In general terms, platelet agonists suppress cAMP formation by inhibiting adenylyl cyclase. Others can accelerate cAMP metabolism by activating cAMP phosphodiesterase. When cAMP is elevated in platelets, calcium is sequestered in the dense tubular system. This also results in inhibition of phospholipase activity and subsequent release of arachidonate (44).

G-PROTEINS: MEDIATORS OF PLATELET ACTIVATION

The group of highly homologous guanine nucleotide-binding regulatory proteins are known as G-proteins. They control interactions between agonist receptors on the cell surface and effector molecules in the cells (43,44,98,145). This includes enzymes involved in generating second messengers and which control ion channels. The G-proteins are heterotrimers consisting of α and $\beta\gamma$ subunits. Each subunit can exist in multiple forms. The α subunits are the most diverse and often account for the major activities of G-proteins (Fig. 9). In the resting cell, the α subunit contains bound guanosine diphosphate (GDP) and association of α and $\beta\gamma$ subunits is favored. When the G-protein binds GTP (rather than GDP) it becomes activated. Interaction with receptors is most efficient with the heterotrimeric form of G-protein. When the rate of dissociation of GDP increases, activation is accelerated, thereby enhancing association with GTP. During the activation process, affinity between the α and $\beta\gamma$ subunits of G-proteins is decreased. This promotes dissociation of the subunits and generation of two pathways for further regulation [α(GTP) and free $\beta\gamma$ subunits] (44,146).

Platelets contain at least nine different G-proteins. In common with other cells, they are critical in signal transduction because they mediate interactions between agonist receptors and enzymes which modulate second messengers (Fig. 11). Among these are G_q, G_{11}, G_{12}, G_{13}, G_z, G_i with its three components, and a variant of G_s. Enzymes interacting with platelet G-proteins include phospholipase C, phospholipase A_2, and adenylyl cyclase (43,44,57) (Fig. 10). Receptors on platelets which can couple to G-proteins have been cloned. Examples are the receptors for epinephrine, thrombin, thromboxane A_2 (TXA_2), vasopressin, and platelet-activating factor (PAF) (44). These receptors are structurally single peptides and contain the classic seven transmembrane do-

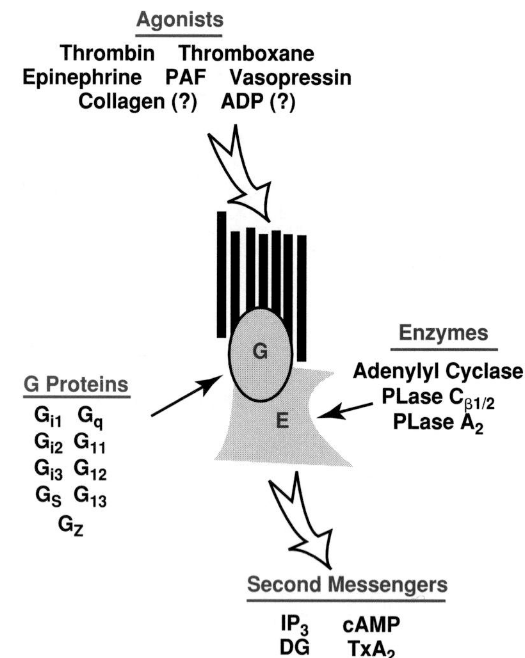

FIG. 11. Guanine nucleotide-regulatory proteins (G-proteins) identified in platelets. G-proteins serve as mediators of interactions between receptors for at least five different agonists and four second messenger generating systems as depicted. (From refs. 42, 43, and 57, courtesy of Dr. Lawrence F. Brass.)

mains and an extracellular N-terminus. The receptor is activated upon agonist binding, except in the case of thrombin, where thrombin as a proteolytic enzyme cleaves the receptor, unmasking a new N-terminus which now functions as a "tethered" ligand (75). In addition to signal–response coupling, G-proteins play a role in megakaryocyte development, platelet formation, and secretion from intracellular platelet granules (44,57).

The proteins G_s and G_i were the first G-proteins to be biochemically and functionally described. G_s stimulates adenylyl cyclase, thereby raising platelet cAMP levels, inhibiting platelet activation. $G_{i\alpha}$ exists in three forms ($G_{i\alpha 1}$, $G_{i\alpha 2}$, and $G_{i\alpha 3}$). These G-proteins are substrates for pertussis toxin, which blocks their ability to interact with receptors, due to ADP-ribosylation. As mentioned, G-proteins are involved in regulation of potassium and calcium channels, hydrolysis of phosphatidylcholine, and activation of phospholipases A_2 and C as well as cGMP phosphodiesterase. The platelet G-proteins identified in accordance with the α-subunit structure are shown in Table 6 (44,57).

In summary, our concepts of early events involving signal transduction in platelets have evolved considerably. During a thrombotic diathesis platelet reactivity is excessive and difficult to reverse. Eventually, we may be able to modify therapeutically signal transduction systems in platelets so that an occlusive lesion could be reversed. Thus, we now know that guanine nucleotide-binding regulatory proteins

TABLE 6. *G-protein α subunits in platelets*

G-protein	M_r (kDa)	Toxin	Phosphorylated?	Enzyme	Function
$G_{i\alpha2} \gg G_{i\alpha3} > G_{i\alpha1}$	40–41	Pertussis	No	Adenylyl cyclase, phospholipase C?	↓ cAMP, ↑ IP_3/DAG?
$G_{2\alpha}$	41	Neither	Yes	?	?
$G_{q\alpha}$, $G_{11\alpha}$	42	Neither	No	Phospholipase C	↑ IP_3/DAG
$G_{12\alpha}$, $G_{13\alpha}$	44	Neither	?	?	?
$G_{s\alpha}$	45	Cholera	No	Adenylyl cyclase	↑ cAMP

(G-proteins) modulate interactions between receptors on the platelet surface and intracellular enzymes which act as second messengers. G-proteins act on phospholipases A_2 and C as well as adenylyl cyclase (Fig. 10). Cloning of several receptors which link to G-proteins has improved our understanding of their mechanisms of action. The common theme is that these receptors consist of a single polypeptide chain with seven transmembrane domains and an extracellular N-terminus (44,77).

PARTICIPATION OF PLATELETS IN FIBRIN FORMATION

Centrifugation of native whole blood (at 4°C) to remove platelets results in a prolonged coagulation time. If the platelets are added back to the blood sample, coagulation takes place within 5–6 s. This demonstrates the remarkable contribution of platelets to coagulation. Is this due to the entire platelet or to a fraction derived therefrom? Specifically, a total phospholipid extract or certain lipids purified therefrom can replace the platelet in an in vitro coagulation system. This is essentially the basis of the partial thromboplastin time (PTT) (89). If the clot-promoting activity of the phospholipid is compared to that of isolated platelet membranes or intact platelets, at least 20 times more phospholipid is required to achieve the same coagulation time as induced by the isolated platelet membrane. In hemostasis and thrombosis, activated platelets promote coagulation via the phospholipoprotein component of the plasma membrane, which undergoes a rearrangement favoring it as a "catalytic lipoprotein platform" for assembly of coagulation factors.

The rearranged platelet surface catalyzes conversion of prothrombin to thrombin through exposure of high-affinity receptors for activated coagulation factor V. Factor V can originate via α-granule release or factor V in the plasma milieu. Bound, activated factor V in the presence of calcium becomes a receptor for activated coagulation factor X (Xa). Activated factor V can bind to either resting or activated platelets. This is probably related to the fact that it is virtually impossible to prepare a totally quiescent platelet suspension. Even gently washed platelets develop procoagulant activity as a consequence of the maneuver. Interestingly, platelet transfusions can improve hemostasis in patients with factor V deficiency. Thus, factor V must have been bound to the surface of the infused platelets. Activated platelets are also involved in factor X activation by providing their phospholipoprotein surface for factor IXa in the presence of factor VIII and calcium (the "tenase" system) (147).

A link between hemostasis and coagulation has been demonstrated by Walsh (87,148). Thus, ADP-stimulated platelets can induce activation of factor XII (Hageman factor). This is defined as "contact product-forming activity" and represents one of the earliest stages in the hemostatic and/or thrombotic process. Activation of factor XI by collagen-stimulated platelets has also been reported by Walsh (87,148).

As coagulation proceeds, platelet-bound factors Xa and XIa are protected from inactivation by natural inhibitors in plasma. These prothrombotic effects of platelets on coagulation may explain why hemostatic defects in patients with thromboasthenia (deficiency in GPIIb/IIIa) and hemophilia are variable. Also, it is anecdotally reported that patients with hemophilia can develop coronary thrombosis. Furthermore, the platelet procoagulant activities discussed may be responsible for the absence of spontaneous hemorrhage in patients with factor XII, prekallikrein, and high-molecular-weight kininogen deficiencies. Activated, procoagulant platelets can bypass components of the early contact system and activate factors XII and XI directly.

As the platelet thrombus expands, it occludes the lumen of the blood vessel and undergoes contraction and consolidation, leading to retraction under the influence of evolving thrombin (7,149). Plasma and platelets contain "thromboregulators" which inhibit activated coagulation factors (9). Further thrombin formation and activation are inhibited so that its action is limited to the injury site ("late thromboregulation"). For example, antithrombin III inactivates serine proteases such as thrombin via peptide binding, creating stable high-molecular-weight complexes. Heparin will strongly potentiate the action of antithrombin III. This is also true of heparin cofactor II—a thrombin inhibitor—as well as α_2-macroglobulin, α_2-antiplasmin, and α_2-antitrypsin. Late thromboregulation is probably very important, given increasing evidence for continuing activation of the coagulation system in patients with unstable angina and myocardial infarction (150).

There is also an inhibitor system which blocks action of coagulation cofactors V and VII (130). Concomitant with thrombin formation, it binds to a receptor on the surface of endothelial cells known as thrombomodulin. The thrombin–thrombomodulin complex activates a vitamin K-dependent serine protease, protein C. Activated protein C, in the presence of its cofactor protein S, inactivates factors Va and VIIIa on the platelet surface. In addition, activated protein C increases fibrinolysis.

Another component of the late thromboregulation system is the tissue factor pathway inhibitor (TFPI). The TFPI complexes with factors VIIa and IXa as well as tissue factor in order to block this pathway. All of these plasma inhibitors of activated coagulation factors are categorized as "late thromboregulators" because they operate *after* thrombin has formed (9,130).

CONTROL SYSTEMS FOR PLATELET REACTIVITY

During the early phases of hemostasis and thrombosis, agonist systems are in place to expand and consolidate the platelet mass in order to arrest bleeding. Even under these hemostatic conditions, control systems are brought into play which confine the hemostatic plug to the local site of injury. In coronary atherosclerosis, where plaque rupture will expose collagen to flowing blood, platelet aggregation and thrombus formation are uncontrolled and lead to occlusive thrombi which obstruct the coronary artery and lead to myocardial infarction. Therapeutic endeavors must be developed in the future to reverse platelet accumulation and bring platelets back to resting levels (as in the case of the endothelial cell ectoADPase) (22,46,71,151).

There are negatively charged proteoglycans on the vessel surface which will repel platelets electrostatically (platelets are also negatively charged). Under in vivo hemostatic (and probably thrombotic) conditions, blood flow with its inherent shear force represents an important modality for controlling the platelet response to injury (11,123). The quantity of platelets arriving at the injury site and the duration of time they adhere to the damaged surface or fissure influence formation of a cohesive aggregate with other platelets. This is directly related to velocity of blood flow. The flow of blood will also determine the shear rate to which platelets are subjected as they adhere to the vessel wall. Shear rate is a manifestation of forces induced by relative velocities in laminar flow of parallel, adjacent layers of a fluid entity. Erythrocytes geographically occupy the center of the axial stream in blood vessels. Thereby they mechanically increase the quantity of platelets directed proximally to the vessel wall. If the platelets have been activated, erythrocytes will further promote platelet reactivity (51). Velocity of flow decreases proximal to the vessel wall. This decreases the flow rate of platelets. Erythrocytes and platelets are in collision at all times (107). As mentioned, such collision allows erythrocytes to respond to the presence of a platelet releasate by production of proaggregatory material which will enhance platelet reactivity (52). Low-dose aspirin therapy does not reduce this erythrocyte activity ex vivo (152).

Platelets in the circulation are not activated as long as the endothelial lining of blood vessels is biochemically and physically intact. Proof of this is that such platelets maintain their disk form—the criterion for the resting state. It would appear that platelets produce and/or transport a substance(s) which maintains the integrity of the vasculature. This substance(s) appears to be inhibitory for spontaneous nontraumatic hemorrhage and probably accounts for the therapeutic effect of platelet transfusions (2).

When platelets are activated as a consequence of injury, intact endothelial cells respond by attempting to limit or reverse the accumulating platelet mass. The platelets are in a state of active recruitment via their releasate. We have defined this endothelial response to platelet activation, adhesion, and aggregation as *thromboregulation* (9,153). Systems have been developed to study thromboregulation in vitro. Experiments are carried out using combined suspensions of cultured human umbilical vein endothelial cells and human platelets in motion in aggregometer cuvettes (73,154). A high degree of cell density is achieved, thereby maximizing biochemical events that result from cell–cell interactions. Functional and biochemical parameters are measured simultaneously. All experiments culminate in a constant result: When in proximity to endothelial cells, platelets are unresponsive to all agonists. Our current experimental data indicate that this unresponsiveness is due to at least three individual endothelial cell regulatory systems: the eicosanoids, endothelium-derived relaxing factor or nitric oxide (EDRF/NO) (74,155,156), and an ectonucleotidase on the surface of the endothelial cell (ATP-diphosphohydrolase, ATPDase). This enzyme can metabolize ADP and ATP, both of which are released from activated platelets (46,157,158). We believe that the thrombotic complications of atherosclerosis can be interpreted as a pathologic breakdown of these defense systems (4,159).

Eicosanoid metabolism in endothelial cells can be induced experimentally by natural agonists such as thrombin and collagen or the model agonist ionophore A23187. Prostacyclin is the most important biologically active product of eicosanoid metabolism in endothelial cells. PGI_2 is derived from the same endoperoxide (PGH_2) which in platelets is transformed to thromboxane A_2 (Fig. 2). PGI_2 released from activated endothelial cells reacts with the platelet surface domain of its receptor, which then initiates a G-protein-linked signal transduction pathway, culminating in activation of adenylyl cyclase. The cyclase catalyzes formation of the second messenger cAMP from ATP (44,57). In contrast to most other cells, where cAMP promotes reactivity, an increase of cAMP in platelets evokes strong inhibition. Importantly, elevated cAMP blocks calcium-mediated responsiveness (58,136). The overall platelet-inhibitory effects of elevated cAMP are mediated by a cAMP-dependent protein kinase(s) (44,58). The action of these mediators is classified as "early thromboregulation," i.e., their effects take place *prior* to thrombin formation. We believe that control of early thromboregulatory events constitutes the most favorable form of antithrombotic and antiatherosclerotic therapeutics. Research efforts in our laboratory are now geared toward upregulation of endothelial cell ectoADPase activity.

Endothelin is a peptide with extremely powerful vasoconstrictor properties. It was initially isolated from supernatants of cultured aortic endothelial cells. A precursor peptide, preproendothelin, is processed proteolytically to endothelin itself. Intravenous injection of endothelin results in a sustained rise in arterial blood pressure which persists for 40–60 min. Structurally, endothelin demonstrates regional homologies to several peptide neurotoxins. Induction of biologic activity requires calcium influx and endothelin production is regulated at the mRNA transcriptional level. Vascular endothelium contains two different endothelin receptors: ET-1 and ET-2. These are selective vasoconstrictor receptors, demonstrating selectivity and located on vascular smooth muscle. In addition, there are two nonselective endothelin receptors on vascular endothelium which, paradoxically, mediate vasodilatation, ET_A and ET_B (160). However, the mechanism by which ET_B induces vasodilatation is not known (160). Thus, endothelin has not yet been placed into direct or indirect perspective with regard to thrombosis and atherosclerosis. Endothelin does not appear to be involved in autacoid responses, but rather appears to be involved in changes of long duration. This might include hypertension, ulcerogenic disease, and toxicity to drugs such as cyclosporine (161).

THERAPEUTIC APPROACHES TO OCCLUSIVE VASCULAR DISEASES VIA INHIBITION OF PLATELET REACTIVITY

Since platelets are the critical component of arterial thrombi, it is natural to assume that inhibition of platelet function could have a protective effect in prevention and/or treatment of cardiovascular events. A daily dose of aspirin (325–650 mg, high dose), ingested by 8,000 males without symptoms protected participants from a detectable episode of coronary or cerebral thrombosis (reviewed in ref. 162). At these levels of aspirin no prostacyclin would have been produced. Thus, beneficial results can be obtained in the absence of a ''protective effect'' of prostacyclin.

Subsequent observations on prolongation of the bleeding time by aspirin led to the conclusion that platelets were involved as target compounds for the drug. In particular, the platelets had been acetylated by the acetyl group from aspirin. The salicylate moiety was not involved in the therapeutic effect (162). The next major step involved the demonstration that aspirin had blocked formation of thromboxane A_2 (34,162). We can broadly summarize all of the randomized clinical trials involving aspirin by saying that 20–30% of patients treated with aspirin will experience a significant reduction of vascular events. The fact that about 70% of patients who are treated with aspirin do not benefit from it indicates that although such therapy is a step forward and constitutes the best we have, it is far from satisfactory, mainly because not enough patients on aspirin receive therapeutic benefit and/or protection.

In Vitro Observations Involving Eicosanoid–Platelet Interactions

It has not been possible to test thromboxane A_2 as a platelet agonist, because of its extremely short half-life. However, purified endoperoxides and endoperoxide analogs which presumably act on the thromboxane receptor have been tested as platelet agonists in our own and other laboratories. As mentioned, these compounds induce a full aggregation curve, but serotonin release amounts to approximately 28%. This would fall into our classification as a weak agonist (collagen and thrombin, strong agonists, induce 60–85% serotonin release). We have concluded that aspirin is actually inhibiting a relatively weak agonist. Results of most randomized clinical trials of aspirin as an antithrombotic agent show that this medication is of definite benefit in about 30% of patients who are treated (10,151,162–166). Since aspirin therapy inhibits cyclooxygenase 100% of the time, why do 70% of the patients receive no benefit? Perhaps it is because thromboxane A_2 is a weak agonist. Alternatively, it might mean that the protective effect of aspirin involves other metabolic pathways which have not yet been elucidated. These comments are in no way derogatory, because aspirin remains one of the best therapeutic modalities yet developed for myocardial infarction, stroke, and alleviation of pathologic effects of vascular events in general (10,162).

Ex Vivo Studies of Aspirin-Treated Platelets

If we isolate platelets from a volunteer who ingested aspirin, several interesting phenomena occur. If we stimulate the platelets alone or in suspension with neutrophils (5,56,73), several biochemical events occur. When the aspirin-treated platelets are activated, they release large quantities of arachidonic acid which can then interact with other cells such as neutrophils and become processed by their 5-lipoxygenase enzyme. These 5-lipoxygenase metabolites may play a role in vascular disease which has not yet been defined. In addition, aspirin-treated platelets release 12-hydroxyeicosatetraenoic acid (12-HETE) and continue to do so as long as free arachidonate is available. 12-HETE penetrates other cells and is also metabolized to new compounds (transcellular metabolism) (112,154). Thus, aspirin-treated platelets constitute a viable metabolic entity which may result in additional protective mechanisms, unrelated to cyclooxygenase inhibition (10,151).

Current Concepts of Aspirin Therapy in Cardiovascular Disease

1. Acute myocardial infarction. When patients are seen well within 12 h of onset of symptoms, intravenous thrombo-

lytic therapy is the treatment of choice. In most clinical trials, aspirin has been administered simultaneously in chewable form (a loading dose of 325 mg followed by maintenance with 160 mg). In relation to thrombolysis, there may be active thrombin adsorbed to the fibrin or elaborated from the clot (10,70,151). Aspirin may reduce platelet reactivity in these circumstances. When aspirin is used as an adjuvant to thrombolysis, the beneficial effects are enhanced in a manner which is unrelated to the specific thrombolytic agent employed. The reocclusion rate and incidence of recurrent ischemia are markedly reduced with this therapeutic regime (10).

2. Aspirin in unstable angina. These patients have transient episodes of coronary vasoconstriction, probably related to intermittent disruption or fissuring of atherosclerotic plaques. Although results reported by different investigators have not been in complete agreement, aspirin is indicated for all patients. Heparin is useful during the acute phase and aspirin (75–325 mg/day) should be continued on a long-term basis (10).

3. Aspirin as secondary prophylaxis following an acute myocardial infarction. Since many of these patients have a lower threshold for ventricular arrhythmia, dysfunction of the left ventricle, and subsequent reinfarction, evaluation of therapeutic results is difficult. Many clinical trials have been carried out to evaluate this question. The general consensus, based on meta-analysis of several published trials, was that inhibition of platelet reactivity by aspirin reduced cardiovascular mortality by 13%, nonfatal reinfarction by 31%, nonfatal stroke by 42%, and all significant vascular events by 25%. High-dose aspirin (900–1,500 mg/day) was no more effective than 325 mg/day. This, again, rules out a protective effect of prostacyclin. Importantly, it could be concluded that aspirin therapy could reduce the risk of fatal and nonfatal cardiovascular events by 25% in patients who survive an initial myocardial infarction (10,163).

4. Aspirin therapeutics in stable angina. We now know that atherosclerotic plaques can continue to expand by virtue of gradual mural thrombosis and fibromuscular proliferation of the unstable type, and may progress to myocardial infarction. Several studies have concluded that if these patients are identified, a single daily dose of 160 mg aspirin effectively reduced the occurrence of myocardial infarction and sudden death by 34% (10,163).

5. Aspirin for primary prevention of cardiovascular disease. As mentioned, when all studies are taken together, aspirin is effective in reducing cardiovascular events by almost 25%. Examination of aspirin's effectiveness in volunteers is a more difficult task. Five thousand English physicians took 500 mg aspirin daily for a period of 6 years (164–166). At that time point, there was no significant difference between the treated groups and controls with regard to cardiovascular events, myocardial infarction, stroke, and total cardiovascular mortality. The incidence of stroke was slightly increased in the treated group. In contrast, 22,000 American physicians who took 325 mg aspirin every other day for 4.8 years demonstrated a 44% reduction in the incidence of myocardial infarction from 0.44% to 0.24% per year. There was also an increase in hemorrhagic stroke in the aspirin-treated group. Summarizing both studies: Aspirin ingestion resulted in a 32% reduction in nonfatal infarction and a 13% decrease in cardiovascular events. There was no difference in total mortality. An increase in the risk of stroke was present but not significant (10,163).

6. Prevention of vascular occlusion during and after percutaneous transluminal coronary angioplasty and coronary artery bypass surgery. Although aspirin therapy has been effective in preventing periprocedural acute occlusive events and ischemic complications, therapy to reduce platelet reactivity or even anticoagulants has not reduced rates of restenosis. This is especially true after coronary angioplasty.

Following coronary angioplasty, there is frequently a somewhat symmetrical smooth muscle proliferative response that leads to restenosis of the vessel lumen. Speir and associates recently examined this question in detail (167). Their results suggest that in some angioplasty patients, restenosis may be triggered by activation of latent human cytomegalovirus (HCMV), an organism which had been previously associated with the development of atherosclerosis in animal models. The virus expresses a protein known as 1E84 which binds to smooth muscle cell p53, a protein known to suppress tumor growth and block progression of the cell cycle. This binding inactivates the p53 by blocking its ability to activate transcriptionally a reporter gene. This confers a selective growth advantage on the infected smooth muscle cells. These interesting early conclusions were drawn from a study of 60 human restenosis lesions, in 38% of which large quantities of measurable p53 protein correlated with the presence of HCMV. In normal cells p53 has a short half-life and is immunohistochemically undetectable. However, in cases where p53 loses its inhibitory function, such as by mutation in malignancies or when bound by inhibitory proteins such as 1E84, p53 protein often displays enhanced stability and is detectable by immunostaining. Culture of smooth muscle cells from lesions revealed that they were expressing 1E84. HCMV infection of normal cultured smooth muscle cells also enhanced p53 accumulation which correlated temporally with 1E84 expression. These initial experiments of Speir et al. indicate that HCMV, through 1E84-mediated inhibition of p53, could contribute to restenosis (167,168). Thus, we now have at least one tentative explanation for the disturbing occurrence of restenosis following coronary angioplasty. This also may provide an additional hypothesis as to why no therapeutic modalities have been successful in preventing restenosis. Follow-up studies extending this concept will be of great interest.

With regard to prevention of early vein graft occlusion, it is now recommended that aspirin be initiated immediately after surgery (within 48 h) and that aspirin be continued indefinitely (10,163).

CLINICAL TRIALS INVOLVING GPIIB/IIIA RECEPTOR BLOCKADE WITH A MONOCLONAL ANTIBODY: RESULTS IN PATIENTS UNDERGOING CORONARY ANGIOPLASTY

As already discussed, following injury to normal vessels or fracture of an atherosclerotic plaque, adhesive glycoproteins which are recognized by specific platelet receptors are exposed. The initial layer of adherent platelets is activated and recruits additional platelets into the evolving thrombus. Platelet aggregation (cohesion) itself is modulated by the GPIIb/IIIa receptor interacting with the adhesive glycoprotein fibrinogen and/or von Willebrand factor. The adhesion process itself as well as shear forces can serve as activating agents for platelets (19). Furthermore, we know that proteins of the thrombolytic system can activate platelets in their own right or via promotion of plasmin or thrombin formation (107,169).

Coller and associates developed a monoclonal antibody 7E3 which could block the GPIIb/IIIa receptor and inhibit platelet reactivity ex vivo (17–19). Studies in animal models of myocardial infarction managed with thrombolytic agents revealed that 7E3 induced rapid reperfusion and blocked reocclusion of the vessel. Platelet-rich thrombi which had resisted lysis by thrombolytic agents by themselves were also dispersed by the antibody. Reduction in dosage of the thrombolytic agent was also possible. Subsequently, a chimeric variant of the Fab fragment of 7E3 was developed (c7E3 Fab) for human volunteers. At a dose of 0.25 mg/kg the antibody blocks 80% of the GPIIb/IIIa receptors and virtually eliminates platelet aggregation. Recently, a prospective, randomized, double-blind study was carried out on 2,099 patients in 56 institutions (18,19,108). The patients were candidates for coronary angioplasty or atherectomy and were clinically at high risk. The risk situations included severe unstable angina, evolving acute myocardial infarction, or angiographic evidence of high-risk coronary artery disease. The time frame of the study was 30 days following randomization and endpoints included any of the following events: death, nonfatal myocardial infarction or urgent requirement for surgical revascularization, repeat percutaneous angioplasty, implantation of a coronary stent, or insertion of an intraaortic balloon pump for untreatable ischemia.

The bolus of c7E3 Fab followed by infusion induced a 35% reduction in the rate of the primary endpoint. With c7E3 Fab bolus alone, the reduction was 10%, which did not differ significantly from placebo controls. Hemorrhage with a transfusion requirement was more frequent in the patients receiving the c7E3 Fab bolus and infusion than in other groups. Bleeding at the femoral puncture site was most common. All patients were treated with aspirin and heparin. The aspirin was given 2 h prior to angioplasty or atherectomy and daily thereafter (325 mg). A bolus dose of heparin was given intravenously (10,000–12,000 units) followed by incremental doses of bolus up to 3,000 units at 15-min intervals. The maximal dose of heparin administered during the procedure was 20,000 units.

Results of the study after 6 months were reported (108). There was a reduction in requirement for subsequent revascularization procedures, therefore implying less occurrence of clinical restenosis. It was also reported that although the infusion was maintained for 12 h, inhibition of platelet reactivity extended over a period of days. This suggested that the antibody had "passivated" the vessel surface in a manner which decreased its thrombogenicity. It will be of interest to correlate these results with those reported by Speir and associates (167,168) concerning the cytomegalovirus–p53 interaction as an explanation for restenosis. In the Speir series of 60 patients, 23 (38%) were p53-immunopositive. Perhaps the remainder of the patients might have responded to c7E3 Fab therapy.

Results of these trials verify that activated platelets accumulating on the vessel wall and recruiting other platelets into the expanding mass are the major offenders in restenosis and subsequent ischemic events.

ACKNOWLEDGMENTS

I wish to thank Dr. M. J. Broekman, Evelyn M. Ludwig, Lenore B. Safier, and Dr. Joan H. Fliessbach for their critical review and comments during the preparation of this chapter.

REFERENCES

1. Sixma JJ. Interaction of blood platelets with the vessel wall. In: Bloom AL, Forbes CD, Thomas DP, Tuddenham EGD, eds. *Haemostasis and Thrombosis,* 3rd ed, Vol 1. Edinburgh: Churchill Livingstone; 1994;259–285.
2. Marcus AJ. Platelets and their disorders. In: Ratnoff OD, Forbes CD, eds. *Disorders of Hemostasis,* 3rd ed. Philadelphia: Saunders; 1994.
3. Ross R. The pathogenesis of atherosclerosis: A perspective for the 1990s. *Nature* 1993;362:801–809.
4. Ross R. Atherosclerosis: A defense mechanism gone awry. *Am J Pathol* 1993;143:987–1002.
5. Marcus AJ. Cellular interactions of platelets in thrombosis. In: Loscalzo J, Schafer AI, eds. *Thrombosis and Hemorrhage.* Boston: Blackwell Scientific; 1994;279–289.
6. Marcus AJ, Hajjar DP. Vascular transcellular signalling. *J Lipid Res* 1993;34:2017–2032.
7. Harker LA. Platelets and vascular thrombosis. *N Engl J Med* 1994; 330:1006–1007.
8. Hathaway WE, Goodnight SH Jr. *Disorders of Hemostasis and Thrombosis. A Clinical Guide.* New York: McGraw-Hill; 1993.
9. Marcus AJ, Safier LB. Thromboregulation: Multicenter modulation of platelet reactivity in hemostasis and thrombosis. *FASEB J* 1993; 7:516–522.
10. Stein B. Antithrombotic therapy in cardiovascular disease: In: Loscalzo J, Schafer AI, eds. *Thrombosis and Hemorrhage.* Boston: Blackwell Scientific; 1994;1253–1274.
11. Ruggeri ZM. Mechanisms of shear-induced platelet adhesion and aggregation. *Thromb Haemostasis* 1993;70:119–123.
12. Ruggeri ZM, Ware J. von Willebrand factor. *FASEB J* 1993;7: 308–316.
13. Roth GJ. Developing relationships: Arterial platelet adhesion, glycoprotein Ib, and leucine-rich glycoproteins. *Blood* 1991;77:5–19.
14. Rabinowitz I, Randi AM, Shindler KS, et al. Type IIb mutation His-505 → Asp implicates a new segment in the control of von Willebrand

factor binding to platelet glycoprotein Ib. *J Biol Chem* 1993;268: 20497–20501.
15. Hickey MJ, Hagen FS, Yagi M, et al. Human platelet glycoprotein V: Characterization of the polypeptide and the related Ib-VI-IX receptor system of adhesive, leucine-rich glycoproteins. *Proc Natl Acad Sci USA* 1993;90:8327–8331.
16. Plow EF, Ginsberg MH. The molecular basis of platelet function. In: Hoffman R, Benz EJ Jr, Shattil SJ, Furie B, Cohen HJ, eds. *Hematology. Basic Principles and Practice*. New York: Churchill Livingstone; 1991;1165–1176.
17. Coller BS, Kutok JL, Scudder LE, et al. Studies of activated GPIIb/IIIa receptors on the luminal surface of adherent platelets. Paradoxical loss of luminal receptors when platelets adhere to high density fibrinogen. *J Clin Invest* 1993;92:2796–2806.
18. EPIC Investigators. Use of a monoclonal antibody directed against the platelet glycoprotein IIb/IIIa receptor in high-risk coronary angioplasty. *N Engl J Med* 1994;330:956–961.
19. Coller BS. Platelet GPIIb/IIIa inhibition by monoclonal antibodies, with observations on blood vessel wall passivation after angioplasty injury. 1994 *[unpublished]*.
20. Sadler JE. von Willebrand Factor. *J Biol Chem* 1991;266: 22777–22780.
21. Fressinaud E, Federici AB, Castaman G, et al. The role of platelet von Willebrand factor in platelet adhesion and thrombus formation: A study of 34 patients with various subtypes of type I von Willebrand disease. *Br J Haematol* 1994;86:327–332.
22. Flores NA, Sheridan DJ. The pathophysiological role of platelets during myocardial ischaemia. *Cardiovasc Res* 1994;28:295–302.
23. Packham MA. Role of platelets in thrombosis and hemostasis. *Can J Physiol Pharmacol* 1994;72:278–284.
24. Berman CL, Yeo EL, Wencel-Drake JD, et al. A platelet alpha granule membrane protein that is associated with the plasma membrane after activation. Characterization and subcellular localization of platelet activation-dependent granule-external membrane protein. *J Clin Invest* 1986;78:130–137.
25. McEver RP. Leukocyte interactions mediated by selectins. *Thromb Haemostasis* 1991;66:80–87.
26. Bevilacqua MP, Nelson RM. Selectins. *J Clin Invest* 1993;91: 379–387.
27. Johnston GI, Cook RG, McEver RP. Cloning of GMP-140, a granule membrane protein of platelets and endothelium: Sequence similarity to proteins involved in cell adhesion and inflammation. *Cell* 1989; 56:1033–1044.
28. Lorant DE, Topham MK, Whatley RE, et al. Inflammatory roles of P-selectin. *J Clin Invest* 1993;92:559–570.
29. Crovello CS, Furie BC, Furie B. Rapid phosphorylation and selective dephosphorylation of P-selectin accompanies platelet activation. *J Biol Chem* 1993;268:14590–14593.
30. Mayadas TN, Johnson RC, Rayburn H, et al. Leukocyte rolling and extravasation are severely compromised in P selectin-deficient mice. *Cell* 1993;74:541–554.
31. Kramer RM, Roberts EF, Manetta JV, et al. Thrombin-induced phosphorylation and activation of Ca^{2+}-sensitive cytosolic phospholipase A_2 in human platelets. *J Biol Chem* 1993;268:26796–26804.
32. Majerus PW. Platelets. In: Stamatoyannopoulos G, Nienhuis AW, Majerus PW, Varmus H, eds. *The Molecular Basis of Blood Diseases*, 2nd ed. Philadelphia: Saunders; 1994;753–785.
33. Meade EA, Smith WL, DeWitt DL. Differential inhibition of prostaglandin endoperoxide synthase (cyclooxygenase) isozymes by aspirin and other nonsteroidal anti-inflammatory drugs. *J Biol Chem* 1993; 268:6610–6614.
34. Lecomte M, Laneuville O, Ji C, et al. Acetylation of human prostaglandin endoperoxide synthase-2 (cyclooxygenase-2) by aspirin. *J Biol Chem* 1994;269:13207–13215.
35. Ohashi K, Ruan K-H, Kulmacz RJ, et al. Primary structure of human thromboxane synthase determined from the cDNA sequence. *J Biol Chem* 1992;267:789–793.
36. Smith WL. Prostanoid biosynthesis and mechanisms of action. *Am J Physiol* 1992;263:F181–F191.
37. Funk CD, Funk LB, FitzGerald GA, et al. Characterization of human 12-lipoxygenase genes. *Proc Natl Acad Sci USA* 1992;89:3962–3966.
38. Chen X-S, Funk CD. Structure–function properties of human platelet 12-lipoxygenase: Chimeric enzyme and *in vitro* mutagenesis studies. *FASEB J* 1993;7:694–701.
39. Rao AK. Congenital disorders of platelet function. *Hematol Oncol Clin N Am* 1990;4:65–86.
40. Hourani SMO, Hall DA. Receptors for ADP on human blood platelets. *Trends Pharmacol Sci* 1994;15:103–108.
41. Marcus AJ. Platelet arachidonic acid metabolism. In: Harker LA, Zimmerman TS, eds. *Methods in Hematology*. Vol 8. *Measurements of Platelet Function*. New York: Churchill Livingstone; 1983;126–143.
42. Brass LF. The biochemistry of platelet activation. In: Hoffman R, Benz EJ Jr, Shattil SJ, Furie B, Cohen HJ, eds. *Hematology. Basic Principles and Practice*. New York: Churchill Livingstone; 1991; 1176–1197.
43. Brass LF, Hoxie JA, Manning DR. Signaling through G proteins and G protein-coupled receptors during platelet activation. *Thromb Haemostasis* 1993;70:217–223.
44. Brass LF, Hoxie JA, Kieber-Emmons T, et al. Agonist receptors and G proteins as mediators of platelet activation. *Adv Exp Med Biol* 1993; 344:17–36.
45. Cristalli G, Mills DCB. Identification of a receptor for ADP on blood platelets by photoaffinity labelling. *Biochem J* 1993;291:875–881.
46. Marcus AJ, Safier LB, Hajjar KA, et al. Inhibition of platelet function by an aspirin-insensitive endothelial cell ADPase. Thromboregulation by endothelial cells. *J Clin Invest* 1991;88:1690–1696.
47. Zucker MB, Katz IR. Platelet factor 4: Production, structure, and physiologic and immunologic action. *Proc Soc Exp Biol Med* 1991; 198:693–702.
48. Niewiarowski S. Secreted platelet proteins. In: Bloom AL, Forbes CD, Thomas DP, Tuddenham EGD, eds. *Haemostasis and Thrombosis*, 3rd ed. Vol 1. Edinburgh: Churchill Livingstone; 1994;167–181.
49. Holmsen H. Platelet secretion and energy metabolism. In: Colman RW, Hirsh J, Marder VJ, Salzman EW, eds. *Hemostasis and Thrombosis: Basic Principles and Clinical Practice*, 3rd ed. Philadelphia: Lippincott; 1994;524–545.
50. Furman MI, Gardner TM, Goldschmidt-Clermont PJ. Mechanisms of cytoskeletal reorganization during platelet activation. *Thromb Haemostasis* 1993;70:229–232.
51. Santos MT, Valles J, Marcus AJ, et al. Enhancement of platelet reactivity and modulation of eicosanoid production by intact erythrocytes. *J Clin Invest* 1991;87:571–580.
52. Valles J, Santos MT, Aznar J, et al. Erythrocytes metabolically enhance collagen-induced platelet responsiveness via increased thromboxane production, ADP release, and recruitment. *Blood* 1991;78: 154–162.
53. Serhan CN. Components of the arachidonic acid signalling cascade: A brief update and hypothesis. In: Hedqvist P, Kalden JR, Muller-Peddinghaus R, Robinson DR, eds. *Bayer Rheuma Workshop: Trends in RA-Research*. Basel: Eular; 1991;141–153.
54. Serhan CN. Lipoxin biosynthesis and its impact in inflammatory and vascular events. *Biochim Biophys Acta* 1994;1212:1–25.
55. Serhan CN. Eicosanoids in leukocyte function. *Curr Opin Hematol* 1994;1:69–77.
56. Marcus AJ. Multicellular eicosanoid and other metabolic interactions of platelets and other cells. In: Colman RW, Hirsh J, Marder VJ, Salzman EW, eds. *Hemostasis and Thrombosis: Basic Principles and Clinical Practice*, 3rd ed. Philadelphia: Lippincott; 1994;590–602.
57. Brass LF, Poncz M, Manning DR. G proteins and the early events of platelet activation. In: Lapetina EG, Bittar EE, eds. *The Platelet*; 1993.
58. Kroll MH. Mechanisms of platelet activation. In: Loscalzo J, Schafer AI, eds. *Thrombosis and Hemorrhage*. Boston: Blackwell Scientific; 1994;247–277.
59. Hla T, Neilson K. Human cyclooxygenase-2 cDNA. *Proc Natl Acad Sci USA* 1992;89:7384–7388.
60. Jones DA, Carlton DP, McIntyre TM, et al. Molecular cloning of human prostaglandin endoperoxide synthase type II and demonstration of expression in response to cytokines. *J Biol Chem* 1993;268: 9049–9054.
61. Vane JR, Mitchell JA, Appleton I, et al. Inducible isoforms of cyclooxygenase and nitric-oxide synthase in inflammation. *Proc Natl Acad Sci USA* 1994;91:2046–2050.
62. Masferrer JL, Zweifel BS, Manning PT, et al. Selective inhibition of inducible cyclooxygenase 2 *in vivo* is antiinflammatory and nonulcerogenic. *Proc Natl Acad Sci USA* 1994;91:3228–3232.
63. O'Neill GP, Ford-Hutchinson AW. Expression of mRNA for cyclooxygenase-1 and cyclooxygenase-2 in human tissues. *FEBS Lett* 1993; 330:156–160.

64. Packham MA, Kinlough-Rathbone RL. Mechanisms of atherogenesis and thrombosis. In: Bloom AL, Forbes CD, Thomas DP, Tuddenham EGD, eds. *Haemostasis and Thrombosis,* 3rd ed, Vol 2. Edinburgh: Churchill Livingstone; 1994;1107–1138.
65. Stary HC, Chandler AB, Glagov S, et al. A definition of initial, fatty streak, and intermediate lesions of atherosclerosis. A report from the committee on vascular lesions of the Council on Arteriosclerosis, American Heart Association. *Circulation* 1992;89:2462–2478.
66. Coughlin SR, Vu T-KH, Hung DT, et al. Characterization of a functional thrombin receptor. Issues and opportunities. *J Clin Invest* 1992; 89:351–355.
67. George JN, Torres MM. Thrombin decreases von Willebrand factor binding to platelet glycoprotein Ib. *Blood* 1988;71:1253–1259.
68. Woolf N. Thrombosis. In: McGee JO, Isaacson PG, Wright NA, eds. *Oxford Textbook of Pathology.* Oxford: Oxford University Press; 1992;509–519.
69. Craig EA, Weissman JS, Horwich AL. Heat shock proteins and molecular chaperones: Mediators of protein conformation and turnover in the cell. *Cell* 1994;78:365–372.
70. Szczeklik A, Dropinski J, Radwan J, et al. Persistent generation of thrombin after acute myocardial infarction. *Arterioscler Thromb* 1992; 12:548–553.
71. DiCorleto PE. Cellular mechanisms of atherogenesis. *Am J Hypertens* 1993;6(Suppl):314S–318S.
72. Pearson JD. Endothelial cell biology. In: Bloom AL, Forbes CD, Thomas DP, Tuddenham EGD, eds. *Haemostasis and Thrombosis,* 3rd ed, Vol 1. Edinburgh: Churchill Livingstone; 1994;219–232.
73. Marcus AJ. Eicosanoid interactions between platelets, endothelial cells, and neutrophils. *Meth Enzymol* 1990;187:585–598.
74. Broekman MJ, Eiroa AM, Marcus AJ. Inhibition of human platelet reactivity by endothelium-derived relaxing factor from human umbilical vein endothelial cells in suspension. Blockade of aggregation and secretion by an aspirin-insensitive mechanism. *Blood* 1991;78: 1033–1040.
75. Coughlin SR. Thrombin receptor function and cardiovascular disease. *Trends Cardiovasc Med* 1994;4:77–83.
76. Nelken NA, Soifer SJ, O'Keefe J, et al. Thrombin receptor expression in normal and atherosclerotic human arteries. *J Clin Invest* 1992;90: 1614–1621.
77. Coughlin SR. Thrombin receptor structure and function. *Thromb Haemostasis* 1993;70:184–187.
78. Gewirtz AM, Poncz M. Megakaryocytopoiesis and platelet function. In: Hoffman R, Benz EJ Jr, Shattil SJ, Furie B, Cohen HJ, eds. *Hematology. Basic Principles and Practice.* New York: Churchill Livingstone; 1991;1148–1157.
79. Isenberg WM, Bainton DF. Megakaryocytes and platelet structure. In: Hoffman R, Benz EJ Jr, Shattil SJ, Furie B, Cohen HJ, eds. *Hematology. Basic Principles and Practice.* New York: Churchill Livingstone; 1991;1157–1165.
80. Metcalf D. Thrombopoietin—at last. *Nature* 1994;369:519–520.
81. Souyri M, Vigon I, Penciolelli JF, et al. A putative truncated cytokine receptor gene transduced by the myeloproliferative leukemia virus immortalizes hematopoietic progenitors. *Cell* 1990;63:1137–1147.
82. de Sauvage FJ, Hass PE, Spencer SD, et al. Stimulation of megakaryocytopoiesis and thrombopoiesis by the c-Mpl ligand. *Nature* 1994; 369:533–538.
83. Kaushansky K, Lok S, Holly RD, et al. Promotion of megakaryocyte progenitor expansion and differentiation by the c-Mpl ligand thrombopoietin. *Nature* 1994;369:568–571.
84. Wendling F, Maraskovsky E, Debill N, et al. c-Mpl ligand is a humoral regulator of megakaryocytopoiesis. *Nature* 1994;369:571–574.
85. Lok S, Kaushansky K, Holly RD, et al. Cloning and expression of murine thrombopoietin cDNA and stimulation of platelet production *in vivo. Nature* 1994;369:565–568.
86. Lind SE. Platelet morphology. In: Loscalzo J, Schafer AI, eds. *Thrombosis and Hemorrhage.* Boston: Blackwell Scientific; 1994;201–218.
87. Ahmad SS, Rawala-Sheikh R, Walsh PN. Components and assembly of the factor X activating complex. *Semin Thromb Hemostasis* 1992; 18:311–323.
88. Zwaal RFA, Comfurius P, Bevers EM. Mechanisms and function of changes in membrane-phospholipid asymmetry in platelets and erythrocytes. *Biochem Soc Trans* 1993;21:248–253.
89. Marcus AJ, Zucker-Franklin D, Safier LB, et al. Studies on human platelet granules and membranes. *J Clin Invest* 1966;45:14–28.
90. Farkouh ME, Lang JD, Sackett DL. Thrombolytic agents: The science of the art of choosing the better treatment. *Ann Intern Med* 1994;120: 886–888.
91. Phillips DR, Charo IF, Parise LV, et al. The platelet membrane glycoprotein IIb–IIIa complex. *Blood* 1988;71:831–843.
92. Hynes RO. Integrins: Versatility, modulation, and signaling in cell adhesion. *Cell* 1992;69:11–25.
93. Kunicki TJ. Human platelet antigens. In: Benz EJ Jr, Cohen HJ, Furie B, Hoffman R, Shattil S, eds. *Hematology: Basic Principles and Practice.* New York: Churchill Livingstone; 1991;1556–1565.
94. Gralnick HR, Williams S, McKeown LP, et al. High-affinity α-thrombin binding to platelet glycoprotein Ibα: Identification of two binding domains. *Proc Natl Acad Sci USA* 1994;91:6334–6338.
95. Clemetson KJ. Biochemistry of platelet membrane glycoproteins. In: Jamieson GA, ed. *Platelet Membrane Receptors: Molecular Biology, Immunology, Biochemistry, and Pathology.* New York: Liss; 1988; 35–75.
96. Ware J, Russell SR, Marchese P, et al. Point mutation in a leucine-rich repeat of platelet glycoprotein Ibα resulting in the Bernard-Soulier syndrome. *J Clin Invest* 1993;92:1213–1220.
97. Lanza F, Morales M, De la Salle C, et al. Cloning and characterization of the gene encoding the human platelet glycoprotein V. A member of the leucine-rich glycoprotein family cleaved during thrombin-induced platelet activation. *J Biol Chem* 1993;268:20801–20807.
98. Vu T-KH, Hung DT, Wheaton VI, et al. Molecular cloning of a functional thrombin receptor reveals a novel proteolytic mechanism of receptor activation. *Cell* 1991;64:1057–1068.
99. Bray PF. Inherited diseases of platelet glycoproteins: Considerations for rapid molecular characterization. *Thromb Haemostasis* 1994;72: 492–502.
100. Shattil SJ. Regulation of platelet anchorage and signaling by integrin $\alpha_{IIb}\beta_3$. *Thromb Haemostasis* 1993;70:224–228.
101. Nurden AT. Human platelet membrane glycoproteins. In: Bloom AL, Forbes CD, Thomas DP, Tuddenham EGD, eds. *Haemostasis and Thrombosis,* 3rd ed, Vol 1. Edinburgh: Churchill Livingstone; 1994; 115–165.
102. Shulman NR, Reid DM. Platelet immunology. In: Colman RW, Hirsh J, Marder VJ, Salzman EW, eds. *Hemostasis and Thrombosis: Basic Principles and Clinical Practice.* 3rd ed. Philadelphia: Lippincott; 1994;414–468.
103. Mosesson MW. Thrombin interactions with fibrinogen and fibrin. *Semin Thromb Hemostasis* 1993;19:361–367.
104. Pierschbacher MD, Ruoslahti E. Influence of stereochemistry of the sequence Arg-Gly-Asp-Xaa on binding specificity in cell adhesion. *J Biol Chem* 1987;262:17294–17298.
105. Ruoslahti E, Pierschbacher MD. New perspectives in cell adhesion: RGD and integrins. *Science* 1987;238:491–497.
106. Leung LLK. Role of thrombospondin in platelet aggregation. *J Clin Invest* 1984;74:1764–1777.
107. Coller BS. Platelets and thrombolytic therapy. *N Engl J Med* 1990; 322:33–42.
108. Topol EJ, Califf RM, Weismann HF, et al. Randomised trial of coronary intervention with antibody against platelet IIb/IIIa integrin for reduction of clinical restenosis: Results at six months. *Lancet* 1994; 343:881–886.
109. Haskard DO. Adhesive proteins. In: Bloom AL, Forbes CD, Thomas DP, Tuddenham EGD, eds. *Haemostasis and Thrombosis,* 3rd ed, Vol 1. Edinburgh: Churchill Livingstone; 1994;233–257.
110. Albelda SM, Smith CW, Ward PA. Adhesion molecules and inflammatory injury. *FASEB J* 1994;8:504–512.
111. Ross R. The role of T lymphocytes in inflammation. *Proc Natl Acad Sci USA* 1994;91:2879.
112. Maclouf J. Transcellular biosynthesis of arachidonic acid metabolites: From *in vitro* investigations to *in vivo* reality. *Bailliere's Clin Haematol* 1993;6:593–608.
113. Vasconcellos CA, Lind SE. Coordinated inhibition of actin-induced platelet aggregation by plasma gelsolin and vitamin D-binding protein. *Blood* 1993;82:3648–3657.
114. Stossel TP. The machinery of blood cell movements. *Blood* 1994;84: 367–379.
115. Aderem A. The MARCKS brothers: A family of protein kinase C substrates. *Cell* 1992;71:713–716.
116. Tate BF, Rittenhouse SE. Thrombin activation of human platelets

causes tyrosine phosphorylation of PLC-gamma$_2$. *Biochim Biophys Acta Mol Cell Res* 1993;1178:281–285.
117. Hartwig JH. Mechanisms of actin rearrangements mediating platelet activation. *J Cell Biol* 1992;118:1421–1442.
118. Burridge K, Petch LA, Romer LH. Signals from focal adhesions. *Curr Biol* 1992;2:537–539.
119. Golden A, Brugge JS, Shattil SJ. Role of platelet membrane glycoprotein IIb–IIIa in agonist-induced tyrosine phosphorylation of platelet proteins. *J Cell Biol* 1990;111:3117–3127.
120. Lipfert L, Haimovich B, Schaller MD, et al. Integrin-dependent phosphorylation and activation of the protein tyrosine kinase pp125^{FAK} in platelets. *J Cell Biol* 1992;119:905–912.
121. Torti M, Lapetina EG. Structure and function of rap proteins in human platelets. *Thromb Haemostasis* 1994;71:533–543.
122. Torti M, Ramaschi G, Sinigaglia F, et al. Glycoprotein IIb–IIIa and the translocation of Rap2B to the platelet cytoskeleton. *Proc Natl Acad Sci USA* 1994;91:4239–4243.
123. Weiss HJ, Hawiger J, Ruggeri ZM, et al. Fibrinogen-independent platelet adhesion and thrombus formation on subendothelium mediated by glycoprotein IIb–IIIa complex at high shear rate. *J Clin Invest* 1989;83:288–297.
124. Weiss HJ. Inherited abnormalities of platelet granules and signal transduction. In: Colman RW, Hirsh J, Marder VJ, Salzman EW, eds. *Hemostasis and Thrombosis: Basic Principles and Clinical Practice.* 3rd ed. Philadelphia: Lippincott; 1994;673–684.
125. Broekman MJ, Westmoreland NP, Cohen P. An improved method for isolating alpha granules and mitochondria from human platelets. *J Cell Biol* 1974;60:507–519.
126. Broekman MJ, Handin RI, Cohen P. Distribution of fibrinogen, and platelet factors 4 and XIII in subcellular fractions of human platelets. *Br J Haematol* 1975;31:51–55.
127. Kaplan KL, Broekman MJ, Chernoff A, et al. Platelet alpha-granule proteins: Studies on release and subcellular localization. *Blood* 1979; 53:604–618.
128. Zucker MB. Platelet aggregation measured by the photometric method. *Meth Enzymol* 1989;169A:117–133.
129. Agbanyo FR, Sixma JJ, De Groot PG, et al. Thrombospondin–platelet interactions. Role of divalent cations, wall shear rate, and platelet membrane glycoproteins. *J Clin Invest* 1993;92:288–296.
130. Esmon CT. Molecular events that control the protein C anticoagulant pathway. *Thromb Haemostasis* 1993;70:29–35.
131. Bevilacqua MP, Butcher EC, Furie BC, et al. Selectins: A family of adhesion receptors. *Cell* 1991;67:233.
132. Law JH, Ribeiro JMC, Wells MA. Biochemical insights derived from insect diversity. *Annu Rev Biochem* 1992;61:87–111.
133. Gebrane-Younès J, Cramer EM, Orcel L, et al. Gray platelet syndrome. Dissociation between abnormal sorting in megakaryocyte α-granules and normal sorting in Weibel–Palade bodies of endothelial cells. *J Clin Invest* 1993;92:3023–3028.
134. Holmsen H. Biochemistry of the platelet: Energy metabolism. In: Colman RW, Hirsh J, Marder VJ, Salzman EW, eds. *Hemostasis and Thrombosis: Basic Principles and Clinical Practice.* 2nd ed. Philadelphia: Lippincott; 1987;631–643.
135. Holmsen H. Platelet secretion. In: Colman RW, Hirsh J, Marder VJ, Salzman EW, eds. *Hemostasis and Thrombosis: Basic Principles and Clinical Practice.* Philadelphia: Lippincott; 1987;606–617.
136. Kroll MH, Schafer AI. Biochemical mechanisms of platelet activation. *Blood* 1989;74:1181–1195.
137. White JG, Krumwiede M. Further studies on the secretory pathway in thrombin-stimulated platelets. *Blood* 1987;69:1196.
138. Brune B, Dimmeler S, Lapetina EG. NADPH: A stimulatory cofactor for nitric oxide-induced ADP-ribosylation reaction. *Biochem Biophys Res Commun* 1992;182:1166–1171.
139. Brass LF, Pizzaro S, Ahuja M, et al. Changes in the structure and function of the human thrombin receptor during receptor activation, internalization, and recycling. *J Biol Chem* 1994;269:2943–2952.
140. Ware JA, Johnson PC, Smith M, et al. Effect of common agonists on cytoplasmic ionized calcium concentration in platelets. Measurement with 2-methyl-6-methoxy 8-nitroquinoline (Quin2) and aequorin. *J Clin Invest* 1986;77:878–886.
141. Berridge MJ. Inositol trisphosphate and calcium signaling. *Nature* 1993;361:315–325.
142. Murad F, Forstermann U, Nakane M, et al. The nitric oxide–cyclic GMP signal transduction system for intracellular and intercellular communication. *Adv Second Messenger Phosphoprotein Res* 1993; 28:101–109.
143. Änggård E. Nitric oxide: Mediator, murderer, and medicine. *Lancet* 1994;343:1199–1206.
144. Nathan C, Xie Q-W. Regulation of biosynthesis of nitric oxide. *J Biol Chem* 1994;269:13725–13728.
145. Spiegel AM, Weinstein LS, Shenker A. Abnormalities in G protein-coupled signal transduction pathways in human disease. *J Clin Invest* 1993;92:1119–1125.
146. Sternweis PC, Smrcka AV. Regulation of phospholipase C by G proteins. *TIBS* 1992;17:502–506.
147. Ichinose A, Davie EW. The blood coagulation factors: Their cDNAs, genes, and expression. In: Colman RW, Hirsh J, Marder VJ, Salzman EW, eds. *Hemostasis and Thrombosis: Basic Principles and Clinical Practice.* 3rd ed. Philadelphia: Lippincott; 1994;19–54.
148. Walsh PN. Platelet–coagulant protein interactions. In: Colman RW, Hirsh J, Marder VJ, Salzman EW, eds. *Hemostasis and Thrombosis: Basic Principles and Clinical Practice.* 3rd ed. Philadelphia: Lippincott; 1994;629–651.
149. Bick RL, Pegram M. Syndromes of hypercoagulability and thrombosis: A review. *Semin Thromb Hemostasis* 1994;20:109.
150. Merlini PA, Bauer KA, Oltrona L, et al. Persistent activation of the coagulation mechanisms in unstable angina and myocardial infarction. *Circulation* 1994;89.
151. Fernández-Ortiz A, Jang I-K, Fuster V. Antiplatelet and antithrombin therapy. *Coron Artery Dis* 1994;5:297–305.
152. Vanin AF. Endothelium-derived relaxing factor is a nitrosyl iron complex with thiol ligands. *FEBS Lett* 1991;289:1–3.
153. Key NS. Scratching the surface: Endothelium as a regulator of thrombosis, fibrinolysis, and inflammation. *J Lab Clin Med* 1992;120: 184–186.
154. Marcus AJ, Weksler BB, Jaffe EA, et al. Synthesis of prostacyclin from platelet-derived endoperoxides by cultured human endothelial cells. *J Clin Invest* 1980;66:979–986.
155. Knowles RG, Moncada S., Nitric oxide synthases in mammals. *Biochem J* 1994;298:249–258.
156. Lowenstein CJ, Dinerman JL, Snyder SH. Nitric oxide: A physiologic messenger. *Ann Intern Med* 1994;120:227–237.
157. Côté YP, Picher M, St-Jean P, et al. Identification and localization of ATP-diphosphohydrolase (apyrase) in bovine aorta: Relevance to vascular tone and platelet aggregation. *Biochim Biophys Acta* 1991; 1078:187–191.
158. Bakker WW, Poelstra K, Barradas MA, et al. Platelets and ectonucleotidases. *Platelets* 1994;5:121–129.
159. Gibbons GH, Dzau VJ. The emerging concept of vascular remodeling. *N Engl J Med* 1994;330:1431–1438.
160. White DG, Mundin JW, Sumner MJ, et al. The effect of endothelins on nitric oxide and prostacyclin production from human umbilical vein, porcine aorta and bovine carotid artery endothelial cells in culture. *Br J Pharmacol* 1993;109:1128–1132.
161. Miller RC, Pelton JT, Huggins JP. Endothelins—from receptors to medicine. *Trends Pharmacol Sci* 1993;14:54–60.
162. Bertelé V, Cerletti C, De Gaetano G. Antiplatelet agents. In: Bloom AL, Forbes CD, Thomas DP, Tuddenham EGD, eds. *Haemostasis and Thrombosis,* 3rd ed, Vol 2. Edinburgh: Churchill Livingstone; 1994;1473–1477.
163. Patrono C. Aspirin as an antiplatelet drug. *N Engl J Med* 1994;330: 1287–1294.
164. AntiPlatelet Trialists' Collaboration. Collaborative overview of randomised trials of antiplatelet therapy—I: Prevention of death, myocardial infarction, and stroke by prolonged antiplatelet therapy in various categories of patients. *Br Med J* 1994;308:81–106.
165. AntiPlatelet Trialists' Collaboration. Collaborative overview of randomised trials of antiplatelet therapy—II: Maintenance of vascular graft or arterial patency by antiplatelet therapy. *Br Med J* 1994;308: 159–168.
166. AntiPlatelet Trialists' Collaboration. Collaborative overview of randomised trials of antiplatelet therapy—III: Reduction in venous thrombosis and pulmonary embolism by antiplatelet prophylaxis among surgical and medical patients. *Br Med J* 1994;308:235–246.
167. Speir E, Modali R, Huang E-S, et al. Potential role of human cytomegalovirus and p53 interaction in coronary restenosis. *Science* 1994;265: 391–394.

168. Marx J. CMV-p53 interaction may help explain clogged arteries. *Science* 1994;265:320.
169. Coller BS. Antiplatelet agents in the prevention and therapy of thrombosis. *Annu Rev Med* 1992;43:171–180.
170. Ford-Hutchinson AW, Gresser M, Young RN. 5-Lipoxygenase. *Annu Rev Biochem* 1994;63:383–417.
171. Colgan SP, Serhan CN, Parkos CA, et al. Lipoxin A_4 modulates transmigration of human neutrophils across intestinal epithelial monolayers. *J Clin Invest* 1993;92:72–85.
172. Levy BD, Romano M, Chapman HA, et al. Human alveolar macrophages have 15-lipoxygenase and generate 15(S)-hydroxy-5,8,11-*cis*-13-*trans*-eicosatetraenoic acid and lipoxins. *J Clin Invest* 1993;92:1572–1579.
173. Beckman BS, Despinasse BP, Spriggs L. Actions of lipoxins A_4 and B_4 on signal transduction events in Friend erythroleukemia cells. *Proc Soc Exp Biol Med* 1992;201:169–173.
174. McGiff JC. Cytochrome P-450 metabolism of arachidonic acid. *Annu Rev Pharmacol Toxicol* 1991;31:339–369.
175. Hill E, Fitzpatrick F, Murphy RC. Biological activity and metabolism of 20-hydroxyeicosatetraenoic acid in the human platelet. *Br J Pharmacol* 1992;106:267–274.
176. Valles J, Santos MT, Marcus AJ, et al. Down-regulation of human platelet reactivity by neutrophils. Participation of lipoxygenase derivatives and adhesive proteins. *J Clin Invest* 1993;92:1357–1365.
177. Hoxie JA, Ahuja M, Belmonte E, et al. Internalization and recycling of activated thrombin receptors. *J Biol Chem* 1993;268:13756–13763.
178. Valenzuela MA, López J, Mancilla M, et al. Comparative subcellular distribution of apyrase from animal and plant sources. Characterization of microsomal apyrase. *Comp Biochem Physiol [B]* 1989;93B:911–919.
179. Katayama M, Handa M, Araki Y, et al. Soluble P-selectin is present in normal circulation and its plasma level is elevated in patients with thrombotic thrombocytopenic purpura and haemolytic uraemic syndrome. *Br J Haematol* 1993;84:702–710.
180. Strader CD, Fong TM, Tota MR, et al. Structure and function of G protein-coupled receptors. *Annu Rev Biochem* 1994;63:101–132.
181. White JG. Platelet granule disorders. *CRC Crit Rev Oncol Hematol* 1986;4:337.

Atherosclerosis and Coronary Artery Disease,
edited by V. Fuster, R. Ross, and E. J. Topol.
Lippincott-Raven Publishers, Philadelphia © 1996.

CHAPTER 36

Interaction of Platelet Activation and Coagulation

Lina Badimon and J. J. Badimon

Key Words: Platelets; Coagulation; Thrombosis; Thrombin; Platelet receptors; Fibrin(ogen); Vessel wall; Blood flow; Stenosis.

INTRODUCTION

Numerous pathologic and angiographic and several angioscopic and intravascular ultrasound reports have documented the presence of intraluminal thrombi both in unstable angina and in acute myocardial infarction. In contrast with the very high incidence of thrombi in acute myocardial infarction, the incidence in unstable angina varied significantly among different studies, related in part to the interval between the onset of symptoms and the angiographic study. Accordingly, when cardiac catheterization was delayed for weeks, the incidence of thrombi was low; on the other hand, angiography early after the onset of symptoms revealed the presence of thrombi in approximately two-thirds of cases. Presumably, the thrombus is occlusive at the time of anginal pain and later may become subocclusive and slowly lysed or digested. Local and systemic ''thrombogenic risk factors'' at the time of coronary plaque disruption may influence the degree and duration of thrombus deposition and hence the different pathologic and clinical syndromes. Some of the local and systemic factors that contribute to the degree of thrombogenicity at a molecular level following plaque rupture are described in this chapter.

The concept of vascular injury and local geometry as triggers and modulators of a thrombotic event is relevant to the pathogenesis of different cardiovascular disorders, including the initiation and progression of atherosclerosis, acute coronary syndromes, vein graft disease, and restenosis following coronary angioplasty. The unveiling of the molecular interactions prevalent in thrombosis will serve the development of more accurate strategies of pharmacologic intervention.

PATHOGENESIS OF ARTERIAL THROMBOSIS

In the initial stages of endothelial injury, with functional alterations but without major morphologic changes, no significant platelet deposition or thrombus formation can be demonstrated. A few scattered platelets may interact with such subtly injured endothelium and contribute, by the release of growth factors, to very mild intimal hyperplasia. In contrast, with endothelial denudation and mild intimal injury, from a monolayer to a few layers of platelets may deposit on the lesion, with or without mural thrombus formation. The release of platelet growth factors may contribute significantly to an accelerated intimal hyperplasia, as it occurs in the coronary vein graft within the first postoperative year. In severe injury, with exposure of components of deeper layers of the vessel, as in spontaneous plaque rupture or in angioplasty, marked platelet aggregation with mural thrombus formation follows. Vascular injury of this magnitude also stimulates thrombin formation through both the

L. Badimon: Cardiovascular Research Center, CSIC-HSCSP-UAB, Jordi Girona, 18-26, 08034 Barcelona, Spain.
J.J. Badimon: Cardiovascular Institute, Mount Sinai Medical Center, New York, New York 10029.

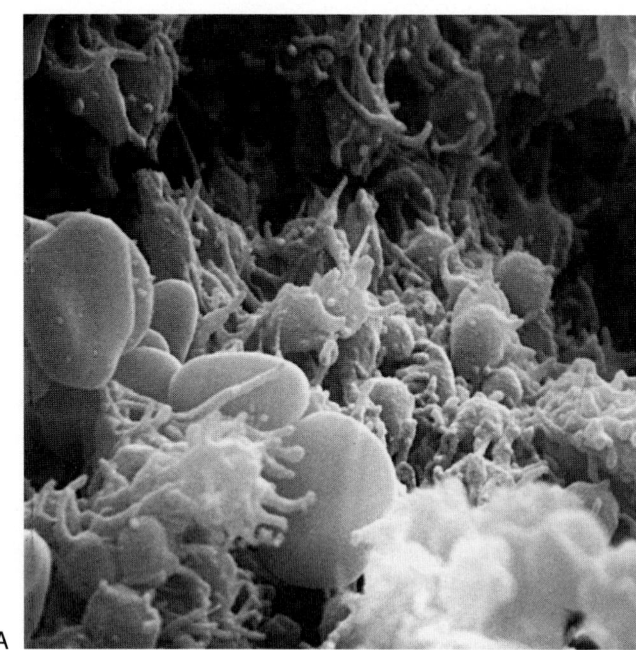

A

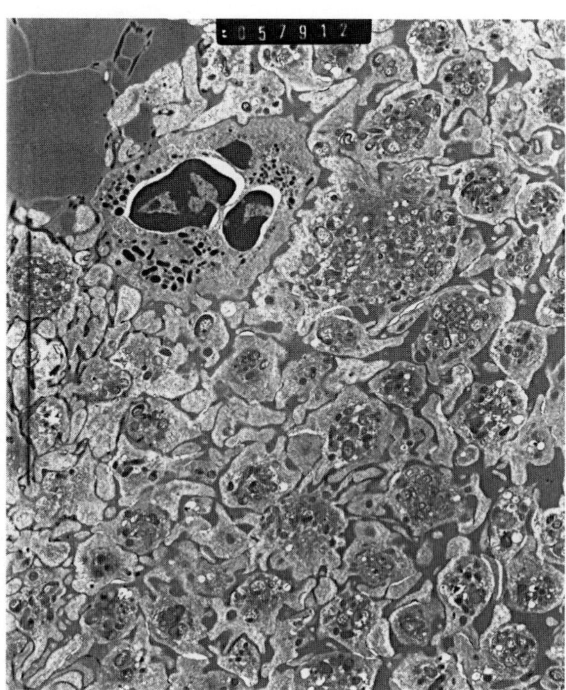

B

FIG. 1. Ultrastructural features of thrombi. **A:** Scanning electron microscopy micrograph of a thrombus showing platelet aggregates, fibrin strands, and red blood cells. **B:** Transmission electron microscopy micrograph of a thrombus showing a platelet aggregate with some completely degranulated platelets, red blood cells, and a leukocyte.

intrinsic (surface-activated) and extrinsic (tissue-factor-dependent) coagulation pathways, in which the platelet membrane facilitates interactions between clotting factors. This concept of vascular injury as a trigger of the platelet coagulation response is important in understanding the pathogenesis of various vascular diseases associated with atherosclerosis and coronary artery disease.

Growing thrombi may locally occlude the lumen, or embolize and be washed away by the blood flow to occlude distal vessels (Fig. 1). However, thrombi may be physiologically and spontaneously lysed by mechanisms that block thrombus propagation. Thrombus size, location, and composition are regulated by hemodynamic forces (mechanical effects), thrombogenicity of exposed substrate (local molecular effects), relative concentration of fluid phase and cellular blood components (local cellular effects), and the efficiency of the physiologic mechanisms of control of the system, mainly fibrinolysis (1–4).

Platelets

After plaque rupture, the exposed vessel structures induce platelet aggregation and thrombosis by mechanisms in some instances different from those prevalent in hemostatic plug formation. The ulcerated atherosclerotic plaque may contain a disrupted fibrous cap, a lipid-rich core, abundant extracellular matrix, and inflammatory cells. Such structures exhibit a potent activating effect on platelets and coagulation. The understanding of the biochemical events involved in platelet activation has progressed significantly (5–7). Most platelet aggregation agonists seem to act through the hydrolysis of platelet membrane phosphatidylinositol by phospholipase C, which results in the mobilization of free calcium from the platelet-dense tubular system (8,9). Exposed matrix from the vessel wall and thrombin generated by the activation of the coagulation cascade as well as circulating epinephrine are powerful platelet agonists. Adenosine diphosphate (ADP) is a platelet agonist that may be released from hemolyzed red cells in the area of vessel injury. Each agonist stimulates the discharge of calcium from the platelet-dense tubular system and promotes the contraction of the platelet, with the subsequent release of its granule contents. Platelet-related adenosine diphosphate and serotonin stimulate adjacent platelets, further enhancing the process of platelet activation. Arachidonate, which is released from the platelet membrane by the stimulatory effect of collagen, thrombin, adenosine diphosphate, and serotonin, is another platelet agonist. Arachidonate is converted to thromboxane A_2 by the sequential effects of cyclooxygenase and thromboxane synthetase. Thromboxane A_2 not only promotes further platelet aggregation, but is also a potent vasoconstrictor (2,3) (Fig. 2).

Signal transduction mechanisms initiated upon binding of agonists to membrane-spanning receptors on the platelet surface have been partially elucidated (5). Agonist binding triggers cascades of intracellular second messengers, including inositol 1,4,5-triphosphate (IP_3) and diacylglycerol (DG). IP_3 releases Ca^{2+} from the platelet-dense tubular sys-

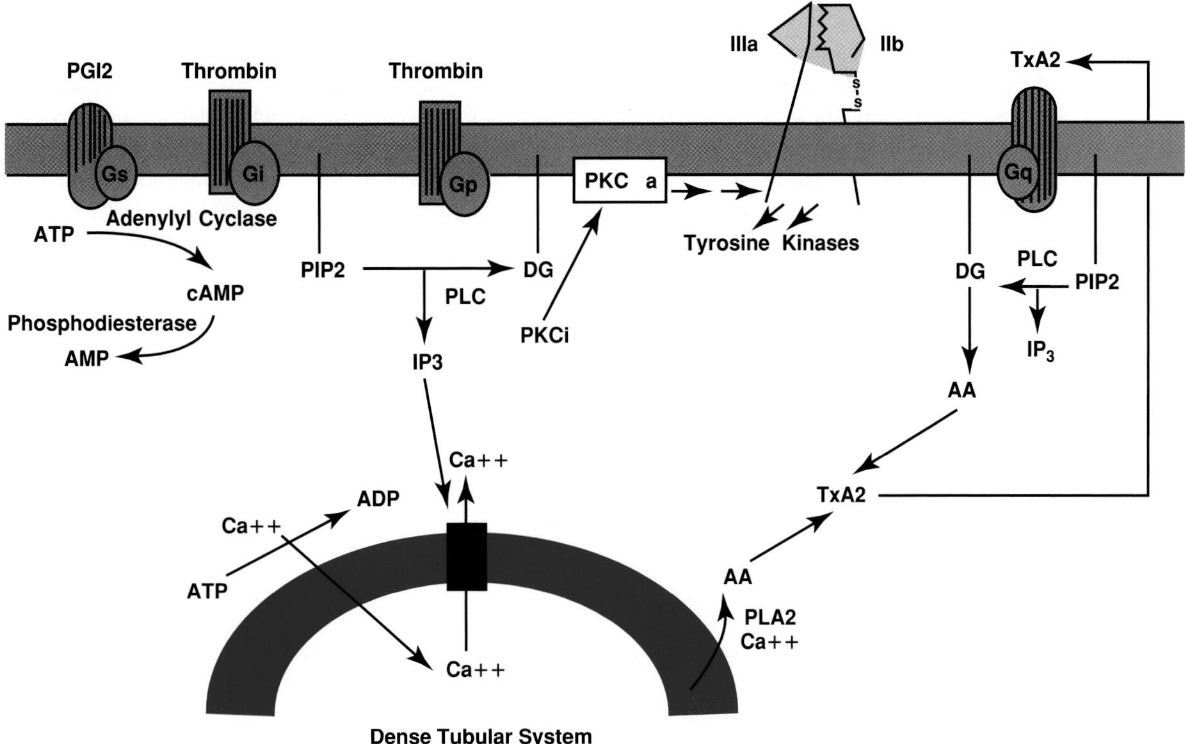

FIG. 2. Signal transduction mechanisms initiated upon binding of agonists to platelet membrane receptors. Binding activates G-proteins and triggers intracellular second messengers such as IP_3 and DG. The final outcome is the activation of the platelet with secretion, further fibrinogen receptor exposure, and aggregation. *PGI_2*, Prostacyclin; *TxA_2*, thromboxane A_2; *PIP_2*, phosphoinositol diphosphate; *PLC*, phospholipase C; *PKC_i* and *PKC_a*, protein kinase C inactivated and activated; *DG*, diacylglycerol; *IP_3*, inositol 1,4,5-triphosphate; *AA*, arachidonic acid; *PLA_2*, phospholipase A_2; *G_s, G_i, G_p, G_q*, guanine nucleotide-binding regulatory proteins; *IIb/IIIa*, receptor glycoprotein for adhesive protein ligands (mainly fibrinogen and vWF), which supports platelet aggregation (receptor occupancy triggers tyrosine kinase activation). (Modified from Marcus and Safier, ref. 5, and Brass, ref. 7.)

tem, raising the cytosolic free Ca^{2+} concentration. Diacylglycerol activates the serine/threonine kinase, protein kinase C, translocating it to the plasma membrane and triggering granule secretion and fibrinogen receptor exposure (glycoprotein IIb–IIIa complex). At the same time, the rising cytosolic free Ca^{2+} concentration facilitates arachidonate (AA) release from phospholipids by phospholipase A_2, a process that may occur at both the plasma membrane and the dense tubular system membrane. Arachidonate is metabolized to thromboxane A_2 (TxA_2), which diffuses out of the cell, interacts with receptors on the platelet surface, and causes further platelet activation. At some point during this process, tyrosine kinases, including members of the src family, are activated in platelets and cause the phosphorylation on tyrosine of multiple platelet proteins, most of which have not been identified. Tyrosine kinase activation in platelets appears to occur predominantly as a consequence of fibrinogen receptor expression and platelet aggregation, but can also occur as an early step in platelet activation. In many cases, the interactions between agonists and the enzymes responsible for second messenger generation are mediated by a guanine nucleotide-binding regulatory protein (G-protein). In platelets, G-proteins have been shown to regulate phosphoinositide hydrolysis and cAMP formation, and are probably involved in the activation of phospholipase A_2. Phospholipase C (presumably phospholipase C_β) is activated in a pertussis toxin-sensitive manner by the still-unidentified G-protein G_p and in a pertussis toxin-resistant manner by the G-protein G_q. Adenylyl cyclase is stimulated by the G-protein G_s and inhibited by the G-protein G_i. The G-protein that regulates phospholipase A_2 activity remains to be characterized. Platelet receptors for thrombin, epinephrine, thromboxane A_2, and platelet-activating factor have been cloned and shown to resemble other G-protein-coupled receptors with a characteristic structure comprised of a single polypeptide with seven transmembrane domains. The low-molecular-weight GTP-binding protein Rap1B has recently been shown to form a complex with phospholipase C_γ and Ras-GAP, supplying a potential mechanism for regulating phospholipase C_{γ} activity. Other low-molecular-weight GTP-binding proteins may be involved in the regulation of vesicular transport and granule secretion in platelets (5,7). (For further details see the chapter by Marcus in this volume.)

The initial recognition of damaged vessel wall by platelets involves (a) adhesion, activation, and adherence to recognition sites on the thromboactive substrate (extracellular matrix proteins; e.g., von Willebrand factor, collagen, fibronectin, vitronectin, laminin), (b) spreading of the platelet on the surface, and (c) aggregation of platelets with each other to form a platelet plug or white thrombus. The efficiency of the platelet recruitment will depend on the underlying substrate and local geometry. A final step of recruitment of other blood cells also occurs; erythrocytes, neutrophils, and occasionally monocytes are found on evolving mixed thrombus (Fig. 3).

Platelet function depends on adhesive interactions and most of the glycoproteins on the platelet membrane surface are receptors for adhesive proteins. Many of these receptors have been identified, cloned, sequenced, and classified within large gene families that mediate a variety of cellular interactions (10,11) (Table 1), (Fig. 2). The most abundant is the integrin family, which includes GPIIb–IIIa, GPIa–IIa,

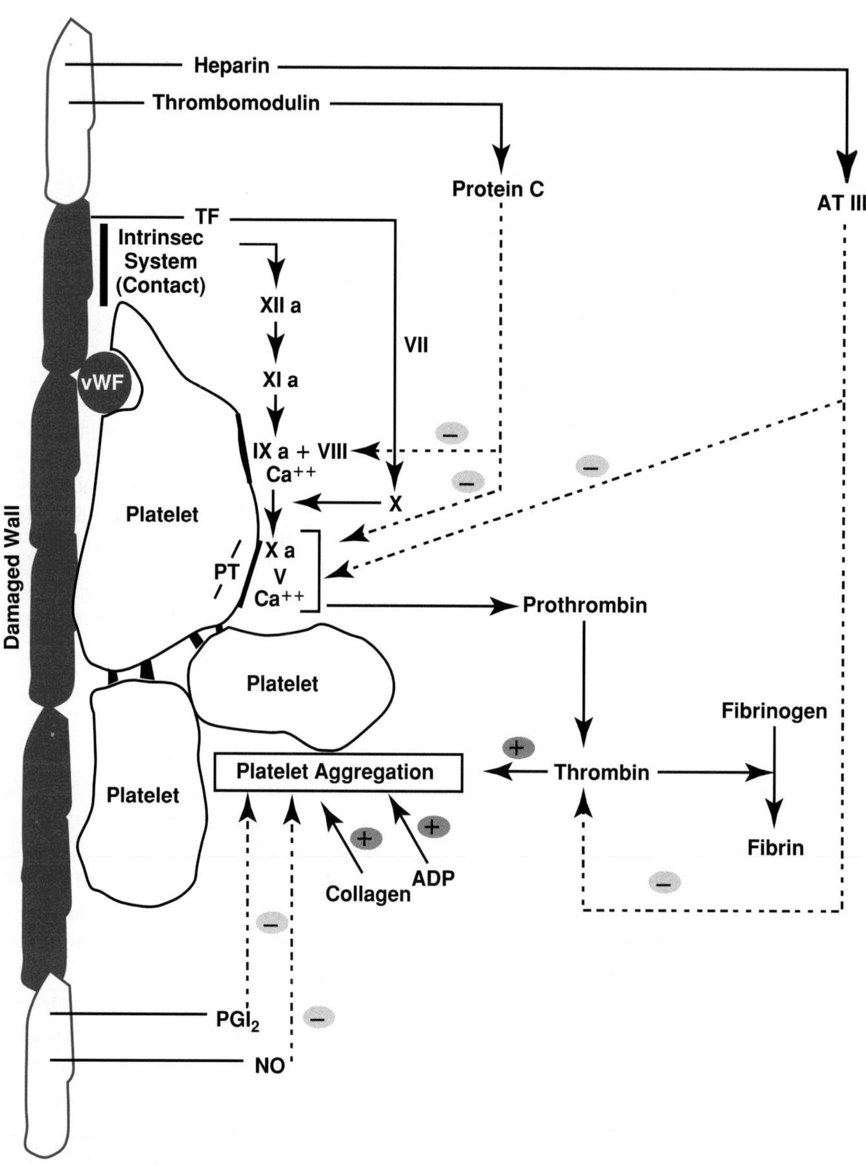

FIG. 3. Simplified diagram of platelet–vessel wall interaction and coagulation enzymes. Platelet adhesion to recognition sites occurs in lesioned areas of the endothelium. Adhesion, spreading, and aggregation of new platelets contribute to mural thrombus formation. Platelet aggregation is enhanced by agonists present in the microenvironment *(arrows with (+) signs)*, while there are spontaneous pathways of inhibition *(arrows with (−) signs)* derived from neighboring normal endothelium. *TF,* Tissue factor; *ATIII,* antithrombin III; *NO,* nitric oxide; *PT,* prothrombinase complex.

TABLE 1. *Platelet membrane glycoprotein receptors*

Glycoprotein receptor	Ligand	Function
GPIIb–IIIa	Fg, vW, Fn, Ts, Vn	Aggregation, adhesion at high shear rate
Receptor Vn	Vn, vW, Fn, Fg, Ts	Adhesion
GPIa–IIa	C	Adhesion
GPIc–IIa	Fn	Adhesion
GPIc′–IIa	Ln	Adhesion
GPIb–IX	vW, T	Adhesion
GPV	Substrate T	Unknown
GPIV (GPIIIb)	Ts, C	Adhesion
GMP-140 (PADGEM)	Unknown	Interaction with leucocytes
PECAM-1 (GPIIa)	Unknown	Unknown

Fg, Fibrinogen; vW, von Willebrand factor; Fn, fibronectin; Ts, thrombospondin; Vn, vitronectin; C, collagen; Ln, laminin; T, thrombin; PECAM-1, platelet/endothelial cell adhesion molecule 1.

GPIc–IIa, the fibronectin receptor, and the vitronectin receptor, in decreasing order of magnitude. Another gene family present in the platelet membrane glycocalyx is the leucine-rich glycoprotein family represented by the GPIb–IX complex, receptor for von Willebrand factor (vWF) on unstimulated platelets that mediates adhesion to subendothelium and GPV. Other gene families include the selectins (such as GMP-140) and the immunoglobulin domain protein (HLA class I antigen and platelet/endothelial cell adhesion molecule 1, PECAM-1). Unrelated to any other gene family is the GPIV (IIIa) (10) (Table 1).

The GPIb–IX complex consist of two disulfide-linked subunits (GPIbα and GPIbβ) tightly (not covalently) complexed with GPIX in a 1:1 heterodimer. GPIbβ and GPIX are transmembrane glycoproteins and form the larger globular domain. The elongated, protruding part of the receptor corresponds to GPIbα. The major role of GPIb–IX is to bind immobilized vWF on the exposed vascular subendothelium and initiate adhesion of platelets. GPIb does not bind soluble vWF in plasma; apparently it undergoes a conformation change upon binding to the extracellular matrix and then exposes a recognition sequence for GPIb–IX. The vWF-binding domain of GPIb–IX has been narrowed to amino acids 251–279 on GPIbα (12). The GPIbα-binding domain of vWF resides in a tryptic fragment extending from residue 449 to 728 of the subunit that does not contain a RGD sequence (13). The cytoplasmic domain of GPIb–IX has a major function in linking the plasma membrane to the intracellular actin filaments of the cytoskeleton and functions to stabilize the membrane and to maintain the platelet shape (14,15).

Randomly distributed on the surface of resting platelets are about 50,000 molecules of GPIIb–IIIa. The complex is composed of one molecule of GPIIb (disulfide-linked large and light chains) and one of GPIIIa (single polypeptide chain). It is a Ca^{2+}-dependent heterodimer, noncovalently associated on the platelet membrane (16). Calcium is required for maintenance of the complex and for binding of adhesive proteins (17,18). On activated platelets, the GPIIb–IIIa is a receptor for fibrinogen, fibronectin, vWF, vitronectin, and thrombospondin (19). The receptor recognition sequences are localized to small peptide sequences (Arg–Gly–Asp [RGD]) in the adhesive proteins (20). Fibrinogen contains two RGD sequences in its α chain, one near the N-terminus (residues 95–97) and a second near the C-terminus (residues 572–574) (21). Fibrinogen has a second site of recognition for GPIIb/IIIa that is the 12-amino acid sequence located at the carboxyl-terminus of the γ chain of the molecule (22). This dodecapeptide is specific for fibrinogen and does not contain the RGD sequence, but competes with RGD-containing peptides for binding to GPIIb/IIIa (10,23,24).

Thrombin plays an important role in the pathogenesis of arterial thrombosis (Fig. 4). It is one of the most potent known agonists for platelet activation and recruitment. The thrombin receptor has 425 amino acids with seven transmembrane domains and a large NH_2-terminal extracellular extension that is cleaved by thrombin to produce a ''tethered'' ligand that activates the receptor to initiate signal transduction (25,26). Thrombin is a critical enzyme in early thrombus formation, cleaving fibrinopeptides A and B from fibrinogen to yield insoluble fibrin, which effectively anchors the evolving thrombus. Both free and fibrin-bound fibrin thrombin are able to convert fibrinogen to fibrin, allowing propagation of thrombus at the site of injury.

Therefore, platelet activation triggers intracellular signaling and expression of platelet membrane receptors for adhesion and initiation of cell contractile processes that induce shape change and secretion of the granular contents. The expression of the integrin IIb/IIa ($\alpha IIb\beta_3$) receptors for adhesive glycoprotein ligands (mainly fibrinogen and von Willebrand factor) in the circulation initiates platelet-to-platelet interaction. The process becomes perpetuated by the arrival of platelets brought by the circulation. Most of the glycoproteins in the platelet membrane surface are receptors for adhesive proteins or mediate cellular interactions.

The receptor-mediated mechanisms related to platelet interaction in the thrombotic process around stenosis have not been directly studied; however, in laminar parallel flow conditions, platelet glycoprotein Ib is necessary for normal platelet adhesion to subendothelium at high shear rates (27,28) through its interaction with von Willebrand factor (vWF) (29,30). Von Willebrand factor has been shown to bind to platelet membrane glycoproteins in both adhesion (platelet–substrate interaction) and aggregation (platelet–platelet interaction), leading to thrombus formation in perfusion studies conducted at high shear rates (27,31–36). The present consensus is that, at high-shear-rate conditions, platelet glycoproteins Ib and IIb–IIIa both appear to be involved in the events of platelet adhesion, whereas glycoprotein IIb–IIIa may be involved predominantly in plate-

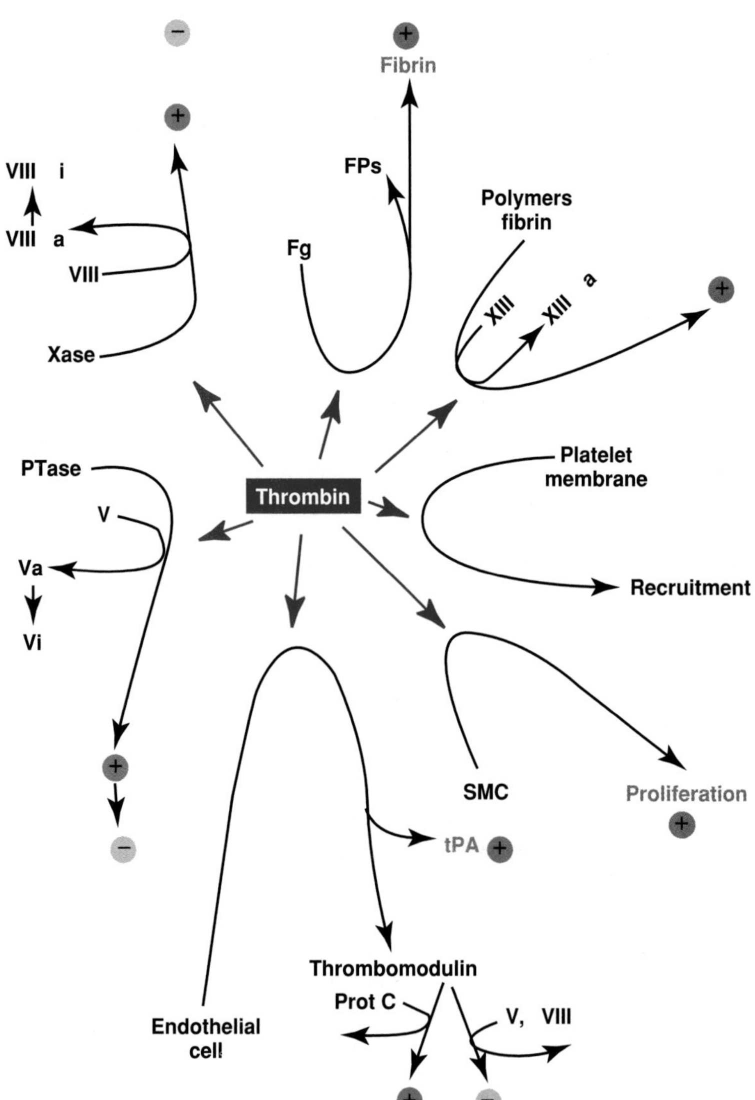

FIG. 4. Role of thrombin in the pathogenesis of arterial thrombosis. Positive signs (+) indicate reactions stimulated by thrombin, while negative signs (−) indicate reactions inhibited by it. In addition to its effects on the activation of coagulation factors and fibrin formation and stabilization, thrombin activates platelets, induces proliferation of smooth muscle cells *(SMC)*, and contributes to the activation of the spontaneous anticoagulant pathway of normal endothelium. *FPs*, Fibrinopeptides; *Fg*, fibrinogen.

let–platelet interaction. These mechanisms have not been evaluated with respect to events in the vicinity of stenosis.

The specific plasma proteins which are predominantly involved in platelet–platelet interactions under various shear conditions and triggering atherosclerotic substrates remain to be determined. The absence of platelet aggregation in thrombasthenia (observed using low-shear and nonflow systems) has been ascribed to the inability of platelets to bind fibrinogen, since platelets are known to require fibrinogen for aggregation in plasma or buffer; however, this requirement is not absolute (37,38). In perfusion studies platelet attachment or aggregate buildup (thrombus formation) on subendothelium was shown to be normal in afibrinogenemia under a wide variety of shear conditions (28,39,40). Antibodies to fibrinogen, even when added to afibrinogenemic blood in order to remove any small trace of residual fibrinogen, did not inhibit platelet interaction with the vessel wall (41), although they did reduce aggregation with adenosine diphosphate and collagen when tested in an aggregometer.

Blocking the glycoprotein IIb–IIIa receptor site on platelets with either an antibody (LJ-CP8) which blocks the general binding of adhesive proteins or with various peptides which simulate the sequence Arg–Gly–Asp (RGD) inhibits both platelet adhesion and thrombus formation in flowing blood at high shear rates. These findings reinforce the importance of the glycoprotein IIb–IIIa site in platelet–vessel wall interaction and suggest that fibrinogen is not always a necessary component for such interactions. Moreover, the results are also consistent with previous perfusion studies which demonstrated the relatively low importance of fibrinogen in favor of vWF in both platelet–platelet and platelet–vessel wall interactions at certain rheological conditions in an in vivo ^{111}In-platelet thrombosis porcine system (27,28, 32–34,42). Additional direct support for the ability of adhesive proteins other than fibrinogen to participate in platelet–platelet interactions has been obtained from studies conducted with a monoclonal antibody (LJ-P5) to glycoprotein IIb–IIIa which blocks the binding of von Willebrand factor

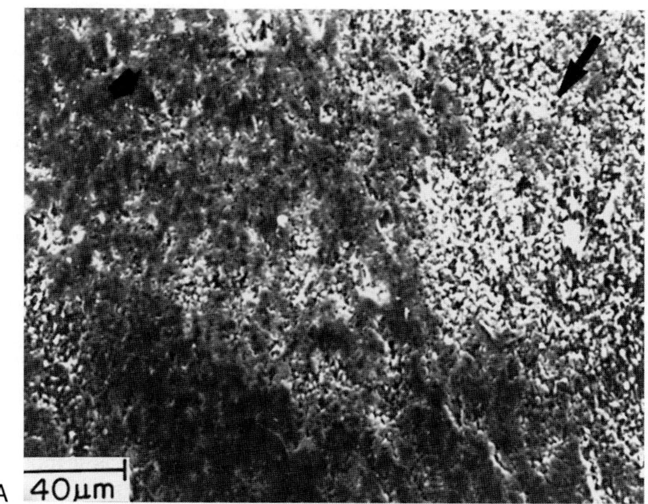

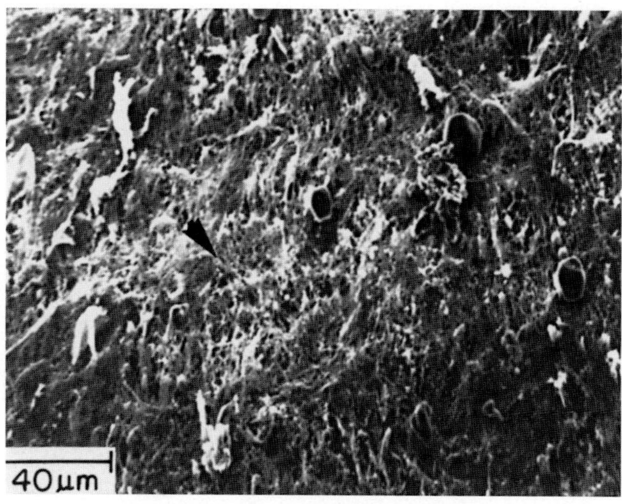

FIG. 5. Ultrastructural analysis by scanning electron microscopy of platelet interaction with subendothelium (model of mild injury). Blood derived from a catheterized carotid artery of heparinized normal **(A)** and homozygous von Willebrand disease (vWD) **(B)** pigs was perfused at high local shear rate (1,690 sec^{-1}) for 10 min through the Badimon perfusion chamber containing the deendothelialized vessel wall. Platelets formed a mural carpet covering the vessel (normal blood); however, blood from homozygous vWD (devoid of vWF) induced very little deposition of platelets. *(Arrows:* thin, isolated platelets; thick, mural carpet of platelets; *head,* matrix not covered by platelets). (Modified from Badimon et al., ref. 32.)

and other adhesive proteins, but not of fibrinogen, to platelets (43). In the presence of this antibody, levels of both platelet–vessel wall and platelet–platelet interaction on subendothelium were reduced, suggesting that von Willebrand factor participates in the thrombotic events occurring in flowing blood.

A peptide-specific monoclonal antibody that inhibits von Willebrand factor binding to glycoprotein IIb–IIIa (152B6) without affecting the binding of other RGD-dependent glycoproteins has been also shown to inhibit significantly platelet deposition to human atherosclerotic vessel wall (44). Pigs that have normal fibrinogen levels but are congenitally deficient in von Willebrand factor showed a significantly reduced ability to deposit platelets in subendothelium, severely damaged vessel wall, and collagen type I bundles using a variety of in vivo and in vitro perfusion conditions at high and low local shear rates in native (nonanticoagulated) and anticoagulated blood (45) (Figs. 5 and 6).

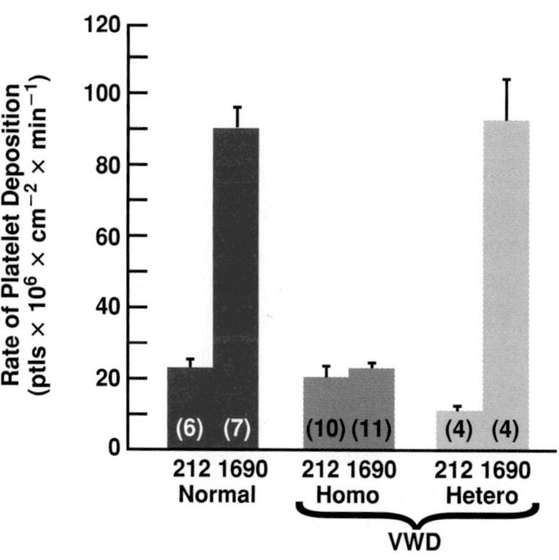

FIG. 6. Rate of platelet deposition on native fibrillar collagen type I bundles (model of severe injury to the vessel wall). Results are expressed as millions of platelets deposited per surface area and per unit time. Nonanticoagulated blood derived from a catheterized carotid artery of normal, homozygous vWD and heterozygous vWD pigs was perfused at low (212 sec^{-1}) and high (1,690 sec^{-1}) local shear rates through the Badimon perfusion chamber containing the collagen substrate. Platelet deposition at high shear rate was significantly increased in normal and heterozygous vWD, but not in homozygous vWD (devoid of vWF). Parentheses give the numbers of experiments. Heterozygous vWD with intermediate levels of plasma vWF showed normal platelet deposition at high shear rate. The three genotypes showed normal fibrinogen levels; therefore, in vivo vWF has an important function in binding GPIIb/IIIa, mainly at areas with high shear, and supports thrombus formation. (From Badimon, et al., ref. 33).

Activation of the Coagulation System

During plaque rupture, in addition to platelet deposition in the injured area, the clotting mechanism is activated by the exposure of the deendothelialized vascular surface. Blocking tissue factor (TF) by a monoclonal antibody has reduced thrombus formation in a rabbit model of angioplasty, and thus TF may be exposed upon vessel injury and contribute to thrombosis (46). The activation of the coagulation cascade leads to the generation of thrombin, which, as mentioned before, is a powerful platelet agonist that contributes to platelet recruitment in addition to catalyzing the formation and polymerization of fibrin. Fibrin is essential in the stabilization of the platelet thrombus and its withstanding removal forces by flow, shear, and high intravascular pressure. These basic concepts have clinical relevance in the context of the acute coronary syndromes where plaque rupture exposes vessel wall matrix and plaque core materials, which by activating platelets and the coagulation system results in the formation of a fixed and occlusive platelet-fibrin thrombus (Fig. 3).

The efficacy of fibrinolytic agents pointedly demonstrates the importance of fibrin-related material in the thrombosis associated with myocardial infarction (47). However, few studies have considered the influence of flow on procoagulant activity either in laminar or nonparallel streamline conditions. The observation that fibrin formation seems to be diminished at increasing shear rates (30) is currently unexplained and needs to be confirmed. While dilution of procoagulant moieties has generally been proposed as the mechanism by which flow minimizes clotting events at surfaces, such a mechanism has never been verified experimentally and in fact there are theoretical grounds to suspect the validity of such a hypothesis (48). It is quite plausible to suspect that flow may have direct effects on certain enzyme or polymerization kinetics involved in thrombosis, in addition to the well-defined effect that flow has in enhancing transport of reactants and products to and from the vessel wall (49). Such effects of flow on immobilized enzymes have been occasionally observed, but never studied with respect to coagulative processes (50,51). However, the regulation of blood coagulation is dependent on processes which take place on membrane surfaces. The proteins which compose the clotting enzymes do not collide and interact on a random basis in the plasma, but interact in complexes in a highly efficient manner on platelet and endothelial surfaces. The major regulatory events in the coagulation (activation, inhibition, generation of anticoagulant proteins) occur on membrane surfaces.

It is interesting to note that venous thrombosis, which is predominantly constituted by fibrin clots, occurs in areas of stasis and low-shear-rate conditions typical of the venous system. Therefore, the low local-shear-rate conditions and flow recirculations developing in the poststenotic areas may explain fibrin accumulation. Vascular subendothelium (mildly injured vessel wall) which is completely devoid of endothelial cells is able to clot whole plasma and more specifically activate factor X in the presence of factor VII (52). This activity results in the deposition of fibrin on the subendothelium at low shear conditions which can be blocked by monoclonal antibody to tissue factor (52). Thus, tissue factor appears to be a major procoagulant factor in the vascular space immediately underlying the endothelial lining of arteries, a site which might be readily accessible upon local injury or upon rupture of an atherosclerotic plaque.

Recently, using an original stenotic perfusion chamber (Fig. 7), we have shown that local fibrin formation on damaged vessel wall is dependent on the severity of the lesion and that fibrin formation also occurs at high shear rate (Fig. 8). The exposure of deep layers of the vessel wall to blood will stimulate local fibrin formation also at the apex of stenotic narrowings even in the presence of a significant amount of systemic heparin (1–2 international units [IU] heparin/ml plasma) (53,54) (Fig. 8). We investigated the effect of a severe (80%), eccentric stenosis (Fig. 7) on fibrin(ogen) interaction with a deeply damaged vessel wall, its relationship to platelet deposition in thrombus formation, and the influence of time on thrombus growth. Porcine ^{125}I-fibrinogen and autologous ^{111}In-platelets were injected into pigs instrumented for extracorporeal circulation and treated with low-dose heparin (activated partial thromboplastin time [aPTT] ratio <1.5) that has been shown not to affect platelet and/or fibrin(ogen) attachment. Tunica media, as a model of severely injured vessel wall, was mounted in a tubular perfusion chamber containing an eccentric axisymmetric sinusoidal stenosis obstructing the lumen, and exposed for 1, 5, and 10 min to perfusing blood. A shear rate of 424 sec^{-1} at the laminar, parallel, parabolic local flow-perfused segments, and of one to two orders of magnitude greater at the apex of the stenosis, was achieved. Fibrin(ogen) deposition, its axial distribution with respect to the apex, and its relationship to platelet deposition were determined by an ex vivo analysis of the test substrates. Fibrin(ogen) and platelet deposition were both significantly higher at the apex of the stenosis than at either the prestenotic or poststenotic area at all the studied perfusion times ($p < 0.02$). However, fibrin(ogen) deposition demonstrated a significantly smaller degree of increase from the prestenotic area to the apex, as well as a smaller degree of decrease from the latter to the poststenotic region, compared to platelet deposition ($p < 0.05$). Although both fibrin(ogen) and platelet deposition increased over time, the ratio of fibrin(ogen) to platelet showed a progressive decrease which became significant from 5 to 10 min ($p < 0.03$) at either low or high shear rate. The rate of platelet deposition was relatively constant; however, fibrin(ogen) deposition progressively decreased, especially at the apex. On severely damaged vessel wall, fibrin(ogen) and platelet deposition is maximal at the apex of the stenosis where shear rate is extremely high and parallel streamlines deformed. Nevertheless, fibrin(ogen) deposition is significantly less dependent on high shear rate than platelets, and the pattern is not influenced by time. Fibrin(ogen) deposition seems to be predominant in the thrombus layers adjacent to a severely damaged vessel wall regardless of the local shear stress levels and flow conditions (54).

The blood coagulation system involves a sequence of reactions integrating zymogens (proteins susceptible to be activated to enzymes via limited proteolysis) and cofactors (nonproteolytic enzyme activators) in three groups: (a) the contact activation (generation of factor XIa via the Hageman factor), (b) the conversion of factor X to factor Xa in a complex reaction requiring the participation of factors IX and VIII, and (c) the conversion of prothrombin to thrombin and fibrin formation (55) (Fig. 9).

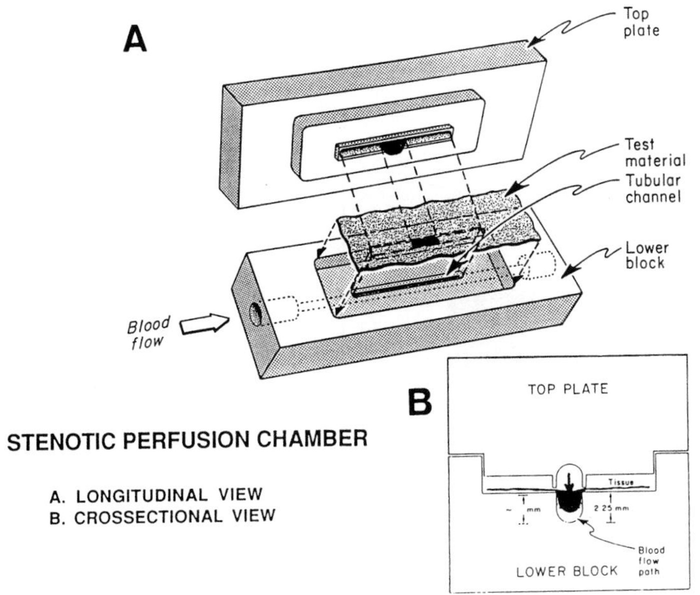

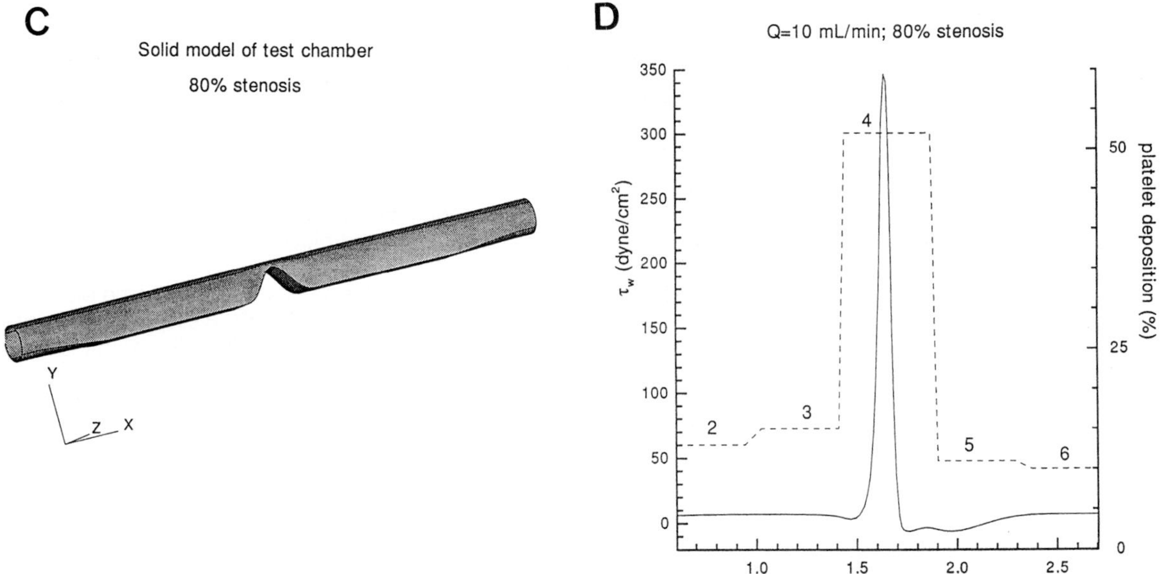

FIG. 7. (A) Longitudinal general external view and **(B)** cross-sectional view of the Badimon stenotic perfusion chamber. **(C)** Computer solid model of the test chamber with 80% stenosis by A. S. Dvinsky, Data Research. **(D)** Double graph of calculated shear stresses along the chamber longitudinal *X* axis *(continuous line)* (finite number analysis, A. S. Dvinsky) and platelet deposition *(dashed line)* on the substrate divided accordingly to the shear stenosis located in segment 4.

The triggering surfaces for in vivo initiation of contact activation have been suggested to be sulfatides and glycosaminoglycans of the vessel wall. The physiologic role of this system is unclear, however, because the absence of Hageman factor, prekallikrein, or high-molecular-weight kininogen does not induce a clinically apparent pathology. Factor XI deficiency is associated with abnormal bleeding. Activated factor XI induces the activation of factor IX in the presence of Ca^{2+}. Factor IXa forms a catalytic complex with factor VIII on a membrane surface and efficiently activates factor X in the presence of Ca^{2+}. Factor IX is a vitamin K-dependent enzyme, as are factor VII, factor X, prothrombin, and protein C (Table 2).

In citrated plasma, an anticoagulant often used in studies on platelet vessel wall interaction, the coagulation reactions do not proceed further than the activation of factor XI because of their dependence on Ca^{2+}. Platelets may provide the membrane requirements for the activation of factor X, although the participation of other cells of the vessel wall (in exposed injured vessels) has not been excluded (55). As

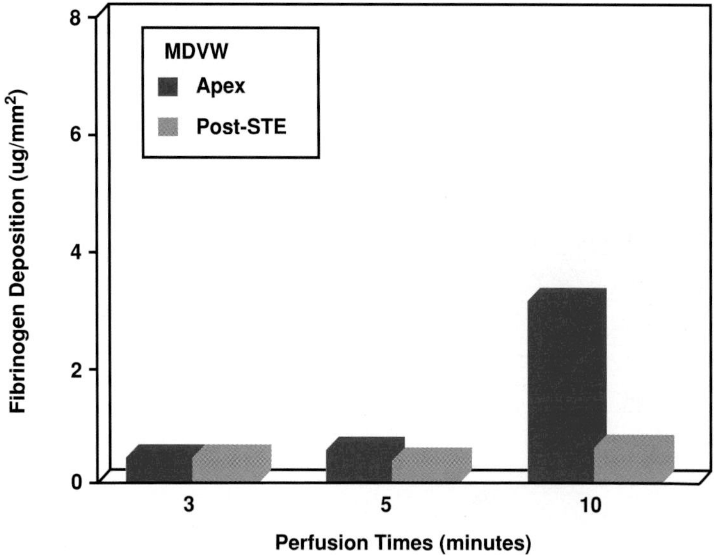

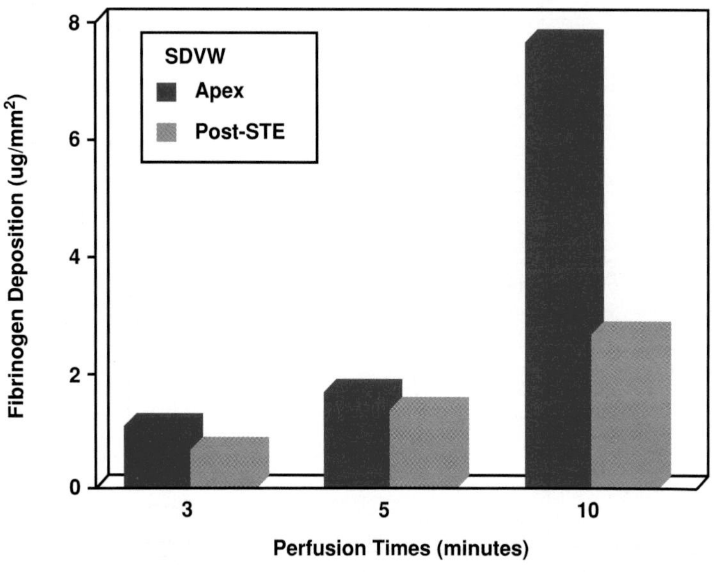

FIG. 8. Deposition of ^{125}I-fibrin(ogen) on mildly damaged vessel wall (MDVW) and severely damaged vessel wall (SDVW) analyzed by perfusing heparinized blood derived from a catheterized carotid artery of a normal pig through the Badimon stenotic perfusion chamber containing MDVW (subendothelium) or SDVW (vessel wall tunica media matrix). Fibrin(ogen) depositions on the apex of the stenosis (80%) and on the neighboring poststenotic zone where flow recirculation develops were compared. Fibrinogen deposition is substrate dependent, since it is always higher in SDVW than in MDVW and it is also flow dependent, because it is also higher in the apex of the stenosis than in the recirculation zone (lower shear rate). (Modified from Badimon et al., ref. 97.)

such, endothelial cells in culture have been shown to support the activation of factor X (56). Factor VIII forms a noncovalent complex with vWF in plasma and its function in coagulation is the acceleration of the effects of IXa on the activation of X to Xa. Absence of factor VIII or IX produces the hemophilic syndromes (57) (Fig. 9).

The tissue factor (TF) pathway, previously known as extrinsic coagulation pathway, through the TF–factor VII complex in the presence of Ca^{2+} induces the formation of Xa. A second TF-dependent reaction catalyzes the transformation of IX into IXa. Tissue factor is an integral membrane protein that serves to initiate the activation of factors IX and X and to localize the reaction to cells on which TF is expressed. Other cofactors include factor VIIIa, which binds to platelets and forms the binding site for IXa, thereby forming the machinery for the activation of X, and factor Va, which binds to platelets and provides a binding site for Xa (Table 2). The human genes for these cofactors have been cloned and sequenced. In physiologic conditions, no cells in contact with blood contain TF, although cells such as monocytes and polymorphonuclear leukocytes can be induced to synthesize and express TF (55).

Activated Xa converts prothrombin into thrombin. The complex which catalyzes the formation of thrombin consists of factors Xa and Va in a 1 : 1 complex. The activation results in the cleavage of fragment 1.2 and formation of thrombin from fragment 2. The interaction of the four components of the ''prothrombinase complex'' (Xa, Va, phospholipid, and Ca^{2+}) yield a more efficient reaction (58).

Activated platelets provide procoagulant surface for the

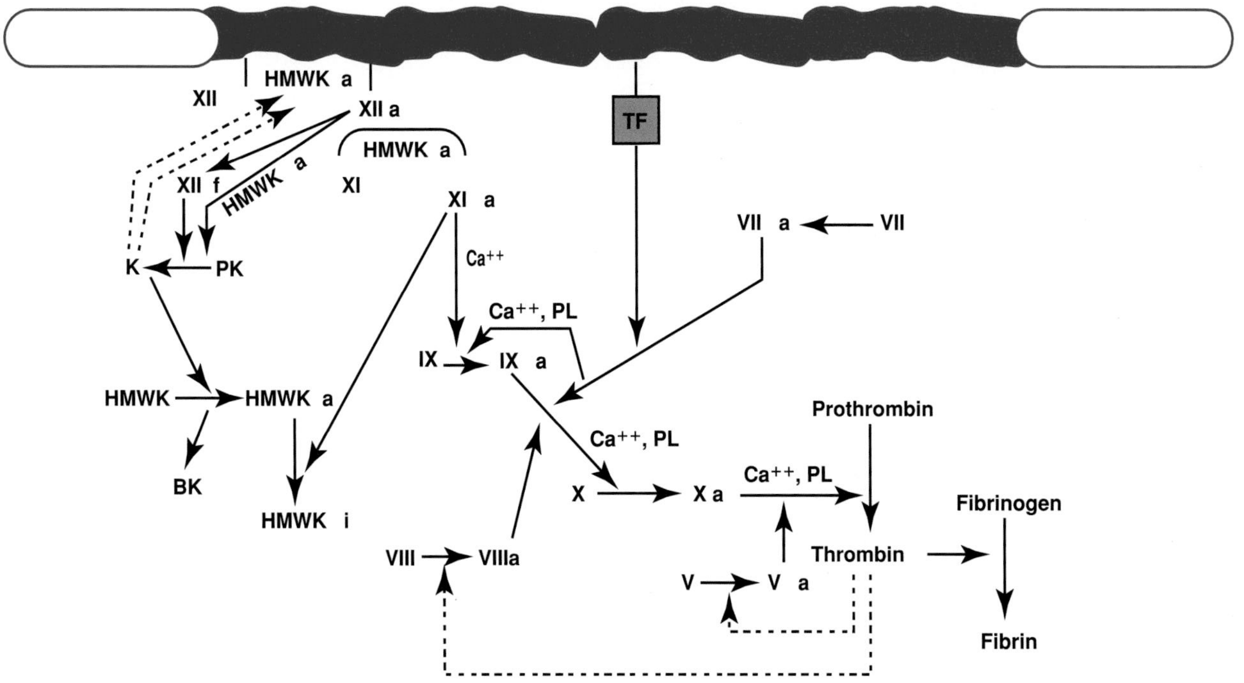

FIG. 9. Simplified diagram of the blood coagulation system integrating the contact activation or generation of factor XIa via Hageman factor, the conversion of factor X to Xa with the participation of factors IX and VIII, and the conversion of prothrombin into thrombin and fibrin formation. *HMWK,* High-molecular-weight kininogen; *PK,* prekallikrein; *K,* kallikrein; *TF,* tissue factor; *BK,* bradykinin; *PL,* phospholipids; *subscript a,* activated factor.

assembly and expression of both intrinsic Xase and prothrombinase enzymatic complexes (59–63). These complexes respectively catalyze the activation of factor X to factor Xa and prothrombin to thrombin. The expression of activity is associated with the binding of both the proteases factor IXa and factor Xa and the cofactors VIIIa and Va to procoagulant surfaces. The binding of IXa and Xa is promoted by VIIIa and Va, respectively, such that Va and likely VIIIa provide the equivalent of receptors for the proteolytic enzymes (64–66). The surface of the platelet expresses the procoagulant phospholipids that bind coagulation factors and contribute to the procoagulant activity of the cell. Whether specific receptors are expressed on the platelet surface for Va and VIIIa is not known, however, although the factors bind to platelets (64).

Blood clotting is blocked at the level of the prothrombinase complex by the physiologic anticoagulant-activated protein C and oral anticoagulants (Fig. 10). Oral anticoagulants prevent posttranslational synthesis of γ-carboxyglutamic acid groups on the vitamin K-dependent clotting factors, preventing binding of prothrombin and Xa to the membrane surface. Activated protein C cleaves factor Va to render it functionally inactive. Loss of Va decreases the role of thrombin formation to negligible levels (67).

TABLE 2. *Coagulation system*

Cofactor	Enzyme	Zymogen	Product
Tissue factor	VIIa	IX	IXa
Tissue factor	VIIa	X	Xa
VIIIa	IXa	X	Xa
Va	Xa	Prothrombin	Thrombin

Thrombin acts on multiple substrates, including fibrinogen, factor XIII, factors V and VIII, and protein C, in addition to its effects on platelets (Fig. 3). It plays a central role in hemostasis and thrombosis. The catalytic transformation of fibrinogen into fibrin is essential in the formation of the hemostatic plug and in the formation of arterial thrombi. It binds to the fibrinogen central domain and cleaves fibrinopeptides A and B, resulting in fibrin monomer and polymer formation (68). The fibrin mesh holds the platelets together and contributes to the attachment of the thrombus to the vessel wall.

The control of the coagulation reactions occurs by diverse mechanisms, such as hemodilution and flow effects, proteolytic feedback by thrombin, inhibition by plasma proteins (such as antithrombin III [ATIII]) and endothelial cell-localized activation of an inhibitory enzyme (protein C), and fibrinolysis (Fig. 10). Although ATIII readily inactivates thrombin in solution, its catalytic site is inaccessible while bound to fibrin, and it may still cleave fibrinopeptides even in the presence of heparin. Thrombin has a specific receptor in endothelial cell surfaces, thrombomodulin, that triggers a physiologic anticoagulative system (69). The thrombin–thrombomodulin complex serves as a receptor for the vitamin K-dependent protein C which is activated and re-

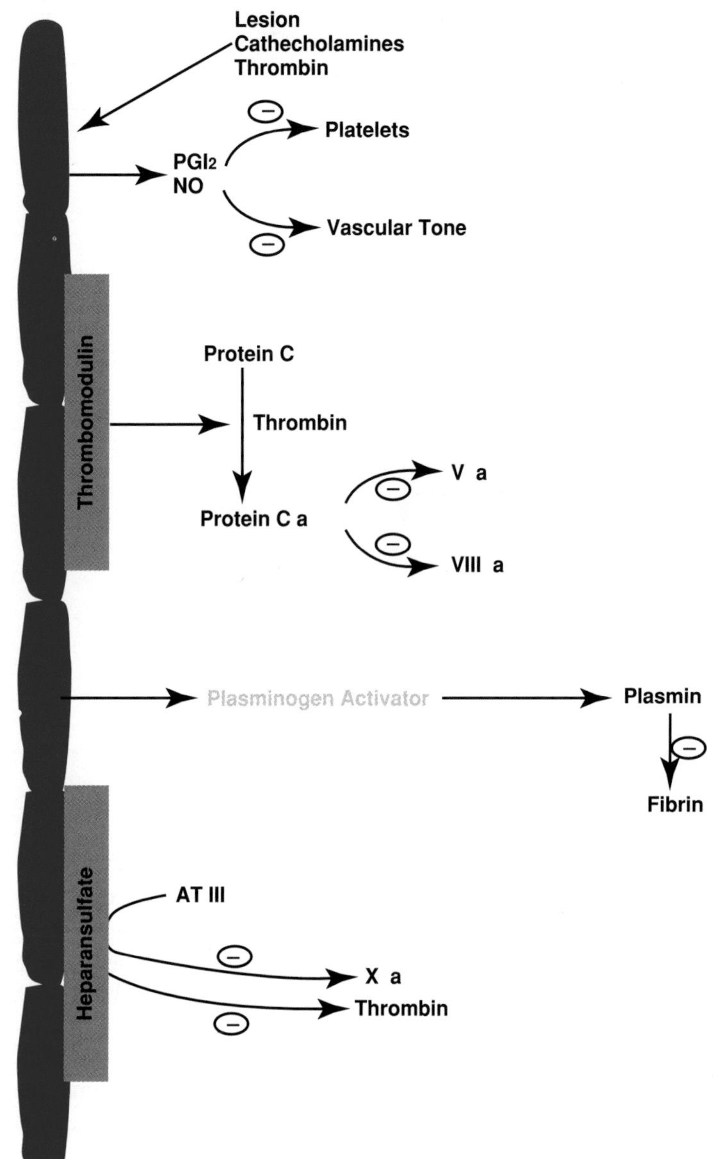

FIG. 10. Simplified diagram of the endothelium physiologic anticoagulant system. The thrombomodulin and heparan sulfate systems work as controllers of the coagulation reaction. Endothelial release of PGI_2 and NO also inhibit platelet activation and reduce the vascular tone.

leased from the endothelial cell surface. Activated protein C blocks the effects of factors V and VIII and limits thrombin effects (Fig. 10). Endogenous fibrinolysis represents a repair mechanism, such as endothelial cell regrowth and vessel recanalization. Fibrinolysis involves catalytic activation of zymogens, positive and negative feedback control, and inhibitor blockade (70,71).

Effects of the Severity of Vessel Wall Damage and Local Geometry on the Thrombotic Response to Atherosclerosis

The dynamics of platelet deposition and thrombus formation following vascular damage are modulated by the type of injury and the local geometry at the site damage (degree of stenosis) (33,72–74). Exposure of deendothelialized vessel wall (mimicking mild vascular injury) to blood at high shear rate (mimicking a stenosed artery) induced significant platelet deposition to the exposed vessel (72). The deposition of platelet reached a maximum within 5–10 min of exposure; however, the evolving aggregates could be dislodged from the substrate by the flowing blood. Exposure of native fibrillar collagen type I bundles with a rough surface (mimicking type III injury) to blood produced platelet deposition of more than two orders of magnitude greater than on subendothelium (33). Even at high shear rate, the thrombus was not dislodged, but remained adherent to the surface. Similar experimental quantitative information on the importance of the degree of vascular damage on the degree and stability of thrombus formation has now been documented by varying degrees of stenosis and with severely damaged vessel wall (exposing medial matrix structures to blood) (73,74). Importantly, besides fibrillar collagen (33), exposed thromboplastin or tissue factor (75,76) seems also to contribute to the high thrombogenicity when deep or severe injury to the vessel wall occurs. Overall, it is likely that when injury to the vessel wall is mild, the thrombogenic stimulus is relatively limited, and the resulting thrombotic occlusion is transient, as occurs in unstable angina. On the other hand, deep vessel injury secondary to plaque rupture or ulceration results in exposure of collagen, tissue factor, and other elements of the vessel matrix, leading to relatively persistent thrombotic occlusion and myocardial infarction (77).

It is likely that the nature of the substrate exposed after spontaneous or angioplasty-induced plaque rupture is one factor determining whether an unstable plaque proceeds rapidly to an occlusive thrombus or persists as nonocclusive mural thrombus. Although observational data show that plaque rupture is a potent stimulus for thrombosis and exposed collagen is suggested to have a predominant role in thrombosis, the relative thrombogenicity of different components of human atherosclerotic plaques is not well established. We have studied the relative contribution of different components of human atherosclerotic plaques to acute thrombus formation after 5-min blood perfusions. Foam-cell-rich matrix (obtained from fatty streaks), collagen-rich matrix (from sclerotic plaques), collagen-poor matrix without cholesterol crystals (from fibrolipid plaques), atheromatous core with abundant cholesterol crystals (from atheromatous plaques), highly cellular plaque (hyperplasic), and segments of normal intima derived from human aortas at necropsy were compared (Fig. 11; see Colorplate 28). Specimens were mounted in the Badimon chamber placed within an ex vivo extracorporeal perfusion system and exposed to heparinized porcine blood (aPTT ratio 1.5 ± 0.04) for 5 min at high-shear-rate conditions mimicking medium-grade stenosis. Thrombus was quantitated by measurement of indium-labeled platelets and morphometric analysis (Fig. 12). Under similar conditions, substrates were perfused with heparinized human blood (2 IU/ml) in an in vitro system and thrombus formation was similarly evaluated. Thrombus formation on atheromatous core was up to sixfold greater than on other substrates, including collagen-rich matrix, in both heterologous and homologous systems (Figs. 11 and 13). Although the atheromatous core had a more irregular exposed surface and thrombus formation tended to increase with increasing roughness, the atheromatous core remained the most thrombogenic substrate when the substrates were normalized by the degree of irregularity as defined by the roughness index. The atheromatous core is the most thrombogenic component of human atherosclerotic plaques, and therefore plaques with a large atheromatous core content are at high risk to lead to acute coronary syndromes after spontaneous or mechanically induced rupture due to the increased thrombogenicity of their contents (78).

Platelet deposition is directly related to the degree of stenosis in the presence of the same degree of injury, indicating a shear-induced platelet activation (73,74). In addition, analysis of the axial distribution of platelet deposition indicates that the apex, and not the flow recirculation zone distal to the apex, is the segment of greatest platelet accumulation. These data suggest that the severity of the acute platelet response to plaque disruption depends in part on the sudden changes in geometry following rupture (3) (Figs. 7 and 14).

Spontaneous lysis of thrombus does occur, not only in unstable angina (77), but also in acute myocardial infarction. In these patients, as well as in those undergoing thrombolysis for acute infarction, the presence of a residual mural thrombus predisposes to recurrent thrombotic vessel occlusion (79–83). Two main contributing factors for the development of rethrombosis have been identified. First, a residual mural thrombus may encroach into the vessel lumen resulting in increased shear rate, which facilitates the activation and deposition of platelets on the lesion. As mentioned previously, using an experimental animal model of ex vivo perfusion, it has been shown that platelet deposition is higher with increasing degrees of vessel stenosis (73,74). Second, the presence of a fragmented thrombus appears to be one of the

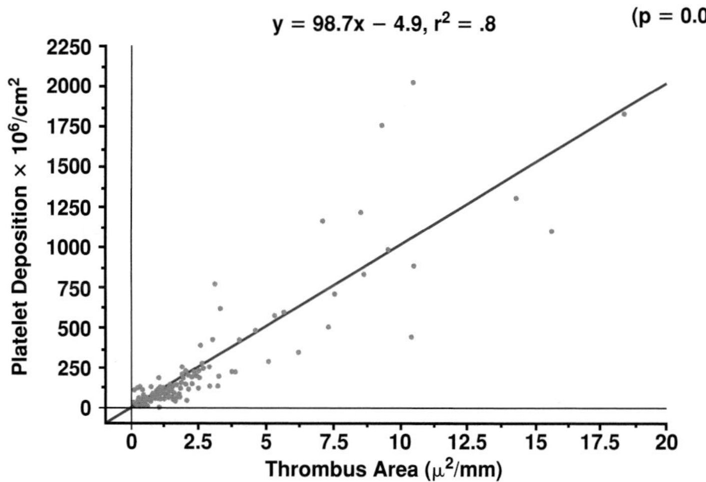

FIG. 12. Morphometric evaluation of thrombus deposited on severely injured vessel wall showing a highly significant correlation with values of platelet deposition obtained by ^{111}In-labeling of platelets. (From Fernández-Ortiz, et al., ref. 78.)

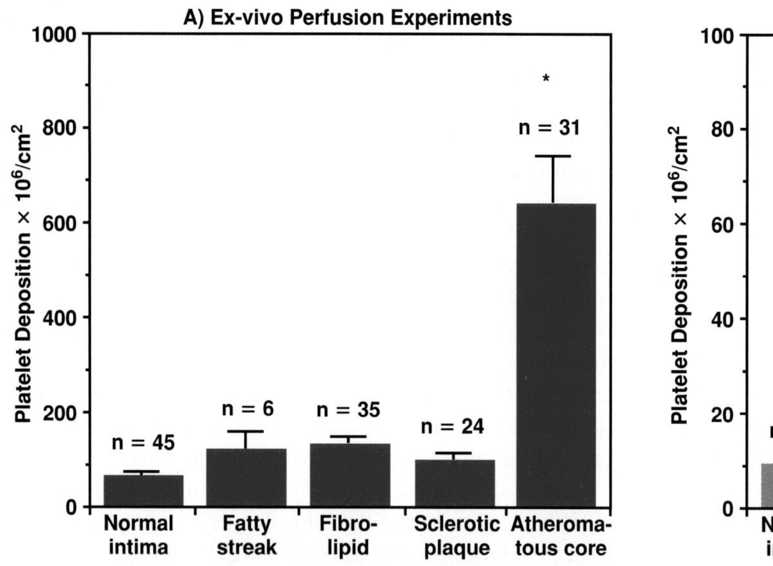

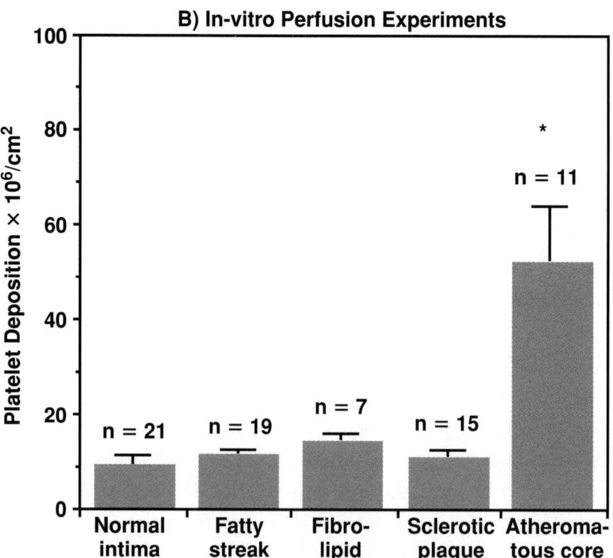

FIG. 13. Platelet deposition on atherosclerotic substrates (as in Fig. 10) evaluated by perfusing blood with ^{111}In-labeled platelets. Experiments were performed using citrated human blood **(A)** and heparinized porcine blood in an extracorporeal in vivo experiment **(B).** (For details see Fernández-Ortiz, et al., ref. 78.)

most powerful thrombogenic surfaces. This was also evaluated in the ex vivo Badimon perfusion chamber model, where platelet deposition was assessed by continuous scintigraphic imaging of ^{111}In-labeled platelets. A gradual increase in platelet deposition in the area of maximal stenosis was observed, followed by an abrupt drop, probably owing to spontaneous thrombus emobilization or platelet deaggregation. This was immediately followed by a rapid increase in platelet deposition, suggesting that the remaining thrombus was markedly thrombogenic. In fact, platelet deposition is increased two to four times on residual thrombus compared with deeply injured arterial wall; and thrombus continues to grow during heparin therapy, but is inhibited by specific antithrombin treatment (84,85).

r-Hirudin, a recombinant molecule that blocks both the catalytic site and the anion-exosite of the thrombin molecule, inhibited significantly the secondary growth (84). In a canine model of coronary thrombolysis, reocclusion of a recanalized artery was mainly related to the high local thrombin activity on the surface of the fragmented thrombus (86). Indeed, experimentally, when thrombus breaks, thrombin bound to fibrin becomes exposed (87). Thus, following lysis, thrombin becomes exposed to the circulating blood, leading to activation of the platelets and coagulation, further enhanc-

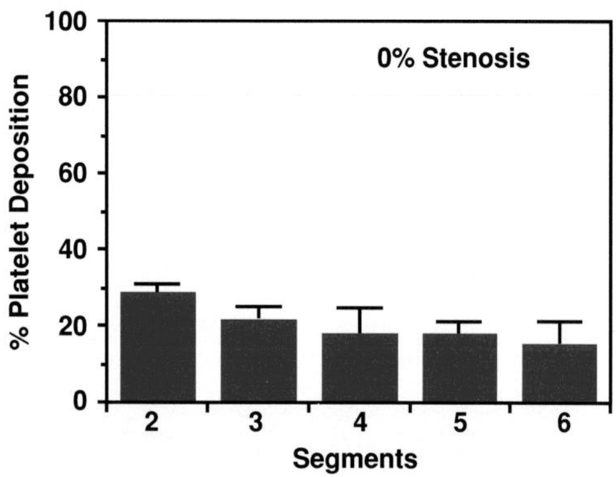

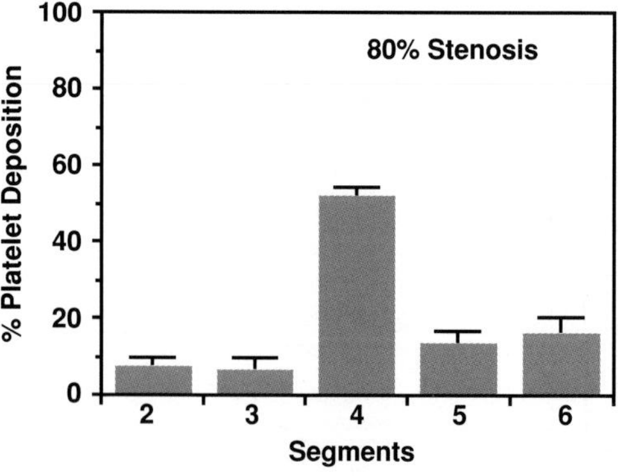

FIG. 14. Platelet deposition on severely injured vessel wall with a sinusoidal eccentric 80% stenosis measured by ^{111}In-labeling of platelets. Maximal deposition was in segment 4, where the apex of the 80% stenosis was localized, and not in the flow recirculation zone next to the apex (segments 5–6). Laminar flow profile (0% stenosis) results in the absence of the stenosis are also shown. The presence of stenosis induces local flow disturbances with blood acceleration (increase in shear rate) at the apex and deceleration at the recirculation zone distal to the apex (eddies and decrease in local shear rate).

ing thrombosis. The antithrombin activity of heparin is limited for three main reasons (85–88). First, a residual thrombus contains active thrombin bound to fibrin, which is thus poorly accessible to the large heparin–antithrombin III complexes; second, a platelet-rich arterial thrombus releases large amounts of platelet factor 4, which may inhibit heparin; third, fibrin II monomer, formed by the action of thrombin on fibrinogen, may also inhibit heparin. Conversely, molecules of hirudin and other specific antithrombins are at least ten times smaller than the heparin–antithrombin III complex, have no natural inhibitors, and therefore have greater accessibility to thrombin bound to fibrin. These experimental results clarify the clinical observations in patients with acute myocardial infarction undergoing thrombolysis, which have shown that residual stenosis is in part related to residual nonlysed thrombus (82,89).

The effects of different antithrombotic treatment regimens on thrombus formation triggered by a residual mural thrombus have been evaluated and specific thrombin inhibition has been shown to be the most effective in inhibiting the progression of thrombus growth when compared to aspirin, heparin, or both (90).

As mentioned before, in addition to these prothrombotic effects, thrombin generates a series of reactions that activate the endogenous anticoagulant system (Fig. 10). Thrombin generated at the site of injury binds to thrombomodulin, an endothelial surface membrane protein, initiating activation of protein C, which in turn (in the presence of protein S) inactivates factors Va and VIIIa. Thrombin stimulates successive release of both tissue plasminogen activator (tPA) and plasminogen-activator inhibitor type 1 from endothelial cells, thus initiating endogenous lysis through plasmin generation from plasminogen by tPA with subsequent modulation through plasminogen-activator inhibitor type 1. Thrombin therefore plays a pivotal role in maintaining the complex balance of initial prothrombotic reparative events and subsequent endogenous anticoagulant and thrombolytic pathways (69,91) (Fig. 4).

The importance of thrombin lies not just in acute thrombus formation following arterial injury, but also in its contribution to smooth muscle cell proliferation by stimulating platelet secretion of growth factors (especially platelet-derived growth factor) and directly acting on smooth muscle cells (Fig. 4). Thus, thrombin has direct effects on cell proliferation and influences the cellular synthetic mechanisms responsible for matrix protein and collagen production (92). The role of thrombin as a possible mitogen for vascular cells has gained support with the identification of the cellular thrombin receptor (64) and with the recent detection of mRNA for this receptor in human atherosclerotic plaques (93). When thrombin is neutralized by complex formation with antithrombin III, thrombin-induced DNA synthesis and cell proliferation in human arterial smooth muscle cells are completely inhibited (94). Since mural thrombosis is usually associated with rescue coronary revascularization procedures, we studied how platelet activation with different agonists may affect smooth muscle cell (SMC) proliferation. Platelet release products from activation with ADP, collagen, and thrombin were incubated with quiescent synchronized coronary smooth muscle cells and ^{3}H-thymidine incorporation into newly formed DNA measured. Thrombin was the only agonist that showed direct proliferative effects on SMC and it also induced significantly higher proliferative effects than the other platelet agonists when platelet release products were coincubated with SMC (Fig. 15). Therefore,

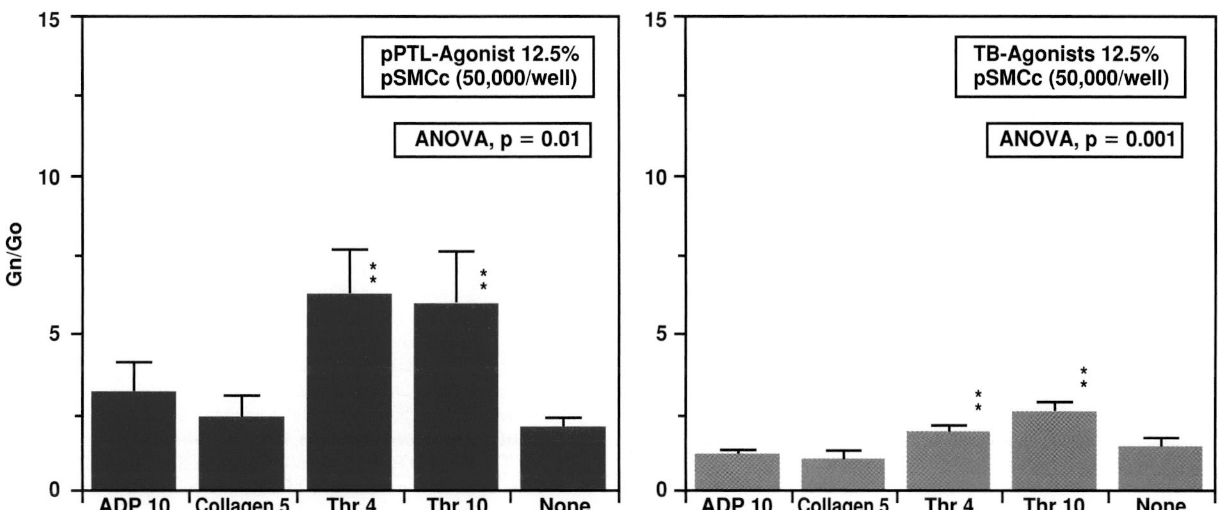

FIG. 15. Subconfluent porcine coronary smooth muscle cells (pSMC) were synchronized for 48 h in serum-free media and coincubated with porcine platelet release products of isolated platelet activation induced by ADP, collagen, and thrombin (Thr). ^{3}H-Thymidine incorporation was measured as an index of DNA synthesis (normalized by ^{3}H-thymidine incorporation in G_o). Thrombin was the agonist that induced the highest response in proliferation. Results are normalized per well protein content. TB, tyrode buffer; pPTL, porcine platelets. (From Varela et al., ref. 95.)

in severe wall injury, when there is significant in situ thrombin generation, platelets will generate a more significant proliferative stimulus for the subjacent SMC than when other agonists for platelet monolayer formation are prevalent (95). Specific thrombin inhibition may also have a potential impact on the relative proliferative response of endothelial and smooth muscle cells after arterial injury such as due to percutaneous transluminal coronary angioplasty by preventing restenosis (96).

SUMMARY

Arterial thrombus formation seems to be an important factor in the conversion of chronic to acute atherosclerotic coronary events after plaque rupture, in the progression of coronary disease, and in the acute phase of revascularization interventions. The knowledge gained (and studies now in progress) on the mechanisms of platelet activation, signal transduction, receptor binding, zymogen activation and function, substrate recognition, and adhesive events will help to design promising approaches for intervention. Receptors originally thought to be involved only in anchoring functions are also important factors in the transduction of information from the extracellular compartment to the inner cell and they are involved in governing cell function, shape, proliferation, and differentiation. The availability of monoclonal antibodies and molecular biology techniques applied to the field of thrombosis and blood cell–vessel wall interaction will provide tools to explore specific pathways of cell activation and cell–cell interaction. These studies together with those to find the most prevalent agonist and substrate to trigger and perpetuate a thrombotic event in every clinical situation will help to establish strategies of prevention of clinical events and to reduce their associated morbidity and mortality.

ACKNOWLEDGMENTS

This article was supported by grants CICYT SAF 712/94, FIS 92-0114, and Cardiovascular Research Foundation-Catalana Occidente, Spain. The authors thank Silvia Morató for the preparation of the manuscript. The original contributions mentioned in the article were generated in a long-standing collaboration with Dr. V. Fuster from the Cardiovascular Institute, Mount Sinai Medical Center.

REFERENCES

1. Fuster V, Badimon L, Badimon JJ, Chesebro JH. The pathogenesis of coronary artery disease and the acute coronary syndromes. (Part I). *N Engl J Med* 1992;326:242–250.
2. Fuster V, Badimon L, Badimon JJ, Chesebro JH. The pathogenesis of coronary artery disease and the acute coronary syndromes. (Part II). *N Engl J Med* 1992;326:310–318.
3. Badimon L, Chesebro JH, Badimon JJ. Thrombus formation on ruptured atherosclerotic plaques and rethrombosis on evolving thrombi. *Circulation* 1992;86(Suppl III):III-74–III-85.
4. Badimon JJ, Fuster V, Chesebro JH, Badimon L. Coronary atherosclerosis. *Circulation* 1993;87:(Suppl II):II-3–II-16.
5. Marcus A, Safier LB. Thromboregulation: Multicellular modulation of platelet reactivity in hemostasis and thrombosis. *FASEB J* 1993;7: 516–522.
6. Kroll MH, Schafer AI. Biochemical mechanisms of platelet activation. *Blood* 1989;74:1181–1195.
7. Brass LF. The biochemistry of platelet activation. In: Hoffman R, Benz EJ Jr, Shattil SJ, Furie B, Cohen HJ, eds. *Hematology: Basic Principles and Practice*. New York: Churchill Livingstone; 1991;1176–1197.
8. Colman RW, Walsh PN. Mechanisms of platelet aggregation. In: Colman RW, Hirsh J, Marder VJ, Salzman E, eds. *Hemostasis and Thrombosis: Basic Principles and Clinical Practice,* 2nd ed. Philadelphia: Lippincott; 1987;594–605.
9. Huang EM, Detwiler TC. Stimulus–response coupling mechanisms. In: Philips DR, Shuman MC, eds. *Biochemistry of Platelets*. New York: Academic Press; 1986;1–68.
10. Kieffer N, Phillips DR. Platelet membrane glycoproteins: Functions in cellular interactions. *Annu Rev Biol* 1990;6:329–357.
11. Kunicki TJ. Organization of glycoproteins within the platelet plasma membrane. In: George JN, Nurden AT, Philips DR, eds. *Platelet Membrane Glycoproteins*. New York: Plenum Press; 1985;87–101.
12. Vicente V, Houghten RA, Ruggeri ZM. Identification of a site in the α chain of platelet glycoprotein Ib that participates in von Willebrand factor binding. *J Biol Chem* 1990;265:274–280.
13. Fujimura Y, Titani K, Holland LZ, Russell SR, Roberts JR, et al. von Willebrand factor. A reduced and alkylated 52/48-kDa fragment beginning at amino acid residue 449 contains the domain interacting with platelet glycoprotein Ib. *J Biol Chem* 1986;261:381–385.
14. Fox JEB, Boyles JK, Berndt MC, Steffen PK, Anderson LK. Identification of a membrane skeleton in platelets. *J Cell Biol* 1988;106: 1525–1538.
15. Meyer D, Girma JP. von Willebrand factor: Structure and function. *Thromb Haemostasis* 1993;70:99–104.
16. Fitzgerald LA, Phillips DR. Calcium regulation of the platelet membrane glycoprotein IIb–IIIa complex. *J Biol Chem* 1985;260: 11366–11376.
17. Calvete JJ, Henschen A, Gonzalez-Rodriguez J. Complete localization of the intrachain disulphide bonds and the N-glycosylation points in the α subunit of human platelet glycoprotein IIb. *Biochem J* 1989;261: 561–568.
18. Beer J, Coller BS. Evidence that platelet glycoprotein IIIa has a large disulfide bonded loop that is susceptible to proteolytic cleavage. *J Biol Chem* 1989;264:17564–17573.
19. Plow EF, Ginsberg MH, Marguerie GA. Expression and function of adhesive proteins on the platelet surface. In: Phillips DR, Shuman MA, eds. *Biochemistry of Platelets*. New York: Academic Press; 1986; 225–256.
20. Ruoslahti E, Pierschbacher MD. New perspectives in cell adhesion: RGD and integrins. *Science* 1987;238:491–497.
21. Doolittle RF, Watt KWK, Cottrell BA, Strong DD, Riley M. The amino acid sequence of the α-chain of human fibrinogen. *Nature* 1979;280: 464–467.
22. Kloczewiak M, Timmons S, Lukas TJ, Hawiger J. Platelet receptor recognition site on human fibrinogen. Synthesis and structure–function relationship of peptides corresponding to the carboxyterminal segment of the γ chain. *Biochemistry* 1984;23:1767–1774.
23. Ginsberg MH, Xiaoping D, O'Toole TE, Loftus JC, Plow EF. Platelet integrins. *Thromb Haemostasis* 1993;70:87–93.
24. Shattil SJ. Regulation of platelet anchorage and signaling by integrin αIIbβ_3. *Thromb Haemostasis* 1993;70:224–228.
25. Vu TH, Hung DT, Wheaton VI, Coughlin SR. Molecular cloning of a functional thrombin receptor reveals a novel proteolytic mechanism of receptor activation. *Cell* 1991;64:1057–1068.
26. Coughlin SR. Thrombin receptor structure and function. *Thromb Haemostasis* 1993;70:184–187.
27. Sakariassen KS, Nievelstein PF, Coller BS, Sixma JJ. The role of platelet membrane glycoproteins Ib and IIb/IIIa in platelet adherence to human artery subendothelium. *Br J Haematol* 1986;63:681–691.
28. Weiss HJ, Turitto VT, Baumgartner HR. Effect of shear rate on platelet interaction with subendothelium in citrated and native blood. I. Shear

rate-dependent decrease of adhesion in von Willebrand's disease and the Bernard–Soulier syndrome. *J Lab Clin Med* 1978;92:750–754.
29. Sixma JJ, Sakariassen KS, Beeser-Vesser NH, et al. Adhesion of platelets to human artery subendothelium: Effects of factor VIII–von Willebrand factor of various multimeric composition. *Blood* 1984;63:128.
30. Turitto VT, Baumgartner HR. Platelet–surface interactions. In: Colman R, Hirsh J, Marder V, Salzman E, eds. *Hemostasis and Thrombosis: Basic Principles and Clinical Practice,* 2nd ed. Philadelphia: Lippincott; 1987;555–571.
31. Sakariassen K, Bolhuis PA, Sixma J. Human blood platelet adhesion to artery subendothelium is mediated by factor VIII–von Willebrand factor bound to the subendothelium. *Nature* 1979;279:636–638.
32. Badimon L, Badimon JJ, Turitto VT, Fuster V. Platelet deposition in von Willebrand factor deficient vessel wall. *J Lab Clin Med* 1987;110: 634–647.
33. Badimon L, Badimon JJ, Turitto VT, Vallabhajosula S, Fuster V. Platelet thrombus formation on collagen type I. Influence of blood rheology, von Willebrand factor and blood coagulation. *Circulation* 1988;78: 1431–1442.
34. Badimon L, Badimon JJ, Chesebro JH, Fuster V. Inhibition of thrombus formation: Blockage of adhesive glycoprotein mechanism versus blockage of the cyclooxygenase pathway. *J Am Coll Cardiol* 1988;11: 30A.
35. Badimon L, Badimon JJ, Turitto VT, Fuster V. Platelet interaction to vessel wall and collagen. Study in homozygous von Willebrand's disease associated with abnormal collagen aggregation in swine. *Thromb Haemostasis* 1989;61:57–64.
36. Badimon L, Badimon JJ, Turitto VT, Fuster V. Role of von Willebrand factor in mediating platelet–vessel wall interaction at low shear rate; the importance of perfusion conditions. *Blood* 1989;73:961–967.
37. Cattaneo M, Kinlough-Rathbone R, Lecchi A, Bevilacqua C, Packham MA, Mustard JF. Fibrinogen-independent aggregation and deaggregation of human platelets: Studies in two afibrinogenemic patients. *Blood* 1987;70:221–226.
38. Soria J, Soria C, Borg JY, et al. Platelet aggregation occurs in congenital afibrinogenaemia despite the absence of fibrinogen or its fragments in plasma and platelets, as demonstrated by immunoenzymology. *Br J Haematol* 1985;60:503–510.
39. Turitto VT, Weiss JH, Baumgartner HR. Platelet interaction with rabbit subendothelium in von Willebrand's disease: Altered thrombus formation distinct from defective platelet adhesion. *J Clin Invest* 1984;74: 1730–1741.
40. Weiss HJ, Turitto VT, Vicic WJ, Baumgartner HR. Fibrin formation, fibrinopeptide A release, and platelet thrombus dimensions on subendothelium exposed to flowing native blood: Greater in factor XII and XI than in factor VIII and IX deficiency. *Blood* 1984;63:1004–1014.
41. Weiss HJ, Hawiger J, Ruggeri ZM, Turitto VT, Thiagarajan I, Hoffman T. Fibrinogen-independent interaction of platelets with subendothelium mediated by glycoprotein IIb–IIIa complex at high shear rate. *J Clin Invest* 1989;83:288–297.
42. Badimon L, Badimon JJ, Cohen M, Chesebro J, Fuster V. Thrombosis in stenotic and laminar flow conditions: Effect of an antiplatelet GPIIb/IIIa monoclonal antibody fragment (7E3F(ab′)$_2$). *Circulation* 1989; 80(Suppl):II-422(abst).
43. Lombardo VT, Hodson E, Roberts JR, Kunicki TJ, Zimmerman TS, Ruggeri ZM. Independent modulation of von Willebrand factor and fibrinogen binding to the platelet membrane glycoprotein IIb/IIIa complex as demonstrated by monoclonal antibody. *J Clin Invest* 1985;76: 1950–1958.
44. Badimon L, Badimon JJ, Ruggeri Z, Fuster V. A peptide-specific monoclonal antibody that inhibits von Willebrand factor binding to GPIIb/IIa (152B6) inhibits platelet deposition to human atherosclerotic vessel wall. *Circulation* 1990;82(4):III-370(abst).
45. Badimon L, Badimon JJ, Chesebro JH, Fuster V. von Willebrand factor and cardiovascular disease. *Thromb Haemostasis* 1993;70:111–118.
46. Pawashe A, Guth BD, Muller TH, Migliaccio F, Ezekowitz MD. Inhibition of experimental thrombosis with monoclonal antibody against rabbit tissue factor. *J Am Coll Cardiol* 1993;21(2):466A.
47. Rentrop KP, Feit F, Blanke H, et al. Effects of intracoronary streptokinase and intracoronary nitroglycerin infusion on coronary angiographic patterns and mortality in patients with acute myocardial infarction. *N Engl J Med* 1984;311:1457–1463.
48. Basmadjian D, Sefton MV. A model of thrombin inactivation in heparinized and non-heparinized tubes with consequences for thrombus formation. *J Biomed Mater Res* 1986;20:633–651.
49. Goldsmith HL, Turitto VT. Rheological aspects of thrombosis and haemostasis: Basic principles and applications. *Thromb Haemostasis* 1986; 55:415–436.
50. Charm SE, Wong BL. Enzyme inactivation with shearing. *Biotechnol Bioeng* 1970;12:1103–1109.
51. Charm SE, Lai CJ. Comparison of ultrafiltration systems for concentration of biologicals. *Biotechnol Bioeng* 1971;12:185–202.
52. Weiss HJ, Turitto VT, Baumgartner HR, Nemerson Y, Hoffman T. Evidence for the presence of tissue-factor activity on subendothelium. *Blood* 1989;73:968–975.
53. Badimon L, Badimon JJ, Lassila R, Heras M, Chesebro JH, Fuster V. Thrombin regulation of platelet interaction with damaged vessel wall and isolated collagen type I at arterial flow conditions in a porcine model. Effects of hirudins, heparin and calcium chelation. *Blood* 1991; 78:423–434.
54. Mailhac A, Badimon JJ, Fallon JT, Fernández-Ortiz A, Meyer B, Chesebro JH, Fuster V, Badimon L. Effect of an eccentric severe stenosis on fibrin(ogen) deposition on severely damaged vessel wall in arterial thrombosis. Relative contribution of fibrin(ogen) and platelets. *Circulation* 1994;90:988–996.
55. Nemerson Y. Mechanism of coagulation. In: Williams WJ, Beutler E, Erslev AJ, Lichtman MA, eds. *Hematology.* New York: McGraw-Hill; 1990;1295–1304.
56. Rimon S, Melamed R, Savion N, et al. Identification of a factor IX/IXa binding protein on the endothelial cell surface. *J Biol Chem* 1987; 262:6023–6031.
57. Colman RW, Marder VJ, Salzman EW, Hirsh J. Overview of hemostasis. In: Colman RW, Hirsh J, Marder VJ, Salzman EW, eds. *Hemostasis and Thrombosis: Basic Principles and Clinical Practice.* Philadelphia: Lippincott; 1987;3–17.
58. Mann KG. Membrane-bound enzyme complexes in blood coagulation. In: Spaet TH, ed. *Progress in Hemostasis and Thrombosis.* New York: Grune & Stratton; 1984;1–23.
59. Tracy PB. Regulation of thrombin generation at cell surfaces. *Semin Thromb Haemostasis* 1988;14:227–233.
60. Mann KG, Nesheim ME, Church WR, Haley P, Krishnaswamy S. Surface dependent reactions of the vitamin K dependent enzyme complexes. *Blood* 1990;76:1–16.
61. Rawala-Sheikh R, Ahmad SS, Ashby B, Walsh PN. Kinetics of coagulation factor X activation by platelet bound factor IXa. *Biochemistry* 1990;29:2606–2611.
62. Tracy PB, Eide LL, Mann KG. Human prothrombinase complex assembly and function on isolated peripheral blood cell populations. *J Biol Chem* 1985;260:2119–2124.
63. Rosing J, van Rijn JLML, Bevers EM, van Dieijen G, Comfurius P, Zwaal RFA. The role of activated human platelets in prothrombin and factor X activation. *Blood* 1985;65:319–332.
64. Nesheim ME, Furmaniak-Kazmierczak E, Henin C, Côté G. On the existence of platelet receptors for factor Va and factor VIIIa. *Thromb Haemostasis* 1993;70:80–86.
65. Tracy PB, Nesheim ME, Mann KG. Coordinate binding of factor Va and factor Xa to the unstimulated platelet. *J Biol Chem* 1981;256: 743–751.
66. Ahmad SS, Rawala-Sheikh R, Monroe DM, Roberts HR, Walsh PN. Comparative platelet binding and kinetic studies with normal and variant factor IXa molecules. *J Biol Chem* 1990;265:20907–20911.
67. Comp PC. Kinetics of plasma coagulation factors. In: Williams WJ, Beutler E, Erslev AJ, Lichtman MA, eds. *Hematology.* New York: McGraw-Hill; 1990;1285–1290.
68. Nemerson Y, Williams WJ. Biochemistry of plasma coagulation factors. In: Williams WJ, Beutler E, Erslev AJ, Lichtman MA, eds. *Hematology.* New York: McGraw-Hill; 1990;1267–1284.
69. Esmon NL, Owen WG, Esmon CT. Isolation of a membrane-bound co-factor for thrombin-catalyzed activation of protein C. *J Biol Chem* 1982;257:859–864.
70. Francis CW, Marder VJ. Physiologic regulation and pathologic disorders of fibrinolysis. In: Colman RW, Hirsh J, Marder VJ, Salzman EW, eds. *Hemostasis and Thrombosis: Basic Principles and Clinical Practice.* Philadelphia: Lippincott; 1987;358–379.
71. Collen D, Lijnen HR. Molecular and cellular basis of fibrinolysis. In: Hoffman R, Benz EJ Jr, Shattil SJ, Furie B, Cohen HJ, eds. *Hematology: Basic Principles and Practice.* New York: Churchill Livingstone; 1991;1232–1242.
72. Badimon L, Badimon JJ, Galvez A, Chesebro JH, Fuster V. Influence

of arterial damage and wall shear rate on platelet deposition. *Ex vivo* study in swine model. *Arteriosclerosis* 1986;6:312–320.
73. Badimon L, Badimon JJ. Mechanism of arterial thrombosis in nonparallel streamlines: Platelet grow at the apex of stenotic severely injured vessel wall. Experimental study in the pig model. *J Clin Invest* 1989;84:1134–1144.
74. Lassila R, Badimon JJ, Vallbhajosula S, Badimon L. Dynamic monitoring of platelet deposition on severely damaged vessel wall in flowing blood. Effects of different stenosis on thrombus growth. *Arteriosclerosis* 1990;10:306–315.
75. Drake TA, Morrissey JH, Edgington TS. Selective cellular expression of tissue factor in human tissues: Implication of hemostasis and thrombosis. *Am J Pathol* 1989;134:1087–1097.
76. Wilcox JN, Smith SM, Schwartz SM, Gordon D. Localization of tissue factor in the normal vessel wall and atherosclerotic plaque. *Proc Natl Acad Sci USA* 1989;2839–2843.
77. Fuster V, Chesebro JH. Mechanisms of unstable angina. *N Engl J Med* 1986;315:1023–1025.
78. Fernández-Ortiz A, Badimon JJ, Falk E, Fuster V, Meyer B, Mailhac A, Weng D, Shah PK, Badimon L. Characterization of the relative thrombogenicity of atherosclerotic plaque components: Implications for consequences of plaque rupture. *J Am Coll Cardiol* 1994;23:1562–1569.
79. Van de Werf F, Arnold AER, and the European Cooperative Study Group for Recombinant Tissue-Type Plasminogen Activator (rt-PA). Effect of intravenous tissue plasminogen activator on infarct size, left ventricular function and survival in patients with acute myocardial infarction. *Br Med J* 1988;297:374–379.
80. Van Lierde, De Geest H, Verstraete M, et al. Angiographic assessment of the infarct-related residual coronary stenosis after spontaneous or therapeutic thrombolysis. *J Am Coll Cardiol* 1990;16:1545–1549.
81. Fuster V, Stein B, Badimon L, Badimon JJ, Ambrose JA, Chesebro JH. Atherosclerotic plaque rupture and thrombosis: Evolving concepts. *Circulation* 1990;82(Suppl II):47–59.
82. Davies SW, Marchant B, Lyon JP, et al. Coronary lesion morphology in acute myocardial infarction: Demonstration of early remodeling after streptokinase treatment. *J Am Coll Cardiol* 1990;16:1079–1086.
83. Gulba DC, Barthels M, Westhoff-Bleck M, et al. Increased thrombin levels during acute myocardial infarction. Relevance for the success of therapy. *Circulation* 1991;83:937–944.
84. Badimon L, Badimon JJ, Lasilla R, Heras M, Chesebro JH, Fuster V. Thrombin inhibition by hirudin decreases platelet thrombus growth on areas of severe vessel wall injury. *J Am Coll Cardiol* 1989;13:145A.
85. Weitz JI, Hudoba M, Massel D, Maragamore J, Hirsh J. Clot-bound thrombin is protected from inhibition by heparin-antithrombin III but is susceptible to inactivation by antithrombin III-independent inhibitors. *J Clin Invest* 1990;86:385–391.
86. Fitzgerald DJ, Fitzgerald GA. Role of thrombin and thromboxane A_2 in reocclusion following coronary thrombolysis with tissue-type plasminogen activator. *Proc Natl Acad Sci USA* 1989;86:7585–7589.
87. Francis CW, Markham RE, Barlow GH, Florack TM, Dobrzynski DM, Marder VJ. Thrombin activity of fibrin thrombi and soluble plasmic derivatives. *J Lab Clin Med* 1983;102:220–230.
88. Hogg PJ, Jackson CM. Fibrin monomer protects thrombin from inactivation by heparin-antithrombin III: Implications for heparin efficacy. *Proc Natl Acad Sci USA* 1989;86:3619–3623.
89. Waller BF, Rothbaum DA, Pinkerton CA, et al. Status of the myocardium and infarct-related coronary artery in 19 necropsy patients with acute recanalization using pharmacologic (streptokinase, r-tissue plasminogen activator), mechanical (percutaneous transluminal coronary angioplasty) or combined types of reperfusion therapy. *J Am Coll Cardiol* 1987;9:785–801.
90. Meyer BJ, Badimon JJ, Mailhac A, Fernández-Ortiz A, Chesebro JH, Fuster V, Badimon L. Inhibition of growth of thrombus on fresh mural thrombus: Targeting optimal therapy. *Circulation* 1994;90:2432–2438.
91. Badimon L, Meyer BJ, Badimon JJ. Thrombin in arterial thrombosis. *Haemostasis* 1994;24:69–80.
92. Graham DJ, Alexander JJ. The effects of thrombin on bovine aortic endothelial and smooth muscle cells. *J Vasc Surg* 1990;11:307–313.
93. Nelken NA, Soifer SJ, O'Keefe J, Vu TH, Charo IF, Coughlin SR. Thrombin receptor expression in normal and atherosclerotic human arteries. *J Clin Invest* 1992;90:1614–1621.
94. Hedin U, Frebelius S, Sanchez J, Dryjski M, Swedenborg J. Antithrombin III inhibits thrombin-induced proliferatioon in human arterial smooth muscle cells. *Arterioscler Thromb* 1994;14:254–260.
95. Varela O, Royo T, Badimon L. Agonist-induced platelet secretion and coronary smooth muscle cell proliferation. *Eur J Clin Invest* 1994;24(Suppl 2):59A (abst).
96. Sarembock IJ, Gertz SD, Gimple LW, Owen RM, Powers ER, Roberts WC. Effectiveness of recombinant desulphatohirudin in reducing restenosis after balloon angioplasty of atherosclerotic femoral arteries in rabbits. *Circulation* 1991;84:232–243.
97. Badimon L, Ruster V, Chesebro JH, Badimon JJ. Kinetics of fibrogen deposition on stenotic damaged vessel wall in arterial thrombosis. *Thromb Haemostasis* 1993;69(6):813 (abst).

Atherosclerosis and Coronary Artery Disease,
edited by V. Fuster, R. Ross, and E. J. Topol.
Lippincott-Raven Publishers, Philadelphia © 1996.

CHAPTER 37

Coronary Spasm and Atherosclerosis

Thomas F. Lüscher, G. Noll, and Carl J. Pepine

Key Words: Atherosclerosis; Coronary spasm; Endothelium; Vascular smooth muscle; Vasomotion; Vasospasm.

INTRODUCTION

In 1959, Prinzmetal and colleagues described a new syndrome consisting of chest pain that developed at rest and very often occurred in the early morning hours (1,2). The pain was associated with ST segment elevations in the electrocardiogram and was relieved by nitroglycerin. They named the syndrome ''variant angina'' and suggested that it was caused by a spasm of a major epicardial coronary artery.

Subsequently, coronary spasm has been documented angiographically in most patients with variant angina (3–7). In addition, coronary constriction has been recognized as an important factor in the pathogenesis of many other ischemia-related coronary syndromes (8,9). Although the phenomenon has been well characterized clinically and angiographically, the cause of coronary spasm remains enigmatic. Moreover, it even appears uncertain whether all increases in coronary vascular tone occurring in acute ischemic syndromes can be explained by a single factor or rather represent a heterogeneous entity ranging from normal coronary vasomotion in a narrowed vascular segment to ''true spasm'' with total or near-total occlusion of an angiographically normal or mildly atherosclerotic coronary artery (8).

In patients with variant angina, vasospasm is often, but not always, a localized phenomenon that repeatedly affects the same coronary vascular segment either spontaneously or after provocation (Fig. 1). Thus, a local dysfunction of the blood vessel wall at the site of spasm must be involved. Accordingly, alterations of local neurogenic control, vascular smooth muscle function, the endothelium, or even blood cells have been implicated. Sometimes, however, spasm may affect multiple sites in the same or different arteries, diffuse sites, or even migrate from site to site. These cases are difficult to explain by a local dysfunction theory.

CORONARY VASOMOTION AND VASOSPASM

As can all blood vessels, coronary arteries are able to contract and relax via various mechanisms. Normally, even in vitro coronary arteries exhibit spontaneous tone; i.e., the vascular smooth muscle is contracted to some degree, a phenomenon that can be demonstrated in vitro or in vivo by application of vasodilators such as nitroglycerin or papaverine. Constriction therefore is a normal phenomenon in the coronary circulation and not necessarily pathological (Fig.

T. F. Lüscher and G. Noll: Division of Cardiology, Cardiovascular Research, University Hospital CH-3010 Bern, Switzerland.
C. J. Pepine: Department of Medicine, University of Florida, Gainesville, Florida 32610.

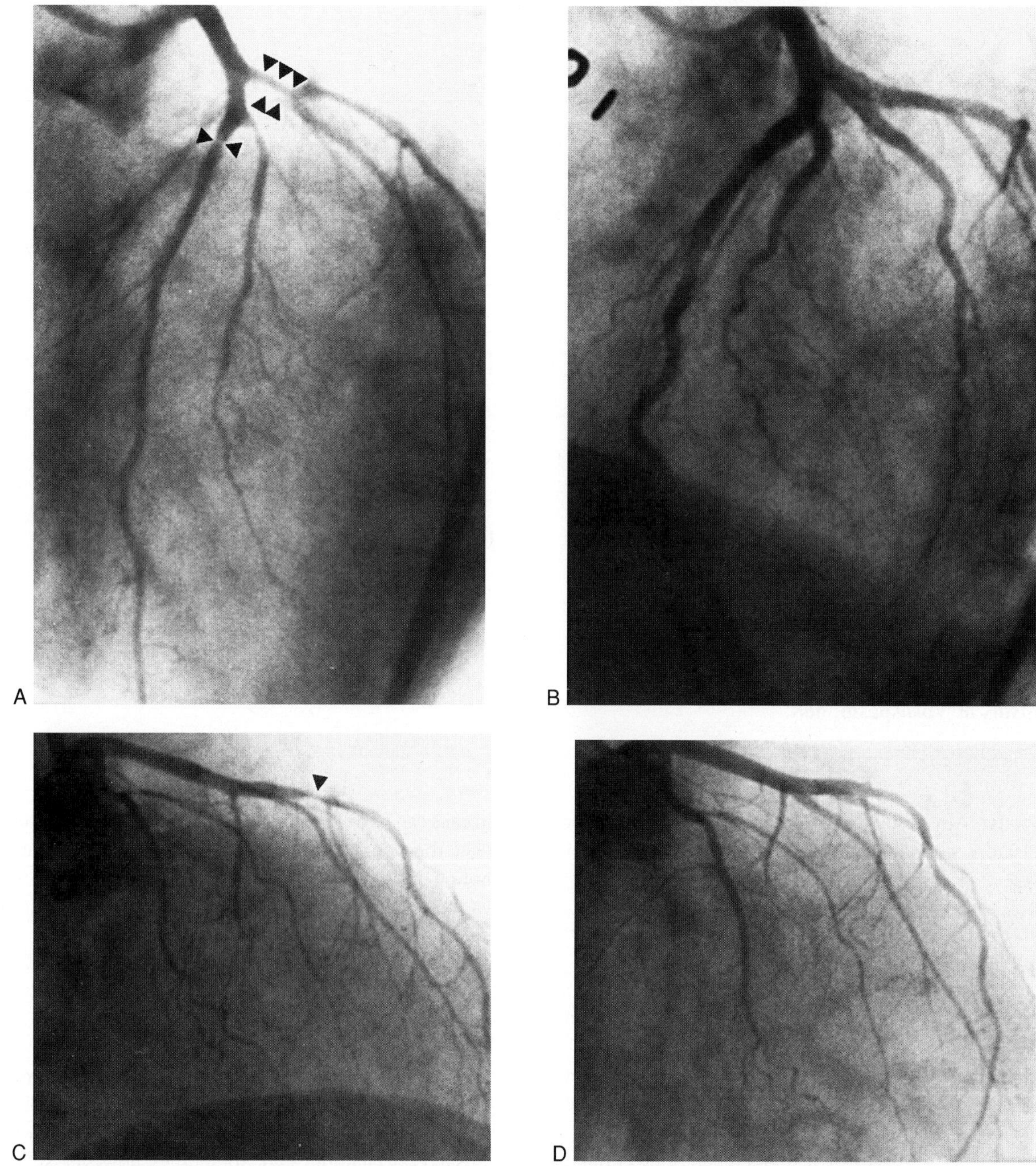

FIG. 1. Examples of coronary spasm. **Top row:** Multivessel spasm. **Left panel:** Spontaneously occurring spasm involving the proximal left anterior descending (single pair of *arrows*), first diagonal branch *(double arrows),* and second diagonal branch (no arrows) as well as the proximal portion of the left circumflex artery *(triple arrows).* **Right panel:** Resolution of spasm at these sites following intracoronary nitroglycerin. **Bottom row:** Single-vessel spasm. **Left panel:** Ergonovine-induced spasm localized to a single site in the mid–left anterior descending artery *(arrow).* **Right panel:** Resolution after nitroglycerin.

2). Under certain disease conditions, however, vasoconstriction becomes more dominant than in the healthy population and may contribute to symptoms such as angina pectoris. The degree of vasoconstriction occurring under these conditions, however, may differ considerably in different syndromes and different patients. Indeed, in certain patients coronary constriction may be only slightly increased and hence may not bother the patient under resting conditions; however, the increased coronary vascular tone may significantly alter the threshold for angina during exercise in these patients (Fig. 2). The fact that most coronary lesions are eccentric (10) may explain why diseased segments are also able to relax and constrict to various stimuli. On the other end of this spectrum are patients in whom coronary constriction is

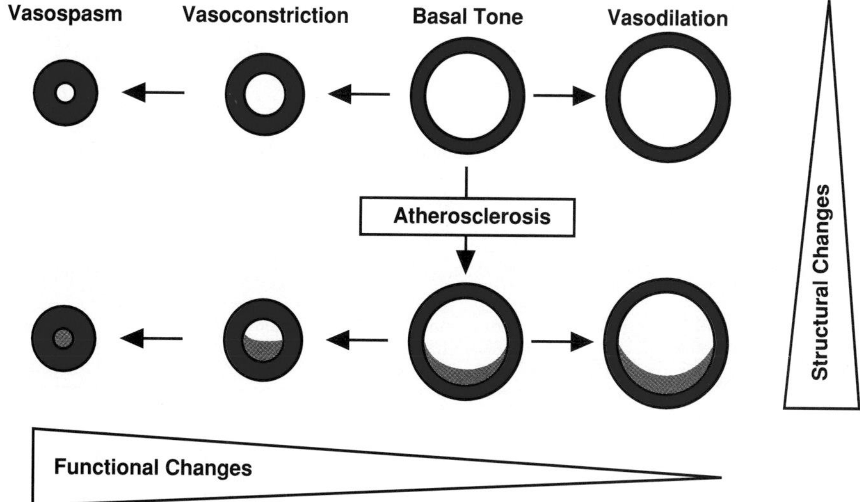

FIG. 2. Role of structural and functional changes of the coronary artery as a determinant of coronary obstruction. Coronary diameter can change as a result of vasoconstriction and vasodilation of normal **(upper line)** and atherosclerotic vessels **(lower line).** "True" coronary spasm is the extreme of the responses.

so severe that angina occurs even under resting conditions. Under these conditions, a near-total or total occlusion of the coronary artery can be demonstrated angiographically (Figs. 1 and 2).

Some authors have emphasized the difference between increased constriction and total occlusion of a coronary artery and have restricted the expression "coronary spasm" to the latter conditions. However, more recent studies clearly suggest that increased constriction contributes to a large variety of coronary syndromes [although total occlusion occurs less commonly (11,12)] and that the difference between hyperconstriction and true coronary spasm is gradual. The distinction between true coronary spasm and hyperconstriction seems artificial because, at this time, there is no definitive evidence for different pathogenetic mechanisms.

CONTROL OF CORONARY VASCULAR TONE

The coronary circulation is regulated by endothelial mediators, neurotransmitters, and the response of vascular smooth muscle cells to these agents (see ref. 13). The contribution of each mechanism to coronary vascular tone differs in large epicardial and intramyocardial coronary arteries. Also, although these mechanisms are important in the control of any circulation in the body, the contribution of certain mediators and the expression of receptors may differ in the coronary circulation as compared to other parts of the body.

Endothelial Mediators

Nitric Oxide

Endothelium-dependent relaxations occur in vitro and in vivo; neurotransmitters, hormones, and substances derived from platelets and the coagulation system can elicit these responses (Fig. 3; 13–19). Furthermore, mechanical factors such as shear stress induce endothelium-dependent vasodilation (20,21). The relaxations are mediated by a diffusible substance with a half-life of a few seconds (15,22), the so-called endothelium-derived relaxing factor (EDRF; 15), which has been identified as nitric oxide (NO; 23–25).

Endothelium-derived nitric oxide (EDNO) is formed from L-arginine by oxidation of its guanidine nitrogen terminal (26). The catalyzing enzyme NO synthase has recently been cloned (27); it is a primarily cytosolic enzyme requiring calmodulin, Ca^{2+}, and NADPH and has similarities with cytochrome P-450 enzymes. Several isoforms of the enzyme have been described, occurring not only in endothelial cells but also in platelets (28), macrophages (29), vascular smooth muscle cells (30–32), and in the brain (33). In addition, an inducible enzyme exists in vascular smooth muscle, endothelium, and macrophages. The enzyme is induced by cytokines such as endotoxin, interleukin-1β, and tumor necrosis factor and hence may be activated in inflammatory processes and endotoxin shock.

In porcine coronary arteries, endothelium-dependent relaxations to serotonin are inhibited by analogs of L-arginine such as L-N^G-monomethyl arginine (L-NMMA) and are restored by L- but not D-arginine (Fig. 4; 34). In quiescent arteries, L-NMMA causes endothelium-dependent contractions (35,36). In intact organs such as the perfused porcine eye or isolated perfused heart, inhibition of nitric oxide formation by L-arginine methyl ester (L-NAME) markedly decreases local blood flow (37). In humans, local infusion of L-NMMA into the brachial artery induces an increase in forearm vascular resistance. When infused intravenously in rabbits as well as in humans, L-NMMA induces long-lasting increases in blood pressure that are reversed by L-arginine

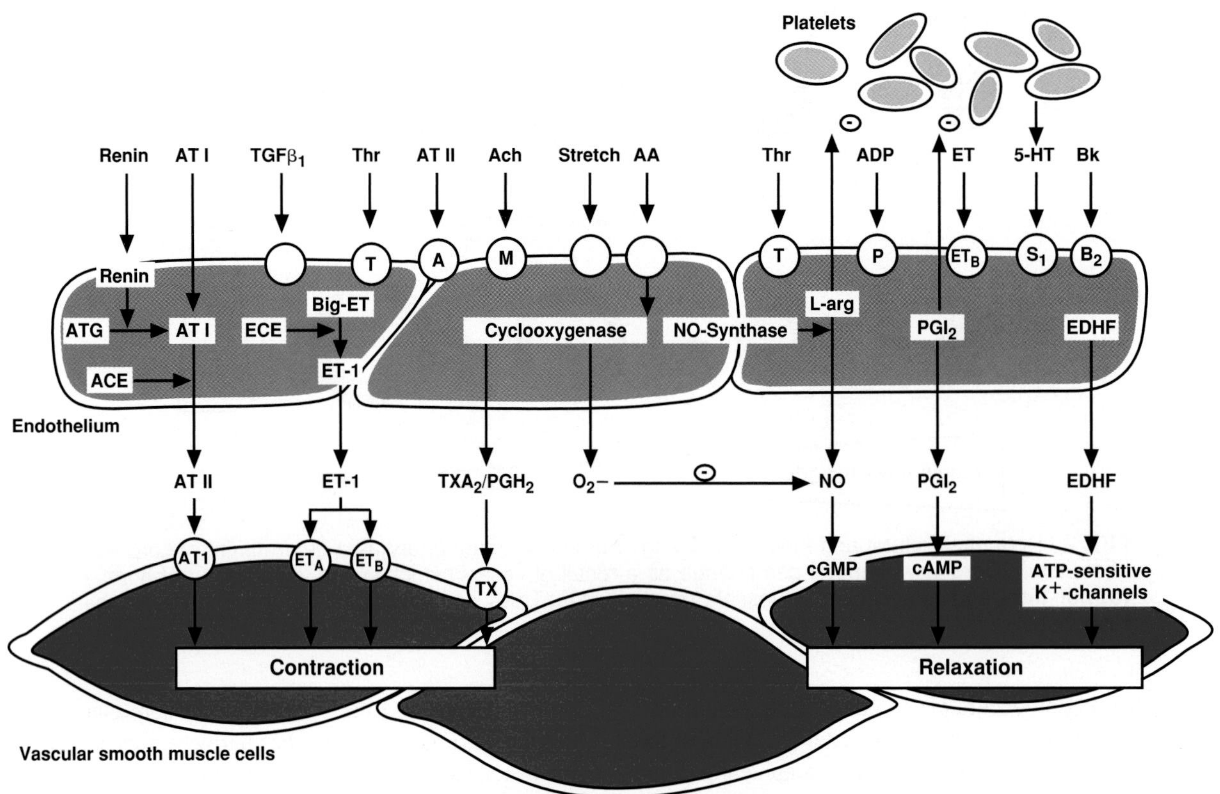

FIG. 3. Endothelium-derived vasoactive substances. The endothelium is a source of relaxing **(right part)** and contracting factors **(left part).** AA, arachidonic acid; ATG, angiotensinogen; AT, angiotensin; ACE, angiotensin converting enzyme; Ach, acetylcholine; ADP, adenosine tri- and diphosphate; Bk, bradykinin; cAMP/cGMP, cyclic adenosine/guanosine monophosphate; ECE, endothelin converting enzyme; EDHF, endothelium-derived hyperpolarizing factor; 5-HT, 5-hydroxytryptamine (serotonin); ET, endothelin-1; L-arg, L-arginine; NO, nitric oxide; O_2^-, superoxide radical; PGH_2, protacyclin H_2; PGI_2, prostacyclin; TGFβ_1, transforming growth factor β_1; Thr, thrombin; TXA_2, thromboxane A_2. *Circles* represent receptors. (Modified from Lüscher et al., ref. 56, by permission fo the American Heart Association.)

(38). This demonstrates that the vasculature is in a constant state of dilation as a result of continuous basal release of NO from endothelium. As judged from the porcine coronary circulation, a relaxing factor distinct from nitric oxide contributes to the relaxations to bradykinin and serotonin, particularly in intramyocardial vessels (35).

Of particular physiological and pathophysiological interest is the recently discovered endogenous inhibitor of the L-arginine nitric oxide pathway, asymmetric dimethylarginine (ADMA; 39). This indicates that there is also an endogenous inhibitory factor that could regulate the activity of the L-arginine NO pathway, both locally and, as it is also detected

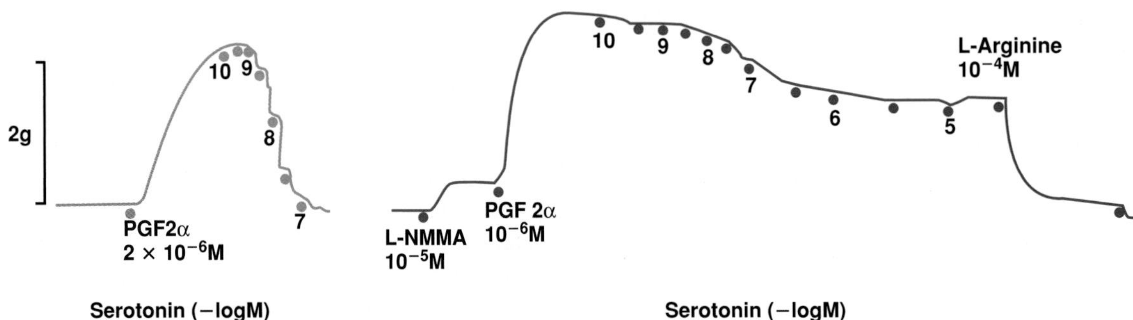

FIG. 4. Response of the isolated porcine coronary artery to serotonin (5-hydroxytryptamine, 5-HT) under control conditions **(left)** and after inhibition of nitric oxide formation by L-N^G-monomethylarginine (L-NMMA; **right**). (Data from Richard et al., ref. 34, by permission.)

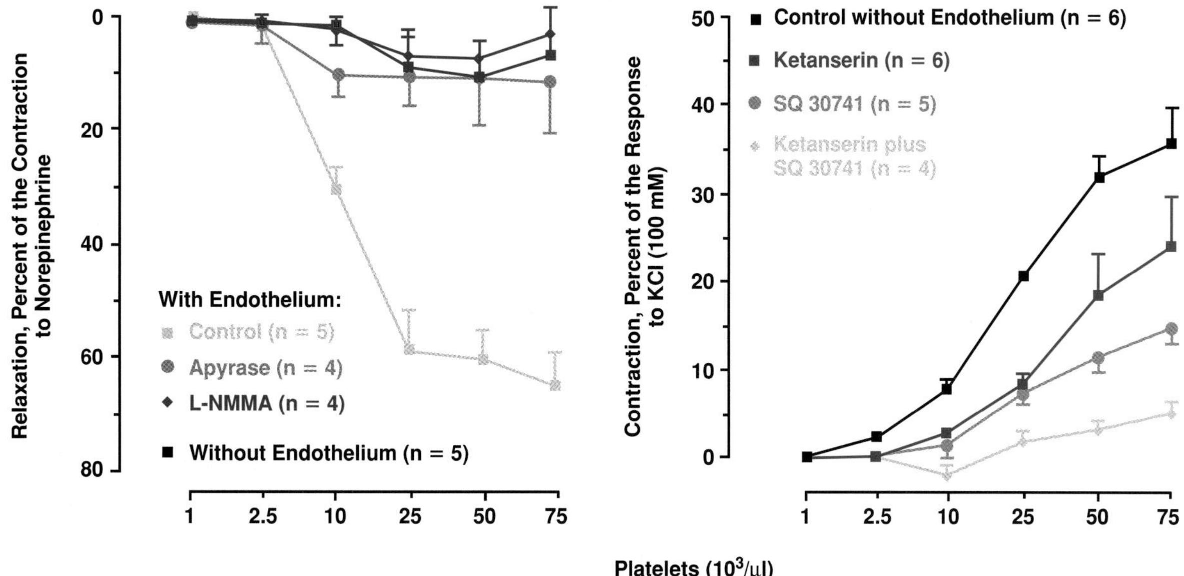

FIG. 5. Effects of aggregating platelets in human internal mammary artery. In vessels contracted with norepinephrine **(left panel),** aggregating platelets cause endothelium-dependent relaxations that are prevented by L-NMMA (an inhibitor of NO formation) or apyrase (an enzyme that breaks down ATP/ADP). In quiescent preparations without endothelium **(right panel),** platelets cause only contractions that are reduced by ketanserin (an antagonist of the 5-HT_2 receptor) or SQ30741 (a thromboxane receptor antagonist). (Modified from Yang et al., ref. 18, by permission.)

in plasma, systemically. Hence, an increased production and/or elimination of this endogenous inhibitor could profoundly affect the function of the cardiovascular system, for instance, in patients with renal failure (39).

Endothelium-derived NO leads to an increase in cyclic 3′,5′-guanosine monophosphate (cGMP) in vascular smooth muscle cells and platelets through activation of soluble guanylate cyclase (40). Methylene blue, an inhibitor of this enzyme, prevents production of cGMP and inhibits endothelium-dependent relaxations (13).

In platelets, an increase of intracellular cGMP is associated with reduced adhesion and aggregation. Therefore, EDNO causes both vasodilatation and platelet deactivation and thereby represents an important antithrombotic feature of the endothelium. Most interestingly, platelets release substances such as adenosine diphosphate and triphosphate as well as serotonin, which activate the release of nitric oxide and prostacyclin from the endothelium (Fig. 5; 16,18,41). Furthermore, thrombin, the major enzyme of the coagulation cascade, stimulates the formation of nitric oxide and prostacyclin by the endothelium of human arteries (17,42). Hence, at sites where platelets and the coagulation cascade are activated, intact endothelial cells immediately release nitric oxide and prostacyclin and in turn cause vasodilation and platelet inhibition, thereby preventing vasoconstriction and thrombus formation.

Vasodilator Prostaglandins

Prostacyclin is the major product of vascular cyclooxygenase (43). It is formed primarily in the intima but also the media and adventitia in response to shear stress, hypoxia, and several mediators that also lead to the formation of EDNO. However, in most blood vessels, the contribution of prostacyclin to endothelium-dependent relaxations is negligible (34,36). Prostacyclin increases cyclic 3′,5′-adenosine monophosphate (cAMP) in smooth muscle and platelets (44), where it inhibits platelet aggregation (Fig. 3). In human platelets EDNO and prostacyclin synergistically inhibit aggregation (45).

Endothelium-Derived Hyperpolarizing Factor

Soon after discovery of nitric oxide as the mediator of endothelium-dependent relaxations, it became obvious that EDNO could not explain all endothelium-dependent responses (13,46). In the porcine coronary artery, endothelium-dependent relaxations to serotonin are inhibited by L-NMMA, hemoglobin, or methylene blue, but the response to bradykinin is only partially affected by the inhibitors of the L-arginine pathways (Fig. 6; 34,35). Relaxations resistant to inhibitors of the nitric oxide pathway are even more prominent in intramyocardial vessels (35). In the canine coronary and mesenteric artery, acetylcholine causes endothelium-dependent hyperpolarization, an effect not shared by nitric oxide (47–49). Although under certain conditions nitric oxide may also hyperpolarize cells (50–52), it appears that it can not explain all endothelium-dependent relaxations in all blood vessels. Hence, an endothelium-dependent hyperpolarizing factor of unknown chemical structure has been proposed (Fig. 3; 13,46). Indirect evidence suggests that it

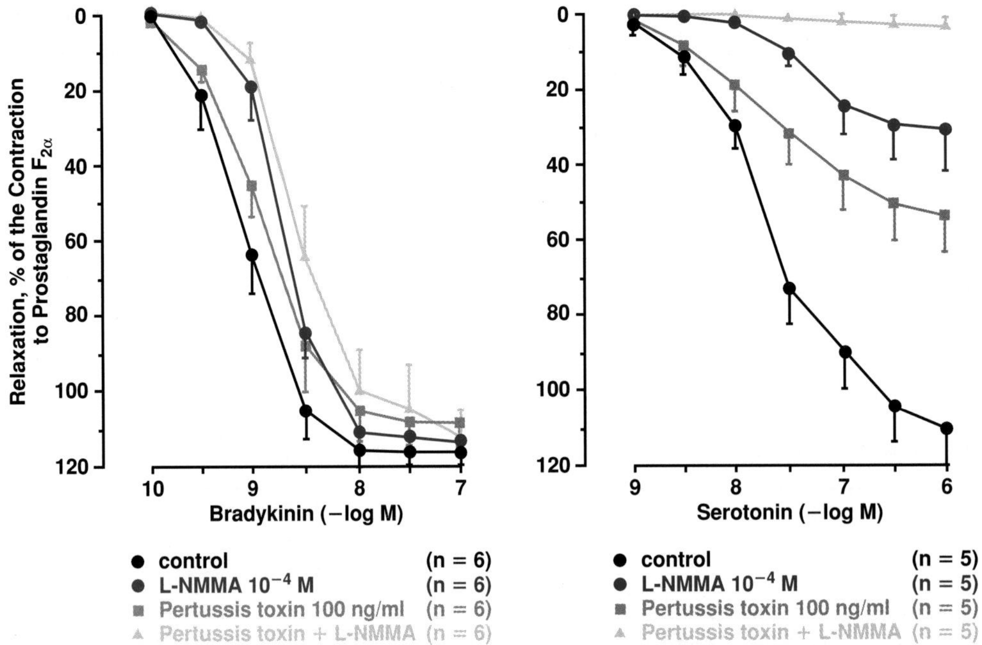

FIG. 6. Endothelium-dependent relaxations to bradykinin in porcine coronary arteries. Bradykinin causes relaxations that are only minimally inhibited by the inhibitor of nitric oxide formation L-N^G-monomethylarginine (L-NMMA; **right**) and by inactivation of G_i proteins by pertussis toxin. In contrast, serotonin (5-hydroxytryptamine; 5-HT) is sensitive to both interventions. (From Richard et al., ref. 34, by permission.)

may be a product of the cytochrome P-450 pathway, but C-type natriuretic peptide (CNP) may also be a candidate (53).

Endothelins

Endothelial cells produce the 21-amino-acid peptide endothelin (54–56). Among the peptides endothelin-1, endothelin-2, and endothelin-3, endothelial cells appear to produce exclusively endothelin-1.

Translation of messenger RNA generates preproendothelin, which is converted to big endothelin (54); its conversion to endothelin-1 by the endothelin-converting enzyme (ECE) is necessary for development of full vascular activity (54–56). Two forms of ECE have recently been cloned; ECE-1 is a phosphoramidone-sensitive enzyme. The expression of messenger RNA and release of the peptide is stimulated by thrombin, transforming growth factor β_1, interleukin-1, epinephrine, angiotensin II, arginine vasopressin, calcium ionophore, and phorbol ester (Fig. 7; 55–59).

Endothelin-1 is a potent vasoconstrictor both in vitro and in vivo (54,60–63). In the coronary and ophthalmic circulation and the human forearm, endothelin causes dilation at lower and marked contractions at higher concentrations (Fig. 8; 37,62,64,65), which in the heart eventually leads to ischemia, arrhythmias, and death. In the porcine coronary circulation, intramyocardial vessels are more sensitive to the vasoconstrictor effects of endothelin-1 than epicardial arteries (66). Also, in human arterial and venous coronary bypass vessels, endothelin causes marked contractions (63). Again, small branches of the internal mammary artery are markedly more sensitive to the contractile effects of endothelin-1 than the main branch of this blood vessel (67). Hence, endothelin appears to be particularly important in small blood vessels, where local blood flow is regulated.

However, circulating levels of endothelin-1 are very low, suggesting that little of the peptide is formed under physiological conditions because of absence of stimuli and/or presence of potent inhibitory mechanisms or that it is released preferentially toward smooth muscle cells (56,68,69). Indeed, three inhibitory mechanisms regulating endothelin production have been delineated: (a) cGMP-dependent inhibition (57,70); (b) cAMP-dependent inhibition (71), and (c) an inhibitory factor produced by vascular smooth muscle cells (68). The cGMP-dependent mechanism can be activated by EDNO, nitroglycerin, linsidomine (SIN-1; 57,58), and atrial natriuretic peptide (which activates particulate guanylate cyclase; 13,71). Thus, after inhibition of the endothelial L-arginine pathway, thrombin-induced production of endothelin is augmented (57); on the other hand, SIN-1 or nitroglycerin prevents thrombin-induced endothelin release via a cGMP-dependent mechanism (58). Endothelin can also release NO and prostacyclin from endothelial cells, which may represent a negative feedback mechanism (60,72). The EDNO also interacts with the effects of endothelin at the level of vascular smooth muscle. Indeed, the contractions to the peptide are enhanced after endothelial removal, indicating that basal production of EDNO reduces its response (63).

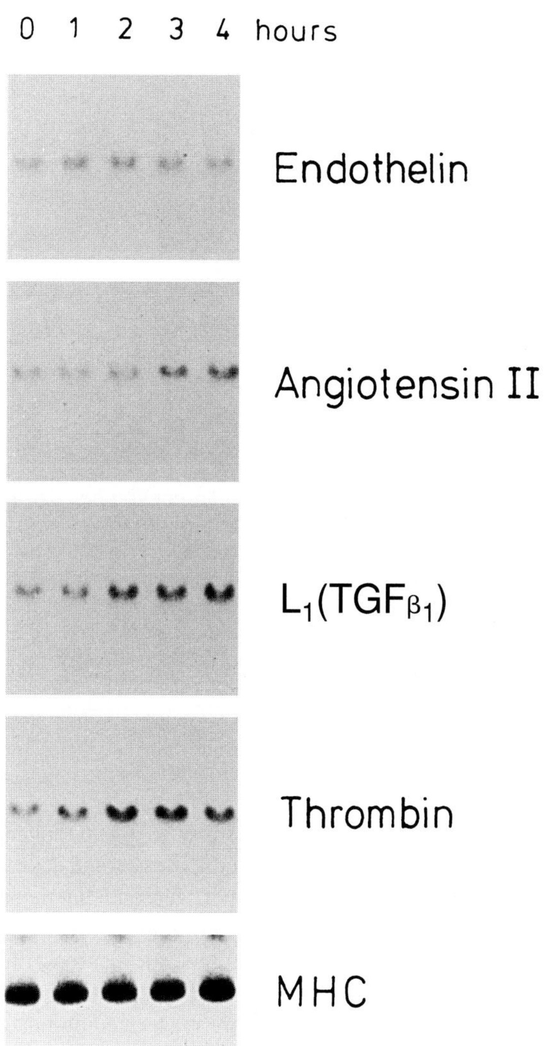

FIG. 7. Expression of endothelin messenger RNA in porcine aortic endothelial cells in culture after exposure to either endothelin, angiotensin II, transforming growth factor L_1 ($TGF_{\beta 1}$, or thrombin. (From Lüscher et al., ref. 205, by permission.)

Stimulation of the formation of EDNO by acetylcholine reverses endothelin-induced contractions in most blood vessels, although this mechanism appears to be less potent in veins (63,73).

Two distinct endothelin receptors have been cloned, the ET_A and ET_B receptor (Fig. 9; 74,75). Endothelial cells express ET_B receptors linked to the formation of NO (72) and prostacyclin (60), which may explain the transient vasodilator effects of endothelin when infused in intact organs or organisms. In vascular smooth muscle, ET_A and in part ET_B receptors are mediating contraction and proliferation (76). ET_B receptors equally bind endothelin-1 and endothelin-3, whereas ET_A receptors preferentially bind endothelin-1. An ET_C receptor also has been cloned in frog tissue (77); its presence and role in the human cardiovascular system however are uncertain.

Several endothelin receptor antagonists have been developed (76,78–81). Most substances are specific ET_A receptor antagonists, but more recently developed molecules also possess combined ET_A and ET_B receptor antagonism (37,76,78,79). In various vascular preparations, the vasoconstrictor effects of endothelin can be potently inhibited by these newly developed molecules. In the human skin microcirculation, the ET_A receptor antagonist FR 139317 increased blood flow and inhibited the endothelin-induced vasoconstriction, indicating that endothelin may play a role in the control of vascular tone (80). Furthermore, the fact that these antagonists do lower blood pressure under certain conditions suggests that endothelin may contribute to blood pressure regulation (78,81,82).

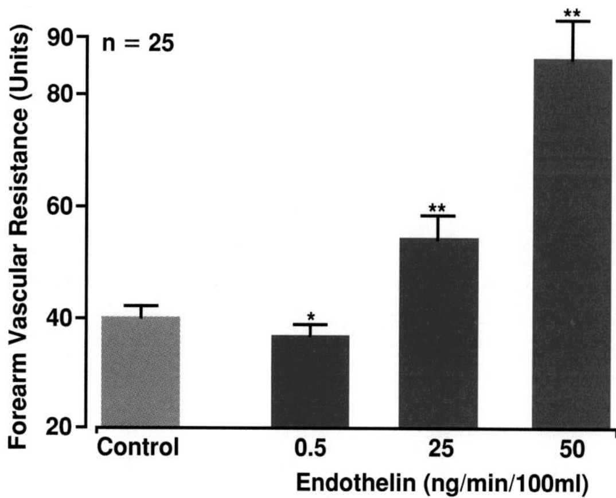

FIG. 8. Effects of intraarterial infusion of endothelin-1 on the forearm circulation of normal human subjects. Endothelin causes a small decrease, followed by marked increases, in forearm vascular resistance. (Modified from Kiowski et al., ref. 62, by permission of the American Heart Association.)

Vasoconstrictor Prostaglandins

Exogenous arachidonic acid can evoke endothelium-dependent contractions prevented by indomethacin (an inhibitor of cyclooxygenase; Fig. 3; 19,83). In humans saphenous vein, acetylcholine and histamine evoke endothelium-dependent contractions; in the presence of indomethacin, however, endothelium-dependent relaxations are unmasked (36). The products of cyclooxygenase mediating the contractions are thromboxane A_2 in the case of acetylcholine and endoperoxides (prostaglandin H_2) in that of histamine (36). Thromboxane A_2 and endoperoxide activate both vascular smooth muscle and platelets and hence counteract effects of NO and prostacyclin.

Furthermore, the cyclooxygenase pathway is a source of superoxide anions, which can break down NO. Besides this indirect effect, superoxide anions can also mediate direct vasoconstriction (84,85). Thus, the cyclooxygenase pathway produces a variety of endothelium-derived contracting factors (Fig. 3); their release appears particularly prominent in veins and in the cerebral and ophthalmic circulation (13).

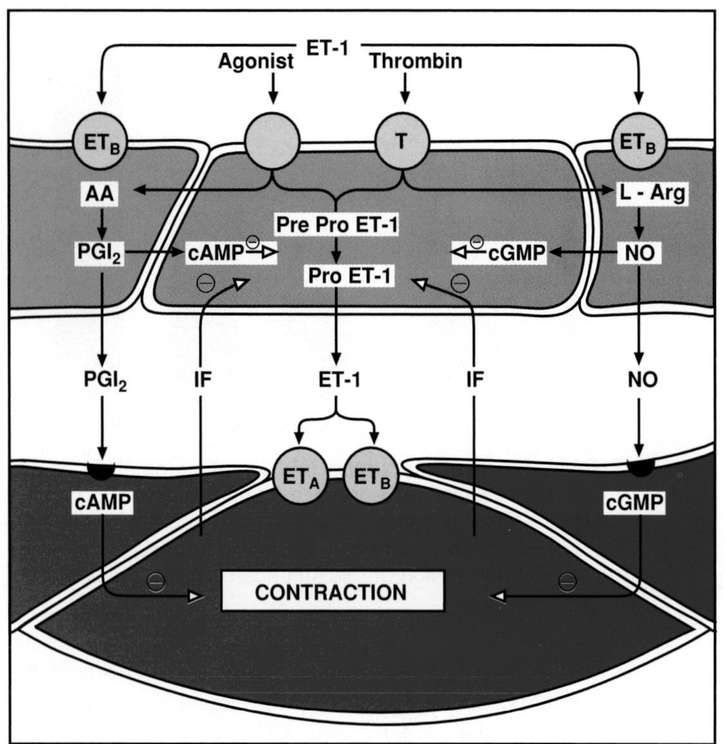

FIG. 9. Regulation of vascular endothelin (ET) production. Endothelin is formed from prepro-ET and big-ET via the endothelin-converting enzymes (ECE) and activates specific receptors *(circles)*. The ET production is stimulated by thrombin (Thr) and many other receptor *(circles)* agonists. Its production is inhibited by nitric oxide (NO) formed from L-arginine (L-Arg), possibly by prostacyclin (PGI_2) and a putative inhibitory factor (IF) produced by vascular smooth muscle cells. (Modified from Lüscher et al., ref. 56, by permission of the American Heart Association.)

Vascular Smooth Muscle

Vascular smooth muscle cells are the responder cells in the regulation of vascular tone as they react to circulating hormones, endothelial mediators, and neurotransmitters released from nerve endings as well as substances released from circulating blood cells such as platelets, leukocytes, and monocytes. The response to such mediators usually involves binding to surface receptors, activation of signal transduction mechanisms, and increases in second messengers, which regulate the intracellular concentration of calcium. Calcium is a crucial ion regulating contractility of vascular smooth muscle cells (86).

Sympathetic Activation

Sympathetic outflow to the resistance vessels is of utmost importance for determination of the level of vascular resistance and, in turn, local blood flow (14,87–92). Sympathetic outflow to blood vessel originates in neurons located in the lateral parts of the reticular formation of the brainstem, i.e., the vasomotor center (14). Activity of the center is governed by the solitary nucleus tract, which relates information from arterial and cardiopulmonary mechanoreceptors (baroreceptors and other afferents; see ref. 14). Axons from neurons of the vasomotor center form the bulbous spinal tract and descend into the intermedial lateral column to the preganglionic neurons of the spinal cord, located in the anterolateral column. Neurons of the bulbospinal tract consist of both excitatory and inhibitory neurons, which innervate preganglionic sympathetic neurons. Outflow to the periphery is determined by interplay between these pressor and depressor neurons. Cholinergic preganglionic neurons interconnect with adrenergic postganglionic neurons in the sympathetic ganglia, and the postganglionic adrenergic neurons finally innervate the heart and the peripheral blood vessels (Fig. 10; 89,91). All mature blood vessels are innervated by postganglionic sympathetic nerves. However, the density of innervation varies. In most arteries the nerves are restricted to the advential–medial border, whereas in veins they usually penetrate into the media. In both animals and humans, the density of adrenergic innervation of blood vessels decreases progressively with age, while sympathetic activity of neurons as measured with microneurography increases with age (87,89–92).

Receptors

Most agonists derived from nerve endings, the circulating blood, platelets, or the endothelium (except nitric oxide; see above) exert their action in vascular smooth muscle by activating specific receptors (Fig. 10; 86). Typically these receptors have seven transmembrane domains and are G protein linked. Important contractile receptors include α_1- and α_2-adrenergic receptors, 5-HT_1- and 5-HT_2-serotonergic receptors (93,94), and thromboxane receptors (both activated after release of the mediators from aggregating platelets), ET_A and ET_B receptors (see above), angiotensin type 1 (AT_1) receptors (95), and V_1 vasopressin receptors (96).

The most important neurotransmitter mediating effects of

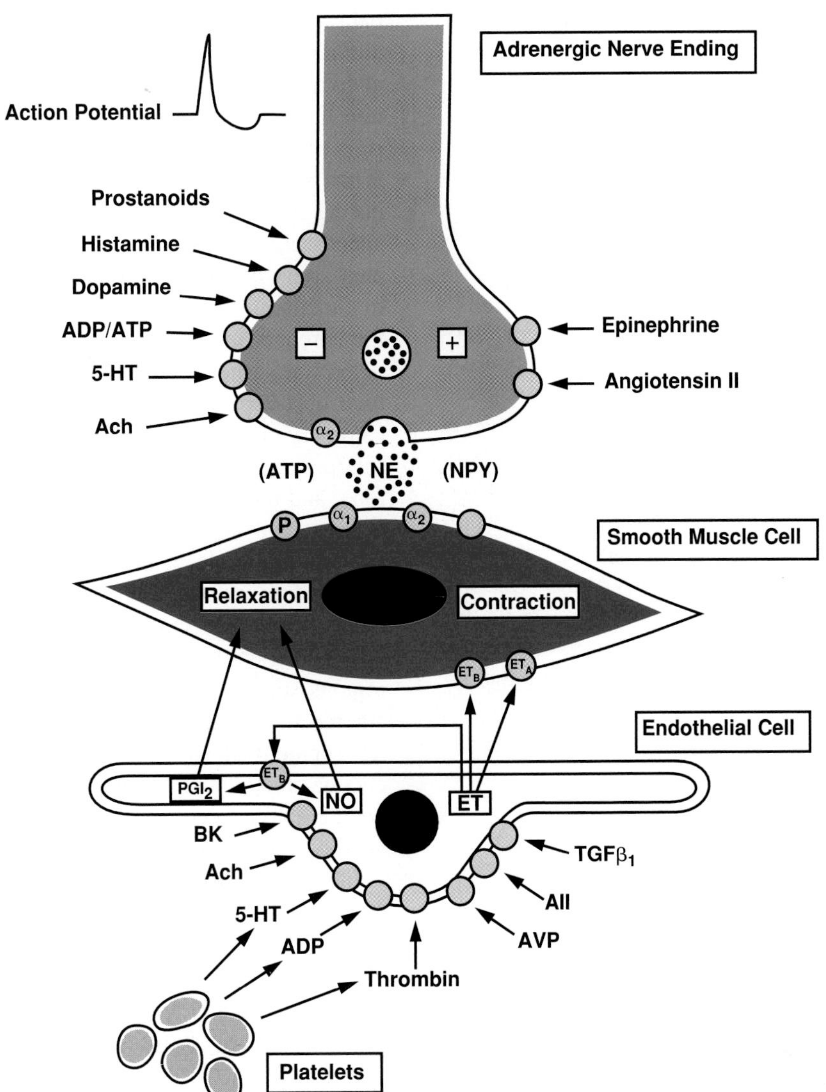

FIG. 10. Regulation of tone of vascular smooth muscle cells by adrenergic nerves and circulating and local factors. AII, angiotensin II; Ach, acetylcholine; ADP/ATP, adenosine di- and triphosphate; AVP, arginine vasopression; Bk, bradykinin; 5-HT, 5-hydroxytryptamine (serotonin); ET, endothelin-1; NO, nitric oxide; NPY, neuropeptide Y; P, purinergic receptor; PGI_2, prostacyclin; TGFβ_1, transforming growth factor-β_1; Thr, thrombin. *Circles* represent receptors. (Modified from T. F. Lüscher, G. Noll, and R. R. Wenzel, *unpublished data*.)

sympathetic neurons in the blood vessel wall is norepinephrine, but adenosine trisphosphate (ATP) and neuropeptide Y also can contribute under certain conditions (Fig. 10; 14,97). Adrenergic neurotransmitters are released after the occurrence of an action potential, and their release is facilitated by epinephrine and angiotensin II but inhibited by norepinephrine itself (via prejunctional α_2-adrenergic receptors), acetylcholine, serotonin (5-hydroxytryptamine), histamine, purines, and prostanoids (98). Released norepinephrine interacts with postjunctional α_1- and α_2-adrenergic receptors. In the coronary circulation, α-adrenergic receptors are sparse, particularly in proximal parts of the epicardial vessels.

Certain receptors on vascular smooth muscle, however, mediate vascular relaxation. Indeed, activation of certain 5-HT_1-serotonergic receptors cause relaxation of human and pig coronary arteries (34,35,99,100). Prostacyclin exerts also relaxation via specific receptors. Finally, epinephrine can activate β_2-adrenergic receptors, which mediate relaxation of epicardial coronary arteries. As judged from the canine coronary circulation, β_2-adrenergic receptors are particularly important in proximal epicardial arteries, whereas the expression of α_1- and α_2-adrenergic receptors is sparse except in distal segments of the coronary vascular tree (101). Normally, although α-adrenergic receptors are activated during stimulation of the sympathetic nervous system (for instance, with exercise or psychological stress), no coronary vasoconstriction occurs because of the increased release of nitric oxide with increased blood flow (i.e., flow-dependent vasodilation; see above; 102,103). Coronary spasm is usually localized to the proximal epicardial arteries.

Signal Transduction Mechanisms

Activation of these receptors activates phospholipase C and in turn leads to formation of inositol trisphosphate (IP_3) and diacylglycerol (DAG; 86,104). While IP_3 releases intracellular calcium from sarcoplasmatic reticulum, DAG activates protein kinase C. Both events allow development of contraction. Activation of sympathetic nerves leads to release not only of norepinephrine but also of neuropeptide Y and adenosine triphosphate (ATP; Fig. 10; 14,97). In particular, neuropeptide Y may contribute importantly to the contractile response as it potentiates the effects of norepinephrine (97). Similarly, endothelin-1 is able to potentiate contractions to serotonin in human coronary arteries (105). This effect occurs even at threshold concentrations of the peptide and is related to an increased calcium sensitivity of the vascular smooth muscle in the presence of endothelin-1 (see below).

Voltage-Operated Calcium Channels

Voltage-operated calcium channels also importantly regulate vascular tone (86). These channels are activated with changes in membrane potential (i.e., depolarization of the cell) and allow extracellular calcium to enter the vascular smooth muscle cell. The channels are blocked by calcium antagonists of the dihydropyridine (e.g., nifedipine, amlodipine), phenylalkalanine (e.g., verapamil, mibefradil), or benzodiazepine type (e.g., diltiazem; 106). Certain receptors, for instance ET receptors on vascular smooth muscle of the porcine coronary artery, are linked via a G_i protein to the channel and thereby can increase influx of extracellular calcium into the cell (107). In the human coronary artery, endothelin-induced contractions are reduced by calcium antagonists, suggesting that similar mechanisms are operative as in the porcine coronary artery (108). The effects of calcium channel blockers appear more pronounced in intramyocardial as compared to epicardial coronary arteries, suggesting that the dependence of calcium-induced contraction on extracellular calcium influx increases as the diameter of porcine coronary arteries decreases (66,109).

CLINICAL ASPECTS

Symptoms and Clinical Presentation

The clinical hallmark of coronary constriction, as well as structural atherosclerotic changes of the blood vessel wall, is angina pectoris. Angina pectoris is caused by myocardial ischemia via only partially understood mechanisms. Anginal pain typically is perceived in the precordial part of the chest, although atypical locations such as the upper part of the abdomen and parts of the back also occur. Radiation of pain into the left shoulder and arm and less frequently into the right arm and jaws is typical for chest pain of cardiac origin. It has become obvious that most cardiac ischemia occurring during life occurs in the absence of angina pectoris (i.e., silent ischemia; 110,111). Ischemia occurs when the coronary artery is not able to maintain an adequate blood supply to functioning myocardium. The degree of obstruction of the coronary lumen, as well as the myocardial O_2 demand, determines whether ischemia occurs at rest (total or near-total obstruction) or only on exertion (partial obstruction). Coronary obstruction is determined by the extent of atherosclerosis of the vascular wall, changes in coronary vascular tone, and thrombus formation within the lumen (Fig. 2).

In variant angina, coronary constriction is the only or overwhelming mechanism. The severity of constriction occurring under these conditions explains why this form of angina typically occurs at rest (1–3). With very severe coronary constriction, myocardial infarction may ensue even in regions supplied by arterial segments with no or minimal atherosclerotic changes (6). The electrocardiogram shows ST segment elevations as a reflection of transmural ischemia. Imaging techniques such as echocardiography or angiography reveal wall motion abnormalities of the involved myocardial segment.

In patients with obstructing coronary atherosclerosis, the structural obstruction per se sets a level of maximal blood flow that limits exercise performance of these patients. However, coronary constriction also contributes importantly (112). The latter explains why the ischemia threshold (i.e., level of exercise above which angina or ischemia occurs) varies in the same patient on different occasions. Indeed, activation of the sympathetic nervous system by cold temperature or psychological stress can cause paradoxical coronary constriction in patients with diseased coronary arteries (113), resulting in symptoms with minimal or no exertion. Vagal stimulation after a heavy meal may also lower the threshold in certain patients. This may be related to decreased vasodilator tone during vagal dominance, although other, less well-defined mechanisms may further contribute. Typically, in patients with obstructive coronary disease, angina occurs on exertion, and the electrocardiogram typically reveals ST segment depression with relief of symptoms at rest. Reversible motion abnormalities in the involved myocardial segment are also typical and are used diagnostically in stress echocardiography (114,115).

Trigger Mechanisms

In the evaluation of patients with nonobstructive coronary disease and angina at rest as well as in patients with normal coronary arteries and ischemia during exercise, several substances have been used in the catheterization laboratory to trigger coronary constriction. Most commonly, acetylcho-

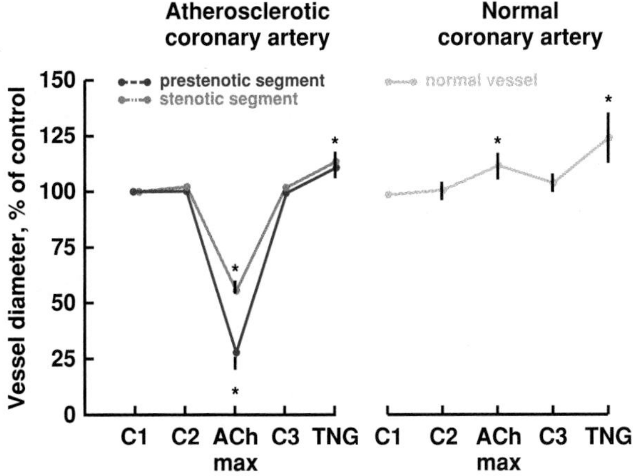

FIG. 11. Effects of intracoronary infusion of acetylcholine (ACh) on the arterial diameter of the left anterior descending coronary artery in normal subjects **(b)** and in patients with coronary artery disease **(a).** The response is expressed as percentage of the control arterial diameter. C1, C2, C3, control periods; TNG, nitroglycerin; *closed circles,* prestenotic or normal segments; *open circles,* stenotic segments. (Modified from Ludmer et al., ref. 11, with permission.)

line, histamine, or ergonovine is infused into the coronary circulation in these patients, and changes in diameter of epicardial coronary arteries are measured at angiography (116).

In patients with variant angina, coronary spasm can be provoked during angiography by methacholine and acetylcholine (117). More recently, however, it has been shown that many patients with coronary artery disease exhibit more or less pronounced coronary constriction after infusion of acetylcholine, whereas mild vasodilation is observed in normals (Fig. 11; 11). Some patients, however, exhibit constriction at one site and dilation at other sites (118). Acetylcholine is the classical muscarinic agonist to elicit endothelium-dependent relaxations in healthy blood vessels of various origins including the human coronary artery (15,17,119). However, in contrast to most other blood vessels, the human coronary artery exhibits marked contractions to acetylcholine after removal of the endothelium because of the presence of excitatory muscarinic receptors on vascular smooth muscle (120).

Others have also used serotonin to evoke coronary constriction. This substance is released from aggregating platelets and may cause ergonovine activating contractile serotonergic receptors and also α-adrenergic receptors. This may explain why it is able to elicit coronary spasm in a considerable number of patients with variant angina not responsive to other tests.

Intracoronary histamine administration leads to dilation in normal humans (121). This can be explained by endothelial H_1-histaminergic receptors linked to release of nitric oxide (119,122). On vascular smooth muscle, however, contractile H_2-histaminergic receptors exist. In one report, in about one-half of the patients with variant angina studied, spasm was provoked by histamine (116).

Natural Course and Prognosis

Atherosclerotic coronary artery disease commonly progresses, although spontaneous regression of existing disease also may occur (123,124). The natural course of atherosclerotic coronary artery disease is determined by lesion progression (which involves lipid accumulation, macrophage invasion and migration, and proliferation of vascular smooth muscle cells; 125,126) and, in particular, plaque rupture, constriction, and thrombus formation leading to prolonged obstruction of a major epicardial coronary artery. Plaque rupture (127,128) appears particularly common in lipid-rich lesions. Immunologic stimuli and physical forces (for instance with strenuous exercise) may also destabilize existing plaques. Plaque rupture and coronary occlusion eventually leads to myocardial infarction with loss of functioning myocardium. Pump failure and arrhythmias are common causes of death under these conditions. Clinically, major determinants of prognosis in patients with coronary artery disease are the extent of coronary artery disease and the degree of functional impairment of the left ventricle.

In patient with variant angina, prognosis may be somewhat more favorable than in those with atherosclerotic coronary artery disease. However, the natural history of coronary spasm is unknown and not likely to become known because therapy alters outcome. The clinical course of patients with objective evidence for transient myocardial ischemia (e.g., ST segment elevation) and angiographically documented coronary spasm is best described as highly variable (129). Periods of exacerbation of transient ischemia (with and without symptoms) and ischemia-related events alternate with remission of ischemia and related events, often without identifiable reason. Long-term data reveal that outcome in the patient with coronary spasm is highly dependent on the presence and severity of associated coronary atherosclerosis (130,131). Over 3 to 5 years, those with coronary spasm and relatively minimal coronary atherosclerosis are at low risk (approximately 5%) for development of death or nonfatal myocardial infarction. Coronary spasm patients who have only one artery showing a 70% or greater ''fixed'' atherosclerotic obstruction are at low to moderate risk. Those with severe multivessel obstructions are at relatively high (approximately 30%) risk for these events. Myocardial infarction occurs most frequently shortly after the patient's initial presentation for rest angina and many times even before the diagnosis of coronary spasm has been given strong consideration. Patients with ventricular dysrhythmias during rest angina have approximately twice the risk of death as those without dysrhythmias, but potentially lethal dysrhythmias are not always dependent on the presence of severe coronary artery disease (132). Retrospective and prospective cohort studies suggest that calcium antagonists seem to have a beneficial effect on risk for adverse outcome events (130,133). Ischemia-related events may continue to occur, however, even when calcium antagonist therapy appears to control rest angina, and events tend to cluster in those with severe multivessel coronary disease (133,134).

MECHANISMS OF VASOSPASM

Although the cause of coronary spasm remains elusive, tremendous progress has been made in understanding local vascular mechanisms capable of causing coronary constriction. Most of these mechanisms involve dysfunction of mediators that are important in regulation of normal coronary vascular tone (see above).

Endothelium

The endothelium may be damaged by a wide variety of factors (e.g., hypertension, smoking, lipids) and even by intense smooth muscle contraction. As indicated above, alterations in the release and/or responsiveness of vascular smooth muscle to substances released by endothelial cells can profoundly affect contractile responses of coronary arteries (Fig. 3; 13). By definition, such endothelial dysfunction could involve local impairment in the release of relaxing factors or increased production of contracting factors by the endothelium. Furthermore, vascular smooth muscle cells may be hyperresponsive to contractile factors released by endothelial cells or lose their responsiveness to the continuous vasodilator tone induced by nitric oxide and/or prostaglandins.

L-Arginine Pathway

In porcine coronary arteries, in vivo denudation of the endothelium with a balloon catheter is followed by a rapid regeneration of the endothelial layer within days (100). Also endothelium-dependent relaxations to bradykinin, serotonin, and aggregating platelets recover at this point. However, 4 weeks after denudation (and lasting up to 5 months at least), the number of endothelial cells per given area is increased, and (Fig. 12; 100) endothelium-dependent relaxations to serotonin, α_2-adrenergic agonists (i.e., UK 14304), and aggregating platelets are reduced (Fig. 13; 100). In contrast, endothelium-dependent relaxations to other agonists such as bradykinin, adenosine diphosphate, thrombin, platelet-activating factor, and the calcium ionophore A23187 are maintained. This indicates a very selective defect of certain receptor-operated mechanisms for release of nitric oxide in regenerated endothelial cells. Interestingly, this defect involves endothelial receptors that are sensitive to pertussis toxin (135), suggesting that in regenerated coronary endothelial cells, expression or function of G_i proteins linked to 5-HT_1-serotonerigic and α_2-adrenergic receptors is defective (136). More recent studies in the porcine coronary circulation demonstrated that ergonovine elicits similar responses as serotonin and that regenerated endothelial cells also exhibit abnormal responses to this agonist (100,137,138). This is of particular interest as ergonovine is the most reliable substance to provoke vasospasm in patients with variant angina (116). Indeed, a loss of nitric oxide release from endothelium, with overwhelming effects on vascular smooth muscle contractile receptors, could explain the constrictor response to ergonovine in coronary segments prone to spasm as well as rapid reversal by low doses of intracoronary nitrate. Structural changes at sites of mechanical endothelial denudation may also contribute. Indeed, myointimal thickening invariably occurs at sites of endothelial denudation (138). The increased muscle mass may further increase vasoconstrictor responses. The response to potassium chloride of denuded and regenerated canine coronary segments is indeed increased (138).

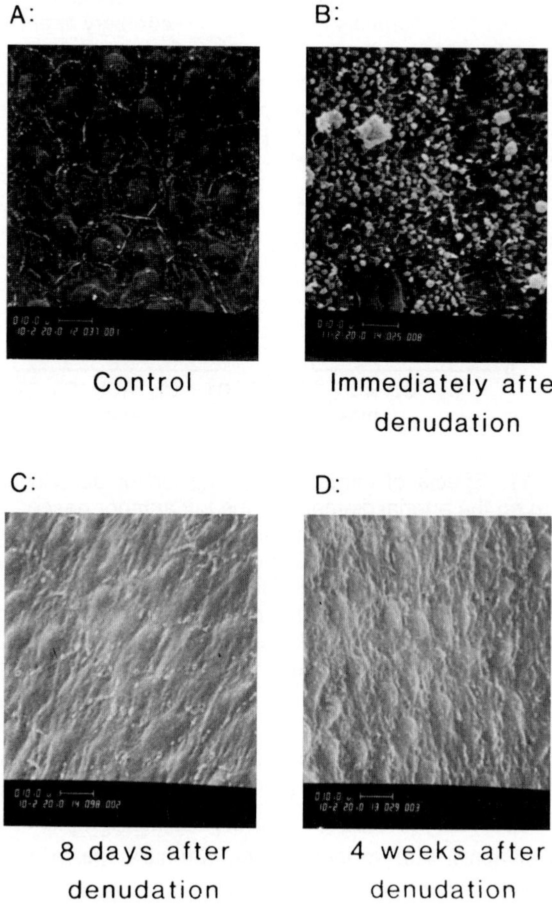

FIG. 12. Scanning electron microscopy of porcine coronary arteries immediately **(B),** 8 days **(C),** and 4 weeks **(D)** after the endothelium had been removed in vivo with a balloon catheter. Note the adhesion of circulating blood cells in **B** and the increased number of endothelial cells in **D** as compared to **C.** (From Shimokawa et al., ref. 100, by permission of the American Heart Association.)

In the pig, coronary spasm can be provoked with histamine several weeks after in vivo endothelial denudation in

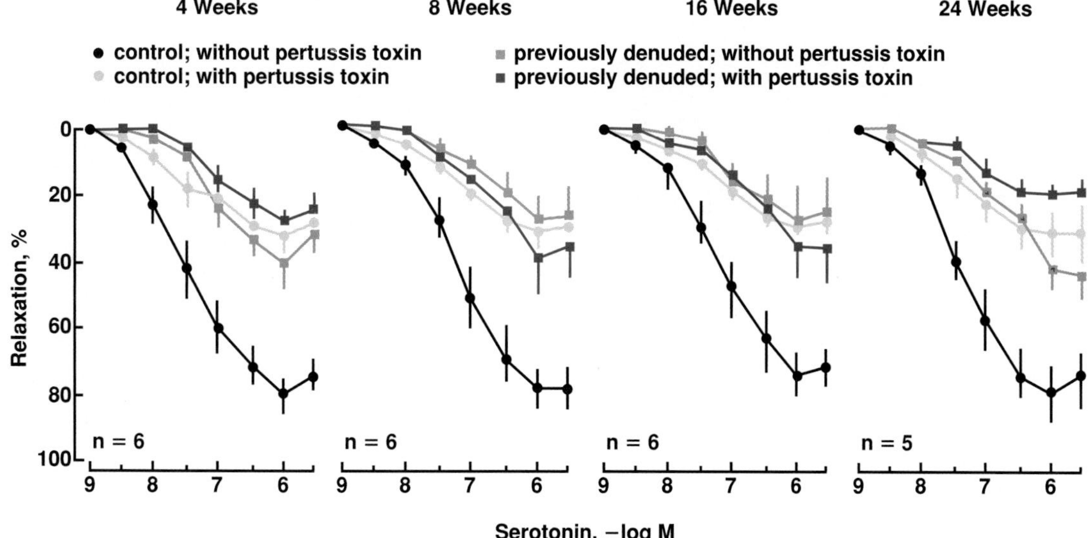

FIG. 13. Endothelium-dependent relaxations of porcine coronary arteries to serotonin in control preparations *(circles)* and arteries in which the endothelium had been previously denuded with a balloon catheter. The effect of pertussis toxin, an inhibitor of G_i proteins, is also shown. (From Shimokawa et al., ref. 136, by permission of the American Heart Association.)

conjunction with an atherogenic diet (100). An increased number of adventitial mast cells, a major source of histamine, has been documented in a patient with coronary spasm (139). Also, coronary arteries from patients with coronary artery disease contain higher amounts of histamine, and they respond with vasoconstriction to the amine (140). As histamine also has a bimodal action in normal coronary arteries (i.e., release of endothelium-derived nitric oxide via H_1-histaminergic receptors and direct vasoconstriction via H_2-histaminergic receptors (119,122); endothelial dysfunction leaving dominant activation of smooth muscle cells could explain some of these findings.

Abnormal coronary vasomotion in response to endothelial vasodilators also has been demonstrated with atherosclerotic coronary artery disease and no signs of variant angina. Indeed, acetylcholine causes vasoconstriction in most patients with coronary artery disease (see Fig. 11; 11,141). Also, intracoronary infusion of serotonin elicits vasodilation in patients with normal coronary arteries but profound contraction in patients with coronary artery disease (Fig. 14; 12) or variant angina (142). In patients with coronary artery disease, the vasoconstriction to serotonin can be inhibited with the 5-HT_2-serotonergic antagonist ketanserin (12). In contrast, ketanserin does not prevent ergonovine-induced coronary spasm in patients with variant angina (143). Hence, either 5-HT_2-serotonergic receptors are not involved in variant angina or ergonovine predominantly activates other serotonergic or adrenergic receptors. Recent in vitro studies indeed demonstrated that contractile 5-HT_1-serotonergic receptors on vascular smooth muscle may importantly contribute to the response to serotonin in human coronary arteries (93).

Prostacyclin

Prostacyclin is a vasodilator in the coronary circulation. However, at least in the pig, prostacyclin contributes very little to endothelium-dependent relaxations of coronary arteries (34). In most patients with variant angina, intravenous prostacyclin does not influence the number, severity, or duration of spontaneous or provoked coronary vasospasm (144).

Vasoconstrictor Prostaglandins

In isolated quiescent porcine coronary arteries studied as ring preparations in organ chambers, serotonin causes contractions with or without endothelium (34,35,100). In arteries with regenerated endothelium, contractions to serotonin are enhanced as compared to preparations with either normal endothelium or those without endothelium (100). These findings suggest that endothelium produces a contracting factor under these conditions, most likely one derived from the cyclooxygenase pathway.

Endothelin

Endothelin does have the capacity of causing profound constriction of coronary arteries (see above). However, the time course of its response is slow but sustained and does not resemble the rapid vasoconstriction elicited in patients with variant angina after mechanical stimulation or activation with acetylcholine, histamine, or ergonovine (54). However, endothelin, particularly low and threshold concentra-

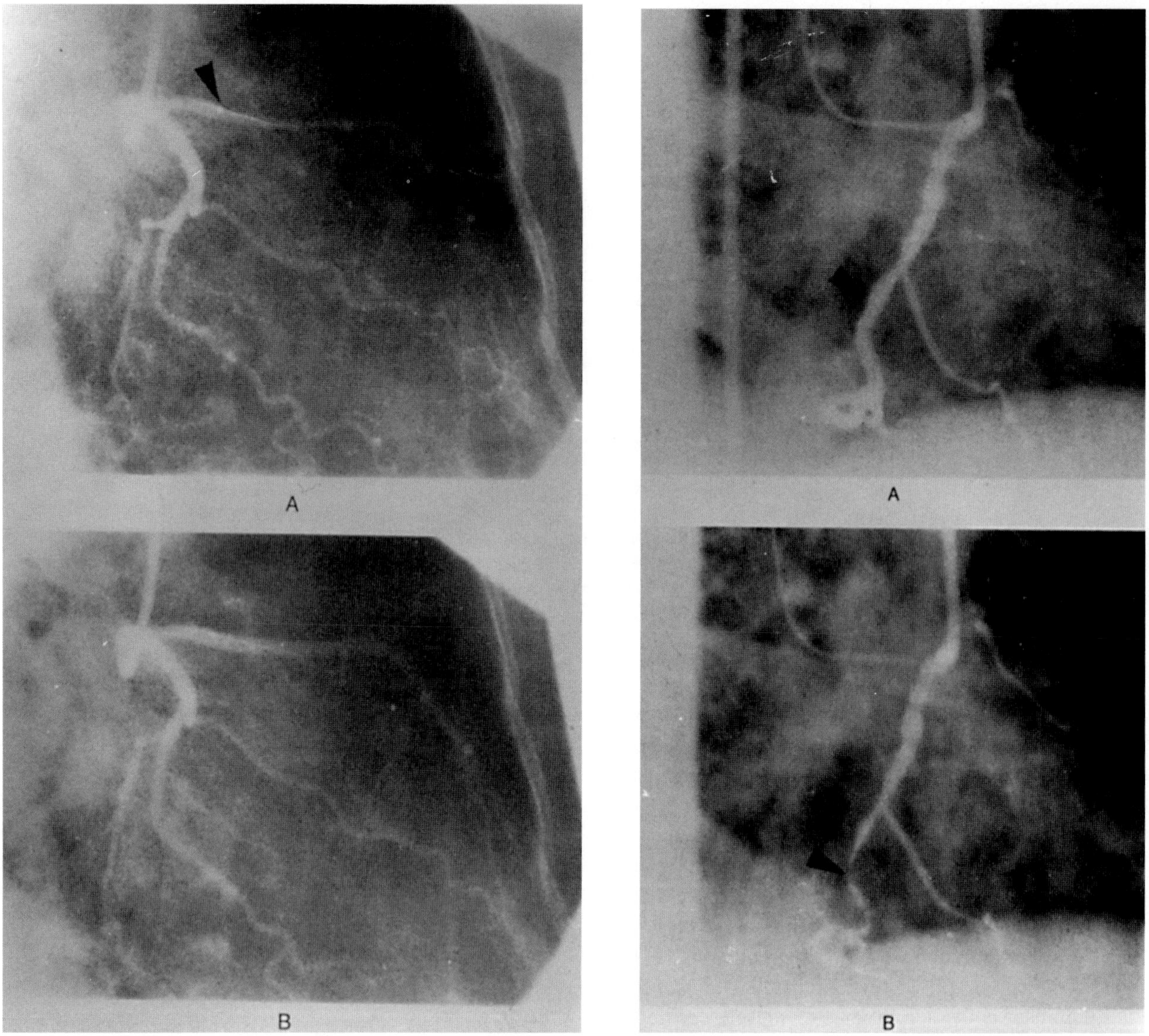

FIG. 14. Effects of intracoronary infusion of serotonin on the arterial diameter of the left anterior descending coronary artery in a patient with normal coronary arteries *(left)* before **(top)** and after **(bottom)** application of the drug. Note the small vasodilation in response to serotonin. In contrast, in a patient with coronary artery disease *(right),* serotonin causes contraction **(bottom).** (Modified from Golino et al., ref. 12, by permission.)

tions, at which its own contractile effects are absent or negligible, is able to potentiate contractions to serotonin of human coronary arteries (Fig. 15; 105). Endothelin appears to increase the sensitivity of vascular smooth muscle to calcium. This could explain the generalized hypercontractility that occurs in certain patients with coronary artery disease and in selected variant angina patients.

In patients with variant angina, circulating levels of endo-

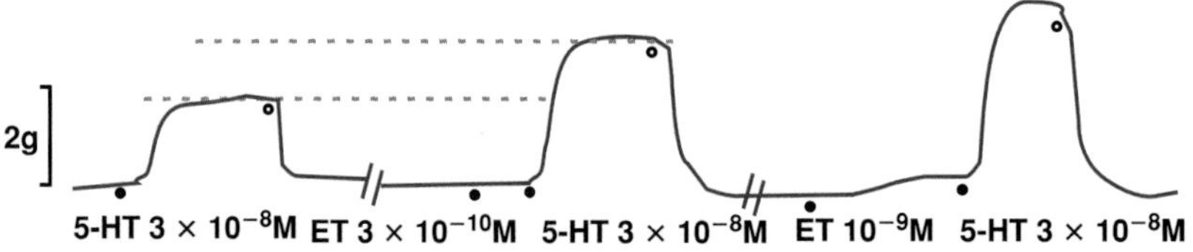

FIG. 15. Potentiating effects of threshold concentrations of endothelin-1 on contractions induced by serotonin (5-hydroxytryptamine; 5-HT) in human coronary artery. (From Yang et al., ref. 105, by permission of the American Heart Association.)

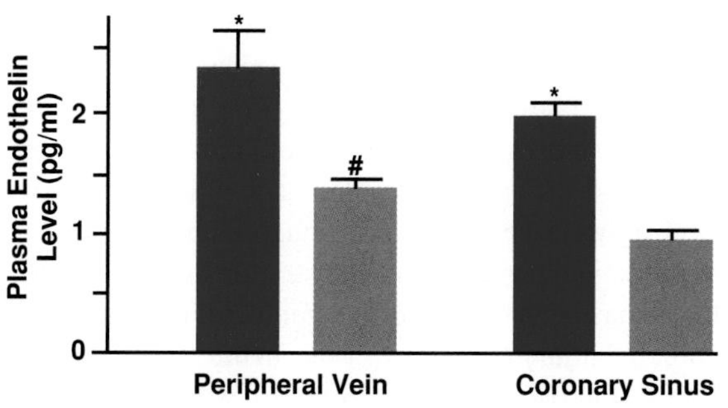

FIG. 16. Endothelin levels in the coronary sinus and peripheral vein in patients with *(hatched bars)* or without *(open bars)* provokable coronary spasm at angiography. (Data from Toyooka et al., ref. 145, by permission of the American Heart Association.) *, significant difference vs. patients without spasms; #, significant difference vs. coronary sinus data.

thelin plasma and in samples obtained in the coronary sinus have been measured. Toyo-oka et al. found increased venous and coronary sinus levels of endothelin-1 in patients with variant angina and provokable coronary vasospasm at angiography (Fig. 16; 145). Interestingly, endothelin plasma levels in the coronary sinus decreased rather than increased during the attack, possibly as a result of reduced flow in the affected coronary segment. In contrast, in patients with clinical findings consistent with variant angina but not provokable vasospasm, systemic venous plasma levels of the peptide were within the normal range. Interestingly, not only in coronary sinus but also in venous samples endothelin levels were twice as high in provokable than in nonprovokable patients (145). If one considers coronary spasm as a very local vascular event, in most cases this is surprising. Indeed, to fully explain local coronary constriction, one would assume a local vascular overproduction of endothelin-1 at the site of spasm with an exclusive paracrine action of the peptide. However, patients with coronary spasm do have a higher incidence of Raynaud's phenomenon, migraine (145), and ocular vasospasm (146) than those without the disease, suggesting some generalized tendency of the vascular system to react with organ-specific focal contraction in response to certain stimuli. This observation would indicate that endothelin may contribute to a generalized vasoconstrictor tendency and that the local trigger mechanism may not necessarily be directly related to the action of the peptide. Development of specific endothelin receptor antagonists (Table 1) will allow determination of whether or not pharmacological blockade of effects of endothelin in coronary vascular smooth muscle is effective in patients with variant angina.

Endothelin may also be important in the pathogenesis of atherosclerotic vascular disease. In atherosclerotic human blood vessels, endothelin production is increased (Fig. 17 see Colorplate 29 for 17B; 147–149), but expression of endothelin receptors is down-regulated (148). A most likely stimulus is oxidized low-density lipoprotein (oxLDL), which increases endothelin gene expression and release of the peptide from porcine and human aortic endothelial cells (Fig. 18; 150). Because the effects of oxLDL are not shared by native LDL, it appears that oxidation of the lipoprotein as occurs in atherosclerotic human arteries is crucially involved in the activation of this local vascular pressor system. In line with these observations, both plasma endothelin levels and vascular endothelin production are increased in patients with hyperlipidemia. In addition to endothelial cells, vascular smooth muscle cells, particularly those that migrated into the intima during the atherosclerotic process, also produce endothelin. In cultured vascular smooth muscle cells, endothelin can be released by growth factors such as platelet-derived growth factor, transforming growth factor β_1, and vasoconstrictors such as arginine vasopressin (151). Hence, several mediators involved in atherosclerosis do stimulate vascular endothelin production. This may explain why plasma endothelin levels are indeed increased in patients with clinically relevant atherosclerosis, and the degree of the increase appears positively correlated with the extent of the atherosclerotic process (147). Furthermore, it appears that lesions removed from the coronary circulation (by atherectomy) of patients with coronary artery disease do exhibit marked staining for endothelin-1 (149). The degree of staining for endothelin-1 appears to be particularly pronounced in patients with unstable angina, suggesting that endothelin

TABLE 1. *Specific endothelin receptor antagonists*

Drug	Receptor
BE-18257 A/B	ET_A
BQ-162	ET_A
BQ-123	ET_A
BQ-153	ET_A
PD 147953 (=FR 139317)	ET_A
RO-462005	ET_A/ET_B
RO-470203 (Bosentan)	ET_A/ET_B
SB 209670	ET_A/ET_B
PD 142893	ET_A/ET_B
PD 145065	ET_A/ET_B

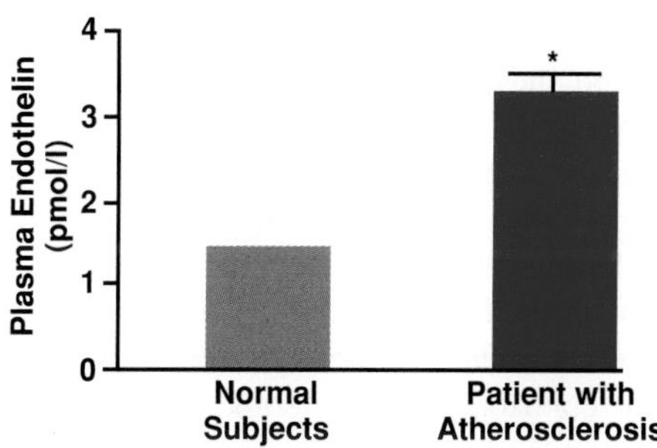

FIG. 17. Endothelin in patients with arteriosclerosis. Plasma levels of endothelin-1 are significantly higher in patients with arteriosclerosis **(A).** Endothelin-1 can be detected immunohistochemically in endothelial cells as well as in the intima and media of arteries of patients with arteriosclerosis **(B).** (See **Colorplate** Section for **B.**) (Modified from Lerman et al., ref. 147, by permission.)

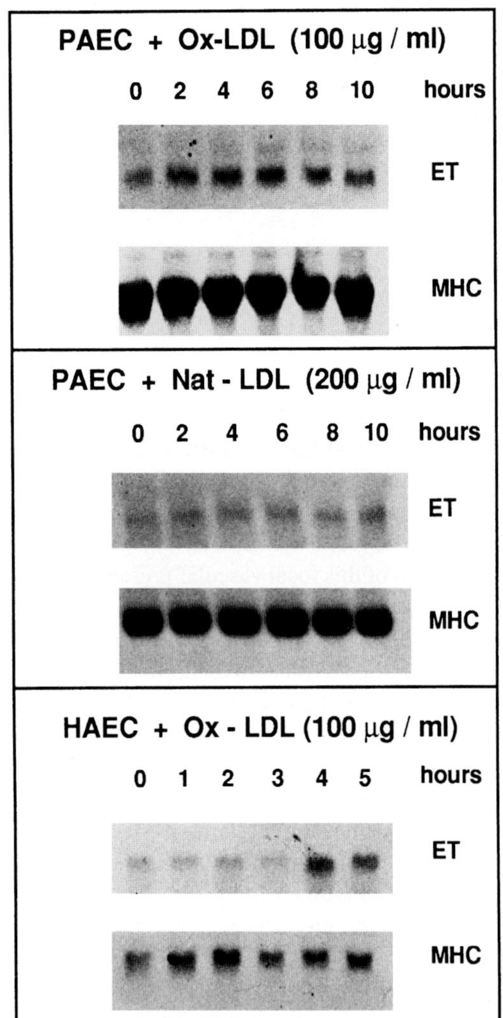

FIG. 18. Stimulation of endothelin (ET) gene expression by oxidized low-density lipoproteins (ox-LDL), but not native LDL (Nat-LDL). Shown is a Northern blot with a cDNA probe for ET in endothelial cells in culture from the porcine aorta (PAEC) and human aorta (HAEC). MHC, major histocompatibility complex served as control. (Modified from Boulanger et al., ref. 150, by permission of the American Heart Association.)

contributes to the abnormal vasomotion in these patients (152). Triggers of endothelin production in patients with acute coronary syndromes might be ischemia (153) and thrombin (54–58). The exact biological role of endothelin in atherosclerotic vascular disease remains to be determined. It may explain the hypervasoconstriction of atherosclerotic blood vessels, particularly at early stages of the disease process and/or contribute to proliferation of vascular smooth muscle cells and in turn to the development of atherosclerotic lesions.

Vascular Smooth Muscle

Hypercontractility of vascular smooth muscle may arise at sites where the continuous vasodilator tone of endothelium-derived nitric oxide is lacking (see above) or in segments in which the responsiveness of vascular smooth muscle cells to contractile stimuli is increased. The latter phenomenon could occur with an increased smooth muscle cell mass and/or increased efficacy of receptor activation. An increased smooth muscle cell mass with augmented contractions to a receptor-independent vasoconstrictor such as potassium chloride has been observed in canine coronary arteries after endothelial injury (see above; 138). In the rabbit, cholesterol-induced atherosclerosis is associated with increased vasoconstrictor responses to serotonin. Oxidized LDL may cause contraction not only via inactivation of the L-arginine/nitric oxide pathway but also through direct stimulation of vascular smooth muscle (154).

Neuronal Mechanisms

Overactivity of the sympathetic nervous system as a cause of variant angina has been suspected by several investigators. However, in patients with coronary spasm, the response to the α_1-adrenergic agonist phenylephrine is normal, and α-adrenergic antagonists are ineffective in experimental models as well as in patients (144,155). Furthermore, sympathetic activation, such as during exercise, is not a typical trigger mechanism in patients with coronary spasm. Hence, it is unlikely that the sympathetic nervous system is importantly involved in variant angina.

The sympathetic nervous system, however, does contribute to the ischemia threshold in patients with coronary atherosclerosis. For example, the cold pressor test (a strong activator of the sympathetic nervous system) causes no change or a small increase in coronary vascular diameter in cases without atherosclerosis, but marked constriction is observed in patients with coronary atherosclerosis (113). During bicycle exercise, flow-dependent vasodilation of normal coronary segments occurs, but diseased segments exhibit paradoxical vasoconstriction (112). In the human forearm circulation, flow-dependent vasodilation can be transformed into paradoxical vasoconstriction after inhibition of nitric oxide synthesis by intraarterial administration of L-NMMA (103). Hence, it appears that lack of nitric oxide production in diseased coronary segments unmasks a vasoconstrictor mechanism. Because the paradoxical vasoconstriction during exercise can be blocked by phentolamine or a calcium antagonist (156), this vasoconstrictor mechanism is likely to be mediated by activation of the sympathetic nervous system. Abnormal coronary vasomotion during exercise may importantly contribute to exercise-induced angina in patients with atherosclerotic coronary disease.

THERAPEUTIC ASPECTS

General Considerations

Certain general considerations should be taken into account when treating patients with coronary artery spasm in any setting. Contributing factors that have been associated with precipitation of exacerbation of coronary artery spasm include exposure to cold, smoking, and emotional stress. These factors should be removed whenever possible. Known vasoconstrictors should be avoided, and patients should be cautioned against use of over-the-counter sympathomimetics. Recent withdrawal of nitrates or calcium or calcium antagonists should be sought as a possible exacerbating factor. Recent institution of β-adrenergic blocking agents should also be considered in the patient with worsening symptoms. Factors contributing to either precipitation or exacerbation of coronary spasm include exposure to cold, smoking, and emotional stress and should be removed whenever possible. Cocaine and other illicit drugs have become an increasingly important cause of vasomotor-related myocardial ischemia in recent years (157).

In patients with variant angina, therapy primarily aims at preventing or reversing coronary constriction. Currently available drugs that relax coronary vascular smooth muscle effectively are nitrates and calcium antagonists (106). Other vasodilators such as potassium channel openers and hydralazine have been for use in susceptible patients, but these have largely been abandoned because they cause a reflex tachycardia, which may aggravate myocardial ischemia. Newer drugs such as endothelin receptor antagonists (see Table 1; 158) or angiotensin type 1 receptor (AT_1) antagonists (95) have not been evaluated yet in patients with known or suspected spasm.

In patients with atherosclerotic coronary artery disease and increased vasomotion, nitrates and calcium antagonists are also very useful in reversing coronary constriction and relieving angina pectoris and signs of ischemia (159,160). Rarely, the angina threshold of patients with coronary spasm may also be lowered by drugs with little vascular action that lower heart rate and myocardial oxygen consumption (i.e., β-blockers), but when a fixed obstruction coexists with spasm, these patients are often benefited. Furthermore, the antianginal effects of nitrates are not only related to coronary dilation but also to reduction in preload of the ventricle. Inhibition of platelet function or coagulation is an important part of therapy of patients with atherosclerotic coronary artery disease, as these drugs have been shown to reduce the risk of myocardial infarction and death (161–165). Ideally, drugs should be able to interfere with the atherosclerotic process itself. This, however, is much more difficult to achieve, although calcium antagonists (166–168) and angiotensin-converting enzyme inhibitors do exert some inhibitory effects on plaque formation (169).

Specific Drugs

Calcium Channel Blockers

Calcium channel blockers inhibit inflow of extracellular calcium through voltage-operated calcium channels into the smooth muscle cell and thereby cause profound vasodilation (see above). Three different classes of calcium channel blockers exist: (a) phenylalkalanines, (b) dihydropyridines, and (c) benzodiazepines (106). The prototype of phenylalkalanines is verapamil, whereas mibefradil, a newly developed compound, interferes not only with L-type, but also with T-type calcium channels (170). Furthermore, although verapamil exhibits negative inotropic and electrophysiological effects, mibefradil lacks these properties. Nifedipine is the classical dihydropyridine; newer compounds such as amlodipine, felodipine, isradipine and nicardipine exhibit marked vascular selectivity (i.e, they are more potent vasodilators and lack negative inotropic effects at clinically used dosages; 106). Finally, diltiazem is the representative of the benzodiazepines and exhibits both vasodilation and negative inotropism. The fact that the three classes of calcium channel blockers bind to different and distinct parts of the L-type calcium channel may explain why, under certain conditions, for instance in patients with severe coronary spasm, combi-

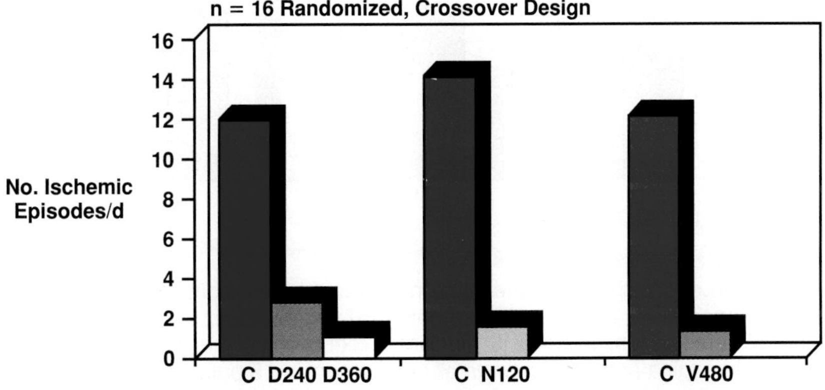

FIG. 19. Comparison of diltiazem (240 and 360 mg/day), nifedipine (120 mg/day), and verapamil (480 mg/day) given to the same patients with variant angina. Note that each of the first-generation calcium antagonists decreased the number of ischemic episodes per day in a similar fashion in this randomized crossover design. (From Turitto et al, ref. 180, with permission.)

nation therapy may be useful. The drugs have been used successfully in patients with both variant angina (alone or in combination) and exercise-induced angina to relieve symptoms.

Short-term controlled trials have demonstrated that calcium antagonists used alone or in combination are very effective for management of recurrent ischemic episodes in the early phase of illness (171–179) (Fig. 19). Comparison studies (180–182) showed similar responses to prevent ischemic episodes among the three first-generation calcium antagonists (diltiazem, nifedipine, verapamil) when the same patients are exposed to the different agents in adequate doses; however, adverse experiences were less frequent with diltiazem (181) (Fig. 20). When the patient is nonresponsive, addition of another calcium antagonist may be helpful, but the risk of side effects may also increase (172,181).

The long-term implications of treatment were evaluated in a prospective study by Walling et al. (130). Treatment consisted of calcium antagonists (diltiazem, nifedipine, verapamil), β-blockers, and long-acting oral or topical nitrates. During follow-up of 65 months, Cox analysis identified left ventricular function and initial treatment as the two strongest predictors of survival without infarction. The other predictors were disease extent score, duration of angina at rest, and disease activity. Treatment with diltiazem, nifedipine, or verapamil improved survival with infarction compared with other medical treatment ($p = 0.002$). Beneficial effects were exerted within the first 3 months after diagnosis (Fig. 21).

Whether or not prognosis of patients after myocardial infarction is favorably affected is uncertain. Indeed, a large trial with diltiazem showed no benefit (183), and another with verapamil found a favorable response only in patients without heart failure (184).

Nitrates

Ever since Thomas Lauder Brunton successfully used nitrate of amyl in patients with angina pectoris (185), nitrates have been a standard therapy in patients with atherosclerotic coronary artery disease and also in those with variant angina. The drugs act by releasing nitric oxide from their molecule (186), which in turn activates guanylate cyclase and leads to the formation of cGMP (Fig. 3; see above). Hence, nitrates act similarly to endothelium-derived nitric oxide and are a substitute for the endogenous nitrovasodilator in disease states with reduced formation of nitric oxide in the blood vessel wall.

In vessels without endothelium, or after inhibition of the endogenous nitric oxide formation, nitrovasodilators are particularly effective vasodilators (187,188). With progressing atherosclerotic coronary artery disease, the response of vascular smooth muscle to nitrates usually is reduced (41).

The potency of nitrovasodilators on a molar basis is related to the number of nitric oxide molecules the compounds are able to release (186). Trinitrates release three, dinitrates two, and mononitrates one nitric oxide molecule. Clinically, however, these differences are not important, as the dosage (on a milligram basis) of the compounds corrects for these differences. However, the potency of nitrates is reduced by

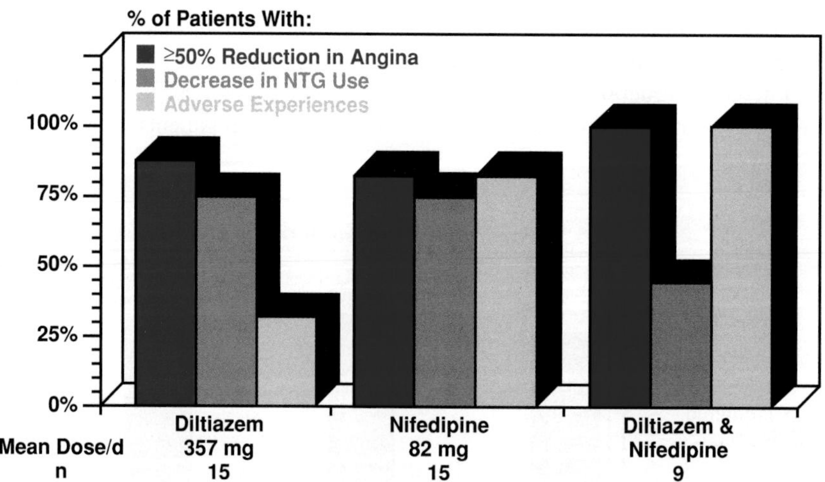

FIG. 20. Comparison of diltiazem and nifedipine monotherapy and combination therapy in the same patients with coronary spasm. Diltiazem (mean dose 357 mg/day) and nifedipine (mean dose 82 mg/day) monotherapy were both associated with significant reductions in the proportion of patients showing a ≥50% reduction in angina *(left hand column of each group)* in 15 patients. Likewise, the decrease in nitroglycerin use paralleled this antianginal effect. Frequency of adverse experiences, however, was higher with nifedipine monotherapy than with diltiazem monotherapy. When diltiazem and nifedipine were combined in nine patients *(bars to the right),* there was an increase in the proportion of patients with reduction in angina, but adverse experiences occurred in every patient exposed to the combination. (From Prida et al., ref. 181, with permission.)

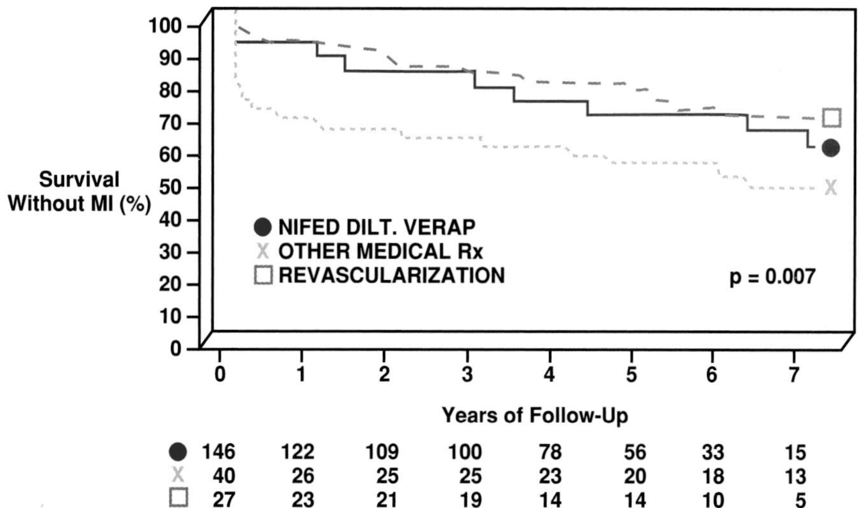

FIG. 21. Survival without myocardial infarction in 217 consecutive patients with variant angina. Patients treated with calcium antagonists *(closed circles)* had a better outcome than patients receiving other medical treatment *(X)*. Too few patients underwent bypass surgery or coronary angioplasty *(open square)* to assess the value of these interventions. (From Walling et al., ref. 130, with permission.)

nitrate tolerance (i.e., the loss of vasodilator effects with prolonged application of the drugs; 189). Nitrate tolerance can occur as a result of counterregulatory mechanisms stimulated by the drugs (i.e., activation of the sympathetic nervous system and the renin–angiotensin system), decreased biotransformation of organic nitrates (because of reduced availability of sulfhydryl groups and other mechanisms), and possibly a reduced activity of guanylate cyclase (189). Nitrovasodilators that do not require enzymatic biotransformation and spontaneously release nitric oxide from their molecule (i.e., molsidomine) appear to be less prone to tolerance (190). Clinically, intermittent therapy with a nitrate-free window of at least 8 h has been recommended.

In patients with variant angina occurring in the catheterization laboratory, intracoronary nitroglycerin rapidly reverses spasm and associated ischemia. Intravenous nitrates are useful for patients with spasms that frequently recur. Sublingual and oral preparations are useful for relieving an acute episode and/or preventing episodes that cluster into one portion of the day (usually the early morning). But in general, when used in dosing schedule that is designed to limit tolerance, nitrates should be combined with calcium antagonists for maximal benefit to control spasm.

New Compounds

Newly developed compounds that may be promising in patients with abnormal coronary vasoconstriction are endothelin receptor antagonists and angiotensin receptor antagonists.

Endothelin binds to specific receptors on vascular smooth muscle and in turn provokes pronounced vasoconstriction (see above; Fig. 9; 74,75). Recently, specific antagonists interfering with ET_A, ET_A/ET_B, or ET_B receptors have been synthesized (Table 1; 158). Some of these compounds are active orally [in particular, bosentan (78), SB209670, and PD 142893 (80,158)] and potent inhibitors of endothelin-induced vasoconstriction in man (80,191). Phase I studies have already been performed, but data in patients with variant angina or atherosclerotic coronary artery disease are lacking. The fact that plasma levels of endothelin are increased in patients with variant angina (Fig. 16; 138) and also in patients with atherosclerosis (Fig. 17; 147–153) strongly suggests that the drugs might be useful tools to interfere with increased coronary vasoconstriction.

Angiotensin II is a potent vasoconstrictor that binds to specific receptors on vascular smooth muscle cells to exert its effects. Up to four angiotensin receptors exist (95), but it appears that in vascular smooth muscle cells, vasoconstriction as well as migration and proliferation are exclusively mediated by angiotensin receptor subtype 1 (AT_1). Losartan and valsartan are specific AT_1 receptor antagonists. Losartan is already used for treatment of hypertension in several countries (192,193), but data in patients with atherosclerotic coronary artery disease or variant angina are lacking.

Current Recommendations

Acute Setting

As noted above, coronary spasm can play an important role in the pathogenesis of unstable or periinfarction angina syndromes. Thus, spasm should be considered in the treatment strategies employed for management of all coronary care unit patients presenting with myocardial ischemia at rest in whom spasm has not been excluded. Accordingly, in the acute setting the initial agent of choice is intravenous nitroglycerin. We initiate therapy with an intravenous bolus of 400 μg followed by an infusion. The infusion rate is started at 5 to 10 μg/min and titrated to achieve resolution of signs and symptoms of ischemia. The infusion should not be targeted to any arbitrary reduction in blood pressure because, potentially, such a strategy may provoke ischemia by reducing coronary perfusion pressure while causing a reflex increase in heart rate in patients with fixed obstructive lesions (194). Acute ischemia caused by coronary spasm is very rapidly relieved by intravenous nitroglycerin, and coronary spasm is very sensitive to nitrates; thus, continuous high blood levels are neither needed nor desirable if tolerance is to be minimized (130). We anticoagulate with intravenous heparin, based on the association of thrombus formation with acute ischemic syndromes and the proven beneficial effect of heparin in such patient groups (195). We also add low-dose aspirin (160 mg/day).

Shortly after parenteral nitrates are started, oral calcium antagonists should also be instituted. Such a combination is logical in view of their complementary mechanisms of action. In the one case, vasodilation in a manner analogous to that of endothelium-derived relaxing factor and, in the other, blockade of calcium-regulated smooth muscle contraction. Both of the primary activation mechanisms (tonic and phasic) in vascular smooth muscle are thereby inhibited.

The choice of calcium antagonist is usually not critical. Verapamil and diltiazem are more potent negative inotropes than the dihydropyridines and should be avoided in patients with either bradydysrhythmias or severe impairment of left ventricular function (194). Dihydropyridine compounds are more potent peripheral vasodilators than either verapamil or diltiazem and should not be used in patients who are hypotensive (194).

In the rare instance in which acute ischemia caused by coronary spasm appears refractory to intravenous nitroglycerin and a calcium anatagonist, a second calcium antagonist may be added. Logic would dictate combining a dihydropyridine with a heart-rate-slowing compound (diltiazem or verapamil). Intravenous administration of either diltiazem or verapamil can be utilized (196,197), although care must be taken to avoid systemic hypotension in this setting. However, if hypotension occurs, restoration of blood pressure may be achieved by fluid administration and down-titration of the dose of nitroglycerin. We have, on rare occasion, given calcium antagonists directly into a coronary artery when spasm has been refractory to all other measures.

When acute ischemia is controlled in the critical care setting, parenteral nitrates should be changed to oral or topical preparations, administered on an eccentric dosing schedule with a 10- to 12-h nitrate-free window (194). Because attacks tend to cluster between midnight and 8 AM (198,199), the nitrate-free window should be positioned during the afternoon and early evening hours.

Some patients with coronary spasm, initially well controlled, may have recurrent ischemia while receiving the measures cited above. When recurrent episodes are either frequent or prolonged, and sufficient time has elapsed since the first angiogram for possible changes in anatomy, repeat coronary angiography may be considered to define the coronary anatomy and guide other therapy if indicated. If the episodes are frequent or prolonged, placement of an intraaortic balloon pump may be useful while the patient is prepared for coronary angiography. When refractory spasm is associated with intracoronary thrombus, thrombolytic therapy may be helpful. When refractory spasm is associated with severe atherosclerotic stenosis adjunct revascularization may be considered.

Adjunctive Revascularization

Coronary artery bypass surgery can be an effective adjunct to calcium antagonist therapy in selected patients with recurrent spasm limited to the site of an important atherosclerotic narrowing (200,201). However, if spasm involves multiple vessels, is diffuse in the same vessel, is migrating to different vessels, or is not associated with important atherosclerotic obstruction, coronary bypass surgery is not indicated. In any patient with suspected coronary spasm undergoing operation, it is essential to provide effective pharmacological prophylaxis against coronary spasm before, during, and after surgery (200). The frequency of graft occlusion and perioperative myocardial infarction is higher in patients with spasm than in those without spasm. Coronary bypass surgery has been combined with denervation (plexectomy), but there is no objective evidence from controlled trials that this improves results.

Infrequently, percutaneous transluminal coronary angioplasty (PTCA) may be an adjunct to pharmacological therapy in managing selected patients with coronary spasm limited to the site of an important atherosclerotic narrowing (202). Angioplasty is not indicated if spasm involves multiple sites or different vessels. Care should be exercised in patients with dynamic stenosis because of a risk for restenosis (203).

Ambulatory Setting

Treatment principles for coronary spasm in ambulatory patients are similar to those outlined in the acute setting and differ only in the routes by which medications are administered. Oral nitrates and calcium antagonists remain the mainstays of chronic ambulatory treatment, with sublingual nitroglycerin used to relieve acute episodes. At our institution, we have found that after several months of combination treatment some patients do well with only calcium antagonist monotherapy. However, because the clinical course of patients with coronary spasm is highly variable and typically displays periods of exacerbation and remission even with seemingly optimal therapy, regular evaluation of treatment regimens is necessary. During flares of activity, our approach is to increase doses of calcium antagonists and nitrates; several different calcium antagonists may be used in combination to take advantage of each agent's different properties and to minimize side effects seen when very large doses of a single agent are employed. Sublingual nitroglycerin is used to relieve acute episodes. After several symptom-free months, one calcium antagonist is discontinued, and, with continued remission, the second is discontinued.

Monitoring Therapy

Following institution of an effective ambulatory treatment regimen, several options are available to follow patients with coronary spasm. Monitoring symptoms may be sufficient for many patients, but there is evidence that as many as 90% of all ischemia-related episodes in coronary spasm patients may be asymptomatic (204). In addition, the natural history of Prinzmetal's angina may be difficult to predict. Thus, it is helpful to attempt a more objective assessment of therapeutic efficacy, especially in patients with severe ischemia or ischemia-related sequelae such as tachydysrhythmias, pump dysfunction, or conduction disturbances related to coronary spasm. Repeat catheterization with ergonovine provocation during therapy to assess efficacy could be considered, but this strategy has not been compared with a less invasive strategy documenting therapeutic success and has obvious disadvantages with regard to costs, risks, and discomfort. Repeated ambulatory ECG monitoring of the ST segment is probably the best current objective method to follow therapy in patients with coronary spasm. If spasm-related dysrhythmias are present in a given patient, these too can be used to follow the adequacy of therapy and the possibility for spontaneous remission. Clearly, ischemia-associated dysrhythmias should be managed by prevention of ischemia rather than by attempting to suppresses the rhythm disturbance with antiarrhythmic agents.

FUTURE DIRECTIONS

Coronary vasomotion is an important regulatory mechanism that allows the coronary circulation to adapt blood flow to the oxygen requirements of the myocardium under different physiological conditions. In disease states such as variant angina as well as exercise-induced angina, the regulation of coronary vascular tone becomes abnormal. Abnormal coronary vasomotion importantly contributes to symptoms and prognosis of these patients. The understanding of the cellular and molecular mechanisms regulating coronary tone has improved dramatically in the last decade. This allowed for the development of new and more dynamic concepts of atherosclerotic coronary artery disease as well as variant angina. This should lead to more effective drugs, some of which are already in clinical development, to treat these patients. At this point, nitrates and calcium channel blockers alone or in combination are most effective to relieve vasospasm in patients with variant angina or increased vasoconstriction in patients with atherosclerotic coronary artery disease.

REFERENCES

1. Prinzmetal M, Kennamer R, Merliss R, Wada T, Bor N. A variant form of angina pectoris. *Am J Med* 1959;27:375–388.
2. Prinzmetal M, Ekmekci A, Kennamer R, Kwocynski JK, Shubin H, Toyoshima H. Variant form of angina pectoris. *JAMA* 1960;174:1794–1800.
3. Wiener L, Kasparian H, Duca PR, Walinsky P, Gottlieb RS, Hanckel F, Brest AN. Spectrum of coronary arterial spasm. Clinical, angiographic and myocardial metabolic experience in 29 cases. *Am J Cardiol* 1976;38:945–955.
4. Dhurandhar RW, Watt DL, Silver MD, Trimble AS, Adelman AG. Prinzmetal's variant form of angina with arteriographic evidence of coronary arterial spasm. *Am J Cardiol* 1972;30:902–905.
5. Oliva PB, Potts DE, Pluss RG. Coronary arterial spasm in Prinzmetal angina. Documentation by coronary arteriography. *N Engl J Med* 1973;288:745–751.
6. Maseri A, L'Abbate A, Baroldi G, Chierchia S, Marzilli M, Ballestra AM, Severi S, Parodi O, Biagini A, Distante A, Pesola A. Coronary vasospasm as a possible cause of myocardial infarction. A conclusion derived from the study of "preinfarction" angina. *N Engl J Med* 1978;299:1271–1277.
7. Vincent GM, Anderson JL, Marshall HW. Coronary spasm producing coronary thrombosis and myocardial infarction. *N Engl J Med* 1983;309:220–223.
8. Hillis LD, Braunwald E. Coronary-artery spasm. *N Engl J Med* 1978;299:695–702.
9. Maseri A, Severi S, Nes MD, L'Abbate A, Chierchia S, Marzilli M, Ballestra AM, Parodi O, Biagini A, Distante A. "Variant" angina: One aspect of a continuous spectrum of vasospastic myocardial ischemia. Pathogenetic mechanisms, estimated incidence and clinical and coronary arteriographic findings in 138 patients. *Am J Cardiol* 1978;42:1019–1035.
10. Rafflenbeul W, Nellessen U, Galvao P, Kreft M, Peters S, Lichtlen P. Progression and regression of coronary sclerosis in the angiographic image. *Z Kardiol* 1984;73(Suppl 2):33–40.
11. Ludmer PL, Selwyn AP, Shook TL, Wayne RR, Mudge GH, Alexander RW, Ganz P. Paradoxical vasoconstriction induced by acetylcholine in atherosclerotic coronary arteries. *N Engl J Med* 1986;315:1046–1051.
12. Golino P, Piscione F, Willerson JT, Cappelli BM, Focaccio A, Villari B, Indolfi C, Russolillo E, Condorelli M, Chiariello M. Divergent effects of serotonin on coronary-artery dimensions and blood flow in patients with coronary atherosclerosis and control patients. *N Engl J Med* 1991;324:641–648.
13. Lüscher TF, Vanhoutte PM. *The Endothelium: Modulator of Cardiovascular Function.* Boca Raton, FL: CRC Press; 1990.
14. Vanhoutte PM, Lüscher TF. Peripheral mechanisms in cardiovascular regulation: Transmitters, receptors and the endothelium. In: Tarazini RC, Zanchetti A, eds. *Handbook of Hypertension* Vol. 8, *Physiology and Pathophysiology of Hypertension—Regulatory Mechanisms.* Amsterdam: Elsevier; 1986:96–123.
15. Furchgott RF, Zawadzki JV. The obligatory role of endothelial cells in the relaxation of arterial smooth muscle by acetylcholine. *Nature* 1980;299:373–376.
16. Cohen RA, Shepherd JT, Vanhoutte PM. Inhibitory role of the endothelium in the response of isolated coronary arteries to platelets. *Science* 1983;221:273–274.
17. Lüscher TF, Diederich D, Siebenmann R, Lehmann K, Stulz P, von SL, Yang ZH, Turina M, Grädel E, Weber E, Bühler FR. Difference between endothelium-dependent relaxation in arterial and in venous coronary bypass grafts. *N Engl J Med* 1988;319:462–467.
18. Yang Z, Stulz P, Von SL, Bauer E, Turina M, Lüscher TF. Different interactions of platelets with arterial and venous coronary bypass vessels. *Lancet* 1991;337:939–943.
19. De Mey JG, Claeys M, Vanhoutte PM. Endothelium-dependent inhibitory effects of acetylcholine, adenosine diphosphate, thrombin and arachidonic acid in the canine femoral artery. *J Pharmacol Exp Ther* 1982;222:166–173.
20. Rubanyi GM, Romero JC, Vanhoutte PM. Flow-induced release of

endothelium-derived relaxing factor. *Am J Physiol* 1988;250: H1145–H1149.
21. Pohl U, Holtz J, Busse R, Bassenge E. Crucial role of endothelium in the vasodilator response to increased flow in vivo. *Hypertension* 1986;8:37–44.
22. Rubanyi GM, Vanhoutte PM. Superoxide anions and hyperoxia inactivate endothelium-derived relaxing factor. *Am J Physiol* 1986;250: H822–H827.
23. Furchgott RF. Studies on relaxation of rabbit aorta by sodium nitrite: The basis for the proposal that acid-activable inhibitory factor from bovine retractor penis is inorganic nitrite and the endothelium-derived relaxing factor is nitric oxide. In: Vanhoutte PM, ed. *Vasodilation: Vascular Smooth Muscle, Peptides, Autonomic Nerves and Endothelium.* New York: Raven Press; 1988:401–414.
24. Palmer RM, Ferrige AG, Moncada S. Nitric oxide release accounts for the biological activity of endothelium-derived relaxing factor. *Nature* 1987;327:524–526.
25. Ignarro LJ, Byrns RE, Buga GM, Wood KS, Chaudhuri G. Pharmacological evidence that endothelium-derived relaxing factor is nitric oxide: Use of pyrogallol and superoxide dismutase to study endothelium-dependent and nitric oxide-elicited vascular smooth muscle relaxation. *J Pharmacol Exp Ther* 1988;244:181–189.
26. Palmer RM, Ashton DS, Moncada S. Vascular endothelial cells synthesize nitric oxide from L-arginine. *Nature* 1988;333:664–666.
27. Bredt DS, Hwang PM, Glatt CE, Lowenstein C, Reed RR, Snyder SH. Cloned and expressed nitric oxide synthase structurally resembles cytochrome P-450 reductase. *Nature* 1991;351:714–718.
28. Radomski MW, Palmer RW, Moncada S. An L-arginine/nitric oxide pathway present in human platelets regulates aggregation. *Proc Natl Acad Sci USA* 1990;87:5193–5197.
29. Hibbs J Jr, Taintor RR, Vavrin Z, Rachlin EM. Nitric oxide: A cytotoxic activated macrophage effector molecule. *Biochem Biophys Res Commun* 1988;157:87–94.
30. Bernhardt J, Tschudi MR, Dohi Y, Gut I, Urwyler B, Bühler FR, Lüscher TF. Release of nitric oxide from human vascular smooth muscle cells. *Biochem Biophys Res Commun* 1991;180:907–912.
31. Julou-Schaeffer G, Gray GA, Fleming I, Schott C, Parratt JR, Stoclet JC. Loss of vascular responsiveness induced by endotoxin involves L-arginine pathway. *Am J Physiol* 1990;259:1038–1043.
32. Wright CE, Rees DD, Moncada S. Protective and pathological roles of nitric oxide in endotoxin shock. *Cardiovasc Res* 1992;26:48–57.
33. Knowles RG, Palacios M, Palmer RM, Moncada S. Formation of nitric oxide from L-arginine in the central nervous system: A transduction mechanism for stimulation of the soluble guanylate cyclase. *Proc Natl Acad Sci USA* 1989;86:5159–5162.
34. Richard V, Tanner FC, Tschudi M, Lüscher TF. Different activation of L-arginine pathway by bradykinin, serotonin, and clonidine in coronary arteries. *Am J Physiol* 1990;259:H1433–H1439.
35. Tschudi M, Richard V, Bühler FR, Lüscher TF. Importance of endothelium-derived nitric oxide in porcine coronary resistance arteries. *Am J Physiol* 1991;260:H13–H20.
36. Yang ZH, von Segesser L, Bauer E, Stulz P, Turina M, Lüscher TF. Different activation of the endothelial L-arginine and cyclooxygenase pathway in the human internal mammary artery and saphenous vein. *Circ Res* 1991;68:52–60.
37. Meyer P, Flammer J, Lüscher TF. Endothelium-dependent regulation of the ophthalmic microcirculation in the perfused porcine eye: Role of nitric oxide and endothelins. *Invest Ophthalmol Vis Sci* 1993;34: 3614–3621.
38. Rees DD, Palmer RMJ, Moncada S. Role of endothelium-derived nitric oxide in the regulation of blood pressure. *Proc Natl Acad Sci USA* 1989;86:3375–3378.
39. Vallance P, Leone A, Calver A, Collier J, Moncada S. Accumulation of an endogenous inhibitor of nitric oxide synthesis in chronic renal failure. *Lancet* 1992;339:572–575.
40. Rapoport RM, Draznin MB, Murad F. Endothelium-dependent relaxation in rat aorta may be mediated through cyclic GMP-dependent protein phosphorylation. *Nature* 1983;306:174–176.
41. Förstermann U, Mügge A, Bode SM, Frölich JC. Response of human coronary arteries to aggregating platelets: Importance of endothelium-derived relaxing factor and prostanoids. *Circ Res* 1988;63:306–312.
42. Yang Z, Arnet U, Bauer E, von Segesser L, Siebenmann R, Turina M, Lüscher TF. Thrombin-induced endothelium-dependent inhibition and direct activation of platelet-vessel wall interaction. Role of prostacyclin, nitric oxide, and thromboxane A_2. *Circulation* 1994;89: 2266–2272.
43. Moncada S, Vane VR. Pharmacology and endogenous roles of prostaglandin endoperoxides, thromboxane A_2 and prostacyclin. *Pharmacol Rev* 1979;30:293–331.
44. Nakahata N, Suzuki T. Effects of prostaglandin E_1, I_2 and isoproterenol on the tissue cyclic AMP content in longitudinal muscle of rabbit intestine. *Prostaglandins* 1981;22:159–165.
45. Radomski MW, Palmer RW, Moncada S. Comparative pharmacology of endothelium-derived relaxing factor, nitric oxide and prostacyclin in platelets. *Br J Pharmacol* 1987;92:181–187.
46. Vanhoutte PM. Vascular physiology: The end of the quest? *Nature* 1987;327:459–460.
47. Feletou M, Vanhoutte PM. Endothelium-dependent hyperpolarization of canine coronary smooth muscle. *Br J Pharmacol* 1988;93:515–524.
48. Nagao T, Vanhoutte PM. Hyperpolarization contributes to endothelium-dependent relaxations to acetylcholine in femoral veins of rats. *Am J Physiol* 1991;261:H1034–H1037.
49. Nagao T, Vanhoutte PM. Hyperpolarization as a mechanism for endothelium-dependent relaxations in the porcine coronary artery. *J Physiol* 1992;445:355–367.
50. Tare M, Parkington HC, Coleman HA, Neild TO, Dusting GJ. Hyperpolarization and relaxation of arterial smooth muscle caused by nitric oxide derived from the endothelium. *Nature* 1990;346:69–71.
51. Archer SL, Huang JM, Hampl V, Nelson DP, Shultz PJ, Weir EK. Nitric oxide and cGMP cause vasorelaxation by activation of a charybdotoxin-sensitive K channel by cGMP-dependent protein kinase. *Proc Natl Acad Sci USA* 1994;91:7583–7587.
52. Bolotina VM, Najibi S, Palacino JJ, Pagano PJ, Cohen RA. Nitric oxide directly activates calcium-dependent potassium channels in vascular smooth muscle. *Nature* 1994;368:850–853.
53. Nakao K, Ogawa Y, Suga S, Imura H. Molecular biology and biochemistry of the natriuretic peptide system. I: Natriuretic peptides. *J Hypertens* 1992;10:907–912.
54. Yanagisawa M, Kurihara H, Kimura S, Tomobe Y, Kobayashi M, Mitsui Y, Yazaki Y, Goto K, Masaki T. A novel potent vasoconstrictor peptide produced by vascular endothelial cells. *Nature* 1988;332: 411–415.
55. Yanagisawa M, Masaki T. Molecular biology and biochemistry of the endothelins. *Trends Pharmacol Sci* 1989;10:374–378.
56. Lüscher TF, Boulanger CM, Dohi Y, Yang ZH. Endothelim-derived contracting factors. *Hypertension* 1992;19:117–130.
57. Boulanger C, Lüscher TF. Release of endothelin from the porcine aorta. Inhibition of endothelium-derived nitric oxide. *J Clin Invest* 1990;85:587–590.
58. Boulanger CM, Lüscher TF. Hirudin and nitrates inhibit the thrombin-induced release of endothelin from the intact porcine aorta. *Circ Res* 1991;68:1768–1772.
59. Dohi Y, Hahn AW, Boulanger CM, Bühler FR, Lüscher TF. Endothelin stimulated by angiotensin II augments contractility of spontaneously hypertensive rat resistance arteries. *Hypertension* 1992;19: 131–137.
60. Dohi Y, Lüscher TF. Endothelin in hypertensive resistance arteries. Intraluminal and extraluminal dysfunction. *Hypertension* 1991;18: 543–549.
61. Clarke JG, Larkin SW, Benjamin N, Keogh BE, Chester A, Davies GJ, Taylor KM, Maseri A. Endothelin-1 is a potent long-lasting vasoconstrictor in dog peripheral vasculature in vivo. *J Cardiovasc Pharmacol* 1989;13:S211–S212.
62. Kiowski W, Lüscher TF, Linder L, Bühler FR. Endothelin-1-induced vasoconstriction in humans. Reversal by calcium channel blockade but not by nitrovasodilators or endothelium-derived relaxing factor. *Circulation* 1991;83:469–475.
63. Lüscher TF, Yang Z, Tschudi M, Von SL, Stulz P, Boulanger C, Siebenmann R, Turina M, Bühler FR. Interaction between endothelin-1 and endothelium-derived relaxing factor in human arteries and veins. *Circ Res* 1990;66:1088–1094.
64. Neubauer S, Ertl G, Haas U, Pulzer F, Kochsiek K. Effects of endothelin-1 in isolated perfused rat heart. *J Cardiovasc Pharmacol* 1990; 16:1–8.
65. Zaugg CE, Zhu P, Simper D, Lüscher TF, Allegrini PR, Buser PT. Differential effects of endothelin-1 on normal and postischemic reperfused myocardium. *J Cardiovasc Pharmacol* 1993;22(Suppl 8): S367–S370.
66. Küng CF, Tschudi MR, Noll G, Clozel J-P, Lüscher TF. Differential effects of calcium antagonism in epicardial and intramyocardial coronary arteries. *J Cardiovasc Pharmacol [inpress].*
67. Tschudi MR, Lüscher TF. Characterization of contractile endothelin

and angiotensin receptors in human resistance arteries: Evidence for two endothelin and one angiotensin receptor. *Biochem Biophys Res Commun* 1994;204:685–690.
68. Stewart DJ, Langleben D, Cernacek P, Cianflone K. Endothelin release is inhibited by coculture of endothelial cells with cells of vascular media. *Am J Physiol* 1990;259:H1928–H1932.
69. Wagner OF, Christ G, Wojta J, Vierhapper H, Parzer S, Nowotny PJ, Schneider B, Waldhausl W, Binder BR. Polar secretion of endothelin-1 by cultured endothelial cells. *J Biol Chem* 1992;267:16066–16068.
70. Saijonmaa O, Ristimaki A, Fyhrquist F. Atrial natriuretic peptide, nitroglycerine, and nitroprusside reduce basal and stimulated endothelin production from cultured endothelial cells. *Biochem Biophys Res Commun* 1990;173:514–520.
71. Yokokawa K, Kohno M, Yasunari K, Murakawa K, Takeda T. Endothelin-3 regulates endothelin-1 production in cultured human endothelial cells. *Hypertension* 1991;18:304–315.
72. Warner TD, Mitchell JA, de Nucci G, Vane JR. Endothelin-1 and endothelin-3 release EDRF from isolated perfused arterial vessels of the rat and rabbit. *J Cardiovasc Pharmacol* 1989;13:S85–S858.
73. Miller VM, Komori K, Burnett JJ, Vanhoutte PM. Differential sensitivity to endothelin in canine arteries and veins. *Am J Physiol* 1989; 257:H1127–H1131.
74. Arai H, Hori S, Aramori I, Ohkubo H, Nakanishi S. Cloning and expression of a cDNA encoding an endothelin receptor. *Nature* 1990; 348:730–732.
75. Sakurai T, Yanagisawa M, Takuwa Y, Miyazaki H, Kimura S, Goto K, Masaki T. Cloning of a cDNA encoding a non-isopeptide-selective subtype of the endothelin receptor. *Nature* 1990;348:732–735.
76. Seo B-G, Siebenmann R, von Segesser L, Lüscher TF. Both ETA- and ETB-receptors mediate endothelin-induced contractions in human blood vessels. *Circulation.*
77. Karne S, Jayawickreme CK, Lerner MR. Cloning and characterization of an endothelin-3 specific receptor (ETC receptor) from *Xenopus laevis* dermal melanophores. *J Biol Chem* 1993;268:19126–19133.
78. Clozel M, Breu V, Burri K, Cassal J-M, Fischli W, Gray GA, Hirth G, Löffler B-M, Müller M, Neidhart W, Ramuz H. Pathophysiologic role of endothelin revealed by the first orally active endothelin receptor antagonist. *Nature* 1993;365:759–761.
79. Bazil MK, Lappe RW, Webb RL. Pharmacologic characterization of an endothelin A (ET_A) receptor antagonist in conscious rats. *J Cardiovasc Pharmacol* 1992;20:940–948.
80. Wenzel RR, Noll G, Lüscher TF. Endothelin receptor antagonists inhibit endothelin in human skin microcirculation. *Hypertension* 1994; 23:581–586.
81. Nishikibe M, Tsuchida S, Okada M, Fukuroda T, Shimamoto K, Yano M, Ishikawa K, Ikemoto F. Antihypertensive effect of a newly synthesized endothelin antagonist, BQ-123, in a genetic hypertensive model. *Life Sci* 1993;52:717–724.
82. Lüscher TF, Seo BG, Bühler FR. Potential role of endothelin in hypertension. Controversy on endothelin in hypertension. *Hypertension* 1993;21:752–757.
83. Miller VM, Vanhoutte PM. Endothelium-dependent contractions to arachidonic acid are mediated by products of cyclooxygenase. *Am J Physiol* 1985;248:H432–H437.
84. Vanhoutte PM, Katusic ZS. Endothelium-derived contracting factor: Endothelin and/or superoxide anion? *Trends Pharmacol Sci* 1988;9: 229–230.
85. Katusic ZS, Vanhoutte PM. Superoxide anion is an endothelium-derived contracting factor. *Am J Physiol* 1989;257:H33–H37.
86. Somlyo AP, Somlyo AV. Signal transduction and regulation in smooth muscle. *Nature* 1994;372:231–236.
87. Wallin BG, Sundlöf G, Eriksson BM, Dominiak P, Grobecker H, Lindblad LE. Plasma noradrenaline correlates to sympathetic muscle nerve activity in normotensive man. *Acta Physiol Scand* 1981;111: 69–73.
88. Goldstein DS, Horwitz D, Keiser HR, Polinsky RJ, Kopin IJ. Plasma *l*-[^{3}H]norepinephrine, *d*-[^{14}C]norepinephrine, and *d,l*-[^{3}H]isoproterenol kinetics in essential hypertension. *J Clin Invest* 1983;72:1748–1758.
89. Frewin DB, Hume WR, Waterson JG, Whelan RF. The histochemical localisation of sympathetic nerve endings in human gingival blood vessels. *Aust J Exp Biol Med Sci* 1971;49:573–580.
90. Waterson JG, Frewin DB, Soltys JS. Age-related differences in catecholamine fluorescence of human vascular tissue. *Blood Vessels* 1974; 11:79–85.
91. Gerke DC, Frewin DB, Soltys JS Adrenergic innervation of human mesenteric blood vessels. *Aust J Exp Biol Med Sci* 1975;53:241–243.
92. Berkowitz BA, Kohler C. Vascular catecholamines and aging. In: Bevan JA, Maxwell RA, Godfraind T, Vanhoutte PM, eds. *Vascular Neuroeffector Mechanisms.* New York: Raven Press; 1980:335.
93. Kaumann AJ, Frenekn M, Brown AM, Posival H. Variable participation of 5-HT_1-like receptors and 5-HT_2 receptors in serotonin-induced contractions of human isolated coronary arteries: 5-HT_1-like receptors resemble cloned 5-HT_{1Db} receptors. *Circulation [in press].*
94. Cohen RA. Contractions of isolated canine coronary arteries resistant to S2-serotonergic blockade. *J Pharmacol Exp Ther* 1986;237: 548–552.
95. Timmermans PB, Chiu AT, Herblin WF, Wong PC, Smith RD. Angiotensin II receptor subtypes. *Am J Hypertens* 1992;5:406–410.
96. Katusic ZS, Shepherd JT, Vanhoutte PM. Oxytocin causes endothelium-dependent relaxations of canine basilar arteries by activating V_1-vasopressinergic receptors. *J Pharmacol Exp Ther* 1986;236: 166–270.
97. Ekblad E, Edvinsson L, Wahlestedt C, Uddman R, Hakanson R, Sundler F. Neuropeptide Y co-exists and co-operates with noradrenaline in perivascular nerve fibers. *Regul Pept* 1984;8:225–235.
98. Vanhoutte PM, Lüscher TF. Perpheral mechanisms in cardiovascular regulation: Transmitter receptors and the endothelium. In: Tarazi RC, Zanchetti A, eds. *Handbook of Hypertension,* Vol. 8, *Physiology and Pathophysiology of Hypertension—Regulatory Mechanisms.* Amsterdam: Elsevier; 1986:96–123.
99. Cohen RA, Shepherd JT, Vanhoutte PM. 5-Hydroxytryptamine can mediate endothelium-dependent relaxation of coronary arteries. *Am J Physiol* 1983;245:H1077–H1080.
100. Shimokawa H, Aarhus LL, Vanhoutte PM. Porcine coronary arteries with regenerated endothelium have a reduced endothelium-dependent responsiveness to aggregating platelets and serotonin. *Circ Res* 1987; 61:256–270.
101. Cohen RA, Shepherd JT, Vanhoutte PM. Neurogenic cholinergic prejunctional inhibition of sympathetic beta adrenergic relaxation in the canine coronary artery. *J Pharmacol Exp Ther* 1984;229:417–421.
102. Cox DA, Vita JA, Treasure CB, Fish RD, Alexander RW, Ganz P, Selwyn AP. Atherosclerosis impairs flow-mediated dilation of coronary arteries in humans. *Circulation* 1989;80:458–465.
103. Joannides R, Haefeli WE, Linder L, Richard V, Bakkali EH, Thuillez C, Lüscher TF. Nitric oxide is responsible for flow-dependent dilation of human peripheral conduit arteries in vivo. *Circulation* 1995;91: 1314–1319.
104. Resink TJ, Scott-Burden T, Bühler FR. Endothelin stimulates phospholipase C in cultured vascular smooth muscle cells. *Biochem Biophys Res Commun* 1988;157:1360–1368.
105. Yang Z, Richard V, Von SL, Bauer E, Stulz P, Turina M, Lüscher TF. Threshold concentrations of endothelin-1 potentiate contractions to norepinephrine and serotonin in human arteries. A new mechanism of vasospasm? *Circulation* 1990;82:188–195.
106. Opie LH, Bühler FR, Fleckenstein A, Hansson L, Harrison DC, Poole-Wilson PA, Schwartz A, Vanhoutte PM, Braunwald E, Nayler WG, et al. International Society and Federation of Cardiology: Working Group on Clasification of Calcium Antagonists for Cardiovascular Disease. *Am J Cardiol* 1987;60:630–632.
107. Goto K, Kasuya Y, Matsuki N, Takuwa Y, Kurihara H, Ishikawa T, Kimura S, Yanagisawa M, Masaki T. Endothelin activates the dihydropyridine-sensitive, voltage-dependent Ca^{2+} channel in vascular smooth muscle. *Proc Natl Acad Sci USA* 1989;86:3915–3918.
108. Godfraind T, Mennig D, Bravo G, Chalant C, Jaumin P. Inhibition by amlodipine of activity evoked in isolated human coronary arteries by endothelin, prostaglandin F_{2alpha} and depolarization. *Am J Cardiol* 1989;64:58I–64I.
109. Cauvin C, Tejerina M, Hwang O, Kai-Yamamaoto M, van Breemen C. The effects of Ca^{2+} antagonists on isolated rat and rabbit mesenteric resistance vessels. What determines the sensitivity of agonist-activated vessels to Ca^{2+} antagonists? *Ann N Y Acad Sci* 1988;522: 338–350.
110. Stern S, Tzivoni D. Early detection of silent ischaemic heart disease by 24-hour electrocardiographic monitoring of active subjects. *Br Heart J* 1974;36:481–486.
111. Schang SJ Jr, Pepine CJ. Transient asymptomatic S-T segment depression during daily activity. *Am J Cardiol* 1977;39:396–402.
112. Gage JE, Hess OM, Murakami T, Ritter M, Grimm J, Krayenbuehl HP. Vasoconstriction of stenotic coronary arteries during dynamic exercise in patients with classic angina pectoris: Reversibility by nitroglycerin. *Circulation* 1986;73:865–876.

113. Zeiher AM, Drexler H, Wollschlaeger H, Saurbier B, Just H. Coronary vasomotion in response to sympathetic stimulation in humans: Importance of the functional integrity of the endothelium. *J Am Coll Cardiol* 1989;14:1181–1190.
114. Picano E. Stress echocardiography. From pathophysiological toy to diagnostic tool. *Circulation* 1992;85:1604–1621.
115. Picano E, Lattanzi F. Dipyridamole echocardiography. A new diagnostic window on coronary artery disease. *Circulation* 1991;83(Suppl III):III-19–III-26.
116. Kaski JC, Crea F, Meran D, Rodriguez L, Araujo L, Chierchia S, Davies G, Maseri A. Local coronary supersensitivity to diverse vasoconstrictive stimuli in patients with variant angina. *Circulation* 1986; 74:1255–1265.
117. Yasue H, Horio Y, Nakamura N, Fujii H, Imoto N, Sonoda R, Kugiyama K, Obata K, Morikami Y, Kimura T. Induction of coronary artery spasm by acetylcholine in patients with variant angina: Possible role of the parasympathetic nervous system in the pathogenesis of coronary artery spasm. *Circulation* 1986;74:955–963.
118. El Tamimi H, Mansour M, Wargovich T, Hill J, Conti CR, Pepine CJ. Constrictor and dilator responses in adjacent segments of the same coronary artery to intracoronary acetylcholine in patients with coronary artery disease; the endothelial function revisited. *Circulation* 1994;89:45–51.
119. Bossaller C, Habib GB, Yamamoto H, Williams C, Wells S, Henry PD. Impaired muscarinic endothelium-dependent relaxation and cyclic guanosine 5′-monophosphate formation in atherosclerotic human coronary artery and rabbit aorta. *J Clin Invest* 1987;79: 170–174.
120. Kalsner S. Coronary artery reactivity in human vessels: Some questions and some answers. *Fed Proc* 1985;44:321–325.
121. Vigorito C, Poto S, Picotti GB, Triggiani M, Marone G. Effect of activation of the H_1 receptor on coronary hemodynamics in man. *Circulation* 1986;73:1175–1182.
122. Yang Z, Diederich D, Schneider K, Siebenmann R, Stulz P, Von SL, Turina M, Bühler FR, Lüscher TF. Endothelium-derived relaxing factor and protection against contractions induced by histamine and serotonin in the human internal mammary artery and in the saphenous vein. *Circulation* 1989;80:1041–1048.
123. Blankenhorn DH, Nessim SA, Johnson RL, Sanmarco ME, Azen SP, Cashin-Hemphill L. Beneficial effects of combined colestipol–niacin therapy on coronary atherosclerosis and coronary venous bypass grafts. *JAMA* 1987;257:3233–3240.
124. Brown G, Albers JJ, Fisher LD, Schaefer SM, Lin JT, Kaplan C, Zhao XQ, Bisson BD, Fitzpatrick VF, Dodge HT. Regression of coronary artery disease as a result of intensive lipid-lowering therapy in men with high levels of apolipoprotein B. *N Engl J Med* 1990;323: 1289–1298.
125. Ross R. The pathogenesis of atherosclerosis: A perspective for the 1990s. *Nature* 1993;362:801–809.
126. Lüscher TF, Espinosa E, Dubey RK, Yang Z. Vascular biology of human coronary and bypass graft disease. *Curr Opin Cardiol* 1993; 8:969–974.
127. Richardson PD, Davies MJ, Born GV. Influence of plaque configuration and stress distribution on fissuring of coronary atherosclerotic plaques. *Lancet* 1989;2:941–944.
128. Lendon CL, Davies MJ, Born GV, Richardson PD. Atherosclerotic plaque caps are locally weakened when macrophages density is increased. *Atherosclerosis* 1991;87:87–90.
129. Rutherford JD, Braunwald E. Chronic ischemic heart disease. In: Braunwald E, ed. *Heart Disease,* 4th ed. Philadelphia: WB Saunders; 1992:1292–1364.
130. Walling A, Waters DD, Miller D, et al. Long term prognosis of patients with variant angina. *Circulation* 1987;76:990–997.
131. Nakamura M, Takesshita A, Nose Y. Clinical characteristics associated with myocardial infarction, arrhythmias, and sudden death in patients with vasospastic angina. *Circulation* 1987;75:110–116.
132. Myerburg RJ, Kessler KM, Mallon SM, et al. Life threatening ventricular arrhythmias in patients with silent myocardial ischemia due to coronary artery spasm. *N Engl J Med* 1992;326:1451.
133. Schroeder JS, Lamb IH, Bristow MR, Ginsburg R, Hung J, McAuley BJ. Prevention of cardiovascular events in variant angina by long-term diltiazem therapy. *J Am Coll Cardiol* 1983;1:1507–1511.
134. Pepine CJ, Feldman RL, Hill JA, et al. Clinical outcome after treatment of rest angina with calcium blockers: Comparative experience during the initial year of therapy with diltiazem, nifedipine, and verapamil. *Am Heart J* 1983;106:1341–1347.
135. Flavahan NA, Shimokawa H, Vanhoutte PM. Pertussis toxin inhibits endothelium-dependent relaxations to certain agonists in porcine coronary arteries. *J Physiol* 1989;408:549–560.
136. Shimokawa H, Flavahan NA, Vanhoutte PM. Natural course of the impairment of endothelium-dependent relaxations after balloon endothelium removal in porcine coronary arteries. Possible dysfunction of a pertussis toxin-sensitive G protein. *Circ Res* 1989;65:740–753.
137. Shimokawa H, Flavahan NA, Shepherd JT, Vanhoutte PM. Endothelium-dependent inhibition of ergonovine-induced contraction is impaired in porcine coronary arteries with regenerated endothelium. *Circulation* 1989;80:643–650.
138. Kawachi Y, Tomoike H, Maruoka Y, Kikuchi Y, Araki H, Ishii Y, Tanaka K, Nakamura M. Selective hypercontraction caused by ergonovine in the canine coronary artery under conditions of induced atherosclerosis. *Circulation* 1984;69:441–450.
139. Forman MB, Oates JA, Robertson D, Robertson RM, Roberts LJD, Virmani R. Increased adventitial mast cells in a patient with coronary spasm. *N Engl J Med* 1985;313:1138–1141.
140. Kalsner S, Richard R. Coronary arteries of cardiac patients are hyperreactive and contain stores of amines: A mechanism for coronary spasm. *Science* 1984;223:1435–1437.
141. Zeiher AM, Drexler H, Saurbier B, Just H. Endothelium-mediated coronary blood flow modulation in humans. Effects of age, atherosclerosis, hypercholesterolemia, and hypertension. *J Clin Invest* 1993;92: 652–662.
142. McFadden EP, Clarke JG, Davies GJ, Kaski JC, Haider AW, Maseri A. Effect of intracoronary serotonin on coronary vessels in patients with stable angina and patients with variant angina. *N Engl J Med* 1991;324:648–654.
143. Freedman SB, Chierchia S, Rodriguez-Plaza L, Bugiardini R, Smith G, Maseri A. Ergonovine-induced myocardial ischemia: No role for serotonergic receptors? *Circulation* 1984;70:178–183.
144. Chierchia S, Davies G, Berkenboom G, Crea F, Crean P, Maseri A. Alpha-adrenergic receptors and coronary spasm: An elusive link. *Circulation* 1984;69:8–14.
145. Toyo-oka T, Aizawa T, Suzuki N, Hirata Y, Miyauchi T, Shin WS, Yanagisawa M, Masaki T, Sugimoto T. Increased plasma level of endothelin-1 and coronary spasm induction in patients with vasospastic angina pectoris. *Circulation* 1991;83:476–483.
146. Guthauser U, Flammer J, Mahler F. The relationship between digital and ocular vasospasm. *Graefes Arch Clin Exp Ophthalmol* 1988;226: 224–226.
147. Lerman A, Edwards BS, Hallett JW, Heublein DM, Sandberg SM, Burnett JJ. Circulating and tissue endothelin immunoreactivity in advanced atherosclerosis. *N Engl J Med* 1991;325:997–1001.
148. Winkles JA, Alberts GF, Brogi E, Libby P. Endothelin-1 and endothelin receptor mRNA expression in normal and atherosclerotic human arteries. *Biochem Biophys Res Commun* 1993;191:1081–1088.
149. Zeiher AM, Ihling C, Pistorius K, Schächinger V, Schaefer H-E. Increased tissue endothelin immunoreactivity in atherosclerotic lesions associated with acute coronary syndromes. *Lancet* 1994;344: 1405–1406.
150. Boulanger CM, Tanner FC, Bea ML, Hahn AW, Werner A, Lüscher TF. Oxidized low density lipoproteins induce mRNA expression and release of endothelin from human and porcine endothelium. *Circ Res* 1992;70:1191–1197.
151. Hahn AW, Resink TJ, Scott-Burden T, Powell J, Dohi Y, Bühler FR. Stimulation of endothelin mRNA and secretion in rat vascular smooth muscle cells: A novel autocrine function. *Cell Regul* 1990;1:649–659.
152. Zeiher AM, Ihling C, Pistorius K, Schächinger V, Schaefer H-E. Increased tissue endothelin immunoreactivity in atherosclerotic lesions associated with acute coronary syndromes. *Lancet* 1994;344: 1405–1408.
153. Rakugi H, Tabuchi Y, Nakamaru M, Nagano M, Higashimori K, Mikami H, Ogihara T, Suzuki N. Evidence for endothelin-1 release from resistance vessels of rats in response to hypoxia. *Biochem Biophys Res Commun* 1990;169:973–977.
154. Galle J, Bassenge E, Busse R. Oxidized low density lipoproteins potentiate vasoconstrictions to various agonists by direct interaction with vascular smooth muscle. *Circ Res* 1990;66:1287–1293.
155. Winniford MD, Filipchuk N, Hillis LD. Alpha-adrenergic blockade

for variant angina: A long-term, double-blind, randomized trial. *Circulation* 1983;67:1185–1188.
156. Vasalli A, Oh H. Mechanisms of flow-dependent vasodilation in the human coronary circulation in vivo. *Circulation [in press].*
157. Lambert CR, Pepine CJ. Angina pectoris: Variant Prinzmetal syndrome. In: Willis Hurst J, ed. *Current Therapy in Cardiovascular Disease,* 4th ed. St. Louis: Mosby Year Book; 1994:157–160.
158. Lüscher TF. Do we need endothelin antagonists? *Cardiovasc Res* 1993;27:2089–2093.
159. Yusuf S, Held P, Furberg C. Update of effects of calcium antagonists in myocardial infarction or angina in light of the second Danish Verapamil Infarction Trial (DAVIT-II) and other recent studies. *Am J Cardiol* 1991;67:1295–1297.
160. Taylor SH. Therapeutic targets in ischaemic heart disease. *Drugs* 1992;43:1–8.
161. Lewis HD Jr, Davis JW, Archibald DG, Steinke WE, Smitherman TC, Doherty JEd, Schnaper HW, Le Winter MM, Linares E, Pouget JM, Sabharwal SC, Chesler E, De Mots H. Protective effects of aspirin against acute myocardial infarction and death in men with unstable angina. Results of a Veterans Administration Cooperative Study. *N Engl J Med* 1983;309:396–403.
162. Cairns JA, Gent M, Singer J, Finnie KJ, Froggatt GM, Holder DA, Jablonsky G, Kostuk WJ, Melendez LJ, Myers MG, et al. Aspirin, sulfinpyrazone, or both in unstable angina. Results of a Canadian multicenter trial. *N Engl J Med* 1985;313:1369–1375.
163. Group TR. Risk of myocardial infarction and death during treatment with low dose aspirin and intravenous heparin in men with unstable coronary artery disease. *Lancet* 1990;336:827–830.
164. Theroux P, Ouimet H, McCans J, Latour JG, Joly P, Levy G, Pelletier E, Juneau M, Stasiak J, de Guise P, et al. Aspirin, heparin, or both to treat acute unstable angina. *N Engl J Med* 1988;319:1105–1111.
165. Resnekov L, Chediak J, Hirsh J, Lewis HD Jr. Antithrombotic agents in coronary artery disease. *Chest* 1989;95:52S–72S.
166. Henry PD, Bentley KI. Suppression of atherogenesis in cholesterol-fed rabbit treated with nifedipine. *J Clin Invest* 1981;68:1366–1369.
167. Loaldi A, Polese A, Montorsi P, De Cesare N, Fabbiocchi F, Ravagnani P, Guazzi MD. Comparison of nifedipine, propranolol and isosorbide dinitrate on angiographic progression and regression of coronary arterial narrowings in angina pectoris. *Am J Cardiol* 1989;64: 433–439.
168. Lichtlen PR, Hugenholtz PG, Rafflenbeul W, Hecker H, Jost S, Deckers JW. Retardation of angiographic progression of coronary artery disease by nifedipine. Results of the International Nifedipine Trial on Antiatherosclerotic Therapy (INTACT). INTACT Group Investigators. *Lancet* 1990;335:1109–1113.
169. Chobanian AV, Haudenschild CC, Nickerson C, Hope S. Trandolapril inhibits atherosclerosis in the Watanabe heritable hyperlipidemic rabbit. *Hypertension* 1992;20:473–477.
170. Mishra SK, Hermsmeyer K. Selective inhibition of T-type Ca^{2+} channels by Ro 40-5967. *Circ Res* 1994;75:144–148.
171. Rosenthal SJ, Ginsburg R, Lamb IH, Baim DS, Schroeder JS. Efficacy of diltiazem for control of symptoms of coronary artery spasm. *Am J Cardiol* 1980:46:1027–1032.
172. Pepine CJ, Feldman RL, Whittle J, Curry RC, Conti CR. Effect of diltiazem in patients with variant angina: A randomized double-blind trial. *Am Heart J* 1981;101:719–725.
173. Johnson SM, Maurtison DR, Willerson JT, Hillis LD. A controlled trial of verapamil for Prinzmetals' variant angina. *N Engl J Med* 1980; 304:862–866.
174. Ginsburg R, Lamb IH, Schroeder JS, Hu M, Harrison DC. Randomized double-blind comparison of nifedipine and isosorbide dinitrate therapy in variant angina pectoris due to coronary artery spasm. *Am Heart J* 1982;103:44–48.
175. Parodi O, Maseri A, Simonetti I. Management of unstable angina at rest by verapamil: A double-blind crossover study in coronary care unit. *Br Heart J* 1979;41:167–174.
176. Chimienti M, Negroni MS, Pussineri E, et al. Once daily felodipine in preventing ergonovine-induced myocardial ischaemia in Prinzmetal's variant angina. *Eur Heart J* 1994;15:389–393.
177. Kishida H, Kato K, Toyama S, Ikeda M, Yamaga T, Suzuki K. Clinical effects of nitrendipine on variant angina pectoris. *Jpn Heart J* 1991; 32:297–305.
178. Sorkin EM, Clissold SP. Nicardipine. A review of its pharmacodynamic and pharmacokinetic properties, and therapeutic efficacy, in the treatment of angina pectoris, hypertension and related cardiovascular disorders. *Drugs* 1987;33:296–345.
179. McGibney D. The efficacy of amlodipine in the management of ischaemic heart disease. *Postgrad Med J* 1991;67(Suppl 3):S24–S28.
180. Turitto G, Pezella A, Prati PL. Diltiazem in spontaneous angina: Comparison with nifedipine and verapamil. *G Ital Cardiol* 1985;15: 1079–1084.
181. Prida XE, Gelman JS, Feldman RL, Hill JA, Pepine CJ, Scott E. Comparison of diltiazem and nifedipine alone in combination in patient with coronary artery spasm. *J Am Coll Cardiol* 1987;9:412–419.
182. L'Abbate A, Parodi O, Salerno JA, et al. Comparison of calcium antagonists as therapy for rest angina. *Cardiol Board Rev* 1989;6: 50–54.
183. The Multicenter Diltiazem Postinfarction Trial Research Group. The effect of diltiazem on mortality and reinfarction after myocardial infarction. *N Engl J Med* 1988;319:385–392.
184. The Danish Verapamil Infarction Trial II—DAVIT II. Effect of verapamil on mortality and major events after acute myocardial infarction. *Am J Cardiol* 1990;66:779–785.
185. Brunton TL. On the use of nitrite of amyl in angina pectoris. *Lancet* 1867;2:97–98.
186. Feelisch M, Noack EA. Correlation between nitric oxide formation during degradation of organic nitrates and activation of guanylate cyclase. *Eur J Pharmacol* 1987;139:19–30.
187. Busse R, Pohl U, Mulsch A, Bassenge E. Modulation of the vasodilator action of SIN-1 by the endothelium. *J Cardiovasc Pharmacol* 1989;14(Suppl 11):S81–S85.
188. Lüscher TF, Richard V, Yang ZH. Interaction between endothelium-derived nitric oxide and SIN-1 in human and porcine blood vessels. *J Cardiovasc Pharmacol* 1989;14(Suppl 11):S76–S80.
189. Abrams J. Clinical aspects of nitrate tolerance. *Eur Heart J* 1991; 12(Suppl E):42–52.
190. Rudolf W, Dirschinger J. Clinical comparison of nitrates and sydnonimines. *Eur Heart J* 1991;12(Suppl E):33–41.
191. Haynes WG, Webb DJ. Contribution of endogenous generation of endothelin-1 to basal vascular tone. *Lancet* 1994;344:852–854.
192. Brown MJ. Angiotensin receptor blockers in essential hypertension. *Lancet* 1993;342:1374–1375.
193. Brunner HR, Nussberger J, Burnier M, Waeber B. Angiotensin II antagonists. *Clin Exp Hypertens* 1993;15:1221–1238.
195. Theroux P, Ouimet H, McCans J, et al. Aspirin, heparin or both to treat acute unstable angina. *N Engl J Med* 1988;319:1105–1111.
196. Schameoth L. The clinical use of intravenous verapamil. *Am Heart J* 1980;100(6 pt 2):1070–1075.
197. Joyal M, Feldman RL, Cremer K, Pieper J, Hill JAA, Pepine CJ. Systemic and coronary hemodynamic effects of combined intravenous diltiazem and nitroglycerin administration. *Am Heart J* 1987;113: 1376–1382.
198. Ogawa H, Yasue H, Oshima S, et al. Circadian variant of plasma fibrinopeptide A level in patients with variant angina. *Circulation* 1989;80:1617–1626.
199. Waters DD, Muller D, Bruchard A, et al. Circadian variation in variant angina. *Am J Cardiol* 1984;54:61–64.
200. Katsumoto K, Nibori T. Prevention of coronary spasm during aorto-coronary (A–C) bypass surgery for variant angina and effort angina with ST elevation. *J Cardiovas Surg* 1988;29:343–348.
201. Kitamura S, Morita R, Kawachi K, et al. Different responses of coronary artery and interval mammary artery bypass grafts to ergonovine and nitroglycerin in variant angina. *Ann Thorac Surg* 1989;47: 756–760.
202. Corcos T, David PR, Bourassa MG, et al. Percutaneous transluminal coronary angioplasty for the treatment of variant angina. *J Am Coll Cardiol* 1985;5:1046–1054.
203. Bertrand ME, LaBlanche JM, et al. Comparative results of percutaneous transluminal coronary angioplasty in patients with dynamic versus fixed coronary stenosis. *J Am Coll Cardiol* 1986;8:504–508.
204. Curry RC Jr, Pepine CJ, Conti CR. Ambulatory monitoring to evaluate therapy in variant angina pectoris. *Circulation* 1979;60(Suppl III):II-90.
205. Lüscher TF, Oemar BS, Boulanger CM, Hahn AW. Molecular and cellular biology of endothelin and its receptors—Part I. *J Hypertens* 1993;11:7–11.

Atherosclerosis and Coronary Artery Disease,
edited by V. Fuster, R. Ross, and E. J. Topol.
Lippincott-Raven Publishers, Philadelphia © 1996.

CHAPTER 38

Differences Between Atherosclerosis and Restenosis

Erling Falk and Masakiyo Nobuyoshi

Key Words: Atherosclerosis; Restenosis; Remodeling; Proliferation; Neointima; Thrombosis; Coronary intervention; Percutaneous transluminal coronary angioplasty; Risk factors.

INTRODUCTION

Arteriosclerosis, literally ''arterial hardening,'' includes three pathogenetically different arterial diseases: atherosclerosis, Mönckeberg's medial sclerosis, and arteriolosclerosis. The term atherosclerosis was introduced by the German pathologist Marchand in 1904 for that particular type of arterial hardening characterized by intimal plaques composed of both a soft (Greek *athere,* gruel) and a hard (Greek *skleros,* hard) component (1). Like cardiac transplant-associated coronary artery disease (2), postinterventional restenosis may be included in the broad term arteriosclerosis, but the question is whether restenosis qualifies also for the term atherosclerosis, just representing an accelerated form of that disease (3). Let us first look at the characteristic features of atherosclerosis and restenosis, and thereafter try to answer the question.

Erling Falk: DHF Cardiovascular Pathology Unit, Skejby University Hospital, 8200 Aarhus N, Denmark.
Masakiyo Nobuyoshi: Department of Cardiology, Kokura Memorial Hospital, Kitakyushu 802, Japan.

ATHEROSCLEROSIS

Atherogenesis

Only four cell types play a role in atherogenesis: endothelial cells, monocyte-derived macrophages, smooth muscle cells (SMCs), and lymphocytes (4). Activated endothelium and monocytes/macrophages constitute the very early and persisting lipid-related *inflammatory component* of atherosclerosis (5–7), but a SMC-related *proliferative component* evolves simultaneously or subsequently (4,8) and a *thrombotic component* may later be added (9,10).

In lesion-prone areas, frequently characterized by preexisting adaptive intimal thickening and probably related to local hemodynamic factors (low and/or oscillating shear forces) (11), increased endothelial permeability leads to increased influx of plasma constituents into the intima, including enhanced transcytosis of low-density lipoproteins (LDL) (12). Blood monocytes stick to activated endothelium via adhesion molecules (6,13,14), pass between endothelial cells, and enter the intima, where they differentiate into macrophages which endocytose the retained LDL, probably via the scavenger receptor after oxidative modification (5), giving rise to the ''hallmark cell'' in atherogenesis: the lipid-filled foam cell. Focal collections of such foam cells may be seen macroscopically as yellow fatty dots or streaks barely raised above the intimal surface. A few T-lymphocytes may also be present early during lesion formation (7). Endothelial cells, adhering platelets, macrophages, lymphocytes, and intimal SMCs interact through cytokines and growth factors which control SMC proliferation, migration, and extracellular matrix synthesis, eventually leading to an elevated and mature atherosclerotic plaque: the advanced fibrolipid plaque (4,15). The endothelium is intact but activated and dysfunctioning during the early phase of atherogenesis. Later it may be lost focally, frequently related to superficial macrophage foam-cell infiltration (15), and platelets may adhere to the denuded surface (15,16). Incorporation of microthrombi and thrombus-related factors [e.g., platelet-derived growth factors, fibrin(ogen) and its degradation products, and thrombin] may now contribute to the progressive growth of the lesion (4,9,17–20). Eventually, a soft and vulnerable atheromatous plaque may evolve, it may rupture, and a complicating thrombus may occlude the lumen (21,22).

Plaque Composition: Atherosis and Sclerosis

Typically, mature atherosclerotic plaques are composed of *soft,* lipid/macrophage-related atheromatous gruel and *hard,* SMC-related sclerotic tissue (Fig. 1; see Colorplate 30). Calcification or ossification may occur in both components (23). Atherosclerosis is from its initiation a multifocal disease process, but the coronary arteries are generally ''diffusely'' involved with confluent plaquing in patients with ischemic heart disease (24). The composition of individual plaques varies greatly without any obvious relation to clinical risk factors or clinical presentation, except that a significant atheromatous component is usually present in culprit lesions responsible for acute coronary syndromes (10,15). The most voluminous plaque component is the SMC-related sclerotic one (25–28), and it may, of course, give rise to chronic angina pectoris, but it is otherwise relatively innocuous. On the contrary, the soft lipid/macrophage-related atheromatous plaque component is dangerous, because it makes plaques vulnerable to rupture with superimposed thrombosis, a process that is responsible for the great majority of acute ischemic syndromes (9).

Atherosis: Macrophage-Related?

Plaque lipid is predominantly blood-derived, located intracellularly within foam cells (mainly cholesteryl esters) or extracellularly (mainly free cholesterol and its esters) (29,30). The former prevails in early lesions (fatty streaks), while the latter accumulates later and constitutes the main lipid component of the advanced fibrolipid plaque. The macrophage foam cells in early lesions are located superficially in the plaque, while extracellular lipid predominantly is retained and begins to accumulate at the plaque base (31). Very little specific is known about the relation between lipid-filled foam cells, extracellular lipids, and the SMC-related sclerotic plaque component, but macrophages are probably critical for plaque softening, leading to formation of a soft atheromatous cavity or core within the plaque (12,15,29). The atheromatous gruel has a consistency like toothpaste at room temperature postmortem and it is even softer at body temperature in vivo (30). The atheromatous core is rich in extracellular lipid, and it is avascular and nearly acellular except for its periphery, where lipid-filled foam cells are frequently found. The extracellular plaque lipid may accumulate via different pathways; it may be trapped by matrix binding and then be deposited directly within the extracellular space, or extracellular accumulation may follow cellular uptake, foam cell formation, and cell death (due to cytotoxic oxidized LDL?) with subsequent extracellular release of foam cell lipids. The latter macrophage-related pathway is widely believed to play the main role in the atheromatous process, eventually leading to the formation of a soft, lipid-rich atheromatous core, also called plaque necrosis, atheronecrosis, or necrotic core formation (12,15,29,32).

Atherosis: The Dangerous Component

The lipid/macrophage-related atheromatous plaque component, though frequently small, is most dangerous because it softens plaques, making them vulnerable to rupture with subsequent thrombus formation, a life-threatening event. There is no obvious relation between plaque size, stenosis severity, and plaque composition (vulnerability to rupture) (22). Nevertheless, nonstenotic vulnerable plaques are more dangerous than stenotic ones, because myocardial infarction is usually the result of sudden occlusion of the former (9,33) while stenotic lesions promote collateral development and therefore are protected and frequently occlude silently (34). A vulnerable fibrolipid plaque consists of an atheromatous core separated from the vascular lumen by a cap of fibrous tissue which may be infiltrated with macrophage foam cells. The size and consistency of the atheromatous core and the thickness and strength of the fibrous cap and its cellular contents, particularly the presence of activated macrophages indicating ongoing inflammation, are probably major determinants of a plaque's vulnerability to rupture (35–43).

Plaque rupture occurs most frequently where the cap is thinnest and most heavily macrophage infiltrated and therefore probably weakest, namely at the cap's shoulders (22). But the shoulder regions are not only weak points, they are also points where the circumferential tensile stress usually is maximal during systole (44–46). Coronary plaques are constantly under the influence of various biomechanical and hemodynamic stresses (47–50). Therefore, the propensity for plaque rupture is a function of both internal plaque changes (vulnerability) and external stresses (triggers) (51). As the presence of a vulnerable plaque is a prerequisite for plaque rupture, vulnerability is probably more important than triggers in determining the risk of a future heart attack. If no vulnerable plaques are present in the coronary arteries, there is no rupture-prone substrate for a potential trigger to work on.

Plaque Progression and Remodeling

It takes many years to develop a mature atherosclerotic plaque in native coronary arteries by lipid accumulation, macrophage infiltration, and SMC proliferation and matrix synthesis. Then, however, further progression may occur rapidly due to complicating thrombosis. During early plaque growth, compensatory dilatation prevents luminal narrowing (52–55). With disease progression, confluent plaquing may cause diffuse narrowing and advanced plaques may give rise to localized stenoses and, rarely, aneurysmal dilatations. Because of compensatory dilatation and confluent plaquing, angiography will always underestimate the severity of vessel wall disease, and new high-grade lesions often develop in arterial segments that appeared normal at previous angiographic examination (33,56). This unpredictable and nonlinear (episodic) progression can be explained by plaque rupture with subsequent hemorrhage into the plaque and/or mural thrombosis leading to stepwise plaque growth (57,58), also explaining why plaque irregularity (plaque composition) rather than stenosis severity (plaque volume) determine progression to infarct-related occlusion (59). Serial coronary angiographic examination of 239 patients demonstrated that patients with myocardial infarction often showed a "jump-up" phenomenon in which a minimal coronary stenosis progressed to total occlusion (33). The study also suggested that coronary spasticity, evaluated by a concomitant ergonovine provocation test, could play a significant role in plaque progression (33), which, however, was not confirmed in a smaller study on Prinzmetal's variant angina pectoris (60). The pathoanatomic substrate for vasospasm is unknown but could be related to endothelial dysfunction (61), mural thrombosis (62), plaque hemorrhages (63), and/or inflammatory changes (64). Importantly, plaque progression documented by serial angiography is a powerful predictor of subsequent clinical events such as cardiac death, myocardial infarction, and need for revascularization (65).

Plaque progression due to SMC proliferation and matrix synthesis is probably episodic with periods of slow indolent growth punctuated by brief episodes of greater proliferative activity causing accelerated growth (66), like the proliferative healing response after angioplasty where severe renarrowing may evolve over a few months. Such an accelerated SMC-related plaque progression has been suggested to underlie primary unstable angina in patients without major luminal thrombosis (67). A SMC-rich plaque component, histologically indistinguishable from postangioplasty neointima, is reportedly present in nearly half of primary lesions debulked by coronary atherectomy (58,68–71) and is also found in plaques from clinically stable patients and may be related to young age of lesions or patients (58,71–73). The proliferative activity within such plaques is usually very low despite high cellularity and irrespective of clinical presentation, as evaluated by immunohistochemistry for proliferating cell nuclear antigen (PCNA) (66,74–76). No evidence of cell replication was found in 82% of 118 primary coronary atherectomy specimens, and only a modest number of PCNA-positive cells (usually less than 1%) were found in the majority of the remaining specimens, although nearly half of the patients had unstable angina pectoris (75). However, a smaller study using the same technique to gauge cell proliferation within plaques found 4% PCNA-positive cells (77). Of note, not only SMCs but also macrophages and endothelial cells may replicate within atherosclerotic plaques (66,75).

Complicating Thrombosis

Autopsy data indicate that plaque rupture occurs frequently during plaque growth (15,22). It is probably the most significant mechanism underlying rapid progression of coronary lesions. Importantly, rupture with nonocclusive rapid progression is clinically silent in the majority of cases. A person will experience new or changing symptoms only if a major luminal thrombus evolves at the rupture site causing flow obstruction. About three-fourths of thrombi responsible for acute ischemic syndromes are precipitated by plaque rupture, exposing the very thrombogenic atheromatous gruel to the flowing blood (10,78). Minor and only superficial injury [endothelial denudation due to ongoing inflammation? (15)] but no frank rupture, i.e., no deep injury, are found beneath the rest of the thrombi, usually in combination with a severe atherosclerotic stenosis (21).

Risk Factors

Male sex, aging, dyslipoproteinemia, arterial hypertension, and diabetes mellitus accelerate the atherosclerotic process, without any obvious differences in plaque composition related to specific risk factors other than calcification [and sclerosis? (27)] increases with age (23). Of note, the soft, lipid-rich atheromatous component is not particularly prominent in plaques from patients with hypercholesterolemia (27,79). Cigarette smoking is in particular related to the rupture/thrombus-dependent rapid plaque progression responsible for acute myocardial infarction (80) and to spasm (81).

Endothelial dysfunction, even in plaque-free arterial segments, correlates with the presence of most if not all of the well-known risk factors for ischemic heart disease (82,83), and, importantly, lowering of a raised serum cholesterol may restore normal endothelial-dependent vasodilatation (84,85). Therefore, intact but dysfunctioning (activated) endothelium may play an important role in the initiation and progression of atherosclerosis.

RESTENOSIS

Since the introduction of percutaneous transluminal coronary angioplasty (PTCA) in the late 1970s, renarrowing after successful dilatation has plagued this and other coronary interventional procedures developed to enlarge a narrowed lumen. Despite intensive research and many clinical trials, the restenosis rate is still very high (30–50%) (86,87), except after stenting (88,89).

Angioplasty-Induced Injury

Successful enlargement of a stenotic lumen will, irrespective of procedure used, cause deep vessel wall injury and extensive deendothelialization. Lumen enlargement may be accomplished by plaque reduction (debulking effect) and/or vessel expansion (balloon effect) with splitting of the plaque at its thinnest (weakest) point separating the plaque from underlying media (dissection), accompanied by stretching of media and adventitia beneath the detached plaque and of the more distensible plaque-free wall segment, if present (32,90–94). While the interior of plaques is exposed by debulking procedures, this is not always the case with balloon dilatation. For example, dilatation of eccentric plaques usually splits them at their edges, often leaving the plaque itself intact, unless it was already disrupted spontaneously before dilatation (95). In the latter situation, dilatation tends to widen the preexisting spontaneous rupture further, exposing more of the thrombogenic gruel but often without causing deeper or additional tearing of the plaque or wall (95). Therefore, spontaneous plaque rupture, balloon-induced vessel wall splitting (with or without plaque rupture), and debulking procedures may expose quite different surfaces, some of which may be very thrombogenic, while others may be more SMC-reactive.

Response to Injury

Neointima formation (intimal hyperplasia) after angioplasty should not be equated with restenosis. Successful angioplasty is always followed by a healing response which needs to be exuberant to be held responsible for restenosis. Restenosis may have other causes (see below), but because injury-induced neointima formation usually is considered to play the main role, its pathogenesis will be considered first. Evaluated by postmortem examination of 34 lesions dilated several hours to 4 years before death in 20 patients (35% underwent emergency angioplasty for refractory angina), the healing response after coronary angioplasty evolves in the following way (96).

Acute Thrombosis

Acute thrombosis was present in one of three lesions examined within 10 days (96). No new tissue (neointima) was seen. Angioscopically, thrombus is frequently found at the angioplasty site early after intervention (97).

Neointima Formation

In 20 lesions examined 10 days to 6 months after PTCA, thrombus and new tissue (neointima) were identified in 6 and 18 lesions, respectively (96). The incidence of thrombus after 1 month was extremely low. The hypercellular neointima consisted of SMCs, predominantly stellate-shaped with large oval nuclei and abundant cytoplasm (synthetic phenotype), surrounded by an abundant loose, proteoglycan-rich (myxoid-like) stroma.

Garratt et al. analyzed tissue obtained from restenotic lesions by directional atherectomy, and they found, besides old plaque tissue, new loose, fibroproliferative SMC-rich tissue and only rarely thrombus (98). Immunostaining for leukocyte common antigen identified only a few inflammatory cells and they tended to be localized in dense, ''necrotic'' areas that appeared to represent the primary atheromatous plaque rather than the postinterventional healing process (69). Lipid-filled foam cells and extracellular lipid deposits (apolipoproteins or cholesterol crystals) are not found in the newly formed tissue within the critical timespan for the development of restenosis, i.e., within the first 3–6 months after angioplasty (99). However, foam cells and extracellular lipid accumulation have been described already 3 and 6 months, respectively, after stenting of coronary vein grafts (100).

Neointima Maturation

Neointimal tissue was found in all eight lesions examined 6 months to 2 years after PTCA (96). With time, the SMCs became more spindle-shaped with elongated nuclei and less cytoplasmlike medial SMCs (contractile phenotype), and the surrounding connective tissue matrix became more collagen-rich, condensed, and appeared less voluminous (Fig. 2; see Colorplate 31).

In three lesions examined after 2 years, angioplasty-related changes were hardly identifiable and the lesions were almost indistinguishable from conventional atherosclerotic plaque (96). With healing, the fibrocellular reparative tissue becomes less cellular and more collagen-rich and dense (fibrotic) (101), but it may still be clearly identified, distinct from preexisting atherosclerotic plaque, even years after angioplasty (92).

Origin of Neointimal SMCs

Microscopic examination of serial step sections cut at close intervals through eight angioplasty sites revealed that the exposed tunica media was the most likely source of the reparative SMCs responsible for healing (102). Medial SMCs seemed to spread to the intima through the disrupted internal elastic membrane, most frequently through breaks in the plaque-free or less-disease wall segment, and extending proximal and distal into adjacent nondisrupted portions of the dilated vessel. Gravanis and Roubin also noticed a more pronounced SMC response over plaque-free wall segments than over plaques themselves (91). The abundant medial SMCs in plaque-free wall segments are probably much more reactive with greater growth potential than the senescent and much fewer SMCs within old plaque tissue (103,104).

Endothelium

Only very sparse human data exist on the state of the endothelium after angioplasty. Atherectomized tissues usually lack endothelial covering (105–107), probably because the procedure used for tissue retrieval destroys the delicate endothelium, if present [many advanced coronary lesions are only incompletely covered by endothelium (15,16)]. Gravanis and Roubin evaluated autopsy specimens after endothelial labeling with antihuman factor VIII-related antigen and Ulex Europeus Agglutinin I, and they concluded that complete restoration of the endothelial lining after angioplasty takes at least 1 month (91). Ueda et al. also studied autopsy specimens after immunostaining for factor VIII-related antigen (101). They identified no endothelium on two lesions studied 20 days after angioplasty, only incomplete reendothelialization on one 5-month-old lesion, and a continuous endothelial covering over two lesions studied 1½ years after angioplasty. One coronary stent was reportedly completely endothelialized without thrombosis when examined 21 days after implantation (108), while incomplete endothelial lining and abnormal platelet/leukocyte adherence were observed as late as 10 months after stenting of saphenous vein bypass grafts (100). Thus, complete endothelial regeneration after angioplasty may take months, and the state of the endothelium could be critical in reversing the SMC phenotype back to the quiescent contractile state. Evaluated angiographically, endothelium-dependent vasodilation may be impaired [or vasoconstriction enhanced (109)] for months *after* angioplasty, but its relation to restenosis is not clear (110–112). The presence of abnormal endothelial-dependent vasomotion *before* angioplasty may, however, identify subgroups of patients at high risk for restenosis (110,113).

Injury–Response Relationship

After arterial injury, an acute thrombotic response is always followed by an SMC-related healing response. Though temporally related, these two phenomena are not necessarily pathogenetically related.

Thrombotic Versus SMC Response

Although the notion is not universally accepted (114), the lipid-rich atheromatous gruel appears to be the most thrombogenic component of advanced atherosclerotic lesions (78,115). Our data indicate that the atheromatous gruel is much more thrombogenic than both the collagen-rich sclerotic plaque component and the SMC-rich tunica media (78,115). The gruel is, however, nearly totally devoid of SMCs and therefore has very little reparative potential, contrary to tunica media, where SMCs are abundantly present. Accordingly, the reactive SMC response after angioplasty seems to evolve much more rapidly and become more extensive where tunica media rather than plaque tissue has been exposed (91,102,116). Depending on plaque composition and procedure used to enlarge the lumen, vessel wall components of differing thrombogenicity and reactivity may be exposed during interventions, explaining why abrupt closure (thrombus-dependent) and late restenosis (SMC-dependent) have different risk profiles, and why they may not necessarily be related (117).

Depth of Injury and SMC Response

In the study referred to above (96), angioplasty-induced intimal, medial, and adventitial tears were identified in 30 of the 34 lesions (88%), and the depth of injury correlated with the healing response; more neointima formation was found in lesions with medial or adventitial tears (deep injury) than in lesions with no or only intimal tears (superficial injury). The existence of a direct injury–response relationship is supported by angiographic follow-up studies after coronary interventional procedures showing that the acute gain in lumen diameter (injury-related) correlates with the subsequent late loss (neointima-related), expressed as "the more you gain, the more you lose" (118). The amount of late loss constitutes, however, only a fraction of the acute gain (approximately 0.4, called the "loss index"), suggesting that "the bigger is the better" irrespective of procedure used to enlarge the lumen (119). Directional coronary atherectomy with deep wall excision, i.e., deep injury but probably also associated with better acute gain, was first reported to increase (120) and then to decrease (118,121,122) the risk of subsequent restenosis.

Experimentally, the depth (123) and length (124,125) of vessel wall injury correlate with the subsequent proliferative healing response in the oversized balloon or stented pig coronary models. The extent of endothelial denudation and the rapidity of subsequent endothelial regeneration could, however, be more important for healing than the depth of injury produced (126–128). In the pig carotid model, extensive deendothelialization with a soft balloon caused as much neointima formation as did angioplasty-induced deep medial injury (127). Similar results have been obtained in rabbit and rat models of arterial injury, where gentle endothelial denudation led to significant neointima formation, which was not observed after even extensive medial injury if the endothelium survived the procedure (126,128). Of notice, the endothelium may easily be scraped or rubbed off during interventional procedures, but it resists dilatation/stretch very well, contrary to medial smooth muscle cells, which are very sensitive to dilatation/stretch (126).

Quiescence After Injury

Eventually the healing process terminates spontaneously, and the reason for that is not entirely clear. SMCs continue to replicate within neointima for weeks after experimental balloon injury (129–132), preferentially along the luminal border (130,131), suggesting that the proliferative activity is driven by blood components or controlled by cells at the blood–neointima interface. Injured or regenerating endothelial cells may stimulate SMC proliferation, while intact confluent and quiescent endothelium has the opposite effect (107). The presence and state of the endothelium could be critical in controlling proliferative stimuli, while the extracellular matrix could regulate cell responsiveness, eventually reverting the SMCs back to the quiescent contractile state. Activated SMCs become suppressed by the matrix they secrete (133), but a quiescent state is apparently not reached before the cells are surrounded by a large and rather predictable amount of extracellular matrix (fourfold more matrix than cells) (130,134). Therefore, the ultimate neointimal mass may be given already by the magnitude of the proliferative response. Of notice, the reparative process stops early and never becomes exuberant in the balloon-damaged but not disrupted tunica media with its preserved extracellular matrix (135), while proliferative and synthetic activities may continue for weeks in the adjacent immature neointima.

Restenosis: A Time-Related Phenomenon

Postinterventional restenosis is a time-dependent and self-limited vascular response with delayed onset, evolving predominantly between 1 and 3 months after the procedure (86,136–139). Serial coronary angiography performed in 229 patients on day 1 and at 1, 3, 6, and 12 months after successful balloon angioplasty revealed the following restenosis rates: 13% at 1 month, 43% at 3 months, 49% at 6 months, and 53% at 1 year (Fig. 3A) (86). Obviously, restenosis most commonly develops between the first and third month postangioplasty. During the first month, lesion regression (thrombus resolution and/or favorable remodeling?) was in fact more prevalent than lesion progression (renarrowing), but the latter was highly predictive of late restenosis (86). Renarrowing already at day 1 (recoil and/or thrombus) and late restenosis did not correlate well, contrary to the result of a recent study (140). A long-term serial follow-up study revealed that 4%, 0.8%, and 0% of the studied patients developed restenosis 3–12 months, 1–3 years, and 3–5 years, respectively, after the intervention (139). Serruys et al. studied 342 patients by quantitative coronary angiography performed at a single predetermined follow-up time of 1, 2, 3, or 4 months (136) (Fig. 3B). The most substantial change in lumen diameter occurred between the second and third months. After 6 months without restenosis, later follow-up rarely reveals restenosis (138,139,141,142) and many lesions apparently regress, leading to a bigger lumen (141).

A similar time relation has been found for restenosis after successful directional coronary atherectomy (143), direct angioplasty for acute myocardial infarction (144), and stenting (145,146). In the last situation, the progressive loss in lumen diameter starts, however, already during the first month and continues, although at a lower pace, beyond 3 months, reaching a stable and quiescent state around 6 months after stent implantation (145,146).

To summarize, the restenosis process (a) peaks between 1 and 3 months after the procedure, (b) becomes quiescent after 3–6 months, and (c) stabilizes or regresses beyond 6 months after intervention. Any theory trying to explain the mechanisms underlying restenosis should conform to this time table.

Restenosis: Causes

Two different phenomena contribute to luminal narrowing and restenosis after angioplasty:

Remodeling: (a) early recoil, (b) vasoconstriction or impaired vasodilation, and (c) late contraction or failed compensatory enlargement.

New mass: (a) thrombosis, which may become organized, and (b) neointima formation, caused by SMC proliferation and matrix synthesis.

Acute thrombosis, elastic recoil, dissection, intimal flaps, vasospasm, and incomplete stent expansion are the key players in abrupt closure and early recurrent stenosis after otherwise successful lumen enlargement (117,140,147–152). In late restenosis, neointima formation (intimal hyperplasia) is usually considered to play the main role. Indeed, neointima formation appears to be the far most important mechanism of in-stent restenosis after Palmaz–Schatz stenting (153),

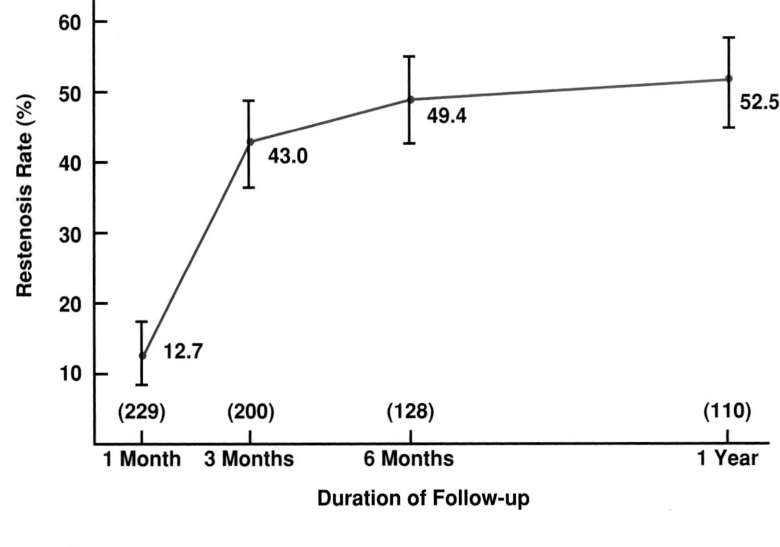

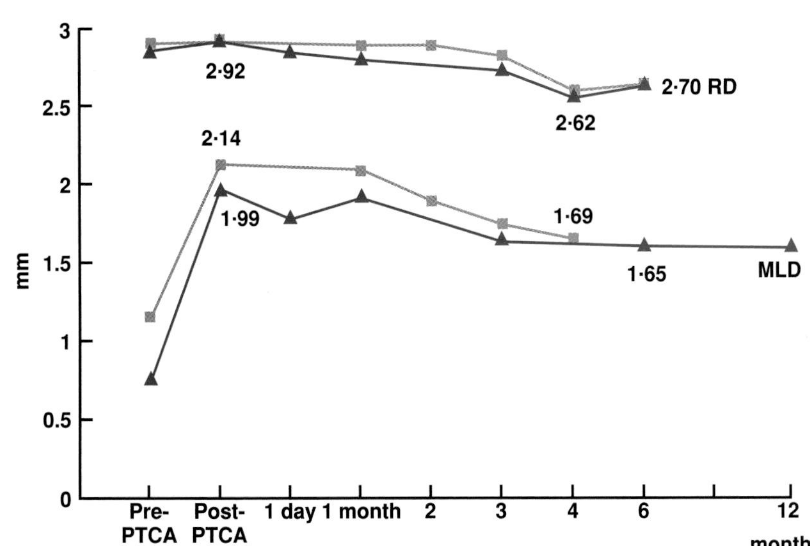

FIG. 3. A: The restenosis rate after successful percutaneous transluminal coronary angioplasty (PTCA), determined by serial angiographic follow-up of 229 patients at 1, 3, 6, and 12 months after the procedure (86). These data suggest that restenosis most commonly develops between the first and third months post-PTCA. (From Nobuyoshi et al., ref. 86, with permission). **B:** Virtually identical time-related loss in minimal luminal diameter (MLD) after PTCA has been reported in two different angiographic follow-up studies; ▲, Nobuyoshi et al., ref. 86; and ■, Serruys et al., ref. 136. RD, Reference diameter. (Adapted from Serruys et al., ref. 246.)

but preliminary human data derived from serial quantitative intracoronary ultrasound measurements suggest that late restenosis after angioplasty may be mediated not only by addition of new tissue (neointima formation), but also by vascular remodeling, i.e., redistribution of existing tissue (154–157). Recent experimental data indicate that unfavorable remodeling, probably related to scar contraction and impaired endothelial function, may be even more important in restenosis than neointima formation (158–162).

Acute Thrombus

Neointima formation after angioplasty is probably platelet-dependent but not necessarily dependent on the mass of thrombus present early after the procedure (117). Thrombus formation after arterial injury peaks very early, after which the thrombus usually is lysed and disappears. Persisting thrombi may, however, provide a provisional matrix for the subsequent proliferative healing response, becoming organized and incorporated into the vessel wall. Because organization usually is associated with and followed by shrinkage, such a mechanism does not fit the observed time relation for restenosis with its 1-month delayed and progressive luminal loss (86). Furthermore, capillaries or other evidence of "organization" are rarely found in the myxoid-like neointima formed after angioplasty (101). Nevertheless, the thrombus burden may be important in late restenosis by constituting a reservoir for active substances such as platelet-derived growth factors, thrombin, and fibrin(ogen) and related degradation products which may influence the proliferative response (19). In pig coronary models of "restenosis," thrombus organization plays no major role in neointima formation after balloon dilatation injury (163) (E. Falk et al., *unpublished observations*) or after stenting (164–166), unless the stent is considerably oversized resulting in both a huge acute luminal gain and extensive vessel wall injury (167–171).

Anticoagulants and weak platelet inhibitors (e.g., aspirin) reduce acute thrombus-related complications after angioplasty without influencing the late restenosis rate (87). If thrombus burden or platelet turnover is important for late restenosis, more potent antithrombotic agents such as platelet GPIIb/IIIa receptor blockers and antithrombins could prove successful, particularly in patients with acute coronary syndromes where culprit lesions frequently are very thrombogenic and contain thrombus already before intervention (151). For stenting, optimal expansion (152) and proper antithrombotic therapy (172) are important to prevent stent thrombosis, but the impact on late restenosis is unknown.

Proliferation

Experimental balloon injury consistently gives rise to early waves of SMC proliferation and migration, followed by matrix synthesis (129,134,173). In humans, however, contradictory results have been reported in two atherectomy studies evaluating the proliferative activity in restenotic lesions, using the proliferating cell nuclear antigen (PCNA) as marker for cell replication. One study of 19 restenotic specimens found proliferating cells in all lesions, even as late as 1 year after angioplasty, with 21% and 15% of the cells showing evidence of proliferation evaluated by in situ hybridization and immunohistochemistry, respectively (77). In contrast, the other study found no evidence of cell replication in 74% of 100 restenotic coronary atherectomy specimens examined, and only a modest number of PCNA-positive cells (usually less than 1%) were found in the majority of the remaining specimens with no obvious proliferative peak, i.e., without evidence of time relation (75). Only 12 of 30 specimens obtained within 60 days of the initial interventional procedure had one or more PCNA-positive nuclei per slide (>4,000 cells per slide). Also a few atherectomy specimens from renarrowed stents have been evaluated for proliferating cells; no PCNA-positive cells were found in the newly formed neointima (174). These data do not, however, rule out a potential role of early and/or low protracted cell proliferation in late restenosis (75,175).

Matrix

SMC migration, proliferation, and matrix synthesis are individually regulated and may occur independently (107). Nevertheless, resting SMCs are nearly always surrounded by a large and predictable volume of extracellular matrix. As mentioned, the activated SMCs do not seem to return to the quiescent state until the ratio of matrix to cell volume approaches 4:1 (130,134). The time relation observed for human postinterventional restenosis conforms much better with progressive matrix accumulation (and remodeling) than with cell proliferation, but the latter may be the major determinant of the former. Angiographically, some nonrestenotic lesions appear to regress beyond 6 months after intervention, which could be due to maturation (collagenization and shrinkage) of the extracellular matrix (141). Transforming growth factor-beta (TGF-beta), which is present in high concentration within platelet granules, is believed to be the principal regulator of matrix production and has been identified in SMCs within restenotic coronary lesions (176) and could be critical in regulating the new mass component of such lesions. However, as with PCNA-gauged cell proliferation, TGF-beta mRNA does not appear to show for restenosis the expected postinterventional time relation or peak expression (177).

Inflammation

Inflammatory cells are rarely seen in restenotic tissue obtained beyond 3–6 months after intervention (69,177), but they might have been present earlier (178). During wound healing, macrophages phagocytose debris and provide degradative enzymes and cytokines essential for early stages of tissue repair (179). If the same occurs after coronary interventional procedures, macrophages could be "good," participating in the removal of necrotic material and thrombi at injury sites promoting normal healing, rather than being "bad," stimulating an exuberant and unfavorable healing response, as frequently suggested (180–186). Of note, anti-inflammatory therapy with steroid has been tested clinically in two restenosis trials with negative result (87).

Remodeling

Redistribution of existing material (remodeling) (187,188) is the way balloon dilatation works, and it may also explain its failure. Elastic recoil (early remodeling) may contribute to late restenosis without influencing the processes responsible for the subsequent protracted luminal narrowing (189). The latter could be due to a protracted return to preinterventional vessel size caused by contraction or failed compensatory enlargement (chronic remodeling) rather than by addition of new mass (neointima formation). Old atherosclerotic plaque and not neointima constitutes the main obstructive component of many restenotic lesions (190), indicating that remodeling may be more important in restenosis than proliferation. Preliminary data derived from serial intracoronary ultrasound examinations agree with these pathologic observations (154–157). The healing response after angioplasty has been likened aptly by Forrester et al. to wound healing with a contracted scar (restenosis?) as the final outcome (179). The endothelium may play a role in both acute and chronic vascular remodeling, influencing both vasomotion and proliferation after arterial injury (188).

Restenosis: Risk Factors

Many studies of multiple-lesion procedures have shown that some lesions may restenose while other lesions in the same patient will not, indicating that restenosis after angioplasty is more lesion-specific than patient-specific (191). Although poorly defined, patient-related factors may, however, also play a role in the restenosis process (192). Similarly, in the pig coronary model, multiple angioplasty sites behave differently, depending much more on local factors (depth and extent of injury) than on systemic factors (125).

Patient-Related Factors

Restenosis after successful coronary angioplasty is a process that cannot be accurately predicted by simple clinical data (193,194). Most of the standard risk factors for atherosclerosis and ischemic heart disease such as aging, male sex, arterial hypertension, dyslipidemia [total cholesterol, LDL-C, HDL-C, apolipoprotein A-1 or B, or lipoprotein(a)], plasma fibrinogen, and continued smoking after angioplasty have no great impact on restenosis rate, and only diabetes mellitus may be of some importance (193–199). Measurements of late lumen loss after stenting [no recoil, spasm, or late contraction (153)] indicate that the diabetic state or diabetic plaques are associated with more exuberant neointima formation after arterial injury (200). No specific diabetic plaque features have been identified.

Primary unstable angina, known frequently to be precipitated by plaque rupture and luminal thrombosis, carries an increased risk of postangioplasty complications [acute closure and probably also late restenosis (193)], particularly in the presence of abnormal coronary vasoconstriction (113). Also, unstable angina due to restenosis is associated with an increased risk of acute complications and recurrent restenosis after repeat angioplasty (201).

Lesion-Related Factors

The architecture (e.g., eccentricity), composition, vulnerability, thrombogenicity, and SMC-reactivity of individual target lesions are important for the immediate outcome (success versus failure), the type, degree, and extent of arterial injury sustained, and, consequently, the subsequent thrombotic (abrupt closure) and healing (restenosis) responses (202,203). Coronary lesions with increased propensity to spasm (unstable and variant angina) are prone to restenose after angioplasty (110,113), and early repeat angioplasty (within 3 months of previous procedure) seems to be associated with a particularly high recurrence rate (204,205). Lesions located in smaller vessels (206,207) and in the left anterior descending coronary artery (207,208) may have increased restenosis rates, but conflicting results have been reported for both vessel size and lesion location (206–210). Long stenoses and severe stenoses may be particularly prone to restenose (207,211).

The presence of thrombus, inflammation (212), high cellularity or neointima-like tissue (71,213–216), and activated or proliferating SMCs (212,217) in atherectomy specimens and the readiness of the retrieved SMCs to grow in culture (216) have in some (212–215,217) but not all (71,212,216) studies correlated positively with subsequent development of late restenosis. Complex lesions (thrombi?) responsible for unstable angina are associated with increased risk of post-interventional abrupt closure, but whether the long-term non-occlusive restenosis rate is also increased remains controversial (117,193). So far, restenosis cannot be predicted reliably from the actual knowledge of target lesion characteristics. The magnitude of acute luminal gain and the injury created during intervention are probably much more important for restenosis than the character of the stenotic lesion present before the procedure.

Tool-Related Factors

New devices for percutaneous transluminal coronary lumen enlargement such as atherectomy devices (directional, extractional, rotational) and lasers have failed to reduce the late restenosis rate. Only stenting has proved successful, sustaining the acute luminal gain by preventing unfavorable remodeling (recoil) (88,89). Relatively more narrowing may occur after atherectomy than after balloon dilatation alone (218), but the data are inconclusive (119).

Interventions

Numerous drugs have been evaluated to reduce postinterventional restenosis. None has proven successful, including antiplatelet agents, anticoagulants, spasmolytica (calcium channel blockers), angiotensin-converting enzyme inhibitors, antiinflammatory agents, antiproliferative agents, growth factor antagonists, and fish oils (87,219–220). Nitric oxide donors have in a single study reduced the restenosis rate without preventing the late loss in lumen diameter (221). Even profound lowering of total and LDL cholesterol by drugs has not proved effective (222,223), but a possible effect of HDL, lipoprotein(a), and antioxidants on restenosis needs to be evaluated further (224–227), as do calcium antagonists (228). Acute-phase profound platelet GPIIb/IIIa receptor blockade has recently been reported to reduce acute complications and clinical restenosis after coronary interventions in high-risk patients, but it remains to be shown whether such a regimen also will reduce the angiographic restenosis rate (151). Stents reduce restenosis by preventing postinterventional recoil, not be reducing new tissue formation (88,89). Compared with balloon angioplasty, the much larger lumen obtained by Palmaz–Schatz stenting is maintained and results in a lower restenosis rate (145).

ATHEROSCLEROSIS AND RESTENOSIS: DIFFERENCES

The following excerpt is from a recent review article on atherosclerosis, written by two distinguished pathologists,

TABLE 1. *Differences between atherosclerosis and restenosis*

	Atherosclerosis	Restenosis
Risk factors	Sex, age, lipids, smoking, blood pressure, diabetes, etc.	Diabetes
Injury	Chronic and superficial	Acute and deep
Early lesion		
Endothelium	+ (activated)	−
Plts/thrombus	−	+
Mono/macrph	+	?
Lipid deposits	+	−
SMC activation	?	+
Mature lesion		
Composition		
Sclerosis	+	+
Atherosis	+/−	−
Foam cells	+	−
Inflammation	+	−
Vulnerability	Stable/unstable	Stable
Complications		
Rupture	+	−
Hemorrhages	+	−
Thrombosis	+	−
Calcification	+	−
Evolution	Slow (decades)	Rapid (few months)
Remodeling	Enlargement	Contraction?
Manifestations	+AMI/SCD	−AMI/SCD
Lipid lowering	Slows progression	No effect

Plts, platelets; Mono, monocytes; macrph, macrophages; SMC, smooth muscle cells; AMI, acute myocardial infarction; SCD, sudden coronary death.

who have been deeply engaged in the study of human and experimental atherosclerosis for many years:

> Isolated intimal smooth muscle proliferation is not atherosclerosis. Smooth muscle proliferation is a general response to injury by the arterial wall and does occur in atherosclerosis. But it is neither unique to nor specific for atherosclerosis. Many animal models of arterial disease have been created in which vascular damage is induced by intraluminal balloon injury or external compression. A localised intimal smooth muscle proliferation occurs which simulates one component of the human atherosclerotic plaque. Post angioplasty stenosis in humans is an example of such a response to injury by an atherosclerotic vessel but the lesion created is different from a human plaque (15).

We totally agree with this viewpoint and will in the following try to specify some of the major differences between atherosclerosis and restenosis (Table 1).

Risk Factors

Of the traditional risk factors for atherosclerosis and ischemic heart disease, only diabetes has rather consistently been related to restenosis (193). Multiple lesions treated in a single patient frequently behave differently (191,192), indicating that lesion-related factors rather than systemic risk factors play the main role in restenosis.

Injury

Both atherosclerosis and restenosis represent responses to arterial injury. During atherogenesis, the endothelium is initially intact and activated (chronic nondenuding injury), playing an active role in recruiting monocyte-derived macrophages and producing cytokines and growth-modulating factors. Later it may be lost focally over established plaques (denuding injury) and eventually plaque rupture (deep injury) may supervene. In contrast, deep injury and extensive deendothelialization, not endothelial activation, initiate the restenotic process that eventually leads to a stable and endothelialized lesion.

Response

The histology of restenosis differs significantly from that of atherosclerosis. The restenotic neointima is monomorphous, consisting of SMCs (cellularity decreases with time) and matrix (collagen increases with time). On the contrary, atherosclerosis is very heterogeneous with plaques composed of a variable mixture of cells (SMCs, macrophages, lymphocytes), connective tissue (usually dense and hypocellular), intracellular lipid (foam cells), extracellular lipids (amorphous and crystalline), cellular debris, calcification/ossification, hemorrhage, and thrombus.

Composition

Atherosis and Sclerosis

For survival, the most important difference between atherosclerosis and restenosis is that the latter lacks the vulnerable lipid/macrophage-related atheromatous component. Both atherosclerosis and restenosis contain, however, a stable SMC-related sclerotic component. As mentioned, many atherosclerotic plaques harbor cellular neointima-like areas (58,67–70) which probably represent an early and possibly accelerated stage in the development of the mature sclerotic plaque component (67). Despite similar morphology, very different cellular interactions, cytokines, and growth factors could, however, underlie the development of sclerotic plaque tissue and restenotic neointima.

SMC Activation, Growth Factors, and Proliferation

Compared to normal arterial tissue, both atherosclerotic and restenotic coronary tissues contain increased amounts of many potent growth factors and cytokines (184). SMCs within restenotic lesions express more human nonmuscle myosin heavy-chain mRNA (considered a marker of cell activation) (229) and more transforming growth factor-beta mRNA and protein (176,177) than do SMCs within atherosclerotic plaques. Evaluated by cell culturing techniques, SMCs obtained from restenotic lesions are more easily cultivated and they proliferate and migrate faster than do cells originating from atherosclerotic plaques (105,106,230,231). Apparently, restenotic SMCs are very ''reactive,'' while plaque cells appear senescent and/or ''exhausted.'' Recently, the expression of acidic and basic fibroblast growth factors was detected in 80–100% of unstable angina (n = 11) and restenosis (n = 10) atherectomy specimens, but in only 1 of 5 stable angina specimens (67).

Evaluated by PCNA staining, both atherosclerotic and restenotic coronary lesions exhibit no or only very low proliferative activity, usually with 0% and only very rarely >1% replicating cells (66,74–76,232). However, a single study which also included peripheral lesions but used the same technique reported very high proliferative activity in both atherosclerotic (4% positive cells) and restenotic (15% positive cells) lesions (77). The reason for these conflicting results is not obvious.

Lipid

Intracellular lipid (foam cells) and extracellular lipid deposits (cholesterol crystals) are not present in neointima responsible for restenosis.

Inflammation

Inflammatory changes (endothelial activation, macrophages, and T-lymphocytes) are present in many early as well as mature atherosclerotic plaques. In contrast, inflammatory cells are rarely found in mature neointima responsible for restenosis (69,177,233), which, however, does not exclude a possible early critical role of inflammation in the late outcome after angioplasty (180,181). If monocytes/macrophages are recruited early after angioplasty (little human data exist on early changes), they apparently leave the lesion again spontaneously, probably in contrast to macrophages of atherosclerotic plaques (233).

Thrombosis

Thrombus after angioplasty is an early phenomenon which may give rise to abrupt closure, but the mature restenotic lesion does not thrombose (144). In contrast, thrombus plays no role early during atherogenesis, but very frequently complicates mature plaques, being responsible for the great majority of acute coronary syndromes.

Speed of Development

It takes many years to develop mature atherosclerotic plaques, while restenosis develops in less than 6 months. A mature atherosclerotic plaque may, however, grow rapidly due to plaque rupture, plaque hemorrhage, and/or luminal thrombosis or at accelerated speed due to bursts of SMC activation, apparently like postinterventional neointima formation (67).

Remodeling

Atherosclerosis is associated with compensatory dilatation early during plaque growth (favorable remodeling), while restenosis frequently is associated with and partly due to vessel contraction (unfavorable remodeling).

Coexisting Atherosclerosis and Restenosis

Evaluated in the same patient, coronary atherosclerosis and restenosis progress independently, suggesting dissimilar processes (234–238). Although angioplasty is followed by short-term renarrowing, this reparative process may, in fact, protect against long-term lesion progression (237,238). New ischemic symptoms are already after 6 months caused by progression of native rather than treated lesions (142,234,237–241), explaining the unchanged long-term prognosis after otherwise successful angioplasty; infarction rate and mortality are not reduced to any extent just by eliminating one or a few angina-producing stenoses in coronary arteries that are diffusely affected by confluent plaquing (34).

Clinical Manifestations

Postinterventional restenosis may give rise to recurrent and sometimes clinically aggressive angina pectoris (237,242). Contrary to atherosclerosis, restenosis rarely causes myocardial infarction or sudden death, probably because neointima lacks the vulnerable atheromatous component.

The Rat Experience

Normal rats are relatively resistant to atherogenesis (243). Nevertheless, balloon deendothelialization of the rat carotid artery is rapidly followed by platelet adhesion forming a monolayer, with subsequent intimal thickening due to SMC proliferation, migration, and matrix synthesis, which, in the course of just a few weeks, leads to the formation of a thick neointima (134). A huge proliferative healing response may thus occur in arteries of animals that are resistant to atherosclerosis, and simultaneous hypercholesterolemia leads to lesions with a composition that indicates that ''atherosis'' and ''sclerosis'' progress and regress independently (244,245). Resistance to atherosclerosis does not protect against restenosis.

FUTURE DIRECTIONS

Until now, proliferation of SMCs has been a focus for restenosis research, considered to be mainly responsible for postinterventional luminal renarrowing. If exuberant, SMC-related neointima formation may cause restenosis, but matrix synthesis could prove to be more important for the final outcome than cell proliferation in providing new mass to the restenotic lesion. More needs to be known about the cellular mechanisms controlling matrix production.

Furthermore, recent data indicate that remodeling (redistribution of existing tissue rather than addition of new tissue) may play an even more important role in restenosis than neointima formation. We need to know more about the basic mechanisms underlying vascular remodeling, which may be both beneficial, with compensatory vessel dilatation during lesion growth and thus maintaining a good lumen (e.g., early atherogenesis), and harmful, causing luminal narrowing without significant intimal growth (may be important in restenosis). Recoil and unfavorable vascular remodeling are important in restenosis, documented by recent stent trials. Ongoing stent research will probably soon lead to lower acute complication rates and improve the long-term results.

SUMMARY

Although both atherosclerosis and restenosis evolve as the result of arterial injury followed by healing (response to injury), their pathogeneses differ significantly. For prevention and treatment it may be more rewarding to consider the two responses as representing two different disease processes than just consider one of them, restenosis, as being an accelerated form of the other, atherosclerosis.

REFERENCES

1. Gotto AM. Some reflections on arteriosclerosis: Past, present, and future. *Circulation* 1985;72:8–17.
2. Schoen FJ, Libby P. Cardiac transplant graft arteriosclerosis. *Trends Cardiovasc Med* 1991;1:216–223.
3. Ip JH, Fuster V, Badimon L, Badimon J, Taubman MB, Chesebro JH. Syndromes of accelerated atherosclerosis: Role of vascular injury and smooth muscle cell proliferation. *J Am Coll Cardiol* 1990;15: 1667–1687.
4. Ross R. The pathogenesis of atherosclerosis: A perspective for the 1990s. *Nature* 1993;362:801–809.
5. Ylä-Herttuala S. Macrophages and oxidized low density lipoproteins in the pathogensis of atherosclerosis. *Ann Med* 1991;23:561–567.
6. Faruqi RM, DiCorleto PE. Mechanisms of monocyte recruitment and accumulation. *Br Heart J* 1993;69:S19–S29.
7. Hansson GK. Immune and inflammatory mechanisms in the development of atherosclerosis. *Br Heart J* 1993;69:S38–S41.
8. Raines EW, Ross R. Smooth muscle cells and the pathogensis of the lesions of atherosclerosis. *Br Heart J* 1993;69:S30–S37.
9. Fuster V, Badimon L, Badimon J, Chesebro JH. The pathogenesis of coronary artery disease and the acute coronary syndromes. *N Eng J Med* 1992;326:242–250, 310–318.
10. Falk E. Coronary thrombosis: Pathogenesis and clinical manifestations. *Am J Cardiol* 1991;68:28B–35B.
11. Stary HC, Blankenhorn DH, Chandler AB, Glagov S, Insull W, Richardson M, Rosenfeld ME, Schaffer SA, Schwartz CJ, Wagner WD, Wissler RW. A definition of the intima of human arteries and of its atherosclerosis-prone regions. A report from the Committee on Vascular Lesions of the Council on Arteriosclerosis, American Heart Association. *Circulation* 1992;85:391–405.
12. Schwartz CJ, Valente AJ, Sprague EA, Kelley JL, Nerem RM. The pathogenesis of atherosclerosis: An overview. *Clin Cardiol* 1991;14: I-1–I-16.
13. van der Wal AC, Das PK, Tigges AJ, Becker AE. Adhesion molecules on the endothelium and mononuclear cells in human atherosclerotic lesions. *Am J Pathol* 1992;141:1427–1433.
14. Wood KM, Cadogan MD, Ramshaw AL, Parums DV. The distribution of adhesion molecules in human atherosclerosis. *Histopathology* 1993;22:437–444.
15. Davies MJ, Woolf N. Atherosclerosis: What is it and why does it occur? *Br Heart J* 1993;69(Suppl):S3–S11.
16. Bürrig K-F. The endothelium of advanced arteriosclerotic plaques in humans. *Arterioscler Thromb* 1991;11:1678–1689.
17. Valenzuela R, Shainoff JR, DiBello PM, Urbanic DA, Anderson JM, Matsueda GR, Kudryk BJ. Immunoelectrophoretic and immunohistochemical characterizations of fibrinogen derivatives in atherosclerotic aortic intimas and vascular prosthesis pseudointimas. *Am J Pathol* 1992;141:861–880.
18. Zhang Y, Cliff WJ, Schoefl GI, Higgins G. Plasma protein insudation as an index of early coronary atherogenesis. *Am J Pathol* 1993;143: 496–506.
19. Wilcox JN. Thrombotic mechanisms in atherosclerosis. *Coron Artery Disease* 1994;5:223–229.
20. Nelken NA, Solfer SJ, O'Keefe J, Vu T-KH, Charo IF, Coughlin SR. Thrombin receptor expression in normal and atherosclerotic human arteries. *J Clin Invest* 1992;90:1614–1621.
21. Falk E. Plaque rupture with severe pre-existing stenosis precipitating coronary thrombosis. Characteristics of coronary atherosclerotic plaques underlying fatal occlusive thrombi. *Br Heart J* 1983;50: 127–134.
22. Falk E. Why do plaques rupture? *Circulation* 1992;86(Suppl III):III-30–III-42.
23. Demer LL, Watson KE, Boström K. Mechanism of calcification in atherosclerosis. *Trends Cardiovasc Med* 1994;4:45–49.
24. Roberts WC. Diffuse extent of coronary atherosclerosis in fatal coronary artery disease. *Am J Cardiol* 1990;65:2F–6F.
25. Kragel AH, Reddy SG, Wittes JT, Roberts WC. Morphometric analysis of the composition of atherosclerotic plaques in the four major epicardial coronary arteries in acute myocardial infarction and in sudden coronary death. *Circulation* 1989;80:1747–1756.
26. Kragel AH, Reddy SG, Wittes JT, Roberts WC. Morphometric analysis of the composition of coronary arterial plaques in isolated unstable angina pectoris with pain at rest. *Am J Cardiol* 1990;66:562–567.
27. Cannistra AJ, Jacobs AK, Horten K, Callum MG, Cupples LA, Currier JW, Faxon DP, Ryan TJ. Quantitative coronary histopathology: Clinical correlates. *Circulation* 1993;88:(Suppl I):I-589(abst).
28. Rosenschein U, Ellis SG, Haudenschild CC, Yakubov S, Muller DWM, Dick RJ, Topol EJ. Comparison of histopathologic coronary lesions obtained from directional atherectomy in stable angina versus acute coronary syndromes. *Am J Cardiol* 1994;73:508–510.
29. Small DM. Progression and regression of atherosclerotic lesions. Insights from lipid physical biochemistry. *Arteriosclerosis* 1988;8: 103–129.
30. Lundberg B. Chemical composition and physical state of lipid deposits in atherosclerosis. *Atherosclerosis* 1985;56:93–110.
31. Bocan TM, Brown SA, Guyton JR. Human aortic fibrolipid lesions. Immunochemical localization of apolipoprotein B and apolipoprotein A. *Arteriosclerosis* 1988;8:499–508.
32. Virmani R, Farb A, Burke AP. Coronary angioplasty from the perspective of atherosclerotic plaque: Morphologic predictors of immediate success and restenosis. *Am Heart J* 1994;127:163–179.
33. Nobuyoshi M, Tanaka M, Nosaka H, Kimura T, Yokoi H, Hamasaki N, Kim K, Shindo T, Kimura K. Progression of coronary atherosclerosis: Is coronary spasm related to progression? *J Am Coll Cardiol* 1991; 18:904–910.
34. Danchin N. Is myocardial revascularisation for tight coronary stenoses always necessary? [Viewpoint]. *Lancet* 1993;342:224–225.
35. Davies MJ, Richardson PD, Woolf N, Katz DR, Mann J. Risk of thrombosis in human atherosclerotic plaques: Role of extracellular

lipid, macrophage, and smooth muscle cell content. *Br Heart J* 1993; 69:377–381.

36. van der Wal AC, Becker AE, van der Loos CM, Das PK. Site of intimal rupture or erosion of thrombosed coronary atherosclerotic plaques is characterized by an inflammatory process irrespective of the dominant plaque morphology. *Circulation* 1994;89:36–44.
37. Buja LM, Willerson JT. Role of inflammation in coronary plaque disruption [Editorial]. *Circulation* 1994;89:503–505.
38. Moreno PR, Falk E, Palacios IF, Newell JB, Fuster V, Fallon JT. Macrophage infiltration in acute coronary syndromes: Implications for plaque rupture. *Circulation* 1994;90:775–778.
39. Henney AM, Wakeley PR, Davies MJ, Foster K, Hembry R, Murphy G, Humphries S. Localization of stromelysin gene expression in atherosclerotic plaques by *in situ* hybridization. *Proc Natl Acad Sci USA* 1991;88:8154–8158.
40. Galis ZS, Sukhova GK, Lark MW, Libby P. Increased expression of matrix metalloproteinases and matrix degrading activity in vulnerable regions of human atherosclerotic plaques. *J Clin Invest* 1994;94: 2493–2503.
41. Shah PK, Falk E, Badimon JJ, Levy G, Fernandez-Ortiz A, Fallon J, Fuster V. Human monocyte-derived macrophages express collagenase and induce collagen breakdown in atherosclerotic fibrous caps: Implications for plaque rupture. *Circulation* 1993;88:I-254(abst).
42. Loree HM, Tobias BJ, Gibson LJ, Kamm RD, Small DM, Lee RT. Mechanical properties of model atherosclerotic lesion lipid pools. *Arterioscler Thromb* 1994;14:230–234.
43. Brown DL, Hibbs MS, Kearney M, Loushin C, Isner JM. Identification of 92-kD gelatinase in human coronary atherosclerotic lesions. Association of active enzyme synthesis with unstable angina. *Circulation* 1995;91:2125–2131.
44. Richardson PD, Davies MJ, Born GVR. Influence of plaque configuration and stress distribution on fissuring of coronary atherosclerotic plaques. *Lancet* 1989;2:941–944.
45. Loree HM, Kamm RD, Stringfellow RG, Lee RT. Effects of fibrous cap thickness on peak circumferential stress in model atherosclerotic vessels. *Circ Res* 1992;71:850–858.
46. Cheng GC, Loree HM, Kamm RD, Fishbein MC, Lee RT. Distribution of circumferential stress in ruptured and stable atherosclerotic lesions. A structural analysis with histopathological correlation. *Circulation* 1993;87:1179–1187.
47. Gertz SD, Roberts WC. Hemodynamic shear force in rupture of coronary arterial atherosclerotic plaques. *Am J Cardiol* 1990;66: 1368–1372.
48. Mizushige K, Reisman M, Buchbinder M, Dittrich H, DeMaria AN. Atheroma deformation during the cardiac cycle: Evaluation by intracoronary ultrasound. *Circulation* 1993;88:I–550(abst).
49. Stein PD, Hamid MS, Shivkumar K, Davis TP, Khaja F, Henry JW. Effects of cyclic flexion of coronary arteries on progression of atherosclerosis. *Am J Cardiol* 1994;73:431–437.
50. Ku DN, McCord BN. Cyclic stress causes rupture of the atherosclerotic plaque cap. *Circulation* 1993;88(No 4, Part 2):I-254(abst).
51. Muller JE, Abela GS, Nesto RW, Tofler GH. Triggers, acute risk factors and vulnerable plaques: The lexicon of a new frontier. *J Am Coll Cardiol* 1994;23:809–813.
52. Glagov S, Weisenberg E, Zarins CK, Stankunavicius R, Kolettis GJ. Compensatory enlargement of human atherosclerotic coronary arteries. *N Engl J Med* 1987;316:1371–1375.
53. Zarins CK, Weisenberg E, Kolettis G, Stankunavicius R, Glagov S. Differential enlargement of artery segments in response to enlarging atherosclerotic plaques. *J Vasc Surg* 1988;7:386–394.
54. Stiel GM, Stiel LS, Schofer J, Donath K, Mathey DG. Impact of compensatory enlargement of atherosclerotic coronary arteries on angiographic assessment of coronary artery disease. *Circulation* 1989; 80:1603–1609.
55. Gerber TC, Erbel R, Görge G, Ge J, Rupprecht HJ, Meyer J. Extent of atherosclerosis and remodeling of the left main coronary artery determined by intravascular ultrasound. *Am J Cardiol* 1994;73: 666–671.
56. Bruschke AVG, Kramer JR, Bal ET, Haque IU, Detrano RC, Goormastic M. The dynamics of progression of coronary atherosclerosis studied in 168 medically treated patients who underwent coronary arteriography three times. *Am Heart J* 1989;117:296–305.
57. Falk E. Unstable angina with fatal outcome: Dynamic coronary thrombosis leading to infarction and/or sudden death. Autopsy evidence of recurrent mural thrombosis with peripheral embolization culminating in total vascular occlusion. *Circulation* 1985;71:699–708.
58. Escaned J, van Suylen RJ, Macleod DC, Umans VAWM, de Jong M, Bosman FT, de Feyter PJ, Serruys PW. Histologic characteristics of tissue excised during directional coronary atherectomy in stable and unstable angina pectoris. *Am J Cardiol* 1993;71:1442–1447.
59. Tousoulis D, Crake T, Rosen S, Uren N, Haider AW, Davies G. Coronary stenosis angiographic findings before and after acute myocardial infarction in patients with angina pectoris. *J Am Coll Cardiol* 1994;23:146A(abst).
60. Kaski JC, Tousoulis D, McFadden E, Crea F, Pereira WI, Maseri A. Variant angina pectoris. Role of coronary spasm in the development of fixed coronary obstructions. *Circulation* 1992;85:619–626.
61. Yamagishi M, Miyatake K, Tamai J, Nakatani S, Koyama J, Nissen SE. Intravascular ultrasound detection of atherosclerosis at the site of focal vasospasm in angiographically normal or minimally narrowed coronary segments. *J Am Coll Cardiol* 1994;23:352–357.
62. Zeiher AM, Schachinger V, Weitzel SH, Wollschlager H, Just H. Intracoronary thrombus formation causes focal vasoconstriction of epicardial arteries in patients with coronary artery disease. *Circulation* 1991;83:1519–1525.
63. Etsuda H, Mizuno K, Arakawa K, Satomura K, Shibuya T, Isojima K. Angioscopy in variant angina: Coronary artery spasm and intimal injury. *Lancet* 1993;342:1322–1324.
64. Kohchi K, Takebayashi S, Hiroki T, Nobuyoshi M. Significance of adventitial inflammation of the coronary artery in patients with unstable angina: Results at autopsy. *Circulation* 1985;71:709–716.
65. Waters D, Craven TE, Lespérance J. Prognostic significance of progression of coronary atherosclerosis. *Circulation* 1993;87: 1067–1075.
66. Gordon D, Reidy MA, Benditt EP, Schwartz SM. Cell proliferation in human coronary arteries. *Proc Natl Acad Sci USA* 1990;87: 4600–4604.
67. Flugelman MY, Virmani R, Correa R, Yu Z-X, Farb A, Leon MB, Elami A, Fu Y-M, Casscells W, Epstein SE. Smooth muscle cell abundance and fibroblast growth factors in coronary lesions of patients with nonfatal unstable angina. A clue to the mechanism of transformation from the stable to the unstable clinical state. *Circulation* 1993; 88:2493–2500.
68. Safian RD, Gelbfish JS, Erny RE, Schnitt SJ, Schmidt DA, Baim DS. Coronary atherectomy. Clinical, angiographic, and histological findings and observations regarding potential mechanisms. *Circulation* 1990;82:69–79.
69. Garratt KN, Edwards WD. Directional coronary atherectomy: Histopathologic studies. In: Holmes DR, Garratt KN, eds. *Atherectomy.* Boston: Blackwell; 1992:106–131.
70. Schnitt SJ, Safian RD, Kuntz RE, Schmidt DA, Baim DS. Histologic findings in specimens obtained by percutaneous directional coronary atherectomy. *Hum Pathol* 1992;23:415–420.
71. Miller MJ, Kuntz RE, Friedrich SP, Leidig GA, Fishman RF, Schnitt SJ, Baim DS, Safian RD. Frequency and consequences of intimal hyperplasia in specimens retrieved by directional atherectomy of native primary coronary artery stenoses and subsequent restenoses. *Am J Cardiol* 1993;71:652–658.
72. Corrado D, Basso C, Poletti A, Angelini A, Valente M, Thiene G. Sudden death in the young. Is acute coronary thrombosis the major precipitating factor? *Circulation* 1994;90:2315–2323.
73. Corrado D, Thiene G, Buja GF, Pantaleoni A, Maiolino P. The relationship between growth of atherosclerotic plaques, variant angina and sudden death. *Int J Cardiol* 1990;26:361–367.
74. O'Brien ER, Stewart DK, Tran N, Hinohara T, Simpson JB, Alpers CE, Schwartz SM. Cellular proliferation in primary coronary artery lesions. *Circulation* 1992;86(Suppl I):I-157(abst).
75. O'Brien ER, Alpers CE, Stewart DK, Ferguson M, Tran N, Gordon D, Benditt EP, Hinohara T, Simpson JB, Schwartz SM. Proliferation in primary and restenotic coronary atherectomy tissue. Implications for antiproliferative therapy. *Circ Res* 1993;73:223–231.
76. Katsuda S, Coltrera MD, Ross R, Gown AM. Human atherosclerosis. IV. Immunocytochemical analysis of cell activation and proliferation in lesions of young adults. *Am J Pathol* 1993;142:1787–1793.
77. Pickering JG, Weir L, Jekanowski J, Kearney MA, Isner JM. Proliferative activity in peripheral and coronary atherosclerotic plaque among patients undergoing percutaneous revascularization. *J Clin Invest* 1993;91:1469–1480.

78. Fernandez-Ortiz A, Badimon JJ, Falk E, Fuster V, Meyer B, Mailhac A, Weng D, Shah PK, Badimon L. Characterization of the relative thrombogenicity of atherosclerotic plaque components: Implications for consequences of plaque rupture. *J Am Coll Cardiol* 1994;23: 1562–1569.
79. Kragel AH, Roberts WC. Composition of atherosclerotic plaques in the coronary arteries in homozygous familial hypercholesterolemia. *Am Heart J* 1991;121:210–211.
80. Kannel WB, McGee DL, Castelli WP. Latest perspectives on cigarette smoking and cardiovascular disease: The Framingham Study. *J Card Rehabil* 1984;4:267–277.
81. Nobuyoshi M, Abe M, Nosaka H, Kimura T, Yokoi H, Hamasaki N, Shindo T, Kimura K, Nakamura T, Nakagawa Y, Shiode N, Sakamoto A, Kakura H, Iwasaki Y, Kim K, Kitaguchi S. Statistical analysis of clinical risk factors for coronary artery spasm: Identification of the most important determinant. *Am Heart J* 1992;124:32–38.
82. Celermajer DS, Sorensen KE, Gooch VM, Spiegelhalter DJ, Miller OI, Sullivan ID, Lloyd JK, Deanfield JE. Non-invasive detection of endothelial dysfunction in children and adults at risk of atherosclerosis. *Lancet* 1992;340:1111–1115.
83. Reddy KG, Nair RN, Sheehan HM, Hodgson JM. Evidence that selective endothelial dysfunction may occur in the absence of angiographic or ultrasound atherosclerosis in patients with risk factors for atherosclerosis. *J Am Coll Cardiol* 1994;23:833–843.
84. Leung W-H, Lau C-P, Wong C-K. Beneficial effect of cholesterol-lowering therapy on coronary endothelium-dependent relaxation in hypercholesterolaemic patients. *Lancet* 1993;341:1496–1500.
85. Gould KL, Martucci JP, Goldberg DI, Hess MJ, Edens RP, Latifi R, Dudrick SJ. Short-term cholesterol lowering decreases size and severity of perfusion abnormalities by positron emission tomography after dipyridamole in patients with coronary artery disease. *Circulation* 1994;89:1530–1538.
86. Nobuyoshi M, Kimura T, Nosaka H, Mioka S, Ueno K, Yokoi H, Hamasaki N, Horiuchi H, Ohishi H. Restenosis after successful percutaneous transluminal coronary angioplasty: Serial angiographic follow-up of 229 patients. *J Am Coll Cardiol* 1988;12:616–623.
87. Faxon DP. Restenosis after angioplasty: What have we learned from clinical trials? *Cardiol Rev* 1993;1(4):209–217.
88. Serruys PW, de Jaegere P, Kiemeneij F, Macaya C, Rutsch W, Heyndrickx G, Emanuelsson H, Marco J, Legrand V, Materne P, Belardi J, Sigwart U, Colombo A, Goy JJ, van den Heuvel P, Delcan J, Morel M-A, for the Benestent Study Group. A comparison of balloon-expandable-stent implantation with balloon angioplasty in patients with coronary artery disease. *N Engl J Med* 1994;331:489–495.
89. Fischman DL, Leon MB, Baim DS, Schatz RA, Savage MP, Penn I, Detre K, Veltri L, Ricci D, Nobuyoshi M, Cleman M, Heuser R, Almond D, Teirstein PS, Fish RD, Colombo A, Brinker J, Moses J, Shaknovich A, Hirshfeld J, Bailey S, Ellis S, Rake R, Goldberg S, for the Stent Restenosis Study Investigators. A randomized comparison of coronary-stent placement and balloon angioplasty in the treatment of coronary artery disease. *N Engl J Med* 1994;331:496–501.
90. Block PC, Myler RK, Stertzer S, Fallon JT. Morphology after transluminal angioplasty in human beings. *N Engl J Med* 1981;305:382–385.
91. Gravanis MB, Roubin GS. Histopathologic phenomena at the site of percutaneous transluminal coronary angioplasty: The problem of restenosis. *Hum Pathol* 1989;20:477–485.
92. Naruko T, Ueda M, Becker AE, Tojo O, Teragaki M, Tekeuchi K, Takeda T. Angiographic-pathologic correlations after elective percutaneous transluminal coronary angioplasty. *Circulation* 1993;88: 1558–1568.
93. Kovach JA, Mintz GS, Pichard AD, Kent KM, Popma JJ, Satler LF, Leon MB. Sequential intravascular ultrasound characterization of the mechanisms of rotational atherectomy and adjunct balloon angioplasty. *J Am Coll Cardiol* 1993;22:1024–1032.
94. Braden GA, Herrington DM, Downes TR, Kutcher MA, Little WC, Qualitative and quantitative contrasts in the mechanisms of lumen enlargement by coronary balloon angioplasty and directional coronary atherectomy. *J Am Coll Cardiol* 1994;23:40–48.
95. Kohchi K, Takebayashi S, Block PC, Hiroki T, Nobuyoshi M. Arterial changes after percutaneous transluminal coronary angioplasty: Results at autopsy. *J Am Coll Cardiol* 1987;10:592–599.
96. Nobuyoshi M, Kimura T, Ohishi H, Horiuchi H, Nosaka H, Hamasaki N, Yokoi H, Kim K. Restenosis after percutaneous transluminal coronary angioplasty: Pathologic observations in 20 patients. *J Am Coll Cardiol* 1991;17:433–439.
97. den Heijer P, van Dijk RB, Pentinga ML, Lie KI. Serial angioscopy during the first hour after successful PTCA. *Circulation* 1992;86(No 4, Suppl I):I-458(abst).
98. Garratt KN, Edwards WD, Kaufmann UP, Vlietstra RE, Holmes DR. Differential histopathology of primary atherosclerotic and restenotic lesions in coronary arteries and saphenous vein bypass grafts: Analysis of tissue obtained from 73 patients by directional atherectomy. *J Am Coll Cardiol* 1991;17:442–448.
99. Austin GE, Ratliff NB, Hollman J, Tabei S, Phillips DF. Intimal proliferation of smooth muscle cells as an explanation for recurrent coronary artery stenosis after percutaneous transluminal coronary angioplasty. *J Am Coll Cardiol* 1985;6:369–375.
100. van Beusekom HM, van der Giessen WJ, van Suylen R, Bos E, Bosman FT, Serruys PW. Histology after stenting of human saphenous vein bypass grafts: Observations from surgically excised grafts 3 to 320 days after stent implantation. *J Am Coll Cardiol* 1993;21:45–54.
101. Ueda M, Becker AE, Tsukada T, Numano F, Fujimoto T. Fibrocellular tissue response after percutaneous transluminal coronary angioplasty: An immunocytochemical analysis of the cellular composition. *Circulation* 1991;83:1327–1332.
102. Morimoto S, Yamada K, Hiramitsu S, Uemura A, Kubo N, Kimura K, Yamaguchi T, Watanabe S, Mizuno Y. Fragmentation of internal elastic lamina and spread of smooth muscle cell proliferation induced by percutaneous transluminal coronary angioplasty. *Jpn Circ J* 1993; 57:388–394.
103. Ross R, White T, Strandness E, Thiele B. Human atherosclerosis. I. Cell constitution and characterization of advanced lesions of superficial femoral arteries. *Am J Pathol* 1984;114:79–93.
104. Liu MW, Roubin GS, King SB. Restenosis after coronary angioplasty. Potential biologic determinants and role of intimal hyperplasia. *Circulation* 1989;79:1374–1387.
105. Dartsch PC, Voisard R, Bauriedel G, Hofling B, Betz E. Growth characteristics and cytoskeletal organization of cultured smooth muscle cells from human primary stenosing and restenosing lesions. *Arteriosclerosis* 1990;10:62–75.
106. Bauriedel G, Windstetter U, DeMaio SJ, Kandolf R, Hofling B. Migratory activity of human smooth muscle cells cultivated from coronary and peripheral primary and restenotic lesions removed by percutaneous atherectomy. *Circulation* 1992;85:554–564.
107. Casscells W. Migration of smooth muscle and endothelial cells. Critical events in restenosis. *Circulation* 1992;86:723–729.
108. Anderson PG, Bajaj RK, Baxley WA, Roubin GS. Vascular pathology of balloon-expandable flexible coil stents in humans. *J Am Coll Cardiol* 1992;19:372–381.
109. McFadden EP, Bauters C, Lablanche JM, Quandalle P, Leory F, Bertrand ME. Response of human coronary arteries to serotonin after injury by coronary angioplasty. *Circulation* 1992;88:2076–2085.
110. Bertrand ME, Lablanche JM, Fourrier JL, Gommeaux A, Ruel M. Relation to restenosis after percutaneous transluminal coronary angioplasty to vasomotion of the dilated coronary arterial segment. *Am J Cardiol* 1989;63:277–281.
111. Kirigaya H, Aizawa T, Ogasawara K, Hirosaka A, Sakuma T, Tabuchi T, Mogami H, Ohta A, Kato K. Coronary vasospastic activity at sites of percutaneous transluminal coronary angioplasty: Evaluation using intracoronary acetylcholine administration. *J Cardiol* 1991;21: 869–877.
112. Kirigaya H, Aizawa T, Ogasawara K, Sato H, Nagashima K, Onoda M, Ogawa K, Yabe A, Kato K. Incidence of acetylcholine-induced spasm of coronary arteries subjected to balloon angioplasty. *Jpn Circ J* 1993;57:883–890.
113. Ardissino D, Barberis P, De Servi S, Merlini PA, Bramucci E, Falcone C, Specchia G. Abnormal coronary vasoconstriction as a predictor of restenosis after successful coronary angioplasty in patients with unstable angina pectoris. *N Engl J Med* 1991;325:1053–1057.
114. van Zanten GH, de Graaf S, Slootweg PJ, Heijnen HFG, Connolly TM, de Groot PG, Sixma JJ. Increased platelet deposition on atherosclerotic coronary arteries. *J Clin Invest* 1994;93:615–632.
115. Fernandez-Ortiz A, Badimon J, Falk E, Fuster V, Chesebro J, Badimon L. Thrombogenicity of human arterial wall: Implications for vascular interventions. *J Am Coll Cardiol* 1994;23:184A(abst).
116. Ueda M, Becker AE, Fujimoto T, Tsukada T. The early phenomena of

restenosis following percutaneous transluminal coronary angioplasty. *Eur Heart J* 1991;12:937–945.

117. Violaris AG, Herrman JPR, Melkert R, Foley DP, Keane D, Serruys PW. Does local thrombus formation increase long term luminal renarrowing following PTCA? A quantitative angiographic analysis. *J Am Coll Cardiol* 1994;23:139A(abst).
118. Umans VAWM, Robert A, Foley D, Wijns W, Haine E, DeFeyter PJ, Serruys PW. Clinical, histologic and quantitative angiographic predictors of restenosis after directional coronary atherectomy: A multivariate analysis of the renarrowing process and late outcome. *J Am Coll Cardiol* 1994;23:49–58.
119. Kuntz RE, Gibson CM, Nobuyoshi M, Baim DS. Generalized model of restenosis after conventional balloon angioplasty, stenting and directional atherectomy. *J Am Coll Cardiol* 1993;21:15–25.
120. Garratt KN, Holmes DR, Bell MR, Bresnahan JF, Kaufmann UP, Vlietstra RE, Edwards WD. Restenosis after directional coronary atherectomy: Differences between primary atheromatous and restenosis lesions and influence of subintimal tissue resection. *J Am Coll Cardiol* 1990;16:1665–1671.
121. Yakubov SJ, Dick RJ, Haudenschild CC, Rosenschein U. Deep tissue retrieval with coronary atherectomy is paradoxically associated with less restenosis. *Circulation* 1991;84(Suppl II):II-520(abst).
122. Kuntz R, Hinohara T, Safian R, Selmon MR, Simpson JB, Baim DS. Restenosis after directional coronary atherectomy: Effects of luminal diameter and deep wall excision. *Circulation* 1992;86:1394–1399.
123. Schwartz RS, Huber KC, Murphy JG, Edwards WD, Camrud AR, Vlietstra RE, Holmes DR. Restenosis and the proportional neointimal response to coronary artery injury: Results in a porcine model. *J Am Coll Cardiol* 1992;19:267–274.
124. Bonan R, Paiement P, Scortichini D, Cloutier MJ, Leung TK. Coronary restenosis: Evaluation of a restenosis injury index in a swine model. *Am Heart J* 1993;126:1334–1340.
125. Humphrey WR, Simmons CA, Toombs CF, Shebuski RJ. Induction of neointimal hyperplasia by coronary angioplasty balloon overinflation: Comparison of feeder pigs to Yucatan minipigs. *Am Heart J* 1994; 127:20–31.
126. Jamal A, Bendeck M, Langille BL. Structural changes and recovery of function after arterial injury. *Arterioscler Thromb* 1992;12:307–317.
127. Lam JYT, Lacoste L, Bourassa MG. Cilazapril and early atherosclerotic changes after balloon injury of porcine carotid arteries. *Circulation* 1992;85:1542–1547.
128. Clowes AW, Clowes MM, Fingerle J, Reidy MA. Kinetics of cellular proliferation after arterial injury. V. Role of acute distension in the induction of smooth muscle proliferation. *Lab Invest* 1989;60: 360–364.
129. Clowes AW, Clowes MM, Fingerle J, Reidy MA. Regulation of smooth muscle cell growth in injured artery. *J Cardiovasc Pharmacol* 1989;14(Suppl 6):S12–S15.
130. Kraiss LW, Kirkman TR, Kohler TR, Zierler B, Clowes AW. Shear stress regulates smooth muscle proliferation and neointimal thickening in porous polytetrafluoroethylene grafts. *Arterioscler Throm* 1991; 11:1844–1852.
131. Wilcox JN, Rodriguez JC, Hanson SR, Harker LA, Lumsden AB, Kelly A. Is non-muscle myosin heavy chain expression a marker for activated smooth muscle cells? *Circulation* 1993;88(Suppl I):I-619(abst).
132. Stadius ML, Gown AM, Kernoff R, Collins CL. Cell proliferation after balloon injury of iliac arteries in the cholesterol-fed New Zealand white rabbit. *Arterioscler Thromb* 1994;14:727–733.
133. Thie M, Harrach B, Schönherr E, Kresse H, Robenek H, Rauterberg J. Responsiveness of aortic smooth muscle cells to soluble growth mediators is influenced by cell-matrix contact. *Arterioscler Thromb* 1993;13:994–1004.
134. Ferns GA, Stewart Lee AL, Anggard EE. Arterial response to mechanical injury: Balloon catheter de-endothelialization. *Atherosclerosis* 1992;92:89–104.
135. Schwartz SM, Reidy MA. Common mechanisms of proliferation of smooth muscle in atherosclerosis and hypertension. *Hum Pathol* 1987; 18:240–247.
136. Serruys PW, Luijten HE, Beatt KJ, Geuskens R, DeFeyter PJ, Brand M, Reiber JHC, Katen HJ, Es GA, Hugenholtz PG. Incidence of restenosis after successful coronary angioplasty: A time-related phenomenon. A quantitative angiographic study in 342 consecutive patients at 1, 2, 3, and 4 months. *Circulation* 1988;77:361–371.
137. Kaltenbach M, Kober G, Scherer D, Vallbracht C. Recurrence rate after successful coronary angioplasty. *Eur Heart J* 1985;6:276–281.
138. Nobuyoshi M, Tanaka M. Nosaka H, Kimura T. Late restenosis after successful percutaneous transluminal coronary angioplasty. *J Am Coll Cardiol* 1991;17(No. 6):198B(abst).
139. Shindo T, Nobuyoshi M, Nosaka H, Kimura T, Yokoi H, Abe M, Kim K, Nakagawa Y, Iwasaki Y, Kaburagi S, Tamura T, Shinoda E, Kashima K, Ojio S, Hinoi T, Sato K. Angiographic follow-up after successful PTCA. *Jpn J Interv Cardiol* 1994;97:71–79.
140. Rodriguez A, Santaera O, Larribeau M, Sosa MI, Palacios IF. Early decrease in minimal luminal diameter after successful percutaneous transluminal coronary angioplasty predicts late restenosis. *Am J Cardiol* 1993;71:1391–1395.
141. Rosing DR, Cannon RO, Watson RM, Bonow RO, Mincemoyer R, Ewels C, Leon MB, Lakatos E, Epstein SE, Kent KM. Three year anatomic, functional and clinical follow-up after successful percutaneous transluminal coronary angioplasty. *J Am Coll Cardiol* 1987;9: 1–7.
142. King SB, Schlumpf M. Ten-year completed follow-up of percutaneous transluminal coronary angioplasty: The early Zurich experience. *J Am Coll Cardiol* 1993;22:353–360.
143. Medina A, Suarez de Lezo J, Hernandez E, Pan M, Ortega JR, Romero M, Melian F, Pavlovic D, Morales J, Marrero J, Cabrera JA. Serial angiographic observations after successful directional coronary atherectomy. *Am Heart J* 1993;125:1217–1221.
144. Nakagawa Y, Iwasaki Y, Nosaka H, Kimura T, Nobuyoshi N. Serial angiographic follow-up after successful direct angioplasty for acute myocardial infarction; single center experience. *Circulation* 1993; 88(Suppl I):I-106(abst).
145. Kimura T, Nosaka H, Yokoi H, Iwabuchi M, Nobuyoshi M. Serial angiographic follow-up after Palmaz–Schatz stent implantation: Comparison with conventional balloon angioplasty. *J Am Coll Cardiol* 1993;21:1557–1563.
146. Kastrati A, Schomig A, Dietz R, Neumann FJ, Richardt G. Time course of restenosis during the first year after emergency coronary stenting. *Circulation* 1993;87:1498–1505.
147. Rensing BJ, Hermans WRM, Beatt KJ, Laarman GJ, Suryapranata H, van den Brand M, de Feyter PJ, Serruys PW. Quantitative angiographic assessment of elastic recoil after percutaneous transluminal coronary angioplasty. *Am J Cardiol* 1990;66:1039–1044.
148. Hjemdahl-Monsen RE, Ambrose JA, Borrico S, Cohen M, Sherman W, Alexopoulos D, Gorlin R, Fuster V. Angiographic patterns of balloon inflation during percutaneous transluminal coronary angioplasty: Role of pressure–diameter curves in studying distensibility and elasticity of the stenotic lesion and the mechanism of dilation. *J Am Coll Cardiol* 1990;16:569–575.
149. Fischell TA, Derby G, Tse TM, Stadius ML. Coronary artery vasoconstriction routinely occurs after percutaneous transluminal coronary angioplasty. A quantitative arteriographic analysis. *Circulation* 1988; 78:1323–1334.
150. Schatz RA, Penn IM, Baim DS. Nobuyoshi M, Colombo A, Ricci DR, Cleman MW, Goldberg S, Heuser RR, Almond D, Fish D, Moses J, Gallup D, Detre K, Leon MB. STent REStenosis Study (STRESS): Analysis of in-hospital results. *Circulation* 1993;88(Suppl I):I-594(abst).
151. Topol EJ, Califf RM, Weisman HF, Ellis SG, Tcheng JE, Worley S, Ivanhoe R, George BS, Fintel D, Weston M, Sigmon K, Anderson KM, Lee KL, Willerson JT. Randomised trial of coronary intervention with antibody against platelet IIb/IIIa integrin for reduction of clinical restenosis: Results at six months. *Lancet* 1994;343:881–886.
152. Colombo A, Hall P, Almagor Y, Malello L, Gaglione A, Nakamura S, Borrione M, Goldberg SL, Finci L, Tobis J. Results of intravascular ultrasound guided coronary stenting without subsequent anticoagulation. *J Am Coll Cardiol* 1994;23:335A(abst).
153. Gordon PC, Gibson CM, Cohen DJ, Carrozza JP, Kuntz RE, Baim DS. Mechanisms of restenosis and redilation within coronary stents—quantitative angiographic assessment. *J Am Coll Cardiol* 1993;21:1166–1174.
154. Mintz GS, Kovach JA, Javier SP, Ditrano CJ, Leon MB. Geometric remodeling is the predominant mechanism of late lumen loss after coronary angioplasty. *Circulation* 1993;88(Suppl I):I-654(abst).
155. Mintz GS, Kovach JA, Pichard AD, Kent KM, Satler LF, Popma JJ, Painter JA, Morgan K, Leon MB. Geometric remodeling is the

predominant mechanism of clinical restenosis after coronary angioplasty. *J Am Coll Cardiol* 1994;23:138A(abst).

156. Bier JD, Kakuta T, Currier JW, Mukjurjee S, Levine GN, Chodos AP, Ryan TJ, Faxon DP. Arterial remodeling: Importance in primary versus restenotic lesions. *J Am Coll Cardiol* 1994;23:139A(abst).
157. Mintz GS, Matar FA, Kent KM, Pichard AD, Satler LF, Harvey M, Ditrano CJ, Prunka N, Popma JJ, Leon MB. Chronic compensatory arterial dilatation following coronary angioplasty: An intravascular ultrasound study. *J Am Coll Cardiol* 1994;23:139A(abst).
158. Nunes GL, Sgoutas DS, Redden RA, Sigman SR, Gravanis MB, King SB III, Berk BC. Combination of vitamins C and E alters the response to coronary balloon injury in the pig. *Arterioscler Thromb Vasc Biol* 1995;15:156–165.
159. Lafont AM, Chisolm GM, Whitlow PL, Goormastic M, Cornhill JF. Post-angioplasty restenosis in the atherosclerotic rabbit: Proliferative response or chronic constriction? *Circulation* 1993;88(Suppl I):I-521(abst).
160. Kakuta T, Currier JW, Haudenschild CC, Ryan TJ, Faxon DP. Differences in compensatory vessel enlargement, not intimal formation, account for restenosis after angioplasty in the hypercholesterolemic rabbit model. *Circulation* 1994;89:2809–2815.
161. Brott BC, Labinaz M, Culp SC, Zidar JP, Fortin DF, Virmani R, Phillips HR, Stack RS. Vessel remodeling after angioplasty: Comparative anatomic studies. *J Am Coll Cardiol* 1994;23:138A(abst).
162. Post MJ, Borst C, Kuntz RE. The relative importance of arterial remodeling compared with intimal hyperplasia in lumen renarrowing after balloon angioplasty. A study in the normal rabbit and the hypercholesterolemic Yucatan micropig. *Circulation* 1994;89:2816–2821.
163. Santoian EC, Gravanis MB, Karas SP, Schneider JE, Anderberg KA, Scott NA, Cipolla G, King SB. Sequence of the reparative phenomena and development of smooth muscle proliferation following coronary angioplasty in a swine restenosis model. *Clin Res* 1992;40:364A(abst).
164. van der Giessen WJ, Serruys PW, van Beusekom HM, van Woerkens LJ, van Loon H, Soei LK, Strauss BH, Beatt KJ, Verdouw PD. Coronary stenting with a new, radiopaque, balloon-expandable endoprosthesis in pigs. *Circulation* 1991;83:1788–1798.
165. Bär FW, van Oppen J, de Swart H, van Ommen V, Havenith M, Daemen M, Leenders P, van der Veen FH, van Lankveld M, Verduin M, Braak L, Wolff R, Wellens HJJ. Percutaneous implantation of a new intracoronary stent in pigs. *Am Heart J* 1991;122:1532–1541.
166. Rodgers GP, Minor ST, Robinson K, Cromeens D, Stephens LC, Woolbert SC, Guyton JR, Wright K, Siegel R, Roubin GS, et al. The coronary artery response to implantation of a balloon-expandable flexible stent in the aspirin- and non-aspirin-treated swine model. *Am Heart J* 1991;122:640–647.
167. Schwartz RS, Edwards WD, Murphy JG, Camrud AR, Holmes DR. Restenosis develops in four stages: Serial histologic studies in a coronary injury model. *J Am Coll Cardiol* 1991;71(Suppl A):52A(abst).
168. Schwartz RS, Huber KC, Edwards WD, Bowie EJW, Nichols WL, Camrud AR, Jorgenson MA, Holmes DR. Restenosis and homozygous von Willebrand's disease: Studies in a porcine coronary model. *J Am Coll Cardiol* 1992;19(No 3):328A(abst).
169. Schwartz RS, Edwards WD, Camrud AR, Jorgenson MA, Holmes DR, Jr, Johnson RG. Tick anticoagulant peptide (TAP) inhibits neointimal thickening in a porcine coronary artery injury model. *Circulation* 1993;88:I-656(abst).
170. Simari RD, Camrud AR, Jorgenson MA, Edwards WD, Schwartz RS. Ancrod and heparin reduce reactive neointimal hyperplasia in a porcine coronary injury model. *Circulation* 1993;88(Suppl I):I-657(abst).
171. Schwartz RS, Holmes DR, Topol EJ. The restenosis paradigm revisited: An alternative proposal for cellular mechanisms [Editorial]. *J Am Coll Cardiol* 1992;20:1284–1293.
172. Ueda Y, Nanto S, Komamura K, Kodama K. Neointimal coverage of stents in human coronary arteries observed by angioscopy. *J Am Coll Cardiol* 1994;23:341–346.
173. Windsor JH, Santoian EC, Tarazona N, Robinson KA, Gu J, Dennis CA, King III SB, Heart D. Smooth muscle proliferation during neointimal development after PTCA in swine: Identification of site and sequence using proliferating cell nuclear antigen staining. *J Am Coll Cardiol* 1994;23:235A(abst).
174. Strauss BH, Umans VA, van Suylen RJ, de Feyter PJ, Marco J, Robertson GC, Renkin J, Heyndrickx G, Vuzevski VD, Bosman FT, Serruys PW. Directional atherectomy for treatment of restenosis within coronary stents: Clinical, angiographic and histologic results. *J Am Coll Cardiol* 1992;20:1465–1473.
175. Schwartz RS, Srivatsa SS, Camrud AR, Isner JM. Smooth muscle cell proliferation in coronary restenosis is limited to a few generations: Cell kinetic model implications. *J Am Coll Cardiol* 1994;23:20A(abst).
176. Nikol S, Isner JM, Pickering JG, Kearney M, Leclerc G, Weir L. Expression of transforming growth factor-beta 1 is increased in human vascular restenosis lesions. *J Clin Invest* 1992;90:1582–1592.
177. Nikol S, Weir L, Sullivan A, Sharaf B, White CJ, Zemel G, Hartzler G, Stack R, Leclerc G, Isner JM. Persistently increased expression of the transforming growth factor-beta1 gene in human vascular restenosis: Analysis of 62 patients with one or more episodes of restenosis. *Cardiovasc Pathol* 1994;3:57–64.
178. Haudenschild CC. Pathobiology of restenosis after angioplasty. *Am J Med* 1993;94:40S–44S.
179. Forrester JS, Fishbein M, Helfant R, Fagin J. A paradigm for restenosis based on cell biology: Clues for the development of new preventive therapies. *J Am Coll Cardiol* 1991;17:758–769.
180. Libby P, Schwartz D, Brogi E, Tanaka H, Clinton SK. A cascade model for restenosis. A special case of atherosclerosis progression. *Circulation* 1992;86:III47–III52.
181. Miller DD, Karim MA, Edwards WD, Schwartz RS. Subendothelial lymphoid cell infiltration is a prominent early response to porcine coronary artery injury: Relationship to resolution of neointimal fibrin. *Circulation* 1992;86(Suppl I):I-800(abst).
182. Rogers C, Karnovsky MJ, Edelman ER. Heparin's inhibition of monocyte adhesion to experimentally injured arteries matches its antiproliferative effects. *Circulation* 1993;88(No 4, Part 2):I-370(abst).
183. Guzman LA, Whitlow PL, Beall CJ, Kolattakudy P. Monocyte chemotactic protein antibody inhibits restenosis in the rabbit atherosclerotic model. *Circulation* 1993;88:I-371(abst).
184. Lundergan CF, Phillips T, Chmielinska JJ, Eisenhower E, Katz RJ. Quantitative growth factor and cytokine profile in human primary atheroma and restenosis tissue. *J Am Coll Cardiol* 1994;23:123A(abst).
185. Rao RS, Factor SM, Menegus MA, Monrad ES, Sherry B, Greenberg MA, Berman JW. Increased expression of chemokine-beta proteins in human restenotic coronary artery lesions following angioplasty. *J Am Coll Cardiol* 1994;23:123A(abst).
186. Clausell N, Lima VC, Molossi S, Turley E, Gotlieb A, Rabinovitch M, Liu P, Adelman A. Restenosis following directional coronary atherectomy is associated with inflammation and increased fibronectin. *J Am Coll Cardiol* 1994;23:124A(abst).
187. Mulvany MJ. Remodeling of resistance vessel structure in essential hypertension. *Curr Opin Nephrol Hypertens* 1993;2:77–81.
188. Gibbons GH, Dzau VJ. The emerging concept of vascular remodeling. *N Engl J Med* 1994;330:1431–1438.
189. Ardissino D, Di Somma S, Kubica J, Barberis P, Merlini PA, Eleuteri E, De Servi S, Bramucci E, Specchia G, Montemartini C. Influence of elastic recoil on restenosis after successful coronary angioplasty in unstable angina pectoris. *Am J Cardiol* 1993;71:659–663.
190. Waller BF, Johnson DE, Schnitt SJ, Pinkerton CA, Simpson JB, Baim DS. Histologic analysis of directional coronary atherectomy samples. A review of findings and their clinical relevance. *Am J Cardiol* 1993;72:80E–87E.
191. Gibson CM, Kuntz RE, Nobuyoshi M, Rosner B, Baim DS. Lesion-to-lesion independence of restenosis after treatment by conventional angioplasty, stenting, or directional atherectomy. Validation of lesion-based restenosis analysis. *Circulation* 1993;87:1123–1129.
192. Weintraub WS, Brown CL, Liberman HA, Morris DC, Douglas JS Jr, King SB. Effect of restenosis at one previously dilated coronary site on the probability of restenosis at another previously dilated coronary site. *Am J Cardiol* 1993;72:1107–1113.
193. Rensing BJ, Hermans WRM, Vos J, Tijssen JGP, Rutch W, Danchin N, Heyndrickx GR, Mast EG, Wijns W, Serruys PW, on Behalf of the Coronary Artery Restenosis Prevention on Repeated Thromboxane Antagonism (CARPORT) Study Group. Luminal narrowing after percutaneous transluminal coronary angioplasty. A study of clinical, procedural, and lesional factors related to long-term angiographic outcome. *Circulation* 1993;88:975–985.
194. Weintraub WS, Kosinski AS, Brown CL, King SB. Can restenosis after coronary angioplasty be predicted from clinical variables? *J Am Coll Cardiol* 1993;21:6–14.

195. Austin GE. Lipids and vascular restenosis [Editorial]. *Circulation* 1992;85:1613–1615.
196. Rozenman Y, Gilon D, Welber S, Sapoznikov D, Lotan C, Geist M, Weiss AT, Hasin Y, Gotsman MS. Plasma lipoproteins are not related to restenosis after successful coronary angioplasty. *Am J Cardiol* 1993;72:1206–1207.
197. Johansson SR, Wiklund O, Emanuelsson H. Lack of correlation between the serum level of lipoprotein (a) and restenosis after coronary angioplasty. *Coron Artery Disease* 1992;3:839–845.
198. Tenda K, Saikawa T, Maeda T, Sato Y, Niwa H, Inoue T, Yonemochi H, Maruyama T, Shimoyama N, Aragaki S, et al. The relationship between serum lipoprotein(a) and restenosis after initial elective percutaneous transluminal coronary angioplasty. *Jpn Circ J* 1993;57: 789–795.
199. Eber B, Schumacher M. Fibrinogen. Its role in the hemostatic regulation in atherosclerosis. *Semin Thromb Hemostasis* 1993;19:104–107.
200. Carrozza JP Jr, Kuntz RE, Fishman RF, Baim DS. Restenosis after arterial injury caused by coronary stenting in patients with diabetes mellitus. *Ann Intern Med* 1993;118:344–349.
201. Bauters C, Lablanche JM, McFadden EP, Leroy F, Bertrand ME. Repeat percutaneous coronary angioplasty; clinical and angiographic follow-up in patients with stable or unstable angina pectoris. *Eur Heart J* 1993;14:235–239.
202. Ryan TJ, Bauman WB, Kennedy JW, Kereiakes DJ, King SB, McCallister BD, Smith SC, Ullyot DJ. Guidelines for percutaneous transluminal coronary angioplasty: A report of the American College of Cardiology/American Heart Association task force on assessment of diagnostic and therapeutic cardiovascular procedures (Committee on Percutaneous Transluminal Coronary Angioplasty). *J Am Coll Cardiol* 1993;22:2033–2054.
203. Myler RK, Shaw RE, Stertzer SH, Hecht HS, Ryan C, Rosenblum J, Cumberland DC, Murphy MC, Hansell HN, Hidalgo B. Lesion morphology and coronary angioplasty: Current experience and analysis. *J Am Coll Cardiol* 1992;19:1641–1652.
204. Bauters C, McFadden EP, Lablanche JM, Quandalle P, Bertrand ME. Restenosis rate after multiple percutaneous transluminal coronary angioplasty procedures at the same site. A quantitative angiographic study in consecutive patients undergoing a third angioplasty procedure for a second restenosis. *Circulation* 1993;88:969–974.
205. Bauters C, Lablanche JM, Leroy F, Bertrand ME. Treatment of first restenosis by recurrent angioplasty. Immediate results and angiographic follow-up after 6 months. *Arch Mal Coeur Vaiss* 1992;85: 1515–1520.
206. Myler RK, Shaw RE, Stertzer SH, Hecht H, Ryan C, Cumberland DC. Restenosis after coronary angioplasty: Pathophysiology and therapeutic implications. *J Invasive Cardiol* 1993;5:278–284, 319–333.
207. Hirshfeld JW Jr, Schwartz JS, Jugo R, MacDonald RG, Goldberg S, Savage MP, Bass TA, Vetrovec G, Cowley M, Taussig AS, et al. Restenosis after coronary angioplasty: A multivariate statistical model to relate lesion and procedure variables to restenosis. The M-HEART Investigators. *J Am Coll Cardiol* 1991;18:647–656.
208. Kuntz RE, Hinohara T, Robertson GC, Safian RD, Simpson JB, Baim DS. Influence of vessel selection on the observed restenosis rate after endoluminal stenting or directional atherectomy. *Am J Cardiol* 1992; 70:1101–1108.
209. Hermans WR, Rensing BJ, Kelder JC, de Feyter PJ, Serruys PW. Postangioplasty restenosis rate between segments of the major coronary arteries. *Am J Cardiol* 1992;69:194–200.
210. Barasch E, Wilson JM, Ferguson JJ. Do vessel size and balloon artery ratio influence restenosis after PTCA. *J Am Coll Cardiol* 1994;23: 70A(abst).
211. Yokoi H, Nobuyoshi M, Kimura T, Iwabuchi M, Taniguchi C. Relation of lesion morphology and restenosis after coronary angioplasty: A quantitative angiographic analysis in 368 lesions. *Circulation* 1992; 86(Suppl I):I-530(abst).
212. Gonschior P, Nerlich A, Mack B, Fleuchaus M, Höfling B. Immunohistologic features in CAVEAT biopsies from directional atherectomy prone to restenosis. *J Am Coll Cardiol* 1994;23:124A(abst).
213. Johnson D, Hinohara T, Selmon MR, Robertson GC, Braden LJ, Simpson JB. Histologic predictors of restenosis after directed coronary atherectomy. *J Am Coll Cardiol* 1991;17(2):53A(abst).
214. Backa D, Nerlich A, Mack B, Höfling B. Histological predictors for restenoses after vascular interventions in primary arteriosclerotic lesions. *J Am Coll Cardiol* 1992;19:170A(abst).
215. Suarez de Lezo J, Romero M, Medina A, Pan M, Pavlovic D, Vaamonde R, Hernandez E, Melian F, Lopez Rubio F, Marrero J, Segura J, Irurita M, Cabrera JA. Intracoronary ultrasound assessment of directional coronary atherectomy: Immediate and follow-up findings. *J Am Coll Cardiol* 1993;21:298–307.
216. Escaned J, Violaris A, deJong M, Umans VA, deFeyter PJ, Serruys PW. A biological paradox of restenosis after directional coronary atherectomy: Enhanced smooth muscle cell outgrowth and high cellularity of retrieved specimens is associated with less luminal loss. *Circulation* 1993;88(Suppl I):I-651(abst).
217. Simons M, Leclerc G, Safian RD, Isner JM, Weir L, Baim DS. Relation between activated smooth-muscle cells in coronary-artery lesions and restenosis after atherectomy. *N Engl J Med* 1993;328:608–613.
218. Umans VA, Hermans W, Foley DP, Strikwerda S, van den Brand M, de Jaegere P, de Feyter PJ, Serruys PW. Restenosis after directional coronary atherectomy and balloon angioplasty: Comparative analysis based on matched lesions. *J Am Coll Cardiol* 1993;21:1382–1390.
219. Leaf A, Jorgensen MB, Jacobs AK, Cote G, Schoenfeld DA, Scheer J, Weiner BH, Slack JD, Kellett MA, Raizner AE, Weber PC, Mahrer PR, Rossouw JE. Do fish oils prevent restenosis after coronary angioplasty? *Circulation* 1994;90:2248–2257.
220. Emanuelsson H, Beatt KJ, Bagger J-P, Balcon R, Heikkilä J, Piessens J, Schaeffer M, Suryapranata H, Foegh M, for the European Angiopeptin Study Group. Long-term effects of angiopeptin treatment in coronary angioplasty. Reduction of clinical events but not angiographic restenosis. *Circulation* 1995;91:1689–1696.
221. The ACCORD Study Investigators U Lille. Nitric oxide donors reduce restenosis after coronary angioplasty: the ACCORD Study. *J Am Coll Cardiol* 1994;23:59A(abst).
222. Weintraub WS, Boccuzzi SJ, Klein JL, Kosinski AS, King SB III, Ivanhoe R, Cedarholm JC, Stillabower ME, Talley JD, DeMaio SJ, O'Neill WW, Frazier JE II, Cohen-Bernstein CL, Robbins DC, Brown CL III, Alexander RW, and the Lovastatin Restenosis Trial Study Group. Lack of effect of lovastatin on restenosis after coronary angioplasty. *N Engl J Med* 1994;331:1331–1337.
223. Freed MS, Safian MA, Safian RD, Jones DE, O'Neill WW, Grines CI. An intensive poly-pharmaceutical approach to the prevention of restenosis: the Mevacor, ACE-inhibitor, Colchicine (BIG-MAC) Pilot Trial. *J Am Coll Cardiol* 1993;21(Suppl A):33A(abst).
224. Shah PK, Amin J. Low high density lipoprotein level is associated with increased restenosis rate after coronary angioplasty. *Circulation* 1992;85:1279–1285.
225. Donohue B, Lasorda D, Barker E, Begg R, Vido D, Ergina F, Incorvati D, Farah T, Sgoutas D. Lp(a) correlates with restenosis after PTCA. *J Am Coll Cardiol* 1993;21:33A(abst).
226. Setsuda M, Inden M, Hiraoka N, Okamoto S, Tanaka H, Okinaka T, Nishimura Y, Okano H, Kouji T, Konishi T, et al. Probucol therapy in the prevention of restenosis after successful percutaneous transluminal coronary angioplasty. *Clin Ther* 1993;15:374–382.
227. Cooke T, Sheahan R, Foley D, Reilly M, D'Arcy G, Jauch W, Gibney M, Gearty G, Crean P, Walsh M. Lipoprotein(a) in restenosis after percutaneous transluminal coronary angioplasty and coronary disease. *Circulation* 1994;89:1593–1598.
228. Hillegass WB, Ohman EM, Leimberger JD, Califf RM. A meta-analysis of randomized trials of calcium antagonists to reduce restenosis after coronary angioplasty. *Am J Cardiol* 1994;73:835–839.
229. Leclerc G, Isner JM, Kearney M, Simons M, Safian RD, Baim DS, Weir L. Evidence implicating nonmuscle myosin in restenosis. Use of *in situ* hybridization to analyze human vascular lesions obtained by directional atherectomy. *Circulation* 1992;85:543–553.
230. Pickering JG, Weir L, Rosenfield K, Stetz J, Jekanowski J, Isner JM. Smooth muscle cell outgrowth from human atherosclerotic plaque: Implications for the assessment of lesion biology. *J Am Coll Cardiol* 1992;20:1430–1439.
231. MacLeod DC, Strauss BH, de Jong M, Escaned J, Umans VA, van Suylen RJ, Verkerk A, de Feyter PJ, Serruys PW. Proliferation and extracellular matrix synthesis of smooth muscle cells cultured from human coronary atherosclerotic and restenotic lesions. *J Am Coll Cardiol* 1994;23:59–65.
232. Foegh ML, Virmani R. Molecular biology of intimal proliferation. *Curr Opin Cardiol* 1993;8:938–950.
233. Haudenschild CC. Restenosis: Basic considerations. In: Topol EJ, ed. *Textbook of Interventional Cardiology*. Philadelphia: Saunders; 1990: 344–362.

234. Cequier A, Bonan R, Crepeau J, Cote G, De Guise P, Joly P, Lesperance J, Waters DD. Restenosis and progression of coronary atherosclerosis after coronary angioplasty. *J Am Coll Cardiol* 1988;12:49–55.
235. Le Feuvre C, Bonan R, Lespérance J, Gosselin G, Joyal M, Crépeau J. Predictive factors of restenosis after multivessel percutaneous transluminal coronary angioplasty. *Am J Cardiol* 1994;73:840–844.
236. Nguyen KP, Shaw RE, Myler RK, Webb JG, Stertzer SH. Does percutaneous transluminal coronary angioplasty accelerate atherosclerotic lesions? *Cathet Cardiovasc Diagn* 1990;21:1–6.
237. Sharaf B, Riley RS, Drew TM, Williams DO. Late (five to eight years) clinical and angiographic assessment of patients undergoing successful percutaneous transluminal coronary angioplasty. *Am J Cardiol* 1992;69:965–967.
238. Chenu PC, Schroeder E, Kremer R, Marchandise B. Long-term outcome of patients with asymptomatic restenosis after percutaneous transluminal coronary angioplasty. *Am J Cardiol* 1993;72: 1209–1211.
239. Weintraub WS, Ghazzal ZM, Cohen CL, Douglas JS, Jr, Liberman H, Morris DC, King SB. Clinical implications of late proven patency after successful coronary angioplasty. *Circulation* 1991;84:572–582.
240. Fishman RF, Kuntz RE, Carrozza JP Jr, Miller MJ, Senerchia CC, Schnitt SJ, Diver DJ, Safian RD, Baim DS. Long-term results of directional coronary atherectomy: Predictors of restenosis. *J Am Coll Cardiol* 1992;20:1101–1110.
241. Ghazzal ZMB, King III SB, Douglas Jr Js, Weintraub WS. Late angiographic status of coronary angioplasty site which was <50% narrowed 4 to 12 months after successful angioplasty. *Am J Cardiol* 1994;73: 892–894.
242. Foley JB, Chisholm RJ, Common AA, Langer A, Armstrong PW. Aggressive clinical pattern of angina at restenosis following coronary angioplasty in unstable angina. *Am Heart J* 1992;124:1174–1180.
243. Gross DR. *Animal Models in Cardiovascular Research.* Boston: Martinus Nijhoff; 1985:537–547.
244. Clowes AW, Ryan GB, Breslow JL, Karnovsky MJ. Absence of enhanced intimal thickening in the response of the carotid arterial wall to endothelial injury in hypercholesterolemic rats. *Lab Invest* 1976; 35:6–17.
245. Clowes AW, Breslow JL, Karnovsky MJ. Regression of myointimal thickening following carotid endothelial injury and development of aortic foam cell lesions in long term hypercholesterolemic rats. *Lab Invest* 1977;36:73–81.
246. Serruys PW, et al. Restenosis after coronary angioplasty: A proposal of new comparative approaches based on quantitative angiography. *Br Heart J* 1992;68:417–424.

Atherosclerosis and Coronary Artery Disease,
edited by V. Fuster, R. Ross, and E. J. Topol.
Lippincott-Raven Publishers, Philadelphia © 1996.

CHAPTER 39

Restenosis

An Assessment of Factors Important in Arterial Occlusion

Stephen M. Schwartz and Michael A. Reidy

Key Words: Angiotensin-converting enzyme; Basic fibroblast growth factor; Intima; Lumen; Neointima; Plasminogen Activator; Platelet-derived growth factor; Proliferating cell nuclear antigen; Restenosis; Transforming growth factor-β.

INTRODUCTION

In this chapter we attempt to compare and contrast current concepts of vascular narrowing following angioplasty, a phenomenon called ''restenosis.'' Most articles about restenosis proceed from the assumption that luminal narrowing occurs as a result of an accumulation of proliferative smooth muscle cells in the pathological intima (1–4). To a large extent, this view is derived from two sources of conventional wisdom. First, for the last 20 years, the most popular concept of vascular response to injury has been that put forward by Ross (5,6). In brief, this model emphasizes smooth muscle proliferation as a dominant component of atherosclerosis in terms of both lesion formation and progression. It seems only reasonable to imagine that the same process(es) would play key roles in the accelerated narrowing of the lumen seen after angioplasty. Second, animal models of response to injury have shown a dramatic proliferative response to vascular injury with balloon catheters. Sophisticated methods have been developed in an attempt to determine the mechanisms underlying the smooth muscle proliferative response. These animal models use catheters similar to the angioplasty devices used in humans. It seems reasonable, therefore, to proceed on the assumption that the exuberant smooth muscle cell proliferation seen following injury to either normal or previously atherosclerotic animal vessels also happens in human vessels following therapeutic angioplasty.

This view of restenosis could be erroneous. Clinical trials in humans based on successful animal studies have not led to a reduction in the incidence or extent of restenosis following angioplasty (7). This lack of success could result from species differences or a lack of adequate understanding of the pharmacology involved in restenosis. However, the lack of

S. M. Schwartz and M. A. Reidy: Department of Pathology, University of Washington School of Medicine, Seattle, Washington 98195.

success in clinical trials of drugs may also indicate that animal studies have modeled the wrong process or at least not all the processes that occur in human restenosis. Indeed, it is intriguing to note that a recent study in the swine-stent model actually showed an increase in restenosis when an injured wall was irradiated to prevent cell proliferation (8).

SPECIAL PROPERTIES OF THE ATHEROSCLEROTIC INTIMA

In examining the process of restenosis, it is important to realize that atherosclerosis is a process specifically localized to the intima of blood vessels, and the special properties of the intima must be taken into account in considering the problem of plaque progression or the responses of plaques to angioplasty. The properties of most relevance to restenosis presumably are those that characterize intimal smooth muscle cells, including their contractile mechanisms, receptors controlling movement and growth, synthesis of extracellular matrix, and adherence molecules, among other critical features (Table 1). Such properties could reflect genetic differences between plaque and medial smooth muscle cells (9) or the effects of chronic inflammatory events occurring within the plaque (10).

As can be seen in the short list in Table 1, human plaques overexpress a large number of genes that are generally not seen in the normal wall or even in the injured wall of an animal model. Many of these are molecules that might positively or negatively affect the proliferative response to injury. In the absence of direct evidence, it may be incorrect to assume that such abnormal tissue will respond as do relatively healthy walls, even in an atherosclerotic animal.

TABLE 1. *Intimal versus medial genes*

Intima	Media
Thrombin receptor	Integrin-α_1
PDGF-β receptor	Integrin-$\alpha_1\beta_3$
PDGF B chain	SM myosin SM1
ACE	Phosphoglucomutase
Tissue factor	*meta*-Vinculin
Osteopontin	SM myosin SM2
ICAM	Calponin
Lipoprotein lipase	Desmin
Cytokeratin 8	IGF-1
VCAM	SM α-actin
PAI-1	Integrin-$\alpha^{v}\beta_1$
Fibronectin, EDA form	
Tenascin	
BMP	
MCSF-1	
Laminin B chain	
PDGF A chain	
Nonmuscle myosin	
Elastin	
AT1 receptor	
H-19 mRNA	

MECHANISM OF LUMEN OCCLUSION IN ATHEROSCLEROSIS

Most investigators believe that neointimal formation is the principal cause of lumen narrowing in atherosclerosis and in the restenosis that occurs after angioplasty (5). Much of this hypothesis is based on the assumption that formation of a neointima implies that this mass intrudes into the lumen. The experimental data supporting the assumption that intimal mass obstructs the lumen or large vessels, however, are confusing. Glagov et al., for example, noted that human vessels can undergo massive accumulations of atherosclerotic plaque with narrowing of the lumen. In this case, the wall compensates for the lesion by remodeling and dilating to permit a normal level of blood flow (11). Compensatory structural change is a normal response that allows the vessel to maintain normal levels of blood flow and wall stress and can be seen in small muscular arteries as well as in large elastic arteries (12,13). Interestingly, when Langille and O'Donnell studied the balloon-injured rabbit carotid artery, they found no narrowing of the lumen despite an increase in wall thickness (14). The same study, however, showed a significant (14%) narrowing in response to an experimental restriction of flow in the vicinity of the thyroid artery, where endothelium had regenerated (13). The effect of the endothelium in an injured vessel was consistent with observations that structural adaptation to changes in flow requires the presence of an endothelium (14). Because reendothelialization generally correlates with a diminution of intimal thickening (15), these data may even imply a *negative* correlation of intimal mass with luminal narrowing. Conversely, the decrease in lumen size in areas where there was an intact endothelium is poorly understood but offers an important alternative mechanism to explain luminal narrowing, especially in human lesions, where there may be extensive vascularization of the plaque by transmural vessels (16). Thus, endothelial-induced remodeling may be as important as intimal thickening in determining lumen size.

The relative role of intimal hyperplasia versus remodeling may relate to the size of the vessel being studied and the extent of the injury, or to other, unknown variables. Drugs that decrease the smooth muscle proliferative response have been shown to decrease the extent of luminal narrowing in at least some models of response to balloon injury (17). As already noted, Glagov et al., studying human coronary artery disease at autopsy, found that vessel lumens showed a compensatory dilation as lesion mass increased, resulting in a maintenance or even dilatation of the lumen as atherosclerosis increased. However, when the lesion mass reached about 40% of the area encompassed by the internal elastic lamina, the ability to compensate was lost, and further increases in lesion size led to a decrease in lumen size (11). Because animal models have generally been created in vessels with an initially normal lumen, the processes involved in narrowing may be very different from those that lead either to the progressive narrowing seen in human atherosclerosis or to changes following angioplasty of a vessel that already has a lesion size beyond Glagov's limit.

RAT CAROTID ARTERY: A SIMPLE MODEL OF NEOINTIMAL FORMATION

Although "intima" may be defined as a normal structure that occurs during development, the term "neointima" refers to a new intimal tissue formed in response to injury. This distinction may be important, because most of our knowledge of the response to balloon injury comes from studies of formation of the neointima in the rat carotid artery.

The rat carotid injury model is appealing because the rat carotid artery is a very simple vessel, consisting only of endothelium and media. There is normally no intima and no penetration of the media by vasa vasorum. Moreover, neointimal formation is a very simple process in the rat, involving only the injured wall and platelets (18,19). No fibrillar fibrin is found at the site of injury, and leukocytes are not attracted to the site. In contrast, arterial injury in larger animals, especially with dietary modifications, can involve leukocytic interactions, fibrin formation, and an angiogenic response that penetrates the media. The simplicity of the rat model has greatly facilitated identification of molecular and pharmacological mechanisms involved in the formation of a neointima.

As we discuss later, we do not know whether the processes involved in forming a neointima are also important in the response of lesions to angioplasty. Human vessels are not identical to those of rats; the atherosclerotic vessel already has an intima before undergoing angioplasty, and the lesions of atherosclerosis have necrosis, inflammation, plaque angiogenesis, and lipid—all properties that could have profound effects on the response to angioplasty. Nevertheless, the rat model is a simple and essential starting point that is useful in understanding the responses of more complex vessels.

It is important to realize that neointimal formation is a general response to a wide range of stimuli, including irradiation, application of turpentine to the adventitia, wrapping the vessel, and electrical stimulation, as well as mechanical injuries, including placement of a suture, scratching with a probe, or dilatation of the common carotid artery with an embolectomy balloon catheter (18,20–26). The best-studied procedure uses a balloon catheter to dilate the vessel. This procedure causes complete destruction of the endothelium over the length of the vessel as well as medial smooth muscle cell death (15% to 25%) from stretching injury (19,27). During the first 24 h after denudation, platelets adhere and form a monolayer on the exposed subendothelial surface (19). Although coagulation enzymes from the plasma are probably activated by exposure to the subendothelium, accumulation of insoluble fibrin is rarely observed by scanning or transmission electron microscopy of injured rat arteries (28). The smooth muscle cell response to balloon injury by replicating and then migrating into the intima ultimately culminates in the formation of a new layer of muscular tissue, the neointima, inside the internal elastic lamina. Luminal narrowing does occur after injury to the rat carotid artery (19). The early stenosis (2 weeks) results from smooth muscle contraction of the vessel and an increase in cell mass, but stenosis seen at late times (12 weeks) results only from intimal thickening or remodeling (Fig. 1).

The smooth muscle cell response to injury follows a pattern that can be conveniently broken down into three phases or waves (Fig. 2a). The first wave is the burst of medial smooth muscle cell proliferation that peaks within a few days after injury and subsides within the next 10 days following repopulation of the media to the preinjury level (Fig. 2a). This proliferative response is caused by the synchronous entry into the cell cycle of 9% to 16% of the smooth muscle

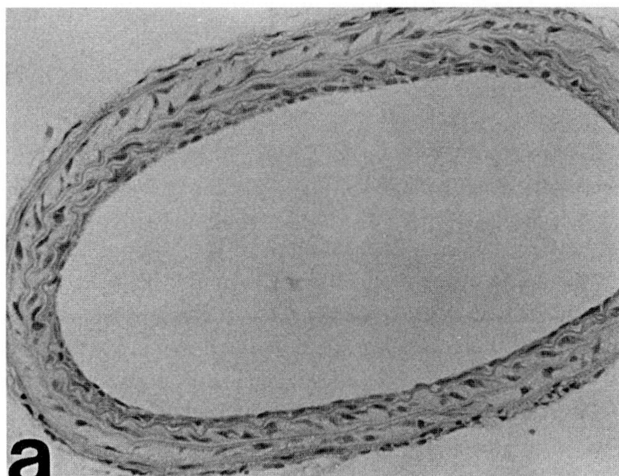

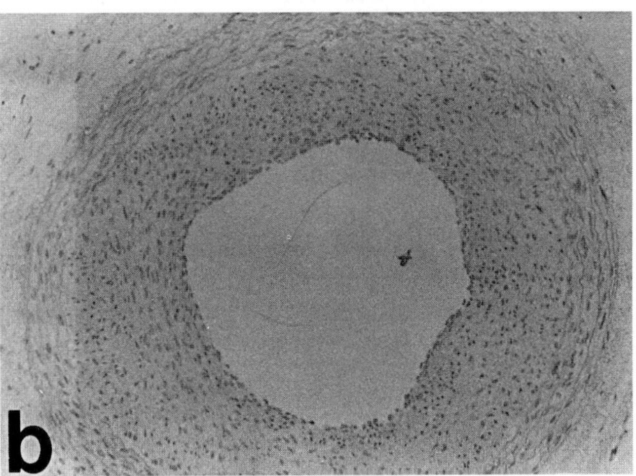

FIG. 1. Rat carotid artery. **(A)** Control uninjured artery; **(B)** artery 6 weeks after balloon catheter injury. Note that the intima is two to three times thicker than the media and that the lumen size is markedly reduced as compared to control.

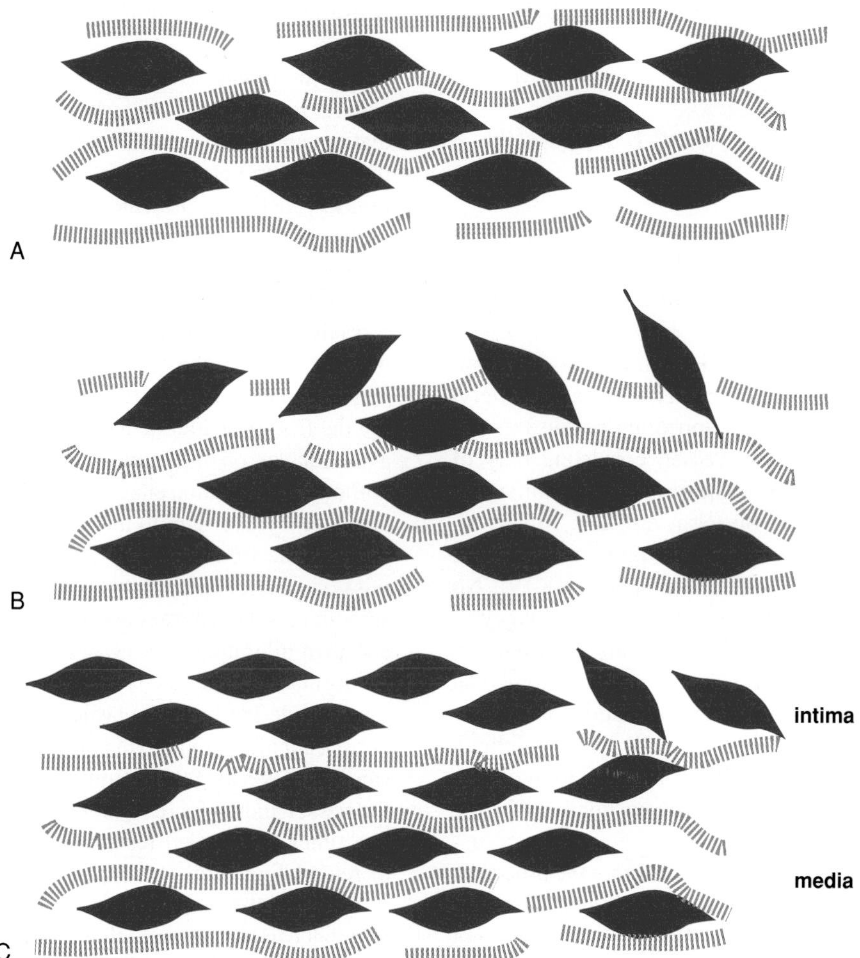

FIG. 2. The three waves. **(A)** First wave. Balloon catheter injury removes the endothelium and causes variable damage to the underlying medial cells. Within 48 h the replication rate of the medial smooth muscle cells of rat carotid artery is frequently increased to 9% to 16%. **(B)** Second wave. Within 4 days after balloon injury, medial smooth muscle cells migrate from the media into the intima, and, in the continued absence of the endothelium, these cells form a pseudoendothelium. The precise duration of migration is not known, but our data with rat arteries suggest that migration is completed after 2 weeks. **(C)** Third wave. Once intimal smooth muscle cells have migrated to the intima, they undergo extensive replication for the next 2 weeks. The increase in size of the intima (see Fig. 1) most probably results from this cell proliferation. After 2 weeks some cells continue to replicate; however, the intima does not enlarge.

cells remaining in the media (19). Replication in the media 2 days after balloon injury is similar whether or not rats are rendered thrombocytopenic with an antibody against circulating platelets (29). This result suggests that platelet-derived products, such as platelet-derived growth factor (PDGF), do not play a major role in initiation of smooth muscle cell proliferation in the media following injury. As discussed below, basic fibroblast growth factor (bFGF) appears to play the central role in the first wave.

The second wave results from migration of smooth muscle cells across the internal elastic lamina to form the intima (Fig. 2b). Smooth muscle cells are readily observed on the luminal side of the internal elastic lamina 4 days after injury. The duration of the second wave in the rat injured carotid is not known, nor do we know whether first-wave replication is required before smooth muscle migration. It is clear, however, that migration can be greatly stimulated without any increase in smooth muscle cell replication (30). Smooth muscle cell migration is probably reduced once medial smooth muscle cells have stopped replicating, because cellular depletion of the media does not occur. Mural thrombosis may be an important contribution to the second wave. Elimination of circulating platelets, a treatment that does not affect the first wave, prevents the appearance of smooth muscle cells on the luminal side of the internal elastic lamina at day 4 after balloon injury (29). Depletion of circulating platelets also significantly reduces the size of the intimal lesion at day 7 after injury. A similar result was obtained when PDGF was blocked by administration of an antibody. Migration of cells into the intima was markedly suppressed at day 4 (31), and the intimal lesion was also reduced (32). This treatment had no effect on smooth muscle cell replication.

The third wave refers to the sustained proliferation of intimal smooth muscle cells, which contributes to the rapid growth of the lesion during the first 4 weeks after injury (Fig. 2c). Chronic proliferation in the intima is particularly striking at the luminal surface of the lesion, where the number of smooth muscle cells incorporating tritiated thymidine is consistently higher than in the deeper layers of the intima as late as 12 weeks after injury (33). The pharmacology of the third wave is still poorly defined. Treatment with an antibody to bFGF 4 and 5 days after injury does not affect intimal smooth muscle cell proliferation (34), although the addition of bFGF does stimulate intimal smooth muscle cell replication (35). Large doses of transforming growth factor-β (TGF-β) given 2 weeks after injury increase modestly the percentage of proliferating cells in the intima (36). In vivo infusion of angiotensin II (AII) in the third and fourth week after injury markedly increased DNA synthesis in intimal and medial smooth muscle cells as well as the cross-sectional area of intimal and medial lesions (37).

A potential "fourth wave" can be considered when the neointima is restimulated. Study of the pharmacology of these responses is only beginning: FGF, AII, and TGF-β are all able to restimulate intimal replication (35–37), although the rates of replication achieved never come close to the values seen in the media soon after balloon injury (35). On the other hand, the fourth wave represents a proliferative response in existing intima and may therefore be more like the proliferative response occurring in the intima of human arteries responding to injury.

Finally, although we have emphasized cell replication, total changes in mass also depend on synthesis of cell matrix. Deposition of extracellular matrix by intimal smooth muscle cells further contributes to the growth of the fibromuscular lesion until 3 months following injury, after which time the intima appears stable (19). Matrix components synthesized in the injured vessel include collagen type I, elastin, osteopontin, and proteoglycans (38–40). Indeed, in injured rat arteries, approximately 80% of the intima is made up of matrix.

CRITICAL MOLECULES IN NEOINTIMAL FORMATION

Fibroblast Growth Factor

Basic FGF is perhaps the best understood mitogen active in the arterial wall (34,35,41). Basic, but not acidic, FGF is normally found in the rat vessel wall and appears to be primarily intracellular. If a vessel is gently denuded so as not to injure medial smooth muscle cells, the first wave is largely abolished (42). If, however, FGF is infused at the time of injury, proliferation still occurs. On the other hand, if the animal is pretreated with an antibody to FGF, the first wave is again abolished (34). Central to the role of bFGF in the arterial wall is its displacement from an intracellular location, where it is inactive, to one where it can interact with the FGF high-affinity receptors on the extracellular side of the cell membrane. This is difficult to demonstrate directly, but we have used heparin, which has a strong affinity for bFGF, to show that bFGF is indeed released after injury (43). Administration of heparin has no effect on bFGF concentration in an uninjured artery, which we believe supports the idea that it is located in an intracellular pool. In contrast, if heparin is given immediately following balloon injury, there is a dramatic loss of bFGF from the arterial wall that coincides with a marked reduction in smooth muscle cell replication. We interpret these data as displacement of bFGF from its intracellular storage pool to the extracellular environment, where it is bound to heparin and so transported away from the artery. Thus, FGF is present in the artery, can be released from injured cells, and is sufficient to account for the first wave of DNA synthesis by medial smooth muscle cells.

Intriguingly, abolishing the first wave by administration of the FGF antibody does not abolish intimal thickening (34). Thus, migration and intimal cell proliferation must be critical parts of lesion formation and seem to be controlled by factors different from those important for the first wave (34,36,37). These studies differ from experiments in which antisense has been used to block neointimal lesion growth, and in some circumstances medial cell replication was reduced by this procedure (44,45). One possible explanation for this finding is that antisense treatment affects multiple targets in these injured arteries by some unknown mechanism.

Platelet-Derived Growth Factor

In vitro studies have emphasized that multipotential role of PDGF as a stimulant of smooth muscle proliferation, migration, and matrix synthesis. The PDGF seems to play a more limited role in vivo, at least in the rat. We know, for example, that PDGF has very little mitogenic effect in the first wave but does appear to increase the numbers of cells that cross the internal elastic lamella (30,32). Other molecules, including FGF, also stimulate migration (46), and the relative contributions of different molecules remain to be explored. Platelet-derived growth factor has little detectable effect on replication in the third wave, but overexpression of PDGF A chain is prominent in areas of the neointima that show elevated replication (47). In contrast, PDGF is a consistent mitogen for smooth muscle in vitro but is only a weak mitogen in vivo (30). The contrast between observations in vivo and in vitro casts some doubt on the validity of in vitro assays of smooth muscle growth control. A recent report from Lindner et al. (48) indicates that a percentage of smooth muscle cells in both normal and injured arteries express PDGF B chain as well as the β-receptor in vivo, which agrees with an older report showing that intimal smooth muscle cells in vitro express PDGF B chain (49). Unfortunately, these new data still do not suggest a role for PDGF in the injured artery because, as stated above, PDGF is at best a weak mitogen in the response of the rat carotid artery. One possibility is that local release of PDGF B chain from these smooth muscle cells in the intima may stimulate chronic migration of cells into the intima, but without a marker for migration, these data are difficult to obtain.

Transforming Growth Factor-β

The potential role of TGF-β in these processes is very intriguing: TGF-β may contribute to connective tissue accumulation as well as to cell proliferation (50).

Transforming growth factor-β is present in the neointima of balloon-injured rats. Infusion of TGF-β causes a restimulation of replication in the neointima (36). Moreover, when TGF-β is overexpressed within the vessel wall, the result is a remarkable increase in connective tissue matrix formation in the neointima (51). Finally, antibody to TGF-β inhibits neointima formation in the rat model (52). All of this suggests a potentially central role for TGF-β in plaque progression or restenosis.

Most studies in vitro have argued for a role for TGF-β as an inhibitor of smooth muscle proliferation. In part, this set of studies may be confusing because the ability of TGF-β to act as a mitogen appears to be complicated by the strain of smooth muscle cells studied, the population density, and the availability of other mitogens (53,54). Gibbons and coworkers showed that the mitogenic effects of AII were enhanced by a TGF-β inhibitory antibody. These authors noted the sometimes contradictory literature on AII as an in vitro mitogen and proposed that the variability had to do with the ability of these cells to synthesize and activate autocrine TGF-β (55).

An intriguing indication for a potential role for TGF-β comes from a recent report that the activity of this growth factor in atherosclerosis may be influenced by a major risk factor, lipoprotein (a) [Lp(a)]. The Lp(a) levels in humans correlate highly with atherosclerosis risk (56). A recent study, moreover, suggests that apolipoprotein [apo (a)] levels may also correlate with increased incidence of restenosis (56). The apoprotein for this lipoprotein, apo (a), is highly homologous with plasminogen activator (PA) and is believed to have a procoagulant effect by inhibiting the formation of plasmin. Current theory suggests that the proatherosclerotic effect is the result of deficient clot lysis. Grainger and his colleagues, however, have pointed out that plasmin, besides its role as a thrombolytic enzyme, is essential to the activation of TGF-β. Apolipoprotein (a) competes with PA for membrane sites required for the latter's activity. Grainger and his colleagues found that apo (a) was mitogenic for smooth muscle cells in culture but that this effect resulted from prevention of the activation of TGF-β as an endogenous growth inhibitor (57). In this view, the predominant role of TGF-β would be as an endogenous inhibitor of lesion formation at sites of active coagulation. Apolipoprotein (a) would enhance lesion formation by diminishing the production of activated TGF-β. On the other hand, as already noted, not all in vitro studies find that TGF-β is inhibitory. Battegay et al. (54) showed that TGF-β, under several circumstances, is mitogenic in vitro, consistent with Majesky's observation (36) that TGF-β is mitogenic for the neointima following balloon injury in the rat.

Proteases

Much of the work on restenosis has focused on the early replication of smooth muscle cells following injury, the "first wave." Inhibition of the first wave, however, will not inhibit growth of intimal lesions. Following the replication of medial smooth muscle cells in the rat injured artery, there is a period when smooth muscle cells move to the intima and thus form the beginnings of a lesion. As mentioned above, PDGF and bFGF stimulate smooth muscle cell migration in injured rat arteries, and inhibition of either factor will significantly suppress migration (31,46). Critical to the process is the expression of proteases that cause matrix digestion and thereby permit cell movement. Work on the molecules that control this process in the arterial wall is in its infancy, but recent data have implicated both PA and certain matrix metalloproteinases (MMP) in lesion development (31,58).

Balloon catheter injury induces expansion of both u-PA and t-PA in rat arteries and a marked increase in plasmin activity at day 3 after injury, which is sustained for approximately another 10 days (31). This time sequence is interesting because the earliest time smooth muscle cells are found in the intima is 4 days after injury. Plasmin can be blocked in vivo with the inhibitor transexamic acid (31), which binds to the lysine binding site of both plasminogen and plasmin. In these studies, a significant reduction in the rate of smooth muscle cell migration in ballooned arteries was found after treatment with this drug, with no concomitant change in cell replication. An interesting finding is that heparin, a well-documented inhibitor of intimal lesion growth, also inhibits arterial plasmin activity and cell migration (59). Thus, the ability of heparin to inhibit intimal hyperplasia (60) may result from an effect on migration as well as replication.

Another group of proteolytic enzymes, MMP, are important for smooth muscle migration. The MMP are found in both normal tissues and metastatic tumors, which have the ability to degrade a variety of matrix molecules. Recently, two gelatinases, MMP2 and MMP9, have been reported to be present in injured rat arteries (58). Within 6 h after balloon injury, a significant increase in mRNA of an 88-kDa gelatinase (MMP9) is observed, which remained elevated for approximately 6 days. Expression was not seen in the intima, nor was it correlated with the presence of smooth muscle cell replication. The transcript for 72-kDa gelatinase (MMP2) was present in normal arteries and showed little change after injury. The activity of MMP in balloon-injured rat arteries was assessed by zymography, and within 1 day an increase in 88-kDa activity was observed. Both inactive and active MMP2 were observed in control arteries, but by day 4 a marked increase in active MMP2 was noted (58). Thus, there is a correlation in balloon-injured arteries between the expression of MMP9 and activities of MMP9 and MMP2 and the migration of smooth muscle cells into the intima. The importance of these proteases for the development of arterial lesions is currently not well understood, but using a metalloprotease inhibitor blocked the migration of smooth muscle cells into the intima and markedly reduced intimal lesion size by day 10 (58). These data illustrate that migration is a critical event in lesion growth in rat arteries and that proteases that facilitate the breakdown of matrix proteins are necessary.

Although these data show that migration is critical for lesion growth in normal arteries, the question arises whether cell migration is necessary or important for lesion growth in arteries that already possess intimal smooth muscle cells. In such arteries, one possibility is that intimal lesion growth occurs solely by replication of the existing intimal cells. Currently there are no reliable markers for cell migration, and therefore, we are not able to answer this question. It will be important to determine the answer, because thus far many successful protocols for inhibiting intimal lesions in the rat use agents that inhibit smooth muscle cell migration (61–63). Both PDGF antibodies and the angiotensin-converting enzyme inhibitors fall into this category, and these treatments were found to have no effect on intimal cell replication, yet they successfully inhibit lesion growth in the rat. The process of smooth muscle cell migration has not thus far been shown to be important in humans.

CRITICAL MOLECULES IN PROCESSES MORE COMPLEX THAN NEOINTIMAL FORMATION

Coagulation

Animal model studies in systems more complex than the rat, especially of stent models in the pig, suggest that thrombosis may well play a key role in the early events leading to restenosis (64), and, of course, the observation that advanced atherosclerotic plaques show repeated thrombotic-coagulative events is an old finding.

Evidence for thrombin is critical to this argument for intramural coagulation in restenosis in the forming intima. Hatton et al. showed that thrombin activity remains elevated over balloon-injured vessels in animals for weeks after injury (65); in contrast, the platelet response is over in 1 to 2 days (19). Moreover, indirect evidence implies that thrombin is functioning in vivo after balloon injury. We showed that the pattern of gene expression for the PDGF receptors and PDGF A chain following balloon injury in vivo closely follows the pattern seen when cultured smooth muscle cells are treated with thrombin (66). Other growth factors and vasoactive molecules do not reproduce this pattern. Activation by thrombin might also explain the synthesis of PDGF B chain by endothelial cells and by macrophages within advanced atherosclerotic plaques (67,68). A thrombin pathway is of special interest because many other pathways may be activated via proteolytic activity, and thrombin may activate or deactivate other molecules implicated in the response of thrombin to injury, including plasmin (31,59). Moreover, there is evidence that nonproteolytic domains of thrombin have their own activities (69,70), and the protease itself may have different substrate specificities depending on occupation of thrombin's allosteric binding sites by heparin, thrombomodulin, the hirudin-like sequence of the thrombin receptor, or perhaps as-yet undefined protease nexins within the vessel wall.

Analyses of the possible role of coagulation in lesions may depend on the use of thrombin inhibitors. For example, animal model studies of thrombus formation following deep arterial injury suggest that anticoagulants are more effective than agents directed at platelets (71). Moreover, hirudin, a potent thrombin inhibitor, significantly inhibited arterial smooth muscle replication when administered locally in high concentrations. Thrombin may be important not only in terms of coagulation and mitogenesis but also directly via its effects on platelets; in this way, thrombin could control a wide range of components of the proliferative response of vessels to injury. Mitogenesis, moreover, is only one of the possible direct actions of thrombin on the vessel wall in restenosis. Thrombin could play a major role in remodeling if remodeling is the result of chronic stimulation of smooth muscle contraction. Thrombin stimulates endothelial cells to produce EDRF, and EDRF results in smooth muscle relaxation and possibly growth inhibition. In contrast, thrombin acts directly on the smooth muscle cells as a vasoconstrictor. It seems likely that such a mechanism plays an important role in the ability of small vessels to contract at sites of vascular injury while neighboring vessels, their endothelium still intact, are stimulated to increase their blood flow. Similar mechanisms might contribute on the one hand to vasospasm and on the other hand to control of blood flow through the adventitial vessels that supply the base of the atherosclerotic plaque (72). Finally, the contractile effect of α-thrombin may be synergistically increased in the presence of epidermal growth factor (EGF), suggesting that the combination of α-thrombin and EGF-like material derived from platelets (e.g., TGF-α) may contribute to vasospasm in vessels where the endothelium is absent (73).

Angiotensin

The renin–angiotensin system is worthy of special attention because of the apparent failure of angiotensin-converting enzyme (ACE) inhibitors as restenosis antagonists in humans (7) despite extensive studies in experimental animal models of restenosis (61,62,74–76).

The first issue may be the mechanism of action. Evidence that angiotensin can act as a mitogen for smooth muscle in vitro is contradictory (55,77,78). In vivo, however, angiotensin is mitogenic and is most effective on neointima cells (37). The reasons for this special property of the neointima are not clear. Because angiotensin I generation by renin is submaximal at normal plasma concentrations of angiotensinogen, higher levels of angiotensinogen in the vasculature are likely to result in a higher rate of angiotensin I generation and an increase in local levels of AII (79). Whether vascular ACE is up-regulated following injury is still a matter of controversy. Rakugi et al. (80) reported that, 2 weeks after injury, the carotid expressed increased levels of ACE activity as well as immunoreactivity using a polyclonal human and monoclonal rat ACE antibody. Viswanathan et al. (81), however, used quantitative autoradiography and reported that binding to ACE in the aortic neointima 15 days after injury was not different from binding in the underlying media or the media of sham-operated animals. Taken together, these observations suggest that ACE activity per unit of wall mass is not increased in the vascular wall 2 weeks after injury. Whether ACE activity is acutely increased earlier after injury remains to be determined. Preliminary data from Fishel et al. (82) suggest that ACE activity in cultured smooth muscle cells is stimulated by bFGF, a growth factor that has been associated with the first wave of smooth muscle cell proliferation after vascular injury. Finally, Viswanathan et al. have shown elevated levels of AT1 receptor binding in the neointima (81). In summary, AII is a mitogen in vivo, the neointima may be able to generate elevated levels of AII, and the neointima overexpresses receptors for AII. Thus, inhibitors of AII formation or blockers for the angiotensin receptor might be expected to be effective against neointimal formation.

The critical issue of clinical relevance is the effect of ACE inhibitors on the three waves. The rat model produces a new intima within 2 weeks after injury. Because restenosis in humans may take months to produce a significant occlusion, we need to consider which waves are affected by ACE inhibitors and are most likely to be effective in humans. The ACE inhibitors affect smooth muscle cell migration in response to injury. Prescott et al. (62) reported that the ACE inhibitor benazeprilat reduced intimal lesion size by 35% 12 days after balloon catheterization of the rat carotid. Treatment with benazeprilat did not affect medial smooth muscle cell proliferation at day 2 after injury but reduced by 68% the number of smooth muscle cells appearing on the luminal side of the internal elastic lamina at day 4, suggesting that smooth muscle cell migration was suppressed. Interestingly, AII has been shown to stimulate migration of cultured smooth muscle cells in an in vitro wound assay system (83). Effects on the replicative component of the lesion are less clear, especially in the more chronic stages of the third wave.

The neointima in rats remains replicative at low but elevated levels for months after injury (33). Moreover, the neointima is hyperresponsive to AII. In vivo infusion of a hypertensive dose of AII during the third and fourth weeks after injury induces smooth muscle cell proliferation in the normal and injured arterial wall (37). The mitogenic effect of hypertension induced by AII appears to depend on the proliferative status of vascular smooth muscle cells, as it was more marked in smooth muscle cells from the neointima than in those from the underlying media. The cumulative labeling fraction of the injured carotid artery was increased from 5% to 20% in the intima, whereas it was increased from 0.2% to 2.5% in the underlying media. The reasons for the increased propensity of smooth muscle cells to proliferate in the neointima are not known, but this property may reflect the altered phenotype of intimal smooth muscle cells, which include increased levels of AT1 receptor expression in vivo (81) or the modulating influence of local factors such as matrix components or growth factors. Infusion of AII during the first 2 weeks of lesion development increases intimal lesion size and seems to reverse at least partially the suppressive effect of cilazapril (63). Increased responsiveness to exogenous AII, however, may not imply that the endogenous replication is caused by the angiotensin system.

Suppression of intimal thickening by ACE inhibitors depends on when and for how long the drug is administered. Lesion size 2 weeks after injury to the rat carotid artery was significantly reduced when daily administration of cilazapril was started 6 days before injury (77% inhibition of intima to media area ratio), but also when daily treatment was initiated as late as 1 h before injury (58% inhibition) or even 2 days after injury (58% inhibition). The increased effectiveness of the earlier administration of the drug may reflect the time needed to achieve complete inhibition of ACE. Intimal thickening at 2 weeks was not affected by a single administration of cilazapril 1 h before injury or when the drug was given 6 days before until 2 days after injury. Finally, prolongation of the treatment with cilazapril for 8 weeks after injury did not result in better inhibition as compared with a 2-week treatment followed by six weeks of placebo (61,63). Taken together, these data suggest that the vascular response to injury is particularly sensitive to ACE inhibitors at the time of intense smooth muscle cell migration and proliferation shortly after trauma rather than at later times, when smooth muscle cell contribution to intimal lesion growth is mainly through extracellular matrix production. Thus, the failure to suppress restenosis with ACE inhibitors in humans may occur because such late events, not the first three waves, are critical to human restenosis. Finally, trials with ACE inhibitors in humans may be misleading for other reasons. Angiotensin-converting enzyme has substrates other than angiotensin I, and these substrates, including bradykinin, may also play a role in neointimal formation or stenosis. Effective doses for inhibition of intima formation greatly exceed the dose required to treat hypertension and therefore the dose used in clinical trials. A second problem with the use of ACE inhibitors in humans as compared to rats is that human chymase is able to convert angiotensin I to AII (84). Thus, in humans, there is a second ACE that is not sensitive to the usual "ACE inhibitors."

PROLIFERATION IN HUMAN RESTENOTIC CORONARY ARTERY LESIONS

In contrast to the wealth of information that is available on the proliferation kinetics in animal models of arterial injury and repair, little is known about the proliferative profile of human restenotic coronary artery lesions. To begin with, it is important to point out that most studies that have described proliferation in human restenotic coronary arteries have not used an objective measurement of replication. For example, Nobuyoshi et al. examined the histological findings in 39 dilated lesions from 20 patients who had undergone antemortem coronary angioplasty (85). The extent of intimal proliferation, defined by the presence of these stellate-shaped cells of the so-called synthetic smooth muscle cell phenotype, was significantly greater in lesions with evidence of medial or adventital tears than in those without tears or with tears limited to the intima. Nobuyoshi assumed that cells with this morphology has recently proliferated. Unfortunately, these "proliferative-like" stellate cells are commonly seen in primary atherosclerotic coronary artery lesions that have never been exposed to an interventional device (86,87). Similar morphology is also seen in normal intima if one selectively looks just beneath the endothelium of human arteries (88,89).

Because stellate cells are seen in normal arterial wall and in plaque, their apparent increase in number might be an artifactual result of a change in the sampling of cells already in the wall as a result of the redistribution of cell types secondary to the dilatation. For example, it is conceivable that primary coronary atherectomy specimens may include more of the superficial luminal layer. Typically this is the fibrous cap. With subsequent restenotic biopsies, deeper layers of the plaque may be removed. Alternatively, the stellate cells could represent a phenotypic change in preexisting cells. In either case, one must be careful not to assume that differences in histology between primary and restenotic coronary atherectomy specimens, which may have been longstanding and preceded the initial procedure, are necessarily caused by a difference in vessel wall biology that occurred with the so-called restenotic process.

Two other approaches have been used to attempt to determine the role of proliferation in restenosis. Recently, we have used immunocytochemical labeling for the proliferating cell nuclear antigen (PCNA) to determine the proliferative profile of 100 restenotic coronary atherectomy specimens (90). The PCNA is regulated at both the pre- and posttranscriptional levels, and the protein is expressed during S phase (as well as G_1 and G_2) of the cell cycle (91). To our surprise, the vast majority of the restenotic specimens (74%) had no evidence of PCNA labeling. The majority of the remaining specimens had only a modest number of PCNA-positive cells per slide (typically <50 cells per slide). On the basis of the mean number of nuclei per slide, the vast majority of these specimens had ≤1% of all cells labeled PCNA-positive. Labeling for PCNA was detected over a wide time interval after the initial procedure (e.g., 1 to 390 days) with no obvious proliferative peak. There was no difference in the proliferative profile of restenotic specimens collected in the first 3 months, 4 to 6 months, 7 to 9 months, or >9 months after the initial interventional procedure (Spearman rank correlation coefficient = 0.081, p = 0.43). Furthermore, only 12 of 30 specimens obtained within 60 days of the initial coronary interventional procedure had one or more PCNA-positive nuclei per slide (including nine specimens collected within 6 days of the initial procedure, only three of which had immunolabeling of 1, 7, and 20 cells per slide) (90). Moreover, a recent preliminary report of in vitro bromodeoxyuridine labeling of restenotic atherectomy specimens also found low levels of proliferation (92). Similarly, Strauss et al. found no PCNA-positive cells in four postmortem stented vessels (93).

The failure to see either elevated replication or a pattern of early replication decreasing with time is contrary to what was expected from animal models. Pickering et al. detected high levels of proliferation in restenotic atherectomy tissue (94). All restenotic coronary and peripheral arterial specimens had surprisingly high percentages of cells that were considered PCNA-positive as measured by either immunocytochemistry (15.2 ± 13.6%), or in situ hybridization (20.6 ± 18.2%). However, only four of the 19 restenotic atherectomy specimens were obtained from coronary artery lesions, and none were obtained within 1 month of the initial interventional procedure (e.g., 1.6, 5.2, 6.1, and 7.9 months). Overall, the labeling indices reported by Pickering et al. seem exceptionally high (e.g., as many as 59% of cells being PCNA-positive) and resemble those of malignant neoplasms (95). Furthermore, unlike our own study, which used intestinal crypt epithelium, the Pickering study lacked a reference tissue with a known replication rate, thereby making the subjective interpretation of PCNA positivity difficult. Pickering's study also did not show evidence of change of replication over time. It is unlikely that mean PCNA labeling indices of 15% to 20% are physically possible in atherosclerotic coronary arteries, where small changes in vessel wall mass can result in dramatic changes in residual luminal diameter.

A likely explanation for the discrepancy in the proliferation data centers around the adequacy of PCNA control experiments. By immunocytochemistry, proliferating cells show increased PCNA labeling as compared with mitotically quiescent cells (91,96). Previous studies of injured arterial tissue using the same protocol that was used in our studies have shown good correlation of PCNA immunolabeling with thymidine or bromodeoxyuridine incorporation (97,98). The inclusion of rat small intestine as positive control tissue with each PCNA immunocytochemistry run in our study provided evidence that the antibody was routinely labeling the nuclei of highly proliferating crypt epithelium PCNA-positive. Moreover, our PCNA index for primary atherosclerotic tissue is in close agreement with the tritiated thymidine labeling index determined by incubating atherosclerotic tissue in vitro (99). By this criterion replication in primary and restenotic tissue is very low, but by the same set of criteria, identical PCNA immunolabeling of rapidly stenosing human arteriovenous hemodialysis arteriovenous fistulas shows high levels of replication (100). Finally, one criticism of PCNA labeling relative to other proliferative measurements is that it is likely to be oversensitive in detecting proliferative cells, because PCNA is expressed through a broader period of cell cycle traverse (97). Therefore, if anti-PCNA antibodies are overlabeling proliferating cells, the degree of proliferation in these atherectomy specimens may actually be lower than the already minimal levels that we have measured.

It is also worth noting that PCNA does pick up replicating cells with a high labeling frequency in plaque. These cells, however, are not the expected smooth muscle cells. By use of cell-specific immunohistochemical markers and a double-labeling technique. PCNA-positive cells were identified as smooth muscle cells, macrophages, and endothelial cells. The relative abundance of each cell type was studied in a selected number of specimens that were positive for PCNA immunolabeling. All fragments had evidence of PCNA-positive smooth muscle cells and macrophages, and approximately 50% of tissue fragments had PCNA-labeled endothelial cells. The percentage of PCNA-positive cells that were endothelial cells was surprisingly high (e.g., 14 ± 15%).

Finally, independent clinical evidence suggests that hyperplasia is not a sufficient explanation of restenosis. Analysis of the vessel wall growth has begun to be possible because of advances in intravascular ultrasound (IVUS). Unlike angiography, IVUS images the full cross-sectional thickness of the vessel wall. Furthermore, IVUS can be performed serially, before and after an interventional procedure in vivo, to determine the mechanisms by which the intervention enlarges the vessel lumen. Recent preliminary information on vessel wall dimensions with IVUS before and after balloon dilatation, as well as crude measurements of vessel wall composition, are promising. Mintz et al. (101) report that increases in plaque area with restenosis are actually small (5% to 7%). The clinical significance of this small increase in plaque mass in an artery that is already severely diseased is unknown. The authors speculate that intimal hyperplasia may not be a dominant factor in the restenotic lesion, and that, instead, "chronic recoil" may account for most of the progressive luminal narrowing. The idea of "chronic recoil" is remarkably similar to the observations of remodeling as described by Langille and O'Donnell (14) and by Folkow (12). Given the modest and relatively infrequent proliferation that we have detected by PCNA immunolabeling in restenotic coronary atherectomy specimens, these imaging data are complementary evidence that proliferation is only one of several important events in the biology of restenosis.

FUTURE DIRECTIONS

We need to think more broadly about mechanisms that may contribute to restenosis. Figure 3 illustrates the problem in a schematic fashion. Rather than real data, the figure shows several possible outcomes of angioplasty.

The simplest clinically desired result, indicated by arrow a in Fig. 3, is that the dilated vessel remains at its dilated diameter indefinitely. It is important to realize that this represents a failure of the vessel to heal after dilation but is the desired nonrestenotic result. The second result, contrary to the desired clinical outcome, is that the dilated vessel heals; that is, the vessel simply returns to its preangioplasty dimensions. This possibility, indicated by arrow b in Fig. 3, could result in loss of the gain in lumen size seen in angioplasty without any requirement for formation of a new intima. In the terminology used in the cardiology literature, this result might be called remodeling, because there is no net increase in intimal mass (pre- and postinjury).

It is very important to realize that these first two possibilities are quite different from most animal models. In animal models, a normal vessel is dilated, and stenosis is measured as a change in the final diameter of the vessel as compared with its preangioplasty dimensions. It is therefore remarkable that the majority of angioplasty-dilated human vessels probably show no actual restenosis. Result c in Fig. 3 represents the typical animal study with loss of lumen size as a result of gain in intimal mass. The last possible result, indicated by arrow d in Fig. 3, shows a vessel with neointimal mass. In this case, the gain in lumen size has been maintained by dilation of the artery wall; i.e., true remodeling.

In summary, restenosis is being defined only by somewhat problematic arteriographic criteria (102). One cannot draw conclusions about what is happening in the wall from assessment of the lumen. Nonetheless, some interesting data are emerging on the timing of luminal loss. Kuntz et al. have used a continuous regression model to examine the results of quantitative follow-up coronary angiographic studies on patients who have undergone either angioplasty, directional atherectomy, or stenting (103). Luminal diameter was measured immediately before and after coronary intervention in 524 consecutive lesions. Three- to six-month follow-up angiography was obtained in 91% of patients. Restenosis was found to depend solely on the extent of residual stenosis immediately after the procedure, regardless of the device employed. Moreover, the loss index (late loss of lumen size divided by acute gain in lumen), a measurement that corrects for differences in acute gain, was not significantly different for all three types of intervention. This result is somewhat surprising; one would expect with animal models that atherectomy, being more invasive, and stenting, being more intrusive, would result in more "intimal hyperplasia." What this

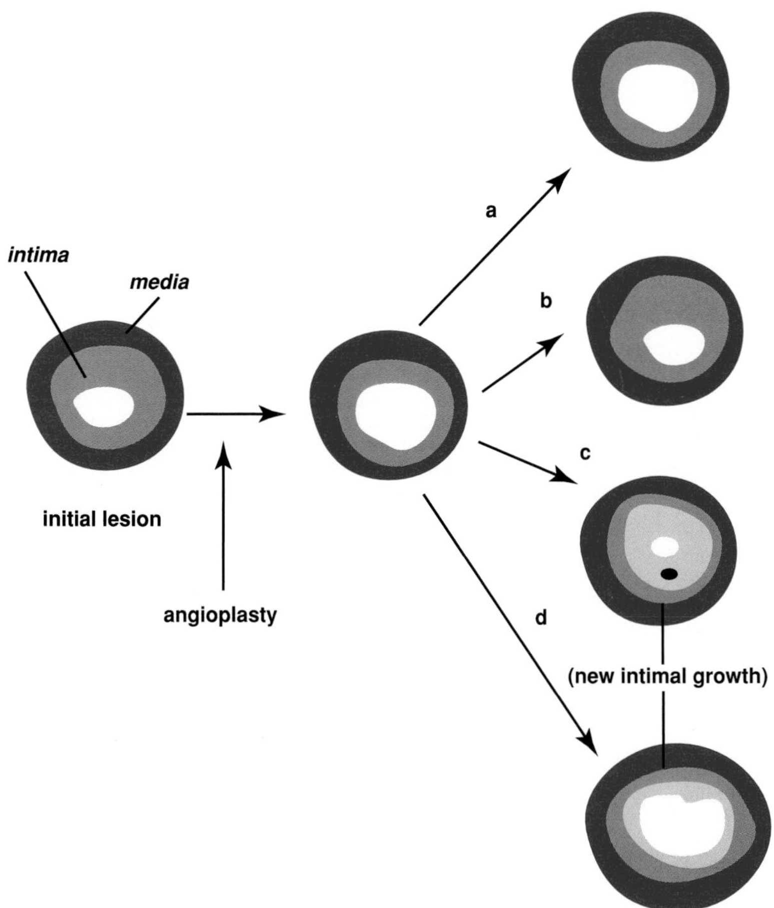

FIG. 3. Proposed outcomes after angioplasty of human atherosclerotic coronary arteries. With angioplasty, the lumen of the diseased artery is increased in size. Following this acute change in lumen size, there are four possible outcomes: **(A)** lumen stays dilated—successful outcome; **(B)** lumen returns to original size without new growth—poor outcome; **(C)** angioplasty stimulates new growth–poor outcome; **(D)** angioplasty stimulates new growth; however, redistribution of wall mass maintains large lumen—successful outcome.

study highlights is the importance of achieving the largest acute luminal gain possible—the so-called ''bigger is better hypothesis'' (104). The mechanisms that result in loss of acute lumen gain are unclear but have been lumped into the term ''recoil.'' This is perhaps illustrated in situation b of Fig. 3, although we suggest that such a healed vessel might result either from an early event, i.e., elastic recoil, or from a more prolonged process comparable with wound healing and wound retraction. Recoil may be something as simple as the elastic properties of the artery returning the artery to its preprocedural dimensions.

Vasospasm may be another contributor to restenosis that has been generally overlooked. Earlier reports suggest that balloon angioplasty routinely causes severe smooth muscle cell injury, thereby disabling the artery into a state of paralysis (105,106). Certainly studies by Fischell et al., using a perfused whole-vessel ex vivo model, indicate that severe arterial stretching is required before smooth muscle vasoconstriction is impaired (107). Chronic vasospasm occurs for several weeks after balloon catheter-induced injury to the rat carotid artery (18). Based on geometric models, medial stretching of critically stenosed human coronary arteries in vivo is probably only modest (e.g., 15% to 40%) and not sufficient to cause severe smooth muscle injury and arterial paralysis. In fact, the same authors used quantitative coronary arteriography and documented the routine occurrence of vasospasm at, and distal to, the site of dilatation in ten patients after coronary angioplasty (108). Furthermore, Nobuyoshi et al. performed angiography on 185 patients 24 h after balloon angioplasty and found restenosis (>50% loss of gain in absolute diameter) already present in 14% of patients (109). Undoubtedly, this form of ''restenosis'' represented mechanical recoil, spasm, or possibly even platelet deposition and organized mural thrombus accumulation. However, because recoil can be documented with IVUS immediately on balloon deflation of combined balloon ultrasound imaging catheters, it is likely that recoil is an instantaneous event (110). One must consider the possibility that early recoil combined with a more chronic process such as intimal hyperplasia or wound healing could account for the more drawn-out process occurring over the next 1 to 6 months (109).

Finally, we also need to consider the molecules that are likely targets for restenosis therapy. Of course, those targets depend on our notions of what restenosis is. Growth factors, for example, become less obvious targets if smooth muscle replication is not a dominant factor of this lesion (90). The term growth factors, however, is misleading: TGF-β, often lumped together with PDGF or FGF, could play a major role in the formation of extracellular matrix as well as in wound contraction. The list of potential roles for thrombin, in addition to coagulation, include vasospasm, cell migration, and growth. Other candidates include vasoactive factors derived perhaps from the endothelium in plaque vessels. Progress in assigning significance to this range of potential mediators will depend on new animal models, ideally models that allow us to isolate mechanisms to stenosis and failure of remodeling as well as formation of intimal mass.

REFERENCES

1. Essed CD, Brand MVD, Becker AE. Transluminal coronary angioplasty and early restenosis. *Br Heart J* 1983;49:393–396.
2. Austin GE, Ratliff NB, Hollman J, Tabei S, Phillips DF. Intimal proliferation of smooth muscle cells as an explanation for recurrent coronary artery stenosis after percutaneous transluminal coronary angioplasty. *J Am Coll Cardiol* 1985;6:369–375.
3. Waller BF, Pinkerton CA, Foster LN. Morphologic evidence of accelerated left main coronary artery stenosis: A late complication of percutaneous transluminal balloon angioplasty of the proximal left anterior descending coronary artery. *J Am Coll Cardiol* 1987;9:1019–1023.
4. Liu MW, Roubin GS, King SB. Restenosis after coronary angioplasty: Potential biologic determinants and role of intimal hyperplasia. *Circulation* 1989;79:1374–1387.
5. Ross R. The pathogenesis of atherosclerosis. A perspective for the 1990s. *Nature* 1993;362:801–813.
6. Ross R. The pathogenesis of atherosclerosis—an update. *N Engl J Med* 1986;314:488–500.
7. MERCATOR Study Group. Does the new angiotensin-converting enzyme inhibitor cilazapril prevent restenosis after percutaneous transluminal coronary angioplasty? *Circulation* 1992;86:100–110.
8. Schwartz RS, Koval TM, Edwards WD, Camrud AR, Bailey KR, Browne K, Vlietstra RE, Holmes DR Jr. Effect of external beam irradiation on neointimal hyperplasia after experimental coronary artery injury. *J Am Coll Cardiol* 1992;19:1106–1113.
9. Schwartz SM, Campbell GR, Campbell JH. Replication of smooth muscle cells in vascular disease. *Circ Res* 1986;58:427–444.
10. Libby P, Schwartz D, Brogi E, Tanaka H, Clinton SK. A cascade model for restenosis. A special case of atherosclerosis progression. *Circulation* 1992;86(Suppl 6):III47–III52.
11. Glagov S, Weisenberg E, Zarins CK, Stankunavicius R, Kolettis GJ. Compensatory enlargement of human atherosclerotic coronary arteries. *N Engl J Med* 1987;316:1371–1375.
12. Folkow B. Physiological aspects of primary hypertension. *Physiol Res* 1982;62:347–504.
13. Jamal A, Bendeck M, Langille BL. Structural changes and recovery of function after arterial injury. *Arterioscler Thromb* 1992;12:307–317.
14. Langille BL, O'Donnell F. Reductions in arterial diameter produced by chronic diseases in blood flow are endothelium-dependent. *Science* 1986;231:405–407.
15. Haudenschild CC, Schwartz SM. Endothelial regeneration. II. Restitution of endothelial continuity. *Lab Invest* 1979;41:407–418.
16. Barger AC, Beeuwkes RI, Lainey LL, Silverman KJ. Vasa vasorum and neovascularization of human coronary arteries. *N Engl J Med* 1984;310:175–177.
17. O'Malley MK, McDermott EWM, Mehigan D, O'Higgins NJ. Role for prazosin in reducing the development of rabbit intimal hyperplasia after endothelial denudation. *Br J Surg* 1989;76:936–938.
18. Clowes AW, Reidy MA, Clowes MM. Mechanisms of stenosis after arterial injury. *Lab Invest* 1983;49:208–215.
19. Clowes AW, Clowes MM, Reidy MA. Kinetics of cellular proliferation after arterial injury. I. Smooth muscle growth in the absence of endothelium. *Lab Invest* 1983;49:327–333.
20. Friedman RJ, Stemerman MB, Wenz B, Moore S, Gauldie J, Gent M, Tiell ML, Spaet TH. The effect of thrombocytopenia on experimental atherosclerotic lesion formation in rabbits. Smooth muscle cell proliferation and re-endothelialization. *J Clin Invest* 1977;60:1191–1201.
21. Bjorkerud S, Bondjers G. Arterial repair and atherosclerosis after mechanical injury. Part 5. Tissue response after induction of a large superficial transverse injury. *Atherosclerosis* 1973;18:235–255.
22. Schwartz SM, Stemerman MB, Benditt EP. The aortic intima. II. Repair of the aortic lining after mechanical denudation. *Am J Pathol* 1975;81:15–42.
23. Betz E, Schlote W. Response of vessel walls to chronically applied electrical stimuli. *Basic Res Cardiol* 1979;74:10–20.
24. French JE. Atherosclerosis in relation to the structure and function of the arterial intima, with special reference to the endothelium. *Int Rev Exp Pathol* 1966;5:253–354.
25. Baumgartner HR. Eine neue Methode zur Erzeugung der Thromben durch gezielte Uberdehnung der Gefasswand. *Z Ges Exp Med* 1963; 137:227.
26. Stemerman MB, Spaet TH, Pitlick F, Clintron J, Lejneks I, Tiell ML. Intimal healing: The pattern of reendothelialization and intimal thickening. *Am J Pathol* 1972;87:125.
27. Clowes AW, Clowes MM, Fingerle J, Reidy MA. Kinetics of cellular proliferation after arterial injury. V. Role of acute distention in the induction of smooth muscle proliferation. *Lab Invest* 1989;60: 360–364.
28. Clowes AW, Reidy MA. Prevention of stenosis after vascular reconstruction: Pharmacologic control of intimal hyperplasia—A review. *J Vasc Surg* 1991;13:885–891.
29. Fingerle J, Johnson R, Clowes AW, Majesky MW, Reidy MA. Role of platelets in smooth muscle cell proliferation and migration after vascular injury in rat carotid artery. *Proc Natl Acad Sci USA* 1989; 86:8412–8416.
30. Jawien A, Bowen-Pope DF, Lindner V, Schwartz SM, Clowes AW. Platelet-derived growth factor promotes smooth muscle migration and intimal thickening in a rat model of balloon angioplasty. *J Clin Invest* 1992;89:507–511.
31. Jackson CL, Raines E, Ross R, Reidy MA. Role of endogenous platelet-derived growth factor in arterial smooth muscle cell migration after balloon catheter injury. *Arterioscler Thromb* 1993;13:1218–1226.
32. Ferns GAA, Raines EW, Sprugel KH, Motani AS, Reidy MA, Ross R. Inhibition of neointimal smooth muscle accumulation after angioplasty by an antibody to PDGF. *Science* 1991;253:1129–1132.
33. Clowes AW, Clowes MM, Reidy MA. Kinetics of cellular proliferation after arterial injury. III. Endothelial and smooth muscle growth in chronically denuded vessels. *Lab Invest* 1986;54:295–303.
34. Lindner V, Reidy MA. Proliferation of smooth muscle cells after vascular injury is inhibited by an antibody against basic fibroblast growth factor. *Proc Natl Acad Sci USA* 1991;88:3739–3743.
35. Lindner V, Lappi DA, Baird A, Majack RA, Reidy MA. Role of basic fibroblast growth factor in vascular lesion formation. *Circ Res* 1991; 68:106–113.
36. Majesky MW, Lindner V, Twardzik DR, Schwartz SM, Reidy MA. Production of transforming growth factor-β-1 during repair of arterial injury. *J Clin Invest* 1991;88:904–910.
37. Daemen MJAP, Lombardi DM, Bosman FT, Schwartz SM. Angiotensin II induces smooth muscle cell proliferation in the normal and injured arterial wall. *Circ Res* 1991;68:450–456.
38. Majesky MW, Giachelli CM, Schwartz SM. Rat carotid neointimal smooth muscle cells reexpress a developmentally regulated phenotype during repair of arterial injury. *Circ Res* 1992;71:759–768.
39. Giachelli CM, Bae N, Almeida M, Denhardt DT, Alpers CE, Schwartz SM. Osteopontin is elevated during neointima formation in rat arteries and is a novel component of human atherosclerotic plaques. *J Clin Invest* 1993;92:1686–1696.
40. Snow AD, Bolender RP, Wight TN, Clowes AW. Heparin modulates the composition of the extracellular matrix domain surrounding arterial smooth muscle cells. *Am J Pathol* 1990;137:313–333.
41. Olson NE, Chao S, Lindner V, Reidy MA. Intimal smooth muscle cell proliferation after balloon catheter injury. The role of basic fibroblast growth factor. *Am J Pathol* 1992;140:1017–1023.
42. Fingerle J, Au YP, Clowes AW, Reidy MA. Intimal lesion formation in rat carotid arteries after endothelial denudation in absence of medial injury. *Arteriosclerosis* 1990;10:1082–1087.
43. Lindner V, Olson NE, Clowes AW, Reidy MA. Inhibition of smooth muscle cell proliferation in injured rat arteries. Interaction of heparin with basic fibroblast growth factor. *J Clin Invest* 1992;90:2044–2049.
44. Morishita R, Gibbons GH, Ellison KE, Nakajima M, Zhang L, Kaneda Y, Ogihara T, Dzau VJ. Single intraluminal delivery of antisense cdc2 kinase and proliferating cell nuclear antigen oligonucleotides results in chronic inhibition of neointimal hyperplasia. *Proc Natl Acad Sci USA* 1993;90:8474–8478.
45. Simons M, Edelman ER, Rosenberg RD. Antisense proliferating cell

nuclear antigen oligonucleotides inhibit intimal hyperplasia in a rat carotid artery injury model. *J Clin Invest* 1994;93:2351–2356.
46. Jackson CL, Reidy MA. Basic fibroblast growth factor. Its role in the control of smooth muscle cell migration. *Am J Pathol* 1993;143:1024–1031.
47. Majesky MW, Reidy MA, Bowen-Pope DF, Wilcox JN, Schwartz SM. Platelet-derived growth factor (PDGF) ligand and receptor gene expression during repair of arterial injury. *J Cell Biol* 1990;111:2149–2158.
48. Lindner V, Giachelli CM, Schwartz SM, Reidy MA. A subpopulation of smooth muscle cells in rat arteries express PDGF-B chain mRNA. *Circ Res [in press].*
49. Walker LN, Bowen-Pope DF, Ross R, Reidy MA. Production of platelet-derived growth factor-like molecules by cultured arterial smooth muscle cells accompanies proliferation after arterial injury. *Proc Natl Acad Sci USA* 1986;83:7311–7315.
50. Roberts AB, Sporn MB. Physiological actions and clinical applications of transforming growth factor-β (TGF-β). *Am J Physiol* 1993;264:G179–G186.
51. Pompili VJ, Shun L, Yang ZY, San H, Liptay S, Gordon D, Derynck R, Nabel GJ, Nabel EG. Direct gene transfer of transforming growth factor-β-1 in the arterial wall stimulates fibrocellular hyperplasia. *Circulation* 1993;88(4, Part 2):I-468.
52. Wolf YG, Rasmussen LM, Ruoslahti E. Antibodies against transforming growth factor-β1 suppress intimal hyperplasia in a rat model. *J Clin Invest* 1994;93:1172–1178.
53. Majack RA, Majesky MW, Goodman LV. Role of PDGF-A expression in the control of vascular smooth muscle cell growth by transforming growth factor-β. *J Cell Biol* 1990;111:239–247.
54. Battegay E, Raines E, Seifert RA, Bowen-Pope DF, Ross R. TGF-BB induces bimodal proliferaiton of connective tissue cells via complex control of an autocrine PDGF loop. *Cell* 1990;63:515–524.
55. Gibbons G, Pratt R, Dzau V. Vascular smooth muscle cell hypertrophy vs. hyperplasia. Autocrine TGF-BB-1 expression determines growth response to angiotensin II. *J Clin Invest* 1992;90:456–461.
56. Hearn JA, Donohue BC, Ba'albaki H, Douglas JS, King SBI, Lembo NJ, Roubin GS, Sgoutas DS. Usefulness of serum lipoprotein (a) as a predictor of restenosis after percutaneous transluminal coronary angioplasty. *Am J Cardiol* 1992;70:1514.
57. Grainger DJ, Kirschenlohr HL, Metcalfe JC, Weissberg PL. Proliferation of human smooth muscle cells promoted by lipoprotein (a). *Science* 1993;260:1655–1658.
58. Bendeck MP, Zempo N, Clowes AW, Galardy RE, Reidy MA. Smooth muscle cell migration and matrix metalloproteinase expression after arterial injury in the rat. *Circ Res* 1994;75:539–545.
59. Clowes AW, Clowes M, Kirkman T, Jackson C, Au Y, Kenagy R. Heparin inhibits the expression of tissue-type plasminogen activator by smooth muscle cells in injured rat carotid artery. *Circ Res* 1992;70:1128–1136.
60. Clowes AW, Karnovsky MJ. Suppression by heparin of smooth muscle cell proliferation in injured arteries. *Nature* 1977;265:625–626.
61. Powell J, Clozel J, Muller R, Kuhn H, Hefti F, Hosang M, Baumgartner H. Inhibitors of angiotensin-converting enzyme prevent myointimal proliferation after vascular injury. *Science* 1989;245:186–188.
62. Prescott M, Webb R, Reidy MA. Angiotensin-converting enzyme inhibitors versus angiotensin II, AT1 receptor antagonist: Effects on smooth muscle cell migration and proliferation after balloon catheter injury. *Am J Pathol* 1991;139:1291–1302.
63. Powell JS, Muller RKM, Rouge M, Kuhn H, Hefti F, Baumgartner HR. The proliferative reponse to vascular injury is suppressed by angiotensin-converting enzyme inhibition. *J Cardiovasc Pharmacol* 1990;16(Suppl 4):S42–S49.
64. Schwartz RS, Edwards WD, Huber KC, Antoniades LC, Bailey KR, Camrud AR, Jorgenson MA, Holmes DR. Coronary restenosis: Prospects for solution and new perspectives from a porcine model. *Mayo Clin Proc* 1993;68:54–62.
65. Hatton MW, Moar SL, Richardson M. De-endothelialization in vivo initiates a thrombogenic reaction at the rabbit aorta surface. *Am J Pathol* 1989;135:499–508.
66. Okazaki H, Majesky MW, Harker LA, Schwartz SM. Regulation of platelet-derived growth factor ligand and receptor gene expression by thrombin in vascular smooth muscle cells. *Circ Res* 1992;71:1285–1293.
67. Wilcox JN, Smith KM, Williams LT, Schwartz SM, Gordon D. Platelet-derived growth factor mRNA detection in human atherosclerotic plaques by in situ hybridization. *J Clin Invest* 1988;82:1134–1143.
68. Ross R, Masuda J, Raines EW, Gown AM, Katsuda S, Sasahara M, Malden LT, Masuko H, Sato H. Localization of PDGF-B protein in macrophages in all phases of atherogenesis. *Science* 1990;248:1009–1012.
69. Carney DH, Mann R, Redin WR, Pernia SD, Berry D, Heggers JP, Hayward PG, Robson MC, Christie J, Annable C, Fenton JWI, Glenn KC. Enhancement of incisional wound healing and neovascularization in normal rats by thrombin and synthetic thrombin receptor-activating peptides. *J Clin Invest* 1992;89:1469–1477.
70. Bar-Shavit R, Benezra M, Eldor A, Hy-Am E, Fenton JWI, Wilner GD. Thrombin immobilized to extracellular matrix is a potent mitogen for vascular smooth muscle cells: Nonenzymatic mode of action. *Cell Regul* 1990;1:453–463.
71. Lam JYT, Chesebro JH, Steele PM, Heras M, Webster MWI, Badimon L, Fuster V. Antithrombotic therapy for deep arterial injury by angioplasty: Efficacy of common platelet inhibition compared with thrombin inhibition in pigs. *Circulation* 1991;84:814–820.
72. Williams JK, Armstrong ML, Heistad DD. Vasa vasorum in atherosclerotic coronary arteries: Responses to vasoactive stimuli and regression of atherosclerosis. *Circ Res* 1988;62:515–523.
73. deBlois D, Drapeau G, Petitclerc E, Marceau F. Synergism between contractile effect of epidermal growth factor and that of des-Arg^9-bradykinin or of -thrombin in rabbit aortic rings. *Br J Pharmacol* 1992;105:959–967.
74. Kauffman RF, Bean JS, Zimmerman KM, Brown RF, Steinberg MI. Losartan, a nonpeptide AII receptor antagonist, inhibits neointima formation following balloon injury to rat carotid arteries. *Life Sci* 1991;49:PL223–PL228.
75. Farhy RD, Ho KL, Carretero OA, Scicli AG. Kinins mediate the antiproliferative effect of ramipril in rat carotid artery. *Biochem Biophys Res Commun* 1992;182:283–288.
76. Huber KC, Schwartz RS, Edwards WD, Camrud AR, Bailey KR, Jorgenson MA, Holmes DR. Effects of angiotensin converting enzyme inhibition on neointimal proliferation in a porcine coronary injury model. *Am Heart J* 1993;125:695–701.
77. Griffin S, Brown W, MacPherson F, McGrath J, Wilson V, Korsgaard N, Mulvany M, Lever A. Angiotensin II causes vascular hypertrophy in part by a non-pressor mechanism. *Hypertension* 1991;17:626–635.
78. Geisterfer AA, Peach MJ, Owens GK. Angiotensin II induces hypertrophy, not hyperplasia, of cultured rat aortic smooth muscle cells. *Circ Res* 1988;62:749–756.
79. Poulsen K, Jacobsen J. Enzymic reactions of the renin–angiotensin system. In: Robertson JI, Nicholls MG, eds. *The Renin–Angiotensin System,* Vol. I. New York: Gower Medical Publishing; 1993:5.1–5.12.
80. Rakugi H, Krieger J, Wang DS, Dzau VJ, Pratt RE. Induction of angiotensin-converting enzyme in neointima after balloon injury. *Arterioscler Thromb* 1991;11:1396a.
81. Viswanathan M, Stromberg C, Seltzer A, Saavedra JM. Balloon angioplasty enhances the expression of angiotensin II AT1 receptors in neointima of rat aorta. *J Clin Invest* 1992;90:1707–1712.
82. Fishel RS, Redden RA, Bernstein KE, Berk BC. Angiotensin-converting enzyme and vascular injury: Synergistic upregulation by stress steroids and basic fibroblast growth factor. *Circulation* 1992;86(Suppl I):I-85.
83. Bell L, Madri JA. Influence of the angiotensin system on endothelial and smooth muscle cell migration. *Am J Pathol* 1990;137:7–12.
84. Kaartinen M, Penttila A, Kovanen PT. Mast cells of the two types differing in neutral protease composition in the human aortic intima. Demonstration of trypase- and trypase/chymase-containing mast cells in normal intimas, fatty streaks and the shoulder region of the atheromas. *Arterioscler Thromb* 1994;14:966–972.
85. Nobuyoshi M, Kimura T, Ohishi H, Horiuchi H, Nosaka H, Hamasaki N, Yokoi H, Kim K. Restenosis after percutaneous transluminal coronary angioplasty: Pathologic observations in 20 patients. *J Am Coll Cardiol* 1991;17:433–439.
86. Miller MJ, Kuntz RE, Friedrich SP, Leidig GA, Fishman RF, Schnitt SJ, Baim DS, Safian RD. Frequency and consequences of intimal hyperplasia in specimens retrieved by directional atherectomy of native primary coronary artery stenoses and subsequent restenoses. *Am J Cardiol* 1993;71:652–658.
87. Schnitt SJ, Safian RD, Kuntz RE, Schmidt DA, Baim DS. Histologic

findings in specimens obtained by percutaneous directional coronary atherectomy. *Hum Pathol* 1992;23:415–420.

88. Orekhov AN, Ankarpova II, Tertov VV, Rudchenko SA, Addreeva ER, Krushinsky AV, Smirnov RN. Cellular composition of atherosclerotic and uninvolved human aortic subendothelial intima: Light-microscopic study of dissociated aortic cells. *Am J Pathol* 1984;115: 17–24.
89. Andreeva ER, Rekhter MD, Romanov YA, Antonova GM, Antonov AS, Mironov AA, Orekhov AN. Stellate cells of aortic intima: II. Arborization of intimal cells in culture. *Tissue Cell* 1992;24:697–704.
90. O'Brien ER, Alpers CE, Stewart DK, Ferguson M, Tran N, Gordon D, Benditt EP, Hinohara T, Simpson JB, Schwartz SM. Proliferation in primary and restenotic coronary atherectomy tissue: Implications for antiproliferative therapy. *Circ Res* 1993;73:223–231.
91. Fairman MP. DNA polymerase delta/PCNA: Actions and interactions. *J Cell Sci* 1990;95:1–4.
92. Leclerc G, Kearney M, Schneider D, Rosenfield K, Losordo DW, Isner JM. Assessment of cell kinetics in human restenotic lesions by in vitro bromodeoxyuridine labeling of excised atherectomy specimens. *Clin Res* 1993;41:343A.
93. Strauss BH, Umans VA, VanSuylen RJ, deFeyter PJ, Marco J, Robertson GC, Renkin J, Heyndrickx G, Vuzevski VD, Bosman FT. Directional atherectomy for treatment of restenosis within coronary stents: Clinical, angiographic and histological results. *J Am Coll Cardiol* 1992;20:1465–1473.
94. Pickering JG, Weir L, Jekanowski J, Kearney MA, Isner JM. Proliferative activity in peripheral and coronary atherosclerotic plaque among patients undergoing percutaneous revascularization. *J Clin Invest* 1993;91:1469–1480.
95. Garcia RL, Coltrera MD, Gown AM. Analysis of proliferative grade using anti-PCNA/cycin monoclonal antibodies in fixed, embedded tissues: Comparison with flow cytometric analysis. *Am J Pathol* 1989; 134:733–739.
96. Celis JE, Bravo R, Larsen PM, Fey SJ. A nuclear protein whose level correlates directly with the proliferative state of normal as well as transformed cells. *Leuk Res* 1984;8:143.
97. Gordon D, Reidy MA, Benditt EP, Schwartz SM. Cell proliferation in human coronary arteries. *Proc Natl Acad Sci USA* 1990;87: 4600–4604.
98. Zeymer U, Fishbein MC, Forrester JS, Cercek B. Proliferating cell nuclear antigen immunohistochemistry in rat aorta after balloon denudation: Comparison with thymidine and bromodeoxyuridine labeling. *Am J Pathol* 1992;141:685–690.
99. Spagnoli LG, Villaschi S, Neri L, Palmieri G, Taurino M, Faraglia V, Fiorani P. Autoradiographic studies of the smooth muscle cells in human arteries. *Arterial Wall* 1981;7:107–112.
100. Rekhter M, Nicholls S, Ferguson M, Gordon D. Cell proliferation in human arteriovenous fistulas used for hemodialysis. *Arterioscler Thromb* 1993;13:609–617.
101. Mintz GS, Douek PC, Bonner RF, Kent KM, Pichard AD, Satler LF, Leon MB. Intravascular ultrasound comparison of de novo and restenotic coronary artery lesions. *J Am Coll Cardiol* 1993;21:118A.
102. Lesperance J, Bourassa MG, Schwartz L, Hudon G, Laurier J, Eastwood C, Kazin F. Definition and measurement of restenosis after successful coronary angioplasty: Implications for clinical trials. *Am Heart J* 1993;125:1394–1408.
103. Kuntz RE, Gibson M, Nobuyoshi M, Baim DS. Generalized model of restenosis after conventional balloon angioplasty, stenting and directional atherectomy. *J Am Coll Cardiol* 1993;21:15–25.
104. Penny WF, Schmidt DA, Safian RD, Erny RE, Baim DS. Insights into the mechanism of luminal improvement after directional coronary atherectomy. *Am J Cardiol* 1991;67:435–437.
105. Faxon DP, Weber VJ, Haudenschild C, Gottsman SB, McGovern WA, Ryan TJ. Acute effects of angioplasty in three experimental models of atherosclerosis. *Arteriosclerosis* 1982;2:125–133.
106. Sanborn TA, Faxon DP, Haudenschild C, Gottsman SB, Ryan TJ. The mechanism of transluminal angioplasty: Evidence for formation of aneurysms in experimental atherosclerosis. *Circulation* 1983;68: 1136–1140.
107. Fischell TA, Grant G, Johnson DE. Determinants of smooth muscle injury during balloon angioplasty. *Circulation* 1990;82:2170–2184.
108. Fischell TA, Derby G, Tse TM, Stadius ML. Coronary artery vasoconstriction routinely occurs after percutaneous transluminal coronary angioplasty: A quantitative arteriographic analysis. *Circulation* 1988; 78:1323–1334.
109. Nobuyoshi M, Kimura H, Nosaka H, Mioka S, Ueno K, Hamasaki N, Horiuchi H, Oshishi H. Restenosis after successful percutaneous transluminal coronary angioplasty: Serial angiographic follow-up of 299 patients. *J Am Coll Cardiol* 1988;12:616–623.
110. Isner JM, Rosenfield K, Losordo DW, Rose L, Langevin REJ, Razvi S, Kosowsky BD. Combination balloon–ultrasound imaging catheter for percutaneous transluminal angioplasty. Validation of imaging, analysis of recoil, and identification of plaque fracture. *Circulation* 1991;84:739–754.

Atherosclerosis and Coronary Artery Disease,
edited by V. Fuster, R. Ross, and E. J. Topol.
Lippincott-Raven Publishers, Philadelphia © 1996.

CHAPTER 40

Transplant Arteriosclerosis

David Gordon

Key Words: Adventitia; Arteriosclerosis; Endothelialitis; Lumen; Macrophages; Transplantation.

INTRODUCTION AND DEFINITIONS

Transplant arteriosclerosis is a diffuse and progressive thickening of the arterial intima that develops in the major and minor arteries of transplanted solid organs. Other commonly used synonyms for this disease include "graft arteriosclerosis," "accelerated atherosclerosis," "allograft arteriopathy," and "chronic rejection." The term "transplant arteriosclerosis" is to be strongly preferred, because this refers to the specific arterial intimal lesions that develop in transplanted organs. In contrast, "graft arteriosclerosis" could also refer to the intimal thickening that occurs in bypass grafts (tissue and prosthetic grafts); some have used "accelerated arteriosclerosis" to refer to bypass graft lesions as well as to the restenosis lesions that follow angioplasty; and "chronic rejection" also encompasses other nonarterial lesions (e.g., loss of bile ducts and interstitial fibrosis in the liver, tubular atrophy and interstitial fibrosis in the kidney).

Transplant arteriosclerotic lesions are progressive and too often eventually lead to severe arterial stenoses and occlusions. The result is sudden and/or progressive ischemic damage to the transplanted organ, with its eventual functional failure. This disease has become a major clinical problem with organ transplants, and at least for hearts, it is the major cause of graft failure (and too often patient death) 1 year after transplantation (1,2). This progressive disease occurs to variable degrees in all types of human solid organs that have been transplanted, including hearts (Fig. 1; see Colorplate 32), kidneys, livers, pancreases, and bowel transplants. The pathology of this lesion is essentially the same in all of these organs, although quantitative differences may exist [e.g., lipid-laden foam cells appear to be more commonly seen the arteries of transplanted livers (3)]. We will refer to the atherosclerosis that occurs in humans unrelated to transplantation, which is generally well modeled by animal models of hypercholesterolemia-induced arterial lesions, as "ordinary atherosclerosis." Because several topographical and cellular similarities exist between transplant arteriosclerosis and ordinary atherosclerosis, many of the theories and ideas concerning ordinary atherosclerosis are now being applied to transplant arteriosclerosis. Finally, this disease has probably been most heavily studied in reference to heart transplants, probably because of causing sudden or eventual death of the affected patients, given the lack of available transplant donors for retransplantation and the lack of suitable life-sustaining alternatives for the affected patients (unlike hemodialysis for renal transplant failures). Thus, this chapter will focus primarily on heart transplant arteriosclerosis, with specific mention of other organs as appropriate. We will also focus on the cell biology and pathology issues of this disease rather than on the detailed immunologic aspects. Several recent literature reviews of transplant arteriosclerosis are available (4–11).

D. Gordon: Department of Pathology, University of Michigan, Ann Arbor, Michigan 48109.

HUMAN PATHOLOGY

General Description and Cell Composition

Historically, transplant arteriosclerosis was first noticed in renal transplants, because kidney transplants were the first solid organ transplants generally performed (7,12). However, as transplants of other organs became more prevalent, this disease has become a recognized clinical problem in all of these organ areas. Cell suspension transplants, such as those of bone marrow, do not appear to be associated with transplant arteriosclerosis, even in the face of recognized graft-versus-host disease (13–15).

Transplant arteriosclerosis has basically the same pathology in all affected transplant organs. In the heart, this manifests grossly as diffuse arterial narrowing that extends far down the arterial tree, involving second- and higher-order arterial branches. Thus, in addition to the surface epicardial coronary arteries, this also involves the penetrating intramyocardial branches. Histological sections generally reveal a circumferentially uniform (''concentric'') thickening of the intima that diffusely involves the affected arteries (Fig. 1). Although more prominent in size, its appearance is much like the diffuse intimal thickening that occurs normally in human epicardial coronary arteries (15–18) and may indeed be difficult to distinguish from the normal aging process in the earliest stages. Failure to recognize diffuse intimal thickening as a normal process in the epicardial coronary arteries may lead to an overestimation of how soon after transplantation actual transplant arteriosclerosis starts. True early transplant arteriosclerosis is probably better appreciated in the penetrating intramyocardial arteries, which normally do not display such a prominent intima.

Despite the diffuse nature of transplant arteriosclerosis seen on angiography and in pathological specimens, there is quite a variable degree of involvement within any one heart (and frequently on the same microscopic section), with some arteries of comparable size appearing normal, and others only minimally diseased. This variability in arterial involvement has not been adequately explained, and we are not aware of any detailed topographic studies relating such lesions to the sites of features such as arterial branch points (as is the case for ordinary atherosclerosis) (19). Animal models of heart transplants also frequently reveal a similar variable involvement of coronary arteries despite presumably all arterial branches being exposed to the same plasma and blood-borne cellular factors that might be responsible for this disease (Fig. 2; see Colorplate 33).

Comparisons with Ordinary Atherosclerosis

Similarities

A number of pathological features exist in common between human transplant arteriosclerosis and human ordinary atherosclerosis (4,7,20–28). These similarities and differences are summarized in Table 1. In regard to general topography, both processes primarily involve the arterial intima, causing its expansion. Although there may be variable fragmentation of the internal elastic lamina, this lamina is generally preserved in both lesion types, with relative sparing of the underlying media. Duplication of the internal elastica may be more common with ordinary atherosclerosis. Both diseases also have variable numbers of inflammatory cells (lymphocytes, monocyte/macrophages) in the surrounding adventitia (3,29). Finally, with the possible exception of transplanted kidneys, there is generally a more prominent involvement of the proximal, large and medium-sized arteries, with decreasing involvement of third- and fourth-order branches down to the arteriole level (3). This is particularly the case with the heart, in which the epicardial coronary arteries and their first-order branches are the ones most likely to be affected, whereas the arterioles seen on endomyocardial biopsy are only rarely affected (20,29). Despite occasional reports (30), most investigators feel that the presence of significant cardiac transplant arteriosclerosis cannot be reliably detected based on endomyocardial biopsy (2), and thus most heart transplant centers perform periodic coronary angiograms on their patients to detect this disease. Some endomyocardial biopsy findings such as focal vasculitis or arterial intimal thickening are felt by some to be predictive of later-developing clinically significant transplant arteriosclerosis (30), and Häyry et al. (11) have reported that several biopsy findings can at least be statistically correlated with the prevalence of this disease, although the predictive value in the individual patient is not clear.

The similarities at the cellular level are also striking (1,4, 6,7,29,31–38). At the well-developed, clinically significant stage, both types of human lesions are composed of numerous smooth muscle cells with their associated extracellular matrix (collagen, proteoglycans, etc.). Additionally, a significant population of monocyte/macrophages are present in both, and foam cells (macrophages with much lipid engorgement) can also be seen in both, especially if the transplant patient is hypercholesterolemic. Prominent foam cell intimal infiltrates have also been described with liver transplants (3). Significant populations of T lymphocytes are present in both, with a relative paucity of B lymphocytes (39). The presence of dendritic cells, which may be important antigen-presenting cells, has been described for human transplant arteriosclerosis (29,32). These are probably also present in ordinary atherosclerotic lesions, although less effort has gone into seeking their presence here. Finally, although it is sometimes difficult to ascertain in human samples, both lesions are also generally felt to be covered by luminal endothelial cells. Certainly focal breaks in the endothelial integrity, or in the fibrous cap, are felt to predispose to coronary thrombosis with ordinary coronary atherosclerosis, and thrombotic occlusions of transplant arteriosclerotic arteries certainly occurs, often leading to silent myocardial infarcts in these patients with denervated hearts. Thus, from a cellular

TABLE 1. *Comparison of pathological features of ordinary atherosclerosis with transplant arteriosclerosis in human organs*

Features	Ordinary atherosclerosis	Transplant arteriosclerosis
Predilection for arterial branches	+++	−
Involves 2nd- and 3rd-order branches	+/−	+++
Concentric lesion morphology	+	+++
Eccentric lesion morphology	+++	+
Subendothelial inflammatory cell concentration	−	+/−
Fragmentation of the internal elastic lamina	++	+/−
Presence of necrotic core with cholesterol crystals	+++	+
Medial necrosis	+	+
Smooth muscle cells	+++	+++
Monocyte/macrophages	+++	+++
Foam cells	+++	+
T lymphocytes	+++	+++
B lymphocytes	+/−	+/−
Chronic inflammatory infiltrate in adventitia	+	++

composition point of view, there are probably no significant *qualitative* differences between ordinary atherosclerosis and transplant arteriosclerosis. This has also been borne out in animal models of these two diseases (hypercholesterolemia-induced atherosclerosis versus transplanted heart or aortic arteriosclerosis; see below). Indeed, except for some mostly statistical and distributional differences described below, the pathologist is often unable to distinguish transplant arteriosclerosis from ordinary atherosclerosis on the basis of inspection of single arterial sections alone.

The sequence of cellular events in the development of the transplant arteriosclerotic lesion is less clearly described in humans than in animal models. However, here again, the general impression is that of an early inflammatory infiltration of the arterial intima by T lymphocytes and monocytes (Fig. 3; see Colorplate 34), with later expansion of the intima by these cells. Subsequent increases in the smooth muscle and extracellular matrix components occur with time. Of note, early inflammatory infiltrates are also often seen in the arterial adventitia, which suggests that the adventitia may be an additional portal of entry of inflammatory cells into the artery wall (29). Lesions such as the fatty streak are considered precursors of ordinary atherosclerosis, and in transplant arteriosclerosis, an influx of monocyte/macrophages and T lymphocytes also precedes the further intimal elaboration of smooth muscle and extracellular matrix components. One confusing issue here is that the human coronary arteries normally start with some diffuse intimal thickening on which either ordinary atherosclerosis or transplant arteriosclerosis occurs. This is unlike most animal models of this disease, which generally use arteries with no preexisting intimal smooth muscle cells.

Differences

Significant differences do exist in the morphology of ordinary atherosclerosis versus transplant arteriosclerosis; however, these tend to be more quantitative than qualitative. Thus, as far as arterial topography is concerned, ordinary atherosclerosis tends to involve the artery wall very focally and has a predilection for arterial branch points, particularly the low-shear-stress regions just beyond and on the lateral aspects of arterial branch bifurcations (19). Second- and third-order arterial branches and penetrating intramyocardial branches tend not to be involved. In contrast, although we are not aware of any detailed three-dimensional reconstructions of the topography of transplant arteriosclerosis lesions, most observers report no such branch point predilection. Instead, in humans and in animal models, the intimal involvement with transplant arteriosclerosis is described as being diffuse, often involving long segments of affected arteries, and extending into second- and third-order branches (3,4, 20,40). Needless to say, several transplanted hearts do exhibit focal lesions as well (4,40).

On arterial cross sections, ordinary atherosclerosis usually involves one part of the arterial more heavily than other parts, producing prominent ''eccentric'' lesions. In contrast, transplant arteriosclerosis is usually described as a diffuse, ''concentric'' intimal thickening (4,20,29). Although this generally is the case, there are certainly numerous examples of ''concentric'' ordinary atherosclerosis, and it is not uncommon to find prominent eccentric lesions in transplanted hearts. In the latter situation, there is often an argument as to whether or not the ''eccentric'' transplant lesion represents transplant arteriosclerosis superimposed on a previously existing ordinary atherosclerotic lesion. However, because one cannot know what the pretransplant morphology was as such sites in humans, this hypothesis cannot be substantiated or disproved. The occasional finding of focal lesions in rat models of this disease (Fig. 2), suggests that focal transplant intimal lesions can be produced by a transplant environment (41–43).

Finally, the features usually associated with complications of ordinary atherosclerotic plaques—calcification, a large necrotic core with an overlying fibrous cap, neovascularization, and intraplaque hemorrhage—are generally absent from transplant arteriosclerotic lesions. Again, one can occasionally see such lesions in transplanted hearts, but the issue of the preexisting lesions at such sites remains. One potentially distinguishing feature is the occurrence in some (but not all) early transplant arteriosclerotic lesions of a marked concentration of lymphocytes and monocyte/macrophages in the immediate subendothelial space (Figs. 3–5; see Colorplates 35, 36, and 37). This prominent collection of mononuclear inflammatory cells has been termed ''endothelialitis'' by some investigators (39), although whether or not there is actual destruction or damage to the overlying endothelial cells suggesting that the inflammatory infiltrate is indeed directed towards the endothelium has not been clarified in human material (33). We have not seen this particular morphology in samples of ordinary atherosclerosis, although again, it is not present in all cases of transplant arteriosclerosis.

EPIDEMIOLOGY

Incidence of the Human Disease

As a direct result of the orthotopic heart transplantation procedure in which the native heart is removed and a donor heart is sutured into its place, the new heart is necessarily denervated, because all of the nerve connections have been cut. Although some mostly anecdotal evidence of partial reinnervation is occasionally mentioned, most of these transplanted hearts remain functionally denervated for the lifetime of the graft (and patient). As a result, patients with significant transplant arteriosclerotic disease do not experience the common clinical warning symptom of angina that patients with ordinary coronary atherosclerosis experience (40). They may begin to experience some signs of congestive heart failure (shortness of breath, fatigue, poor exercise tolerance); however, these may also be produced by acute rejection of the myocardium or by fluid overload, particularly in patients with some degree of renal failure (e.g., from hypertension and cyclosporine effects). When these other disease processes are ruled out, the clinician may suspect significant transplant arteriosclerosis by exclusion. Unfortunately, sudden death is all too often the first distinct clinical manifestation of this disease.

Primarily for this reason, most transplant centers perform periodic coronary angiograms on heart transplant patients (e.g., annually) to assess this disease (40), making *coronary* transplant arteriosclerosis development far better studied clinically than that occurring in other solid organ transplants. From such serial angiographic studies, it has been estimated that the general incidence in transplanted hearts increase approximately 10% per year after transplantation (9,11, 44–46). At 5 years after transplantation, approximately one-half of the transplanted hearts have some evidence of this disease (40,45,47). The angiographic description is usually one of very diffuse involvement along the courses of the major epicardial coronary arteries and their first-order branches. Pruning and/or obliteration of smaller branches is also seen.

Unfortunately, angiography, which has been the mainstay of clinical assessments of coronary arterial narrowing for many years, is not by any means perfect and essentially provides an image of only the lumen and not the arterial wall. Indeed, angiographic estimates of the onset and prevalence of transplant arteriosclerosis probably represent underestimates of the actual pathologically determined disease, primarily for three reasons. (a) The earliest small lesions are not angiographically detectable. (b) Angiographic degrees of stenosis are usually based on comparisons with so called ''normal'' coronary artery segments; such segments are often difficult to find because of the diffuse nature of the disease, and undoubtedly many segments designated ''normal'' are in fact narrowed (40). Indeed, this is a recognized problem even with ordinary atherosclerosis (48). Quantitative angiographic measurements of lumen diameters, especially when there is a baseline angiogram for comparison, is an improvement in this regard. (c) As has been shown at least for ordinary coronary atherosclerosis, the artery wall is able to undergo a considerable amount of remodeling by expanding the contour of the media in order to maintain lumen dimensions in the face of an increasing volume of atherosclerotic intima (49,50). Thus, even quantitative angiography would be expected to underestimate the amount of intimal disease. The extent to which such arterial remodeling occurs during the evolution of human transplant arteriosclerosis needs study. Finally, intravascular ultrasound has the promise of showing lumen diameters as well as arterial layer dimensions and is rapidly becoming the technique of choice for following the clinical development of this disease (40).

As discussed above, there may also be problems in identifying the onset of this disease pathologically, because in humans, variable degrees of progressive diffuse intimal thickening of at least the epicardial coronary arteries is a universal finding, even among nontransplanted and nonatherosclerotic hearts. Finally, some investigators have demonstrated ''endothelial dysfunction,'' defined as abnormal vasoreactivity in response to acetylcholine, in transplanted human hearts. This is felt to be caused by defective nitric oxide physiology in the arterial wall, similar to what is seen with ordinary atherosclerotic arteries, and may be an early indication of this disease before clinically significant stenoses develop (51). However, this does not appear to be a routinely used method of detection of this disease.

Risk Factors for Cardiac Transplant Arteriosclerosis

Several risk factors have been sought in relation to transport arteriosclerosis, without much consistent success (8,9,11). Indeed, most studies have shown no significant risk factor associations other than with the survival time of the graft, as discussed above (9,39,52). With heart transplants, the vast majority are done either for end-stage ordinary coronary atherosclerotic disease or for idiopathic dilated cardiomyopathies (in which the coronary arteries are usually normal or only minimally affected by atherosclerosis). However, transplant arteriosclerosis appears in both groups of patients with similar incidence; thus, the original disease does not predict risk (4). Similarly, sex and age of the patient have not been well correlated with this disease (52); however, some have reported that the age of the *donor* heart may be related to disease development once this heart is transplanted (4,11,53). The degree of tissue mismatch has also been studied, and although some studies have suggested a relationship between HLA or ABO mismatch degree (53,54), others have not found such associations (4,31,52).

Because some of the transplanted patients have hypercholesterolemia, either endogenously, or as a complication of cyclosporine treatment, lipid profile factors that are risk factors for ordinary atherosclerosis have been studied. Yet even here, except for occasional mention of hypertriglyceridemia as being statistically associated with transplant arteriosclerosis, these factors (e.g., LDL cholesterol) have not been found to be predictors of the transplant disease (4,52,55). Although foam cell macrophage infiltrates are occasionally described in human transplant arteriosclerotic lesions, based on animal model studies, this may be more a case of coexisting hyperlipidemia giving a foam-cell character to lesions that would likely develop anyway in the absence of hyperlipidemia (56–58). These studies indicate that in the rabbit, hypercholesterolemia may exacerbate transplant arteriosclerosis in terms of the number and size or arterial lesions, but hypercholesterolemia is not a requirement for the development of this disease (56–58), as also evidenced by rat models of transplant arteriosclerosis (9–11).

Some reports have indicated that the number of biopsy-demonstrated acute cellular rejection episodes in the myocardium experienced by heart transplant patients correlated positively with the incidence of transplant arteriosclerosis (8,11,44,53). This is important because it may reflect suboptimal immunosuppressive control of acute cellular rejection, with a similar immunologic injury affecting the arteries. However, other studies have reported no such positive correlation between transplant arteriosclerosis and frequency of acute rejection episodes (8,20,51). This has recently been restudied by Häyry et al. in a Finnish clinical study, and they do report a positive correlation. However, they admit that the more genetically homogeneous population of Finland seems to exhibit a lower frequency of acute cellular rejection episodes than those reported elsewhere, and their experience may not be generalizable to other populations (11). Thus, this area remains controversial.

An interesting area of investigation has been on the role of cytomegalovirus (CMV) infection. Several groups have reported striking positive correlations between the incidence of acute CMV viral infections (detected by rising anti-CMV viral titers or by use of endomyocardial biopsies with immunocytochemical or polymerase chain reaction techniques) and transplant arteriosclerosis (11,40,52,59,60). This is of particular interest in view of the work of Hajjar, the Fabricants, and others suggesting that herpes viruses can be causative of ordinary human atherosclerosis as well (61–68) (see also the chapter by Kaner and Hajjar, *this volume*). The potential roles played by CMV in the development of transplant arteriosclerosis have, however, not been elucidated, and few studies have found the CMV organism directly in involved arteries (60). Of interest, Häyry and colleagues have reported that a rat form of cytomegalovirus induces PDGF gene expression associated with increased smooth muscle cell proliferation in their rat model of transplant arteriosclerosis (69,70). It should be noted that most of the general population has had previous exposure to CMV and that many cases of active infection following transplantation probably reflect a resurgence of endogenous virus on immunosuppression, as opposed to truly new infections. It is also of interest that CMV infections have been correlated with the number of acute cellular rejection episodes, and it is unclear whether or not the positive association between rejection episodes and transplant arteriosclerosis reported by some investigators could have CMV infections as a basis. Finally, the causal role of CMV in transplant arteriosclerosis is not without controversy.

CELLULAR PATHOBIOLOGY AND EXPERIMENTAL STUDIES

Animal Models Used

A number of animal models have been used to study transplant arteriosclerosis. Most of these have involved either the rat (9–11,71–75) or the rabbit (56,57,76–85); however, most recently, mouse models of this disease are being described (86,87). All of these model systems appear to reproduce the basic pathology of this lesion as seen in humans. Rats have probably been the most studied with respect to immune system mechanisms and have the advantage over rabbits of having several well-defined and truly syngeneic strains. The rat, however, is not well suited for studies of the effects of hypercholesterolemia, at least compared to the rabbit or mouse. Rabbits appear to generate arterial lesions faster than rats but suffer somewhat from the decreased availability of reagents for study (e.g., cell type- and subtype-specific antibodies, cloned genes). They are, however, good for hypercholesterolemia studies as they are with ordinary atherosclerosis. With the increasing availability of transgenic mice and specific gene knockouts in the mouse, mouse models are likely to receive a great deal of attention in the coming years, particularly in elucidating molecular mechanisms and the importance of specific gene expressions in the evolution of this disease. Certainly the mouse has been the most heavily studied from a basic immunology point of view, and the availability of reagents for study is probably best with this species. The surgery for arterial or heart transplantation, however, is considerably more challenging in these small animals, compared to rats and rabbits.

In all animal systems, two primary models of transplantation have been used. In *heterotopic heart transplantation,* the recipient's heart is left *in situ,* and a donor heart is transplanted into the abdomen (or the neck). The groups led by Minick (56,85) and separated by Laden (88,89) were among the first to pursue transplant arteriosclerosis studies using these whole-heart transplantation systems. In this procedure, the donor heart's aorta is anastomosed to the abdominal aorta (or common carotid artery in the neck), the right atrial vena cava inflows are tied off, and for transplanted heart venous outflow the pulmonary artery is anastomosed to the inferior vena cava (or jugular vein in the neck). Such hearts are thus perfused through their coronary arteries but, given their heterotopic nature, are not truly working hearts, because the recipient animal's own heart still supports the cardiac output for the whole animal. Whether or not this lack of ''working heart'' physiology has any bearing on the rate of development and/or character of transplant arteriosclerosis is unclear; however, such hearts certainly do develop transplant-associated arterial lesions. The left ventricular cavity, being a blind pouch with respect to blood flow, usually thromboses. Finally, most heart transplants require some sort of immunosuppression therapy to allow the heart to survive long enough to develop significant arterial lesions (usually a few to several weeks of transplantation). Otherwise uncontrolled acute rejection usually supervenes and destroys the heart within a few days.

In *straight arterial segment transplants,* a segment of straight artery (usually aorta) is anastomosed end-to-end to the arterial circulation, usually in the abdominal aortic position but sometimes in the common carotid position. The advantages of straight artery segment transplants over heart transplants include: (a) there is no whole organ to protect, and thus the sequence of cellular events can be studied in the absence of immunosuppressions; (b) the straight segment allows for easier en face assessment of early leukocyte adhesion to the endothelial surface using techniques such as scanning electron microscopy, which is technically much more difficult in the curved and tortuous coronary arteries; (c) similarly, the straight segment allows for easier morphometric quantitation of the area or volume of intimal thickening that develops, compared to the tortuous coronary arteries, which are frequently cut tangentially on tissue sections. As a result, much of the whole-heart transplant data are in the form of semiquantitative assessments of arterial involvement over different-sized arteries (e.g., ''present/absent'' percentage of vessels involved, or qualitative scores of degree of involvement). (d) Straight artery segments are more amenable to bulk biochemical studies of transplanted arterial tissue not including surrounding organ tissue (e.g., RNA extraction for Northern blotting).

The disadvantages of using straight arterial segments include the following: (a) The commonly used straight segments are usually elastic arteries such as the aorta and not the more muscular arteries of the heart. (b) Coronary flow patterns differ from straight artery segments and could conceivably have an effect on the development of transplant arteriosclerosis. (c) Whole-heart preparations allow a comparison of the inflammatory events occurring at the artery wall with those occurring in the microvasculature and parenchymal cells of the transplanted organ. And although these studies usually employ some immunosuppression, this is more analogous to the actual human situation in which all patients are on multiple-drug immunosuppression regimens. (d) Finally, a potentially important difference that occurs in the straight-artery-segment models, but not to a significant degree in the whole-heart transplants, is a progressive loss of smooth muscle cells from the media of the transplanted segment, frequently with replacement by monocyte/macrophages (75,77,86,90). This finding has raised concern about the representatives of such straight artery segments to the actual human disease. However, this loss of medial smooth muscle cells is generally reported when no immunosuppression is used and appears not to occur when immunosuppression with agents such as cyclosporine is used (91–93). Additionally, some focal medial necrosis can be seen even in human cases on immunosuppression, although this may be called ''vasculitis'' as opposed to transplant arteriosclerosis (1,2,4,6,20,29). Since a prominent inflammatory infiltrate of the artery wall is clearly involved in the evolution of transplant arteriosclerosis, where ''vasculitis'' ends and ''true transplant arteriosclerosis'' begins is quite unclear. It is conceivable, however, that the development of transplant-associated intimal thickening may represent a balance between immune-mediated cell death of arterial wall cells and arterial smooth muscle proliferation. Intense vasculitic responses tend to promote arterial destruction without much proliferation, whereas more moderate rejection responses may allow the intimal proliferative and extracellular matrix aspects to predominate.

Cellular Sequence of Events

Despite the several models, species used, and laboratories involved in the study of transplant arteriosclerosis, there is a general consensus on the cellular sequence of events. Most of the early sequence of events, as well as measures of cell proliferation, have necessarily come from animal experimental work, with some corroborative observations in human material. Although the general sequence of events here is the same across various models, the times of occurrence vary depending on the model used (immunologic cross variable) and on the type of immunosuppressive treatment (if any) used.

Endothelium

The earliest change after transplantation appears to be increased adhesion of mononuclear inflammatory cells to the luminal surface of the arterial endothelium. This has been shown most graphically by the scanning electron microscopy studies of Reidy et al., in which straight artery segments of rabbit aorta were transplanted (78,94). This early leukocyte adhesion becomes noticeable within 24 h of transplantation, and a progressively increasing density of these cells is seen from that time onward. Morphologically, many of the cells appear to be monocytes and probably lymphocytes, although careful immunocytochemical typing of such early surface cells appears to be lacking. As for the role of cell adhesion molecules, although this has been extensively studied in the myocardial and renal microvasculature during acute cellular rejection, there has been much less work done in the arteries. However, most relevant studies suggest an early increase in VCAM-1 and increased ICAM-1 expression in such model systems (8,10,58,82,95). Both of these cell adhesion molecules are clearly relevant to the adhesion of lymphocytes and monocytes, but whether or not leukocyte adhesion precedes or follows the initial increased expression of these adhesion ligands (as has been suggested for the hypercholesterolemic rabbit model of ordinary atherosclerosis) is not clear (96). Additionally, very few cell adhesion-blocking experiments in an attempt to inhibit transplant arteriosclerosis have yet been done (81), whereas such blocking studies have shown a prolongation of heart graft survival from acute cellular rejection (97–99). When looked for, up-regulation of MHC class I antigens and early expression of MHC class II antigens by the endothelium are also seen, as is class II expression in transplanted artery smooth muscle (6,33, 81,100).

These attached mononuclear inflammatory cells appear to migrate rapidly between the endothelial cells to gain access to the subendothelial space. This secondarily gives the endothelial surface a very irregular contour, as seen on scanning electron microscopy, again not unlike that described for hypercholesterolemia models of ordinary atherosclerosis. However, the fate of the allografted endothelium is much less clear. Although some human studies have mentioned that the arterial endothelium is (101) or is not damaged (33), this cannot be easily studied in human material, because good endothelial preservation for detailed study requires en face techniques and perfusion fixation, which is usually not possible with human samples. Reidy et al. reported eventual loss of the arterial endothelium in rabbit aortic allografts (78), but in retrospect, Reidy has suggested that the resolution of the scanning electron microscopy used could not clearly separate the loss of the initial smooth endothelial surface from actual endothelial cell loss and population of the luminal surface by other cell types *(personal communication)*. Some other animal studies have indicated that focal or diffuse endothelial damage does occur (72,80,102,103), but the majority of animal studies do not report significant endothelial cell death alterations in transplanted arteries (43,58,82,83,86,92,102,104). Careful studies specifically looking at endothelial cell death and proliferation indices, as have been done for nontransplant animal studies (105–109), are needed here.

Finally, studies that try to determine clearly whose endothelium (recipient or host) populates the luminal surface are lacking. A couple of human studies using either sex chromatin identification (in cases in which donor and recipient were of a different sex) (31) or specific anti-HLA antibodies (110) have suggested that whereas the inflammatory component in transplanted arteries is of recipient origin, most mesenchymal cells appear to be of allograft origin. However, these have not been of an appropriate resolution to address the endothelial origin question. It is perhaps hard to conceive of all of the allografted heart endothelium (arterial and microvascular) being destroyed and/or replaced and the heart remaining viable. Thus, although it is conceivable that, similar to hypercholesterolemia models of ordinary atherosclerosis, the endothelium remains largely intact until either significant subendothelial deposits of cells and/or lesion complications such as thrombosis occur, this area clearly needs much further investigation.

Intima

The intima, which is usually just the potential space between the endothelium and the internal elastic lamina, soon becomes expanded by rapidly accumulating numbers of monocyte/macrophages and predominantly T lymphocytes. These progressively expand the intima by both a process of continued cellular influx as well as in situ proliferation as determined by thymidine labeling or other proliferation markers such as the proliferating cell nuclear antigen (PCNA) (11,75,86,89,111). This inflammatory cell proliferation is later followed by some proliferative activity among smooth muscle cells within the media, associated with subsequent migration of smooth muscle cells from the media into the intima. Once in the intima, these smooth muscle cells also continue to divide and begin elaborating extracellular matrix (including fibronectin and collagen), particularly in those intimal regions closest to the media. Thus, with time, the cellular character of the intima changes from a closely packed, inflammatory-rich cell mass to a later one enriched with smooth muscle cells, extracellular matrix, and a progressively decreasing cell density.

The time course of cell proliferation after transplantation has been best studied in the straight-artery-segment transplant models without immunosuppression (11,75,86,111) and appears to be self-limited, with peak proliferative indices occurring at approximately 15 to 30 days after transplantation, depending on the model. Of note, in our own studies (75) many of the proliferating cells did not mark with any of our available cell type markers and could therefore represent "dedifferentiated" smooth muscle cells or undefined cell types that are important to the development of this lesion. Thus, the overall pattern of smooth muscle proliferative activity has similarities to that described after mechanical injury to the artery wall, in which there is a brief early burst in proliferative activity, followed by migration of cells into the intima and continued cell proliferation, followed by a prominent extracellular matrix synthesis and an expansion phase (112–114).

Thus, overall proliferative activity, despite transplant arteriosclerosis being viewed as a chronically progressive lesion (''chronic rejection''), may be characterized by an initial self-limited burst of proliferative activity, followed by mostly extracellular matrix expansion in its later stages. Compared to the balloon injury rat carotid artery model, this transplant arteriosclerosis lesion develops over a longer period of time and has a much smaller peak in proliferative activity (6–7% versus 30–50% in the rat balloon injury model), but the sequence of early proliferation and later extracellular matrix expansion appears to be similar. This may have treatment ramifications if it can be shown that an abrogation of this early proliferative wave can inhibit this intimal thickening, just as has been shown for models of mechanical arterial injury.

The types of extracellular matrix molecules synthesized in transplant arteriosclerotic lesions have not received much direct attention, but by extrapolation from morphology and a few direct studies, type I collagen, elastin, fibronectin, and probably several proteoglycans are among the newly formed intimal matrix constituents. Rabinovitch et al. have recently drawn attention to the importance of endogenously synthesized fibronectin in pig and rabbit models of transplant arteriosclerosis (100). This molecule appears to have chemotactic activity for monocyte/macrophages and smooth muscle cells and thus may serve to attract and trap both cell types within the developing neointima (100). This transplant intimal thickening can also be inhibited by infusion of soluble TNF receptor *(personal communication).*

Finally, the growth factors that drive this proliferative activity of inflammatory cells and smooth muscle cells are not fully known. However, several growth factors have been described. In human transplant arteriosclerosis lesions, we have seen intimal immunoreactivity for basic fibroblast growth factor (bFGF) (115) and the B form of platelet-derived growth factor (PDGF). Our limited human observations could be consistent with either growth factor promoting cell proliferation and are complicated by the finding of proliferating monocyte/macrophages in these lesions and signs of PCNA immunoreactivity *(unpublished observations).* Others have also found evidence for other growth factors in transplant arteriosclerotic lesions, including PDGF, IL-1, and TNF (10,11,58,100).

Adventitia

The adventitia also develops a chronic inflammatory infiltrate after transplantation. This is seen in hearts (58) and is particularly prominent in straight-artery-segment transplants (75). The minimal to absent chronic inflammatory infiltrate in the adventitia associated with isografts further indicates that such lymphocyte and monocyte/macrophage infiltration of the adventitia is indeed transplant mediated and not simply a reaction to the trauma of surgery. With time, as the intima is being infiltrated by similar inflammatory cells, penetration of the media from the adventitia is also seen. Thus, at least for arteries, the transplant-associated cellular immune response appears to have two portals of entry into the artery wall: (a) via the surface endothelium and (b) via the adventitia. Although the adventitia is a relatively neglected area in both ordinary atherosclerosis and transplant arteriosclerosis studies, we have certainly seen prominent proliferative activity and type I collagen gene expression in this region (unpublished observations). Progressive scarring of the adventitia could conceivably affect arterial wall compliance and possibly interfere with the kind of compensatory dilatation described for ordinary atherosclerosis to minimize encroachment on the lumen.

Media

In most heart models of transplant arteriosclerosis, the media is described as relatively undisturbed save for focal breaks in the internal elastica. However, as mentioned above, some human hearts do show focal destruction of the media and/or replacement by inflammatory cells and fibrosis. In the straight-artery-segment models of transplant arteriosclerosis, if no immunosuppression is given, progressive necrosis of the media with loss of smooth muscle elements and often replacement by inflammatory cells is seen. This may lead to some degree of arterial dilatation. As discussed above, this is frequently prevented by immunosuppression (e.g., cyclosporine), which is usually used for the heart transplants.

Immunologic Aspects

A historical debate that remains unresolved is whether or not transplant arteriosclerosis is the result of a humoral or a cell-mediated immunologic attack on the arterial wall. The similarity between these lesions and those induced experimentally in the arteries of serum sickness models [e.g., Minick et al. studies in which bovine serum albumin was injected into rabbits, with or without coincident hypercholesterolemia (116,117)] would argue for a humorally mediated arm. Support for this view also comes from the observations that immunosuppressive treatments such as cyclosporine, which are successful in treating cellular rejection, generally do not prevent transplant arteriosclerosis (43,44,91,93), although some inhibition of transplant arteriosclerosis with cyclosporine has been reported in rabbits (79). Some agents such as imuran, which are better at inhibiting the humoral immune response, can reportedly inhibit transplant arteriosclerosis (88). Finally, as mentioned previously, in humans there does not appear to be a good correlation between HLA mismatch and the development of cardiac transplant arteriosclerosis.

Arguments in favor of a cell-mediated response include the finding of numerous activated T cells and up-regulation of MHC class II expression within the transplanted arterial wall (3,6,10,32,33,39,58,75,81,86,91,95,100,118,119). Additionally, studies in rats in which the degree of MHC mismatch has been varied have been done at least for whole-heart transplants. However, here the complication appears to be survival of the myocardium from cellular rejection for a long enough period that one can see the later arterial changes (9,71). Thus, most such heart transplant models employ minimal MHC differences and do not truly answer the question. The kinds of lymphocyte-type reconstruction studies that have been used to discern the cellular immune components necessary for myocardial rejection appear lacking in relation to transplant arteriosclerosis (120–122). With the current availability of a mouse straight-artery-segment model of transplant arteriosclerosis (86), the way is now open for dissecting this issue via the use of specific knockout mouse strains for transplantation.

TREATMENT

Currently, there are no clinical treatments for transplant arteriosclerosis causing transplant organ failure, short of retransplantation. As discussed above, although modern immunosuppressive therapy is quite effective in controlling cellular rejection of the organ parenchyma, this has not significantly decreased the incidence of transplant arteriosclerosis. Because of the markedly growing disparity between the demand for transplanted organs and their supply, this is becoming an increasingly critical problem. For heart transplant patients, this often means death of the patient while waiting for a second donor, and discussions continue on the ethics of providing a failing transplant patient with a second donor heart, often at the expense of providing that same donor heart to a needy individual who has not yet had the chance of survival through transplantation. Thus, effective treatments are being actively sought.

Some encouraging potential treatments have been reported in animal model studies. Foegh et al. reported that the administration of estrogens to a rabbit straight-artery-segment model could reduce the amount of transplant intimal thickening seen (80,102). This is interesting in light of the lack of a sex predilection for this disease. These same investigators have also reported that a somatostatin analog, angiopeptin, can inhibit transplant intimal thickening, and clinical trials with this agent have been ongoing (41,123). Others have reported that whereas cyclosporine A alone does not have much inhibitory effect on a rat model of transplant arteriosclerosis, when used in combination with low-molecular-weight heparin, it can inhibit transplant intimal thickening (43,93). Whether or not any of these treatments gain clinical applicability remains to be seen.

Many of the proposed treatments have been aimed at inhibiting smooth muscle proliferation. The early burst in cell proliferation and subsequent phase of extracellular matrix synthesis may have important treatment ramifications in that inhibition of these rather early processes could conceivably inhibit the progressive intimal thickening seen in "chronic rejection." Perhaps self-limited treatments that abrogate early arterial wall proliferation, such as thymidine kinase gene expression with ganciclovir administration, may soon prove effective in this regard, similar to their demonstrated effectiveness in reducing intimal thickening after arterial injury (124). Similarly, increased focus should be directed at separately inhibiting the extracellular matrix synthesis phase of this disease.

FUTURE DIRECTIONS

As highlighted above, although we have learned a great deal about human and animal models of transplant arteriosclerosis, several unresolved issues remain with respect to how this disease develops. In humans and in rat hearts, the lesions are frequently spotty, as seen on histological sections. Are there specific anatomic predilections? Could a superimposed injury such as ischemia/reperfusion at the time of transplantation act synergistically with allograft immune rejection to account for some of this focal nature and to exacerbate transplant arteriosclerosis? Most investigators have found no correlation between human donor heart ischemic time and who develops the disease (9,125). However, all such hearts are necessarily ischemic to some degree, and at least one investigator has presented rat data in favor of such a synergism (126). Perhaps a look at agents that minimize ischemia/reperfusion injuries should be done for transplant arteriosclerosis. Several growth factors have been identified in transplanted arterial tissue, but their direct correlation with ongoing cell proliferation needs to be determined. Additionally, specific blocking experiments are need to test their significance, as has been done for mechanical injury models of intimal thickening. Similar studies need to be done to elucidate the controls of extracellular matrix synthesis and to clarify the roles of specific cytokines in this disease.

The nature of solid organ transplantation, specifically placing the organ in a holding solution before transplantation, would seem to be particularly amenable to gene transfer methods aimed at immunosuppression or inhibition of the proliferative events leading to arterial occlusion. It is hoped that further elucidation of the growth factors and cytokines involved will help in this endeavor and open the way for more localized treatment of transplant patients without many of the systemic effects of current immunosuppressive therapy.

REFERENCES

1. Uys CJ, Rose AG. Pathologic findings in long-term cardiac transplants. *Arch Pathol Lab Med* 1984;108:112–116.

2. Chomette G, Auriol M, Cabrol C. Chronic rejection in human heart transplantation. *J Heart Transplant* 1988;7:292–297.
3. Demetris AJ, Zerbe T, Banner B. Morphology of solid organ allograft arteriopathy: Identification of proliferating intimal cell populations. *Transplant Proc* 1989;21:3667–3669.
4. Billingham ME. Cardiac transplant atherosclerosis. *Transplant Proc* 1987;19:19–25.
5. Libby P, Salomon RN, Payne DD, Schoen FJ, Pober JS. Functions of vascular wall cells related to development of transplantation-associated coronary arteriosclerosis. *Transplant Proc* 1989;21:3677–3684.
6. Schoen FJ, Libby P. Cardiac transplant graft arteriosclerosis. *Trends Cardiovasc Med* 1991;1:216–223.
7. Vollmer E, Roessner A. Renal transplant arteriopathy: Similarities to atherosclerosis. In: Robenek H, Severs NJ, eds. *Cell Interactions in Atherosclerosis.* Boca Raton, FL: CRC Press; 1992:71–100.
8. Tilney NL, Whitley WD, Diamond JR, Kupiec-Weglinski JW, Adams DH. Chronic rejection—An undefined conundrum. *Transplant* 1991; 52:389–398.
9. Cramer D. *Graft Arteriosclerosis in Heart Transplantation.* Austin, TX: R.G. Landes; 1993:1–95.
10. Adams DH, Russell ME, Hancock WW, Sayegh MH, Wyner LR, Karnovsky MJ. Chronic rejection in experimental cardiac transplantation: Studies in the Lewis-F344 model. *Immunol Rev* 1993;5:19.
11. Häyry P, Isoneimi H, Yilmaz S, Mennander A, Lemström K, Räisänen-Sokolowski A, Koskinen P, Ustinov P, Lautenschlager I, Taskinen E, Krogerus L, Aho P, Paavonen T. Chronic allograft rejection. *Immunol Rev* 1993;134:33–81.
12. Hume DM, Merrill JP, Miller BF, Thorn GW. Experiences with renal homotransplantation in the human: Report of nine cases. *J Clin Invest* 1955;34:327–382.
13. Sale GE. Bone marrow and thymic transplantation. In: Sale GE, ed. *The Pathology of Organ Transplantation.* Boston: Butterworths; 1990:229–259.
14. Armitage JO. Bone marrow transplantation. *N Engl J Med* 1994;330: 827–838.
15. Stary HC. Macrophages, macrophage foam cells, and eccentric intimal thickening in coronary arteries of young children. *Atherosclerosis* 1987;64:91–108.
16. Velican C, Velican D. Intimal thickening in developing coronary arteries and its relevance to atherosclerotic involvement. *Atherosclerosis* 1976;23:345–355.
17. Hartman JD. Structural changes within the media of coronary arteries related to intimal thickening. *Am J Pathol* 1977;89:13–34.
18. Sims FH. A comparison of coronary and internal mammary arteries and implications of the results in the etiology of arteriosclerosis. *Am Heart J* 1983;105:560–566.
19. Glagov S, Zarins C, Giddens DP, Ku DN. Hemodynamics and atherosclerosis. Insights and perspectives gained from studies of human arteries. *Arch Pathol Lab Med* 1988;112:1018–1031.
20. Rose AG, Viviers L, Odell JA. Pathology of chronic cardiac rejection: An analysis of the epicardial and intramyocardial coronary arteries and myocardial alterations in 43 human allografts. *Cardiovasc Pathol* 1993;2:7–19.
21. McGill HC. Persistent problems in the pathogenesis of atherosclerosis. *Arteriosclerosis* 1984;4:443–451.
22. Wissler RW. The evolution of the atherosclerotic plaque and its complications. In: Connor WE, Bristow JD, eds. *Coronary Heart Disease.* Philadelphia: J.B. Lippincott; 1985:193–214.
23. Ross R. The pathogenesis of atherosclerosis—an update. *N Engl J Med* 1986;314:488–500.
24. Velican C, Velican D. Natural history of coronary atherosclerosis as related to age. In: Velican C, Velican D, eds. *Natural History of Coronary Atherosclerosis.* Boca Raton, FL: CRC Press; 1989: 279–352.
25. Stary HC. The sequence of cell and matrix changes in atherosclerotic lesions of coronary arteries in the first forty years of life. *Eur Heart J* 1990;11(Suppl E):3–19.
26. Libby P, Hansson GK. Involvement of the immune system in human atherogenesis: Current knowledge and unanswered questions. *Lab Invest* 1991;64:5–15.
27. Ross R. The pathogenesis of atherosclerosis: A perspective for the 1990s. *Nature* 1993;362:801–809.
28. Davies MJ, Woolf N. Atherosclerosis: what is it and why does it occur? *Br Heart J* 1993;69(Suppl):S3–S11.
29. Gravanis MB. Allograft heart accelerated atherosclerosis: Evidence for cell-mediated immunity in pathogenesis. *Mod Pathol* 1989;2: 495–505.
30. Palmer DC, Tsai CC, Roodman ST, Codd JE, Miller LW, Sarafian JE, Williams GA. Heart graft aretriosclerosis: An ominous finding on endomyocardial biopsy. *Transplant* 1985;39:385–388.
31. Beiber CP, Stinson EB. Cardiac transplantation in man. VII. Cardiac allograft pathology. *Circulation* 1970;41:753–772.
32. Oguma S, Banner B, Zerbe T, Starzl T, Demetris AJ. Participation of dentritic cells in vascular lesions of chronic rejection of human allografts. *Lancet* 1988;2:933–936.
33. Salomon RN, Hughes CCW, Schoen FJ, Payne DD, Pober JS, Libby P. Human coronary transplantation-associated arteriosclerosis: Evidence for a chronic immune reaction to activated graft endothelial cells. *Am J Pathol* 1991;138:791–798.
34. Jahn L, Kreuzer J, von Hodenberg E, Kübler W, Franke WW, Allenberg J, Izumo S. Cytokeratins 8 and 18 in smooth muscle cells: Detection in human coronary artery, peripheral vascular, and vein graft disease and in transplantation-associated arteriosclerosis. *Arterioscler Thromb* 1993;13:1631–1639.
35. Hansson GK, Jonasson L, Holm J, Claesson-Welsh L. Class II MHC antigen expression in the atherosclerotic plaque: Smooth muscle cells express HLA-DR, HLA-DQ and the invariant gamma chain. *Clin Exp Immunol* 1986;64:261–268.
36. Gown AM, Tsukada T, Ross R. Human atherosclerosis. II. Immunocytochemical analysis of the cellular composition of human atherosclerotic lesions. *Am J Pathol* 1986;125:191–207.
37. Hansson GK, Holm J, Jonasson L. Detection of activated T lymphocytes in the human atherosclerotic plaque. *Am J Pathol* 1989;135: 169–175.
38. Katsuda S, Coltrera MD, Ross R, Gown AM. Human atherosclerosis: IV. Immunocytochemical analysis of cell activation and proliferation in lesions of young adults. *Am J Pathol* 1993;142:1787–1793.
39. Hruban RH, Beschorner WE, Baumgartner WA, Augustine SM, Ren H, Reitz BA, Hutchins GM. Accelerated arteriosclerosis in heart transplant recipients is associated with a T-lymphocyte-mediated endothelialitis. *Am J Pathol* 1990;137:871–882.
40. Schroeder JS, Gao S, Hunt SA, Stinson EB. Accelerated graft coronary artery disease: Diagnosis and prevention. *J Heart Lung Transplant* 1992;11:S258–S266.
41. Foegh ML. Accelerated cardiac transplant atherosclerosis/chronic rejection in rabbits: Inhibition by angiopeptin. *Transplant Proc* 1993; 25:2095–2097.
42. Sarris GE, Mitchell RS, Billingham ME, Glasson JR, Cahill PD, Miller DC. Inhibition of accelerated cardiac allograft arteriosclerosis by fish oil. *J Thorac Cardiovasc Surg* 1989;97:841–855.
43. Aziz S, Tada Y, Gordon D, McDonald TO, Fareed J, Verrier ED. A reduction in accelerated graft coronary disease and an improvement in cardiac allograft survival using low molecular weight heparin in combination with cyclosporine. *J Heart Lung Transplant* 1993;12: 634–643.
44. Uretsky BF, Murali S, Reddy PS, Rabin B, Lee A, Griffith BP, Hardesty RL, Trento A, Bahnson HT. Development of coronary artery disease in cardiac transplant patients receiving immunosuppressive therapy with cyclosporine and prednisone. *Circulation* 1987;76: 827–834.
45. Paul LC. Chronic rejection of organ allografts: Magnitude of the problem. *Transplant Proc* 1993;25:2024–2025.
46. Gao SZ, Schroeder JS, Alderman EL, Hunt SA, Silverman JF, Wiederhold V, Stinson EB. Clinical and laboratory correlates of accelerated coronary artery disease in the cardiac transplant patient. *Circulation* 1987;76:V56–V61.
47. Pascoe EA, Barnhart GR, Carter WH, Thompson JA, Hess ML, Hastillo A, Szentpetery S, Lower RR. The prevalence of cardiac allograft arteriosclerosis. *Transplant* 1987;44:838–839.
48. Roberts WC. Coronary heart disease: A review of abnormalities observed in the coronary arteries. *Cardiovasc Med* 1977;2:29–48.
49. Glagov S, Weisenberg E, Zarins CK, Stankunavicius R, Kolettis GJ. Compensatory enlargement of human atherosclerotic coronary arteries. *N Engl J Med* 1987;316:1371–1375.
50. Clarkson TB, Prichard RW, Morgan TM, Petrick GS, Klein KP. Remodeling of coronary arteries in human and nonhuman primates. *JAMA* 1994;271:289–294.
51. Fish RD, Nabel EG, Selwyn AP, Ludmer PL, Mudge GH, Kirshen-

baum JM, Schoen FJ, Alexander RW, Ganz P. Responses of coronary arteries of cardiac transplant patients to acetylcholine. *J Clin Invest* 1987;81:21–31.

52. McDonald K, Rector TS, Braunlin EA, Kubo SH, Olivari T. Association of coronary artery disease in cardiac transplant recipients with cytomegalovirus infection. *Am J Cardiol* 1989;64:359–362.
53. Almond PS, Matas AJ, Gillingham K, Dunn DL, Payne WD, Gores P, Gruessner R, Najarian JS. Predictors of chronic rejection in renal transplant recipients. *Transplant Proc* 1993;25:936.
54. Nakatani T, Aida H, Frazier OH, Macris MP. Effect of ABO blood type on survival of heart transplant patients treated with cyclosporine. *J Heart Transplant* 1989;8:27–33.
55. Hess MJ, Hatillo A, Mohanakumar T, Cowley MJ, Vetrovac G, Szentpetery S, Wolfgang TC, Lower RR. Accelerated atherosclerosis in cardiac transplantation: role of cytotoxic B-cell antibodies and hyperlipidemia. *Circulation* 1983;68(Suppl II):II-94–II-101.
56. Alonso DR, Starek PK, Minick CR. Studies on the pathogenesis of atheroarteriosclerosis induced in rabbit cardiac allografts by the synergy of graft rejection and hypercholesterolemia. *Am J Pathol* 1977; 87:415–422.
57. Laden AMK. Experimental atherosclerosis in rat and rabbit cardiac allografts. *Arch Pathol* 1972;93:240–245.
58. Tanaka H, Sukhova GK, Libby P. Interaction of the allogeneic state and hypercholesterolemia in arterial lesion formation in experimental cardiac allografts. *Arterioscler Thromb* 1994;14:734–745.
59. Grattan MT, Moreno-Cabral CE, Starnes VA, Oyer PE, Stinson EB, Shumway NE. Cytomegalovirus infection is associated with cardiac allograft rejection and atherosclerosis. *JAMA* 1989;261:3561–3566.
60. Wu T, Hruban RH, Ambinder RF, Pizzorno M, Cameron DE, Baumgartner WA, Reitz BA, Hayward GS, Hutchins GM. Demonstration of cytomegalovirus nucleic acids in the coronary arteries of transplanted hearts. *Am J Pathol* 1992;140:739–747.
61. Hajjar DP. Viral pathogenesis of atherosclerosis: Impact of molecular mimicry and viral genes. *Am J Pathol* 1991;139:1195–1211.
62. Hajjar DP, Pomerantz KB, Falcone DJ, Weksler BB, Grant AJ. Herpes simplex virus infection in human arterial cells: Implications in arteriosclerosis. *J Clin Invest* 1987;80:1317–1321.
63. Melnick JL, Dreesman GR, McCollum CH, Petrie BL, Burek J, DeBakey ME. Cytomegalovirus antigen within human arterial smooth muscle cells. *Lancet* 1983;2:644–647.
64. Yamashiroya HM, Ghosh L, Yang R, Robertson AL. Herpesviridae in the coronary arteries and aorta of young trauma victims. *Am J Pathol* 1988;130:71–79.
65. Melnick JL, Adam E, DeBakey ME. Possible role of cytomegalovirus in atherogenesis. *JAMA* 1990;263:2204–2207.
66. Hendrix MGR, Salimans MMM, van Boven CPA, Bruggeman CA. High prevalence of latently present cytomegalovirus in arterial walls of patients suffering from grade III atherosclerosis. *Am J Pathol* 1990; 136:23–28.
67. Benditt EP, Barrett T, McDougall JK. Viruses in the etiology of atherosclerosis. *Proc Natl Acad Sci USA* 1983;80:6386–6389.
68. Hendrix MGR, Dormans PHJ, Kitslaar P, Bosman F, Bruggeman CA. The presence of cytomegalovirus nucleic acids in arterial walls of atherosclerotic and nonatherosclerotic patients. *Am J Pathol* 1989; 134:1151–1157.
69. Lemström KB, Bruning JH, Bruggeman CA, Lautenschlager IT, Häyry PJ. Cytomegalovirus infection enhances smooth muscle cell proliferation and intimal thickening of rat aortic allografts. *J Clin Invest* 1993;92:549–558.
70. Lemström KB, Aho PT, Bruggeman CA, Häyry PJ. Cytomegalovirus infection enhances mRNA expression of platelet-derived growth factor-BB and transforming growth factor-β_1 in rat aortic allografts: Possible mechanism for cytomegalovirus-enhanced graft arteriosclerosis. *Arterioscler Thromb* 1994;14:2043–2052.
71. Cramer DV, Qian S, Harnaha J, Chapman FA, Estes LW, Starzl TE, Makowka L. Cardiac transplantation in the rat. I. The effect of histocompatibility differences on graft arteriosclerosis. *Transplant* 1989; 47:414–419.
72. Laden AMK, Sinclair RA. Thickening of arterial intima in rat cardiac allografts. *Am J Pathol* 1971;63:69–84.
73. Lurie KG, Billingham ME, Jamieson SW, Harrison DC, Reitz BA. Pathogenesis and prevention of graft arteriosclerosis in an experimental heart transplant model. *Transplant* 1981;31:41–47.
74. Halttunen J, Partanen T, Leszczynski D, Rinta K, Häyry P. Rat aortic allografts: A model for chronic vascular rejection. *Transplant Proc* 1990;22:125.
75. Isik FF, McDonald TO, Ferguson M, Yamanaka E, Gordon D. Transplant arteriosclerosis in a rat aortic model. *Am J Pathol* 1992;141: 1139–1149.
76. Sasaguri S, Tsukada T, Hosoda Y. Immunocytochemical investigations of vessel allograft arteriosclerosis using smooth muscle cell- and macrophage-specific monoclonal antibodies. *Transplant* 1990;50: 898–901.
77. Reddy GSR, Cliff WJ. Morphologic changes in arterial grafts in rabbit ears. *Lab Invest* 1979;40:109–121.
78. Bowyer DE, Reidy MA. Scanning electron miscroscope studies of the endothelium of aortic allografts in the rabbit: Morphological observations. *J Pathol* 1977;123:237–245.
79. Andersen H, Madsen G, Nordestgaard BG, Hansen BF, Kjeldsen K, Stender S. Cyclosporin suppresses transplant arteriosclerosis in the aorta-allografted, cholesterol-clamped rabbit: Suppression preceded by decrease in arterial lipoprotein permeability. *Arterioscler Thromb* 1994;14:944–950.
80. Cheng LP, Kuwahara M, Jacobson J, Foegh MI. Inhibition of myointimal hyperplasia and macrophage infiltration by estradiol in aorta allografts. *Transplant* 1991;52:967–972.
81. Sadahiro M, McDonald TO, Allen MD. Reduction in cellular and vascular rejection by blocking leukocyte adhesion molecule receptors. *Am J Pathol* 1993;142:675–683.
82. Tanaka H, Sukhova GK, Swanson SJ, Cybulsky MI, Schoen FJ, Libby P. Endothelial and smooth muscle cells express leukocyte adhesion molecules heterogeneously during acute rejection of rabbit cardiac allografts. *Am J Pathol* 1994;144:938–951.
83. Eich DM, Nestler JE, Johnson DE, Dworkin GH, Ko D, Wechsler AS, Hess ML. Inhibition of accelerated coronary atherosclerosis with dehydroepiandrosterone in the heterotopic rabbit model of cardiac transplantation. *Circulation* 1993;87:261–269.
84. Hjelms E, Stender S. Accelerated cholesterol accumulation in homologous arterial transplants in cholesterol-fed rabbits: A surgical model to study transplantation atherosclerosis. *Arterioscler Thromb* 1992; 12:771–779.
85. Minick CR, Murphy GE. Immunologic injury and atherosclerosis. *Adv Exp Med Biol* 1974;43:355–376.
86. Shi C, Russell ME, Bianchi C, Newell JB, Haber E. Murine model of accelerated transplant arteriosclerosis. *Circ Res* 1994;75:199–207.
87. Russell PS, Chase CM, Winn HJ, Colvin RB. Coronary atherosclerosis in transplanted mouse hearts: III. Effects of recipient treatment with a monoclonal antibody to the interferon-γ. *Transplant* 1994;57: 1367–1371.
88. Laden AMK. The effects of treatment on the arterial lesions of rat and rabbit cardiac allografts. *Transplant* 1972;13:281–290.
89. Laden AMK. Autoradiographic evidence for the origin of cells constituting arterial intimal thickening in experimental cardiac allografts. *J Reticuloendothel Soc* 1972;11:524–533.
90. Häyry P, Mennander A, Tiisala S, Halttunen J, Yilmaz S, Paavonen T. Rat aortic allografts: An experimental model for chronic transplant arteriosclerosis. *Transplant Proc* 1991;23:611–612.
91. Schmitz-Rixen T, Megerman J, Colvin RB, Williams AM, Abbott WM. Immunosuppressive treatment of aortic allografts. *J Vasc Surg* 1988;7:82–92.
92. Mennander A, Paavonen T, Häyry P. Intimal thickening and medial necrosis in allograft arteriosclerosis (chronic rejection) are independently regulated. *Arterioscler Thromb* 1993;13:1019–1025.
93. Plissonnier D, Amichot G, Lecagneux J, Duriez M, Gentric D, Michel J. Additive and synergistic effects of a low-molecular-weight, heparin-like molecule and low doses of cyclosporin in preventing arterial graft rejection in rats. *Arterioscler Thromb* 1993;13:112–119.
94. Reidy MA, Bowyer DE. Scanning electron-microscope studies of the endothelium of aortic allografts in the rabbit: Effect of azathioprine, prednisolone, and promethazine on early cellular invasion. *J Pathol* 1978;124:1–5.
95. Tilney NL, Whitley WD, Tullius SG, Heemann UW, Wasowska B, Baldwin WM, Hancock WW. Serial analysis of cytokines, adhesion molecule expression, and humoral responses during development of chronic kidney allograft rejection in a new rat model. *Transplant Proc* 1993;25:861–862.
96. Li H, Cybulsky MI, Gimbrone MA, Libby P. An atherogenic diet rapidly induces VCAM-1, a cytokine-regulatable mononuclear leuko-

cyte adhesion molecule, in rabbit aortic endothelium. *Arterioscler Thromb* 1993;13:197–204.

97. Cosimi AB, Conti D, Delmonico FL, Preffer FI, Wee S, Wothlein R, Faanes R, Colvin RB. In vivo effects of monoclonal antibody to ICAM-1 (CD54) in nonhuman primates with renal allografts. *J Immunol* 1990;144:4604–4612.
98. Isobe M, Yagita H, Okumura K, Ihara A. Specific acceptance of cardiac allograft after treatment with antibodies to ICAM-1 and LFA-1. *Science* 1992;255:1125–1127.
99. Orosz CG, Ohye RG, Pelletier RP, Van Buskirk AM, Huang E, Morgan C, Kincade PW, Ferguson RM. Treatment with anti-vascular cell adhesion molecule 1 monoclonal antibody induces long-term murine cardiac allograft acceptance. *Transplant* 1993;56:453–460.
100. Clausell N, Molossi S, Rabinovitch M. Increased interleukin-1β and fibronectin expression are early features of the development of the postcardiac transplant coronary arteriopathy in piglets. *Am J Pathol* 1993;142:1772–1786.
101. Yowell RL, Hammond EH, Bristow MR, Watson FS, Renlund DG, O'Connell JB. Acute vascular rejection involving the major coronary arteries of a cardiac allograft. *J Heart Transplant* 1988;7:191–197.
102. Jacobsson J, Cheng L, Lyke K, Kuwahara M, Kagan E, Ramwell PW, Foegh ML. Effect of estradiol on accelerated atherosclerosis in rabbit heterotopic aortic allografts. *J Heart Lung Transplant* 1992;11: 1188–1193.
103. Kosek JC, Beiber C, Lower RR. Heart graft arteriosclerosis. *Transplant Proc* 1971;3:512–514.
104. Kuwahara M, Jacobsson J, Kagan E, Ramwell PW, Foegh Ml. Coronary artery ultrastructural changes in cardiac transplant atherosclerosis in the rabbit. *Transplant* 1991;52:759–765.
105. Hansson GK, Chao S, Schwartz SM, Reidy MA. Aortic endothelial cell death and replication in normal and lipopolysaccharide-treated rats. *Am J Pathol* 1985;121:123–127.
106. Schwartz SM, Lombardi DM. Effect of chronic hypertension and antihypertensive therapy on endothelial cell replication in the spontaneously hypertensive rat. *Lab Invest* 1982;47:510–515.
107. Walker LN, Reidy MA, Bowyer DE. Morphology and cell kinetics of fatty streak lesion formation in the hypercholesterolemic rabbit. *Am J Pathol* 1986;125:450–459.
108. Reidy MA, Yoshida K, Harker LA, Schwartz SM. Vascular injury: Quantification of experimental focal endothelial denudation in rats using indium-111-labeled platelets. *Arteriosclerosis* 1986;6:305–311.
109. Hansson GK, Schwartz SM. Evidence for cell death in the vascular endothelium in vivo and in vitro. *Am J Pathol* 1983;112:278–286.
110. Kennedy LJ, Weissman IL. Dual origin of intimal cells in cardiac-allograft arteriosclerosis. *N Engl J Med* 1971;285:884–887.
111. Mennander A, Tiisala S, Halttunen J, Yilmaz S, Paavonen T, Häyry P. Chronic rejection in rat aortic allografts: An experimental model for transplant arteriosclerosis. *Arterioscler Thromb* 1991;11:671–680.
112. Clowes AW, Reidy MA, Clowes MM. Mechanisms of stenosis after arterial injury. *Lab Invest* 1983;49:208–215.
113. Clowes AW, Reidy MA, Clowes MM. Kinetics of cellular proliferation after arterial injury. I. Smooth muscle growth in the absence of endothelium. *Lab Invest* 1983;49:327–333.
114. Snow AD, Bolender RP, Wight TN, Clowes AW. Heparin modulates the composition of the extracellular matrix domain surrounding arterial smooth muscle cells. *Am J Pathol* 1990;137:313–330.
115. Isik FF, Valentine HA, McDonald TO, Baird A, Gordon D. Localization of bFGF in human transplant coronary atherosclerosis. *Ann NY Acad Sci* 1991;638:487–488.
116. Minick CR, Murphy GE, Campbell WG. Experimental induction of athero-arteriosclerosis by the synergy of allergic injury to arteries and lipid-rich diet. I. Effect of repeated injections of horse serum in rabbits fed a dietary cholesterol supplement. *J Exp Med* 1966;124:635–652.
117. Hardin NJ, Minick CR, Murphy GE. Experimental induction of atheroarteriosclerosis by the synergy of allergic injury to arteries and lipid-rich diet. III. The role of earlier acquired fibromuscular intimal thickening in the pathogenesis of later developing atherosclerosis. *Am J Pathol* 1973;73:301–327.
118. Gravanis MB, Ansari AA, Neckelman N, Zaki S. Evidence of cell-mediated immunity in the pathogenesis of allograft heart arteriosclerosis. *J Am Coll Cardiol* 1990;15:127a.
119. Hancock WW, Whitley WD, Baldwin WM, Tilney NL. Cells, cytokines, adhesion molecules, and humoral responses in a rat model of chronic renal allograft rejection. *Transplant Proc* 1992;24: 2315–2316.
120. Hall BM, Dorsch S, Roser B. The cellular basis of allograft rejection in vivo. 1. The cellular requirements for first-set rejection of heart grafts. *J Exp Med* 1978;148:878–889.
121. Hall BM, Dorsch S, Roser B. The cellular basis of allograft rejection in vivo. II. The nature of memory cells mediating second set heart graft rejection. *J Exp Med* 1978;148:890–902.
122. Hall BM, Saxe I, Dorsch S. The cellular basis of allograft rejection in vivo. III. Restoration of first-set rejection of heart grafts by T helper cells in irradiated rats. *Transplant* 1983;36:700–705.
123. Foegh ML, Khirabadi BS, Chambers E, Ramwell PW. Peptide inhibition of accelerated transplant atherosclerosis. *Transplant Proc* 1989; 21:3674–3676.
124. Ohno T, Gordon D, San H, Pompili VJ, Imperiale MJ, Nabel GJ, Nabel EG. Gene therapy for vascular smooth muscle cell proliferation after arterial injury. *Science* 1994;265:781–784.
125. Masetti P, DiSesa VJ, Schoen FJ, Sun S, Byrne JG, Appleyard RF, Laurence R, Cohn LH. Ischemic injury before heart transplantation does not cause coronary arteriopathy in experimental isografts. *J Heart Transplant* 1991;10:597–599.
126. Wanders A, Akyürek ML, Waltenberger J, Ren ZP, Stafberg C, Funa K, Larsson E, Fellström B. Ischemia-induced transplant arteriosclerosis in the rat. *Arterioscler Thromb* 1995;15:145–155.

Atherosclerosis and Coronary Artery Disease,
edited by V. Fuster, R. Ross, and E. J. Topol.
Lippincott-Raven Publishers, Philadelphia © 1996.

CHAPTER 41

Vascular Grafts and Their Sequelae

Larry W. Kraiss and Alexander W. Clowes

Key Words: Intimal hyperplasia; Fluid shear stress; Wall stress; Growth factor; Endothelial dysfunction; Nitric oxide.

INTRODUCTION

Surgical revascularization of the coronary arteries is usually accomplished with autogenous bypass conduits, most commonly the internal mammary artery (IMA) or the saphenous vein. These grafts are readily available, have been extensively studied, are clinically durable, and constitute the gold standards by which all other bypass conduits are compared.

Much evidence suggests that the IMA is the superior bypass vessel, with long-term patency surpassing that of saphenous veins by up to 30% (1–4). Patients receiving an IMA graft have better survival than patients treated only with vein grafts (4–6). Despite widespread preference for the IMA [especially for revascularizing the territory of the left anterior descending (LAD) artery], saphenous vein bypasses are frequently performed, primarily because of logistic considerations such as emergent operation or the need to bypass multiple vessels.

This chapter will focus on the biology of the IMA and the saphenous vein as the preferred conduits for coronary bypass. In particular, reasons for the apparent superiority of the IMA over the saphenous vein will be explored.

Larry W. Kraiss and Alexander W. Clowes: Department of Surgery, Box 356410, University of Washington School of Medicine, Seattle, Washington 98195-6410.

THE INTERNAL MAMMARY ARTERY AND SAPHENOUS VEIN COMPARED

Clinical Experience and Patency Rates

The excellent patency of IMA grafts to the coronary arteries is well established, with numerous groups reporting late (5- to 10-year) patency of well over 90% (1–4) (Fig. 1). Late saphenous vein graft patency over the same period is much poorer (only 40–70%) (1,2,7). The improved patency of IMA grafts translates into better long-term survival and increased freedom from later cardiac morbidity (1,5,6).

Use of the IMA as a graft carries a certain price. Experimental surgical mobilization of the IMA significantly impairs sternal perfusion (8) and may predispose patients to sternal nonunion and subsequent mediastinitis, especially if both IMAs are utilized (9,10). Yet some groups have reported no overall differences in perioperative morbidity and mortality between patients receiving an IMA graft or exclusively vein grafts (11).

Comparative Histology and Physiology

The prominent histologic features of the IMA and saphenous veins are compared in Table 1.

The IMA is a muscular artery with a well-developed media composed of many circumferentially oriented smooth muscle cells (SMC) embedded in an extracellular matrix containing collagen, elastin, and proteoglycans (12). The in-

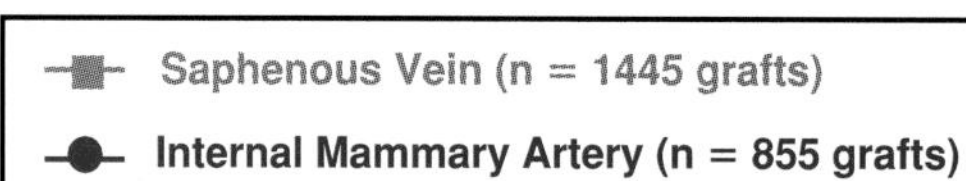

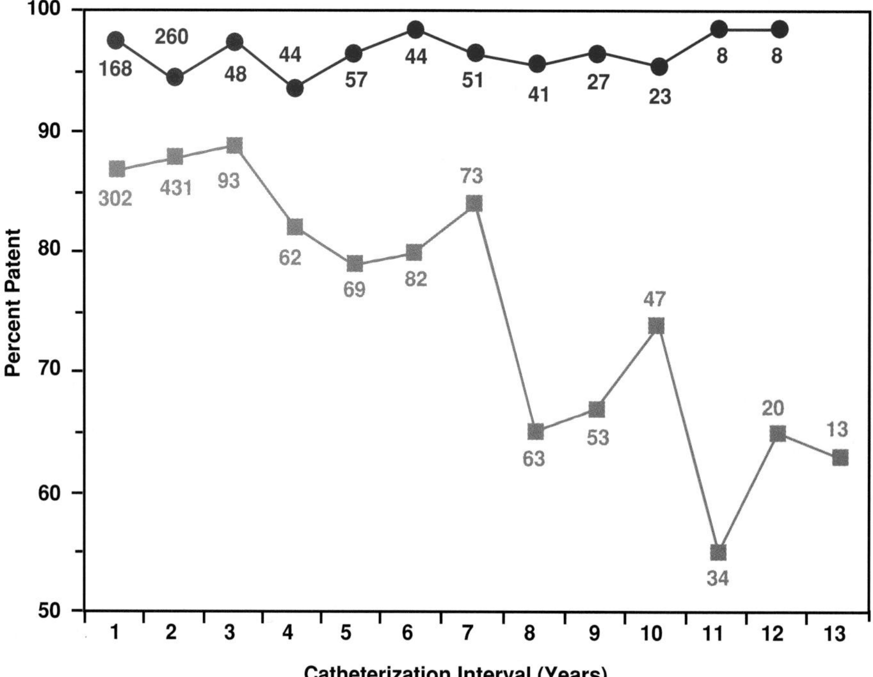

FIG. 1. Patency of internal mammary artery (*circles; n* = 855 grafts) and saphenous vein (*squares; n* = 1,445 grafts) grafts at 1-year intervals. The number of patients restudied at each interval is noted. (From Loop et al., ref. 1, with permission.)

timal compartment is separated from the media by a distinct internal elastic lamina (IEL) rich in laminin, type IV collagen, and heparan sulfate proteoglycans (13).

In contrast, the saphenous vein media is relatively thin, containing fewer SMC, which tend to assume a more random orientation than in the IMA. The IEL is less well defined in the vein than in the IMA. This difference may be important, since a prominent component in the IEL is heparan sulfate proteoglycan, a molecule with known antithrombotic and antiproliferative properties (13). Compared to the IMA, heparin sulfate is less prominent in the media of saphenous veins (14). Thus, the saphenous vein may be more prone to intimal SMC hyperplasia, thrombus formation, or both.

Ultrastructural differences between arterial and venous endothelium also exist (15,16). Arterial endothelial cells appear to be smaller with more cellular processes extending deep into the subendothelial space compared to venous endothelium (15). It is possible that arterial endothelium is more resistant to the trauma of surgical preparation than venous endothelium. The intercellular junctions in venous endothelium tend to be more permeable than arterial intercellular junctions (16) and this may be an important factor contribut-

TABLE 1. *Histologic comparison of veins and arteries*

	Vein	Artery
Endothelial cells	Larger, thinner, less firmly anchored to subendothelium	Smaller, thicker, more firmly anchored to subendothelium
Tunica intima	More permeable	Less permeable
Internal elastic membrane	Poorly defined	Well defined
Media	Thin	Thick
Elastic lamellae	Absent	Present
Medial smooth muscle cells	Few, circular, and longitudinal in arrangement, widely separated by collagen	Circular arrangement, orderly array with collagen, elastic fibers, and matrix
Vasa vasorum	More anastomoses	Less anastomoses
Valves	Present	Absent

Adapted from Cox et al., ref. 12.

ing to the propensity of saphenous vein grafts to become atherosclerotic in the arterial circulation (17).

Another obvious difference between veins and arteries is the presence of venous valves. To prevent obstruction to arterial blood flow, saphenous vein grafts must be reversed, often resulting in a significant size mismatch between the graft and target artery. This mismatch may accentuate hemodynamic abnormalities and flow disturbances at the distal anastomosis. The valves themselves may cause flow disturbances in the body of the graft, especially if scarring is present from preexisting venous disease.

The saphenous vein and IMA also differ significantly in vasoactive responsiveness to various agonists (18). Endothelium-dependent relaxing activity appears much more pronounced in arteries than veins (19,20). These differences are due to reduced production by the veins of the endothelium-derived relaxing factor nitric oxide (NO) (20). In particular, thrombin evokes much greater relaxation in IMA grafts than in saphenous vein grafts. NO is a potent inhibitor of platelet activation, so this difference in NO production may make saphenous vein grafts more prone to thrombosis than IMA grafts (21).

These intrinsic structural and physiologic differences provide a basis for a discussion of the different ways saphenous veins and the IMA respond to being grafted into the coronary circulation.

Pathophysiologic Changes After Grafting

IMA Grafts

IMA grafts appear to undergo few if any significant degenerative changes after functioning for many years as coronary bypasses and are particularly resistant to the development of atherosclerosis (22,23). In selected retrospective series of patients who died or underwent reoperation, up to 40% of IMA grafts displayed identifiable intimal hyperplasia: an accumulation of SMC, and extracellular matrix in the intimal compartment (24). In these patients, the areas of intimal hyperplasia correlated with known sites of angiographic stenosis. The true prevalence of intimal hyperplasia in IMA grafts in a large population of unselected patients is unknown, so it is difficult to determine the clinical importance of this lesion or its relationship to subsequent IMA graft failure.

Saphenous Vein Grafts

Veins grafted into the arterial circulation, whether coronary or peripheral, do not transform themselves into arteries. In this sense, use of the popular term "arterialization" to describe the adaptive changes in vein grafts is inaccurate. While the walls of the veins do thicken after grafting, the ultimate histologic appearance is much different from that of an artery (12). However, the basic concept that a vein transplanted from a low-flow, low-pressure system into a high-flow, high-pressure system must somehow adapt to the radically different hemodynamic environment is fundamental (25). Whether this process is termed "arterialization" or "arterial adaptation" or something else is less important than the realization that the hemodynamic differences between the venous and arterial circuits are profound and probably underly many if not most of the changes that develop in saphenous vein grafts.

Many saphenous veins have preexisting abnormalities at the time they are harvested (26,27). While fibrotic narrowing of ≥25% luminal diameter is unusual (<15% of patients) (27), more than 90% of vein samples contain recognizable intimal hyperplasia (26). Thus, not all pathologic abnormalities found in saphenous vein grafts can be attributed to changes induced by grafting.

A widely recognized sequence of histopathologic changes occur in saphenous vein grafts (7,12,28,29) (Figs. 2, 3; see colorplates 37 and 38). The earliest changes are probably the result of manipulation during harvest and preparation, a process that requires complete dissection and removal of the vein from its native bed as well as some degree of hydrostatic distention. Focal, but not extensive, loss of endothelial cells is fairly common in carefully harvested human saphenous veins (30,31) as well as in experimental situations (32).

Thrombosis is the greatest threat to graft patency during the first few weeks and months after grafting and is the most frequent finding in patients suffering fatal cardiac events during the early postoperative period (33). Accumulations of fibrin on the luminal surface associated with variable degrees of endothelial denudation, edema, and inflammation are common early findings in grafts that remain patent (34).

After the initial postoperative period and during the first year, many saphenous vein grafts develop prominent intimal hyperplasia (7,12) (Fig. 2). In its earliest form, this lesion is quite cellular. Later, extracellular matrix forms the bulk of the lesion, especially in the depths of the intima near the IEL. Simultaneous with the appearance of intimal hyperplasia, the media of the vein graft becomes less cellular and progressively more fibrotic. The net effect of these processes is overall thickening of the vein wall, hence the superficial resemblance to an artery and the origin of the term "arterialization." Since the bulk of the thickening occurs in the intima, while the media actually becomes less cellular, the adapted vein graft is actually quite different from a normal artery.

In the absence of superimposed thrombus, luminal occlusion by exuberant intimal hyperplasia is probably a rare event given the widespread prevalence of the process and the relative infrequency of vein graft failure during the period in which the intimal lesion is growing (35) (see Fig. 1). It is also possible that some of the early reports of fibrotic occlusion of the vein graft were actually instances of chronic thrombotic occlusions that had undergone fibrous reorganization (12,36).

Pathologic lesions occurring more than 3 years after grafting are generally atherosclerotic in appearance (12,37) (Fig. 2). All of the recognized preatherosclerotic and atherosclerotic lesions have been observed in vein grafts. Fatty streaks and fibrous plaques are noted first, while lesions with a lipid core and fibrous cap appear later. Late failure of vein grafts during postoperative years 5–10 is often accompanied by the classic pathologic finding of plaque rupture and luminal occlusion by superimposed thrombus (38). Thus, saphenous vein grafts develop an accelerated process that is very similar to arterial atherosclerosis.

Aneurysmal change is another form of late structural degeneration and may be a particular manifestation of vein graft atherosclerosis. Vein grafts with no other stigmata of atherosclerosis rarely develop aneurysms (7).

MECHANISMS OF GRAFT FAILURE

Thrombosis

The most immediate threat to graft patency after coronary bypass, whatever the conduit, is thrombosis. A number of factors favor the activation of platelets and the coagulation cascade in the newly placed graft, but thrombus formation is usually checked before luminal occlusion occurs. When antithrombotic forces are overwhelmed, graft thrombosis and occlusion occurs. Fortunately, this potentially catastrophic event is relatively unusual (39).

The surgeon can help prevent graft thrombosis by preparing the graft and constructing the anastomoses with technical excellence and by exercising good judgment when choosing the site of the distal anastomosis. Widespread endothelial loss from careless or rough graft preparation will predispose the graft to thrombus formation. Anastomotic strictures or poor outflow because of extensive atherosclerosis in the coronary bed distal to the graft will reduce graft flow, produce stasis, and promote thrombus formation.

Under normal conditions, undiseased arteries and veins exert a net anticoagulant influence, preventing platelet activation at the vessel wall as well as inhibiting the coagulation cascade. Thrombus formation occurs as a combined result of platelet and thrombin generation via the intrinsic or extrinsic coagulation pathways ultimately leading to fibrin formation (40). The importance of preserving endothelial integrity is emphasized when the various antithrombotic roles of endothelium are considered. Normally functioning endothelium regulates both platelet activation and thrombin formation as well as fibrinolysis.

The first step in platelet activation is adherence (41). Platelets possess membrane receptors that allow binding to thrombin, fibrin, and subendothelial elements such as fibronectin. An intact endothelial monolayer helps prevent platelet adherence by masking subendothelial binding sites.

Two significant inhibitors of platelet activation, prostacyclin and NO, are synthesized by endothelial cells. Prostacyclin appears to function by increasing production of cyclic adenosine monophosphate (AMP) in platelets, while NO increases cyclic guanosine monophosphate (GMP). Increased levels of these cyclic nucleotides within the platelet cytosol appear to inhibit platelet activation (41). The process of grafting impairs the production of NO by saphenous vein grafts to much greater extent than by IMA grafts (42–44).

Normally functioning endothelium also inhibits the extrinsic coagulation pathway by preventing activation of circulating factor VII to VIIa by tissue factor. An intensely procoagulant molecule, tissue factor is present in the subendothelial space and may be expressed by damaged or diseased endothelium (40). The endothelium also prevents thrombin formation by several mechanisms apart from preventing the interaction between tissue factor and factor VII. It mediates the physiologic effects of the circulating anticoagulants proteins C and S by expressing thrombomodulin, a molecule necessary for activation of protein C (40). Harvest and preparation of a saphenous vein graft has been shown to decrease thrombomodulin activity by about 30% (45). Heparan sulfate, a glycosaminoglycan that potentiates the activity of antithrombin III, is also synthesized and expressed by endothelial cells in the form of cell-surface and interstitial proteoglycans (46). Antithrombin III inhibits every step of the coagulation cascade and its inhibitory activity is potentiated dramatically by heparin or heparan binding (47).

Tissue plasminogen activator (tPA) is synthesized by endothelial cells and converts plasminogen to plasmin, which then lyses fibrin (48). Significant endothelial loss will thus not only promote the formation of thrombus, it will also impair the graft's ability to lyse the clot before complete graft thrombosis occurs.

At least three of these endothelium-based antithrombotic mechanisms are sensitive to blood flow. The production of prostacyclin (49), NO (50), and tPA (51,52) by endothelial cells are all enhanced by increased fluid shear stress. These findings highlight the importance of maintaining the highest possible blood flow in newly placed, carefully prepared grafts and provide a physiologic explanation for the traditional tenet that stasis promotes thrombosis.

A variety of antiplatelet and anticoagulant strategies have been successfully employed to improve early graft patency. Aspirin (ASA) significantly improves early saphenous vein graft patency when given in the perioperative period, but is of no benefit if started after the second postoperative day (39,41). The addition of other antiplatelet agents such as dipyridamole adds little to the effect of ASA (39,41). When ASA is started preoperatively, there is a higher incidence of postoperative hemorrhagic complications (39). These problems are largely eliminated by starting ASA 6 hr postoperatively without any loss in early graft patency (53).

Anticoagulant treatment with vitamin K antagonists such as warfarin also increases postoperative graft patency, particularly in grafts known to have low flow (54). Obviously, such treatment should be initiated in the postoperative period after a careful consideration of the risks of complete anticoagulation.

Intimal Hyperplasia

The pathologic characteristics that define this lesion are an accumulation of SMC and accompanying extracellular matrix in the intimal compartment. Intimal hyperplasia is undesirable to the extent that it contributes to restenosis and the recurrence of ischemic symptoms, although intimal hyperplasia itself may not cause graft failure (35). Intimal hyperplasia may be a precursor lesion to the subsequent development of atherosclerosis, at least in vein grafts (7).

For a vessel without preexisting intimal hyperplasia, the development of this lesion involves a minimum of two separate processes. First, the SMC must migrate into the intima. Second, the surrounding extracellular matrix must be synthesized. It is also likely that SMC proliferation occurring after migration into the intima contributes to intimal growth.

The pathophysiology of intimal hyperplasia has been most extensively studied in the setting of experimental balloon injury of previously normal arteries (55). In these arteries, intimal hyperplasia develops as a result of medial SMC proliferation, migration of SMC from the media into the intima, followed by ongoing proliferation of intimal SMC and accompanying synthesis of extracellular material (56,57). The initial activation and proliferation of medial SMC is probably driven by release of basic fibroblast growth factor (bFGF) from injured or destroyed vascular wall cells (58). Migration of SMC from the media to the intima appears to be dependent upon the platelet-derived growth factor (PDGF) (59,60).

If the segment of balloon-injured artery is sufficiently long, the destroyed endothelium does not completely regenerate (61,62). In the central part of the injured region, SMC migration and intimal SMC proliferation occur in the absence of an endothelial cover; intimal thickening is much more prominent than at either end of the injured segment where endothelium had regenerated. This finding supports the hypothesis that endothelial cells inhibit or prevent intimal thickening in blood vessels (62).

While the growth-inhibitory function of endothelium might be explained in part by exclusion of blood-borne stimulatory elements from the vessel wall, it is probable that endothelial cells play a more active role in controlling vascular SMC behavior. Endothelium is a very dynamic tissue, capable of synthesizing many molecules which regulate SMC growth or migration. Among these are bFGF, PDGF, transforming growth factor-β (TGF-β), heparan sulfate, endothelin, prostacyclin, and NO (63). Since the intima of most normal blood vessels consists only of endothelium without significant thickening or SMC accumulation, it is probable that a basal function of endothelial cells is to help maintain medial SMC quiescence. Loss of this tonic growth-inhibitory influence through endothelial denudation might then permit SMC proliferation and migration to occur.

While much valuable information has been derived from balloon injury experiments, it is very likely that vein grafts develop intimal thickening through different mechanisms (43,55). The extensive endothelial loss that occurs with balloon injury is unusual in carefully harvested and prepared vein grafts. While surgical preparation may produce enough injury to cause an initial round of SMC proliferation (64,65), the focal areas of endothelial denudation are generally replaced within weeks of grafting. Yet the bulk of the intimal hyperplasia in experimental and clinical vein grafts develops after the endothelium has regenerated (7,31,32). Obviously, the mere presence of endothelium in these vessels is insufficient to prevent SMC from migrating into the intima, proliferating, and synthesizing extracellular matrix. The concept of altered or "dysfunctional" endothelium—endothelium that no longer exerts the expected growth inhibition—can be invoked to account for these observations.

Recall that definite morphologic differences exist between arterial and venous endothelium (see Table 1). It is not surprising, then, that venous endothelium might function differently than arterial endothelium. Endothelial cells in vein grafts cannot *a priori* be expected to functionally mimic arterial endothelial cells, especially when one considers the different hemodynamic environments in the venous and arterial systems. It is also possible that vein graft endothelium is not behaving dysfunctionally, but rather is responding to the new surroundings in a way that optimizes the graft's function as a surrogate artery. From this perspective, the altered biology of the endothelium is not "dysfunctional," but is entirely "appropriate."

A wide array of various growth promoters and growth inhibitors are potentially present in the vessel wall. Some of the better-characterized growth regulators are PDGF, bFGF, TGF-β, and NO. Since it is not possible to exhaustively characterize them here, the reader is referred to several excellent reviews (57,63,66). It is important to remember that most of what is known about how these various factors influence SMC biology *in vivo* comes from arterial injury experiments as opposed to vein grafting experiments.

The growth state of intimal SMC (or the degree of intimal hyperplasia) may represent a dynamic balance between growth promoters and growth inhibitors, similar to the equilibrium between procoagulant and anticoagulant forces that govern thrombotic tendency. In the normal, unperturbed state, most blood vessels have little intimal thickening (perhaps indicating a relative predominance of growth-inhibitory factors). When blood vessels are traumatized by balloon injury, ischemia–reperfusion, or exposure to unfamiliar hemodynamic environments, intimal hyperplasia often results, implying a shift in the balance of growth regulation toward SMC migration and proliferation.

In particular, the IMA may display relative overexpression of growth inhibitors compared to saphenous vein. Basal levels of cyclic GMP (a second messenger system activated by the growth-inhibitory nitrovasodilators) are higher in the IMA than in the saphenous vein (67) and, as mentioned previously, the IMA releases larger amounts of endothelium-derived NO than saphenous vein in response to agonists such as thrombin and acetylcholine (18,20).

The endothelium is probably the pivotal cell type in determining the growth state of the intima. A particular pattern of endothelial gene expression is usually associated with the normal, unperturbed state, while an entirely different pattern can be observed in injured or diseased vessels and vein grafts. Normal endothelium is typically antithrombotic, inhibits SMC proliferation, and readily releases NO in response to defined stimuli (acetylcholine or increased shear stress). In contrast, an altered pattern of endothelial physiology often coexists with the hyperplastic response to injury—or the endothelium is not present at all. Injured vessels are frequently prothrombotic, contain actively proliferating SMC and tend to be vasospastic or display attenuated vasodilation in response to the usual vasorelaxants (31,43,55). For example, saphenous vein grafts appear to lose endothelium-dependent relaxing activity, suggesting a predominance of constricting over relaxing factors after grafting. Vasoconstrictors generally possess mitogenic activity for vascular SMC, while vasodilators tend to be cytostatic (68). Thus, it is logical to consider how the endothelium is affected by the process of vein grafting in hopes of gaining insight into how the equilibrium between SMC growth and inhibition might be shifted to promote the development of intimal hyperplasia. In other words, how does grafting promote SMC growth?

Ischemia–Reperfusion Injury

Veins that are completely removed from their usual anatomic site in preparation for grafting necessarily undergo a period of ischemia, then reperfusion once engrafted. Ischemia–reperfusion induces a burst of superoxide radical generation by endothelial cells, followed shortly thereafter by decreased endothelial production of prostacyclin, NO, and adenosine (64). These substances have all been shown to inhibit SMC proliferation (57). Active oxygen species may also instigate the development of intimal hyperplasia by directly activating SMC proliferation (69). Thus, ischemia–reperfusion appears to increase the expression of growth promoters while decreasing expression of growth inhibitors in the vessel wall. Antioxidant therapy prevents the development of intimal hyperplasia in experimental vein grafts, further supporting the concept that free radicals are important in this disease process (70).

Biomechanical and Hemodynamic Considerations

The coronary artery environment, with its increased intraluminal pressure and altered fluid shear stress relative to the venous environment, may predispose vein grafts to intimal hyperplasia. As discussed previously, this adaptive process has been questionably termed ''arterialization.''

The wall stress S experienced by any blood vessel is directly proportional to intraluminal pressure P and vessel radius R, but inversely proportional to vessel wall thickness h: $S = PR/h$ (71). Saphenous veins typically have larger diameters and thinner walls than coronary arteries. Thus, the wall stress experienced by a saphenous vein after coronary grafting is acutely increased.

In experimental situations, overall wall thickening in vein grafts appears to be related to wall stress. Zwolak et al. (32) showed that rabbit vein grafts inserted into the carotid position stop thickening when their radius to wall thickness ratio (a substitute expression for wall stress) approximates that of the carotid artery. When wall stress in rabbit vein grafts is minimized by external support, wall thickening is also reduced (72). The effects of increased wall stress in vein grafts may be sensed more by mural SMC than the endothelial cells. Dobrin et al. (73) have demonstrated that medial thickening (as opposed to intimal thickening) in canine vein grafts is most dependent upon wall stress. *In vitro,* SMC produce increased amounts of collagen when exposed to cyclic stretching (74). Medial SMC experiencing higher levels of wall stress *in vivo* may respond similarly with increased production of extracellular matrix (leading to wall thickening).

In addition to changes in wall stress, it is likely that a vein graft experiences significantly different fluid shear stresses when transplanted into an arterial location. According to the Hagen–Poiseuille relationship

$$\tau \propto Q/\pi r^3$$

shear stress τ is directly proportional to volume flow Q and inversely proportional to the cube of the vessel radius r (71). Volume flow Q is predicted by the product of mean velocity MV and cross-sectional area πr^2. Substituting these terms for Q allows the Hagen–Poiseuille relationship to be reexpressed as

$$\tau \propto MV/r$$

Relative to the venous circulation, arterial blood velocity is higher, a difference that would tend to increase shear stress. However, because of distention by increased intraluminal pressure, the diameter of vein grafts in the arterial position may be significantly greater than their diameter in the venous circuit. This increased diameter would tend to reduce shear stress. Increased vein diameter would also tend to reduce mean blood velocity, since for a given volume flow, vessels of greater cross-sectional area will have lower velocities. When compared to IMA grafts, saphenous vein grafts to single coronary arteries have been shown to have significantly lower blood velocities (75–77). Berceli et al. modeled the change in shear stress experienced by a canine jugular vein transplanted into the carotid position and calculated that shear stress is *reduced* sixfold as a result of grafting (78). Analogous modeling studies have not been performed for saphenous veins transplanted to the coronary position, so it is difficult to know exactly the changes in shear stress that occur with coronary bypass grafting. It seems reasonable to conclude that shear stress in saphenous vein grafts is probably significantly reduced compared to IMA grafts or native coronary arteries (76,77).

There is abundant evidence that intimal thickening is highly regulated by the local fluid shear-stress environment. Numerous experimental studies have shown that vein grafts in high-shear environments develop less intimal thickening than grafts in low-shear environments (73,79,80). Since it is the endothelial cell that is most likely to sense and respond to changes in fluid shear stress, these findings are consistent with the hypothesis that SMC behavior in vein grafts is controlled by the overlying endothelium. How might shear stress affect the way endothelial cells regulate SMC?

Endothelial cells express a wide variety of genes whose protein products may significantly affect the growth state of underlying medial SMC. Many of these gene products are known to be shear-regulated. These include the mitogens PDGF (81–85), bFGF (83), and endothelin-1 (83,86) as well as the growth inhibitors TGF-β (85) and NO (50,87). If the observed shear-dependent pattern of intimal thickening is to be explained through regulation of growth factors, increased shear stress should reduce growth promoter and increase growth inhibitor expression; decreased shear stress should produce a reciprocal pattern of expression. In general, this particular pattern of growth regulation by shear stress has been observed, particularly with endothelin (86,88) and NO (50,87). PDGF expression by endothelial cells *in vitro* appears to be upregulated by exposure to shear stress (81–85) but the experimental conditions may not accurately reflect the response of endothelium *in vivo*. Using an *in vivo* model of prosthetic graft healing, we have developed evidence that expression of PDGF-A by endothelial cells is upregulated by reduced shear stress (L. W. Kraiss et al., unpublished observations) and nitric oxide synthase expression is reduced (E.J.R. Mattsson et al., unpublished observations). This pattern is thus consistent with the idea that increased shear stress inhibits SMC growth.

In summary, vein grafts experience increased wall stress when transplanted into the arterial circulation; wall thickening tends to reduce wall stress and may represent a compensatory response by the vein graft to the new pressure environment. The change in fluid shear stress that accompanies vein grafting is more difficult to estimate, but there are indications that the shear stress in saphenous vein grafts may be significantly less than in the corresponding coronary artery or IMA grafts because of increased vein diameter (78) and lower overall mean blood flow velocity (75). If this is true, then the combined effects of the alterations in wall stress and shear stress might be a powerful influence favoring the development of vein-graft wall thickening. While intimal thickening in and of itself does not appear to predispose a vein graft to failure by thrombosis, it may provide fertile soil for the development of overt atherosclerotic changes (7).

Atherosclerosis

The lesions of atherosclerosis are generally considered to be fatty streaks (focal accumulations of lipid-laden macrophages) and fibrous plaques (areas of intimal thickening secondary to accumulation of layers of SMC with associated leukocytes) which ultimately develop lipid cores and become complicated by either ulceration or intraplaque hemorrhage (63). These complicated plaques are thought to be responsible for the clinical events that accompany end-stage atherosclerosis: thrombosis and embolization.

IMA grafts appear to be particularly resistant to the development of atherosclerotic lesions (24). Even in patients undergoing reoperation for recurrent coronary artery disease, <10% of previously placed IMA grafts displayed atherosclerotic changes.

In contrast, coronary vein grafts develop an accelerated form of atherosclerosis that is histologically similar to that occurring in arteries (7,29,37,89). It is unusual for vein grafts to display atherosclerotic changes in the first few years after bypass grafting, but in patients undergoing reoperation more than 3 years after the initial procedure, more than half of the grafts are involved with atherosclerosis (7,89). Complicated atherosclerotic plaques in saphenous vein grafts are often the sites of superimposed occlusive thrombus (38).

The true incidence of vein graft atherosclerosis is probably underestimated since the published reports arise from series of patients undergoing reoperation—those who have become sufficiently symptomatic again to justify surgical reintervention. Risk factors for development of vein graft atherosclerosis have been identified from these series (7,89). Graft-specific variables associated with atherosclerosis are the age of the graft, increased intimal thickening, enlarged external diameter, and aneurysm formation. Whether severe intimal thickening, enlarged external diameter, and aneurysmal degeneration are causes or effects of the atherosclerotic process is not known.

Patients with recurrent symptoms because of vein graft atherosclerosis are significantly more likely to have hypercholesterolemia when compared to patients who remain asymptomatic (7,89). In addition, aggressive lipid-lowering therapy reduces the rate at which new stenotic lesions appear in coronary vein grafts (90). The impact of diabetes and smoking is less clear, with one study finding an association with vein graft atherosclerosis (89) and another finding no correlation (7).

As in arteries, atherosclerotic changes and aneurysm formation appear to predispose vein grafts to subsequent thrombosis (7,89).

Treatment of the Failing Graft

Clinicians are often confronted with patients who have recurrent ischemia after previously undergoing coronary artery bypass grafting. Given the progressive decline in vein graft patency with time, these symptoms may be due to disease in the vein graft as well as progression within the native circulation (38,91,92). When ischemia is due to vein graft disease, the prognosis is especially poor without intervention, especially if the involved graft is perfusing the LAD territory (92). Reoperation can improve survival of patients with symptoms due to vein graft disease (93), but it is also more morbid than the initial operation. As a result, nonsurgical means of salvaging failing vein grafts have been developed.

Percutaneous transluminal balloon angioplasty of coronary vein grafts has been performed for over 10 years (94–101). These procedures are most often necessary several years after bypass grafting and are directed at lesions located in the body of the graft rather than at the anastomoses. The experience with angioplasty of IMA grafts is much more limited. In general, these procedures are performed earlier than angioplasty of vein grafts and the culprit lesion is more often anastomotic (94,102,103). These data suggest that the process narrowing the IMA is more likely to be intimal hyperplasia, while in vein grafts it is likely to be atherosclerotic change (94).

Dilatation of diseased vein grafts and diseased coronary arteries results in approximately equal rates of immediate success (95–101), but restenosis occurs more frequently in the vein grafts (95–97,99,101). In addition, angioplasty of vein grafts appears to be complicated more often by distal embolization of atherosclerotic debris resulting in non-Q-wave infarcts due to occlusion of small vessels beyond the reach of bypass (104). Patients whose recurrent symptoms are treated solely by vein graft angioplasty may have poorer long-term survival compared to patients who undergo angioplasty of additional native arterial lesions or who undergo reoperation (98,100).

Stenting of the stenotic vein graft has been proposed as a means of preventing later restenosis (105–108). This technique seems promising, as the largest series of 200 lesions reports only a 17% restenosis rate at 6 months (106). Other studies have reported restenosis rates of 25–36% (105,107,108).

In an effort to address the relatively high restenosis rates seen with balloon angioplasty as well as the problem of distal embolization, atherectomy devices have been used to excise or extract occlusive lesions in coronary vein grafts (109–112). The immediate success rates with atherectomy are as good as with angioplasty; however, no appreciable impact has been made on the rate of complications, and restenosis may occur even more frequently.

The increased risk of distal embolization, higher rates of restenosis, and perhaps poorer long-term survival suggest that these nonsurgical techniques designed to salvage failing grafts are most appropriate for patients who are at particularly high risk for surgery (113). It remains to be seen whether the initial results with vein graft stenting (106) will be confirmed by other studies.

ALTERNATIVES TO THE INTERNAL MAMMARY ARTERY OR SAPHENOUS VEIN

While experience is much more limited than with the IMA, reports using other autogenous arterial conduits such as the radial, inferior epigastric, or gastroepiploic arteries are generally positive (114–116). The gastroepiploic artery possesses a vasoreactive profile that resembles the IMA (117), suggesting that these arteries are more likely to function like IMA grafts than saphenous vein grafts. Use of these conduits significantly increases the overall technical complexity of a coronary bypass procedure.

The patency of other autogenous veins such as the cephalic is much poorer than the saphenous vein when used as a coronary graft (118). Similarly dismal results have been noted with cryopreserved venous allografts (119,120) and these conduits cannot be recommended except as an absolute last resort.

Neither xenografts nor prosthetic coronary grafts are currently viable alternatives to autogenous arterial conduits or saphenous vein.

FUTURE DIRECTIONS

The study of biologic vascular grafts is progressively moving from histologic description toward dissection of the cellular and molecular processes that occur in response to grafting. The next few years will probably see further detailed descriptions of the physiologic differences between arterial and venous endothelium and how these differences affect the performance of arteries or veins as vascular grafts.

As more is learned about the molecular differences between vein grafts and arteries, interventions may emerge that are designed to endow vein grafts with "arterial" properties in an effort to improve long-term vein graft function. One possibility includes manipulation of the nitric oxide system in venous endothelium in an attempt to restore some of the "normal" endothelial properties (growth inhibition, antithrombotic influences, vasodilatory tone) that are lost with grafting.

SUMMARY

At the present time, the best available conduit for coronary revascularization appears to be the IMA. It provides better long-term patency and overall survival when compared to saphenous vein bypass grafts. The biologic reasons for this enhanced performance are beginning to be elucidated and may potentially be explained by fundamental differences in arterial and venous endothelial physiology. For these reasons, the IMA should be used as a graft whenever feasible and should preferably revascularize the critical LAD territory.

Saphenous veins will continue to play a large role in coronary revascularization since multiple grafts are often necessary and emergent conditions may preclude preparation of an IMA graft. While long-term performance is inferior to the IMA, saphenous veins are clearly preferred over other venous conduits, autogenous or otherwise.

REFERENCES

1. Loop FD, Lytle BW, Cosgrove DM, Stewart RW, Goormastic M, Williams GW, Golding LA, Gill CC, Taylor PC, Sheldon WC, Proudfit WL. Influence of the internal-mammary-artery graft on 10-year survival and other cardiac events. *N Engl J Med* 1986;314:1–6.
2. Lytle BW, Loop FD, Cosgrove DM, Ratliff NB, Easley K, Taylor PC. Long-term (5 to 12 years) serial studies of internal mammary artery and saphenous vein coronary bypass grafts. *J Thorac Cardiovasc Surg* 1985;89:248–258.
3. Tector AJ, Schmahl TM, Janson B, Kallies JR, Johnson G. The internal mammary artery graft. Its longevity after coronary bypass. *JAMA* 1981;246:2181–2183.
4. Acinapura AJ, Jacobowitz IJ, Kramer MD, Zisbrod Z, Cunningham JN. Internal mammary artery bypass: thirteen years of experience. Influence of angina and survival in 5125 patients. *J Cardiovasc Surg Torino* 1992;33:554–559.
5. Cameron A, Davis KB, Green GE, Myers WO, Pettinger M. Clinical implications of internal mammary artery bypass grafts: the Coronary Artery Surgery Study experience. *Circulation* 1988;77:815–819.
6. Boylan MJ, Lytle BW, Loop FD, Taylor PC, Borsh JA, Goormastic M, Cosgrove DM. Surgical treatment of isolated left anterior descending coronary stenosis. Comparison of left internal mammary artery and venous autograft at 18 to 20 years of follow-up. *J Thorac Cardiovasc Surg* 1994;107:657–662.
7. Solymoss BC, Leung TK, Pelletier LC, Campeau L. Pathologic changes in coronary artery saphenous vein grafts and related etiologic factors. *Cardiovasc Clin* 1991;21:45–65.
8. Seyfer AE, Shriver CD, Miller TR, Graeber GM. Sternal blood flow after median sternotomy and mobilization of the internal mammary arteries. *Surgery* 1988;104:899–904.
9. Kouchoukos NT, Wareing TH, Murphy SF, Pelate C, Marshall WG Jr. Risks of bilateral internal mammary artery bypass grafting. *Ann Thorac Surg* 1990;49:210–217.
10. Grover FL, Johnson RR, Marshall G, Hammermeister KE. Impact of mammary grafts on coronary bypass operative mortality and morbidity. Department of Veterans Affairs Cardiac Surgeons. *Ann Thorac Surg* 1994;57:559–568.
11. Sethi GK, Copeland JG, Moritz T, Henderson W, Zadina K, Goldman S. Comparison of postoperative complications between saphenous vein and IMA grafts to left anterior descending coronary artery. *Ann Thorac Surg* 1991;51:733–738.
12. Cox JL, Chiasson DA, Gotlieb AI. Stranger in a strange land: the pathogenesis of saphenous vein graft stenosis with emphasis on structural and functional differences between veins and arteries. *Prog Cardiovasc Dis* 1991;34:45–68.
13. Carey DJ. Control of growth and differentiation of vascular cells by extracellular matrix proteins. *Annu Rev Physiol* 1991;53:161–177.
14. Sisto T, Yla-Herttuala S, Luoma J, Riekkinen H, Nikkari T. Biochemical composition of human internal mammary artery and saphenous vein. *J Vasc Surg* 1990;11:418–422.
15. Merrilees MJ, Shepphard AJ, Robinson MC. Structural features of saphenous vein and internal thoracic artery endothelium: correlates with susceptibility and resistance to graft atherosclerosis. *J Cardio Surg Torino* 1988;29:639–646.
16. Simionescu M, Simionescu N, Palade GE. Segmental differentiations of cell junctions in the vascular endothelium. Arteries and veins. *J Cell Biol* 1976;68:705–723.
17. Berceli SA, Borovetz HS, Sheppeck RA, Moosa HH, Warty VS, Armany MA, Herman IM. Mechanisms of vein graft atherosclerosis: LDL metabolism and endothelial actin reorganization. *J Vasc Surg* 1991; 13:336–347.
18. Luscher TF, Tanner FC, Tschudi MR, Noll G. Endothelial dysfunction in coronary artery disease. *Annu Rev Med* 1993;44:395–418.
19. De Mey JG, Vanhoutte PM. Heterogeneous behavior of the canine arterial and venous wall. Importance of the endothelium. *Circ Res* 1982;51:439–447.
20. Luscher TF, Diederich D, Siebenmann R, Lehmann K, Stulz P, von Segesser L, Yang ZH, Turina M, Gradel E, Weber E. Difference between endothelium-dependent relaxation in arterial and in venous coronary bypass grafts. *N Engl J Med* 1988;319:462–467.
21. Moncada S, Palmer RMJ, Higgs EA. Nitric oxide: physiology, pathophysiology, and pharmacology. *Pharmacol Rev* 1991;43:109–142.
22. Grondin CM, Campeau L, Lesperance J, Enjalbert M, Bourassa MG. Comparison of late changes in internal mammary artery and saphenous vein grafts in two consecutive series of patients 10 years after operation. *Circulation* 1984;70:i208–i212.
23. Bourassa MG, Campeau L, Lesperance J. Changes in grafts and coronary arteries after coronary bypass surgery. *Cardiovasc Clin* 1991; 21:83–100.
24. Shelton ME, Forman MB, Virmani R, Bajaj A, Stoney WS, Atkinson JB. A comparison of morphologic and angiographic findings in long-term internal mammary artery and saphenous vein bypass grafts. *J Am Coll Cardiol* 1988;11:297–307.
25. Carrel A, Guthrie CC. Results of the biterminal transplantation of veins. *Am J Med Sci* 1906;132:415–422.
26. Sayers RD, Jones L, Varty K, Allen K, Morgan JDT, Bell PRF, London NJM. The histopathology of infrainguinal vein graft stenoses. *Eur J Vasc Surg* 1993;7:16–20.
27. Waller BF, Roberts EC. Remnant saphenous veins after aortocoronary bypass grafting: analysis of 3,394 centimeters of unused vein from 402 patients. *Am J Cardiol* 1985;55:65–71.
28. Batayias GE, Barboriak JJ, Korns ME, Pintar K. The spectrum of pathologic changes in aortocoronary saphenous vein grafts. *Circulation* 1977;56:iI18–iI22.
29. Barboriak JJ, Pintar K, Van HDL, Batayias GE, Korns ME. Pathologic findings in the aortocoronary vein grafts. A scanning electron microscope study. *Atherosclerosis* 1978;29:69–80.
30. Sayers RD, Watt PA, Muller S, Bell PR, Thurston H. Structural and functional smooth muscle injury after surgical preparation of reversed and non-reversed *(in situ)* saphenous vein bypass grafts. *Br J Surg* 1991;78:1256–1258.
31. Davies MG, Hagen PO. Structural and functional consequences of bypass grafting with autologous vein. *Cryobiology* 1994;31:63–70.
32. Zwolak RM, Adams MC, Clowes AW. Kinetics of vein graft hyperplasia: association with tangential stress. *J Vasc Surg* 1987;5: 126–136.
33. Vlodaver Z, Edwards JE. Pathologic analysis in fatal cases following saphenous vein coronary arterial bypass. *Chest* 1973;64:555–563.
34. Spray TL, Roberts WC. Changes in saphenous veins used as aortocoronary bypass grafts. *Am Heart J* 1977;94:500–516.
35. Lawrie GM, Lie JT, Morris GC Jr, Beazley HL. Vein graft patency and intimal proliferation after aortocoronary bypass: early and long-term angiopathologic correlations. *Am J Cardiol* 1976;38:856–862.
36. Kern WH, Dermer GB, Lindesmith GG. The intimal proliferation in aortic-coronary saphenous vein grafts. Light and electron microscopic studies. *Am Heart J* 1972;84:771–777.
37. Lie JT, Lawrie GM, Morris GC Jr. Aortocoronary bypass saphenous vein graft atherosclerosis. Anatomic study of 99 vein grafts from normal and hyperlipoproteinemic patients up to 75 months postoperatively. *Am J Cardiol* 1977;40:906–914.
38. Qiao JH, Walts AE, Fishbein MC. The severity of atherosclerosis at sites of plaque rupture with occlusive thrombosis in saphenous vein coronary artery bypass grafts. *Am Heart J* 1991;122:955–958.
39. Goldman S, Copeland J, Moritz T, Henderson W, Zadina K, Ovitt T, Doherty J, Read R, Chesler E, Sako Y, Lancaster L, Emery R, Sharma GVRK, Josa M, Pacold I, Montoya A, Parikh D, Sethi G, Holt J, Kirklin J, Shabetai R, Moores W, Aldridge J, Masud Z, DeMots H, Floten S, Haakenson C, Harker LA. Improvement in early saphenous vein graft patency after coronary artery bypass surgery with antiplatelet therapy: results of a Veterans Administration Cooperative Study. *Circulation* 1988;77:1324–1332.
40. Nachman RL, Silverstein R. Hypercoagulable states. *Ann Intern Med* 1993;119:819–827.
41. Stein B, Fuster V, Israel DH, Cohen M, Badimon L, Badimon JJ, Chesebro JH. Platelet inhibitor agents in cardiovascular disease: an update. *J Am Coll Cardiol* 1989;14:813–836.
42. Yang Z, Luscher TF. Endothelium-dependent regulatory mechanisms in human coronary bypass grafts: possible clinical implications. *Z Kardiol* 1989;78:80–84.

43. Yang Z, Luscher TF. Basic cellular mechanisms of coronary bypass graft disease. *Eur Heart J* 1993;14:193–197.
44. Yang ZH, Stulz P, von Segesser L, Bauer E, Turina M, Luscher TF. Different interactions of platelets with arterial and venous coronary bypass vessels. *Lancet* 1991;337:939–943.
45. Cook JM, Cook CD, Marlar R, Solis MM, Fink L, Eidt JF. Thrombomodulin activity on human saphenous vein grafts prepared for coronary artery bypass. *J Vasc Surg* 1991;14:147–151.
46. Marcum JA, Atha DH, Fritze LM, Nawroth P, Stern D, Rosenberg RD. Cloned bovine aortic endothelial cells synthesize anticoagulantly active heparan sulfate proteoglycan. *J Biol Chem* 1986;361: 7507–7517.
47. Marcum JA, McKenney JB, Rosenberg RD. Acceleration of thrombin–antithrombin complex formation in rat hindquarters via heparinlike molecules bound to the endothelium. *J Clin Invest* 1984;74: 341–350.
48. Van Hinsbergh VW. Regulation of the synthesis and secretion of plasminogen activators by endothelial cells. *Haemostasis* 1988;18: 307–327.
49. Frangos JA, Eskin SG, McIntire LV, Ives CL. Flow effects on prostacyclin production by cultured human endothelial cells. *Science* 1985; 227:1477–1479.
50. Rubanyi GM, Romero JC, Vanhoutte PM. Flow-induced release of endothelium-derived relaxing factor. *Am J Physiol* 1986;250: h1145–h1149.
51. Diamond SL, Eskin SG, McIntire LV. Fluid flow stimulates tissue plasminogen activator secretion by cultured human endothelial cells. *Science* 1989;243:1483–1485.
52. Diamond SL, Sharefkin JB, Dieffenbach C, Frasier-Scott K, McIntire LV, Eskin SG. Tissue plasminogen activator messenger RNA levels increase in cultured human endothelial cells exposed to laminar shear stress. *J Cell Physiol* 1990;143:364–371.
53. Goldman S, Copeland J, Moritz T, Henderson W, Zadina K, Ovitt T, Kern KB, Sethi G, Sharma GV, Khuri S, Richards K, Grover F, Morrison D, Whitman G, Chesler E, Sako Y, Pacold I, Montoya A, DeMots H, Floten S, Doherty J, Read R, Scott S, Spooner T, Masud Z, Haakenson C, Harker LA, Department of Veterans Affairs Cooperative Study Group. Starting aspirin therapy after operation: effects on early graft patency. Department of Veterans Affairs Cooperative Study Group. *Circulation* 1991;84:520–526.
54. Gohlke H, Gohlke-Barwolf C, Sturzenhofecker P, Gornandt L, Ritter B, Reichelt M, Buchwalsky R, Schmuziger M, Roskamm H. Improved graft patency with anticoagulant therapy after aortocoronary bypass surgery: a prospective, randomized study. *Circulation* 1981;64: iI22–iI27.
55. Clowes AW. Intimal hyperplasia and graft failure. *Cardiovasc Pathol* 1993;2:179S–186S.
56. Clowes AW, Clowes MM, Fingerle J, Reidy MA. Regulation of smooth muscle cell growth in injured artery. *J Cardiovasc Pharmacol* 1989;14:S12–S15.
57. Jackson CL, Schwartz SM. Pharmacology of smooth muscle cell replication. *Hypertension* 1992;20:713–736.
58. Lindner V, Reidy MA. Proliferation of smooth muscle cells after vascular injury is inhibited by an antibody against basic fibroblast growth factor. *Proc Natl Acad Sci USA* 1991;88:3739–3743.
59. Jawien A, Bowen-Pope DF, Lindner V, Schwartz SM, Clowes AW. Platelet-derived growth factor promotes smooth muscle migration and intimal thickening in a rat model of balloon angioplasty. *J Clin Invest* 1992;89:507–511.
60. Ferns GA, Raines EW, Sprugel KH, Motani AS, Reidy MA, Ross R. Inhibition of neointimal smooth muscle accumulation after angioplasty by an antibody to PDGF. *Science* 1991;253:1129–1132.
61. Clowes AW, Reidy MA, Clowes MM. Kinetics of cellular proliferation after arterial injury. I. Smooth muscle growth in the absence of endothelium. *Lab Invest* 1983;49:327–333.
62. Clowes AW, Clowes MM, Reidy MA. Kinetics of cellular proliferation after arterial injury. III. Endothelial and smooth muscle growth in chronically denuded vessels. *Lab Invest* 1986;54:295–303.
63. Ross R. The pathogenesis of atherosclerosis: a perspective for the 1990s. *Nature* 1993;362:801–809.
64. Holt CM, Francis SE, Newby AC, Rogers S, Gadsdon PA, Taylor T, Angelini GD. Comparison of response to injury in organ culture of human saphenous vein and internal mammary artery. *Ann Thorac Surg* 1993;55:1522–1528.
65. Soyombo AA, Angelini GD, Bryan AJ, Newby AC. Surgical preparation induces injury and promotes smooth muscle cell proliferation in a culture of human saphenous vein. *Cardiovasc Res* 1993;27: 1961–1967.
66. Schwartz SM, Heimark RL, Majesky MW. Developmental mechanisms underlying pathology of arteries. *Physiol Rev* 1990;70: 1177–1209.
67. Tadjkarimi S, O'Neil GS, Luu TN, Allen SP, Schyns CJ, Chester AH, Yacoub MH. Comparison of cyclic GMP in human internal mammary artery and saphenous vein: implications for coronary artery bypass graft patency. *Cardiovasc Res* 1992;26:297–300.
68. Berk BC, Alexander RW. Vasoactive effects of growth factors. *Biochem Pharmacol* 1989;38:219–225.
69. Rao GN, Berk BC. Active oxygen species stimulate vascular smooth muscle cell growth and proto-oncogene expression. *Circ Res* 1992; 70:593–599.
70. Hagen PO, Davies MG, Schuman RW, Murray JJ. Reduction of vein graft intimal hyperplasia by *ex vivo* treatment with desferrioxamine manganese. *J Vasc Res* 1992;29:405–409.
71. Milnor WR. *Hemodynamics,* 2nd ed. Baltimore: Williams and Wilkins; 1989.
72. Kohler TR, Kirkman TR, Clowes AW. The effect of rigid external support on vein graft adaptation to the arterial circulation. *J Vasc Surg* 1989;9:277–285.
73. Dobrin PB, Littooy FN, Endean ED. Mechanical factors predisposing to intimal hyperplasia and medial thickening in autogenous vein grafts. *Surgery* 1989;105:393–400.
74. Sumpio BE, Banes AJ, Link WG, Johnson G Jr. Enhanced collagen production by smooth muscle cells during repetitive mechanical stretching. *Arch Surg* 1988;123:1233–1236.
75. Bandyk DF, Galbraith TA, Haasler GB, Almassi GH. Blood flow velocity of internal mammary artery and saphenous vein grafts to the coronary arteries. *J Surg Res* 1988;44:342–351.
76. Fusejima K, Takahara Y, Sudo Y, Murayama H, Masuda Y, Inagaki Y. Comparison of coronary hemodynamics in patients with internal mammary artery and saphenous vein coronary artery bypass grafts: a noninvasive approach using combined two-dimensional and Doppler echocardiography. *J Am Coll Cardiol* 1990;15:131–139.
77. Bach RG, Kern MJ, Donohue TJ, Aguirre FV, Caracciolo EA. Comparison of phasic blood flow velocity characteristics of arterial and venous coronary artery bypass conduits. *Circulation* 1993;88:II-133–II-140.
78. Berceli SA, Showalter DP, Sheppeck RA, Mandarino WA, Borovetz HS. Biomechanics of the venous wall under simulated arterial conditions. *J Biomech* 1990;23:985–989.
79. Berguer R, Higgins RF, Reddy DJ. Intimal hyperplasia: an experimental study. *Arch Surg* 1980;115:332–335.
80. Rittgers SE, Karayannacos PE, Guy JF, Nerem RM, Shaw GM, Hostetler JR, Vasko JS. Velocity distribution and intimal proliferation in autologous vein grafts in dogs. *Circ Res* 1978;42:792–801.
81. Hsieh H-J, Li N-Q, Frangos JA. Shear-induced platelet-derived growth factor gene expression in human endothelial cells is mediated by protein kinase C. *J Cell Physiol* 1992;150:552–528.
81. Hsieh H-J, Li N-Q, Frangos JA. Shear stress increases endothelial platelet-derived growth factor mRNA levels. *Am J Physiol* 1991;260: H642–H646.
83. Malek AM, Gibbons GH, Dzau VJ, Izumo S. Fluid shear stress differentially modulates expression of genes encoding basic fibroblast growth factor and platelet-derived growth factor B chain in vascular endothelium. *J Clin Invest* 1993;92:2013–2021.
84. Mitsumata M, Fishel RS, Nerem RM, Alexander RW, Berk BC. Fluid shear stress stimulates platelet-derived growth factor expression in endothelial cells. *Am J Physiol* 1993;265:H3–H8.
85. Resnick N, Collins T, Atkinson W, Bonthron DT, Dewey CF Jr, Gimbrone MA Jr. Platelet-derived growth factor B chain promoter contains a *cis*-acting fluid shear-stress-responsive element. *Proc Natl Acad Sci USA* 1993;90:4591–4595.
86. Sharefkin JB, Diamond SL, Eskin SG, McIntire LV, Dieffenbach CW. Fluid flow decreases preproendothelin mRNA levels and suppresses endothelin-1 peptide release in cultured human endothelial cells. *J Vasc Surg* 1991;14:1–9.
87. Buga GM, Gold ME, Fukuto JM, Ignarro LJ. Shear stress-induced release of nitric oxide from endothelial cells grown on beads. *Hypertension* 1991;17:187–193.

88. Malek A, Izumo S. Physiological fluid shear stress causes downregulation of endothelin-1 mRNA in bovine aortic endothelium. *Am J Physiol* 1992;263:C389–C396.
89. Neitzel GF, Barboriak JJ, Pintar K, Qureshi I. Atherosclerosis in aortocoronary bypass grafts. Morphologic study and risk factor analysis 6 to 12 years after surgery. *Arteriosclerosis* 1986;6:594–600.
90. Cashin-Hemphill L, Mack WJ, Pogoda JM, Sanmarco ME, Azen SP, Blankenhorn DH. Beneficial effects of colestipol–niacin on coronary atherosclerosis. A 4-year follow-up. *JAMA* 1990;264:3013–3017.
91. Singh RN, Sosa JA, Green GE. Long-term fate of the internal mammary artery and saphenous vein grafts. *J Thorac Cardiovasc Surg* 1983;86:359–363.
92. Lytle BW, Loop FD, Taylor PC, Simpfendorfer C, Kramer JR, Ratliff NB, Goormastic M, Cosgrove DM. Vein graft disease: the clinical impact of stenoses in saphenous vein bypass grafts to coronary arteries. *J Thorac Cardiovasc Surg* 1992;103:831–840.
93. Lytle BW, Loop FD, Taylor PC, Goormastic M, Stewart RW, Novoa R, McCarthy P, Cosgrove DM. The effect of coronary reoperation on the survival of patients with stenoses in saphenous vein bypass grafts to coronary arteries. *J Thorac Cardiovasc Surg* 1993;105:605–612.
94. Waters D, Cote G. Angioplasty of bypass grafts and native arteries. *Cardiovasc Clin* 1991;21:241–256.
95. Pinkerton CA, Slack JD, Orr CM, Vantassel JW, Smith ML. Percutaneous transluminal angioplasty in patients with prior myocardial revascularization surgery. *Am J Cardiol* 1988;61:15G–22G.
96. Cote G, Myler RK, Stertzer SH, Clark DA, Fishman RJ, Murphy M, Shaw RE. Percutaneous transluminal angioplasty of stenotic coronary artery bypass grafts: 5 years' experience. *J Am Coll Cardiol* 1987;9: 8–17.
97. Douglas JS Jr, Gruentzig AR, King SB III, Hollman J, Ischinger T, Meier B, Craver JM, Jones EL, Waller JL, Bone DK, Guyton R. Percutaneous transluminal coronary angioplasty in patients with prior coronary bypass surgery. *J Am Coll Cardiol* 1983;2:745–754.
98. Dorros G, Iyer S, Mathiak LM, Anderson AJ. The impact of balloon angioplasty of coronary artery and/or vein bypass graft lesion(s) upon the survival of patients > or = 5 years after their last bypass surgery. *Eur Heart J* 1993;14:1354–1364.
99. Meester BJ, Samson M, Suryapranata H, Bonsel G, van den Brand M, de Feyter PJ, Serruys PW. Long-term follow-up after attempted angioplasty of saphenous vein grafts: the Thoraxcenter experience 1981–1988. *Eur Heart J* 1991;12:648–653.
100. Morrison DA, Crowley ST, Veerakul G, Barbiere CC, Grover F, Sacks J. Percutaneous transluminal angioplasty of saphenous vein grafts for medically refractory unstable angina. *J Am Coll Cardiol* 1994;23: 1066–1070.
101. Platko WP, Hollman J, Whitlow PL, Franco I. Percutaneous transluminal angioplasty of saphenous vein graft stenosis: long-term follow-up. *J Am Coll Cardiol* 1989;14:1645–1650.
102. Pinkerton CA, Slack JD, Orr CM, Van Tassel JW. Percutaneous transluminal angioplasty involving internal mammary artery bypass grafts: a femoral approach. *Cathet Cardiovasc Diagn* 1987;13:414–418.
103. Shimshak TM, Giorgi LV, Johnson WL, McConahay DR, Rutherford BD, Ligon R, Hartzler GO. Application of percutaneous transluminal coronary angioplasty to the internal mammary artery graft. *J Am Coll Cardiol* 1988;12:1205–1214.
104. Liu MW, Douglas JS Jr, Lembo NJ, King SB III. Angiographic predictors of a rise in serum creatine kinase (distal embolization) after balloon angioplasty of saphenous vein coronary artery bypass grafts. *Am J Cardiol* 1993;72:514–517.
105. Pomerantz RM, Kuntz RE, Carrozza JP, Fishman RF, Mansour M, Schnitt SJ, Safian RD, Baim DS. Acute and long-term outcome of narrowed saphenous venous grafts treated by endoluminal stenting and directional atherectomy. *Am J Cardiol* 1992;70:161–167.
106. Piana RN, Moscucci M, Cohen DJ, Kugelmass AD, Senerchia C, Kuntz RE, Baim DS, Carrozza JPJ. Palmaz–Schatz stenting for treatment of focal vein graft stenosis: immediate results and long-term outcome. *J Am Coll Cardiol* 1994;23:1296–1304.
107. Eeckhout E, Goy JJ, Vogt P, Stauffer JC, Sigwart U, Kappenberger L. Complications and follow-up after intracoronary stenting: critical analysis of a 6-year single-center experience. *Am Heart J* 1994;127: 262–272.
108. Strauss BH, Serruys PW, de Scheerder IK, Tijssen JGP, Bertrand ME, Puel J, Meier B, Kaufmann U, Stauffer JC, Rickards AF, Sigwart U. Relative risk analysis of angiographic predictors of restenosis within the coronary Wallstent. *Circulation* 1991;84:1636–1643.
109. Popma JJ, De Cesare NB, Pinkerton CA, Kereiakes DJ, Whitlow P, King SB III, Topol EJ, Holmes DR, Leon MB, Ellis SG. Quantitative analysis of factors influencing late lumen loss and restenosis after directional coronary atherectomy. *Am J Cardiol* 1993;71:552–557.
110. Kaufmann UP, Garratt KN, Vlietstra RE, Holmes DR Jr. Transluminal atherectomy of saphenous vein aortocoronary bypass grafts. *Am J Cardiol* 1990;65:1430–1433.
111. Hong MK, Popma JJ, Pichard AD, Kent KM, Satler LF, Chuang YC, Mintz GS, Keller MB, Leon MB. Clinical significance of distal embolization after transluminal extraction atherectomy in diffusely diseased saphenous vein grafts. *Am Heart J* 1994;127:1496–1503.
112. Safian RD, Grines CL, May MA, Lichtenberg A, Juran N, Schreiber TL, Pavlides G, Meany TB, Savas V, O'Neill WW. Clinical and angiographic results of transluminal extraction coronary atherectomy in saphenous vein bypass grafts. *Circulation* 1994;89:302–312.
113. De Feyter PJ, van Suylen RJ, de Jaegere PP, Topol EJ, Serruys PW. Balloon angioplasty for the treatment of lesions in saphenous vein bypass grafts. *J Am Coll Cardiol* 1993;21:1539–1549.
114. Acar C, Jebara VA, Portoghese M, Beyssen B, Pagny JY, Grare P, Chachques JC, Fabiani JN, Deloche A, Guermonprez JL, Carpentier AF. Revival of the radial artery for coronary artery bypass grafting. *Ann Thorac Surg* 1992;54:652–659.
115. Beretta L, Antonacci C, Santoli C. Gastroepiploic artery free graft for coronary bypass. *Eur J Cardiothorac Surg* 1991;5:110–111.
116. Suma H, Amano A, Fukuda S, Kigawa I, Horii T, Wanibuchi Y, Nabuchi A. Gastroepiploic artery graft for anterior descending coronary artery bypass. *Ann Thorac Surg* 1994;57:925–927.
117. Ochiai M, Ohno M, Taguchi J, Hara K, Suma H, Isshiki T, Yamaguchi T, Kurokawa K. Responses of human gastroepiploic arteries to vasoactive substances: comparison with responses of internal mammary arteries and saphenous veins. *J Thorac Cardiovasc Surg* 1992;104: 453–458.
118. Wijnberg DS, Boeve WJ, Ebels T, van Gelder IC, van den Toren EW, Lie KI, Homan van der Heide JN. Patency of arm vein grafts used in aorto-coronary bypass surgery. *Eur J Cardiothorac Surg* 1990;4: 510–513.
119. Sellke FW, Stanford W, Rossi NP. Failure of cryopreserved saphenous vein allografts following coronary artery bypass surgery. *J Cardiovasc Surg Torino* 1991;32:820–823.
120. Laub GW, Muralidharan S, Clancy R, Eldredge WJ, Chen C, Adkins MS, Fernandez J, Anderson WA, McGrath LB. Cryopreserved allograft veins as alternative coronary artery bypass conduits: early phase results. *Ann Thorac Surg* 1992;54:826–831.

Atherosclerosis and Coronary Artery Disease,
edited by V. Fuster, R. Ross, and E. J. Topol.
Lippincott-Raven Publishers, Philadelphia © 1996.

CHAPTER 42

Gene Transfer

Elizabeth G. Nabel and Gary J. Nabel

Key Words: vascular disease; gene transfer; gene therapy; molecular biology; vectors; growth factors; endothelial cells; smooth muscle cells; antisense oligonucleotides.

INTRODUCTION

Gene transfer is the introduction and expression of recombinant genes in mammalian cells. In the past 10 years, major advances have been made in the field of gene transfer, including vector design and development of animal models of human disease. Genetic models of human disease have been created and employed to study the pathophysiology of these diseases and to design gene-based therapeutics. Many of the advances in recombinant DNA technology that affect the clinical management of patients have involved the development of new molecular techniques for the diagnosis of disorders. The concept that human disease might be treated by the transfer of genetic material into specific cells of a patient, rather than by conventional drugs, is straightforward and appealing. However, the technical challenges of gene transfer are significant, and this research requires the coordinated development of many new technologies and the establishment of collaborative interactions between basic scientists and clinical investigators.

In this chapter, we review the field of gene transfer in relation to cardiovascular disease. The principles of gene transfer are defined. Viral and nonviral vectors used to transduce vascular cells are discussed, and animal models of vascular disease created by gene transfer methods are presented. Although advances in the application of these methods to the treatment of human vascular diseases have been made, a number of parameters must yet be optimized with respect to efficiency of gene delivery, achievement of high level, stable and targeted gene expression, and design of vectors that are safe for human administration.

E. G. Nabel and G. J. Nabel: Departments of Internal Medicine and Biological Chemistry, Cardiovascular Research Center, Howard Hughes Medical Institute, University of Michigan, Ann Arbor, Michigan 48109.

PRINCIPLES OF GENE TRANSFER

The goal of gene transfer is to introduce recombinant genes, genes that have been modified in the laboratory to incorporate foreign DNA or gene sequences of interest, into target cells to study the mechanisms and consequences of gene expression. An initial step in this approach is the construction of gene transfer vectors. The coding region of the recombinant gene (the DNA containing the nucleotide sequence that is transcribed and translated into the corresponding protein) is inserted or ligated into a vector for its return to host cells. Genes are transfected into cells using vectors (1,2), including defective viruses, such as retroviruses, adenoviruses, adeno-associated viruses, or herpesviruses, and nonviral vectors such as cationic liposomes, viral liposome complexes, or physical injection. Vectors are used to transfer genes into cells because most cells are resistant to the uptake of foreign DNA. Vectors penetrate the host cell with varying efficiency, depending on the cell type. In general, vectors enter target cells by receptor-mediated endocytosis or pH-independent fusion with the cell membrane. In the cytoplasm, the foreign DNA is released from endosomes and is transported to the nucleus. The foreign DNA integrates into the host genome or is maintained in the nucleus as an episome without integration. The recombinant gene undergoes transcription into RNA and is translated into protein by host enzymes, culminating in the expression of the recombinant protein. The recombinant protein may remain intracellular or be secreted into the extracellular space or circulation. Gene expression can be transient or stable, depending on whether integration into chromosomes occurs. The efficiency of DNA uptake and gene expression, often referred to as transfection efficiency, is dependent on many factors, including delivery of DNA to the cell, uptake of DNA into the cytoplasm, degradation of DNA in endosomes, release of DNA from endosomes into the cytoplasm, transport to the nucleus, and persistence in the nucleus.

Following construction of a vector encoding a recombinant gene, the vector generally is tested in vascular endothelial or smooth muscle cells in culture, and animal models are then developed in vivo. In vivo gene transfer animal models are established by two approaches: ex vivo gene transfer and direct in vivo gene transfer. Cell-mediated or ex vivo gene transfer involves removing autologous cells from the host and transfecting the cells with the vector in vitro (3,4). The genetically modified cells are reintroduced into the host by infusion or injection. Ex vivo gene transfer permits the introduction of recombinant genetic material into a specific cell, for example, endothelial or smooth muscle cells, and analysis of recombinant gene expression within that cell type. Ex vivo gene transfer, however, is a complex procedure, requiring the establishment and modification of patient cells in the laboratory. In addition, there are many instances in which cell lines cannot be established in the laboratory from patients or in animal models.

In vivo gene transfer employs the direct introduction of recombinant genes into target cells and tissues. This approach is straightforward, and direct in vivo gene transfer in the vasculature has been achieved by catheter gene delivery (5). Direct gene transfer in the vasculature, however, is currently limited by a lack of targeted gene expression to either endothelial cells or smooth muscle cells. Following in vivo gene transfer, recombinant genes are expressed in multiple cells, including endothelial cells, smooth muscle cells, and macrophages. An additional limitation is that gene expression cannot be precisely regulated. The development of cell-specific and regulated promoters may alleviate this difficulty. Both ex vivo and in vivo gene transfer approaches have been employed in the development of animal models of vascular disease and in clinical trials of gene transfer to the cardiovascular system.

VECTOR SYSTEMS

Viral Vectors

Transfection of appropriate target cells represent the critical first step in gene transfer. As a result, development of gene transfer methods has represented a significant area of research in the field. Both viral and nonviral vectors have been employed in vascular gene transfer studies (Table 1). A common feature of these methods is the efficient delivery of genes into cells. Vectors differ, however, in the processing of foreign DNA and the frequency of integration into chromosomal DNA. In the case of retroviral vectors, the transferred sequences are stably integrated into the chromosomal DNA of the target cell. These vectors have been considered most often for ex vivo gene therapy. Other methods of gene transfer result primarily in the introduction of foreign DNA into target cell nucleus in an unintegrated form. These methods result in high, but transient, gene expression. These vectors, including adenovirus and cationic liposomes, have been employed predominantly in in vivo gene transfer studies

Retroviruses

Retroviruses were the first vectors employed in gene transfer studies in the 1980s (6–8). Interest in retroviruses as vectors stemmed from the observation that these vectors can stably transduce up to 100% of target cells in culture (9). The life cycle of a retrovirus is characterized by binding of virus to a retroviral receptor, entry into a cell, with introduction of genetic material (RNA) and proteins into the cyto-

TABLE 1. *Vectors used in catheter gene transfer to arteries in vivo*[a]

	Efficiency	Integration	Stability	Toxicity
Viral				
Retrovirus	Low	High	Months	Minimal
Adenovirus	High	Low	Weeks	Immunity
Adenovirus-augmented, receptor-mediated gene delivery	Unknown	Low	Unknown	Unknown
Nonviral				
Cationic liposomes	Low–moderate	Low	Weeks to months	Minimal
HVJ liposomes	Low–moderate	Low	Weeks to months	Minimal
DNA gel	Low	Low	Weeks to months	Minimal
Naked DNA	Low	Low	Weeks to months	Minimal

[a] From Nabel and Nabel (189), with permission.

plasm (10). Retroviral RNA includes three major coding regions: *gag,* which encodes proteins of the viral core; *pol,* which encodes the enzyme reverse transcriptase; and *env,* which encodes the constituents of the envelope coat. In the cytoplasm, reverse transcriptase converts RNA into DNA, and proviral DNA migrates to the nucleus and integrates into chromosomes. The provirus DNA directs the synthesis of viral RNA and proteins. The proteins enclose the RNA, forming viral particles that bud from the cell.

Investigators have taken advantage of retroviral replication in host cells, including integration of viral DNA into chromosomes, in the design of retroviral vectors (Fig. 1). Retroviral vectors are constructed to express the recombinant gene within the cell and to be replication incompetent, thus limiting subsequent viral replication after delivery of the foreign gene to the host cell. Retroviruses are modified for use as vectors by removal of the viral structural genes necessary for viral replication while leaving the packaging signal intact (11,12). This renders the retrovirus replication incompetent so that wild-type retroviruses cannot be produced in the target cell (13). The altered retrovirus is transfected into a packaging cell line. This packaging cell line contains plasmids encoding all of the retroviral structural genes under control of the regulatory sequences of the viral promoter but lacks the packaging signal (14). The vector transcripts are recognized by the viral proteins involved in packaging, and a replication-deficient virion is produced. The viral particles carry foreign gene sequences and not viral replication genes. These virions are collected and concentrated from culture supernatant and used in gene transfer studies. The virions enter target cells and insert the foreign gene into cellular DNA, but they cannot reproduce. Introduction of multiple modifications of the helper provirus have been made so that more than one recombination event is required to generate wild-type virus (14–16). This provides further protection to the host.

Retroviral vectors have been employed in many early in vitro (17,18) and in vivo (3,19) demonstrations of vascular gene transfer. In addition, retroviral vectors were employed in gene transfer approaches in other target cells, including skin fibroblasts (20,21), bone marrow progenitor cells (22–24), and hepatocytes (25,26). Stable retroviral infection has been accomplished in many cell types, predominantly those characterized by high proliferative indices. In vascular cells, however, the efficiency of gene transfer is lower. Approximately 5–10% of rat, porcine, or bovine endothelial cells are routinely transfected in vitro, while 0.1 to 1% of endothelial cells have been transfected in vivo (27,28). Because replication of the target cell is necessary to proviral integration to occur (29), the quiescent state of most vascular cells in intact arteries in vivo probably accounts for this difference. Successful retroviral gene transfer depends on the ability to induce proliferation of the target cell, at least for a short period of time. However, following stable integration of recombinant gene sequences, gene expression in vascular cells is stable over several months' duration (5). Problems encountered in transfecting vascular endothelial and smooth muscle cells with retroviral vectors may result in part from the lack of expression of appropriate viral receptors. An additional concern is that the retroviral particle is relatively labile in comparison to other viruses. Attempts to purify or concentrate retroviruses can lead to significant loss of infectivity, partly as a result of loss of the viral *env* product. In addition, retroviral particles are rapidly inactivated in the presence of serum, probably by a complement-mediated process.

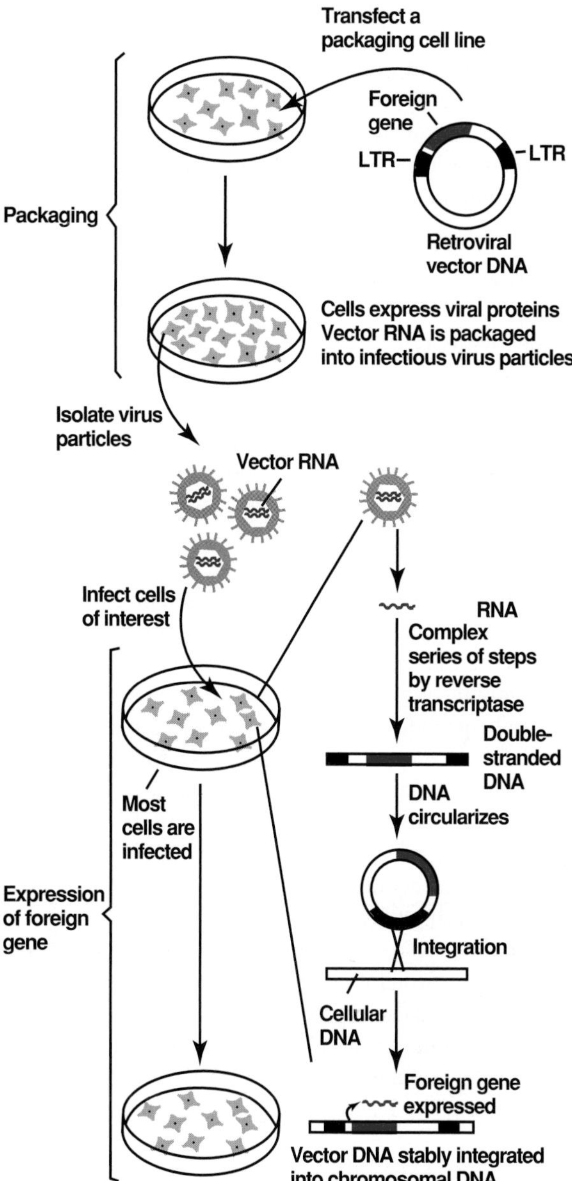

FIG. 1. Retroviral vectors for cell transfection. The gene is cloned into a retroviral vector. The vector DNA is transfected into a packaging cell line, and the cells express viral proteins. Vector RNA is packaged and virus particles are isolated. Cells are infected with viral particles, and the foreign gene is expressed. (From Watson et al., ref. 2, p. 227, with permission.)

The development of specialized cell lines or packaging

cells for the generation of retroviral vectors was an important advance in vector technology and permitted the production of high titers of replication-defective recombinant virus (14,15). In theory, because no genetic information for virus production is transferred from the packaging cells into recombinant virions, transfected cells are unable to perpetuate an infection and spread virus to other cells.

Adenovirus

Adenovirus type 2 (Ad-2) and type 5 (Ad-5) have been developed for use as viral vectors in gene therapy. The adenovirus genome is composed of linear, double-stranded DNA approximately 36 kb in length, which is divided into 100 map units, each of which is 360 base pairs in length (30). The DNA contains short inverted terminal repeats (ITRs) at the end of the genome that are required for viral DNA replication. The gene products are organized into early (E1–E4) and late (L1–L5) regions, based on expression before or after initiation of DNA replication. Adenoviruses have a lytic life cycle that is characterized by attachment to an adenoviral glycoprotein receptor on mammalian target cells and entry into cells by receptor-mediated endocytosis. Adenoviruses escape lysosomal degradation by adenoviral capsid proteins, and viral DNA translocates to the nucleus. Expression of viral genes depends on cellular transcription factors and expression of the adenoviral E1 region (early region), which encodes a transactivator of viral gene expression (31). During lytic infection, the viral genome replicates to several thousand copies per cell. The viral genome associates with core proteins and is packaged into capsids by self-assembling of major capsid proteins.

Replication-deficient adenoviral vectors developed for gene transfer contain deletions of the E1A and E1B regions (32) (Fig. 2). The E1 region regulates adenoviral transcription and is required for viral replication. Foreign cDNAs inserted into the adenoviral genome as a replacement for the E1 region result in a replication-defective adenovirus. Adenoviral vectors are produced by homologous recombination in 293 cells or any cell line that contains an integrated copy of the adenoviral E1 region (33). A foreign cDNA with appropriate eukaryotic regulatory sequences is introduced into a bacterial plasmid that contains a small region of the left adenoviral genome (type 2 or type 5) that has been deleted of the native E1 gene. The bacterial plasmid is cotransfected into 293 cells with an incomplete adenoviral genome. Homologous recombination between the two DNAs generates a recombinant genome in which the E1 region is replaced by the foreign gene. Viral stock is propagated in 293 cells to high titer, generally 10^9 to 10^{10} plaque-forming units (pfu) per milliliter.

Adenovirus type 2 and type 5 produce a respiratory disease in humans. These subclasses of adenovirus are not associated with human malignancies (34). Live adenovirus vaccines have been used safely in human populations (34,35). Adenoviral vectors have several additional advantages, including efficient infection of mammalian cells and expression in nondividing cells in vitro and in vivo. These vectors are relatively stable and can be grown and concentrated to a high titer. Extrachromosomal replication of the vector greatly reduces the chance of mutation by random integration and dysregulation of host cellular genes.

Despite these advantages, there are several limitations to the use of adenoviral vectors for gene transfer experiments. Gene expression in vascular and myocardial cells following adenoviral infection usually persists for only several weeks (36–39). Although transient gene expression may be desirable for some vascular therapies, other vascular diseases may require long-term gene expression. Loss of foreign gene sequences has been observed in the liver (40), muscle (41),

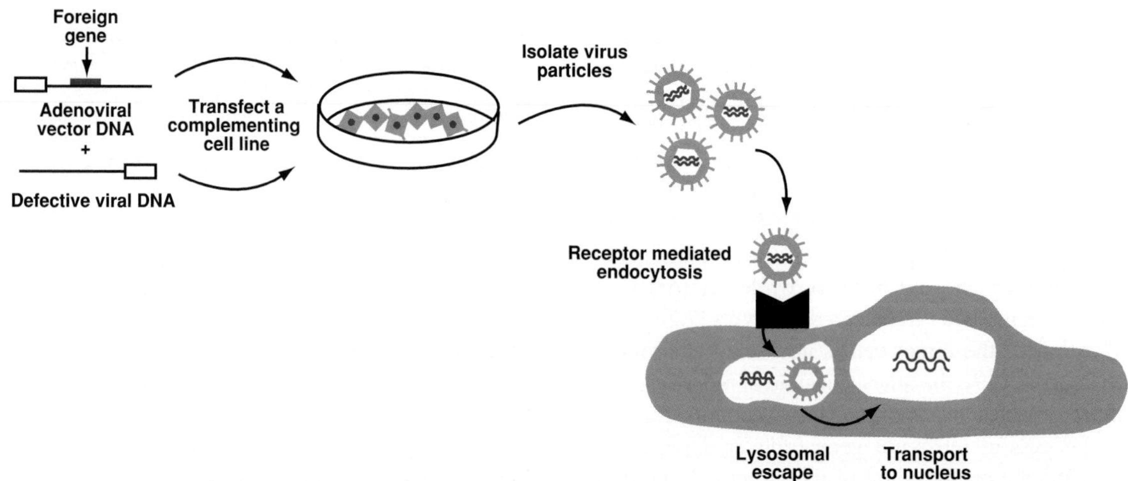

FIG. 2. Adenoviral vectors. Adenoviral vectors are constructed by homologous recombination between adenoviral plasmid DNA and modified adenoviral genome. Adenoviral particles are isolated and used to infect mammalian cells. (From: Nabel and Nabel, ref. 189, p. 22, with permission.)

and other tissues following adenoviral infection. Transient expression may result from loss of viral genomic DNA, promoter extinction, or host immune responses.

The development of host immune response to adenoviral proteins has been a major limitation to use of these vectors in vivo (42). Most adults have neutralizing antibodies to one or more adenoviral serotypes. Viral infection of experimental animals results in neutralizing antibody titers directed against adenoviral capsid proteins (43,44). Serum neutralizing antibodies have also been detected following adenoviral infection of synovium (45). Although low levels of neutralizing antibodies do not appear to have adverse clinical effects, it remains to be determined whether host immune responses to the adenovirus will preclude repeated administrations of the same serotype of adenovirus (46,47). First-generation recombinant adenoviral vectors (deletion of E1A and E1B genes and partial deletion of E3 genes) have been used for in vivo gene therapy treatments for cystic fibrosis (42,48,49); however, in animal models, gene expression has been transient and often associated with tissue inflammation, particularly in the liver and lung (50–52). These inflammatory changes in murine lung are diminished when recombinant adenoviruses with E2A and E1 deletions are employed. Inactivation of the E2A gene is associated with longer gene expression and less inflammation in lung (53) and liver (54). In arterial gene transfer studies employing adenoviral vectors, mononuclear inflammatory cell infiltrates have been observed in the adventitia of peripheral (55) and pulmonary (39) arteries, but no necrosis or vasculitis was observed. Infection of pulmonary arteries with adenovirus was associated with mild degrees of perivascular inflammation; however, pulmonary arteries instilled with saline or liposomes also exhibited mild accumulation of perivascular mononuclear cells (39). Further studies are required to determine the utility of these first-generation adenoviral vectors for vascular gene transfer studies. It is likely that further modification in these vectors, including deletions in the E2 and E4 regions, will alter host immune responses.

Recombinant adenoviral vectors have been employed to introduce genes into multiple cell lines in vitro and into tissue in vivo. These include cardiac and skeletal muscle (38,56), arteries (36–39,57), brain (58–60), lung (61–66), synovium (45), and liver (52,54,67). Despite the current problems with generation of immune response to adenoviral capsid proteins, the adenoviral vectors are attractive vehicles for in vivo gene transfer because of their efficient infection of many mammalian cells, including nondividing quiescent cells.

Adenovirus-Augmented, Receptor-Mediated Gene Delivery

A potentially promising vector for vascular gene transfer is receptor-mediated gene delivery using ligand DNA complexes linked to inactivated adenovirus. Although these vectors have not been well characterized in vascular cells, investigations have been conducted in other cell types, including hepatocytes (68) and fibroblasts (69). These vectors consist of two parts. DNA condenses with polylysine, which is bound to inactivated virus (70,71). A ligand, most commonly transferrin, is conjugated to the virus complex (72). The DNA–polylysine–adenovirus conjugate enter cells by transferrin ligand binding to transferrin receptors. The complex is internalized by receptor-mediated endocytosis. The inactivated adenovirus functions to disrupt endosomes, limiting degradation of DNA (73). DNA is maintained as an episome. Potential advantages of these vectors in the use of cell-specific receptors and ligands in order to achieve cell targeting. These vectors have not been explored extensively in the vasculature.

Nonviral Vectors

In the late 1980s, concerns about potential hazards of direct viral infection in vivo led to the development of nonviral vectors. Several nonviral vectors have been employed in the vasculature, including cationic liposomes, viral liposome conjugates, and polymers.

Cationic Liposomes

Cationic lipids are preparations of positively charged lipids that spontaneously complex with negatively charged DNA to form DNA–lipid conjugates. The lipid component facilitates delivery of DNA to cells by fusion with plasmid membrane or with endosomal membranes after endocytosis. Following release from endosomes, plasmid DNA is maintained in an extrachromosomal form.

Cationic liposomes were developed in the 1980s in part to overcome some of the deficiencies of neutral and anionic liposomes (74,75). Problems associated with neutral and anionic liposomes for DNA delivery were low encapsulation efficiency and lysosomal degradation of liposomes and DNA (76). DNA encapsulated by cationic liposomes achieve a much higher concentration in target tissues than the same agent incorporated in neutral or anionic liposomes (77). Cationic liposomes have a geometry and physical properties conducive to stable bilayer formation. The entrapment of DNA into cationic liposomes is not dependent on or limited by the DNA. Cationic liposomes are small in size, approximately 250–500 nm, and are homogeneous, thereby delivering polynucleotide uniformly to target cells.

Cationic liposomes interact spontaneously and rapidly with polyanions, such as DNA and RNA, to form liposome complexes (Fig. 3). One of the first reagents was DOTMA/DOPE {*N*-[1-(2,3-dioleyloxy)propyl]-*N*,*N*,*N*-trimethylammonium chloride/dioleoyl phosphatidylethanolamine} mixed in equal molar ratios (Lipofectin) (74). Additional cationic liposome reagents used in vascular gene transfer

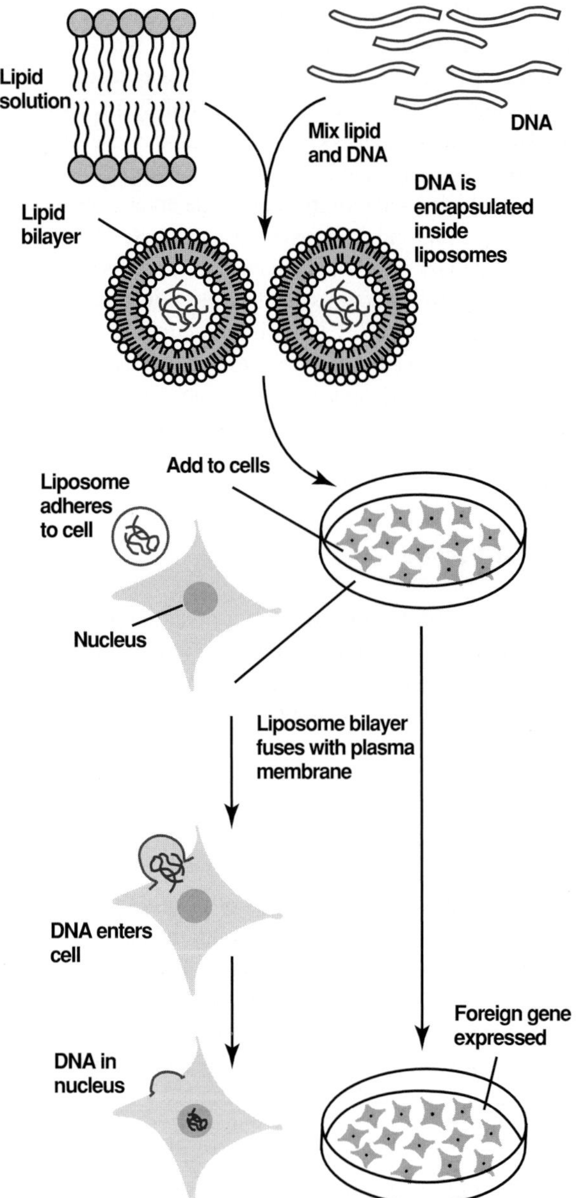

FIG. 3. Liposome gene transfer. Cationic liposomes are mixed with plasmid DNA, and DNA is incorporated into the liposome complex. Cells are transfected with these DNA–liposome conjugates. The liposomes fuse spontaneously to cell membranes, releasing contents into the cytoplasm. (From Watson et al., ref. 2, p. 222, with permission.)

studies include DC-cholesterol {dioleoyl phosphatidylethanolamine 3b[*n*-(*N*′,*N*′-dimethylaminoethane)carbamoyl]-cholesterol} (78); DOSPA/DOPE {2,3-dioleyloxy-*N*-[2(spermine carboxamido)ethyl]-*N*,*N*-dimethyl-1-propanaminiumtrifluoroacetate/dioleoyl phosphatidylethanolamine} (Lipofectamine) (35); and DMRIE/DOPE (1,2-dimyristyloxypropyl-3-dimethylhydroxyethyl ammonium bromide/dioleoyl phosphatidylethanolamine) (79).

Cationic liposomes have been employed in arterial gene transfer studies in vivo in several animal models, including rats (80), rabbits (27,81), dogs (82,83), and pigs (5,84). There are several advantages of cationic liposomes, including a favorable safety profile. Liposome vectors contain no viral coding sequences. There are fewer cDNA size constraints in vector construction. Cationic liposomes have been administered intravenously and intraarterially with minimal biochemical, hemodynamic, or cardiac toxicity in animals or humans (78,79). Cationic liposome vectors are straightforward to prepare for experimental and clinical use.

In vitro, approximately 5–15% of endothelial cells and smooth muscle cells are transfected with liposome vectors (39). In porcine arteries in vivo, the efficiency of gene transfer is 0.1% to 1% of cells (5,27). Following liposomal transfection, gene expression persists for approximately 1 month (39). Cell division is not required for liposome transfection, although the efficiency appears to be increased in proliferating vascular cells (81). Further modifications to the chemical formulations of cationic liposomes appear promising (85).

Hemagglutinating Virus of Japan Liposome Complexes

Another liposome vector involves the encapsulation of plasmid DNA and nuclear protein in liposomes fused with a heat-inactivated hemagglutinating virus of Japan (HVJ) (Fig. 4). The HVJ virus is used to fuse DNA-loaded liposome vesicles with cell membranes. A nuclear protein, high mobility group I (HMG 1), is often included to facilitate migration of plasmid DNA to the nucleus. HVJ liposomal transfection has resulted in increased expression of DNA in adult rat liver (86,87) and kidney (88). The HVJ liposome gene transfer has also been employed in rat arterial models to investigate the function of angiotensin-converting enzyme and renin genes (80). In the rat carotid artery, this vector yields an efficiency greater than or equal to 30% of vascular cells without local toxicity. In addition, HVJ liposomes have been used to deliver antisense oligonucleotides to rat carotid arteries, to inhibit vascular cell proliferation (89,90). It is likely that further modifications to vectors employed for vascular gene transfer will include components of viral and nonviral vectors that optimize delivery, improve gene expression, and minimize toxic side effects (91).

Polymers

Nucleic acids have been applied to polymer gels that are coated onto balloon catheters or directly applied to arteries. One example is a hydrogel catheter that consists of an angioplasty balloon coated with a hydrophilic polyacrylic acid polymer (92). Plasmid DNA is applied to the gel-coated balloon. When the balloon is inflated in an artery, the nucleic acid is pressed into the arterial wall. This method has been employed to deliver recombinant DNA to rabbit arteries in vivo (92) and recently has been proposed for a human gene therapy trial to increase collateral circulation in patients with

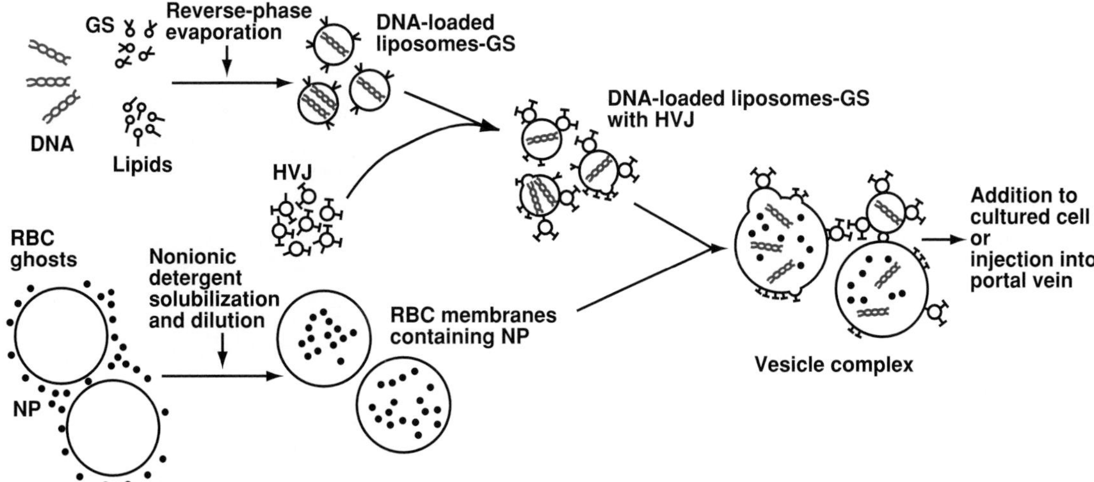

FIG. 4. HVJ liposome vectors. Plasmid DNA and high-mobility group I (HMG1) protein are encapsulated in liposomes by agitation and cointroduced into cells by hemagglutinating virus of Japan (HVJ)-mediated cell membrane fusion. (From Kaneda et al., ref. 86; copyright 1989, AAAS, with permission.)

peripheral vascular disease. One disadvantage of the hydrogel catheter is that nucleic acid can be rapidly washed off the balloon after exposure to the bloodstream, such that protective sheaths are often employed to protect the balloon catheter until deployment. Pluronic gels have also been employed to deliver antisense oligonucleotides to the adventitia of rat carotid arteries (93,94). Although the pharmacokinetics of oligonucleotide delivery and persistence have not been precisely defined, the data suggest that *c-myb* (93) and PCNA (94) RNA is inhibited 24 h after injury.

VASCULAR GENE TRANSFER

Development of Animal Models

During the past 5 years, there has been considerable interest in developing methods for introducing and expressing recombinant DNA and other nucleic acids in the vasculature in vivo. The goals of these studies have been to define gene function and to develop potential new therapeutic strategies for vascular proliferative disorders. Two approaches have been employed: ex vivo and in vivo gene transfer.

Ex Vivo Gene Transfer

Ex vivo gene transfer in the vasculature is the seeding of transduced cells onto denuded arteries or vascular prostheses. The feasibility of ex vivo gene transfer has been demonstrated in several animal models. Transfected autologous endothelial cells have been seeded onto denuded porcine (3) and rabbit (95) iliofemoral arteries. Genetically modified vascular smooth muscle cells have also been seeded onto denuded porcine iliofemoral arteries (4) and rat carotid arteries (96). Seeding of autologous transfected endothelial cells into rat skeletal muscle capillaries has also been demonstrated (97). Clowes and colleagues investigated the viability of retrovirally transduced smooth muscle cells seeded onto rat carotid arteries and found that these cells are not phenotypically altered or transformed 1 year after initial seeding. These cells stop replicating after 1 month and continue to express recombinant genes (98). Their studies show that secretion of a human adenosine deaminase gene from transduced smooth muscle cells is detectable both early (1 month) (96) and late (12 months) (98) following cell seeding. Additional studies have improved conditions for increasing protein expression from retrovirally transduced endothelial cells (99).

One application of ex vivo gene transfer technology is the seeding of vascular prostheses, such as synthetic grafts and stents, with endothelial cells transduced to optimize fibrinolysis and/or thrombolysis. A major complication of vascular devices is thrombosis. The local continuous secretion of thrombolytic or fibrinolytic proteins from transduced cells offers a potential approach to minimizing intravascular thrombosis. The feasibility of seeding prosthetic grafts was demonstrated in studies examining genetically modified canine endothelial cells seeded onto Dacron grafts (19). These grafts were implanted in canine carotid arteries, and reporter gene expression was observed for at least 5 weeks. Intravascular stents have also been seeded with genetically modified sheep endothelial cells in vitro (18), although reimplantation of seeded stents in vivo has not been demonstrated. Current investigations are examining prosthetic devices seeded with endothelial cells infected with adenoviral vectors encoding fibrinolytic genes such as t-PA and u-PA. The level of recombinant proteins secreted from infected cells and the duration of protein secretion have not been determined. Further studies are required to define the usefulness of this approach.

Direct in Vivo Gene Transfer

Direct gene transfer into arteries has been demonstrated in normal, injured, and atherosclerotic vessels of rats, rabbits, dogs, and pigs. Initial studies employed retroviral and cationic liposome vectors. Studies in normal arteries of pigs (5), dogs (82,83), and rabbits (27) suggested an efficiency of gene transfer of approximately 0.1% to 1% of cells. Gene transfer into balloon-injured arteries was higher, suggesting that ongoing cell proliferation at the time of transfection may improve the frequency of gene expression (100). Iliofemoral arteries in hyperlipidemic rabbits with early foam cell lesions also express reporter genes following direct gene transfer. Several conclusions can be derived from these studies. First, following transfer of reporter genes, multiple layers in arteries are transfected, including the intima, media, and adventitia. However, regions of highest gene expression are endothelial and smooth muscle cells in the intima, smooth muscle cells in the luminal region of the media, and connective tissues and capillary endothelial cells in the adventitia. Simple infusion of vector into normal arteries results in transfection of primarily intimal cells; the application of pressure to the vector infusate results in delivery of DNA vector transmurally with gene expression in the media. Several delivery catheters have been employed in gene transfer studies, and the patterns of gene expression within an artery may differ depending on the design of the catheter (101,102). These catheters include the double-balloon catheter, porous balloon catheter, hydrogel catheter, and simple ligation techniques (Fig. 5). Finally, vascular gene transfer studies employing liposome vectors demonstrate rare gene expression in systemic organs following local arterial delivery, suggesting that gene expression is local in nature without systemic toxicities (78,79).

In order to improve gene transfer frequencies and expression in the vasculature, adenoviral vectors have been employed more recently. These first-generation adenoviral vectors, characterized by deletion of E1A and E1B genes and partial deletion of E3 genes, result in a higher efficiency of gene transfer and expression in arteries in vivo. Adenoviral vectors encoding reporter genes have been infused in direct gene transfer experiments in the peripheral, coronary, and pulmonary vasculature in several species, including sheep (36), rabbits (38), pigs (39,55), and rats (57,103). Adenoviral infection of injured rat and porcine arteries results in reporter gene expression in endothelial cells as well as smooth muscle cells in the intima and media (55,57,103). The efficiency of gene transfer in intimal smooth muscle cells of injured rat arteries was reported to be 10–75% (103), and other reports suggest that approximately 30% of smooth muscle cells in the media of rat injured arteries are transduced (57). A common finding in these studies is the transient nature of gene expression following adenoviral injection. Gene expression, measured by mRNA and protein expression, generally peaks at 1 to 2 weeks and is lost by 1 month (36,38,39).

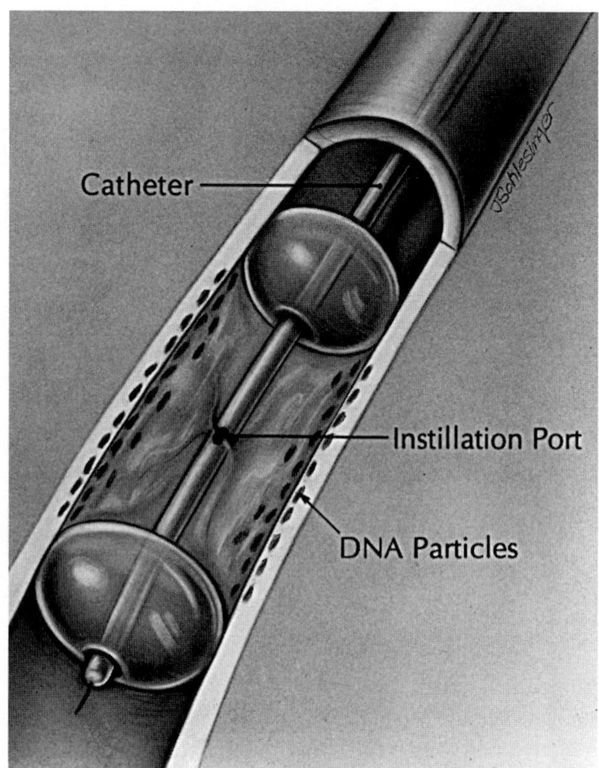

FIG. 5. Catheter delivery of recombinant DNA and vector for direct gene transfer into arteries in vivo. Proximal and distal balloon inflation isolates a central space within the artery, allowing for instillation of DNA and vector. (From Nabel and Nabel, ref. 190, p. 1107, with permission.)

Catheter infusion of adenoviral vectors encoding reporter genes has been shown to be an efficient method for induction of gene expression in coronary arteries and the myocardium of rabbits (38). A single intracoronary infusion of adenovirus resulted in recombinant gene expression in coronary arteries and surrounding myocardium of rabbits at 2 weeks. Inflammatory cells and necrosis were not observed in the vasculature or myocardium. Gene expression again was transient, and reporter gene expression was lost in the coronary arteries and myocardium within 1 month.

The safety and toxicity of these first-generation adenoviral vectors is being defined. In our studies in porcine iliofemoral arteries, we have noted mononuclear cell infiltrates in the adventitia following adenoviral infection (55). These inflammatory cell infiltrates have not been associated with the necrosis characteristic of vasculitis. Local delivery of adenovirus with a double-balloon catheter is rarely associated with spread of adenovirus to systemic organs. We occasionally had detected adenoviral sequences by PCR in systemic organs within the first week following gene transfer, but not at later time points. This PCR signal has not been associated with organ pathology determined by light microscopy studies or with serum biochemical or hematological abnormalities (55). The type of delivery catheter employed may be an important determinant of systemic spread of adenovirus.

Catheters in which adenovirus is infused through the end hole result in greater systemic dissemination of the adenovirus compared with local delivery with a double-balloon catheter in which adenovirus is removed from the central space after delivery. Finally, the local toxicities of adenoviral infection on endothelial and smooth muscle cells have not been determined. For example, it is not known whether adenoviral infection of endothelial cells may up-regulate expression of adhesion molecules such as VCAM-1 or ICAM-1 or cytokines such as IL-1, IL-2, or TNF. The cellular effects of adenoviral infection require further exploration.

Studies of Gene Expression and Function

Direct gene transfer has been employed as a somatic transgenic model to define gene function in the vessel wall. In this system, recombinant genes are expressed in local arterial segments, and their biological function is investigated. This approach has proved useful for the investigation of growth regulatory and cytokine genes, whose direct in vivo effects have been difficult to analyze (104).

Our laboratory has been interested in investigating the pathogenesis of smooth muscle cell proliferation in vivo, and we have examined the expression of growth factor genes in porcine arteries. These recombinant growth factor genes include platelet-derived growth factor B (PDGF B) (84), the secreted form of fibroblast growth factor 1 (FGF-1) (105), and a secreted form of active transforming growth factor β1 (TGF-β1) (106). These plasmid expression vectors were transfected into porcine peripheral arteries. For each factor, expression of mRNA was confirmed by reverse transcriptase (RT) PCR, and protein expression in transduced cells was identified by immunohistochemistry. Arteries transfected with a PDGF B gene demonstrated severe intimal thickening, characterized by increased intima-to-media area ratios, compared with control vessels transfected with a reporter gene (84). Smooth muscle cell proliferation in the intima was observed within 4 days following gene transfer and peaked at 7–14 days. After 14 days, expansion of the intima continued with a decrease in density of cell nuclei, suggesting synthesis of extracellular matrix. These findings were confirmed by immunohistochemical studies demonstrating procollagen and other extracellular matrix synthesis in the intima. These data support the hypothesis that PDGF B gene expression in vivo stimulates smooth muscle cell proliferation early after gene transfer and that collagen and extracellular matrix synthesis is a later feature of these lesions. The role of a PDGF B gene in promoting smooth muscle migration and/or proliferation is difficult to distinguish in porcine arteries because the intima of these arteries contains smooth muscle cells. It is possible that expression of a PDGF B gene in smooth muscle cells results in both migration of smooth muscle cells from the media to the intima as well as proliferation of smooth muscle cells within the intima.

The heparin-binding fibroblast growth factor family has proliferative and angiogenic properties in vivo (107,108). To investigate the role of FGF-1 in vascular pathology, a eukaryotic plasmid expression vector encoding a secreted form of FGF-1 was transfected into porcine arteries (105). Expression of recombinant FGF-1 was confirmed by RT PCR and immunohistochemical studies. Expression of secreted FGF-1 was associated with expansion of the intima as well as intimal angiogenesis (Fig. 6; see Colorplate 39). The source of the intimal capillaries is proposed to be luminal endothelial cells, because immunohistochemical studies identifying endothelial cells using vWF antibody revealed vWF staining in adventitial capillaries but not in luminal endothelial cells or in intimal capillary endothelial cells. Further studies are investigating the pathogenesis of these intimal capillaries, including the role of hypoxia, VEGF, and other cofactors that may contribute to capillary formation.

Transforming growth factor β1 is a secreted multifunctional protein that plays an important role in wound repair and embryonic development (109,110). The role of TGF-β1 in the pathophysiology of intimal and medial hyperplasia was investigated using a plasmid expression vector encoding a secreted active form of TGF-β1 (106). Arteries transfected with a human TGF-β1 gene demonstrated increased procollagen synthesis in the intima and media as early as 4 days following gene transfer, compared with control arteries transfected with a reporter gene. Procollagen synthesis in TGF-β1-transfected arteries occurred at earlier times compared with arteries transfected with a PDGF B gene, and in addition, the number of intimal procollagen-expressing cells per high-power field at all time points after gene transfer were higher in TGF-β-transduced cells compared with PDGF-B-transduced arteries. These findings suggest differential patterns of gene expression following transfection of TGF-β1 and PDGF B genes in arteries. Although these recombinant growth factor genes, PDGF B, FGF-1, and TGF-β1, each stimulate vascular cell proliferation in vivo, they otherwise exert different effects on smooth muscle cell proliferation, angiogenesis, and procollagen synthesis. These findings suggest that intimal thickening is a common response to the expression of many growth factors and cytokines.

One approach to investigating the pathogenesis of vascular cell proliferation in vivo is to examine gene products that inhibit cell proliferation. Molecular genetic approaches to limit smooth muscle cell proliferation or extracellular matrix synthesis at sites of vascular injury might also provide insight into the pathophysiology of vascular proliferative disorders such as restenosis. Local delivery of an antiproliferative agent during the peak of smooth muscle cell proliferation or collagen matrix synthesis following balloon injury might limit expansion of the intima. Several molecular approaches have been explored in this setting, including recombinant chimeric toxins (111–113), antisense oligonucleotide strategies (89,93), and gene transfer (55,114).

One approach to the selective elimination of dividing cells

is to express a herpes virus thymidine kinase (HSV-*tk*) gene in smooth muscle cells following balloon injury. Thymidine kinase, when expressed in transduced cells, converts ganciclovir, a nucleoside analog, into an active toxic form (115–117). Incorporation of phosphorylated ganciclovir into cellular DNA induces chain termination in dividing cells, which induces cell death (118–120). A bystander effect, which has been demonstrated in smooth muscle cells and endothelial cells in vitro (55), inhibits cell growth in non-transduced neighboring cells as well. A metabolite of phosphorylated ganciclovir is presumably diffusable to adjacent cells, and neighboring dividing cells are rendered sensitive to ganciclovir. This strategy has been employed in gene transfer approaches to tumor therapy including glioma (59,121), mesothelioma (122), and adenocarcinoma (123).

To develop an approach to gene transfer in a porcine balloon injury model, the kinetics of smooth muscle cell proliferation in the intima following balloon injury were defined (55). Proliferation was observed within 24 h after injury, was maximal after 7 days, and subsided by 14 days as determined by immunohistochemical studies of 5-bromo-2′-deoxycytosine (BrdC) labeling. Continued expansion of the arterial intima occurred by deposition of extracellular matrix through 21 days. Additional pilot studies were performed in balloon-injured porcine arteries to determine cell types transduced following adenoviral infection. Using a human placental alkaline phosphatase gene, we found that intimal and medial smooth muscle cells as well as intimal endothelial cells were primary targets for adenoviral infection. The period of gene expression following adenoviral infection was sufficient to express recombinant genes during the peak of proliferation.

The efficacy of an adenoviral vector encoding a herpes virus *tk* gene (ADV-*tk*) in altering the development of intimal hyperplasia after balloon injury was then tested (Fig. 7; see Colorplate 40). The ADV-*tk* vector was transfected into balloon-injured porcine arteries, and ganciclovir or saline treatment was administered 36 h later. Arteries were analyzed 3 or 6 weeks later. A significant reduction in the intima-to-media (I/M) area ratio was observed in vessels subjected to mild (87%) or severe (54–59%) injury in animals transduced with ADV-*tk* and treated with ganciclovir, compared with control groups: animals infected with ADV-*tk* treated with saline (ADV-*tk*/-GC), a control vector ADV-ΔE1 treated with ganciclovir (ADV-ΔE1/+GC) and a control vector treated with saline (ADV-ΔE1/-GC). A 40% reduction in BrdC labeling in intimal cells was observed in ADV-*tk*/+GC-treated animals compared with ADV-*tk*/-GC-treated animals 7 days after gene transfer, suggesting that inhibition of smooth muscle cell proliferation contributed to the effect. A 46% reduction in I/M area ratio was observed between experimental and treatment groups 6 weeks following balloon injury, suggesting that the reduction in intimal thickening was a prolonged effect. In balloon-injured rat carotid arteries, introduction of adenoviral vectors encoding HSV-*tk* immediately (124) or 7 days later (114) treatment with ganciclovir results in 46–58% (124) and 48% (114) reductions in intima-to-media area ratios.

There are several interesting features of these studies that require further examination. The HSV-*tk* gene selectively eliminates dividing cells, including smooth muscle and endothelial cells. A bystander effect has been demonstrated for both cell types in vitro. The endothelial surface in arteries has regenerated at 3 to 6 weeks, determined by scanning electron microscopy studies and by vWF immunohistochemistry. Although reendothelialization may be delayed by HSV-*tk* infection and ganciclovir treatment, intravascular thrombosis was not observed. Infiltration of mononuclear inflammatory cells in the adventitia of adenoviral-infected animals was observed, regardless of vector or treatment. This mononuclear cell infiltrate was not associated with vasculitis or necrosis. Tissues from systemic organs, including non-transfected artery, heart, lung, liver, kidney, spleen, skeletal muscle, and ovaries, demonstrated no pathological changes by light microscopy, and standard biochemical parameters were within normal range. Thus, significant toxicity was not observed. In this model, proliferating smooth muscle cells were probably eliminated early following vascular injury, prior to establishment of an neointima. Therefore, expansion of the intima was prevented rather than reversed by lysis of a developed neointima.

Additional approaches to limit smooth muscle cell proliferation following vascular injury could potentially include targeting of nuclear cell cycle regulatory pathways including the retinoblastoma gene product *(Rb)* (125–128), p21 (129–132), p53 (133–135), or protooncogenes such as *c-myb* and *c-myc* (136). Studies in injured rat carotid and porcine femoral artery models suggest that expression of a non-phosphorylatable, constitutively active form of *Rb* following adenoviral infection limits migration of medial smooth muscle cells to the intima and intimal smooth muscle cell proliferation 21 days following vascular injury (137).

Gene expression and function of vascular angiotensin-converting enzyme (ACE) has also been explored in rat carotid artery models using HVJ liposome vectors (80,138). Because the effects of circulating and local vascular ACE can be difficult to identify, local gene transfer provides one approach to discerning the function of vascular ACE in situ. Expression of a human ACE gene within rat carotid arteries promotes angiotensin-II-mediated vascular hypertrophy. An increase in vascular ACE activity was associated with an increase in DNA synthesis, measured by BrdU immunohistochemistry. Increases in DNA synthesis were abolished by infusion of angiotensin II receptor-specific antagonist. These findings demonstrated that angiotensin II exerts a direct effect on vascular hypertrophy, independent of systemic effects on blood pressure. These data suggest that vascular ACE and local production of an angiotensin II can produce vascular hypertrophy independent of hemodynamic or systemic factors.

The role of constitutive or endothelium-derived nitric oxide synthase (NOS) in the regulation of smooth muscle cell proliferation has been studied in vivo (139). Transfection of HVJ liposome vectors encoding endothelial-cell-derived NOS (ec-NOS) in injured rat carotid arteries was associated with local nitric oxide generation and a reduction in intimal thickening in ec-NOS-transfected vessels compared with control vessels transfected with a reporter gene. These studies have provided insight into the regulation of local nitric oxide generation in vascular lesion formation.

Antisense Oligonucleotides

Antisense oligonucleotides are another approach to use of recombinant genes or oligonucleotides to suppress the function of specific gene products. Antisense oligonucleotides are single-stranded DNA molecules, typically 15–30 base pairs in length (140). The sequence of the oligonucleotide is dictated by the sequence of the specific target molecule. Oligonucleotides that are targeted to inhibit RNA molecules are synthesized with a base pair sequence reversibly complementary to the mRNA sequence of a cellular gene (141,142). Standard or unmodified oligonucleotides (phosphodiester oligonucleotides) have a short half life (1–3 h) in tissue cells because of nuclease degradation (143,144). Chemical modifications in the nucleotide backbone have prolonged survival of oligonucleotides. Several modifications directed to the phosphodiester nucleotide backbone include phosphorothioates (sulfur replacing oxygen) (145,146) and methylphosphonates (methyl group replacing oxygen) (147,148). These phosphorothioates and methylphosphonates have increased survival in tissues, with a half-life greater than 24 h in some cases.

Oligonucleotides can inhibit the normal pathway of protein synthesis at several steps. Normally, genetic information encoded in a double-stranded DNA molecule is transcribed into a single-stranded messenger RNA chain (sense), which in turn is translated into protein. One approach to interrupt protein synthesis is an anti-DNA strategy. Transcription can be inhibited by designing oligonucleotides that bind to specific DNA elements. These oligonucleotides prevent DNA unwinding, interaction with transcription factors, or the action of RNA polymerase. Oligonucleotides can also target RNA molecules, by binding specifically to the coding or sense RNA strand. These antisense oligonucleotides target mRNA by degradation of RNase binding to 5′ cap sites, preventing translation, disrupting mRNA splicing, or blocking mRNA transport from the nucleus.

Antisense oligonucleotides have been studied in animal models of vascular disease, primarily to inhibit smooth muscle cell proliferation. The regulation of smooth muscle cell proliferation is likely associated with altered expression of tumor suppressor genes and protooncogenes (137). Antisense oligonucleotides targeted to cell cycle genes have been employed in studies in vitro and in vivo to inhibit smooth muscle cell proliferation. The administration of antisense oligonucleotides to the protooncogene *c-myb,* a DNA-binding protein, leads to a reduction in the targeted mRNA level, a decrease in protein expression, and dose-dependent suppression of cellular proliferation (149). Other studies in vitro have employed antisense oligonucleotides targeted to *c-myc* (150–152); proliferating cell nuclear antigen (PCNA), a subunit of DNA polymerase (153); and nonmuscle myosin heavy chain (149), a gene thought to be involved in mitosis.

These studies demonstrated the feasibility of targeting cell cycle genes involved in smooth muscle cell proliferation in vitro. Further in vivo studies have been performed in injured rat carotid and porcine coronary arteries. In these studies, antisense oligonucleotides have been delivered to arteries by local extravascular delivery, intravascular catheter delivery, or intravascular infusion. A pluronic gel has been used to deliver antisense *c-myb* oligonucleotides to the adventitia of injured rat carotid arteries (Fig. 8; see Colorplate 41) (93). These investigators demonstrated a reduction in *c-myb* RNA, which was associated with a decrease in intimal-to-medial area ratio and diminished intimal formation. Although the application of oligonucleotides to the gel probably resulted in exposure to the artery for less than 3 hr, the reduction in neointimal formation was prolonged at least 2 weeks. A similar approach was used to delivery antisense *c-myc* (154) and *cdc2* and *cdk2* (155) oligonucleotides to the adventitia of injured rat carotid arteries. Similar reductions in neointimal formation were seen. A single local intraluminal administration of antisense *cdc2* kinase and PCNA oligonucleotides in the presence of HVJ liposomes resulted in prolonged suppression of neointimal formation for 6 weeks (89). These investigators have shown similar effects in rat carotid arteries using antisense *cdk2* kinase oligonucleotides (90). Intraluminal delivery of antisense PCNA oligonucleotides has also reduced intimal thickening following balloon injury (94). More recently, a single administration of antisense *c-myc* oligonucleotides to injured porcine coronary arteries resulted in a reduction in intimal area (156). These results suggest that an antisense oligonucleotide approach to inhibit cell proliferation may be applicable to several animal species.

Despite the appeal of antisense oligonucleotides, there are a number of technical issues and challenges that must be considered. These include specificity of effect, local delivery, and oligonucleotide toxicity (157,158). Ideally, antisense oligonucleotides employed in anti-RNA strategies would disrupt a specific targeted mRNA, would not affect other RNAs, and would not be cytotoxic. However, oligonucleotides can potentially affect other mRNAs because of incomplete sequence matches or other secondary protein interactions producing unpredictable phenotypes and toxic effects. The production of RNA–DNA hybrids can potentially inactivate other enzymes, including kinases, that affect protein synthesis. Therefore, careful controls must be performed in these studies. Such controls include the use of multiple antisense sequences that produce the same phenotype and minimize the chance that the observed effect was a nonspecific interaction; scrambled sequences, that is, oligonucleotides of the same base pair composition as the antisense sequence but synthesized in a different order that demonstrate no biological effect and do not effect targeted gene RNA and protein levels; and sense controls. Local delivery catheters are as important for antisense oligonucleotide studies as they are for gene transfer studies. It remains to be determined whether antisense oligonucleotides can be delivered in sufficient quantity in atherosclerotic lesions to affect or disrupt targeted genes. The pharmacokinetics, including optimum conditions for delivery, timing and duration of administration, and delivery vectors, need to be carefully investigated (159). Finally, antisense oligonucleotides can result in cytotoxicity from nonspecific effects. These effects can include cellular metabolism of antisense structures as well as direct toxicity from the chemical backbones of the oligonucleotide. Oligonucleotide preparations are currently being evaluated in a number of animal species.

LIPOPROTEIN TRANSPORT AND METABOLISM

Gene transfer, in combination with transgenic technology and homologous recombination, has lead to the development of murine models of atherosclerosis that have been employed to investigate lipoprotein transport and metabolism. In the 1980s, murine atherosclerosis was investigated by identifying susceptible strains of mice, developing atherogenic high-fat diets, and quantitating lesion area in murine aorta (160,161). These studies established the difference in atherosclerosis susceptibility of inbred laboratory strains (162). Transgenic techniques have allowed single genes to be either overexpressed or eliminated (163). For complex diseases such as atherosclerosis, this allows the assessment of the action of individual molecules on the disease process, permitting the testing of hypotheses, developed by human epidemiologic studies, in complex models in vivo. The subsequent development of homologous recombination technology (164), permitting the inactivation of single genes, has advanced the field to where specific overexpression or knockout of genes can now be investigated in animal models (165,166). Examples of the applications of transgenic techniques to atherosclerosis research include the overexpression of the human LDL receptor in transgenic mice (167) and the production of LDL receptor knockout mice (168). These studies were followed by reconstitution of LDL receptor function following delivery of adenoviral vectors encoding the human LDL receptor gene into LDL receptor knockout mice (Fig. 9) (169). These studies confirmed the key role in this receptor and lipoprotein metabolism in the control of hypercholesterolemia, defined the feasibility of replacing LDL receptor function by virus-mediated gene delivery, and permitted in vivo determination of structure–function relationships. Other areas in which adenoviral gene delivery in transgenic or homologous recombination murine models is likely to prove useful include the analysis of apolipoprotein(a) (170,171), Lp(a) (172), apolipoprotein E (165,166, 173–175), apolipoprotein A-I (176,177), and apolipoprotein A-II (178).

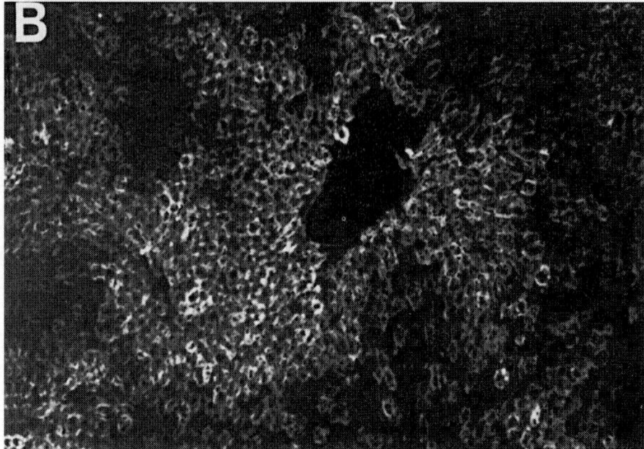

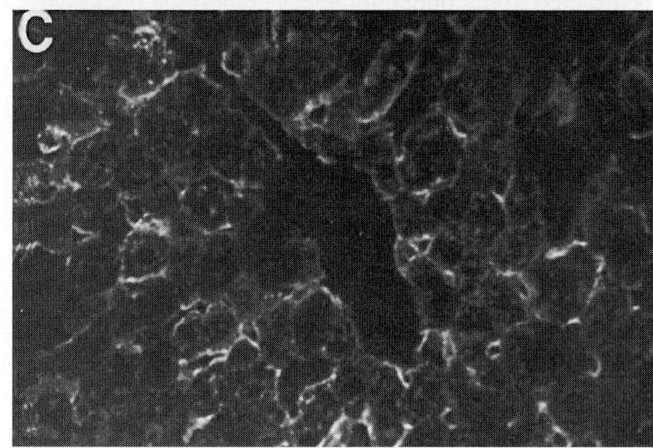

FIG. 9. Reconstitution of LDL receptors in the liver of LDL-*R*-deficient mouse after infection with adenoviral vectors encoding human LDL receptor cDNA. Homozygous LDL-receptor-negative mice were injected with control adenovirus **(A)** or adenovirus encoding human LDL receptor cDNA **(B).** Immunohistochemical studies for LDL receptor were performed (Magnification **A,B** ×25; **C** ×100). (From Ishibashi et al., ref. 169, with permission.)

Adenoviral gene delivery has been employed to study inhibition of hepatic chylomicron remnant uptake. The hypothesis that low-density lipoprotein receptor-related proteins (LRP) mediate the uptake of dietary lipoprotein into hepatocytes with the LDL receptor was tested by transient inactivation of LRP in vivo (179). A dominant negative regulator of LRP was transferred by an adenoviral vector to LDL receptor knockout mice. The inactivation of LRP by the dominant negative regulator was associated with a marked accumulation of chylomicron remnants in these LDL receptor knockout mice and, to a lesser degree, in normal mice. These findings suggest that both the LDL receptor and LRP are involved in remnant clearance.

The role of the LDL receptor in the regulation of cholesterol metabolism in LDL receptor-deficient animals and humans has also been investigated using gene transfer approaches. Wilson and colleagues have demonstrated that the hypercholesterolemia in the Watanabe rabbit (LDL receptor deficient) can be reversed following reconstitution of LDL receptors using genetically modified hepatic cells (180,181) or direct viral-mediated gene transfer (182). The successful demonstration of reconstitution of LDL receptor function in these animal models has led to a human gene therapy trial for patients with familial hypercholesterolemia (183,184).

It is likely that gene transfer, in combination with transgenic and homologous recombination technology, will be increasingly employed to investigate the role of specific genes in lipoprotein transport and metabolism.

CLINICAL TRIALS

The number of human gene therapy protocols initiated in the United States has grown rapidly over the past 5 years (185). Since 1989, more than 100 gene-marking and gene therapy protocols have been approved by the Recombinant DNA Advisory Committee of the National Institutes of Health and the Food and Drug Administration (186). The majority of these protocols are designed to treat cancer, AIDS, and inherited single-gene disorders. The application of gene transfer to human therapies for cardiovascular diseases has proceeded at a slower rate. The risk-to-benefit ratio for cardiovascular patients is higher compared with other diseases such as cancer and AIDS, in which treatment options are more limited. Most cardiovascular diseases are polygenic disorders, and identification of candidate genes to treat vascular or myopathic disorders has been difficult. Nonetheless, with recent advances made in gene transfer and antisense oligonucleotides, potential candidate genes to treat vascular proliferative disorders, for example, have been identified. Issues, such as catheter delivery, gene expression and vector pharmacokinetics, are being considered. Finally, safety issues related to use of viral and nonviral vectors in the vasculature are being addressed.

Several human therapy trials completed or in progress are applicable to the cardiopulmonary field. The safety of direct DNA introduction into humans, both by direct injection and catheter infusion into the vasculature, has been demonstrated in a trial of direct DNA liposome transfection from immunotherapy against melanoma (187,188). In this trial, the gene encoding a major histocompatibility complex protein, HLA-B7, was introduced into HLA-B7-negative patients with advanced melanoma by injection of DNA liposome into subcutaneous tumor nodules (187) and by catheter into pulmonary lesions in the lung (188). Recombinant HLA-B7 mRNA and protein expression were demonstrated in tumor biopsy tissue in all patients. Immune response to HLA-B7 and autologous tumors were also detected. One patient demonstrated regression of injected tumors on two independent treatments, one of which was accompanied by regression of tumors at distant sites. Catheter delivery of HLA-B7 DNA liposomes was safely carried out and well tolerated in one patient with lesions in the right lower lobe of the lung (Fig. 10). These studies demonstrated the feasibility, safety, and therapeutic potential of direct gene transfer in humans by direct injection and percutaneous catheter delivery.

In a trial for homozygous familial hypercholesterolemia, patients with inherited deficiencies of LDL receptor function have undergone partial hepatectomy (183). Autologous hepatocytes were transduced with a retroviral vector encoding a human LDL receptor gene. Transduced hepatocytes expressing human LDL receptors are reinfused into the liver via the portal vein. In one patient, an approximate 20% reduction of serum cholesterol in combination with HMG-CoA reductase therapy was observed (184).

Several trials have been approved to treat cystic fibrosis in which a first-generation adenoviral vector encoding the cystic fibrosis transmembrane regulator (CFTR) gene, which

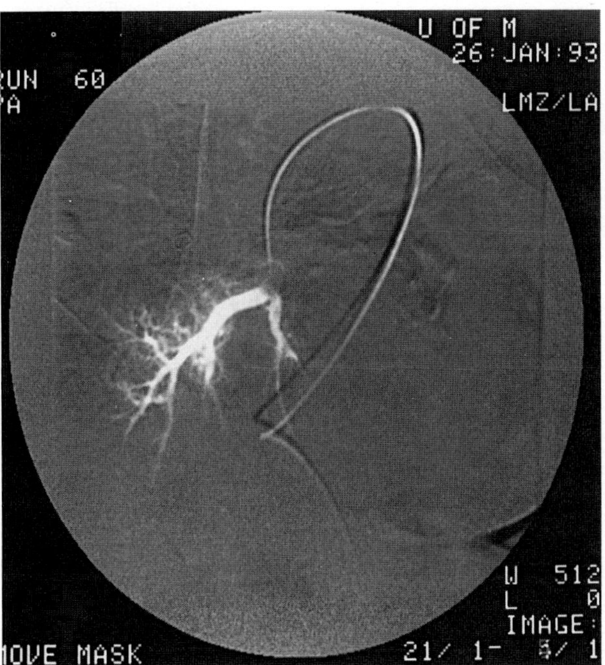

FIG. 10. Digital subtraction angiogram of a pulmonary artery in a patient undergoing catheter gene delivery to the pulmonary vasculature for treatment of metastatic melanoma. The intravenous contrast agent demonstrates arteries proximal to the tumor transduced with DNA–liposome complexes. Plasmid HLA-B7 DNA and cationic liposomes were instilled into the pulmonary artery. (From Nabel et al., ref. 188, with permission.)

is introduced into the nasal mucosa or airway epithelium in patients by bronchoscopy (42,48,49). The safety of these first-generation adenoviral vectors is being evaluated, and several groups have made modifications in these vectors by mutations in the E2, E3, or E4 regions (52,54). Studies with modified or second-generation adenoviral vectors are beginning. The feasibility of adenoviral-mediated gene therapy for inherited disorders such as cystic fibrosis, in which repeated administration of a vector are likely to be needed, is being investigated.

A cardiovascular gene therapy protocol applicable to the vasculature was approved by the NIH Recombinant DNA Advisory Committee and the FDA. In this protocol, patients with peripheral vascular disease will be treated by percutaneous catheter delivery of a VEGF plasmid expression vector coated onto a hydrogel balloon into the femoral artery. The hypothesis that expression of VEGF will result in increased collateral circulation in the femoral artery will be tested.

FUTURE DIRECTIONS

These studies suggest that gene transfer, alone or in combination with other genetic technologies, is proving useful in creating complex animal models of vascular disease in which the function of gene products in vivo can be investigated. It is likely that gene transfer and other recombinant DNA technologies will contribute to our understanding of gene expression and function in cardiovascular systems. These technologies also show promise for the treatment of human cardiovascular diseases, despite remaining technical issues. In the field of coronary artery disease and atherosclerosis, basic questions regarding the pathophysiology of atherosclerosis and restenosis must be addressed. The feasibility and efficiency of gene transfer in atherosclerotic vessels requires further investigation. Whether gene delivery also requires appropriate, regulated expression of recombinant genes in atherosclerotic tissues is unknown. Other synthetic nucleic acids, such as ribozymes, might be useful in these genetic approaches. New research opportunities present a challenge for basic scientists and clinical investigators to explore the possibilities of molecular genetics to further the understanding and treatment of cardiovascular diseases.

REFERENCES

1. Mulligan RC. The basic science of gene therapy. *Science* 1993;260: 926–932.
2. Watson J, Gilman M, Witkowsk J, Zoller M. *Recombinant DNA*, 2nd ed. New York: W. H. Freeman and Company; 1992.
3. Nabel EG, Plautz G, Boyce FM, Stanley JC, Nabel GJ. Recombinant gene expression in vivo within endothelial cells of the arterial wall. *Science* 1989;244:1342–1344.
4. Plautz G, Nabel EG, Nabel GJ. Introduction of vascular smooth muscle cells expressing recombinant genes in vivo. *Circulation* 1991;83: 578–583.
5. Nabel EG, Plautz G, Nabel GJ. Site-specific gene expression in vivo by direct gene transfer into the arterial wall. *Science* 1990;249: 1285–1288.
6. Anderson WF. Prospects for human gene therapy. *Science* 1984;226: 401–409.
7. Eglitis MA, Anderson WF. Retroviral vectors for introduction of genes into mammalian cells. *BioTechniques* 1988;6:608–614.
8. Friedman T. Progress toward human gene therapy. *Science* 1989;244: 1275–1281.
9. Miller AD. Retroviral vectors. *Curr Top Microbiol* 1992;158:1–24.
10. Varmus H. Retroviruses. *Science* 1988;240:1427–1435.
11. Verma IM. Gene therapy. *Sci Am* 1990;Nov:68–84.
12. Danos O. Construction of retroviral packaging cell lines. *Methods Mol Biol* 1991;8:17–27.
13. Cone RD, Mulligan RC. High-efficiency gene transfer into mammalian cells: Generation of helper-free recombinant retrovirus with broad mammalian host range. *Proc Natl Acad Sci USA* 1984;81:6349–6353.
14. Danos O, Mulligan RC. Safe and efficient generation of recombinant retroviruses with amphotropic and ectropic host ranges. *Proc Natl Acad Sci USA* 1988;85:6460–6464.
15. Miller AD, Buttimore C. Redesign of retrovirus packaging cell lines to avoid recombination leading to helper virus production. *Mol Cell Biol* 1986;6:2895–2902.
16. Tolstoshev P. Retroviral-mediated gene therapy—safety considerations and preclinical studies. *Bone Marrow Transplant* 1992;1: 148–150.
17. Zwiebel JA, Freeman SM, Kantoff PW, Cornetta K, Ryan US, Anderson WF. High-level recombinant gene expression in rabbit endothelial cells transduced by retroviral vectors. *Science* 1989;243:220–222.
18. Dichek DA, Neville RF, Zwiebel JA, Freeman SM, Leon MB, Anderson WF. Seeding of intravascular stents with genetically engineered endothelial cells. *Circulation* 1989;80:1347–1353.
19. Wilson JM, Birinyi LK, Salomon RN, Libby P, Callow AD, Mulligan RC. Implantation of vascular grafts lined with genetically modified endothelial cells. *Science* 1989;244:1344–1346.
20. Eglitis MA, Kantoff PW, Gilboa E, Anderson WF. Gene expression in mice after high efficiency retroviral-mediated gene transfer. *Science* 1985;230:1395–1398.
21. Morgan JR, Barrandon Y, Green H, Mulligan RC. Expression of an exogenous growth hormone gene by transplantable epidermal cells. *Science* 1987;237:1476–1479.
22. Hock RA, Miller AD. Retrovirus-mediated transfer and expression of drug resistance genes in human haemotopoietic progenitor cells. *Nature* 1986;320:275–277.
23. Keller G, Paige C, Gilboa E, Wagner EF. Expression of a foreign gene in myeloid and lymphoid cells derived from multipotent haematopoietic precursors. *Nature* 1985;318:149–154.
24. Kwok WW, Scheuning F, Stead RB, Miller AD. Retroviral transfer of genes into canine hemopoietic progenitor cells in culture: A model for human gene therapy. *Proc Natl Acad Sci USA* 1986;83: 4552–4555.
25. Ledley FD, Darlington GJ, Tahn T, Woo SLC. Retrovirus gene transduction into primary hepatocytes: Implications for genetic therapy of liver-specific functions. *Proc Natl Acad Sci USA* 1987;84:5335–5339.
26. Wilson JM, Jefferson DM, Chowdhury JR, Novikoff PM, Johnston DE, Mulligan RC. Retrovirus-mediated transduction of adult hepatocytes. *Proc Natl Acad Sci USA* 1988;85:3014–3018.
27. Leclerc G, Gal D, Takeshita S, Nikol S, Weir L, Isner JM. Percutaneous arterial gene transfer in a rabbit model. Efficiency in normal and balloon-dilated atherosclerotic arteries. *J Clin Invest* 1992;90: 936–944.
28. Flugelman MY, Jaklitsch MT, Newman KD, Casscells W, Bratthauer GL, Dichek DA. Low level in vivo gene transfer into the arterial wall through a perforated balloon catheter. *Circulation* 1992;3:1110–1117.
29. Miller DG, Adam MA, Miller AD. Gene transfer by retrovirus vectors occurs only in cells that are actively replicating at the time of infection. *Mol Cell Biol* 1990;10:4239–4242.
30. Graham FL, Prevec L. Adenovirus-based expression vectors and recombinant vaccines. In: Ellis RW, ed. *Vaccines: New Approaches to Immunological Problems.* Boston: Butterworth-Heinemann; 1992: 363–390.
31. Nevins JR. Adenovirus E1A-dependent trans-activation of transcription. *Cancer Biol* 1990;1:59–68.
32. Berkner KL. Expression of heterologous sequences in adenoviral vectors. *Curr Top Microbiol* 1992;58:39–66.

33. Graham FL, Smiley J, Russel WC, Nairu R. Characteristics of a human cell line transformed by DNA from human adenovirus type 5. *J Gen Virol* 1977;36:59–72.
34. Straus SE. Adenovirus infections in man. In: Ginsburg HS, ed. *The Adenoviruses*. New York: Plenum Press; 1984:451–496.
35. Chanock RM, Ludwig W, Heubner RJ, Cate TR, Chu L-W. Immunization by selective infection with type 4 adenovirus grown in human diploid tissue culture I. Safety and lack of oncogenicity and tests for potency in volunteers. *JAMA* 1966;195:151–165.
36. Lemarchand P, Jones M, Yamada I, Crystal RG. In vivo gene transfer and expression in normal uninjured blood vessels using replication-deficient recombinant adenovirus vectors. *Circ Res* 1993;72: 1132–1138.
37. Guzman RJ, Lemarchand P, Crystal RG, Epstein SE, Finkel T. Efficient gene transfer into myocardium by direct injection of adenovirus vectors. *Circ Res* 1993;73:1202–1207.
38. Barr E, Carroll J, Kalynych AM, Tripathy SK, Kozarsky K, Wilson JM, Leiden JM. Efficient catheter-mediated gene transfer into the heart using replication-defective adenovirus. *Gene Ther* 1994;1: 51–58.
39. Muller DW, Gordon D, San H, Yang Z, Pompili VJ, Nable GJ, Nabel EG. Catheter-mediated pulmonary vascular gene transfer and expression. *Circ Res* 1994;75:1039–1049.
40. Jaffe HA, Danel C, Longenecker G, Metzger M, Setoguchi Y, Rosenfeld MA, Gant TW, Thorgeirsson SS, Stratford-Perricaudet LD, Perricaudet M, Pavirani A, Lecocq JP, Crystal RG. Adenovirus-mediated in vivo gene transfer and expression in normal rat liver. *Nature Genet* 1992;1:372–378.
41. Stratford-Perricaudet LD, Makeh I, Perricaudet M, Briand P. Widespread long-term gene transfer to mouse skeletal muscles and heart. *J Clin Invest* 1992;90:626–630.
42. Crystal RG, McElvaney NG, Rosenfeld MA, Chu C-S, Mastrangeli A, Hay JG, Brody SL, Jaffe HA, Eissa NT, Danel C. Administration of an adenovirus containing the human CFTR cDNA to the respiratory tract of individuals with cystic fibrosis. *Nature Genet* 1994;8:42–50.
43. Prevec L, Schneider M, Rosenthal KL, Belbeck LW, Derbyshire JB, Graham FL. Use of human adenovirus-based vectors for antigen expression in animals. *J Gen Virol* 1989;70:429–434.
44. Natuk RJ, Chanda PK, Lubeck MD, Davis AR, Wilhelm J, Hjorth R, Wade MS, Bhat BM, Mizutani S, Lee S, Eichberg J, Gallo RC, Hung PP, Robert-Guroff M. Adenovirus-human immunodeficiency virus (HIV) envelope recombinant vaccines elicit high-titered HIV-neutralizing antibodies in the dog model. *Proc Natl Acad Sci USA* 1992; 89:7777–7781.
45. Roessler BJ, Allen ED, Wilson JM, Hartman JW, Davidson BL. Adenoviral-mediated gene transfer to rabbit synovium in vivo. *J Clin Invest* 1993;92:1085–1092.
46. Zabner J, Petersen DM, Puga AP, Graham SM, Couture LA, Keyes LD, Lukason MJ, St. George JA, Gregory RJ, Smith AE, Welsh MJ. Safety and efficacy of repetitive adenovirus-mediated transfer of CFTR cDNA to airway epithelia of primates and cotton rats. *Nature Genet* 1994;6:75–83.
47. Yei S, Mittereder N, Tang K, O'Sullivan C, Trapnell BC. Adenovirus-mediated gene transfer for cystic fibrosis: Quantitative evaluation of repeated in vivo vector administration to the lung. *Gene Ther* 1994; 1:192–200.
48. Zabner J, Couture LA, Gregory RJ, Graham SM, Smith AE, Welsh MJ. Adenovirus-mediated gene transfer transiently corrects the chloride transport defect in nasal epithelia of patients with cystic fibrosis. *Cell* 1993;75:207–216.
49. Wilson JM, Engelhardt JF, Grossman M, Simon RH, Yang Y. Gene therapy of cystic fibrous lung disease using E1 deleted adenoviruses: A phase I trial. *Gene Ther* 1994;5:501–519.
50. Ginsberg HS, Moldawer LL, Sehgal PB, Redington M, Kilian PL, Chanock RM, Prince GA. A mouse model for investigating the molecular pathogenesis of adenovirus pneumonia. *Proc Natl Acad Sci USA* 1991;88:1651–1655.
51. Prince GA, Porter DD, Jenson AB, Horswood RL, Chanock RM, Ginsberg HS. Pathogenesis of adenovirus type 5 pneumonia in cotton rats *(Sigmodon hispidus)*. *J Virol* 1993;67:101–111.
52. Yang Y, Nunes FA, Berencsi K, Furth EE, Gonczol E, Wilson JM. Cellular immunity to viral antigens limits E1-deleted adenoviruses for gene therapy. *Proc Natl Acad Sci USA* 1994;91:4407–4411.
53. Yang Y, Nunes FA, Berencsi K, Gonczol E, Engelhardt JF, Wilson JM. Inactivation of E2a in recombinant adenoviruses improves the prospect for gene therapy in cystic fibrosis. *Nature Genet* 1994;7: 362–369.
54. Engelhardt JF, Ye X, Doranz B, Wilson JM. Ablation of E2A in recombinant adenoviruses improves transgene persistence and decreases inflammatory response in mouse liver. *Proc Natl Acad Sci USA* 1994;91:6196–6200.
55. Ohno T, Gordon D, San H, Pompili VJ, Imperiale MJ, Nabel GJ, Nabel EG. Gene therapy for vascular smooth muscle cell proliferation after arterial injury. *Science* 1994;265:781–784.
56. Tripathy SK, Goldwasser E, Lu MM, Barr E, Leiden JM. Stable delivery of physiological levels of recombinant erythropoietin to the systemic circulation by intramuscular injection of replication-defective adenovirus. *Proc Natl Acad Sci USA* 1994;91:11557–11561.
57. Lee SW, Trapnell BC, Rade JJ, Virmani R, Dichek DA. In vivo adenoviral vector-mediated gene transfer into balloon-injured rat carotid arteries. *Circ Res* 1993;273:797–807.
58. Davidson BL, Allen ED, Kozarsky KF, Wilson JM, Roessler BJ. A model system for in vivo gene transfer into the central nervous system using an adenoviral vector. *Nature Genet* 1993;3:219–223.
59. Chen S-H, Shine HD, Goodman JC, Grossman RG, Woo SLC. Gene therapy for brain tumors: Regression of experimental gliomas by adenovirus-mediated gene transfer in vivo. *Proc Natl Acad Sci USA* 1994; 91:3054–3057.
60. Akli S, Caillaud C, Vigne E, Stratford-Perricaudet LD, Poenaru L, Perricaudet M, Kahn A, Peschanski MR. Transfer of a foreign gene into the brain using adenovirus vectors. *Nature Genet* 1993;3: 224–228.
61. Rosenfeld MA, Siegfried W, Yoshimura K, Yoneyama K, Fukayama M, Stier LE, Paakko P, Gilardi P, Stratford-Perricaudet LD, Perricaudet M, Jallat WS, Pavarani A, Lecocq J-P, Crystal RG. Adenovirus-mediated transfer of a recombinant 1-antitrypsin gene to the lung epithelium in vivo. *Science* 1991;252:431–434.
62. Rosenfield MA, Yoshimura K, Trapnell BC, Yoneyama K, Rosenthal ER, Dalemans W, Fukayama M, Bargon J, Stier LE, Stratford-Perricaudet L, Perricaudet M, Guggiono WB, Pavarani A, Lecocq J-P, Crystal RG. In vivo transfer of the human cystic fibrosis transmembrane conductance regulator gene to the airway epithelium. *Cell* 1992; 68:143–155.
63. Mastrangeli A, Danel C, Rosenfeld MA, Stratford-Perricaudet L, Perricaudet M, Pavirani L, Lecocq J-P, Crystal RG. Diversity of airway epithelial cell targets for in vivo recombinant adenovirus-mediated gene transfer. *J Clin Invest* 1993;91:225–234.
64. Engelhardt JF, Yang Y, Stratford-Perricaudet LD, Allen ED, Kozarsky K, Perricaudet M, Yankaskas JR, Wilson JM. Direct gene transfer of human CFTR into human bronchial epithelia of xenografts with E1-deleted adenoviruses. *Nature Genet* 1993;4:27–34.
65. Engelhardt JF, Yankaskas JR, Ernst SA, Yang Y, Marino CR, Boucher RC, Cohn JA, Wilson JA. Submucosal glands are the predominant site of CFTR expression in the human bronchus. *Nature Genet* 1992; 2:240–248.
66. Engelhardt JF, Zepeda M, Cohn JA, Yankaskas JR, Wilson JM. Expression of the cystic fibrosis gene in adult human lung. *J Clin Invest* 1994;93:737–749.
67. Yang Y, Raper SE, Cohn JA, Engelhardt JF, Wilson JM. An approach for treating the hepatobiliary disease of cystic fibrosis by somatic gene transfer. *Proc Natl Acad Sci USA* 1993;90:4601–4605.
68. Wu GY, Wilson JM, Shalaby F, Grossman M, Shafritz DA, Wu CH. Receptor-mediated gene delivery in vivo. Partial correction of genetic analbuminemia in Nagase rats. *J Biol Chem* 1991;266:14338–14342.
69. Zatloukal K, Cotten M, Berger M, Schmidt W, Wagner E, Birnstiel ML. In vivo production of human factor VII in mice after intrasplenic implantation of primary fibroblasts transfected by receptor-mediated, adenovirus-augmented gene delivery. *Proc Natl Acad Sci USA* 1994; 91:5148–5152.
70. Wagner E, Zatloukal K, Cotten M, Kirlappos H, Mechtler K, Curiel DT, Birnstiel ML. Coupling of adenovirus to transferrin-polylysine/ DNA complexes greatly enhances receptor-mediated gene delivery and expression of transfected genes. *Proc Natl Acad Sci USA* 1992; 89:6099–6103.
71. Curiel DT, Agarwal S, Wagner E, Cotten M. Adenovirus enhancement of transferrin-polylysine-mediated gene delivery. *Proc Natl Acad Sci USA* 1991;88:8850–8854.
72. Wagner E, Zenke M, Cotten M, Beug H, Birnstiel ML. Transferrin-

polycation conjugates as carriers for DNA uptake into cells. *Proc Natl Acad Sci USA* 1990;87:3410–3414.

73. Cotten M, Wagner E, Zatloukal K, Phillips S, Curiel DT, Birnstiel ML. High-efficiency receptor-mediated delivery of small and large (48 kilobase) gene constructs using the endosome-disruption activity of defective or chemically inactivated adenovirus particles. *Proc Natl Acad Sci USA* 1992;89:6094–6098.
74. Felgner PL, Gadek TR, Holm M, Roman R, Chan HW, Wenz M, Northrop JP, Ringold GM, Danielsen M. Lipofection: A highly efficient, lipid-mediated DNA-transfection procedure. *Proc Natl Acad Sci USA* 1987;84:7413–7417.
75. Felgner PL. Particulate systems and polymers for in vitro and in vivo delivery of polynucleotides. *Adv Drug Deliv Rev* 1990;5:163–187.
76. Felgner PL, Holm M, Chan H. Cationic liposome mediated transfection. *Proc West Pharmacol Soc* 1989;32:115–121.
77. Felgner PL, Ringold GM. Cationic liposome-mediated transfection. *Nature* 1989;337:387–388.
78. Nabel EG, Gordon D, Xang Z-Y, Xu L, San H, Plautz GE, Gao X, Huang L, Nabel GJ. Gene transfer in vivo with DNA–liposome complexes: Lack of autoimmunity and gonadal localization. *Hum Gen Ther* 1992;3:649–656.
79. San H, Yang ZY, Pompili VJ, Jaffe ML, Plautz GE, Xu L, Felgner JH, Wheeler CJ, Felgner PL, Gao X, Huang L, Gordon D, Nabel JG, Nabel EG. Safety and short-term toxicity of a novel cationic lipid formulation for human gene therapy. *Hum Gene Ther* 1993;4: 781–788.
80. Morishita R, Gibbons GH, Kaneda Y, Ogihara T, Dzau VJ. Novel and effective gene transfer technique for study of vascular renin angiotensin system. *J Clin Invest* 1993;91:2580–2585.
81. Takeshita S, Gai D, Leclerc G, Pickering JG, Riessen R, Weir L, Isner JM. Increased gene expression after liposome-mediated arterial gene transfer associated with intimal smooth muscle gene proliferation. *J Clin Invest* 1994;93:652–661.
82. Lim CS, Chapman GD, Gammon RS, Muhlestein JB, Bauman RP, Stack RS, Swain JL. Direct in vivo gene transfer into the coronary and peripheral vasculatures of the intact dog. *Circulation* 1991;83: 2007–2011.
83. Chapman GD, Lim CS, Gammon RS, Culp SC, Desper S, Bauman RP, Swain JL, Stack RS. Gene transfer into coronary arteries of intact animals with a percutaneous balloon catheter. *Circ Res* 1992;71: 27–33.
84. Nabel EG, Yang Z, Liptay S, San H, Gordon D, Haudenschild CC, Nabel GJ. Recombinant platelet-derived growth factor B gene expression in porcine arteries induces intimal hyperplasia in vivo. *J Clin Invest* 1993;91:1822–1829.
85. Felgner J, Bennett F, Felgner PL. Cationic lipid-mediated delivery of polynucleotides. *Methods* 1993;5:67–75.
86. Kaneda Y, Iwai K, Uchida T. Increased expression of DNA cointroduced with nuclear protein in adult rat liver. *Science* 1989;243: 375–378.
87. Kato K, Nakanishi M, Kaneda Y, Uchida T, Okada Y. Expression of hepatitis B virus surface antigen in adult rat liver. *J Biol Chem* 1991; 266:3361–3364.
88. Tomita N, Higaki J, Morishita R, Kato K, Mikami H, Kaneda Y, Ogihara T. Direct in vivo gene introduction into rat kidney. *Biochem Biophys Res Commun* 1992;186:129–134.
89. Morishita R, Gibbons GH, Ellison KE, Nakajima M, Zhang L, Kaneda Y, Ogihara T, Dzau VJ. Single intraluminal delivery of antisense cdc2 kinase and proliferating-cell nuclear antigen oligonucleotides results in chronic inhibition of neointimal hyperplasia. *Proc Natl Acad Sci USA* 1993;90:8474–8478.
90. Morishita R, Gibbons GJ, Ellison KE, Nakajima M, von der Leyen H, Zhang L, Kaneda Y, Ogihara T, Dzau VJ. Intimal hyperplasia after vascular injury is inhibited by antisense cdk 2 kinse oligonucleotides. *J Clin Invest* 1994;93:1458–1464.
91. Wagner E, Plank C, Zatloukal K, Cotten M, Birnstiel ML. Influenza virus hemagglutinin HA-2 N-terminal fusosgenic peptides augment gene transfer by transferrin-polylysine-DNA complexes: Toward a synthetic virus-like gene-transfer vehicle. *Proc Natl Acad Sci USA* 1992:89:7934–7938.
92. Riessen R, Rahimizadeh H, Blessing E, Takeshita S, Barry JJ, Isner JM. Arterial gene transfer using pure DNA applied directly to a hydrogel-coated angioplasty balloon. *Hum Gene Ther* 1993;4:749–758.
93. Simons M, Edelman ER, DeKeyser JL, Langer R, Rosenberg RD. Antisense *c-myb* oligonucleotides inhibit intimal arterial smooth muscle cell accumulation in vivo. *Nature* 1992;359:67–70.
94. Simons M, Edelman ER, Rosenberg RD. Antisense proliferating cell nuclear antigen oligonucleotides inhibit intimal hyperplasia in a rat carotid artery injury model. *J Clin Invest* 1994;93:2351–2356.
95. Conte MS, Birinyi LK, Miyata T, Fallon JT, Gold HK, Whittemore AD, Mulligan RC. Efficient repopulation of denuded rabbit arteries with autologous genetically modified endothelial cells. *Circulation* 1994;89:2161–2169.
96. Lynch CM, Clowes MM, Osborne WR, Clowes AW, Miller AD. Long-term expression of human adenosine deaminase in vascular smooth muscle cells of rats: A model for gene therapy. *Proc Natl Acad Sci USA* 1992;89:1138–1142.
97. Messina LM, Podrazik RM, Whitehill TA, Ekhterae D, Brothers TE, Wilson JM, Burkel WE, Stanley JC. Adhesion and incorporation of *lac-Z*-transduced endothelial cells into the intact capillary wall in the rat. *Proc Natl Acad Sci USA* 1992;89:12018–12022.
98. Clowes MM, Lynch CM, Miller AD, Miller DG, Osborne WRA, Clowes AW. Long-term biological response of injured rat carotid artery seeded with smooth muscle cells expressing retrovirally introduced human genes. *J Clin Invest* 1994;93:644–651.
99. Podrazik RM, Whitehill TA, Ekhterae D, Williams WD, Messina LM, Stanley JC. High-level expression of recombinant human tPA in cultivated canine endothelial cells under varying conditions of retroviral gene transfer. *Ann Surg* 1992;216:233–240.
100. Takeshita S, Gal D, Leclerc G, Pickering JG, Riessen R, Weir L, Isner JM. Increased gene expression following liposome-mediated arterial gene transfer associated with intimal smooth muscle cell proliferation. In vitro and in vivo findings in a rabbit model of vascular injury. *J Clin Invest* 1994;93:652–661.
101. Willard JE, Landau C, Glamann B, Burns D, Jessen ME, Pirwitz MJ, Gerard RD, Meidell RS. Genetic modification of the vessel wall. Comparison of surgical and catheter-based techniques for delivery of recombinant adenovirus. *Circulation* 1994;89:2190–2197.
102. Riessen R, Isner JM. Prospects for site-specific delivery of pharmacologic and molecular therapies. *J Am Coll Cardiol* 1994;23:1234–1244.
103. Guzman RJ, Lemarchand P, Cystsal RG, Epstein SE, Finkel T. Efficient and selective adenovirus-mediated gene transfer into vascular neointima. *Circulation* 1993;88:2838–2848.
104. Nabel EG, Plautz G, Nabel GJ. Transduction of a foreign histocompatibility gene into the arterial wall induces vasculitis. *Proc Natl Acad Sci USA* 1992;89:5157–5161.
105. Nabel EG, Yang Z, Plautz G, Forough R, Zhan X, Haudenschild CC, Maciag T, Nabel GJ. Recombinant fibroblast growth factor-1 promotes intimal hyperplasia and angiogenesis in arteries in vivo. *Nature* 1993;362:844–846.
106. Nabel EG, Shum L, Pompili VJ, Yang ZY, San H, Shu HB, Liptay S, Gordon D, Derynck R, Nabel GJ. Direct gene transfer of transforming growth factor $\beta1$ into arteries stimulates fibrocellular hyperplasia. *Proc Natl Acad Sci USA* 1993;90:10759–10763.
107. Burgess WH, Maciag T. The heparin-binding (fibroblast) growth factor family of proteins. *Annu Rev Biochem* 1989;58:575–606.
108. Brogi E, Winkles JA, Underwood R, Clinton SK, Alberts GF, Libby P. Distinct patterns of expression of fibroblast growth factors and their receptors in human atheroma and nonatherosclerotic arteries. *J Clin Invest* 1993;92:2408–2418.
109. Massague J. The transforming growth factor-β family. *Annu Rev Cell Biol* 1990;6:597–641.
110. Roberts A, Sporn MB. The transforming growth factor-betas. In: Sporn MB, Roberts A, eds. *Peptide Growth Factors and Their Receptors. Handbook for Experimental Pharmacology.* Heidelberg: Springer-Verlag; 1990:419–472.
111. Epstein SE, Siegall CB, Biro S, Fu YM, FitzGerald D, Pastan I. Cytoxic effects of a recombinant chimeric toxin on rapidly proliferating vascular smooth muscle cells. *Circulation* 1991;84:778–787.
112. Biro S, Siegall CB, Fu YM, Speir E, Pastan I, Epstein SE. In vitro effects of a recombinant toxin targeted to the FGF receptor on rat vascular smooth muscle and endothelial cells. *Circ Res* 1992;71: 640–645.
113. Casscells W, Lappi DA, Olwin BB, Wai C, Siegman M, Speir EH, Sasse J, Baird A. Elimination of smooth muscle cells in experimental restenosis: Targeting of fibroblast growth factor receptors. *Proc Natl Acad Sci USA* 1992;89:7159–7163.
114. Guzman RJ, Hirschowitz EA, Brody SL, Crystal RG, Epstein SE,

Finkel T. In vivo suppression of injury-induced vascular smooth muscle cell accumulation using adenovirus-mediated transfer of herpes simplex thymidine kinase gene. *Proc Natl Acad Sci USA* 1994;91: 10732–10736.

115. Gordon JW, Scangos GA, Plotkin DJ, Barbosa JA, Ruddle FH. Genetic transformation of mouse embryos by microinjection of purified DNA. *Proc Natl Acad Sci USA* 1980;77:7380–7384.
116. Borrelli E, Heyman R, Hsi M, Evans RM. Targeting of an inducible toxic phenotype in animal cells. *Proc Natl Acad Sci USA* 1988;85: 7572–7576.
117. Heyman RA, Borrelli E, Lesley J, Anderson D, Richman DD, Baird SM, Hyman R, Evans RM. Thymidine kinase obliteration: Creation of transgenic mice with controlled immune deficiency. *Proc Natl Acad Sci USA* 1989;86:2698–2702.
118. Moolten FL, Wells JM. Curability of tumors bearing herpes thymidine kinase genes transferred by retroviral vectors. *J Natl Cancer Inst* 1990; 82:297–300.
119. Smith KO, Galloway KS, Kennell WL, Ogilvie KK, Radatus BK. A new nucleoside analog, 9-[[2-hydroxy-1-(hydroxymethyl)ethoxyl]-methyl]guanine, highly active in vitro against herpes simplex virus types 1 and 2. *Antimicrob Agents Chemother* 1982;22:55–61.
120. Field AK, Davies ME, DeWitt C, Perry HC, Liou R, Germershausen J, Karkas JD, Ashton WT, Johnston DB, Tolman RL. 9-([2-Hydroxy-1-(hydroxymethyl)ethyxyl]methyl)guanine: A selective inhibitor of herpes group virus replication. *Proc Natl Acad Sci USA* 1983;80: 4139–4143.
121. Culver KW, Ram Z, Wallbridge S, Ishii H, Oldfield EH, Blaese RM. In vivo gene transfer with retroviral vector-producer cells for treatment of experimental brain tumors. *Science* 1992;256:1550–1552.
122. Smythe WR, Hwang HC, Amin KM, Eck SL, Wilson JM, Kaiser LR, Albelda SM. Successful treatment of experimental human mesothelioma using adenovirus transfer of the herpes simplex-thymidine kinase gene. *Ann Thorac Surg* 1994;57:1383–1384.
123. Plautz G, Nabel EG, Nabel GJ. Selective elimination of recombinant genes in vivo with a suicide retroviral vector. *New Biol* 1991;3: 709–715.
124. Chang MW, Ohno T, Gordon D, Lu MM, Nabel GJ, Nabel EG, Leiden JM. Adenovirus-mediated transfer of the herpes simplex virus thymidine kinase gene inhibits vascular smooth muscle cell proliferation and neointima formation following balloon angioplasty of the rat carotid artery. *Mol Med* 1995;1:172–181.
125. Hollingsworth RE Jr, Hensey CE, Lee WH. Retinoblastoma protein and the cell cycle. *Curr Opin Genet Dev* 1993;3:55–62.
126. Qian YW, Wang YC, Hollingsworth RE Jr, Jones D, Ling N, Lee E. A retinoblastoma-binding protein related to a negative regulator of *Ras* in yeast. *Nature* 1993;364:648–652.
127. Johnson DG, Schwarz JK, Cress WD, Nevins JR. Expression of transcription factor E2F1 induces quiescent cells to enter S phase. *Nature* 1993;365:349–352.
128. Nevins JR. E2F. A link between the Rb tumor suppressor protein and viral oncoproteins. *Science* 1992;258:424–429.
129. Waga S, Hannon GJ, Beach D, Stillman B. The p21 inhibitor of cyclin-dependent kinases controls DNA replication by interaction with PCNA. *Nature* 1994;369:574–578.
130. el-Deiry WS, Tokino T, Velculescu VE, Levy DB, Parson R, Trend JM, Lin D, Mercer WE, Kinzler KW, Vogelstein B. WAF1, a potential mediator of p53 tumor suppression. *Cell* 1993;75:817–825.
131. Gu Y, Turck CW, Morgan DO. Inhibition of CDK2 activity in vivo by an associated 20K regulatory subunit. *Nature* 1993;366:707–710.
132. Xiong, Y, Hannon JG, Zhang H, Casso D, Kobayashi R, Beach D. p21 is a universal inhibitor of cyclin kinases. *Nature* 1993;366:701–704.
133. Antoniades HN, Galanopoulos T, Neville-Golden J, Kiritsy CP, Lynch SE. p53 expression during normal tissue regeneration in response to acute cutaneous injury in swine. *J Clin Invest* 1994;93:2206–2214.
134. White E. p53, guardian of Rb. *Nature* 1994;371:21–22.
135. Yonish-Rouach E, Grunwald D, Wilder S, Kimchi A, May E, Lawrence JJ, May P, Oren M. p53-mediated cell death: Relationship to cell cycle control. *Mol Cell Biol* 1993;13:1415–1423.
136. Luscher B, Wisenman RN. New light on *myc* and *myb*. Part II. *myb*. *Genes Dev* 1990;4:2235–2241.
137. Chang MW, Barr E, Seltzer J, Jiang J-Q, Nabel GJ, Nabel EG, Parmacek MS, Leiden JM. Cytostatic gene therapy for vascular proliferative disorders using a constitutively active form of Rb. *Science* 1995; 267:518–522.
138. Morishita R, Gibbons GH, Ellison KE, Lee W, Zhang L, Yu H, Kaneda Y, Ogihara T, Dzau VJ. Evidence for direct local effect of angiotensin in vascular hypertrophy: In vivo gene transfer of angiotensin converting enzyme. *J Clin Invest* 1994;94:978–984.
139. von der Leyen H, Gibbons GH, Morishita R, Lewis NP, Zhang L, Kaneda Y, Cooke JP, Dzau VJ. In vivo gene transfer to prevent hyperplasia after vascular injury: Effect of overexpression of constitutive nitric oxide synthase. *Proc Natl Acad Sci USA* 1995;92:1137–1141. *J* 1994;8:A802.
140. Weintraub HM. Antisense RNA and DNA. *Sci Am* 1990;262:40–46.
141. Toulme JJ, Helene C. Antimessenger of oligodeoxyribonucleotides: An alternative to antisense RNA for artificial regulation of gene expression: A review. *Gene* 1988;72:51–58.
142. van der Krol AR, Mol JN, Stuitje AR. Modulation of eukaryotic gene expression by complementary RNA or DNA sequences. *BioTechniques* 1988;6:958–976.
143. Zon G. Oligonucleotide analogues as potential chemotherapeutic agents. *Pharm Res* 1988;5:539–549.
144. Marcus-Sekura CJ. Techniques for using antisense oligodeoxyribonucleotides to study gene expression. *Anal Biochem* 1988;172: 289–295.
145. Bielinska A, Shivdasani RA, Zhang L, Nabel GJ. Regulation of gene expression with double-stranded phosphorothioate oligonucleotides. *Science* 1990;250:997–1000.
146. Agrawal S, Temsamani J, Tang HY. Pharmacokinetics, biodistribution, and stability of oligodeoxynucleotide phosphorothioates in mice. *Proc Natl Acad Sci USA* 1991;88:7595–7599.
147. Marcus-Sekura CJ, Woerner AM, Shinozuka K, Zon G, Quinnan GV Jr. Comparative inhibition of chloramphenicol acetyltransferase gene expression by antisense oligonucleotide analogues having alkyl phosphotriester, methylphosphonate and phosphorothioate linkages. *Nucleic Acids Res* 1987;15:5749–5763.
148. Sarin PS, Agrawal S, Civeira MP, Goodchild J, Ikeuchi T, Zamecnik PC. Inhibition of acquired immunodeficiency syndrome virus by oligodeoxynucleoside methylphosphonates. *Proc Natl Acad Sci USA* 1988;85:7448–7451.
149. Simons M, Rosenberg RD. Antisense nonmuscle myosin heavy chain and *c-myb* oligonucleotides suppress smooth muscle cell proliferation in vitro. *Circ Res* 1992;70:835–843.
150. Biro S, Fu YM, Yu ZX, Epstein SE. Inhibitory effects of antisense oligodeoxynucleotides targeting *c-myc* mRNA on smooth muscle cell proliferation and migration. *Proc Natl Acad Sci USA* 1993;90: 654–658.
151. Shi Y, Hutchinson HG, Hall DJ, Zalewski A. Down regulation of *c-myc* expression by antisense oligonucleotides inhibits proliferation of human smooth muscle cells. *Circulation* 1993;88:1190–1195.
152. Ebbecke M, Unterberg C, Buchwald A, Stohr S, Wiegand V. Antiproliferative effects of a *c-myc* antisense oligonucleotide on human arterial smooth muscle cells. *Basic Res Cardiol* 1992;87:585–591.
153. Speir E, Epstein SE. Inhibition of smooth muscle cell proliferation by an antisense oligodeoxynucleotide targeting the messenger RNA encoding proliferating cell nuclear antigen. *Circulation* 1993;86: 538–547.
154. Bennett MR, Anglin S, McEwan JR, Jagoe R, Newby AC, Evan GI. Inhibition of vascular smooth muscle cell proliferation in vitro and in vivo by *c-myc* antisense oligonucleotides. *J Clin Invest* 1994;93: 820–828.
155. Abe J, Zhou W, Taguchi J, Takuwa N, Miki K, Okazaki H, Kurokawa K, Kumada M, Takuwa Y. Supression of neointimal smooth muscle cell accumulation in vivo by antisense cdc2 and cdk2 oligonucleotides in rat carotid artery. *Biochem Biophys Res Commun* 1994;198:16–24.
156. Shi Y, Fard A, Galeo A, Hutchinson HG, Vermani P, Dodge GR, Hall DJ, Shabeen F, Zalewski A. Transcatheter delivery of *c-myc* antisense oligomers reduces neointimal formation in a porcine model of coronary artery balloon injury. *Circulation* 1994;90:944–951.
157. Epstein SE, Speir E, Finkel T. Do antisense approaches to the problem of restenosis make sense? *Circulation* 1993;88:1351–1353.
158. Stein CA, Cheng Y-C. Antisense oligonucleotides as therapeutic agents—is the bullet really magical? *Science* 1993;261:1004–1012.
159. Edelman ER, Simons M, Rosenberg RD. mRNA burden and duration of gene expression determine the vasculo-proliferative inhibitory effects of antisense oligonucleotides. *Circulation* 1993;88:I-81.
160. Paigen B, Morrow A, Brandon C, Mitchell D, Holmes P. Variation in

susceptibility to atherosclerosis among inbred strains of mice. *Athero* 1985;57:65–73.

161. Paigen B, Morrow A, Holmes PA, Mitchell D, Williams RA. Quantitative assessment of atherosclerotic lesions in mice. *Athero* 1987;68: 231–240.
162. Paigen B, Mitchell D, Rueu K, Morrow A, Lusis AJ, LeBouef RC. *Ath-1,* a gene determining atherosclerosis susceptibility and high density lipoprotein levels in mice. *Proc Natl Acad Sci USA* 1987;84: 3763–3767.
163. Breslow JL. Transgenic mouse models of lipoprotein metabolism and atherosclerosis. *Proc Natl Acad Sci USA* 1993;90:8314–8318.
164. Capecchi MR. Altering the genome by homologous recombination. *Science* 1989;244:1288–1292.
165. Plump AS, Smith JD, Hayek T, Aalto-Setala K, Walsh A, Verstuyft JG, Rubin EM, Breslow JL. Severe hypercholesterolemia and atherosclerosis in apolipoprotein E-deficient mice created by homologous recombination in ES cells. *Cell* 1992;71:343–353.
166. Zhang ZH, Reddick RL, Piedrahita JA, Maeda N. Spontaneous hypercholesterolemia and arterial lesions in mice lacking apolipoprotein E. *Science* 1992;258:468–471.
167. Hofmann SL, Russell DW, Brown MS, Goldstein JL, Hammer RE. Overexpression of low density lipoprotein (LDL) receptor eliminates LDL from plasma in transgenic mice. *Science* 1988;239:1277–1281.
168. Ishibashi S, Goldstein JL, Brown MS, Herz J, Burns D. Massive xanthomatosis and atherosclerosis in cholesterol-fed low density lipoprotein receptor-negative mice. *J Clin Invest* 1994;93:1885–1893.
169. Ishibashi S, Brown MS, Golstein JL, Gerardx RD, Hammer RE, Herz J. Hypercholesterolemia in low density lipoprotein receptor knockout mice and its reversal by adenovirus-mediated gene delivery. *J Clin Invest* 1993;92:883–893.
170. Chiesa G, Hobbs HH, Koschinsky ML, Lawn RM, Maika SD, Hammer RE. Reconstitution of lipoprotein(a) by infusion of human LDL in transgenic mice expressing human apolipoprotein(a). *J Biol Chem* 1992;267:24369–24374.
171. Lawn RM, Wade DP, Hammer RE, Chiesa G, Verstuyft JG, Rubin EM. Atherogenesis in transgenic mice expressing human apolipoprotein(a). *Nature* 1992;360:670–672.
172. Grainger DJ, Kirschenlohr HL, Metcalfe JC, Weissberg PL, Wade DP, Lawn RM. Proliferation of human smooth muscle cells promoted by lipoprotein(a). *Science* 1993;260:1655–1658.
173. Nakashima Y, Plump AS, Raines EW, Breslow J, Ross R. ApoE-deficient mice develop lesions of all phases of atherosclerosis through the arterial tree. *Arterioscler Thromb* 1994;14:133–140.
174. Reddick RL, Zhang SJ, Maeda N. Atherosclerosis in mice lacking Apo E. Evaluation of lesional development and progression. *Arterioscler Thromb* 1994;14:141–147.
175. Ishibashi S, Herz J, Maeda N, Goldstein JL, Brown MS. The two-receptor model of lipoprotein clearance: Tests of the hypothesis in "knockout" mice lacking the low denity lipoprotein receptor, apolipoprotein E, or both proteins. *Proc Natl Acad Sci USA* 1994;91: 4431–4435.
176. Rubin EM, Krauss RM, Spangler EA, Verstuyft JG, Clift SM. Inhibition of early atherogenesis in transgenic mice by human apolipoprotein AI. *Nature* 1991;353:265.
177. Kopfler WP, Willard M, Betz T, Willard JE, Gerard RD, Meidell RS. Adenovirus-mediated transfer of a gene encoding human apolipoprotein A-I into normal mice increases circulating high-density lipoprotein cholesterol. *Circulation* 1994;90:1319–1327.
178. Warden CH, Hedrick CC, Qiao JH, Castellani LW, Lusis AJ. Atherosclerosis in transgenic mice overexpressing apolipoprotein A-II. *Science* 1993;261:469–472.
179. Willnow TE, Sheng Z, Ishibashi S, Herz J. Inhibition of hepatic chylomicron remnant uptake by gene transfer of a receptor antagonist. *Science* 1994;264:1471–1474.
180. Wilson JM, Chowdhury NR, Grossman M, Wajsman R, Epstein A, Mulligan RC, Chowdhury JR. Temporary amelioration of hyperlipidemia in low density lipoprotein receptor-deficient rabbits transplanted with genetically modified hepatocytes. *Proc Natl Acad Sci USA* 1990; 87:8437–8441.
181. Chowdhury JR, Grossman M, Gupta S, Chowdhury NR, Baker JR Jr, Wilson JM. Long-term improvement of hypercholesterolemia after ex vivo gene therapy in LDLR-deficient rabbits. *Science* 1991;254: 1802–1805.
182. Kozarsky KF, McKinley DR, Austin LL, Raper SE, Stratford-Perricaudet LD, Wilson JM. In vivo correction of low density lipoprotein receptor deficiency in the Watanabe heritable hyperlipidemic rabbit with recombinant adenoviruses. *J Biol Chem* 1994;269:13695–13702.
183. Wilson JM, Grossman M, Raper SE, Baker JR, Newton RS, Thoene JG. Ex vivo gene therapy of familial hypercholesterolemia. *Hum Gen Ther* 1992;3:179–222.
184. Grossman M, Raper SE, Kozarsky K, Stein EA, Engelhardt JF, Muller D, Lupien PJ, Wilson JM. Successful ex vivo gene therapy directed to liver in a patient with familial hypercholesterolaemia. *Nature Genet* 1994;6:335–341.
185. Miller AD. Human gene therapy comes of age. *Nature* 1992;357: 455–460.
186. Human gene marker/therapy clinical protocol. *Hum Gene Ther* 1994; 5:787–789.
187. Nabel GJ, Nabel EG, Yang Z, Fox B, Plautz G, Gao X, Huang L, Shu S, Gordon D, Chang AE. Direct gene transfer with DNA liposome complexes in melanoma: Expression, biologic activity and lack of toxicity in humans. *Proc Natl Acad Sci USA* 1993;90:11307–11311.
188. Nabel EG, Yang ZY, Muller D, Change AE, Gao X, Huang L, Cho KJ, Nabel GJ. Safety and toxicity of catheter gene delivery to the pulmonary vasculature in a patient with metastatic melanoma. *Hum Gene Ther* 1994;5:1089–1094.
189. Nabel EG, Nabel GJ. Gene therapy for cardiovascular diseases: Potential applications. In: Braunwald E, ed. *Heart Disease Update.* Philadelphia: WB Saunders; 1994:1–12.
190. Nabel EG, Nabel GJ. Molecular genetic interventions for cardiovascular disease. In: Topol EJ, ed. Textbook of Interventional Cardiology, 2nd ed. Philadelphia: WB Saunders; 1994:1006–1019.

Atherosclerosis and Coronary Artery Disease,
edited by V. Fuster, R. Ross, and E. J. Topol.
Lippincott-Raven Publishers, Philadelphia © 1996.

CHAPTER 43

Nonatherosclerotic Coronary Artery Disease

Donald C. Harrison

Key Words: Congenital anomalies; Coronary artery aneurysm; Muscle bridges; Coronary arteritis; Myocardial oxygen demand/supply imbalance.

INTRODUCTION

Coronary artery disease caused by nonatherosclerotic processes has been recognized with increasing frequency as a result of the widespread use of new modalities for invasive and noninvasive imaging of the cardiovascular system. Congenital anomalies of the origin of coronary arteries, coronary artery aneurysms, coronary embolization, genetic metabolic disorders, and coronary arteritis are all important causes of nonatherosclerotic disease. With the increasing utilization of catheter-based interventional techniques for treating coronary artery disease, coronary dissection, coronary embolization, and coronary aneurysm are occurring with increasing frequency. Although they occur much less frequently than atherosclerotic processes, the nonatherosclerotic diseases of coronary arteries are particularly important in younger individuals, and it is important for practicing cardiologists to make the correct diagnosis in order to achieve successful therapeutic outcomes.

Ischemic heart disease (angina pectoris, myocardial infarction, and sudden cardiac death) is almost always caused by narrowing of major coronary arteries by atherosclerosis,

D. C. Harrison: University of Cincinnati Medical Center, Cincinnati, Ohio 45267-0663.

TABLE 1. *Nonatherosclerotic coronary artery disease*[a]

1. Congenital anomalies of the coronary circulation
   a. Anomalous origin from the aorta
      (1) Origin from the contralateral sinus of Valsalva
      (2) Single coronary artery
      (3) Atresia of the coronary ostium
   b. Anomalous origin from the pulmonary artery
   c. Coronary artery fistula
   d. Coronary artery aneurysm
2. Mechanical insults to the coronary circulation
   a. Coronary artery embolus
      (1) Thrombus
      (2) Calcium plaques
      (3) Cardiac surgery
      (4) Coronary catheterization
      (5) Coronary angioplasty
      (6) Prosthetic valves
      (7) Paradoxical (venous)
   b. Coronary artery dissection
   c. Coronary artery trauma
      (1) Nonpenetrating trauma
      (2) Penetrating trauma
      (3) Trauma during cardiac catheterization or surgery
   d. Coronary thrombosis (polycythemia and other hypercoagulable states)
3. Progressive nonatherosclerotic coronary occlusive disease
   a. Coronary artery vasculitis
      (1) Polyarteritis nodosa
      (2) Systemic lupus erythematosus
      (3) Wegener's granulomatosis
      (4) Takayasu's disease
      (5) Kawasaki's disease
      (6) Infection
   b. Intimal proliferation or fibrosis
      (1) Ionizing radiation
      (2) Cardiac transplantation
      (3) Coronary angioplasty
      (4) Cocaine
      (5) Treatment with methysergide
   c. Accumulation of metabolic substances
      (1) Inborn errors of metabolism (Hurler, Hunter)
      (2) Amyloid accumulation
      (3) Homocystinuria
   d. Extrinsic coronary compression
      (1) Muscle bridges
      (2) Primary or metastatic tumors
      (3) Aortic aneurysm
4. Miscellaneous causes
   a. Myocardial oxygen demand–supply imbalance
      (1) Aortic stenosis
      (2) CO poisoning
      (3) Severe hypotension (prolonged)
   b. Substance abuse
      (1) Cocaine
      (2) Amphetamines

[a] Adapted from Harrison and Baim (5), Waller (4), and Alpert and Braunwald (6).

but in rare instances it may result from one of a variety of nonatherosclerotic coronary artery pathologies (Table 1) (1–4). In societies outside the United States there appears to be a greater prevalence of the nonatherosclerotic coronary syndromes, and with the recent increase in early interventions in acute infarction, the number of traumatic injuries to coronary arteries has increased. In order to use thrombolytic therapy and advanced interventional techniques appropriately, recognition of these rarer forms of coronary artery disease is essential. However, these relatively uncommon disease processes pose several important problems for the clinician: (a) they often occur in patients in whom ischemic heart disease is uncommon, unsuspected, or masked by an underlying systemic disease; (b) they may occur in association with underlying atherosclerotic coronary artery disease; (c) they may require specialized noninvasive and invasive techniques for diagnosis; and (d) their natural histories, pathophysiologies, and optimal management are frequently incompletely understood. Because specific and potentially life-saving therapies have recently been shown to be effective in these syndromes, the physician should have an overall familiarity with the diagnosis and therapy of these nonatherosclerotic coronary artery diseases.

CLINICAL RECOGNITION OF NONATHEROSCLEROTIC CORONARY DISEASE

The clinical recognition of nonatherosclerotic coronary disease is difficult because the clinical symptoms are quite similar to those occurring with atherosclerotic coronary disease. When the symptoms are chest pain, they are frequently overlooked in teenage and young patients, who may present on multiple occasions, and the diagnosis and definition of a cause occur only after acute myocardial infarction for which no atherosclerotic process can be identified, or after coronary angiography in which no luminal atherosclerotic process can be visualized. The most helpful way for the physician to make the diagnosis is to recognize situations in which atherosclerosis is uncommon and suspect one of the diagnoses listed in Table 1. Clues that can be helpful are symptoms of coronary artery disease in young patients, especially under the age of 30, the absence of routine coronary risk factors, and the recognition and diagnosis of any of the associated diseases or conditions listed in Table 1.

Approximately 5% of all patients with acute myocardial infarction do not have documented atherosclerotic disease at the time of angiography or autopsy (7,8). A number of studies suggest that approximately 95% of all patients with fatal myocardial infarction have at least one major coronary artery with more than 80% narrowing or total occlusion. Approximately 5% of all patients at autopsy have normal coronary arteries. In those patients under the age of 30, there is a three- or fourfold increase in this number to as great as 20%. Of those patients who have acute myocardial infarction with normal or near normal coronary arteries, many probably represent the syndrome of clinical coronary artery spasm (See Luscher and Pepine, *this volume*).

CORONARY ARTERY SPASM

The frequency of coronary artery spasm in coronary arteries that are not involved with the atherosclerotic process is unknown. Recent studies have documented that myocardial infarction may occur in this syndrome, and it appears to be higher in Oriental populations. Recent pathophysiological studies have defined alterations in endothelial function as a signaling mechanism for the constriction of coronary arteries, but much remains to be identified for a full definition of coronary artery spasm's pathophysiology. The clinical syndrome and pathophysiology are presented extensively by Luscher and Pepine *(this volume)*.

CONGENITAL ANOMALIES OF THE CORONARY CIRCULATION

Coronary artery anomalies—variations in the origin, course, and distribution of the coronary arteries—are present in 1–2% of the population (7–11). Ostial lesions, passage of a major artery between the walls of the pulmonary trunk and the aorta, the origin of a major artery from the pulmonary trunk, and myocardial bridges appear to produce more symptoms of ischemia and subsequent myocardial infarction (12). These anomalies may make angiographic visualization of the coronary circulation more difficult and probably increase the risk of coronary artery trauma during cardiac surgery. Only a fraction of the patients in whom these congenital anomalies are present experience myocardial ischemia. The absence or presence of symptoms of ischemia depend on the origin of the coronary artery, the direction of blood flow at rest, and the alterations in flow that result during physical exertion, which in some cases may produce a true "coronary steal" syndrome. The anatomy and physiology of anomalies of the coronary arteries that produce the "coronary steal" syndrome have been defined. For a "coronary steal," it is required to have a common coronary vessel have a resistance to flow that supplies two myocardial regions in parallel and vasodilatation that is greater in one of the two parallel regions (13). The conditions are met when there is a single coronary artery. Drug therapy that results in differential vasodilatation in the two parallel vascular beds appears to be the mechanism for producing this phenomenon (14). If one vascular bed is already maximally dilated because of myocardial ischemia, and a coronary vasodilator drug is administered, there is an increase in coronary blood flow, but the increase to the normal vascular bed is greater, and the "steal" occurs because blood is differentially shunted from the ischemic area.

Evaluation of each patient with a coronary anomaly must therefore include an anatomic classification, recognition of the particular anomaly as one capable of producing myocardial ischemia, and documentation that true ischemia is present by symptomatic or biochemical studies. In many symptomatic patients with coronary anomalies in whom ischemia can be documented by exercise testing, isotopic myocardial perfusion scanning, or transmyocardial metabolic testing, effective corrective cardiac surgery can usually be performed.

Anomalous Origin from the Aorta

In normal coronary circulation, the right coronary artery originates from a single ostium within the right sinus of Valsalva, and the left coronary artery originates from a single ostium within the left sinus of Valsalva (Fig. 1A) (7,15). Abnormally high or low locations of the coronary ostia and the presence within the appropriate sinus of Valsalva of sepa-

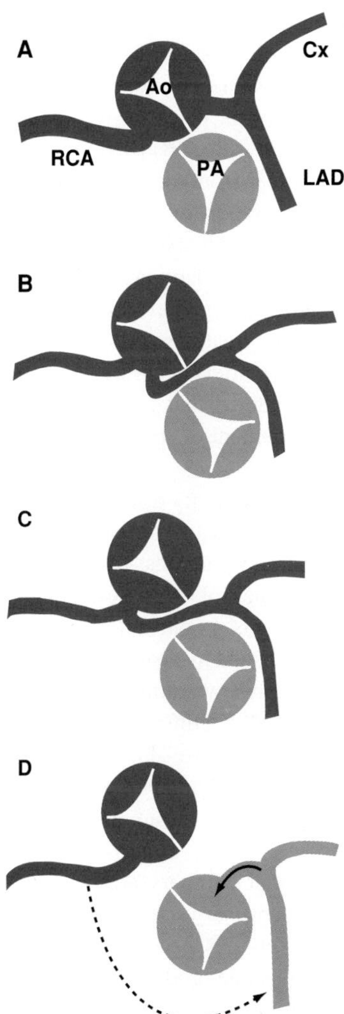

FIG. 1. Representative patterns of anomalous coronary artery origin. **A:** Normal coronary circulation with origin of the right coronary artery (RCA) from the right sinus of Valsalva and origin of the left coronary artery from the left sinus of Valsalva. The aorta (Ao), pulmonary artery (PA), and left anterior descending (LAD) and circumflex (Cx) branches of the left coronary artery are shown. **B:** Anomalous origin of the left coronary artery from the right sinus of Valsalva, with passage of the left main coronary artery between the aorta and pulmonary artery. **C:** Single coronary artery originating from the right sinus of Valsalva, with passage of the left main coronary artery between the aorta and pulmonary artery. **D:** Origin of the left coronary artery from the pulmonary artery, showing the development of collateral flow *(dotted arrow)* from the right coronary artery and the associated left-to-right shunt into the pulmonary artery *(solid arrow)*.

rate ostia from the left anterior descending and circumflex coronary artery branches, or for the right coronary artery and its conus branch, are common minor variations that do not result in myocardial ischemia. Other anomalous patterns of coronary artery origin from the aorta are potential causes of myocardial ischemia even in the absence of atherosclerosis.

Origin from the Contralateral Sinus of Valsalva

When one of the coronary arteries originates from the contralateral sinus of Valsalva, this anomalous vessel must traverse the base of the heart to reach its territory of distribution, passing anterior to, posterior to, or between the aorta and pulmonary artery (Fig. 1B) (8–15). Acute angulation at the origin of the artery from the aorta may result in anatomic or functional constriction of the proximal portion of the anomalous coronary artery. Anomalous vessels passing between the aorta and pulmonary artery seem to carry an additional risk of ischemia, possibly as a result of being compressed between the great vessels, although this is unlikely at normal pulmonary artery pressure. Abnormal mechanical stresses or flow patterns that produce internal injury may enhance the development of coronary atherosclerosis in the anomalous segment.

Origin of the left coronary artery from the right sinus of Valsalva with passage of the proximal left coronary artery between the aorta and pulmonary artery is associated with an increased incidence of exercise-related sudden cardiac death in young patients. In one autopsy study of 33 patients with this anomaly, sudden death occurred in nine (27%), generally without prior warning symptoms (15). Autopsy studies in sudden death victims without known atherosclerosis occurring during exercise show a high incidence of this syndrome. Some even recommend prophylactic coronary artery bypass surgery when this anomaly is detected in young patients (12,15).

In patients without coronary atherosclerosis, passage of the anomalous left coronary artery either anterior or posterior to both great vessels has been associated with pacing-induced myocardial lactate production and angina pectoris but does not seem to carry a significant risk of sudden death. Angina pectoris has also been reported in patients in whom the right coronary artery originates from the left sinus of Valsalva, but confirmation of myocardial ischemia has been less complete in these patients than in patients with anomalous origin of the left coronary artery. The most common pattern of anomalous aortic origin, origin of the circumflex coronary artery from the right sinus of Valsalva or proximal right coronary artery, does not seem to impose independent ischemic risk.

Single Coronary Artery

Derivation of the entire coronary circulation from a single ostium is a rare coronary anomaly (Fig. 1C). In a study of 50,000 consecutive coronary angiograms, only 33 cases of a single coronary artery were described, yielding an incidence of 0.066% (16). Approximately 40% of patients with this anomaly have an associated congenital cardiac defect, i.e., tetralogy of Fallot, transposition of the great vessels, or improper division of the truncus arteriosus (17). There is no clear sex predominance for this condition, and the frequency of occurrence of single left and single right coronary arteries is approximately equal (18). As in the case of anomalous origin from the contralateral sinus of Valsalva, one or more components of the coronary circulation system must cross the base of the heart to reach its territory of distribution, passing anterior to, posterior to, or between the great vessels. These transposed vessels may thereby be exposed to the risks of angulation, compression, and accelerated atherosclerosis. Because the entire myocardium is supplied by way of the single coronary artery, proximal coronary atherosclerosis poses the risk of global myocardial ischemia and death. Coronary atherosclerosis frequently develops in the single coronary artery syndrome but probably does not differ in incidence from the normal population.

Clinical manifestations of the single coronary artery anomaly depend in part on associated cardiac defects and atherosclerosis, but up to 15% of patients with only this anomaly develop severe cardiac complications by age 40 (17). Angina pectoris and myocardial lactate production have been demonstrated in patients with a single coronary artery in the absence of coronary atherosclerosis or vessel passage between the aorta and pulmonary artery (18).

Atresia of the Coronary Ostium

Atresia or severe stenosis of one of the coronary ostia, often associated with hypoplasia of the proximal coronary artery, is a rare congenital coronary anomaly, with only seven reported cases (9,19). The absence of a second coronary ostium may lead to the incorrect diagnosis of a single coronary artery. Myocardial perfusion studies will differentiate inadequate flow to segments of the myocardium and establish the diagnosis. Because the involved vessel is dependent on collateral flow from the contralateral coronary artery, myocardial ischemia or infarction may develop during infancy. In this sense, patients with ostial atresia bear an angiographic and clinical resemblance to patients with anomalous origin of a coronary artery from the pulmonary artery (see below). Successful coronary artery bypass grafting has been reported in a patient as young as 10 years old with ostial atresia (19).

Anomalous Origin from the Pulmonary Artery

Origin of a coronary artery from the pulmonary artery rather than from the aorta is a relatively uncommon but severe coronary anomaly. It should be recognized by pediatric cardiologists because it is generally treatable with surgery.

In more than 90% of cases, it is the left coronary artery that originates from the pulmonary artery, generally from the left posterior pulmonary sinus (9). Generally, it is the left main coronary artery with an anomalous origin and the right coronary arising correctly from the aorta (9) (Fig. 1D). Origin of the right coronary artery, an accessory coronary artery, and both coronary arteries from the pulmonary artery have been described, the last of which is invariably fatal in the neonatal period (9,10,20).

As the pulmonary artery pressure falls during the first weeks of life, perfusion of the anomalous coronary artery from the pulmonary artery decreases. Unless adequate collateral flow develops from the contralateral coronary artery, the territory of the anomalous vessel becomes ischemic. Angina pectoris or congestive heart failure with mitral regurgitation may then develop, often accompanied by electrocardiographic manifestations of myocardial ischemia or infarction. This clinical picture, the infantile syndrome, develops in approximately 80% of affected patients, usually within the first 4 months of life (9,21,22). In the absence of surgical correction, this syndrome has an 80% first-year mortality, although the mortality is somewhat lower with anomalous origin of the right coronary artery (20). Those who do not develop the infantile syndrome may present during childhood or adult life with one of the following: congestive heart failure, asymptomatic murmur, mitral regurgitation, angina pectoris, or sudden death (9,21).

Patients surviving infancy tend to have extensive intercoronary collateral flow, with dilatation of both the normal and the anomalous vessels. This collateral flow reverses the direction of blood flow in the anomalous coronary artery, constituting a left-to-right shunt into the pulmonary artery. Despite extensive collateralization, electrocardiographic evidence of ischemia and pathological evidence of subendocardial fibrosis usually persist.

Surgical correction of anomalous coronary artery origin from the pulmonary artery seeks to eliminate the left-to-right shunt and to establish an independent arterial blood supply to the anomalous vessel. Ligation of the anomalous vessel at its origin in combination with saphenous vein aortocoronary bypass grafting has been performed, but it is technically difficult in children under 2 years of age and is associated with a high rate of graft failure (22). The alternative method of correction, reimplantation of the anomalous vessel with the subclavian artery, seems more successful in infants. This anomaly is associated with high morbidity and mortality rates, and because suitable techniques are available, early surgical correction appears to be the treatment of choice.

Coronary Artery Fistula

The most common hemodynamically significant coronary artery anomaly is a direct anastomosis between a major coronary artery and one of the cardiac chambers or major great vessels, such as the superior vena cava, coronary sinus, or pulmonary artery. Fistulas from the right coronary artery are slightly more common than those from the left coronary artery, and bilateral fistulas are present in 4% to 5% of cases (Fig. 2) (23,24). Fistulas are recognized with increasing frequency because of the greater utilization of coronary angiography, three-dimensional echocardiographic studies, and MRI imaging technologies. Over 90% of the fistulas drain into the venous circulation (the right ventricle in 41%; the right atrium in 26%; pulmonary artery in 17%; coronary

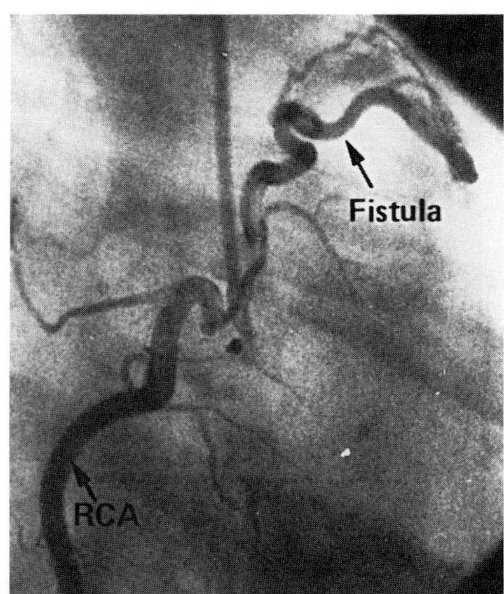

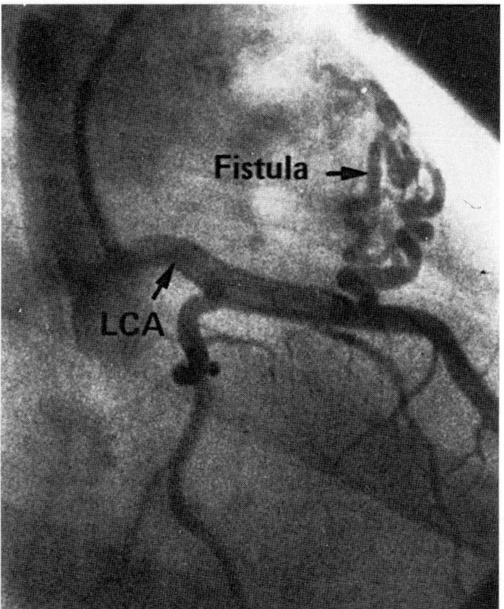

FIG. 2. Bilateral coronary artery to pulmonary artery fistula, originating from the proximal right coronary artery (RCA) and the left anterior descending branch of the left coronary artery (LCA), in an asymptomatic 29-year-old woman with a continuous heart murmur. No left-to-right shunt was detected by oximetry.

sinus in 7%; superior vena cava in 1% (5). The remaining fistulas drain into the arterial circulation (left atrium in 5%; left ventricle in 3%) (5). Multiple anastomoses between the involved coronary artery and the structure within the heart or great vessels into which it drains are possible. The involved coronary artery proximal to the fistula is markedly dilated, and flow through the fistula may be several times that delivering oxygen to the myocardium. When the fistula drains into the venous circulation, a significant left-to-right shunt may be present.

Runoff through a fistula may lower intracoronary diastolic pressure and produce myocardial ischemia in some patients by a "coronary steal" phenomenon (9,10). Physical examination often reveals a continuous heart murmur, which brings approximately one-half of patients with coronary artery fistulas to medical attention. In one series of 58 patients, 21 had associated cardiac defects that brought them to diagnostic study (25).

In a large study of 171 neonates with pulmonary atresia, coronary artery–right ventricular fistulas were found in 45% of the patients, and right ventricular dependency was severe in nine. This again demonstrates the frequency of fistula associated with other congenital abnormalities of the heart.

The chest X-ray is usually normal but may show evidence of pulmonary overcirculation when a large left-to-right shunt is present, mimicking a patent ductus arteriosus. Electrocardiographic abnormalities are uncommon. Diagnosis is best made by selective coronary angiography, particularly when catheterization to evaluate a continuous murmur has failed to disclose the expected anatomic abnormality. Similar fistulas may result from cardiac trauma.

This is the most clinically recognized nonatherosclerotic coronary syndrome and merits understanding by all cardiologists. The great majority of patients with coronary fistulas are asymptomatic and may be detected only by the presence of a murmur or an abnormal ECG, so the decision regarding surgical correction of a fistula is complex. Ischemia has been documented in some patients with coronary fistulas and no atherosclerosis (9,10), and there is evidence that the majority of patients do become symptomatic with advancing age (24). In addition to angina and myocardial infarction, congestive heart failure, bacterial endocarditis, and fistula rupture have been described. Because spontaneous fistula closure is rare, and the risk of surgical closure of the fistula is significantly lower in patients under age 20, some authorities have suggested elective fistula ligation in young patients, including those who are asymptomatic (24). A recent report of 58 patients showed surgery to be safe and effective with long-term good results (25). No deaths occurred in patients with isolated fistulas and no other congenital heart lesions. Antibiotic prophylaxis against bacterial endocarditis is recommended for all patients (23).

Muscle Bridge: Tunneling of Coronary Arteries into the Myocardium

In some patients, the major epicardial coronary arteries penetrate into the myocardium to be covered over with muscle bands. The intramyocardial segments of the large coronary arteries, particularly the left anterior descending artery, may be subject to systolic compression with cardiac contraction, or "milking" (Fig. 3). This pathological finding has been known for several centuries, but only recently has it

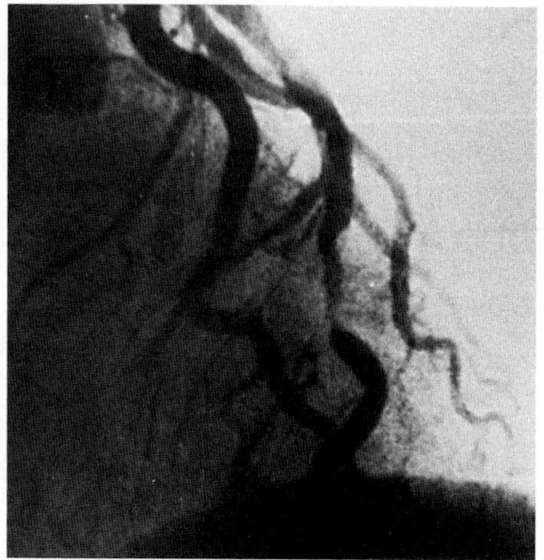

Systole

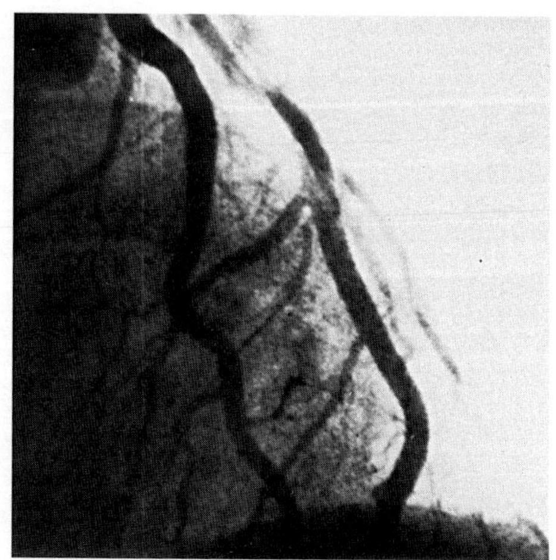

Diastole

FIG. 3. Systolic compression of the midleft anterior descending coronary artery by a muscle bridge with restoration of the normal coronary artery diameter during diastole in a young man with exercise-induced ventricular tachycardia. Treated with oral propranolol, the patient was free of both arrhythmia and electrocardiographic evidence of myocardial ischemia during maximal treadmill exercise testing. (Courtesy of Dr. John A. Michal, Santa Barbara, CA.)

been shown to be of clinical relevance. Intramyocardial segments of the coronary arteries are present in approximately 20% of autopsied hearts (4,26), but angiographic evidence of systolic compression is reported in only 0.5% of patients undergoing coronary angiography for chest pain (27). In most cases angiographic compression is a benign finding, but when a long vessel segment demonstrates systolic compression to less than 25% of its diastolic diameter, ischemia may be revealed by exercise, by ^{201}TL myocardial perfusion scanning, or by coronary sinus pacing metabolic evaluation, even in the absence of coronary atherosclerosis (27).

Because most coronary flow takes place during diastole, it is not clear how systolic compression alone results in myocardial ischemia. One possibility is that the compression results in abnormal vascular tone in the segment and coronary spasm. In some symptomatic patients, coronary compression may extend into early diastole, and excessive myocardial oxygen demand may be present as the result of associated left ventricular hypertrophy (27). Although muscle bridges are a congenital anomaly, symptoms of ischemia may not develop until middle age, which is likely because of associated changes in vascular tone.

Angina pectoris resulting from systolic coronary artery compression may respond to therapy with β-adrenergic blocking drugs and/or calcium channel-blocking agents. When symptoms are refractory to medical therapy, and when inducible ischemia has been unequivocally demonstrated, coronary bypass grafting or simple unroofing of the bridged coronary segment has resulted in relief of symptoms and normalization of myocardial perfusion and metabolism (27,28).

In a recent study, nine patients with obstruction to coronary artery flow caused by myocardial bridging underwent surgery after failure of medical therapy. Postoperative scintigraphic and angiographic studies demonstrated restoration of normal coronary flow and myocardial perfusion in all nine of these patients. The impaired flow occurred in the distribution of the left coronary descending artery in seven patients and in a diagonal branch in two. All patients are alive and asymptomatic (29).

CORONARY ARTERY ANEURYSM

Coronary artery aneurysms, localized areas of coronary dilatation relative to adjacent normal arterial segments, occur in approximately 1.5% of patients studied by autopsy or coronary angiography (30). Acquired causes (Table 2) frequently result from intrinsic pathology of the arterial wall media or damage to it during a procedure. The aneurysms are frequently multiple, may attain a diameter of several centimeters, involve the right coronary artery more frequently than the left (31), and may be either congenital or acquired. Atherosclerosis, either by stenosis with poststenotic dilatation or by primary destruction of the coronary intima and media, accounts for a large percentage of coronary aneurysms in Western populations. Atherosclerotic damage may also produce diffuse coronary ectasia rather than focal coronary aneurysm (2). Other pathological processes that damage the arterial wall, including dissection, trauma, coronary angioplasty, vasculitis, mycotic emboli, syphilis, and mucocutaneous lymph node syndrome, may also lead to aneurysm formation (30,31). Coronary aneurysms may also be congenital in origin. The largest cause of coronary aneurysms in Oriental populations is Kawasaki disease (see below), but many cases are reported in U.S. pediatric populations as well. Early therapy with aspirin in Kawasaki's disease was reported to prevent the occurrence of coronary aneurysms (32), but this has been largely replaced with treatment with other antiinflammatory agents. Aneurysms are frequently detected with echocardiographic techniques, and treatment of the inflammatory disease frequently results in resolution of the aneurysms (33). Similar resolution has been noted in 188 cases followed with serial angiograms (34).

TABLE 2. *Causes of coronary aneurysms*[a]

Atherosclerosis with vessel ectasia
Atherectomy
Dissection of coronary arteries
Angioplasty
Mycotic emboli
Kawasaki's disease
Arteritis
Trauma
Congenital

[a] Adapted from Waller (4).

There are no reliable clinical features of coronary artery aneurysm, although a diastolic or continuous heart murmur may occasionally be present (30). The chest X-ray may show a pericardiac mass or calcification, and although echocardiography may detect the largest and most proximal coronary aneurysms, coronary angiography is required for accurate diagnosis. The most frequent way in which they are diagnosed is repeat coronary angiography after angioplasty or atherectomy.

The clinical course of patients with coronary artery aneurysms usually depends on the severity of the associated atherosclerotic stenoses. Even in the absence of stenosis, abnormal flow patterns within the aneurysm may lead to thrombus formation with subsequent vessel occlusion, distal thromboembolization, or myocardial infarction (30). One case has been reported in which a large intramyocardial aneurysm resulted in angina by a coronary steal mechanism. Rupture of a coronary aneurysm is a rare but serious complication.

Surgical therapy of combined stenotic and aneurysmal atherosclerosis consists of ligation of the involved vessel immediately beyond the aneurysm (to eliminate subsequent emboli) and aortocoronary bypass grafting to the distal vessel. Similar surgery has been suggested in patients without stenotic lesions and even in asymptomatic patients with coronary aneurysms (30). Anticoagulant or antiplatelet therapy may also be of value in this condition (2). Because aneurysmal changes are frequently present in other vessels, particularly the abdominal aorta, comprehensive arteriographic evaluation is recommended in patients with coronary artery aneurysms (30,31).

In inflammatory etiologies such as Kawasaki's, surgery is generally not indicated because response to antiinflammatory drugs is usually good. Surgical correction with aortocoronary bypass and ligation of large aneurysms is indicated only with persistent myocardial ischemia.

MECHANICAL INSULTS TO THE CORONARY ARTERY CIRCULATION

Mechanical injury to coronary arteries has been recognized for centuries, but with the more widespread application of catheter-based interventions in coronary artery disease, the prevalence of these types of injuries has markedly increased. Early recognition of mechanical injury to coronary arteries may permit early thrombolytic therapy or surgical intervention to salvage viable myocardium.

Coronary Artery Embolus

The coronary arteries may be partially protected from embolic events by the acute angulation of the coronary ostia relative to the aortic stream and by their position behind the aortic valve leaflets during systole. When coronary artery emboli do occur (Table 3), the outcome is dictated by the size of the embolus and its position of impaction in the coronary circulation, which determines the magnitude of the ensuing infarctions. Small emboli tend to produce occlusion of a distal branch of one of the coronary arteries (most commonly the left anterior descending artery), resulting in a small area of myocardial necrosis that may not be clinically evident (35,36). These small emboli appear to be relatively frequent. In one autopsy series they were found in 13% of patients with histologically evident myocardial necrosis (36). Quite possibly these small emboli may trigger sudden death by producing small areas of ischemia that are arrhythmogenic. Larger coronary artery emboli are relatively less frequent but generally result in clinically apparent myocardial infarction.

TABLE 3. *Causes of coronary arterial emboli*

Infective endocarditis (native or artificial valves)
Cardiac cavitary thrombus
Left ventricle (MI, cardiomyopathies, ventricular aneurysms)
Left atrium (mitral stenosis, atrial fibrillation)
Cardiac tumors (myxomas)
Metastatic cancer
Calcific aortic or mitral valves
Coronary plaques or aneurysms
Coronary artery trauma
Cardiac surgery
Angioplasty
Atherectomy
During cardiac catheterization and angioplasty
Paradoxical
Atrial septal defect with pulmonary hypertension
Patent foramen ovale from thrombophlebitis
Congenital heart disease

Coronary artery emboli should be considered in the differential diagnosis of acute myocardial ischemia in patients whose clinical condition predisposes them to arterial emboli, including patients with valvular heart disease (endocarditis, noninfected abnormal valve, prosthetic valve), mural thrombus (congestive cardiomyopathy, previous myocardial infarction, atrial fibrillation), left-sided catheterization, or the anatomic potential for paradoxical embolization (35,36). Coronary emboli of a variety of materials, including tumor, myocardial or skeletal muscle, and materials used in cardiac surgery, have also been reported. Extracardiac emboli may also be present. In patients sustaining coronary emboli, prompt coronary angiography may show occlusion of the involved vessel, but restudy as soon as 1 month following the acute event may show renewed vessel patency as the result of lysis or recanalization of the embolus (35).

In the past 12 years, coronary embolism occurring with attempted transluminal angioplasty or the introduction of thrombolytic agents (streptokinase, t-PA, etc.) into coronary arteries has been noted with increasing frequency. During the past several years with newer invasive techniques to treat coronary atherosclerosis such as atherectomy, rotobladers, stents, and lasers, emboli to the coronary arteries are more frequently reported. Because these patients have fresh thrombus in their coronary arteries and are undergoing acute infarction, it is difficult to separate the effects of progressive disease from the effects of embolizing the thrombus more distally. In such instances, where distal embolic material is noted with persistent symptoms, the administration of additional thrombolytic therapy is suggested. If flow is not restored promptly and loss of significant myocardium seems likely, bypass surgery is indicated.

The role of cardiac surgery in the treatment of acute coronary emboli has become commonplace when they occur during interventional cardiac procedures and threaten large segments of myocardium. When emboli occur during cardiac surgery, embolectomy appears to correct the myocardial ischemia. Embolectomy performed for emboli associated with endocarditis (37) or cardiac catheterization seems to have less influence on the evolution of myocardial infarction. If the embolus is a result of thrombotic material dislodged from more proximal sites, thrombolytic therapy is indicated.

Coronary Artery Dissection

Hemorrhage into the coronary artery wall, with or without an associated intimal tear, forces the intima into the coronary lumen and may produce distal myocardial ischemia or frank infarction. Coronary artery dissections may occur by extension of aortic root dissection (secondary dissection) or may be limited to the coronary artery (primary dissection). Primary coronary artery dissections may occur as the result of diagnostic coronary angiography, coronary angioplasty, cardiac surgery, or chest trauma (see below), or they may occur spontaneously. Angiographically evident localized coronary dissection occurs in at least 30% of patients undergoing coronary angioplasty and may progress to abrupt vessel reclosure in the first hour following the procedure in 2% to 3% of patients (38). These percentages appear to be decreasing with better prediction of patients who require atherectomy as compared to standard balloon angioplasty. In the remaining patients, dissection is not progressive, does not lead to myocardial ischemia, and heals within 2 to 3 months to produce a vessel that appears angiographically patent.

During the past decade, the technologies available for treating coronary artery obstructions caused by atherosclerosis have improved significantly. There have been major modifications of the catheters and the balloon profiles, and the ability to visualize the placement of angioplasty catheters has undergone a major revolution. In addition, new interventional cardiology procedures utilizing lasers, high-frequency rotobladers, and several techniques for atherectomy have been introduced (41). The choices of technologies available to the interventional cardiologist to remove obstructions in coronary arteries have expanded considerably during the past decade. Matching the correct lesion with the best technology available has resulted in these devices being used in place of balloon angioplasty in patient groups where experience has taught that coronary artery dissection might commonly occur. With these approaches, the frequency of dissections resulting in coronary artery occlusion and/or surgical intervention has decreased. Several long-term studies have recently been published to support the use of directional atherectomy as a safe and effective method to remove obstructions in coronary arteries (42,43). In addition, rotational atherectomy has recently been reported in a multicenter trial to be safe and as affective as balloon angioplasty (44). In this study, angiographic evidence of dissection occurred in 10.5% and abrupt occlusion in 3.1% of patients. Restenosis occurred within 6 months in 37.7% of those treated. These figures do not differ from those of balloon angioplasty or directional atherectomy. However, the exact place for these procedures in the treatment of coronary artery disease is still being defined. Whether or not the total number of surgical interventions for coronary artery dissections has decreased is open to question, since the number of procedures on coronary arteries has increased markedly.

As the number of coronary angioplasty procedures increased to a projected level of 125,000 in 1987, the frequency of coronary artery dissections reported also increased (39,40). In the 1990s, coronary angioplasty procedures have increased to approximately 400,000 annually. The frequency of dissections of the coronary arteries has decreased progressively with the introduction of new technologies such as the low-profile balloon, smaller catheters, and techniques for better visualization of the placement of angioplasty catheters (41). In the NHLBI angiographic registry experience, 6.6% of patients required emergency surgery, among which 46% were operated on for coronary dissection (39). These figures have also decreased markedly as new technologies for angioplasty and other approaches in interventional cardiology were developed during the 1990s. Bypass surgery has a three to four times higher mortality in those patients requiring emergency surgery than in those having elective surgery (41,45), while coronary dissection is a major cause of early occlusion of a successfully dilated coronary artery by percutaneous transluminal coronary angioplasty (PTCA). Some cardiologists believe that dissection is necessary to achieve a satisfactory long-term result (46,47). A careful study in postmortem hearts showed angiographic evidence of dissection in 47% of vessels studied (46). Histological evidence for tears was noted for the intima, media, and adventitia involving more than one-fourth the circumference of the vessels (46). These results suggested that intimal and media tears were necessary for success of the procedure. Although tears in all layers of the coronary artery occur frequently during the course of angioplasty, directional atherectomy and rotational atherectomy healing occurs, and endothelial growth over the lesion results. It is not possible to determine whether or not the tears promote healing and whether or not restenosis is more common if there is extensive smooth muscle damage in the media of the treated coronary artery.

Most spontaneous dissections occur in women, particularly in the peripartum period (44,49). Hypertension and coronary atherosclerotic involvement are infrequent, but changes resembling cystic medial necrosis may be present (48–50). The involved vessel is enlarged and ecchymotic and may rupture. The left anterior descending artery is involved in three-fourths of cases, usually within 2 cm of its origin (50).

The diagnosis of coronary artery dissection during life relies on coronary angiography showing extravasation or delayed clearance of contrast, an intimal flap, or the presence of true and false lumina, but dissection may present simply as occlusion of the involved vessel (49,50).

CORONARY ARTERY TRAUMA

Nonpenetrating Blunt Trauma

Chest-wall impact, frequently the result of vehicular trauma, of being thrown against the steering device, may lead to myocardial necrosis by direct myocardial contusion or by occlusive injury to the coronary arteries. This occlusive injury may be the result of coronary artery dissection, thrombosis, or rupture (51,52). Coronary artery fistulas or aneurysms may develop as late sequelae (53,54). The left anterior descending and right coronary arteries are most frequently involved. The electrocardiogram usually shows a pattern of acute myocardial infarction, but this finding does not distinguish between coronary occlusion and myocardial contusion. This distinction can be made by prompt coronary angiography, which should be performed promptly and followed by immediate revascularization (bypass surgery, thrombolytic therapy, or angioplasty performed on an emergency basis). Recovery is the rule, although left ventricular aneurysm formation is common.

Penetrating Trauma

Laceration of a coronary artery, as in a stab wound or small-caliber gunshot wound, may cause acute myocardial ischemia, although the immediate presentation is generally that of acute pericardial tamponade. The left anterior descending and right coronary arteries are most frequently involved. Laceration of small coronary artery branches may be treated with simple ligation without producing significant myocardial ischemia, but ligation of larger vessels often results in a large area of myocardial ischemia (manifested as immediate myocardial discoloration and hypokinesis), necessitating coronary artery bypass grafting (55). Development of a loud continuous murmur days to months after the original injury may signal the development of a coronary artery fistula. Surgical repair of these fistulas is often only transiently successful, with return of the murmur in the postoperative period; thus, surgery should be reserved for patients with evidence of hemodynamic compromise (53).

Trauma During Cardiac Catheterization or Surgery

Catheterization of the left side of the heart, particularly selective cannulation of the coronary arteries, is associated with a 0.1% to 0.2% incidence of myocardial infarction as the result of coronary artery embolization (thrombus, dislodged plaque, air) or coronary artery dissection (56,57). Coronary artery dissection (particularly that which occurs during percutaneous transluminal angioplasty) and embolization have been reported without ischemic sequelae, but when they result in acute myocardial infarction with hypotension or refractory arrhythmia, urgent coronary artery bypass surgery may be life-saving (see Dissection of Coronary Arteries, above). Careful flushing technique and systemic heparinization during coronary angiography have minimized these complications. Laceration of a coronary artery is a potential but rare complication during pericardiocentesis.

CORONARY THROMBOSIS

Coronary thrombosis clearly plays an important role in the evolution of myocardial infarction. When myocardial infarction develops in the setting of coronary atherosclerosis, superimposed coronary thrombosis is nearly always present. In certain disorders involving thrombocytosis or platelet activation, including polycythemia vera, idiopathic thrombocytosis, thrombotic thrombocytopenia purpura, and multiple myeloma (58,59), acute myocardial infarction has occurred in the absence of significant underlying atherosclerosis. Although this circumstantial evidence points toward primary coronary thrombosis as the cause of infarction, the differentiation between in situ thrombosis and thromboembolus may be difficult. Although acute infarction as a complication of these diseases is rare, it should be considered by expert clinicians when the clinical symptoms appear.

PROGRESSIVE NONATHEROSCLEROTIC CORONARY OCCLUSIVE DISEASE

There are a number of conditions that develop as progressive nonatherosclerotic coronary occlusion and that may result from coronary artery vasculitis (60), intimal proliferation or fibrosis, abnormal accumulation of metabolic substances (2), or extrinsic coronary artery compression. If large proximal coronary arteries are involved, angina pectoris or acute myocardial infarction may result, but clinical, angiographic, and even histological differentiation of progressive nonatherosclerotic coronary occlusion from occlusive atherosclerosis may be difficult. When the small coronary vessels (0.1 to 1.0 mm in diameter) are involved, as they may be in diabetes mellitus, collagen vascular disease, cardiac transplantation, neuromuscular diseases (Friedreich's ataxia and progressive muscular dystrophy), rheumatoid arthritis, hypertrophic cardiomyopathy, thrombotic thrombocytopenic purpura, or homocystinuria, the patient may develop arrhythmias, conduction defects, chest pain, or sudden death despite angiographic normality of the large coronary arteries (61). A special syndrome of small-vessel coronary disease has been postulated, and patients with unexplained "ischemia" pain have been so categorized based on endomyocardial biopsy studies. These unexplained ischemic syndromes have been called "syndrome X." Mosseri and colleagues (62) have studied ten autopsied patients with typical pictures of acute myocardial infarction who died within 25 days of the onset of symptoms. The coronary arterial system showed little luminal narrowing, and no thrombotic material was observed in the coronary arteries, despite the fact that the acute myocardial infarction was only 2 days old in five of the patients. A number of theories have been proposed to explain the occurrence of infarction, which has been reported with increasing frequency, in these types of patients. These include coronary artery disease in vessels too small to be visualized angiographically or a severe form of coronary artery spasm. These studies have shown intimal and medial changes in vessels 20 to 50 μm in diameter, but because there are changes from aging in the same vessels, the relationship of pathology to a specific disease entity has been difficult to establish (62). The overall prevalence of

TABLE 4. *Conditions producing coronary vasculitis*[a]

Rheumatic fever
Giant cell arteritis
Polyarteritis nodosa
Tuberculosis
Leprosy
Mucocutaneous lymph node syndrome
Takayasu's disease
Typhus
Infective endocarditis
Rheumatoid arthritis
Syphilis
Wegener's granulomatosis
Salmonella infections
Systemic lupus erythematosus
Ankylosing spondylitis

[a] From Waller (4), reproduced with permission.

small-vessel disease and the frequency with which it leads to clinical sequelae are not known, but cases of this "syndrome X" are being reported with increasing frequency.

Coronary Artery Vasculitis

Major coronary artery vasculitis is a rare event and may occur in conjunction with several medical conditions (Table 4). The coronary artery lesion may lead directly to myocardial ischemia and infarction with or without associated coronary artery thrombosis. A useful classification of arteritis conditions based on the type of coronary artery pathology has recently been proposed by Baroldi (63). Arteritis of the coronary arteries may result from direct extension from adjacent organs or tissue infections involving the heart, such as myocardial abscess from aortic valve endocarditis or pericardial tuberculosis. The coronary artery adventitial layer is involved directly in these cases. On the other hand, coronary arteritis may develop from hematogenous spread through the coronary lumen or through the vasa vasorum. In this case, the intimal layer of the coronary artery is involved in the process. Baroldi (63) proposed the following morphological and histological findings as signs of coronary arteritis. First, focal artery necrosis with or without calcification; second, coronary artery thrombosis or recanalization of thrombus associated with underlying arteriosclerotic plaques; third, rupture of vessel walls that are not associated with trauma or interventional procedures; fourth, coronary artery wall thickening with secondary luminal narrowing; and fifth, wall thickening with aneurysm formation. There may be specific causes for the coronary arteritis, as is discussed below.

Tuberculosis

Tuberculous arteritis is most often noted in patients with pericardial or myocardial lesions (63,64). Tuberculous granulomas may also involve the adventitia, the intima, or the entire wall of the coronary artery. With the emergence of resistant forms of tuberculosis in patients with depressed immune systems, physicians should consider the possibility of this form of arteritis when patients with tuberculosis present with chest pain.

Polyarteritis Nodosa

Polyarteritis nodosa is probably the most common cause of coronary vasculitis. It is a systemic necrotizing vasculitis that affects the media and small arteries and is most prevalent in men aged 30 to 60. Of 66 cases of polyarteritis nodosa reported by Holsinger et al. (65), 41 (62%) had involvement of epicardial coronary arteries, and 41 also had myocardial infarctions of various sizes. The coronary lesions resemble necrotizing vascular lesions found elsewhere in the body with the demonstration of acute cellular-phase destruction of media and internal elastic membranes together with subsequent intimal proliferation and scars in the muscle of the heart. In these patients coronary aneurysm formation or occlusion may lead to myocardial infarction (52,65).

Systemic Lupus Erythematosus

Systemic lupus erythematosus is a chronic multisystem disease that most commonly affects women between the ages of 20 and 40. Pericarditis and myocarditis are common and may lead to chest pain and electrocardiographic abnormalities. In addition, several young patients with lupus erythematosus have developed acute myocardial infarction despite the absence of conventional coronary atherosclerosis risk factors (59,66). Pathological examination in these cases showed intimal fibrosis of the coronary arteries, but to what degree this was the result of coronary arteritis rather than atherosclerosis accelerated by the underlying disease or corticosteroid therapy is unclear. In one reported case, however, progressive coronary occlusion was observed on sequential coronary angiograms performed several days apart and was attributed to coronary vasculitis (65). Coronary vasculitis has also been reported in pathological studies of patients with rheumatoid arthritis and acute rheumatic fever (59).

Bürger's Disease (Thromboangiitis Obliterans)

In Bürger's disease the epicardial coronary arteries have been shown to be involved with focal polymorphonuclear infiltrates, histiocytes, and giant cells with or without coronary thrombosis (67) or with only coronary thrombosis. In 30 cases studied by Sophir (67), only one patient had coronary involvement, whereas in 19 cases studied by others (68), six patients had coronary thrombosis.

Wegener's Granulomatosis

Wegener's granulomatosis is a necrotizing vasculitis that most commonly affects the respiratory tract and kidney. Cardiac involvement is rare, but fibrinoid necrosis of the small and medium-sized coronary arteries has been described (60). One case of large-vessel coronary occlusion with myocardial infarction has been reported (69).

Takayasu's Disease (Pulseless Disease)

Takayasu's disease is predominantly a disease of young Oriental women. Granulomatous panarteritis and fibrosis of the aorta and its large branches lead to stenosis of these vessels, associated with decreased pulse amplitude and vascular bruits. Involvement of the coronary ostia and proximal coronary arteries, which has been described in 16 patients, may lead to angina pectoris or myocardial infarction (60). This disease is seen with greater frequency in areas such as the west coast with large Oriental populations. Successful coronary artery bypass grafting has been performed for this condition.

Kawasaki's Disease (Mucocutaneous Lymph Node Syndrome)

This clinical syndrome, first described by Kawasaki in 1967, appears much more prevalent than first suspected (32,33,34). It is a febrile illness of infants and young children producing sterile conjunctivitis, oral pharyngeal erythema, desquamative reaction of the extremities, and nonpurulent cervical adenopathy. In more than 20% of patients, intense vasculitis of the coronary vasa vasorum leads to inflammation of coronary arteries, coronary artery aneurysm, thrombosis, and severe stenotic scarring. The etiology of the disease has been considered immunologic because of the nature of the vasculitis and the infiltration of mononuclear cells in the area of panvasculitis. Several studies have identified abnormalities in T lymphocytes and in various ratios of $OKT3^+$, $OKT4^+$, and $OKT8^+$ cells in those patients with and without vasculitis (70). These abnormalities may identify those patients likely to develop coronary involvement and to need intense immune suppression. Other studies have suggested that a retrovirus may be the pathogenic agent for Kawasaki's disease (71,72).

Death from Kawasaki's may result from myocardial ischemia or arrhythmias, frequently during the recovery phase. Coronary aneurysm or diffuse stenosis may present as myocardial ischemia in the later course of the disease. Early recognition and intense therapy with aspirin and immunosuppression has been postulated to reduce the sequelae of the active process. Coronary bypass grafting has been performed successfully on these patients, although continued scarring and aneurysm formation may occur (59,73,74). This disease appears to be becoming more prevalent and is of great interest at this time.

Infection

Syphilis is the most common infectious disease affecting the coronary arteries. Up to one-fourth of patients with tertiary cardiovascular syphilis may have ostial stenosis of one or both coronary arteries in addition to involvement of the ascending aorta or aortic valve. The right coronary artery is most frequently affected. Angina and myocardial infarction have resulted from syphilitic coronary disease (75).

Other infections that cause coronary arteritis only rarely include *Salmonella,* tuberculosis, and leprosy (1). Viral infections have caused abnormalities of the coronary intima in experimental animals and have been proposed as a cause of myocardial infarction in young patients (76).

Intimal Proliferation or Fibrosis

Coronary arteries may be narrowed severely by a fibrous hyperplasia that produces myocardial ischemia and infarction. This condition may be associated with fibromuscular hyperplasia of the renal arteries, the use of methysergide, ostial cannulation during cardiac surgery or angioplasty, and following aortic valve replacement (77,78). As many as 50% of patients undergoing cardiac transplantation develop significant epicardial coronary artery narrowing or total occlusion by intimal fibrous proliferation within 3 to 5 years after transplantation. Myocardial infarction and sudden death have resulted from this type of chronic rejection. This process is thought to be related to the cardiac rejection process, which serves as the basis for the fibrous hyperplasia. A similar process has been noted following balloon angioplasty (77,78). Waller and associates (79) recently reported a case of left main coronary fibrous proliferation occurring after balloon angioplasty of a lesion in the left anterior descending coronary artery. They postulated that this process resulted from the angioplasty procedure.

Ionizing Radiation

Therapeutic doses of ionizing radiation delivered to the heart may cause pericarditis or myocardial fibrosis. The level necessary to cause arteritis exceeds 6,000 rads. Animal experimentation suggests that cardiac radiation may also injure capillary walls and enhance the development of lesions resembling atherosclerotic plaque in animals fed lipid-rich diets. In a small number of young patients with no conventional risk factors for coronary atherosclerosis, acute myocardial infarction has been reported at varying intervals following therapeutic cardiac radiation (80). The relation between radiation and coronary atherosclerosis in these patients has not been established (81).

CARDIAC TRANSPLANTATION

A number of patients develop significant coronary fibrosis or atherosclerosis within 3 years of cardiac transplantation. The disease is almost always diffusely distributed in large and small coronary arteries. It is not usually treatable with angioplasty or bypass surgery, and it is not symptomatic with angina because of cardiac denervation, so it must be followed by periodic angiography. The lesions differ from native-vessel atherosclerosis. This is discussed in detail in the chapter by Gordon, this volume. It may be immunologically mediated and probably related to chronic rejection occurring in the intima (82). Myocardial rejection is frequently associated with the graft atherosclerosis as demonstrated by endomyocardial biopsy (83). Better means of immunosuppression with cyclosporine and its analogs have reduced the incidence of atherosclerosis following successful cardiac transplantation. Angina pectoris is absent because of cardiac denervation, but myocardial infarction or sudden death may result. This process usually involves the epicardial coronary arteries and is therefore evident on coronary arteriography. Selective fibrosis of the smaller coronary vessels has also been reported. Intimal damage resulting from immunologic rejection is believed to be the initiating injury causing coronary artery disease following cardiac transplantation (84). In patients who do not experience clinical or biopsy evidence for rejection, there appears to be a smaller prevalence of coronary atherosclerosis. Studies using diet, lipid-lowering drugs, and exercise programs appear to show a longer survival for patients undergoing cardiac transplantation.

ACCUMULATION OF METABOLIC SUBSTANCES

Specific metabolic substances may accumulate in various body tissues as the result of an inborn error of metabolism. Deposition of these substances in the walls of large and small coronary arteries may narrow the vessel lumen and lead to myocardial ischemia. These diseases include the mucopolysaccharidoses [Hunter's and Hurler's diseases (85)], gangliosidoses (Sandhoff's disease and G_{M1}), primary oxalosis, alkaptonuria, and Fabry's disease. Accentuated intimal proliferation of the coronary arteries has been reported in patients with homocystinuria and Friedreich's ataxia (1–5).

In patients with systemic amyloidosis, amyloid may be deposited in the walls of both large and small coronary arteries and may lead to focal myocardial necrosis. The clinical importance of such small areas of necrosis is unclear, but they may contribute to the myocardial dysfunction that results from extensive deposits of myeloid in the myocardium (86).

EXTRINSIC CORONARY ARTERY COMPRESSION

External compression of the coronary artery may cause progressive narrowing of the vessel lumen. This has been reported in patients with aneurysms of the sinus of Valsalva and in patients with epicardial tumor metastases (80). Systolic coronary compression by muscle bridges has been discussed previously.

SUBSTANCE ABUSE: COCAINE

Reports have documented that cocaine abuse may result in myocardial ischemia and infarction in the absence of coronary artery disease. Both coronary artery thrombosis and coronary artery spasm have been reported in patients with cocaine abuse (87–92). A number of physiological studies using coronary artery segments in vivo have also demonstrated the coronary constrictive capacity of cocaine. In some instances there is underlying atherosclerotic plaque disease, but in many others the coronary arteries are totally normal. The syndrome has been associated with cocaine-induced coronary artery spasm or possibly primary thrombogenicity produced by cocaine and its metabolites.

Cocaine may also have progressive and long-term effects on coronary arteries. Simpson and Edwards (93) have reported severely narrowed coronary arteries by fibrointimal proliferation that was caused by focal vessel endothelial injury and platelet adherence and aggregation. Platelets liberate platelet-derived growth factors, which can produce intimal proliferative lesions similar to those seen in restenosis after angioplasty. Thus, it appears that cocaine-induced coronary spasm may produce endothelial disruption and promote platelet aggregation and further vasoconstriction, which can lead to myocardial infarction.

MYOCARDIAL OXYGEN DEMAND–SUPPLY IMBALANCE

An abnormality of myocardial oxygen demand–supply balance is the basis for much of the reported chest pain in all types of atherosclerosis. But in some instances an imbalance may result without obstructive coronary artery disease. The classic example of a failure to deliver adequate oxygen supplies to the myocardium has been noted in carbon monoxide poisoning (94). This condition has been associated with extensive focal infarction in the presence of normal coronary arteries. Prolonged hypotensive shock may also produce extensive nontransmural necrosis, especially of papillary muscles.

The classic example of a situation in which there is increased myocardial wall tension requiring increased coronary oxygen supply, producing an imbalance, is aortic stenosis or hypertrophic obstructive cardiomyopathy. These increased myocardial oxygen demands, frequently associated with increased muscle mass of the heart, result in a limited blood supply and poor perfusion of the myocardium. This may result in decreased myocardial function and a syndrome known as the ''stone heart syndrome'' when it is of prolonged duration. Thyrotoxicosis has also been shown to result occasionally in fibrosis in the myocardium, which is likely the result of an imbalance in myocardial oxygen demands as compared to the supply available (95).

FUTURE DIRECTIONS

Congenital anomalies of the coronary artery origin and course will be diagnosed with increasing frequency as noninvasive and invasive imaging technology improves and is more widely used. Acquired coronary aneurysm, coronary artery dissection, and coronary embolization will be noted with increasing frequency as catheter-based interventional cardiology becomes more commonly employed. Weakening of the medial layer of the wall of the coronary artery by atherectomy and laser technology may also result in a greater prevalence of coronary aneurysm.

As cardiac transplantation becomes more widely performed, a better understanding of the immune injury to the coronary arteries, and ways to modify or prevent it, will be developed. These observations may also increase our understanding of the common variety of atherosclerosis. Coronary arteritis, which develops in the course of many collagen vascular diseases and in association with some metabolic diseases, will likely be recognized with increasing frequency as clinicians appreciate the importance of nonatherosclerotic artery disease in these patients.

Many studies that are now under way to determine the function of the endothelium and how it is involved in regulating vascular tone in coronary arteries will lead to a greater understanding of and treatment for coronary artery spasm and the regulation of coronary blood flow in other forms of coronary artery disease. Endothelial injury to coronary arteries that occurs during interventional cardiologic procedures may hold a key to understanding the process of atherosclerosis as a reaction to injury and thus lead to new avenues for prevention and treatment.

ACKNOWLEDGMENT

This work was supported in part by a gift from the Eugene Fife Family Foundation.

REFERENCES

1. Cheitlin MD, McAllister HA, DeCastro CM. Myocardial infarction without atherosclerosis. *JAMA* 1975;231:951–959.
2. Rozavi M. Unusual forms of coronary artery disease. *Cardiovasc Clin* 1975;7:25.
3. Neufeld HN, Blieden LC. Coronary artery disease in children. *Postgrad Med J* 1978;54:163–170.
4. Waller BF. Nonatherosclerotic coronary heart disease. In: Hurst JW, ed. *The Heart.* New York: McGraw-Hill; 1994:1239–1261.
5. Harrison DC, Baim DS. Nonatherosclerotic coronary heart disease. In: Hurst JW, eds. *The Heart,* 6th ed. New York: McGraw-Hill; 1990: 1130–1139.
6. Alpert JS, Braunwald E. Acute myocardial infarction: Pathological, pathophysiological and clinical manifestations. In: Braunwald E, ed. *Heart Disease. A Textbook of Cardiovascular Medicine.* Philadelphia: WB Saunders; 1984:1262–1300.
7. Waller BF. Atherosclerotic and nonatherosclerotic coronary artery factors in acute myocardial infarction. In: Pepine CF, ed. *Acute Myocardial Infarction.* Philadelphia: FA Davis; 1989:29–104.
8. Engel HJ, Torres C, Page HL Jr. Major variations in anatomical origin of the coronary arteries: Angiographic observations in 4,250 patients without associated congenital heart disease. *Cathet Cardiovasc Diagn* 1975;1:157–161.
9. Levin DC, Fellows KE, Abrams HL. Hemodynamically significant primary anomalies of the coronary arteries: Angiographic aspects. *Circulation* 1978;58:25–34.
10. Roberts WC. Major anomalies of coronary arterial origin seen in adulthood. *Am Heart J* 1986;111:941–963.
11. Kimbiris D, Iskandrian AS, Segal B, Bemis CE. Anomalous aortic origin of coronary arteries. *Circulation* 1978;58:606–615.
12. Liberthson RR, Dinsmore RE, Fallon JT. Aberrant coronary artery origin from the aorta. Report of 18 patients, review of literature and delineation of natural history and management. *Circulation* 1979;59: 748–754.
13. Becker LC. Conditions for vasodilatory-induced coronary steal in experimental myocardial ischemia. *Circulation* 1978;57:1103.
14. Muller JE, Gunther SJ. Nifedipine therapy for Prinzmetal angina. *Circulation* 1978;57:137.
15. Chaitman BR, Lesperance J, Saltiel J. Clinical, angiographic, and hemodynamic findings in patients with anomalous origin of the coronary arteries. *Circulation* 1976;53:122–131.
16. Desmet W, Vanhaecke J, Vrolix M, Van-de-Werf F, Piessens J, Willems J, de-Geest H. Isolated single coronary artery: A review of 50,000 consecutive coronary angiographies. *Eur Heart J* 1992;13:1637–1640.
17. Sharbaugh AH, White RS. Single coronary artery. Analysis of the anatomic variation, clinical importance, and report of five cases. *JAMA* 1974;230:243–246.
18. Joswig BC, Warren SE, Vieweg WV, Hagan AD. Transmural myocardial infarction in the absence of coronary arterial luminal narrowing in a young man with single coronary arterial anomaly. *Cathet Cardiovasc Diagn* 1978;4:297–301.
19. Byrum CJ, Blackman MS, Schneider B, Sondheimer HM, Kavey RE. Congenital atresia of the left coronary ostium and hypoplasia of the left main coronary artery. *Am Heart J* 1980;99:354–358.
20. Lerberg DB, Ogden JA, Zuberbuhler JR, Bahnson HT. Anomalous origin of the right coronary artery from the pulmonary artery. *Ann Thorac Surg* 1979;27:87–94.
21. Wesselhoeft H, Fawcett JS, Johnson AL. Anomalous origin of the left coronary artery from the pulmonary trunk. *Circulation* 1968;38: 403–425.
22. Richardson JV, Doty DB. Correction of anomalous origin of the left coronary artery. *J Thorac Cardiovasc Surg* 1979;77:699–703.
23. Baim DS, Kline H, Silverman JF. Bilateral coronary–pulmonary artery fistulae: Report of five cases and review of the literature. *Circulation* 1982;65:810–815.
24. Liberthson RR, Sagar K, Berkoben JP, Weintraub RM, Levine FH. Congenital coronary arteriovenous fistula: Report of 13 patients. Review of the literature and delineation of the management. *Circulation* 1979;59:849–854.
25. Urrutia-S CO, Falaschi G, Ott DA, Cooley DA. Surgical management of 56 patients with congenital coronary artery fistulas. *Ann Thorac Surg* 1983;35:300–307.
26. Geiringer E. The mural coronary artery. *Am Heart J* 1951;41:359–368.
27. Noble J, Bourassa MG, Petitclerc R, Dyrda I. Myocardial bridging and milking effect of the left anterior descending coronary artery: Normal variant or obstruction. *Am J Cardiol* 1976;37:993–999.
28. Grondin P, Bourassa MG, Noble J, Petitclerc R, Dydra I. Successful course after supra-arterial myotomy for myocardial bridging and milking effect of the left anterior descending artery. *Ann Thorac Surg* 1977; 24:422–429.
29. Iversen S, Hake U, Mayer E, Erbel R, Deifenbach C, Oelert H. Surgical treatment of myocardial bridging causing coronary artery obstruction. *Scand J Thorac Cardiovasc Surg* 1992;26:107–111.
30. Glickel SZ, Maggs PR, Ellis FH Jr. Coronary artery aneurysm. *Ann Thorac Surg* 1978;25:372–376.
31. Befeler B, Aranda JM, Embi A, Mullin FL, El-Sherif N, Lazzara R. Coronary artery aneurysms: Study of the etiology, clinical course and

effect on left ventricular function and prognosis. *Am J Med* 1977;62: 597–607.
32. Daniels SR, Specker B, Capannari TE, Schwartz DC, Burke MJ, Kaplan S. Correlates of coronary artery aneurysm formation in patients with Kawasaki disease. *Am J Dis Child* 1987;141:205–207.
33. Takahashi M, Mason W, Lewis AB. Regression of coronary aneurysms in patients with Kawasaki syndrome. *Circulation* 1987;75:387–394.
34. Kato H, Ichinose E, Kawasaki T. Myocardial infarction in Kawasaki disease: Clinical analyses in 195 cases. *J Pediatr* 1986;108:923–927.
35. Roberts WC. Coronary embolism: A review of causes, consequences, and diagnostic considerations. *Cardiovasc Med* 1978;3:699–703.
36. Prizel KR, Hutchins GM, Bulkley BH. Coronary artery embolism and myocardial infarction. *Ann Intern Med* 1978;88:155–161.
37. Pfeifer JF, Lipton MJ, Oury JH. Acute coronary embolism complicating bacterial endocarditis: Operative treatment. *Am J Cardiol* 1976;37: 920–922.
38. Baim DS. Percutaneous transluminal coronary angioplasty: Analysis of unsuccessful procedures as a guide toward improved results. *Cardiovasc Intervent Radiol* 1982;5:186–193.
39. Cowley MJ, Dorris G, Kelsey SF, Van Raden M, Detre KM. Emergency coronary bypass surgery after coronary angioplasty: The National Heart, Lung and Blood Institute's percutaneous transluminal coronary angioplasty registry experience. *Am J Cardiol* 1984;53:22C–26C.
40. Ischinger T, Gruentzig AR, Meier B, Galan K. Coronary dissection and total coronary occlusion associated with percutaneous transluminal coronary angioplasty: Significance of initial angiographic morphology of coronary stenoses. *Circulation* 1986;74:1371–1378.
41. Bell MR, Garratt KN, Bresnahan JF, Edwards WD, Holmes DR Jr. Relation of deep arterial resection and coronary artery aneurysms after directional coronary atherectomy. *J Am Coll Cardiol* 1992;20: 1474–1481.
42. Topol EJ, Leya F, Piinkerton CA, Whitlow PL, Hofling B, Simonton CA, Masden RR, Serruys PW, Leon MB, Williams DO, King SB, Mark DB, Isner JM, Holmes DR, Ellis SG, Lee KL, Keeler GP, Berdan LG, Hinohara T, Califf RM. A comparison of directional atherectomy with coronary angioplasty in patients with coronary artery disease. *N Engl J Med* 1993;329:221–227.
43. Adelman AG, Cohen M, Kimball BP, Bonan R, Ricci DR, Webb JB, Larame L, Barbeau G, Traboulsi M, Cornett BN, Schwartz L, Logan AG. Canadian Coronary Atherectomy Trial. A randomized comparison of directional coronary atherectomy and percutaneous transluminal coronary angioplasty for lesions of the proximal left anterior descending artery. *N Engl J Med* 1993;329:228–234.
44. Warth DC, Martin BL, O'Neil W, Zacca N, Polissar NL, Buchbinder M. Rotational atherectomy multicenter registry: Acute results, complications and 6-month angiographic follow-up in 709 patients. *J Am Coll Cardiol* 1994;24:641–648.
45. Brahos GJ, Baker NH, Ewy HG, Moore PJ, Thomas JW, Sanfelippo PM, McVicker RF, Fankhauser DJ. Aortocoronary bypass following unsuccessful PTCA: Experience in 100 consecutive patients. *Ann Thorac Surg* 1985;40:7–10.
46. Hoshino T, Yoshida H, Takayama S, Iwase T, Sakata K, Shingu T, Yokoyama S, Mori N, Kaburagi T. Significance of intimal tears in the mechanism of luminal enlargement in percutaneous transluminal coronary angioplasty: Correlation of histolic and angiographic findings in postmortem human hearts. *Am Heart J* 1987;114:503–510.
47. Spring DA. Coronary artery dissection during PTCA: A necessary evil? *Cath Cardiovasc Diagn* 1985;11:1–3.
48. Claudon DG, Claudon DB, Edwards JE. Primary dissecting aneurysm of coronary artery. *Circulation* 1972;45:259–266.
49. Shaver PJ, Carrig TF, Baker WP. Postpartum coronary artery dissection. *Br Heart J* 1978;40:83–86.
50. Smith JC. Dissecting aneurysms of coronary arteries. *Arch Pathol* 1975; 99:117–121.
51. Ciraulo DA, Chesne RB. Coronary arterial dissection: An unrecognized cause of myocardial infarction, with subsequent coronary arterial patency. *Chest* 1978;73:677–679.
52. Allen RP, Liedtke AJ. The role of coronary artery injury and perfusion in the development of cardiac contusion secondary to nonpenetrating chest trauma. *J Trauma* 1979;19:153–156.
53. Cheitlin MD. Cardiovascular trauma (parts I and II). *Circulation* 1982; 65:1529–1532; 66:244–247.
54. Austin SM, Applefeld MM, Turney SZ, Mech KF Jr. Traumatic left anterior descending coronary artery to right ventricle fistula: Report of two cases. *South Med J* 1977;70:581–584.
55. Espada R, Whisennand HH, Mattox KL, Beall AC Jr. Surgical management of penetrating injuries to the coronary arteries. *Surgery* 1975;78: 755–760.
56. Sethi GK, Scott SM, Takaro T. Iatrogenic coronary artery stenosis following aortic valve replacement. *J Thorac Cardiovasc Surg* 1979; 77:760–767.
57. Kennedy JW. Complications associated with cardiac catheterization and angiography. *Cathet Cardiovasc Diagn* 1982;8:5–11.
58. Virmani R, Popovsky MA, Roberts WC. Thrombocytosis, coronary thrombosis and acute myocardial infarction. *Am J Med* 1979;67: 498–506.
59. Ridolfi RL, Hutchins GM, Bell WR. The heart and cardiac conduction system in thrombotic thrombocytopenia purpura. A clinicopathologic study of 17 autopsied patients. *Ann Intern Med* 1979;91:357–363.
60. Parillo JE, Fauci AS. Necrotizing vasculitis, coronary angiitis and the cardiologist. *Am Heart J* 1980;99:547–554.
61. James TN. Small arteries of the heart. *Circulation* 1977;56:2–14.
62. Mosseri M, Yarom R, Gotsman MS, Hasin Y. Histologic evidence for small-vessel coronary artery disease in patients with angina pectoris and patent large coronary arteries. *Circulation* 1986;74:964–972.
63. Baroldi G. Diseases of the coronary arteries. In: Silver MD, ed. *Cardiovascular Pathology*. New York: Churchill Livingstone; 1983:341.
64. Gouley BA, Bellet S, McMillan TM. Tuberculosis of the myocardium: Report of six cases, with observations on involvement of coronary arteries. *Arch Intern Med* 1933;51:244–263.
65. Holsinger DR, Osmundson PJ, Edwards JE. The heart in periarteritis nodosa. *Circulation* 1962;25:610–618.
66. Meller J, Conde CA, Deppisch LM. Myocardial infarction due to coronary atherosclerosis in three young adults with systemic lupus erythematosus. *Am J Cardiol* 1975;35:309–314.
67. Sophir O. Thromboangiitis obliterans of the coronary arteries and its relation to atherosclerosis. *Am Heart J* 1936;12:521–535.
68. Averbuck SH, Silbert S. Thromboangiitis obliterans: Cause of death. *Arch Intern Med* 1934;54:436–465.
69. Gatenby PA, Lytton DG, Bulteau VG, et al. Myocardial infarction in Wegener's granulomatosis. *Aust NZ J Med* 1976;6:336–340.
70. Terai M, Kohno Y, Niwa K, Toba T, Sakurai N, Nakajima H. Imbalance among T-cell subsets in patients with coronary arterial aneurysms in Kawasaki disease. *Am J Cardiol* 1987;60:555–559.
71. Shulman ST, Rowley AH. Does Kawasaki disease have a retroviral aetiology? *Lancet* 1986;2:545–546.
72. Burns JC, Geha RS, Schneeberger EE, Newburger JW, Rosen FS, Glezen LS, Huang AS, Natale J, Leung DYM. Polymerase activity in lymphocyte culture supernatants from patients with Kawasaki disease. *Nature* 1986;323:814–816.
73. Onouchi Z, Shinichiro S, Kiyosawa N, Takamtsu T, Hamaoka K. Aneurysms in the coronary arteries in Kawasaki disease—an angiographic study of 30 cases. *Circulation* 1982;66:6–13.
74. Fukushige J, Nihill MR, McNamara DG. Spectrum of cardiovascular lesions in mucocutaneous lymph node syndrome. *Am J Cardiol* 1980; 45:98–107.
75. Holt S. Syphilitic ostial occlusion. *Br Heart J* 1977;39:469–470.
76. Burch GE, Shewey LL. Viral coronary arteritis and myocardial infarction. *Am Heart J* 1976;92:11–14.
77. Brill IC, Brodeur MTH, Oyama AA. Myocardial infarction in two sisters less than 20 years old. *JAMA* 1971;217:1345–1348.
78. Trimble AS, Bigelow WG, Wigle ED. Coronary ostial stenosis: A late complication of coronary perfusion in open-heart surgery. *J Thorac Cardiovasc Surg* 1969;57:792–795.
79. Waller BF, Pinkerton CA, Foster LN. Morphologic evidence of accelerated left main coronary artery stenosis: A late complication of percutaneous transluminal angioplasty of the proximal left anterior descending coronary artery. *J Am Coll Cardiol* 1987;9:1019–1023.
80. Kopelson G, Herwig KJ. The etiologies of coronary artery disease in cancer patients. *Int J Radiat Oncol Biol Phys* 1978;4:895–906.
81. Fajardo LF. Radiation-induced coronary artery disease (editorial). *Chest* 1977;71:563–564.
82. Frist WH, Oyer PE, Baldwin JC, Stinson EB, Shumway NE. HLA antigen compatibility and cardiac transplant recipient survival. *Ann Thorac Surg* 1987;44:242–246.
83. Narrod J, Kormos R, Armitage J, Hardesty R, Ladowski J, Griffith B.

Acute rejection and plantation (abstract). *J Heart Transplant* 1988;7: 71.
84. Mason JW, Strefling A. Small vessel disease of the heart resulting in myocardial necrosis and death despite angiographically normal coronary arteries. *Am J Cardiol* 1979;44:171–176.
85. Brosius FC, Roberts WC. Coronary artery disease in the Hurler syndrome. *Am J Cardiol* 1981;47:649–653.
86. Smith RR, Hutchins GM. Ischemic heart disease secondary to amyloidosis of intramyocardial arteries. *Am J Cardiol* 1979;44:413–417.
87. Isner JM, Estes NAM III, Thompson PD, Costanzo-Nordin MR, Subramanian R, Miller G. Acute cardiac events temporally related to cocaine abuse. *N Engl J Med* 1986;315:1438–1443.
88. Simpson RW, Edwards WD. Pathogenesis of cocaine-induced ischemic heart disease. *Arch Pathol Lab Med* 1986;110:479–484.
89. Zimmerman FH, Gustafson GM, Kemp HG. Recurrent myocardial infarction associated with cocaine abuse in a young man with normal coronary arteries: Evidence for coronary artery spasm culminating in thrombosis. *J Am Coll Cardiol* 1987;9:964–978.
90. Smith HWB, Liberman HA, Brody SL, Battey LL, Donohue BC, Morris DC. Acute myocardial infarction temporarily related to cocaine use. Clinical, angiographic and pathophysiologic observations. *Ann Intern Med* 1987;107:13–18.
91. Patel R, Haider B, Ahmed S, Regan TJ. Cocaine-related myocardial infarction: High prevalence of occlusive coronary thrombi without significant obstructive atherosclerosis (abstract). *Circulation* 1988; 78(suppl II):II-436.
92. Lange RA, Cigarroa RG, Yancy CW, et al. Cocaine-induced coronary artery vasoconstriction. *N Engl J Med* 1989;321:1557–1562.
93. Simpson RW, Edwards WD. Pathogenesis of cocaine-induced ischemic heart disease. Autopsy finding in a 21-year-old man. *Arch Pathol Lab Med* 1986;110:479–484.
94. Cheitlin MD, McAllister HA, deCastro CM. Myocardial infarction without atherosclerosis. *JAMA* 1975;231:951–959.
95. Gross II, Stenberg WH. Myocardial infarction without significant lesions of coronary arteries. *Arch Intern Med* 1939;64:249–267.

Atherosclerosis and Coronary Artery Disease,
edited by V. Fuster, R. Ross, and E. J. Topol.
Lippincott-Raven Publishers, Philadelphia © 1996.

The Microcirculation in Atherosclerotic Coronary Artery Disease

Richard O. Cannon III

Key Words: Angiogenesis; Collaterals; Coronary microcirculation; Endothelium; Hypercholesterolemia; Hypertension; Myocardial ischemia; Nitric oxide.

INTRODUCTION

Although the focus of clinical and experimental attention in myocardial ischemic syndromes has been on the role of atherosclerosis in epicardial coronary arteries, there is increasing evidence that disease or dysfunction of the coronary microcirculation may cause or contribute to myocardial ischemia. Conditions commonly associated with epicardial coronary atherosclerosis may adversely affect the coronary microcirculation. Limited pharmacological flow reserve has been demonstrated in animal models of hypertension and in hypertensive patients, especially those with left ventricular hypertrophy. Small intramural arteries from hypertensive animals and patients have shown morphological changes, including media hypertrophy and smooth muscle hypoplasia with luminal narrowing. Small arteries from hypercholesterolemic animals have shown evidence of microvascular endothelial dysfunction in the absence of overt atherosclerosis of the microcirculation. Studies performed in humans with early atherosclerosis of epicardial arteries but without obstructive lesions have shown evidence of coronary microvascular endothelial dysfunction. Coronary microvascular endothelial dysfunction is also present in humans with hypertension with or without associated left ventricular hypertrophy. Recent studies indicate that coronary microvascular dysfunction may be reversible with pharmacological interventions. Collateral growth may be stimulated with angiogenic factors in patients with coronary artery disease, which may represent a novel therapeutic approach to relieving ischemia and preventing myocardial infarction in patients with advanced disease.

The association of angina pectoris and evidence for myocardial ischemia with atherosclerotic disease of the epicardial coronary arteries is supported by a wealth of clinical experience and clinicopathological observations. Further, in dogs, the coronary flow response to drugs that maximally

R. O. Cannon III: Clinical Service and Cardiovascular Diagnosis Section, Cardiology Branch, NHLBI, National Institutes of Health, Bethesda, Maryland 20892.

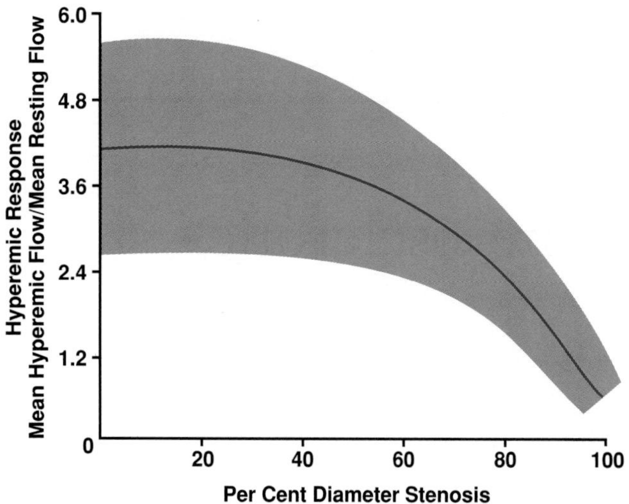

FIG. 1. Relationship of percentage diameter narrowing of a single stenosis of the circumflex artery to hyperemic responses after intracoronary injection of contrast medium in ten consecutive dogs. Hyperemic responses are expressed as the ratio of hyperemic mean flow after injection of contrast medium to resting basal mean flow before each injection. The *shaded area* indicates the limits of the relations plotted for individual dogs. (From Gould and Lipscomb, ref. 1, with permission.)

dilate the microcirculation is compromised only with epicardial coronary artery stenoses greater than 50% luminal diameter narrowing, and resting flow is compromised only with stenoses greater than 90% luminal diameter narrowing (Fig. 1) (1). Indeed, until recently, the coronary microcirculation has generally been considered to have only an indirect role in the induction of myocardial ischemia by exhaustion of vasodilator capacity in the presence of stenotic atherosclerotic epicardial coronary arteries. However, animal and clinical studies in recent years suggest that coronary arteries too small to be imaged angiographically, diseased or dysfunctional as a consequence of the same conditions associated with atherosclerosis of the epicardial arteries, may contribute to or cause myocardial ischemia.

In this chapter, the coronary microcirculation is defined as vessels too small to be imaged angiographically: intermediate-sized intramural arteries 100 to 300 μm diameter, arterioles and collateral arteries 20 to 100 μm diameter, and capillaries and venules <20 μm in diameter. This chapter initially presents animal investigations of the coronary microcirculation, followed by animal studies of the effects of hypertension and hypercholesterolemia on the coronary microcirculation. Human studies of coronary microvascular flow dynamics are discussed, with an emphasis on potential mechanisms for myocardial ischemia independent of significant obstructive disease of the epicardial arteries by atherosclerosis. Finally, new research suggesting novel strategies for improving microvascular function and stimulating collateral growth will be presented.

STUDIES OF THE CORONARY MICROCIRCULATION IN ANIMALS

Until recently, only the smallest component of the coronary microcirculation, arterioles approximately 20 to 30 μm diameter, were believed to ordinarily impose any significant resistance to coronary flow. In response to surrounding myocardial metabolic conditions, arterioles could dilate or constrict in order to match flow appropriate to myocardial oxygen demands. However, Chilian et al. (2,3), using an epicardial imaging system and micropuncture measurements of pressure in small subepicardial arteries of the beating cat heart, showed that 40% to 50% of the total coronary resistance is imposed by small arteries between 100 and 300 μm in diameter (Fig. 2). In contrast, the arterioles accounted for only about 10% of the total basal coronary vascular resistance. This group also showed that coronary microvessels within the subepicardium may not respond uniformly to stimuli or agonists that affect coronary flow. For example, in response to reduction of coronary perfusion pressure, only arteries less than 100 μm in diameter dilated (larger vessels actually constricted) (4), whereas in response to the myocardial oxygen demands of pacing, all levels of microvessels dilated (5). The level of microvascular response to many neural, humoral, and pharmacological agents has been determined by this group (6) and is summarized in Table 1. The heterogeneity of microvascular responses may result from variability in the distribution of receptors, myogenic tone, and innervation as well as other considerations (6). For technical reasons, these studies have been limited to the subepicardial microcirculation; the microvasculature at deeper levels within the myocardium may differ both in the relative contribution of small intramural arteries to resistance to coronary flow and in the vasomotor responses to neurohumoral stimuli.

The discovery of endothelium-derived relaxing factors (7), nitric oxide in particular (8), has resulted in numerous studies of the role of nitric oxide in the coronary microcirculation. Inhibition of nitric oxide synthesis with N^G-monomethyl-L-arginine (L-NMMA) increases basal coronary vascular resistance and blunts the vasodilator response to the endothelium-dependent agonists acetylcholine and bradykinin in isolated perfused hearts (9,10). These responses to nitric oxide inhibition are reversible by addition of L-arginine, the substrate for nitric oxide synthesis within the endothelium by the enzyme nitric oxide synthase (9,10). L-NMMA administered systemically to the awake dog at doses that increase systemic blood pressure by blocking nitric oxide production in the systemic circulation also increases basal coronary vascular resistance (11). L-NMMA inhibits vasodilation of subepicardial arteries greater than 120 μm in diameter by the endothelium-dependent vasodilator acetylcholine, with partial inhibition of this response by L-NMMA in arteries less than 120 μm in diameter (12). In the anesthetized dog, nitric oxide inhibition with N-nitro-L-arginine attenuates acetylcholine-induced increases in coro-

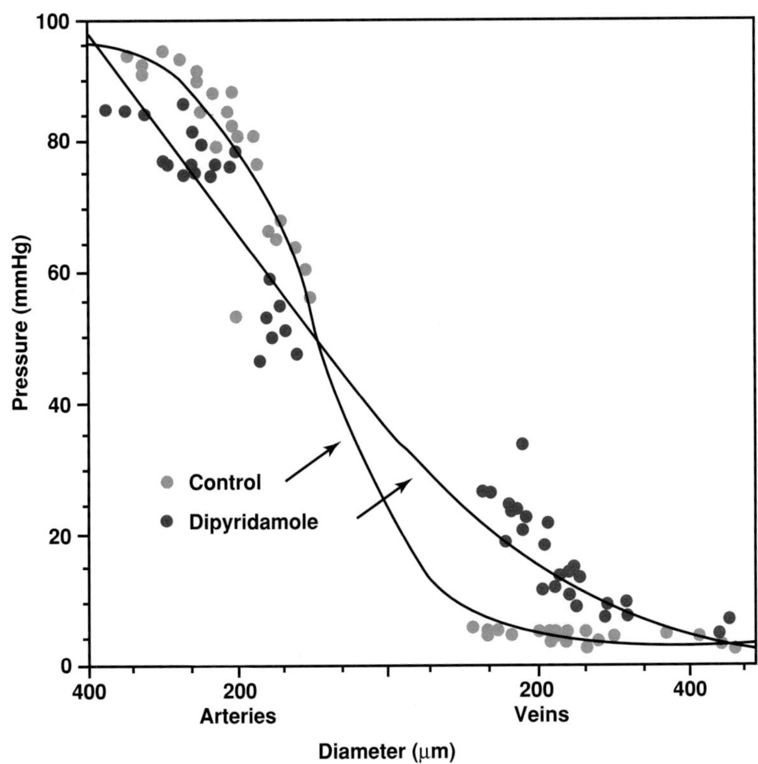

FIG. 2. Distribution of microvascular pressure as a percentage of aortic pressure in different-sized coronary arteries and venules in the normal left ventricle in pentobarbital-anesthetized cats during control conditions (●) and intravenous administration of dipyridamole (0.4 mg·kg^{-1}·min^{-1}) (○). During infusion of dipyridamole, there is a redistribution of microvascular resistance such that larger arteries and veins account for a greater portion of resistance. (From Chilian et al., ref. 3, with permission.)

nary flow (13,14). Thus, animal studies indicate that coronary vascular resistance is decreased or increased by agonists that augment or inhibit nitric oxide production, respectively. Because the majority of coronary resistance is mediated by intramyocardial small arteries and arterioles, it seems likely that microvascular endothelial release of relaxant factors such as nitric oxide is important in regulating basal and agonist-stimulated coronary flood flow. However, in all these studies, the contribution of epicardial coronary artery vasomotor responses to changes in coronary vascular resistance was not assessed.

TABLE 1. *Distribution of coronary microvascular responses to neural, humoral, and pharmacological stimuli*[a]

	Coronary microvascular diameter	
	<100 μm	>100 μm
α-adrenergic stimulation (with β-blockade)	Dilate	Constrict
Vagal stimulation	Dilate	Dilate
thromboxane mimetic	Constrict	Constrict
Endothelium-dependent vasodilators		
Acetylcholine	Dilate	Dilate
Serotonin	Dilate	Constrict
Vasopressin	Constrict	±Dilate
Endothelium-independent vasodilators		
Nitroglycerin	No effect	Dilate
S-Nitrosocysteine	Dilate	Dilate
Nifedipine	Dilate	Dilate

[a] Data from Marcus et al. (6).

Hypertension and the Coronary Microcirculation

Several studies in animal models of hypertension have shown the coronary flow reserve of hypertrophied hearts in response to a potent arteriolar dilator such as adenosine to be reduced compared with nonhypertrophied hearts (15–17). Limited coronary flow reserve may be a consequence of elevated absolute flow requirements secondary to increased oxygen demands of pressure-induced hypertrophy, with partial exhaustion of arteriolar dilator capacity (especially in the endocardium, where wall stress is highest). However, the limited flow reserve could also result from limitation in either absolute or relative (to the mass of the myocardium) maximum vasodilator capacity. Indeed, several studies suggest that impairment in peak flow capacity may be particularly important in hypertensive left ventricular hypertrophy. Morphometric and microsphere studies have demonstrated absent or insufficient neovascularization in response to pressure load (18–20). This could lead to insufficient oxygen delivery during stress as a consequence of a relative paucity of microvessels and capillaries, with attendant increases in diffusion distances (21).

Abnormalities in vascular and perivascular morphology accompanying left ventricular hypertrophy have also been described, including interstitial fibrosis, vascular media hypertrophy, and smooth muscle hyperplasia (22–25). Consequences of these morphological alterations might include compromise of the vascular lumen, limitations in vasodilator capacity, and heightened sensitivity of microvascular smooth muscle to neurohumoral constrictor stimuli. Experimental imposition of left ventricular pressure overload in older animals produces more coronary microvascular changes associated with hypertrophy in contrast to left ventricular pressure overload with hypertrophy in younger animals (26). Dogs with long-standing hypertension-induced left ventricular hypertrophy have been shown to have abnormal transmural distribution of coronary flow, with relative subendocardial underperfusion (27). Impaired autoregulation, particularly at lower systemic pressures, has been demonstrated in experimental left ventricular hypertrophy (28). All of these deleterious effects of hypertension on coronary flow reserve and flow distribution may explain the observation that coronary occlusion in dogs with experimental hypertensive left ventricular hypertrophy results in larger infarcts for a given risk area and higher mortality than coronary occlusion in dogs without left ventricular hypertrophy (29).

Regression of Left Ventricular Hypertrophy and Coronary Flow Dynamics

Therapeutic studies in animal models of hypertensive left ventricular hypertrophy provide evidence that many of the abnormalities resulting in impaired myocardial perfusion are reversible. Antihypertensive therapy resulting in regression of left ventricular hypertrophy can increase coronary flow reserve in animals (22,24,30–33). Further, myocardial collagen content is reduced along with left ventricular hypertrophy regression in treated animals, an effect that could improve myocardial perfusion by improving diastolic effects on intramyocardial coronary flow (24,34,35). Nonpharmacological reversal of pressure overload has been found to regress left ventricular hypertrophy and improve coronary flow dynamics in rats following 4 weeks of aortic banding, along with improved autoregulatory control of myocardial blood flow (36,37) with less improvement in coronary flow dynamics in animals with 10 weeks of banding (38). Thus, at least in animal models, the beneficial impact of regression of hypertrophy on the coronary flow dynamics may in part depend on the duration of pressure-induced hypertrophy.

Atherosclerosis and the Coronary Microcirculation

Vascular strips or rings from large arteries of animals fed high-cholesterol diets exhibit impaired responses to endothelium-dependent vasodilators such as acetylcholine, with endothelium-independent vasodilator responses to drugs such as nitroglycerin unaffected by atherosclerosis (39–41). The precise mechanism underlying this defective endothelial function in hypercholesterolemia and atherosclerosis is unknown, but recent investigations indicate that endothelial dysfunction may be selective for certain signal transduction pathways that link receptor activation on the endothelial cell surface to activation of nitric oxide synthase (42,43). For example, despite impaired vasodilator responses of vascular rings from hypercholesterolemic pigs to acetylcholine, an endothelium-dependent vasodilator that likely activates nitric oxide production via a pertussis-toxin-sensitive G_i-protein-dependent signal transduction pathway, the responses to other endothelium-dependent vasodilators such as bradykinin, which utilizes a different signal transduction pathway that is unaffected by pertussin toxin, are unimpaired, at least in animals with early atherosclerosis (43). Oxidatively modified low-density lipoproteins, especially lysolecithin in the oxidized particle, may be responsible for inhibition of nitric oxide production (44,45). Nitric oxide may also be degraded to biologically inactive nitrogen oxide compounds by the action of superoxide anions, which appear to be increased in activity in hypercholesterolemia (46). Thus, nitric oxide bioavailability may be reduced in atherosclerotic animal models by a combination of reduced production (which may be selective for some signal transduction pathways; there may be augmented production of nitric oxide by other pathways (46) and accelerated degradation of nitric oxide, resulting in impaired endothelium-dependent vascular relaxation and vasodilation. The acute or chronic administration of L-arginine, the substrate for nitric oxide synthesis, improves endothelium-dependent relaxation of large arteries from animals fed atherogenic diets but not arteries from untreated animals [47–49]). These experiments suggest that hypercholesterolemia may be associated with a relative deficiency in the substrate for nitric oxide production, possibly because of enhanced nitric oxide synthase activity.

Animal models of atherosclerosis have also revealed endothelial dysfunction of the small arteries of the heart. Small subepicardial arteries approximately 300 μm in diameter from cholesterol-fed rabbits contracted in vitro in response to doses of acetylcholine that produced relaxation in similar-sized small arteries from control animals, despite equal degrees of relaxation to a nitric oxide donor in the two groups of animals (50). Microscopic examination of the vascular segments used in the study showed the endothelium of the small arteries from hypercholesterolemic rabbits to be structurally intact and free of atherosclerosis, although small lipid deposits were seen within endothelial cells. The media of the arteries appeared unaltered by hypercholesterolemia. This observation of impaired endothelium-dependent function in small coronary arteries is consistent with earlier work showing impaired dilator responses of arterioles from cremasteric muscle of atherosclerotic rabbits to acetylcholine compared to control animals, with responses to the endothelium-independent vasodilator nitroprusside unaffected (51). Microscopic examination of the cremasteric arterioles showed no differences between cholesterol-fed and control animals. Small epicardial coronary arteries (122 to 222 μm in diameter) dissected from the hearts of cynomolgus monkeys fed an atherogenic diet were found to contract in response to acetylcholine, with impaired dilator responses to other endo-

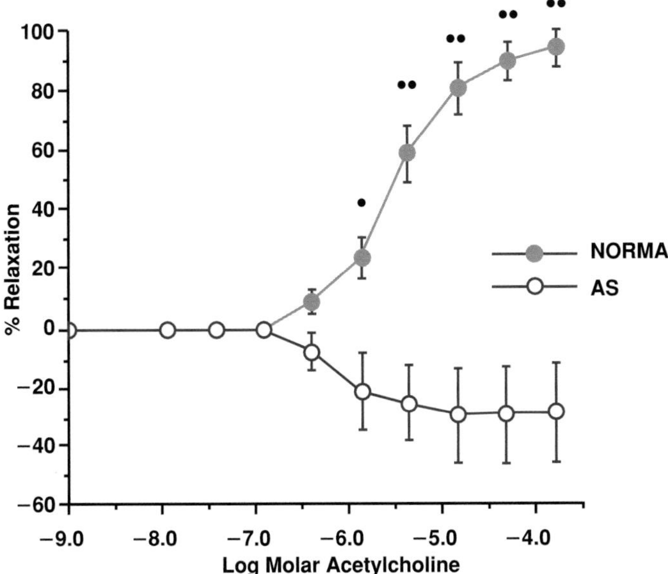

FIG. 3. Plot of responses of coronary microvessels (122–220 μm) from normal (n = 6) and atherosclerotic monkeys (n = 6) to acetylcholine. Vessels were preconstricted to 30–70% of the baseline diameter with U46619. Acetylcholine was administered extraluminally. Values less than zero indicate constriction. $^{*}p < 0.01$, $^{**}p < 0.001$. (From Selke et al., ref. 52, with permission.)

thelium-dependent vasodilator agonists such as bradykinin and calcium ionophore (which stimulates nitric oxide production within the endothelium without activation of cell surface receptors), compared to similar-sized small arteries from control animals, which dilated to all endothelium-dependent agonists (Fig. 3) (52). These responses were not affected by indomethacin, which blocks the synthesis of vasodilating prostaglandins. The responses of the small arteries to the endothelium-independent vasodilators adenosine and nitroprusside were no different between cholesterol-fed and control monkeys in this study. Histological examination of the vascular segments showed no atherosclerosis involving the small arteries of the cholesterol-fed animals despite extensive atherosclerosis of the large arteries, although intracellular vacuoles were noted in the endothelium of small arteries from cholesterol-fed animals.

Recently, even smaller coronary arteries (30 to 70 μm diameter) have been isolated from cholesterol-fed pigs and studied in vitro (53). Compared to similar-sized microvessels from control animals, these vascular segments exhibited impaired responses to the endothelium-dependent vasodilators histamine, serotonin, and ADP and to increases in flow (shear stress), also an endothelium-dependent vasodilator stimulus. These abnormal responses were normalized by exposure of the vascular segments to L-arginine, the precursor for nitric oxide synthesis. Consistent with other studies, the microvascular endothelium from the cholesterol-fed animals often contained large lipid-laden vacuoles.

Thus, animal studies have consistently shown that the coronary microcirculation of animals fed an atherogenic diet exhibits impaired endothelium-dependent vasodilation in the absence of overt atherosclerosis despite the presence of atherosclerosis in the large arteries of these animals. Consistent with vasomotor responses in large arteries from animals fed atherogenic diets, the response of small arteries and arterioles to endothelium-independent vasodilators is unimpaired, indicating normal smooth muscle responsiveness. Similar to the effect on large arteries, L-arginine, the precursor to nitric oxide synthesis, can normalize the impaired endothelium-dependent responses of small arteries from hearts of animals fed atherogenic diets, indicating that microvascular endothelial dysfunction may be reversible.

Summary

Animal studies have shown that conditions commonly associated with atherosclerosis in humans can affect the coronary microcirculation, either by means of left ventricular hypertrophy and morphological and functional alterations of small intramural arteries by hypertension or by virtue of the deleterious impact of hypercholesterolemia on endothelium-dependent vasodilator function. Accordingly, it is possible that hypertension and hypercholesterolemia might have deleterious effects on coronary microvascular structure and function in humans prior to the development of significant atherosclerotic disease of the epicardial coronary arteries or may coexist with significant atherosclerotic disease of the epicardial coronary arteries and contribute to limitation in appropriate coronary flow responses and myocardial ischemia during stress.

CORONARY VASCULAR STUDIES IN HUMANS

Methodological Considerations

Unlike many of the animal studies described above, in which small arteries were directly visualized in beating hearts or studied in vitro, the coronary microcirculation in humans can be assessed only indirectly. Changes in coronary flow in response to an agonist in the absence of obstructive epicardial coronary artery disease or significant changes in epicardial coronary artery luminal diameter are generally interpreted to reflect vasomotor changes of the coronary microcirculation. These assumptions immediately raise several concerns. For example, what quantity of atherosclerotic disease or changes in luminal diameter in the epicardial coronary arteries can be considered "insignificant" and thus not limit coronary flow during stress? The important studies of Gould showed that focal stenoses of greater than 50% luminal diameter narrowing are required to affect pharmacologically stimulated coronary flow adversely (Fig. 1) (1). In humans, however, atherosclerosis may be diffuse, and lesions may be multiple and in series, thus making the detection of "significance" by a simple percentage stenosis at a given lesion site problematic. Indeed, a "50% stenosis" in humans may or may not adversely affect coronary flow responses to coronary microvascular vasodilators such as papaverine, suggesting that visual assessment of lesions "intermediate" in severity is often inaccurate (54). With regard to changes in luminal diameter of epicardial arteries, the resistance to coronary flow is inversely related to the diameter of the epicardial artery to the fourth power and directly related to the length of the arterial segment analyzed. For a normal epicardial artery, small changes in the diameter will have little impact on coronary resistance (ignoring compensatory changes in microvascular tone) (55). However, diffuse narrowing of an epicardial vessel in response to an agonist may result in some resistance to coronary flow, especially if superimposed on "insignificant" coronary artery disease. Accordingly, the contribution of the epicardial coronary arteries to coronary resistance can be confidently excluded only in the absence of coronary artery disease (other than minimal plaquing) and in the absence of constriction of epicardial arteries in response to an agonist.

With regard to measurement of coronary flow, necessary for assessment of microvascular function, all methodologies available for humans are less accurate and precise than those modalities used in animals. For example, thermodilution measurements of coronary venous outflow can be affected by right atrial reflux and catheter movement and may underestimate the magnitude of high flows after pharmacological stimulation. Inert gas saturation or washout techniques require multiple blood samples over a period of time, which makes accurate measurement of peak flows difficult after pharmacological vasodilators that have a variable time of onset, duration of maximum affect, and relative potency in humans. In recent years intracoronary Doppler measurements of flow velocity have been utilized, a technique thoroughly validated in animals and experimental flow models (56,57). A Doppler catheter (56) or the newer Doppler guidewire (57) can be positioned in a coronary artery of interest and measure phasic flow velocity patterns in humans during cardiac catheterization. Instantaneous changes in flow velocity can be recorded following administration of a vasoactive agonist such as acetylcholine or adenosine. Flow velocity measurements require simultaneous quantitative angiography in order to derive volume flow. Quantitative angiography, even if it utilizes computerized edge detection techniques, necessitates geometric assumptions about the artery, which may not be valid in patients with coronary artery disease.

Positron emission tomography (PET) provides measurement of regional myocardial perfusion using flow tracers such as ^{115}O-labeled water and ^{13}N-labeled ammonia and can be used to assess coronary flow reserve in response to vasodilators such as dipyridamole and adenosine (58,59). However, in addition to limited availability, PET cannot be used to assess endothelium-dependent agonists such as acetylcholine that require administration into a coronary artery. Further, interpretation of a limited flow response to a vasodilator or stress as being caused by microvascular dysfunction requires knowledge of the absence of obstructive atherosclerotic disease or vasoconstriction of the epicardial coronary arteries.

Additional methodological concerns regarding studies of coronary flow dynamics in humans include the fact that patients undergoing cardiac catheterization are commonly on therapy prior to study, with potential residual effects on coronary flow responses despite cessation of drugs for several pharmacological half-lives before performance of the study (for example, up-regulation of β receptors following discontinuation of β-blocker therapy). Also, assessment of coronary microvascular morphology in living humans is limited to endocardial biopsies, which sample only the smallest intramyocardial vessels. Finally, no true "normal controls" can be studied in the catheterization laboratory; all patients have chest pain syndromes justifying an invasive study.

Hypertension and Coronary Flow in Humans

Several studies suggest that although resting coronary flow per unit mass may be normal in hypertensive patients with left ventricular hypertrophy and normal systolic function, coronary flow reserve may be markedly limited. Strauer (60) performed studies of coronary flow (inert gas method) in 114 patients with hypertension and normal coronary angiograms and found significant reduction in coronary flow reserve in response to dipyridamole 0.5 mg/kg compared to normotensive controls. Opherk et al. (61) reported that 16 hypertensive patients with chest pain, normal coronary angiograms, and ECG evidence of left ventricular hypertrophy had a significantly higher minimum coronary resistance (i.e., less vasodilation of the coronary microcirculation) following dipyridamole, 0.5 mg/kg (flow measured by inert gas method), compared to normotensive controls. Left ventricular biopsies performed in seven patients showed myocyte hypertrophy but no vascular abnormalities or interstitial fibrosis. Vogt et al. (62) measured coronary flow reserve (inert gas method) following dipyridamole, 0.5 mg/kg, in 54 hypertensive patients with chest pain and normal coronary angiograms. These patients were found to have resting coronary flow and myocardial oxygen consumption per unit mass similar to 12 normotensive controls. However, there was a significant reduction in the flow response to dipyridamole, with elevation of minimum coronary resistance compared to normotensive controls. The authors found no significant correlation between minimum coronary resistance or coronary flow reserve responses to dipyridamole and left ventricular mass or diastolic wall stress, concluding that coronary microvascular structural abnormalities might have contributed to impaired coronary flow reserve independent of left ventricular hypertrophy.

Houghton et al. (63) performed intracoronary Doppler flow velocity measurements in 40 hypertensive patients with chest pain and no or ''minor'' coronary artery disease, some of whom had thallium scintigraphic abnormalities following exercise stress. Flow reserve was assessed following dipyridamole (average dose 0.59 mg/kg). The authors found that patients with thallium perfusion abnormalities were more likely to have a limited flow velocity response to dipyridamole than those with normal thallium perfusion scans (Fig. 4) and that patients with thallium defects were more likely to have a greater degree of left ventricular hypertrophy than those with normal thallium scans. However, the decrement in flow reserve in response to dipyridamole was not linearly related to the magnitude of left ventricular hypertrophy, suggesting that structural changes in intramyocardial small arteries might have contributed to the limitation in dipyridamole-stimulated flow.

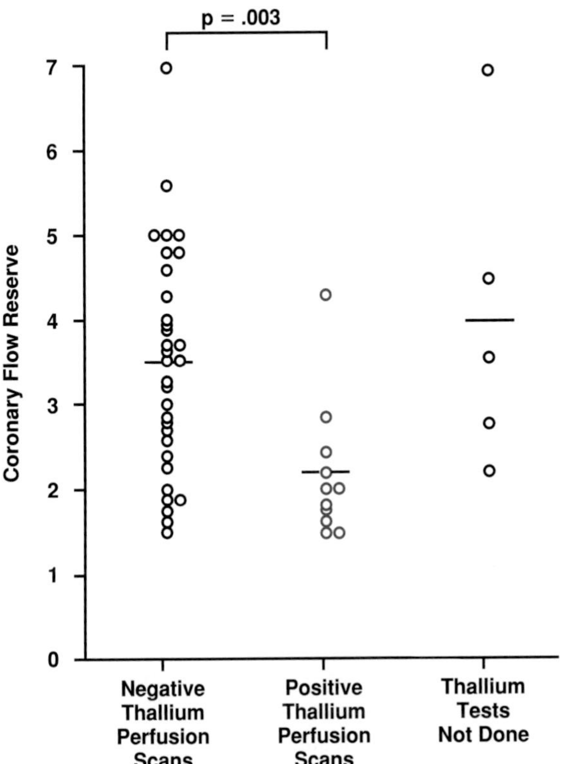

FIG. 4. Coronary flow reserve following dipyridamole administration in 32 hypertensive patients without thallium defects *(negative scans)* and 11 with thallium defects *(positive scans)* and in 5 patients who did not undergo or complete thallium testing. (From Houghton et al., ref. 63, with permission.)

Additional studies indicate that morphological abnormalities in microvascular density and structure may limit appropriate coronary flow in humans with pressure-induced left ventricular hypertrophy. Anatomic studies by Rakusan showed substantial reduction in capillary density in hypertrophied human hearts (19). Tanaka et al. found medial thickening with luminal narrowing of intramyocardial small arteries in hearts of patients with left ventricular hypertrophy at necropsy (64). Schwartzkopff et al. found luminal narrowing in intramural arteries from right ventricular septal biopsies performed in patients with chest pain, hypertension, and normal coronary angiograms (65). They found a correlation between the minimum coronary resistance following dipyridamole, 0.5 mg/kg (inert gas method), and the arterial medial wall area. No correlation was found between left ventricular mass index by echocardiography and the minimum coronary resistance. They concluded that the wall thickening was causally related to the diminished coronary reserve and partly independent of myocardial hypertrophy.

Functional abnormalities of coronary microvascular function may also be important in hypertension. Brush et al. reported that 12 hypertensive patients without significant left ventricular hypertrophy and normal coronary angiograms had a coronary microvascular constrictor response to ergonovine, 0.15 mg intravenously (flow measured by thermodilution) (66). In contrast, 13 normotensive subjects had a dilator response to ergonovine, an endothelium-dependent vasodilator that also has direct smooth muscle constrictor properties. More recently, Treasure et al. (67) reported that endothelium-dependent relaxation to acetylcholine was impaired in the microcirculation of ten hypertensive patients with left ventricular hypertrophy and normal coronary angiograms, with flow velocity measured by an intracoronary Doppler catheter, compared to nine normotensive subjects also undergoing cardiac catheterization (Fig. 5). In contrast to impaired responses to acetylcholine in the hypertensive patients, the responses to the endothelium-independent vasodilator adenosine were no different between the two groups. Brush et al., using similar doses of intracoronary acetylcholine, observed an actual fall in coronary flow (intracoronary Doppler flow velocity measurement) in eight hypertensive patients compared to a slight increase in flow in six normotensive patients, accompanied by an almost 50% reduction in epicardial coronary artery diameter in the hypertensive group (68). Quyyumi et al. (69) found that the coronary flow response (thermodilution method) to pacing stress correlated with the flow response to intracoronary acetylcholine in 20 hypertensive patients with normal epicardial coronary arteries and no or minimal left ventricular hypertrophy (69). These findings suggest that microvascular endothelial dys-

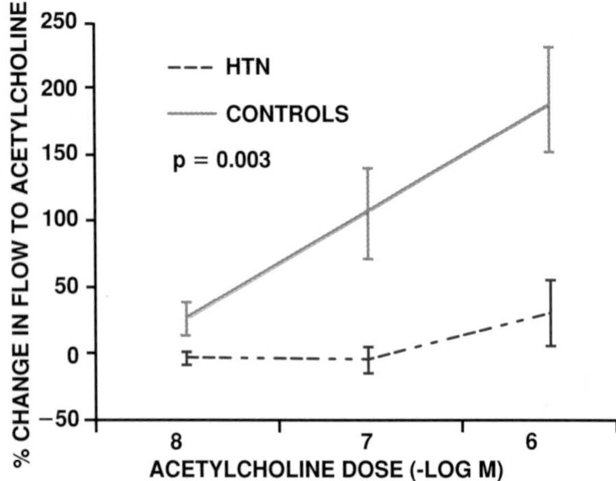

FIG. 5. Coronary flow responses to serial infusions of acetylcholine expressed as percentage change from baseline flow. Flow response to acetylcholine was markedly impaired in patients with hypertension (HTN) and ventricular hypertrophy. Probability value refers to comparison of dose–response curves using ANOVA for repeated measures; *error bars* represent mean ± SEM. (From Treasure et al., ref. 67, with permission.)

function may contribute to abnormal flow responses to stress.

Thus, patients with hypertension commonly have abnormal pharmacological flow reserve or abnormal flow responses to stress despite normal coronary angiograms, with several studies suggesting an independent contribution of the coronary microcirculation, possibly because of structural disease and luminal narrowing or endothelial dysfunction. Abnormal structure and function of the coronary microcirculation and left ventricular hypertrophy may contribute to impaired autoregulation of coronary flow with reduction in systemic pressure, as reported by Polese et al. (70).

The Coronary Microcirculation in Diabetes Mellitus

Diabetes mellitus is commonly associated with microangiopathy of many organ systems, including the glomerulus of the kidney and the retina of the eye. Morphologically abnormal small arteries, arterioles, and capillaries have been described within the heart, especially in tissue from insulin-dependent juvenile-onset diabetics (71–74). However, the severity and extent of microvascular abnormalities within the heart was commonly found to be minimal in these studies, even in tissue from patients who died in heart failure. Indeed, one group found no difference in the prevalence of morphologically abnormal small arteries in hearts from diabetic patients at necropsy compared with nondiabetic controls (75). Further, it has not been shown that small vessel disease in diabetics, if present, causes impaired coronary flow responses and myocardial ischemia during stress. Abnormal endothelial function has been shown in the forearm circulation of diabetics (76,77), but analogous studies have not been reported in the coronary circulation of humans. The interpretation of such studies might be confounded by the common coexistence of hypertension and hypercholesterolemia with diabetes, which could independently produce adverse effects in microvascular endothelial function.

Hyperinsulinemia is commonly demonstrated in adult-onset diabetics, and the association with hypertension (78) has raised the possibility that insulin might raise arterial blood pressure by augmenting sodium reabsorption in the kidney and by increasing sympathetic activity (79). However, studies have shown that although insulin infusion increases sympathetic activity in muscle, the net result is vasodilation (80). Nonetheless, the possibility that hyperinsulinemia might produce vasoconstriction in the setting of endothelial dysfunction in either the systemic or the coronary circulation has not been investigated.

Atherosclerosis and the Coronary Circulation in Humans

As discussed previously in this chapter, atherosclerosis can impair endothelium-dependent vasodilator responses in large arteries (including coronary arteries) of animals fed high-cholesterol diets. Ludmer et al. reported that epicardial coronary arteries in humans with significant coronary artery disease constricted both at sites of significant disease and at sites of plaquing in response to acetylcholine, as opposed to vasodilation in coronary arteries of patients without any evidence of coronary artery disease (81). In contrast to the different responses of these two patient groups to acetylcholine, the response to nitroglycerin was similar, indicating unimpaired smooth muscle function in atherosclerotic arteries. Patients without atheromatous plaquing only or with "nonsignificant" coronary artery disease also exhibit constrictor responses of epicardial arteries to intracoronary acetylcholine (82–84). Other studies have shown that angiographically normal coronary arteries of patients with significant atherosclerotic disease involving other arteries also constrict in response to intracoronary acetylcholine in doses that cause dilation of epicardial arteries in patients with entirely normal coronary angiograms (85). Even risk factors for atherosclerosis such as hypercholesterolemia, male gender, age, and family history of coronary artery disease have been associated with constrictor responses of the epicardial coronary arteries to acetylcholine in patients with normal-appearing coronary angiograms (83,86).

These observations are compatible with the concept that endothelial dysfunction of epicardial coronary arteries may precede development of atherosclerotic disease that is either angiographically apparent or of sufficient obstructive severity to cause myocardial ischemia and angina pectoris. However, because acetylcholine also stimulates muscarinic receptors on smooth muscle that result in constriction, vasoconstrictor responses to acetylcholine could indicate vascular smooth muscle hyperplasia or hypersensitivity to the muscarinic effects of acetylcholine and not defective release of nitric oxide from the endothelium. Indeed, substance P, an endothelium-dependent vasodilator that has no smooth muscle effects, dilates epicardial coronary arteries that constrict in response to relatively high doses of intracoronary acetylcholine (87) and dilates atheromatous epicardial coronary arteries in patients with coronary artery disease (88). Smooth muscle constrictor responses to acetylcholine may explain why in one study epicardial coronary arteries in patients with hypercholesterolemia constricted in response to acetylcholine but dilated in response to two other endothelium-dependent vasodilator stimuli; coronary flow increase (shear stress) and cold pressor testing (83). On the other hand, studies of epicardial coronary arteries from explanted hearts at time of cardiac transplantation have shown that atherosclerotic arteries dilate less in response to the endothelium-dependent vasodilators substance P, bradykinin, and calcium ionophore than do nondiseased arteries. Further, these vasodilator responses were blocked by inhibition of nitric oxide synthesis (89,90).

Several studies of epicardial coronary responses to endothelium-dependent and endothelium-independent vasodilators in patients with early atherosclerosis also reported the effects of these agonists on coronary blood flow. Zeiher et al. (83) found a smaller decrease in coronary resistance (coronary flow derived from intracoronary Doppler flow velocity measurement) in response to intracoronary acetylcholine (range 0.72 to 7.2 μg/min) in nine patients with hypercholesterolemia (average cholesterol 281 mg/dl) but smooth epicardial coronary arteries, compared to 29 normocholesterolemic patients either without angiographic evidence for coronary artery disease or with "early" atherosclerosis only. Coronary resistance responses to the endothelium-independent vasodilator papaverine were unaffected by hypercholesterolemia. In the hypercholesterolemic patients, acetylcholine resulted in a 35% decrease in epicardial coronary artery area. Egashira et al. (84) reported that coronary flow (intracoronary Doppler flow velocity measurement) responses to intracoronary acetylcholine (range 1–30 μg/min) in 12 patients with "mild" (less than 40% stenosis) epicardial coronary atherosclerosis were impaired compared to 16 patients with normal coronary angiograms and similar responses to the endothelium-independent vasodilator papaverine (Fig. 6). The highest dose of acetylcholine used in this study was associated with a 26% reduction in arterial cross-sectional area in the patients with atherosclerosis. By univariate analysis, hypertension, hypercholesterolemia, age greater than 50 years, and total number of coronary risk factors were associated with the impaired increase in coronary flow in response to acetylcholine. Endothelial dysfunction of the coronary microcirculation may coexist with endothelial dysfunction of the peripheral microvascular endothelium. Quyyumi et al. found a significant correlation between the flow (intravascular Doppler flow velocity measurement) responses to acetylcholine in the coronary and lower extremity vascular beds but no correlation between nitroprusside responses (91). The

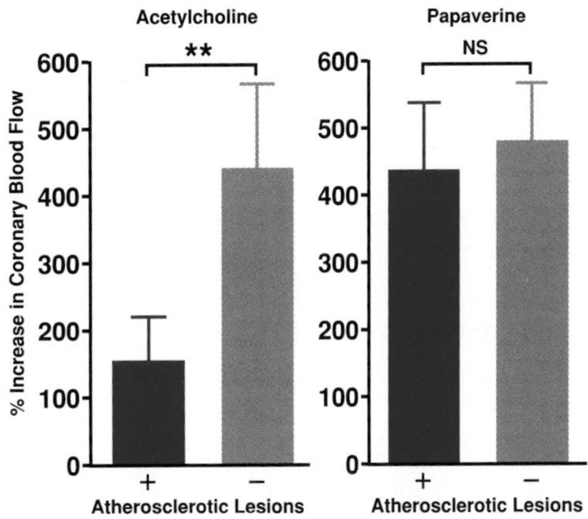

FIG. 6. Summary of the percentage increases in coronary blood flow in response to acetylcholine and to papaverine in patients with and without atherosclerotic lesions (<40% stenoses) in the study artery. $^{**}p < 0.001$ by unpaired t test. (From Egashira et al., ref. 84, with permission.)

number of risk factors for atherosclerosis correlated significantly with these flow responses to acetylcholine (92).

The authors of these studies concluded that risk factors for atherosclerosis may cause microvascular endothelial dysfunction. Although the reduction in epicardial cross-sectional area in response to acetylcholine might have contributed to the limited flow increase in response to acetylcholine in these studies, the results are consistent with the animal studies described earlier in this chapter regarding the impact of hypercholesterolemia on the coronary microcirculation. Further, the results are also consistent with responses to the same agonists in the forearms of hypertensive and hypercholesterolemic patients, a vascular bed generally spared from large artery atherosclerosis (93–95).

Implications of Human Studies

Although observations from these studies are compatible with microvascular endothelial dysfunction in patients with risk factors for coronary artery disease with or without angiographic evidence of early atherosclerosis of the epicardial coronary arteries, the implication of these findings is uncertain. That is, no study determined whether endothelial dysfunction of the coronary microcirculation in the absence of "significant" disease of the epicardial coronary arteries can cause myocardial ischemia, either at rest or during stress. Presumably, all patients underwent cardiac catheterization because of chest pain syndromes. However, in none of the studies discussed above were the results of noninvasive testing reported, indicating the presence (or absence) of myocardial ischemia during stress. Thus, the chest pain that warranted cardiac catheterization could have been entirely unrelated to the determination of endothelial dysfunction in the coronary circulation (large or small arteries), which may only represent a marker of early vascular disease.

Activities commonly encountered by patients with coronary artery disease may adversely affect the coronary microcirculation. Yeung et al. reported that arithmetic mental stress produced a 24% constriction in stenosed epicardial coronary arteries but no change in the diameter of smooth arteries (96). In seven patients with stenosed or plaqued arteries, coronary flow (intracoronary Doppler flow velocity measurement) decreased by 27%, as opposed to minimal changes in the flow in smooth arteries. Intracoronary acetylcholine also caused similar degrees of constriction of epicardial coronary arteries at the same sites that constricted during mental stress, although blood flow increased by 51%. These data suggest that mental stress may have deleterious effects on the coronary microcirculation, resulting in a decrease in flow, additional to the effects on epicardial coronary arteries. Quillen et al. reported that cigarette smoking produced a 21% increase in coronary vascular resistance (intracoronary Doppler flow velocity measurement) in eight patients with either smooth or ''nonstenotic'' atherosclerotic arteries, despite an increase in heart rate and blood pressure (97). Because smoking provoked less than 10% epicardial luminal narrowing, the increase in coronary resistance likely represented coronary microvascular constriction. Pupita et al. performed exercise testing in 11 patients with a total occlusion of single coronary artery, with that vascular territory supplied by collaterals (98). The exercise ischemic threshold of these patients was enhanced by nitroglycerin and reduced by ergonovine. Ergonovine administration to these same patients in the catheterization laboratory produced ST segment depression with reduced filling of collateral and collateralized arteries. The authors concluded that vasomotion of small coronary arteries (e.g., collateral vessels) may result in variation in the ischemic threshold, a conclusion supported by their observations of variations in heart rate at the onset of ischemia during ambulatory monitoring in these same patients. Thus, mental stress, cigarette smoking, and exercise may have constrictor effects on the coronary microcirculation that might contribute to or aggravate myocardial ischemia.

Reversibility of Coronary Microvascular Dysfunction

Three groups have reported improvement in acetylcholine-stimulated coronary blood flow in patients with ''nonstenotic'' atheroma or normal-appearing epicardial coronary arteries following intracoronary infusion of L-arginine, the precursor to nitric oxide synthesis, in hypercholesterolemic patients (Table 2; Fig. 7) (99–101). Reis et al. reported that intravenous ethinyl estradiol increased basal coronary flow and epicardial coronary artery diameter in postmenopausal women and prevented acetylcholine-induced decreases in coronary artery diameter and coronary flow (102). Intracoronary 17β-estradiol administration achieving physiological levels in the coronary sinus was shown by Gilligan et al. to improve epicardial and microvascular endothelium-dependent vasomotor responses to acetylcholine in estrogen-deficient postmenopausal women without altering endothelium-independent vasodilator responses (103). Dakak et al. reported that α-adrenergic blockade with phentolamine prevented the constrictor effects of mental stress on the coronary microcirculation of six patients with coronary atherosclerosis (104). Egashira and co-workers administered the HMG-CoA reductase inhibitor pravastatin, 10 to 20 mg daily, to hypercholesterolemic patients with coronary artery disease following coronary angioplasty (105). At the follow-up study approximately 6 months later, epicardial and microvascular endothelium-dependent vasomotor responses to acetylcholine were improved compared to the pretreatment study. The coronary flow response to the endothelium-independent vasodilator papaverine was unaltered by treatment. Thus, impaired microvascular endothelial function may be reversible in humans.

TABLE 2. *Pharmacological enhancement of coronary microvascular endothelium-dependent vasodilation*[a]

Reference	No. patients	Condition	Drug	Administration
Drexler et al. (99)	8CAD/7 normals	Hypercholesterolemia	L-Arginine	Acute IC
Duboid-Rande et al. (100)	13 CAD	Hypercholesterolemia	L-Arginine	Acute IC
Quyyumi et al. (101)	9 CAD/11 normals	Hypercholesterolemia	L-Arginine	Acute IC
Reis et al. (102)	7 CAD/8 normals	Postmenopausal	Ethinyl estradiol	Acute IV
Gilligan et al. (103)	7 CAD/13 normals	Postmenopausal	17β-Estradiol	Acute IC
Dakak et al. (104)	6 CAD	Mental stress	Phentolamine	Acute IC
Egashira et al. (105)	9 CAD	Hypercholesterolemia	Pravastatin	3–12 months

[a] CAD, coronary artery disease; IC, intracoronary; IV, intravenous. In all reports, the coronary artery studied had <50% obstruction, and flow measurements were made by intracoronary Doppler technique.

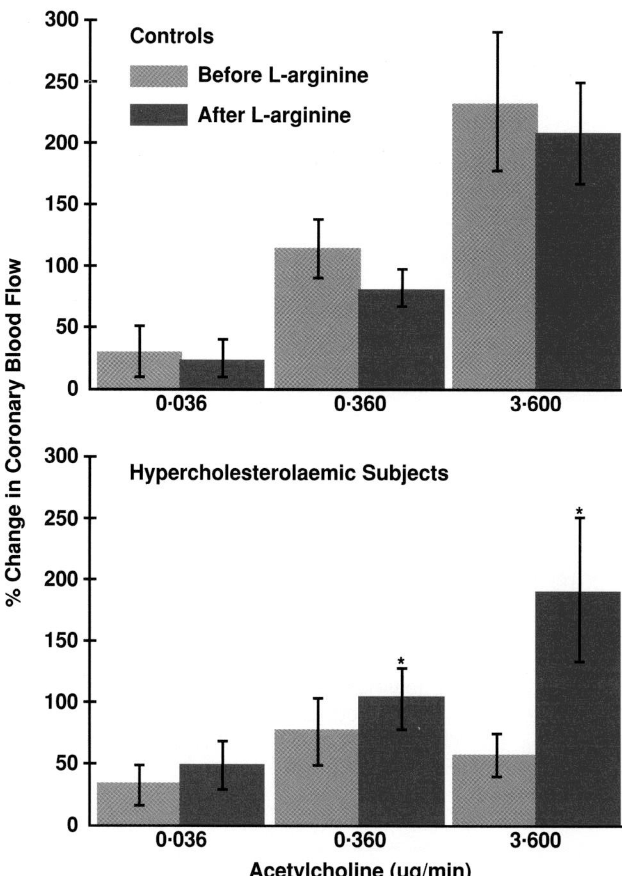

FIG. 7. Acetylcholine-induced changes in coronary blood flow before and after L-arginine in controls **(upper)** and hypercholesterolemic subjects **(lower).** Change in flow (mean ± SEM) expressed as a percentage of the baseline value. **p* < 0.05 compared with infusion of acetylcholine before L-arginine. (From Drexler et al., ref. 99, with permission.)

THE CORONARY MICROCIRCULATION FOLLOWING ACUTE AND CHRONIC ISCHEMIA

Reperfusion following prolonged ischemia in animals is associated with limitation in myocardial perfusion, likely in part as a result of injury to the coronary microcirculation (106,107). Impairment in microvascular endothelial function was suggested by the studies of Mehta et al., in which coronary flow responses to acetylcholine and to bradykinin were attenuated in open-chest dogs following 1 h of coronary occlusion and 1 h of reperfusion, compared to the flow responses to these same endothelium-dependent vasodilator agonists prior to occlusion (108). Indeed, the microvascular endothelium may be more vulnerable to the effects of ischemia and reperfusion than the epicardial coronary artery endothelium. Quillen et al. found depressed relaxation of preconstricted coronary microvessels (110 to 220 μm diameter) isolated from dogs to the endothelium-dependent vasodilator agonists acetylcholine, ADP, and calcium ionophore following 1 h of coronary artery occlusion and 1 h of reperfusion compared to preocclusion responses, with unaltered vasorelaxant responses to nitroglycerin (109). Ischemia alone produced less depression in the responses of the microvessels to these agonists. The endothelium-dependent and endothelium-independent vasodilator responses of epicardial coronary artery rings were unaltered by ischemia, with or without reperfusion.

Damaged endothelium may limit vasodilation or promote vasoconstriction in response to circulating and platelet-derived substances, permit adhesion and ingress of inflammatory cells into the vessel wall, promote platelet activation, promote the release of superoxide anions, activate local procoagulant mechanisms, and contribute to the formation of microthrombi (Fig. 8) (110,111). All of these deleterious effects could exacerbate ischemic myocardial injury and necrosis and contribute to or prolong impaired myocardial systolic function (stunning), thus compromising the success of thrombolytic or mechanical reperfusion in humans. Several interventions, such as inhibition of superoxide free radical and thrombin formation, have been shown to benefit coronary flow and left ventricular functional responses to ischemia–reperfusion in animal models (112,113).

Persistent limitation in pharmacological coronary flow reserve has been noted in humans following successful coronary angioplasty (114). The mechanism of this response is unclear, but it could be related to ischemic injury to the microcirculation following repetitive balloon inflation, activation of platelets in response to balloon injury-induced vascular trauma with vasoconstrictor effects on the microcirculation, down-regulation of microvascular receptors and activity as a consequence of chronic reduction in coronary flow, or simply an artifact of procedure-related increases in basal flow giving the appearance of a reduction in pharmacological flow reserve (114,115). Regardless of the mechanism, flow reserve improves in the weeks following angioplasty (114). Nonetheless, in some patients, abnormal microvascular function may account for persistent symptoms and evidence for ischemia despite angiographic evidence of successful angioplasty (116,117).

ANGIOGENESIS AND THE COLLATERAL CIRCULATION

Vascular connections (collaterals) between branches of the same or different coronary arteries are commonly visible during angiography of patients with coronary artery disease. These vessels may arise from microscopic nonfunctional vessels within the myocardium or develop de novo as a result of an angiogenic stimulus such as repetitive myocardial ischemia. Because extensive collaterals between diseased and nondiseased coronary arteries may convey sufficient blood flow to prevent ischemia or infarction in the diseased vascular territory, much research has been directed at experimentally promoting collateral growth in animals and humans with the hope that such effects could be of therapeutic benefit

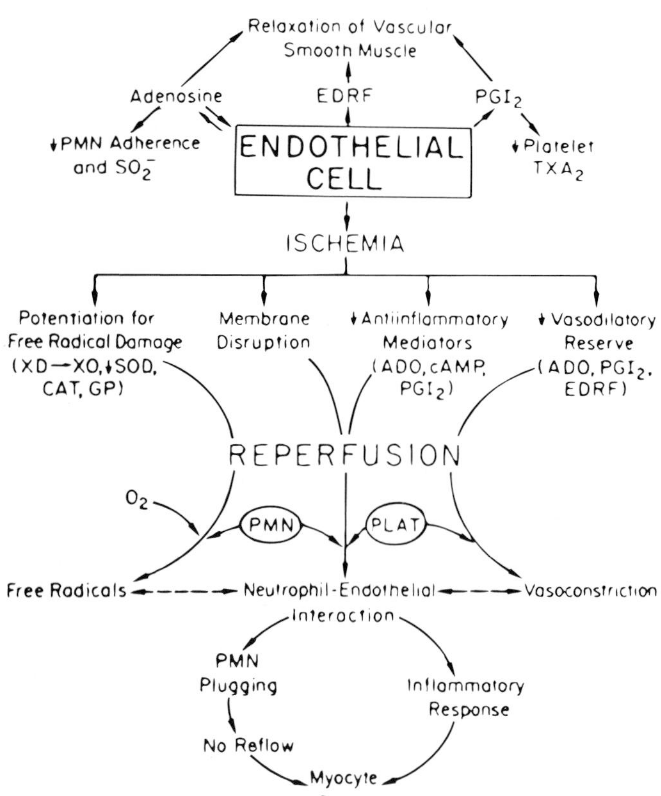

FIG. 8. Schematic diagram illustrating the potential role of the endothelial cell in myocardial reperfusion injury. ADO, adenosine; cAMP, cyclic adenosine monophosphate; CAT, catalase; EDRF, endothelial-derived relaxing factor; GP, glutathione peroxidase; PGI_2, prostacyclin; PLAT, platelet; PMN, polymorphonuclear leukocyte; SO_2, superoxide anion; ↓SOD, reduction in superoxide dismutase; TXA_2, thromboxane A_2; XD, xanthine dehydrogenase; XO, xanthine oxidase. (From Forman et al., ref. 110, with permission.)

to patients with coronary artery disease. Based on the observation that heparin accelerates collateral development in response to repetitive ischemia in conscious dogs (118), Fujita et al. administered intravenous heparin, 5,000 units, to ten patients with coronary artery disease prior to each of two daily exercise treadmill tests for 10 days (119). They reported that following this regimen, exercise duration, rate–pressure product at end-exercise, time to onset of angina, and time to onset of ST segment depression were all prolonged compared to pretreatment exercise. Further, repeat coronary angiography showed increased opacification of collaterals compared to baseline angiograms. In contrast, six patients who underwent twice-daily treadmill exercise testing for 10 days but did not receive heparin showed no difference in their exercise parameters compared to baseline exercise. Quyyumi et al. recently reported that low-molecular-weight, nonanticoagulant fragments of heparin (Fragmin) also appeared to possess angiogenic properties in humans (120). In 23 patients with coronary artery disease, the ten patients receiving Fragmin for 4 weeks demonstrated an increase in rate–pressure product at the onset of ST segment depression, greater exercise duration during treadmill exercise, and decreased frequency of ST segment depression on ambulatory monitoring than placebo-treated patients.

Growth factors have also been investigated as potential angiogenic agents in promoting collateral growth. Yanagisawa-Miwa and co-workers reported that basic fibroblast growth factor (bFGF) administered intracoronarily into a canine myocardial infarct model reduced infarct size and improved cardiac systolic function, associated with an increase in the number of arterioles and capillaries in the infarct region (121). Unger et al. administered bFGF as a daily bolus injection directly into a collateral-dependent zone of a canine model 10 days following placement of an ameroid constrictor on the circumflex artery (122). Compared to saline-treated animals, bFGF-treated dogs demonstrated a significantly greater increase in the collateral-zone-to-normal-zone flow ratio, associated with a significant increase in the density and distribution of vessels within the collateral zone (Fig. 9). The same group has recently reported that vascular endothelial growth factor also appears to have angiogenic effects in the collateral zone of dogs using the same experimental model of chronic circumflex occlusion (123).

Thus, pharmacological enhancement of collateral growth may represent a novel therapeutic approach for the treatment of patients with coronary artery disease. This approach may have particular appeal to patients who are not candidates for revascularization procedures and who continue to be symptomatic despite optimal medical management.

FUTURE DIRECTIONS

Future research directions include proving a link between coronary microvascular dysfunction and inducible myocardial ischemia and acute and chronic impairment in left ventricular function. Therapies that might improve microvascu-

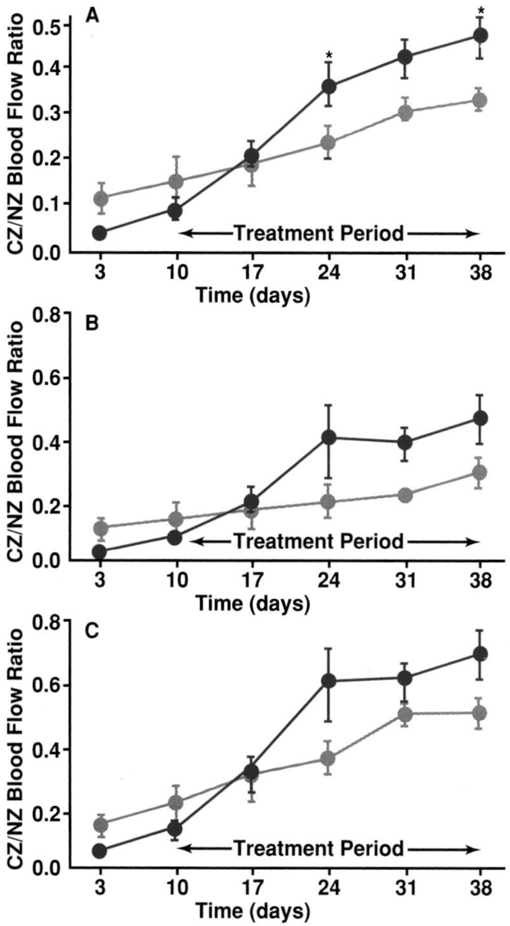

FIG. 9. Collateral blood flow as a function of time. Collateral flow is expressed as collateral-dependent zone-to-normal zone (CZ/NZ) ratio during maximal vasodilatation (means ± SE). Treatment was begun following blood flow measurement on day 10. *Closed circles,* basic fibroblast growth factor (FGF)-treated dogs; *open circles,* controls. During the first 2 weeks of drug administration (days 10–24), the slope of the CZ/NZ versus time relationship increased significantly in basic FGF-treated dogs compared with control dogs. Differences in transmural collateral blood flow at days 24 and 38 are significant ($p \leq 0.001$, **A**). Improvement in flow related to basic FGF was apparent in the epicardium **(C)** as well as the endocardium **(B)**. (Adapted from Unger et al., ref. 122, with permission.)

lar endothelial vasomotor responsiveness, such as cholesterol reduction therapy, antioxidant therapy, estrogen replacement, L-arginine supplementation, nitric oxide donors, and antiplatelet therapy, should be tested in patients with evidence of microvascular dysfunction, especially those with evidence of ischemia during stress. Additionally, studies of the microvascular endothelium with regard to properties other than vasomotor regulation, such as control of local hemostasis, will be important to understand more fully the potential role of the coronary microcirculation in myocardial ischemia. Finally, pharmacological stimulation of coronary microvessels may one day provide sufficient collateral blood flow to prevent ischemia and infarction in patients with coronary artery disease.

SUMMARY

The coronary microcirculation, which cannot be assessed angiographically, contributes importantly to coronary flow regulation. Conditions such as hypertension, hypercholesterolemia, and diabetes mellitus, commonly associated with atherosclerotic disease of the epicardial coronary arteries, may have harmful effects on the coronary microcirculation as well despite the absence of atherosclerotic involvement of these small arteries. Atherosclerosis of the epicardial coronary arteries may coexist with evidence of microvascular dysfunction in humans. In addition to impaired microvascular vasomotor regulation as a result of endothelial dysfunction, other properties of endothelium may also be adversely affected by hypercholesterolemia, such as the release of anticoagulant factors and inhibition of platelet activation. Common activities such as mental stress, smoking, and exercise may have adverse effects on the coronary microcirculation and contribute to myocardial ischemia. Finally, acute and chronic ischemia, especially when associated with reperfusion, may have adverse effects on coronary microvascular function that may compromise the therapeutic success of revascularization with acute and chronic adverse effects on left ventricular function.

REFERENCES

1. Gould KL, Lipscomb K. Effects of coronary stenosis on coronary flow reserve and resistance. *Am J Cardiol* 1974;34:48–55.
2. Chilian WM, Eastham CL, Marcus ML. Microvascular distribution of coronary vascular resistance in beating left ventricle. *Am J Physiol* 1986;251:H779–H788.
3. Chilian WM, Layne SM, Klausner EC, Eastham CL, Marcus ML. Redistribution of coronary microvascular resistance produced by dipyridamole. *Am J Physiol* 1989;256:H383–H390.
4. Kanatsuka H, Lamping KG, Eastham CL, Marcus ML. Heterogeneous changes in epimyocardial microvascular size during graded coronary stenosis. Evidence of the microvascular site for anticoagulation. *Circ Res* 1990;66:389–396.
5. Kanatsuka H, Lamping KG, Eastham CL, Dellsperger KC, Marcus MC. Comparison of the effects of increased myocardial oxygen consumption and adenosine on the coronary microvascular resistance. *Circ Res* 1989;65:1296–1305.
6. Marcus ML, Chilian WM, Kanatsuka H, Dellsperger KC, Eastham CL, Lamping KG. Understanding the coronary circulation through studies at the microvascular level. *Circulation* 1990;82:1–7.
7. Furchgott RF, Zawadzki JV. The obligatory role of endothelial cells in the relaxation of arterial smooth muscle by acetylcholine. *Nature* 1980;288:373–376.
8. Palmer RMJ, Ferrige AG, Moncada S. Nitric oxide release accounts for the biological activity of endothelium-derived relaxant factor. *Nature* 1987;327:524–526.
9. Amezcua JL, Palmer RMJ, de Souza BM, Moncado S. Nitric oxide synthesized from L-arginine regulates vascular tone in the coronary circulation of the rabbit. *Br J Pharmacol* 1989;97:1119–1124.
10. Levi R, Gross SS, Lamparter B, Fasehun OA, Aisaka K, Jaffe EA, Griffith OW, Stuehr DJ. Evidence that L-arginine is the biosynthetic

precursor of vascular and cardiac nitric oxide. In: Moncada S, Higgs EA, eds. *Nitric Oxide from L-Arginine: A Bioregulatory System*. Amsterdam: Exerpta Medica; 1990:35–45.

11. Chu A, Chambers DE, Lin CC, Kuehl WD, Palmer RMJ, Moncada S, Cobb FR. Effects of inhibition of nitric oxide formation on basal vasomotion and endothelium-dependent responses of the coronary arteries in awake dogs. *J Clin Invest* 1991;87:1964–1968.
12. Komaru T, Lamping KG, Eastham CL, Harrison DG, Marcus ML, Dellsperger KC. Effect of an arginine analogue on acetylcholine-induced coronary microvascular dilatation in dogs. *Am J Physiol* 1991; 261:H2001–H2007.
13. Woodman OL, Dusting GJ. N-Nitro-L-arginine causes coronary vasoconstriction and inhibits endothelium-dependent vasodilatation in anesthetized greyhounds. *Br J Pharmacol* 1991;103:1407–1410.
14. Broten TP, Miyashiro JK, Moncada S, Feigl EO. Role of endothelium-derived relaxing factor in parasympathetic coronary vasodilation. *Am J Physiol* 1992;262:H1579–H1584.
15. Mueller TM, Marcus ML, Kerber RE, Young JA, Barnes RW, Abboud FM. Effect of renal hypertension and left ventricular hypertrophy on the coronary circulation in dogs. *Circ Res* 1978;42:543–549.
16. O'Keefe DD, Hoffman JIE, Chietlin M, O'Neill JO, Allard JR, Shapkin E. Coronary blood flow in experimental canine left ventricular hypertrophy. *Circ Res* 1978;43:43–51.
17. Rembert JC, Kleinman LH, Fedor JM, Wechsler AS, Greenfield JC. Myocardial blood flow distribution in concentric left ventricular hypertrophy. *J Clin Invest* 1978;62:379–386.
18. Wearn JT. The extent of the capillary bed of the heart. *J Exp Med* 1928;47:273–292.
19. Rakusan K. Quantitative morphology of capillaries of the heart. Number of capillaries in animal and human hearts under normal and pathological conditions. *Methods Achiev Exp Pathol* 1971;5:272–286.
20. Tomanek RJ, Searls JC, Lachenbruch PA. Quantitative changes in the capillary bed during developing, peak, and stabilized cardiac hypertrophy in the spontaneously hypertensive rat. *Cir Res* 1982;51: 295–304.
21. Henquell L, Odoroff CC, Honig CR. Intercapillary distance and capillary reserve in hypertrophied rat hearts beating in situ. *Circ Res* 1977; 41:400–408.
22. Bostrom SL, Fryklund J. Protein synthesis and composition of cardiac and vascular tissue in spontaneously hypertensive rats and the effects of beta-adenergic antagonist treatment. *Clin Sci* 1979;57:39–41.
23. Yamori Y, Mori C, Nishio T, Ooshima A, Horie R, Ohtaka M, Soeda T, Saito M, Abe K, Nara Y, Nakao Y, Kihara M. Cardiac hypertrophy in early hypertension. *Am J Cardiol* 1979;44:964–969.
24. Brilla CG, Janicki JS, Weber KT. Impaired diastolic function and coronary reserve in genetic hypertension. Role of interstitial fibrosis and medial thickening of intramyocardial coronary arteries. *Circ Res* 1991;69:107–115.
25. Klepzig M, Eisenlohr H, Steindl J, Schmiebusch H, Strauer BE. Media hypertrophy in hypertensive coronary resistance vessels. *J Cardiovasc Pharmacol* 1987;10(Suppl 6):S97–S102.
26. Isoyama S, Sato F, Takashima T. Effect of age on coronary circulation after imposition of pressure-overload in rats. *Hypertension* 1991;17: 369–377.
27. Holtz J, Restorff WV, Bard P, Bassenge E. Transmural distribution of myocardial blood flow of coronary reserve in canine left ventricular hypertrophy. *Basic Res Cardiol* 1977;72:286–292.
28. Harrison DG, Florentine MS, Brooks LA, Copper SM, Marcus ML. The effect of hypertension and left ventricular hypertrophy on the lower range of coronary autoregulation. *Circulation* 1988;77: 1108–1115.
29. Koyanagi S, Eastham CL, Harrison DG, Marcus ML. Increased size of myocardial infarction in dogs with chronic hypertension and left ventricular hypertrophy. *Circ Res* 1982;50:55–62.
30. Lundin SA, Hallback-Norlander M. Regression of structural cardiovascular changes by antihypertensive therapy in spontaneously hypertensive rats. *J Hypertens* 1984;2:11–18.
31. Sano T, Tarazi RC. Differential structural responses of small resistance vessels to antihypertensive therapy. *Circulation* 1987;75: 618–626.
32. Sen S, Tarazi RC, Bumpus FM. Reversal of cardiac hypertrophy in renal hypertensive rats: Medical versus surgical therapy. *Am J Physiol* 1981;240:H408–H412.
33. Warshaw DM, Root DT, Halpern W. Effects of antihypertensive drug therapy on the morphology and mechanics of resistance arteries from spontaneously hypertensive rats. *Blood Vessels* 1980;17:257–270.
34. Cutilletta AF, Dowell RT, Rudnik M, Arcilla RA, Zak R. Regression of myocardial hypertrophy. I. Experimental model, changes in heart weight, nucleic acids and collagen. *J Mol Cell Cardiol* 1975;7: 767–781.
35. Motz W, Strauer BE. Left ventricular function and collagen content after regression of hypertensive hypertrophy. *Hypertension* 1989;13: 43–50.
36. Isoyama S, Ito N, Kuroha M, Takashima T. Complete reversibility of physiological coronary vascular abnormalities in hypertrophied hearts produced by pressure overload in the rat. *J Clin Invest* 1989;84: 288–294.
37. Sato F, Isoyama S, Takishima T. Normalization of impaired coronary circulation in hypertrophied rat hearts. *Hypertension* 1990;16:26–34.
38. Ito N, Isoyama S, Kuroha M, Takashima T. Duration of pressure overload alters regression of coronary circulation abnormalities. *Am J Physiol* 1990;258:H1753–H1760.
39. Habib JR, Bossaler C, Wells G, Williams C, Morrisett JD, Henry PD. Preservation of endothelium-dependent vascular relaxation in cholesterol-fed rabbit by treatment with the calcium channel blocker PN 200110. *Circ Res* 1986;58:305–309.
40. Verbeuren TJ, Jordaens FH, Zonnekeyn LL, VanHove CE, Coene MC, Herman AG. Effect of hypercholesterolemia on vascular reactivity in the rabbit: I. Endothelium-dependent and endothelium-independent contractions and relaxations in isolated arteries of control and hypercholesterolemic rabbits. *Circ Res* 1986;58:552–564.
41. Freiman PC, Mitchell GC, Heistad DD, Armstrong ML, Harrison DG. Atherosclerosis impairs endothelium-dependent vascular relaxation to acetylcholine and thrombin in primates. *Circ Res* 1986;58:783–789.
42. Cohen RA, Zitnay KM, Haudenschild CC, Cunningham LD. Loss of selective endothelial cell vasoactive functions caused by hypercholesterolemia in pig coronary arteries. *Circ Res* 1988;63:903–910.
43. Shimokawa H, Flavahan NA, Vanhoutte PM. Loss of endothelial pertussis toxin-sensitive G protein function in atherosclerotic porcine coronary arteries. *Circulation* 1991;83:652–660.
44. Kugiyama K, Kerns SA, Morrisett JD, Roberts R, Henry PD. Impairment of endothelium-dependent arterial relaxation by lysolecithin in modified low-density lipoproteins. *Nature* 1990;344:160–162.
45. Flavahan NA. Atherosclerosis or lipoprotein-induced endothelial dysfunction: Potential mechanisms underlying reduction in EDRF/nitric oxide activity. *Circulation* 1992;85:1927–1938.
46. Minor RL, Myers PR, Guerra R, Bates JN, Harrison DG. Diet-induced atherosclerosis increases the release of nitrogen oxides from rabbit aorta. *J Clin Invest* 1990;86:2109–2116.
47. Girerd XL, Hirsch AT, Cooke JP, Dzau VJ, Creagher MA. L-Arginine augments endothelium-dependent vasodilation in cholesterol-fed rabbits. *Circ Res* 1990;67:1301–1308.
48. Cooke JP, Andon NA, Girerd XJ, Hirsch AJ, Creagher MA. Arginine restores choleinergic relaxation of hypercholesterolemic rabbit thoracic aorta. *Circulation* 1991;83:1057–1062.
49. Cooke JP, Singer AH, Tsau P, Zera P, Rowson RA, Billingham ME. Antiatherogenic effects of L-arginine in the hypercholesterolemic rabbit. *J Clin Invest* 1992;90:1168–1172.
50. Osborne JA, Siegman MJ, Sedar AW, Mooers SV, Lefer AM. Lack of endothelium-dependent relaxation in coronary resistance arteries of cholesterol-fed rabbits. *Am J Physiol* 1989;256:C591–C597.
51. Yamamoto H, Bossaller C, Cartwright J Jr, Henry PD. Videomicroscopic demonstration of defective cholinergic arteriolar vasodilation in atherosclerotic rabbit. *J Clin Invest* 1988;81:1752–1758.
52. Selke FW, Armstrong ML, Harrison DG. Endothelium-dependent vascular relaxation is abnormal in the coronary microcirculation of atherosclerotic primates. *Circulation* 1990;81:1586–1593.
53. Kuo L, Davis MJ, Cannon MS, Chilian WM. Pathophysiological consequences of atherosclerosis extend into the coronary microcirculation. Restoration of endothelium-dependent responses by L-arginine. *Circ Res* 1992;70:465–476.
54. White CW, Wright CB, Doty DB, Hiratza LF, Eastham CL, Harrison DG, Marcus ML. Does visual interpretation of the coronary arteriogram predict the physiologic importance of a coronary stenosis? *N Engl J Med* 1984;310:819–824.
55. Epstein SE, Talbot TL. Dynamic coronary tone in precipitation, exacerbation, and relief of angina pectoris. *Am J Cardiol* 1981;48: 797–803.

56. Wilson RF, Laughlin DE, Ackell PH, Chilian WM, Holida MD, Hartley CJ, Armstrong ML, Marcus ML, White CW. Transluminal, subselective measurement of coronary artery blood flow velocity and vasodilator reserve in man. *Circulation* 1985;72:82–92.
57. Doucette JW, Corl PD, Payne HM, Flynn AE, Goto M, Nassi M, Segal J. Validation of a Doppler guide wire for intravascular measurement of coronary artery flow velocity. *Circulation* 1992;85:1899–1911.
58. Demer LL, Gould KL, Goldstein RA, Kirkeeide RL, Mullani NA, Smalling RW, Nishikawa A, Merhige ME. Assessment of coronary artery disease severity by positron emission tomography. Comparison with quantitative arteriography in 193 patients. *Circulation* 1989;79:825–835.
59. Uren NG, Melin JA, De Bruyne B, Wijns W, Baudhuin T, Camici PG. Relation between myocardial blood flow and the severity of coronary artery stenoses. *N Engl J Med* 1994;330:1782–1788.
60. Strauer BE. Ventricular function and coronary hemodynamics in hypertensive heart disease. *Am J Cardiol* 1979;44:999–1002.
61. Opherk D, Mall G, Zebe H, Schwarz F, Weihe E, Manthey J, Kubler W. Reduction of coronary reserve: A mechanism for angina pectoris in patients with arterial hypertension and normal coronary arteries. *Circulation* 1984;69:1–7.
62. Vogt M, Motz W, Schwartzkopff B, Strauer BE. Coronary microangiopathy and cardiac hypertrophy. *Eur Heart J* 1990;II(Suppl B):133–138.
63. Houghton JL, Frank MJ, Carr AA, Von Dohlen TW, Prisant LM. Relations among impaired coronary flow reserve, left ventricular hypertrophy, and thallium perfusion defects in hypertensive patients without obstructive coronary artery disease. *J Am Coll Cardiol* 1990;15:43–51.
64. Tanaka M, Fujiwara H, Onodera T, Wu D-J, Matsuda M, Hamashima Y, Kawai C. Quantitative analysis of narrowings of intramyocardial small arteries in normal hearts, hypertensive hearts, and hearts with hypertrophic cardiomyopathy. *Circulation* 1987;75:1130–1139.
65. Schwartzkopff B, Vogt M, Knauer S, Motz W, Strauer BE. Medial hypertrophy of intramural coronary arteries in patients with reduced coronary reserve in hypertensive heart disease. *Circulation* 1991;84:II-479 (abstr).
66. Brush JE, Cannon RO, Schenke WH, Bonow RO, Leon MB, Maron BJ, Epstein SE. Angina due to coronary microvascular disease in hypertensive patients without left ventricular hypertrophy. *N Engl J Med* 1988;319:1302–1307.
67. Treasure CB, Klein JL, Vita JA, Manoukian SV, Renwick GH, Selwyn AP, Ganz P, Alexander RW. Hypertension and left ventricular hypertrophy are associated with impaired endothelium-mediated relaxation in human coronary resistance vessels. *Circulation* 1993;87:86–93.
68. Brush JE, Faxon DP, Salmon S, Jacobs AK, Ryan TJ. Abnormal endothelium-dependent coronary vasomotion in hypertensive patients. *J Am Coll Cardiol* 1992;19:809–815.
69. Quyyumi AA, Cannon RO, Panza JA, Diodati JG, Epstein SE. Endothelial dysfunction in patients with chest pain and normal coronary arteries. *Circulation* 1992;86:1864–1871.
70. Polese A, De Cesare N, Montorsi P, Fabbiocchi F, Guazzi M, Loaldi A, Guazzi MD. Upward shift of the lower range of coronary flow autoregulation in hypertensive patients with hypertrophy of the left ventricle. *Circulation* 1991;83:845–853.
71. Ledet T. Diabetic cardiopathy. Quantitative histological studies of the heart from young juvenile diabetics. *Acta Pathol Microbiol Scand* 1976;84:421–428.
72. Crall FV, Roberts WC. The extramural and intramural coronary arteries in juvenile diabetes mellitus. *Am J Med* 1978;64:221–230.
73. Zoneraich S, Silverman G, Zoneraich O. Primarial myocardial disease, diabetes mellitus and small vessel disease. *Am Heart J* 1980;100:754–755.
74. Sutherland CGG, Fisher BM, Frier BM, Dargie HJ, More JAR, Lindop GBM. Endomyocardial biopsy pathology in insulin-dependent diabetic patients with abnormal ventricular function. *Histopathology* 1989;14:593–602.
75. Sunni S, Bishop SP, Kent SP, Greer JC. Diabetic cardiomyopathy. A morphologic study of intramyocardial arteries. *Arch Pathol Lab Med* 1986;110:375–381.
76. Calver AC, Collier JG, Vallance PJT. Inhibition and stimulation of nitric oxide synthesis on the human forearm arterial bed of patients with insulin-dependent diabetes. *J Clin Invest* 1992;90:2548–2554.
77. Johnstone MT, Creager SJ, Scales KM, Cusco JA, Lee BK, Creager MA. Impaired endothelium-dependent vasodilation in patients with insulin-dependent diabetes mellitus. *Circulation* 1993;88:2510–2516.
78. Ferrannini E, Buzzigoli G, Bonadonna R, Giorico MA, Oleggini M, Graziadei L, Pedrinelli R, Brandi L, Bevilacqua S. Insulin resistance in essential hypertension. *N Engl J Med* 1987;15:350–357.
79. Reaven GM. Role of insulin resistance in human disease. *Diabetes* 1988;37:1595–1609.
80. Anderson EA, Mark AL. The vasodilator action of insulin. Implications for the insulin hypothesis of hypertension. *Hypertension* 1993;21:136–141.
81. Ludmer PL, Selwyn AP, Shook TL, Wayne RR, Mudge GH, Alexander RW, Ganz P. Paradoxical vasoconstriction induced by acetylcholine in atherosclerotic coronary arteries. *N Engl J Med* 1986;315:1046–1051.
82. Hodgson JMcB, Marshall JJ. Direct vasoconstriction and endothelium-dependent vasodilation. Mechanisms of acetylcholine effects on coronary flow and arterial diameter in patients with nonstenotic coronary arteries. *Circulation* 1989;79:1043–1051.
83. Zeiher AM, Drexler H, Wollschlager H, Just H. Modulation of coronary vasomotor tone in humans. Progressive endothelial dysfunction with different early stages of coronary atherosclerosis. *Circulation* 1991;83:391–401.
84. Egashira K, Inou T, Hirooka Y, Yamada A, Maruoka Y, Kai H, Sugimachi M, Suzuki S, Takeshita A. Impaired coronary blood flow response to acetylcholine in patients with coronary risk factors and proximal atherosclerotic lesions. *J Clin Invest* 1993;91:29–37.
85. Werns SW, Walton JA, Hsia HH, Nabel EG, Sanz ML, Pitt B. Evidence of endothelial dysfunction in angiographically normal coronary arteries of patients with coronary artery disease. *Circulation* 1989;79:287–291.
86. Vita JA, Treasure CB, Nabel EG, McLenachan JM, Fish RD, Yeung AC, Vekshtein VI, Selwyn AP, Ganz P. Coronary vasomotor response to acetylcholine relates to risk factors for coronary artery disease. *Circulation* 1990;81:491–497.
87. Egashira K, Inou T, Yamada A, Hirooka Y, Urabe Y, Nagasawa K, Takeshita A. Heterogeneous effects of the endothelium-dependent vasodilators acetylcholine and substance P on the coronary circulation of patients with angiographically normal coronary arteries. *Coron Artery Dis* 1992;3:945–952.
88. Crossman DC, Larkin SW, Dashwood MR, Davies GJ, Yacoub M, Maseri A. Responses of atherosclerotic human coronary arteries in vivo to the endothelium-dependent vasodilator substance P. *Circulation* 1991;84:2001–2010.
89. Forstermann U, Mugge A, Alheid U, Haverich A, Frolich JC. Selective attenuation of endothelium-mediated vasodilation in atherosclerotic coronary arteries. *Circ Res* 1988;62:185–190.
90. Chester AH, O'Neil GS, Moncada S, Tadjkarimi S, Yacoub MH. Low basal and stimulated release of nitric oxide in atherosclerotic epicardial coronary arteries. *Lancet* 1990;336:897–900.
91. Quyyumi AA, Dakak N, Gilligan DM, Andrews NP, Diodati JG, Panza JA, Cannon RO. Peripheral vascular endothelial dysfunction in syndrome X patients and endothelial dysfunction of the coronary microvasculature. *Circulation* 1993;88:I-369 (abstr).
92. Dakak N, Gilligan DM, Andrews NP, Diodati JG, Panza JA, Schenke WH, Cannon RO. Peripheral vascular endothelial dysfunction in patients with multiple coronary risk factors. *Circulation* 1993;88:I-618 (abstr).
93. Creager MA, Cooke JP, Mendelsohn ME, Gallagher SJ, Coleman SM, Loscalzo J, Dzau VJ. Impaired vasodilation of forearm resistance vessels in hypercholesterolemic humans. *J Clin Invest* 1990;86:228–234.
94. Casino PR, Kilcoyne CM, Quyyumi AA, Hoeg JM, Panza JA. The role of nitric oxide in the endothelium-dependent vasodilation of hypercholesterolemic patients. *Circulation* 1993;88:2541–2547.
95. Panza JA, Quyyumi AA, Brush JE Jr, Epstein SE. Abnormal endothelium-dependent vascular relaxation in patients with essential hypertension. *N Engl J Med* 1990;323:22–27.
96. Yeung AC, Vekshtein VI, Krantz DS, Vita JA, Ryan TJ, Ganz P, Selwyn AP. The effect of atherosclerosis on the vasomotor response of coronary arteries to mental stress. *N Engl J Med* 1991;325:1551–1556.
97. Quillen JE, Rossen JD, Oskarsson HJ, Minor RL, Lopez AG, Winniford MD. Acute effect of cigarette smoking on the coronary circulation: Constriction of epicardial and resistance vessels. *J Am Coll Cardiol* 1993;22:642–647.

98. Pupita G, Maseri A, Kaski JC, Galassi AR, Gavrielides S, Davies G, Crea F. Myocardial ischemia caused by distal coronary artery constriction in stable angina pectoris. *N Engl J Med* 1990;323:514–520.
99. Drexler H, Zeiher AM, Meinzer K, Just H. Correction of endothelial dysfunction in coronary microcirculation of hypercholesterolemic patients by L-arginine. *Lancet* 1991;338:1546–1550.
100. Dubois-Rande J-L, Zelinsky R, Roudot F, Chabrier DE, Castaigne A, Geschwind H, Adnot S. Effects of infusion of L-arginine into the left anterior descending coronary artery on acetylcholine-induced vasoconstriction of human atheromatous coronary arteries. *Am J Cardiol* 1992;70:1269–1275.
101. Quyyumi AA, Dakak N, Gilligan DM, Diodati JG, Panza JA, Cannon RO. Effects of L-arginine, the substrate for nitric oxide, on endothelium-dependent vasodilation of the coronary microvascular. *J Am Coll Cardiol* 1993;21:151 (abstr).
102. Reis SE, Gloth ST, Blumenthal RS, Resar JR, Zacur HA, Gerstenblith G, Brinker JA. Ethinyl estradiol acutely attenuates abnormal coronary vasomotor responses to acetylcholine in postmenopausal women. *Circulation* 1994;89:52–60.
103. Gilligan DM, Quyyumi AA, Cannon RO. Effects of physiological levels of estrogen on coronary vasomotor function in postmenopausal women. *Circulation* 1994;89:2545–2551.
104. Dakak N, Quyyumi AA, Eisenhofer G, Goldstein DS, Cannon RO. Effects of cardiac α-adrenergic blockade on coronary vasomotor responses and cardiac norepinephrine kinetics during mental stress in patients with coronary artery disease. *Circulation* 1993;88:I-494 (abstr).
105. Egashira K, Hirooka Y, Kai H, Sugimachi M, Suzuki S, Inou T, Takeshita A. Reduction in serum cholesterol with pravastatin improves endothelium-dependent vasomotion in patients with hypercholesterolemia. *Circulation* 1994;89:2519–2524.
106. Kloner RA, Ganote CE, Jennings RB. The ''no-reflow'' phenomenon after temporary occlusion in the dog. *J Clin Invest* 1974;54: 1496–1508.
107. Braunwald E, Kloner RA, Myocardial reperfusion: A double edged sword. *J Clin Invest* 1985;76:1713–1719.
108. Mehta JL, Nichols WW, Donnelly WH, Lawson DL, Saldeen TGP. Impaired canine coronary vasodilatory response to acetylcholine and bradykinin after occlusion–reperfusion. *Circ Res* 1989;64:43–54.
109. Quillen JE, Selke FW, Brooks LA, Harrison DG. Ischemia–reperfusion impairs endothelium-dependent relaxation of coronary microvessels but does not affect large arteries. *Circulation* 1990;82:586–594.
110. Forman MB, Puett DW, Virmani R. Endothelial and myocardial injury during ischemia and reperfusion: Pathogenesis and therapeutic implications. *J Am Coll Cardiol* 1989;13:450–459.
111. Berk BC. The microcirculation in coronary ischemia. Are native anticoagulant mechanisms a path to new therapies? *Circulation* 1991;84: 439–441.
112. Snow TR, Deal MT, Dickey DT, Esmon CT. Protein C activation following coronary artery occlusion in the in situ porcine heart. *Circulation* 1991;84:293–299.
113. Shlafer M, Kane PF, Wiggins VY, Kirsh MM. Possible role for cytotoxic oxygen metabolites in the pathogenesis of cardiac ischemic injury. *Circulation* 1982;66(Suppl I):I-85–I-139.
114. Wilson RF, Johnson MR, Marcus ML, Aylward PEG, Skorton DJ, Collins S, White CW. The effect of coronary angioplasty on coronary flow reserve. *Circulation* 1988;77:873–885.
115. Kern MJ, Deligonul U, Vandormael M, Labovitz A, Gudipati CV, Gabliani G, Bodet J, Shah Y, Kennedy HL. Impaired coronary vasodilator reserve in the immediate postcoronary angioplasty period: Analysis of coronary artery flow velocity indexes and regional cardiac venous efflux. *J Am Coll Cardiol* 1989;13:860–872.
116. El-Tamimi H, Graham JD, Sritara P, Hackett D, Crea F, Maseri A. Inappropriate constriction of small coronary vessels as a possible cause of a positive exercise test early after successful coronary angioplasty. *Circulation* 1991;84:2307–2312.
117. Joelson JM, Most AS, Williams DO. Angiographic findings when chest pain recurs after successful percutaneous transluminal coronary angioplasty. *Am J Cardiol* 1987;60:792–795.
118. Fujita M, Mikuniya A, Takahashi M, Gaddis R, Hartley J, McKown D, Franklin O. Acceleration of coronary collateral development by heparin in conscious dogs. *Jpn Circ J* 1987;51:395–402.
119. Fujita M, Sasayama S, Asanoi H, Nakajima H, Sakai O, Ohno A. Improvement of treadmill capacity and collateral circulation as a result of exercise with heparin pretreatment in patients with effort angina. *Circulation* 1988;77:1022–1029.
120. Quyyumi AA, Diodati JG, Lakatos E, Bonow RO, Epstein SE. Angiogenic effects of low molecular weight heparin in patients with stable coronary artery disease: A pilot study. *J Am Coll Cardiol* 1993; 22:635–641.
121. Yanagisawa-Miwa A, Uchida Y, Nakamura F, Tomaru T, Kido H, Kamijo T, Sugimoto T, Kaji K, Utsoyama M, Kurashima C, Ito H. Salvage of infarcted myocardium by angiogenic action of basic fibroblast growth factor. *Science* 1992;257:1401–1403.
122. Unger EF, Banai S, Shou M, Lazarous DF, Jaklitsch MT, Scheinowitz M, Correa R, Klingbeil C, Epstein SE. Basic fibroblast growth factor enhances myocardial collateral flow in a canine model. *Am J Physiol* 1994;266:H1588–H1595.
123. Banai S, Jaklitsch MT, Shou M, Lazarous DF, Scheinowitz M, Biro S, Epstein SE, Unger EF. Angiogenic-induced enhancement of collateral blood flow to ischemic myocardium by vascular endothelial growth factor in dogs. *Circulation* 1994;89:2183–2189.

PART III

Acute Myocardial Infarction

Pathophysiology

Atherosclerosis and Coronary Artery Disease,
edited by V. Fuster, R. Ross, and E. J. Topol.
Lippincott-Raven Publishers, Philadelphia © 1996.

CHAPTER 45

Pathology of Myocardial Infarction and Reperfusion

John T. Fallon

Key Words: Coagulation necrosis; Infarct; Ischemia; Myocardial infarction; Reperfusion.

INTRODUCTION

Myocardial infarction is defined as the necrosis of cardiac tissue due to ischemia that results in the replacement of myocardium by dense fibrotic scar. The major functional consequence of myocardial infarction is a decrease of systolic compliance, i.e., pump function, for the chamber in whose wall the loss of muscle occurs. In addition, myocardial infarction often results in electrical instability within the heart muscle and the generation of fatal arrhythmias. Myocardial infarction is a common occurrence and is a major cause of morbidity and mortality throughout the Western world. While myocardial infarction is most often a sequelae of atherosclerotic disease of the epicardial coronary arteries, there are many other diseases which cause myocardial ischemia and result in myocardial infarction (see other chapters in this book). This chapter focuses on the pathologic aspects of myocardial infarction from its inception through the healing process.

ISCHEMIA

Myocardial infarction is not a primary event, but is always due to ischemia. Ischemia is defined as an imbalance between oxygen supply and oxygen demand. Actively contracting myocardial tissue is exquisitely sensitive to oxygen supply and myocardial ischemia is often caused by a decrease in oxygen supply secondary to impaired coronary artery blood flow, e.g., as seen in the clinical syndrome of angina at rest. Likewise, coronary blood flow may be inadequate to meet the oxygen demands of a stressed myocardium, also resulting in ischemia, e.g., stable angina pectoris.

Thus, ischemia is produced in the myocardium as a result of either a decreased oxygen supply or an increased oxygen demand. The imbalance created is not an all-or-nothing phenomenon. Ischemia occurs as a continuum of degrees between none and complete. Myocardial infarction occurs when ischemia of any degree occurs for a length of time sufficient to cause irreversible injury, i.e., necrosis of myocytes. Furthermore, the degree of ischemia and the length of time of ischemia necessary to cause the necrosis of myocardium are not fixed. This phenomenon was first shown by the experimental studies of Reimer and Jennings on ''the wavefront of infarction'' (1). Briefly, coronary occlusion was performed creating a region of complete ischemia (an area at risk) in the left ventricle. At varying times after the onset of ischemia, the coronary occlusion was released and coronary reflow allowed to occur, thus interrupting and reversing the ischemic insult. Following reflow, animals were allowed to recover and then killed at a later time and the hearts examined pathologically for the presence of myocardial infarction. The results of such experiments reveal that short periods of complete ischemia produce necrosis of subendocardial myocardium. Increasing the ischemic time re-

J. T. Fallon: Cardiovascular Institute and Department of Pathology, Mount Sinai School of Medicine, New York, New York 10029.

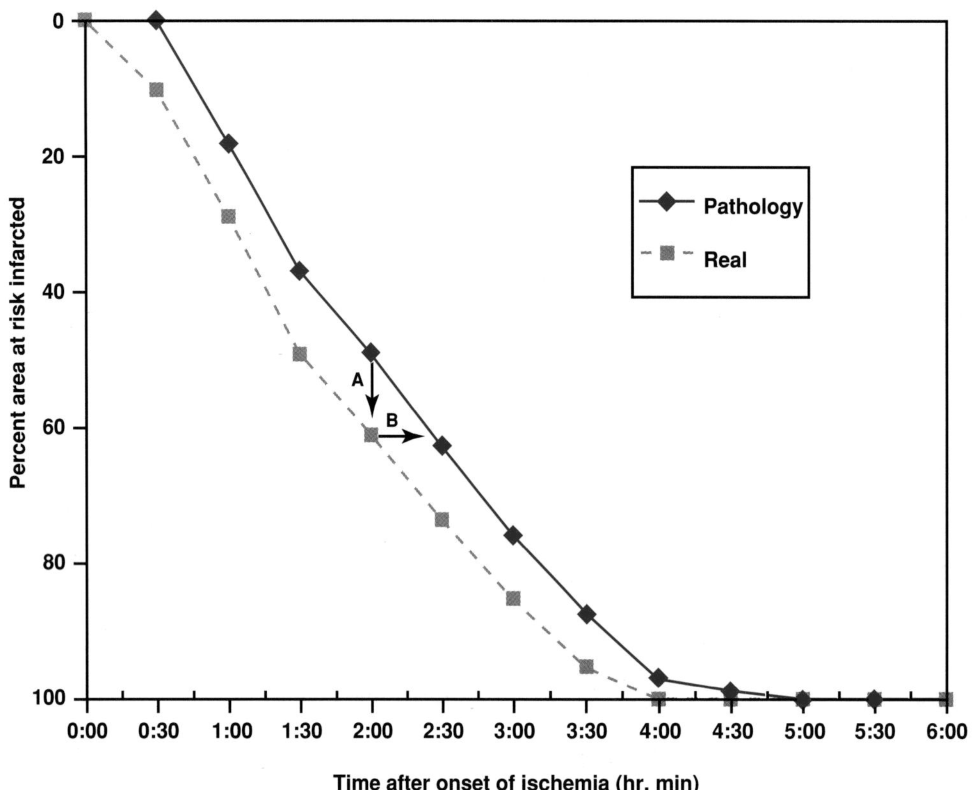

FIG. 1. Hypothetical curves showing the development of myocardial infarction in a 100% ischemic zone at risk. *Upper solid curve:* the pathologically discernible curve; *lower dashed curve:* the true irreversible injury curve. If an infarct is examined after 2 hr of ischemia by even the most sensitive and specific pathologic techniques, an infarct of 50% of the area at risk will be demonstrated. However, the true infarct size is closer to 60% *(arrow A).* Reperfusion at 2 hr with survival and then pathologic assessment results in an infarct of 60% of the area at risk. This represents the "real" infarct size at 2 hr. The 10% difference in infarct sizes is often referred to as due to "reperfusion injury," but probably represents the portion of the infarct that cannot be seen by current pathologic methods for discerning irreversible cell injury.

sults in progression of necrosis from the subendocardium toward the epicardium and laterally toward the borders of the area at risk. It takes several hours for complete infarction of the area at risk (Fig. 1). Thus, the process of myocardial infarction in a completely ischemic area at risk occurs over time as a wavefront from subendocardium outward toward the borders of the area at risk. The rate of progression of infarction varies among species and for the location of the area at risk within the heart. Extrapolation of these experimental studies to humans is the basis for the success of current early reperfusion therapies of the treatment of acute myocardial infarction (2).

REPERFUSION

In humans, myocardial necrosis begins in the subendocardium 30–40 min after the onset of coronary occlusion and it takes approximately 4 hr of coronary occlusion to infarct completely an area at risk. However, the exact time to complete infarction is influenced by a number of other factors including collateral circulation, prior ischemic events, neurologic reflexes, metabolic state, activity level, and concurrent drug therapy.

Restoration of coronary flow at any time prior to complete infarction results in sparing of myocardium within the zone at risk. Whether or not the reestablishing coronary flow also causes ''reperfusion injury'' is controversial (3,4). Reperfusion injury is the increase in infarct volume caused by restoration of flow. Theoretically, reperfusion is thought to produce more myocardial cell necrosis by causing formation of free radicals in noninfarcted but ischemic myocardium (3). However, experimental studies using agents that scavenge free radicals do not significantly reduce infarct size (4). Figure 1 depicts a more likely scenario to explain what has been called reperfusion injury, suggesting that reperfusion injury is really an artifact of the pathologic evaluation of myocyte necrosis, i.e., the lack of a gold standard.

TYPES OF INFARCTS

The major types of ventricular myocardial infarction are regional transmural (Q-wave infarction), regional subendocardial (non-Q-wave infarction), and circumferential subendocardial infarction. The former two types of infarcts are usually the result of occlusive lesions in one of the major epicardial coronary arteries, whereas the latter is often the sequelae of a hypotensive event. Pathologically, a transmural infarction is defined as an area of myocardial necrosis involving more than half of the ventricular wall thickness and a subendocardial or nontransmural infarction is defined as the involvement of less than half the wall thickness. Transmural infarcts are usually large contiguous zones of infarction with relatively sharply defined borders, whereas subendocardial infarcts are often patchy and irregular in their involvement of the inner ventricular wall with intercourant myocardium that is not infarcted.

Regional infarcts are also defined by their location in the ventricular wall. The common forms of regional infarcts are anterior, apical, lateral, posterior, and inferior. There is often some confusion in the naming of infarcts by location because of the lack of common clinical, i.e., electrocardiographic, and pathologic terms for the same location. However, understanding the relationship of an infarct to the etiologic epicardial coronary lesion is the most important pathophysiologic aspect for both clinicians and pathologists.

Myocardial ischemia may occur at any site within the heart and, depending on its degree and length of time, may result in myocyte necrosis. Regional infarcts are one end of the spectrum of ischemic heart disease, but it should also be noted that ischemia may produce less pathologically apparent infarction and fibrosis in areas of the heart that are nonetheless vital to cardiac function and survival. For example, ischemia of the sinoatrial node may result in dysfunction, if not infarction, and clinically produce the sick sinus syndrome. Similarly, inadequate blood supply in the atrioventricular nodal artery may give rise to ischemia and even infarction with fibrosis of the atrioventricular node or its proximal branches, leading to varying degrees of clinically apparent atrioventricular conduction blocks. Likewise, ischemia or isolated infarction of a papillary muscle of the mitral valve may result in mitral regurgitation without other clinical signs or symptoms of ischemic heart disease. Finally, subclinical subendocardial infarcts that result in small foci of fibrosis in the ventricular myocardium may result in a lethal outcome due to arrhythmia.

PHASES OF INFARCTION

The pathologic process of myocardial infarction may be divided into four major phases: (a) ischemic insult, (b) coagulation necrosis, (c) healing, and (d) scarring.

Ischemic Insult

The *first phase* of myocardial infarction is the period of acute ischemia insult between 0 and 4 h following coronary occlusion. As noted above, coronary occlusion may result in complete ischemia to a region of myocardium at risk. Within a few beats after cessation of coronary flow, the ischemic myocardium stops beating (loss of systolic function) and shortly thereafter the ischemic region becomes relatively electrically silent (ST changes on EKG). However, irreversible changes indicative of necrosis, such as leakage of cytoplasmic enzymes and ultrastructural demonstration of sarcoplasmic disruption, are not evident until complete ischemia is about 40 min in duration (5,6). Even then, the morphologic changes of irreversible myocytic injury are only evident in the subendocardial myocytes. If reperfusion occurs prior to this time, infarction does not occur, although the contractile function of the ischemic myocardial cells may not return for several hours after such an ischemic insult. The latter phenomenon is termed ''myocardial stunning'' (7). Interestingly, Caulfield et al. *(personal communication,* 1994) have demonstrated a rapid loss of the normal extracellular connective tissue support structures within ischemic myocardium following even brief periods of ischemia. They hypothesize that stunning is a result of this loss. Experimentally and now clinically, reperfusion at any time before approximately 4 hr after onset results in salvage of myocardium within the epicardial and lateral borders of the zone at risk, as predicted from the experimental studies of Reimer and Jennings. After 4 hr of complete ischemia, the zone at risk of myocardium is essentially totally infarcted. Vascular endothelial integrity is also lost with time, resulting in diapedis of red blood cells into the interstitial spaces or occlusion of the small arteries and arterioles by swollen endothelial cells and platelet plugs at the periphery of an infarct zone. Reperfusion of such an infarct zone within the next few hours results in either ''hemorrhagic'' infarction or a ''no-reflow'' phenomenon, depending on the integrity and/or the ability of blood to enter the capillaries and veins of the infarct zone, respectively.

Gross and histologic examinations of hearts after 4 hr of complete regional ischemia show virtually no pathologic changes indicative of myocardial infarction. Electron microscopic studies reveal evidence of myocyte necrosis such as sarcolemmal disruption (8), mitochondrial matrix granules, and clumping of nuclear chromatin. Histochemical studies using a tetrazolium dye are useful in delineating regional infarcts of this age (9). In the presence of an appropriate substrate, these dyes are reduced to a colored formazan that stains noninfarcted myocardium. With the impairment of the reducing enzyme systems in irreversibly injured myocardium, there is no staining of the infarct. Careful histologic examination of sections of myocardium, taken with the guidance of tetrazolium staining, often reveal ''contraction band necrosis'' in a narrow band of myocytes at the periphery of an infarct. In addition, careful examination of viable myocardium at the peripheral region may also reveal the presence of dilated venules containing neutrophils beginning to marginate prior to emigrating into the neighboring necrotic region. The myocardium in the center of an infarct most often appears histologically normal at this time. However, in large transmural regional infarcts the so-called "wavy fiber" change may be seen in histologic sections taken parallel to the long axis of the myocytes (10). Wavy myocytes are characterized by thinning of individual cells and undulations of individual cells, groups of cells, and bundles of myocytes. This histologic feature is diagnostic of myocardial infarction, but unfortunately is not always present. "Wavy fibers" result from stretching of the nonfunctional infarcted myocardium by either neighboring contracting muscle or the dyskinetic motion of the infarcted myocardium during ventricular systole. In either case, this histologic feature is also an early indicator of "infarct expansion," a process that results in thinning of the infarcted ventricular wall and area enlargement of the infarct zone (11). Both "wavy fibers" and "infarct expansion" may occur as the result of an acute loss of compliance resulting from the dissolution of the normal interstitial connective tissue support structure in the ischemically injured myocardium.

Coagulation Necrosis

The *second phase* of myocardial infarction is the development of coagulation necrosis and the onset of acute inflammation, which occurs between 4 and 48 hr following coronary occlusion. In contrast to the first phase, neither this phase nor subsequent phases are interrupted or reversed by the process of reperfusion.

As mentioned above, reperfusion after 4 hr of complete ischemia may result in either a hemorrhagic infarct or no reflow. However, clinical thrombolysis studies have shown a long-term functional benefit of coronary reperfusion successfully performed as late as 12 hr after onset. The pathologic basis for this is not known, although it is presumed that late reperfusion may hasten the healing process. Reperfusion of an established myocardial infarct, at any time results in an accentuated release of myocytic cytoplasmic enzymes, e.g., creatine kinase-MB, and the subsequent appearance of large concentration peaks of these enzymes in the blood.

Routine histologic sections of myocardial infarcts early (6–12 hr) in the second phase reveal hypereosinophilia of myocytes and prominent margination of neutrophils in venules at the periphery of the infarct. The hypereosinophilia represents a loss of basophilic staining components of the myocyte sarcoplasm, in particular, RNA. The nuclei of the myocytes also become pyknotic, i.e., shrunken and deeply stained. These histologic features are classically termed coagulation necrosis and are seen in all organs and tissues as a result of ischemia injury. The pathology of human myocardial infarction and the process of coagulation necrosis are described in exquisite detail in the classic paper from 1939 by Mallory et al. (12).

At autopsy, a myocardial infarct is grossly appreciated only if the patient survives for at least 12 hr after onset. On cut section, infarcted myocardium of 12–24 hr appears as a pale, slightly discolored region sometimes with a thin border of red tissue which represents vascular congestion in the peripheral intact myocardium.

A very common problem for the pathologist is dating or timing of myocardial infarcts. This important question is often raised by clinicians, family, and forensic investigators. Precise dating is an extremely difficult proposition, but there are a few hallmarks of the coagulation necrosis process that are helpful in pinpointing the time of onset of a myocardial infarction (Fig. 2). Disappearance of myocyte nuclei is a common feature of infarcts that are 24 hr or older; thus, histologic sections of hypereosinophilic myocardium showing intact nuclei are less than 24 hr old, but greater than 6 hr. In contrast, hypereosinophilic myocardium without nuclei represents an infarction process greater than 24 hr old. After 24 hr, dating of infarcts is less precise and is based on the histologic character of the inflammatory healing process at the periphery of the infarct. The presence of large numbers of neutrophils at the periphery is indicative of an infarct that is less than 72 hr old, whereas the presence of predominantly mononuclear inflammatory cells in this location suggests an infarct greater than 72 hr. The presence of neutrophils in myocardial infarcts is rather brief. These cells degranulate and disintegrate within just a few hours. The neutrophilic response occurs at the periphery of infarcts, producing enzymatic dissolution of cells and extracellular matrix confined to the infarcted region. In large regional infarcts, neutrophilic infiltration does not penetrate into the central portions of the infarcted tissue. The central portions of an infarct are thus not dissolved by the enzymatic activity of neutrophils, but are rather removed by the activity of macrophages over the course of weeks and even months. The central area of such an infarct is often referred to as "mummified." Contrary to classical descriptions, infarcted myocytes often do maintain cross-striations, a feature that has been said to be lost early in the infarct process.

Healing

The *third phase* of myocardial infarction is the healing phase, which begins at about 72 hr. Gross observation in the autopsy room of hearts with a regional, transmural infarction may show a zone of shaggy fibrinous exudate on the epicardial surface overlying the infarct region. This represents extension of the acute inflammatory reaction to the epicardium and is the basis for the early infarct-related pericarditis (13). Grossly, an infarct of this age may also show evidence of mural thrombus on the endocardial surface of the infarcted region. In subendocardial infarcts and even in large transmural infarcts, the immediately subjacent endocardial myocytes are usually spared from the infarction process probably because they are able to derive enough oxygen supply directly from the ventricular blood. In infarcts with this spared endocardial zone, mural thrombus is usually not present. However, in large transmural infarcts, necrosis may extend to

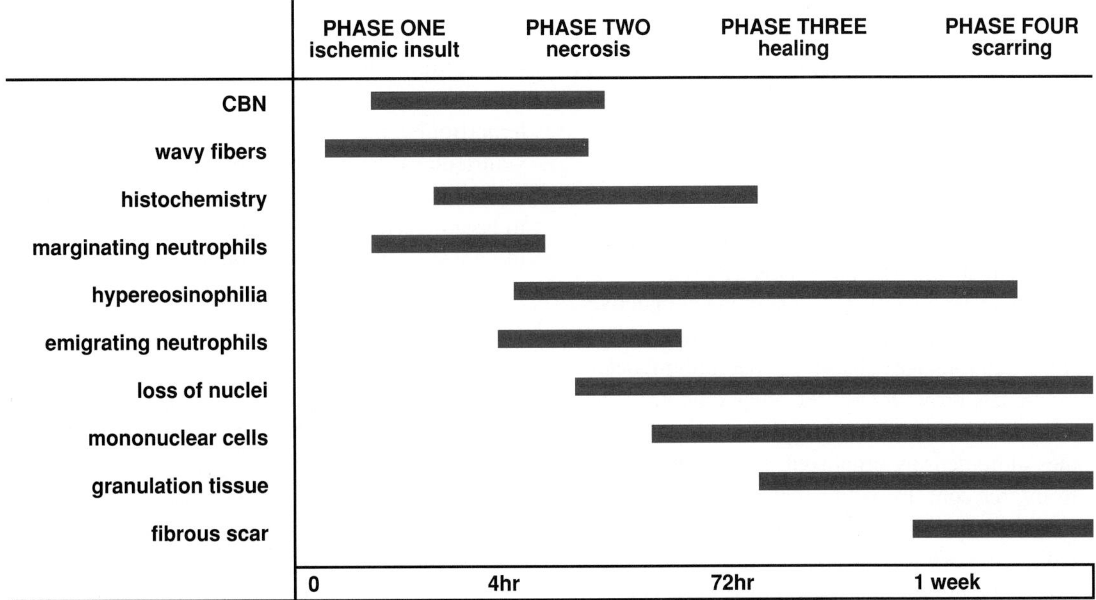

FIG. 2. Major morphologic features of each phase of myocardial infarction that may be helpful in dating an infarct. The best site to observe these findings is at the periphery of the infarct zone. CBN, Contraction band necrosis.

involve the endocardium and thus promote mural thrombus formation due to a local inflammatory activation of coagulation.

Gross observation of the cut section of infarcted myocardium during this phase shows a yellow coloration of the infarct and a distinct red border zone. The yellow color has been ascribed to neutrophilic infiltration, but is actually due to a loss of the normal brown color of myocardium secondary to the breakdown and loss of myoglobin from the necrotic myocytes in the infarct. Histologic sections of the infarct border show that the grossly visible red border consists of a mononuclear cell infiltrate containing macrophages, T cells, and plasma cells, with dilation of the small vessels of the adjacent intact myocardium and interstitial edema. This process continues and is well established by 96 hr as the nuclear remnants of the early neutrophilic infiltration are resolved.

During the early portion of the healing phase (48–96 hr), the infarcted myocardium is most susceptible to rupture. The muscle is necrotic and the supporting interstitial connective tissues are destroyed. The tensile strength of the wall is lost and its integrity depends solely on the ability of the surrounding intact myocardium and epicardial tissues to hold the infarcted tissue together. Fortunately, even for large, regional transmural infarcts, an epicardial border zone of intact tissue often exists and is apparently compliant enough to withstand the increased wall stresses since only 10–15% of such infarcts rupture. While most ruptures occur during this time, they may also occur earlier or slightly later, but all ruptures occur within infarcted myocardium usually via serpiginous tears near the border of the infarct. Depending on the regional location of the infarct, ruptures may result in acute onset of mitral regurgitation due to papillary muscle rupture, a predominantly left-to-right shunt secondary to ventricular septal rupture (14), or sudden death due to free wall rupture, hemopericardium, and resulting pericardial tamponade. Rarely, a free wall rupture is contained by the overlying pericardium that is adherent to the epicardium secondary to the early inflammatory reaction of the infarction process. Such a contained rupture is the basis for development of a ventricular pseudoaneurysm in which the wall of the aneurysm body is composed only of parietal pericardium and connects to the ventricular chamber via a thin neck which was the original rupture site in the ventricular free wall.

The process of infarct expansion that begins in the earliest phase of myocardial infarction continues into the healing phase. Large, regional transmural infarcts, particularly those involving the apex or anterolateral wall of the left ventricle, commonly undergo the process of expansion due to the loss of tensile strength within the infarcted tissue. The necrotic muscle is stretched, resulting in thinning of the wall and enlargement of the infarct area, but not its volume. The end result of this expansion process is a true aneurysm of the ventricular wall. Such aneurysm formation is often accompanied by variable amounts of mural thrombus on the endocardial wall.

As the healing phase continues past 96 hr following onset of the ischemic injury, the mononuclear inflammatory infiltration continues at the periphery of the infarct, slowly progressing inward into the necrotic muscle. Capillary sprouts and fibroblasts are present at the border and with increasing time these are also seen to progress further into the infarct region. Grossly, at this time, the central portion of the infarct is yellow and border zones have a gelatinous appearance due to the presence of granulation tissue composed as noted above. Large transmural infarcts may take weeks to months for the granulation tissue to replace completely the necrotic myocardium.

Scarring

The *fourth phase* begins approximately 1 week after the onset of the ischemic insult. The advancing granulation tissue begins to be replaced by collagen-containing connective tissue. Initially a loose network of collagen is laid down by fibroblasts as the macrophages absorb the necrotic myocardium and new vessels grow in with the advancing granulation tissue. As more necrotic tissue is replaced, the collagen matrix becomes more densely organized, eventually replacing the entire infarct zone by white scar. By 2 weeks the scarring phase is usually well established. If the infarct is relatively small, dense white scar tissue is seen grossly replacing a region of the myocardial wall. If the infarct is large and expansion with aneurysm formation has occurred, the wall becomes a thin fibrous capsule bulging outward. Unorganized mural thrombus and dystrophic calcification are common features of such ventricular aneurysm walls. Over time, ventricular aneurysms may slowly expand, but in contrast to either vascular "true" aneurysms or the rare ventricular pseudoaneurysm, such ventricular aneurysms do not rupture. Occasionally, ventricular mural thrombus either overlying a healing infarct or within an aneurysm is a source of systemic thromboemboli.

In contrast to the dense scars and fibrotic aneurysms of the large transmural infarcts, subendocardial infarcts and to some extent small regional infarcts, particularly those of the inferior wall, may undergo a remodeling process that results in their virtual disappearance with time. Scar tissue in the myocardium is like scar tissue elsewhere in the body in that it is constantly, albeit slowly, undergoing change. Over the course of months to years, an infarct scar may be completely resorbed. This is accomplished by the process of fatty metamorphosis of the scar and by compensatory hypertrophy of neighboring intact myocytes. Years after a well-documented inferior myocardial infarction, the pathologist examining the heart at autopsy may see no gross evidence of old myocardial infarction. Histologically, the only telltale signs are the presence of small interstitial islands of fatty tissue among hypertrophied myocytes: thus, the disappearing infarct.

Compensatory hypertrophy of myocytes also occurs in the surviving myocardium after a large transmural myocardial infarction. This myocyte hypertrophy is usually of the eccentric type and occurs in response to ventricular volume overload resulting from loss of ventricular systolic function and the secondary ventricular increase of diastolic volume. This hypertrophy may initially prevent further deterioration in ventricular function following myocardial infarction, but as with other forms of myocardial hypertrophy, often gives rise to later deterioration of ventricular function and the inevitable onset of chronic heart failure.

REFERENCES

1. Reimer KA, Jennings RB. The "wavefront phenomenon" of myocardial ischemic cell death: II. Transmural progression of necrosis within the framework of ischemic bed size (myocardium at risk) and collateral flow. *Lab Invest* 1979;40:633–644.
2. Gold HK, Fallon JT, Yasuda T, Leinbach RC, Khaw BA, Newell JB, Guerrero JL, Vislosky FM, Hoyng CF, Grossbard E, Collen D. Coronary thrombolysis with recombinant human tissue-type plasminogen activator. *Circulation* 1984;70:700–707.
3. Ambrosio G, Becker LC, Hutchins GM, Weisman HF, Weisfeldt ML. Reduction in experimental infarct size by recombinant human superoxide dismutase: insights into the pathophysiology of reperfusion injury. *Circulation* 1986;74:1424–1433.
4. Nejima J, Knight DR, Fallon JT, Uemura N, Manders WT, Canfield DR, Cohen MV, Vatner SF. Superoxide dismutase reduces reperfusion arrhythmias but fails to salvage regional function or myocardium at risk in conscious dogs. *Circulation* 1989;79:143–153.
5. Vatner ST, Heyndrickx GR, Fallon JT. Effects of brief periods of myocardial ischemia on regional myocardial function and creatine kinase release in conscious dogs and baboons. *Can J Cardiol* 1986;(SupplA): 19–24.
6. Fulghum TG, McMahon M, Aretz T, Khaw BA, Fallon JT, Haber E, Powell WJ. The time course of canine ischemic myocardial necrosis evaluated by immunocytochemistry using cardiac myosin specific monoclonal antibodies *in vivo*. *J Appl Cardiol* 1986;1:385–401.
7. Patel B, Kloner RA, Przyklenk K, Braunwald E. Postischemic myocardial "stunning": a clinically relevant phenomenon. *Ann Intern Med* 1988;108:626–628.
8. Frame LH, Lopez A, Khaw BA, Fallon JT, Haber E, Powell WJ. Early membrane damage during coronary reperfusion in dogs. Detection by radiolabelled anticardiac myosin $(Fab')_2$). *J Clin Invest* 1983;72: 535–544.
9. Fallon JT. Postmortem histochemical techniques. In: Wagner GS, ed. *Myocardial infarction: measurement and intervention.* Boston: Martinus Nijhoff; 1982:373–384.
10. Bouchardy B, Majno G. Histopathology of early myocardial infarcts. A new approach. *Am J Pathol* 1974;74:301–330.
11. Weiss JL, Marino PN, Shapiro EP. Myocardial infarct expansion: recognition, significance and pathology. *Am J Cardiol* 1991;68:35D–40D.
12. Mallory GK, White PD, Salcedo-Salgar J. The speed and healing of myocardial infarction. *Am Heart J* 1939;18:647–658.
13. Waller BF. The pathology of acute myocardial infarction: definition, location, pathogenesis, effects of reperfusion, complications, and sequelae. *Cardiol Clin* 1988;6:1–28.
14. Radford MJ, Johnson RA, Daggett WM, Fallon JT, et al. Ventricular septal rupture: a review of clinical and physiologic features and an analysis of survival. *Circulation* 1981;64:545–553.

Atherosclerosis and Coronary Artery Disease,
edited by V. Fuster, R. Ross, and E. J. Topol.
Lippincott-Raven Publishers, Philadelphia © 1996.

CHAPTER 46

Coronary Pathophysiology and Angiographic Correlations in Acute Myocardial Infarction

John A. Ambrose

Key Words: Angiography; Myocardial infarction; Non-Q-wave infarction; Occlusion; Reperfusion.

INTRODUCTION

Since its inception, coronary angiography has been the "gold standard" for the in vivo diagnosis of coronary artery disease. The presence and extent of coronary artery disease as determined by angiography directly correlate with the presence of symptoms and/or noninvasive evidence of ischemia (1–3). The extent of coronary artery disease also correlates with the short- and long-term prognosis of the patient (4,5). Angiography has also been essential for the development of major therapeutic advances in cardiology. Without angiography, coronary bypass surgery, angioplasty, and thrombolytic therapy would have been impossible. In addition, because coronary angiography is "a window inside the heart," it has provided great insight into the pathophysiology of various clinical syndromes such as acute myocardial infarction, unstable angina, Prinzmetal's angina, and sudden death.

In this chapter we consider the coronary pathophysiology of acute myocardial infarction as defined by angiographic techniques. However, before considering this topic, we must briefly discuss angiography and its limitations in assessing the presence and extent of atherosclerosis. Some of these aspects are also discussed in other chapters.

ANGIOGRAPHIC ANALYSIS OF CORONARY ARTERY DISEASE

Atherosclerosis and Nonluminal Narrowing

When performing an angiogram one commonly assumes that an artery or segment without luminal narrowing is free of atherosclerosis and that the severity of a focal lesion can be measured by comparison with an adjacent, nondiseased portion. In validating these assumptions, early investigators compared pre- or postmortem angiographic assessment to postmortem analysis of the coronary arteries. Some studies showed, overall, a good correlation between angiography

J. A. Ambrose: Cardiac Catheterization Laboratory, Mount Sinai Hospital, New York, New York 10029.

and postmortem analysis, but many other studies indicated significant underestimation of atherosclerosis by angiography (6–8). However, these morphological studies did not pressure-fix the arteries at normal perfusion pressures. Lack of pressure fixation may overestimate the degree of narrowing detected pathologically (in comparison to angiography) by collapsing the lumen. Even with pressure fixation, later investigators showed overestimation with angiography in a substantial portion of segments (9–11). Because angiography visualizes only the lumen and not the thickness of the wall, it is easy to see how it might underestimate the degree of atherosclerosis. When atherosclerosis is diffuse, angiography may be analogous to visualizing the hole in a donut. One cannot determine the size of the donut (the degree of atherosclerosis) by examining the hole. More recent information with other techniques such as intravascular ultrasound also corroborates this underestimation by angiography of the amount of atherosclerotic narrowing (12–14).

Vessel Remodeling

This represents another potential source of error in angiographic analysis. Histological analysis of pressure-fixed arteries indicates that the lumen of a human coronary artery enlarges in relation to plaque area, and the appearance of functionally important luminal stenoses may be delayed until lesions occupy about 40% of the internal elastic lamina area (15). This enlargement represents a compensation to maintain a normal luminal opening. Additionally, postmortem angiographic comparisons to histological cross sections of proximal arteries indicate that compensatory enlargement of the lumen is a significant cause of angiographic underestimation of atherosclerotic lesions (16). This may particularly affect eccentric lesions, which geometrically represent about 75% of all atherosclerotic plaques as detected at autopsy (17). Atrophy of the media overlying an eccentric plaque and resulting in its outward displacement represents one of the mechanisms whereby luminal opening is maintained during the development of these lesions. With intravascular ultrasound, the increase in total arterial area is proportional to the amount of plaque, and compensatory enlargement is a focal process that does not affect the normal adjacent arterial segments (18) (Fig. 1).

Intravascular Ultrasound and Angioscopy as Adjuncts to Angiography

The use of intravascular ultrasound and percutaneous angioscopy that do not rely on postmortem comparisons have given us a reliable and more easily accessible method of studying the relationship of angiography to the degree of atherosclerosis and the presence of intraluminal thrombus. As was noted for postmortem studies, angiography tends to underestimate atherosclerosis in comparison to ultrasound, although minimal lumen diameter correlates better between these two techniques than does the amount of atherosclerosis. In one study of mildly diseased arteries by angiography, Porter et al. found, in 67 segments in 37 vessels, a mean arterial area narrowing by ultrasound of 36 ± 20% compared to a mean percentage area stenosis by quantitative angiography of 19 ± 23% ($p < 0.001$) (13). Minimal lumen diameters were closer (3.3 ± 0.9 mm by ultrasound and 2.7 ± 0.8 mm by angiography), although there was still a tendency to underestimate with angiography.

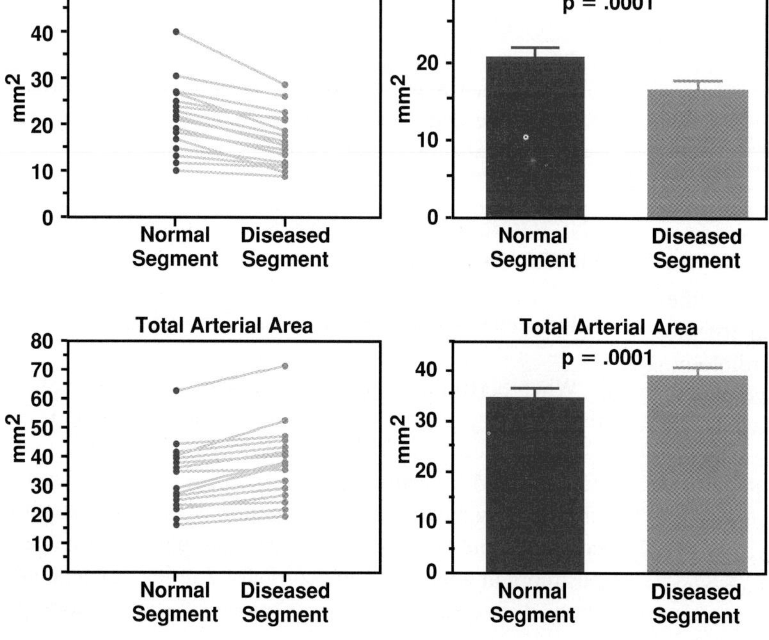

FIG. 1. *Plots* and *bar graphs* of luminal cross-sectional area **(top)** and total arterial area **(bottom)** of paired normal and atherosclerotic vessel segments in superficial femoral arteries examined with intravascular ultrasound (IVUS). **Top left:** Dimensions of paired segments from individual arteries demonstrating the expected decrease in luminal area in the diseased segments. **Bottom left:** Change in total arterial area in the same vessel segments, disclosing an associated consistent increase in total arterial area. The graphs on the **right** show the mean change in luminal area and total arterial area in the same superficial femoral artery segments studies with IVUS. (From Losordo et al., ref. 18, with permission.)

Percutaneous coronary angioscopy is another in vivo technique for evaluating the coronary arteries (19). Here, the intimal surface may be visualized so that plaque may be differentiated from thrombus, and in some cases plaque ulceration may be identified. Following angioplasty, angioscopy may easily identify intimal dissection. Thrombus is noted more frequently with angioscopy than with angiography. Both sensitivity and specificity for thrombus detection are higher with angioscopy in comparison to angiography (20,21).

ANGIOGRAPHIC FINDINGS IN ACUTE MYOCARDIAL INFARCTION

In spite of these limitations of angiography in the assessment of atherosclerosis and in some cases thrombosis, angiography has been vital in understanding coronary anatomy and pathophysiology within the first few hours following myocardial infarction. Although acute myocardial infarction had previously been considered a contraindication to performing coronary arteriography (22), DeWood et al. and other investigators studied early angiographic findings in acute myocardial infarction in the late 1970s (23,24). The incidence of total coronary occlusion of the infarct lesion within the first 12 h of infarction ranges between 66% and 86%. The incidence of total occlusion for patients presenting with transmural ischemia was higher within the first 6 h following infarction than in the subsequent hours after presentation. In the study by DeWood et al., total occlusion was found in 87% within 4 h; this dropped to 68% between 6 and 12 h and to 65% from 12 to 24 h after onset of symptoms (23). Angiographic features of total occlusion suggesting coronary thrombosis included persistent staining of intraluminal material by the contrast agent and a convex border at the site of occlusion. In patients with definite angiographic features of thrombus, DeWood et al. recovered thrombi surgically in 88% of arteries (23). Intracoronary infusions of thrombolytic agents were able to open totally occluded arteries in approximately 70% of cases, which also indicated the presence of acute thrombus at the site of coronary occlusion (24,25).

In patients presenting with non-Q-wave infarction, the incidence of total coronary occlusion before hospital discharge averages about 50% (26). This was significantly higher than the incidence of total occlusion before hospital discharge in Q-wave infarction. Two other studies reported an incidence of total occlusion between 20% and 40% after non-Q infarction (27,28). In patients with non-Q-wave infarction and total occlusion, coronary collaterals can frequently be demonstrated. These collaterals are infrequently present within the first 12 h following Q-wave myocardial infarction. In only about 30% of patients presenting with transmural infarction can collaterals to the distal vessel be demonstrated angiographically (29). In contrast to the above findings in acute myocardial infarction, the incidence of total coronary occlusion of the culprit vessel in unstable angina in patients presenting even with rest angina is in the range of 10% to 15% (30,31). As in non-Q-wave infarction, most patients with total coronary occlusion and unstable angina have collaterals present that fill the vessel distal to the obstruction (32). Previous data indicate that collaterals provide similar perfusion to a patent vessel with a 90% obstruction. These collaterals can maintain viability and limit or prevent myocardial necrosis (33).

LATE ANGIOGRAPHIC FOLLOW-UP AFTER MYOCARDIAL INFARCTION: THE FATE OF THE THROMBUS

The percentage of patients with occluded infarct-related arteries following infarction is about 50% in patients studied between 2 weeks and 1 year after the event (34). This lower percentage likely represents endogenous thrombolysis, although a survival benefit for the open artery is probably also present because patients with persistently closed infarct-related arteries may be more likely to succumb following infarction than those with open arteries. In favor of the importance of spontaneous thrombolysis are serial angiographic studies in the same patient following myocardial infarction showing a progressive decrease in percentage diameter stenosis and increase in minimal luminal diameter of the culprit lesion following successful reperfusion. With reperfusion of a totally occluded artery, residual thrombus is initially present, and this requires time for further lysis. Brown et al. found that the recanalized lumen forms along an interface between thrombus and vessel wall, progressively enlarging over time. At 3 to 5 weeks in a group of patients studied serially, there was a 0.34-mm increase in luminal diameter and a 13% decrease in diameter stenosis of the culprit lesion compared to the initial postinfarction open vessel. These changes were statistically significant (35). Progressive decreases in lesion irregularity as well as decreases in percentage diameter stenosis have also been documented to occur following infarction and are potentiated by the use of antithrombotic and anticoagulant therapy after myocardial infarction (36,37).

CORONARY MORPHOLOGY AFTER Q-WAVE AND NON-Q-WAVE MYOCARDIAL INFARCTION

When the infarct-related artery is not totally occluded, the morphology of the lesion is similar to that seen in the culprit lesion in unstable angina (38). These lesions are complex; i.e., they have angiographic features suggesting the presence of intracoronary thrombus and or plaque ulceration or fissuring. The angiographic features of a complex lesion include lesions that have irregular borders, overhanging edges, ulcerations, and/or filling defects (39,40) (Fig. 2). In unselected patients studied following myocardial infarction, the incidence of a complex lesion in the patent infarct-related artery

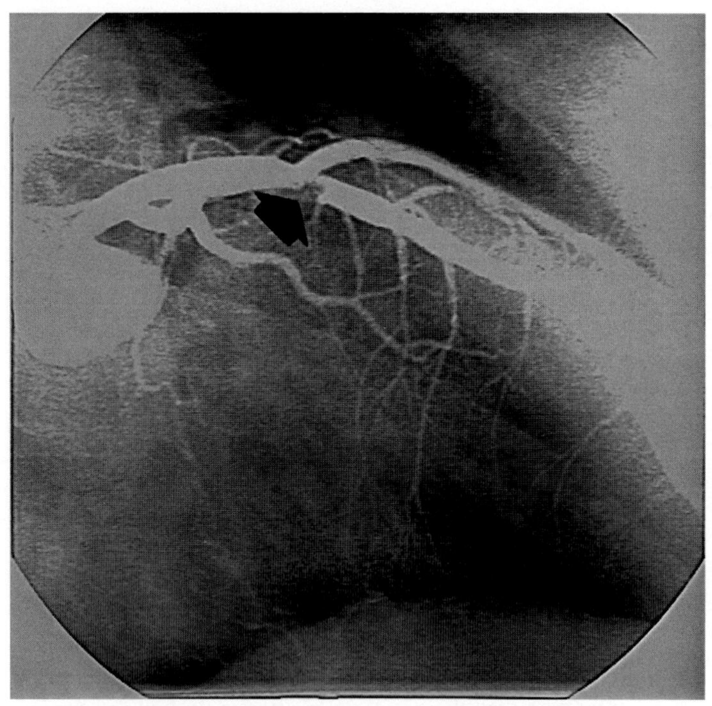

FIG. 2. The *arrow* points to a lesion in the midportion of the left anterior descending artery in a patient who presented with acute myocardial infarction. Angiography was performed on day 3 after infarction for recurrent pain. The lesion has the typical characteristics of a complex lesion: eccentric with irregular borders and overhanging edges.

is about 70% (35). In patients with both Q-wave myocardial infarction and non-Q-wave myocardial infarction, these lesions can be demonstrated in approximately equal percentages. This morphology is similar to that present in unstable angina, although it has been our impression that filling defects proximal and particularly distal to a significant lesion are seen more commonly in patent infarct arteries than in complex lesions in unstable angina (29). Immediately following thrombolysis, when there is successful reperfusion, lesion irregularity can be seen in nearly all patients. At a mean interval of 3 days following intravenous streptokinase for acute myocardial infarction, Davies et al. found that 89% of culprit lesions in the infarct-related artery were irregular (complex), and 91% were eccentric (36). On follow-up angiography (Table 1) performed during the same admission, there were significant differences in the morphology of the culprit lesion. There were significant decreases in the number of lesions appearing complex as well as significant decreases in the number of lesions with globular filling defects. The ulceration index, a semiquantitative measure of lesion irregularity, also decreased significantly on the second study.

In a preliminary report from the APRICOT study there were significant decreases in lesion irregularity of the culprit lesion as well as increases in percentage diameter stenosis on 3-month follow-up after myocardial infarction. These differences in lesion irregularity were enhanced by the use of antithrombotic and anticoagulant therapy following infarction (37).

POSTMORTEM ANGIOGRAPHIC CORRELATIONS OF LESION MORPHOLOGY

Levin and Fallon correlated postmortem coronary angiographic morphology with histological sections in 73 localized subtotal coronary stenoses that were 50% to 99% occlusive (41). Postmortem arteriograms were performed by perfusing the right and left coronaries at 150 mm Hg. Lesions were classified angiographically into smooth and irregular. Histologically, lesions were divided into uncomplicated stenoses and complicated stenoses that manifested plaque rupture, plaque hemorrhage, superimposed partially occlusive

TABLE 1. *Analysis of morphological features of coronary lesions at first and second catheter studies after streptokinase*[a]

	First study	Second study	*p* Value[b]
Smooth versus irregular	29 irr/31	17 irr/31	<0.001 (FE)
Globular filling defect present	8/35	0/35	<0.005 (FE)
Contrast staining present	5/35	0/55	<0.05 (FE)
Ulceration index	7.4 ± 10.4	3.0 ± 1.6	<0.001 (Wil)

[a] Modified from Davies et al. (37), with permission.
[b] FE, Fischer's exact test; Wil, Wilcoxon test.

TABLE 2. *Angiographic/pathological correlations of directional atherectomy thrombus angiographic findings*[a]

	Angiographic findings	
Study	Complex lesion/ + thrombus	Simple lesion/ − thrombus
Isner et al. (43)	24 (54%)	258 (39%)
Christou et al. (44)	44 (78%)	12 (25%)
Sharma et al. (45)	79 (65%)	106 (28%)

[a] Numbers and percentages reflect incidence of thrombus detected by directional atherectomy.

thrombus, or recanalized thrombus. Among 35 lesions that angiographically demonstrated a smooth, noncomplex morphology, 11.4% were complicated lesions histologically. Among 38 stenosis that were angiographically consistent with complex lesions, 78.9% were complicated lesions histologically. This study, which preceded the later angiographic data on morphology, laid the groundwork for the clinical–angiographic correlations in acute syndromes. These findings were reconfirmed by Onodera et al., who studied 21 patients who died 1 h to 7 days after selective intracoronary thrombolysis (42). Cineangiographic findings were compared to the histological findings at postmortem of 17 lesions that were classified as irregular or with intraluminal filling defects. Eighty-two percent demonstrated ruptured atheroma and/or thrombus. On the other hand, of 21 angiographic lesions that were classified as smooth, only 10% demonstrated these findings.

Recently, angiographic findings prior to coronary atherectomy have been compared to the histological detection of thrombus retrieved by the atherocath (43–45). In three preliminary studies reported, lesions classified as complex or thrombus-containing on angiography demonstrated thrombus in 54% to 78% of cases. In lesions classified angiographically as simple or without thrombus, the incidence of thrombus on histology was between 25% and 39% (Table 2). Although this type of investigation may be hampered by sampling error and inadequate detection of platelet thrombus (46), it supports the postmortem analyses indicating that lesion irregularity and complexity are generally associated with histological features of thrombus.

SERIAL ANGIOGRAPHY AND ACUTE MYOCARDIAL INFARCTION

Angiographic studies of coronary artery disease indicate that progression of disease is neither linear nor predictable. Several angiographic studies in which the same patient underwent serial angiography prior to and after myocardial infarction suggest that it is often the mild to moderate lesion that is the site of subsequent myocardial infarction rather than lesions that are necessarily severe before the event (47–51). Likewise, angiographic studies performed following infarction have shown that the percentage diameter stenosis of a patent infarct-related artery is often less than severe (52,53). Although the limitations of angiography have been considered in a previous section and indicate that angiography may underestimate the degree of atherosclerosis, it is improbable that this limitation negates the importance of these studies in myocardial infarction. One may be underestimating the amount of narrowing in the artery, but most of the studies indicate that the most severe angiographic stenoses are unlikely to be responsible for the subsequent infarction. For example, Little et al. found that in only 38% was the most severe angiographic stenosis the site of subsequent infarction (48).

Retrospective Studies

At least five serial angiographic studies have been reported that retrospectively analyzed the coronary anatomy prior to and following myocardial infarction (47–51) (Table 3). In all of these studies, patients were selected on the basis of having had at least two angiograms and having sustained a myocardial infarction between the two studies. Patients with angioplasty or bypass surgery in the intervening interval were excluded. In these five studies in total, 193 pairs of angiograms were analyzed. In 134 (69.4%) the site of subsequent infarction demonstrated a percentage diameter stenosis of ≤50% in the culprit lesion on the first angiogram. In only 28 (14.5%) was the culprit lesion >70% on the first angiogram. Even in angiograms performed <1 year apart, the site of subsequent infarction was ≤50% in over 50% of cases. In the study by Little et al. (48), the most stenotic lesion on the first angiogram was usually not the site of subsequent infarction. In 66% the artery that subsequently occluded was <50% on the first angiogram. Analysis of angiographic severity on the first angiogram could not predict the time or location of subsequent infarction. In all five studies, the findings were all concordant in showing that lesions ≤50% were predominantly present at the site of subsequent infarction.

Not all serial angiographic data are completely consistent with this hypothesis. In a review of 313 patients undergoing two angiograms, Moise et al. found a new total occlusion in 37% at the time of the second angiogram (54). The presence of a high-grade stenosis was an important predictor of the development of a new coronary artery occlusion, and occlusions were strongly associated with interim infarctions.

TABLE 3. *Angiographic evolution to myocardial infarction*

		Initial angiographic stenosis		
Study	*n*	≤50%	51–70%	>70%
Ambrose et al. (47)	23	48	30	22
Little et al. (48)	29	66	31	3
Nobuyoshi et al. (49)	39	59	15	26
Giroud et al. (50)	92	78	9	13
Hackett et al. (51)	10	90	10	0

However, analysis of their data as reported by Little et al. indicated that 72% of occlusions previously contained <75% stenoses on the initial angiogram (55). In another study, Ellis et al. analyzed patients in the CASS Registry with left anterior descending coronary artery lesions (56). A severe lesion in the left anterior descending was the most important factor related to subsequent anterior infarction. Repeat angiography, however, was not performed, and the culprit lesion responsible for anterior infarction could not be accurately determined. In addition, in this study nearly half of the patients with myocardial infarction had sustained a non-Q-wave infarction. Although there are limited data on serial angiographic finding in non-Q-wave infarction, at least in some patients a severe narrowing on an initial angiogram may precede non-Q-wave infarction. In these patients, total occlusion occurred, and collaterals developed or increased, acutely limiting the amount of myocardial necrosis (46). However, in contrast to the above, Little found no difference in percentage diameter stenosis of the culprit lesion before non-Q-wave in comparison to Q-wave myocardial infarction (57).

Taeymans et al. assessed hemodynamic and rheological factors related to subsequent thrombotic occlusion (58). In an angiographic analysis of 38 lesions that occluded within 3 years, causing acute infarction, the authors observed that occlusion at the site of an atherosclerotic plaque is not completely random but is related to plaque geometry and local blood flow. The presence of a branch originating within a lesion, the severity of the lesion (averaging 47.5 ± 17.8% diameter reduction), and the steepness of the stenosis inflow and outflow angles were all related to subsequent infarction and indicated that particularly high shear stress was an important rheological determinant of occlusion leading to subsequent infarction.

Prospective Studies

In a prospective angiographic trial, 370 patients with a baseline angiogram were followed for 5 years, and angiography was repeated (59). The results substantiated the findings of the retrospective analyses. In 30 patients who developed acute infarction, the preexisting lesion in the infarct-related artery was ≤50% in 52% of patients. The lesion was ≤75% in 85% of patients. On the other hand, asymptomatic coronary occlusion occurred in 62 patients, and in these patients a preceding stenosis of 76% to 99% was found in 56% whereas only 32% in this group had a preceding stenosis <50%. These data are consistent with the retrospective study of Ambrose et al., who, in addition to analyzing serial angiograms in patients who sustained infarction, also analyzed a group of patients who presented with a new total occlusion but had not sustained infarction (47). In this latter group of patients, 61% of the lesions that progressed to total occlusion were initially >70% on the first angiogram (Fig. 3). In these patients, collaterals prevented myocardial necrosis. Autopsy data also indicate that thrombotic occlusion does not necessarily lead to acute myocardial infarction. Evidence of prior thrombotic occlusion can be demonstrated in a majority of patients with stable angina, and it is found equally in patients with and without old infarction (60).

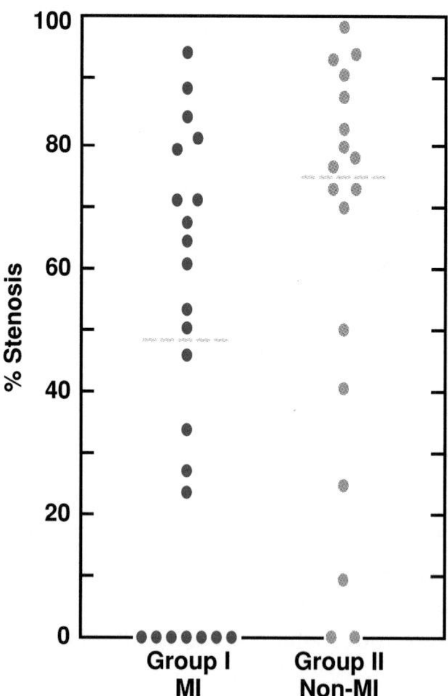

FIG. 3. Initial percentage stenosis of infarct-related artery at restudy in 23 group I patients with myocardial infarction (MI) or new total occlusions in 18 group II patients without myocardial infarction. Median values *(dashed line)* for each group are included. (From Ambrose et al., ref. 47, with permission.)

The Culprit Lesion Following Infarction: Residual Stenosis

In several studies the severity of residual coronary stenoses after successful thrombolytic recanalization has been studied. As mentioned earlier, depending on the timing of angiography following infarction, it is likely that residual thrombus may still be present. For example, in the APRICOT Study, 3 months following infarction there were significant increases in minimal luminal diameter of the culprit lesion compared to the angiogram performed immediately postinfarct (37). In spite of the fact that angiograms performed immediately after thrombolysis may, therefore, overestimate lesion severity prior to infarction because of residual thrombus formation, Hackett et al. found residual stenoses of <60% (diameter obstruction) in 47% immediately after thrombolysis (52). Likewise, Serruys et al. found that following intracoronary streptokinase or intravenous tissue-type plasminogen activator, the residual stenosis of the infarct lesion following infarction averaged 50% by quantitative analysis (53).

A UNIFYING CONCEPT OF ACUTE CORONARY SYNDROMES BASED ON ANGIOGRAPHIC CORRELATIONS

The above data suggest that in a majority of cases of acute myocardial infarction presenting with transmural ischemia, the cause is total and sustained thrombotic occlusion. Prior to occlusion, the lesion responsible for the infarct contained a narrowing that was not severe enough once the vessel occluded acutely to immediately recruit collateral vessels. Based on the serial angiographic studies, the angiographic narrowing of the future infarct lesion was, therefore, not severe (>70% obstructive) prior to infarction. Despite the underestimation of angiography in terms of defining the amount of atherosclerosis, this hypothesis seems plausible to explain the majority of patients presenting with large myocardial infarctions. Once occlusion occurs, the red-cell–fibrin thrombus may be modulated in most cases by acute thrombolytic interventions.

In patients presenting with non-Q-wave infarction, several possibilities are present. In about one-quarter of patients, a new and persistent total occlusion is present. These patients will usually have collateral vessels, and most had prior lesions that were severely stenotic prior to infarction. In the majority, non-Q-wave patients may be not unlike those with unstable angina, in whom there was only a mild to moderate lesion present prior to infarction. In these patients it is likely that non-Q-wave infarction was precipitated by a new nontotal occlusion of the culprit vessel or a total occlusion that spontaneously reperfuses (61). Spontaneous reperfusion is suggested by transient ST segment elevation in about 40% of patients with non-Q-wave infarction on the initial electrocardiogram and an early peak of creatine kinase in the blood (62,63). In a small percentage of patients, total occlusion of small branch vessels, even with a prior insignificant lesion, is probably responsible for the clinical syndrome.

In unstable angina, most patients present with a new lesion that is not totally occluded. In these patients the process that is responsible for the onset of unstable angina leads to a significant narrowing in the artery that alters the balance between supply and demand, leading to myocardial ischemia. Based on all of the pathological data presented in other chapters, it is reasonable to postulate that in the vast majority of cases of acute myocardial infarction and unstable angina, the acute process leading to thrombotic occlusion is associated with a fissuring or disruption of an atherosclerotic plaque that is usually lipid-laden. Exposure of the fatty gruel under the plaque leads to acute thrombotic occlusion in myocardial infarction. In unstable angina, plaque fissuring leads to a mural rather than an occlusive thrombus or a thrombus that is transient and spontaneously lyses or embolizes.

SUMMARY AND FUTURE DIRECTIONS

Angiographic analysis of the coronary anatomy prior to, during, and immediately following acute myocardial infarction has provided great insight into the pathogenesis of myocardial infarction. Angiography has confirmed the previously reported pathological studies indicating the importance of acute thrombosis as the primary cause of myocardial infarction. Serial angiographic analyses in the same patient prior to and following infarction indicate the importance of the mild to moderate lesion as the precursor of acute myocardial infarction in a majority of cases.

Further prospective angiographic data are needed to ascertain the true incidence of the mild lesion as the precursor to acute myocardial infarction. It is likely that within 10 years diagnostic coronary angiography will be performed noninvasively with magnetic resonance imaging. Serial studies before and after infarction in certain high-risk subgroups (e.g., those with multiple risk factors) will be required for this type of analysis. Only when large groups of patients are followed serially can we be sure that the angiographic observations presented in this chapter apply to more nonselected groups.

REFERENCES

1. Rutherford JD, Braunwald E. Chronic ischemic heart disease. In: Braunwald E, ed. *Heart Disease*. Philadelphia: WB Saunders; 1992.
2. Bruschke AVG, Proudfit WL, Sones FM Jr. Clinical course of patients with normal and slightly or moderately abnormal coronary arteriograms. A follow up study on 500 patients. *Circulation* 1973;47: 936–945.
3. Burggraf GW, Parker JO. Prognosis in coronary artery disease. Angiographic, hemodynamic and clinical factors. *Circulation* 1975;51: 146–156.
4. Conti CR. Coronary arteriography. *Circulation* 1977;55:227–237.
5. Guidelines for coronary arteriography. A report of the American College of Cardiology/American Heart Association Task Force on Assessment of Diagnostic and Therapeutic Cardiovascular Procedures (Subcommittee on Coronary Angiography). *Circulation* 1987;76:963A.
6. Eusterman JH, Achor RWP, Kincaid OW, Brown AL Jr. Atherosclerotic disease of the coronary arteries. A pathologic–radiologic correlative study. *Circulation* 1962;26:1288–1295.
7. Kemp HG, Evans H, Elliott WC, Gorlin R. Diagnostic accuracy of selective coronary cinearteriography. *Circulation* 1967;36:526–533.
8. Hutchins GM, Bulkley BH, Ridolfi RL, et al. Correlation of coronary arteriograms and left ventriculograms with postmortem studies. *Circulation* 1977;56:32–37.
9. Gray CR, Hoffman HA, Hammond WS, Miller KL, Oseasohn RO. Correlation of arteriographic and pathologic findings in the coronary arteries in man. *Circulation* 1962;26:494–499.
10. Schwartz JN, Kong Y, Hackel DB, Bartel AG. Comparison of angiographic and postmortem findings in patients with coronary artery disease. *Am J Cardiol* 1975;36:174–178.
11. Joseph A, Ackerman D, Talley JD, Johnstone J, Kupersmith J. Manifestations of coronary atherosclerosis in young trauma victims—an Autopsy study. *J Am Coll Cardiol* 1993;22:459–467.
12. Nissen SE, Gurley JC, Grines CL, Booth DC, McClure R, Berk M, Fischer C, DeMaria AN. Intravascular ultrasound assessment of lumen Size and wall morphology in normal subjects and patients with coronary artery disease. *Circulation* 1991;84:1087–1099.
13. Porter TR, D'Sa A, Turner C, Jones LA, Minisi AJ, Mohanty PK, Vevtrovec GW, Nixon JV. Myocardial contrast echocardiography for the assessment of coronary blood flow reserve: Validation in humans. *J Am Coll Cardiol* 1993;21:349–355.
14. Waller BF, Pinkerton CA, Slack JD. Intravascular ultrasound: A histological study of vessels during life: The new "gold standard" for vascular imaging. *Circulation* 1992;85:2305–2310.
15. Glagov S, Weisenberd E, Zairns CK, Stankunavicius R, Kolettis GJ. Compensatory enlargement of human coronary arteries. *N Engl J Med* 1987;316:1371–1375.
16. Stiel GM, Stiel LSG, Schofer J, Donath K, Mathey DG. Impact of

compensatory enlargement of atherosclerotic coronary arteries on angiographic assessment of coronary artery disease. *Circulation* 1989; 80:1603–1609.
17. Freudenberg H, Lichtlen PR. The normal wall segment in coronary stenosis—a postmortem study. *Z Kardiol* 1981;70:863–869.
18. Losordo DW, Rosenfield K, Kaufman J, Pieczek A, Isner JM. Focal compensatory enlargement of human arteries in response to progressive atherosclerosis; in vivo documentation using intravascular ultrasound. *Circulation* 1994;89:2570–2577.
19. Sherman CT, Litvak F, Grundfest W, Lee M, Hickey A, Chaux A, Kass R, Blanche C, Matloff J, Morgenstern L, Ganz W, Swan HJC, Forrester J. Coronary angioscopy in patients with unstable angina pectoris. *N Engl J Med* 1986;315:913–919.
20. White CJ, Ramee SR, Collins TJ, Mesa JE, Jain A. Percutaneous angioscopy of saphenous vein coronary bypass grafts. *J Am Coll Cardiol* 1993;21:1181–1185.
21. den Heijer P, Foley DP, Escaned J, Hillege HL, van Dijk RB, Serruys PW, Lie KI. Angioscopic versus angiographic detection of intimal dissection and intracoronary thrombus. *J Am Coll Cardiol* 1994;24: 649–654.
22. Baltaxe HA, Levin DC. Coronary angiography; its role in the management of the patient with angina pectoris. *Circulation* 1972;46: 1161–1172.
23. DeWood MA, Spores J, Notske R, Mouser LT, Burroughs R, Golden MS, Lang HT. Prevalence of total coronary occlusion during the early hours of transmural myocardial infarction. *N Engl J Med* 1980;303: 897–902.
24. Kennedy WJ, Ritchie JL, Davis KB, Fritz JK. Western Washington randomized trial of intracoronary streptokinase in acute myocardial infarction. *N Engl J Med* 1983;309:1477–1482.
25. Rentrop KP. Thrombolytic therapy in patients with acute myocardial infarction. *Circulation* 1985;71:627–631.
26. Gibson RJ. Non-Q wave myocardial infarction: Diagnosis, prognosis and management. *Curr Prob Cardiol* 1988;13:(1)9–72.
27. DeWood MA, Stifler WF, Simpson CS, et al. Coronary arteriographic findings soon after non-Q wave myocardial infarction. *N Engl J Med* 1986;315:417–523.
28. Ambrose JA, Monsen CE, Borrico S, Gorlin R, Fuster V. Angiographic demonstration of a common link between unstable angina pectoris and non-Q wave acute myocardial infarction. *Am J Cardiol* 1988;61: 244–247.
29. Rentrop KP, Feit F, Blanke H, Stecy P, Schneider R, Rey M, Horowitz S, Goldman M. Effects of intracoronary streptokinase and intracoronary nitroglycerin infusion on coronary angiographic patterns and mortality in patients with acute myocardial infarction. *N Engl J Med* 1984;311: 1456–1463.
30. Ambrose JA, Israel DH. Angiography in unstable angina. *Am J Cardiol* 1991;68:78B–84B.
31. Cowley MJ, DiSciascio G, Rehr RB, Vetrovec GW. Angiographic observations and clinical relevance of coronary thrombus in unstable angina pectoris. *Am J Cardiol* 1989;63:108E–113E.
32. Ambrose JA, Hjemdahl-Monsen C. Acute ischemic syndromes: Coronary pathophysiology and angiographic correlations. In: Gersh BJ, Rahimtoola SH, eds. *Acute Myocardial Infarction.* Amsterdam: Elsevier; 1991.
33. Cohen M, Rentrop KP. Limitation of myocardial ischemia by collateral circulation during controlled coronary artery occlusion in human subjects: A prospective study. *Circulation* 1986;74:469–476.
34. de Feyter PJ, van den Brand M, Serruys PW, Wijns W. Early angiography after myocardial infarction: What have we learned? *Am Heart J* 1985;109:194–199.
35. Brown BG, Gallery CA, Badger RS, Kennedy JW, Mathey D, Bolson EL, Dodge HT. Incomplete lysis of thrombus in the moderate underlying atherosclerotic lesion during intracoronary infusion of streptokinase for acute myocardial infarction: Quantitative angiographic observations. *Circulation* 1986;73:653–661.
36. Davies SW, Marchant B, Lyons JP, Timmis AD, Rothman MT, Layton CA, Balcon R. Coronary lesion morphology in acute myocardial infarction: Demonstration of early remodeling after streptokinase treatment. *J Am Coll Cardiol* 1990;16:1079.
37. Veen G, Meijer A, Werter CJPJ, et al. Dynamic changes of culprit lesion morphology and severity after successful thrombolysis for acute myocardial infarction: An angiographic follow up study. *J Am Coll Cardiol* 1994;23:147A.
38. Ambrose JA, Winters S, Arora R, Haft JI, Goldstein J, Gorlin R, Fuster V. Coronary angiography morphology in myocardial infarction—a link between the pathogenesis of unstable angina and myocardial infarction. *J Am Coll Cardiol* 1985;6:1233–1238.
39. Ambrose JA, Winters SL, Stern A, Eng A, Teicholz LE, Gorlin R, Fuster V. Angiographic morphology and the pathogenesis of unstable angina pectoris. *J Am Coll Cardiol* 1985;5:609–616.
40. Bresnahan DR, Davis DR, Holmes DR Jr, Smith HC. Angiographic occurrence and clinical correlates of intraluminal coronary artery thrombus; Role of unstable angina. *J Am Coll Cardiol* 1985;6:285–289.
41. Levin DC, Fallon JT. Significance of the angiographic morphology of localized coronary stenoses: Histopathologic correlations. *Circulation* 1982;66:316–320.
42. Onodera T, Fujiwara H, Tanaka M, Wu DJ, Matsuda M, Takemura G, Ishida M, Kawamura A, Kawai C. Cineangiographic and pathological features of the infarct related vessel in successful and unsuccessful thrombolysis. *Br Heart J* 1989;61:385–389.
43. Isner JM, Brinker JA, Gottlieb RS, Leya F, Masden RR, Shani J, Kearney M, Topol EJ, for CAVEAT. Coronary thrombus: Clinical features and angiographic diagnosis in 370 patients studied by directional atherectomy. *Circulation* 1992;86:I-649.
44. Christou CP, Haft JI, Goldstein JE, Carnes RE. Correlation of ischemic coronary syndromes with angiographic morphology and lesion histology. *J Am Coll Cardiol* 1992;19:375A.
45. Sharma SK, Israel DH, Fyfe B, Lotvin A, Torre SR, Kushner AL, McMurtry K, Marmur J, Cocke T, Almeida OD, Ambrose JA. Coronary thrombus: Clinical and angiographic correlates in 185 lesions undergoing directional coronary atherectomy. *Circulation* 1993;88:I-208.
46. Mizuno K, Satomuro K, Miyamato A, et al. Angioscopic evaluation of the character of coronary thrombi in acute coronary syndromes. *N Engl J Med* 1992;326:287–291.
47. Ambrose JA, Tannenbaum MA, Alexopoulos D, Hjemdahl-Monsen CE, Leavy J, Weiss M, Borrico S, Gorlin R, Fuster V. Angiographic progression of coronary artery disease and the development of myocardial infarction. *J Am Coll Cardiol* 1988;12:56–62.
48. Little WC, Constantinescu MD, Applegate RJ, Kutcher MA, Burrows MT, Kahl FR, Santamore WP. Can coronary angiography predict the site of a subsequent myocardial infarction in patients with mild to moderate coronary artery disease? *Circulation* 1988;78:1157–1166.
49. Nobuyoshi M, Tanaka M, Mosaka H, et al. Progression of coronary atherosclerosis: Is coronary spasm related to progression? *J Am Coll Cardiol* 1991;18:904–910.
50. Giroud D, Li JM, Urban P, Meier B, Rutishauser W. Relation of the site of acute myocardial infarction to the most severe coronary arterial stenosis at prior angiography. *Am J Cardiol* 1992;69:729–732.
51. Hackett D, Verwilghen J, Davies G, Maseri A. Coronary stenoses before and after acute myocardial infarction. *Am J Cardiol* 1989;63: 1517–1518.
52. Hackett D, Davies G, Maseri A. Pre-existing coronary stenoses in patients with first myocardial infarction are not necessarily severe. *Eur Heart J* 1988;9:1317–1323.
53. Serruys PW, Arnold AER, Brower RW, DeBono DP, Bokslag M, Lusben J, Reiber JHC, Rutsch WR, Uebis R, Vahanian A, Verstraete M, for the European Co-operative Study Group for Recombinant Tissue-type Plasminogen Activator. Effect of continued rt-PA administration on the residual stenosis after initially successful recanalization in acute myocardial infarction—a quantitative coronary angiography study of a randomized trial. *Eur Heart J* 1987;8:1172–1181.
54. Moise A, Lesperance J, Theroux P, Taeymans Y, Goulet C, Bourassa MG. Clinical and angiographic predictors of new total coronary occlusion in coronary artery disease; analysis of 313 nonoperated patients. *Am J Cardiol* 1984;54:1176–1181.
55. Little WC, Downes TR, Applegate RJ. The underlying coronary lesion in myocardial infarction: Implications for coronary angiography. *Clin Cardiol* 1991;14:868–874.
56. Ellis S, Alderman E, Cain K, Fisher L, Sanders W, Bourassa M, the CASS Investigators. Prediction of risk of anterior myocardial infarction by lesion severity and measurement method of stenoses in the left anterior descending coronary distribution: A CASS Registry Study. *J Am Coll Cardiol* 1988;11:908–916.
57. Little WC. Angiographic assessment of the culprit coronary artery lesion before acute myocardial infarction. *Am J Cardiol* 1990;66: 44G–47G.

58. Taeymans Y, Theroux P, Lesperance J, Waters D. Quantitative angiographic morphology of the coronary artery lesions at risk of thrombotic occlusion. *Circulation* 1992;85:78–85.
59. Chesebro JH, Webster MWI, Zoldhelyi P, Roche PC, Badimon L, Badimon JJ. Antithrombotic therapy and progression of coronary artery disease; antiplatelet versus antithrombins. *Circulation* 1992;86(Suppl III):III-100–III-111.
60. Handgartner JRW, Charleston AJ, Davies MJ, Thomas AC. Morphological characteristics of clinically significant coronary artery stenoses in stable angina. *Br Heart J* 1986;56:501–508.
61. Gorlin R, Fuster V, Ambrose JA. Anatomic–physiologic links between acute coronary syndromes. *Circulation* 1986;74:6–9.
62. Gibson RS, Beller GA, Gheorghiade M, et al. The prevalence and clinical significance of residual myocardial ischemia two weeks after uncomplicated non-Q wave infarction: A prospective natural history study. *Circulation* 1986;73:1186–1198.
63. Huey BL, Gheorghiade M, Crampton RS, et al. Acute non-Q wave myocardial infarction associated with early ST segment elevation: Evidence for spontaneous reperfusion and implications for thrombolytic trials. *J Am Coll Cardiol* 1987;9:18–25.

Atherosclerosis and Coronary Artery Disease,
edited by V. Fuster, R. Ross, and E. J. Topol.
Lippincott-Raven Publishers, Philadelphia © 1996.

CHAPTER 47

The Pathophysiology and Biochemistry of Myocardial Ischemia, Necrosis, and Reperfusion

Yoshifumi Naka, David M. Stern, and David J. Pinsky

Key Words: Ischemia; myocardial stunning; myocyte; necrosis; neutrophils; no-reflow phenomenon; reperfusion; reperfusion arrhythmias; vascular homeostasis; vascular reperfusion injury.

INTRODUCTION

The heart is an organ which, like all organs, is critically dependent upon a continual supply of fresh blood to perform its vital functions. Interruption of this blood supply, even for very brief periods, sets a panoply of homeostatic mechanisms into motion, which serve to limit the resulting damage. Because of the heart's rich vascular supply, however, a number of vascular homeostatic mechanisms are perturbed which can lead to irreversible myocardial damage. Even upon reestablishment of blood flow in the large conduit epicardial arteries, further damage may ensue due to reperfusion injury, which shares many features characteristic of the inflammatory response. Reperfusion injury comes about because of interactions of a number of different cell types as well as components of the coagulation and complement systems, which combine to form a toxic milieu in which myocytes may not survive. Understanding the mechanisms which lead to myocyte death has led to the development of novel therapeutic interventions designed to mitigate the pathophysiologic processes which accompany myocardial ischemia and reperfusion.

Yoshifumi Naka, David M. Stern, and David J. Pinsky: Department of Physiology, College of Physicians and Surgeons of Columbia University, New York, New York 10032.

PATHOLOGIC SUBSTRATE

There are numerous possible mechanisms whereby myocytes may die during a period of cardiac ischemia and reperfusion. *Myocardial ischemia* is defined simply as an arterial oxygen supply which is insufficient to meet the metabolic demands of the tissue (1). Shortly after cessation of blood flow to a region of the heart, tissue myoglobin oxygen stores are consumed, the partial pressure of oxygen in the region declines (2), and that region of cardiac muscle which is ischemic loses its ability to maintain its normal (negative) resting membrane potential (3). Adenosine triphosphate (ATP) stores are depleted (4), mechanical contraction ceases (3), and cardiac myocytes arrest in the relaxed state, perhaps as the result of passive stretch imposed by adjacent nonischemic (contracting) muscle (5). These changes are accompanied by increases in tissue lactate (4,6), H^+ ions (7), phosphate (6), and potassium (8,9). During ischemia, cytosolic calcium levels are only slightly elevated, although mitochondrial calcium is increased (10). Arterioles become maximally dilated (11), but if blood flow is insufficient for as little as 20 min, early stages of myocardial necrosis may be observed (12). If early reperfusion ensues, however, mechanical function can return (13).

The earliest structural changes seen in the heart following a period of ischemia are a decrease in the size and number of glycogen granules present within the myocytes, consumed by the relatively inefficient processes of anaerobic metabolism (14–16). Microscopic examination reveals that myofibrils are relaxed, presumably stretched by the tugging of adjacent nonischemic cells (17). Intracellular edema develops, with concomitant swelling of the t-tubules, sarcoplasmic reticulum, and mitochondria (14–16). This edema is manifest as an increase in myocardial water content, small during the first 15 min following coronary artery occlusion, but increasing by nearly 50% by 75 min in an in situ model of coronary occlusion in the pig (18,19). Part of this increased myocardial water content during ischemia is the result of interstitial edema (20), which has been interpreted as resulting from increased microvascular permeability (21) as a consequence of the retraction of the lateral margins of vascular endothelial cells, thereby enlarging intercellular spaces (22).

IRREVERSIBLE MYOCYTE DEATH

These pathologic processes occur incrementally over the early minutes to hours of ischemia, and it is difficult to define exactly when myocytes cross the threshold of irreversibility, i.e., the degree of ischemia which makes it inevitable that they will die. A working definition of *irreversibility* has been proposed as an ischemic insult of such severity that cells will continue to degenerate/necrose even after restoration of blood flow (23). The degree of ischemia and the duration of ischemia are both important factors in determining the point of irreversibility, with severe reductions of arterial flow causing irreversibility as early as 20 min following onset (23). Histologically, irreversible cell death is characterized by ultrastructural changes which include the development of contraction bands (24–26) as well as amorphous densities within the mitochondria (24). Numerous plasma markers of myocyte death have been used with varying degrees of success to quantify the degree of myocardial necrosis in patients. In addition to traditional markers such as lactate dehydrogenase, creatinine phosphokinase, and serum glutamic oxaloacetic transaminase, myoglobin, troponins T and I, and cardiac-specific myosin light chains have been investigated (27). Although the kinetics of release and detection vary among these different markers, they share in common the feature that their elevations in plasma reflect a loss of myocyte membrane integrity. Reperfusion of an ischemic area may also contribute to a rapid washout of these markers into peripheral blood, resulting in earlier peaks, complicating an analysis of extent of infarction (28).

REPERFUSION

Definitions

Restoration of blood flow to a previously ischemic zone causes profound physiologic changes in both myocytes and the local vasculature in the reperfused zone. Collectively, these changes may promote further tissue damage in a process called *reperfusion injury*. Although there are numerous experimental models of reperfusion injury, it has been impossible to define exactly those cells which were otherwise destined to live following ischemia alone, but were killed by the process of reperfusion (29). Reperfusion of ischemic myocardium halts the advancing wavefront of ischemic myocyte death, with an exponential decay in the number of myocytes that may be salvaged as ischemic time lengthens (30), so that clinical reperfusion should be attempted even in the face of potential reperfusion injury. Clinical trials of patients receiving thrombolytic therapy for acute myocardial infarction have repeatedly demonstrated that timely reperfusion is beneficial (14). That is not to say that improving the reperfusion milieu is of little added benefit, however; in fact, substantial evidence exists to the contrary (see below), suggesting that future therapy for acute myocardial infarction will consist of timely reperfusion and an optimal reperfusion milieu.

The term reperfusion injury encompasses a spectrum of changes, which has been recently categorized into four separate components (29). *Lethal reperfusion injury* refers to the death of myocytes which is attributed to reperfusion per se, rather than to the preceding period of ischemia. *Vascular reperfusion injury* includes a progressive deterioration of blood flow secondary to vascular damage, thrombosis, and neutrophil plugging during reperfusion, which is accompanied by a deterioration of the normal ability of the coronary vasculature to dilate in times of need, referred to as coronary flow reserve. This latter aspect may be largely secondary to the production of reactive oxygen intermediates, which rapidly quench available nitric oxide, leading to a failure of endothelium-dependent vasodilation (31,32). *Myocardial stunning* comprises a third category of reperfusion injury, representing a delayed failure of return of normal myocardial contractility, even when blood flow has been adequately restored. Ventricular tachycardia or fibrillation may herald the onset of reperfusion, and represents a final form of reperfusion injury termed *reperfusion arrhythmias* (33,34).

Mechanisms

Reoxygenation of endothelial cells is associated with a burst of oxygen free radical production both from endothelial cells (32) as well as from the heart itself (35–37). This oxygen free radical production appears to peak within minutes of reperfusion, and continues for hours at lower levels (38–40), producing such toxic species as superoxide, hydroxyl anion, and hydrogen peroxide. These highly reactive molecules may result in lipid peroxidation, membrane dysfunction, and further increases in membrane permeability beyond those observed during ischemia alone (41). The biochemical source of these free radicals remains controversial, however. While xanthine oxidase has been repeatedly implicated in their production (42), this enzyme is virtually undetectable in human myocardial tissue (43–45). Other likely sources include mitochondria (46), recruited neutrophils (47), or transition-metal-catalyzed formation of hydroxyl radical by the Haber–Weiss pathway (48).

Evidence for the formation of reactive oxygen intermediates in the human heart also abounds. Malondialdehyde, a detectable by-product of lipid peroxidation (49), has been shown to increase in coronary sinus blood following percutaneous coronary angioplasty (50). When peripheral venous blood was sampled in the setting of myocardial infarction 2 hr following streptokinase administration, levels of thiobarbituric acid-reactive substances (a measure of malondialdehyde levels) increased only in those patients in whom coronary artery patency was reestablished (51). Although there is little controversy regarding the generation of oxygen free radicals during reperfusion, there remains some skepticism regarding the clinical benefits of scavenging these free radicals as adjunctive therapy in managing clinical reperfusion. Although canine studies have demonstrated benefit by the use of superoxide dismutase linked to polyethylene glycol to prolong its half-life in the circulation (52), the effectiveness of this strategy may be improved by adding catalase (53) to eliminate the hydrogen peroxide generated by the dismutation of superoxide.

At a cellular level, reperfusion of an ischemic zone results in an explosive increase in intracellular sodium and calcium, with a concomitant abrupt cellular swelling (54–56). A *calcium paradox* has been described, wherein there is little increase in free intracellular calcium during ischemia, but a tenfold rise within 10 min of reperfusion (57). These processes appear to accelerate myocyte necrosis, although this may occur only in cells otherwise destined to die (56). The end result is that calcium precipitates in mitochondria (56), intracellular vesicles and subsarcolemmal blebs form (54,56), and contraction bands appear (56). Reperfusion injury is not limited to cardiac myocytes, however, as there is significant vascular involvement as well. Thrombosis and hemorrhage are seen in areas of reperfused myocardium (58) as well as neutrophil adhesion to the reperfused endothelium (32,59,60). Edema of microvascular endothelial cells is observed, with endothelial blebs and gaps which may expose blood to the tissue-factor-rich procoagulant subendothelium, accelerating thrombosis (58).

These processes contribute to the *no-reflow phenomenon,* wherein blood flow does not return to preischemic levels even following release of the coronary artery occlusion (29,58). In fact, no-reflow worsens as time elapses after reperfusion (61), suggesting an important role for recruited effector mechanisms, such as progressive microcirculatory thrombosis, vasomotor dysfunction, and neutrophil recruitment (29). The no-reflow phenomenon is more than simply a laboratory observation. Thallium-201- and Tc-99m-labeled microsphere studies in humans show that perfusion defects persist even for several weeks after successful thrombolysis of coronary artery occlusions in humans (62).

Following successful reperfusion, often myocytes do not immediately regain normal contractile function. This postischemic dysfunction of viable myocytes is called *myocardial stunning* (63). Even if flow is adequately restored, myocardial stunning reflects the presence of a flow/function mismatch (64,65), the discussion of which is beyond the scope of this chapter.

MECHANISMS OF ISCHEMIA-REPERFUSION-INDUCED MYOCYTE DEATH

Numerous mechanisms have been proposed to explain the final common pathway by which myocytes die during ischemia and reperfusion. Because of the unavailability of molecular oxygen during the period of ischemia, maintaining the myocyte energy charge of ATP is relegated to relatively inefficient glycolytic processes. As ATP demands overtake ATP supply, cellular energy charge is depleted, resulting in an inability of metabolic pumps to maintain normal ion gradients (4). Cytosolic calcium overload is thought to be an important mediator of ischemic contracture (66) and myocyte death (67). Depletion of ATP can also result in depletion of the reduced form of glutathione (GSH), which serves as a physiologic defense against cellular oxidant stress (67). Depletion of GSH, with the concomitant accumulation of the oxidized form of glutathione (GSSG), impairs the detoxifying functions of glutathione peroxidase (68), which normally removes hydrogen peroxide (10,67,68). Protons are generated (6,69), which also may contribute to the toxic intracellular milieu. Activation of phospholipase A_2 by ischemia can turn membrane phospholipids such as lecithin into highly detergent-like lysophospholipid micelles (70). Oxygen-derived free radicals may not only directly oxidize membrane lipids and cause membrane dysfunction, but may further inhibit glycolysis and contribute to calcium overload (71). Recent evidence suggests that reperfused myocytes may undergo programmed cell death *(apoptosis),* a process wherein endogenous nucleases are activated by specific genes within the cardiac myocytes, cleaving DNA into characteristic 200-base-pair fragments (72). These diverse mechanisms probably all contribute to some degree to irreversible myocyte death.

ROLE OF THE ENDOTHELIUM

Considerations of the biochemistry of myocardial ischemia and reperfusion would be incomplete without specific attention to the important role of the vasculature in these processes. There is a great deal of evidence to support the cardinal role of endothelial cells in orchestrating the complex vascular processes which maintain *vascular homeostasis,* wherein nutrient supply and waste elimination are in balance, and leukocyte traffic is maintained in a steady state. Endothelial cells line both the cardiac macro- and microvasculature, providing the nonwetting surface over which blood must continually flow. Endothelial cells do not simply serve as passive conduits for blood, but have a cardinal role in maintaining normal barrier properties of the blood vessel wall, maintaining blood fluidity by preventing coagulation, regulating blood vessel lumenal diameter by modulating vasomotor tone of the underlying vascular smooth muscle, and regulating neutrophil adhesion and egress into the underlying tissue. Dysfunction of any of these important endothelial functions may be observed in the setting of cardiac ischemia and reperfusion, where it may lead to the characteristic highly permeable, prothrombotic, and proinflammatory phenotype of the ischemic and reperfused vascular wall. Because the period of hypoxia is an important component of the ischemic period, many laboratories (including our own) have studied the responses of endothelial cells to hypoxia and reoxygenation, which has helped to elucidate mechanisms of endothelial cell dysfunction that are relevant to the period of cardiac ischemia and reperfusion.

Barrier Function

Under physiologic conditions, endothelial cells are normally tightly adherent to one another, forming the characteristic cobblestone appearance of unperturbed endothelium. This endothelial surface forms a barrier to the passage of solutes as well as the cellular components of the blood. Endothelial barrier function has been demonstrated by studies of electrical conductivity of endothelial cell monolayers as well as by studies in which the passage of radiolabeled solutes of various sizes across endothelial cell monolayers may be quantified. When endothelial cells are exposed to a period of hypoxia of the same severity as accompanies cardiac ischemia, they undergo changes in their actin-based cytoskeleton, leading to retraction of their lateral margins (73). This forms large gaps (1–3 μM) between apposing endothelial cells (73,74) through which large solutes may readily pass. Permeability to small molecules such as sorbitol increases, and even large molecules such as albumin have higher permeability across the hypoxic endothelial cell monolayer (73). This may be manifest as leakage of large intravascular proteins into the interstitial space, similar to the transvascular protein leakage observed in the lungs of rats exposed to hypoxia (75). The loss of endothelial barrier function is dependent both on the duration of exposure of the monolayer to hypoxia as well as to the absolute level of hypoxia (73,74).

When the relationship between levels of hypoxia and endothelial cell hyperpermeability was explored further, it was determined that the increased permeability only occurred at lower oxygen tensions. In parallel with the increased endothelial cell permeability as oxygen tension declined, a fall in cyclic adenosine monophosphate (cAMP) levels within the endothelial cells was noted, due to a reduction of both basal and stimulated adenylate cyclase activity (76). Restoration of levels of the second messenger cyclic nucleotide cAMP using a membrane-permeable cAMP analog, dibutyryl-cAMP, restored endothelial barrier function in a dose-dependent manner (76). Similarly, other disparate means of increasing the activity of the cAMP second messenger pathway, such as protein kinase A activation or pertussis toxin treatment, likewise normalized endothelial cell permeability under conditions of hypoxia (76,77). Studies in other laboratories support these observations (78–81), with phosphodiesterase inhibition being particularly effective at reducing capillary hyperpermeability in an isolated perfused rabbit lung model (82).

Vasomotor Tone

Not only does the hypoxia-induced fall in endothelial cell cAMP levels have implications with respect to endothelial cell barrier function, but cAMP serves as an important vasodilator in vascular smooth muscle (83). When vascular smooth muscle was studied under hypoxic conditions, a similar fall in cAMP levels was noted, although in these cells, it appears that this was due to increased activity of types III and IV phosphodiesterase (60). These observations may have important implications for the no-reflow phenomenon, especially when one considers that reactive oxygen intermediates increase the activity of phosphodiesterases in vitro (84), which may compound the vasoconstrictive effects of low vascular cAMP levels during reperfusion. In a global cardiac model of ischemia and reperfusion in the rat, restoration of the cAMP second messenger pathway using cAMP analogs, phosphodiesterase inhibitors, or activators of the cAMP-dependent protein kinase enhanced cardiac preservation in parallel with improving blood flow following reperfusion (60), suggesting the potential relevance of these observations to the heart.

In addition to cAMP, endothelium-derived relaxation factor [EDRF-identified as nitric oxide (85)] subserves a critical vasodilatory role that is under endothelial control. Although during hypoxic exposure, nitric oxide synthesis proceeds unabated, reoxygenation results in a rapid decline in available nitric oxide levels, largely due to the rapid quenching effects of superoxide anion generated during reoxygenation (32). These observations are entirely consistent with the rapid decline of coronary vascular EDRF bioactivity (31) or nitric oxide levels by direct measurement (32) observed within minutes of reperfusion. Similarly, endocardial nitric oxide

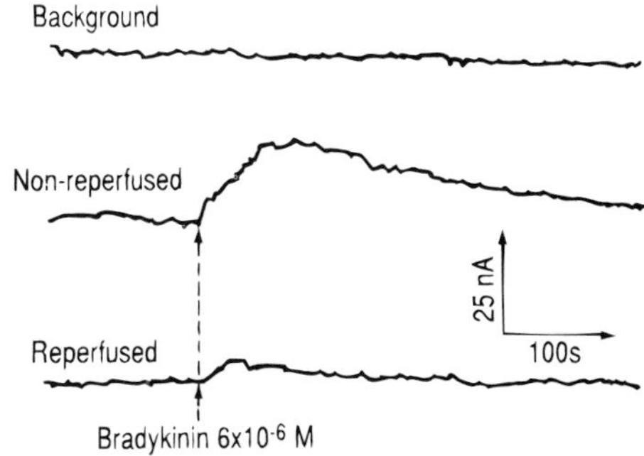

FIG. 1. Endocardial nitric oxide levels measured in situ following ischemia and reperfusion. A porphyrinic microsensor which is highly sensitive and specific for nitric oxide (143) was embedded in the septal endocardium, and bradykinin was applied. Nitric oxide levels are significantly lower following a period of ischemia and reperfusion than in nonreperfused endocardium (peak levels at the endocardial surface were ≈0.65 μM following bradykinin challenge in the nonreperfused endocardium). Application of superoxide dismutase increased endocardial nitric oxide levels, suggesting that superoxide quenches available nitric oxide during reperfusion. (Adapted from Pinsky et al., ref. 32.)

levels also plummet during reperfusion (32) (Fig. 1). This rapid decline in available nitric oxide levels has far-ranging implications beyond simple vasoconstriction, as nitric oxide also serves to attenuate neutrophil adhesion to the endothelium (86), prevent platelet aggregation (87), and maintain endothelial barrier function (88).

To demonstrate the potential relevance of these observations to human cardiac preservation, a preservation solution was designed which incorporated dibutyryl-cAMP as well as nitroglycerin, to augment both the cAMP and NO/cyclic guanosine monophosphate second messenger pathways. These experiments enabled unprecedented 24-h preservation of primate hearts with simple ex vivo hypothermic storage (89), suggesting the potential clinical relevance of these observations to human cardiac preservation. While the mechanisms of benefit continue to be evaluated, it appears as if augmentation of blood flow (32,60), reduction of neutrophil infiltration (32,60), reduction of oxidant stress *[unpublished observation]*, and reduction of platelet aggregation *[unpublished observation]* during reperfusion are of paramount importance.

Procoagulant/Anticoagulant Balance

Quiescent endothelium maintains an anticoagulant phenotype by a number of different mechanisms, which serve to maintain blood fluidity. The nonwetting endothelial surface prevents contact of the coagulation system with highly procoagulant subendothelial matrix, rich in collagen and tissue factor (90). Under physiologic conditions, quiescent endothelial cells (EC) constitutively express the membrane-spanning protein thrombomodulin, which binds to thrombin to accelerate local production of the anticoagulant protein C (91). In addition, local production of nitric oxide potently inhibits platelet aggregation (87,92).

Hypoxic exposure activates endothelium to shift the balance to the procoagulant phenotype. Gaps which form between apposing endothelial cells are sufficiently large to permit contact of the blood-borne coagulation elements with procoagulant subendothelial collagen and tissue factor. Hypoxia selectively modulates endothelial cell expression of certain proteins such as thrombomodulin, which is significantly reduced (both message and activity) following endothelial cell exposure to hypoxia (73). Decreased thrombomodulin elicited by a period of oxygen deprivation would be expected to prime the vessel wall for procoagulant events, as an antithrombotic mechanism is compromised. De novo synthesis of interleukin-1 by hypoxic macrophages (93) or endothelial cells (94) within the heart can promote endothelial cell expression of procoagulant tissue factor (95). In addition, there is increased secretion of the procoagulant polypeptide von Willebrand factor in endothelial cells exposed to hypoxia, as well as in the vasculature of human hearts during myocardial preservation (96). Finally, the marked depression of nitric oxide levels during reperfusion (31,32), brought about because of rapid quenching by superoxide anion, would also be expected to contribute to the prothrombotic state by fostering platelet aggregation.

Cytokine Production/Adhesion Molecule Expression

Leukocytes have been ascribed a central role in the tissue damage which occurs in ischemic syndromes (97–101). Multiple cytokines act synergistically to draw leukocytes into loci of hypoxic vascular injury. These proinflammatory cytokines include interleukin-1 (IL-1) (102,103), tumor necrosis factor (TNF) (104), and interleukin-8 (104,105). Endothelial cells exposed to hypoxia demonstrate de novo synthesis of IL-1, with steadily increasing levels peaking within 16 h of hypoxic exposure in in vitro experiments, with increased plasma levels in mice exposed to hypoxia reaching a peak within 6–8 h of hypoxic exposure (94). In similar experiments, IL-8 transcripts as well as antigen and activity were increased in endothelial cell culture supernatants as well as in blood vessels exposed to a hypoxic environment (106) (Fig. 2). In addition, reoxygenated human mononuclear phagocytes, present in abundance in the reperfused heart, likewise synthesize and release interleukin-1 (93).

Both IL-1 and TNF have the potential to set in motion events resulting in increased expression of leukocyte adherence molecules on the endothelial cell surface (95) as well as the further production of neutrophil chemoattractant substances (104). The IL-1 synthesis is specifically associated with endothelial expression of intracellular adhesion molecule-1 (ICAM-1) and E-selectin, both of which can be blocked by preventing IL-1 synthesis (using antisense oligomers for IL-1α) or blocking it at the ligand-receptor level

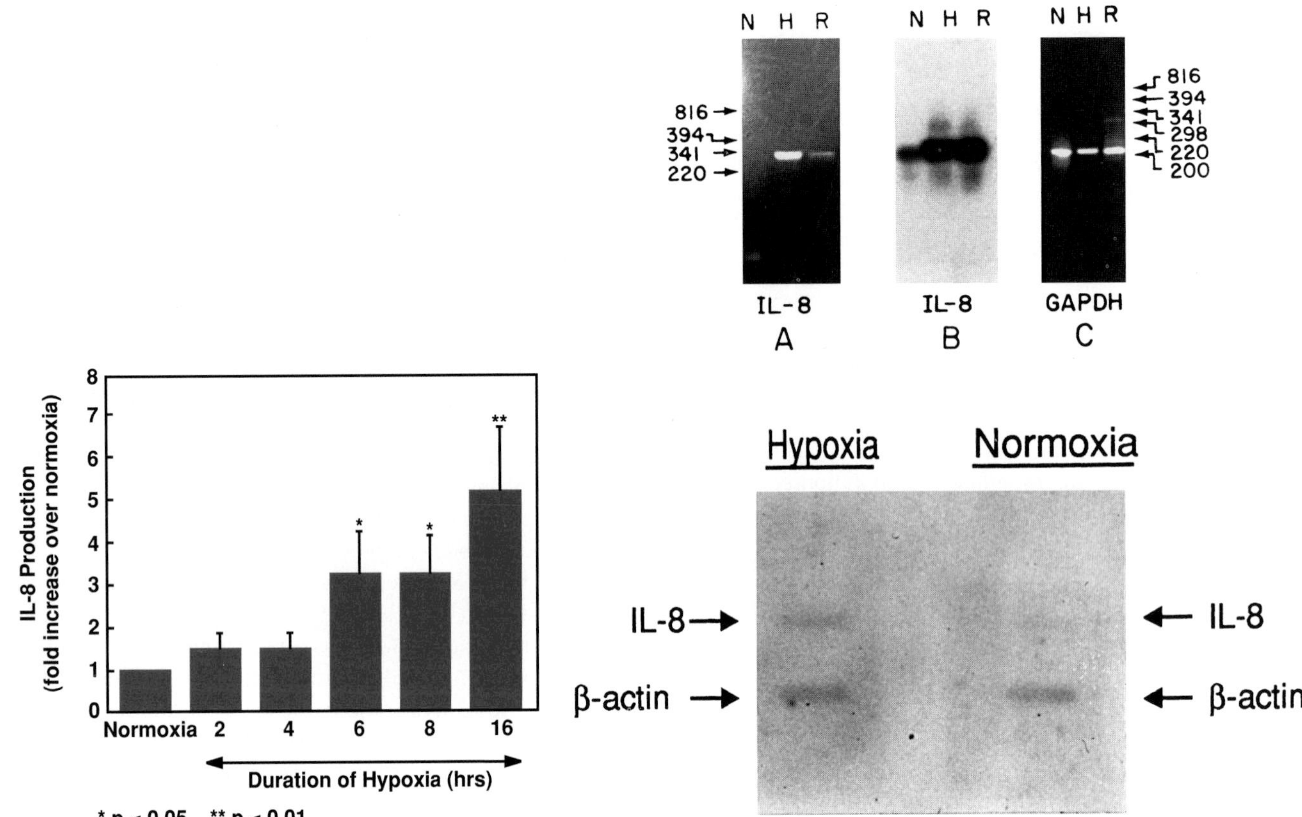

FIG. 2. Hypoxia-induced production of endothelial interleukin-8. **A:** Enzyme-linked immunosorbent assay demonstrates an increase in IL-8 antigen following hypoxic exposure of human umbilical vein endothelial cells. **B:** IL-8 message is likewise increased in hypoxia, as demonstrated by polymerase chain reaction **(left),** and Southern blotting of amplicons to confirm their identity **(middle),** compared with control glyceraldehyde phosphate dehydrogenase (GAPDH) message **(right).** *N,* Normoxia; *H,* hypoxia; *R,* reoxygenation. **C:** Nuclear run-on assay further confirming an upregulation of IL-8 transcripts in hypoxia **(left)** compared with control β-actin transcripts **(right).** (Adapted from Karakurum et al., ref. 106.)

(using blocking antibodies or IL-1 receptor antagonist) (94). These results have been corroborated by other investigators, who have shown that anoxia/reoxygenation induces neutrophil adherence to cultured endothelial cells (107) and that platelet activating factor may also play a role in this neutrophil adherence (108,109).

As a final ischemia/reperfusion-driven mechanism which promotes neutrophil adhesion, consideration must be given to EC surface expression of P-selectin expression. Along with von Willebrand factor, P-selectin is stored in subplasmalemmal granules within endothelial cells, called Weibel–Palade bodies (110–112). Increases in calcium within endothelial cells, such as occur with thrombin or histamine stimulation (113), promote rapid surface expression of P-selectin (114). Exposure of endothelial cells to reactive oxygen intermediates, such as are formed in abundance during coronary reperfusion (35,36), promotes expression of P-selectin at the endothelial cell surface (115), which may rapidly cause neutrophil adhesion (116) during reperfusion. The importance of P-selectin in cardiac ischemia and reperfusion has been recently verified in a feline model (117) (Fig. 3).

ROLE OF NEUTROPHILS AND PROINFLAMMATORY CYTOKINES

Neutrophils (polymorphonuclear leukocytes, PMNs) play a cardinal role in reperfusion-induced tissue damage in the heart (118–124). It is not surprising that neutrophils may be toxic to tissues in which they accumulate, as they serve an important role in the initial clearing of debris following an ischemic event. Upon recruitment to ischemic/reperfused tissue, they release numerous cytotoxic lysosomal enzymes with which to carry out these functions, including elastase, the metalloproteases collagenase and gelatinase, neutral proteases, and heparinase (125). In addition, recruited neutrophils may be activated by cytokines and chemotactic factors to undergo a respiratory burst, which elicits a sudden release of toxic reactive oxygen metabolites such as superoxide anion, chloramine, hypochlorous acid, hydroxyl radical, and hydrogen peroxide (125). Multiple studies have demonstrated that either depleting neutrophils prior to ischemia/reperfusion (118) or interfering with neutrophil adhesion to the endothelium can limit infarct size in experimental ani-

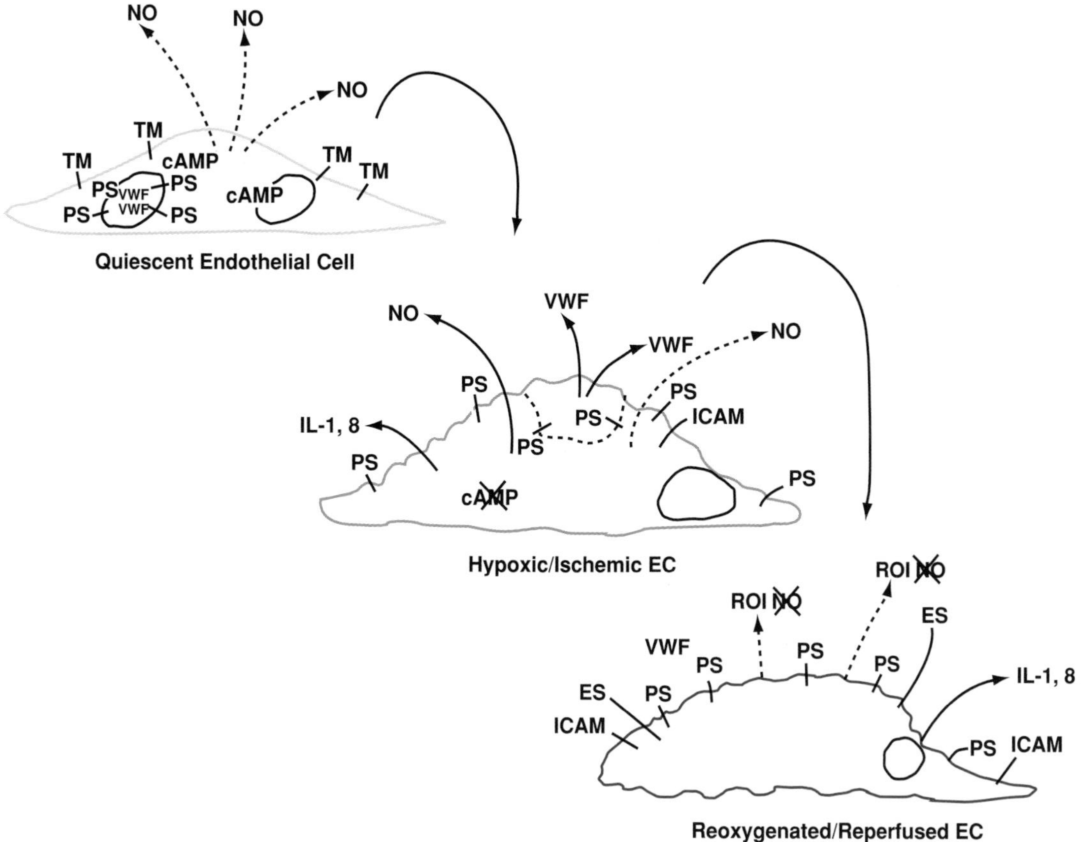

FIG. 3. Schematic representation of endothelial perturbations during hypoxia and reoxygenation. During hypoxia and reoxygenation, endothelial cAMP levels fall *(cAMP)* and endothelial cells secrete proinflammatory cytokines such as interleukins-1 and -8 *(IL-1, IL-8)* and procoagulant von Willebrand factor *(VWF),* and express neutrophil adhesion molecules on their surface (E-selectin, *ES;* P-selectin, *PS;* intracellular adhesion molecule-1, *ICAM*). In addition, surface expression of the anticoagulant cofactor thrombomodulin *(TM)* is reduced. Reoxygenation is association with the production of reactive oxygen intermediates *(ROI)* which can rapidly quench nitric oxide *(NO),* making it unavailable to perform its vasodilatory, antiplatelet, antipermeability, and antineutrophil functions.

mals (126,127). Even in models of global cardiac ischemia/reperfusion, such as occurs during heart transplantation, therapies which interfere with neutrophil adhesion and reduce the extent of graft myeloperoxidase activity (a specific marker of the presence of neutrophils) are associated with improved graft survival (32,60) (Fig. 4).

The process of PMN recruitment into the ischemic and reperfused vasculature occurs in several phases, largely controlled by endothelial cell/PMN interactions. Neutrophils are first attracted into an ischemic or reperfused milieu by specific chemoattractants, such as the activated complement components C3a and C5a (125), as well as the recently identified specific neutrophil chemoattractant interleukin-8 (128), which not only recruits neutrophils, but also activates them (129,130) and promotes their emigration from the vasculature (128). Circulating neutrophils which localize to an ischemic and reperfused area first adhere to the activated endothelial surface in a decelerating, rolling type of adhesive process mediated by endothelial P-selectin and its carbohydrate counterligand (sialyl-Lewis^x) on the neutrophil (131). This interaction brings the neutrophils into close approximation with the endothelial surface, to promote firmer adhesive interactions mediated by such molecules as L-selectin, platelet activating factor, ICAM-1 on the endothelial cell, and the neutrophil β_2 integrins (CD11/CD18) (125). The hypoxic/ischemic, proinflammatory milieu includes such cytokines as interleukin-1, which upregulates endothelial cell expression of ICAM-1 (132) and E-selectin (94), which further support PMN adhesion.

Recent strategies to block neutrophil adhesion have met with similar successes in experimental models of ischemia and reperfusion, although none is at present used clinically as adjunctive therapy with thrombolysis. Antibody to IL-8 administered to rabbits limits pulmonary reperfusion injury (133). Anti-P-selectin treatment not only attenuates reperfusion injury in the rabbit ear (134), but limits myocardial infarct size in a feline model (117). In other models of cardiac ischemia and reperfusion, anti-β_2 integrin (98,127) or anti-ICAM-1 (126) therapy has been shown to be similarly effective. Although antibody therapy is cumbersome and

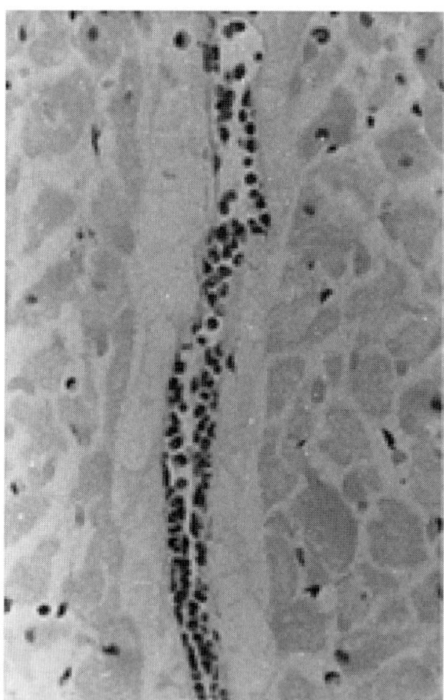

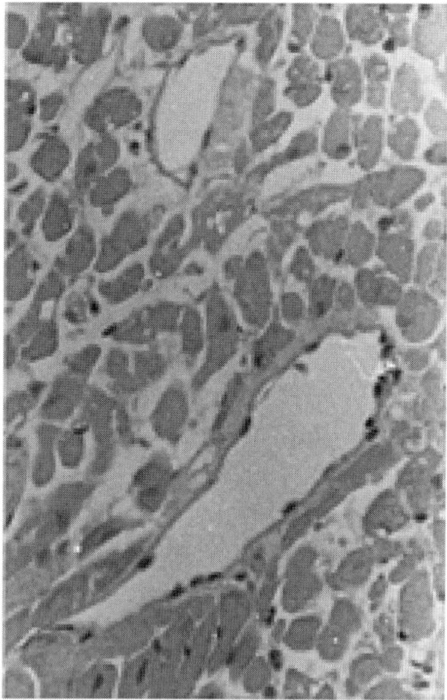

FIG. 4. Neutrophil infiltration into the heart following reperfusion. Using a model of global cardiac ischemia and reperfusion, one can see neutrophils adhere to the endothelial lining of blood vessels as early as 10 min following reperfusion **(left).** This neutrophil recruitment can be blocked by using nitroglycerin during the ischemic period, which acts as a nitric oxide donor to reduce neutrophil adherence to the reperfused vasculature **(right).** These results were corroborated by tissue myeloperoxidase activity, measured by a chromogenic assay which quantifies the presence of the neutrophil-specific enzyme myeloperoxidase. (Adapted from Pinsky et al., ref. 32.)

probably will be of limited clinical use, novel antiadhesion strategies are currently under study, such as administration of the oligosaccharide counterligand for P-selectin (sialyl-Lewis^{x}) (135), which may be of significant clinical benefit in the future.

ROLE OF THE COMPLEMENT CASCADE

Initial study of the role of the complement system in myocardial infarction in rats (136) led to subsequent studies in which decomplementation of experimental animals by administration of cobra venom factor reduced myocardial necrosis following ischemia and reperfusion (123,137). Briefly, the complement system consists of two components, the classical and the alternative pathways, which are activated by a proteolytic cascade in a similar fashion to the activation of coagulation. The two pathways converge at complement component C3, the cleavage of which leads to the formation of anaphylatoxins (C3a and C5a) as well as the amphiphilic membrane attack complex (MAC), consisting of complement components C5b–C9. The membrane attack complex adheres to membrane phospholipids and essentially punches gaping holes in cells, resulting in rapid target-cell lysis.

It is not surprising that ischemia and reperfusion may likewise result in complement activation, which may be deleterious to myocytes both by amplification of the inflammatory milieu by way of further neutrophil recruitment and activation, or by local generation and insertion of the membrane attack complex into bystander myocytes. Deposition of MAC has been noted in areas of myocardial infarction, with relatively little deposition in adjacent nonischemic areas (138). Even sublytic amounts of C5b–C9 may trigger endothelial cell Weibel–Palade body exocytosis, with concomitant translocation of P-selectin to the endothelial surface, which may further contribute to neutrophil adhesion (139). Local activation of complement is deleterious to the heart, as has been shown in a number of studies (123,140,141). Complement blockade has shown promise in recent trials in which soluble complement receptor type 1 (SCR1), which lacks cytosolic and transmembrane domains, has protected against postischemic myocardial inflammation and necrosis (142).

CONCLUSION

The pathophysiology and biochemistry of cardiac ischemia, necrosis, and reperfusion can be seen as a complex interplay between myocytes and the surrounding tissue. Various proinflammatory and procoagulant effector mechanisms contribute to the ultimate outcome following myocardial infarction. Cellular effector mechanisms (including neutrophils) as well as humoral mechanisms (including the complement and coagulation cascades) are activated during the processes of ischemia and reperfusion. The cardiac vasculature plays a critical modulatory role in these events, with the period of hypoxia/ischemia emerging as an important priming event for the subsequent endothelial cell dysfunction and proinflammatory milieu which follows a period of myocardial ischemia and reperfusion. Novel strategies designed to abrogate endothelial dysfunction and to limit the consequences of neutrophil adhesion and complement activation are likely to play important adjunctive roles along with thrombolytic therapy in the future treatment of acute myocardial infarction.

REFERENCES

1. Jennings RB. Myocardial ischemia observations, definitions, and speculations [Editorial]. *J Mol Cell Cardiol* 1970;1:345–349.

2. Sayen JJ, Sheldon WF, Pierce G, Kuo PT. Polarigraphic oxygen, the epicardial electrocardiogram and muscle contraction in experimental acute regional ischemia of the left ventricle. *Circ Res* 1958;6: 779–798.
3. Jennings RB. Early phase of myocardial ischemic injury and infarction. *Am J Cardiol* 1969;24:753–765.
4. Braasch W, Gudbjarnason S, Puri PS, Ravens KG, Bing RJ. Early changes in energy metabolism in the myocardium following acute coronary artery occlusion in anesthetized dogs. *Circ Res* 1968;23: 429–438.
5. Kloner RA, Ellis SG, Lange R, Braunwald E. Studies of experimental coronary artery reperfusion: Effects on infarct size, myocardial function, biochemistry, ultrastructure, and microvascular damage. *Circulation* 1983;68(Suppl I):8–15.
6. Hersdon PB, Katzenbach JP, Jennings RB. Fine structural and biochemical changes in dog myocardium during autolysis. *Am J Pathol* 1969;57:539–557.
7. Krug A. Der Fruhnachweis des Herzinfarktes durch Bestimmung der Wasserstoffionenkonzentration im Hertzmuskel mit Idicatorpapier. *Virchows Arch [Pathol Anat]* 1965;338:339–341.
8. Harris AS, Bisteni A, Russell RA, Brigham JC, Firestone JE. Excitatory factors in ventricular tachycardia resulting from myocardial ischemia: Potassium is a major excitant. *Science* 1954;119:200–203.
9. Case RB, Nasser MG, Crampton RS. Biochemical aspects of early myocardial ischemia. *Am J Cardiol* 1969;24:766–775.
10. Ferrari R, Ceconi C, Curello S, Alfieri O, Visioli O. Myocardial damage during ischemia and reperfusion. *Eur Heart J* 1993;14(Suppl G): 25–30.
11. Berne RM, Rubio R. Acute coronary occlusion: Early changes that induce coronary dilatation and the development of collateral circulation. *Am J Cardiol* 1969;24:776–781.
12. Jennings RB, Sommers HM, Smyth GA, Flack HA, Linn H. Myocardial necrosis induced by temporary occlusion of a coronary artery in the dog. *AMA Arch Pathol* 1960;70:68–78.
13. Tennant R, Wiggers CJ. The effect of coronary occlusion on myocardial contraction. *Am J Physiol* 1935;112:351–361.
14. Sobel BE. Acute myocardial infarction. In Pasternak RC, Braunwald E, eds. *Heart Disease, A Textbook of Cardiovascular Medicine*. Philadelphia: Saunders; 1992:1200–1272.
15. Kloner RA, Rude RE, Carlson N, Maroko PR, Deboer LW, Braunwald E. Ultrastructural evidence of microvascular damage and myocardial cell injury after coronary artery occlusion: Which comes first? *Circulation* 1980;62:945–952.
16. Kloner RA, DeBoer LW, Carlson N, Braunwald E. The effect of verapamil on myocardial ultrastructure during and following release of coronary artery occlusion. *Exp Mol Pathol* 1982;36:277–286.
17. Jennings RB, Reimer KA. Salvage of ischemic myocardium. *Mod Concepts Cardiovasc Dis* 1974;43:125–130.
18. Garcia-Dorado D, Oliveras J. Myocardial oedema: A preventable cause of reperfusion injury? *Cardiovasc Res* 1993;27:1555–1563.
19. Garcia-Dorado D, Theroux P, Munoz R, Alonso J, Elizada J, Fernandez-Aviles F, Botas J, Solares J, Soriano J, Duran JM. Favorable effects of hyperosmotic reperfusion on myocardial edema and infarct size. *Am J Physiol* 1992;262:H17–H22.
20. Steenbergen CH, Hill ML, Jennings RB. Volume regulation and plasma membrane injury in aerobic, anaerobic, and ischemic myocardium *in vitro*. *Circ Res* 1985;57:864–875.
21. Dauber IM, Vanbenthuysen KM, McMurtry IF, Wheeler GS, Lesnefsky EJ, Horwitz LD, Weil JV. Functional coronary microvascular injury evident as increased permeability due to brief ischemia and reperfusion. *Circ Res* 1990;66:986–998.
22. Pilati CE. Macromolecular transport in canine coronary microvasculature. *Am J Physiol* 1990;258:H748–H753.
23. Jennings RB, Ganote CE, Reimer KA. Ischemic tissue injury. *Am J Pathol* 1975;81:179–198.
24. Jennings RB, Schaper J, Hill ML, Steenbergen C Jr, Reimer KA. Effects of reperfusion late in the phase of reversible ischemic injury: Changes in cell volume, electrolytes, metabolites, and ultrastructure. *Circ Res* 1985;56:262–278.
25. Baroldi G. Different types of myocardial necrosis in coronary heart disease: A pathophysiologic review of their functional significance. *Am Heart J* 1975;89:742–752.
26. Hutchins GM, Bulkley BH. Correlation of myocardial contraction band necrosis and vascular patency: A study of coronary artery bypass graft anastomoses at branch points. *Lab Invest* 1977;36:642–648.
27. Adams JE III, Abendschein DR, Jaffe AS. Biochemical markers of myocardial injury: Is MB creatine kinase the choice for the 1990s? *Circulation* 1993;88:750–763.
28. Devries SR, Jaffe AS, Geltman EM, Sobel BE, Abendschein DR. Enzymatic estimation of the extent of irreversible myocardial injury early after reperfusion. *Am Heart J* 1989;177:31–36.
29. Kloner RA. Does reperfusion injury exist in humans? *J Am Coll Cardiol* 1993;21:537–545.
30. Reimer KA, Vander-Heide RS, Richard VJ. Reperfusion in acute myocardial infarction: Effect of timing and modulating factors in experimental models. *Am J Cardiol* 1993;72:13G–21G.
31. Lefer AM, Tsao PS, Lefer DJ, Ma X-L. Role of endothelial dysfunction in the pathogenesis of reperfusion injury after myocardial ischemia. *FASEB J* 1991;5:2029–2034.
32. Pinsky DJ, Oz MC, Koga S, Taha Z, Broekman MJ, Marcus AJ, Liao H, Naka Y, Brett J, Cannon PJ, Nowygrod R, Malinski T, Stern DM. Cardiac preservation is enhanced in a heterotopic rat transplant model by supplementing the nitric oxide pathway. *J Clin Invest* 1994;93: 2291–2297.
33. Manning AS, Hearse DJ. Reperfusion-induced arrhythmias: Mechanisms and prevention. *J Mol Cell Cardiol* 1984;16:497–518.
34. Hale SL, Lange R, Alker KJ, Kloner RA. Correlates of reperfusion ventricular fibrillation in dogs. *Am J Cardiol* 1984;53:1397–1400.
35. Zweier JL. Measurement of superoxide-derived free radicals in the reperfused heart: Evidence for a free-radical mechanism of injury. *J Biol Chem* 1988;263:1353–1357.
36. Babbs C, Cregor M, Turek J, Badylak S. Endothelial superoxide production in the isolated rat heart during early reperfusion after ischemia. *Am J Pathol* 1991;139:1069–1080.
37. Kramer JH, Arroyo CM, Dickens BF, Wglicki WB. Spin trapping evidence that graded myocardial ischemia alters post-ischemic superoxide production. *Free Radic Biol Med* 1987;3:153–159.
38. McCord JM. Free radicals and myocardial ischemia: Overview and outlook. *Free Radic Biol Med* 1988;4:9–14.
39. Zweier JL, Rayburn NK, Flaherty JT, Weisfeldt ML. Recombinant superoxide dismutase reduces oxygen free radical concentrations in reperfused myocardium. *J Clin Invest* 1987;80:1728–1734.
40. Bolli R, Patel BS, Jeroudi MO, Lai EK, McCay PB. Demonstration of free radical generation in "stunned" myocardium of intact dogs with the use of the spin traps alpha-phenyl *N-tert*-butyl nitrone. *J Clin Invest* 1988;82:476–485.
41. McCord JM. Oxygen-derived free radicals in post-ischemic tissue. *N Engl J Med* 1985;312:159–163.
42. McCord JM, Roy RS, Schaffer SW. Free radicals in myocardial ischemia. The role of xanthine oxidase. *Adv Myocardial* 1985;5: 183–189.
43. Eddy J, Stewart R, Jones H, Yellon D, McCord JM, Downey J. Xantine oxidase is detected in ischemic rat heart but not in human hearts. *Physiologist* 1986;29:166.
44. Eddy LJ, Stewart JR, Jones H, Engerson TD, McCord JM, Downey MJ. Free radical-producing enzyme, xanthine oxidase, is undetectable in human hearts. *Am J Physiol* 1987;253:H709–H711.
45. Muxfeldt M, Schaper W. The activity of xanthine oxidase in hearts of pigs, guinea pigs, rats, and humans. *Basic Res Cardiol* 1987;82: 486–492.
46. Boveris A, Chance B. The mitochondrial generation of hydrogen peroxide: General properties and effects of hyperbaric oxygen. *Biochem J* 1986;134:707–716.
47. Lucchesi BR, Werns SW, Fantone JC. The role of the neutrophil and free radicals in ischemic myocardial injury. *J Mol Cell Cardiol* 1989; 21:1241–1251.
48. Halliwell B. Oxidants and human disease: Some new concepts. *FASEB J* 1987;1:358–364.
49. Gutteridge JMC. Aspects to consider when detecting and measuring lipid peroxidation. *Free Radic Res Commun* 1986;1:173–184.
50. Roberts MJD, Young IS, Trouton TG, Trimble ER, Khan MM, Webb SW, Wilson CM, Patterson GC, Adger AA. Transient release of lipid peroxides after coronary artery balloon angioplasty. *Lancet* 1990;336: 143–145.
51. Davies SW, Ranjadayalan K, Wickens DG, Dorurandy TL, Timmis AD. Lipid peroxidation associated with successful thrombolysis. *Lancet* 1990;335:741–743.

52. Tamura Y, Chi L, Driscoll EM, Hoff PT, Freeman BA, Gallagher KP, Lucchesi BR. Superoxide dismutase conjugated to polyethylene glycol provides sustained protection against myocardial ischemia/reperfusion injury in the canine heart. *Circ Res* 1988;63:944–959.
53. Jolly SR, Kane WJ, Bailie MB, Abrams GD, Lucchesi BR. Canine myocardial reperfusion injury: Its reduction by the combined administration of superoxide dismutase and catalase. *Circ Res* 1984;54: 277–285.
54. Whalen DA Jr, Hamilton DG, Canote CE, Jennings RB. Effect of a transient period of ischemia on myocardial cells. I. Effects on cell volume regulation. *Am J Pathol* 1974;74:381–398.
55. Schen AC, Jennings RB. Kinetics of calcium accumulation in acute myocardial ischemic injury. *Am J Pathol* 1972;67:449–452.
56. Kloner RA, Glanote CE, Whalen DA Jr, Jennings RB. Effect of a transient period of ischemia on myocardial cells. II. Fine structure during the first few minutes of reflow. *Am J Pathol* 1974;74:399–420.
57. Schen AC, Jennings RB. Myocardial calcium and magnesium in acute ischemic injury. *Am J Pathol* 1972;67:417–434.
58. Kloner RA, Ganote CE, Jennings RB. The ''no-reflow'' phenomenon after temporary coronary occlusion in the dog. *J Clin Invest* 1974;54: 1496–1508.
59. Engler RL, Schmid-Schonbein GW, Pavelec RS. Leukocyte capillary plugging in myocardial ischemia and reperfusion in the dog. *Am J Pathol* 1983;111:98–111.
60. Pinsky D, Oz M, Liao H, Morris S, Brett J, Morales A, Karakurum M, Van Lookeren Campagne M, Nowygrod R, Stern D. Restoration of the cyclic AMP second messenger pathway enhances cardiac preservation for transplantation in a heterotopic rat model. *J Clin Invest* 1993;92:2994–3002.
61. Komamura K, Kitakaze M, Nishida K, Naka M, Tamai J, Uematsu M, Kovetsune Y, Nanto S, Hori M, Inoue M. Progressive decreases in coronary vein flow during reperfusion in acute myocardial infarction: clinical documentation of the no-reflow phenomenon after successful thrombolysis. *J Am Coll Cardiol* 1994;24:370–377.
62. Schofer J, Montz R, Mathey DG. Scintigraphic evidence of the ''no reflow'' phenomenon in human beings after coronary thrombolysis. *J Am Coll Cardiol* 1985;5:593–598.
63. Braunwald E, Kloner RA. The stunned myocardium: Prolonged, postischemic ventricular dysfunction. *Circulation* 1982;66:1146–1149.
64. Takeishi Y, Tono-oka I, Kubota I, Ikeda K, Masakone I, Chiba J, Abe S, Tuiki K, Komatani A, Yamaguchi I. Functional recovery of hibernating myocardium after coronary bypass surgery: Does it coincide with improvement in perfusion? *Am Heart J* 1991;122:665–670.
65. Stack RS, Phillips HR, Grierson DS, Behar VS, Kong Y, Peter RH, Swain JL, Grenfield JC Jr. Functional improvement of jeopardized myocardium following intracoronary streptokinase infusion in acute myocardial infarction. *J Clin Invest* 1983;72:84–95.
66. Owen P, Dennis S, Opie LH. Glucose flux rate regulates onset of ischemic contracture in globally underperfused rat hearts. *Circ Res* 1990;66:344–354.
67. Opie LH. The mechanism of myocyte death in ischemia. *Eur Heart J* 1993;14(Suppl G):31–33.
68. Ferrari R, Alfieri O, Currello S, Ceconi C, Cargnoni A, Marzollo P. Occurrence of oxidative stress during reperfusion of the human heart. *Circulation* 1990;81:201–211.
69. Dennis SC, Gevers W, Opie LH. Protons in ischemia: Where do they come from, where do they go? *J Mol Cell Cardiol* 1991;23: 1077–1086.
70. Corr PB, Gross RW, Sobel BE. Arrhythmogenic amphiphilic lipids and the myocardial cell membrane. *J Mol Cell Cardiol* 1982;14: 619–626.
71. Corretti MC, Koretsune Y, Kusuoka H, Chacko VP, Zweier JL, Marban E. Glycolytic inhibition and calcium overload as consequences of exogenously generated free radicals in rabbit hearts. *J Clin Invest* 1991;88:1014–1025.
72. Gottlieb RA, Burleson KO, Kloner RA, Babior BM, Engler RL. Reperfusion injury induces apoptosis in rabbit cardiomyocytes. *J Clin Invest* 1994;94:1621–1628.
73. Ogawa S, Gerlach H, Esposito C, Pasagian-Macaulay A, Brett J, Stern D. Hypoxia modulates the barrier and coagulant function of cultured bovine endothelium. *J Clin Invest* 1990;85:1090–1098.
74. Ogawa S, Shreeniwas R, Brett J, Clauss M, Furie M, Stern D. The effect of hypoxia on capillary endothelial cell function: modulation of barrier function and coagulant function. *Br J Haematol* 1990;75: 517–524.
75. Stelzner T, O'Brien R, Sato K, Weil J. Hypoxia-induced increases in pulmonary transvascular protein escape in rats. *J Clin Invest* 1988; 82:1840–1847.
76. Ogawa S, Koga S, Kuwabara K, Morris S, Bilezikian J, Silverstein S, Stern D. Hypoxia-induced increased permeability and lowering of cellular cAMP levels. *Am J Physiol* 1992;262:C546–C554.
77. Beebe S, Corbin J. Cyclic nucleotide-dependent protein kinases. In: *The Enzymes*. New York: Academic Press; 1986:43–111.
78. Minnear F, Johnson A, Malik A. Beta-adrenergic modulation of pulmonary transvascular fluid and protein exchange. *J Appl Physiol* 1986; 60:266–274.
79. Minnear F, DeMichele M, Moon D, Rieder C, Fenton J. Isoproterenol reduces thrombin-induced pulmonary endothelial permeability *in vitro*. *Am J Physiol* 1989;257:H1613–H1623.
80. Farrukh I, Gurtner G, Michael J. Pharmacological modification of pulmonary vascular injury: Possible role of cAMP. *J Appl Physiol* 1987;62:47–54.
81. Stelzne T, Weil J, O'Brien R. Role of cyclic adenosine monophosphate in the induction of endothelial barrier properties. *J Cell Physiol* 1989;139:157–166.
82. Adkins W, Barnard J, May S, Seiber A, Haynes J, Taylor A. Compounds that increase cAMP prevent ischemia-reperfusion pulmonary capillary injury. *J Appl Physiol* 1992;72:492–497.
83. Haynes J, Robinson J, Saunders L, Taylor A, Strada S. Role of cAMP-dependent protein kinase in cAMP-mediated vasodilation. *Am J Physiol* 1992;262:H511–H516.
84. Suttorp N, Weber U, Welsch T, Schudt C. Role of phosphodiesterases in the regulation of endothelial permeability in vitro. *J Clin Invest* 1993;91:1421–1428.
85. Feelisch M, te Poel M, Zamora R, Deussen A, Moncada S. Understanding the controversy over the identity of EDRF. *Nature* 1994; 368:62–65.
86. Kubes P, Suzuki M, Granger D. NO: Modulator of leukocyte adhesion. *Proc Natl Acad Sci USA* 1991;88:4651–4655.
87. Radomski M, Palmer R, Moncada S. Endogenous nitric oxide inhibits human platelet adhesion to vascular endothelium. *Lancet* 1987;ii: 1057–1058.
88. Kubes P, Granger D. NO modulates vascular permeability. *Am J Physiol* 1992;262:H611–H615.
89. Oz M, Pinsky D, Koga S, Marboe C, Han D, Kline R, Jeevanandam V, Williams M, Morales A, Popilskis S, Nowygrod R, Stern D, Rose E, MIchler R. Novel preservation solution permits 24 hours preservation in rat and baboon cardiac transplant models. *Circulation* 1993; 88(5, pt 2):291–297.
90. Gerlach H, Clauss M, Ogawa S, Stern D. Perturbation of endothelial barrier and coagulant properties by environmental factors. In: *Endothelial Cell Dysfunction*. New York: Plenum Press; 1991:525–545.
91. Esmon C. The regulation of natural anticoagulant pathways. *Science* 1987;235:1348–1352.
92. Broekman M, Eiroa A, Marcus A. Inhibition of human platelet reactivity by endothelium-derived relaxing factor from human umbilical vein endothelial cells in suspension. *Blood* 1991;78:1033–1040.
93. Koga S, Ogawa S, Kuwabara K, Brett J, Leavy J, Ryan J, Koga Y, Plockinski J, Benjamin W, Burns D, Stern D. Synthesis and release of interleukin-1 by reoxygenated human mononuclear phagocytes. *J Clin Invest* 1992;90:1007–1015.
94. Shreeniwas R, Koga S, Karakurum M, Pinsky D, Kaiser E, Brett J, Wolitzky B, Norton C, Plocinski J, Benjamin W, Burns D, Goldstein A, Stern D. Hypoxia-mediated induction of endothelial interleukin-1 alpha. *J Clin Invest* 1992;90:2333–2339.
95. Pober J. Warner-Lambert Parke-Davis Award Lecture. Cytokine-mediated activation of vascular endothelium. *Am J Pathol* 1988;133: 426–433.
96. Oz M, Rose E, Michler R, Spotnitz H, Smith C, Liao H, Stern D, Pinsky D. Coronary vascular endothelium may release contents of Weibel–Palade bodies but does not shed membrane proteins during cardiac surgery. *Circulation* 1993;88(4, pt 2):I-247.
97. Horgan M, Wright S, Malik A. Antibody against leukocyte integrin (CD18) prevents reperfusion-induced lung injury. *Am J Physiol* 1990; 259:L315–L319.
98. Simpson P, Todd R III, Fantone J, Michelson J, Griffin J, Lucchesi B. Reduction of experimental canine myocardial reperfusion injury by

a monoclonal antibody (anti-Mol, anti-CD11b) that inhibits leukocyte adhesion. *J Clin Invest* 1988;81:624–629.

99. Repine J, Cheronis J, Rodell T, Linas S, Patt A. Pulmonary oxygen toxicity and ischemia-reperfusion injury. A mechanism in common involving xanthine oxidase and neutrophils. *Am Rev Respir Dis* 1987; 136:483–485.
100. Colletti L, Remick D, Burtch G, Kunkel S, Strieter R, Campbell D. Role of tumor necrosis factor alpha in the pathophysiologic alterations after hepatic ischemia/reperfusion injury in the rat. *J Clin Invest* 1990; 85:1936–1943.
101. Dreyer W, Michael L, West M, Smith C, Rothlein R, Rossen R, Anderson D, Entman M. Neutrophil accumulation in ischemic canine myocardium: Insights into time course, distribution, and mechanism of localization during early reperfusion. *Circulation* 1988;84:400–411.
102. Dinarello C. Interleukin-1 and its biologically related cytokines. *Adv Immunol* 1989;44:153–205.
103. Sherry B, Cerami A. Cachectin/tumor necrosis factor exerts endocrine, paracrine, and autocrine control of inflammatory responses. *J Cell Biol* 1988;107:1269–1277.
104. Strieter R, Kunkel S, Showell H, Remick D, Phan S, Ward P, Marks R. Endothelial cell gene expression of a neutrophil chemotactic factor by TNF-alpha, LPS, and IL-1 beta. *Science* 1989;243:1467–1469.
105. Baggiolini M, Walz A, Kunkel S. Neutrophil-activating peptide-1/Il-8, a novel cytokine that activates neutrophils. *J Clin Invest* 1989;84: 1045–1049.
106. Karakurum M, Shreeniwas R, Chen J, Pinsky D, Yan S-D, Anderson M, Sunouchi K, Major J, Hamilton T, Kuwabara K, Rot A, Nowygrod R, Stern D. Hypoxic induction of interleukin-8 gene expression in human endothelial cells. *J Clin Invest* 1994;93:1564–1570.
107. Yoshida N, Granger D, Anderson D, Rothelein R, Lane C, Kvietys P. Anoxia/reoxygenation-induce neutrophil adherence to cultured endothelial cells. *Am J Physiol* 1992;262:H1891–H1898.
108. Arnould T, Michiels C, Remacle J. Increased PMN adherence on ECs after hypoxia: Involvement of PAF, CD18/CD11B, and ICAM-1. *Am J Physiol* 1993;264:C1102–1110.
109. Kubes P, Ibbotson G, Russel JM, Wallace JL, Granger DN. Role of platelet-activating factor in ischemia-reperfusion induced leukocyte adherence. *Am J Physiol* 1990;259:G300–G305.
110. Hattori R, Hamilton K, Fugate R, McEver R, Sims P. Stimulated secretion of endothelial vWF is accompanied by rapid redistribution to the cell surface of the intracellular granule membrane protein GMP-140. *J Biol Chem* 1989;264:7768–7771.
111. McEver RP, Beckstead JH, Moore KL, Marshall-Carlson L, Bainton DF. GMP-140, a platelet α-granule membrane protein, is also synthesized by vascular endothelial cells and is localized in Weibel–Palade bodies. *J Clin Invest* 1989;84:92–99.
112. Ewenstein B, Warhol M, Handin R, Pober J. Composition of the vWF storage organelle isolated from cultured human umbilical vein endothelial cells. *J Cell Biol* 1987;104:1423–1433.
113. Birch K, Pober J, Zavoico G, Means A, Ewenstein B. Calcium/calmodulin transduces thrombin-stimulated secretion: Studies in intact and minimally permeabilized human umbilical vein endothelial cells. *J Cell Biol* 1992;118:1501–1510.
114. Lorant DE, Patel KD, McIntyre TM, McEver RP, Prescott SM, Zimmerman GA. Coexpression of GMP-140 and PAF by endothelium stimulated by histamine or thrombin: a juxtacrine system for adhesion and activation of neutrophils. *J Cell Biol* 1991;115:223–234.
115. Patel KD, Zimmerman GA, Prescott SM, McEver RP, McIntyre TM. Oxygen radicals induce human endothelial cells to express GMP-140 and bind neutrophils. *J Cell Biol* 1991;112:749–759.
116. Geng J-G, Bevilacqua MP, Moore KL, McIntyre TM, Prescott SM, Kim JM, Bliss GA, Zimmerman GA, McEver RP. Rapid neutrophil adhesion to activated endothelium mediated by GMP-140. *Nature* 1990;343:757–760.
117. Weyrich AS, Ma X-L, Lefer DJ, Albertine KH, Lefer AM. *In vivo* neutrolization of P-selectin protects feline heart and endothelium in myocardial ischemia and reperfusion injury. *J Clin Invest* 1993;91: 2620–2629.
118. Romson JL, Hook BG, Kunsel SL, Abrams GD, Schork MA, Lucchesi BR. Reduction of the extent of ischemic myocardial injury by neutrophil depletion in the dog. *Circulation* 1983;67:1016–1023.
119. Mullane KM, Read M, Salmon JA, Moncada S. Role for leukocytes in acute myocardial infarction in anesthetized dogs: Relationship of myocardial salvage by antiinflammatory drugs. *J Pharmacol Exp Ther* 1984;228:510–522.
120. Lucchesi B, Mullane K. Leukocytes and ischemia induced myocardial injury. *Annu Rev Pharmacol Toxicol* 1986;26:201–224.
121. Dreyer WJ, Michael LH, West MS, Smith CW, Rothlein R, Rossen RD, Anderson DC, Entman ML. Neutrophil accumulation in ischemic canine myocardium. Insights into time course, distribution, and mechanism of localization during early reperfusion. *Circulation* 1991;84: 400–411.
122. Entman ML, Michael L, Rossen RD, Dreyer WJ, Anderson DC, Taylor AA, Smith CW. Inflammatory in the course of early myocardial ischemia. *FASEB J* 1991;5:2529–2537.
123. Crawford M, Grover F, Kolb W, McMahan C, O'Rourke R, McManus L, Pinckard R. Complement and neutrophil activation in the pathogenesis of ischemic myocardial injury. *Circulation* 1988;78:1449–1458.
124. Granger D. Role of xanthine oxidase and granulocytes in ischemia-reperfusion injury. *Am J Physiol* 1988;255:H1269–H1275.
125. Kilgore KS, Lucchesi BR. Reperfusion injury after myocardial infarction: The role of free radicals and the inflammatory response. *Clin Biochem* 1993;26:359–370.
126. Ma X-L, Lefer D, Lefer A, Rothlein R. Cardiac protective effects of a monoclonal antibody to intercellular adhesion molecule-1 in myocardial ischemia and reperfusion. *Circulation* 1992;86:937–946.
127. Ma X, Tsao P, Lefer A. Antibody to CD18 exerts endothelial and cardiac protective effects in myocardial ischemia and reperfusion. *J Clin Invest* 1991;88:1237–1243.
128. Rot A. Endothelial cell binding NAP-1/IL-8: Role in neutrophil emigration. *Immunol Today* 1992;13:291–294.
129. Peveri P, Walz A, DeWald B, Baggiolini M. A novel neutrophil-activating factor produced by human mononuclear phagocytes. *J Exp Med* 1988;167:1547–1559.
130. Detmers PA, Lo SK, Olsen-Egbert E, Walz A, Baggiolini M, Cohn ZA. Neutrophil activating protein 1-interleukin-8 stimulates binding activity of the leukocyte adhesion receptor CD11b/CD18 on human neutrophils. *J Exp Med* 1990;171:1155–1162.
131. Mayadas TN, Johnson RC, Rayburn H, Hynes RO, Wagner DD. Leukocyte rolling and extravasation are severely compromised in P selectin deficient mice. *Cell* 1993;74:541–554.
132. Vadas MA, Gamble JR. Regulation of the adhesion of neutrophils to endothelium. *Biochem Pharmacol* 1990;40:1683–1688.
133. Sekido N, Mukaida N, Harada A, Nakanishi I, Watanabe Y, Matsushima K. Prevention of lung reperfusion injury in rabbits by a monoclonal antibody against interleukin-8. *Nature* 1993;365:654–657.
134. Winn RK, Liggitt D, Vedder NB, Paulson JC, Harlan JM. Anti-P-selectin monoclonal antibody attenuates reperfusion injury to the rabbit ear. *J Clin Invest* 1993;92:2042–2047.
135. Mulligan MS, Paulson JC, De Frees S, Lowe JB, Ward PA. Protective effects of oligosaccharides in P-selectin-dependent lung injury. *Nature* 1993;364:149–151.
136. Hill JH, Ward PA. The physiologic role of C3 leukotactic fragments in myocardial infarcts of rats. *J Exp Med* 1971;133:885–900.
137. Maroko PR, Carpenter CB, Chiareillo M, Fishbein MC, Radvany P, Knostman JD, Hale SL. Reduction by cobra venom factor of myocardial necrosis after coronary artery occlusion. *J Clin Invest* 1978;61: 661–670.
138. Schafer H, Mathey D, Hugo F, Bhakdi S. Deposition of the terminal C5b-9 complex in infarcted areas of human myocardium. *J Immunol* 1986;137:1945–1949.
139. Hattori R, Hamilton KK, McEver RP, Sims PJ. Complement proteins C5b-9 induce secretion of high molecular weight multimers of endothelial von Willebrand factor and translocation of granule membrane protein GMP-140 to the cell surface. *J Biol Chem* 1989;264: 9053–9060.
140. Homeister JW, Satoh P, Lucchesi PS. Effects of complement activation in the isolated heart: Role of the terminal complement components. *Circ Res* 1992;71:303–319.
141. Homeister JW, Satoh PS, Kilgore KS, Lucchesi BR. Soluble complement receptor type 1 prevents human complement-mediated damage of the rabbit isolated heart. *J Immunol* 1993;150:1055–1064.
142. Weisman HF, Bartow T, Leppo MK, Marsh HC Jr, Carson GR, Cocino MF, Boyle MP, Roux KH, Weisfeldt ML, Fearon DT. Soluble human complement receptor type 1: *In vivo* inhibitor of complement suppressing post-ischemic myocardial inflammation and necrosis. *Science* 1990;249:146–151.
143. Malinski T, Taha Z. Nitric oxide release from a single cell measured *in situ* by a porphyrinic-based microsensor. *Nature* 1992;358:676–678.

Atherosclerosis and Coronary Artery Disease,
edited by V. Fuster, R. Ross, and E. J. Topol.
Lippincott-Raven Publishers, Philadelphia © 1996.

CHAPTER 48

Triggering of Onset of Myocardial Infarction and Sudden Cardiac Death

James E. Muller, Geoffrey H. Tofler, and Murray Mittleman

Key Words: Arrhythmia; Circadian rhythm; Endothelium; Myocardial infarction; Plaques; Sudden cardiac death; Thrombosis; Triggering.

INTRODUCTION

Over the past decade, substantial information has been obtained indicating that the onset of myocardial infarction, as well as sudden cardiac death, is often triggered by activities of the patient (1–3). This information is now helping to illuminate the mechanisms linking a previously quiescent atherosclerotic plaque to the acute coronary syndromes (4). Exploration of this relatively unstudied aspect of coronary artery disease is of great importance, not because triggers could be identified and avoided but because a better understanding of mechanism of onset would create new opportunities for prevention. The method of prevention would be to develop pharmacological and other strategies to interrupt the linkage between a trigger and its pathological consequences.

The relative position of this new field of research into triggering of coronary thrombosis is shown in Fig. 1. The arrow in the center of the figure indicates the onset of coronary thrombosis causing nonfatal myocardial infarction or sudden cardiac death. The four columns represent research areas focusing on the different stages of coronary artery disease. Chronic risk factors, acute treatment, and prognosis have already been areas of intense research interest and considerable progress. In contrast, the events occurring in the hours and minutes prior to the onset of thrombosis—the causes of conversion of chronic to acute disease—have received relatively little attention.

The increased prospects for success in this hitherto difficult and relatively unapproachable field of study result from the multiple advances in understanding of acute coronary artery disease achieved during the 1980s. The work of DeWood et al. (5) clearly established that acute thrombosis causes myocardial infarction. Davies and Thomas (6), Falk (7), and others, building on the pioneering studies of Con-

J. E. Muller, G. H. Tofler, and M. Mittleman: Institute for Prevention of Cardiovascular Disease, Deaconess Hospital, Boston, Massachusetts 02215.

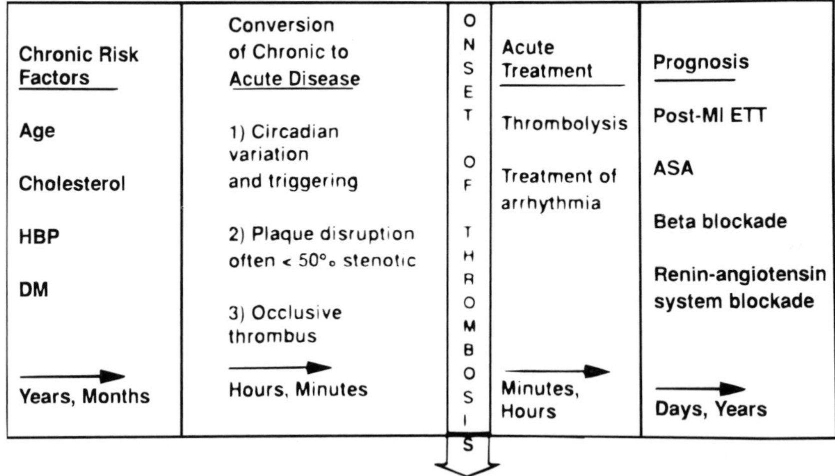

FIG. 1. The relation of the relatively undeveloped area of research on conversion of chronic to acute disease to the traditional areas of research on coronary artery disease.

stantinides in the 1960s (8), identified the pathoanatomic role of plaque disruption and thrombosis in sudden death and unstable angina as well as in myocardial infarction. Fuster and colleagues characterized the types of arterial injury likely to produce thrombosis (9), and Willerson et al. (10) identified interventions capable of modifying conversion of chronic to acute disease in experimental animals. Randomized clinical trials have demonstrated that aspirin (11), β-adrenergic blocking agents (12), lipid-lowering regimens (13), and, more recently, angiotensin-converting enzyme inhibitors (14) can prevent myocardial infarction, but the mechanisms of the beneficial effects are not fully explained.

Plaques that are disrupted and cause disease onset have been found to contain higher concentrations of lipids and macrophages that nondisrupted plaques (15,16). Finally, it is now recognized that the entire sequence of plaque disruption and occlusive thrombosis often begins in lesions previously causing less than 50% reduction of the diameter of the arterial lumen, as judged by prior angiograms (17) and from angiographic assessment following thrombolysis of degree of original stenosis (18).

Although these gains in understanding are impressive, the field of triggering remains relatively unexplored, and only a small fraction of its potential benefit has yet been realized. Heart attack, the term for the combined disorders of myocardial infarction and sudden cardiac death, continues to account for an estimated 500,000 deaths per year in the United States (19). Even the optimal utilization of thrombolytic therapy for myocardial infarction—the advance on which the greatest attention has been focused—could prevent only 25,000 deaths acutely, or 5% of the total, because most deaths occur suddenly, before any type of treatment can be initiated (20).

Improved understanding of triggering could lead to far more effective means to reduce morbidity and mortality from cardiovascular disease.

HISTORY OF THE TRIGGERING CONCEPT

Although triggering and circadian variation appear to be new topics of interest, the concepts have strong historical roots. In their original clinical description of acute myocardial infarction (MI) in 1910, Obraztsov and Strazhesko noted, "Direct events often precipitated the disease; the infarct began in one case on climbing a high staircase, in another during an unpleasant conversation, and in a third during emotional distress associated with a heated card game" (21). In the 1930s, studies in larger numbers of patients revealed that myocardial infarction often occurred without an obvious precipitating event, thus challenging their view. Authors argued for (22,23) and against (24,25) the belief that triggers were frequent. The controversy was eventually suspended for many years as Master's conclusion, based on retrospective questionnaires and no control data, that "Coronary occlusion takes place irrespective of the physical activity being performed or the type of rest taken," gained widespread acceptance (26). However, studies conducted with modern epidemiologic methods and with the insight provided by new understanding of the pathogenesis of myocardial infarction indicate the validity of the original concept of Obraztsov and Strazhesko.

MORNING INCREASE OF MYOCARDIAL INFARCTION

The evidence that MI does not occur randomly throughout the day but shows a prominent increased morning frequency supports the concept that daily activities are important triggers. Data indicating that the onset of MI is more likely to occur in the morning come from two studies that determined the time of onset of infarction objectively with creatine kinase timing (1,27) and by other studies (28,29) that used onset of pain as the marker for time of myocardial infarction

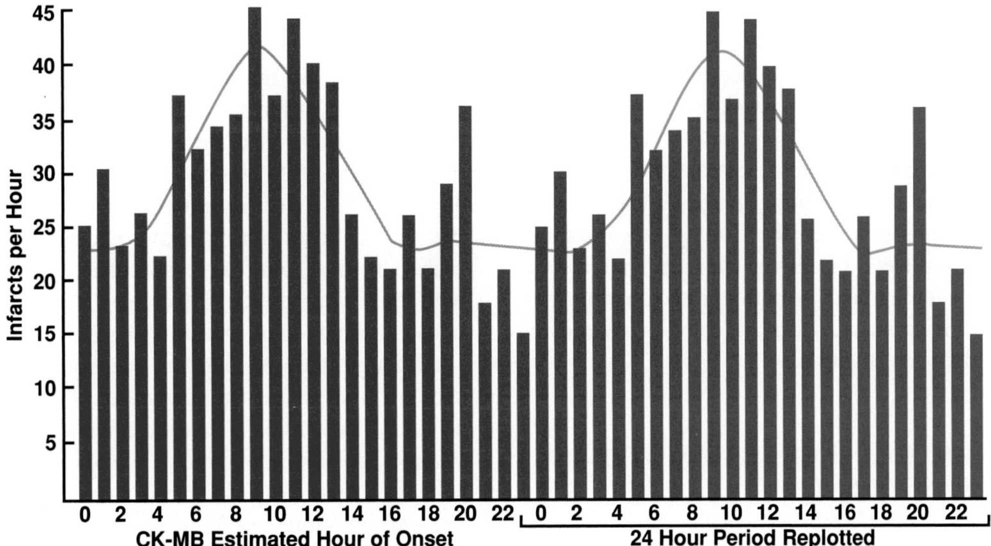

FIG. 2. Hourly frequency of onset of myocardial infarction as determined by the creatine kinase-MB method. The number of infarctions beginning during each of the 24 hours of the day is plotted on the left side of the figure. On the right, the identical data are plotted again to permit appreciation of the relationship between the end and the beginning of the day. A two-harmonic regression equation for the frequency of onset of myocardial infarction has been fitted to the data *(curved line).* A primary peak incidence of infarction occurs at 9 AM, and a secondary peak occurs at 8 PM. (From Muller et al., ref. 1, with permission.)

onset. In the Multicenter Investigation of Limitation of Infarct Size (MILIS) (1), numerous creatine kinase MB determinations were made to obtain an objective determination of the time of onset of MI in 849 patients. The onset of MI was considered to have occurred 4 h before the initial elevation of creatine kinase. The time of day of onset of MI in the 703 patients for whom complete creatine kinase timing was available is shown in Fig. 2. The abscissa shows the hour of the day with the same data replotted for a second day to permit appreciation of the relationship between the end of one day and the beginning of the next. The ordinate shows the number of infarcts per hour. A marked daily variation is present, with a maximum of 45 infarcts between 9 and 10 AM and a minimum of 15 between 11 PM and midnight. This objective evidence obtained in the MILIS data base was confirmed in the data base (1,741 patients) from the Intravenous Streptokinase in Acute Myocardial Infarction (ISAM) Study (27) demonstrating that MI was four times more likely to occur between 8 and 9 AM than between midnight and 1 AM.

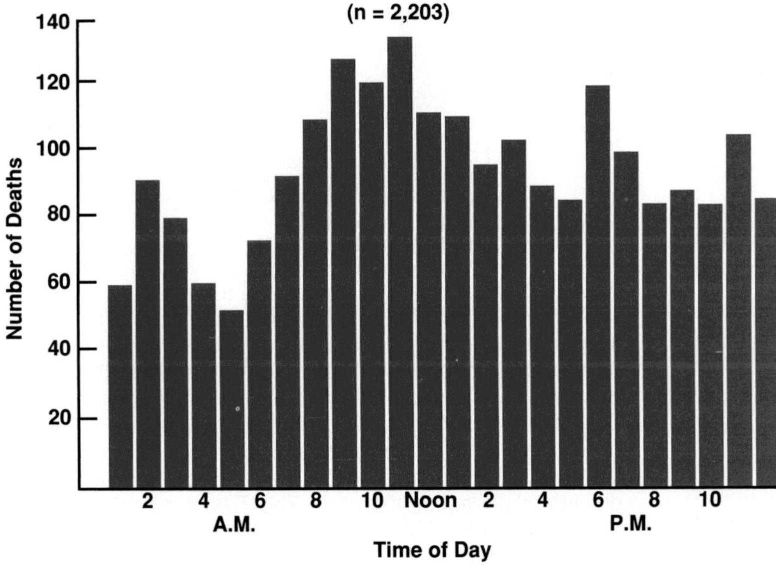

FIG. 3. The time of day of out-of-hospital sudden cardiac death (ICD-410 ≤1 h from onset of symptoms to death) for 2,203 individuals dying in Massachusetts in 1983. A statistically significant ($p < 0.001$) circadian rhythm is present with a primary peak between 7 and 11 AM and a secondary peak between 5 and 6 PM. (From Willich et al., ref. 2, with permission.)

The finding of these two studies is further supported by Goldberg et al., who have subsequently refined this evidence by reporting that the increased incidence of myocardial infarction occurs in the first 4 h after awakening and onset of activity (29).

Two other major cardiovascular diseases, sudden cardiac death and stroke, also show morning increases (2,33) (Fig. 3). These observations reinforce the finding that nonfatal myocardial infarction has a prominent morning increase in onset. A smaller, evening peak of both MI and sudden cardiac death appears in some data bases; its cause is not known and requires further investigation.

EPIDEMIOLOGIC EVIDENCE THAT ACTIVITIES TRIGGER DISEASE ONSET

Increasingly convincing evidence has been obtained indicating that certain activities trigger disease onset. Observational studies without control data suggested the relationships that have now been confirmed with controlled studies.

Observational data on possible triggering activities collected from 849 patients enrolled in the MILIS Study (34) suggested frequent triggering. Possible triggers were reported by 48.5% of patients, 13.6% of whom reported two or more triggers. The triggers included emotional upset (18.8%), moderate physical activity (14.4%), heavy physical activity (8.7%), lack of sleep (8.0%), overeating (6.9%), sexual activity (1.2%), surgery (0.4%), and miscellaneous (6.6%). These data are similar to those reported by Sumiyoshi et al. (35).

The level of physical activity at onset of MI was determined in 3,339 patients entered into the Thrombolysis in Myocardial Infarction (TIMI) II Study (36). Moderate or marked physical activity occurred at onset of MI in 18.7% of patients, more than could be expected from the proportionally much smaller fraction of the 24 h that the subjects engage in moderate or marked activity.

Although these and other studies suggest that triggers of MI are present, the abovementioned studies suffer from a lack of control data. To assess the relative risk of an MI occurring following a common stressor such as physical exercise, it is essential to estimate the expected level of activity in the hours before the MI. Adjustment for usual exposure is also needed for comparisons of possible triggering between groups because differences clearly exist in the likelihood of patients with specific characteristics, such as older age, performing activities such as heavy physical exertion.

These and other methodological limitations of earlier studies have been addressed in the Determinants of Onset of Myocardial Infarction Study (ONSET), in which over 1,800 patients have been interviewed to identify possible triggers of their MI. For the ONSET Study, a case-crossover study design developed by Maclure (37) and Mittleman et al. (38) has enabled estimation of the relative risk of an MI following a trigger. This risk is calculated as the observed frequency of the activity during a designated hazard period (the hour prior to the MI) compared with its expected frequency based on the individual's usual frequency of exertion. By the use of this method, it has now been demonstrated that heavy exertion (exertion estimated to be ≥6 METS) produced a 5.9-fold increase in risk (95% confidence interval 4.6–7.7) of MI in the subsequent hour (38) (Fig. 4). The risk of MI onset during heavy exertion was significantly higher in those who were sedentary (107-fold) compared with those who regularly exercised (twofold) (Fig. 5). Willich et al. found similar results in a German population (39).

Although there is abundant anecdotal evidence that psychological stress may trigger onset of MI, there have been no controlled studies of this acute phenomenon. Prior studies of anger, hostility, and type A personality as risk factors for MI have focused on chronic risk and have yielded controversial and sometimes contradictory results (40). In the ONSET study, data on outbursts of anger were collected in 1,623 patients. Anger corresponding to levels greater than 4 in a 7-level self-report anger scale was reported by 14% of patients within 26 h prior to MI onset. Using the same study design described above for the study of physical exertion, we found that the risk of MI onset was significantly elevated in the 2 h following an outburst of anger, with a relative risk of 2.3 (95% confidence interval 1.7–3.2) (41).

Sexual activity has also been documented to trigger myocardial infarction (42). The relative risk of an MI occurring in the hour after sexual activity is 2.1 compared to baseline risk. Although this documentation of an elevated relative

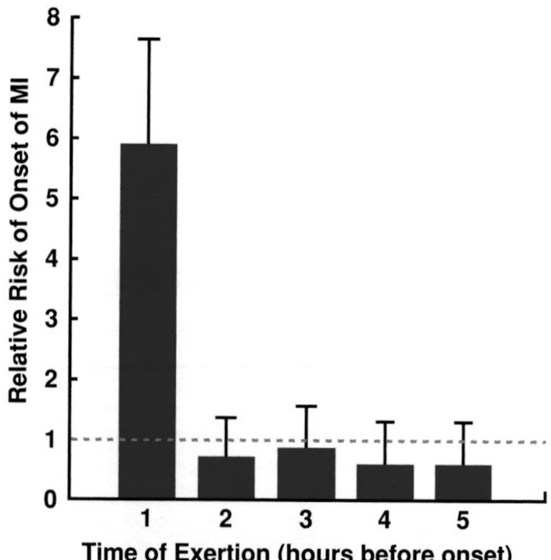

FIG. 4. Time of onset of myocardial infarction after an episode of heavy physical exertion (induction time). Each of the five hours before the onset of myocardial infarction was assessed as an independent hazard period, and exertion during each hour was compared with that during the control period. Only exertion during the hour immediately before the onset of myocardial infarction was associated with an increase in the relative risk, suggesting that the induction time for myocardial infarction is less than 1 h. The *T bars* indicate the 95% confidence limits. The *dotted line* indicates the baseline risk. (From Mittleman et al., ref. 38, with permission.)

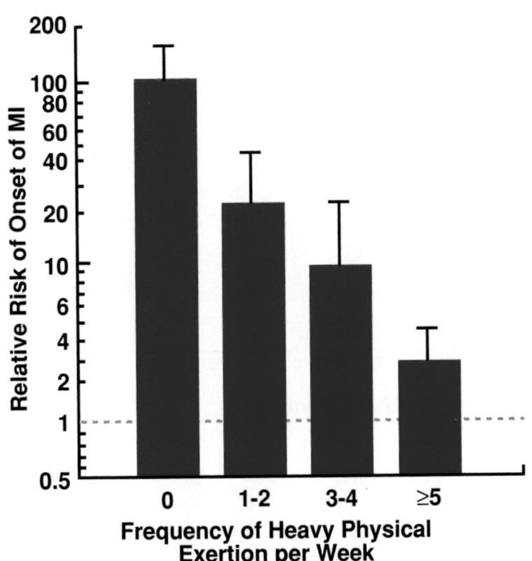

FIG. 5. Modification of the relative risk of myocardial infarction by usual frequency of heavy exertion (defined as ≥6 METS). The relative risks for heavy physical exertion are shown for subgroups of patients whose habitual frequency of heavy physical exertion is less than 1, 1 to 2, 3 to 4, and 5 or more episodes per week. Note that the relative risk is presented on a logarithmic scale. Sedentary individuals experienced an extreme relative risk (107), while those who exerted themselves five or more times per week had an increase in risk only 2.4 times over baseline ($p < 0.001$). *Error bars* indicate 95% confidence intervals. (From Mittleman et al., ref. 38, with permission.)

risk might lead to concern over sexual activity in patients in rehabilitation programs, the data actually provide grounds for reassurance of such patients. The relative risk was not elevated in those with a history of cardiac disease compared to those without. In addition, because the baseline absolute risk of an MI in any given hour is extremely low (approximately 10 chances in 1 million per hour for a patient with a prior MI), doubling of baseline risk would produce only a small increase in absolute risk and should not be a factor in the decision of an asymptomatic cardiac patient to engage in sexual activity.

Finally, the progress made in identifying triggers of MI in controlled studies makes it possible to estimate the percentage of all infarctions that are triggered. As shown in Fig. 6, the recognized triggers of awakening, physical exertion, anger, and sexual activity account for 15% to 20% of MIs, or almost 250,000 MIs annually in the United States. This undoubtedly represents an underestimate of triggering and indicates the importance of understanding triggering mechanisms.

AUTOPSY AND ANGIOGRAPHIC DATA PERTINENT TO TRIGGERING MECHANISMS

In 1980, DeWood et al. demonstrated that occlusive coronary artery thrombosis is the cause of most Q-wave myocardial infarctions (5). Furthermore, coronary angiographic and angioscopic studies have demonstrated a high frequency of nonocclusive coronary thrombosis in patients with unstable angina (43,44). Constantinides observed that thrombus had formed over a ruptured atherosclerotic plaque in all the cases of occluded coronary arteries that he examined (8). The angiographic finding that contrast medium outpouching, indicative of plaque rupture, was observed in patients who had undergone successful thrombolysis supports the importance of plaque rupture in acute coronary syndromes (45).

Although autopsy studies generally reveal severe atherosclerotic stenosis at the base of a fatal coronary thrombus (7), there is angiographic evidence that in many patients surviving a myocardial infarction, the degree of stenosis is relatively mild, and obstructive thrombus accounts for the majority of the obstruction to blood flow (17,18,46). These findings may explain the absence of prior symptoms in many patients presenting with acute myocardial infarction. Intrinsic plaque characteristics and extrinsic factors that predispose and initiate plaque disruption remain areas of intense investigation. Richardson and co-workers have reported that in 63% of cases, plaque disruption occurred at the junction of a lipid pool with normal tissue (15). A lipid core, a thin fibrous cap, and macrophage activity seem to be important factors that predispose an atherosclerotic plaque to disrupt (47). The recent finding that there is a spectrum of lesions from fibrous plaques composed predominantly of smooth muscle cells to lipid-rich lesions with numerous macrophages leads to the concept that inflammatory mechanisms modulate plaque morphology (48–50).

MORNING INCREASE OF PHYSIOLOGICAL PROCESSES THAT MIGHT TRIGGER MYOCARDIAL INFARCTION

A variety of mechanisms, alone or in combination, could account for the morning increase in myocardial infarction

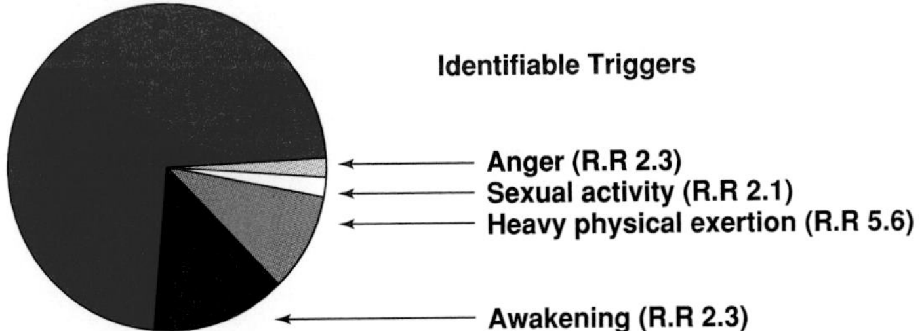

FIG. 6. Percentage of MIs that are triggered.

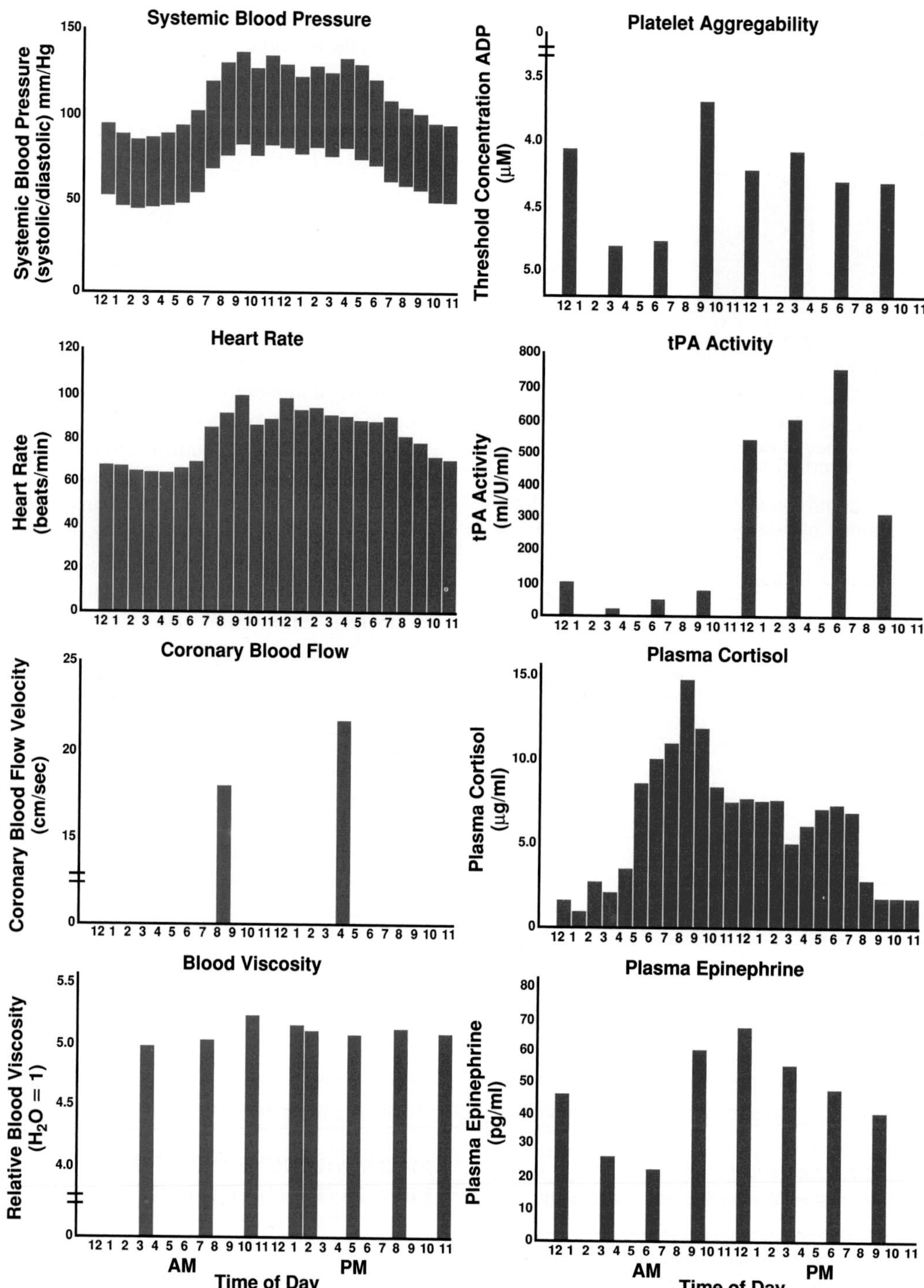

FIG. 7. Bar graphs of variation during a 24-h period of eight physiological processes possibly contributing to the increased morning frequency of disease onset: systemic blood pressure and heart rate measured intraarterially in five normotensive ambulant subjects, coronary blood flow velocity measured by Doppler ultrasonic flow probe in 21 dogs, whole blood viscosity measured by Ostwald-capillary viscometer in eight normal male volunteers, platelet aggregability measured by in vitro platelet aggregometry in 15 normal male volunteers, tissue-type plasminogen activity (t-PA) measured by spectrophotometric assay in six normal volunteers (four men, two women), plasma cortisol measured by competitive protein binding method in six normal male volunteers, and plasma epinephrine measured by a radioisotope method in 15 normal male volunteers. (From Muller et al., Ref. 3, with permission.)

onset (Fig. 7). A morning arterial pressure surge could initiate plaque disruption. An increase in coronary arterial tone could worsen the flow reduction produced by a fixed stenosis. The combination of increases in arterial pressure and coronary tone increase could result in increased shear stress (force directed against the endothelium resulting from increased coronary blood flow velocity), thus predisposing a vulnerable plaque to disrupt. Other prothrombotic processes, including increased platelet adhesion, increased blood viscosity, and increased platelet aggregability (51,52), have been implicated in the morning increase in ischemic events. Such a thrombotic tendency added to a reduced fibrinolytic activity in the morning (53) could increase the likelihood that an otherwise harmless mural thrombus overlying a small plaque fissure would propagate and occlude the coronary lumen.

OTHER POTENTIAL TRIGGERING CYCLES

The circadian (24-h) cycle is not the only cycle that may provide clues to triggering of disease onset; seasonal variation and increases around the time of holidays and birthdays have also been reported. Mortality from ischemic heart disease shows an annual cycle with an increase in the winter (56). It is interesting to note that in the Southern Hemisphere seasonal variation in heart disease mortality has been confirmed, with peak mortality occurring during the Southern Hemisphere winter months of June, July, and August.

TIMING AND TRIGGERS OF TRANSIENT MYOCARDIAL ISCHEMIA

Transient myocardial ischemia, a phenomenon that is more frequent than myocardial infarction, sudden cardiac death, and stroke, has been studied using Holter monitoring. This method allows precise timing of ischemic periods. Such studies have consistently demonstrated a peak incidence of ischemic episodes between 6 AM and 12 noon (57). In addition to demonstrating this morning peak, investigations using Holter ST-segment analysis have also provided insight into the possible triggers of transient ischemia. Such studies demonstrate that over half of transient ischemic episodes are preceded by possible triggers such as mental or physical stress (57). A recent study by Parker et al. has shown that delay of morning activity delays the onset of the transient ischemia peak (58).

Although a 24-h periodicity of disease onset (Figs. 2 and 3) and physiological processes (Fig. 7) is well established, it remains unclear if this periodicity results from a true endogenous circadian rhythm or from the daily rest–activity cycle. Cortisol secretion, for example, is well known to be an endogenous circadian process not dependent on daily activity (54), whereas the morning platelet aggregability increase is abolished if the subjects remain at bed rest (55). There may also be an interaction between circadian and rest–activity cycles; e.g., assumption of the upright posture leading to sympathetic activation may be more likely to cause intense vasoconstriction when endogenously controlled cortisol levels are high. This concept is controversial because circadian stage and sleep–wake cycles with posture change are highly correlated in all epidemiologic studies of infarction timing thus far reported. Investigations analyzing the relationship between an unusual wake time on the day of myocardial infarction and standard wake time on other days could potentially separate the wake–sleep cycle from the underlying cortisol rhythm, but such studies have not been reported.

Although the peak incidence of disease onset occurs in the morning, it is likely that similar physiological processes trigger disease onset at other times of the day. The peak morning incidence of infarct onset probably results from the synchronization of potential triggers in the morning, whereas a secondary evening peak in infarct onset observed in the MILIS data may result from synchronization of the population for an additional potential trigger, such as the evening meal. For other periods of the day, exposure of the population to potential triggers is sporadic, and no other prominent peaks of incidence are observed.

EFFECT OF DRUG THERAPY ON CIRCADIAN VARIATION OF DISEASE

As the field of study of circadian variation of cardiovascular disease has progressed, investigators have attempted to determine if various types of drug therapy alter the timing of cardiovascular events. For nonfatal myocardial infarction and sudden cardiac death, the conditions that have received the most attention, there is strong evidence that β-adrenergic blockade, a therapy well-documented to prevent the occurrence of these disorders, selectively decreases the morning peak of events.

The evidence supporting this effect of β-blockade is of two types. First, studies determining the timing of infarction have shown a flattening of the morning peak in patients who happened to be receiving β-adrenergic blocking agents prior to their infarct (1). Because β-blockers were not randomly assigned, these studies are open to the criticism that the absence of the morning peak resulted from confounding by factors other than the therapy. The second type of evidence, which is not subject to the concerns over confounding, comes from the Beta Blocker Heart Attack Trial (BHAT), in which patients were randomly assigned to β-blockade or placebo. β-Blockade demonstrated a selective beneficial effect against the occurrence of sudden cardiac death in the morning (59).

Evidence indicating a selective benefit of aspirin therapy in the morning has been less impressive than that for β-blockade. Observations of the timing of infarction in patients taking aspirin therapy, but not by random assignment, prior to their infarction have yielded mixed results. However, the single randomized study in which the effect has been studied has demonstrated a selective morning decrease in nonfatal myocardial infarction in patients receiving aspirin therapy (60). It is possible that the randomized study is powerful enough to detect a small beneficial effect that cannot be detected by the nonrandomized, observational studies.

Studies of silent myocardial ischemia have demonstrated that β-blockade, but not a short-acting calcium channel blocker, attenuates the morning increase in silent myocardial ischemia (61). A recent study has demonstrated that the morning increase in silent ischemia can be prevented by nadolol therapy (58).

These studies indicate that pharmacological therapy can affect the time of day of cardiac events. However, these observations have not yet been complemented by studies of the ability of therapy to prevent triggering of events by activities such as heavy exertion. Data have been obtained indicating that aspirin may diminish the ability of anger to trigger infarction (41).

GENERAL THEORY OF TRIGGERING OF CORONARY THROMBOSIS

The new information on triggering has provided the basis for a general theory of onset of coronary thrombosis (62). The hypothesis presented in Fig. 8 adds the concept of triggering activities to the general scheme of the role of thrombosis in the acute coronary syndromes advanced by Falk, Davies and Thomas, Fuster, Willerson, and others (6,7,9,10, 63,64). It involves several important new concepts—triggers, acute risk factors, and vulnerable plaques—that contribute to three processes central to the development of coronary thrombosis.

The first process is disruption of an atherosclerotic plaque. This may be caused by systemic factors, such as an increase in systemic arterial pressure causing hemodynamic stress on the plaque, or by local factors, such as increased macrophage activity and vasoconstriction. The second process is thrombus formation, which may be mural or occlusive depending on local and systemic factors. Finally, postdisruption vasoconstriction, which is dependent on the thrombus itself and

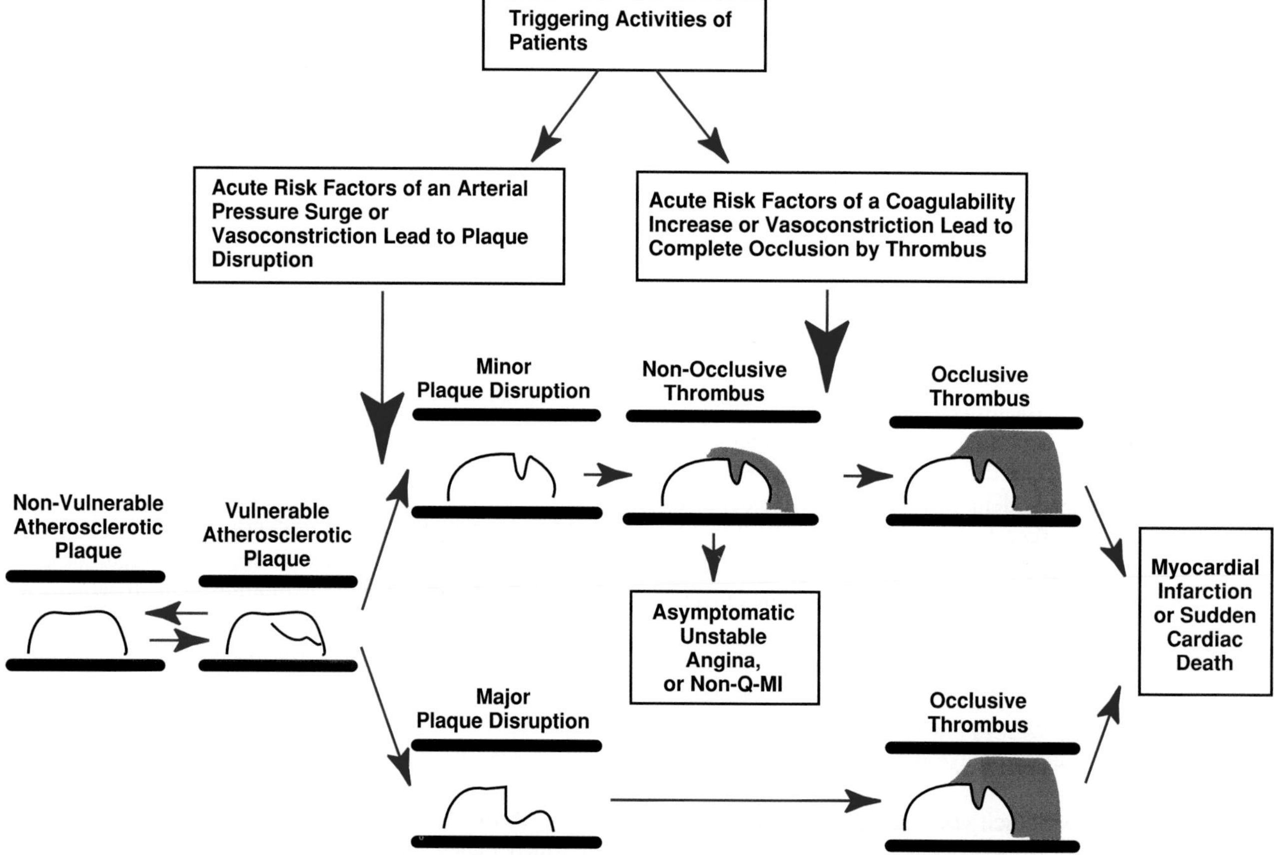

FIG. 8. Illustration of a hypothetical method by which daily activities may trigger coronary thrombosis. Three triggering mechanisms are presented: (1) physical or mental stress producing hemodynamic changes leading to plaque rupture, (2) activities causing a coagulability increase, and (3) stimuli leading to vasoconstriction. The scheme depicting the role of coronary thrombosis in unstable angina, myocardial infarction, and sudden cardiac death has been well described by numerous authors. The novel portion of this figure is the addition of triggers. See text for detailed discussion. (From Muller et al., ref. 62, with permission.)

the degree of endothelial dysfunction, may determine if the thrombus occludes the artery. With these three processes in mind, it is possible to examine the potential mechanisms of the various triggers of disease onset.

It is proposed that the initial step in the process leading to disease onset is the development, with advancing age, of a vulnerable atherosclerotic plaque. Plaque vulnerability is defined functionally as the susceptibility of a plaque to disruption. Development of such vulnerability is a poorly understood process but is presumably a dynamic, potentially reversible disorder caused by several factors including changes in plaque constituents or its blood supply via vasa vasorum and/or changes in the functional integrity of the overlying endothelium, in part from increased macrophage activity and thinning of the plaque collagen cap. The new catheterization laboratory techniques of intracoronary angioscopy and ultrasound may, in the future, permit detection of vulnerable plaques before their disruption.

Onset of MI might begin when a physical or mental stress produces a hemodynamic change that is sufficient to disrupt a vulnerable plaque. Vasoconstrictive and thrombogenic forces might then lead to coronary occlusion. Shear forces may also play an important role in thrombus formation, as suggested by Coller et al. (63) and others.

The finding that disrupted plaques without thrombi are sometimes observed at autopsy in patients dying of noncardiac disease suggests that, in some cases, acute plaque disruption may not be the initial step in disease onset (65). In such patients the trigger may lead to occlusive thrombosis by causing an increase in thrombotic tendency or vasoconstriction in the presence of a previously nonthrombogenic plaque. It is also possible that the plaques became disrupted at the time of death, an occurrence perhaps more likely during a violent death. These possibilities underscore the need for studies of the lesions causing disease onset in living patients.

A synergistic combination of triggering activities may account for thrombosis in a setting in which each activity alone may not exceed the threshold for causation of infarction. For example, the combination of physical exertion (producing a minor plaque disruption) followed by cigarette smoking (producing an increase in coronary artery vasoconstriction and a relatively hypercoagulable state) (66) may be needed to cause occlusive thrombosis and disease onset. Also, the response of a healthy individual to a potential trigger may differ from that observed in an individual with a condition predisposing to MI. Exaggerated or paradoxical responses may be observed. For example, hypertensives demonstrate a greater increase in forearm vascular resistance after infusion of norepinephrine than normals (67). Patients with atherosclerosis may demonstrate a paradoxical vasoconstrictor response in response to acetylcholine infusion (68), and an impaired increase in fibrinolytic potential with exercise (69).

The findings of circadian variation and triggering have also led to the concept of an acute risk factor that supplements the traditional concept of a chronic risk factor. The acute risk factor is defined as the pathophysiological change (vasoconstrictive, hemodynamic, or hemostatic) potentially leading to occlusive coronary thrombosis. It results from a combination of an external stress (physical or mental) and the individual's reactivity to that stress. Although the extent of atherosclerosis changes slowly with time (chronic risk factor), hemodynamic, vasoconstrictive, and prothrombotic forces (acute risk factors) may be rapidly generated by external stresses.

SUDDEN CARDIAC DEATH

The findings described above for nonfatal myocardial infarction caused by coronary thrombosis are of great importance for the larger problem of sudden cardiac death. Although nonfatal myocardial infarction causes considerable morbidity, the problem of sudden cardiac death is of greater significance because it leads to the death of over 250,000 individuals each year in the United States alone (70–73). Furthermore, effective treatment of sudden cardiac death requires a preventive approach because, by definition, the deaths occur, in most cases, before intervention is feasible.

Discussion of triggering of sudden cardiac death must begin with consideration of the relationship between nonfatal myocardial infarction and sudden cardiac death. From autopsy data, it is apparent that approximately one-third of sudden cardiac deaths are caused by acute total coronary occlusion by thrombosis (74–78). Findings in patients resuscitated from sudden cardiac death support these pathological findings (79). Thus, in many cases, the only difference between nonfatal infarction and sudden cardiac death is that the patients dying suddenly experienced a fatal arrhythmia or immediate pump failure during what would otherwise have been a nonfatal infarction.

In addition to this one-third of sudden cardiac death patients clearly sharing a common mechanism with nonfatal myocardial infarction, there is evidence that intracoronary thrombosis may play a role in a far greater proportion of sudden cardiac death patients. Davies and Thomas (77) found that in ≥90% of patients dying of sudden cardiac death, there were signs of rupture of an atherosclerotic plaque associated with thrombosis. In 44% of the patients, there was intracoronary thrombus, defined as ≥50% luminal obstruction, associated with the site of plaque rupture. An additional 30% of patients showed evidence of a recent nonobstructive coronary thrombus.

In addition to these sudden cardiac deaths associated with occlusive or nonocclusive coronary thrombosis, there are sudden cardiac deaths caused by primary electrical abnormalities, valvular disorders, hypertrophic cardiomyopathy, and abnormalities of the conducting system. All of these causes are likely to experience a certain amount of triggering by external activities.

Although the field of triggering of nonfatal myocardial infarction has advanced rapidly, there are greater difficulties in the study of triggering of sudden cardiac death. By definition, the patients do not survive the disorder; therefore, information about potential triggering activities must be obtained from witnesses, if they are available. Witnesses often have difficulty recounting the exact activities of the patient prior to the event.

Despite these difficulties, a considerable amount of evidence is now available and has been summarized in a recent review article (80). The first direct evidence of circadian variation of sudden cardiac death, cited earlier, was reported in 1987 from an analysis of mortality records of the Massachusetts population (2). Sudden cardiac death was defined as death from cardiac disease occurring within 1 h after onset of symptoms. A total of 2,203 individuals were identified who presumably died of sudden cardiac death outside of the hospital or nursing home. The time of day of death in this population showed a distinct circadian variation with a primary peak in the late morning from 9 to 11 AM and a minor secondary peak in the late afternoon, similar to the pattern described for nonfatal myocardial infarction (Fig. 2). A limitation of this study is that it was based on information obtained from death certificates. Therefore, further study of time of day of sudden cardiac death was performed in subjects enrolled in the prospective Framingham Heart Study (30). A total of 264 subjects (11% of all deaths among subjects of the original cohort of the Framingham Heart Study) had experienced a definite sudden cardiac death. Analysis of the time of death in these individuals demonstrated circadian variation with approximately a threefold increased risk of sudden cardiac death during the morning and a low incidence during the night. This finding in a carefully monitored population firmly established the morning increase in sudden cardiac death.

In a study conducted in Germany, Arntz et al. (80) reported preliminary findings on the time of day of sudden cardiac death in groups of patients characterized by ECG recordings obtained by emergency physicians. Patients demonstrating an initial rhythm of ventricular tachycardia or ventricular fibrillation showed a marked circadian variation in occurrence. The time of death of patients whose initial finding was electromechanical dissociation or asystole was relatively evenly distributed throughout the day.

A circadian variation of ventricular tachycardia has been documented by Hausmann et al. (81). An increased morning risk was observed in patients with poor left ventricular function or prolonged tachycardia.

More recent studies have demonstrated that the increase in sudden cardiac death appears to be concentrated in the hours after awakening, as observed for nonfatal myocardial infarction. Peters et al. (82) reported preliminary findings that sudden death of 37 patients in the CAST study began most frequently within the 2 h after awakening. A recent study by Willich et al. demonstrated similar results in the general population (83). The increased availability of implantable cardioverter defibrillators provides an opportunity to better characterize the timing and triggers of potentially lethal tachyarrhythmias. Recent data obtained by our group and others have confirmed the increased morning frequency of ventricular tachyarrhythmias.

ACTIVITY PRIOR TO SUDDEN CARDIAC DEATH

Although controlled studies of triggering activities are limited for sudden cardiac death, there are several observational studies suggesting that either physical or mental stress may trigger sudden cardiac death. Moritz and Zamcheck (84) observed in soldiers of World War II that sudden death of unknown cause frequently occurred during or shortly after strenuous exertion. In a controlled study, Thompson et al. identified an age-adjusted risk of sudden cardiac death during jogging of 7 (95% CI 4 to 26) compared with the estimated rate during sedentary activities (85). Siscovick et al. found that among men with low levels of habitual activity, the relative risk of sudden cardiac death during vigorous activity was 56 (95 CI 23 to 31); among men with high levels of habitual activity, it was 5 (95 CI 2 to 14) (86).

Mental stress has also been implicated as a trigger of sudden cardiac death. A major review of this issue has recently been published by Kamarack and Jennings (87). The difficulties of identifying triggering by physical exertion are magnified for mental stress, because it is difficult to determine the amount of stress associated with potential psychological triggers.

Myers and Dewar reported in 1975 that in 40 of 100 cases, sudden death occurred within 24 h after acute psychological stress (88). Appropriate control data were not presented. In the Cardiac Arrhythmia Pilot Study (CAPS), a high level of depression, type A behavior pattern, and low pulse rate reactivity to challenge were significant predictors of subsequent cardiac arrest (89). In the Recurrent Coronary Prevention Project, a type A behavior pattern was a significant predictor for sudden cardiac death during follow-up of patients post-MI (90).

INCREASED AUTONOMIC NERVOUS SYSTEM ACTIVITY IN SUDDEN CARDIAC DEATH

The extensive evidence suggesting that both physical exertion and mental stress can lead to sudden cardiac death suggests a prominent role for the autonomic nervous system in triggering the disease. There are laboratory findings supporting this linkage. In experimental animals, an increase in basal tone or acute stimulation of the central nervous system by drugs or electrical stimuli lowers the threshold for cardiac electrical instability and may invoke a variety of arrhythmias, including ventricular fibrillation in experimental animals (91,92). Studies in experimental animals have demonstrated a reduced threshold for ventricular fibrillation in dogs subjected to acute psychological stress (93). The relationship between platelet activity and sympathetic activation has been investigated in an animal model developed by Folts et al.

(94). Thrombotic tendency can be increased by epinephrine infusion and decreased by sympatholytic interventions. This model exemplifies the importance of sympathetic activity in the pathogenesis of sudden cardiac death and suggests a possible physiological link between physical or psychosocial stressors causing sympathetic activation and the occurrence of fatal arrhythmias.

HYPOTHETICAL MODEL OF TRIGGERING OF SUDDEN CARDIAC DEATH

The model presented above for the occurrence of thrombotic coronary occlusion leading to nonfatal MI also serves as the mechanism through which thrombosis produces sudden cardiac death (SCD). In addition, it is likely that triggers cause sudden cardiac death through several other mechanisms. First, the trigger and increased sympathetic activation may decrease the threshold of the myocardium for a fatal arrhythmia. Second, the trigger may act on the conducting system of the heart, thereby predisposing to a fatal arrhythmia. Third, in conditions with hypertrophic cardiomyopathy or significant valvular disease, a triggering activity may lead to death through hemodynamic mechanisms. Thus, it is likely that the triggering mechanisms for SCD will include, but not be limited to, those responsible for total thrombotic coronary occlusion. In addition, the adequacy of the collateral circulation and the condition of the microcirculation may play critical roles in determining whether a total coronary occlusion leads to a lethal cardiac arrhythmia (95,96). Collateral flow can equal that provided by a major epicardial vessel with a 90% occlusion. Hence, if a severely stenotic lesion adequate to stimulate collateral development suddenly occludes, there may be adequate collateral flow to prevent development of a malignant ventricular arrhythmia (97).

CLINICAL IMPLICATIONS OF CIRCADIAN VARIATION AND TRIGGERING OF MYOCARDIAL INFARCTION AND SUDDEN CARDIAC DEATH

The current state of knowledge of the morning increase and triggering of disease onset raises the question as to whether pharmacological therapy should be altered to prevent triggering.

For β-blockade, the data appear sufficient to justify selection of an agent that will provide adequate 24-h protection, particularly in the morning hours. This recommendation is based on substantial evidence, but it is important to note that there has not been, and is unlikely to be, a randomized trial comparing the ability of a long-acting β-blocker versus a shorter-acting agent to prevent cardiovascular events.

For aspirin, the issue of morning protection is moot because a single dose of aspirin provides suppression of morning platelet activity for approximately 3 days. For other agents, such as coronary vasodilators and antihypertensive agents, the issue is unresolved. It seems reasonable that pharmacological protection should be provided during the morning hours for patients already receiving antiischemic and antihypertensive therapy. However, studies documenting that such a regimen is more likely to prevent myocardial infarction or sudden death than a regimen providing less morning protection have not been reported and, to our knowledge, are not in progress or planned.

Because infarcts are more frequent in the morning and can be triggered by exertion, questions about the relative risk of morning exercise versus afternoon or evening exercise have been raised. It is clear that exercise is beneficial in reducing the risk of infarction, and, although theoretical concerns can be raised, there is no evidence that exercise in the morning is more hazardous than exercise at other times of the day. On the contrary, recent data from the ONSET Study indicate that the relative risk of exertion in the morning is not substantially greater than the risk of exertion at other times of the day. A study by Murray et al. excluded a relative risk above 6 for morning versus afternoon exertion (98).

The difference between the relative risk and the absolute risk of experiencing an event during exertion, or any other potential trigger, is also important. Although there may exist a sixfold increase in the relative risk of an infarction during exercise in the morning hours, this translates to only a very small increase in absolute risk because baseline risk is low. The absolute risk that an individual would experience an MI in the hour after exertion might rise from approximately five in one million for afternoon exercise to thirty in one million for morning exercise. Therefore, there does not appear to be a major risk associated with morning versus afternoon exertion. The well-recognized benefits of regular exertion support a recommendation to patients that they exercise regularly regardless of the time of day (99).

FUTURE STUDIES

The primary significance of the recognition of triggering and circadian variation of disease onset are the clues provided for understanding of disease onset and the new opportunities for prevention that such knowledge would provide. These clues suggest value for studies ranging from the epidemiologic to the molecular level.

On the epidemiologic level, studies must be conducted in which patients who have experienced a nonfatal myocardial infarction are interviewed to determine if the event had an identifiable trigger. Because potentially triggering activities often occur without producing an event, the studies must be controlled for the frequency of potential triggers at times when an event did not occur. The modifiers of triggering must also be determined. Similar epidemiologic studies of potential triggers of sudden cardiac death are also needed.

The certainty with which an activity can be identified as a trigger will also vary in individual cases. In a patient whose plaque is only slightly vulnerable, the activity required to produce disease onset may be extreme, and the activity can be recognized as a trigger by its intensity. Other features that may aid in the recognition of an activity as a trigger are its occurrence immediately before the event, its ability to produce physiological changes likely to trigger thrombosis, and its absence as part of the patient's routine activity. However, in a patient with an extremely vulnerable plaque, even nonstrenuous, routine, daily activities such as eating a heavy meal may be sufficient to trigger the cascade leading to infarction. In such instances, it may be impossible to identify the triggering activity even though it was present. Thus, the group of patients with identifiable triggers will be a subset of those in whom external triggering actually occurred.

On the clinical level, increased study of the relationship between daily activities and potentially triggering physiological responses could clarify the manner in which these processes cause disease onset. The catheterization laboratory techniques of coronary angioscopy, characterization of plaque composition by intracoronary ultrasound, and atherectomy should be used to characterize the plaques responsible for disease onset. Such studies might lead to the possibility that vulnerable plaques could be recognized before their disruption.

On the basic science level, there is a need for complete characterization of the control mechanisms of potentially adverse and beneficial physiological processes pertinent to triggering. With improved understanding of these mechanisms, clinicians may eventually be able to eliminate unnecessary and potentially detrimental surges in arterial pressure, vasoconstriction, and coagulability that contribute to disease onset, and to increase the activity of potentially beneficial processes such as the fibrinolytic system.

The factors determining plaque vulnerability also require further characterization. The reduction in clinical events recently achieved by marked lowering of plasma cholesterol might result not only from reduction of coronary artery stenosis but also from a reduction in the formation of lipid pools within plaques, which might decrease plaque vulnerability.

Studies of plaque disruption can utilize an atherosclerotic rabbit model developed in 1964 by Dr. Paris Constantinides, which subsequently received very little attention because of lack of appreciation of the clinical importance of plaque disruption (100). We have recently reestablished this rabbit model in our laboratories (101). Following 8 months on an intermittent cholesterol-feeding atherogenic diet, Russell viper venom (a proteolytic procoagulant) and histamine (a pressor in rabbits) are injected into the rabbits to attempt to trigger plaque disruption and thrombosis. Constantinides has documented that this regimen produced localized platelet-rich thrombi overlying disrupted aortic atherosclerotic plaques in approximately 30% of the rabbits. This animal model will be used to test many of the hypotheses generated by the new findings regarding disease onset.

Greater understanding of triggering mechanisms should facilitate progress in the prevention of clinical coronary artery disease. The means of prevention would not be to eliminate potential triggering activities—an undesirable and unattainable goal—but to design regimens that can be evaluated in randomized studies for their ability to sever the linkage between a potential triggering activity and development of myocardial infarction and sudden cardiac death.

REFERENCES

1. Muller JE, Stone PH, Turi ZG, Rutherford JD, Czeisler C, Parker C, Poole WK, Passamani E, Roberts R, Robertson T, Sobel BE, Willerson JT, Braunwald E, the MILIS Study Group. Circadian variation in the frequency of onset of acute myocardial infarction. *N Engl J Med* 1985;313:1315–1322.
2. Muller JE, Ludmer PL, Willich SN, Tofler GH, Aylmer G, Klangos I, Stone PH. Circadian variation in the frequency of sudden cardiac death. *Circulation* 1987;75:131–138.
3. Muller JE, Tofler GH, Stone PH. Circadian variation and triggers of onset of acute cardiovascular disease. Clinical progress series. *Circulation* 1989;79:733–743.
4. MacIsaac AI, Thomas JD, Topol EJ. Toward the quiescent coronary plaque. *J Am Coll Cardiol* 1993;22:1228–1241.
5. DeWood MA, Spores J, Notske R, et al. Prevalence of total coronary occlusion during the early hours of transmural myocardial infarction. *N Engl J Med* 1980;303:897–902.
6. Davies MJ, Thomas AC. Thrombosis and acute coronary artery lesions in sudden cardiac ischemic death. *N Engl J Med* 1984;310:1137–1140.
7. Falk E. Plaque rupture with severe pre-existing stenosis precipitating coronary thrombosis: Characteristics of coronary atherosclerotic plaques underlying fatal occlusive thrombi. *Br Heart J* 1983;50: 127–134.
8. Constantinides P. Plaque fissure in human coronary thrombosis. *J Atheroscler Res* 1966;1:1–17.
9. Ip JH, Fuster V, Badimon L, Badimon J, Taubman MB, Chesebro JH. Syndromes of accelerated atherosclerosis: Role of vascular injury and smooth muscle cell proliferation. *J Am Coll Cardiol* 1990;15: 1667–1687.
10. Willerson JT, Campbell WB, Winniford MD, et al. Conversion from chronic to acute coronary artery disease: Speculation regarding mechanisms (editorial). *Am J Cardiol* 1984;54:1349–1354.
11. The Steering Committee of the Physicians' Health Study Research Group. *N Engl J Med* 1988;318:262–264.
12. Peters RW, Muller JE, Goldstein S, Byington R, Friedman LM. Propranolol and the morning increase in the frequency of sudden cardiac death (BHAT Study). *Am J Cardiol* 1989;63:1518–1520.
13. The Lipid Research Clinics Coronary Primary Prevention Trial results. I. Reduction in incidence of coronary heart disease. *JAMA* 1984;251: 351–364.
14. Pfeffer MA, Braunwald E, Moye LA, et al. Effect of captopril on mortality and morbidity in patients with left ventricular dysfunction after myocardial infarction. Results of the survival and ventricular enlargement trial. *N Engl J Med* 1992;327:669–677.
15. Richardson PD, Davies MJ, Born GVR. Influence of plaque configuration and stress distribution on fissuring of coronary atherosclerotic plaques. *Lancet* 1989;2:941–944.
16. Jonasson L, Holm J, Skalli O, Bondjers G, Hansson GK. Regional accumulation of T cells, macrophages, and smooth muscle cells in the human atherosclerotic plaque. *Arteriosclerosis* 1986;6:131–138.
17. Little WC, Constantinescu M, Applegate RJ, et al. Can coronary angiography predict the site of a subsequent myocardial infarction in patients with mild-to-moderate coronary artery disease. *Circulation* 1988;78:1157–1166.
18. Brown BG, Gallery CA, Badger RS, et al. Incomplete lysis of thrombus in the moderate underlying atherosclerotic lesion during intracoronary infusion of streptokinase for acute myocardial infarction: Quantitative angiographic observations. *Circulation* 1986;73:635–661.
19. *1992 Heart and Stroke Facts*. American Heart Association.
20. Muller JE, Tofler GH. Circadian variation and cardiovascular disease (editorial). *N Engl J Med* 1991;325:1038–1039.
21. Obraztsov VP, Strazhesko ND. The symptomatology and diagnosis

of coronary thrombosis. In: Vorobeva VA, Konchalovski MP, eds. *Works of the First Congress of Russian Therapists*. Comradeship Typography of A.E. Mamontov, 1910:26–43.

22. Fitzhugh G, Hamilton BE. Coronary occlusion and fatal angina pectoris. Study of the immediate causes and their prevention. *JAMA* 1933; 100:475–480.
23. Sproul J. A general practitioner's views on the treatment of angina pectoris. *N Engl J Med* 1936;215:443–452.
24. Parkinson J, Bedford DE. Cardiac infarction and coronary thrombosis. *Lancet* 1928;1:4–11.
25. Phipps C. Contributory causes of coronary thrombosis. *JAMA* 1936; 106:761–762.
26. Master AM. The role of effort and occupation (including physicians) in coronary occlusion. *JAMA* 1960;174:942–948.
27. Willich SN, Linderer T, Wegscheider K, Leizorovicz MD, Alamercery I, Schroder R, the ISAM Study Group. Increased morning incidence of myocardial infarction in the ISAM Study: Absence with prior beta-adrenergic blockade. *Circulation* 1989;80:853–858.
28. Thompson DR, Blandford RL, Sutton TW, Marchant PR. Time of onset of chest pain in acute myocardial infarction. *Int J Cardiol* 1985; 7:139–146.
29. Goldberg R, Brady P, Muller JE, et al. Time of onset of symptoms of acute myocardial infarction. *Am J Cardiol* 1990;66:140–144.
30. Willich SN, Levy D, Rocco MB, Tofler GH, Stone PH, Muller JE. Circadian variation in the incidence of sudden cardiac death in the Framingham Heart Study population. *Am J Cardiol* 1987;60:801–806.
31. French AJ, Dock W. Fatal coronary arteriosclerosis in young soldiers. *JAMA* 1944;124:1233–1237.
32. Tsementzis SA, Gill JS, Hitchcock ER, Gill SK, Beevers DG. Diurnal variation of and activity during the onset of stroke. *Neurosurgery* 1985;17:901–904.
33. Marler JR, Price TR, Clark GL, et al. Morning increase in onset of ischemic stroke. *Stroke* 1989;20:473–476.
34. Tofler GH, Stone PH, Maclure M, et al. Analysis of possible triggers of acute myocardial infarction (MILIS Study). *Am J Cardiol* 1990; 66:22–27.
35. Sumiyoshi T, Haze K, Saito M, Fukami K, Goto Y, Hiramori K. Evaluation of clinical factors involved in onset of myocardial infarction. *Jpn Circ J* 1986;50:164–173.
36. Tofler GH, Muller JE, Stone PH, et al. Modifiers of timing and possible triggers of acute myocardial infarction in the Thrombolysis in Myocardial Infarction Study (TIMI II) population. *J Am Coll Cardiol* 1992;20:1045–1055.
37. Maclure M. The case-crossover design: A method for studying transient effects on the risk of acute events. *Am J Epidemiol* 1991;133: 144–153.
38. Mittleman MA, Maclure M, Tofler GH, Sherwood JB, Goldberg RJ, Muller JE, for the Determinants of Myocardial Infarction Onset Study Investigators. Triggering of acute myocardial infarction by heavy physical exertion: Protection against triggering by regular exertion. *N Engl J Med* 1993;329:1677–1683.
39. Willich SN, Lewis SM, Lowel H, Arntz HR, Schubert F, Schroder R. Physical exertion as a trigger of acute myocardial infarction. Triggers and mechanisms of Myocardial Infarction Study Group. *N Engl J Med* 1993;329:1684–1690.
40. Eaker ED. Use of questionnaires, interviews and psychological tests in epidemiologic studies of coronary heart disease. *Eur Heart J* 1988; 9:698–704.
41. Mittleman MA, Maclure M, Sherwood JB, Mulry RP, Tofler GH, Jacobs SC, Friedman R, Benson H, Muller JE. Triggering of myocardial infarction onset by episodes of anger. *Circulation* 1995 (*in press*).
42. Muller JE, Maclure M, Mittleman M, Sherwood J, Tofler GH, for the ONSET Study Investigators. Risk of myocardial infarction doubles in the two hours after sexual activity but absolute risk remains low. *Circulation* 1993;88(Suppl I):I-509.
43. Ambrose JA, Winters SL, Stern A, et al. Angiographic morphology and the pathogenesis of unstable angina pectoris. *J Am Coll Cardiol* 1985;5:609–616.
44. Sherman CT, Litvack F, Grundfest W, et al. Coronary angioscopy in patients with unstable angina pectoris. *N Engl J Med* 1986;315: 913–919.
45. Nakagawa S, Hanada Y, Koiwaya Y, Tanaka K. Angiographic features in the infarct-related artery after intracoronary urokinase followed by prolonged anticoagulation: Role of ruptured atheromatous plaque and adherent thrombus in acute myocardial infarction in vivo. *Circulation* 1988;78:1335–1344.
46. Haft JI, Haik BJ, Goldstein JE. Catastrophic progression of coronary artery lesions, the common mechanism for coronary disease progression. *Circulation* 1987;76(Suppl IV):IV-168(abstr).
47. Falk E. Why do plaques rupture? *Circulation* 1992;86(Suppl III):III-30–III-42.
48. van der Wal AC, Becker AE, van der Loos CM, Das PK. Site of intimal rupture or erosion of thrombosed coronary atherosclerotic plaques is characterized by an inflammatory process irrespective of the dominant plaque morphology. *Circulation* 1994;89:36–44.
49. Fernandez-Ortiz A, Badimon JJ, Falk E, Fuster V, Meyer B, Mailhac A, Weng D, Shah PK, Badimon L. Characterization of the relative thrombogenicity of atherosclerotic plaque components: Implications for consequences of plaque rupture. *J Am Coll Cardiol* 1994;23: 1562–1569.
50. Alexander RW. Inflammation and coronary artery disease. *N Engl J Med* 1994;331:468–469.
51. Tofler GH, Brezinski DA, Schafer AI, Czeisler CA, Rutherford JD, Willich SN, Gleason RE, Williams GH, Muller JE. Concurrent morning increase in platelet aggregability and the risk of myocardial infarction and sudden cardiac death. *N Engl J Med* 1987;316:1514–1518.
52. Rocco MB, Barry J, Campbell S, Nabel E, Cook EF, Goldman L, Selwyn AP. Circadian variation of transient myocardial ischemia in patients with coronary artery disease. *Circulation* 1987;75:395–400.
53. Jimenez AH, Tofler GH, Chen X, Stubbs ME, Solomon HS, Muller JE. Effects of nadolol on hemodynamic and hemostatic responses to potential mental and physical triggers of myocardial infarction in subjects with mild systemic hypertension. *Am J Cardiol* 1993;72: 47–52.
54. Weitzman ED, Fukushima D, Nogeire C, Roffwarg H, Gallagher TF, Hellman L. Twenty-four hour pattern of the episodic secretion of cortisol in normal subjects. *J Clin Endocrinol* 1971;33:14–22.
55. Winther K, Hillegass W, Tofler GH, Jimenez A, Brezinski DA, Schafer AI, Loscalzo J, Williams GH, Muller JE. Effects of platelet aggregation and fibrinolytic activity during upright posture and exercise in healthy men. *Am J Cardiol* 1992;70:1051–1055.
56. Rose G. Cold weather and ischaemic heart disease. *Br J Prev Soc Med* 1966;20:97–100.
57. Rocco MB, Barry J, Campbell S, Nabel E, Cook EF, Goldman L, Selwyn AP. Circadian variation of transient myocardial ischemia in patients with coronary artery disease. *Circulation* 1987;75:395–400.
58. Parker JD, Testa MA, Jimenez AH, Tofler GH, Muller JE, Parker JO, Stone PH. Morning increase in ambulatory ischemia in patients with stable coronary artery disease. Importance of physical activity and increased cardiac demand. *Circulation* 1994;89:604–614.
59. Peters RW, Muller JE, Goldstein S, Byington R, Friedman L. Propranolol and the morning increase in the frequency of sudden cardiac death (The BHAT Study). *Am J Cardiol* 1989;63:1518–1520.
60. Ridker PM, Manson JE, Buring JE, Muller JE, Hennekens CH. Circadian variation of acute myocardial infarction and the effect of low-dose aspirin in a randomized trial of physicians. *Circulation* 1990; 82:897–902.
61. Mulcahy D, Keegan J, Cunningham D, Quyyumi A, Crear P, Park A, Wright C, Fox K. Circadian variation of total ischemic burden and its alteration with anti-anginal agents. *Lancet* 1988;2:755–759.
62. Muller JE, Abela GS, Nesto RW, Tofler GH. Triggers, acute risk factors, and vulnerable plaques: The lexicon of a new frontier. *J Am Coll Cardiol* 1994;23:809–813.
63. Coller BS, Folts JD, Smith SR, Scudder LE, Jordan R. Abolition of in vivo platelet thrombus formation in primates with monoclonal antibodies to the platelet GPIIb/IIIA receptor. Correlation with bleeding time, platelet aggregation, and blockade of GPIIb/IIIa receptors. *Circulation* 1989;80:1766–1774.
64. Fuster V, Badimon L, Badimon JJ, Chesebro JH. The pathogenesis of coronary artery disease and the acute coronary syndromes. *N Engl J Med* 1992;326:242–250.
65. Arbustini E, Grass M, Diegoli M, Morbini P, Aguzzi A, Fasani R, Specchia G. Coronary thrombosis in non-cardiac death. *Coron Artery Dis* 1993;4:751–759.
66. Belch JJF, McArdle BM, Burns P, Lowe GDO, Forbes CD. The effects of acute smoking on platelet behaviour, fibrinolysis, and haemorheology in habitual smokers. *Thromb Haemostas* 1984;51:6–8.
67. Egan B, Schork N, Panis R, Hinderliter A. Vascular structure enhances

regional resistance responses in mild essential hypertension. *J Hypertens* 1988;6:41–48.
68. Ludmer PL, Selwyn AP, Shook TL, et al. Paradoxical vasoconstriction induced by acetylcholine in atherosclerotic coronary arteries. *N Engl J Med* 1986;315:1046–1051.
69. Khann PK, Seth HN, Balasubramanian V, Hoon RS. Effect of submaximal exercise on fibrinolytic activity in ischemic heart disease. *Br Med J* 1975;2:910–912.
70. Gillum RF. Sudden coronary death in the United States, 1980–1985. *Circulation* 1989;79:756–765.
71. Goldberg J. Declining out-of-hospital sudden coronary death rates: Additional pieces of the epidemiologic puzzle. *Circulation* 1989;79: 1369–1373.
72. Myerburg RJ, Kessler KM, Castellanos A. Sudden cardiac death: Structure, function, and time dependence of risk. *Circulation* 1992; 85(Suppl I):2–10.
73. Lown B. Sudden cardiac death: The major challenge facing contemporary cardiology. *Am J Cardiol* 1979;41:313–328.
74. Hinkle LE, Thaler HT. Clinical classification of cardiac death. *Circulation* 1982;65:457–464.
75. Lovegrove T, Thompson P. The role of acute myocardial infarction in sudden cardiac death: A statistician's nightmare. *Am Heart J* 1978; 96:711–713.
76. Goldstein S. Toward a new understanding of the mechanism and prevention of sudden death in coronary heart disease. *Circulation* 1990; 82:284–288.
77. Davies MJ. Anatomic features in victims of sudden coronary death: Coronary artery pathology. *Circulation* 1992;85(Suppl I):19–24.
78. Goldstein S, Landis JR, Leighton R, Ritter G, Vasu CM, Lantis A, Serokman R. Characteristics of the resuscitated out-of-hospital cardiac arrest victim with coronary heart disease. *Circulation* 1981;64: 977–984.
79. Willich SN, Maclure M, Mittleman M, Arntz HR, Muller JE. Sudden cardiac death. Support for a role of triggering in causation. *Circulation* 1993;87:1442–1450.
80. Arnst HR, Willich SN, Oeff M, Bruggemann T, Stern R, Heinzmann A, Matenaer B, Schroder R. Circadian variation of sudden cardiac death reflects age-related variability in ventricular fibrillation. *Circulation* 1993;88:2284–2289.
81. Hausmann D, Trappe HJ, Bargheer K, Daniel WG, Wenzlaff P, Lichtlen PR. Circadian variation of ventricular tachycardia in patients after myocardial infarction. *J Am Coll Cardiol* 1992;19(Suppl A):368A.
82. Peters RW, Mitchell LB, Pawitan Y, Barker AH, Capone RJ, Echt DS, CAST Investigators. Circadian pattern of sudden arrhythmic death in patients receiving encainide or flecainide in the Cardiac Arrhythmia Suppression Trial (CAST). *Circulation* 1990;82(Suppl III):III-138.
83. Willich SN, Goldberg RJ, Maclure M, Perriello L, Muller JE. Increased onset of sudden cardiac death in the first 3 hours after awakening. *Am J Cardiol* 1992;70:65–68.
84. Moritz AR, Zamcheck N. Sudden and unexpected deaths of young soldiers: Diseases responsible for such deaths during World War II. *Arch Pathol* 1946;42:459–494.
85. Thompson PD, Funk EJ, Carleton RA, Sturner WQ. Incidence of death during jogging on Rhode Island from 1975 through 1980. *JAMA* 1982;247:2535–2538.
86. Siscovick DS, Weiss NS, Fletcher RH, Lasky T. The incidence of primary cardiac arrest during vigorous exercise. *N Engl J Med* 1984; 311:874–877.
87. Kamarch T, Jenning JR. Biobehavioral factors in sudden cardiac death. *Psychol Bull* 1991;109:42–75.
88. Myers A, Dewar HA. Circumstances attending 100 sudden deaths from coronary artery disease with coroner's necropsies. *Br Heart J* 1975;37:1133.
89. Ahern DK, Gorkin L, Anderson JL, Tierney C, Hallstrom A, Ewart C, Capone RJ, Schron E, Kornfeld D, Herd JA, Richardson DW, Follik MJ, CAPS Investigators. Biobehavioral variables and mortality or cardiac arrest in the Cardiac Arrhythmias Pilot Study (CAPS). *Am J Cardiol* 1990;66:59–62.
90. Brackett CD, Powell LH. Psychosocial and physiological predictors of sudden cardiac death after healing of acute myocardial infarction. *Am J Cardiol* 1990;66:59–62.
91. Karch SB, Billingham ME. The pathology and etiology of cocaine-induced heart disease. *Arch Pathol Lab Med* 1988;112:225–230.
92. de Silva RA. Central nervous system risk factors for sudden cardiac death. In: Greenberg HM, Dwyer EM, eds. *Sudden Coronary Death.* New York: New York Academy of Sciences; 1982:143–160.
93. Corbalan R, Verrier R, Lown B. Psychological stress and ventricular arrhythmias during myocardial infarction in the conscious dog. *Am J Cardiol* 1974;36:692–696.
94. Folts JD, Stamler J, Loscalzo J. Intravenous nitroglycerin infusion inhibits cyclic blood flow responses caused by periodic platelet thrombus formation in stenosed canine coronary arteries. *Circulation* 1991; 83:2122–2127.
95. Fuster V. Mechanisms leading to myocardial infarction: Insights from studies of vascular biology. Clinical cardiology frontiers. *Circulation* 1994;90:2126–2146.
96. Fuster V, Stein B, Ambrose JA, Badimon L, Badimon JJ, Chesebro J. Atherosclerosis plaque rupture and thrombosis: Evolving concepts. *Circulation* 1990;86(Suppl III):47–59.
97. Fuster V, Frye RL, Kennedy MA, Connolly DC, Makin HT. The role of collateral circulation in the various coronary syndromes. *Circulation* 1979;59:1137–1144.
98. Murray PM, Herrington DM, Pettus CW, Miller HS, Cantwell JD, Little WC. Should patients with heart disease exercise in the morning or afternoon. *Arch Intern Med* 1993;153:833–836.
99. Muller JE, Tofler GH. Morning vs afternoon exertion. Both are safe, but which is safer? *Arch Intern Med* 1993;153:803–804.
100. Constantinides P. *Experimental Atherosclerosis.* Amsterdam: Elsevier; 1965:27–34,41.
101. Abela GS, Picon PD, Fried SE, Gebara OC, Miyamoto A, Federman M, Toffler GH, Muller JE. Triggering of plaque disruption and arterial thrombosis in an atherosclerotic model. *Circulation* 1995;91: 776–784.

Index

Index

E

J

K

L

M

N

Q

R